EPILEPSY

A Comprehensive Textbook

Second Edition

EPILEPSY
A Comprehensive Textbook

SECOND EDITION

VOLUME III

Editors

Jerome Engel, Jr., MD, PhD

Jonathan Sinay Distinguished Professor of Neurology
Neurobiology, and Psychiatry and Behavioral Sciences
Director of the UCLA Seizure Disorder Center
David Geffen School of Medicine at UCLA
Los Angeles, California

Timothy A. Pedley, MD

Henry and Lucy Moses Professor of Neurology
and Chairman, Department of Neurology
College of Physicians and Surgeons of Columbia University
Neurologist-in-Chief
The Neurological Institute of New York
The New York-Presbyterian Hospital at
Columbia University Medical Center
New York, New York

Associate Editors

Jean Aicardi, MD, FRCP

Professor of Neurology
University Hospital Robert Debre
Epilepsy Unit
Child Neurology and Metabolic Disease
Paris, France

Marc A. Dichter, MD, PhD

Professor of Neurology and Pharmacology
University of Pennsylvania School of Medicine
Philadelphia, Pennsylvania

Emilio Perucca, MD, PhD, FRCP

Professor, Clinical Pharmacology Unit
Department of Internal Medicine and Therapeutics
University of Pavia
Director, Laboratories for Diagnostics and
Applied Biological Research
Institute of Neurology IRCCS C. Mondino Foundation
Pavia, Italy

Solomon L. Moshé, MD

Vice Chair and Professor of Neurology,
Neuroscience and Pediatrics
Albert Einstein College of Medicine of Yeshiva University
Director of Child Neurology and Clinical Neurophysiology
Department of Neurology and Pediatric Neurology
Montefiore Medical Center
Bronx, New York

Michael R. Trimble, MD

Professor of Behavioral Neurology
Institute of Neurology
London, United Kingdom

Wolters Kluwer | Lippincott Williams & Wilkins
Health

Philadelphia • Baltimore • New York • London
Buenos Aires • Hong Kong • Sydney • Tokyo

Acquisitions Editor: Frances DeStefano
Managing Editor: Leanne McMillan
Developmental Editor: Dovetail Content Solutions, Keith Donnellan
Production Editor: Bridgett Dougherty
Manufacturing Manager: Benjamin Rivera
Design Coordinator: Stephen Druding
Compositor: Aptara, Inc.

530 Walnut Street
Philadelphia, PA 19106 USA
LWW.com

Printed in the USA

Library of Congress Cataloging-in-Publication Data

Epilepsy : a comprehensive textbook / editors, Jerome Engel Jr., Timothy A. Pedley ; associate editors, Jean Aicardi ... [et al.]. — 2nd ed.
p. ; cm.
Includes bibliographical references and index.
ISBN-13: 978-0-7817-5777-5 (alk. paper)
ISBN-10: 0-7817-5777-0 (alk. paper)
1. Epilepsy. I. Engel, Jerome. II. Pedley, Timothy A.
[DNLM: 1. Epilepsy. WL 385 E6025 2008]
RC372.E657 2008
616.8′53—dc22

2007032096

Care has been taken to confirm the accuracy of the information presented and to describe generally accepted practices. However, the authors, editors, and publisher are not responsible for errors or omissions or for any consequences from application of the information in this book and make no warranty, expressed or implied, with respect to the currency, completeness, or accuracy of the contents of the publication. Application of this information in a particular situation remains the professional responsibility of the practitioner.

The authors, editors, and publisher have exerted every effort to ensure that drug selection and dosage set forth in this text are in accordance with current recommendations and practice at the time of publication. However, in view of ongoing research, changes in government regulations, and the constant flow of information relating to drug therapy and drug reactions, the reader is urged to check the package insert for each drug for any change in indications and dosage and for added warnings and precautions. This is particularly important when the recommended agent is a new or infrequently employed drug.

Some drugs and medical devices presented in this publication have Food and Drug Administration (FDA) clearance for limited use in restricted research settings. It is the responsibility of the health care provider to ascertain the FDA status of each drug or device planned for use in their clinical practice.

To purchase additional copies of this book, call our customer service department at (800) 638-3030 or fax orders to (301) 223-2320. International customers should call (301) 223-2300.

Visit Lippincott Williams & Wilkins on the Internet: at LWW.com. Lippincott Williams & Wilkins customer service representatives are available from 8:30 am to 6 pm, EST.

10 9 8 7 6 5 4 3 2 1

WE DEDICATE THIS EDITION TO OUR WIVES, CATHERINE AND BARBARA, AND THE OTHERS IN OUR FAMILIES WHO ALL TOO OFTEN LOST US TO THESE VOLUMES. ABOVE ALL, THIS BOOK IS FOR PERSONS WITH EPILEPSY AND THEIR FAMILIES, WHO DAILY GIVE MEANING TO OUR WORK.

CONTENTS OVERVIEW

VOLUME I

VOLUME II

VOLUME III

VOLUME I

VOLUME II

VOLUME III

CONTENTS

VOLUME I

VOLUME II

SECTION V ■ GENERAL TREATMENT CONSIDERATIONS

Section Editors: Elinor Ben-Menachem, David W. Chadwick, Solomon Moshé, John Pellock, Emilio Perucca, and Timothy A. Pedley

SECTION VII ■ SURGICAL THERAPY

Section Editors: Emilio Perucca, Dennis D. Spencer, Heinz Gregor Wieser, and Jerome Engel, Jr.

SECTION VIII ■ CLINICAL BIOLOGY OF EPILEPSY

Section Editors: Michael J. Aminoff, Marc A. Dichter, Emilio Perucca, and Timothy A. Pedley

VOLUME III

SECTION IX ■ PSYCHIATRIC AND SOCIAL ISSUES

Section Editors: Joan K. Austin, Robert T. Fraser, Andres M. Kanner, Michael R. Trimble, and Jerome Engel, Jr.

PSYCHIATRIC ISSUES

SOCIAL ISSUES

SECTION X ■ EPILEPSY SYNDROMES

Section Editors: Jean Aicardi, Warren T. Blume, Olivier Dulac, Natalio Fejerman, Masakazu Seino, Peter Wolf, and Jerome Engel, Jr.

NEONATAL SYNDROMES

SYNDROMES OF INFANCY AND EARLY CHILDHOOD

SPECIALIZED CENTERS FOR EPILEPSY

COST AND ALLOCATION OF RESOURCES

CONTRIBUTING AUTHORS

Eric Abadie
Director, Therapeutic Evaluation
Agence Francaise de Secunte Sanitaire des Products de Sante
Paris, France

Carlos Acevedo, MD, Sch
Professor of Pediatric Neurology
Universidad de los Andes
Department of Pediatric Neurology
Clinica Alemana de Santiago
Santiago, Chile

Keryma A. Acevedo, MD
Assistant Professor
Department of Pediatrics, Northern Campus
University of Chile
Staff of Pediatric Neurology
Emergency Department
Clinica Alemana de Santiago
Santiago, Chile

Bola Adamolekun, MD, FWACP
Director of Epilepsy
Department of Neurology
University of Tennessee Health Science Center
Memphis, Tennessee

Jean Aicardi, MD, FRCP
Department
University Hospital Robert Debre
Epilepsy Unit
Children Neurology and Metabolic Disease
Paris, France

Fiorenzo Albini, MD
Laboratory of Clinical Neuropharmacology
University of Bologna
Bologna, Italy

Albert P. Aldenkamp, PhD
Professor of Epileptology
Department of Neurology
University of Maastricht
University Hospital Maastricht
Head Department of Behavioural Sciences
Epilepsy Centre Kempenhaeghe
Heeze, The Netherlands

Brian K. Alldredge, Pharm.D
Professor of Clinical Pharmacy and Neurology
University of California
San Francisco, California

Abdul Aziz Al Semari, MD
Director, Comprehensive Epilepsy Program
Chairman, Epilepsy Support and Information Center and Head, Section of Neurology
Department of Neurosciences
King Faisal Specialist Hospital and Research Center
Kingdom of Saudi Arabia

Michael J. Aminoff, MD, DSc, FRCP
Professor and Executive Vice Chair of Neurology
University of California School of Medicine
Attending Physician
Department of Neurology
University of Calfornia Medical Center
San Francisco, California

Eva Andermann, MD, PhD
Professor of Neurology and Neurosurgery
Montreal Neurological Institute and Hospital
McGill University
Montreal, Canada

Frédérick Andermann, MD, FRCPC
Professor of Neurology and Neurosurgery
Montreal Neurological Institute and Hospital
McGill University
Montreal, Canada

V. Elving Anderson, PhD
Professor Emeritus
Department of Genetics, Cell Biology, and Development
University of Minnesota
Minneapolis, Minnesota

Santiago Arroyo, MD, PhD
Clinical Discovery Neurosciences
Bristol-Myer-Squibb
Lawrenceville, New Jersey

Alexis Arzimanoglou, MD
CTRS-IDEE
University of Lyon
Lyon, France
Head, Department of Neurology
University Hospital Robert Debré
Paris, France

Joan K. Austin, DNS
Department of Environments for Health
Indiana University School of Nursing
Indianapolis, Indiana

Giuliano G. Avanzini, MD
Professor of Neurology
Division of Clinical Epileptology and Experimental Neurophysiology
Istituto Nazionale Neurologico
Milano, Italy

Thomas L. Babb, PhD
Professor of Pediatrics and Neurology
Children's Hospital of Michigan
Wayne State University
Detroit, Michigan

Torbjörn Backström, MD, PhD
Professor
Department of Clinical Sciences
Umeå University
Consultant
Department of Obstetrics and Gynecology
Norrlands University Hospital
Umeå, Sweden

Gus A. Baker, PhD, FBPsS
Professor of Clinical Neuropsychology
Consultant Clinical Neuropsychologist
Division of Neurosciences
University of Liverpool
Walton Centre for Neurology & Neurosurgery
Liverpool, United Kingdom

Poonam Nina Banerjee, PhD
Department of Neurology and Sergievsky Center
College of Physicians and Surgeons
Department of Epidemiology
Mailman School of Public Health
Columbia University
New York, New York

Tallie Z. Baram, MD, PhD
Professor of Pediatrics, Anatomy/Neurobiology, and Neurology
Scientific Director
Comprehensive Epilepsy Program
University of California, Irvine
Irvine, California

Amit Bar-Or, MD, FRCPC
Associate Professor of Neurology and Neurosurgery
Associate, Microbiology and Immunology
McGill University
Director, Program in Experimental Therapeutics
Scientific Director, Clinical Research Unit
Montreal Neurological Institute
Montreal, Quebec
Canada

William B. Barr, PhD
Comprehensive Epilepsy Center
New York University Medical Center
New York, New York

Shehzad Basaria, MD
Assistant Professor of Internal Medicine
Johns Hopkins University School of Medicine
Johns Hopkins Bayview Medical Center
Baltimore, Maryland

Agatino Battaglia, MD
Stella Maris Clinical Research Institute for Child and Adolescent Neuropsychiatry
Calambrone, Pisa
Italy

Dina Battino, MD
Division of Neurophysiology and Epileptology
Carlos Besta, National Neurological Institute
Milan, Italy

Michel Baulac, MD
Professor
University Pierre et Marie Curie (Paris VI)
INSERM Unit U739 Cortex and Epilepsy
CHU Pitie-Salpetriere
Physician and Chief of Department
Unit of Epileptology
Hôpital Salpêtrière
Batiment Paul Castaigne
Paris, France

Christoph Baumgartner, MD
Associate Professor of Neurology
Head, Comprehensive Epilepsy Program
Medical University of Vienna
Vienna, Austria

Carl W. Bazil, MD, PhD
Associate Professor of Neurology
Columbia University Medical Center
Attending Neurologist
New York-Presbyterian Hospital
New York, New York

Heinz Beck, MD
Head, Laboratory of Experimental Epileptology
Professor, Department of Epileptology
University of Bonn Medical Center
Bonn, Germany

Ettore Beghi, MD
Epilepsy Center
Ospedale "San Gerardo" Monza
Monza, Milan, Italy

Elinor Ben-Menachem, MD, PhD
Sahlgren University Hospital
Department of Neurology
Institute of Clinical Neuroscience
Goteborg, Sweden

Roy G. Beran, MD, FRACP, FRCP, FRACGP, FACLM, B Leg S, MHL
Conjoint Associate Professor
University of New South Wales
Professor School of Medicine
Griffith University
Chatswood, New South Wales
Australia

Anne T. Berg, PhD
Associate Professor
Department of Biology
Northern Illinois University
DeKalb, Illinois

Gregory K. Bergey, MD
Professor of Neurology
Department of Neurology
Director, Johns Hopkins Epilepsy Center
Johns Hopkins School of Medicine and Hospital
Baltimore, Maryland

Samuel F. Berkovic, MD, FRS
Professor
Epilepsy Reseach Centre
University of Melbourne
Director of Comprehensive Epilepsy Program
Austin Health
Heidelberg, Victoria
Australia

Christophe Bernard, PhD
Professor
Inserm U751
Université de la Mediterranee
Marseille, France

Gianna Bertani, MD
Physician
Child Neurology Unit
Arcispedale s. Maria Nuova
Reggio Emilia, Italy

Edward H. Bertram, MD
Professor of Neurology
Department of Neurology
University of Virginia
Charlottesville, Virginia

Frank M.C. Besag, MB, ChB, FRCP, FRCPsych, FRCPCH
Visiting Professor of Neuropsychiatry
Faculty of Health and Social Sciences
University of Bedfordshire
Luton, Beds
Consultant Neuropsychiatrist
Child and Adolescent Mental Health Services
Bedfordshire and Luton Partnership NHS Trust
Bedford, Beds
United Kingdom

Tim Betts
Seizure Clinic and Epilepsy Liaison
Birmingham University, Edgbaston
Queen Elizabeth Psychiatric Hospital
Birmingham, United Kingdom

Ahmad A. Beydoun, MD
Professor of Neurology
Department of Internal Medicine
American University of Beirut Medical Center
Beirut, Lebanon

Nadir E. Bharucha, MD
Bombay Hospital Medical Research
Department of Neuroepidemiology
Mumbai, India

Meir Bialer, PhD, MBA
David H. Eisenberg Professor of Pharmacy
Department of Pharmaceutics
School of Pharmacy, Faculty of Medicine
Hebrew University of Jerusalem
Jerusalem, Israel

Christian G. Bien, MD
Senior Neurologist and Leading Assistant Medical Director
Department of Epileptology
University of Bonn
Bonn, Germany

Devin K. Binder, MD, PhD
Assistant Professor
Department of Neurological Surgery
University of California, Irvine
Orange, California

Gretchen L. Birbeck, MD, MPH, DTMH
Director and Associate Professor
International Neurologic and Psychiatric Epidemiology
Michigan State University
East Lansing, Mississippi
Director
Epilepsy Care Team
Chikankata Health Services
Mazabuka, Zambia

Jonathan M. Bird, MD
Burden Centre for Neuropsychiatry
Frenchay Hospital
United Kingdom

Angela K. Birnbaum, PhD
Associate Professor
Experimental and Clinical Pharmacology
University of Minnesota
Minneapolis, Minnesota

Peter F. Bladin, MD, BS, BSc, FRACP, FRACPEd
Professor
Faculty of Medicine, Dentistry, Health Sciences
University of Melbourne
Neurologist, Comprehensive Epilepsy
Austin Hospital
Melbourne, Victoria
Australia

Thomas P. Bleck, MD, FCCM
Professor of Neurology and Neurosurgery
The Ruth Cain Ruggles Chairman of Neurology
Northwestern University Feinberg School of Medicine
Evanston Northwestern Healthcare
Chicago, Illinois

Ingmar Blümcke, MD
Department of Neuropathology
Friedrich Alexander University
Erlangen, Germany

Warren T. Blume, MD
Professor of Neurology Emeritus
Clinical Neurological Sciences
University of Western Ontario
London, Ontario
Canada

Hal Blumenfeld, MD, PhD
Director of Medical Studies
Clinical Neurosciences
Associate Professor
Departments of Neurology, Neurobiology, Neurosurgery
Yale University School of Medicine
New Haven, Connecticut

Dietrich Blumer, MD
Professor of Psychiatry
Head of Neuropsychiatry
University of Tennessee
Memphis, Tennessee

Joshua L. Bonkowsky, MD, PhD
Department of Pediatrics
University of Utah School of Medicine
Salt Lake City, Utah

Harold E. Booker, MD
Carolina Neurological Clinic
Charleston, South Carolina

Susan Y. Bookheimer, PhD
University of California at Los Angeles Department of Psychiatry and Biobehavioral Sciences
Los Angeles, California

Paul Boon, MD, PhD
Professor and Chairman, Department of Neurology
University Hospital
Ghent, Belgium

Carmel H. Bouclaous, MD
Division of Neurosurgery
American University of Beirut
Beirut, Lebanon

Blaise F. D. Bourgeois, MD
Professor of Neurology
Harvard Medical School
Director
Division of Epilepsy and Clinical Neurophysiology
Children's Hospital
Boston, Massachusetts

Martin J. Brodie, MD, FRCP
Professor of Medicine and Clinical Pharmacology
Division of Cardiovascular and Medical Sciences
University of Glasgow
Consultant Physician and Clinical Pharmacologist
Division of Cardiovascular and Medical Sciences
Western Infirmary
Glasgow, United Kingdom

Eylert Brodtkorb
Department of Neurology and Clinical Neurophysiology
Trondheim University Hospital
Trondheim, Norway

Edward B. Bromfield, MD
Chief, Division of Epilepsy and EEG
Division of Neurology
Brigham & Women's Hospital
Associate Professor of Neurology
Harvard Medical School
Boston, Massachusetts

Richard J. Brown, PhD, Clin. Psy. D
Lecturer in Clinical Psychology
University of Manchester
Clinical Psychologist
Department of Clinical and Health Psychology
Manchester, United Kingdom

Stephen W. Brown, FRCPsych
The David Lewis Centre for Epilepsy
Cheshire, United Kingdom
Clinical Director, Learning Disabilities Service
Norwich Community Health
Norwich, Norfolk, United Kingdom

Thomas R. Browne, MD
Boston University School of Medicine
Fairmouth, Massachusetts

John C. M. Brust, MD
Professor of Clinical Neurology
Columbia University College of Physicians and Surgeons
Director, Department of Neurology
Harlem Hospital Center
New York, New York

Michelle Bureau, MD
Head of Neurophysiology (emer.)
EEG Laboratory
Centre Saint Paul
Marseille, France

György Buzsáki, MD, PhD
Center for Molecular and Behavioral Neuroscience, Rutgers
The State University of New Jersey
Newark, New Jersey

Carol S. Camfield, MD, FRCP(C)
Professor of Pediatrics
Dalhousie University
Halifax, Nova Scotia, Canada

Peter R. Camfield, MD
Professor of Pediatrics
Dalhousie University
Halifax, Nova Scotia, Canada

Rochelle Caplan, MD
Semel Institute for Neuroscience and Behavior
Los Angeles, California

Roberto Caraballo, MD
Department of Neurology
Hospital de Pediatria
Buenos Aires, Argentina

Arturo Carpio, MD
Professor of Neurology
School of Medicine
University of Cuenca
Neurologist
Comprehensive Epilepsy Center
Hospital "Vicente Corral M."
Cuenca, Ecuador

Romeo Carrozzo, MD
Medical Genetics and General Pediatrics
National Health Service
Milan, Italy

Gregory D. Cascino, MD
Department of Neurology
Mayo Clinic
Rochester, Minnesota

Idil Cavus, MD, PhD
Assistant Professor of Psychiatry and Neurosurgery
Assistant Professor of Psychiatry
Yale University School of Medicine
Connecticut Mental Health Center
New Haven, Connecticut

Jennifer Cavitt, MD
Assistant Professor of Neurology
University of Cincinnati
Cincinnati, Ohio

Fernando Cendes, MD, PhD
Associate Professor of Neurology
University of Campinas
Campinas, Brazil

David W. Chadwick, DM, FRCP, FMedSci
Professor of Neuroscience
University of Liverpool
Walton Centre
Liverpool, United Kingdom

Roukoz B. Chamoun, MD
Division of Neurosurgery
American University of Beirut
Beirut, Lebanon

Gian-Emillio Chatrian, MD
Professor Emeritus
Department of Neurology
University of Washington Medical Center
Seattle, Washington

Patrick Chauvel, MD
Service de Neurophysiologie Clinique et Epileptologie
CHU Timone et Universite de la Mediterranee
Marseille, France

Catherine Chiron, MD
Service de Neurologie et Metablolisme
Hopital Necker
Paris, France

Dan Chisholm
Department of Health Systems Financing
World Health Organization
Geneva, Switzerland

Harry T. Chugani, MD
Children's Hospital of Michigan
Detroit, Michigan

Maria Roberta Cilio, MD, PhD
Attending Physician
Department of Neurology
Bambino Gesu Children's Hospital
Rome, Italy

Robert R. Clancy, MD
Professor of Neurology and Pediatrics
University of Pennsylvania School of Medicine
Director, Pediatric Regional Epilepsy Program
Division of Neurology
The Children's Hospital of Philadelphia
Philadelphia, Pennsylvania

David C. Clemmons, PhD
Vocational Services
University of Washington Regional Epilepsy Center
Seattle, Washington

Mark S. Cohen, PhD
Professor-in-Residence
Department of Psychiatry, Neurology, Radiology, Psychology, Biomedical Physics
University of California at Los Angeles
Los Angeles, California

Youssef G. Comair, MD, FRCP
Department of Neurosurgery
Cleveland Clinic Foundation
Cleveland, Ohio

Barry W. Connors, PhD
Professor and Chair
Department of Neuroscience
Brown University
Providence, Rhode Island

Douglas A. Coulter, PhD
Department of Pediatric Neruology
University of Pennsylvania
Children's Hospital of Philadelphia
Philadelphia, Pennsylvania

Joyce A. Cramer, BS
Associate Research Scientist
Department of Psychiatry
Yale University School of Medicine
West Haven, Connecticut

Peter B. Crino, MD, PhD
Assistant Professor
Department of Neurology
University of Pennsylvania
Philadelphia, Pennsylvania

J. Helen Cross, MB, ChB, PhD, FRCP, FRCPCH
Professor
Neurosciences Unit
UCL-Institute of Child Health
Honorary Consultant/Clinical Lead
Paediatric Neurology (Epilepsy)
Great Ormond St Hospital for Children NHS Trust
London, United Kingdom

Patricia K. Crumrine, MD
Professor of Pediatrics
Director of Pediatric Epilepsy and EEG
Department of Child Neurology
University of Pittsburgh
Children's Hospital of Pittsburgh
Pittsburgh, Pennsylvania

Bernardo Dalla Bernardina, MD, PhD
Professor and Director
Service of Child Neuropsychiatry
University of Verona
Policlinico G.B. Rossi
Verona, Italy

Michael D. Daras, MD, PhD
Clinical Professor of Neurology
Department of Neurology
Columbia University
Attending Neurologist
New York Presbyterian Hospital
New York, New York

Hanneke M. de Boer
Senior Officer International Relations
Epilepsy Centres of The Netherlands Foundation
Haarlem, The Netherlands

Nihal C. De Lanerolle, DPhil, DSc
Associate Professor of Neurosurgery
Yale University School of Medicine
New Haven, Connecticut

Oscar H. Del Brutto, MD
Department of Neurological Sciences
Hospital-Clínica Kennedy
Guayaquil, Ecuador

Robert J. DeLorenzo, MD, PhD, MPH
Professor of Neurology
Biochemistry, Pharmacology and Toxicology
Virginia Commonwealth University
Richmond, Virginia

John De Toledo, MD
International Center for Epilepsy
University of Miami
Miami, Florida

John A. Devereux, BA, LLB, DPhil
Professor of Common Law
T.C. Beirne School of Law
University of Queensland
Brisbane, Queensland
Australia

Orrin Devinsky, MD
Professor of Neurology
Director, New York University Epilepsy Center
New York University Medical Center
New York University School of Medicine

Darryl C. De Vivo, MD
Sidney Carter Professor of Neurology and Pediatrics
Neurological Institute of New York
New York, New York

Marc A. Dichter, MD, PhD
Departments of Neurology and Pharmacology
University of Pennsylvania School of Medicine
Philadelphia, Pennsylvania

Salvatore DiMauro, MD
Lucy G. Moses Professor of Neurology
H. Houston Merritt Clinical Research Center for Muscular Dystrophy and Related Diseases
Department of Neurology
College of Physicians and Surgeons
New York, New York

Raymond Dingledine, PhD
Professor and Chair
Department of Pharmacology
Emory University School of Medicine
Atlanta, Georgia

Amadou Gallo Diop, MD, PhD
Clinique Neurologique
Hopital Universitaire de Fann
Dakar, Senegal

Aleksandra Djukic, MD, PhD
Assistant Professor
Department of Neurology
Albert Einstein College of Medicine
Attending Physician of Neurology
Montefiore Medical Center
Bronx, New York

W. Edwin Dodson, MD
Professor of Neurology and Pediatrics
Washington University School of Medicine
Neurologist
Division of Pediatric Neurology
St. Louis Children's Hospital
St. Louis, Missouri

Werner Doyle, MD
Department of Neurosurgery
New York University Medical School
New York, New York

Charlotte Dravet, MD
Honorary Consultant Ospedale A. Gemelli
Department of Child Neurology and Psychiatry
Catholic University School of Medicine
Rome, Italy
Honorary Consultant IRCCS, Stella Maris Foundation
Epilepsy, Neurophysiology, Neurogenetics Unit
IRCCS, Stella Maris Foundation
Calambrone, Pisa
Italy

Frank W. Drislane, MD
Associate Professor of Neurology
Harvard Medical School
Neurologist, Comprehensive Epilepsy Center
Department of Neurology
Beth Israel Deaconess Medical Center
Boston, Massachusetts

Maurice L. Druzin, MD
Department of Gynecology and Obstetrics
Stanford University School of Medicine
Stanford University Medical Center
Stanford, California

François Dubeau, MD
Associate Professor of Neurology and Neurosurgery
McGill University
Staff and Chief of EEG
Department of Neurology and Neurosurgery
Montreal Neurological Hospital and Institute
Montreal, Quebec
Canada

Michael S. Duchowny, MD
Comprehensive Epilepsy Center
Miami Children's Hospital
Miami, Florida

Olivier Dulac, MD
Neuropediatric Department
Hôpital Necker
Paris, France

John S. Duncan, MA, DM, FRCP
Professor of Neurology
Department of Clinical and Experimental Epilepsy
Institute of Neurology UCL
London, United Kingdom
Medical Director
National Society for Epilepsy
Chalfont Centre for Epilepsy
Bucks, United Kingdom

David W. Dunn, MD
Division of Child and Adolescent Psychiatry
Departments of Psychiatry and Neurology
Indiana University School of Medicine
Indianapolis, Indiana

Mervyn J. Eadie, AO, MD, PhD, FRCP, FRACP
Department of Medicine
University of Queensland
Brisbane, Australia

John S. Ebersole, MD
Professor of Neurology
Director, Adult Epilepsy Service
Co-Director, Comprehensive Epilepsy Center
Department of Neurology
The University of Chicago
Chicago, Illinois

Orvar Eeg-Olofsson, MD PhD
Professor of Neuropediatrics
Department of Women's and Children's Health
Uppsala University
Consultant of Neuropediatrics
University Children's Hospital
Uppsala, Sweden

Jerome Engel, Jr. MD, PhD
Jonathan Sinay Distinguished Professor of Neurology, Neurobiology and Psychiatry and Behavioral Sciences
Director of the UCLA Seizure Disorder Center
David Geffen School of Medicine at UCLA
Los Angeles, California

Leon Eisenberg, MD
Professor of Child Psychiatry and Social Medicine, Emeritus
Department of Social Medicine
Harvard Medical Science
Honorary Psychiatrist
Department of Psychiatry
Massachusetts General Hospital
Boston, Massachusetts

Frances Elmslie, MD, FRCP
Consultant Clinical Geneticist
Department of Medical Genetics
St. George's University of London
London, United Kingdom

Charles M. Epstein, MD
Professor of Neurology
Emory University School of Medicine
Attending Physician
Emory University Hospital
Atlanta, Georgia

Kai J. Eriksson, MD, PhD
Chief, Department of Pediatric Neurology
Tampere University Hospital
Tampere, Finland

Alan B. Ettinger, MD
Department of Neurology
North Shore-LIJ Comprehensive Epilepsy Centers
New Hyde Park, New York

Stanley Fahn, MD
H. Houston Merritt Professor of Neurology
Department of Neurology
Columbia University Medical Center
Neurological Institute or New York
New York, New York

Johan Falk-Pedersen, Esq.
A/S Forretningsadvokatene
Solli, Norway

Erika E. Fanselow, PhD
Postdoctoral Associate
Department of Neuroscience
Brown University
Providence, Rhode Island

Kevin Farrell, MB, ChB, FRCPC
Professor
Division of Neurology
Department of Pediatrics
University of British Columbia
British Columbia's Children's Hospital
Vancouver, Canada

Michael A. Farrell, MB
Department of Neuropathology
Beaumont Hospital
Dublin, Ireland

Edward Faught, MD
Professor and Vice Chairman
Department of Neurology
Director, Division of Epilepsy
University of Alabama at Birmingham Epilepsy Center
Birmingham, Alabama

Natalio Fejerman, MD
Hospital de Pediatria "Juan P. Garrahan"
Beunos Aires, Argentina

Evan J. Fertig, MD
Assistant Professor of Neurology, Neurosurgery, and Pediatrics
Yale University School of Medicine
New Haven, Connecticut

Alexandra Finucane, Esq.
Epilepsy Foundation of America
Landover, Maryland

Bruce J. Fisch, MD
Professor of Neurology
Director
LSU Epilepsy Center of Excellance School of Medicine
Louisiana State University
New Orleans, Louisiana

Robert S. Fisher, MD, PhD
Maslah Saul MD Professor of Neurology
Department of Neurology and Neurological Sciences
Stanford University School of Medicine
Stanford, California

Robert T. Fraser, PhD, CRC
Department of Neurology
University of Washington Epilepsy Center
Harborview Medical Center
Seattle, Washington

Jeremy L. Freeman, MBBS, FRACP
Honorary Lecturer of Pediatrics
Monash University
Clayton, Victoria
Neurologist
Department of Neurology
The Royal Children's Hospital
Parkville, Victoria
Australia

John M. Freeman, MD
Lederer Professor of Pediatric Epilepsy Emeritus
Director, Pediatric Epilepsy Center Emeritus
Professor of Neurology and Pediatrics
Johns Hopkins Medical Institutions
Baltimore, Maryland

Jacqueline A. French, MD
Professor, Assistant Dean for Clinical Trials
Department of Neurology
University of Pennsylvania
Chief, Epilepsy Section
Department of Neurology
Hospital of the University of Pennsylvania
Philadelphia, Pennsylvania

Itzhak Fried, MD, PhD
Division of Neurosurgery
University of California Los Angeles School of Medicine
Los Angeles, California
Functional Neurosurgery Unit
Tel-Aviv Medical Center and Sackler School of Medicine
Tel-Aviv University
Tel-Aviv, Israel

James D. Frost, Jr., MD
Professor of Neurophysiology
Department of Neurology and Neuroscience
Baylor College of Medicine
St. Luke's Episcepal Hospital
Houston, Texas

Steven J. Frucht, MD
Associate Professor of Clinical Neurology
Associate Attending Neurologist
Department of Neurology
Columbia University Medical Center
New York, New York

Cheryl A. Frye, PhD
Departments of Psychology, Biology, and Centers for Neuroscience and Life Sciences Research
The University at Albany-State University of New York
Albany, New York

Lucia Fusco, MD, PhD
Section of Neurophysiology
Bambino Gesu Children's Hospital
Rome, Italy

Eija Gaily
Associate Professor of Pediatric Neurology
Helsinki University
Chief of Epilepsy Unit
Pediatric Neurology
Hospital for Children and Adolescents
Helsinki, Finland

Karen Gale, PhD
Department of Pharmacology
Georgetown University Medical Center
Washington, DC

Elena Gardella, MD, PhD
Research Fellow
Department of Neurosciences
University of Bologna
Bellaria Hospital
Bologna, Italy

Pierre Genton, MD
Neurologist
Centre Saint Paul Hospital
Marseille, France

Mark S. George, MD
Distinguished Professor of Psychiatry, Radiology and Neurosciences
Medical University of South Carolina
Charleston, South Carolina

Barry E. Gidal, PharmD
Professor
School of Pharmacy and Department of Neurology
University of Wisconsin
Madison, Wisconsin

Christopher Gillberg, MD
Section of Child and Adolescent Psychiatry
Department of Clinical Neuroscience
Annedals Clinics
Göteborg, Sweden

Frank Gilliam, MD
Caitlin Tynan Doyle Professor of Neurology
Director, Comprehensive Epilepsy Center
The Neurological Institute
Columbia University
NewYork, NewYork

Michael Glantz, MD
University of Massachusetts
Berkshire Medical Center
Pittsfield, Massachusetts

Tracy A. Glauser, MD
Professor of Pediatrics and Neurology
University of Cincinnati College of Medicine
Director, Comprehensive Epilepsy Program
Division of Child Neurology
Cincinnati Children's Hospital Medical Center
Cincinnati, Ohio

Giuseppe Gobbi, MD
Chief of Child Neurology and Psychiatry
Ospedale Maggiore "Pizzardi" Hospital
Bologna, Italy

David B. Goldstein, MD
Department of Molecular Genetics and Microbiology
Duke University Medical Center
Durham, North Carolia

Jeffrey H. Goodman, PhD
Research Scientist
Center for Neural Recovery and Rehabilitation Research
Helen Hayes Hospital
West Haverstraw, New York

Robert R. Goodman, MD, PhD
Associate Professor
Department of Neurological Surgery
Columbia University College of Physicians and Surgeons
New York, New York

Jean Gotman, PhD
Professor
Department of Neurology and Neurosurgery
McGill University and Montreal Neurological Institute
Montreal, Quebec
Canada

Salvatore Grosso, MD, PhD
Researcher and Assistant
Department of Pediatrics
SS. Maria alle Scotte Hospital
University of Siena
Siena, Italy

Carlos A. M. Guerreiro, MD, PhD
Professor of Neurology
State University of Campinas
Campinas, Brazil

Renzo Guerrini, MD
Professor
University of Florence
Director of Child Neurology Unit
AOU Meyer
Florence, Italy

Robert J. Gumnit, MD
Clinical Professor of Neurology, Neurosurgery and Pharmacy
University of Minnesota
President
MINCEP Epilepsy Care
Minneapolis, Minnesota

Houda Hachad, PharmD
Senior Research Scientist
Department of Pharmaceutics
University of Washington
Seattle, Washington

Michael M. Haglund, MD, PhD
Department of Neurosurgery
Duke University Medical Center
Durham, North Carolina

Mark Hallett, MD
Chief, Human Motor Control Section
National Institute of Neurological Disorders and Stroke
National Institute of Health
Bethesda, Maryland

Marla Hamberger, PhD
Associate Professor of Clinical Neuropsychology
Department of Neurology
Chief Neuropsychologist
Comprehensive Epilepsy Center
The Neurological Institute
New York, New York

Cynthia L. Harden, MD
Professor of Neurology
Weill Medical College of Cornell University
Attending Neurologist
New York-Presbyterian Hospital
New York, New York

A. Simon Harvey, MD
Department of Neurology
Children's Epilepsy Program
Royal Children's Hospital
Melbourne, Australia

W. Allen Hauser, MD
Professor of Epidemiology and Neurology
G. H. Dergievsky Center
Associate Director
College of Physicians and Surgeons and Mailman School of Public Health
Columbia University Medical Center
Attending Neurologist
Neurological Institute
New York, New York

Sheryl Haut, MD
Associate Professor of Clinical Neurology
Director, Adult Epilepsy Service
Albert Einstein College of Medicine
Bronx, New York

Philip G. Haydon, PhD
Professor and Director
Silvio Conte Center for Integration at the Tripartite Synapse
Director, Center for Dynamic Imaging of Nervous System Function
Department of Neuroscience
University of Pennsylvania School of Medicine
Philadelphia, Pennsylvania

Liyun He, MD
Associate Professor
Clinical Evaluation Center
China Academy of Chinese Medicine Sciences
Beijing, China

Uwe Heinemann, PhD
Head of Institute of Neurophysiology
Charite Medical University Berlin
Berlin, Germany

Christoph Helmstaedter, PhD
Associate Professor of Clinical Neuropsychology
Department of Epileptology
University of Bonn
Bonn, Germany

Thomas R. Henry, MD
Professor of Neurology
University of Minnesota
Minneapolis, Minnesota

Bruce P. Hermann, PhD
Department of Neuropsychology
University of Wisconsin
Madison, Wisconsin

Dale C. Hesdorffer, PhD
Assistant Professor
Gertrude H. Sergievsky Center
Columbia University
New York, New York

Andrew G. Herzog, MD, MSc
Professor of Neurology
Harvard Medical School
Director of Neuroendocrine Unit
Beth Israel Deaconess Medical Center
Boston, Massachusetts

Michio Hirano, MD
Associate Professor of Neurology
H. Houston Merritt Clinical Research Center for Muscular Dystrophy and Related Diseases
Department of Neurology
College of Physicians and Surgeons of Columbia University
New York, New York

Edouard Hirsch, MD
Professor of Neurology
HUS Strasburg
IDEE
Strasburg, France

Lawrence J. Hirsch, MD
Associate Clinical Professor
Department of Neurology
Columbia University Medical Center
Associate Attending Neurologist
New York-Presbyterian Hospital
New York, New York

Daryl Hochman, PhD
Department of Neurosurgery
Duke University Medical Center
Durham, North Carolina

Gregory L. Holmes, MD
Professor of Neurology and Pediatrics
Neuroscience Center at Dartmouth
Dartmouth Medical School
Hanover, New Hampshire
Chief, Section of Neurology
Dartmouth-Hitchcock Medical Center
Lebanon, New Hampshire

Mark D. Holmes, MD
Professor of Neurology
University of Washington
Director, Clinical Neuropyhsiology
Regional Epilepsy Center
Harborview Medical Center
Seattle, Washington

Richard A. Hrachovy, MD
Professor of Neurolgoy
Baylor College of Medicine
Associate Chief of EEG
Department of Neurophysiology
St. Luke's Episcopal Hospital
Houston, Texas

Yushi Inoue, MD, PhD
Vice-director
National Epilepsy Center
Shizuoka Institute of Epilepsy and Neurological Disorders
Shizuoka, Japan

Graeme D. Jackson, MD
Brain Research Institute
West Heidelberg, Australia

Ann Jacoby, PhD
Professor of Medical Sociology
Division of Public Health, School of Population, Community and Behavioral Sciences
University of Liverpool
Liverpool, United Kingdom

Satish Jain, MD, DM
Director, Indian Epilepsy Center
New Delhi, India

Pierre Jallon, MD
Epilepsy and EEG Unit
University Hospital
Geneva, Switzerland

Damir Janigro, PhD
Professor, Molecular Medicine
Department of Neurosurgery and Molecular Medicine
Cleveland Clinic Foundation
Cleveland, Ohio

Prasanna Jayakar, MD, PhD
Chair
Brain Institute
Miami Children's Hospital
Miami, Florida

John G. R. Jefferys, FMedSci
Professor of Neuroscience
Division of Neuroscience
School of Medicine
University Birmingham
Birmingham, United Kingdom

Frances E. Jensen, MD
Professor of Neurology
Director of Epilepsy Research
Department of Neurology
Children's Hospital
Boston, Massachusetts

Svein I. Johannessen, PhD
Director of Research
The National Center for Epilepsy, Sandvika
Division of Clinical Neuroscience, Rikshospitalet, Oslo
Sandvika, Norway

Marilyn Jones-Gotman, PhD
Professor of Neurology and Neurosurgery
McGill University
Coordinator, Neuropsychology Epilepsy Service
Montreal Neurological Institute
Montreal, Quebec
Canada

Philippe Kahane, MD, PhD
Neurophysiopathologie de l'Epilepsie
Clinique Neurologique
Grenoble, France

Ellie Kalichi, RN
Chikankata Epilepsy Care Team Coordinator
Mazabuka, Zambia

Reetta Kälviäinen, MD, PhD
Docent/Associate Professor of Neurology
University of Kuopio Academic Institution
Director of Neurology
Kuopio Epilepsy Center
Kuopio University Hospital
Kuopio, Finland

Anna Kaminska
Department of Pediatric Neurophysiology
Groupe Hospitalier Cochin-Saint
Vincent de Paul and Necker Enfant
Paris, France

Kousuke Kanemoto
Department of Neuropsychiatry
Aichi Medical University
Nagakute, Aichi, Japan

Andres M. Kanner, MD
Department of Neurology
Rush University Medical Center
Chicago, Illinois

Peter W. Kaplan, MBBS
Professor of Neurology
Director of Epilepsy and Electrophysiology
Bayview Medical Center
Johns Hopkins University School of Medicine
Baltimore, Maryland

Russell Katz, MD
U.S. Food and Drug Administration
Division of Neuropharmacological Drug Products
Rockville, Maryland

Noojan J. Kazemi, MBBS
Doctorial Student
Department of Surgery
University of Melbourne
Registrar
Department of Neurosurgery
The Royal Melbourne Hospital
Parkville, Victoria
Australia

Michael P. Kerr, MBChB, MRCEP, MRCPsych, MSc in Psychiatry
Professor of Learning Disability Psychiatry
Psychological Medicine
Cardiff University School of Medicine
Cardiff, United Kingdom

Sonia Khan, FRCP (Lond), FRCP (Edin)
Director and Consultant
Department of Neurosciences
Riyadh Military Hospital
Riyadh, Kingdom of Saudi Arabia

Negar Khanlou,
Section of Neuropathology
UCLA Medical Center
Los Angeles, California

Eliane Kobayashi, MD, PhD
Assistant Professor
Department of Neurology and Neurosurgery
Montreal Neurological Institute and Hospital
McGill University
Montreal, Quebec
Canada

Steffi C. Koch-Stoecker, MD
Head of Psychiatric Outpatient Clinic
Psychiatric Consultant of Epilepsy Center
Ev. Krankenhaus Bielefeld
Bielefeld, Germany

Barbara S. Koppel, MD
Professor of Clinical Neurology
New York Medical College
Valhalla, New York
Chief, Neurology Service
Metropolitan Hospital
New York, New York

Maria D. Kostka-Rokosz, Pharm D
Department of Pharmacy Practice
Massachusetts College of Pharmacy and Health Sciences
Boston, Massachusetts

Prakash Kotagal, MD
Head, Pediatric Epilepsy
Epilepsy Center
Cleveland Clinic
Cleveland, Ohio

Dimitri M. Kullmann, DPhil, FRCP
Professor
Institute of Neurology
University College London
Consultant Neurologist
National Hospital for Neurology and Neurosurgery
London, United Kingdom

Wolfram S. Kunz, PhD
Divison of Neurochemistry
Department of Epileptology
University of Bonn Medical Center
Bonn, Germany

Harvey J. Kupferberg, PhD, PharmD,
Kupferberg Consultants, LLC
Chief, Preclinical Pharmacology Section (retired)
Epilepsy Branch
National Institute of Neurological Disorders and Stroke
National Institutes of Health
Bethesda, Maryland

Ruben I. Kuzniecky, MD
New York University Epilepsy Center
New York, New York

Patrick Kwan, MB, BChir, MRCP, PhD
Division of Neurology
Department of Medicine
The Chinese University of Hong Kong
Prince of Wales Hospital
Hong Kong, China

W. Curt LaFrance, Jr. MD
Departments of Psychiatry and Neurology
Rhode Island Hospital
Providence Rhode Island

Chi-Wan Lai, MD
Professor of Neurology
Tzu Chi University Medical School
Hualien, Taiwan
Staff Neurologist
Department of Medicine
Sun Yat-Sen Cancer Center
Taipei, Taiwan

Frederick G. Langendorf, MD
Associate Professor
Department of Neurology
University of Minnesota
Assistant Chief of Neurology
Hennepin County Medical Center
Minneapolis, Minnesota

John T. Langfitt, PhD
Associate Professor of Neurology and Psychiatry
University of Rochester Medical Center
Rochester, New York

Barbara W. LeDuc
Assistant Professor
Department of Pharmacology
Massachusetts College of Pharmacology and Health Sciences
Boston, Massachusetts

Gabriel Lee, MBS (Hons), MS, FRACS
Consultant Neurosurgeon
Department of Neurosurgery
Sir Charles Gairdner Hospital
Perth, Western Australia

Alan D. Legatt, MD, PhD
Professor of Clinical Neurology
Department of Neurology
Albert Einstein College of Medicine
Director, EEG Laboratory
Department of Neurology
Montefiore Medical Center
Bronx, New York

Cynthia Lehman, Esq
Epilepsy Foundation of America
Landover, Maryland

Klaus Lehnertz, PhD
Associate Professor of Physics
Faculty of Mathematics and Natural Science
Head Neurophysics Group
Department of Epileptology
University of Bonn Medical Center
Bonn, Germany

Matilde Leonardi, MD
Head, Department of Neurology
Public Health and Disability Unit (HEADNET)
Neurological Institute Carlo Besta IRCCS Foundation
Milan, Italy

Ilo E. Leppik, MD
Professor of Neurology and Pharmacy
University of Minnesota
Minneapolis, Minnesota

Ronald P. Lesser, MD
Professor of Neurology and Neurosurgery
Member, Zanvyl Krieger Mind/Brain Institute
Department of Neurology
Johns Hopkins Medical Institutions
Baltimore, Maryland

Pierre LeVan, M.Eng.
Graduate Student
Biomedical Engineering
McGill University
Department of Electroencephalogram
Montreal Neurological Institute
Montreal, Quebec
Canada

Michel Le Van Quyen, PhD
INSERM Researcher
French National Institute for Health and Medical Research
Laboratory of Brain Imaging and Cognitive Neuroscience
Hopital de la Salpetriere
Paris, France

René H. Levy, PhD
Department of Pharmaceutics
University of Washington
Seattle, Washington

Darrell V. Lewis, MD
Professor of Pediatrics
Division of Pediatric Neurology
Duke University Medical Center
Durham, North Carolina

Samden D. Lhatoo, MD
Department of Neurology
Institute of Clinical Neurosciences
Frenchay Hospital
University of Bristol
Bristol, United Kingdom

Shichuo Li, MD
President
China Association Against Epilepsy
Beijing, People's Republic of China

Weiping Liao, MD
Professor
Neuroscience Institute
Guangzhou Medical College
Guangzhou, China

Jack J. Lin, MD
Assistant Professor of Neurology
Director, Clinical Neurophysiology Fellowship
University of California, Irvine
Irvine, California

Richard B. Lipton, MD
Professor and Vice Chair of Neurology,
Professor of Epidemiology and Population Health
Albert Einstein College of Medicine
Director, Montefiore Headache Unit
Innovative Medical AECOM
Bronx, New York

Brian Litt, MD
Associate Professor
Department of Neurology and Bioengineering
University of Pennsylvania
Philadelphia, Pennsylvania

Iscia Lopes-Cendes, MD, PhD
Associate Professor
Medical Genetics
University of Campinas
Campinas, Brazil

Fernando H. Lopes da Silva, MD
Emeritus Professor
Center of Neuroscience
Swammerdam Institute for Life Sciences
University of Amsterdam
Amsterdam, The Netherlands

David W. Loring, PhD
Professor of Neurology
Department of Neurology
McKnight Brain Institute
Gainesville, Florida

Wolfgang Löscher,
Department of Pharmacology, Toxicology & Pharmacy
University of Veterinary Medicine, Hannover
Hannover, Germany

Daniel H. Lowenstein, MD
Professor of Neurology
Director, Epilepsy Center
Department of Neurology
University of California
San Francisco, California

Guoming Luan, MD
Professor of Neurosurgery
San Bo Brain Sciences Institute of Beijing
Beijing, China

Hans O. Lüders, MD
Professor of Neurology
Director, Epilepsy Center
Case Western Reserve Medical Center
Cleveland, Ohio

Katarzyna Lukasiuk, PhD
Associate Professor
Department of Molecular and Cellular Neurobiology
The Nencki Institute of Experimental Biology
Warsaw, Poland

Robert L. Macdonald, MD, PhD
Professor and Chair of Neurology
Vanderbilt University Medical Center
Nashville, Tennessee

Mark W. Mahowald, MD
Minnesota Regional Sleep Disorders Center
Hennepin County Medical Center
Minneapolis, Minnesota

Beth A. Malow, MD, MS
Associate Professor
Department of Neurology
Medical Director
Vanderbilt Sleep Disorders Center
Vanderbilt University Medical Center
Nashville, Tennessee

Gary W. Mathern, MD
Professor and Attending Physician
Department of Neurosurgery
David Geffen School of Medicine
University of California Los Angeles
Los Angeles, California

Richard H. Mattson, MD
Department of Neurology
Yale Medical Center
New Haven, Connecticut

John C. Mazziotta, MD, PhD
Chair, Department of Neurology
Pierson-Lovelace Investigator
Stark Chair in Neurology
Director, Brain Mapping Center
Associate Director, Neuropsychiatric Institute
David Geffen School of Medicine at UCLA
Los Angeles, California

Dan C. McIntyre, PhD
Chancellor's Professor
Department of Psychology, Institute of Neuroscience
Carleton University
Ottawa, Ontario
Canada

Guy M. McKhann, II, MD
Florence Irving Associate Professor of Neurological Surgery
The Neurological Institute
Columbia University Medical Center
New York, New York

William McLin
Merriman and Co.
Washington, DC

Kimford J. Meador, MD
Professor of Neurology
Melvin Greer
University of Florida
Gainesville, Florida

Harry Meinardi, MD
Professor of Epileptology (Retired)
Department of Neurology
Medical Director
Instituut voor Epilepsiebestrijding
Heenstede, The Netherlands

Brian S. Meldrum, MD, PhD
King College London
GKT School of Medicine
Hodgkin House
London, England

Roberto Michelucci, MD, PhD
Director of Neurology Unit
Department of Neurosciences
Bellaria Hospital
Bologna, Italy

David Millett
Clinical Fellow
Department of Neurology
University of California Los Angeles
Los Angeles, California

Hajime Miyata, MD, PhD
Department of Neuropathology
Institute of Neurological Sciences
Faculty of Medicine
Totori University
Yonago, Tottori
Japan

Eli M. Mizrahi, MD
Head, Peter Kellaway Section of Neurophysiology
Vice-Chairman, Department of Neurology
Professor of Neurology and Pediatrics
Baylor College of Medicine
Chief, Neurophysiology Services
St. Luke's Episcopal Hospital
Texas Children's Hospital
Houston, Texas

Istvan Mody, PhD
Professor
Departments of Neurology and Physiology
The David Geffen School of Medicine at UCLA
Los Angeles, California

Georgia D. Montouris, MD
Assistant Professor
Department of Neurology
Boston University School of Medicine
Director of Epilepsy Services
Boston Medical Center
Boston, Massachusetts

Joan T. Moroney, MD, MRCPI
Beaumont Hospital
Department of Neurology
Dublin, Ireland

Martha J. Morrell, MD
Clinical Professor of Neurology
Stanford University Medical Center
Stanford, California

Solomon L. Moshé, MD
Vice Chair and Professor of Neurology, Neuroscience and Pediatrics
Albert Einstein College of Medicine of Yeshiva University
Director of Child Neurology and Clinical Neurophysiology
Department of Neurology and Pediatric Neurology
Montefiore Medical Center
Bronx, New York

Marco Mula, MD, PhD
Research Fellow
Department of Clinical & Experimental Medicine, Section of Neurology
Amedeo Avogadro University
Novara, Italy
Department of Psychiatry, Neurobiology, Pharmacology and Biotechnology
University of Pisa
Pisa, Italy

Karl O. Nakken, MD, PhD
Chief Physician
Division of Clinical Neuroscience
The National Center for Epilepsy
Sandvika, Norway

Martha A. Nance, MD
Adjunct Associate Professor
Department of Neurology
University of Minnesota
Minneapolis, Minnesota

Lina Nashef, MBChB, MRCP, MD, FRCP
Honorary Senior Lecturer
Department of Clinical Neuroscience
King's College London, Institute of Psychiatry
Consultant Neurologist
Department of Neurology
King's College Hospital
London, United Kingdom

Wassim M. Nasreddine, MD
Chief and Head, Neurology Division
Beirut Governmental University Hospital
Jnah, Beirut
Lebanon

Ibrahima Pierre Ndiaye, MD
Department of Neurology
University Hospital of Fann
Dakar, Senegal

Astrid Nehlig, PhD
Research Director
French National Institute for Health and Medical Research
Faculty of Medicine
Strasbourg, France

Brian G. Neville, MD
The Wolfson Centre
London, United Kingdom

Jeffrey L. Noebels, MD, PhD
Professor of Neurology, Neuroscience and Molecular Genetics
Baylor College of Medicine
Houston, Texas

Douglas R. Nordli, Jr., MD
Associate Professor of Neurology and Pediatrics
Northwestern University Feinberg School of Medicine
Lorna S. and James P. Langdon Chair of Pediatric Epilepsy
Director, Epilepsy Center
Children's Memorial Hospital
Chicago, Illinois

Marc R. Nuwer, MD, PhD
Professor of Neurology
Head, Department of Clinical Neurophysiology
Univeristy of California Los Angeles
Los Angeles, California

Terence J. O'Brien, MBBS
St. Vincent Hospital
Department of Clinical Neurosciences
Victoria, Australia

Shunsuke Ohtahara, MD, PhD
Professor Emeritus
Department of Child Neurology
Okayama University Graduate School of Medicine, Dentistry and Pharmaceutical Sciences
Shikatacho, Okayama
Japan

Yoko Ohtsuka, MD, PhD
Professor
Department of Child Neurology
Okayama University Graduate School of Medicine, Dentistry and Pharmaceutical Sciences
Shikatacho, Okayama
Japan

George A. Ojemann, MD
University of Washington
Regional Epilepsy Center
Harborview Medical Center
Seattle, Washington

Ruth Ottman, PhD
Professor of Epidemiology
Sergievsky Center
Columbia University
New York, New York

Christoph Pachlatko, Dr. oec. Pfr.
Managing Director
Swiss Epilepsy Center
Zürich, Switzerland

Alison M. Pack, MD
Assistant Professor of Clinical Neurology
Department of Neurology
Columbia University
New York Presbyterian Hospital
New York, New York

Chrysostomos P. Panayiotopoulos, MD, PhD
Consultant Emeritus
Department of Clinical Neurophysiology and Epilepsies
St. Thomas' Hospital
London, United Kingdom

Jack M. Parent, MD
Associate Professor of Neurology
University of Michigan
Ann Arbor, Michigan

Elena Parrini, PhD
Molecular Biologist
Neurogenetics Lab
Child Neurology Unit
AOU Meyer
Florence, Italy

Philip N. Patsalos, FRCPath, PhD
Professor
Department of Clinical and Experimental Epilepsy
Institute of Neurology
London, United Kingdom
Professor
Pharmacology and Therapeutics Unit
Chalfont Centre for Epilepsy
Chalfont St. Peter, Buckinghamshire
United Kingdom

Timothy A. Pedley, MD
Henry and Lucy Moses Professor of Neurology
Chairman, Department of Neurology
Columbia University
Neurologist-in-Chief
The Neurological Institute of New York
The New York-Presbyterian Hospital
Columbia University Medical Center
New York, New York

John M. Pellock, MD
Division of Child Neurology
Medical College of Virginia
Richmond, Virginia

Jukka Peltola, MD, PhD
Deputy Chief
Department of Neurology
Tampere University Hospital
Tampere, Finland

Emilio Perucca, MD, PhD, FRCP(Edin)
Professor, Clinical Pharmacology Unit
Department of Internal Medicine and Therapeutics
University of Pavia
Director, Laboratories for Diagnostics and Applied Biological Research
Institute of Neurology IRCCS C. Mondino Foundation
Pavia, Italy

Ognen A. C. Petroff, MD
Associate Professor of Neurology
Director of EEG and Attending Physician
Department of Neurology
Yale University
Yale-New Haven Hospital
New Haven Connecticut

Margarete Pfäfflin
Epilepsy-Center Bethel
Bielefeld, Germany

Fabienne Picard, MD
Department of Neurology
University Hospital of Geneva
Geneva, Switezerland

Demetris K. Pillas, MSc
PhD Candidate
Epidemiology and Public Health Department
Imperial College of London
London, United Kingdom

Antonella Pini, MD
Physician
Child Neurology Unit
Ospedale Maggiore Ca Pizzardi
Bologna, Italy

Munir Pirmohamed, PhD, FRCP, FRCP(E)
Professor of Clinical Pharmacology
Department of Pharmacology and Therapeutics
The University of Liverpool
Consultant Physician
The Royal Liverpool University Hospital
Liverpool, United Kingdom

Asla Pitkänen, MD, PhD, DSc
Professor in Neurobiology
A.I.Virtanen Institute for Molecular Sciences
University of Kuopio
Kuopio, Finland

Perrine Plouin, MD
Head of Clinical Neurophysiology
Necker Enfants Malades Hospital
Paris, France

Charles E. Polkey, MD, FRCS
Professor Emeritus of Functional Neurosurgery
Department of Clinical Neurociences
Institute of Psychiatry
London, United Kingdom

Roger J. Porter, MD
Adjunct Professor of Neurology
University of Pennsylvania
Philadelphia, Pennsylvania
Adjunct Professor of Pharmacology
Uniformed Services University of the Health Sciences
Bethesda, Maryland

Tiziano Pramparo, PhD
Molecular Biologist
Department of Biology and Medical Genetics
University of Pavia
Pavia, Italy

Michael D. Privitera, MD
Professor and Vice Chair Neurology
Director, Cincinnati Epilepsy Center
University of Cincinnati Medical Center
Cincinnati, Ohio

Mark Proctor, MD
Department of Neurosurgery
Brigham and Women's Hospital
Boston, Massachusetts

Mark S. Quigg, MD, MSc
Associate Professor of Neurology
Medical Director
EEG, Intensive Monitoring, Evoked Potential, and Neurological Sleep Laboratories
Health Sciences Center
University of Virginia
Charlottesville, Virginia

Kurupath Radhakrishnan, MD
R. Madhavan Nayar Center for Comprehensive Epilepsy Care
Sree Chitra Tirunal Institute for Medical Sciences and Technology
Trivandrum, Kerala, India

R. Eugene Ramsay, MD
International Center for Epilepsy
Miami, Florida

Peter M. Rankin D. Clin. Psych.
Honorary Senior Lecturer
Institute of Child Health
University College London
Consultant Paediatric Neuropsychologist
Department of Psychological Medicine
Great Ormond Street Hospital For Children NHS Trust
London, United Kingdom

Lawrence D. Recht, MD
Professor of Neurolgoy
Stanford University
Stanford, California

Jean Régis, MD
Professor of Neurosurgery
Stereotatic and Functional Neurosurgery Department
Timone Hospital
Marseille, France

Trevor J. Resnick, MD
Associate Professor
Chief of Neurology
University of Miami, Miller School of Medicine
Miami Children's Hospital
Miami, Florida

Jong M. Rho, MD
Associate Professor
Department of Neurology
University of Arizona College of Medicine
Children's Health Center
St. Joseph's Hospital and Medical Center
Phoenix, Arizona

Kristen A. Richardson, PhD
Postdoctoral Associate
Department of Neuroscience
Brown University
Providence, Rhode Island

David W. Roberts, MD
Section of Neurosurgery
Dartmouth-Hitchcock Medical Center
Lebanon, New Hampshire

Michael A. Rogawski, MD, PhD
Epilepsy Research Section
National Institute of Neurological Disorders and Stroke
National Institutes of Health
Bethesda, Maryland

Guido Rubboli, MD
Attending Physician
Department of Neurosciences
Bellaria Hospital
Bologna, Italy

Zarya A. Rubin, MD, FRCPC
Comprehensive Epilepsy Center
Neurological Institute of New York
Columbia University
New York, New York

Anne Sabers, MD
Chief of the Epilepsy Unit
Department of Neurology
Glostrup University Hospital
Glostrup, Denmark

Ralph L. Sacco, MD
Department of Neurology and the School of Public Health in the Sergievsky Center
Columbia University
Neurological Institute of New York
New York, New York

Noriko Salamon, MD, PhD
Department of Neuroradiology
David Geffen School of Medicine
University of California Los Angeles Medical Center
Los Angeles, California

Josemir W. Sander, MD, PhD, FRCP
Professor of Clinical and Experimental Epilepsy
Honorary Consultant Neurologist
Epilepsy Centre
National Hospital for Neurology and Neurosurgery
London, United Kingdom

Raman Sankar, MD, PhD
Departments of Neurology and Pediatrics
University of California Los Angeles School of Medicine
Los Angeles, California

P. Satishchandra, MBBS, DM (Neurology), FAMS, FIAN
Professor of Neurology
National Institute of Mental Health and Neurosciences (NIMHANS)
Bangalore, Karnataka
India

Steven C. Schachter, MD
Professor of Neurology
Harvard Medical School
Director of Research
Department of Neurology
Beth Israel Deaconess Medical Center
Boston, Massachusetts

Helen E. Scharfman, PhD
Associate Professor
Helen Hayes Hospital Center
New York, New York
Associate Professor of Clinical Pharmacology (in Neurology)
Department of Pharmacology and Neurology
Columbia University
New York, New York
Director
Center for Neural Recovery and Rehabilitation Research
Helen Hayes Hospital, New York State Department of Health
West Haverstraw, New York

Ingrid E. Scheffer, MBBS, PhD, FRACP
Professor of Paediatric Neurology Research
Department of Medicine, Austin Health
Department of Paediatrics, Royal Children's Hospital
The University of Melbourne
Parkville, Victoria
Director of Paediatrics
Department of Medicine
Austin Health Repatriation Hospital
Heidelberg, Victoria
Australia

Carlos H. Schenck, MD
Department of Psychiatry
Hennepin County Medical Center
University of Minnesota Medical Center,
Minneapolis, Minnesota

Mark S. Scher, MD
Professor of Pediatrics and Neurology
Department of Pediatrics
Division Chief, Pediatric Neurology
Director, Pediatric Sleep/Epilepsy & Fetal/Neonatal Neurology Program
Rainbow Babies & Children's Hospital
University Hospital Case Medical Center
Cleveland, Ohio

Bernd Schmidt, MD
Head, Neurology and Psychiatry Outpatient Clinic
Wittnau, Germany

Dieter Schmidt, MD
Emeritus Professor of Neurology
Epilepsy Research Group
Berlin, Germany

Bettina Schmitz
Professor
Charite Neurologie
Berlin, Germany

Donald L. Schomer, MD
Maslah Saul MD Professor of Neurology
Department of Neurology and Neurological Sciences
Stanford University School of Medicine
Stanford, California
Comprehensive Epilepsy Program
Beth Israel Deaconess Medical Center
Boston, Massachusetts

Stephanie Schorge, PhD
Assistant Professor
Institute of Neurology
University College London
London, United Kingdom

Johannes Schramm
Professor and Chairman
Department of Neurosurgery
University of Bonn
Bonn, Germany

Robert Schwarcz, PhD
Professor of Psychiatry
Maryland Psychiatric Research Center
University of Maryland School of Medicine
Baltimore, Maryland

Philip A. Schwartzkroin, PhD
Department of Neurological Surgery
University of California–Davis
Davis, California

Michael Seidenberg, PhD
Department of Psychology
Finch University of Health Sciences
The Chicago Medical School
Chicago, Illinois

Masakazu Seino, MD*
National Epilepsy Center
Shizuoka Medical Institute of Neurologic Diseases
Shizuoka, Japan

Caroline E. Selai, BA(Hons), MSc, PhD, DipPsych, CPsychol.
Senior Lecturer in Clinical Neuroscience
University College London, Institute of Neurology
National Hospital for Neurology and Neurosurgery
London, United Kingdom

Patricia O. Shafer, RN, MN
Division of Public Health
University of Liverpool
Liverpool, United Kingdom

*Deceased

Volney L. Sheen, MD, PhD
Department of Neurology
Harvard Medical School
Beth Israel Deaconess Medical Center
Boston, Massachusetts

D. Alan Shewmon, MD
Department of Neurology
Olive View-UCLA Medical Center
Sylmar, California

Hiroshi Shibasaki, MD, PhD
Consultant
Takeda General Hospital
Kyoto, Japan

W. Donald Shields, MD
University of California Los Angeles Medical Center
Department of Pediatric Neurology
Mattel Children's Hospital
Los Angeles, California

Hideo Shigematsu, MD
Chief
Department of Pediatrics
National Epilepsy Center
Shizouka Medical Institute of Neurological Disorders
Shizouka, Japan

Shlomo Shinnar, MD, PhD
Albert Einstein College of Medicine
Montefiore Medical Center
Bronx, New York

Simon D. Shorvon, MD, FRCP
Professor in Clinical Neurology and Clinical Subdean Consultant Neurologist
University College of London
National Hospital for Neurology and Neurosurgery
London, United Kingdom

Margaret N. Shouse, PhD
Professor
Department of Neurobiology
University of California Los Angeles School of Medicine
Los Angeles, Californina
Chief, Sleep Disturbance Research
VA Greater Los Angeles Healthcare System
North Hills, California

Stephen D. Silberstein, MD
Professor of Neurology
Jefferson Medical College
Director, Jefferson Headache Center
Thomas Jefferson University Hospital
Philadelphia, Pennsylvania

Sanjay M. Sisodiya, MBBChir, MA, PhD, FRCP
Professor
Department of Clinical and Experimental Epilepsy
UCL Institute of Neurology
Honorary Consultant Neurologist
Division of Neurology
National Hospital for Neurology and Neurosurgery
London, United Kingdom

Mary Lou Smith, PhD
Professor of Psychology
University of Toronto Mississauga
Mississaugo, Ontario
Psychologist
Department of Psychology and Neurology
Hospital for Sick Children
Toronto, Ontario
Canada

Michael C. Smith, MD
Department of Neurological Sciences
Rush Epilepsy Center
Chicago, Illinois

Dee Snape
Division of Public Health
University of Liverpool
Liverpool, United Kingdom

O. Carter Snead, III, MD
Head, Division of Neurology
Hospital for Sick Children
Toronto, Ontario
Canada

Elson L. So, MD
Professor of Neurology
Consultant and Director of Neurology
Section of Electroencephalography
Mayo Clinic College of Medicine
Rochester, Minnesota

Luigi Specchio, MD
Clinic of Nervous System Diseases
University of Foggia
Foggia, Italy

Nicola Specchio, MD
Section of Neurophysiology
Bambino Gesu Children's Hospital
Rome, Italy

Sarah J. Spence, MD, PhD
UCLA Department of Psychiatry & Biobehavioral Sciences
Medical Director UCLA Autism Evaluation Clinic
Medical Director of the Autism Genetic Resource Exchange
Los Angeles, California

Dennis D. Spencer, MD
Yale University
School of Medicine Neurosurgery
New Haven Connecticut

Susan S. Spencer, MD
Professor of Neurology
Yale University School of Medicine
Attending Director, Epilepsy Unit
Department of Neurology
Yale New Haven Hospital
New Haven, Connecticut

Michael R. Sperling, MD
Professor of Neurology
Thomas Jefferson University
Director, Jefferson Comprehensive Epilepsy Center
Thomas Jefferson University Hospital
Philadelphia, Pennsylvania

Carl E. Stafstrom, MD, PhD
Professor of Neurology and Pediatrics
Chief, Section of Pediatric Neurology
University of Wisconsin
Madison, Wisconsin

Hermann Stefan, Prof.Dr.Med.
Professor
Epilepsy Center
University Erlangen
Director of Epilepsy Center
University Hospital Erlangen
Erlangen, Bavaria
Germany

Christian Steinhäuser, PhD
Professor and Director
Institute of Cellular Neurosciences
University of Bonn Medical School
Bonn, Germany

Ortrud K. Steinlein, MD
Head of Department
Institute of Human Genetics
University of Munich
Munchen, Germany

Linda J. Stephen, MBChB
Honorary Senior Lecturer
Division of Cardiovascular and Medical Sciences
University of Glasgow
Associate Specialist
Division of Cardiovascular and Medical Sciences
Western Infirmary
Glasgow, Scotland
United Kingdom

John B. P. Stephenson, MA, DM
Honorary Professor in Pediatric Neurology
University of Glasgow
Fraser of Allander Neurosciences Unit
Royal Hospital for Sick Children
Glasgow, Scotland
United Kingdom

John M. Stern, MD
Associate Professor of Neurology
David Geffen School of Medicine at UCLA
Los Angeles, California

Mark Stewart, MD, PhD
Associate Professor
Department of Physiology and Pharmacology Neurology
State University of New York Downstate Medical Center
Brooklyn, New York

John W. Swann, PhD
Professor
Department of Pediatric and Neuroscience
Baylor College of Medicine
Scientific Director
The Cain Foundation Laboratories
Texas Children's Hospital
Houston, Texas

Chong Tin Tan, MD, FRCP
University of Malaya
Chair of the Commission on Asian and Oceanian Affairs
International League Against Epilepsy
Kuala Lumpur, Malaysia

Carlo Alberto Tassinari, MD
Professor of Neurological Sciences
University of Bologna
Consultant
Department of Neurosciences
Bellaria Hospital
Bologna, Italy

David C. Taylor, MD, MSc, FRCP, FRCPsych
Institute of Child Health and Great Ormond Street Hospital
The Wolfson Centre
London, United Kingdom

Joanne Taylor, BSc
Postgraduate Research Student
Department of Neurological Science
The University of Liverpool
Clinical Science Centre for Research and Education
Liverpool, United Kingdom

Ludger Tebartz van Elst, MD, PhD
Professor of Psychiatry and Psychotherapy
Consultant Psychiatrist
University of Freiburg
Freiburg, Germany

Nancy R. Temkin, PhD
Professor
Departments of Neurological Surgery and Biostatistics
University of Washington
Seattle, Washington

Kiyohito Terada, MD, PhD
Chief
Department of Neurology
National Epilepsy Center
Shizuoka Institute of Epilepsy and Neurological Disorders
Shizuoka, Japan

William H. Theodore, MD
Chief, Clinical Epilepsy Section
National Institute of Neurological Disorders and Stroke
National Institute of Health
Bethesda, Maryland

Pierre Thomas, MD, PhD
Professor of Neurology
Department of Medicine
University of Nice-Sophia-Antipolis
Chief
Department of Epileptology and Clinical Neurology
Hopital Pasteur
Nice, France

Rupprecht Thorbecke
Epilepsy Center Bethel
Klinik Mara
Bielefeld, Germany

Arthur W. Toga, PhD
Professor of Neurology
University of California Los Angeles School of Medicine
Los Angeles, California

Torbjörn Tomson, MD
Department of Clinical Neuroscience
Karolinska Institutet
Stockholm, Sweden

Roger D. Traub, MD
Department of Physiology and Pharmacology, and Neurology
SUNY Downstate Medical Center
Brooklyn, New York

David M. Treiman, MD
Newsome Chair in Epileptology
Vice Chair, Neurology
Director, Epilepsy Program
Barrow Neurological Institute
Phoenix, Arizona
Research Professor
Harrington Department of Bioengineering
Arizona State University
Tempe, Arizona

Andrew J. Trevelyan, MD
Department of Biological Sciences
Columbia University
New York, New York

Michael R. Trimble, MD
Professor of Behavioral Neurology
Institute of Neurology
London, United Kingdom

John D. Van Horn, PhD, MEng
Assistant Professor
Department of Neurology
University of California Los Angeles School of Medicine
Los Angeles, California

Paul C. Van Ness, MD
Associate Professor of Neurology
University of Texas Southwestern Medical Center
Director, UT Southwestern Epilepsy Center
Department of Neurology
Parkland Memoral Hospital
Dallas, Texas

Faraneh Vargha-Khadem, PhD
Professor of Developmental Cognitive Neuroscience/
Head of Unit
Institute of Child Health
University College London
Consultant Paediatric Neuropsychologist
Department Neuropsychology
Great Ormond Street Hospital for Children NHS Trust
London, United Kingdom

Jana Velíšková, MD, PhD
Assistant Professor
Department of Neurology and Neuroscience
Albert Einstein College of Medicine
Rose F. Kennedy Center
Bronx, New York

Paul M. Vespa, MD
Associate Professor of Neurology in Neurosurgery
University of California, Los Angeles
Los Angeles California

Annamaria Vezzani, PhD
Head of Experimental Neurology Laboratory
Department of Neuroscience
Mario Negri Institute for Pharmacological Research
Milano, Italy

Barbara G. Vickrey, MD, MPH
Professor and Vice Chair
Department of Neurology
University of California, Los Angeles
Physician of Neurology
VA Greater Los Angeles Healthcare System
Los Angeles, California

Federico Vigevano, MD
Professor of Neurology
Departments of Neurology and Neurophysiology
Bambino Gesu Children's Hospital
Rome, Italy

Flavio Villani, MD
Staff Neurologist
Division of Clinical Epileptology and Experimental Neurophysiology
Fondazione IRCCS Istituto Nazionale Neurologico "C. Besta"
Milano, Italy

Eileen P. G. Vining, MD
Professor of Neurology and Pediatrics
Johns Hopkins University School of Medicine
Baltimore, Maryland

Harry V. Vinters, MD
Section of Neuropathology
Brain Research Institute
Mental Retardation Research Center
University of California Los Angeles Medical Center
Los Angeles, California

Kenneth Vives, MD
Chief of Stereotactic and Functional Neurosurgery
Department of Neurosurgery
Yale University School of Medicine
New Haven, Connecticut

Charles Vorkas, MD
New York University Epilepsy Center
New York, New York

Thaddeus S. Walczak, MD
Adjunct Professor
Department of Neurology
University of Minnesota
Director, Clinical Neurophysiology
MINCEP Epilepsy Care
Minneapolis, Minnesota

Nicole Walley
Institute for Genome Sciences and Policy
Center for Population Genomics and Pharmacogenetics
Duke University
Durham, North Carolina

Christopher A. Walsh, MD, PhD
Bullard Professor of Neurology
Howard Hughes Medical Institute
Harvard Medical School
Chief of Genetics
Children's Hospital Boston
Boston, Massachusetts

Wenzhi Wang, MD
Professor
Neuroepidemiology Department
Beijing Neurosurgical Institute
Beijing, China

Braxton B. Wannamaker, MD
Clinical Professor
Department of Neurosciences
Medical University of South Carolina
Charleston, South Carolina

Claude G. Wasterlain, MD
Chair, Department of Neurology
VA Greater Los Angeles Health Care System
Professor and Vice-Chair, Department of Neurology,
David Geffen School of Medicine at UCLA,
West L.A. VA Medical Center
Los Angeles, California

Kazuyoshi Watanabe, MD, PhD
Faculty of Medical Welfare
Aichi Shukutoku University
Chikusa-ku, Nagoya, Japan

Donald F. Weaver, MD, PhD
Departments of Medicine
Chemistry and Biomedical Engineering
Dalhousie University
Halifax, Nova Scotia, Canada

Peter J. West, MD
Anticonvulsant Drug Development Program
Department of Pharmacology and Toxicology
University of Utah
Salt Lake City, Utah

H. Steve White, PhD
Anticonvulsant Drug Development Program
University of Utah
Salt Lake City, Utah

Samuel Wiebe, MD, MSc(Epidemiol.), FRCPC
Professor of Clinical Neurosciences
University of Calgary
Head, Division of Neurology
Foothills Medical Centre
Calgary, Alberta
Canada

Heinz Wiendl, MD
Department of Neurology
University of Wuerzburg
Wuerzburg, Germany

Heinz Gregor Wieser, MD
Professor of Neurology
Chief, Department of Epileptology and Electroencephalography
Neurology Clinic
University Hospital
Zurich, Switzerland

Karen S. Wilcox, PhD
Department of Pharmacology & Toxicology
University of Utah
Salt Lake City, Utah

Alan J. Wilensky, MD
Regional Epilepsy Center
Harborview Medical Center
Seattle, Washington

Peter D. Williamson, MD
Department of Neurology
Dartmouth Medical School
Dartmouth-Hitchcock Medical Center
Lebanon, New Hampshire

L. James Willmore, MD
Professor of Neurology and Pharmacology and Physiology Neurology
Saint Louis University School of Medicine
Attending Neurologist
Saint Louis University Hospital
St. Louis, Missouri

Charles L. Wilson, PhD
Professor Emeritus
Department of Neurology
David Geffen School of Medicine
University of California Los Angeles
Los Angeles, California

Melodie R. Winawer, MD, MS
Assistant Professor
Attending Physician
Department of Neurology
Columbia University Medical Center
New York, New York

Peter Wolf, MD, PhD
Professor of Neurology
Copenhagen University
Copenhagen, Denmark
Physician
Danish Epilepsy Hospital
Dianalund, Denmark

Peter K. H. Wong, B.Eng, MD
Professor of Pediatrics
University of British Columbia
Director
Department of Diagnostic Neurophysiology
Children's Hospital
Vancouver, British Columbia
Canada

Clinton B. Wright, MD
Assistant Professor of Neurology
Columbia University
Assistant Attending
Department of Neurology
New York Presbyterian Hospital
Columbia University Medicine Center
New York, New York

Jianzhong Wu, MD
Professor
Beijing Neurosurgical Institute
Beijing, China

Liwen Wu, MD
Professor of Neurology
Peking Union Medical College Hospital
Beijing, China

Elaine Wyllie, MD
Departments of Neurology and Pediatrics
Cleveland Clinic
Cleveland, Ohio

Yoel Yaari, PhD
Faculty of Medicine
The Hebrew University
Jerusalem, Israel

Kazuichi Yagi, MD
Shizuoka Higashi Hospital
National Epilepsy Center
Shizuoka, Japan

Yasuko Yamatogi, MD
Faculty of Health and Welfare Science of Okayama
Prefectural University
Soja-shi, Okayama, Japan

E. Ann Yeh, MA, MD
Assistant Professor of Neurology
SUNY at Buffalo
Attending in Child Neurology
Clinical Co-Director, Pediatric MS and Demyelinating Disorders Center
Division of Child Neurology
Women and Children's Hospital of Buffalo
Buffalo, New York

Mark S. Yerby, MD
North Pacific Epilepsy Research,
Associate Clinical Professor of Public Health, Neurology and Obstetrics and Gynecology
Oregon Health Sciences University
Director, Epilepsy Program Providence St. Vincent's Medical Center
Portland, Oregon

Rafael M. Yuste, MD, PhD
HHMI Investigator
Professor
Department of Biological Sciences
Columbia University
New York, New York

Benjamin G. Zifkin, MD, CM, FRCPC
Epilepsy Clinic
Montreal Neurological Hospital
Montreal, Canada

Orsatta Zuffardi, PhD
Professor
Department of Biology and Medical Genetics
University of Pavia
Director of Medical Genetics
IRCCS Policlinico San Matteo
Pavia, Italy

PREFACE TO THE FIRST EDITION

Epilepsy is the most common primary disorder of the brain, and, according to the World Health Organization, second only to depression as the leading cause of neuropsychiatric disability worldwide. The causes and manifestations of epilepsy are so diverse and multifaceted that it impinges on virtually every aspect of modern biomedical science, from molecular biology to vocational rehabilitation. The pathophysiological mechanisms of epilepsy encompass all aspects of basic neuroscience, and every health care professional can expect to become involved in the diagnosis or treatment of epilepsy or its consequences. For this reason, a great number of excellent books have been written on various aspects of epilepsy, some of them intended as general references for nonspecialists and others as sources of detailed information on specific topics for specialists. However, there is no single comprehensive textbook for the international community of practicing physicians and other professionals to whom persons with epilepsy are most likely to be referred. These volumes, therefore, are intended primarily for neurologists, psychiatrists, and pediatricians, who bear the major burden of diagnosis and treatment of epilepsy, although we hope that they will also be a useful reference for all who concern themselves with human illness, whether they themselves are specialists in some aspect of epileptology or are only occasionally likely to encounter a patient who suffers from epileptic seizures.

This textbook has been in preparation for over five years. The ambitious intent to create a truly comprehensive and definitive work required the collaboration of a large number of associate editors and section editors with both an overlapping expertise covering the entire field of epileptology and a perspective that was international rather than regional or parochial. The editors held several meetings with the associate and section editors to plan the organization of each of the three volumes, as well as to identify, and later recruit, leaders in each field to write the individual chapters. In most cases, two or more authors representing different points of view were selected in order for each chapter to be as authoritative as possible. These early organizational efforts, which were necessary to avoid inadvertent omissions on the one hand and unnecessary redundancy on the other, were made possible, in large part, by generous educational grants from a number of pharmaceutical companies.

The three volumes of this textbook contain 12 major topic areas, beginning with factors that contribute to the occurrence of epilepsy, basic mechanisms, phenomenology of epileptic seizures, and diagnosis in Volume I; treatment, clinical biology, and psychiatric and social issues in Volume II; and descriptions of specific epileptic disorders, conditions that mimic epilepsy, and socioeconomic considerations in Volume III. The authors of the 289 chapters are major contributors of original papers for each of their topics and, therefore, have an intimate knowledge of the latest developments, often citing papers and books that were still in press at the time their chapters were being typeset.

The extent to which this textbook has achieved the original goals of being both comprehensive and definitive will be determined by how well it meets the needs of those who use it. We recognize that in a project as large as this, with the inevitable unforeseen mishaps that seemed to expand exponentially with the number of authors involved, the end result is bound to be less than perfect. The concept of this textbook, however, is that it should be seen as a work in progress, where we can learn by our mistakes so that subsequent editions, anticipated at fairly frequent intervals, can more closely approximate the ideal initially envisioned. In addition, there will be a CD-ROM version that can be updated regularly and ultimately linked with original research publications and more specialized texts. We welcome suggestions and constructive criticism, which will be of great importance to us in crafting later versions of this work.

Jerome Engel, Jr., MD, PhD
Los Angeles
Timothy A. Pedley, MD
New York

PREFACE TO THE SECOND EDITION

A decade has intervened between the first and second editions of *Epilepsy: A Comprehensive Textbook*. The process of revision afforded a unique opportunity to observe the extraordinary advances in research and the great improvements in clinical care that have occurred during this time. New insights into the basic mechanisms of seizures and epilepsy can be attributed largely to the increased application of cellular and molecular biology to the study of epileptic phenomena. In addition, there have been more direct investigations of patients using the tools of genetics and various brain imaging techniques. All aspects of treatment have improved, and both seizure control and quality of life for people with epilepsy are better today than ever before.

This progress is symbolized by noting that the second edition contains 20 more chapters than the first, of which 42 are completely new and 251 have been extensively rewritten. There were 351 contributors in the first edition; there are 444 in the second, of whom 225 are returning authors and 219 are new. As a result, although the book's outline follows that of the first edition, this is essentially an entirely new textbook.

As with the first edition, our objective with the second is to create a comprehensive textbook that addresses all aspects of epilepsy, from basic pathophysiology at cellular, molecular and organ levels to clinical phenomenology, diagnostic evaluation, treatment options, comorbidities, psychosocial rehabilitation and health care delivery. All chapters are written by distinguished experts in each field, and most have two or more authors representing different points of view to provide an authoritative consensus on each topic. Selection of editors and authors was designed to assure a perspective that is truly international. Therapeutic recommendations are evidence-based to the extent that is currently possible.

With completion of the second edition, we are acutely aware how much we owe to the section editors and, especially, our associate editors, all of whom are themselves internationally recognized experts in epilepsy. Without their help, chapters would not have been as consistently rigorous, balanced or current.

We also note with sadness the passing of colleagues who participated in the first edition, many of whom also contributed, or were scheduled to contribute, to the second. They include John Fred Annegers, Frank Benson, Fritz E. Dreifuss, John R. Gates, Richard W. Homan, Peter Kellaway, Pierre Loiseau, Eric Lothman, K. S. Mani, Frank Morrell, Claudio Munari, J. Kiffen Penry, Luis Felipe Quesney, A. James Rowan, Masakazu Seino, Arthur Sonnen and Sheila J. Wallace. We miss them, but they live on through their work and accomplishments, and the fond memories we have of them.

The first edition of *Epilepsy: A Comprehensive Textbook* was intended to be a work in progress, a basis for developing a comprehensive reference resource in a format that had the potential to be updated regularly. A CD-ROM was subsequently prepared that included additional materials and revisions of some chapters. The second edition will have a digital version that is Internet based for inclusion of additional figures and images, more color illustrations, and other enhancements, as well as advanced search capabilities. The Internet version of the textbook affords an opportunity for all authors to update their chapters on an ongoing basis, to ensure that the electronic version remains current with the very latest information.

As always, we welcome suggestions and constructive criticism from readers. This input will not only assist in improving future hard copy editions but also help us to provide an Internet-based digital version that is as useful as possible.

Jerome Engel, Jr., MD, PhD
Los Angeles, California
Timothy A. Pedley, MD
New York, New York

ACKNOWLEDGMENTS

Once again, we gratefully acknowledge the vital contributions of the associate and section editors, whose work and effort were instrumental in producing this second edition. We also thank our chapter authors, who tolerated constant badgering, criticisms (we hope helpful), and many editorial changes, all with good humor. A textbook of this size cannot be created without the committed efforts of a large number of individuals, including Keith Donnellan, our Development Editor at Dovetail Content Solutions, who worked with authors, kept track of submissions and the many revisions, and greatly assisted in keeping everything organized; the staff at Lippincott Williams & Wilkins, especially Leanne McMillan, our Managing editor and Chris Miller from Aptara who provided excellent service at the key points; and our own office staff, especially Malinda Walford and Grissel Coplin in New York, and Dale Booth and Sabrina Hubbard in Los Angeles, who daily - for nearly two years - bore the brunt of our overly ambitious goals.

Jerome Engel Jr., MD, PhD
Timothy A. Pedley, MD

CHAPTER 199 ■ OVERVIEW: PSYCHIATRIC ISSUES

MICHAEL R. TRIMBLE

INTRODUCTION

The links between epilepsy and psychiatry have a long and respectable history, but for reasons best deliberated on by historians, the growing gap between neurology and psychiatry in the 20th century led to a considerable divergence of opinion as to the relationships between psychiatric disorders and epilepsy. Part of this confusion was due to the eventually almost exclusive psychological approach taken to neuropsychiatric disorders by psychiatrists, and the relative neglect by neurologists of behavior problems that could be associated with neurologic disorders. Further, in the field of epilepsy there was confusion over the distinction between seizures and epilepsy. Many people equated the two, but seizures as signs and causing symptoms are quite distinct from the underlying pathologic process of the epilepsy. The ongoing interictal electrophysiologic disturbances, which presumably reflect on underlying electrochemical aberrations within the brain that are easily identifiable by various imaging techniques, may be expected to lead to continuing disturbances of cerebral function. If these occur in areas of the central nervous system that have an impact on emotion and behavior, then psychiatric disturbances may be the expected outcome of at least some people with epilepsy, depending upon the site and type of the underlying epileptic discharge.

By the midpoint of the 20th century, it was a strongly held view, particularly in the United States, that people with epilepsy, if they had psychiatric difficulties, had them because of secondary factors. These included not only the stigmatization of having a terrible condition such as epilepsy, with such a poor quality of life and considerable social disadvantage (which was known to occur then and still occurs now), but also drug factors (remembering that phenobarbitone was commonly employed in those times) or, for example, cerebral trauma from head injuries following seizures. The concept that the underlying neurologic disturbance that led to the epileptic seizures could also provoke psychiatric problems was hard for many to accept.

There was, however, a slowly growing literature that emphasized not only the possible neurologic underpinnings of psychiatric disorders generally, but also the psychiatric complications of neurologic disorders, including epilepsy. From a purely anatomic point of view, the unraveling of the concept of the limbic system, from the earlier circuitry proposed by Papez to the later, more sophisticated elaborations of people such as MacLean, emphasized that within the brain there were neuronal structures and circuits that had specifically to do with modulation of emotion. This was a new idea, because before the development of the limbic system concept, there was no clear cerebral framework for an understanding of how the brain felt and expressed emotion. It was crucial to elaborating on the link between epilepsy and emotion to realize that two key limbic structures, the hippocampus and the amygdala, were frequently involved in the underlying pathology of epilepsy, particularly in the localization-related epilepsies, and newly developed techniques of recording from sites within the brain revealed that in between seizures, interictal abnormalities were recorded from such structures. More recently, the uncovering and elaboration of the direct associations between medial temporal structures and limbic forebrain structures and the unraveling of the neuroanatomy of the limbic forebrain by authors such as Heimer et al. have given clear neurologic underpinnings for an understanding of the behavioral consequences of neurologic disorders, epilepsy being no exception.[1]

However, understanding the neuroanatomy in more detail is not sufficient. It is clear that people with epilepsy, like anybody else, can have a straightforward psychiatric problem. A number of these are classifiable in terms of standardized diagnostic schedules (for example DSM-VI or ICD-10) and, when present in people with epilepsy, should receive the same amount of attention for management as they would if the patient did not have epilepsy. However, the contention of the last 30 or so years has been that there are some psychiatric problems that are more intimately imbedded within the context of the underlying neurobiologic process of the epilepsy.

This underlying neurobiology of the behavior disorders is discussed at the very outset of this section. The first chapter essentially makes the point that at least some of the psychiatric presentations are potentially directly interwoven with either the ictus or the interictal neurologic changes, this underlying neurology giving a particular stamp to the clinical presentations that lead them to differ somewhat from the psychiatric presentations diagnosed in the absence of the underlying neurologic disorder.

A further complication arises from the fact that the patients with epilepsy who are most liable to psychiatric disorders are those who are treated with antiepileptic medications chronically, often with polytherapy, and the medications themselves can contribute considerably to some of the ongoing symptomatology. This includes not only some of the more florid psychotic presentations, but also one of the most interesting phenomena in neuropsychiatry, namely, the precipitation of a psychiatric disorder when an antiepileptic drug is prescribed and seizures are suddenly turned off (referred to as forced normalization—the Landolt phenomenon). Equally important, however, are the subtle changes of mood and cognition that can be induced by antiepileptic medications. These matters are noted in several of the following chapters, but need specific highlighting for certain populations, such as those with learning disorders. They form a vulnerable group for the development of behavior disorders, but often their management falls short of the optimum. This may be due to some physicians failing to recognize that patients with learning disorders and seizures do have epilepsy! It may be missed or dismissed on the grounds that this population of patients somehow lies outside of the neurologic limit. With language and motor abnormalities, their psychopathology is sometimes simply not recognized. A second group that requires special consideration is children. The spectrum of clinical psychopathology is different in younger patients with epilepsy, and the management of such patients also requires different treatment strategies and agencies.

Some of the psychiatric disorders seen in people with epilepsy (e.g., the postictal psychoses) are simply not found in standardized diagnostic manuals for psychiatric disorders, and yet their presentation is highly characteristic and will be found only in people with seizure disorders. Other more subtle neuropsychiatric complications of epilepsy, including the schizophrenialike interictal psychoses (of Slater) and the interictal dysphoric disorder (of Kraepelin and Blumer), have been harder to define, but are now recognized as epilepsy-specific presentations, even if still requiring more elaboration and validity testing. To a large extent, these presentations no longer arouse the controversies that they used to in the past. A more vexed problem is the issue of the interictal personality disorder, particularly as it was described by Waxman and Geschwind in the 1970s.[3] At that time neurologists were becoming cognizant of the fact that patients with frontal lobe damage could develop personality changes reflective of the injuries, and the term *frontal lobe personality disorder* began to appear in neurologic texts. Further, with regard to the temporal lobes, the Klüver-Bucy Syndrome was described, initially in animals but then in patients, with central features to this being alterations of personality with taming of the emotions, alteration of spontaneity, and changes of mood and social behaviors. Thus, it does not seem out of keeping with the growing knowledge of clinical behavioral neurology, and the elaborations of the neuroanatomy of the limbic system, that an interictal personality syndrome may be defined and consequent of temporal/limbic/neuroanatomic/neurophysiologic disturbances. In fact, descriptions of an interictal personality syndrome can be found in the European literature from well over a hundred years ago, but it was well codified by Gastaut and Geschwind. The main features of the disorder, such as hypergraphia and hyperreligiosity, are discussed in the relevant chapter, but other, perhaps even more controversial topics such as the links between aggression and epilepsy are given appropriate space.

Geschwind et al. and followers gave to us the term *behavioral neurology*, essentially an offshoot of 19th-century neuropsychiatry. The paper that introduced the interictal personality syndrome pushed the field in new directions, as it touched on behaviors not usually discussed in neurologic circles (e.g., creativity and religiosity). Although the characteristics of the interictal personality disorder are now very well known, there are still many neurologists, even epileptologists, who find it hard to see the specimen when it flutters before them to be pinned down. In part, this still reflects on that confusion between seizures and epilepsy, which still in the minds of many remains conceptually muddled.

It is important that whatever the clinical problem, patients receive appropriate psychiatric care where necessary. At least part of this will involve psychopharmacology, and therefore, chapters on management and treatment of these problems are also included. All the chapters in this section emphasize the importance of recognizing c-morbid psychopathology in people with epilepsy. If the seizure is considered to be the only problem that patients face and the comorbidities are ignored, then an appropriate schedule of management cannot evolve, and the patient's untreated psychopathology may well undermine the ongoing attempts to manage the epileptic seizures.

David Taylor, in his overview on psychiatric issues of the first edition of this textbook,[2] pointed out that there had been an overcorrection of emphasis from the epoch of psychoanalysis, with the rise of biologic psychiatry, and noted the complexity of trying to disentangle brain–behavior relationships in epilepsy. While the lesion within the developing brain, present at a time when the anlage of the developing personality is being laid down, will be influenced and in turn influences interpersonal and familial relationships, he noted how accommodation and compensation within a brain, which has such developmental skews, may appear to lead to effective ways of coping at certain stages of development but not at others. There is, as he said, "a need to consider the complex interaction, over the course of the development of the individual, among impairments of cerebral structure, disorders of cerebral function, psychological deficits, and the sort of family and peer group functioning within which these deficits interact." He drew clear distinctions between diseases, illnesses, and predicaments, which bear not only on common sense, but also on our clinical experience. By disease he meant evidence of dysfunctions that are more often nowadays revealed through, for example, brain imaging than through postmortem analysis. By illness, he referred to the limitations of functioning and suffering that people experience as a consequence of the underlying disease, and he noted that psychiatric problems essentially are illnesses rather than diseases. The importance is to understand the illnesses and the predicaments that they present to the person who is ill and his or her family. Helping people with their predicaments, trying to understand their illnesses, and attending to their underlying discernible disease are all parts of the complexity of the neuropsychiatry of epilepsy.

SUMMARY AND CONCLUSIONS

In the 21st century we now have a much clearer understanding of the underlying neuroanatomy and neurochemistry of psychiatric disorders in general, but also of why a number of neurologic disorders, in which neuroanatomic changes are identifiable in limbic and forebrain structures, may lead to a susceptibility to the development of psychiatric syndromes. There is an overlap between psychiatry and neurology, and epilepsy has always been central to discussions about this interface. Most neurologists now accept that psychopathology is an integral part of some epilepsy syndromes, whether it be memory disturbances and other cognitive difficulties or more florid psychopathologies as one may see, for example, in the psychoses. A substantial portion of this comprehensive textbook has been devoted to these behavioral problems, and it is hoped that the chapters in this section will be of interest and importance to both neurologists seeking understanding and psychiatrists seeking enlightenment.

References

1. Heimer L. A new anatomical framework for neuropsychiatric disorders and drug abuse. *Am J Psychiatry*. 2003;160:1726–1739.
2. Taylor D. Overview: psychiatric issues. In: Engel J, Pedley TA, eds. *Epilepsy: A Comprehensive Textbook*. Philadelphia: Lippincott-Raven Publishers; 1997: 2039–2043.
3. Waxman SG, Geschwind N. Hypergraphia in temporal lobe epilepsy. *Neurology*. 1974;24:629–636.

CHAPTER 200 ■ NEUROBIOLOGY OF BEHAVIORAL DISORDERS

JEROME ENGEL, JR., DAVID C. TAYLOR, AND MICHAEL R. TRIMBLE

INTRODUCTION

Many persons with epilepsy suffer from interictal disturbances in behavior* that can contribute significantly to their illness and in some cases constitute the major disability. Although there remains some controversy on this subject, it is generally accepted by most workers in the field that the degree of behavioral problems associated with epilepsy is greater than would be expected on the basis of the existence of a chronic illness alone, both in adults[40] and in children.[64] To a certain extent, the psychiatric consequences of epilepsy can be attributed to external factors, specifically the predicament imposed by epilepsy not only as a traditionally stigmatizing disorder but also because the unpredictable nature of recurrent ictal events allows society to impose rather severe limitations on activities of daily living.[63] In addition, however, there are legitimate neurobiologic explanations for interictal behavioral disturbances in this patient population, including (a) nonepileptic factors, such as effects of the underlying pathologic substrate itself; (b) the unwanted effects of medical and surgical treatment on cerebral function; (c) epileptic mechanisms consisting of unrecognized prolonged ictal events that are witnessed as interictal behavioral disturbances; and (d) the ability of recurrent epileptic activity to cause enduring changes in neuronal function.

The concept that epileptic seizures themselves can effect a persistent disruption of normal neuronal function leading to the appearance of interictal behavioral disorders is not new[10,17,18,20,21,54,59] but is still not completely accepted and is even adamantly rejected by many. One socially sensitive justification for the contrasting point of view is that there are already too many negative associations with epilepsy, so that to add the fear of becoming "insane," without definitive proof, would impose a further unnecessary burden. On the other hand, formal recognition that epileptic mechanisms *might* contribute to transient and enduring changes of both function and structure in the brain is necessary before investigation of this possibility can begin. Appropriately designed clinical and animal research could lead to interventions that would reverse or prevent a major cause of epilepsy-associated disability.

NONEPILEPTIC ORGANIC CAUSATIVE FACTORS

Symptomatic epilepsies result from a variety of underlying pathologic processes that might be localized or diffuse, unilateral or bilateral, static or progressive. These can produce epileptic seizures as their only clinically apparent manifestation. However, they might also give rise to chronic neurologic or psychiatric deficits related to (a) the nature of the pathophysiologic substrate, (b) its precise location in the brain, and (c) the time of its occurrence with respect to brain development. In idiopathic epilepsies, there is no obvious structural pathology, but the genetic defect responsible for the spontaneous recurrence of epileptic seizures presumably produces a disturbance in neuronal responsivity, transmission, or wiring that is continuously present between seizures and could have other, nonepileptic functional consequences manifesting as deficits in learning and skills, as well as interictal behavioral disturbances. Although focused research on this subject cannot begin until the specific defective gene or its aberrant products have been identified, this hypothesis offers a plausible explanation for the association of certain mild behavioral disturbances with some of the idiopathic generalized epilepsy syndromes that have been supposed to be only epilepsy and nothing more.[28,52] All current antiepileptic drugs act nonspecifically to alter excitatory or inhibitory influences or reduce neuronal synchronization, processes that are critical to normal cerebral function.[32] It is not surprising, therefore, that pharmacotherapy can be associated with sedation, cognitive impairment, and a range of psychiatric disturbances.

A hitherto unanswered question is whether psychiatric syndromes associated with antiepileptic drugs are a function of prior risk (i.e., faulty organization): Why are some, but not all, persons affected? Among a group of affected persons, a variety of psychiatric disorders might be associated with the use of any particular medication. This suggests that the specific disorder induced in an individual is that to which they are most genetically liable. Monitoring of these responses on a multicenter basis could be helpful in elucidating not only the problem of drug-induced disorders, but also the mechanism of the psychiatric disorders concerned. Surgical treatment, whether resection, ablation, or disconnection, also disrupts normal neuronal integration and new neurologic or psychiatric disturbances can emerge subsequently, either at the point in development when they normally occur (e.g., schizophrenia) or in direct reaction to tissue damage (e.g., specific learning deficits). Effects of pharmacotherapy and surgical therapy on behavior are dealt with in Chapters 208 and 209 and are not considered further here.

Nature of the Lesion

Epilepsy that is attributed to a lesion typically develops after a prolonged latent period, although brain organization could be adversely affected much earlier. Discrete, well-localized structural epileptogenic lesions in so-called silent brain areas may cause no perceptible disturbances other than recurrent ictal events, but more extensive lesions are likely to impinge on critical cortical areas and be associated with some degree of

*Behavior disorder is used here as a broad term encompassing phenomena that might, but might not, reach criteria for psychiatric illness. In this text, behavior is the manifest aspect of psychic life, and aberrations of behavior are usually attributed to some form of abnormal mental state.

interictal impairment. Consequently, cognitive deficits and neurologic signs and symptoms commonly accompany epileptogenic substrates that tend to be diffuse or multifocal. Disorders such as tuberous sclerosis or cortical dysplasia can be sufficiently mild that only a single localized lesion is identified on magnetic resonance imaging (MRI), but chronic behavioral impairment could suggest, in these cases, the presence of much more widespread aberrations in neuronal migration and differentiation that are beyond the resolution of current imaging techniques. For other lesions, disturbances in cerebral function could reflect distant cerebral abnormalities of a related disorder; for instance, the high incidence of schizophrenia reported to occur in women with hamartomas and gangliogliomas[61] was postulated to be caused by a karyotype abnormality associated with ectodermal dysplasias and abnormal behavior.[49] Progressive lesions that continue to destroy or disrupt neuronal function are clearly more likely to give rise to interictal behavioral problems than static lesions, the latter of which permit recovery of function through compensatory mechanisms. For the same reason, rapidly progressive disease processes cause more interictal disturbances than slowly progressive ones. It is also conceivable that some neoplastic lesions could secrete neuroactive substances that influence interictal behavior, and some vascular lesions can cause nonepileptic signs or symptoms by bleeding or a steal phenomenon. Lesions that were thought to be static, such as hippocampal sclerosis, are now reported to be common sequelae of stress in its widest sense.[56] Thus, stress would be an important factor in the epilepsies and in psychiatric disorders.

The Location of the Lesion

The neurologic signs and symptoms produced by focal structural lesions depend on the function of the brain area involved. Discrete neocortical lesions in primary areas produce very localized deficits, whereas diffuse bilateral abnormalities cause cognitive impairment and more global dysfunction. Lesions of the limbic system are of particular interest in epileptology because they are the most likely to produce epileptic seizures and because these lesions are associated with much more varied interictal behavioral disturbances than lesions of neocortex.[35]

The most common deficit associated with lesions of the mesial temporal limbic system is impairment of episodic memory, which is usually material specific for the hemisphere involved.[41] This is more noticeable, and therefore more disabling, when the lesion is in the language-dominant temporal lobe, and there is usually an associated verbal learning disturbance. The limbic system, however, also plays a key role in modulating mood and affect, basic drives (including sexual function), and motivation, functions that, when distorted by structural or functional lesions, could conceivably give rise to virtually every behavioral aberration attributed to epilepsy, including specific psychiatric illnesses.

It is important to note that lesions in certain locations that are epileptogenic might be more likely to cause enduring disturbances referable to the normal function of that area than lesions that are purely ablative.[61] Because there is a certain degree of plasticity of brain tissue, even in the adult, destructive lesions can cause transient deficits that eventually recover as other brain areas take over the function. When the neuronal disruption is intermittent, however, as with epileptic seizures, it is possible that natural compensatory mechanisms are not activated, and recovery of function does not occur. Furthermore, epileptic discharges propagate and can disrupt function at a distance from the primary epileptogenic region, including contralateral structures. Consequently, specific temporal lobe or frontal lobe signs and symptoms that require bilateral homotopic dysfunction would not occur with a nonepileptic destructive lesion in one hemisphere but are commonly seen with unilateral epileptogenic lesions. The existence of secondary bilateral involvement and its reversibility are readily demonstrated following successful anterior temporal lobectomy, when material-specific memory referable to the contralateral temporal lobe subsequently improves and patients may experience an overall increase in IQ.[47,62]

Developmental Considerations

Classical neurology has an adult perspective. Its premise is of some fault or accident that disrupts a previously normally functioning central nervous system (CNS). The lesson of epilepsy has been that the faults are often early prenatal or late prenatal or early postnatal, but the problem of interest (the epilepsy or the cognitive capacities or the behavior) becomes "eloquent" at some later stage. Models of this exist in syphilis, encephalitis, rheumatic heart disease, Huntington chorea, and many other conditions. The developmental perspective is to consider the possibility that the lesion or fault could have been "eloquent" in other ways before the condition of interest arose or could become "eloquent" in those ways later in development. This removes a need for thinking that a chronic lesion that arose in embryonal life has somehow acquired new powers at age 14 (or whenever) because "it has started to cause epilepsy." It allows consideration that the condition of interest (e.g., epilepsy) arises from a constellation of circumstances that have not existed previously, a combination of aging and maturation together with hormonal and psychosocial factors.

Ordinarily, localized destructive cortical lesions that occur early in the course of development are less likely to cause lasting deficits than lesions occurring in later life because of the increased plastic potential of the immature brain. For instance, patients with extensive damage to the left hemisphere incurred within the first few years of life usually have a pathologic compensatory shift of language dominance to the right hemisphere, with little or no disturbance in speech or language.[48] On the other hand, more diffuse bilateral lesions occurring early in life are usually accompanied by a developmental delay that persists into adulthood. Taylor,[62] however, challenged functional shift as the only basis of handedness change, because alien tissue lesions are associated with left handedness whether they are in the left or right hemisphere. He suggested that an alien tissue lesion could act by reducing the effect of the gene for right-handedness bias. If this is confirmed in other studies, it would help our understanding of prenatal organization of cerebral functions.

As mentioned in the previous section, epileptogenic lesions may be more likely to produce a lasting effect on behavior than destructive lesions because intermittent disturbances could confound compensatory recovery processes. This appears to be particularly true during the period of cerebral development. Furthermore, the widespread electrical epileptiform electroencephalogram (EEG) abnormalities that characterize certain epileptic syndromes in infancy and early childhood, such as West syndrome, can reflect propagation of discharges from a localized epileptogenic lesion that also produces the same global behavioral disturbances usually associated with a diffuse bilateral destructive lesion. The evidence for this comes from the observation that some infants and small children with developmental delay who initially appear to have catastrophic secondary generalized epilepsy actually have a single lesion localized to one hemisphere, and surgical removal of this area not only eliminates the ictal events, but also helps to reverse the developmental delay.[53]

EPILEPTIC CAUSATIVE FACTORS

Unrecognized simple partial status epilepticus causes behavioral disturbances that can be mistakenly labeled "interictal," and prolonged convulsive status epilepticus can cause brain damage. There is an abundance of evidence for epilepsy-induced enduring functional disturbances from well-described phenomena in experimental animals.[10,14] The confounding effects of the pathologic process responsible for the epileptic condition on behavior and the effects of antiepileptic drugs, which are invariably present, make it extremely difficult to demonstrate, in a clinical setting, that recurrent, transient epileptic events alone can cause interictal behavioral disturbances.[59] If such changes do occur in patients, undoubtedly they are more likely to result from some types of epileptic abnormalities than others, and conceivably there are also ictal and interictal epileptiform events that pose no risk for persistent dysfunction. For this reason, it would be inappropriate to suggest that all epileptiform abnormalities are capable of inducing enduring neuronal dysfunction or that all epilepsies have the potential of being progressive in some way. On the other hand, it is of great practical importance to make every effort to document the occurrence of such epilepsy-induced behavioral disorders in patients in order to determine what types of seizures and epileptic syndromes are likely to give rise to persistent problems and at what point in the course of these conditions the disturbance might become irreversible. Such information would provide essential guidelines for early aggressive intervention in patients who are deemed to be at risk.

Unrecognized Prolonged Ictal Events

One inarguable cause of an inappropriate diagnosis of "interictal" behavioral disturbances, although perhaps rare, is nonconvulsive status epilepticus. Simple partial seizures of limbic origin can cause virtually any psychiatric sign or symptom in clear consciousness, and the scalp EEG in this condition is almost always normal.[71] Sensory symptoms caused by simple partial status epilepticus of neocortical origin can give rise to bizarre experiences that are acted on in strange ways to create a persistent interictal behavioral disturbance. These forms of simple partial status epilepticus (also called aura continua) are easy to recognize when they occur in patients with known epilepsy, and the ongoing signs and symptoms match those of the habitual simple partial seizures (auras) that usually precede more obvious ictal events. In patients who have never had an obvious epileptic seizure and who have a normal EEG, this diagnosis would be exceedingly difficult. Rapid reversal of signs and symptoms with intravenous benzodiazepines suggests, but in no way proves, a diagnosis of epilepsy because many nonepileptic conditions can also transiently respond to this treatment. Complex partial status epilepticus and absence status can also rarely be mistaken for a psychiatric condition when the clouding of consciousness is subtle. EEGs in these conditions, however, reveal the diagnosis, although sometimes only after extreme persistence.[2]

In patients with known epilepsy and well-documented, frequent interictal EEG abnormalities, the only surface EEG correlate of a simple partial seizure is, classically, disappearance of the interictal EEG spike. For instance, in temporal lobe epilepsy, a simple partial seizure is associated with an ictal discharge in mesial temporal lobe structures, which are then no longer able to generate interictal spikes that ordinarily would propagate to temporal neocortex and appear on the scalp EEG. Consequently, disappearance of the typical interictal EEG spike pattern in a patient with persistent behavioral disturbances could be used as supportive evidence for simple partial status epilepticus. Indeed, one postulated explanation for Landolt's so-called "forced normalization"[31] (the occasional observation that the EEGs of some patients with known epilepsy normalize during episodes of psychosis) is that the behavioral disturbance is actually simple partial status epilepticus.[72]

Epileptic Brain Damage

Another incontestable consequence of epileptic seizures is cell death from the excitotoxic effect of excessive release of excitatory amino acids during status epilepticus.[59] It is well known that susceptible cerebral structures, particularly the hippocampus, undergo irreversible damage in patients after prolonged convulsive status epilepticus, and studies in experimental animal models show that this occurs even when cerebral perfusion, ventilation, and normothermia are preserved.[39] Much is now known about the cellular mechanisms of excitotoxic cell death, but it is unclear whether (and if so, to what extent) this occurs in human epilepsy apart from the severe insult associated with convulsive status epilepticus.[59] Excitotoxic effects are associated with massive calcium influx, which may be insufficient to cause cells to die but, rather, turns on genetic mechanisms that could profoundly alter cell structure or function, perhaps inducing transsynaptic changes at a distance from the epileptogenic lesion. Such a mechanism could provide a ready substrate for persistent interictal behavioral disturbances.

Hippocampal sclerosis, believed to result, at least in part, from processes inducing excitotoxic cell death, has been associated with behavioral disturbances described mainly in terms of effects on personality, with evidence of immaturity, irritability, and trivial aggression, at that time recorded as psychopathy.[60,66] Hippocampal sclerosis has been shown to follow from conditions other than prolonged febrile convulsions, such as trauma, that occur early in life.[36] It is intriguing that there is now also considerable literature on the deleterious effect of high levels of cortisol, produced in response to stress, on the developing hippocampus.[56] It is possible that hippocampal sclerosis arising from prolonged febrile convulsions is a unique syndrome. Various other mental states have been associated with hippocampal sclerosis, including schizophrenia[7,42,58,69] and depression.[33,60] The behavioral syndrome associated with mesial temporal lobe epilepsy is subtle and deserves more research.[5,70] The immaturity, irritability, rigidity, stickiness, hypergraphia, and hyperreligiosity that most often are mentioned with this syndrome are, importantly, relieved by successful mesial temporal resection and disappear rapidly over the first 2 or 3 postoperative years.[66] Because the treatment is ablative, the effect must be through relief of seizures and/or obliging the rest of the limbic system to take over the tasks of the ablated tissue. Psychological evidence[47,62] suggests that successful surgery leads to generally improved functioning in other domains, too.

Kindling and Secondary Epileptogenesis

Although kindling[23] and secondary epileptogenesis[43] are extremely well documented in the animal laboratory, their relevance to human epilepsy remains controversial.[24,44] In virtually all vertebrate animals tested, from frogs to subhuman primates, subthreshold stimulation of susceptible limbic and neocortical structures, when repeated at appropriate intervals, gives rise to epileptiform EEG and behavioral abnormalities that become increasingly prolonged and severe, and eventually, spontaneous seizures occur. This phenomenon has been demonstrated with both electrical and chemical stimulation; there is crossover from one stimulation modality to the other, and the effect is persistent, at least to some degree, for as long as the animal is subsequently tested. The kindling paradigm brings under experimental control the more naturally occurring process of mirror focus development,[43] whereby a region capable of generating spontaneous epileptic seizures gradually develops contralateral and homotopic to an experimental epileptic focus, presumably as a result of continuous bombardment of epileptiform discharges across the corpus callosum. Nevertheless, despite years of research, there remains debate about the existence of significant secondary epileptogenesis in humans.

Some studies of patients undergoing surgical treatment for brain tumors provide evidence for mirror focus development,[44] and similar secondary epileptogenesis may account for the inverse relationship between duration of epilepsy and surgical outcome reported for anterior temporal lobectomies.[15] But the abrupt cessation of seizures and abnormal electrical discharges after successful surgery on patients who have had years of apparent provocation of secondary foci requires us to keep the issue open. There are a few scattered reports of seizures in patients following repeated brain stimulation that might mimic electrical kindling.[55] In a more general sense, the latent period between the occurrence of an epileptogenic insult and the appearance of spontaneous epileptic seizures that commonly occurs in humans,[29] what Penfield and Jasper[45] referred to as "ripening of the scar," has been taken as evidence that some kindling process is necessary for seizures to occur spontaneously.[22] In some cases, however, this could reflect the time required to reach the stage of cerebral and physical development necessary to support the manifestations of seizures.

Whether or not kindling and secondary epileptogenesis occur in the human brain to produce additional independent epileptogenic areas, the fact that such activity-induced changes occur at all in the mammalian brain strongly suggests that they could also exist to some extent in the human epileptic brain. The exact mechanisms underlying these functional or structural transsynaptic changes are unknown; however, they must have some effect on normal neuronal function and certainly could provide a substrate for the development of interictal behavioral disturbances.[16]

One example of how kindlinglike modulatory influences could alter interictal behavior comes from studies of defensive rage in cats.[3] This is a stereotyped behavior that can be induced by electrical stimulation of hypothalamus or periaqueductal gray. The manifestations of stimulation-induced defensive rage can be modified by stimulation of the amygdala and hippocampus, and establishment of an experimental hippocampal epileptic focus not only exacerbated stimulation-induced defensive rage, but also caused this behavior to appear spontaneously in response to rough handling.[25] In the human, such "hard-wired" affective displays come under cortical control and may be more likely to manifest not as rage but as modified responses such as impulsiveness, depression, or other more socially acceptable, albeit disturbing, behaviors.

Another experimental example of kindling-induced interictal behavioral disturbances also derives from studies of cats that showed an enduring enhancement of methamphetamine-induced stereotypy following amygdala kindling.[51] This observation was interpreted to reflect a persistent up-regulation of dopamine receptors that could be another mechanism for the development of psychiatric disorders in patients with epilepsy.

The effect of kindling may depend upon the pre-existing affective state. For instance, amygdala kindling can reduce the manifestations of anxiety in high-anxiety rats, but exacerbates anxiety in low-anxiety rats.[1] The kindling effects of epileptiform discharges in patients with epilepsy, therefore, may depend not only on the location and type of the epileptogenic abnormality, but also on the predisposing behavioral state of the patient.

Some of the personality traits attributed in the literature to patients with temporal lobe epilepsy, such as hyposexuality and emotionality,[5,6,70] have been interpreted as being the opposite of the Klüver-Bucy syndrome[20]; changes in behavior, including taming and loss of affective responses, caused in primates by bilateral amygdalectomies; and seen in humans sometimes following head injuries or with certain dementias. One explanation for this effect could be a kindlinglike enhancement along amygdala projection fields.

Behavioral Effects of Natural Seizure-suppressing Influences

There are numerous inhibitory processes and other seizure-suppressing mechanisms that develop as a homeostatic reaction to the occurrence of epileptic seizures and presumably act to maintain the interictal state. These include the so-called inhibitory surround that limits the spread of localized epileptic activity,[46] the interhemispheric interference that opposes the development of secondary epileptogenesis,[38] and a variety of active mechanisms that terminate epileptic seizures.[8,12] These protective mechanisms persist between seizures and undoubtedly affect normal neuronal activity, conceivably contributing to the development of interictal behavioral disturbances.

Clinically, postictal changes are well documented, ranging from localized Todd paralysis[13] to profound global dysfunction following a generalized convulsion. In some patients, postictal behavior can involve complicated actions, such as the reactive automatisms that follow complex partial seizures, and may result in inappropriate semidirected responses, such as aggression toward someone attempting restraint. Other patients experience postictal psychosis.[6] It is easy to see how these behaviors, if persistent, could explain certain interictal disturbances. Such manifestations were evident in Hughlings Jackson's paradigmatic case of temporal lobe epilepsy, Dr. Z,[67] who diagnosed "pneumonia at the left base" in one of his own patients while totally amnesic after a seizure, a diagnosis that proved correct when he re-examined the child later.

Endogenous opioids are released during some types of epileptic seizures[27] and help to terminate seizures[8] but are also believed to be natural euphorogens, perhaps explaining the therapeutic effect of electroconvulsive shock therapy on clinical depression.[30] Also, there are people who feel much better after they have had a seizure, and parents who, enduring the escalating behavioral problems of their children between seizures, the so-called prodrome, look forward to the positive changes the seizure will bring. Opioid peptides have been shown to mediate several different postictal behaviors in rats, but the mechanisms are complicated. Whereas postictal hypofunction appears to be caused by a direct opioid effect, postictal explosive behavior is more likely the result of opioid withdrawal.[8] Different postictal behaviors appear to be mediated by different cerebral structures because seizures in rats increase opiate release in some brain areas and decrease opioid release in others.[50] Enduring changes in opiate mechanisms clearly occur in some patients with epilepsy, as shown by positron emission tomography (PET) evidence of increased μ-opiate-receptor binding in the neocortex of the epileptogenic temporal lobe.[19] If endogenous opioids are released in some brain structures during seizures and contribute to the appearance of postictal behaviors, it is conceivable that some patients could become dependent on high levels of endogenous opiates when they are having seizures and experience some degree of withdrawal when seizures stop. This might explain the transient depression that is often seen following successful surgical treatment of epilepsy.[14] The fact that depression can also be a side effect of antiepileptic drug treatment suggests that the same withdrawal phenomenon following successful pharmacotherapy could contribute to what has largely been interpreted as a direct effect of medication on mood and affect.

Developmental Factors

Recurrent epileptiform discharges that disrupt function at a distance in the immature brain might interfere with critical phases of development and result in lasting behavioral disturbances.[16] Experimental evidence for epilepsy-induced disruption of normal development derives from a series of elegant experiments that demonstrated that lateral geniculate neurons in rabbits fail to acquire normal visual receptive properties when a chronic epileptic focus is created in the visual cortex to which they project.[4,9] Whether normal neuronal functional integration of the lateral geniculate body is disrupted by antidromic "backfiring" of the epileptiform discharges from visual cortex or orthodromic propagation from cortical neurons that feed back on the geniculate is not known. Conceivably, both mechanisms can influence behavior transiently and presumably effect more persistent functional or even structural changes. The reversibility of the noxious effect of epileptogenic tissue in the immature brain on distant normal structures, at least early in the course of the process, has been demonstrated by the observation that developmental delay is reversed in patients with infantile spasms caused by a unilateral localized lesion when resection of this lesion eliminates the habitual seizures,[53] as discussed earlier in this chapter.

There is a long history to the relationship between epilepsy and psychosis, particularly schizophrenia. Nonpsychiatrists should be aware of major changes in nomenclature, vocabulary, and interpretation that have taken place over the last 50 years when reading older texts.[34,69]

In the 1960s, the dominating influence was a paper by Slater and Beard,[54] some 50 pages long, showing a close association between epilepsy and "schizophrenialike" psychosis. (The label "schizophrenialike" was necessary because everyone important "knew" that schizophrenia was a functional disorder.) Falconer had operated on 16 such patients before deciding that the balance of benefit from surgery was such that it was not appropriate to continue. Taylor[61,62] showed that those patients, with chronic schizophrenic symptoms, were characterized by excesses of (a) females, (b) onsets of epilepsy at ages 5 to 15, (c) left handedness, and (d) alien tissue lesions (e) in the left temporal lobe. This unique material allowed him to suggest that brains that suffered schizophrenia had been biased from embryonal, prenatal life and had required compensations in the organization of speech and language that later proved to be problematic when the normal condensation and shifts in the organization of language occurred. This developmental hypothesis arose from the excess of prenatally acquired lesions, the excess of left handedness, and the relative excess of girls, whose language organization is different from that of boys. The emergence of a neuropathologic basis for schizophrenia in people without epilepsy tends to confirm these findings from patients with epilepsy.

It seems probable, in hindsight, that the benefit of surgery to these patients was underestimated and that their life situations and lack of appropriate modern management contributed to continuing chronicity of their psychoses.

Normally excluded from consideration is the whole issue of autisticlike syndromes and various degrees of language regression associated with Landau-Kleffner syndrome, continuous spikes and waves during slow sleep, and West syndrome. Because about a third of children with autism develop epilepsy, the association deserves urgent research. Taylor et al.[65] reported, in the Great Ormond Street series of patients considered for surgical treatment, a sequence of male children, mostly with dysembryoplastic neuroepithelial tumors of the right temporal lobe, who exhibited marked autistic features. Subsequently, a larger number of children with other lesions have been recruited to that series.[37]

Effects on Sleep and Endocrine Function

There is considerable evidence from both the animal and the clinical literature that certain types of epileptic seizures cause chronic disruption in sleep organization, particularly a reduction in rapid eye movement (REM) sleep.[57] It is well known that REM sleep deprivation can produce behavioral disturbances, including psychosis,[11] so the possibility that this could be an indirect means by which some forms of epilepsy produce lasting interictal disturbances in behavior needs to be further investigated.

Another potential source of epilepsy-induced interictal behavioral problems that has not been adequately pursued relates to the effect chronic epileptic seizures have on endocrine function.[26,68] Seizures are associated with release of prolactin and other hormones, altering diurnal fluctuations and absolute levels in brain and blood, which could have dramatic effects on behavior and might, for instance, account for the sexual dysfunction seen in some patients with epilepsy.

SUMMARY AND CONCLUSIONS

Suffering from epilepsy is not limited to having seizures. Indeed, it has to be emphasized that seizures are not the same as epilepsy, and are but one manifestation of the underlying neuroanatomic/neurophysiologic changes that represent the latter. The brain has a problem to deal with and is dealing with it all the time. Whether by developmental anomaly, scar, tumor, or the effect of trauma, the process by which persons come to declare their brain abnormality by having noticeable epileptic seizures will have originated at some point in time before that manifestation, and it is clearly present between each noted seizure. There are other ways in which the brain problem can manifest itself, such as gross or minor neurologic signs and, we argue, gross (or minor) behavioral signs and learning problems. The various expressions of the brain problem will not be constant over time. Just as seizures are not constant over time and are often reactive to circumstance, so too the behavioral problems are not constant and are reactive. Even severe psychoses can come and go. Medications will also affect the chemical manifestations of the brain problem, but so will other natural physiologic processes. As the brain changes radically over development, and those changes are often reflected in the scale, type, and frequency of seizures, so too the behavioral manifestations will change during the course of development. Furthermore, seizures can alter brain function in a manner that influences behavior just as behavior influences seizures. Behavioral changes are important because they are clinically relevant, but there is important research to be done not just on the mental states of people with epilepsy, but also in understanding these mental states, behavioral changes, serious psychoses in general, and their causes, using the models provided in the animal laboratory and by people with epilepsy.

ACKNOWLEDGMENTS

Original research reported by Dr. Engel was supported in part by Grants NS-02808, NS-15654, NS-33310, and GM-24839 from the National Institutes of Health and Contract DE-AC03-76-SF00012 from the Department of Energy. Professor Trimble is supported by the Raymond-Way Fund.

References

1. Adamec R, Shallow T, Blundell J, et al. Contribution of pre kindling affective state to hemispheric differences in the effects on anxiety of basolateral amygdala kindling. In: Corcoran ME, Moshé S, eds. *Kindling 6*. New York: Springer; 2004:263–271.
2. Aylett S, Cross J, Taylor D, et al. Epileptic akinetic mutism following temporal lobectomy for Rasmussen's syndrome. *Eur Child Adolesc Psychiatry*. 1996;5:222–225.
3. Bandler R. Induction of rage following microinjections of glutamate into midbrain but not hypothalamus of cats. *Neurosci Lett*. 1982;30: 183–188.
4. Baumbach HD, Chow KL. Visuocortical epileptiform discharges in rabbits: differential effects on neuronal development in the lateral geniculate nucleus and superior colliculus. *Brain Res*. 1981;209:61–76.
5. Bear DM, Fedio P. Quantitative analysis of interictal behavior in temporal lobe epilepsy. *Arch Neurol*. 1977;34:454–467.
6. Blumer D, Benson DF. Psychiatric manifestations of epilepsy. In: Benson D, Blumer DF, eds. *Psychiatric Aspects of Neurologic Disease*, Vol II. New York: Grune & Stratton; 1982:25–48.
7. Bruton CJ, Stevens JR, Frith CD. Epilepsy, psychosis, and schizophrenia: clinical neuropathological correlations. *Neurology*. 1994;44:34–42.
8. Caldecott-Hazard S, Engel J Jr. Limbic postictal events: anatomical substrates and opioid receptor involvement. *Prog Neuropsychopharmacol Biol Psychiatry*. 1987;11:389–418.
9. Chow KL, Baumbach HD, Glanzman DL. Abnormal development of lateral geniculate neurons in rabbit subjected to either eyelid closure or corticofugal paroxysmal discharges. *Brain Res*. 1978;146:151–158.
10. Corcoran M, Moshé S, eds. *Kindling 5*. New York: Plenum Press; 1998.
11. Dement W, Henry P, Cohen H, et al. Studies on the effect of REM deprivation in humans and in animals. In: Kety S, Evarts E, Williams H, eds. *Association for Research on Nervous and Mental Diseases, Vol XLV: Sleep and Altered States of Consciousness*. Baltimore: Williams & Wilkins; 1967: 456–468.
12. Dragunov M, Goddard GV, Laverty R. Is adenosine an endogenous anticonvulsant? *Epilepsia*. 1985;26:480–487.
13. Efron, R. Post-epileptic paralysis: theoretical critique and report of a case. *Brain*. 1961;84:381–394.
14. Engel J Jr, Bandler R, Griffith NC, et al. Neurobiological evidence for epilepsy-induced interictal disturbances. In: Smith D, Treiman D, Trimble M, eds. *Advances in Neurology*, Vol 55. New York: Raven Press; 1991:97–111.
15. Engel J Jr, Cahan L. Potential relevance of kindling to human partial epilepsy. In: Wada J, ed. *Kindling 3*. New York: Raven Press; 1986:37–51.
16. Engel J Jr, Shewmon DA. Impact of the kindling phenomenon on clinical epileptology. In: Morrell F, ed. *Kindling and Synaptic Plasticity: The Legacy of Graham Goddard*. Cambridge, MA: Birkhäuser Boston; 1991:195–210.
17. Falret J. De l'état mental des épileptiques. *Arch Gén Méd*. 1860–1861; 16:666–679; 17:461–491; 18:423–443.
18. Flor-Henry P. Epilepsy and psychopathology. In: Granville-Grossman K, ed. *Recent Advances in Clinical Psychiatry—2*. London: Churchill Livingstone; 1976:262–294.
19. Frost JJ, Mayberg HS, Fisher RS, et al. Mu-opiate receptors measured by positron emission tomography are increased in temporal lobe epilepsy. *Ann Neurol*. 1988;23:231–237.
20. Gastaut H, Morin G, Leserre N. Etude du comportement des épileptiques psychomoteurs dans l'intervalle de leurs crises: les troubles de l'activitie globale et de la socialite. *Ann Med Psychol*. 1955;113:1–27.
21. Gibbs FA. Ictal and nonictal psychiatric disorders in temporal lobe epilepsy. *J Nerv Ment Dis*. 1951;113:522–528.
22. Goddard GV. The kindling model of epilepsy. *Trends Neurosci*. 1983;6:275–279.
23. Goddard GV, McIntyre DC, Leech CK. A permanent change in brain function resulting from daily electrical stimulation. *Exp Neurol*. 1969;25:295–330.
24. Goldensohn ES. The relevance of secondary epileptogenesis to the treatment of epilepsy: kindling and the mirror focus. *Epilepsia*. 1984;25(Suppl 2):S156–S173.
25. Griffith N, Engel J Jr, Bandler R. Ictal and enduring interictal disturbances in emotional behaviour in an animal model of temporal lobe epilepsy. *Brain Res*. 1987;400:360–364.
26. Herzog AG, Russell V, Vaitukaitis JL, et al. Neuroendocrine dysfunction in temporal lobe epilepsy. *Arch Neurol*. 1982;39:133–135.
27. Hong JS, Gillin JC, Yang HYT, et al. Repeated ECS and the brain content of endorphins. *Brain Res*. 1979;177:273–278.
28. Janz D, Christian W. Impulsiv-Pet Mal. *Dtsch Z Nervenheilkd*. 1957;176:346–386.
29. Jennet B. *Epilepsy After Non-Missile Head Injuries*. 2nd ed. Chicago: William Heinemann; 1975.
30. Kline NS, Li CH, Lehmann HE, et al. Beta-endorphine-induced changes in schizophrenic and depressed patients. *Arch Gen Psychiatry*. 1977;34:1111–1113.
31. Landolt H. Serial encephalographic investigations during psychotic episodes in epileptic patients and during schizophrenic attacks. In: Lorentz de Haas AM, ed. *Lectures on Epilepsy*. Amsterdam: Elsevier; 1958:91–133.
32. Levy RH, Mattson RH, Meldrum BS, eds. *Antiepileptic Drugs*. 4th ed. New York: Raven Press; 1995.
33. Mace CJ. Epilepsy and schizophrenia. *Br J Psychiatry*. 1993;163:439–445.
34. Mace CJ, Trimble MR. Psychosis following temporal lobe surgery: a report of six cases. *J Neurol Neurosurg Psychiatry*. 1991;54:639–644.
35. Malamud N. Psychiatric disorder with intracranial tumours of the limbic system. *Arch Neurol*. 1967;17:113–123.
36. Mathern GW, Pretorius JK, Babb TL. Influence of the type of initial precipitating injury and at what age it occurs on course and outcome in patients with temporal lobe seizures. *J Neurosurg*. 1995;82:220–227.
37. McCellan A, Davies S, Heyman I, et al. Psychiatric disorders in childhood epilepsy candidates before and after temporal lobe resection. *Dev Med Child Neurol*. 2005;47:666–672.
38. McIntyre DC. Split brain rat: transfer and interference of kindled amygdala convulsions. *Can J Neurol Sci*. 1975;2:429–437.
39. Meldrum BS, Horton RW, Brierley JB. Epileptic brain damage in adolescent baboons following seizures induced by allylglycine. *Brain*. 1974;97:407–418.
40. Mendez MF, Cummings JL, Benson DF. Depression in epilepsy: significance and phenomenology. *Arch Neurol*. 1986;43:766–770.
41. Milner B. Psychological aspects of focal epilepsy and its neurosurgical management. *Adv Neurol*. 1975;8:299–321.
42. Monroe RR. *Episodic Behavioral Disorders. A Psychodynamic and Neurophysiologic Analysis*. Cambridge, MA: Harvard University Press; 1970.
43. Morrell F. Secondary epileptogenic lesions. *Epilepsia*. 1959–1960;1:538–560.
44. Morrell F. Varieties of human secondary epileptogenesis. *J Clin Neurophysiol*. 1989;6:227–275.
45. Penfield W, Jasper H. *Epilepsy and the Functional Anatomy of the Human Brain*. Boston: Little, Brown; 1954.
46. Prince DA, Wilder BJ. Control mechanisms in cortical epileptogenic foci: "surround" inhibition. *Arch Neurol*. 1967;16:194–202.
47. Rausch R, Crandall PH. Psychological status related to surgical control of temporal lobe seizures. *Epilepsia*. 1982;23:191–202.
48. Rausch R, Walsh GO. Right-hemisphere language dominance in right-handed epileptic patients. *Arch Neurol*. 1984;41:1077–1080.
49. Razavi L. Cytogenic and somatic variation in the neurobiology of violence: epidemiological, clinical and morphogenic considerations. In: Fields WS, Sweet WH, eds. *Neural Bases of Violence and Aggression*. St. Louis: WH Green; 1975:205–272.
50. Rocha LL, Maidment NT, Evans CJ, et al. Opioid peptide release and mu receptor binding during amygdala kindling in rats: regional discordances. *Epilepsy Res*. 1996;(Suppl 12):215–228.
51. Sato M. Long-lasting hypersensitivity to methamphetamine following amygdaloid kindling in cats: the relationship between limbic epilepsy and the psychotic state. *Biol Psychiatry*. 1983;18:525–536.
52. Sato S, Dreifuss FE, Penry JK. Prognostic factors in absence seizures. *Neurology*. 1976;26:788–796.
53. Shields WD, Shewmon DA, Chugani HT, et al. The role of surgery in the treatment of infantile spasms. *J Epilepsy [Suppl]*. 1990;3:321–324.
54. Slater E, Beard AW. The schizophrenia-like psychoses of epilepsy. *Br J Psychiatry*. 1963;109:95–150.
55. Sramka M, Sedlack P, Nadvornik P. Observation of the kindling phenomenon in treatment of pain by stimulation in the thalamus. In: Sweet WH, Obrador S, Martin-Rodriguez JG, eds. *Neurosurgical Treatment in Psychiatry, Pain and Epilepsy*. Baltimore: University Park Press; 1977: 651–654.
56. Steckler T, Kalin NH, Reul JMHM, eds. *Handbook of Stress and the Brain (2 vols), Techniques in the Behavioral & Neural Sciences*, V.15. Philadelphia: Elsevier; 2005.
57. Sterman MB, Shouse MN, Passouant P, eds. *Sleep and Epilepsy*. New York: Academic Press; 1982.
58. Stevens JR. Psychiatric implications of psychomotor epilepsy. *Arch Gen Psychiatry*. 1966;14:461–471.
59. Sutula T, Pitkänen A, eds. Do seizures damage the brain? *Progress in Brain Research*, Vol. 135. Amsterdam: Elsevier; 2002.
60. Taylor DC. Mental state and temporal lobe epilepsy. A correlative account of 100 patients treated surgically. *Epilepsia*. 1972;13:727–765.
61. Taylor DC. Factors influencing the occurrence of schizophrenia-like psychosis in patients with temporal lobe epilepsy. *Psychol Med*. 1975;5:249–254.
62. Taylor DC. Developmental stratagems organising intellectual skills: evidence from studies of temporal lobectomy for epilepsy. In: Knight RM, Bakker DJ, eds. *The Neuropsychology of Learning Disorders: Theoretical Approaches*. Baltimore: University Park Press; 1976:149–171.
63. Taylor D. Epilepsy as a chronic sickness: remediating its impact. In: Engel J Jr, ed. *Surgical Treatment of the Epilepsies*. 2nd ed. New York: Raven Press; 1993:11–22.
64. Taylor D. Psychiatric aspects. In: Wallace S, ed. *Epilepsy in Children*. London: Chapman and Hall; 1996:601–616.
65. Taylor DC, Cross HC, Neville BG. Autistic spectrum disorders in childhood epilepsy surgery candidates. *Eur Chid Adolesc Psychiatry*. 1999;8: 189–192.
66. Taylor DC, Falconer MA. Clinical socio-economic and psychological changes after temporal lobectomy for epilepsy. *Br J Psychiatry*. 1968;114: 1247–1261.

67. Taylor DC, Marsh SM. Hughlings Jackson's Dr. Z: the paradigm of temporal lobe epilepsy revealed. *J Neurol Neurosurg Psychiatry*. 1980;43:758–767.
68. Toone B. Sexual disorders in epilepsy. In: Pedley TA, Meldrum BS, eds. *Recent Advances in Epilepsy, 3*. New York: Churchill Livingstone; 1987:233–259.
69. Trimble M. *The Psychoses of Epilepsy*. New York: Raven Press; 1991.
70. Waxman SG, Geschwind N. Hypergraphia in temporal lobe epilepsy. *Neurology*. 1974;24:629–636.
71. Wieser HG, Hailemariam S, Regard M, et al. Unilateral limbic epileptic status activity: stereo EEG behavioral and cognitive data. *Epilepsia*. 1985;26:19–29.
72. Wolf P. Acute behavioral symptomatology at disappearance of epileptiform EEG abnormality: paradoxical, or "forced" normalization. In: Smith D, Treiman D, Trimble M, eds. *Advances in Neurology,* Vol 55. New York: Raven Press; 1991:127–142.

CHAPTER 201 ■ COGNITIVE SIDE EFFECTS OF ANTIEPILEPTIC DRUGS

ALBERT P. ALDENKAMP, JOANNE TAYLOR, AND GUS A. BAKER

INTRODUCTION

Cognitive impairment is the most common comorbid disorder in epilepsy.[13,28] Memory impairments, mental slowing, and attentional deficits are the most frequently reported cognitive disorders.[14,29] Such consequences may be more debilitating for a patient than the seizures; thus, it is worthwhile to explore the factors that lead to cognitive impairment. The exact cause of cognitive impairment in epilepsy has not been explored fully, but three factors clearly are involved: Etiology, the seizures, and the "central" side effects of drug treatment.[3] In this chapter we will concentrate on the unwanted effects of antiepileptic medication on cognitive function. When evaluating this factor separately, it is imperative to realize that in clinical practice most cognitive problems have a multifactorial origin and that, for the most part, the three aforementioned factors, combined, are responsible for the makeup of a cognitive problem in an individual patient. Moreover, the factors are related, which causes therapeutic dilemmas in some patients when seizure control can only be achieved with treatments that are associated with cognitive side effects.

The interest in the cognitive side effects of antiepileptic drug (AED) treatment is of recent origin. The possibility that cognitive impairment may develop as a consequence or aftermath of epilepsy was raised as early as 1885 when Gowers described "epileptic dementia" as an effect of the pathologic sequela of seizures. Nonetheless, the topic was not coupled to AED treatment until the 1970s,[27,38] probably stimulated by the widening range of possibilities for drug treatment during that period (i.e., the introduction of carbamazepine and valproate). Since then, a plethora of studies have been published, the majority on the commonly used AEDs: valproate (VPA), carbamazepine (CBZ), and phenytoin (PHT).

In the last decade, several new AEDs have been introduced. Although it is claimed that these drugs have different efficacy profiles and that some drugs are particularly efficacious in specific syndromes (e.g., vigabatrin [VGB]), head-to-head comparisons between the newer drugs and the commonly used drugs (such as CBZ and VPA) are rare. The types of studies used to investigate the newer AEDs are summarized in Table 1. Nonetheless, meta-analyses such as the influential Cochrane reviews[39,54] do not show significant differences in efficacy between these newer and commonly used drugs. Also, studies analyzing long-term retention do not show differences between the drugs.[78,90] Several studies have shown retention rate to be the best parameter of the long-term clinical usefulness of a particular drug.[47] Retention rate is considered to be a composite of drug efficacy and drug safety and expresses the willingness of patients to continue drug treatment. It is therefore the best standard for evaluating the clinical relevance of side effects. The 1-year retention rate is reported not to be higher than 55% for topiramate (TPM),[41] 60% for lamotrigine (LTG), 58% for VGB, and 45% for gabapentin (GBP).[53] Long-term (mostly 3-year) retention is about 35% for all newer AEDs.[52] Side effects appear to be the major factor affecting long-term retention for most drugs.[4,22] In clinical practice, tolerability is therefore a major issue and the choice of a certain AED is at least partially based on comparison of tolerability profiles of the drugs. Also, the tolerability profiles of the newer drugs have become a more important issue in drug development, stimulated by the interest of regulatory agencies.[4] Cognitive side effects have been demonstrated to be one of the most important tolerability problems in chronic AED treatment.

METHOD

In evaluating studies of the cognitive effects of AEDs, we will follow an evidence-based approach.[12,87] Randomized clinical trials with monotherapy in patients with newly diagnosed epilepsy represent the most accurate procedure for assessing the cognitive impact of AEDs.[4] These studies are not clouded by the effect of concurrent or previous AED use and permit the accurate collection of nondrug baseline data that is required for determining whether a particular treatment affects cognitive processing (i.e., to isolate drug-induced impairments from those due to other sources such as the seizures). Data from such studies can be supplemented with information from studies using add-on or polytherapy designs. In these studies, the use of two AEDs makes identifying the components of the treatment that are responsible for the observed effects more complex. In many cases, however, patients with epilepsy require dual AED therapy before adequate seizure control is obtained; therefore, data from add-on studies does warrant consideration. Also, data from healthy volunteers should be treated with caution. In general, the power of such studies is limited by small sample sizes, and drug exposure periods are typically brief. It is possible that chronic treatment results in entirely different types of cognitive impairment that cannot be observed during short-term treatment. For example, such differences in side effect profile between acute and long-term administration have been found with PHT. Finally, the differing cerebral substrate in patients with epilepsy and healthy volunteers suggests that cognitive responses to AEDs may be different in these populations. Nonetheless, volunteer studies may provide an early insight into the cognitive effects of an AED and therefore provide a foundation for further studies in patients with epilepsy (see reference 87 for a discussion of methodologic aspects of cognitive drug trials in epilepsy).

RESULTS

Phenobarbital

The main anticonvulsant mechanism of action is the increase of the duration (not the frequency) of the γ-aminobutyric acid

TABLE 1

TYPE OF STUDY TO INVESTIGATE THE COGNITIVE SIDE-EFFECTS OF NEWER AEDs

AED	Volunteer studies	Controlled studies in patients with newly diagnosed epilepsy	Add-on clinical studies in patients with epilepsy
OXC	Curran & Java (1993)	Laaksonen et al. (1985) Sabers et al. (1995) Äikiä et al. (1992) McKee et al. (1994)	
TPM	Martin et al. (1999)	Donati et al. (2006)	Meador (1997) Aldenkamp et al. (2000) Burton & Harden (1997) Bootsma et al. (2004) Thompson et al. (2000) Fritz et al. (2005)
LTG	Cohen et al. (1985) Hamilton et al. (1993) Martin et al. (1999) Meador et al. (2000) Aldenkamp et al. (2002)	Gillham et al. (2000)	Smith et al. (1993) Banks and Beran (1991) Aldenkamp et al. (1997)
LEV			Neyens et al. (1995)
TGB		Dodrill et al. (1997)	Kälviäinen et al. (1996) Sveinbjornsdottir et al. (1994)
GBP	Martin et al. (1999) Meador et al. (1999)		Leach et al. (1997)
RUF			Aldenkamp and Alpherts (2006)

AED, antiepileptic drug; GBP, gabapentin; LEV, levetiracetam; LTG, lamotrigine; OXC, oxcarbazepine; RUF, rufinamide; TGB, tiagabine; TPM, topiramate.

(GABA)-activated chloride ion channel opening,[86] hence potentiating GABA-mediated inhibitory neurotransmission. Phenobarbital (PB) can also activate the $GABA_A$ receptor in the absence of GABA, which is sometimes considered to be a mechanism leading to its sedative properties. PB is used for the treatment of epilepsy since the discovery of its antiepileptic effect by Hauptman in 1912.

For PB one study[49] is available allowing the evaluation of the cognitive effects of PB relative to a nondrug condition. This study show relative serious memory impairment (short-term memory recall) in 19 patients with epilepsy.

Comparisons with other AEDs are available from four studies[21,35,60,88] of patients with epilepsy. One of these shows more impairment for PB than for PHT or CBZ on visuomotor and memory tests[35] and two other studies show convincing and clinically highly relevant impairments of intelligence scores after long-term PB treatment in comparison with VPA.[21,88] A randomized, double-blind, crossover study of healthy volunteers also found more impairment on some measures for PB compared to PHT and VPA.[61] Only the study by Meador et al.[60] does not show differences between PB and PHT or CBZ.

Phenytoin

The main anticonvulsant mechanism of action is use-dependent (voltage- and frequency-dependent) sodium channel blocking.[75] It binds to the fast inactivated state of the channel, reducing high-frequency neuronal firing. PHT has a stronger effect on the sodium channel than CBZ, delaying recovery stronger than CBZ. PHT may also have mild effects on the excitatory glutamate system and on the inhibitory GABA system. PHT has been used as an antiepileptic drug since it was introduced for the treatment of epilepsy in 1938 by Merritt and Putnam. For 20 years PHT was (together with PB) the universal treatment of epilepsy. PHT has excellent anticonvulsant properties and is used as a broad-range AED.

For PHT five studies are available[58,59,77,82,83] comparing PHT with a nondrug condition. These studies all reveal PHT-induced cognitive impairment in the areas of attention, memory, and especially mental speed. The magnitude of the reported effects is moderate to large. A caveat is in order, however, as all these studies were carried out in normal volunteers, which opens the possibility that these effects represent short-term outcomes of the drug.

The results of head-to-head comparisons with other AEDs are somewhat more confusing. Using an ingenious long-term treatment and withdrawal design, Gallassi et al.[35] found more cognitive impairment than CBZ. On the other hand, no difference with CBZ, VPA, oxcarbazepine (OXC), and even PB are reported.[2,33,58–60,74]

Ethosuximide

Ethosuximide (ESX) modifies the properties of voltage-dependent calcium channels, reducing the T-type currents and thereby preventing synchronized firing. The reduction is most prominent at negative membrane potentials and less prominent at more positive membrane potentials. Most effect is assumed to take place in thalamocortical relay neurons. ESX was introduced in 1960 and is mainly used for the treatment of generalized absence seizures.

No controlled studies are available to evaluate the cognitive effects of ESX.

Carbamazepine

The main anticonvulsant mechanism of action is similar to that of PHT with a less "slowing" effect in the recovery state than obtained for PHT. The mechanism of action is also voltage and frequency dependent. CBZ was first synthesized in the early 1950s[68,69] and introduced as an antiepileptic drug by Bonduelle in 1964 in Europe. CBZ is used for patients with partial complex seizures, with or without secondary generalization. Approval by the Food and Drug Administration (FDA) for use in the United States followed much later (1978) because of concerns about serious hematologic toxicity (e.g., aplastic anemia).

For CBZ two studies, one in normal volunteers[82] and one in patients with epilepsy,[6] report "no cognitive impairment" compared to a nondrug condition. This is challenged by the group by Meador et al.[58,59] that reported impairments of memory, attention, and mental speed, largely the areas that may also be affected by phenytoin.

When evaluating the comparisons of CBZ with other AEDs, there are the conflicting results of the Italian study by Gallassi et al., showing a more favorable profile compared with PHT and PB[35] and the U.S.-based study by Meador et al.[58–60] that showed no differences compared with PHT and PB.

Valproate

VPA, a fatty acid, is believed to possess multiple mechanisms of action. A number of studies have demonstrated an effect on sodium channels, however, different from PHT and CBZ. An effect on T-type calcium channels has also been demonstrated. Recent studies have, however, demonstrated that a predominant effect concerns the interaction with the GABAergic neurotransmitter system. More precisely, VPA elevates brain GABA levels and potentiates GABA responses, possibly by enhancing GABA synthesis and inhibiting degradation. Furthermore, VPA may augment GABA release and block the reuptake of GABA into glia cells. VPA is one of the most effective drugs against generalized absence seizures. It was introduced in approximately the same period as CBZ.

For VPA, three studies[24,71,84] allow the interpretation of absolute effects and show mild to moderate impairment of psychomotor and mental speed. The comparison with other drugs shows lower performance of memory and visuomotor function compared to CBZ[35] and a favorable profile compared to PHB on tests for intelligence.[21,88] One study does not show a difference with PHT.[33]

Oxcarbazepine

Oxcarbazepine (OXC) is essentially a prodrug, a keto homolog of CBZ, structurally very similar to CBZ, but with a different metabolic profile. In humans, the keto group is rapidly and quantitatively reduced to form a monohydroxy derivative that is the main active anticonvulsant agent during OXC therapy. Metabolism of OXC does not result in the formation of 10,11-epoxy carbamazepine that is sometimes considered to be the main metabolite causing side effects. The mechanism of action is similar to CBZ. However, OXC is also considered to reduce presynaptic glutamate release, possibly by reduction of high-threshold calcium currents. OXC was approved in the European Union in 1999 and is indicated for use as monotherapy or adjunctive therapy for partial seizures with or without secondarily generalized tonic–clonic seizures in patients 6 years of age or older.

The effects of OXC on cognitive function have been evaluated in one study in healthy volunteers and in four studies in patients with epilepsy. A double-blind, placebo-controlled, crossover study was conducted in 12 healthy volunteers.[25] The effects of two doses of OXC (300 mg/day and 600 mg/day) and placebo on cognitive function and psychomotor performance were assessed. The treatment duration for each condition was 2 weeks. Cognitive function tests were administered before treatment initiation and 4 hours after the morning doses on days 1, 8, and 15. In this study, OXC improved performance on a focused attention task, increased manual writing speed, and had no effect on long-term memory processes.

In patients with epilepsy, four monotherapy comparative studies are available to evaluate the effects of OXC on cognitive functions in adult patients with newly diagnosed epilepsy. The first study[44] was a double-blind, active-control study evaluating the effects of CBZ and OXC on memory and attention in 41 patients with newly diagnosed epilepsy. The treatment duration was 1 year. Cognitive function and intelligence tests were administered before treatment initiation and after 1 year of treatment. The results indicated no deterioration of memory or attention with either CBZ or OXC. The second study was an active-control study that evaluated the effects of CBZ, VPA, and OXC on intelligence, learning and memory, attention, psychomotor speed, verbal span, and visuospatial construction in 32 patients with newly diagnosed epilepsy.[73] The treatment duration was 4 months. Cognitive function and intelligence tests were administered before treatment initiation and after 4 months of treatment. The results indicated no deterioration of cognitive function in any treatment group. Significant improvements in learning and memory tests were found for the CBZ- and OXC-treated patients. Improvements were also found in attention and psychomotor speed tests for the VPA-treated patients and partly for the CBZ-treated patients. The third study was a double-blind, randomized, active-control study that evaluated the effects of PHT and OXC on memory, attention, and psychomotor speed in 29 patients with newly diagnosed epilepsy.[2] The treatment duration was 1 year. Cognitive function tests were administered before treatment initiation and after 6 and 12 months of treatment. The results indicated no significant differential cognitive effects between PHT and OXC during the first year of treatment in patients with newly diagnosed epilepsy who achieved adequate seizure control. In the fourth study,[56] three groups of 12 patients taking either CBZ, VPA, or PHT took a single 600-mg dose of OXC followed 7 days later by 3 weeks of treatment with OXC 300 mg thrice daily and matched placebo in random order. Seven untreated patients, acting as controls, were prescribed the single OXC dose and 3 weeks of active treatment only. There were no important changes in cognitive function test results during administration of OXC compared with placebo. Finally a study in newly diagnosed children, randomized to OXC ($n = 55$), CBZ ($n = 28$), and VPA ($n = 21$) was performed showing no differences between the three drugs.[29a]

In summary, the results of these studies indicate that OXC does not affect cognitive function in healthy volunteers and adult patients with newly diagnosed epilepsy. The effects of OXC on cognitive function, however, have not been systematically studied in children and adolescents. In accordance with the latest revision of the Committee for Proprietary Medicinal Products (CPMP) Note of Guidance (CPMP EWP/566/98 rev 1, dated November 16, 2000, Sections 2.5 and 5.2), a study has recently been launched (Protocol #: CTRI476E2337) to investigate the effects of OXC on cognitive function (i.e., psychomotor speed and alertness, mental information processing speed and attention, memory, and learning) in children and adolescents aged 6 to 17 years with partial seizures.

Topiramate

TPM is a sulfamate-substituted monosaccharide that has clearly multiple mechanisms of action.[89] TPM blocks neuronal sodium channels in a voltage- and frequency-dependent manner, inhibits CA, promotes the action of GABA at the $GABA_A$ receptor complex, and elevates GABA brain concentrations by about 60% at 3 and 6 hours after a single dose; this increase was maintained with 4 weeks of TPM administration.[70] TPM is a carbonic anhydrase–inhibiting drug. TPM has proved to be effective in patients with refractory chronic partial epilepsies.[32,72] It was recently introduced in the United States and Europe.

During the initial add-on clinical trials, central nervous system (CNS)-related "cognitive" subjective complaints were frequently reported, including mental slowing, attentional deficits, speech problems, and memory difficulties.[72] It should be mentioned, however, that higher target doses and faster titration schedules were used than are now common in clinical practice (see reference 32 for a discussion of dose and titration speed). Recent studies with TPM-treated patients have confirmed high levels of adverse cognitive effects based on subjective complaints.[42,80] A follow-up study[19] showed long-term retention of 30% for a 4-year follow-up. For about half of the 70% of patients who discontinued treatment, side effects were the major reason, with cognitive side effects being most frequently mentioned.

Only a few studies have psychometrically measured cognitive changes using neuropsychological tests. A study by Martin et al.[55] in six normal volunteers used an acute dose of 2.8 mg/kg (~200 mg/day) followed by a titration to 5.7 mg/kg (~400 mg/day) in 4 weeks, resulting in weekly dose escalations of about 100 mg. The rate at which TPM was escalated in this study was very similar to the dose escalation used in the initial TPM adjunctive therapy trials,[72] in which escalating the TPM dose to 200 or 400 mg/day over 2 to 3 weeks was associated with somnolence, psychomotor slowing, speech disorders, and concentration and memory difficulties.[19] Martin et al. showed neuropsychometric changes commensurate with these CNS effects. The cognitive effects of the acute starting dose of 200 mg/day were impairments of verbal function (word finding and verbal fluency) of approximately two standard deviations (which represents very serious impairment) and of sustained attention. Titration to 400 mg/day in 4 weeks resulted in impairments of verbal memory and mental speed of more than two standard deviations.

Six studies involving patients with epilepsy are available. In a study by Meador[57] with 155 patients with epilepsy, the effects of the gradual introduction of TPM as add-on (a 50-mg starting dose, followed by increments of 50 mg per week over 8 weeks) were compared with those of more rapid dose escalation (initial dose of 100 mg, followed by two consecutive weekly increments of 100 and 200 mg). In a test battery of 23 variables representing selective attention, word fluency, and visuomotor speed, the subjects who were on a slow-titration schedule and treated with one background AED displayed TPM-associated score changes of more than one third but less than one standard deviation. A study by Aldenkamp et al.[10] was specifically designed to compare cognitive effects of TPM and VPA added to therapeutic dosages of CBZ in 59 patients with epilepsy. In this study, a slow titration speed was used with a starting dose of 25 mg/day TPM and weekly increments of 25 mg. Moreover, the average achieved dose (approximately 250 mg) was relatively low. Neuropsychometric testing was conducted 8 weeks after the last dosage increase (20 weeks after the start of TPM therapy). The study therefore used optimal conditions (i.e., slow titration, relatively low dose, and a longer treatment period), allowing for patient habituation to the effects of TPM therapy. Nonetheless, cognitive impairment was found for verbal memory function both during titration and at end-point. In a study by Burton and Harden,[20] attention was assessed weekly in ten subjects receiving TPM over a 3-month period. Four of nine subjects showed significant correlations between TPM dosage and forward digit span measured weekly, such that higher dosage was associated with poorer attention. In a retrospective study by Thompson et al.,[81] the neuropsychological test scores of 18 patients obtained before and after the introduction of treatment with TPM (median dose 300 mg) were compared with changes in test performance of 18 patients who had undergone repeat neuropsychological assessments at the same time intervals. In those patients taking TPM, a significant deterioration in many domains was found. The largest changes were for verbal IQ, verbal fluency, and verbal learning.

A retrospective study by Kockelmann et al.[43] investigated the cognitive profile of 42 patients on AED polytherapy containing TPM compared to 42 patients taking LTG. Patients were assessed on an extensive battery of neuropsychological assessments and blood serum levels were obtained. The TPM-treated patients performed significantly worse on executive functioning measures such as working memory and verbal fluency. Significant correlations with blood serum levels were only evident for verbal fluency, verbal memory span, and verbal memory (delayed recall and recognition). A lack of correlation with other variables may be in part due to the small sample size.[43]

In an open, prospective study, 41 patients with intractable epilepsy initially received either TPM or tiagabine (TGB) as add-on treatment. Of these, 21 patients were assessed at baseline, after a 3-month titration phase, and after a 3-month maintenance phase. The patients were assessed on various aspects of cognitive functioning such as attention, memory, language, and self-report of mood and quality of life. The TPM group performed worse on measures of verbal fluency and working memory and reported more depression than the TGB group. They also felt that they were suffering from more adverse effects due to the TPM medication. However, TPM patients did report an increase in mental flexibility between titration and maintenance phase.[34]

In summary, there is clear clinical evidence for TPM-induced cognitive impairment. Not all studies are comparable because of the confusion about dose and titration speed (see reference 5 for a discussion). Moreover, the complete lack of controlled studies is remarkable.

Lamotrigine

LTG is a phenyltriazine with weak antifolate activity. The main anticonvulsant mechanism of action is to block voltage-dependent sodium channels that result in voltage- and frequency-dependent inhibition of the channel. This suggests that the mechanism of action is similar to that of PHT and CBZ. However, much attention is focused recently on the fact that this mechanism in LTG treatment results in preventing presynaptic excitatory neurotransmitter release. It is still in debate to what extent the mechanisms of action are different from CBZ.[46] Clinical evidence indicates that LTG is effective against partial and secondarily generalized tonic–clonic seizures, as well as idiopathic (primary) generalized epilepsy. LTG was introduced in Europe in 1991 and in the United States in 1994.

A large number of cognitive studies are available for LTG (see reference 11 for an overview). Five volunteer studies have been conducted with LTG. Doses of 120 mg and 240 mg did not produce a significant change in cognitive function compared with baseline when administered to 12 normal volunteers in an acute study of 1 day.[23] Similarly, five volunteers received LTG (acute dose 3.5 mg/kg and then titrated to a maximum of

7.1 mg/kg) in a single-blind manner and were assessed for change in cognitive function after 2 and 4 weeks.[55] There was no significant change in any of the neurocognitive measures relative to baseline performance. LTG and CBZ have been compared in 12 healthy male volunteers and associations were made between the observed cognitive effects and plasma concentrations of these drugs.[37] The effects of these drugs were examined by means of adaptive tracking, which assesses eye–hand coordination and effects of attention, and eye movement tests. LTG treatment was not significantly different from placebo, but increased CBZ saliva concentrations were significantly associated with impaired adaptive tracking and smooth and saccadic eye movements. The long-term effects of LTG and CBZ were compared in 23 volunteers in a 10-week crossover study.[63] The neuropsychological battery in this study consisted of 19 instruments yielding 40 variables, including both subjective and objective measures. LTG showed better performance or fewer side effects in 17 (42%) of the variables, while no statistically significant differences were seen in the remaining variables. Finally, a study by Aldenkamp et al.[8] in 30 volunteers (12 days of treatment, using a daily dose of 50 mg of LTG) showed evidence for a selective positive effect of LTG on cognitive activation, relative to both placebo and VPA. Although the results of these volunteer studies provide us with preliminary insight into the impact of LTG on cognition, the generalizability of the results from these studies to patients with epilepsy receiving long-term AED treatment is limited.

The effects of LTG on cognitive function have been compared with those of CBZ in patients with newly diagnosed epilepsy. Patients completed tests of verbal learning and memory, attention, and mental flexibility at baseline and then periodically for up to 48 weeks. Significant differences favoring LTG over CBZ were observed with semantic processing, verbal learning, and attention.[36] The authors concluded that LTG may have a favorable long-term effect on cognitive function when compared with CBZ. Other studies have reported positive cognitive effects of LTG used as adjunctive therapy. Two independent double-blind, randomized, crossover studies have examined the cognitive effects of LTG used as add-on therapy.[17,76] Both studies included patients with a history of partial seizures (at least once weekly during the preceding 3 months) who had received no more than two other AEDs or VPA monotherapy. Both studies also used two treatment periods (12 and 18 weeks), which were separated by a washout period (4 and 6 weeks). Despite the similarity in trial design and patients, there is some inconsistency between the findings of these two studies. One study showed a marginal reduction in general "cerebral efficiency" (an indirect measure of cognitive function) following LTG treatment.[17] Conversely, significant improvements were reported in the second study.[76] In an uncontrolled add-on study[15] using CBZ as baseline drug, no deterioration on any of the cognitive tests was found after introducing LTG (200 mg). LTG therapy in seven patients with epilepsy and mental retardation caused both positive and negative psychotropic effects.[31] These findings were based on the observations of parents and supervising staff. Positive effects included reduced irritability and increased compliance with simple instructions, while negative effects included behavioral deterioration with temper tantrums, restlessness, and hyperactivity. Similarly, a second study in 67 patients with mental retardation showed that following adjunctive treatment with LTG, social functioning was stable or improved in 90% of patients.[30]

In addition to clinical studies that have assessed the impact of LTG on cognitive function, further evidence can be obtained from examining the effect of LTG on electroencephalographic (EEG) parameters. Overt EEG discharges can occur without any visible clinical correlate in many patients with epilepsy. These epileptiform episodes may be associated with transient deterioration in cognitive function.[1,9] Data from several studies indicate that LTG may reduce spontaneous epileptiform discharges, which may partially explain the favorable cognitive profile of LTG. In five patients displaying spontaneous EEG discharges, a single dose of LTG (120 mg or 240 mg in addition to existing medication) resulted in a substantial reduction in spontaneous interictal discharges within a 24-hour period.[18] The long-term effects of LTG on paroxysmal abnormalities have also been monitored with a computer-based analysis system.[50] Twenty-one patients with intractable epilepsy (20 of whom were receiving multiple AED therapy) were evaluated before and after LTG treatment for EEG ictal events and number of spikes in a 10-minute period. Before LTG treatment, patients typically showed discharges characterized by diffuse spike-wave complexes. However, following a 4-month treatment period with LTG, ictal discharges disappeared and diffuse slow-wave activity was seen with no adverse effect on background activity. Nineteen of the 21 patients also showed a reduction in seizure frequency.

The effect of LTG add-on therapy in 11 patients with refractory partial seizures with or without secondary generalization has also been reported.[51] LTG was added to existing therapy consisting of CBZ with at least one additional AED. EEG recordings were made at rest with eyes closed, during an attentive task (blocking reaction induced by several episodes of eyes open lasting 8 to 9 seconds), during cognitive tasks, and while performing mental arithmetic. In addition, a battery of neuropsychological tests was carried out. Before LTG treatment, EEG data revealed a decrease in fast activity at rest and a reduction in α and β bands during attentive and cognitive tasks. LTG treatment resulted in a selective increase in α reactivity and β power during the attentive tasks with no other detectable changes. During cortical activation, subtle changes were observed that were taken as indicative of a slight improvement in attention. Neuropsychological evaluation revealed that following 3 months of LTG therapy, no deterioration in cognitive function had occurred.

LTG also shows a promising cognitive profile in elderly patients suffering from age-associated memory impairment.[64] A neuropsychological test battery in combination with auditory event-related potentials (ERPs) was used to measure the impact of LTG on cognitive function. LTG treatment caused a reduction in amplitude of the P300 component of the ERP and a corresponding improvement in immediate and delayed visual memory and delayed logical memory. LTG may therefore improve simple memory functions in a memory-impaired elderly population.

Levetiracetam

Levetiracetam (LEV) is a new AED, structurally and mechanistically dissimilar to other AEDs. It is believed to bind to a specific, as yet undetermined, site on the synaptic plasma membrane. Moreover, LEV seems to reduce the GABA turnover in the striatum by reducing GABA synthesis and increasing GABA metabolism. It is effective in reducing partial seizures in patients with epilepsy, both as adjunctive treatment and as monotherapy. LEV has many therapeutic advantages for patients with epilepsy. It has favorable pharmacokinetic characteristics (good bioavailability, linear pharmacokinetics, insignificant protein binding, lack of hepatic metabolism, and rapid achievement of steady-state concentrations) and a low potential for drug interactions. It is licensed for use as adjunctive treatment for partial seizures, with or without secondary generalization, in people aged over 16 years.

For its impact on cognitive function, we only have data from a small pilot study that does not allow definite conclusions.[66] An international (UK/The Netherlands) cognitive study is presently being carried out. In this study a first-line add-on design is used, comparing the cognitive effects of LEV with CBZ and VPA.

Tiagabine

TGB is a GABA uptake inhibitor that is structurally related to the prototypic GABA uptake blocker nipecotic acid, but has an improved ability to cross the blood–brain barrier. TGB temporarily prolongs the presence of GABA in the synaptic cleft by delayed clearance. Clinical trials have shown that TGB is effective as add-on therapy in the management of patients with refractory partial epilepsy. TGB was recently marketed and some aspects of the development program are still not finished.

Three cognitive studies are available. Dodrill et al.[26] included 162 patients who received the following treatments: Placebo ($n = 57$), 16 mg/day TGB ($n = 34$), 32 mg/day TGB ($n = 45$), or 56 mg/day TGB ($n = 26$) at a fixed dose for 12 weeks after a 4-week dose titration period. Eight cognitive tests and three measures of mood and adjustment were administered during the baseline period and again during the double-blind period near the end of treatment (or at the time of dropout). The results showed no cognitive effects of monotherapy with TGB at a low or high dose, but there was some evidence for mood effects of add-on treatment with TGB at higher dosing, possibly related to titration speed. In the add-on polytherapy study by Kälviäinen et al.,[40] 37 patients with partial epilepsy were included. The study protocol consisted of a randomized, double-blind, placebo-controlled, parallel-group add-on study and an open-label extension study. During the 3-month double-blind phase at low doses (30 mg/day), TGB treatment did not cause any cognitive changes as compared with placebo. TGB treatment also did not cause deterioration in cognitive performance during longer follow-up with successful treatment on higher doses after 6 to 12 months (mean 65.7 mg/day, range 30–80 mg/day) and after 18 to 24 months (mean dose 67.6 mg/day, range 24–80 mg/day). Finally, a study by Sveinbjornsdottir et al.[79] was an open trial of 22 adult patients with refractory partial epilepsy followed by a double-blind, placebo-controlled, crossover trial in 12 subjects. Nineteen patients completed the initial open titration and fixed-dose phase of the study and 11 patients completed the double-blind phase. The median daily TGB dose was 32 mg during the open fixed dose and 24 mg during the double-blind period. Neuropsychological evaluation did not show any significant effect on cognitive function in the open or double-blind phase.

Gabapentin

GBP (1-(aminomethyl) cyclohexane-acetic acid) is a novel AED, currently used as add-on therapy in patients with partial and generalized tonic–clonic seizures. GBP is a cyclic GABA analog, originally designed as a GABA agonist.[48] Further research has clearly shown a specific effect of GBP on GABAergic neurotransmitter systems, especially influencing GABA turnover. Investigations using nuclear magnetic resonance imaging spectroscopy have confirmed that GBP elevates GABA concentrations, specifically in the occipital cortex of patients with epilepsy.[70]

Two volunteer studies and one clinical study are available to interpret the cognitive effects.

Martin et al.[55] used an acute dose and rapid titration in six volunteers and did not find cognitive effects of GBP. Meador et al.[62] compared the cognitive effects of GBP and CBZ in 35 healthy subjects by using a double-blind, randomized, crossover design with two 5-week treatment periods. During each treatment condition, subjects received either GBP 2,400 mg/day or CBZ (mean 731 mg/day). Subjects were tested at the end of each AED treatment period and in four drug-free conditions (two pretreatment baselines and two posttreatment washout periods [1 month after each AED]). The neuropsychological test battery included 17 measures yielding 31 total variables. Significantly better performance on eight variables was found for GBP, but on no variables for CBZ. Comparison of CBZ and GBP with the nondrug average revealed significant statistical differences for 15 (48%) of 31 variables. Leach et al.[45] studied GBP in 21 patients in an add-on polytherapy study after 4 weeks of adjunctive therapy and found no change in psychomotor and memory tests. Drowsiness was more often found in higher dosing (2,400 mg). Mortimore et al.[65] did not find a difference between continued polytherapy and an add-on with GBP in measures of quality of life.

Zonisamide

The anticonvulsant properties of zonisamide (ZNS) were discovered through extensive testing of a variety of sulfonamide compounds. Like TPM, it has multiple mechanisms of action: Blocking voltage-gated sodium channels, reducing sustained repetitive firing, blocking T-type calcium channels, and inhibiting ligand binding to the $GABA_A$ receptor. Like TPM, ZNS is a carbonic anhydrase–inhibiting drug. Although there is longer experience with ZNS in Japan (where it was developed), it recently was introduced in the United States and Europe for partial-onset seizures in refractory epilepsy.

Clinical anecdotal information and a pilot study by Ojemann et al.[67] show a cognitive side effect profile very similar to TPM, but no controlled studies are available. Also, no information is available about ongoing studies.

Rufinamide

Rufinamide (RUF 331; 1-(2,6-difluoro-phenyl)methyl-1H-1,2,3-triazole-4-carboxamide) is a structurally novel compound that limits the frequency of sodium-dependent neuronal action potentials. One study is available to assess the cognitive effects.[7] The study used a multicenter, multinational double-blind, randomized, placebo-controlled parallel study design with four different doses of rufinamide (based on prior studies): 200 mg/day, 400 mg/day, 800 mg/day, and 1,600 mg/day as add-on to the existing medication. Cognitive assessments were performed at baseline (before the start with RUF treatment) and at end-point (after 3 months of treatment). The most important finding is that for none of the cognitive tests, a statistically significant worsening occurs for any of the doses of rufinamide when the period after 12 weeks of treatment was compared with the baseline before introducing rufinamide. Also, none of the comparisons between dose and placebo showed a statistically significant difference.

SUMMARY AND CONCLUSIONS

A general conclusion that may be derived from meta-analyses[87] is that polypharmacy shows a relatively severe impact on cognitive function when compared with monotherapy, irrespective of the type of AEDs included. Two drugs that individually have mild cognitive effects may induce serious cognitive impairment when used together, possibly because of potentiation of tolerability problems.[85]

Possibly the most remarkable finding is that, although the severity of cognitive side effects is generally considered to be mild to moderate for most AEDs,[87] all commonly used AEDs have some impact on cognitive function. Such mild impact may be amplified in specific conditions and may become substantial in some patients when crucial functions are involved, such as learning in children[14] or driving capacities in adults (often requiring millisecond precision), or when functions are impaired that are already vulnerable, such as memory function in the elderly.[85] Moreover, the cognitive side effects represent the long-term outcome of AED therapy; therefore, the effects may increase with prolonged therapy, which contributes to the impact on daily life functioning in refractory epilepsies.[16]

Definite evidence for drug-induced cognitive impairment has been established for phenobarbitone (memory impairment), phenytoin (mental slowing), and topiramate (mental slowing and dysphasia). Treatment with these drugs should consider these side effects and patients should be monitored on a regular basis. Mild effects (mostly psychomotor slowing) were found for carbamazepine, oxcarbazepine, valproate, and lamotrigine (with mild cognitive-activating effects). The effects for ethosuximide, tiagabine, gabapentin, levetiracetam, and zonisamide are inconclusive. It is clear, however, from the available evidence that there still exists a need to conduct studies that compare the relative effects of the neuropsychological consequences of AED treatment using standardized protocols. Further, the lack of well-designed studies of the neuropsychological effects of AED treatment means that we must remain cautious about our level of understanding about the impact of the newer drugs.

References

1. Aarts JH, Binnie CD, Smit AM, et al. Selective cognitive impairment during focal and generalized epileptiform EEG activity. *Brain.* 1984;107:293–308.
2. Äikiä M, Kälviäinen R, Sivenius J, et al. Cognitive effects of oxcarbazepine and phenytoin monotherapy in newly diagnosed epilepsy: one year follow-up. *Epilepsy Res.* 1992;11:199–203.
3. Aldenkamp AP. Antiepileptic drug treatment and epileptic seizures–effects on cognitive function. In: Trimble M, Schmitz B, eds. *The Neuropsychiatry of Epilepsy.* New York: Cambridge University Press; 2002:256–267.
4. Aldenkamp AP. Cognitive and behavioural assessment in clinical trials: when should they be done? *Epilepsy Res.* 2001;45:155–159.
5. Aldenkamp AP. Cognitive effects of topiramate, gabapentin and lamotrigine in healthy young adults. *Neurology.* 2000;54:270–272.
6. Aldenkamp AP, Alpherts WCJ, Blennow G, et al. Withdrawal of antiepileptic medication—effects on cognitive function in children: the Multicentre Holmfrid Study. *Neurology.* 1993;43:41–50.
7. Aldenkamp AP, Alpherts WCJ. The effect of the new antiepileptic drug rufinamide on cognitive functions. *Epilepsia.* 2006; 7(7):1153–1159.
8. Aldenkamp AP, Arends J, Bootsma HP, et al. Randomized, double-blind parallel-group study comparing cognitive effects of a low-dose lamotrigine with valproate and placebo in healthy volunteers. *Epilepsia.* 2002;43: 19–26.
9. Aldenkamp AP, Arends J, Overweg-Plandsoen TC, et al. Acute cognitive effects of nonconvulsive difficult-to-detect epileptic seizures and epileptiform electroencephalographic discharges. *J Child Neurol.* 2001;16: 119–123.
10. Aldenkamp AP, Baker G, Mulder OG, et al. A multicentre randomized clinical study to evaluate the effect on cognitive function of topiramate compared with valproate as add-on therapy to carbamazepine in patients with partial-onset seizures. *Epilepsia.* 2000;41:1167–1178.
11. Aldenkamp AP, Baker G. A systematic review of the effects of lamotrigine on cognitive function and quality of life. *Epilepsy Behav.* 2001;2:85–91.
12. Aldenkamp AP, De Krom M, Reijs R. Newer antiepileptic drugs and cognitive issues. *Epilepsia.* 2003;44(Suppl 4):21–29.
13. Aldenkamp AP, Dodson WE, eds. Epilepsy and education; cognitive factors in learning behavior. *Epilepsia.* 1990;31(suppl 4):S9–S20.
14. Aldenkamp AP, Dreifuss FE, Renier WO, et al. *Epilepsy in Children and Adolescents.* Boca Raton, FL: CRC Press; 1995.
15. Aldenkamp AP, Mulder OG, Overweg J. Cognitive effects of lamotrigine as first line add-on in patients with localized related (partial) epilepsy. *J Epilepsy.* 1997;10:117–121.
16. American Academy of Pediatrics. Behavioral and cognitive effects of anticonvulsant therapy. Committee on Drugs. *Pediatrics.* 1985;76:644–647.
17. Banks GK, Beran RG. Neuropsychological assessment in lamotrigine treated epileptic patients. *Clin Exp Neurol.* 1991;28:230–237.
18. Binnie CD, van Emde BW, Kasteleijn-Nolste-Trenite DG, et al. Acute effects of lamotrigine (BW430C) in persons with epilepsy. *Epilepsia.* 1986;27:248–254.
19. Bootsma HP, Coolen F, Aldenkamp AP, et al. Topiramate in clinical practice: long-term experience in patients with refractory epilepsy referred to a tertiary epilepsy center. *Epilepsy Behav.* 2004;5(3):380–387.
20. Burton LA, Harden C. Effect of topiramate on attention. *Epilepsy Res.* 1997;27:29–32.
21. Calandre EP, Dominguez-Granados R, Gomez-Rubio M, et al. Cognitive effects of long-term treatment with phenobarbital and valproic acid in school children. *Acta Neur Scand.* 1990;81:504–506.
22. Chadwick DW, Marson T, Kadir Z. Clinical administration of new antiepileptic drugs: an overview of safety and efficacy. *Epilepsia.* 1996; 37(Suppl 6):S17–22.
23. Cohen AF, Ashby L, Crowley D, et al. Lamotrigine (BW430C), a potential anticonvulsant. Effects on the central nervous system in comparison with phenytoin and diazepam. *Br J Clin Pharmacol.* 1985;20:619–629.
24. Craig I, Tallis R. Impact of valproate and phenytoin on cognitive function in elderly patients: results of a single-blind randomized comparative study. *Epilepsia.* 1994;35:381–390.
25. Curran HV, Java R. Memory and psychomotor effects of oxcarbazepine in healthy human volunteers. *Eur J Clin Pharmacol.* 1993;44:529–533.
26. Dodrill CB, Arnett JL, Sommerville KW, et al. Cognitive and quality of life effects of differing dosages of tiagabine in epilepsy. *Neurology.* 1997;48:1025–1031.
27. Dodrill CB, Troupin AS. Psychotropic effects of carbamazepine in epilepsy: a double-blind comparison with phenytoin. *Neurology.* 1977;27:1023–1028.
28. Dodson WE, Pellock JM. *Pediatric Epilepsy: Diagnosis and Treatment.* New York: Demos Publications; 1993.
29. Dodson WE, Trimble MR. *Epilepsy and Quality of Life.* New York: Raven Press; 1994.

29a. Donati F, Gobbi G, Campistol J, et al. Aldenkamp AP. Effects of oxcarbazepine on cognitive function in children and adolescents with partial seizures. *Neurology.* 2006; 67(4)679–682.

30. Earl N, McKee JR, Sunder TR, et al. Lamotrigine adjunctive therapy in patients with refractory epilepsy and mental retardation [abstract]. *Epilepsia.* 2000;41(Suppl 1):72(abst).
31. Ettinger AB, Weisbrot DM, Saracco J, et al. Positive and negative psychotropic effects of lamotrigine in patients with epilepsy and mental retardation. *Epilepsia.* 1998;39:874–877.
32. Faught E, Wilder BJ, Ramsay RE, et al. Topiramate placebo-controlled dose-ranging trial in refractory partial epilepsy using 200-, 400-, and 600-mg daily dosages. *Neurology.* 1996;46:1684–1690.
33. Forsythe I, Butler R, Berg I, et al. Cognitive impairment in new cases of epilepsy randomly assigned to carbamazepine, phenytoin and sodium valproate. *Dev Med Child Neurol.* 1991;33:524–534.
34. Fritz N, Glogau S, Hoffmann J, et al. Efficacy and cognitive side effects of tiagabine and topiramate in patients with epilepsy. *Epilepsy Behav.* 2005;6(3):373–381.
35. Gallassi R, Morreale A, Di Sarro R, et al. Cognitive effects of antiepileptic drug discontinuation. *Epilepsia.* 1992;33(Suppl 6):S41–44.
36. Gillham R, Kane K, Bryant-Comstock L, et al. A double-blind comparison of lamotrigine and carbamazepine in newly diagnosed epilepsy with health-related quality of life as an outcome measure. *Seizure.* 2000;9:375–379.
37. Hamilton MJ, Cohen AF, Yuen AW, et al. Carbamazepine and lamotrigine in healthy volunteers: relevance to early tolerance and clinical trial dosage. *Epilepsia.* 1993;34:166–173.
38. Ideström CM, Schalling D, Carlquist U, et al. Acute effects of diphenylhydantoin in relation to plasma levels. Behavioral and psychological studies. *Psychol Med.* 1972;2:111–120.
39. Jette NJ, Marson AG, Hutton JL. Topiramate add-on for drug-resistant partial epilepsy. *Cochrane Database Syst Rev.* 2002;(3):CD001417.
40. Kälviäinen R, Äikiä M, Mervaala E, et al. Long-term cognitive and EEG effects of tiagabine in drug-resistant partial epilepsy. *Epilepsy Res.* 1996;25:291–297.
41. Kellet MW, Smith DF, Stockton PA, et al. Topiramate in clinical practice: first year's postlicensing experience in a specialist epilepsy clinic. *J Neurol Neurosurg Psychiatry.* 1999;66:759–763.
42. Ketter TA, Post RM, Theodore WH. Positive and negative psychiatric effects of antiepileptic drugs in patients with seizure disorders. *Neurology.* 1999;53(5 Suppl 2):53–67.
43. Kockelmann E, Elger CE, Hemstaedter C. Cognitive profile of topiramate as compared with lamotrigine in epilepsy patients on antiepileptic drug polytherapy: relationships to blood serum levels and comedication. *Epilepsy Behav.* 2004;5:716–721.
44. Laaksonen R, Kaimola K, Grahn-Teräväinen E, et al. A controlled clinical trial of the effects of carbamazepine and oxcarbazepine on memory and attention [abstract]. 16th International Epilepsy Congress, Hamburg, 1985(abst.)
45. Leach JP, Girvan J, Paul A, et al. Gabapentin and cognition: a double blind, dose ranging, placebo controlled study in refractory epilepsy. *J Neurol Neurosurg Psychiatry.* 1997;62:372–376.

46. Leach MJ, Lees G, Riddall DR. Lamotrigine: mechanisms of action. In: Levy RH, Mattson RH, Meldrum BS, eds. *Antiepileptic Drugs*. 4th ed. New York: Raven Press; 1995:861–869.
47. Lhatoo SD, Wong ICK, Sander JW. Prognostic factors affecting long-term retention of topiramate in patients with chronic epilepsy. *Epilepsia*. 2000;41:338–341.
48. Macdonald RL, Kelly, KM. Antiepileptic drug mechanisms of action. *Epilepsia*. 1995;36(S2):2–12.
49. MacLeod CM, Dekaban AS, Hunt E. Memory impairment in epileptic patients: selective effects of phenobarbital concentration. *Science*. 1978;202:1102–1104.
50. Marciani MG, Spanedda F, Bassetti MA, et al. Effect of lamotrigine on EEG paroxysmal abnormalities and background activity: a computerized analysis. *Br J Clin Pharmacol*. 1996;42:621–627.
51. Marciani MG, Stanzione P, Mattia D, et al. Lamotrigine add-on therapy in focal epilepsy: electroencephalographic and neuropsychological evaluation. *Clin Neuropharmacol*. 1998;21:41–47.
52. Marson AG, Hutton JL, Leach JP, et al. Levetiracetam, oxcarbazepine, remacemide, and zonisamide, for drug resistant localization-related epilepsy: a systematic review. *Epilepsy Res*. 2001;46:259–270.
53. Marson AG, Kadir ZA, Hutton JL, et al. Gabapentin for drug-resistant partial epilepsy. *Cochrane Database Syst Rev*. 2000;(2):CD001415.
54. Marson AG, Kadir ZA, Hutton JL, et al. The new antiepileptic drugs: a systematic review of their efficacy and tolerability. *Epilepsia*. 1997;38:859–880.
55. Martin R, Kuzniecky R, Ho S, et al. Cognitive effects of topiramate, gabapentin, and lamotrigine in healthy young adults. *Neurology*. 1999;52: 321–327.
56. McKee PJ, Blacklaw J, Forrest G, et al. A double-blind, placebo-controlled interaction study between oxcarbazepine and carbamazepine, sodium valproate and phenytoin in epileptic patients. *Br J Clin Pharmacol*. 1994;37:27–32.
57. Meador KJ. Assessing cognitive effects of a new AED without the bias of practice effects [abstract]. *Epilepsia*. 1997;38(Suppl 3):60(abst).
58. Meador KJ, Loring DW, Abney OL, et al. Effects of carbamazepine and phenytoin on EEG and memory in healthy adults. *Epilepsia*. 1993;34(1):153–157.
59. Meador KJ, Loring DW, Allen ME, et al. Comparative cognitive effects of carbamazepine and phenytoin in healthy adults. *Neurology*. 1991;41:1537–1540.
60. Meador KJ, Loring DW, Huh K, et al. Comparative cognitive effects of anticonvulsants. *Neurology*. 1990;40:391–394.
61. Meador KJ, Loring DW, Moore EE, et al. Comparative cognitive effects of Phenobarbital, phenytoin, and valproate in healthy adults. *Neurology*. 1995;45(8):1494–1499.
62. Meador KJ, Loring DW, Ray PG, et al. Differential cognitive effects of carbamazepine and gabapentin. *Epilepsia*. 1999;40:1279–1285.
63. Meador KJ, Loring DW, Ray PG, et al. Differential effects of carbamazepine and lamotrigine [abstract]. *Neurology*. 2000;54(Suppl 3):A84(abst).
64. Mervaala E, Koivista K, Hanninen T, et al. Electrophysiological and neuropsychological profiles of lamotrigine in young and age-associated memory impairment (AAMI) subjects [abstract]. *Neurology*. 1995;45(Suppl 4):A259(abst).
65. Mortimore C, Trimble M, Emmers E. Effects of gabapentin on cognition and quality of life in patients with epilepsy. *Seizure*. 1998;7:359–366.
66. Neyens LGJ, Alpherts WCJ, Aldenkamp AP. Cognitive effects of a new pyrrolidine derivative (levetiracetam) in patients with epilepsy. *Prog Neuropsychopharmacol Biol Psychiatry*. 1995;19:411–419.
67. Ojemann, LM, Ojemann GA, Dodrill CB, et al. Language disturbances as side effects of topiramate and zonisamide therapy. *Epilepsy Behav*. 2001;2:579–584.
68. Parnas J, Flachs H, Gram L. Psychotropic effect of antiepileptic drugs. *Acta Neurol Scand*. 1979;60:329–343.
69. Parnas J, Gram L, Flachs H. Psychopharmacological aspects of antiepileptic treatment. *Prog Neurobiol*. 1980;15:119–138.
70. Petroff OAC, Rothman DL, Behar KL, et al. The effect of gabapentin on brain gamma-aminobutyric acid in patients with epilepsy. *Ann Neurol*. 1996;39:95–99.
71. Prevey ML, Delaney RC, Cramer JA, et al. Effect of valproate on cognitive function. Comparison with carbamazepine. The Department of Veterans Affairs Epilepsy Cooperative Study 264 Group. *Arch Neurol.*, 1996;53(10):1008–1016.
72. Privitera M, Fincham R, Penry J, et al. Topiramate placebo-controlled dose-ranging trial in refractory partial epilepsy using 600-, 800-, and 1000-mg daily dosages. Topiramate YE Study Group. *Neurology*. 1996;46:1678–1683.
73. Sabers A, Moller A, Dam M, et al. Cognitive function and anticonvulsant therapy: effect of monotherapy in epilepsy. *Acta Neurol Scand*. 1995;92:19–27.
74. Salinsky MC, Spencer D, Oken BS, et al. Effects of oxcarbazeoine and phenytoin on the EEG and cognition in healthy volunteers. *Epilepsy Behav*. 2004;5:894–902.
75. Schwartz JR, Grigat G. Phenytoin and carbamazepine: potential- and frequency-dependent black of NA currents in mammalian myelinated nerve fibers. *Epilepsia*. 1989;30:286–294.
76. Smith D, Baker G, Davies G, et al. Outcomes of add-on treatment with lamotrigine in partial epilepsy. *Epilepsia*. 1993;34:312–322.
77. Smith WL, Lowrey JB. Effects of diphenylhydantoin on mental abilities in the elderly. *J Am Geriatr Soc*. 1975;23:207–211.
78. Stefan H, Krämer G, Mamoli B, eds. *Challenge Epilepsy–New Antiepileptic Drugs*. Berlin: Blackwell Science; 1998.
79. Sveinbjornsdottir S, Sander JW, Patsalos PN, et al. Neuropsychological effects of tiagabine, a potential new antiepileptic drug. *Seizure*. 1994;3: 29–35.
80. Tatum WO, French JA, Faught E, et al. Postmarketing experience with topiramate and cognition. *Epilepsia*. 2001;42:1134–1140.
81. Thompson PJ, Baxendale SA, Duncan JS, et al. Effects of topiramate on cognitive function. *J Neurol Neurosurg Psychiatry*. 2000;69:636–641.
82. Thompson PJ, Huppert F, Trimble MR. Anticonvulsant drugs, cognitive function and memory. *Acta Neurol Scand*. 1980;S80:75–80.
83. Thompson PJ, Huppert FA, Trimble MR. Phenytoin and cognitive functions: effects on normal volunteers and implications for epilepsy. *Br J Clin Psychol*. 1981;20:155–162.
84. Thompson PJ, Trimble MR. Sodium valproate en cognitive functioning in normal volunteers. *Br J Clin Pharmacol*. 1981;12:819–824.
85. Trimble MR. Anticonvulsant drugs and cognitive function: a review of the literature. *Epilepsia*. 1987;28(Suppl 3):37–45.
86. Twyman RE, Rogers CJ, Macdonald RL. Differential regulation of gamma-aminobutyric acid receptor channels by diazepam and phenobarbital. *Ann Neurol*. 1989;25:213–220.
87. Vermeulen J, Aldenkamp AP. Cognitive side-effects of chronic antiepileptic drug treatment: a review of 25 years of research. *Epilepsy Res*. 1995;22: 65–95.
88. Vining EP, Mellitis ED, Dorsen MM, et al. Psychologic and behavioral effects of antiepileptic drugs in children: a double-blind comparison between phenobarbital and valproic acid. *Pediatrics*. 1987;80(2):165–174.
89. White HS. Clinical significance of animal seizure models and mechanism of action studies of potential antiepileptic drugs. *Epilepsia*. 1997;38(Suppl 1):S9–S17.
90. Wong IC. New antiepileptic drugs. Study suggests that under a quarter of patients will still be taking the new drugs after six years. *BMJ*. 1997;314:603–604.

CHAPTER 202 ■ LEARNING DISORDERS

MICHAEL P. KERR AND MARY LOU SMITH

INTRODUCTION

The potential impact of epilepsy and its treatment on learning provides a considerable challenge for clinicians, patients, and families alike. In addition, the picture is often complicated by the association between the presence of epilepsy and apparently already coexistent disorders of learning and development. This poses important heuristic questions into the relative impact of epilepsy on the development of learning disorders.

It is beyond the scope of this chapter to address in detail this crucial question in the field of epileptology. For further reading please refer to the chapters on neonatal syndromes and syndromes of childhood and adolescence. This chapter will have as its focus the nature, impact, and management of epilepsy in those with an apparently coexistent intellectual disability (mental retardation). Such an approach helps the clarity of the chapter, yet it is important to reflect on how the populations of people who have intellectual disability are placed within the scope of learning disorders associated with epilepsy. This will be covered initially within our discussion on classification and terminology and later in the chapter within the section on the impact of epilepsy on people with an intellectual disability.

Key themes discussed in the chapter will include the association between certain syndromes of intellectual disability and seizure types, the impact of epilepsy, approaches to management, the association between epilepsy and behavioral disorders, and the multidisciplinary approach to care.

CLASSIFICATION AND TERMINOLOGY OF INTELLECTUAL DISABILITY

Considerable variation occurs in the terminology of intellectual disability. While *intellectual disability* is currently the internationally accepted term, *mental retardation* is favored in the United States and much of Europe, *learning disability* in the United Kingdom, *mental handicap* in much of the world during the 1990s, and *intellectual handicap* in Australia and New Zealand.

Definition of Disability

The American Association for Mental Retardation defines mental retardation as follows:

> "Mental retardation is a disability characterized by significant limitations both in intellectual functioning and in adaptive behavior as expressed in conceptual, social and practical adaptive skills.... The disability originates before the age of 18."

It adds five assumptions, which are essential to the application of the definition:

1. Limitations in present functioning must be considered within the context of community environments typical of the individual's age, peers, and culture.
2. Valid assessment considers cultural and linguistic diversity as well as differences in communication, sensory, motor, and behavioral factors.
3. Within an individual, limitations often coexist with strengths.
4. An important purpose of describing limitations is to develop a profile of needed supports.
5. With appropriate personalized supports over a sustained period, the life functioning of the person with mental retardation generally will improve.

From a clinical viewpoint, particularly in administrative terms, mental retardation is defined using the International Classification of Diseases rubric, currently in its 10th version. All codes for mental retardation are prefixed with F7. Assessment should include clinical findings, adaptive behavior, and the use of psychometric tests.

The range of disability is defined in Table 1.

THE NATURE AND IMPACT OF EPILEPSY IN PEOPLE WITH INTELLECTUAL DISABILITY

Epidemiology

Epidemiologic data for this population are particularly influenced by methodologic and sampling issues, raising concerns regarding the interpretation of results that vary significantly depending on the study's design.[41,91] These concerns focus on the usually selective nature of the population samples and difficulties in allowing for comparative levels of intellectual disability. The prevalence of epilepsy is significantly greater in people with intellectual disability than in the general population,[62] with estimates in intellectual disability populations ranging from 18% to over 60%.

The major influences on prevalence estimates are (a) age; (b) residence, institution, or community; and (c) the severity of disability.[18,57,84]

Cohort effects, due to year of birth, are important in defining prevalence in both intellectual disability[37] and epilepsy.[16]

A comparison between community and institutionally based surveys[67,108] show as much as a 10% discrepancy in the prevalence found. Table 2 describes a range of epidemiologic surveys of the prevalence of epilepsy in people with intellectual disability.

TABLE 1

CLASSIFICATION OF INTELLECTUAL DISABILITY (ICD-10)

Code	Definition	Attributes
F70	Mild mental retardation	1) Ability to use speech 2) Full independence in self-care 3) IQ range between 50 and 69
F71	Moderate mental retardation	1) Slow in comprehension 2) Immobility or restricted mobility 3) Retarded motor skills 4) IQ range between 35 and 49
F72	Severe mental retardation	1) Marked impairment of motor skills 2) Clinically significant damage to CNS 3) IQ range between 20 and 34
F73	Profound mental retardation	1) Severely limited understanding 2) Immobility or restricted mobility 3) Incontinence 4) Requiring constant supervision 5) IQ <20 6) Usually organic etiology

CNS, central nervous system; ICD, International Classification of Diseases.

The increasing prevalence of epilepsy with increasing severity of intellectual disability is well recognized in both children[1] and adults.[4]

Definition of seizure type in populations of people with intellectual disability has proven difficult.[24,57] An example of this is seen in a community study of children with intellectual disability.[90] In this survey, there was evidence of a lack of investigation in the population, with only 10% having had electrophysiologic tests. Despite this, they showed an increase in generalized tonic–clonic and myoclonic seizures and a decrease in partial seizures with increasing handicap. The authors concluded that this increase in generalized seizure disorder was an artifact of the lack of investigation, though other explanations such as genetic causes may be valid.

A Japanese study focusing on people with severe intellectual disability[4] identified cerebral palsy as the most common etiology (42.3%); multiple seizure types were common (almost half had two or more seizures) and paroxysms were found on the electroencephalogram (EEG) in 90.6% of cases and abnormal computed tomography (CT) scan in 82.7% of cases. In a Finnish study in children,[1] prenatal causation was most frequent (47%), and seizures were most frequently partial (72%). As we shall see later, it is unrealistic when considering seizure type to take the intellectual disability population as a whole; individual etiologic characteristics are crucial in syndromal and seizure classification.

TABLE 2

EPIDEMIOLOGIC SURVEYS OF THE PREVALENCE OF EPILEPSY IN PEOPLE WITH INTELLECTUAL DISABILITY (ID)

Sample	Prevalence
Children under age 14 Community SMR[19]	20%
Children up to 22 yr Community[85] Institution[67]	Mild ID 24% Severe ID 44% All 32%
Children 6–13 yr Community[97]	Mild ID 14% Severe ID 24%
Adults, community based[108]	All ID 22.1%
Community identified pediatric sample[1]	All ID: 19% by age 10 years and 21% by age 22 years Severe ID: Fivefold risk as compared with mild ID
All ages, record-linked health data[71]	All ID 18.3%
Primary care health facilities[68]	Down syndrome 13.6% Cerebral palsy 40%

ETIOLOGIC ISSUES

Intellectual disability is caused by a range of pathologic processes, as, of course, is epilepsy. In particular, genetic advances into the individual causes of intellectual disability and of the epilepsies have expanded.[5,21]

It is beyond the scope of this chapter to highlight all the etiologic processes involved in the development of an intellectual disability. Two issues are, however, of particular relevance to this population: (a) are specific etiologies associated with recognizable epilepsy patterns? and (b) what impact do seizures have on development and learning?

Etiology Associated Patterns of Epilepsy

A further approach to investigating the etiology of epilepsy in people with intellectual disability has been to define the nature of the epilepsy in individual disability syndromes. This approach will hopefully lead to the matching of known genetic abnormalities with the individual's epilepsy and thus direct treatment options.

This section includes a brief overview of a select group of syndromes that have intellectual disability as a key feature, and that may also have epilepsy as a concomitant disorder. This section is not intended to provide a detailed analysis of the causes of the syndromes, or the etiology, features, or treatment of the associated epilepsies; these issues are reviewed in depth elsewhere in this textbook. This co-occurrence of epilepsy with these syndromes is important to recognize at a clinical level because the seizures add an additional burden to both the individual with the syndrome and to the caregivers.

Down Syndrome

Down syndrome (DS), or trisomy 21, is the most common genetic cause of intellectual disability.[93] In addition to intellectual disability, of which there is a range in severity, DS is characterized by growth retardation, hypotonia, a number of facial dysmorphologies, hypogonadism, an increased risk of cardiac disease and leukemia, and Alzheimer disease in those over the age of 35 years. A bimodal distribution in age of seizure onset has been described, with peaks in childhood and middle age.[82,98,105] The incidence of epilepsy increases with age, and the increase later in life is thought to be related to the onset and progression of Alzheimer disease.[54,63,105] A variety of seizure types have been reported, including infantile spasms, generalized tonic–clonic seizures, Lennox-Gastaut syndrome, and psychomotor seizures.[44,81,98]

Angelman Syndrome

Angelman syndrome (AS) is a genetic disorder that is estimated to account for up to 6% of all children presenting with severe intellectual disability and epilepsy.[42] Clinical findings present in all patients include developmental delay, which becomes apparent by 6 to 12 months of age; severely impaired expressive language; ataxic ("puppetlike") gait; tremulousness of limbs; and a typical behavioral profile, including a happy demeanor, hypermotor behavior, and low attention span. Although development may appear almost normal or only slightly delayed during the first 6 months of life, all patients eventually develop severe intellectual disability. The typical lack of speech may not be due to the intellectual disability alone; oral motor dyspraxia and deficits in social interaction and attention also contribute to the lack of expressive language.[80] Sleep problems may affect a significant portion of individuals with AS and are persistent; parents report adverse effects of their child's sleep problems on their own well-being.[26,92]

Seizures, abnormal electroencephalography, microcephaly, and scoliosis are observed in >80% of patients, with onset of epilepsy typically occurring in infancy or early childhood.[30,34] A variety of seizure types are seen, including febrile, atypical absence, generalized tonic-clonic, myoclonic, and clonic unilateral seizures.[39,43,106] There are contradictory data on whether the severity of the developmental disturbance in AS is related to the severity of epilepsy,[58,77] and whether there is an improvement in epilepsy with age.[59,92,110]

Fragile X Syndrome

Fragile X syndrome (FXS) is the most common known cause of autism or "autisticlike" behaviors, and the incidence of cognitive impairment is quite high. The clinical phenotype in the male typically also includes tall stature, large testes, relative macrocephaly, characteristic facial features, and delays in speech and language development.[23,100,109] Up to 80% of males with FXS are described as cognitively delayed. In the older studies of males with FXS, almost all were described as having moderate or severe mental retardation. However, many of these studies were based upon institutionalized males, and with better ascertainment studies, it has become clear that 10% to 15% of boys with FXS have a less severe degree of developmental delay, with IQs in the borderline or mild intellectual disability range. A high number of boys with fragile X (80% to 90%) are described as distractible and impulsive, with symptoms of attention deficit hyperactivity disorder, and anxiety is a common personality feature.[38]

Girls with FXS tend to be less severely affected in terms of intellectual disability. Approximately 30% of girls with the full mutation have IQ scores above 85, with the other 70% mostly in the borderline or mild mental intellectual disability range.[23] However, those girls with normal intelligence are at higher risk for specific learning disabilities. The behavioral features in girls include shyness and poor eye contact.[100]

Seizures occur in approximately 15% to 20% of children with FXS.[6,53] Seizure types include absence, partial motor, generalized, and partial complex seizures; benign rolandic epilepsy is found frequently.[6,73,74] Epilepsy in individuals with FXS generally follows a benign course, and in a relatively high number, seizures remit before the age of 20.[86]

Rett Syndrome

In Rett syndrome (RS), there typically is normal development until 6 to 18 months (although as long as 30 months), after which development slows, or even deteriorates. The physical characteristics of RS include scoliosis, gait dyspraxia, and repetitive movements of the hands, often involving hand wringing. Individuals may have autonomic dysfunction, difficulty chewing, and teeth grinding, and eventually show growth failure and deceleration of head growth.[40,45] There is a high prevalence of behavioral and emotional disorders in RS, with anxiety, flat mood, self-injurious behavior, and autism seen frequently.[45,88] Frequently, there is a regression in cognition, behavior, and social and motor skills throughout the lifetime of patients with RS. The degree of developmental delay is usually within the severely to profoundly intellectually disabled range, although there is a spectrum of severity ranging from severe neurologic compromise to only minor neurologic symptoms.[51] There is a preserved speech variant, which shows the same course and stereotypic hand movements, but patients typically recover some hand use and speech; epilepsy is rare in this group.[22]

Epilepsy is common, occurring in between 80% and 95% of cases.[45,96] The severity of epilepsy may decrease with increasing age.[96] A variety of seizure types are found in RS, including generalized tonic–clonic, absence, myoclonic jerk, atonic, and tonic seizures. The incidence of true clinical seizures may be overestimated because the autonomic dysfunction may be incorrectly identified as absence or complex partial seizures.

The Impact of Epilepsy on Development and Learning

It is generally accepted that the causal process of epilepsy follows a path from brain damage through to the development of epilepsy.[57] Cognitive decline, as seen in a few patients with epilepsy, is usually associated with repeated head injury or through anoxic episodes in periods of status epilepticus. Other deterioration may be linked to seizures impacting information processing.[8]

However, increasing knowledge on conditions such as infantile encephalopathy (infantile spasms, myoclonic epilepsy) and the treatments for these devastating conditions seem to imply that epileptic phenomena can be associated with the development of intellectual disability.[27] A recent survey in Atlanta on the epidemiology and outcome of infantile spasms suggests that, at age 10 years, 83% will have intellectual disability.[103] The same survey suggested that 12% of 10-year-old children with profound intellectual disability had a history of infantile spasms.

Impact of Epilepsy

People with an intellectual disability are equally susceptible to the negative impacts of epilepsy on physical and psychological health, cognition, life expectancy, and social factors[10,32] as the general population. This impact should be seen as additional to their other impairments, if present. This is particularly important as underestimating the impact of epilepsy may lead to incomplete attempts at treatment.

Physical Health

The known impact of epilepsy on physical health as seen by an overrepresentation of hospitalization[20] and a range of antiepileptic drug (AED)-related morbidity holds true for people with an intellectual disability. An increase in admissions to accident and emergency rooms and to the hospital in general is seen.[71]

Psychological Health

Studies have found rates of behavior disturbance and psychiatric disorder to be significantly higher in people with epilepsy[24,50,64] and in people with intellectual disability.[11,28,64,66] Furthermore, a study in children[12] was able to identify decreasing IQ as a predictor of increasing mental health problems.

Considering the very strong evidence for an increased prevalence of emotional disturbance in individuals with epilepsy who do not have intellectual disability as compared with nonepilepsy controls,[50,64] it has proved much harder to find a similar link within populations who have epilepsy and intellectual disability. That is, it has been difficult to tease out any additional impact from epilepsy with the already high morbidity present in these populations.

Epidemiologic evidence does not support such a population link in adults or children. Deb and Hunter[25] showed an underlying prevalence of behavior disorder of 52.5% and that in the epilepsy population of 58%. An Australian study[61] showed in an epidemiologic-defined population of children with intellectual disability no difference in "caseness" of behavior and emotional disturbance between those with and without epilepsy. Other work has shown that aggression and self-injury were associated with frequent seizures and polytherapy. This approach is almost certainly missing the potential for epilepsy to impact on individuals' patterns of behavior. In particular, it may be that the particularly high frequency of mental illness, depression, and anxiety seen in general epilepsy populations may be underrecognized in people with an intellectual disability.

A study of a large epilepsy service database of people with intellectual disability[33] explored potential predictors of psychopathology within an epilepsy and intellectual disability group. They concluded that there was a relatively weak input from seizure factors such as frequency on psychopathology and that behavior disorders were more related to general disability factors than to seizure related factors.

The Family

Many factors associated with the burden of caring for someone with intellectual disability have been identified.[34,48] The most robustly replicated factor was behavior disorder. Caregiver burden is an important issue as the well-being of caregivers affects the prognosis of people in their care.[14]

The coexistence of epilepsy also seems to be a factor associated with caregiver burden.[32] Unfortunately, however, we know little about the precise impact of epilepsy on families of individuals who also have intellectual disability. A study of people with epilepsy without intellectual disability[102] found that levels of stress and dissatisfaction with their social situation were high, particularly in primary caregivers (mothers, in most instances). Respite periods away from home were few and the perceived level of support was low. Poor emotional adjustment was associated with severity of tonic and atonic attacks and periods of status epilepticus, and low levels of support were associated with depression.

MORTALITY

Patients with epilepsy are known to have increased risk of mortality over the population in general.[17,47] A recent Dutch cohort study demonstrated that patients with epilepsy have an increased risk ratio of 3.2 for all causes of mortality, and this rose to over 7 in those aged under 20.[89]

This is broadly similar to a Danish study, which demonstrated a standardized mortality ratio (SMR) of 3.6 for all deaths.[76] This excess risk is partly explained by underlying causes of epilepsy such as cerebrovascular disease, injuries, and poisoning. This probably explains the relatively higher SMRs in the year immediately after diagnosis of epilepsy.[17]

Patients with intellectual disability are also known to have a lower life expectancy than the general population[36] and an estimated SMR of 1.6.[35] Not surprisingly, the probability of survival decreases as the severity of intellectual disability increases.[49] This excess is increased for those patients with coexisting epilepsy[35,36] whose SMR may be as high as 5. It is possible that some of this increased mortality may be explained by an increase in sudden unexplained epilepsy death (SUDEP). An institutional review in North America revealed an increase in unexpected death of 1.3 deaths per 1,000 in the nonepilepsy group compared with 3.6 per 1,000 in those with epilepsy.[69] The impact of epilepsy on mortality in people with an intellectual disability appears to hold across all degrees of intellectual impairment.[79]

MANAGEMENT

Epilepsy management requires special skills and competencies for the epileptologist. These include (a) special communication skills specific to this population, (b) analysis of safety and communication of therapeutic interventions, and (c) knowledge of the care environment to work with multidisciplinary teams.

Communication Skills: Management by Proxy

Witness report from a caregiver or family member is common; a report from the individual is less so in people with intellectual disability. Thus, the history and management will commonly progress through, or at least be influenced by, another "management by proxy." The degree of this will increase as the individual's communicative skills decrease.

Notwithstanding the need to manage third-party clinical consultations, a central aim should be to empower the individual to communicate his or her needs. Components of successful communication methods are highlighted below:

1. Nonverbal: Gaze, appropriate touch, use of gesture
2. Vocal: Appropriate tone, intelligibility
3. Verbal: Greeting, using individual's name, balance of communication with caregiver
4. Response: Recognizing the individual's responses and following leads, respecting information from the caregiver
5. Empathy: Showing appropriate respect and empathy

Specific Issues in Differential Diagnosis: Seizures or Behavior Disturbance?

In the majority of cases seizure disorder presents itself as paroxysmal episodes of abnormal behavior. In many cases, for example, a generalized tonic-clonic convulsion, the nature of these behaviors is well defined and cannot be confused with many other conditions. Other seizure disorders, however, are less well defined or are dependent on the verbal description of the individual and witnesses for a diagnosis. An example of the former is the pattern of behavior seen in complex partial seizures, particularly when they are associated with ictal or postictal automatisms. Differentiating these in the general population from psychiatric disturbance or, in some cases, from nonepileptic attack disorder is complex. Communication issues and the high prevalence of behavior and motor disorders in this population further complicate differentiating these in people with intellectual disability.

TABLE 3

DIFFERENTIATING SEIZURE AND BEHAVIOR DISORDER

Seizure	Behavior disturbance
Identical behavior on each occasion	Variation in behavior with circumstances
No precipitant	Commonly that is a precipitant such as demands, need to avoid situation
Unresponsive to communication, calming	Responsive to calming, support, removal from stressor
Investigations:	*Investigations*:
Analysis of behavior: No relationship to behavior and environment	Analysis of behavior: Relationship found
Video: Shows typical seizure features	Video: Atypical picture seen
EEG: Positive interictal EEG	EEG: Negative interictal EEG of some use

EEG, electroencephalogram.

Repetitive episodes of manneristic or stereotyped behavior would be most unusual in many people without handicaps and the diagnosis of epilepsy would be highly likely. However, in a young man with autistic tendencies, for example, such behaviors may be reflections of the cognitive disturbance of the autism and not, in fact, epilepsy. Similarly, brief apparent losses of consciousness can be equally undiscriminating due to concurrent physical illness; an example of Sandifer syndrome misdiagnosed as complex partial seizure would be highly unlikely in an individual who could communicate his or her symptoms.[95] Clinicians need a structured approach to this differentiation. Table 3 highlights guidelines to this differential diagnosis, though in many cases behavioral analysis will be required to sufficiently differentiate the behavior.

THERAPEUTIC INTERVENTIONS

With such a strong case for the negative impact of epilepsy on individuals with an intellectual disability and their caregivers, there would appear to be a mandate for interventions to alleviate seizure-related morbidity. Such interventions should be guided by appropriate evidence and sensitive to the key concerns in this population that, in general, relate to the balance between seizure efficacy and concern over apparent side effects. Aspects of pharmacotherapy with antiepileptic drugs have been covered elsewhere in this book. We therefore will focus on those elements of particular relevance to this population: (a) recognition of the need for therapeutic intervention, (b) choosing an intervention, and (c) assessing therapeutic outcome.

Recognition of Need of Intervention

Seizures have a profound effect on this population, and intervention needs will usually be defined through an assessment that this impact exists and that a reduction would both reduce seizure-related risk and improve quality of life. Domains of impact as already described—physical, psychological, cognitive, and social—should be assessed on an individual basis.

Choosing an Intervention

Treatment guidelines[52] exist and can guide clinicians. As many of these patients already have longstanding complicated treatment histories, treatment choice will be influenced by which therapeutic options, either AEDs or surgical, remain available.

This therapeutic choice is mainly influenced by the same evidence base and decision-making process as in the general epilepsy population. Figure 1 shows a potential treatment pathway for people with intellectual disability who have epilepsy and can be used as a useful marker for judging the options available to an individual on his or her treatment pathway. This pathway relates to the use of AEDs. Surgical options are as relevant for this population both for potentially curative resective seizures and for procedures that may ameliorate the epilepsy, such as vagal nerve stimulation.

There does exist, however, a body of evidence relating to interventional studies in epilepsy and intellectual disability. Such evidence, while frequently hampered by its quality, can provide markers for treatment effect in terms of efficacy and safety.

Quality Evidence?

In general, therapeutic trials of AEDs use measures based on seizure frequency, seizure severity, quality of life, and side effect data. These measures, while appropriate in those without intellectual disability, may not be sufficient or may not be valid in those with intellectual disability.[31,56] It has been suggested that research in this population should use the following standard components:

1. Define the individual—use the Adaptive Behavior Scale.[75]
2. Define the individual epilepsy—etiology of intellectual disability, seizure type, and syndrome.
3. Use measures sensitive to change in the intellectual disability population.
4. Determine seizure frequency using seizure diaries.
5. Assess behavior using validated measure of behavior such as Aberrant Behavior Checklist,[3] or Developmental Behavior Checklist in children.[29]
6. Determine quality of life using specific mental retardation and epilepsy quality-of-life scales—Glasgow Epilepsy Outcome Scale (GEOS).[32]

Learning from the Evidence

Seizure Impact

Several high-quality randomized placebo-controlled trials have been published in populations of people with intellectual disability. The majority of these have been in people with Lennox-Gastaut syndrome. This syndrome is strongly associated with intellectual disability. However, the reproducibility of data from this specific seizure syndrome population into the total intellectual disability population is not proven.

Table 4[55,72,87,101] summarizes the data from these studies.

The advantage of these studies is that the placebo arm may provide some evidence of the natural course of seizure frequency in a trial setting. The studies show variation in seizure change within the placebo arms and by different seizure types. Atonic seizures ranged from a 9% decrease to a 5% increase. Tonic–clonic (recorded in one study) showed a 10% worsening and all seizure types showed from a 9% decrease to a 4% increase.

A published study[7] used a retrospective case note review to assess the use of vigabatrin, lamotrigine, and gabapentin in adults with mental retardation. The study again showed

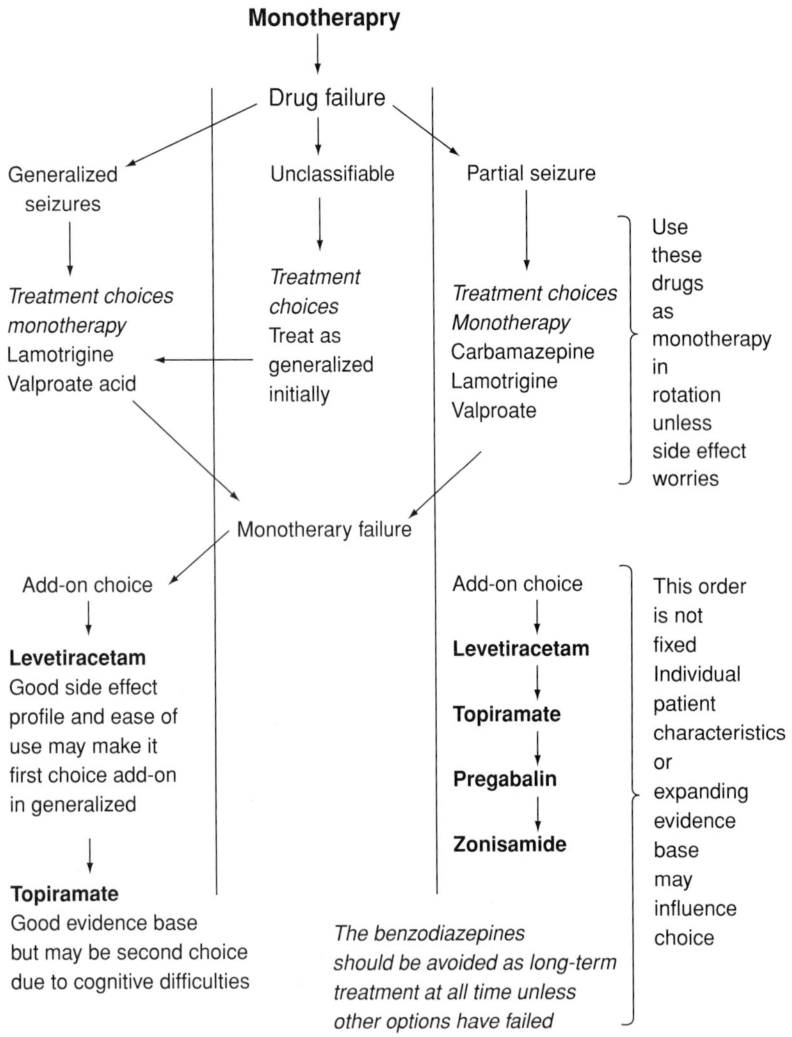

FIGURE 1. A treatment pathway for people with intellectual disability and epilepsy. (Published with permission of Clarion Press.)

variation in the percentage of patients reporting an increase in seizure frequency: Two (8%) of the patients on vigabatrin, six (24%) of the patients on lamotrigine, and zero (0%) of those on gabapentin.

It appears that seizure worsening occurs in Randomised Controlled Trials (RCTs) with novel AEDs in patients with intellectual disability, suggesting an association between seizure increase and natural fluctuation in seizure control.

The Impact of Antiepileptic Drugs on Behavior

Randomized placebo-controlled trials that have been published in populations of people with intellectual disability and Lennox-Gastaut syndrome may again offer some insight into safety issues. However, the reproducibility of data from this specific seizure syndrome population into the total intellectual disability population should again be treated with caution.

The studies showed a relatively high level of behavioral symptoms in placebo arms: Nervousness in 10% to 14%, somnolence in 22%, and "behavioral problems" in 10% (Table 4).

Data from the nonrandomized controlled trials are less valuable. However, a UK-based study[7] using a retrospective case note review showed behavior problems in 5 of 23 patients on vigabatrin, 2 of 25 patients on lamotrigine, and 1 of 23 patients on gabapentin.

The data on behavioral side effects in studies of AEDs in people with intellectual disability are particularly poor. The key problem is nonvalidated definitions of behavior. Where blinded control data do exist, they show that behavioral deterioration can occur and may be—in the case of topiramate—a specific drug effect.

Assessing Therapeutic Outcome

A judgment on treatment outcome has particular importance in people with an intellectual disability; there is certainly no "one size fits all" approach to this. In many instances very individualized approaches will be necessary, particularly in those with multiple physical and intellectual disabilities.

In a clinical context the assessment of treatment outcome will involve a more pragmatic approach. This is likely to have several broad aims. The first will be to analyze accurately any seizure change. To do this, accurate seizure charts are necessary. These will need space to identify several seizure types. Acquiring high-quality seizure frequency data can be a long-term and difficult process. Frequently, parents and caregivers will need guidance into differentiating varying seizure types and in accurate recording.

Secondly, clinicians will have to assess any negative impact from the treatment change. This again can be a challenging task, especially in individuals who may have poor communication and a range of concurrent illnesses, all with symptoms not unlike those of potential drug side effects. Of these, the most concerning to clinicians and caregivers alike is the potential for behavior change. A structured approach is necessary to

TABLE 4

EPILEPSY AND INTELLECTUAL DISABILITY: IMPACT ON SEIZURES AND BEHAVIOR OF AEDs FROM CONTROLLED TRIALS

Trial	N	Seizure outcome	Behavioral outcome
Felbamate[101]	73	*Atonic seizures* Active—34% decrease Placebo—9% *Total seizures* Active—19% decrease Placebo—4% increase	*Nervousness* Active—5 (14%) Control—5 (14%) No other behavioral outcome recorded, possibly due to side effects that occurred less than five times not recorded
Lamotrigine[72]	169	*All seizures* Active—32% decrease Placebo—9% decrease *Tonic-clonic seizures* Active—36% decrease Placebo—10% increase *Atonic seizures* Active—34% decrease Placebo—9% decrease	*Somnolence* Active—3 (4%) Control—4 (4%)
Topiramate[87]	98	*All seizures* Active—20.6% Placebo—8.8% *Atonic seizures* Active—14.8% reduction Placebo—5.1% increase	*Somnolence* Active—42% Control—22% *Nervousness* Active—21% Control—10% *Behavioral problems* Active—21% Control—10%
Topiramate[55]	88	*All seizures* Active—30% decrease Placebo—1% decrease	*Somnolence* Active—32.4% Control—10.8% *Nervousness* Active—2.7% Control—13.5% *Behavioral problems* Baseline change in Aberrant Behavior Checklist Active reduction in 7.3 points Control reduction by 9.3

identify those occasions where behavioral symptoms are likely to be treatment related (Fig. 2).

SURGERY

For many years in the history of epilepsy surgery, patients with low IQ were excluded as candidates. One reason was that low IQ has been thought to be indicative of generalized cerebral dysfunction, suggesting that the prognosis for improvement of seizures after focal resection is low.[30,60,99] It has also been suggested that in patients with low IQ, the integrity of brain outside the area of focus may not be adequate to allow for compensation after surgery, thus making these individuals more prone to cognitive deterioration.[9,83] A third reason was the assumption that some patients with low IQ may be unable to cooperate or tolerate the preoperative procedures necessary for identifying good surgical candidates.[107] Despite these assumptions, present guidelines typically do not include intellectual status as an exclusion criterion for surgery.

Vasconcellos et al.[104] examined intellectual function in pediatric candidates for epilepsy surgery. Younger age at onset was associated with lower IQ, and mean IQ was significantly lower in patients with seizure onset at or before 2 years of age. The frequency of patients with intellectual disability varied with age of seizure onset, with 46% of those with seizure onset at or before 2 years of age having IQs lower than 70, compared with only 12% of those with onset after that age. This difference was independent of etiology of the epilepsy[9] reported on surgical outcome in 31 patients with IQ $\leq$70, approximately 15% of a consecutive surgical series in Norway. Two years after surgery, 52% of those with temporal lobe resections and 38% with extratemporal resections were seizure free. Unfortunately, the authors did not compare outcomes with the other patients in their own series, but comparison with other published series suggested that the seizure outcome was poorer than in patients with higher IQs.[15] An important finding was that the surgical result was related to duration of epilepsy, with greater likelihood of seizure freedom obtained with shorter duration of epilepsy prior to surgery. The authors suggested that when duration was taken into account, the rate of success was comparable to patients with normal intelligence.[60] Cognition did not improve in patients irrespective of IQ, a finding that has been demonstrated in other studies reporting neuropsychological outcomes of surgery in patients of all levels of intellectual

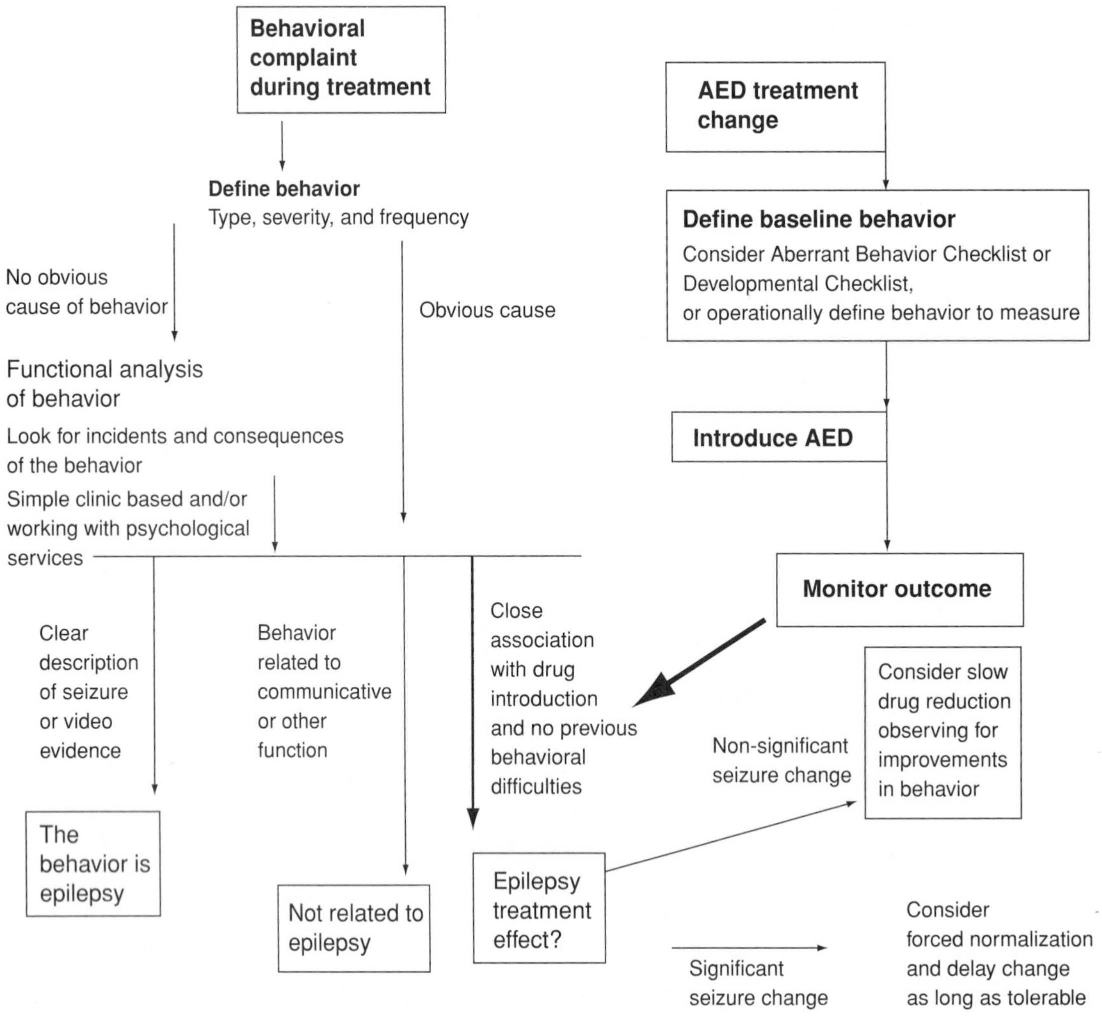

FIGURE 2. Assessing behavioral change during antiepileptic drug treatment. AED, antiepileptic drug. (Published with permission of Clarion Press.)

function.[70,94] A review[60] suggested that with careful presurgical evaluations, outcomes are similar between patients with normal IQ scores and those with low scores.

A high proportion of children with infantile spasms have mental retardation and behavior disorders. The UCLA Pediatric Epilepsy Surgery Research Group has compared surgical outcomes in these children with those of children with other forms of intractable symptomatic epilepsy.[13] At 2-year follow-up assessment, both groups continued to show impaired development of language, cognition, and social communication despite improved seizure control.

VAGAL NERVE STIMULATION

The effects of vagal nerve stimulation (VNS) have been investigated in a number of studies that have included children with intellectual disabilities associated with epileptic syndromes and developmental disorders. Despite reported improvements in seizure frequency and/or severity, mood, and quality of life, changes in cognitive function have not been found.[2,46,65,78] In a series of patients with Lennox-Gastaut syndrome, seizure reduction was highest in patients with highest baseline cognitive function,[2,65] leading these authors to conclude that intellectual disability is a negative prognostic factor for efficacy of VNS.

THE CONTEXT OF CARE

Unfortunately, service delivery to individuals with an intellectual disability who have epilepsy has received little attention from the research community. However, five key areas exist around which multiagency care can be structured: Health advocacy, barriers and safety, quality of care, specialist provision, and the needs of the family (Table 5).

Health Advocacy

Due to the inherent difficulties in communication associated with intellectual disability, both the individual and the clinician can be disadvantaged. Parents frequently provide communication functions. However, when an individual lives in care, the agency will need to ensure that someone can describe the current seizures, their frequency, and the impact epilepsy is having on the individual. Additionally, services should be able to support the individual to make choices over epilepsy management where appropriate.

TABLE 5

MULTIAGENCY AREAS OF NEED FOR INDIVIDUALS WITH LEARNING DISABILITY AND EPILEPSY

Area	Example issues
Health advocacy	Assistance in the communication of an individual's seizures Assistance in communication of an individual's response to treatment and past treatment history
Barriers and safety	Risk assessment of dangers of epilepsy such as bathing Assessment of the impact of epilepsy on an individual's social inclusion
Quality of care	Quality of care environment for individual Ability of environment to supply prescribed treatment Ability to administer rescue medication
Specialist provision	Education, housing Support services such as psychological or behavioral support Investigative services such as EEG and MRI under anesthesia
The family	Respite services Education Training Support

EEG, electroencephalogram; MRI, magnetic resonance imaging.

Barriers and Safety

Services have a responsibility to the safety of their charges; in particular, risk of bathing accidents must be carefully assessed. Additionally, where epilepsy has become a barrier to social inclusion, this should be identified and appropriate remedies sought.

Quality of Care

Any care setting for an individual with an intellectual disability should be able to meet his or her epilepsy management needs. In particular, medication, where prescribed, should be given, and where rescue medication is prescribed, appropriate management plans should exist.

Specialist Provision

The potential for specialist provision can read something like a wish list of potential services. This, of course, merely reflects the diverse needs of this population. An individual may need appropriate housing or education. Specific support services such as psychology or behavior support agencies may be needed. Completion of investigations will need appropriate disability-aware investigative electrophysiologic and imaging services.

The Family

Families provide much of the health advocacy and housing needs of this population. To deliver this, support is needed with education into epilepsy and its treatment, with the emotional effects on the family members, and with adequate respite services.

Coordinating Multiagency Care Delivery

The delivery of multiagency care does, of itself, need coordination. The availability of resources and trained staff will of course influence the ability to provide and coordinate multiagency care. Some of the key themes can be delivered relatively cheaply such as education on safety and education to caregivers. Where resource exists, other agencies can make a large impact into epilepsy care.

SUMMARY AND CONCLUSIONS

The interaction between epilepsy and learning disorder is complex and can be subtle and transient. Notwithstanding this for a large proportion of the population with epilepsy major intellectual disability coexists with severe refractory epilepsy. This combination of morbidities impacts on the individuals in their quality of life, and on the professional, demanding specific skills in assessment and treatment. Such skills include the use of communication strategies, recognition of phenotypes, the assessment of behavioural change, application of AEDs and surgical assessment. Our knowledge of this field is advancing as it is in the general epilepsy population. However this advancement is uneven, our chapter shows how the new genetic and aetiological knowledge can be readily applied to this group; yet there are relatively few data from interventional studies and as such the gap in our knowledge on the application and effectiveness of treatments in this group is widening as compared to the general epilepsy population. The challenge for the professional epilepsy community is to close this gap.

References

1. Airaksinen E, Matilainen R, Mononen T, et al. A population study on epilepsy in mentally retarded children. *Epilepsia*. 2000;41(9):1214–1220.
2. Aldenkamp AP, Majoie HJ, Perfelo MW, et al. Long-term effects of 24-month treatment of vagus nerve stimulation on behavior in children with Lennox-Gastaut syndrome. *Epilepsy Behav*. 2002;3:475–479.
3. Aman MG, Singh NN, Stewart AW, et al. The Aberrant Behaviour Checklist: a behaviour rating scale for the assessment of treatment effects. *Am J Ment Defic*. 1985;89:485–491.
4. Amano K, Takamutso J, Ogata A, et al. Characteristics of epilepsy in severely mentally retarded individuals. *Psychiatry Clin Neurosci*. 2000;54:17–22.
5. Bate L, Gardiner M. Genetics of inherited epilepsies. *Epileptic Disord*. 1999;1(1):7–19.
6. Berry-Kravis E. Epilepsy in fragile X syndrome. *Dev Med Child Neurol*. 2002;44:724–728.
7. Bhaumik S, Branford D, Duggirala C, et al. A naturalistic study of the use of vigabatrin, lamotrigine and gabapentin in adults with learning disabilities. *Seizure*. 1997;6:127–133.
8. Binnie CD, Channon S, Marston D. Learning disabilities in epilepsy: neurophysiological aspects. *Epilepsia*. 1990;31(4):S2–S8.
9. Bjornaes H, Stabell KE, Heminghyt E, et al. Resective surgery for intractable focal epilepsy in patients with low IQ: predictors for seizure control and outcome with respect to seizures and neuropsychological and psychosocial functioning. *Epilepsia*. 2004;45:131–139.
10. Blunden R. Pragmatic features of quality services. In: Janicki MP, Krauss MW, Seltzer MM, eds. *Community Residences for Persons with Developmental Disabilities: Here to Stay*. Baltimore: Paul H Brookes; 1988.
11. Bouras N, Drummond C. Behaviour and psychiatric disorders of people with mental handicaps living in the community. *J Intell Dis Res*. 1992;36:349–357.
12. Buelow J, Austin J, Perkins S, et al. Behavioural and mental health problems in children with epilepsy and low IQ. *Dev Med Child Neurol*. 2003;45:683–692.
13. Caplan R, Siddath P, Mathern, G, et al. Developmental outcome with and without successful intervention. *Int Rev Neurobiol*. 2002;49:269–284.

14. Carnwarth T, Johnson D. Psychiatric morbidity among spouses of patients with stroke. *BMJ*. 1987;294:409–411.
15. Chelune GJ, Nagle RI, Hermann BP, et al. Does presurgical IQ predict seizure outcome after temporal lobectomy? Evidence from the Bozeman Epilepsy Consortium. *Epilepsia*. 1998;39:314–318.
16. Cockerell OC, Eckle I, Goodridge DMG, et al. Epilepsy in a population of 6000 re-examined: secular trends in first attendance rates, prevalence, and prognosis. *J Neurol Neurosurg Psychiatry*. 1995;58:570–576.
17. Cockerell OC, Johnson AL, Sander JWAS, et al. Mortality from epilepsy: results from a prospective population-based study. *Lancet*. 1994;344:918–921.
18. Corbett J. Epilepsy and mental handicap. In: Laidlaw J, Richens A, Oxley J, eds. *A Textbook of Epilepsy*. 3rd ed. Edinburgh: Churchill Livingstone; 1993:631–636.
19. Corbett JA, Harris R, Robinson R. Epilepsy. In: Wortis J, ed. *Mental Retardation and Developmental Disabilities*. Vol VII. New York: Raven Press; 1975:79–111.
20. Currie C, Morgan C, Peters J, et al. The demands for hospital services for patients with epilepsy. *Epilepsia*. 1998;39(5):537–544.
21. Curry CJ, Stevenson RE, Aughton D, et al. Evaluation of mental retardation: recommendations of a consensus conference. *Am J Med Gen*. 1997;72:468–477.
22. De Bona C, Zappella M, Hayek G, et al. Preserved speech variant is allelic of classic Rett syndrome. *Eur J Hum Genet*. 2000;8:325–330.
23. de Vries BB, Robinson H, Stolte-Dijkstra I, et al. General overgrowth in the fragile X syndrome: variability in the phenotypic expression of the FMR1 gene mutation. *J Med Genet*. 1995;32:764–769.
24. Deb S. Mental disorder in adults with mental retardation and epilepsy. *Compr Psychiatry*. 1997;38:179–184.
25. Deb S, Hunter D. Psychology of people with mental handicap and epilepsy. *Br J Psychiatry*. 1991;159:822–826.
26. Didden R, Korzilius H, Smits MG, et al. Sleep problems in individuals with Angelman syndrome. *Am J Ment Retard*. 2004;109:275–284.
27. Dulac O, Chugani HT, Bernardina BD. *Infantile Spasms and West Syndrome*. London: W.B. Saunders Company Ltd; 1994.
28. Eaton LF, Menolascino FJ. Psychiatric disorders in the mentally retarded: types, problems challenges. *Am J Psychiatry*. 1982;139:1297–1303.
29. Einfield SL, Tonge BJ. The Developmental Behaviour Checklist: the development and validation of an instrument to assess behavioural and emotional disturbance in children and adolescents with mental retardation. *J Autism Dev Disord*. 1995;25:81–104.
30. Engel J Jr. Principles of epilepsy surgery. In: Shorvon A, Fish D, Thomas D, eds. *The Treatment of Epilepsy*. Oxford: Blackwell Science; 1996: 519–529.
31. Espie CA, Kerr M, Paul A, et al. Learning disability and epilepsy. 2, a review of available outcome measures and position statement on development priorities. *Seizure*. 1997;6:337–350.
32. Espie CA, Paul A, Graham M, et al. The Epilepsy Outcome Scale: the development of a measure for use with carer's of people with epilepsy plus intellectual disability. *J Intell Dis Res*. 1998;42:90–96.
33. Espie CA, Watkins J, Curtice L, et al. Psychopathology in people with epilepsy and intellectual disability; an investigation of potential explanatory variables. *J Neurol Neurosurg Psychiatry*. 2003;74(11):1485–1492.
34. Eyman RK, Call T. Maladaptive behaviour and community placement of mentally retarded persons. *Am J Ment Retard*. 1977;82:137–144.
35. Forgren L, Edvinsson S, Nystrom L, et al. Influence of epilepsy on mortality in mental retardation: an epidemiological study. *Epilepsia*. 1996;37(10):956–963.
36. Forssman H, Akesson HO. Mortality of the mentally deficient: a study of 12,903 institutionalised subjects. *J Ment Defic Res*. 1970;14: 276–294.
37. Fryers T. Epidemiological issues in mental retardation. *J Ment Defic Res*. 1987;31(Pt 4):365–384.
38. Fryns JP, Jacobs J, Kleckowska A, et al. The psychological profile of the fragile X syndrome. *Clin Genet*. 1984;25:131–134.
39. Galvan-Manso M, Campistol J, Conill J, et al. Analysis of the characteristics of epilepsy in 37 patients with the molecular diagnosis of Angelman syndrome. *Epileptic Disord*. 2005;7:19–25.
40. Glaze DG, Schultz RJ. Rett syndrome: meeting the challenge of this gender-specific neurodevelopmental disorder. *Medscape Womens Health*. 1997;2:3.
41. Goulden KJ, Shinnar S, Koller H, et al. Epilepsy in children with mental retardation: a cohort study. *Epilepsia*. 1991;32(5):690–697.
42. Guerrini R, Carrozzo R, Rinaldi R, et al. Angelman syndrome: etiology, clinical features, diagnosis, and management of symptoms. *Paediatr Drugs*. 2003;5:647–661.
43. Guerrini R, De Lorey TM, Bonanni P, et al. Cortical myoclonus in Angelman syndrome. *Ann Neurol*. 1996;40:39–48.
44. Guerrini R, Gobbi G, Genton P, et al. Chromosomal abnormalities. In: Engel J Jr, Pedley TA, eds. *Epilepsy: A Comprehensive Textbook*. Philadelphia: Lippincott-Raven Publishers; 1997:2533–2546.
45. Hagberg B, Aicardi J, Dias K, et al. A progressive syndrome of autism, dementia, ataxia, and loss of purposeful hand use in girls: Rett's syndrome: report of 35 cases. *Ann Neurol*. 1983;14:471–479.
46. Hallbook T, Lundgren J, Stjernqvist K, et al. Vagus nerve stimulation in 15 children with therapy resistant epilepsy; its impact on cognition, quality of life, behaviour and mood. *Seizure*. 2005;14:503–514.
47. Hauser WA, Annegers JF, Elveback LR. Mortality in patients with epilepsy. *Epilepsia*. 1980;21:399–412.
48. Heller T, Miller A, Factor A. Adults with mental retardation as supports to their parents: effects on parental caregiving appraisal. *Ment Retard*. 1997;35:338–346.
49. Herbst DS, Baird PA. Survival rates and causes of death among persons with non-specific mental retardation. In: Berg JM, ed. *Perspectives and Progress in Mental Retardation. Vol. II. Biomedical Aspects*. Baltimore: University Park Press; 1984:3–15.
50. Hoare P. The development of psychiatric disorder among school children with epilepsy. *Dev Med Child Neurol*. 1984;26:3–13.
51. Huppke P, Held M, Laccone F, et al. The spectrum of phenotypes in females with Rett syndrome. *Brain Dev*. 2003;25:346–351.
52. IASSID Guidelines Group. Clinical guidelines for the management of epilepsy in adults with an intellectual disability. *Seizure*. 2001;10(6):401–409.
53. Incorpora G, Sorge G, Sorge A, et al. Epilepsy in fragile X syndrome. *Brain Dev*. 2002;24:766–769.
54. Johannsen P, Christensen JE, Goldstein H, et al. Epilepsy in Down syndrome-prevalence in three age groups. *Seizure*. 1996;5:121–125.
55. Kerr MP, Baker G, Brodie M. A randomised, double-blind, placebo-controlled trial of Topiramate in adults with epilepsy and intellectual disability: impact on seizures, severity and quality of life. *Epilepsy Behav*. 2005;7:472–480.
56. Kerr MP, Espie CA. Learning disabilities and epilepsy. 1, towards common outcome measures. *Seizure*. 1997;6:331–336.
57. Kerr M, Fraser W, Felce D. Primary health care for people with a learning disability; a keynote review. *Br J Learning Disabil*. 1996;24:2–8.
58. Kumada T, Ito M, Miyajima T, et al. Multi-institutional study on the correlation between chromosomal abnormalities and epilepsy. *Brain Dev*. 2005;27:127–134.
59. Laan LA, Renier WO, Arts WF, et al. Evolution of epilepsy and EEG findings in Angelman syndrome. 13: *Epilepsia*. 1997;38:195–199.
60. Levisohn PM. Epilepsy surgery in children with developmental disabilities. *Semin Pediatr Neurol*. 2000;7:194–203.
61. Lewis JN, Tonge BJ, Mowat DR, et al. Epilepsy and associated psychopathology in young people with intellectual disability. *J Paed Child Health*. 2000;36(2):172–175.
62. Lhatoo SD, Sander JW. The epidemiology of epilepsy and learning disability. *Epilepsia*. 2001;42(Suppl 1):6–9.
63. Lott IT, Lai F. Dementia in Down syndrome: observations from a neurology clinic. *Appl Res Ment Retard*. 1982;3:233–239.
64. Lund J. Epilepsy and psychiatric disorder in the mentally retarded adult. *Acta Psychiatr Scand*. 1985;72:557–562.
65. Majoie H, Berfelo MW, Aldenkamp AP, et al. Vagus nerve stimulation in patients with catastrophic childhood epilepsy, a 2 year follow-up study. *Seizure*. 2005;14:10–18.
66. Mansell JL. *Services for People with Learning Disabilities and Challenging Behaviour or Mental Health Needs*. London: HMSO; 1993.
67. Mariani E, Ferini-Strambi L, Sala M, et al. Epilepsy in institutionalised patients with encephalopathy: clinical aspects and nosological considerations. *Am J Ment Retard*. 1993;98:27–33.
68. McDermott S, Moran R, Platt T, et al. Prevalence of epilepsy in adults with mental retardation and related disabilities in primary care. *Am J Ment Retard*. 2005: 110(1):48–56.
69. McKee JR, Bodfish JW. Sudden unexplained death in epilepsy in adults with mental retardation. *Am J Ment Retard*. 2000;105(4):229–235.
70. Miranda C, Smith ML. Predictors of intelligence after temporal lobectomy in children with epilepsy. *Epilepsy Behav*. 2001;2:1–8.
71. Morgan CL, Baxter H, Kerr MP. Prevalence of epilepsy and associated health service utilization and mortality among patients with intellectual disability. *Am J Ment Retard*. 2003;108(5):293–300.
72. Motte J, Trevathan E, Barrera MN, et al. Lamotrigine for generalized seizures associated with the Lennox-Gastaut syndrome. *N Engl J Med*. 1997;337:1807–1812.
73. Musumeci SA, Ferri R, Elia L. Epilepsy and fragile X syndrome: a follow-up study. *Am J Med Genet*. 1991;38:511–513.
74. Nihira K, Leland H, Lambert N. *Adaptive Behaviour Scales*. Austin, Texas: American Association on Mental Retardation; 1993.
75. Nilsson L, Tomson T, Farahmand BY, et al. Cause-specific mortality in epilepsy: a cohort study of more than 9,000 patients once hospitalised for epilepsy. *Epilepsia*. 1997;38:1062–1068.
76. Ohtsuka Y, Kobayashi K, Yoshinaga H, et al. Relationship between severity of epilepsy and developmental outcome in Angelman syndrome. *Brain Dev*. 2005;27:95–100.
77. Park YD. The effects of vagus nerve stimulation therapy on patients with intractable seizures and either Landau-Kleffner syndrome or autism. *Epilepsy Behav*. 2003;4:286–290.
78. Patja K, Iivanainen M, Vesela H, et al. Life expectancy of people with intellectual disability: a 35 year follow up study. *J Intell Dis Res*. 2000;44(5):591–599.
79. Penner KA, Johnston J, Faircloth BH, et al. Communication, cognition, and social interaction in the Angelman syndrome. *Am J Med Genet*. 1993;46:34–39.

80. Pollack MA, Golden GS, Schmidt R, et al. Infantile spasms in Down syndrome: a report of 5 cases and review of the literature. *Ann Neurol.* 1978;3:406–408.
81. Prasher VP. Epilepsy and associated effects on adaptive behaviour in adults with Down syndrome. *Seizure.* 1995;4:53–56.
82. Rausch R. Factors affecting neuropsychological and psychosocial outcome of epilepsy surgery. In: Luders H, ed. *Epilepsy Surgery.* New York: Raven Press; 1991:487–493.
83. Richardson SA, Katz M, Koller H, et al. Some characteristics of a population of mentally retarded young adults in a British city. A basis for estimating some service needs. *J Ment Defic Res.* 1979;23(4):275–285.
84. Richardson SA, Koller H, Katz M, et al. A functional classification of seizures and its distribution in a mentally retarded population. *Am J Ment Defic.* 1981;85:457–466.
85. Sabaratnam M, Vroegop PG, Gangadharan SK. Epilepsy and EEG findings in 18 males with fragile X syndrome. *Seizure.* 2001;10:60–63.
86. Sachdeo RC, Glauser TA, Ritter F, et al. A double-blind, randomised trial of topiramate in Lennox-Gastaut syndrome. *Neurology.* 1999;52:1882–1887.
87. Sansom D, Krishnan VH, Corbett J, et al. Emotional and behavioural aspects of Rett syndrome. *Dev Med Child Neurol.* 1993;35:340–345.
88. Shackleton DP, Westendorp RG, Trenite DG, et al. Mortality in patients with epilepsy: 40 years of follow up in a Dutch cohort study. *J Neurol Neurosurg Psychiatry.* 1999;66:636–640.
89. Shepherd C, Hosking G. Epilepsy in school children with intellectual impairments in Sheffield: the size and nature of the problem and the implications for service provision. *J Ment Defic Res.* 1989;33:511–514.
90. Sillanpaa M. Epilepsy in the mentally retarded. In: Wallace W, ed. *Epilepsy in Children.* London: Chapman and Hall; 1996:417–427.
91. Smith A, Wiles C, Haan E, et al. Clinical features in 27 patients with Angelman syndrome resulting from DNA deletion. *J Med Genet.* 1996;33:107–112.
92. Smith GF, Berg JM. *Down's Anomaly.* 2nd ed. Edinburgh: Churchill Livingston; 1976.
93. Smith ML, Elliott IM, Lach, L. Cognitive, psychological and family function after pediatric epilepsy surgery. *Epilepsia.* 2004;45:650–660.
94. Somjit S, Lee Y, Berkovic S, et al. Sandifer syndrome misdiagnosed as refractory partial seizures in an adult. *Epileptic Disord.* 2004;6(1):49–50.
95. Steffenburg U, Hagberg G, Hagberg B. Epilepsy in a representative series of Rett syndrome. *Acta Paediatr.* 2001;90:34–39.
96. Steffenburg U, Hagberg G, Videggal G, et al. Active epilepsy in mentally retarded children. I. Prevalence and additional neuro-impairments *Acta Paediatr.* 1995;84(10):1147–1152.
97. Tatsuno M, Hayashi M, Iwamoto H, et al. Epilepsy in childhood Down syndrome. *Brain Dev.* 1984;6:37–44.
98. Taylor DC, Falconer MA. Clinical, socioeconomic and psychological changes after temporal lobectomy for epilepsy. *Br J Psychiatry.* 1968;114:1247–1261.
99. Terracciano A, Chiurazzi P, Neri G. Fragile X syndrome. *Am J Med Genet C Semin Med Genet.* 2005;137:32–37.
100. The Felbamate Study Group. Efficacy of felbamate in childhood epileptic encephalopathy (Lennox-Gastaut syndrome). *N Engl J Med.* 1993;328:29–33.
101. Thompson PJ, Upton D. The impact of chronic epilepsy on the family. *Seizure.* 1992;1(1):43–48.
102. Trevethan E, Murphy CC, Yeargin-Allsopp M. The descriptive epidemiology of infantile spasms among Atlanta children. *Epilepsia.* 1990;40(6):748–751.
103. Vasconcellos E, Wyllie E, Sullivan S, et al. Mental retardation in pediatric candidates for epilepsy surgery: the role of early seizure onset. *Epilepsia.* 2001;42:268–274.
104. Veall RM. The prevalence of epilepsy among Mongols related to age. *J Ment Defic Res.* 1974;18:99–106.
105. Viani F, Romeo A, Viri M, et al. Seizure and EEG patterns in Angelman's syndrome. *J Child Neurol.* 1995;10:467–471.
106. Walker E. Surgery for epilepsy. In: Vinken PJ, Bruyn GW, eds. *Handbook of Clinical Neurology.* 15th ed. Amsterdam: North Holland Publishing; 1974: 739–757.
107. Welsh Office. Welsh Health Survey. Cardiff: Welsh Office; 1995.
108. Wisniewski KE, French JH, Fernando S, et al. Fragile X syndrome: associated neurological abnormalities and developmental disabilities. *Ann Neurol.* 1985;18:665–669.
109. Zori RT, Hendrickson J, Woolven S, et al. Angelman syndrome: clinical profile. *J Child Neurol.* 1992;7:270–280.

CHAPTER 203 ■ PERSONALITY DISORDERS IN EPILEPSY

ORRIN DEVINSKY, CHARLES VORKAS, WILLIAM B. BARR, AND BRUCE P. HERMANN

INTRODUCTION

At the turn of the 20th century, most of the lay and professional communities believed that people with epilepsy had pathologic personality traits and psychopathologic disorders such as aggression, sociopathy, and psychosis. However, from the medical perspective, this was partly an artifact of the main setting from which epilepsy was viewed: Chronically institutionalized patients, many of whom suffered comorbid disorders (e.g., head trauma, neurosyphilis). The concept of an epileptic personality—a ubiquitous and characteristically negative set of behavioral changes in epilepsy patients—was already established in antiquity, but continued to evolve slowly and relentlessly. Simultaneously, more humanistic and balanced views evolved during the 19th century. Based on extensive experience with a private outpatient population with idiopathic epilepsy, Reynolds[87] concluded that epilepsy does not invariably involve abnormal mental change, and Gowers[42] also recognized that many epilepsy patients had normal personality and intellect, but that many others could develop intraparoxysmal behavioral changes. He suggested that these changes resulted from many factors, but mainly from epilepsy.

The early 20th century brought diverse views concerning people with epilepsy and their behaviors. Wilson[121] offered a progressive psychosocial view: "On epileptic temperament inordinate stress has been laid. Life is difficult for these patients, and much that is attributed to temperament can with greater reason be assigned to chronic invalidism and unlucky circumstance." Sjobring[99] adhered to the negative, pervasive view: "A mental change of a specific nature takes place in individuals suffering from epileptic seizures. They become torpid and circumstantial, sticky and adhesive, effectively tense and suffer from explosive outburst of rage, anxiety, etc." Kraepelin[61] reported aggressiveness in some of his outpatient epilepsy patients: "Almost always an intensification of mental irritability occurs." The adhesive or viscous personality traits in which the patient has difficulty in disengaging from interpersonal exchanges was reviewed by many observers in the European literature under various terminologies such as the "enechetic constitution," "ixoid character," and "glischroid trait."

THE MODERN ERA

Early in the 20th century, the term "epileptic personality" was used by psychoanalytic theorists to describe a set of character traits associated with epilepsy that focused on impulsivity, egocentricity, and affective viscosity.[17] These features were considered to result from hereditary factors, directly from seizures or treatment, or a reaction to painful social situations associated with epilepsy. Others believed that these particular personality features, in individuals with or without seizures, were a direct expression of epilepsy itself. Two coincident developments in the middle of the century helped reintroduce the highly controversial concept of personality changes in epilepsy: Identifying the role of the limbic system in emotion and behavior and localizing the onset of many partial seizures to the temporal lobe.

Papez[81] conceived a circuit of interconnected structures comprising the emotion system: Hippocampus—fornix—hypothalamus/mammillary bodies—mammillothalamic tract—anterior thalamic nuclei—thalamocingulate fibers—cingulate cortex—amygdala/hippocampus. This emotion circuit theory was based on anatomic connections, sham rage studies, and lesion studies. Yakovlev[124] conceived a basolateral circuit modulating emotional behavior, including the amygdala, insula, orbitofrontal cortex, and dorsomedial thalamic nucleus. MacLean[67] combined earlier ideas and conceived the limbic system with all the above regions, as well as the septum and nucleus accumbens.

The specific association of temporal lobe epilepsy (TLE) and psychopathology had its major genesis in the 1951 report by Gibbs[40] that up to 33% of patients with "psychomotor seizures" of temporal lobe origin exhibited interictal behavioral changes. Gastaut et al.[36] in 1954 reiterated common observations on the frequency of emotional viscosity, hyposexuality, hypoactivity, and aggressiveness in epilepsy patients, and first suggested that the stereotypic symptom complex was the antithesis of behaviors in the Kluver-Bucy syndrome (KBS). KBS is characterized by oral exploratory behavior, increased sexual appetite, decreased aggressivity, and continuous environmental exploration as a consequence of bilateral anterior temporal destructive lesions.[59]

Waxman and Geschwind[117] proposed a distinct subset of nonpathologic behaviors associated with TLE, which included deepened emotions, circumstantiality, altered religious and sexual concerns, and hypergraphia. They coined the term "interictal behavior syndrome," sometimes referred to as Geschwind syndrome or Gastaut-Geschwind syndrome.[6] Bear and Fedio[4] expanded this syndrome to include the 18 traits based on a literature review. They found an increased frequency of all 18 traits in patients with TLE compared with non-neurologic controls. The interictal behavioral traits described by Bear and Fedio are summarized in Table 1. Some of these traits associated with this syndrome are described below in more detail.

Viscosity

Viscosity is a tendency for prolonged interpersonal contacts; talking repetitively, circumstantially; and pedantically; and not ending conversations and visits after a socially appropriate interval. Bear and Fedio[4] reported viscosity to be significantly elevated in both right and left TLE compared to normal and neurologic controls. Brandt et al.[10] found increased viscosity among left TLE and generalized epilepsy (GE) patients, with no difference between right TLE and controls. Hoeppner et al.[51] presented the "cookie thief" picture from the Boston

TABLE 1

PROPOSED PERSONALITY TRAITS BY BEAR AND FEDIO

Hypergraphia
Hypermoralism
Altered sexuality
Religiosity
Aggression
Obsessionalism
Paranoia
Guilt
Humorlessness
Sadness
Emotionality
Circumstantiality
Philosophical interest
Personal destiny
Viscosity
Dependence
Elation
Anger

Diagnostic Aphasia Examination, which shows a drawing of a boy stealing a cookie, to TLE, GE, and control subjects. Taped responses were reviewed blindly and all four individuals with verbose responses, characterized by trivial, circumstantial, and subjective details, had left temporal foci. A ten-item viscosity scale revealed significantly higher scores in the self-reports of patients with left TLE compared to right or bilateral TLE, absence seizures, panic disorder, or normal subjects.[86] Proxy raters reported a trend for increased viscosity scores in the left TLE group, endorsing items such as "when I have a phone conversation with him/her, I always find I am the one who wants to get off first." Seizure duration and viscosity score were significantly correlated for patients with left TLE.

Viscosity may result from some combination of linguistic impairment, social cohesion, mental slowness, and psychological dependence. Language dysfunction associated with left temporal lobe seizure foci may contribute to a verbal style characterized by circumstantiality and excessive discourse. However, there may be independent effects of left temporal foci on social behavior. Viscosity, the personality trait, may also result from an increased desire for interpersonal closeness, a need for affiliation with another being. Discrete limbic lesions can profoundly alter how animals maintain contacts with other members of their own or other species.[41,60,73] For example, rats with septal lesions will remain in contact with each other in an open field and, if left alone, will actively approach cats despite expressions of fear.[73] It is possible that some biologic effects of the epileptogenic process or recurrent seizures in a minority of patients with temporolimbic epilepsy, especially in the dominant hemisphere, fosters the development of viscosity.

Hyposexuality

Various changes in interictal sexual behavior occur in patients with TLE. Hyposexuality is frequently reported,[7,31,35,83,93,98,101,108] with anecdotal reports of hypersexuality[38,98] and deviant sexual behavior including exhibitionism,[7,52] transvestism,[27,84] transsexualism,[50] and fetishism.[26,74] Isolated cases of unusual sexual behavior occurring in patients with epilepsy could be chance associations. However, some cases develop profound changes in adulthood, shortly after the onset of epilepsy, raising the possibility of an etiologic relationship. Hyposexuality, including decreased libido and impotence, occurs in approximately half of TLE patients without gender bias. In many cases, especially those with seizure onset before puberty, patients may not marry or regard hyposexuality as a problem. Complaints are more likely to come from the spouse or parent who observes lack of interest in the opposite sex. Much of the original literature on hyposexuality from 1954 to 1985 was based on self-report[76] without detailed interviews to assess the relative roles of libido, arousal, erectile dysfunction, anorgasmia, and sexual satisfaction, as well as physiologic measures of endocrine and sexual function.

Most studies found higher rates of hyposexuality and sexual dysfunction in TLE than other epilepsy groups, although Fenwick et al.[31] did not observe any significant difference in sexual activity related to seizure type, type of epilepsy, or seizure frequency. Among those with TLE, no laterality effects were found for sexual behavior in left- versus right-sided seizure foci.[16] A well-designed study of six men with erectile dysfunction found abnormal nocturnal penile tumescence and rigidity in five.[44] The pattern of abnormality was consistent with neurogenic, not vasogenic, erectile dysfunction. In a self-report survey of 116 women with epilepsy, partial epilepsy patients experienced more dyspareunia, vaginismus, arousal insufficiency, and sexual dissatisfaction, whereas primary generalized epilepsy (PGE) patients experienced more anorgasmia and sexual dissatisfaction.[75] Sexual symptoms were not associated with seizure frequency, antiepileptic drug (AED) exposure, sexual experience, depression, or prepubertal seizure onset.

The pathogenetic role of temporal lobe seizures in hyposexuality is supported by animal models[30] and observations that sexual activity can increase following successful seizure control with AEDs[83] and temporal lobectomy.[7] In some postlobectomy subjects, marked hypersexuality similar to the Kluver-Bucy syndrome can develop occasionally.[9] However, AEDs modulate hypothalamic-pituitary-gonadal axis hormone activity and can directly inhibit sexual behavior.[64] Barbiturates may cause the greatest decrease in libido and sexual dysfunction.[70] Other hepatic enzyme–inducing AEDs are also associated with decreased testosterone levels and diminished libido and function.[49] Valproic acid is associated with menstrual disorders, hyperandrogenism, and polycystic ovaries.[54,78]

Religiosity

The ancient association between epilepsy and mystical/religious phenomena is paradigmatic of the difficulty reconciling dramatic anecdotes and long-standing medical opinion with limited clinical studies. Hippocrates began his monograph *On the Sacred Disease* by refuting the association between epilepsy and the divine. Despite his modern insights, religious and magical treatments of epilepsy predominated throughout the Middle Ages and Renaissance.[109] In the 19th century, psychiatrists stressed the religiosity of epilepsy patients and observed that Siberian medicine men preferred epileptic pupils.[64] Classic monographs on religious mysticism noted that "among the dread diseases that afflict humanity there is only one that interests us quite particularly; that disease is epilepsy."[64] Intense religious experiences and beliefs are reported frequently by people with epilepsy. Many prominent religious figures allegedly had epilepsy, including prophets and founders of several religions.[116] The evidence supporting epilepsy in these people varies. Intense religious experiences can occur in association with seizures.[13,25,53,66,102]

Dewhurst and Beard[23] reported six TLE patients who underwent sudden religious conversions. There was a clear temporal relationship between conversion and increased seizure activity in five patients; one patient had a marked decrease in seizure frequency prior to conversion (she attributed her improved seizure disorder to the Almighty). Increased religious conviction and practice is not a consistent behavioral feature in patients with epilepsy. There is little evidence that epilepsy or TLE patients as a group are hyperreligious, although a subgroup may have unusually strong religious beliefs. Two studies with questionnaires on religion failed to differentiate patients with right versus left TLE, TLE versus GE, or epilepsy patients and controls.[110,120] However, one study found that patients with smaller right hippocampi had significantly higher ratings on a religiosity scale.[123]

Hypergraphia

Hypergraphia is not characteristic of interictal behavior among TLE or GE patients. However, several studies support that the subgroup manifesting this behavior most intensely are those with temporal lobe foci. Waxman and Geschwind[116] reported seven TLE patients with hypergraphia, which is a tendency toward extensive and sometimes compulsive writing. There was a striking preoccupation with detail—words were defined and redefined and underlined, parentheses were used to make word meaning absolutely clear—and the writers accorded great importance to their material. In four patients, the writings focused on moral and religious concerns. Hypergraphia was viewed as a component of the deepened emotions and especially viscosity of interictal behavioral changes.

Utilizing a mailed standard questionnaire, Sachdev and Waxman[92] demonstrated that TLE patients responded frequently and extensively (mean 1,301 words) as compared to other epilepsy patients (mean 106 words). Hermann et al.[47] replicated the higher response rates and longest letters in the TLE group, but they did not find that the average response was longer in TLE patients compared to other seizure patients. Duration of epilepsy, hypomania, and number of significant life events during the past year positively correlated with hypergraphia.[47,48] Hypergraphia occurs in 7% to 10% of TLE patients.[47,48]

Dostoyevsky was the most famous hypergraphic TLE patient,[39] although his prolific writing also reflected his pay per page and financial troubles. As a person, he was deeply emotional, irritable, angered over minor provocations, guilt ridden, depressed, and tortured over the question of God's existence. He described the relation between his writing and epilepsy in a letter to his brother (August 27, 1849): "Whenever formerly I had such nervous disturbances, I made use of them for writing; in such a state I could write much more and much better than usual."[24]

Aggression

Interictal violence and aggression is a highly contentious topic, especially the relationship between TLE and aggression. There appears to be a relatively elevated incidence of interictal violence and hostility in patients with epilepsy as compared to healthy controls. The neurosurgical series of Serafetinides[97] and of Taylor[107] demonstrated rates of interictal aggression approaching 30% in TLE patients prior to temporal lobectomy. These studies were criticized for selection bias of refractory patients and those with psychiatric presentations. Rodin[91] identified 5% of patients presenting to an epilepsy center as manifesting aggressive behavior. Seizure type did not distinguish aggressive from nonaggressive patients. Gunn and Fenton[45] documented increased prevalence of epilepsy in British prisons relative to the general population. A study of the Illinois prison system documented a prevalence rate of epilepsy of 2.4%, elevated relative to the U.S. population at the time of the study. However, census of prisoners with epilepsy against matched nonepileptic controls did not reveal more serious violent crimes on the part of the epilepsy group.[118]

Violence and hostility in epilepsy is likely a consequence of an interaction of neurophysiologic as well as social factors. Male sex is a risk factor for violence and epilepsy, and Serafetinides noted that aggressiveness as a personality trait in TLE patients was more likely in those with seizure onset prior to age 10 years. Other risk factors identified in the TLE group include premature interruption of formal schooling, lower intellectual quotient, and lower socioeconomic status. These risk factors are associated with a greater risk of aggression in nonepileptic patients as well. Several studies found that ictal and interictal aggression appear to be more common in children than adults with TLE.[43,80,106] More specific neurobiologic factors were identified in a quantitative magnetic resonance imaging (MRI) analysis of mesial temporal structures in epilepsy patients with and without a history of interictal aggression.[112] Those with interictal aggression had less hippocampal atrophy. Two subgroups of those with aggression were identified: Those with severe amygdala atrophy and a history of encephalitis and those with left temporal lesions affecting the amygdala or periamygdaloid regions.[112]

PROBLEMS OF DEFINITION AND METHODOLOGY

Defining specific personality traits and aberrations in patients with epilepsy is difficult and controversial. From a psychiatric standpoint, studies on interictal behavioral changes in epilepsy have not been "discipline neutral."[2] Over the past decades, stereotyped notions of personality attributes in patients with chronic seizures have been dominated by psychoanalysts and those performing trait analyses within the psychometric tradition of self-report methodologies and multivariate statistics. Debates in the literature center on complex personality concepts (e.g., hyperreligiosity) rather than attempt to integrate "first order" biologic variables that underlie the causality of complex behaviors (vide infra).

Considering the variety of epilepsy syndromes and their many etiologies, correlation of interictal behavior with a specific physiologic process or anatomic locus is difficult. Many studies on behavior and epilepsy were done before video-electroencephalographic (V-EEG) confirmation of a specific ictal onset zone and without high-resolution MRI. Many authors simplistically approach "TLE" as a monolithic entity primarily involving mesiotemporal structures. Analyses and speculations thereby focus exclusively on limbic-affective states. However, subdural grid electrode recordings frequently document TLE seizure onsets from neocortical extralimbic regions in isolation or together with mesial structures.[58,68] Even when invasive monitoring documents a temporal lobe "focus," there often is associated extratemporal glucose hypometabolism as defined by positron emission tomography (PET).[57] In patients with TLE, as an illustration, prefrontal metabolic asymmetry is associated with cognitive impairment and depression.[12,57]

Identifying behavioral changes confined to the interictal period is another methodologic challenge. Preictal (premonitory), postictal, and interictal behavioral alterations are less well circumscribed temporally than ictal changes. In the extreme case of partial status epilepticus, cognitive impairments form a continuum despite EEG evolution from discrete seizures to periodic discharges and finally re-emergence of normal EEG background.[88] For isolated seizures, transitions between ictal, preictal, postictal, and interictal behavioral states can be fluid, and clinical distinctions made may be artificial. These behavioral changes may morph over time and extend from their initial extent during the postictal period to more continuous disorders that fill the interictal periods.[105]

Studies from the pre-MRI/pre–V-EEG era are limited by methodologic issues, including the diagnosis of epilepsy (e.g., nonepileptic events), syndromic diagnosis (e.g., benign rolandic epilepsy vs. TLE in a child), and localization of the seizure focus (e.g., frontal vs. temporal), which may all be more problematic in older than more recent studies. Before high-resolution MRI, structural lesions such as cortical dysplasias, vascular malformations, and low-grade neoplasms were not identified. Studies of TLE patients in the pre-MRI era likely included patients with erroneous localization and lateralization.

Finally, past behavioral analysis of the population with epilepsy focused on personality structure rarely assessed lifetime developmental, antiepileptic drug, or other variables.[14,79,96,104]

INTERICTAL BEHAVIORAL CHANGES IN OTHER EPILEPSY SYNDROMES

Personality Changes in Primary Generalized Epilepsy

Personality changes in epilepsy are not restricted to patients with partial epilepsy; they also occur in patients with PGE syndromes such as juvenile myoclonic epilepsy (JME)[55] and absence epilepsy.[100] In JME, reported traits included irresponsibility and impaired impulse control, neglect of duties, self-interest, emotional instability, exaggeration, inconsiderateness, quick temper, and distractibility. Janz[55] found that many JME patients repeatedly exposed themselves to sleep deprivation and often failed to comply with AEDs, taking their illness lightly. They denied problems and conflicts, or often yielded to temptation against better judgment. There was limited support for Janz's clinical impression,[5] although scientific evidence is sparse and some of these behaviors may reflect adolescence, not JME. Other studies found high rates of psychiatric disorders among patients with JME.[82,113] Gelisse et al.[37] reported 45 (26.5%) of 170 consecutive JME patients with psychiatric disorders. Twenty-four of these 45 patients had personality disorders, including borderline (11 cases), dependent (five cases), histrionic (two cases), obsessive-compulsive (one case), and not otherwise specified (five cases).

Absence epilepsy, long considered one of the most benign forms of epilepsy, recently has been associated with significant behavioral changes in a very well-controlled study. Wirrell et al.[122] compared all children in Nova Scotia with typical absence epilepsy or juvenile rheumatoid arthritis (JRA) diagnosed between 1986 and 1997, who were aged 18 years or older at follow-up (mean age 23 years). Remission occurred in 32 (57%) of the patients with typical absence epilepsy but in only 17 (28%) of the patients with JRA. Five categories of outcome were studied: Academic-personal, behavioral, employment-financial, family relations, and social-personal relations. Patients with typical absence epilepsy had greater difficulties in the academic-personal and in the behavioral categories (p <0.001) than those with JRA. Those with ongoing seizures had the least favorable outcome. Most seizure-related factors showed minimal correlation with psychosocial functioning. Even patients whose epilepsy had remitted had significantly poorer outcomes than the JRA patients in the academic-personal and behavioral domains. Another recent study found that 54% of pediatric patients with PGE had psychiatric disorders.[12] Early age of onset and poor seizure control were significantly associated with the severity of illogical thinking in these children. Thus, the recent literature strongly supports prior research that PGE is a risk factor for cognitive and behavioral problems.

Personality Changes in Patients with Frontal Lobe Epilepsy

The frontal lobes are important in personality, as highlighted by the effects of prefrontal surgeries. Thus, as limbic disorders can alter emotion- and drive-related behavior (e.g., sex and aggression), frontal dysfunction can alter personality, judgment, and executive functions. Further, the posterior orbitofrontal cortex and anterior cingulate gyrus, two critical limbic (paralimbic) areas, are located within the frontal lobe. Patients with anterior cingulate seizure foci can develop interictal psychosis, aggression, sociopathic behavior, sexual deviancy, irritability, obsessive-compulsive disorder, and poor impulse control.[3,19,21,71] Orbitofrontal lesions can cause hyperphagia, failure to use autonomic cues to guide behavior, aberrant emotional responsiveness, increased aggression, dysfunctional social behavior (e.g., case of Phineas Gage[16,97]), behavioral disinhibition, and confabulation.[20] Systematic studies on interictal behavior in patients with orbitofrontal seizure foci are lacking; however, behavioral disorders such as attention deficit hyperactivity disorder can occur.[85] Given the critical role of this limbic cortex in social and emotional behavior, epileptic foci in this site could cause prominent interictal behavioral changes.

In the Vietnam Head Injury Study,[103] patients with tonic–clonic seizures had a higher frequency of psychiatric treatment than those with complex partial seizures, possibly reflecting greater frontal lobe involvement. The role of the frontal lobe in the personality and behavior of epileptic patients deserves greater attention. Functional imaging studies suggest that, even among patients with temporal lobe seizure foci, frontal dysfunction contributes to affective, personality, and cognitive disorders.[11,82,94]

CHARACTERIZING THE INTERICTAL BEHAVIOR SYNDROME

The Bear Fedio Inventory

In the original study using this measure, all 18 self-rated traits were significantly higher in the TLE group than in neurologic and healthy controls. The most significant differences (p <0.0001) were humorlessness, circumstantiality, dependence, and sense of personal destiny. Proxy raters (i.e., family or friends) identified TLE patients as significantly different from controls on 14 traits, most strongly (p <0.0001) for circumstantiality, obsessionalism, and dependence. Patients with right temporal foci reported more emotional traits and minimized their behavioral changes (i.e., polished their image), whereas patients with left temporal foci had more ideational traits and often tarnished their image on self-report relative to proxy reports. The previously reported associations of right hemisphere lesions with denial and neglect syndromes and left hemisphere lesions with depression[33,34,89,90] were consistent with the right/left:polish/tarnish correlation.

Replication studies using the Bear Fedio Inventory (BFI) have produced mixed results.[11,22,46,77] Use of the BFI generally reveals increased rates of these behavioral traits in patients with epilepsy (TLE and GE) in comparison to healthy controls or some medical patients, but it does not distinguish epilepsy (TLE or GE) from psychiatric patients. Findings from TLE versus GE patient comparisons are inconsistent. When differences are present, the TLE group usually has higher scores than the GE group. Left–right differences in TLE are typically minor.

The complicating issue of frontal lobe seizure foci or frontal lobe involvement (e.g., seizure spread or interictal hypometabolism/neuronal dysfunction) should also be considered in patients with TLE. Although personality disorders are highlighted in the literature as elements of TLE, they would be expected to be features of frontal lobe epilepsy (FLE) as well. Indeed, in the literature on the BFI, the study by Wieser[119] was the only one to use invasive electrodes for localization and lateralization, and failed to replicate any laterality effects found by Bear and Fedio.[5] Interestingly, Wieser found a significant increase in humorlessness in the FLE group and a nonsignificant trend for an increase in all BFI behavioral traits in the FLE group.

The studies with the BFI nearly vanished after 1990, just as high-resolution MRI and V-EEG monitoring allowed more confident anatomic and physiologic diagnoses. As the BFI fell out of favor, so did much of the research on personality in epilepsy patients. Consequently, the subject of personality changes in epilepsy warrants further study.

The Neurobehavioral Inventory (NBI) is a more recent tool to specifically assess interictal psychopathology in epilepsy patients.[8] There has been relatively little use of the NBI, but it may prove valuable. In one study, patients with high ratings on the NBI religiosity scale had smaller hippocampi, while in another study, hyposexuality and hypergraphia were associated with bilateral hippocampal atrophy.[111]

Mazzini et al.[72] evaluated 143 patients with traumatic brain injury (TBI), of which 27 developed posttraumatic epilepsy (PTE), using another measure—the Neurobehavioral Rating Scale (NBHRS)—along with the Minnesota Multiphasic Personality Inventory (MMPI), Overt Aggression Scale, Back Depression Inventory (BDI), and *Diagnostic and Statistical Manual of Mental Disorders,* 4th ed. (DSM-IV) definitions for personality disorders. Patients with epilepsy showed a significantly higher incidence of severe personality disorders. Disinhibited behavior, irritability, and agitated and aggressive behavior were significantly more frequent and severe in PTE patients.

Feddersen et al.[29] examined 37 TLE patients, 38 with idiopathic generalized epilepsy with absence and generalized tonic–clonic seizures and 25 healthy controls using the Freiburg Personality Inventory/Form A (FPI-A-H)[28] and the Index of Personality Characteristics (IPC).[62] Patients with left TLE had increased emotional dependency, less externally judged composedness, increased depressive drive and mood, increased nervousness, increased search for information and exchange of disease experience, and greater tendency to persevere ($p < 0.05$). This study supported the differentiation made by Bear and Fedio[4] that patients with left TLE are more rational and tarnish their image, whereas patients with right TLE are more emotional and polish their image.

One study with the Millon Behavioral Health Inventory (MBHI) found that epilepsy patients have deficient coping styles.[115] Patients with epilepsy obtained higher scores on scales assessing inhibition and sensitivity and lower scores on scales evaluating sociability and confidence.

DSM AXIS II Disorders

Another approach to examining personality disorder in epilepsy is to turn to formal DSM-IV Axis II diagnoses. By definition, personality disorders are characterized by long-lasting patterns of thought and behavior that deviate from cultural expectations, inflexible and pervasive in nature, that result in impairment of function. To receive a diagnosis of personality disorder, the pattern of behavior must result in significant distress or impairment in personal, social, or occupational situations. Several criteria must be met in addition to the specific criteria for individually named personality disorders. These include the following:

1. Experience and behavior that deviates markedly from the expectations of the individual's culture. This pattern is manifested in two (or more) areas including cognition, affectivity, interpersonal functioning, and impulse control.
2. The enduring pattern is inflexible and pervasive across a broad range of personal and social situations.
3. The enduring pattern leads to clinically significant distress or impairment in social, occupational, or other important areas of functioning.
4. The pattern is stable and of long duration and its onset can be traced back at least to adolescence or early adulthood.
5. The enduring pattern is not better accounted for as a manifestation or consequence of another mental disorder.
6. The enduring pattern is not due to the direct physiologic effects of a substance or a general medical condition such as head injury.

There are ten specific personality disorders in DSM-IV, which are grouped into three clusters: *Cluster A* (odd or eccentric disorders) includes paranoid personality disorder, schizoid personality disorder, and schizotypal personality disorder; *cluster B* (dramatic, emotional, or erratic disorders) includes antisocial personality disorder, borderline personality disorder, histrionic personality disorder, and narcissistic personality disorder; and *cluster C* (anxious or fearful disorders) includes avoidant personality disorder, dependent personality disorder, and obsessive-compulsive personality disorder. Finally, *personality disorder NOS* is a category for behavior patterns that do not match these ten disorders but have the characteristics of a personality disorder.

A series of investigations have assessed Axis II disorders (not including mental retardation) in patients with epilepsy using contemporary diagnostic procedures. As can be seen in Table 2, the rate of Axis II disorders range from 18% to 61% across studies, with a mean of 31% (median = 21%). Only two studies incorporated controls. These rates are elevated overall and investigations that examined the distribution of clusters A through C reveal that most individuals with epilepsy with Axis II disorders exhibit cluster C disorders. Even biologically oriented researchers recognize that problems associated with living with epilepsy, particularly early-onset epilepsy, may lead to dependant and avoidant personality traits, although this contention has not been examined empirically.

Axis II disorders are probably underrecognized and incompletely addressed in the traditional clinic setting (Table 3). There is little information regarding their consequences, but

TABLE 2

RATE OF PERSONALITY DISORDERS IN EPILEPSY

Schwartz and Cummings (1988)[95]	38% (4% controls)
Fiordelli et al. (1993)[32]	21% (0% controls)
Victoroff (1994)[114]	18%
Manchanda et al. (1996)[69]	18%
Arnold and Privitera (1996)[1]	18%
Lopez-Rodriguez et al. (1999)[65]	21%
Krishnamoorthy et al. (2001)[63]	47%
Koch-Stoecker (2002)[59a]	61%
Galimberti et al. (2003)[33a]	38%

TABLE 3

DISTRIBUTION OF SPECIFIC PERSONALITY DISORDERS IN EPILEPSY

Authors	N	A	B	C	Procedure
Lopez-Rodriguez et al. 1999	52	0.0%	5.8%	15.4%	SCID-II
Galimberti et al. 2003	69	1.4%	10.1%	26.0%	SCID-II
Koch-Stoecker et al. 2002	100	6.0%	15.0%	24.0%	DSM-III-R
Krishnamoorthy et al. 2001	35	17.1%	2.9%	22.9%	SAP

SCID-II Structured Clinical Interview for DSM-IV-TR
DSM-III-R Diagnostic and Statistical Manual of Mental Disorders-III-R
PSE Present State Examination
A Cluster A; odd or eccentric disorders
B Cluster B; dramatic, emotional, or erratic disorders
C Cluster C; anxious or fearful disorders

the evidence available suggests that they are of consequence. Koch-Stoecker examined the predictors of postoperative psychiatric complications in 100 patients who underwent anterior temporal lobectomy (ATL).[59a] Patients were assessed for Axis I and II disorders preoperatively. Fourteen percent of their surgical patients were hospitalized for psychiatric reasons postoperatively and all these patients exhibited Axis II disorders preoperatively, either alone of in combination with Axis I disorders. No patients with just an Axis I disorder underwent postoperative psychiatric hospitalization.

Another indication of the maladaptive consequences associated with adverse personality features is demonstrated by Derry et al., who examined the impact of neuroticism on postoperative course in 45 individual ATL patients.[18] Those who were high in preoperative neuroticism exhibited significantly worse postoperative psychosocial adjustment and quality of life.

SUMMARY AND CONCLUSIONS

Personality disorders and other, less pathologic personality changes are common and often unrecognized in epilepsy patients. These disorders likely result from biologic factors such as structural and physiologic abnormalities as well as social and emotional factors. The specificity of certain personality traits or clusters and anatomic seizure foci (e.g., TLE or FLE) and epilepsy syndromes (e.g., partial vs. generalized) remains controversial, mired in methodologic issues and limited by a literature that often predated MRI and V-EEG studies. However, traits such as hypergraphia, although present in <10% of TLE patients, appear to be much more common in this form of epilepsy than others. Patients with FLE and idiopathic generalized epilepsy can also develop behavioral changes and personality disorders that can significantly impact their lives. The area remains ripe for additional studies using modern psychiatric and neurologic diagnostic tools.

References

1. Arnold LM, Privetera MD. Psychopathology and trauma in epileptic and psychogenic seizure patients. *Psychosomatics*. 1996;37:438–443.
2. Barratt ES, Kent T, Stanford MJ. Biologic variables defining and measuring personality. In: Rately JJ, ed. *Neuropsychiatry of Personality Disorders*. Oxford: Blackwell Science; 1995:36–37.
3. Bear D, Levin K, Blumer D, et al. Interictal behavior. I. Hospitalized temporal lobe epileptics: relationship to idiopathic psychiatric syndrome. *J Neurol Neurosurg Psychiatry*. 1982;45:481–488.
4. Bear DM, Fedio P. Quantitative analysis of interictal behavior in temporal lobe epilepsy. *Arch Neurol*. 1977;34:454–467.
5. Bech P, Pedersen KK, Simonsen N, et al. Personality in epilepsy. *Acta Neurol Scand*. 1976;54:348–358.
6. Benson DF. The Geschwind syndrome. *Adv Neurol*. 1991;55:411–421.
7. Blumer D, Walker EA. Sexual behavior in temporal lobe epilepsy. *Arch Neurol*. 1967;16;37–43.
8. Blumer D. The neurobehavioral inventory: personality disorders in epilepsy. In: Ratey JJ, ed. *Neuropsychiatry of Personality Disorders*. Boston: Blackwell Science; 1995:230–263.
9. Blumer D. Hypersexual episodes in temporal lobe epilepsy. *Am J Psychiatry*. 1970;126:1099–1106.
10. Brandt J, Seidman LJ, Kohl D. Personality characteristics of epileptic patients: a controlled study of generalized and temporal lobe cases. *J Clin Exp Neuropsychol*. 1985;7:25–38.
11. Bromfield EB, Altshuler L, Leiderman DB, et al. Cerebral metabolism and depression in patients with complex partial seizures. *Epilepsia*. 1990;31:625–626.
12. Caplan R, Arbelle S, Guthrie D, et al. Formal thought disorder and psychopathology in pediatric primary generalized and complex partial epilepsy. *J Am Acad Child Adolesc Psychiatry*. 1997;36:1286–1294.
13. Cirignotta F, Todesco CV, Lugaresi E. Temporal lobe epilepsy with ecstatic seizures (so-called Dostoyevsky epilepsy). *Epilepsia*. 1980;21:705–710.
14. Csernansky JG, Leiderman DB, Mandabach M, et al. Psychopathology and limbic epilepsy: relationship to seizure variables and neuropsychological function. *Epilepsia*. 1990;31:275–280.
15. Damasio H, Grabowski T, Frank R, et al. The return of Phineas Gage: clues about the brain from the skull of a famous patient. *Science*. 1994;264:1102–1105.
16. Daniele A, Azzoni A, Bizzi A, et al. Sexual behavior and hemispheric laterality of the focus in patients with temporal lobe epilepsy. *Biol Psychiatry*. 1997;42:617–624.
17. Delay J, Pichot P, Lemperiere T, et al. *The Rorschach and the Epileptic Personality*. New York: Logos Press; 1958.
18. Derry PA, Rose KJ, McLachlan RS. Moderators of the affect of seizure symptoms on MMPI-2 clinical interpretation. *J Clin Psychol*. 2002;58:817–826.
19. Devinsky O, Abramson H, Alper K, et al. Postictal psychosis: a case control series of 20 patients and 150 controls. *Epilepsy Res*. 1995;20:247–253.
20. Devinsky O, D'Esposito M. *The Neurology of Cognition and Behavior*. New York: Oxford University Press; 2004:330–317.
21. Devinsky O, Morrell M, Bogt B. Contribution of anterior cingulate cortex to behavior. *Brain*. 1995;118:279–306.
22. Devinsky O, Theodore WH, eds. *Epilepsy and Behavior*. New York: Wiley-Liss; 1991.
23. Dewhurst K, Beard AW. Sudden religious conversions in temporal lobe epilepsy. *Br J Psychiatry*. 1970;117:497–507.
24. Dostoyevsky FM. *Letters of Fyodor Michailovitch Dostoevsky to His Family and Friends. Mayne EC, translator*. New York: Macmillan; 1915.
25. Dostoyevsky FM. *The Idiot*. Magarshack D, translator. London: Penguin Books; 1955.
26. Epstein AW. Fetishism: a study of its psychopathology with particular reference to a proposed disorder in brain mechanisms as an etiologic factor. *J Nerv Ment Dis*. 1960;23:247–249.
27. Epstein AW. Relationship of fetishism and transvestism to brain and particularly to temporal lobe dysfunction. *J Nerv Ment Dis*. 1961;133:247–253.
28. Fahrenberg J, Selg H, Hempel R. *Das Freiburger Personlichkeitsinventar FPI*. Gottingen: Hogrefe Verlag; 1973.
29. Feddersen B, Herzer R, Hartmann U, et al. On the psychopathology of unilateral temporal lobe epilepsy. *Epilepsy Behav*. 2005;6:43–49.
30. Feeney DM, Gullotta FP, Gilmore W. Hyposexuality produced by temporal lobe epilepsy in the cat. *Epilepsia*. 1998;39:140–149.
31. Fenwick PBC, Toone BK, Wheeler MJ, et al. Sexual behavior in a centre for epilepsy. *Acta Neurol Scand*. 1985;71:428–435.
32. Fiordelli E, Beghi E, Boglium G, et al. Epilepsy and psychiatric disturbance. *Brit J Psychiatry*. 1993;163:446–460.
33. Gainotti G. Emotional behavior and hemispheric side of lesion. *Cortex*. 1972;8:41–45.

33a. Galimberti CA, Ratti MT, Murelli R, et al. Patients with psychogenic nonepileptic seizures, alone or epilepsy-associated, share a psychological profile distinct from that of epilepsy. *J Neurol.* 2003;250:338–346.
34. Galin D. Implications for psychiatry of left and right cerebral specialization. *Arch Gen Psychiatry.* 1974;31:572–583.
35. Gastaut H, Collomb H. Etude du comportement sexuel chez les epileptiques psychomoteurs. *Ann Med Psychol (Paris).* 1954;112:657–696.
36. Gastaut H, Morin G, Leserve N. Etude du comportement des épileptiques psycho-moteurs dans l'intervalle de leurs crises. *Ann Medico-Psychol.* 1955;113:1–27.
37. Gelisse P, Genton P, Samuelian JC, et al. Psychiatric disorders in juvenile myoclonic epilepsy. *Rev Neurol.* 2001;157:2907–2302
38. Geschwind N, Shader RI, Bear D, et al. Behavioral changes with temporal lobe epilepsy: assessment and treatment. *J Clin Psychiatry.* 1980;41:89–95.
39. Geschwind N. Dostoyevsky's epilepsy. In: Blumer D, ed. *Psychiatric Aspects of Epilepsy.* Washington, DC: American Psychiatric Press, 1984:325–334. (Dosteyevsky letter, August 27, 1849.)
40. Gibbs FA. Ictal and non-ictal psychiatric disorders in temporal lobe epilepsy. *Nerv Ment Dis.* 1951;113:522–528.
41. Glendenning KK. Effects of septal and amygdaloid lesions on social behavior of the cat. *J Comp Physiol Psychol.* 1972;80:199–207.
42. Gowers WR. *Epilepsy and Other Chronic Convulsive Disorders.* New York: William Wood & Co.; 1885:101.
43. Guimaraes CA, Franzon RC, Souza EA, et al. Abnormal behavior in children with temporal lobe epilepsy and ganglioglioma. *Epilepsy Behav.* 2004;5:788–791.
44. Guldner GT, Morrell MJ. Nocturnal penile tumescence and rigidity evaluation in men with epilepsy. *Epilepsia.* 1996;37:1211–1214.
45. Gunn J, Fenton G. Epilepsy in prisons: a diagnostic survey. *BMJ.* 1969;4:326–328.
46. Hermann BP, Reil P. Interictal personality and behavioral traits in temporal lobe and generalized epilepsy. *Cortex.* 1981;17:125–128.
47. Hermann BP, Whitman S, Arnston P. Hypergraphia in epilepsy: is there a specificity to temporal lobe epilepsy? *J Neurol Neurosurg Psychiatry.* 1983;46:848–853.
48. Hermann BP, Whitman S, Wyler AR, et al. The neurological, psychosocial and demographic correlates of hypergraphia in patients with epilepsy. *J Neurol Neurosurg Psychiatry.* 1988;51:203–208.
49. Herzog AG, Fowler KM. Sexual hormones and epilepsy: threat and opportunities. *Curr Opin Neurol.* 2005;18:167–172.
50. Hoenig J, Kenna JC. EEG abnormalities and transsexualism. *Br J Psychiatry.* 1979;134:293–300.
51. Hoeppner JB, Garron DC, Wilson RS, et al. Epilepsy and verbosity. *Epilepsia.* 1987;28:35–40.
52. Hooshmand H, Brawley BW. Temporal lobe seizures and exhibitionism. *Neurology.* 1969;19:1119–1124.
53. Howden JC. The religious sentiments in epileptics. *J Ment Sci.* 1872–1873;18:491–497.
54. Isojarvi JI, Laatikainen TJ, Pakarinen AJ, et al. Polycystic ovaries and hyperandrogenism in women taking valproate for epilepsy. *N Engl J Med.* 1993;329:1383–1388.
55. Janz D. *Die epilepsien.* Stuttgart: Georg Thieme; 1969.
56. Jensen I, Larsen JK. Mental aspects of temporal lobe epilepsy. *J Neurol Neurosurg Psychiatry.* 1979;42:256–265.
57. Jokeit H, Seitz RJ, Markowitsch HJ, et al. Prefrontal asymmetric interictal glucose hypometabolism and cognitive impairment in patients with temporal lobe epilepsy. *Brain.* 1997;120:2283–2294.
58. Jung WY, Pacia SV, Devinsky O. Neocortical temporal lobe epilepsy: intracranial EEG features and surgical outcome. *J Clin Neurophysiol.* 1999;16:419–425.
59. Kluver H, Bray PC. Preliminary analysis of functions of the temporal lobe in monkeys. *Arch Neurol Psychiatry.* 1939;42:979–1002.
59a. Koch-Stoecker S. Personality disorders as predictors of severe postsurgical psychiatric complications in epilepsy patients undergoing temporal lobe resections. *Epilepsy Behav.* 2002;3:526–531.
60. Kolb B, Nonneman AJ. Frontolimbic lesions and social behavior in the rat. *Physiol Behav.* 1974;13:637–643.
61. Kraepelin E. *Lectures on Clinical Psychiatry.* 3rd ed. New York: William Wood & Col.; 1913.
62. Krampen G. *IPC-Fragebogen zu Kontrollueberzeugungen.* Gottingen/Toronto/Zurich: Verlag fur Psychologie; 1981.
63. Krishnamoorthy EA, Brown RJ, Trimble MR. Personality and psychopathology in nonepileptic attack disorder and epilepsy. *Epilepsy Behav.* 2001;2:418–422.
64. Leuba JH. *The Psychology of Religious Mysticism.* London: Kegan Paul, Trench, Trubner & Co.; 1925:204.
65. Lopez-Rodriguez F, Altschuler L, Kay J, et al. Personality disorder among medically refractory epileptic patients. *J Neuropsych Clin Neurosci.* 1999;11:464–469.
66. Mabille H. Hallucinations religieuses et delire religieux transitoire dans l'epilepsie. *Ann Medico-Psychol.* 1899;9/10:76–81.
67. MacLean PD. *The Evolution of the Triune Brain.* New York: Plenum; 1990.
68. Maillard L, Vignal JP, Gavaret M, et al. Semiologic and electrophysiologic correlations in temporal lobe seizure subtypes. *Epilepsia.* 2004;45:1590–1599.
69. Manchanda R, Schaefer B, McLachlan RS, et al. Psychiatric disorders in candidates for surgery for epilepsy. *J Neurol Neurosurg Psychiatry.* 1996;61:82–89.
70. Mattson RH, Cramer JA, Collins JF, et al. Comparison of carbamazepine, phenobarbital, phenytoin, and primidone in partial and secondarily generalized tonic-clonic seizures. *N Engl J Med.* 1985;313:145–151.
71. Mazars G. Criteria for identifying cingulate epilepsies. *Epilepsia.* 1970; 11:41–47.
72. Mazzini L, Cossa FM, Angelino E, et al. Posttraumatic epilepsy: neuroradiologic and neuropsychological assessment of long-term outcome. *Epilepsia.* 2003;44(4):569–574.
73. Meyer DR, Ruth RA, Lavond DG. The septal social cohesiveness effect: its robustness and main determinants. *Physiol Behav.* 1978;21:1027–1029.
74. Mitchell W, Falconer MA, Hill D. Epilepsy with fetishism relieved by temporal lobectomy. *Lancet.* 1954;2:626–630.
75. Morrell MJ, Guldner GT. Self-reported sexual function and sexual arousability in women with epilepsy. *Epilepsia.* 1996;37:1204–1210.
76. Morrell MJ. Sexual dysfunction in epilepsy. *Epilepsia.* 1991;32[Suppl 6]: S38–S45.
77. Mungas D. Interictal behavior abnormality in temporal lobe epilepsy: a specific syndrome or nonspecific psychopathology. *Arch Gen Psychiatry.* 1982;39:108–111.
78. Murialdo G, Galimberti CA, Magri F, et al. Menstrual cycle and ovary alterations in women with epilepsy on antiepileptic therapy. *J Endocrinol Invest.* 1997;20:519–526.
79. Nielsen H, Kristensen O. Personality correlates of sphenoidal EEG foci in temporal lobe epilepsy. *Acta Neurol Scand.* 1981;64:289–300.
80. Ounstead C. Aggression and epilepsy: rage in children with temporal lobe epilepsy. *J Psychosom Res.* 1969;13:237–242.
81. Papez JW. A proposed mechanism of emotion. *Arch Neurol Psychiatry.* 1937;38:725–743.
82. Perini GI, Tosin C, Carraro C, et al. Interictal mood and personality disorders in temporal lobe epilepsy and juvenile myoclonic epilepsy. *J Neurol Neurosurg Psychiatry.* 1996;61:601–605.
83. Peters UH. Sexualstorungen bei psychomotorischer Epilepsie. *J Neurovis Relat.* 1971;[Suppl 10]:491–497.
84. Petritzer BK, Foster J. A case study of a male transvestite with epilepsy and juvenile diabetes. *J Nerv Ment Dis.* 1955;121:557–563.
85. Powell AL, Yudd A, Zee P, et al. Attention deficit hyperactivity disorder associated with orbitofrontal epilepsy in a father and a son. *Neuropsychiatry Neuropsychol Behav Neurol.* 1997;10:151–154.
86. Rao SM, Devinsky O, Grafman J, et al. Viscosity in complex partial seizures: relationship to cerebral laterality and seizure duration. *J Neurol Neurosurg Psychiatry.* 1992;55:149–152.
87. Reynolds JR. *Epilepsy: Its Symptoms, Treatment, and Relation to Other Chronic Convulsive Disorders.* London: Churchill; 1861:39–77.
88. Ritaccio AL, March GR. The significance of BIPLEDS in complex partial status epilepticus. *Am J Electroencephalogr Technol.* 1993;33:27–34.
89. Robertson MM, Trimble MR, Townsend HRA. The phenomenology of depression in epilepsy. *Epilepsia.* 1987;28:364–372.
90. Rodin E, Schmaltz S. The Bear-Fedio personality inventory and temporal lobe epilepsy. *Neurology.* 1984;34:591–596.
91. Rodin EA. Psychomotor epilepsy and aggressive behavior. *Arch Gen Psychiatry.* 1973;28:210–213.
92. Sachdev HS, Waxman SG. Frequency of hypergraphia in temporal lobe epilepsy: an index of interictal behavior syndrome. *J Neurol Neurosurg Psychiatry.* 1981;44:358–360.
93. Saunders M, Rawson M. Sexuality in male epileptics. *J Neurol Sci.* 1970;10:577–583.
94. Schmitz EB, Moriarty J, Costa DC, et al. Psychiatric profiles and patterns of cerebral blood flow in focal epilepsy: interactions between depression, obsessionality, and perfusion related to the laterality of the epilepsy. *J Neurol Neurosurg Psychiatry.* 1997;62:458–463.
95. Schwartz, J, Cummings JL. Psychopathology and epilepsy: an outpatient consultation-liaison experience. *Psychosomatics.* 1988;29:295–300.
96. Seidman L. Lateralized cerebral dysfunction, personality, and cognition in temporal lobe epilepsy. Ph.D. thesis, University of Michigan, University Microfilms International, Ann Arbor, MI, 1980.
97. Serafetinides EA. Aggressiveness in temporal lobe epileptics and its relation to cerebral dysfunction and environmental factors. *Epilepsia.* 1965;6:33–42.
98. Shukla GD, Hrivastava ON, Katiyar BC. Sexual disturbances in temporal lobe epilepsy: a controlled study. *Br J Psychiatry.* 1979;134:288–292.
99. Sjobring H. Ixophreni. In: *Psykologisk-pedagogisk uppslagsbok.* Bd. 2. Stockholm; 1944. Quoted and translated by Gudmundsson.
100. Small JG, Milstein V, Stevens JR. Are psychomotor epileptics different? A controlled study. *Arch Neurol.* 1962;7:187–194.
101. Spark RF, Wills CA, Royal H. Hypogonadism, hyperprolactinemia, and temporal lobe epilepsy in hyposexual men. *Lancet.* 1984;1:413–416.
102. Spratling WP. *Epilepsy and Its Treatment.* New York: WB Saunders; 1904:473–474.
103. Swanson SJ, Rao SM, Grafman J, et al. The relationship between seizure type and interictal personality. Results from the Vietnam Head Injury Study. *Brain.* 1995;118:91–103.

104. Swinkels WAM, Duijsens IJ, Spinhoven Ph. Personality disorder traits in patients with epilepsy. *Seizure*. 2003;12:587–594.
105. Tarulli A, Devinsky O, Alper K. Progression of postictal to interictal psychosis. *Epilepsia*. 2001;42:1468–1471.
106. Tassinari CA, Tassi L, Calandra-Buonaura G, et al. Biting behavior, aggression, and seizures. *Epilepsia*. 2005;46:654–663.
107. Taylor DC. Aggression and epilepsy. *J Psychosom Res*. 1969;13:229–236.
108. Taylor DC. Sexual behavior and temporal lobe epilepsy. *Arch Neurol*. 1979;21:510–516.
109. Temkin O. *The Falling Sickness*. 2nd ed. Baltimore: Johns Hopkins University Press; 1971.
110. Tucker DM, Novelly RA, Walker PJ. Hyperreligiosity in temporal lobe epilepsy: redefining the relationship. *J Nerv Ment Dis*. 1987;175: 181–184.
111. van Elst LT, Krishnamoorthy ES, Baumer D, et al. Psychopathological profile in patients with severe bilateral hippocampal atrophy and temporal lobe epilepsy: evidence in support of the Geschwind syndrome? *Epilepsy Behav*. 2003;4:291–297.
112. van Elst LT, Woermann FG, Lemieux L, et al. Affective aggression in patients with temporal lobe epilepsy: a quantitative MRI study of the amygdala. *Brain*. 2000;123:234–243.
113. Vazquez B, Devinsky O, Luciano D, et al. Juvenile myoclonic epilepsy: clinical features and factors related to misdiagnosis. *J Epilepsy*. 1993;6:233–238.
114. Victoroff J. DSM-III-R psychiatric diagnoses in candidates for epilepsy surgery: lifetime prevalence. *Neuropsych Neuropsych Behav Neurology*. 1994;7(2):87–97.
115. Watten VP, Watten RG. Psychological profiles in patients with medically refractory epilepsy. *Seizure*. 1999;8(5):304–309.
116. Waxman SG, Geschwind N. Hypergraphia in temporal lobe epilepsy. *Neurology*. 1974;24:629–631.
117. Waxman SG, Geschwind N. The interictal behavior syndrome in temporal lobe epilepsy. *Arch Gen Psychiatry*. 1975;32:1580–1586.
118. Whitman S, Coleman TE, Patmon C, et al. Epilepsy in prison: elevated prevalence and no relationship to violence. *Neurology*. 1984;6:775–782.
119. Wieser HG. Selective amygdalohippocampectomy: indications, investigative technique and results. *Adv Tech Stand Neurosurg*. 1986;13:39–133.
120. Willmore LJ, Heilman KM, Fennell E, et al. Affects of chronic seizures on religiosity. *Trans Am Neurol Assoc*. 1980;105:85–87.
121. Wilson SAK. *Neurology*. Baltimore: Williams & Wilkins; 1940:1486.
122. Wirrell EC, Camfield CS, Camfield PR, et al. Long-term psychosocial outcome in typical absence epilepsy. Sometimes a wolf in sheep's clothing. *Arch Pediatr Adolesc Med*. 1997;151:152–158.
123. Wuerfel J, Krishnamoorthy ES, Brown RJ, et al. Religiosity is associated with hippocampal but not amygdala volumes in patients with refractory epilepsy. *J Neurol Neurosurg Psychiatry*. 2004;75:640–642.
124. Yakovlev PI. Motility, behavior and the brain: stereodynamic organization and neural coordinates in behavior. *J Nerv Ment Dis*. 1948;107: 313–335.

CHAPTER 204 ■ SCHIZOPHRENIA AND OTHER PSYCHOSES

MICHAEL R. TRIMBLE AND BETTINA SCHMITZ

INTRODUCTION

Because the brain is the central organ that regulates behavior, a change of behavior may come about with disturbances of the brain, either through alteration of its structure or via functional change, functional here being used in its original meaning to emphasize disturbance of brain function.[92] Neurologists interested in behavioral disorders have mainly concerned themselves with patients with lesions that cause structural changes, whereas psychiatrists have dealt more with the consequences of disturbed function, where underlying structural lesions have been more difficult to discern. Epilepsy is one of a number of conditions in which there is often an underlying structural abnormality to be found if the appropriate technique is used (e. g., neuropathology, magnetic resonance imaging), but profound functional changes also occur, either as a consequence or independently. These may be reflected in the seizure, one manifestation of the epilepsy process, but may also be associated with some of the less dramatic but nonetheless clinically significant behavioral manifestations of epilepsy.

DEFINITIONS AND PHENOMENOLOGY

Psychosis, as used in the International Classification of Diseases (ICD)-10,[25] defines a disorder with the presence of "hallucinations, delusions, or a limited number of severe abnormalities of behavior, such as gross excitement and overactivity, marked psychomotor retardation, and catatonic behavior." In the *Diagnostic and Statistical Manual of Mental Disorders,* 4th ed. (DSM-IV), the term psychotic refers to delusions, any prominent hallucinations, disorganized speech, or disorganized or catatonic behavior.[7]

Hallucinations and delusions, the hallmark of psychosis, suggest some deviant neurologic processing, underlying which are usually structural but sometimes solely functional alterations of activity. Although in epilepsy hallucinations and delusions may be experienced in certain settings for which patients have clear insight, in the majority of cases insight is lacking, and the condition is truly psychotic.

HISTORICAL BACKGROUND

In the middle of the 19th century, European psychiatrists noted the high incidence of psychotic episodes in institutionalized patients with epilepsy. Several authors described the specific psychopathology of psychiatric complications occurring in the context of epilepsy using such terms as "épilepsie lavvée,"[50] "grand mal intellectual,"[9] "epileptoid states,"[18] and "epileptic equivalents."[24] Samt[62] put forward the idea that the pathophysiology of certain psychoses occurring in the context of epilepsy, especially episodic twilight states, was identical to the pathophysiology of motor seizures. He suggested that in the absence of epileptic seizures, such epileptic equivalents could be sufficient for a diagnosis of epilepsy.

Some authors in the 19th century explicitly noted the rarity of chronic paranoia or true madness in patients with epilepsy. These observations resulted in intensive discussions on the nature of the relationship between epilepsy and schizophrenia, a subject frequently chosen in theoretical disputes on definitions of terms such as disease and symptom complex in psychiatry at the beginning of the 20th century.[20,30]

Combined seizures and schizophrenialike symptoms have generally been interpreted either as symptomatic seizures secondary to cerebral sequelae of insanity—for example, brain edema in catatonia—or as symptomatic psychoses caused by seizures or the underlying epileptic process.[32,36] In cases with no obvious temporal relationship between epileptic seizures and psychotic symptoms, it was speculated that both were not directly linked but were caused by the same underlying brain pathology.[54,73] Ganter,[13] Krapf,[32] and Glaus[16] published clinical case series with prevalence rates of combinations lower than expected. These studies, together with observations of alternating periods with seizures and seizure-free periods with psychosis in some patients and the improvement of psychotic symptoms after spontaneous seizures in others, led to the theory of functional dependency and biologic antagonism of schizophrenic and epileptic symptoms, a concept that influenced von Meduna[46] to introduce iatrogenic convulsions into the treatment of schizophrenia.

With progress in diagnosis and treatment in epilepsy, epileptology shifted conceptually to the realm of neurologists in many countries. Psychiatric aspects were neglected until they were "rediscovered" in the 1950 s and 1960 s.[14,38,82] American and English authors reported an excess of schizophrenialike psychoses in epilepsy patients, especially in those suffering from temporal lobe epilepsy.[15,55,70]

Slater et al. published a detailed analysis of 69 patients from two London hospitals who suffered from epilepsy and interictal psychoses. On the basis of this case series, the authors challenged the antagonism theory and postulated a positive link between epilepsy and schizophrenia. Although Slater was criticized for drawing conclusions on the basis of insufficient statistics,[77] the temporal lobe hypothesis soon became broadly accepted and stimulated extensive research into the role of temporal lobe pathology in schizophrenia. The use of epileptic psychoses as a biologic model or "mockup" of schizophrenia[59] is largely based on Gibbs and Slater's work.

The possible impact of research into epileptic psychosis on the understanding of the pathophysiology of endogenous psychoses explains the bias in the literature toward study of interictal schizophrenialike psychoses. The spectrum of psychotic syndromes in epilepsy is, however, much more complex, and psychotic complications are not restricted to patients with temporal lobe epilepsy.

EPIDEMIOLOGY

Some of the earlier studies were reviewed in the first edition of this textbook (Chapter 197). The more recent studies have employed an improved methodology. Bredkjaer[2] in a record linkage study looked for associations between epilepsy from the national patient register of Denmark and the equivalent psychiatric register. The incidence of nonorganic, nonaffective psychoses, which included schizophrenia and schizophrenia spectrum disorders, was significantly increased in epilepsy, even when patients with learning disability or substance misuse were excluded.

Stefansson et al.[76] in a case-control study compared the prevalence of nonorganic psychiatric disorders in patients with epilepsy to those with other somatic diseases, the groups being taken from a disability register in Iceland. Although the difference in psychiatric diagnoses overall was not significant, there was a higher rate of psychoses, particularly schizophrenia and paranoid states, among males with epilepsy.

Qin et al.[56] in another study from Denmark have confirmed the increased risk of schizophrenia and schizophrenialike psychoses in epilepsy, and in this study a family history of psychoses and a family history of epilepsy were significant risk factors for psychosis.

Studies from Japan examining new referrals for epilepsy quote a 6% prevalence of psychoses in those with normal intelligence (in contrast to 24% in those with learning disability).[44]

There are several studies of much more selected populations, such as hospital case series. Thus, Gureje,[19] in patients attending a neurologic clinic, quoted that 37% of patients were psychiatric cases and that 29% of these were psychotic. Mendez et al.[48] in a retrospective investigation reported that interictal psychotic disorders were found in over 9% of a large cohort of patients with epilepsy in contrast to just over 1% in patients with migraine. The epilepsy sample had more complex partial seizures, more auras, and less generalized epilepsy.

None of the above studies has been able to examine issues related to epilepsy classification in any detail, cohorts being derived from case registers lacking detailed information from, for example, brain imaging. Certain risk factors have been defined, but not from these data, and are noted below.

CLASSIFICATION

There is no internationally accepted syndromic classification of psychoses in epilepsy. Most of the previously proposed classification systems for these psychoses[3,10,29,85] are based on a combination of psychopathologic, etiologic, longitudinal, and electroencephalographic (EEG) parameters. Unfortunately, because of a lack of taxonomic studies, our knowledge about regular syndromic associations is still limited.

"Atypical" syndromes are not unusual, and presentations such as those associated with forced normalization (see below) and postictal psychoses make simple divisions between what is ictal and what is interictal difficult to discern. In other words, the above two examples are of psychotic states closely tied to the biology of the ictus but which are interictal in their timing. A new multiaxial approach to the classification of psychoses in epilepsy can be found in the proposal by Krishnamoorthy.[33]

It is suggested that patients with epilepsy and psychoses receive two separate diagnoses according to either ICD-10 or DSM-IV,[7] but in addition, the relationships between onset of psychosis and seizure activity, antiepileptic therapy, and changes of EEG findings should be noted.

For pragmatic reasons, however, it remains convenient to group psychoses in epilepsy according to their temporal relationship to seizures.

SYNDROMES OF PSYCHOSES IN RELATION TO SEIZURE ACTIVITY

The various syndromes are described in Table 1. The ictal psychoses are more likely to be linked to complex partial seizure status but have never been examined in any detail. In clinical practice they are not uncommon in seizures of temporal origin, but some of them are secondary to frontal lobe seizures. Simple focal status or aura continua may cause complex hallucinations, thought disorders, and affective symptoms. The continuous epileptic activity is restricted and may escape scalp EEG recordings. Insight usually is maintained, and true psychoses emerging from such a state have not been described. Nonconvulsive status epilepticus requires immediate treatment with intravenous antiepileptic drugs.

Postictal Psychoses

Most postictal psychoses are precipitated by a series or status of generalized tonic–clonic seizures. More rarely, psychoses occur after single grand mal seizures or following a cluster of complex partial seizures.[69] In the elderly, a postictal psychosis may be the first presentation of a new-onset epilepsy disorder.

TABLE 1

CLINICAL CHARACTERISTICS OF PSYCHOSES IN RELATION TO SEIZURE ACTIVITY

	Ictal	Postictal	Parictal	Alternative	Interictal
Relative frequency	~10%	~50%	~10%	~10%	~20%
Consciousness	Impaired	Impaired or normal	Impaired	Normal	Normal
Typical features	Mild motor symptoms	Lucid interval	Occurs often during presurgical evaluation	Initial symptom insomnia	Schizophrenialike psychopathology
Duration	Hours to days	Days to weeks	Days to weeks	Weeks	Months
EEG	Status epilepticus	Increased slowing, increased epileptic	Increased slowing, increased epileptic	Normalized	Unchanged
Treatment	Antiepileptic drugs IV	Spontaneous recovery, benzodiazepines, seizure control	Seizure control	Sleep regulation, reduction of antiepileptic drugs	Antipsychotics

EEG, electroencephalogram.

TABLE 2

DIFFERENCES BETWEEN POSTICTAL PSYCHOSES (PIP) AND INTERICTAL PSYCHOSES (IIP) (STATISTICALLY SIGNIFICANT)

	PIP (n = 45)	IIP (n = 126)
Reduced intelligence (<70 IQ)	4	39
Complex partial seizures	37	84
Déjà vu aura[a]	10 of 43	10 of 103
Temporal MRI lesion	16	25
Temporal lobe epilepsy	39	74
Generalized spike-waves	1	21
Age at epilepsy onset (years)	16	11
Age at psychosis onset (years)	35	25
Interval between onset epilepsy and psychosis (years)	18	13

[a]Calculated for the subgroup of patients with focal epilepsies.
Data from Kanemoto K. Postictal psychosis revisited. In: Trimble MR, Schmitz B, eds. *The Neuropsychiatry of Epilepsy.* Cambridge: Cambridge University Press; 2002:117–134.

Postictal psychoses account for approximately 25% of psychoses in epilepsy.[17,64]

The relationship to the type of epilepsy is not clear. Dongier[8] described a preponderance of generalized epilepsies, and Logsdail and Toone[41] noted a higher frequency of postictal psychosis in patients with focal epilepsies and complex focal seizures. One of the more comprehensive studies has been that of Kanemoto, and his distinction between postictal and interictal psychoses is shown in Table 2. Essentially, the postictal psychoses occur with later age of onset of epilepsy and at a later age than the interictal psychoses. They are significantly associated with temporal lobe epilepsy, complex partial seizures, and magnetic resonance imaging (MRI) temporal plus extratemporal structural lesions. Patients are less likely to have learning disability and are less likely to have generalized spike-wave abnormalities on the EEG. He also noted an association with déjà vu auras.[27] Others have suggested an association between ictal fear and postictal psychosis.[63]

A characteristic lucid interval is described in most patients during which time the mental state appears to be normal. This interval can last from 1 to 6 days between the epileptic seizures and onset of psychosis.[73] Failure to appreciate the presence of this lucid interval can lead to a misdiagnosis of this condition.

The psychopathology of postictal psychosis is polymorphic, but most patients present with abnormal mood and paranoid delusions.[41] Some patients are confused throughout the episode; others present with fluctuating impairment of consciousness and orientation; and sometimes there is no confusion at all. Kanemoto[27] suggests that up to 50% have a psychosis in clear consciousness. Dominant are delusions of grandiosity and religiosity often associated with an elevated mood when compared with interictal psychoses. Patients may also be anxious and a typical symptom is fear of impending death. Because patients often have a clear sensorium and may receive command hallucinations if the latter relate to violence or suicide, it is during such states that violent attacks on the self or others may occur.

The EEG during postictal psychosis is usually deteriorated, with increased epileptic as well as slow-wave activity, but there are few reliable studies since people with acute psychoses are difficult to examine.

The psychotic symptoms spontaneously remit within days or weeks, often without need for psychotropic drug treatment. However, in some cases, chronic psychoses develop from recurrent and even a single postictal psychosis[41,94]; this is estimated to occur in about 25% of cases.

The pathophysiology is not known. Savard et al.[63] noted the clinical analogy of psychoses following complex partial seizures to other postictal phenomena such as Todd paresis or postictal memory loss. Logsdail and Toone hypothesized that postictal psychosis results from increased postsynaptic dopamine sensitivity. Ring et al.[58] have tested this hypothesis using single-photon emission computed tomography (SPECT) and the D_2 ligand [^{123}I] iodobenzamide (IBZM). They noted that patients with epilepsy and psychoses had decreased binding to the ligand, suggesting that there was increased release of endogenous dopamine in the psychotic state. Kanemoto[27] suggested that we are dealing with a restricted limbic status epilepticus, but limited functional imaging studies produced contradictory results.[39]

Parictal Psychosis

Most authors do not distinguish between parictal and postictal psychoses.[63] In parictal psychosis,[94] psychotic symptoms develop gradually and parallel to increases in seizure frequency. The relationship to seizures is easily overlooked if seizure frequency is not carefully documented over prolonged periods. More rapid development of parictal psychoses can be seen, especially during the presurgical assessment of patients with intractable epilepsy, when series of epileptic seizures may be provoked by withdrawal of antiepileptic drugs. Impairment of consciousness is more frequent than in postictal psychosis.

Interictal Psychoses

Interictal psychoses occur between seizures and cannot directly be linked to the ictus. They are less frequent than peri-ictal psychoses, and account for 10% to 30% of diagnoses in unselected case series.[8,64] Interictal psychoses are, however, clinically more significant in terms of severity and duration than peri-ictal psychoses, which usually are brief and often self-limiting.

Slater and Beard stated that, in the absence of epilepsy, the psychoses in their study group would have been diagnosed as schizophrenia, and noted the frequent presence of the First Rank Symptoms of Schneider.[70] However, there have been persistent arguments as to the exact relationship between the two disorders and the phenomenology of the interictal epileptic psychoses. Slater maintained that there was a distinct difference between schizophrenia and the schizophrenialike psychoses associated with epilepsy, and they highlighted the preservation of affect, a high frequency of delusions and religious mystical experiences, and few motor symptoms.

Other authors have stressed the rarity of negative symptoms and the absence of formal thought disorder and catatonic states.[28] McKenna et al.[45] pointed out that visual hallucinations were more prominent than auditory hallucinations. Tellenbach[82] stated that delusions were less well organized, and Sherwin[67] remarked that neuroleptic treatment was less frequently necessary. There have been other authors, however, who denied any clear psychopathologic differences between epileptic psychosis and schizophrenia.[21,31]

Using the Present State Examination and the CATEGO computer program, which is a semistandardized and validated method for quantifying psychopathology, it has been possible to compare the presentation of psychosis in epilepsy with process schizophrenia. Very few significant differences emerged from such studies,[53,84] which suggests that, assuming the patients were representative, a significant number will have a schizophrenialike presentation virtually indistinguishable from schizophrenia in the absence of epilepsy.

Phenomenology apart, Slater argued that long-term prognosis of psychosis in epilepsy was better than that in process schizophrenia. In a follow-up study on his patients, he found that chronic psychotic symptoms tended to remit, and personality deterioration was rare.[17] Other authors have also described the outcome to be more favorable and long-term institutionalization to be less frequent than in schizophrenia.[28,67] Unfortunately, there have been no longitudinal studies comparing the long-term outcome of psychosis in epilepsy and process schizophrenia.

RISK FACTORS

The pathogenesis of psychotic episodes in epilepsy is likely to be heterogeneous. In most patients, a multitude of chronic and acute factors can be identified that are potentially responsible for the development of a psychiatric disorder. These factors are difficult to investigate in retrospect, and the interpretation of them as either causally related or simply intercorrelated is arguable.

The literature on risk factors is highly controversial; studies are difficult to compare because of varying definitions of the epilepsy, the psychiatric disorder, and the investigated risk factors. Most studies are restricted to interictal psychoses. Table 3 summarizes factors that have frequently been described to be associated with the interictal psychosis in epilepsy.[85]

Genetic Predisposition

With few exceptions,[26,56] most authors do not find any evidence for an increased rate of psychiatric disorders in relatives of epilepsy patients with psychoses.[11,53,69] This was one reason why Slater suggested that these psychoses were truly symptomatic, a representative phenotype of the genotype.

Sex Distribution

There has been a bias toward female sex in several case series,[80] but this has not been confirmed in controlled studies.[1,34,35]

TABLE 3

RISK FACTORS ASSOCIATED WITH INTERICTAL PSYCHOSES OF EPILEPSY[a]

Sex	Bias to female patients
Age of onset	Early adolescence
Interval	Onset of seizures to onset of psychosis: Mean 14 years
Epileptic syndrome	Temporal lobe epilepsy
Seizure type	Complex focal
Seizure frequency	Low, diminished
Neurologic findings	Sinistrality
Pathology	Gangliogliomas, hamartomas
EEG	Mediobasal focus, especially left sided

EEG, electroencephalogram.

Duration of Epilepsy

The interval between age at onset of epilepsy and age at first manifestation of psychosis has been remarkably homogeneous, in the region of 11 to 15 years, in many series.[85] This interval has been used to postulate the etiologic significance of the seizure disorder and a kindlinglike mechanism. However, some authors[5,77] have argued that the supposedly specific interval represents an artifact. They have drawn attention to the wide range, with a significantly shorter interval in patients with later onset of epilepsy. They also have pointed out that patients whose psychoses did not succeed their epilepsy were excluded in most series, and that there is a tendency in the general population for the age of onset of epilepsy to have an earlier peak than that of schizophrenia.

Type of Epilepsy

There is a clear excess of temporal lobe epilepsy in almost all case series of patients with epilepsy and psychosis. Among the pooled data of ten studies, 217 (76%) of 287 patients suffered from temporal lobe epilepsy.[85] The preponderance of this type of epilepsy is, however, not a uniform finding; in Gudmundsson's epidemiologic study, for example, only 7% suffered from "psychomotor" epilepsy. However, in many studies, especially the early ones, the classification of seizures and epilepsy is confused, and not supported by neurologic investigations.

The nature of a possible link of psychoses to temporal lobe epilepsy (TLE) is not entirely clear,[65] partly because of ambiguities in the definition of TLE in the literature, based on either seizure symptomatology (psychomotor epilepsy), involvement of specific functional systems (limbic epilepsy), or anatomic localization as detected by depth EEG or neuroimaging (amygdalohippocampal epilepsy). Unfortunately, most authors have not sufficiently differentiated frontal and temporal lobe epilepsy.

The temporal lobe hypothesis, although widely accepted, has been criticized for being based on uncontrolled case series, such as in the studies by Gibbs[15] and Slater and Beard.[70] It was argued that TLE is the most frequent type of epilepsy in the general population and that there is an overrepresentation of this type of epilepsy in patients attending specialized centers. However, there is a general consensus that psychoses are less common in patients with neocortical extratemporal epilepsies.[5,15,17,51,64,66,77] Adachi[1] suggested that psychoses in patients with frontal lobe epilepsy may be overlooked because of a differing psychopathology, hebephrenic symptoms in particular dominating the presentation.

The findings are less unequivocal regarding TLE and generalized epilepsies. Four studies[19,53,66,68] note significant differences in the frequency of psychoses in temporal lobe epilepsy, but several do not.[4,14,49,64,72,75,77] However, many patients with generalized epilepsy show pathology of temporal structures, making classification difficult, and again many reports lack the sophisticated brain imaging that is now required for such hypotheses to be tested.

There are several studies showing that psychoses in generalized epilepsies differ from psychoses in TLE.[85] The former are more likely to be of short duration and confusional.[4,8,77] Alternative psychoses, which are especially common in generalized epilepsy, are usually relatively mild and often remit before any development of paranoid-hallucinatory symptoms. Schneiderian first-rank symptoms and chronicity are more frequent in patients with TLE.[64,86] This has considerable significance for psychiatrists attempting to unravel the underlying "neurology" of schizophrenia, and the findings from epilepsy were instrumental in altering the view of schizophrenia away from a psychosocial to a biologic model.

Type of Seizures

There is evidence from several studies that focal seizure symptoms that indicate ictal mesial temporal or limbic involvement are overrepresented in patients with psychosis. Hermann and Chabria[23] noted a relationship between ictal fear and high scores on paranoia and schizophrenia scales of the Minnesota Multiphasic Personality Inventory (MMPI). Kristensen and Sindrup[34,35] found an excess of dysmnesic and epigastric auras in their psychotic group. They also reported a higher rate of ictal amnesia. In another controlled study, ictal impairment of consciousness was related to psychosis, but simple seizure symptoms indicating limbic involvement were not.[64]

No seizure type is specifically related to psychosis in generalized epilepsies. Most patients with psychosis and generalized epilepsies have absence seizures.[64]

Severity of Epilepsy

The strongest risk factors for psychosis in epilepsy are those that indicate severity of epilepsy. These are long duration of active epilepsy,[70] multiple seizure types,[5,22,40,52,60,64,66] history of status epilepticus,[64] and poor response to drug treatment.[40] Seizure frequency, however, is reported by most authors to be lower in psychotic epilepsy patients than in nonpsychotic patients.[11,66,71,74] It has not been clarified whether seizure frequency was low before or during the psychotic episode. This may represent a variant of forced normalization (see below).

Laterality

Left lateralization of temporal lobe dysfunction or temporal lobe pathology as a risk factor for schizophreniform psychosis was originally suggested by Flor-Henry.[11] Studies supporting the laterality hypothesis have been made using surface EEG,[40] depth electrode recordings,[67] computed tomography,[6,83] neuropathology,[79] neuropsychology,[53] and positron emission tomography (PET),[91] and more recently with MRI. The earlier literature has been summarized by Trimble.[85] In a synopsis of 14 studies with 341 patients, 43% had left, 23% right, and 34% bilateral abnormalities. This is a striking bias toward left lateralization. However, lateralization of epileptogenic foci was not confirmed in all controlled studies.[8,34,35,68] Again, it may be that certain symptoms rather than any syndrome are associated with a specific side of focus. Trimble pointed out that a specific group of hallucinations and delusions, defined by Schneider and referred to as first rank symptoms, which usually (but not exclusively) signifies schizophrenia, may be relevant.[89,90] He suggested that these may be signifiers of temporal lobe dysfunction, representing disturbances of language and symbolic representation. In this sense, he then equated to a Babinski sign for a neurologist (i.e., pointing to a location and lateralization of an abnormality in the central nervous system).

These laterality findings have received support from brain imaging studies, especially SPECT and MRI. Mellers,[47] using a verbal fluency activation paradigm and HMPAO SPECT, compared patients with schizophrenialike psychoses of epilepsy (n = 12), with schizophrenia (n = 11), and epilepsy and no psychoses (n = 16). The psychotic epilepsy patients showed lower blood flow in the superior temporal gyrus during activation than the other two groups. Using MR spectroscopy, Maier et al.[42] were able to compare hippocampal-amygdala volumes and hippocampal *N*-acetyl aspartate (NAA) levels in patients with temporal lobe epilepsy and schizophrenialike psychoses of epilepsy (n = 12), temporal lobe epilepsy and no psychoses (n = 12), schizophrenia and no epilepsy (n = 26), and matched normal controls (n = 38). The psychotic patients showed significant left-sided reduction of NAA, and this was greater in the psychotic epilepsy group. Regional volume reductions were noted bilaterally in this group, and in the left hippocampus-amygdala in the schizophrenic group.

Flugel et al.[12] have recently examined 20 psychotic and 20 nonpsychotic cases with temporal lobe epilepsy using magnetization transfer imaging. They reported significant reductions of the magnetization transfer ratio (an index of signal loss) in the left superior and middle temporal gyri in the psychotic patients; this was unrelated to volume changes and best revealed in the subgroup with no focal MRI lesions.

Structural Lesions

The literature on brain damage and epileptic psychosis is very controversial. Some authors have suggested a higher rate of pathologic neurologic examinations, diffuse slowing on the EEG, and mental retardation,[34,35] but others could not find an association with psychosis.[11,26] Neuropathologic studies of resected temporal lobes from patients with TLE have suggested a link between psychosis and the presence of cerebral malformations such as hamartomas and gangliogliomas as compared with mesial temporal sclerosis.[4,59,80] These findings have been seen as consistent with recent findings of structural abnormalities in the brains of schizophrenic patients without epilepsy that arise during fetal development.

Bruton[4] has noted enlarged ventricles, periventricular gliosis, and an excess of acquired focal damage in brains of institutionalized psychotic epileptic patients compared with nonpsychotic controls. Bruton also reported that schizophrenialike psychoses were also distinguished by an excess of perivascular white matter softenings.

In a study specifically looking at hippocampal and amygdala volumes, Tebartz van Elst et al.[81] examined 26 patients with epileptic psychoses, 24 with temporal lobe epilepsy and no psychosis, and 20 healthy controls. The psychotic patients had significantly increased amygdala sizes in comparison with the other two groups, which were bilateral, not related to the laterality of the focus or length of epilepsy history. No hippocampal differences were noted in this study. In a complementary study on the same groups, Rusch et al.[61] were unable to find any neocortical cortical volumetric differences.

FORCED NORMALIZATION

A full understanding of the relationships between epilepsy and psychosis requires appreciation of this concept.

Earlier this century, reports appeared that suggested that there was some kind of antagonism between epilepsy and psychosis. This was one of the reasons that led von Meduna to introduce convulsive therapy for the treatment of schizophrenia. In the 1950 s, Landolt[37,38] published a series of papers on patients who had epilepsy who became psychotic when their seizures were under control. He defined forced normalization as follows: "Forced normalisation is the phenomenon characterised by the fact that, with the recurrence of psychotic states, the EEG becomes more normal, or entirely normal, as compared with previous and subsequent EEG findings."

Forced normalization was thus essentially an EEG phenomenon. The clinical counterpart of patients becoming psychotic when their seizures became under control and their psychosis resolving with return of seizures was referred to as alternative psychoses by Tellenbach.[82]

These phenomena have now been well documented clinically. The following are important to note, however. First, the EEG does not need to become "normal," but the interictal disturbances decrease and in some cases disappear. Second, the clinical presentation need not necessarily be a psychosis but sometimes is. In childhood or in the mentally handicapped, aggression and agitation are common. Other manifestations include pseudoseizures or other conversion symptoms, depression, mania, and anxiety states. Third, the disturbed behavior may last days or weeks. They may be terminated by a seizure, and the EEG abnormalities then return. Fourthly, Landolt originally associated this phenomenon with focal epilepsies, but with the introduction of the succinimide drugs, he noted an association with the generalized epilepsies. Certainly, forced normalization may be provoked by the administration of anticonvulsants and has been reported with barbiturates, benzodiazepines, ethosuximide, tiagabine, topiramate, vigabatrin, levetiracetam, and more recently lamotrigine[5,85] (see Chapter 208).

The literature on antagonism between epilepsy and psychosis has been held to be incompatible with the suggestions outlined above that there is an increased association between epilepsy and psychosis. This has been resolved by more careful understanding of the original literature.[93] Thus, within the association or link between psychosis and epilepsy, there may be an antagonism of symptoms between seizures and the symptoms of psychosis (i.e., the hallucinations and delusions). It is the longitudinal course of the disorders that has to be followed, and forced normalization, as opposed to alternative psychosis, requires serial EEG recordings before the diagnosis can be made.

It is often denied that forced normalization occurs, probably with good reason. Thus, it is certainly rarer than made out by Landolt, and studies are few and far between. It is difficult to document cases precisely, EEG recordings being difficult to obtain at the right times. However, other less enlightened reasons to ignore such findings relate to the fact that the concept brings psychiatry uncomfortably close to neurology, revealing a close biologic link between seizures and psychosis. It also affects treatment. Thus, if in some patients suppression of seizures provokes psychopathology, it reinforces the fact, often ignored or misunderstood, that seizures and epilepsy are not synonymous, and that an understanding of the epileptic process and its treatment goes far beyond the control of seizures. In clinical practice, to ignore the fact that some patients manifest these problems as their seizures come under control can lead to the continuation of severe behavior disturbances, with all of the social disruption that then emerges, and a failure to manage the epilepsy appropriately.

PSYCHOSIS FOLLOWING SURGERY

Temporal lobectomy is an ever-increasing treatment for patients with intractable epilepsy. Ever since the early series, the possibility that surgery itself may be associated with the development of psychiatric disturbance, in particular psychosis, has been discussed. Some of the best evidence comes from the Maudsley series, initially described by Taylor[78] and more recently by Bruton.[4] Most centers have stopped operating on floridly psychotic patients, based on the observation that psychoses generally do not improve with the operation. A few centers, however, regularly include psychiatric screening as part of their preoperative assessment, but postoperative psychiatric follow-up is often nonexistent. Assessment of psychosocial adjustment is rarely performed, in contrast to the often scrupulous recording of neuropsychological deficits.

The Maudsley series show that some patients develop new psychosis postoperatively, and there is an increased reporting of depression. Bruton[4] has suggested that the development of postoperative psychoses may be more common with certain pathologies (gangliogliomas). Patients with right-sided temporal lobectomies may be more prone to these psychiatric disturbances.[85] In some cases, the sudden relief of seizures that occurs following surgery may suggest a mechanism similar to forced normalization, although no persistent clear relationship emerges between success of operation and the development of psychotic postoperative states. In recent times, there have been several small series reported of patients with psychoses who have been successfully operated on, without worsening of their seizures but with marked improvement in seizure control. This topic is discussed in much more detail in Chapter 209.[57]

DIAGNOSIS

The principles of diagnosis of psychiatric problems in epilepsy are essentially the same as when a patient does not have epilepsy. However, as noted, it is not possible to apply the strict DSM-IV classifications,[7] and in many patients there are subtle aspects to the clinical picture that may suggest the underlying neurologic flavor of the phenomenology. These include in the schizophrenialike psychoses the retention of affective responses, lack of chronic personality and lifestyle deterioration, and development of some of the personality features noted in the interictal personality syndrome. An inclination to mysticism with developing religiosity is one of the most common.

Close attention to the relationship of the development of the psychoses to the seizure pattern is essential if the peri-ictal disorders are to be distinguished from the interictal, although in many patients this is not always clear, and the pattern may change with time. In particular, there are reports of ictally driven psychoses evolving to a chronic interictal syndrome, subtle at first but then more enduring. In other cases, the acute psychoses may erupt in the absence of an obvious cluster of seizures, even though on previous occasions the relationship has been obvious. The EEG in some cases is very important in clarifying the diagnoses, especially for nonconvulsive status and states of forced normalization.

Because many patients with psychoses of epilepsy display prominent affective symptoms, it is important to identify those patients with an affective disorder, as opposed to a schizophrenialike state or a paranoid illness, that may respond initially to effective antidepressant therapy.

TREATMENT

Essentially, management of psychiatric problems in patients with epilepsy is similar to that in patients without epilepsy, with a few caveats. Certainly, a number of nonmedical treatments are available. These should always be thought of in individual cases.

Patients with psychoses should be treated with neuroleptic medications, although these, like most antidepressants, can lower the seizure threshold. To date, all known neuroleptics have this potential, although some more than others; this is covered in more detail in Chapter 214.

Postictal psychoses may occasionally need neuroleptic drugs, although they usually settle rapidly. It is more important to prevent patients from damaging themselves or causing harm to others, but a drug such as haloperidol or one of the newer atypical antipsychotics at regular intervals may control behavior satisfactorily. Interictally, the paranoid or schizophrenialike states need to be evaluated in terms of their relationship to seizure frequency. Thus, in patients who stop having seizures in association with the onset of psychosis, a neuroleptic that increases the seizure threshold (e.g., chlorpromazine or even clozapine) may be the most logical prescription.

Where patients with epilepsy have no alteration of the seizure frequency or the psychosis is occurring in the setting of increased seizure frequency, a neuroleptic less likely to precipitate seizures, such as risperidone, an atypical antipsychotic, is logical. It should be recalled that patients taking anticonvulsants that increase hepatic metabolism will show lower serum levels of neuroleptics and may therefore require somewhat higher doses than patients not on these medications to achieve a similar clinical effect. Occasionally, the addition of an antidepressant or a neuroleptic to a patient's prescription may lead to increases in serum anticonvulsant levels.

Postictal psychoses often do not require psychotropic medication, resolving over a few hours. However, it is important to stress how dangerous these cases can be, and it is essential to take note of any command hallucinations or delusions of harm to the self or others and protect accordingly. In the first instance, treatment with a benzodiazepine is helpful, since there is a risk, especially with some of the antipsychotics, of precipitating further seizures and exacerbating the psychosis. Regular benzodiazepines for perhaps 48 hours are often sufficient. In the longer-term management it is important to realize that postictal psychoses have a tendency to recur. It is therefore important to warn about this, and to try with effective antiepileptic drug therapy to try to prevent clusters of seizures. It is sometimes possible to prevent such a cluster and hence the later psychosis by telling patients to take their benzodiazepine at the onset of any cluster and continue then for about 48 hours. Sometimes all these measures fail, and so intermittent or even continuous antipsychotic treatment becomes important.

As with all psychiatric problems, psychopharmacologic management alone is not sufficient. Although the role of psychotherapy in the management of psychotic conditions has not proven of any substantial value, it is important to acknowledge that epileptic patients with psychosis bear the burden of epilepsy in addition to their psychosis. Patients with intermittent psychotic states are often perplexed and embarrassed about what has happened to them while psychotic and fear further continuing bouts with a descent into insanity. Patients with continuous psychosis require the skills of paramedical intervention, and the full resources of community care may be needed to help them rehabilitate and to assist their families in coping with their difficulties. In many patients with chronic psychoses of epilepsy, the preservation of affect and lack of personality disintegration over years sustains them well in their communities and may enable them to live with their families or even marry. Maintaining them and bringing such support to them is important, sustaining them in the community and preventing their recurrent admission to the hospital. Further, in a good family environment with adequate medical facilities and follow-up care, patient compliance will tend to be good. Deterioration of an otherwise delicate situation induced by poor compliance, leading to more seizures and exacerbation of psychopathology with loss of control by the family and the physician, may thereby be avoided.

SUMMARY AND CONCLUSIONS

There is evidence that psychoses are overrepresented in patients with epilepsy, and few physicians who manage epilepsy have not seen patients with either an ictal, postictal, or interictal psychosis. The link to temporal lobe epilepsy is strong, both clinically and theoretically, because there is an acknowledged link between the limbic system and the modulation of emotional and social behaviors.[88] It has to be of profound interest that epilepsy, which is so often associated with lesions in medial temporal structures that tend to be present from an early phase in life, is linked to psychoses, which often resemble paranoid and schizophreniform states found in the absence of epilepsy. Thus, the latter can also be shown to have pathology in the same areas of the brain,[87] and schizophrenia is now viewed as a developmental disorder associated with anomalous central nervous system development in the fetal or perinatal era of life.

Although the underlying pathology may be different, the absence of gliosis in the hippocampus and related structures characterizing schizophrenia, the site of the pathology, the timing of the lesions, and the consequent functional changes in the brain may all be crucial to the later development of any behavior changes in both epilepsy and schizophrenia. Thus, the behavior changes should be viewed as an integral part of the process of epilepsy that are manifest in some patients. However, the recent evidence, especially from brain imaging studies, suggests that Slater's original hypothesis was part right but part wrong. Thus, the interictal psychoses seem different from schizophrenia, especially with regard to the admixture with affective symptoms and the long-term prognosis. While hippocampal changes may relate to both disorders, the increased amygdala size, bilateral and around 17% to 20%, and the lesser volumetric changes in the hippocampus suggest that the two psychopathologic states are biologically quite different. While the laterality findings with regard to the functioning of the left hemisphere seem to hold up, the data point away from fundamentally cortical abnormalities in these psychoses, and bring the amygdala and related structures as central in pathogenesis. Finally, it has to be repeated that epilepsy is not synonymous with seizures, and the latter are but one manifestation of the disordered cerebral function of patients with epilepsy.

References

1. Adachi N, Onuma T, Nishiwaki S, et al. Inter-ictal and post-ictal psychoses in frontal lobe epilepsy: a retrospective comparison with psychoses in temporal lobe epilepsy. *Seizure*. 2000;9(5):328–335.
2. Bredkjaer SR, Mortensen PB, Parnas J. Epilepsy and non-organic non-affective psychosis. National epidemiologic study. *Br J Psychiatry*. 1998;172: 235–238.
3. Bruens JH. Psychoses in epilepsy. In: Vinken PJ, Bruyn GW, eds. *Handbook of Clinical Neurology, vol 15*. Amsterdam: North Holland; 1974:593–610.
4. Bruton CJ. The neuropathology of temporal lobe epilepsy. In: *Maudsley Monograph No 31*. Oxford: Oxford University Press; 1988.
5. Clemens B. Forced normalisation precipitated by lamotrigine. *Seizure*. 2005;14(7):485–489.
6. Conlon P, Trimble MR, Rogers D. A study of epileptic psychosis using magnetic resonance imaging. *Br J Psychiatry*. 1990;156:231–235.
7. *Diagnostic and Statistical Manual of Mental Disorders, 4th ed (DSM-IV): Draft Criteria*. Washington, DC: American Psychiatric Association; 1993.
8. Dongier S. Statistical study of clinical and electroencephalographic manifestations of 536 psychotic episodes occurring in 516 epileptics between clinical seizures. *Epilepsia*. 1959–1960;1:117–142.
9. Falret J. De l'état mental des epileptiques. *Arch Gen Med*. 1860;16:661–679.
10. Fenton GJ. Psychiatric disorders of epilepsy: classification and phenomenology. In: Reynolds EH, Trimble MR, eds. *Epilepsy and Psychiatry*. Edinburgh: Churchill Livingstone; 1981:12–26.
11. Flor-Henry P. Psychosis and temporal lobe epilepsy. A controlled investigation. *Epilepsia*. 1969;10:363–395.
12. Flugel D, Cercignani M, Symms MR, et al. A magnetization transfer imaging study in patients with temporal lobe epilepsy and interictal psychosis. *Biol Psychiatry*. 2005; Sep 13.
13. Ganter R. Ein mit Schizophrenie kombinierter Fall von Epilepsie. *Arch Psychiatr Nervenkr*. 1925;74:829–837.
14. Gastaut H. Colloque de Marseille, 15–19 Octobre 1956. Compte rendu du colloque sur l'étude electroclinique des episodes psychotiques qui surviennient chez les épileptiques en dehors des crises cliniques. *Rev Neurol*. 1956;95:587–616.
15. Gibbs FA. Ictal and non-ictal psychiatric disorders in temporal lobe epilepsy. *J Nerv Ment Disord*. 1951;113:522–528.
16. Glaus A. Über Kombinationen von Schizophrenie und Epilepsie. *Z Ges Neurol Psychiatr*. 1931;135:450–500.

17. Glithero E, Slater E. The schizophrenia-like psychoses of epilepsy. IV: follow-up record and outcome. *Br J Psychiatry*. 1963;109:134–142.
18. Griesinger W. Über einige epileptoide Zustände. *Arch Psychiatr Nervenkr*. 1868;1:320–333.
19. Gureje O. Interictal psychopathology in epilepsy—prevalence and pattern in a Nigerian clinic. *Br J Psychiatry*. 1991;158:700–705.
20. Gurewitsch M. Zur differentialdiagnose des epileptischen Irreseins. Zugleich ein Beitrag zur Lehre von den kombinierten Psychosen. *Z Ges Neurol Psychiatr*. 1912;9:359–390.
21. Helmchen H. Zerebrale Bedingungkonstellationen psychopathologischer Syndrome bei Epileptikern. In: Helmchen H, Hippius H, eds. *Entwicklungstendenzen biologischer Psychiatrie*. Stuttgart: Thieme; 1975:125–148.
22. Hermann BP, Dikmen S, Schwartz MS, et al. Psychopathology in patients with ictal fear: a quantitative investigation. *Neurology*. 1982;32:7–11.
23. Herrman BP, Chabria S. Interictal psychopathology in patients with ictal fear. *Arch Neurol*. 1980;37:667–668.
24. Hoffmann F. Über die Einteilung der Nervenkrankheiten in Siegburg. *Allg Z Psychiatr*. 1872;19:367–391.
25. International Classification of Diseases—10. *Classification of Mental and Behavioural Disorders*. Geneva: World Health Organization; 1992.
26. Jensen I, Larsen JK. Mental aspects of temporal lobe epilepsy. *J Neurol Neurosurg Psychiatry*. 1979;42:256–265.
27. Kanemoto K. Postictal psychosis revisited. In: Trimble MR, Schmitz B, eds. *The Neuropsychiatry of Epilepsy*. Cambridge: Cambridge University Press; 2002:117–134.
28. Köhler GK. Epileptische Psychosen - Klassifikationsversuche und EEG-Verlaufsbeobachtungen. *Fortschr Neurol Psychiatr*. 1975;43:99–153.
29. Köhler GK. Zur Einteilung der Psychosen bei Epilepsie. Zum Begriff "Psychosen bei Epilepsie" bzw. "epileptische Psychosen." In: Wolf P, Köhler GK, eds. *Psychopathologische und Pathogenetische Probleme Psychotischer Syndrome bei Epilepsie*. Bern: Huber; 1980:11–18.
30. Kraepelin E. *Psychiatrie*. Leipzig: JA Barth; 1903.
31. Kraft AM, Price TRP, Peltier D. Complex partial seizures and schizophrenia. *Compr Psychiatry*. 1984;25:113–124.
32. Krapf E. Epilepsie und Schizophrenie. *Arch Psychiatr Nervenheil*. 1928;83:547–586.
33. Krishnamoorthy ES. An approach to classifying neuropsychiatric disorders in epilepsy. *Epilepsy Behav*. 2000;1(6):373–377.
34. Kristensen O, Sindrup HH. Psychomotor epilepsy and psychosis. I. Physical aspects. *Acta Neurol Scand*. 1978;57:361–369.
35. Kristensen O, Sindrup HH. Psychomotor epilepsy and psychosis. II. Electroencephalographic findings. *Acta Neurol Scand*. 1978;57:370–379.
36. Lachmund. Ueber vereinzelt auftretende Halluzinationen bei Epileptikern. *Monatsschr Psychiatr Neurol*. 1904;15:434–444.
37. Landolt H. Serial electroencephalographic investigations during psychotic episodes in epileptic patients and during schizophrenic attacks. In: Lorentz de Haas AM, ed. *Lectures on Epilepsy*. Amsterdam: Elsevier; 1958:91–133.
38. Landolt H. Some clinical EEG correlations in epileptic psychoses (twilight states). *Electroencephalogr Clin Neurophysiol*. 1953;5:121.
39. Leutmezer F, Podreka I, Asenbaum S, et al. Postictal psychosis in temporal lobe epilepsy. *Epilepsia*. 2003;44(4):582–590.
40. Lindsay J, Ounsted C, Richards P. Long-term outcome in children with temporal lobe seizures. II. Psychiatric aspects in childhood and adult life. *Dev Med Child Neurol*. 1979;21:630–636.
41. Logsdail SJ, Toone BK. Postictal psychoses. A clinical and phenomenological description. *Br J Psychiatry*. 1988;152:246–252.
42. Maier M, Mellers J, Toone B, et al. Schizophrenia, temporal lobe epilepsy and psychosis: an in vivo magnetic resonance spectroscopy and imaging study of the hippocampus/amygdala complex. *Psychol Med*. 2000;30(3):571–581.
43. Mann SC, Caroff SN, Bleier HR, et al. Lethal catatonia. *Am J Psychiatry*. 1986;143:1374–1381.
44. Matsuura M, Adachi N, Muramatsu R, et al. Intellectual disability and psychotic disorders of adult epilepsy. *Epilepsia*. 2005;46(Suppl 1):11–14.
45. McKenna PJ, Kane JM, Parrish K. Psychotic symptoms in epilepsy. *Am J Psychiatry*. 1985;142:895–904.
46. Von Meduna L. Versuche ueber die biologische Beeintlussung des Ablaufes der Schizophrenie. I. Campher- und Cadiazolkraempfe. *Z Ges Neurol Psychiatr*. 1935;152:235–262.
47. Mellers JD, Adachi N, Takei N, et al. SPET study of verbal fluency in schizophrenia and epilepsy. *Br J Psychiatry*. 1998;173:69–74.
48. Mendez MF, Grau R, Doss RC, et al. Schizophrenia in epilepsy: seizure and psychosis variables. *Neurology*. 1993;43(6):1073–1077.
49. Mignone RJ, Donnelly EF, Sadowsky D. Psychological and neurological comparisons of psychomotor and non-psychomotor epileptic patients. *Epilepsia*. 1970;11:345–359.
50. Morel B. D'une forme de delire, suite d'une surexcitation nerveuse se rattachent a une variété non encore d'écrite d'épilepsie. *Gaz Hebd Med Chir*. 1860;7:773–775.
51. Onuma T. Limbic lobe epilepsy with paranoid symptoms: analysis of clinical features and psychological tests. *Fol Psychiatr Neurol Jpn*. 1983;37:253–258.
52. Ounsted C. Aggression and epilepsy. Rage in children with temporal lobe epilepsy. *J Psychosom Res*. 1969;13:237–242.
53. Perez MM, Trimble MR. Epileptic psychosis—diagnostic comparison with process schizophrenia. *Br J Psychiatry*. 1980;137:245–249.
54. Pohl H. Über das Zusammenvorkommen von Epilepsie und originärer Paranoia. *Prager Med Wochenschr*. 1880;35.
55. Pond DA. Discussion remark. *Proc R Soc Med*. 1962;55:316.
56. Qin P, Xu H, Laursen TM, et al. Risk for schizophrenia and schizophrenia-like psychosis among patients with epilepsy: population based cohort study. *BMJ*. 2005;331(7507):23.
57. Reutens DC, Savard G, Andermann F, et al. Results of surgical treatment in temporal lobe epilepsy with chronic psychosis. *Brain*. 1997;120 (Pt 11):1929–1936.
58. Ring HA, Trimble MR, Costa DC, et al. Striatal dopamine receptor binding in epileptic psychoses. *Biol Psychiatry*. 1994;35:375–380.
59. Roberts GW, Done DJ, Bruton C, et al. A "mock up" of schizophrenia: temporal lobe epilepsy and schizophrenia-like psychosis. *Biol Psychiatry*. 1990;28:127–143.
60. Rodin EA, Collomb H, Pache D. Differences between patients with temporal lobe seizures and those with other forms of epileptic attacks. *Epilepsia*. 1976;17:313–320.
61. Rusch N, Tebartz van Elst L, Baeumer D, et al. Absence of cortical gray matter abnormalities in psychosis of epilepsy: a voxel-based MRI study in patients with temporal lobe epilepsy. *J Neuropsychiatry Clin Neurosci*. 2004;16(2):148–155.
62. Samt P. Epileptische Irreseinsformen. *Arch Psychiatr Nervenkr*. 1876;6:110–216.
63. Savard G, Andermann F, Olivier A, et al. Postictal psychosis after partial complex seizures: a multiple case study. *Epilepsia*. 1991;32:225–231.
64. Schmitz B. Psychosen bei Epilepsie. Eine epidemiologische Untersuchung. Thesis, FU Berlin, 1988.
65. Schmitz B. Psychosis and epilepsy. The link to the temporal lobe. In: Trimble MR, Bolwig TG, eds. *The Temporal Lobes and the Limbic System*. Petersfield, UK: Wrightson Biomedical Publishing; 1992:149–167.
66. Sengoku A, Yagi K, Seino M, et al. Risks of occurrence of psychoses in relation to the types of epilepsies and epileptic seizures. *Fol Psychiatr Neurol Jpn*. 1983;37:221–226.
67. Sherwin I. Differential psychiatric features in epilepsy; relationship to lesion laterality. *Acta Psychiatr Scand [Suppl]*. 1984;313:92–103.
68. Shukla GD, Srivastava ON, Katiyar BC, et al. Psychiatric manifestations in temporal lobe epilepsy. A controlled study. *Br J Psychiatry*. 1979;135:411–417.
69. Slater E, Beard AW, Glithero E. The schizophrenia-like psychoses of epilepsy. *Br J Psychiatry*. 1963;109:95–150.
70. Slater E, Beard AW. The schizophrenia-like psychoses of epilepsy. V. Discussion and conclusions. *Br J Psychiatry*. 1963;109:143–150.
71. Slater E, Moran PAP. The schizophrenia-like psychoses of epilepsy: relation between ages of onset. *Br J Psychiatry*. 1969;115:599–600.
72. Small JG, Milstein V, Stevens JR. Are psychomotor epileptics different? *Arch Neurol*. 1962;7:187–194.
73. Sommer W. Postepileptisches Irresein. *Arch Psychiatr Nervenkr*. 1881;11:549–612.
74. Standage KF, Fenton GW. Psychiatric symptom profiles of patients with epilepsy: a controlled investigation. *Psychol Med*. 1975;5:152–160.
75. Standage KF. Schizophreniform psychosis among epileptics in a mental hospital. *Br J Psychiatry*. 1973;123:231–232.
76. Stefansson SB, Olafsson E, Hauser WA. Psychiatric morbidity in epilepsy: a case controlled study of adults receiving disability benefits. *J Neurol Neurosurg Psychiatry*. 1998;64(2):238–241.
77. Stevens JR. Psychiatric implications of psychomotor epilepsy. *Arch Gen Psychiatry*. 1966;14:461–471.
78. Taylor DC. Factors influencing the occurrence of schizophrenia-like psychosis in patients with temporal lobe epilepsy. *Psychol Med*. 1975;5:249–254.
79. Taylor DC. Mental state and temporal lobe epilepsy. A correlative account of 100 patients treated surgically. *Epilepsia*. 1972;13:727–765.
80. Taylor DC. Ontogenesis of chronic epileptic psychoses. A reanalysis. *Psychol Med*. 1971;1:247–253.
81. Tebartz van Elst L, Baeumer D, Lemieux L, et al. Amygdala pathology in psychosis of epilepsy: a magnetic resonance imaging study in patients with temporal lobe epilepsy. *Brain*. 2002;125(Pt 1):140–149.
82. Tellenbach H. Epilepsie als Anfallsleiden und als Psychose. Ueber alternative Psychosen paranoider prägung bei "forcierter Normalisierung" (Landolt) des Elektroencephalogramms Epileptischer. *Nervenarzt*. 1965;36:190–202.
83. Toone B, Dawson J, Driver MV. Psychoses of epilepsy. A radiological evaluation. *Br J Psychiatry*. 1982;140:244–248.
84. Toone B. Psychoses of epilepsy. In: Reynolds EH, Trimble MR, eds. *Epilepsy and Psychiatry*. Edinburgh: Churchill Livingstone; 1981:113–137.
85. Trimble M. *The Psychoses of Epilepsy*. New York: Raven Press; 1991.
86. Trimble MR, Perez MM. The phenomenology of the chronic psychoses of epilepsy. In: Koella WP, Trimble MR, eds. *Temporal Lobe Epilepsy, Mania and Schizophrenia and the Limbic System*. Basel: Karger; 1982: 98–105.
87. Trimble MR. *Biological Psychiatry*. 2nd ed. Chichester: John Wiley & Sons; 1995.
88. Trimble MR. *Biological Psychiatry*. Chichester: John Wiley & Sons; 1988.

89. Trimble MR. First rank symptoms of Schneider, a new perspective. *Br J Psychiatry*. 1990;156:195–200.
90. Trimble MR. Interictal psychoses of epilepsy. In: Smith D, Treiman D, Trimble MR, eds. *Advances in Neurology 55*. New York: Raven Press; 1991:143–152.
91. Trimble MR. PET-scanning in epilepsy. In: Trimble MR, Bolwig TG, eds. *Aspects of Epilepsy and Psychiatry*. Chichester: John Wiley & Sons; 1986:147–162.
92. Trimble MR. Phenomenology of epileptic psychosis: a historical introduction to changing concepts. In: Koella WP, Trimble MR, eds. *Temporal Lobe Epilepsy, Mania and Schizophrenia and the Limbic System*. Basel: Karger; 1982:1–11.
93. Wolf P, Trimble MR. Biological antagonism and epileptic psychosis. *Br J Psychiatry*. 1985;146:272–276.
94. Wolf P. *Psychosen bei Epilepsie. Ihre Bedingungen und Wechselbeziehungen zu Anfaellen*. Freie Universitaet Berlin: Habilitationsschrift; 1976.

CHAPTER 205 ■ AFFECTIVE DISORDERS

ANDRES M. KANNER AND DIETRICH BLUMER

INTRODUCTION

Mood disorders are the most common comorbid psychiatric disorders associated with epilepsy, but their real incidence and prevalence have yet to be established. Some of the primary reasons for the lack of definitive epidemiologic data include the diversity in methodologies and sample populations across studies, the underreporting of symptoms of depression by patients and families, and the underrecognition by clinicians. Population-based studies, however, have clearly shown that the prevalence of depression in people with epilepsy (PWE) is significantly higher than in healthy controls, as well as in people with chronic medical disorders.[59,62,96,104,144]

There is an ongoing debate as to whether depression in PWE differs from that in people with primary mood disorders.[105] Proponents of both schools of thought are probably correct, as a significant percentage of PWE can experience any of the various forms of primary mood disorders (i.e., major depressive disorder, dysthymic disorder, bipolar disorder, cyclothymic disorder) indistinguishable from those described in the *Diagnostic and Statistical Manual of Mental Disorders*, Fourth Edition (DSM-IV).[57] By the same token, several authors have identified atypical clinical manifestations of mood disorders in a significant proportion of PWE that fail to meet any of the diagnostic criteria suggested in the DSM-III, DSM-III-R, and DSM-IV.[19,105,110,134] Kraepelin and Bleuler were the first to recognize a "unique" clinical presentation of mood disorders in PWE consisting of recurrent episodes of "dysphoric symptoms"[18,115]; Gastaut expanded on Kraepelin's initial observations and Blumer coined the term *interictal dysphoric disorder.*[19,74,75] The purpose of this chapter is to provide a comprehensive review of mood disorders in epilepsy. The aim of this chapter is to provide a general review of the different aspects of affective disorder in PWE with special attention to epidemiologic and clinical data, the underlying pathogenic mechanisms with special attention to the existence of common pathogenic mechanisms that may be operant in depression and epilepsy, and the basic principles in their treatment. The chapter concludes with a brief discussion of interictal dysphoric disorder.

EPIDEMIOLOGIC DATA

Lifetime prevalences for major depressive episodes in the general population have been reported to range between 3.7% and 6.7%, for dysthymic and minor depressive disorders between 2.1% and 3.8%, and for manic episodes 0.6% and 1.1%.[111] Recent population-based studies identified significantly higher prevalence rates of depression in PWE. For example, the Canadian Community Health Survey evaluated the existence of mental health problems in a large sample of the population (n = 36,984).[200] A total of 253 subjects were found to have epilepsy (corresponding to a prevalence rate of epilepsy of 0.6%). The investigators used the Composite International Diagnostic Interview (Short Form) to identify a history of depression and found a lifetime prevalence of depression of 22.2% (95% confidence interval [CI], 14.0% to 30.4%) compared with 12.2% in the general population, with higher rates of major depression in younger, but not older (>64 years), age groups. Furthermore, lifetime suicidal ideation was higher in PWE (25.0% [95% CI, 16.6 to 33.3]) than in the general population (13.3% [95% CI, 12.8 to 13.9]). In a separate population-based study, Ettinger et al. investigated the presence of symptoms of depression among 775 PWE, 395 people with asthma, and 362 healthy controls identified from a cohort of 85,358 adults aged 18 years and older using the Centers of Epidemiologic Studies-Depression (CES-D) Instrument.[62] PWE experienced symptoms of depression with a significantly greater frequency (36.5%) and severity than people with asthma (27.8%) and healthy controls (11.8%). Of note, 38.5% of PWE whose score on the CES-D suggested the presence of a depressive disorder and 43.7% of people with asthma and depression were never previously evaluated for depression. The same group of investigators compared the lifetime prevalence rates of bipolar symptoms and past diagnoses of bipolar I and II disorder with the Mood Disorder Questionnaire (MDQ) among subjects who identified themselves as having epilepsy and those with migraine, asthma, or diabetes mellitus or a healthy comparison group.[63] Bipolar symptoms, evident in 12.2% of epilepsy patients, were 1.6 to 2.2 times more common in subjects with epilepsy than with migraine, asthma, or diabetes mellitus, and 6.6 times more likely to occur than in the healthy comparison group. A total of 49.7% of patients with epilepsy who screened positive for bipolar symptoms were diagnosed with bipolar disorder by a physician, nearly twice the rate seen in other disorders. However, 26.3% of MDQ-positive epilepsy subjects carried a diagnosis of unipolar depression, and 25.8% had neither a uni- nor bipolar depression diagnosis.

The impact of seizure control on the prevalence of depression has been investigated in four population-based studies. Using the Hospital Depression and Anxiety Symptoms scale, Jacoby et al.[96] reported that of 168 patients with recurrent seizures, 21% met criteria for clinical depression. Using the same instrument, O'Donoghue et al.[144] showed that among 155 PWE identified through two large primary care practices in the United Kingdom, 33% with recurrent seizures and 6% of those in remission had depression. Edeh and Toone[59] used the Clinical Interview Schedule to demonstrate a depressive disorder in 22% of 88 epilepsy patients identified from general practices in the United Kingdom.

Clearly, the prevalence rates of depression are significantly higher in studies done in tertiary centers. For example, Victoroff et al. assessed the lifetime prevalence of psychiatric disorders meeting DSM-III-R diagnostic criteria by administering the Structured Clinical Interview for DSM-III-R—Patient Version (SCID-P) to 60 patients with medically intractable complex partial seizures.[207] The standard interview was enlarged by explorations of the relationship between psychiatric complaints and course of the epilepsy, of brief periods of depression and elation, and of atypical personality features that had been reported among patients with temporal lobe epilepsy (TLE). Of the 60 patients, 42 (70%) had histories of one or more DSM-III-R axis I diagnoses and 35 (58%) had histories of major depressive episodes or other depressive disorders.

Current diagnoses of depression can also be identified more frequently among patients followed in tertiary centers. In a recently completed study of 199 consecutive outpatients from five epilepsy centers,[103] the presence of an axis I diagnosis was identified according to DSM-IV criteria with the Structured Clinical Interview for DSM-IV diagnosis (SCID) and the Mini International Psychiatric Interview (MINI). Sixty-seven patients (34%) met a DSM-IV criterion of a mood and/or anxiety disorder: 37 (19%) met criteria for major depression, of whom 17 (8.5%) had a mixed major depression and anxiety disorder. Only four patients (2%) met criteria for dysthymic disorder and 27 (13.6%) for an anxiety disorder.

The relation between depression and epilepsy has traditionally been thought to be unidirectional, given the higher incidence and prevalence of depression in PWE and the recognition of several epilepsy-related pathogenic mechanisms, including (a) a reactive process to psychosocial stressors associated with a life with epilepsy, (b) neurophysiologic and neurochemical changes related to the seizure activity, and (c) iatrogenic pharmacologic and surgical factors. Yet, the higher prevalence rates of depression in PWE were based on cross-sectional studies, which do not necessarily establish causality between the two disorders. In fact, three recent population-based studies have questioned this long-held assumption of a unidirectional relation and suggested the existence of a "bidirectional" relation between depression and epilepsy, whereby the presence of a mood disorder can also be associated with an increased risk of developing epilepsy.[20,89,90] Of note, these investigators were not the first ones to suggest the existence of such bidirectional relationship; indeed, 26 centuries ago, Hippocrates wrote: "melancholics ordinarily become epileptics, and epileptics melancholics: what determines the preference is the direction the malady takes; if it bears upon the body, epilepsy, if upon the intelligence, melancholy."[124] Such bidirectional relationship may in fact reflect the existence of common pathogenic mechanisms shared by epilepsy and depression, which facilitate the development of one disorder in the presence of the other (see below).

CLINICAL PRESENTATIONS

Symptoms of mood disorders in epilepsy are classified according to their temporal relation to seizure occurrence into peri-ictal and interictal symptoms. Peri-ictal symptoms include symptoms that precede (preictal), follow (postictal), or are the expression of a seizure (ictal), while interictal symptoms occur independently of seizures. Often, patients may experience symptoms of depression during both peri-ictal and interictal periods.

Peri-ictal Symptoms

Peri-ictal depressive symptoms and episodes are the least well studied with respect to their actual prevalence and are usually ignored by clinicians. Their occurrence has never been factored into any study investigating the prevalence of depressive symptoms/disorders in PWE despite the fact that their existence has been known to neurologists and psychiatrists for a long time.

Ictal Symptoms

It has been estimated that psychiatric symptoms occur in 25% of "auras"; 15% of these involve affect or mood changes.[54,209,212] For example, ictal symptoms of depression ranked second after symptoms of anxiety/fear, which are the most common type of ictal affect in one study. Ictal symptoms of depression are of short duration typically, are stereotypical, occur out of context, and are associated with other ictal phenomena. The most frequent symptoms include feelings of anhedonia, guilt, and suicidal ideation.

Preictal Symptoms

Preictal symptoms or episodes typically present as a dysphoric mood preceding a seizure by several hours to days. The best evidence is presented in the study by Blanchet and Frommer, who investigated mood changes in the course of 56 days in 27 PWE who were asked to rate their mood on a daily basis.[17] Mood ratings pointed to a dysphoric state 3 days prior to a seizure in 22 patients. This change in mood was more accentuated during the 24 hours preceding the seizure.

Postictal Symptoms

Postictal symptoms have been recognized for a very long time, but have been poorly studied in a systematic manner. Their detection can often be elusive as they do not occur necessarily on the same day as the seizure. Rather, symptom-free periods of up to 5 days can exist between the seizure occurrence and onset of psychiatric symptoms. The prevalence of postictal psychiatric symptoms was investigated in a study done at the Rush Epilepsy Center in Chicago in 100 consecutive patients with refractory epilepsy.[107] Only symptoms that occurred following more than 50% of seizures in the previous 3 months were included. In this study, the postictal period was defined as the 72 hours that followed a seizure. Symptoms that occurred during both interictal and postictal periods were also identified and compared in their severity during these periods. Since neurovegetative symptoms and fatigue are common postictal symptoms as well as symptoms of depression, they were analyzed separately so as not to inflate falsely the prevalence of postictal symptoms of depression (PSD).

Among the 100 patients, 43 experienced a mean of 4.8 $\pm$ 2.4 PSD (range 2 to 9; median = 5). The median duration of two thirds of symptoms was 24 hours. Twenty-five had a history of a mood disorder and 11 of an anxiety disorder. Table 1 shows the PSD and their respective median duration.

There was a significant association between a history of depression and the occurrence of the following PSD: Hopelessness, suicidal ideation, self-deprecation, and guilt. Furthermore, there was a significantly greater number of PSD in the presence of a history of depression and anxiety disorders.

Thirteen of these patients experienced a minimum of seven PSD lasting 24 hours or longer. Postictal suicidal ideation was identified in 13 patients. Eight patients experienced passive and active suicidal thoughts, while five only reported passive suicidal ideation. Ten of these 13 patients (77%) had a past history of either major depression or bipolar disorder, and this association was highly significant. Furthermore, the presence of postictal suicidal ideation was also significantly associated with a history of psychiatric hospitalization.

Among these 43 patients, PSD occurred together with postictal symptoms of anxiety (PSA) in 27 patients (63%) and seven other patients reported as well postictal psychotic symptoms. Table 1 shows the types of PSA and their median duration. Furthermore, 37 patients reported interictal symptoms of depression that worsened in severity during the postictal period in 30 patients.

Postictal hypomanic symptoms (PHM) included excessive energy and racing thoughts, which were identified in 22 patients: 15 patients reported racing thoughts and nine reported increased energy, but only two reported both symptoms (see Table 1). The occurrence of PHM only correlated significantly with that of postictal psychotic symptoms. In contrast to PSD, a psychiatric history was not a risk factor of PHM.

TABLE 1

PREVALENCE AND MEDIAN DURATION OF POSTICTAL SYMPTOMS OF DEPRESSION AND ANXIETY

Postictal symptom	Prevalence	Median duration in hours (range)
Symptoms of depression, total	43	
Irritability	30	24 (0.5–108)
Poor frustration tolerance	36	24 (0.1–108)
Anhedonia	32	24 (0.1–148)
Hopelessness	25	24 (1.0–108)
Helplessness	31	24 (1.0–108)
Crying bouts	26	6 (0.1–108)
Suicidal ideation	13	24 (1.0–240)
Active suicidal thoughts	8	
Passive suicidal thoughts	13	
Feelings of self-deprecation	27	24 (1.0–120)
Feelings of guilt	23	24 (0.1–240)
Symptoms of anxiety, total	45	
Constant worrying	33	24 (0.5–108)
Panicky feelings	10	6 (0.1–148)
Agoraphobic symptoms	29	24 (0.5–296)
Due to fear of seizure recurrence	20	
Compulsions	10	15 (0.1–72)
Self-consciousness	26	6 (0.05–108)
Hypomanic symptoms, total	22	
Excessive energy	9	2 (0.15–48)
Thought racing	15	2 (0.1–24)

Clearly, the occurrence of PSD is relatively high among patients with refractory epilepsy. Yet, in none of the studies on the prevalence of depression in epilepsy published so far has any investigator discriminated between an interictal, preictal, or postictal occurrence. The impact that PSD may have in "shaping" the psychiatric clinical phenomena of depression in PWE has yet to be established. Yet, it is likely that preictal symptoms and PSD may account for the frequent "atypical" characteristic of depressive disorders.

Interictal Depressive Disorders

Interictal depressive disorders have been the most commonly recognized. As stated above, there is an ongoing debate as to whether depressive disorders differ between people with and without epilepsy. In fact, some investigators have found that in up to 50% of PWE suffering from a depressive disorder, the depressive disorder failed to meet a DSM-III or -IV diagnostic criteria for one of the listed mood disorders.[134]

The following categories are included in the DSM-IV: Major Depressive Disorder, Dysthymic Disorder, Minor Depression, Bipolar Disorder, and Depressive Disorder Not Otherwise Specified or secondary to a medical condition or substance.[57] The difference between major depressive disorders and dysthymic disorder is based largely on severity, persistence, and chronicity. According to DSM-IV criteria, symptoms in both disorders may include combinations of depressed mood, anhedonia, worthlessness, guilt, decreased concentration ability, recurrent thoughts of death, and neurovegetative symptoms (i.e., weight loss or gain, insomnia or hypersomnia, psychomotor agitation or retardation, fatigue). In patients with a major depressive episode, at least 2 weeks of either a depressed mood or anhedonia must accompany four of these symptoms. In contrast, dysthymic disorder is a more chronic but less intense process with symptoms persistent for more days than not for at least 2 years. Minor depression is a category that is similar to major depressive episode in duration but encompasses at least two but less than five of the depressive symptoms noted above.

Bipolar disorders are of two types, depending on the occurrence of manic (type I) or hypomanic (type II) episodes in addition to major depressive episodes. The DSM-IV diagnosis for manic episodes includes the requirement of a distinct period of abnormally and persistently elevated mood lasting at least 1 week and of sufficient severity to cause marked impairment in social functioning. The diagnosis for a hypomanic episode includes the requirement of a distinct period of persistently elevated mood lasting throughout at least 4 days and observable as a disturbance by others. The diagnosis of a cyclothymic disorder requires the presence of numerous hypomanic and minor depressive episodes for at least 2 years.

Concurrent Psychiatric Symptoms in Depressive Disorders in Epilepsy

Investigators have reported a frequent co-occurrence of mood and anxiety disorders in patients with and without epilepsy, with comorbid rates ranging between 50% and 80% in patients with primary mood disorders. The existence of comorbid anxiety symptoms or disorders has a significant impact on the quality of life of depressed patients and their recognition is of the essence as they significantly increase the suicidal risk of depressed patients.[29] Thus, any evaluation of mood disorders for clinical or research purposes are incomplete in the absence of an investigation of comorbid symptoms of depression and vice versa.

Similar observations have been made in PWE. In a study of 199 patients with epilepsy from five epilepsy centers, 73% of patients with a history of depression met also DSM-IV criteria for an anxiety disorder.[103] Furthermore, several investigators dating back to Kraepelin, Bleuler, Gastaut, and more recently Blumer and Kanner have made a point of emphasizing the pleomorphic nature of the symptomatology in depressive disorders in PWE, which in addition to symptoms of anxiety include irritability, increased energy, and physical symptoms.[18,19,74,75,110,115] To a significant degree, these authors attributed the atypical manifestations of depression in epilepsy to these symptoms. This point is discussed in greater detail in the section on Interictal Dysphoric Disorder.

Nonetheless, recent studies have shown that these additional symptoms can be identified in PWE suffering from depressive disorders that also meet DSM-IV diagnostic criteria. In the study by Jones et al. cited above,[103] a DSM-IV diagnosis of a mood and/or anxiety disorders was established with the MINI and SCID in 199 consecutive outpatients from five epilepsy centers. These patients completed a 46-item self-rating instrument the Mood and Anxiety Symptoms in Epilepsy (MASE), which includes symptoms from eight domains (depression, anxiety, irritability, self-consciousness, physical symptoms, disturbances in socialization, suicidal ideation, and increased energy) on two occasions, 2 weeks apart. Sixty-seven patients met criteria for a DSM-IV axis I diagnosis: Each one of the 37 patients that met criteria for major depression reported symptoms of irritability and anxiety; 36 experienced physical symptoms, primarily fatigue; and 31 reported periods of increased energy. Clearly, these data show that depression in epilepsy in its "typical" manifestations not only consists of symptoms of depression, but is more often than not accompanied by symptoms of anxiety and irritability and, paradoxically, symptoms of increased energy. Whether this pleomorphic semiology is specific to depression in PWE or may be present in other neurologic disorders has yet to be established.

Atypical Expressions of Depression in Epilepsy

As stated above, depressive disorders in PWE often fail to meet any of the DSM-III, -III-R, or -IV criteria. For example, using DSM-III-R criteria, Mendez et al. had to classify almost 50% of depressive disorders as atypical depression.[134] Wiegartz et al. found that the depressive episodes of 25% of PWE were also classified as atypical depression not otherwise specified.[211] The interictal dysphoric disorder is the classic example of the atypical expression of depression in PWE and is reviewed at the end of this chapter.

In a study of the semiology of depressive episodes severe enough to merit pharmacotherapy in 97 consecutive patients with refractory epilepsy, only 28 (29%) met DSM-IV criteria for major depressive disorder.[110] The remaining 69 patients (71%) failed to meet criteria for any of the DSM-IV categories. These 69 patients presented a clinical picture consisting of anhedonia (with or without hopelessness), fatigue, anxiety, irritability, poor frustration tolerance, and mood lability with bouts of crying. Some patients also reported changes in appetite and sleep patterns and problems with concentration. Most symptoms presented with a waxing and waning course, with repeated interspersed symptom-free periods of 1 to several days' duration. Their semiology resembled the most a dysthymic disorder, but the recurrence of symptom-free periods intermittently precluded DSM criteria for this condition. We therefore referred to this form of depression as *dysthymic-like disorder of epilepsy* (DLDE).

In 33 of these 69 patients, the predominant and most disabling symptom was anhedonia, while in the remaining 36 patients irritability and poor frustration tolerance were the most disabling symptoms. Of note, patients with DLDE in whom anhedonia was the predominant symptom (vs. irritability) were significantly more likely to have experienced a prior history of major depressive episodes (45.5% vs. 19.5%). Whether DLDE is a variant of the interictal dysphoric disorder has yet to be established in systematic studies (see below).

Subclinical or subsyndromic forms of depression are another presentation of atypical depression, both in primary mood disorders and in depressive disorders of PWE. In the study of 199 consecutive PWE cited above,[103,109] 132 patients (64%) failed to meet any DSM-IV axis I diagnosis according to the SCID and MINI; yet, using the self-rating instruments Beck Depression Inventory (BDI) or the CES-D, 32 patients (16% of the entire cohort) were also found to have been experiencing symptoms of depression of mild to moderate severity. Furthermore, symptoms of anxiety were identified in 31 of these 32 patients with the MASE, symptoms of irritability in 32, physical symptoms in 24, and symptoms of increased energy in 18.

Suicidality as an Expression of Depression in Epilepsy

The suicide rate in PWE is five times higher than the expected rate in the general population. However, among patients with TLE the suicide rate can be 25 times higher.[77] For example, Robertson reviewed 17 studies pertaining to mortality in epilepsy and found that suicide was ten times more frequent than in the general population.[166] Rafnsson et al. recently reported the results of a population-based incidence cohort study in PWE from Iceland in which suicide had the highest standard mortality rate (5.8) of all causes of death,[158] and it was 3.5 in a Swedish study carried out among 9,000 previously hospitalized PWE.[142] The topic of suicidality in PWE is reviewed in detail in Chapter 211 in this book.

IMPACT ON QUALITY OF LIFE

Depression has been found to yield a significant negative impact on the quality of life of PWE. For example, in a study of 56 consecutive patients with TLE, Lehrner et al.[123] found depression to be the most powerful predictor for each domain of health-related quality of life. Even after controlling for seizure frequency and severity and other psychosocial variables, there remained a significant association between depression and ratings indicative of poor quality of life. In another study of 257 patients with epilepsy, Perrine et al.[150] found that the mood factor had the highest correlations with scales of the Quality of Life in Epilepsy (QOLIE-89) and was the strongest predictor of quality of life in regression analyses, as the mood factor was responsible for 46% of the variance in overall quality of life.

Likewise, in a group of 125 patients who had undergone temporal lobe surgery at least 12 months previously, Gilliam et al. showed that mood status was the most significant predictor of the patients' assessment of their own health status.[78] In another investigation, Gilliam examined the variables responsible for poor quality of life identified with the QOLIE-89 in 194 adult patients with refractory partial epilepsy[80] and found that the only independent variables significantly related to poor quality-of-life scores were high levels of depression and neurotoxicity from antiepileptic drugs. Patients had a median 9.7 seizures/month (range 0.3 to 51), but the author saw no relationship between the type and/or the frequency of seizures and quality-of-life scores. Identical findings were replicated by Boylan et al. in a more recent study.[28] Cramer et al. also found that depression was significantly associated with poor quality-of-life scores on the QOLIE-89 independently of the type of seizures; these investigators found, however, that seizure freedom for the last 3 months increased (i.e., improved) the quality-of-life ratings.[47] In the study of 199 patients described above, Kanner et al. found that the scores of the QOLIE-89 were significantly higher (i.e., better quality of life) among patients who had been seizure free for the last 6 months than those with persistent seizures.[109] These patients, however, were significantly less likely to have experienced a depressive disorder. The presence of a comorbid anxiety disorder with depression has also been associated with worse ratings in the QOLIE-89. In the same study cited above, patients with mixed anxiety/major depression had significantly lower scores than patients with major depression alone and these were in turn lower than those with only anxiety disorder.

Depression in PWE can also have a significant impact on health care costs associated with the management of the seizure disorder. For example, Cramer et al. investigated the impact of comorbid depression on health care utilization and health care coverage by PWE in U.S. communities using a postal survey questionnaire.[46] They found that people whose depression was untreated used significantly more health resources of all types, independently of seizure type and time since the last seizure. Furthermore, people with mild to moderate depression had a twofold and people with severe depression a fourfold higher frequency of medical visits than nondepressed people. Also, the presence and severity of depression was found to be a predictor of worse disability scores (Sheehan's Disability Scale), independently of duration of the seizure disorder. These data highlight the impact of comorbid depression on health care utilization by people with epilepsy.

Pathogenic Mechanisms

Is There a Bidirectional Relationship between Depression and Epilepsy?

Three studies published in the last 15 years have raised the possibility of a bidirectional relation between depression and epilepsy.[69,89,90] In the first study, Forsgren and Nystrom conducted a population-based case-control study of patients with newly diagnosed onset epilepsy in Sweden, and discovered that patients were seven times more likely to have reported a history of depression than were controls.[69] Hesdorffer et al. conducted a second population-based case-control investigation of the prevalence of new onset epilepsy among adults aged 55 and older, and showed that compared to controls, patients were 3.7 more likely to have had a history of depression *prior* to their first seizure.[89] The same authors conducted a population-based study in Iceland that included children and adults with newly diagnosed unprovoked seizures and/or epilepsy.[90] They found that patients with a history of major depression (by DSM-IV criteria) were significantly more likely than controls (odds ratio [OR] 1.7) to suffer from unprovoked seizures and epilepsy. Furthermore, a history of suicidal ideation was associated with a significantly greater risk of developing epilepsy (OR 5.5) independent of a history of major depression. These data do not indicate causality between the two disorders, but rather suggest the existence of common pathogenic mechanisms operant in depression and epilepsy.

Common Pathogenic Mechanisms in Epilepsy and Depression

Two classes of pathogenic mechanisms are likely to be operant in both disorders: (a) abnormal secretion patterns of neurotransmitter systems including serotonin (5HT), norepinephrine (NE), dopamine (DA), γ-aminobutyric acid (GABA), and glutamate; and (b) structural and functional abnormalities of common neuroanatomic structures in limbic structures, particularly in temporal and frontal lobes.

Abnormal Secretion of Neurotransmitters

Data from experimental animal studies. Abnormal serotonergic, noradrenergic, and dopaminergic transmission in the brain has been recognized as a pivotal pathogenic mechanism of mood disorders and has been the basis for the development of antidepressant pharmacologic treatments.[191] By the same token, a decreased serotonergic and noradrenergic activity has been shown to facilitate the kindling of seizures, exacerbate seizure severity, and intensify seizure predisposition in some animal models of epilepsy as shown below.[98] Compelling data are derived from studies with two strains of genetic epilepsy-prone rats (GEPR), GEPR-3 and GEPR-9, which are characterized by genetically determined predisposition to sound-induced generalized tonic–clonic seizures (GTCSs).[44,50,98–100,205] Both strains of rats have innate pre- and postsynaptic noradrenergic and serotonergic transmission deficits, the former resulting from deficient arborization of neurons arising from the locus coeruleus coupled with excessive presynaptic suppression of stimulated NE release in the terminal fields and lack of postsynaptic compensatory up-regulation.[44,50,98–100,205] GEPR-9 rats have a more pronounced NE transmission deficit and, in turn, exhibit more severe seizures than GEPR-3 rats.[215] Abnormal serotonergic arborization has also been identified in the GEPR's brain coupled with deficient postsynaptic serotonin$_{1A}$-receptor density in the hippocampus.[49] Of note, GEPRs display similar endocrine abnormalities to those identified in patients with major depressive disorder (MDD), such as increased corticosterone serum levels, deficient secretion of growth hormone, and hypothyroidism.[101]

Increments of either NE and/or 5HT transmission with the selective serotonin reuptake inhibitor (SSRI) sertraline resulted in a dose-dependent seizure frequency reduction in the GEPR, which correlated with the extracellular thalamic serotonergic thalamic concentration.[213,214] In addition, the 5-HT precursor 5-HTP has been shown to have anticonvulsant effects in GEPRs when combined with a monoamine oxidase inhibitor (MAOI),[98] while SSRIs and MAOIs have been found to exert anticonvulsant effects in genetically prone epilepsy mice and baboons as well as in nongenetically prone cats, rabbits, and rhesus monkeys.[133,152,153,213,217] Conversely, drugs that interfere with the release or synthesis of NE or 5HT exacerbate seizures in the GEPRs.[98,138] These include NE storage vesicle inactivators reserpine or tetrabenazine, the NE false transmitter α-methyl-m-tryosine, the NE synthesis inhibitor α-methyl-Δ-tyrosine, and the 5-HT synthesis inhibitor Δ-chlorophenylalanine, all of which have also been found to facilitate seizure occurrence in humans.[138,143,197]

An anticonvulsant effect of serotonergic activity has been reported in other animal models of epilepsy. Lopez-Meraz et al. studied the impact of two 5HT$_{1A}$ receptor agonists, 8-OH-DPAT and indorenate, in three animal models of epileptic seizures (clonic–tonic induced by pentylenetetrazol [PTZ], status epilepticus of limbic seizures induced by kainic acid [KA], and tonic–clonic seizures induced by amygdala kindling) in Wistar rats.[127] They found that 8-OH-DPAT lowered the incidence of seizures and the mortality induced by PTZ, increased the latency and reduced the frequency of wet-dog shake and generalized seizures induced by KA and at high doses diminished the occurrence and delayed the establishment of status epilepticus. Indorenate increased the latency to the PTZ-induced seizures and decreased the percentage of rats that showed tonic extension and death, augmented the latency to wet-dog shake and generalized seizures, and diminished the number of generalized seizures.

The antiepileptic effect of 5HT$_{1A}$ receptors has been associated with a membrane hyperpolarizing response associated with increased potassium conductance in hippocampal kindled seizures in cats, and in intrahippocampal kainic acid–induced seizures in freely moving rats.[13,148] Furthermore, antiepileptic drugs (AEDs) with established psychotropic effects (carbamazepine [CBZ], valproic acid [VPA], and lamotrigine [LTG]) have been found to cause an increase in 5HT.[41,42,51–53,189,210,216] In fact, the anticonvulsant protection of CBZ can be blocked with 5HT-depleting drugs in GEPRs.[216] Likewise, in a recent study, Clinckers et al. investigated the impact of oxcarbazepine (OXC) infusion on the extracellular hippocampal concentration of 5HT and DA in the focal pilocarpine model for limbic seizures.[41] When OXC was administered together with verapamil or probenecid (so as to ensure its passage through the blood–brain barrier), complete seizure remission was obtained associated with an increase in 5HT and DA extracellular concentrations.[42]

In addition, it has been suggested that the anticonvulsant effect of the vagal nerve stimulator (VNS) in the rat could be mediated by noradrenergic and serotonergic mechanisms, as deletion of noradrenergic and serotonergic neurons in the rat prevents or reduces significantly the anticonvulsant effect of VNS against electroshock- or pentylenetetrazol-induced seizures.[35,139] Furthermore, the effect of VNS on the locus coeruleus and raphe may be responsible for its antidepressant effects identified in humans.[3]

Data from studies in humans. Depression in PWE has been associated more frequently with seizure disorders of temporal and frontal lobe origin, with prevalence rates ranging from 19% to 65% in various patient series.[6,74,75,95,104,163,207] In contrast to animal studies, the impact of pharmacologic augmentation or reduction in 5HT and NE transmission on seizures in humans has been rather sparse and mostly based on uncontrolled data. For example, depletion of monoamines with reserpine has been associated with an increase in frequency and severity of seizures in PWE,[143,197] while the use of reserpine at doses of 2 to 10 mg/day was found to lower the electroshock seizure threshold and the severity of the resulting seizures in patients with schizophrenia.[138] The tricyclic antidepressant imipramine, with reuptake inhibitory effects of NE and 5HT, was reported to suppress absence and myoclonic seizures in double-blind placebo-controlled studies.[71–73] Open trials with the SSRIs fluoxetine and citalopram yielded an improvement in seizure frequency, but no controlled studies with this class of antidepressants have been performed as of yet.[4,65]

Functional Neuroimaging Studies in Epilepsy and Primary Depression. The use of positron emission tomography (PET) and single photon emission computed tomography (SPECT) studies has yielded significant data suggestive of abnormal 5HT activity in primary depressive disorders and in epilepsy, with particular involvement of $5HT_{1A}$ receptors. Deficits in 5HT transmission in human depression is thought to be partially related to a paucity of serotonergic innervation of its terminal areas suggested by a scarcity of 5HT levels in brain tissue, plasma, and platelets and with a deficit in serotonin transporter binding sites in postmortem human brain.[8,30,32,33,38,39,120–122,129,140,145,146,151,167,192,195] Serotonin stores and transporter protein are important components of serotonin terminals so that a combined deficit is a plausible indicator of reduced axonal branching and synapse formation.

With respect to abnormal serotonergic activity in functional neuroimaging studies of patients with primary major depression, Sargent et al. demonstrated a reduced binding potential of $5HT_{1A}$ receptors in frontal, temporal, and limbic cortex with PET studies using [11 C]WAY-100635 in both unmedicated and medicated depressed patients compared with healthy volunteers.[172] Of note, binding potential values in medicated patients were similar to those in unmedicated patients. Drevets et al., using the same radioligand, reported a decreased binding potential of $5HT_{1A}$ receptors in mesial temporal cortex and in the raphe in 12 patients with familial recurrent major depressive episodes compared to controls.[58] A deficit in the density or affinity of postsynaptic $5HT_{1A}$ receptors has been identified in the hippocampus and amygdala of untreated depressed patients who committed suicide.[147] In addition, impaired serotonergic transmission has been associated with defects in the dorsal raphe nuclei of suicide victims with major depressive disorder consisting of an excessive density of serotonergic somatodendritic impulse-suppressing $5HT_{1A}$ autoreceptors.[122]

Similar abnormalities have been reported in patients with epilepsy. In a PET study of patients with TLE using the $5HT_{1A}$ receptor antagonist [18F]trans-4-fluro-N-2-[4-(2-methoxyphenyl)piperazin-1-yl]ethyl-N-(2-pyridyl) cyclohexanecarboxamide reduced $5HT_{1A}$ binding was found in mesial temporal structures ipsilateral to the seizure focus in patients with and without hippocampal atrophy. Reduced serotonergic activity was independent of the presence or absence of hippocampal atrophy on magnetic resonance imaging (MRI), and reduced volume of distribution and binding remained significant after partial volume correction.[201] In addition, a 20% binding reduction was found in the raphe and a 34% lower binding in the ipsilateral thalamic region to the seizure focus. In a separate PET study aimed at quantifying $5HT_{1A}$ receptor binding in 14 patients with TLE, a decreased binding was identified in the epileptogenic hippocampus, amygdala, anterior cingulate, and lateral temporal neocortex ipsilateral to the seizure focus, as well as in the contralateral hippocampi, but to a lesser degree, and in the raphe nuclei.[174] Other investigators using the $5HT_{1A}$ tracer 4,2-(methoxyphenyl)-1-[2-(*N*-2-pyridinyl)-*p*-fluorobenzamido]ethylpiperazine ([^{203}F]MPPF) found that the decrease in binding of $5HT_{1A}$ was significantly greater in the areas of seizure onset and propagation identified with intracranial electrode recordings. As in the other studies, reduction in $5HT_{1A}$ binding was present even when quantitative and qualitative MRIs were normal.[135]

Reduction in $5HT_{1A}$ receptor binding is not restricted to patients with TLE. PET studies with the $5HT_{1A}$ receptor antagonist carbonyl-carbon 11-WAY-100635 ([11c]WAY-100635) found a decreased binding potential in the dorsolateral prefrontal cortex, raphe nuclei, and hippocampus of 11 patients with juvenile myoclonic epilepsy compared to 11 controls.[136]

With respect to abnormal DA activity as a common pathogenic mechanism, Tremblay et al. recently demonstrated abnormal dopaminergic function in the brain of patients with primary major depressive disorders.[203] Using functional MRI blood oxygen level–dependent activation during a controlled task and measurement of dextroamphetamine subjective effects, patients with major depression had a twofold increase in the response to the rewarding effects of dextroamphetamine, compared to a group of 12 healthy controls. Abnormal brain activation was identified in the ventrolateral prefrontal cortex and orbitofrontal cortex as well as in the caudate and putamen in the patient group.

Likewise, abnormal dopamine activity in the brain of patients with refractory epilepsy has been recently suggested in a PET study using 18F-fluoro-DOPA.[27] Three groups of patients were included: One consisted of 16 patients with a ring chromosome 20 (r20); a second group included 10 patients with absence-like epilepsy; and the third group was integrated by nine patients with intractable TLE. Compared to a group of ten healthy volunteers, patients from all three epilepsy groups displayed a decrease of 18F-fluro-DOPA uptake, but only in patients with TLE was the decreased uptake lateralized to the side of the seizure focus. A bilateral uptake was found in the substantia nigra in all three patient groups.

Involvement of frontal lobes in primary depression has also been demonstrated with functional neuroimaging (PET, SPECT) and neuropsychological studies.[11,114] For example, executive abnormalities are consistently found among studies, and are more apparent in more severe depressive disorders. These neuropsychological disturbances correlated with reduced blood flow in mesial prefrontal cortex. Furthermore, in tests demanding executive function, cingulate cortex and striatum could not be activated in patients with major depressive disorders.[125] Functional disturbance of frontal lobe structures has been recognized in TLE and particularly among patients with TLE and comorbid depression, as they have been found to have bilateral reduction in inferofrontal metabolism.[31,102] Likewise, neuropsychological testing with the Wisconsin Card Sorting Test (WCST), which is highly sensitive to executive dysfunction, has revealed poor performance in patients with TLE and comorbid depression.[45,82,83,85–87,94,178] Of note, inferior frontal cortex is the main target of the mesolimbic dopaminergic neurons and provides input to the serotonergic neurons of the dorsal raphe nucleus.

The abnormal serotonergic secretion in the brain of PWE may account for the prominence of comorbid symptoms of anxiety and panic, irritability, and poor frustration tolerance, as well as the increased incidence rates of suicidality. Neumeister et al., using the selective $5HT_{1A}$ radioligand [18F]-FCWAY, found reduced $5HT_{1A}$ receptor binding in the anterior and posterior cingulate in patients with panic disorder with and without comorbid depression.[1] A relationship between abnormal serotonin activity and suicidal behavior associated with several psychiatric diagnoses has been suggested in multiple studies, including quantitative autoradiography studies of brain tissues obtained from suicidal victims, in studies of serotonin transporter sites, and in studies of $5HT_{1A}$ receptor binding, to name a few.[147] These studies suggest abnormal serotonergic function primarily at the ventral prefrontal cortex.

Common Neuroanatomic Structures Involved in Depression and Epilepsy

Structural changes in temporal lobes. Structural neuroimaging studies of patients with major depressive disorders revealed involvement of mesial temporal, orbitofrontal, and mesial frontal structures, as well as subcortical structures including basal ganglia and thalamic nuclei.[185] Sheline et al. reported bilateral smaller hippocampal volumes in two separate studies of patients with a history of primary major depressive disorders in remission when compared to hippocampal volumes of age-, sex-, and height-matched normal controls.[182–184] They also identified large hippocampal low-signal foci ($\geq$4.5 mm in diameter) and their number correlated with the total number of days depressed. A significant inverse correlation between the duration of depression and left hippocampal volume was also demonstrated, suggesting that patients with more chronic and active disease were more likely to have hippocampal atrophy. More recently, Sheline et al. demonstrated that hippocampal atrophy was prevented with antidepressant drug therapy in a study of 38 female patients with a history of major depressive disorders.[180] They found a significant correlation between reduction in hippocampal volume and the duration of depression that went untreated, while there was no correlation between hippocampal volume loss and time depressed while taking antidepressant medication or with lifetime exposure to antidepressants. Similar findings have been reported by other investigators.[206]

Atrophy has also been identified in entorhinal cortex and amygdala.[15,154,185] Furthermore, in a neuropathologic study of amygdala and entorhinal cortex, a significant reduction of glial cells and of the glial/neurons ratio was found in left amygdala and to a lesser degree in left entorhinal cortex of patients with major depressive disorder and bipolar disorder (not treated with lithium and valproic acid) compared to those of controls.[181]

By the same token, abnormalities of mesial temporal structures are among the most frequently identified in PWE and comorbid depression. In three studies of patients with TLE, higher scores of depression were associated with the presence of mesial temporal sclerosis (MTS), decreased temporal lobe and frontal lobe perfusion on (99m) Tc-HMPAO SPECT scans, and greater abnormalities identified with magnetic resonance spectroscopy.[79,157,177]

It is important to notice, however, that the magnitude of hippocampal atrophy in TLE is significantly greater than that in major depressive disorder, while the neuropathologic findings are different. In MTS, neuropathologic findings consist of neuronal cell loss and astrocytosis in hippocampal formation (including areas CA1, CA2, CA3, and CA4, dentate gyrus, and subiculum), amygdala entorhinal cortex, and parahippocampal gyrus.[130]

Unfortunately, there have been very few neuropathologic studies of the human hippocampal formation in patients with primary major depressive disorder. Lucassen et al. carried out a neuropathologic study of 15 hippocampi of patients with a history of major depressive disorder and compared them to those of 16 matched controls and nine steroid-treated patients.[128] In 11 of 15 depressed patients, rare but convincing apoptosis was identified in entorhinal cortex, subiculum, dentate gyrus, CA1, and CA4. Apoptosis was also found in three steroid-treated patients and one control. However, no apoptosis of pyramidal cells in CA3 was identified. Other neuropathologic changes in brains from patients with major depression were reported by Stockheimer et al.[194] These investigators compared the density of pyramidal neurons, dentate granule cell neurons, and glia and the size of the neuronal soma from postmortem sections of right hippocampus obtained from 19 patients with major depressive disorders and 21 aged-matched psychiatrically normal controls. They found that in patients with major depressive disorders, the density of granule cells and glia in dentate gyrus and pyramidal neurons and glia in all cornu ammonis was significantly increased by 30% to 35%, while the average soma size of pyramidal neurons was decreased.

Hippocampal atrophy in primary major depressive disorders has been attributed to two potential pathogenic mechanisms: (a) an alteration in neurotrophic factors resulting from the mood disorder[40,141,187] and (b) high glucocorticoid exposure.[92,93,161,170]

Acute and chronic stress decreases levels of brain-derived neurotrophic factor (BDNF) in the dentate gyrus, pyramidal cell layer of hippocampus, amygdala, and neocortex, which may contribute to structural hippocampal changes.[187] These changes are mediated by glucocorticoids and can be overturned with antidepressant therapy, as chronic administration of antidepressant drugs increased BDNF expression and also prevented a stress-induced decrease in BDNF levels.[40,141] There is also evidence that antidepressant drugs can increase hippocampal BDNF levels in humans.[40,141] These data indicate that antidepressant-induced up-regulation of BDNF can hypothetically repair damage to hippocampal neurons and protect vulnerable neurons from additional damage.

The high glucocorticoid exposure mediating hippocampal atrophy is based on the excessive activation of the hypothalamic-pituitary-adrenal axis identified in almost half of individuals with depression resulting in impaired dexamethasone suppression of adrenocorticotropic hormone (ACTH) and cortisol. These changes are reversible to treatment with antidepressants.[93] In experimental studies with rats and monkeys, prolonged increased concentrations of glucocorticoids have been found to damage hippocampal neurons, particularly CA3 pyramidal neurons, possibly by reduction of dendritic branching and loss of dendritic spines that are included in glutamatergic synaptic inputs.[170] Hypercortisolemia has also been found to interfere with the development of new granule cell neurons in the adult hippocampal dentate gyrus. Deleterious effects of chronic glucocorticoid exposure may lead initially to a transient and reversible atrophy of the CA3 dendritic tree and to an increased vulnerability to a variety of insults and finally result in cell death under extreme and prolonged conditions.[170]

Structural changes in frontal lobes. Likewise, structural changes have been identified in the orbitofrontal and prefrontal cortex and cingulate gyrus, as well as in their white matter, including a smaller volume of orbitofrontal cortex in young adults and geriatric patients with major depressive disorder.[116,117,198,199] Of note, the magnitude of prefrontal volume changes was related to the severity of the depression, as elderly patients with minor depression had lesser changes than those with major depressive disorder.[116]

Neuropathologic studies have also documented structural cortical changes in frontal lobes of depressed patients. Rajkowska et al. found a decrease in cortical thickness, neuronal sizes, and neuronal densities in layers II, III, and IV of the rostral orbitofrontal region in the brains of depressed patients.[159] In the caudal orbitofrontal cortex, there were significant reductions in glial densities in cortical layers V and VI that were also associated with decreases in neuronal sizes. Finally, in the dorsolateral prefrontal cortex, there was a decrease in neuronal and glial density and size in all cortical layers.

Other Pathogenic Mechanisms

Psychosocial causes of depression. For many years, clinicians and patients have, erroneously, attributed and explained their patients' depressed mood solely as a "normal reaction" to the numerous social and personal obstacles resulting from epilepsy. These include (a) the patient's and/or family inability to accept and adjust to a diagnosis of epilepsy; (b) the stigma related to the diagnosis of epilepsy and the well-known discrimination patients face; (c) the lack of control in one's life resulting from the unpredictable occurrence of epileptic seizures; and (d) the patient's lack of social support and the need to make major adjustments in lifestyle, such as giving up driving privileges or changing jobs to maximize seizure precautions.[36,55,56,84,97,175] Any one or combination of these factors could result in an *initial* adjustment reaction with depressive and anxiety features, but they are unlikely *on their own* to result in *chronic* depressive disorder. Also, patients displaying comorbid depression may have less ability to cope with these obstacles. Additionally, even epileptic patients with a normal intelligence have been found to show a lower degree of flexibility of mental processing compared with normal controls in neuropsychological studies.[34,188] Nonetheless, a depressed state that persists after several months can no longer be diagnosed from a clinical standpoint as a "normal" reactive process and warrants a detailed psychiatric evaluation.

Depression as an iatrogenic process. Every AED, including those with positive psychotropic properties, can trigger depressive symptoms in PWE, some more than others.[132] Phenobarbital (PB) can result in depression that may occasionally be complicated with suicidal ideation; primidone (PRM), tiagabine, vigabatrin, felbamate, topiramate (TPM), levetiracetam (LEV), and zonisamide (ZNS) have also been associated with symptoms of depression.[9,29,66,106,131,137,162,186] On the other hand, the presence of a current or prior depressive disorder may increase the risk of cognitive adverse events associated with topiramate.[106,137]

Depression following epilepsy surgery. In the last two decades, depressive disorders have been recognized with increased frequency during the first year following an anterotemporal lobectomy.[23,173] It is common for patients to exhibit "mood lability" within the first 6 weeks after surgery, and usually these symptoms subside; however, overt depressive symptoms become clear within the initial 6 months in up to 30% of patients. Typically, symptoms of depression range in caliber from mild to very severe, including suicidal attempts. In general, pharmacologic treatment with antidepressant drugs is effective. Patients with a past history of depression are at increased risk. In a recent study of 90 consecutive patients that underwent an anterotemporal lobectomy at the Rush Epilepsy Center, 23 exhibited an exacerbation or recurrence of a previous depressive disorder and 11 experienced a de novo depressive disorder.[108] Remission of all symptoms was obtained in 22 patients, while in 12 symptoms persisted despite multiple pharmacologic trials with various antidepressants. There was no difference in the risk of developing a persistent depressive disorder among patients with de novo versus those with a prior history of depression. Postsurgical seizure freedom was associated with a lower likelihood of experiencing a postsurgical depressive episode. Thus, all patients preparing for epilepsy surgery should be warned of this possible risk, *prior to surgery*.

A paradoxic "iatrogenic" cause of psychopathology among epileptic patients includes the phenomenon of "forced normalization," which consists of the development of psychiatric disorders following the cessation of epileptic seizures.[165] An interictal depression, therefore, may exacerbate or present de novo in patients as increased seizure control is attained, although the frequency of this phenomenon remains to be established. This problem is discussed in greater detail in section II.

A genetic predisposition. A common risk to develop a depressive disorder in patients with and without epilepsy is a family history of depression. In fact, over 50% of PWE suffering from depression have been found to show a family history of psychiatric illness, affective disorders being the most frequent condition.[95,163]

Laterality of the seizure focus. Despite having been raised as a potential pathogenic parameter, the laterality of the seizure focus remains a topic of debate. Certain authors have suggested, however, that a left hemispheric focus may be a predisposing factor of depression based on PET and SPECT studies.[165]

TREATMENT

Despite the relatively high comorbidity of mood disorders in epilepsy, they continue to remain unrecognized and untreated in a significant percentage of patients. Indeed, depression in epilepsy remains underrecognized and undertreated. For example, in a study of 97 patients with epilepsy with depressive disorders severe enough to merit pharmacologic treatment, 60% had been symptomatic for more than 1 year before any treatment was suggested.[110] Only one third of the 97 patients had been treated within 6 months of the onset of their symptoms. To our surprise, delay in recognizing the need for therapy was not related to the severity of the depressive disorder, as the proportion of untreated patients for more than 1 year did not differ between patients with major depression and dysthymic disorders. Wiegartz et al.[211] reported similar findings. Thirty percent of 76 patients with partial epilepsy met criteria of a lifetime-to-date diagnosis of major depressive disorder, 9% with a diagnosis of current major depressive episode, and 22% with a lifetime diagnosis of major depressive disorder. Twenty-five percent of these 76 patients reported symptoms of minor depressive disorders (dysthymic disorders, depressive disorder not otherwise specified). None of these patients had received treatment for their dysthymic disorder and commonly had not been trained to understand and treat the psychiatric complications of epilepsy.

Even when recognized, clinicians refrain from considering the use of pharmacologic treatment for (a mistaken) fear of worsening the patient's seizures. The hesitancy of using psychotropic medications in PWE has resulted in the absence of controlled studies on the efficacy and safety of antidepressants in these patients. Indeed, to date there has been only one controlled study published in the literature that compared under blind conditions the efficacy of two antidepressant drugs (amitriptyline and mianserin) to placebo in major depression of PWE.[179] Consequently, the data available for the management of mood disorders in PWE have to be derived from open uncontrolled trials, based on the experience obtained in the treatment of primary depression. Given the relatively high frequency of atypical depressive disorders in PWE, one cannot assume that efficacy in mood disorders in patients without epilepsy may apply to PWE. The absence of methodologically sound data has further compounded the clinician's reluctance to treat patients with psychotropic drugs, and in the end the persistence of a mood disorder ends up having a worse impact on the patient's quality of life than the actual seizures and increases their risk of suicide, which has also clearly surpassed the risk of death from a seizure, as documented in a separated chapter.

Some Preliminary Basic Concepts

Before starting any specific treatment strategy, it is important to consider the following questions:

1. Did the symptoms of depression and anxiety appear following the introduction or increase in the dose of an AED known to cause psychiatric adverse events?
2. Did the psychiatric symptoms follow the discontinuation of an AED with positive psychotropic (mood stabilizing, antidepressant, and anxiolytic) properties (i.e., CBZ, VPA, LTG, OXC)? In this case, the psychiatric symptoms may be the expression of recurrence of a latent psychiatric disorder that had been in remission (or masked) by the AED discontinued.[164] By the same token, it is important to investigate the existence of any psychiatric family history that places the patient at an increased risk when exposed to an AED with negative psychotropic properties (i.e., symptoms of depression following exposure to PB, PRM, or ZNS in patients with a family history of mood disorders).
3. Did the psychiatric symptoms occur after the introduction of an enzyme-inducing AED (CBZ, PHT, PB, PRM, high-dose TPM, or OXC) in a patient who was already taking a psychotropic drug for a previously recognized depression or anxiety disorder? In such case, the symptom recurrence may have resulted from a pharmacokinetic interaction between the AED and the psychotropic drug on board that caused a drop in the psychotropic drug's serum concentration. Accordingly, a readjustment in the dose of the psychotropic drug may be sufficient to induce symptom remission.
4. Are the psychiatric symptoms temporally related to the seizure occurrence? That is, do they precede (preictal), do they follow (postictal), do they precede and follow, are they the expression of an ictal event, or do they occur interictally with a peri-ictal exacerbation in severity? In the case of pre- or postictal without interictal symptoms, pharmacotherapy may fail to yield any benefit. Postictal breakthrough symptoms may occur in patients whose interictal symptoms remitted with pharmacotherapy.
5. Are the psychiatric symptoms related to the remission of seizures following a period of persistent seizures, or are they associated with worsening of the patient's seizure disorder? In the former case, the symptoms may be the expression of the phenomenon known as "forced normalization" or "alternative psychopathology."
6. Is the patient experiencing other psychiatric symptoms (i.e., symptoms of anxiety) that need to be targeted for treatment?

Pharmacotherapy of Depressive Disorders

Today, SSRIs and serotonin norepinephrine reuptake inhibitors (SNRIs) have become the first line of pharmacotherapy for primary major, dysthymic, and minor depressive disorders as well as for the treatment of generalized anxiety and panic disorders (Table 2).[37,112] These drugs are also being advocated for the treatment of these psychiatric disorders in PWE. Furthermore, the use of SSRIs is particularly relevant in PWE given the relatively high comorbidity of anxiety disorders and the prominence of irritability in which these drugs have shown marked efficacy.

Therapeutic Expectations of Pharmacotherapy of Depressive Disorders

A "primary" major depressive episode left untreated may last between 6 and 24 months in 90% to 95% of cases, while the remaining 5% to 10% could last more than 2 years.[37,60,91,112,202] When pharmacotherapy is started, "responders" to pharmacotherapy experience an improvement in their symptomatology (i.e., at least 50% reduction of severity of symptoms measured with a variety of rating scales) during the first 8 weeks. Two thirds of patients are expected to "respond" to antidepressant medication, and in controlled studies, one third are expected to respond to placebo. "Response to therapy," however, does not imply a symptom-free state and persistence of symptoms increases significantly the risk of recurrence of future major depressive episodes. When such symptom-free state is achieved,

TABLE 2

EFFICACY OF SELECTIVE SEROTONIN REUPTAKE INHIBITORS AND SEROTONIN NOREPINEPHRINE REUPTAKE INHIBITORS IN PRIMARY DEPRESSION AND ANXIETY DISORDERS

Antidepressant drug	Depression	Panic disorder	Generalized anxiety	Starting dose	Maximal dose
Paroxetine	+	+	+	10	60
Sertraline	+	+		25	200
Fluoxetine	+	+		10	80
Citalopram	+			10	60
Escitalopram	+	+	+	5	30
Venlafaxine	+	+	+	37.5	300

Fluvoxamine was not included in this table due to the absence of any data in people with epilepsy.

the patient is considered to have entered "remission." It is estimated that approximately 50% of patients will reach remission within the first 6 months and about two thirds within 2 years of the start of therapy. When remission has lasted for a period of 6 to 12 months, the patient is considered to have reached a state of "recovery." Approximately 15% to 20% of patients will fail to respond to any antidepressant trial. It has yet to be established whether pharmacotherapy of major depression in PWE yields the same efficacy as that in primary major depressive disorders.

The variables predictive of relapse include (a) multiple prior episodes; (b) severe episodes; (c) long-lasting episodes; (d) episodes with psychotic or bipolar features; and (e) incomplete recovery between two consecutive episodes. Furthermore, premature discontinuation of antidepressant medication can result in relapse. Indeed, only 10% of patients who had an initial response to antidepressant drugs and who were kept for at least 12 months on the drug are likely to experience a relapse, in contrast to 50% of patients in whom the antidepressant medication was discontinued within 6 to 12 months of the start of therapy. If psychotherapy is considered, patients can be referred to a psychologist or to a local mental health clinic for this type of treatment (see below). Many patients will require a combination of pharmacotherapy and psychotherapy.

Pharmacotherapy of Dysthymic-like Disorders

There are no controlled data available on the treatment of DLDE. In an open trial with the SSRI sertraline carried out at the Rush Epilepsy Center in 67 patients with DLDE, complete symptom remission was reached in 57% of patients. While these results are similar to those reported in primary dysthymia, they need to be replicated in randomized placebo-controlled studies in PWE.[110]

Role of the Neurologist in the Management of Mood Disorders in People with Epilepsy

Given their relatively high prevalence in PWE, neurologists should be able to identify the depressive and bipolar disorders described above. They should know how to *initiate* pharmacotherapy for major, dysthymic, and minor depressive episodes. However, the following are the mood disorders that deserve immediate referral to a psychiatrist: (a) any depressive episode associated with suicidal ideation. (b) Any major depressive disorder with psychotic features. Approximately 25% of major depressive disorders can present with psychotic features. In such cases, pharmacotherapy has to include antipsychotic and antidepressant drugs, and at times, the use of electroshock therapy (ECT) has to be considered. Furthermore, the presence of psychotic symptomatology increases significantly the suicidal risk of these patients. (c) Any major depressive or dysthymic episode that has failed to respond to a prior trial with SSRIs or SNRIs at optimal doses. These patients may require a combination of antidepressant drugs or the addition of lithium, thyroid drugs, or central nervous system stimulants to one or two antidepressants and occasionally ECT to reach a euthymic state. (d) Any bipolar disorder. The management of bipolar disorders is fret with a significantly lower therapeutic success and potential serious complications from an inappropriate use of psychotropic drugs such as the conversion of a bipolar disorder into a rapid cycling disorder.[60] Indeed, clinicians must keep in mind that the use of antidepressant medication in a bipolar disorder can facilitate the development of manic and hypomanic episodes and of a rapid cycling bipolar disorder (defined as the presence of four or more depressive, manic, or hypomanic episodes in a 12-month period). The American Psychiatric Association guidelines for the treatment of acute depression in bipolar disease advise against an initial use of antidepressant drugs.[60,202] Thus, in patients with "apparent" stable bipolar disorders, neurologists should at the least refer the patient for *one* psychiatric consultation to confirm that optimal treatment options are being prescribed.

Choice of Antidepressant Drug

As stated above, there is a general consensus among psychiatrists that SSRIs and/or SNRIs are the drugs of choice to treat the various types of primary depression. However, when choosing an antidepressant drug in PWE, clinicians must also consider the following issues:

1. The potential of the antidepressant drug to worsen seizures
2. The pharmacokinetic and pharmacodynamic interactions of the AEDs with the antidepressant drug
3. The potential of the antidepressant drug to worsen underlying comorbid disorders specific to PWE

Do Selective Serotonin Reuptake Inhibitors and Serotonin Norepinephrine Reuptake Inhibitors Worsen Seizures?

The incidence of seizures in nonepilepsy patients exposed to SSRIs is presented in Table 3.

Clearly, the incidence of seizures is lower than that expected in the general population. Furthermore, in a recent critical review of the literature, Jobe and Browning concluded that not only is the use of SSRIs safe, but also that the proconvulsant effects of antidepressants cannot be accounted by their serotonergic or noradrenergic effects.[156] A recent study supports these conclusions. Khan et al. compared the incidence of seizures among patients randomized to SSRIs (citalopram, fluoxetine, fluvoxamine), the SNRI venlafaxine, and the α2-adrenergic antagonist antidepressant mirtazapine in regulatory trials. They found that patients randomized to the antidepressants were significantly less likely to have had an epileptic seizure than controls[2] (and Alper et al., submitted). These findings support the conclusions of Jobe and Browning as well as the data presented by Forsgren and Nystrom[103] and Hesdorffer et al.[89,90] in the sense that a history of depression increases the

TABLE 3

INCIDENCE OF SEIZURES IN PEOPLE WITHOUT EPILEPSY

Antidepressants	Incidence of seizures
Selective serotonin reuptake inhibitors	
Sertraline	0.08%
Paroxetine	0.1%
Fluoxetine	0.2%
Fluvoxamine	0.2%
Citalopram/escitalopram	<0.1%
Serotonin norepinephrine reuptake inhibitor	
Venlafaxine	0.3%

risk of seizures. These data raise the question of whether the seizures that occur after the start of SSRIs are in fact related to an increased risk associated with the depressive disorder. Yet, this question needs to be examined in prospective and controlled studies, as the occurrence of seizures has been occasionally reported to the introduction of an SSRI (see also Chapter 214).

The use of SSRIs in PWE has been investigated in the case of sertraline, citalopram, and fluoxetine.[4,65,110] In a study from our center, sertraline was found to *definitely* worsen seizures in only 1 of 100 patients.[110] In another five patients, a transient increase in seizure frequency was attributed to this antidepressant drug with a probable, but not definite, causality. Four of these five patients were maintained on sertraline therapy. Following adjustment of the dose of their AED, none of these patients experienced further seizure exacerbation. In the study that investigated the safety of citalopram in 45 PWE, none of the patients experienced a worsening of seizures[4]; in fact the authors noted a reduction in seizure frequency. Similar findings were reported in the study of fluoxetine in PWE.[65]

Blumer has also reported using tricyclic antidepressants (TCAs) alone and TCAs in combination with SSRIs in epileptic patients without seizure exacerbation.[19] No data have been published on the safety of SNRIs in PWE. We have used the SNRI venlafaxine in more than 100 PWE, a significant proportion of whom suffered from intractable epilepsy without observing any worsening in seizure frequency or severity (Kanner, unpublished data).

MAOIs are not known to cause seizures in nonepileptic patients; bupropion, maprotiline, and amoxapine are the antidepressant drugs with the strongest proconvulsant properties and should be avoided in epileptic patients.[48,113]

A review of the literature shows that the variables associated with an increased risk of seizure occurrence following exposure to TCAs in general *in nonepileptic* patients include (a) high plasma serum concentrations; (b) rapid dose increments; and (c) the presence of other drugs with proconvulsant properties.[48,113,196] There are four antidepressant drugs that should be avoided in PWE; these include maprotiline, bupropion, amoxapine, and chlorimipramine. Thus, to minimize the risk of seizures in PWE, antidepressant drugs should be started at low doses with small increments until the desired clinical response is reached; this will minimize the risk of causing and/or exacerbating seizures.

Pharmacokinetic Interactions between Antidepressants and Antiepileptic Drugs

All of the SSRIs and SNRIs are metabolized in the liver via the CP450 system and their metabolism is accelerated in the presence of AEDs with enzyme-inducing properties, which include phenytoin, carbamazepine, phenobarbital, and primidone at regular doses and oxcarbazepine and topiramate at higher doses. This pharmacokinetic effect is not observed with the new AEDs gabapentin, lamotrigine, tiagabine, levetiracetam, and zonisamide. Thus, upon introduction of an enzyme-inducing AED, clinicians need to advise patients to be on the lookout for symptom recurrence, in which case the dose of the SSRI or SNRI may need to be increased.

Conversely, some of the SSRIs are inhibitors of one or more isoenzymes of the CP450 system. These include fluoxetine, paroxetine, and fluvoxamine and, to a lesser degree, sertraline.[81,149,204] Adjustment of some of the AED (primarily carbamazepine and phenytoin) doses may be necessary. Citalopram, escitalopram, venlafaxine, and mirtazapine are the antidepressant drugs with the least impact on CP450 isoenzymes.

Pharmacodynamic Effects of Antidepressant Drugs to Watch for in People with Epilepsy

The acute stimulation of four serotonin receptor subtypes (5HT-2 A, 5HT-2 C, 5HT-3, and 5HT-4) may account for the adverse events associated with SSRIs and SNRIs.[70,80] In addition, adverse events may result from a direct action of serotonin outside the brain, such as the spinal cord and gastrointestinal tract. The adverse events associated with these drugs include anxiety and agitation during the acute phase of treatment; gastrointestinal symptoms including nausea, abdominal cramping, and diarrhea; changes in appetite and weight; sexual disturbances; and, rarely, involuntary movements.[112] Among the SNRIs, hypertension is a potential adverse event identified in patients taking venlafaxine.[112]

A variety of sexual disturbances including decreased libido, anorgasmia, impotence, and disturbances in ejaculation as well as dyspareunia are more frequent among PWE than the general population, either as an expression of an iatrogenic effect of AEDs and/or as a direct impact of the seizure disorder. Adverse effects of SSRIs and SNRIs have been reported in about 20% to 30% of patients.[37,112] Citalopram and its s-enantiomer escitalopram and mirtazapine have the lowest incidence of sexual adverse events. Whether the adverse effects mediated by these drugs worsen already existing sexual disturbances in PWE has yet to be investigated. Patients, nonetheless, should be advised to report any of these adverse events, either whether occurring de novo or as a worsening of pre-existing disturbances. Tolerance may develop over time, and at times lowering of the dose or switching to another SSRI may improve these side effects.

By the same token, some SSRIs can cause changes in weight in the form of weight gain, as in the case of paroxetine, aggravating a weight gain problem triggered by AEDs like valproic acid, gabapentin, and carbamazepine. On the other hand, fluoxetine can cause weight loss in the first 3 months of therapy, but patients regain the weight lost thereafter.[37]

Finally, discontinuation of antidepressant drugs including TCAs, SSRIs, and SNRIs cannot be abrupt as it can result in withdrawal symptoms[70,112] including nausea, vomiting, tremors, and anxiety.

Other Treatments

Mood-stabilizing Agents

In the treatment of bipolar patients, mood-stabilizing agents have become the first line of drugs to prevent recurrence of major depressive and manic/hypomanic episodes. Fortunately for PWE, several of the AEDs, mainly CBZ, VPA, LTG, and OXC, have been found to show efficacy in this respect.[7,64,68,176,190] Often, however, administration of these AEDs may not be sufficient to cause remission of a major depressive disorder. In such cases a short-term use of an antidepressant may have to be considered, but always in the presence of a mood-stabilizing agent to minimize the risk of conversion to a manic or hypomanic episode. Occasionally, the use of lithium may be necessary to render the patient euthymic; this drug can be fraught with several problems including changes in electroencephalographic (EEG) recordings and proconvulsant properties at therapeutic serum concentrations in nonepileptic patients.[10,190] Its neurotoxicity and related increase in seizure risk increases with the concurrent use of neuroleptic drugs, in the presence of EEG abnormalities, and with a history of central nervous system (CNS) disorder, and thus should be used with caution in PWE. Furthermore, lithium can be associated with neurotoxicity (i.e., dizziness, diplopia, blurred vision, ataxia) when given in combination with CBZ, even when the serum concentrations of both drugs are in the therapeutic range, requiring the reduction in the dose of carbamazepine or a switch to another AED.

Electroshock Therapy

Electroshock therapy may need to be considered in very severe and treatment-resistant major depressive episodes.[14] ECT is not contraindicated in patients with epilepsy.[155] It is a well-tolerated treatment and is worth considering in patients with epilepsy with very severe depression or manic episodes that fail to respond to AD. Blackwood et al. found that the incidence of seizures in patients following treatment with ECT was no higher than in the general population.[155] In fact, several studies have shown that ECT increases seizure threshold by 50% to 100%.[5,16,43,168,169,208] Finally, there are case reports of ECT used successfully for the treatment of seizures in patients with epilepsy not responsive to multiple anticonvulsant medications.[160] Hence, it seems clear that ECT is not contraindicated as a treatment for depression in patients with epilepsy.

When Should Patients Be Referred for Psychotherapy?

Often, mood (and anxiety) disorders may benefit from a combination of pharmacotherapy and psychotherapy, above all when patients have been symptomatic for a protracted period of time and when the psychiatric symptoms have interfered with the patients' ability to maintain employment, a social life, etc. In fact, there are several studies that have established the efficacy of cognitive behavior therapy (CBT) for the management of depressive and anxiety disorders, either by themselves or in combination with pharmacotherapy. In general, CBT consists of short-term treatments of 16 to 20 sessions given during 12 weeks on average.[67] They should only be administered by health care professionals that have been trained specifically in this technique.

CONCEPT OF THE INTERICTAL DYSPHORIC DISORDER

Modern studies of the interictal psychiatric disorders have usually attempted to identify their similarity to the psychiatric disorders that meet the current DSM-III/IV criteria. Our careful review has shown this to be a difficult task, particularly in view of the pleomorphic and intermittent presentation of the interictal psychiatric changes.

Modern psychiatry excluded epilepsy from its considerations when establishing the DSM classification; it has also omitted genetic considerations and based its classification on the descriptive symptomatology of psychiatric disorders. Admittedly, the current DSM is a work in progress.

Premodern psychiatry deemed epilepsy one of the major spheres of its interests, distinct by etiology and symptomatology from the spheres of manic depressive, schizophrenic, and sexual disorders. Kraepelin[115] precisely described the psychiatric changes among patients with epilepsy as they presented before the modern era of anticonvulsant therapy: Intermittent dysphoric episodes were characterized by irritability, depressive moods, and anxiety, as well as headaches, insomnia, and at times euphoric moods. These pleomorphic dysphoric episodes would occur every few days to every few months and would last from a few hours up to 2 days. Dysphoric symptoms were also observed in the prodromal and postictal phases of a seizure. Kraepelin identified the dysphoric disorder of epilepsy not by cross-sectional inquiries, but based on the daily observations of long-term inpatients with epilepsy at a university hospital. With an appropriate instrument, longitudinal assessment of the dysphoric symptoms in patients with chronic epilepsy has confirmed the pleomorphic and intermittent pattern of the interictal dysphoric disorder.[22,26]

Compared with the premodern psychiatric description of the dysphoric disorder, presumably as an undesirable result of modern antiepileptic drugs, the dysphoric symptoms now appear to be more protracted; for the same reason, chronic interictal psychoses are now more frequent, and suicidality has become a significant problem. This finding needs an explanation.

In 1951, Gibbs observed that the epileptic and psychiatric components of psychomotor epilepsy appeared to be physiologically antithetical.[207] A few years later, Landolt observed a patient whose epileptiform EEG had normalized each time he was dysphoric, ascribed the finding to a "supernormal braking action," and developed the concept of "forced normalization."[118,119] Related studies focused particularly on the alternating pattern of interictal psychoses and seizures, and the term "forced normalization" came into current use. Trimble, in particular, has emphasized the importance of forced normalization in several studies and a recent monograph.[205] Engel[61] and Stevens[193] postulated that the psychiatric disorders of epilepsy may result from the inhibitory activity that develops in reaction to the excessive excitatory activity of the chronic seizure disorder. The following findings are in accordance with this postulate[25]:

> (1) The development of the interictal dysphoric and psychotic disorders is delayed (by about 2 years and 12 years, respectively) following onset of epilepsy as inhibitory mechanisms become increasingly established. This finding accords with the particular linkage of the psychiatric disorders of epilepsy with its common relatively refractory form, mesial temporal lobe epilepsy. (2) Upon decrease, and particularly upon full control, of seizures, dysphoric or psychotic symptoms tend to be exacerbated or to emerge de novo (forced normalization or alternating psychosis). (3) Psychiatric changes emerge at times when severe exacerbation of the seizure activity engages an enhanced inhibitory response; thus, the prodromal phase of seizures may be associated with dysphoric symptoms (such as elated mood or heightened irritability), and the postictal phase is commonly associated with dysphoric symptoms (such as anergia, pain, depression, and, in rare cases, even suicidality) and at times (usually after a flurry of seizures) with a psychotic episode.

According to the above hypothesis of the pathogenesis of the psychiatric disorders of epilepsy, their pharmacologic treatment has to be directed primarily against the inhibitory mechanisms. Safety and effectiveness of prescribing the SSRI-type antidepressants for the mood disorders of epilepsy have been previously discussed. The more proconvulsant tricyclic antidepressant drugs, at modest doses, appear to serve as effective antagonists to excessive inhibition and, in fact, may be indispensable for successfully treating the interictal dysphoric disorders.[21,24] Gastaut et al.[74] pointed out that, as measured by their response to Metrazol, patients with temporal lobe epilepsy (in contrast to those with primary generalized epilepsy) show, surprisingly, a higher interictal seizure threshold than do persons without epilepsy. The bias against the use of antidepressants for the psychiatric disorders of epilepsy, on the grounds that they may cause seizures, is erroneous on both empirical and theoretical grounds. Modest amounts of tricyclic antidepressant medication do not increase the seizure frequency in patients with chronic epilepsy whose dysphoric disorder indicates the presence of marked inhibition, and the SSRIs, which we commonly use as adjuncts to the tricyclic antidepressants, are not known to lower the seizure threshold significantly. The combination appears more effective than the use of a tricyclic or of an SSRI alone.[24] Variations that may be necessary in the pharmacotherapy of the interictal dysphoric disorder have been described elsewhere.[21]

The mechanism of action of the antidepressant drugs in the interictal dysphoric disorder clearly is different than in traditional depressive disorders. The drugs are effective rapidly at lower doses and have a broad-spectrum effect for the entire range of symptoms of the limbic disorder, not just for depressive moods, anergia, and insomnia, but also for anxiety, fears, irritability, atypical pains, and euphoric moods.

It is of interest that DSM-IV recognizes the common premenstrual dysphoric disorder as an entity presenting with pleomorphic and labile symptomatology identical to that of the interictal dysphoric disorder.[20] More than two thirds of women with epilepsy experience their seizures predominantly or exclusively in a catamenial pattern, and many experience severe premenstrual dysphoria. This finding has been related to a shift in the estradiol/progesterone ratio in favor of the proconvulsant estradiol over the anticonvulsant progesterone.[88] It has been suggested that the premenstrual dysphoric disorder—as a subictal disorder—may be best treated, like the interictal dysphoric disorder, with the combination of an antidepressant and an anticonvulsant.[20]

SUMMARY AND CONCLUSIONS

In conclusion, mood disorders in PWE continue to be underrecognized and undertreated. It is of the essence that double-blind placebo-controlled studies be done in PWE with mood disorders to establish their safety and efficacy as well as ideal doses, more so because of the atypical manifestations exhibited by a significant percentage of patients. After all, as suggested by the data reviewed in this article, depression and epilepsy have a very close relationship, which most likely is bidirectional and not unidirectional, which is the expression of common pathogenic mechanisms shared by the two disorders.

References

1. Neumeister A, Bain E, Nugent AC, et al. Reduced serotonin type 1A receptor binding in panic disorder. *J Neurosci.* 2004;24:589–591.
2. Jobe PC, Browning RA. The serotonergic and noradrenergic effects of antidepressant drugs are anticonvulsant, not proconvulsant. *Epilepsy Behav.* 2005;7(4):602–619.
3. Nahas Z, Marangell LB, Husain MM, et al. Two-year outcome of vagus nerve stimulation (VNS) for treatment of major depressive episodes. *J Clin Psychiatry.* 2005;66(9):1097–1104.
4. Specchio LM, Iudice A, Specchio N, et al. Citalopram as treatment of depression in patients with epilepsy. *Clin Neuropharmacol.* 2004;27(3):133–136.
5. Abrams R. Electroconvulsive therapy in the high-risk patient. In: Abrams R. ed. *Electroconvulsive Therapy*. New York: Oxford University Press; 1997: 81–113.
6. Altshuler LL, Devinsky O, Post RM, et al. Depression, anxiety, and temporal lobe epilepsy. *Arch Neurol.* 1990;47:284–288.
7. Anticonvulsants for the treatment of manic depression. *Cleveland Clin J Med.* 1989;56:756–761.
8. Asberg M, Traskman L, Thoren P. 5-HIAA in the cerebrospinal fluid. A biochemical suicide predictor? *Arch Gen Psychiatry.* 1976;33:1193–1197.
9. Barabas G, Matthews W. Barbiturate anticonvulsants as a cause of severe depression. *Pediatrics.* 1988;82:284–285.
10. Barry JJ, Lembke A, Huynh N. Affective disorders in epilepsy. In: Ettinger AB, Kanner AM, eds. *Psychiatric Issues in Epilepsy: A Practical Guide to Diagnosis and Treatment*. Philadelphia: Lippincott Williams and Wilkins; 2001:45–72.
11. Baxter LR, Schwartz JM, Phelps ME, et al. Reduction in the prefrontal cortex glucose metabolism common to three types of depression. *Arch Gen Psychiatry.* 1989;46:243–250.
12. Beck AT. Cognition, affect and psychopathology. *Arch Gen Psychiatry.* 1971;24:495–500.
13. Beck SG, Choi KC. 5-Hydroxytryptamine hyperpolarizes CA3 hippocampal pyramidal cells through an increase in potassium conductance. *Neurosci Lett.* 1991;133:93–96.
14. Bell AJ, Cole A, Eccleston D, et al. Lithium neurotoxicity at normal therapeutic levels. *Br J Psychiatry.* 1993;162:688–692.
15. Bell-McGinty S, Butters MA, Meltzer CC, et al. Brain morphometric abnormalities in geriatric depression: long term neurobiological effects of illness duration. *Am J Psychiatry.* 2002;159(8):1424–1427.
16. Blackwood DHR, Cull RE, Freeman CP, et al. A study of the incidence of epilepsy following ECT. *J Neurol Neurosurg Psychiatry.* 1980;43:1098–1102.
17. Blanchet P, Frommer GP. Mood change preceding epileptic seizures. *J Nerv Ment Dis.* 1986;174:471–476.
18. Bleuler E. *Lehrbuch der Psychiatrie*. 8th ed. Berlin: Springer; 1949.
19. Blumer D, Altshuler LL. Affective disorders. In: Engel J, Pedley TA, eds. *Epilepsy: A Comprehensive Textbook*. Vol. II. Philadelphia: Lippincott-Raven; 1998:2083–2099.
20. Blumer D, Herzog AG, Himmelhoch J, et al. To what extent do premenstrual and interictal dysphoric disorders overlap? Significance for therapy. *J Affect Disord.* 1998;48:215–225.
21. Blumer D, Montouris G, Davies K. The interictal dysphoric disorder: recognition, pathogenesis, and treatment of the major psychiatric disorder of epilepsy. *Epilepsy Behav.* 2004;5:826–840.
22. Blumer D, Montouris G, Hermann B. Psychiatric morbidity in seizure patients on a neurodiagnostic monitoring unit. *J Neuropsychiatry Clin Neurosci.* 1995;7:445–456.
23. Blumer D, Wakhlu S, Davies K, et al. Psychiatric outcome for temporal lobectomy for epilepsy: incidence and treatment of psychiatric complications. *Epilepsia.* 1998;39:478–486.
24. Blumer D. Antidepressant and double antidepressant treatment for the affective disorder of epilepsy. *J Clin Psychiatry.* 1997;58:3–11.
25. Blumer D. Dysphoric disorders and paroxysmal affects: recognition and treatment of epilepsy related psychiatric disorders. *Harvard Rev Psychiatry.* 2000;8:8–17.
26. Blumer D. Psychiatric issues in epilepsy surgery. In: Ettinger AB, Kanner AM, eds. *Psychiatric Issues in Epilepsy: A Practical Guide to Diagnosis and Treatment*. Philadelphia: Lippincott Williams & Wilkins; 2001:231–249.
27. Bouilleret V, Semah F, Biraben A, et al. Involvement of the basal ganglia in refractory epilepsy: an 18-F-fluoro-L-DOPA PET study using 2 methods of analysis. *J Nucl Med.* 2005;46:540–547.
28. Boylan LS, Flint LA, Labovitz DL, et al. Depression but not seizure frequency predicts quality of life in treatment-resistant epilepsy. *Neurology.* 2004;62(2):258–261.
29. Brent D, Crumrine P, Varma R. Phenobarbital treatment and major depressive disorder in children with epilepsy. *Pediatrics.* 1987;80:909–917.
30. Briley MS, Langer SZ, Raisman R, et al. Tritiated imipramine binding sites are decreased in platelets of untreated depressed patients. *Science.* 1980;209:303–305.
31. Bromfield E, Altshuler L, Leiderman D. Cerebral metabolism and depression in patients with complex partial seizures. *Epilepsia.* 1990;31:625.
32. Brown GL, Ebert MH, Goyer PF, et al. Aggression, suicide, and serotonin: relationships to CSF amine metabolites. *Am J Psychiatry.* 1982;139:741–746.
33. Brown GL, Linnoila MI. CSF serotonin metabolite (5-HIAA) studies in depression, impulsivity, and violence. *J Clin Psychiatry.* 1990;51(Suppl):31–41.
34. Brown S, Reynolds E. Cognitive impairment in epileptic patients. In: Reynolds E, Trimble M, eds. *Epilepsy and Psychiatry*. Edinburgh: Churchill Livingstone; 1981:147.
35. Browning RA, Clark KB, Naritoku, DK, et al. Loss of anticonvulsant effect of vagus nerve stimulation in the pentylenetetrazol seizure model following treatment with 6-hydroxydopamine or 5,7-dihydroxy-tryptamine. *Soc Neurosci.* 1997;23:2424.
36. Chaplin J, Yepez R, Shorvon S. A quantitative approach to measuring the social effects of epilepsy. *Neuroepidemiology.* 1990;9:151–158.
37. Charney DS, Berman RM, Miller HL. Treatment of depression. In: Schatzberg AF, Nemeroff CB, eds. *Textbook of Psychopharmacology*. 2nd ed. Washington, DC: American Psychiatric Association Press; 1998: 705–732.
38. Cheetham SC, Crompton MR, Czudek C, et al. Serotonin concentrations and turnover in brains of depressed suicides. *Brain Res.* 1989;502:332–340.
39. Cheetham SC, Crompton MR, Katona CL, et al. Brain 5-HT1 binding sites in depressed suicides. *Psychopharmacology.* 1990;102:544–548.
40. Chen B, Dowlatshahi D, MacQueen GM, et al. Increased hippocampal BDNF immunoreactivity in subjects treated with antidepressant medication. *Biol Psychiatry.* 2001;50:260–265.
41. Clinckers R, Smolders I, Meurs A, et al. Hippocampal dopamine and serotonin elevations as pharmacodynamic markers for the anticonvulsant efficacy of oxcarbazepine and 10,11-dihydro-10-hydroxicarbamazepine. *Neurosci Lett.* 2005;390:48–53.
42. Clinckers R, Smolders I, Meurs A, et al. Quantitative in-vivo microdialysis study on the influence of multidrug transporters on the blood-brain barrier passage of oxcarbazepine: concomitant use of hippocampal monoamines as pharmacodynamic markers for the anticonvulsant activity. *J Pharmacol Exp Ther.* 2005;314:725–731.
43. Coffey CE, Lucke J, Weiner RD, et al. Seizure threshold in electroconvulsive therapy (ECT) II. The anticonvulsant effect of ECT. *Biol Psychiatry.* 1995;37:777–788.
44. Coffey LL, Reith MEA, Chen NH, et al. Amygdala kindling of forebrain seizures and the occurrence of brainstem seizures in genetically epilepsy-prone rats. *Epilepsia.* 1996;37:188–197.
45. Corcoran R, Upton D. A role for the hippocampus in card sorting? *Cortex.* 1993;29:293–304.

46. Cramer JA, Blum D, Fanning K, et al., and the Epilepsy Impact Project Group. The impact of comorbid depression on health resource utilization in a community sample of people with epilepsy. *Epilepsy Behav.* 2004;5:337–342.
47. Cramer JA, Blum M, Reed M, et al., and Epilepsy Impact Project. The influence of comorbid depression on quality of life for people with epilepsy. *Epilepsy Behav.* 2003;4:515–521.
48. Curran S, DePauw K. Selecting an antidepressant for use in a patient with epilepsy. Safety considerations. *Drug Saf.* 1998;18:125–133.
49. Dailey JW, Mishra PK, Ko KH, et al. Serotonergic abnormalities in the central nervous system of seizure-naive genetically epilepsy-prone rats. *Life Sci.* 1992;50:319–326.
50. Dailey JW, Reigel CE, Mishra PK, et al. Neurobiology of seizure predisposition in the genetically epilepsy-prone rat. *Epilepsy Res.* 1989;3:3–17.
51. Dailey JW, Reith ME, Steidley KR, et al. Carbamazepine-induced release of serotonin from rat hippocampus in vitro. *Epilepsia.* 1998;39(10):1054–1063.
52. Dailey JW, Reith ME, Yan QS, et al. Carbamazepine increases extracellular serotonin concentration: lack of antagonism by tetrodotoxin or zero Ca2+. *Eur J Pharmacol.* 1997;328(2–3):153–162.
53. Dailey JW, Reith MEA, Yan QS, et al. Anticonvulsant doses of carbamazepine increase hippocampal extracellular serotonin in genetically epilepsy-prone rats: dose response relationships. *Neurosci Lett.* 1997;227(1):13–16.
54. Daly D. Ictal affect. *Am J Psychiatry.* 1958;115:97–108.
55. Dell J. Social dimension of epilepsy: stigma and response. In: Whitman S, Hermann B, eds. *Psychopathology in Epilepsy: Social Dimensions.* New York: Oxford University Press; 1986.
56. DeVellis R, DeVellis B, Wallston B. Epilepsy and learned helplessness. *Basic Appl Soc Psychol.* 1980;1:241–253.
57. *Diagnostic and Statistical Manuel of Mental Disorders.* 4th ed. Washington, DC: American Psychiatric Press.
58. Drevets WC, Frank E, Price JC, et al. PET imaging of serotonin 1A receptor binding in depression. *Biol Psychiatry.* 1999;46:1375–1387.
59. Edeh J, Toone B. Relationship between interictal psychopathology and the type of epilepsy. Results of a survey in general practice. *Br J Psychiatry.* 1987;151:95–101.
60. Elkin T, Shea MT, Watkins JT, et al. National Institute of Mental Health Treatment of Depression Collaborative Research Program. General effectiveness of treatment. *Arch Gen Psychiatry.* 1989;46:971–982.
61. Engel J. *Seizures and Epilepsy.* Philadelphia: Davis; 1989.
62. Ettinger A, Reed M, Cramer J, for the Epilepsy Impact Group. Depression comorbidity in community-based patients with epilepsy or asthma. *Neurology.* 2004;63:1008–1014.
63. Ettinger AB, Reed ML, Goldberg JF, et al. Prevalence of bipolar symptoms in epilepsy vs other chronic health disorders. *Neurology.* 2005;65:535–540.
64. Fatemi SH, Rapport DJ, Calabrese JR, et al. Lamotrigine in rapid-cycling bipolar disorder. *J Clin Psychiatry.* 1997;58:522–527.
65. Favale E, Rubino V, Mainardi P, et al. The anticonvulsant effect of fluoxetine in humans. *Neurology.* 1995;45:1926.
66. Ferrari N, Barabas G, Matthews W. Psychological and behavioral disturbance among epileptic children treated with barbiturate anticonvulsants. *Am J Psychiatry.* 1983;140(1):112–113.
67. Fink M, Kellner C, Sackheim HA. Intractable seizures, status epilepticus and ECT. *J ECT Lett.* 1999;15:282–284.
68. Fogelson DL, Sternbach H. Lamotrigine treatment of refractory bipolar disorder. *J Clin Psychiatry.* 1997;58:271–273.
69. Forsgren L, Nystrom L. An incident case referent study of epileptic seizures in adults. *Epilepsy Res.* 1990;6:66–81.
70. Fritze J, Unsorg B, Lanczik M. Interaction between carbamazepine and fluvoxamine. *Acta Psychiatr Scand.* 1991;84:583–584.
71. Fromm GH, Amores CY, Thies W. Imipramine in epilepsy. *Arch Neurol.* 1972;27:198.
72. Fromm GH, Rosen JA, Amores CY. Clinical and experimental investigation of the effect of imipramine on epilepsy. *Epilepsia.* 1971;12:282.
73. Fromm GH, Wessel HB, Glass JD, et al. Imipramine in absence and myoclonic-astatic seizures. *Neurology.* 1978;28:953.
74. Gastaut H, Morin G, Lesèvre N. Étude du comportement des épileptiques psychomoteurs dans l'intervalle de leurs crises: les troubles de l'activité globale et de la sociabilité. *Ann Med Psychol (Paris).* 1955;113:1–27.
75. Gastaut H, Roger J, Lesèvre N. Différenciation psychologique des épileptiques en fonction des formes électrocliniques de leur maladie. *Rev Psychol Appl.* 1953;3:237–249.
76. Gibbs FA. Ictal and non-ictal psychiatric disorders in temporal lobe epilepsy. *J Nerv Ment Dis.* 1951;113:522–528.
77. Gilliam F, Kanner AM. Treatment of depressive disorders in epilepsy patients. *Epilepsy Behav.* 2002;3(5 Suppl 1):S2–9.
78. Gilliam F, Kuzniecky R, Faught E, et al. Patient-validated content of epilepsy-specific quality-of-life measurement. *Epilepsia.* 1997;38(2):233–236.
79. Gilliam F, Maton B, Martin RC, et al. Extent of 1H spectroscopy abnormalities independently predicts mood status and quality of life in temporal lobe epilepsy. *Epilepsia.* 2000;41(suppl):54.
80. Gilliam F. Optimizing health outcomes in active epilepsy. *Neurology.* 2002;58(Suppl 5):S9–S19.
81. Grimsley S, Jann M, Carter J, et al. Increased carbamazepine plasma concentrations after fluoxetine coadministration. *Clin Pharmacol Ther.* 1991;50:10–15.
82. Hempel A, Risse GL, Mercer K, et al. Neuropsychological evidence of frontal lobe dysfunction in patients with temporal lobe epilepsy. *Epilepsia.* 1996;37(Suppl 5):119.
83. Hermann B, Seidenberg M. Executive system dysfunction in temporal lobe epilepsy: effects of nociferous cortex versus hippocampal pathology. *J Clin Exp Neuropsychol.* 1995;17:809–819.
84. Hermann B, Whitman S. Psychosocial predictors of interictal depression. *J Epilepsy.* 1989;2:231–237.
85. Hermann BP, Seidenberg M, Schoenfeld J, et al. Neuropsychological characteristics of the syndrome of mesial temporal lobe epilepsy. *Arch Neurol.* 1997;54:369–376.
86. Hermann BP, Wyler AR, Richey ET. Epilepsy, frontal lobes and personality. *Biol Psychiatry.* 1987;22:1055–1057.
87. Hermann BP, Wyler AR, Richey ET. Wisconsin card sorting test performance in patients with complex partial seizures of temporal-lobeorigin. *J Clin Exp Neuropsychol.* 1988;10:467–476.
88. Herzog AG, Klein P, Ransil BJ. Three patterns of catamenial epilepsy. *Epilepsia.* 1997;38(10):1082–1088.
89. Hesdorffer DC, Hauser WA, Annegers JF, et al. Major depression is a risk factor for seizures in older adults. *Ann Neurol.* 2000;47:246–249.
90. Hesdorffer DC, Hauser WA, Olafsson E, et al. Depression and suicidal attempt as risk factor for incidental unprovoked seizures. *Ann Neurol.* 2006;59:35–41.
91. Hirschfield RMA, Bowden CL, Gitlin MJ, et al. Practice guideline for the treatment of patients with bipolar disorder. *Am J Psychiatry.* 2002;159(Suppl 4):1–15.
92. Holsboer F. Corticotropin-releasing hormone modulators and depression. *Curr Opin Investig Drugs.* 2003;4:46–50.
93. Holsboer F. Stress, hypercortisolism and corticosteroid receptors in depression: implications for therapy. *J Affect Disord.* 2001;62:77–91.
94. Horner MD, Flashman LA, Freides D, et al. Temporal lobe epilepsy and performance on the Wisconsin Card Sorting Test. *J Clin Exp Neuropsychol.* 1996;18:310–313.
95. Indaco A, Carrieri P, Nappi C. Interictal depression in epilepsy. *Epilepsy Res.* 1992;12:45–50.
96. Jacoby A, Baker GA, Steen N, et al. The clinical course of epilepsy and its psychosocial correlates: findings from a U.K. Community study. *Epilepsia.* 1996;37(2):148–161.
97. Jacoby A. Felt versus enacted stigma: a concept revisited. *Soc Sci Med.* 1994;38:269–274.
98. Jobe PC, Dailey JW, Wernicke JF. A noradrenergic and serotonergic hypothesis of the linkage between epilepsy and affective disorders. *Crit Rev Neurobiol.* 1999;13:317–356.
99. Jobe PC, Mishra PK, Browning RA, et al. Noradrenergic abnormalities in the genetically epilepsy-prone rat. *Brain Res Bull.* 1994;35:493–504.
100. Jobe PC, Mishra PK, Dailey JW, et al. Genetic predisposition to partial (focal) seizures and to generalized tonic/clonic seizures: interactions between seizure circuitry of the forebrain and brainstem. In: Berkovic SF, Genton P, Hirsch E, et al., eds. *Genetics of Focal Epilepsies.* Avignon, France: John Libbey & Company, Ltd.; 1999:251.
101. Jobe PC. Affective disorder and epilepsy comorbidity in the genetically epilepsy prone-rat (GEPR). In: Gilliam F, Kanner AM, Sheline YI, eds. *Depression and Brain Dysfunction.* London: Taylor & Francis; 121–157.
102. Jokeit H, Seitz RJ, Markowitsch HJ, et al. Prefrontal asymmetric interictal glucosa hypometabolism and cognitive impairment in patients with temporal lobe epilepsy. *Brain.* 1997;12:2283–2294.
103. Jones JE, Herman BP, Berry JJ, et al. Clinical assessment of axis I psychiatric morbidity in chronic epilepsy: a multicenter investigation. *J Neuropsychiatry Clin Neurosci.* 2005;17(2):172–179.
104. Kanner AM, Balabanov A. Depression in epilepsy: how closely related are these two disorders?. *Neurology.* 2002;58(Suppl 5):S27–39.
105. Kanner AM, Barry JJ. Depression and psychotic disorders associated with epilepsy-are they unique? *Epilepsy Behav.* 2001;2:170–186.
106. Kanner AM, Faught E, French J, et al. Psychiatric adverse events caused by topiramate and lamotrigine: a postmarketing prevalence and risk factor study. *Epilepsia.* 2000;41(Suppl 7):169.
107. Kanner AM, Soto A, Gross-Kanner H. Prevalence and clinical characteristics of postictal psychiatric symptoms in partial epilepsy. *Neurology.* 2004;62:708–713.
108. Kanner AM, Tilwalli S, Byrne R. Psychiatric and neurologic predictors of post-surgical psychiatric complications following a temporal lobectomy. *Neurology.* 2004;64(Suppl 1):A-358.
109. Kanner AM, Wuu J, Barry J, et al. Atypical depressive episodes in epilepsy: a study of their clinical characteristics and impact on quality of life. *Neurology.* 2004;62:(Suppl 5):A249.
110. Kanner, AM, Kozak AM, Frey M. The use of sertraline in patients with epilepsy: is it safe? *Epilepsy Behav.* 2000;1(2):100–105.
111. Kessler RC, McGonagle KA, Zhao S, et al. Life-time and 12 month prevalence of DSM-III-R psychiatric disorders in the United States: results from the National Comorbidity Survey. *Arch Gen Psychiatry.* 1994;51:8–18.
112. Ketter TA, Malow BA, Flamini R, et al. Anticonvulsant withdrawal-emergent psychopathology. *Neurology.* 1994;44:55–61.

113. Khan A, Alper K, Schwartz K, et al. Seizure risk among patients participating in psychopharmacology clinical trials. Poster Session I #148. American College of Neuropsychopharmacology (ACNP) 44th Annual Meeting, Waikoloa, Hawaii; 2005.
114. Kimbrell TA, Ketter TA, George MS, et al. Regional cerebral glucose utilization in patients with a range of severities of unipolar depression. *Biol Psychiatry*. 2002;51:237–252.
115. Kraepelin E. *Psychiatrie* Vol 3. Leipzig: Johann Ambrosius Barth; 1923.
116. Kumar A, Zhisong J, Warren B, et al. Late-onset minor and major depression: early evidence for common neuroanatomical substrates detected by using MRI. *Proc Natl Acad Sci USA*. 1998;95(13):7654–7658.
117. Lai T, Payne ME, Byrum CE, et al. Reduction of orbital frontal cortex volume in geriatric depression. *Biol Psychiatry*. 2000;48(10):971–975.
118. Landolt H. Serial electroencephalographic investigation during psychotic episodes in epileptic patients and during schizophrenic attacks. In: Lorentz de Haas AM, ed. *Lectures on Epilepsy*. Amsterdam: Elsevier; 1958:91–133.
119. Landolt H. Über Verstimmungen, Dämmerzustände und schizophrene Zustandsbilder bei Epilepsie: Ergebnisse klinischer und elektroenzephalographischer Untersuchungen. *Schweiz Arch Neurol Psychiatrie*. 1955;76:313–321.
120. Langer SZ, Galzin AM. Studies on the serotonin transporter in platelets. *Experientia*. 1988;44:127–130.
121. Langer SZ, Zarifian E, Briley M, et al. High-affinity binding of 3H-imipramine in brain and platelets and its relevance to the biochemistry of affective disorders. *Life Sci*. 1981;29:211–220.
122. Leake A, Fairbairn AF, McKeith IG, et al. Studies on the serotonin uptake binding site in major depressive disorder and control post-mortem brain: neurochemical and clinical correlates. *Psychiatry Res*. 1991;39:155–165.
123. Lehrner J, Kalchmayr R, Serles W, et al. Health-related quality of life (HRQOL), activity of daily living (ADL) and depressive mood disorder in temporal lobe epilepsy patients. *Seizure*. 1999;8(2):88–92.
124. Lewis A. Melancholia: a historical review. *J Mental Sci*. 1934;80:1–42.
125. Liotti M, Mayberg H, McGinnis S, et al. Unmasking disease specific cerebral blood flow abnormalities: mood challenge in patients with remitted unipolar depression. *Am J Psychiatry*. 2002;159:1830–1840.
126. Lithium neuroleptic interactions: electroencephalographic studies. *Res Comm Psychol Psychiatry Behav*. 1991; 16(1&2):35–40.
127. Lopez-Meraz ML, Gonzalez-Trujano ME, Neri-Bazan L, et al. 5-HT1A receptor agonists modify seizures in three experimental models in rats. *Neuropharmacology*. 2005;49:367–375.
128. Lucassen PJ, Muller MB, Holsboer F, et al. Hippocampal apoptosis in major depression is a minor event and absent from subareas at risk for glucocorticoid overexposure. *Am J Pathol*. 2001;158:453–468.
129. Malison RT, Price LH, Berman R, et al. Reduced brain serotonin transporter availability in major depression as measured by [123I]-2 beta-carbomethoxy-3 beta-(4-iodophenyl)tropane and single photon emission computed tomography. *Biol Psychiatry*. 1998;44:1090–1098.
130. Mathern GW, Babb TL, Armstrong DL. Hippocampal sclerosis. In: Engel J, Pedley TA, eds. *Epilepsy: A Comprehensive Textbook*. Philadelphia: Lippincott-Raven; 1997:133–155.
131. McConnell H, Duffy J, Cress K. Behavioral effects of felbamate. *J Neuropsychiatry Clin Neurosci*. 1994;6:323.
132. McConnell H, Duncan D. Treatment of psychiatric comorbidity in epilepsy. In: McConnell H, Snyder P, eds. *Psychiatric Comorbidity in Epilepsy*. Washington, DC: American Psychiatric Press; 1998:245–362.
133. Meldrum BS, Anlezark GM, Adam HK, et al. Anticonvulsant and proconvulsant properties of viloxazine hydrohloride: pharmacological and pharmacokinetic studies in rodents and epileptic baboon. *Psychopharmacology (Berlin)* . 1982;76:212.
134. Mendez MF, Cummings J, Benson D, et al. Depression in epilepsy. Significance and phenomenology. *Arch Neurol*. 1986;43:766–770.
135. Merlet I, Ostrowsky K, Costes N, et al. 5-HT1A receptor binding and intracerebral activity in temporal lobe epilepsy: an [18F]MPPF-PET study. *Brain*. 2004;127:900–913.
136. Meschaks A, Lindstrom P, Halldin C, et al. Regional reductions in serotonin 1A receptor binding in juvenile myoclonic epilepsy. *Arch Neurol*. 2005;62:946–960.
137. Mula M, Trimble MR, Yuen A, et al. Psychiatric adverse events during levetiracetam therapy. *Neurology*. 2003;61:704–706.
138. Naidoo D. The effects of reserpine (Serpasil) on the chronic disturbed schizophrenic: a comparative study of rauwolfia alkaloids and electroconvulsive therapy. *J Nerv Ment Dis*. 1956;123.
139. Naritokku DK, Terry WJ, Helfert RH. Regional induction of fos immunoreactivity in the brain by anticonvulsant stimulation of the vagus nerve. *Epilepsy Res*. 1995;22:53.
140. Nemeroff CB, Knight DL, Krishnan RR, et al. Marked reduction in the number of platelet-tritiated imipramine binding sites in geriatric depression. *Arch Gen Psychiatry*. 1988;45:919–923.
141. Nibuya M, Morinobu S, Duman RS. Regulation of BDNF and trkB mRNA in rat brain by chronic electroconvulsive seizure and antidepressant drug treatments. *J Neurosci*. 1995;15:7539–7547.
142. Nilsson L, Tomson T, Farahmand BY, et al. Cause-specific mortality in epilepsy: a cohort study of more than 9,000 patients once hospitalized for epilepsy. *Epilepsia*. 1997;38(10):1062–1068.
143. Noce RH, Williams DB, Rapaport W. Reserpine (Serpasil) in management of the mentally ill. *JAMA*. 1955;158:11.
144. O'Donoghue MF, Goodridge DM, Redhead K, et al. Assessing the psychosocial consequences of epilepsy: a community-based study. *Br J Gen Pract*. 1999;49(440):211–214.
145. Ogilvie AD, Battersby S, Bubb VJ, et al. Polymorphism in serotonin transporter gene associated with susceptibility to major depression. *Lancet*. 1996;347:731–733.
146. Ogilvie AD, Harmar AJ. Association between the serotonin transporter gene and affective disorder: the evidence so far. *Mol Med*. 1997;3:90–93.
147. Oguendo MA, Placidi GP, Malone KM, et al. Positron emission tomography of regional brain metabolic responses to a serotonergic challenge and lethality of suicide attempts in major depression. *Arch Gen Psychiatry*. 2003;60:14–22.
148. Okuhara DY, Beck SG. 5-HT1A receptor linked to inward-rectifying potassium current in hippocampal CA3 pyramidal cells. *J Neurophysiol*. 1994;71:2161–2167.
149. Pearson H. Interaction of fluoxetine and carbamazepine. *J Clin Psychiatry*. 1990;51:126.
150. Perrine K, Hermann BP, Meador KJ, et al. The relationship of neuropsychological functioning to quality of life in epilepsy [see comments]. *Arch Neurol*. 1995;52(10):997–1003.
151. Perry EK, Marshall EF, Blessed G, et al. Decreased imipramine binding in the brains of patients with depressive illness. *Br J Psychiatry*. 1983;142:188–192.
152. Piette Y, Delaunois AL, De Shaepdryver AF, et al. Imipramine and electroshock threshold. *Arch Int Pharmacodyn Ther*. 1963;144:293.
153. Polc P, Schneeberger J, Haefely W. Effects of several centrally active drugs on the sleep wakefulness cycle of cats. *Neuropharmacology*. 1979;18:259.
154. Posener JA, Wang L, Price JL, et al. High-dimensional mapping of the hippocampus in depression. *Am J Psychiatry*. 2003;160:83–89.
155. Post R, Putnam F, Uhde T. Electroconvulsive therapy as an anticonvulsant: implications for its mechanisms of action in affective illness. In: Malitz S, Sackeim H, eds. *Electroconvulsive Therapy: Clinical and Basic Research Issues*. New York: New York Academy of Sciences; 1986.
156. Practice guideline for the treatment of patients with bipolar disorder. *Am J Psychiatry*. 2002;159(Suppl 4):4–15.
157. Quiske A, Helmstaedter C, Lux S, et al. Depression in patients with temporal lobe epilepsy is related to mesial temporal sclerosis. *Epilepsy Res*. 2000;39(2):121–125.
158. Rafnsson V, Olafsson E, Hauser WA, et al. Cause-specific mortality in adults with unprovoked seizures. A population-based incidence cohort study. *Neuroepidemiology*. 2001;20(4):232–236.
159. Rajkowska G, Miguel-Hidalgo JJ, Wei J, et al. Morphometric evidence for neuronal and glial prefrontal cell pathology in major depression. *Biol Psychiatry*. 1999;45(9):1085–1098.
160. Regenold WT, Weintraub D, Taller A. Electroconvulsive therapy for epilepsy and major depression. *Am J Geriatr Psychiatry*. 1998;6:180–183.
161. Reul JM, Holsboer F. Corticotropin-releasing factor receptors 1 and 2 in anxiety and depression. *Curr Opin Pharmacol*. 2002;2:23–33.
162. Ring H, Reynolds E. Vigabatrin and behavior disturbance. *Lancet*. 1990;335:970.
163. Robertson M. Carbamazepine and depression. *Int Clin Psychopharmacol*. 1987;2:23–35.
164. Robertson M. Depression in patients with epilepsy: an overview and clinical study. In: Trimble M, ed. *The Psychopharmacology of Epilepsy*. John Wiley and Sons Ltd; 1985:65.
165. Robertson M. Forced normalization and the aetiology of depression in epilepsy. In: Trimble MR, Schmitz B, eds. *Forced Normalization and Alternative Psychosis of Epilepsy*. Petersfield: Writson Biomedical Publishing Ltd.; 1998:143–168.
166. Robertson MM. Suicide, parasuicide, and epilepsy. In: Pedley T, Engel, J, ed. *Epilepsy: A Comprehensive Textbook*. Philadelphia: Lippincott-Raven; 1997.
167. Roy A, De Jong J, Linnoila M. Cerebrospinal fluid monoamine metabolites and suicidal behavior in depressed patients. A 5-year follow-up study. *Arch Gen Psychiatry*. 1989;46:609–612.
168. Sackeim HA, Decina P, Prohovnik I, et al. Anticonvulsant and antidepressant properties of electroconvulsive therapy: a proposed mechanism of action. *Biol Psychiatry*. 1983;18:1301–1310.
169. Sackeim HA. The anticonvulsant hypothesis of the mechanisms of action of ECT: current status. *J ECT*. 1999;15:5–26.
170. Sapolsky RM. Glucocorticoids and hippocampal atrophy in neuropsychiatric disorders. *Arch Gen Psychiatry*. 2000;57:925–935.
171. Sareen J, Cox BJ, Afifi TO, et al. Anxiety disorders and risk for suicidal ideation and suicide attempts: a population-based longitudinal study of adults. *Arch Gen Psychiatry*. 2005;62:1249–1257.
172. Sargent PA, Kjaer KH, Bench CJ, et al. Brain serotonin1A receptor binding measured by positron emission tomography with [11C]WAY-100635: effects of depression and antidepressant treatment. *Arch Gen Psychiatry*. 2000;57:174–180.
173. Savard G, Andermann LF, Reutens D, et al. Epilepsy, surgical treatment and postoperative psychiatric complications: a re-evaluation of the evidence. In: Trimble MR, Schmitz B, eds. *Forced Normalization and Alternative Psychosis of Epilepsy*. Petersfield: Writson Biomedical Publishing Ltd.; 1998: 179–192.
174. Savic I, Lindstrom P, Gulyas B, et al. Limbic reductions of 5-HT1A receptor binding in human temporal lobe epilepsy. *Neurology*. 2004;62:1343–1351.

175. Scambler G. Sociological aspects of epilepsy. In: Hopkins A, ed. *Epilepsy*. New York: Demos; 1987.
176. Schatzberg AF, Haddad P, Kaplan EM, et al. Serotonin reuptake discontinuation syndrome: a hypothetical definition (discontinuation consensus panel). *J Clin Psychiatry*. 1997;58(Suppl 7):5–10.
177. Schmitz EB, Moriarty J, Costa JC, et al. Psychiatric profiles and patterns of cerebral blood flow in focal epilepsy: interactions between depression, obsessionality, and perfusion related to the laterality of the epilepsy. *J Neurol Neurosurg Psychiatry*. 1997;62(5):458–463.
178. Seidenberg M, Hermann BP, Noe A. Depression in temporal lobe epilepsy: a possible role for associated frontal lobe dysfunction? In: Sackellares JC, Berent S, eds. *Psychological Disturbances in Epilepsy*. Newton, MA: Butterworth-Heinemann; 1996:143–157.
179. Septien L, Giroud M, Didi-Roy R. Depression and partial epilepsy: relevance of laterality of the epileptic focus. *Neurol Res*. 1993;15:136–138.
180. Sheline YI, Gado MH, Kraemer HC. Untreated depression and hippocampal volume loss. *Am J Psychiatry*. 2003;160:1516–1518.
181. Sheline YI, Gado MH, Price JL. Amygdala core nuclei volumes are decreased in recurrent major depression. *Neuroreport*. 1998;9(9):2023–2028.
182. Sheline YI, Sanghavi M, Mintun MA, et al. Depression duration but not age predicts hippocampal volume loss in medically healthy women with recurrent major depression. *J Neurosci*. 1999;19(12):5034–5043.
183. Sheline YI, Sanghavi M, Mintun MA, et al. Depression duration but not age predicts hippocampal volume loss in medically healthy women with recurrent major depression. *J Neurosci*. 1999;19(12):5034–5043.
184. Sheline YI, Wang PW, Gado MH, et al. Hippocampal atrophy in recurrent major depression. *Proc Natl Acad Sci U S A*. 1996;93(9):3908–3913.
185. Sheline YI. Brain structural changes associated with depression. In: Gilliam F, Kanner AM, Sheline YI, eds. *Depression and Brain Dysfunction*. London: Taylor & Francis; 85–104.
186. Smith D, Collins J. Behavioral effects of carbamazepine, phenobarbital, phenytoin and primidone. *Epilepsia*. 1987;28:598.
187. Smith MA, Makino S, Kvetnansky R, et al. Effects of stress on neurotrophic factor expression in the rat brain. *Ann N Y Acad Sci*. 1995;771:234–239.
188. Sorensen A, Hansen H, Hogenhaven H. Ego functions in epilepsy. *Acta Psychiatr Scand*. 1988;78:211–221.
189. Southam E, Kirkby D, Higgins GA, et al. Lamotrigine inhibits monoamine uptake in vitro and modulates 5-hydroxytryptamine uptake in rats. *Eur J Pharmacol*. 1998;358(1):19–24.
190. Sporn J, Sachs G. The anticonvulsant lamotrigine in treatment-resistant manic-depressive illness. *J Clin Psychopharmacol*. 1997;17:185–189.
191. Stahl SM. Depression and bipolar disorders. In: Stahl SM, ed. *Essential Pharmacology: Neuroscientific Basis and Practical Applications*. 2nd ed. New York: Cambridge University Press; 2000:135–197.
192. Stanley M, Virgilio J, Gershon S. Tritiated imipramine binding sites are decreased in the frontal cortex of suicides. *Science*. 1982;216:1337–1339.
193. Stevens JR. Interictal clinical manifestations of complex partial seizures. In: Penry JK, Daly DD, eds. *Advances in Neurology, Vol. 11: Complex Partial Seizures and Their Treatment*. New York: Raven; 1975:85–112.
194. Stockheimer CA, Mahajan GJ, Konic LC, et al. Cellular changes in the postmortem hippocampus in major depression. *Biol Psychiatry*. 2004;56:640–650.
195. Stockmeier CA, Shapiro LA, Dilley GE, et al. Increase in serotonin-1A autoreceptors in the midbrain of suicide victims with major depression-postmortem evidence for decreased serotonin activity. *J Neurosci*. 1998;18:7394–7401.
196. Swinkels J, Jonghe F. Safety of antidepressants. *Int Clin Psychopharmacol*. 1995;9(Supp 4):19–25.
197. Tasher DC, Chermak MW. The use of reserpine in shock-reversible patients and shock-resistant patients. *Ann N Y Acad Sci*. 1955;61:108.
198. Taylor WD, MacFall Jr, Steffens DC, et al. Localization of age-associated white matter hyperintensities in late-life depression. *Prog Neuropsychopharmocol Biol Psychiatry*. 2003;27(3):539–544.
199. Taylor WD, Steffens DC, McQuoid DR, et al. Smaller orbital frontal cortex volumes associated with functional disability in depressed elders. *Biol Psychiatry*. 2003;53(2):144–149.
200. Tellez-Zenteno JSF, Patten SB, Wiebe S. Psychiatric comorbidity in epilepsy: a population-based analysis. *Epilepsia*. 2007.
201. Toczek MT, Carson RE, Lang L, et al. PET imaging of 5-HT1A receptor binding in patients with temporal lobe epilepsy. *Neurology*. 2003;60:749–756.
202. Tollefson GD, Rosenbaum JF. Selective serotonin reuptake inhibitors. In: Schatzberg AF, Nemeroff CB, eds. *Textbook of Psychopharmacology*. 2nd ed. Washinton, DC: American Psychiatric Association Press; 1998:219–237.
203. Tremblay LK, Naranjo CA, Graham SJ, et al. Functional neuroanatomical substrates of altered reward processing in major depressive disorder revealed by a dopamine probe. *Arch Gen Psychiatry*. 2005;62:1228–1236.
204. Tricyclic antidepressant induced seizures and plasma drug concentration. *J Clin Psychiatry*. 1992;53:160–162.
205. Trimble MR, Schmitz B, eds. *Forced Normalization and Alternative Psychoses of Epilepsy*. Petersfield, U.K.: Wrightson Biomedical Publishing Ltd.; 1998.
206. Vakili K, Pillay SS, Lafer B, et al. Hippocampal volume in primary unipolar major depression: a magnetic resonance imaging study. *Biol Psychiatry*. 2000;47(12):1087–1090.
207. Victoroff J, Benson F, Grafton S. Depression in complex partial seizures. Electroencephalography and cerebral metabolic correlates. *Arch Neurol*. 1994;51:155–163.
208. Viparelli U, Viparelli G. ECT and grand mal epilepsy. *Convulsive Ther*. 1992;8:39–42.
209. Weil A. Depressive reactions associated with temporal lobe uncinate seizures. *J Nerv Ment Dis*. 1955;121:505–510.
210. Whitton PS, Fowler LJ. The effect of valproic acid on 5-hydroxytryptamine and 5-hydroxyindoleacetic acid concentration in hippocampal dialysates in vivo. *Eur J Pharmacol*. 1991;200:167–169.
211. Wiegartz P, Seidenberg M, Woodard A, et al. Co-morbid psychiatric disorder in chronic epilepsy: recognition and etiology of depression. *Neurology*. 1999;53(Suppl 2):S3–S8.
212. Williams D. The structure of emotions reflected in epileptic experiences. *Brain*. 1956;79:29–67.
213. Yan QS, Jobe PC, Dailey JW. Evidence that a serotonergic mechanism is involved in the anticonvulsant effect of fluoxetine in genetically epilepsy-prone rats. *Eur J Pharmacol*. 1993;252(1):105–112.
214. Yan QS, Jobe PC, Dailey JW. Further evidence of anticonvulsant role for 5-hydroxytryptamine in genetically epilepsy prone rats. *Br J Pharmacol*. 1995;115:1314–1318.
215. Yan QS, Jobe PC, Dailey JW. Thalamic deficiency in norepinephrine release detected via intracerebral microdialysis: a synaptic determinant of seizure predisposition in the genetically epilepsy-prone rat. *Epilepsy Res*. 1993;14:229–236.
216. Yan QS, Mishra PK, Burger RL, et al. Evidence that carbamazepine and antiepilepsirine may produce a component of their anticonvulsant effects by activating serotonergic neurons in genetically epilepsy-prone rats. *J Pharmacol Exp Ther*. 1992;261:652–659.
217. Yanagita T, Wakasa Y, Kiyohara H. Drug-dependance potential of viloxazine hydrochloride tested in rhesus monkeys. *Pharmacol Biochem Behav*. 1980;12:155.

CHAPTER 206 ■ ANXIETY DISORDERS

ANDRES M. KANNER AND ALAN B. ETTINGER

INTRODUCTION

Anxiety disorders are common in people with chronic medical disorders, including people with epilepsy (PWE). While population-based studies have suggested prevalence rates of 25%, equivalent to almost twice that of the general population, the actual incidence and prevalence rates of anxiety disorders in PWE is yet to be established.[54,96] The lack of such data stems from several methodologic problems including a paucity of population-based studies, the use of *screening* instruments that identify "anxiety symptoms" and not "anxiety disorders" (see section on epidemiology), and, to a large degree, an under-recognition of anxiety disorders by patients and families alike. Indeed, patients often misinterpret symptoms of anxiety as "a normal reaction to a life with epilepsy" or an "expected" response to the stresses associated with the multiple obstacles that PWE have to face, above all when their seizures fail to remit.

Deciding when anxiety symptoms are an appropriate response to stressful experiences or an expression of a pathologic disorder has been the source of debate, with some investigators suggesting a "continuum" between these two extremes. According to Hans Selye, stress is "a nonspecific response of the body to any demand."[156] He added that stressful situations in daily life are not harmful and, in fact, may help individuals to adapt to new life circumstances. In support of these observations, Levine[106] found that young mice exposed to mild stress from time to time consisting of handling or weak electric shocks were better able to handle stressful events and became stronger and larger as adults than the mice that were not subjected to such stressors.

At what point does a "normal" response to stress become pathologic and symptomatic of an anxiety disorder? Selye postulated the existence of a "general adaptation syndrome" that includes three phases:[156] (a) alarm, (b) resistance, and (c) exhaustion. The alarm phase triggers a response of the sympathetic nervous system with activation of corticotrophin-releasing hormone (CRH), which in turn causes secretion of adrenocorticotropic hormone (ACTH), leading to a release of cortisol and norepinephrine (NE) from the adrenal glands. The resistance stage is considered to be aimed at overcoming the stress-producing event, by preparing the animal for fight or flight; during this phase, there is a significant increment of vesicles containing corticosteroids in adrenal glands available for release. According to Selye's theory, if resistance is not successful, the body reaches a state of "exhaustion," during which no further corticosteroid vesicles can be identified, resulting in the animals' death. The corollary of these changes in humans is expressed in the development of mental illness in the form of depression, anxiety, and psychosomatic disorders. Some of these observations may be applicable to the development of anxiety in PWE. For example, Hermann et al. found that psychopathology was associated with poor adjustment to epilepsy, elevated number of stressful life events during the past year, financial stress, vocational problems, external locus of control with increased perceived stigma, and an earlier onset of epilepsy.[71] Multiple regression analyses identified three independent predictors of psychopathology: An increased number of stressful life events in the past year, poor adjustment to epilepsy, and financial stress.

The unpredictability of seizure occurrence can very well play an important role in the generation of anxiety symptoms or full-blown anxiety disorders facilitated by a perception of "loss" of the locus of control. Experimentally, this phenomenon can be studied in the animal model of fear conditioning.[74] This model is based on a classical conditioning paradigm consisting of 20-second conditioning stimulus trials in the animal (using a sound as a conditioning stimulus) that are terminated by onset of an aversive unconditioned stimulus consisting of a footshock of 0.5 second's duration. The resulting conditioned response is expressed by behavioral immobility (freezing) during the 20-second sound-conditioning stimulus. On the first trial, when the sound comes on the animal moves around freely. Within a few trials the animal freezes when the sound comes on, and remains still for most of its duration. The conditioned response—freezing—is used as a measure of fear. The manifestations of the inferred fear state in this animal model closely parallel the clinical criteria of generalized anxiety, as evidenced by increased heart rate and stroke volume, dry mouth/decreased salivation, stomach ulcers/upset stomach, altered respiration, scanning and vigilance, increased urination and defecation, grooming/fidgeting, and freezing/apprehension. Fear conditioning is a strikingly dramatic and reproducible phenomenon and can be elicited among many different animal species.

In addition to the above, it is important to consider the potential pathogenic role of neurophysiologic and neurochemical changes associated with the seizure disorder per se, particularly in temporal lobe epilepsy (TLE). Indeed, mesial temporal structures play a primordial role in the generation of symptoms of anxiety, as exemplified in the animal models of fear sensitization and kindling. Kindling refers to the gradual development and intensification of elicited motor seizures resulting from the repetitive administration of initially subconvulsive stimulations to particular brain regions.[61,87] Kindling of limbic structures has also been shown to effect lasting changes in affect in rodents and cats. For example, kindling of rodents' amygdala facilitates the development of behaviors suggestive of "symptoms of anxiety," and partial kindling of amygdala and ventral hippocampus in cats leads to less predatory behavior. The question is then raised whether fear sensitization may result from hyperexcitation of fear circuits perhaps via long-term potentiation of excitatory amygdala efferents and whether kindling could be comparable to repetitive seizures, thereby inducing interictal anxiety.[1,2] In this chapter we review the available epidemiologic data, clinical manifestations, and treatment of the four most frequent anxiety disorders in PWE: Generalized anxiety disorder (GAD), panic disorder (PD), phobias, and obsessive-compulsive disorder (OCD). We devote a section to the discussion of the most relevant pathogenic mechanisms operant in the development of anxiety disorders in PWE, with special attention to the pathogenic mechanisms that may be shared by anxiety disorders and epilepsy.

EPIDEMIOLOGY

Together with mood disorders, anxiety disorders are the more frequent psychiatric comorbidity in PWE. The *Diagnostic and Statistical Manual of Mental Disorders,* 4th ed., text revision (DSM-IV-TR) lists 11 different types of anxiety disorders: GAD, PD (with and without agoraphobia), OCD, posttraumatic stress disorder (PTSD), acute stress disorder, specific phobias (i.e., to animals, injections, etc.), social phobia, anxiety disorders due to medical conditions, substance-induced anxiety disorder, and anxiety disorders not otherwise specified,[6] which include all those clusters of anxiety symptoms that fail to meet any of the above-cited categories (i.e., subsyndromic types).

As stated in our introduction, the real prevalence of each one of these anxiety disorders in PWE is yet to be established for the following reasons: (a) underrecognition by clinicians and underreporting by patients; (b) paucity of population-based studies; (c) use of diverse methodologies to identify psychiatric semiology, with some of the studies having relied essentially on the use of screening instruments that identify "symptoms," while only a few studies having used structured interviews designed to establish current and past psychiatric syndromes (Axis I diagnoses) according to the DSM criteria; and (d) the use of relatively small case series, often derived from tertiary epilepsy centers, which attract patients with more severe forms of epilepsy and comorbid disorders. To make sense of published prevalence and incidence rates data, it is necessary to review separately those studies that screened for *symptoms* of anxiety from those that identified anxiety *disorders* with structured psychiatric interviews.

Prevalence of Anxiety Symptoms

In a review of the literature, Torta and Keller found anxiety symptoms in up to 66% of patients with epilepsy.[174] Using the Hospital Anxiety and Depression Scale in a study of 201 PWE, Cramer et al. found that 48% reported symptoms of anxiety; in 25% of these patients they were rated as mild, moderate in 16%, and severe in 7%.[36] In this study, anxiety symptoms were more prevalent than depressive symptoms, which were reported in 38% of subjects. Similar findings were reported in studies done in other cultures. For example, Nubukpo et al. investigated the presence of symptoms of depression and anxiety in 281 adults with epilepsy in West Africa using Goldberg's Anxiety and Depression Scale.[120] Compared to a control group, PWE had significantly higher depression and anxiety scores, which correlated with higher seizure frequency and lack of treatment.

Symptoms of OCD have been found to be more frequent among PWE than healthy controls in small case series. For example, Monaco et al.[114] investigated the presence of OCD symptoms among 62 patients with TLE, 20 patients with idiopathic generalized epilepsy, and 82 matched healthy controls. Symptoms of OCD were reported by nine of the TLE patients, none of the idiopathic generalized patients, and one control. In another small study, Isaacs et al. investigated the presence of OCD symptoms in 30 patients with TLE using the Obsessive-Compulsive Inventory (OCI).[75] As a group, patients with TLE had a higher prevalence of obsessive and compulsive symptoms than the nonpatient normative sample. In addition, TLE patients exhibited elevated scores on all but 3 of the 16 OCI scales and subscales.

Symptoms of anxiety disorders have also been found to be relatively frequent in children with epilepsy. For example, in a study of children whose age ranged from 7 to 18 years old, Ettinger et al. found elevated scores on the Revised Child Manifest Anxiety Scale in 16%,[50] while Williams et al. found this to be the case in 23%.[183] Alwash et al. found anxiety symptoms in almost 50% of Jordanian children or adolescents with epilepsy.[5]

Anxiety Disorders

Various studies have estimated the prevalence of anxiety disorders to range from 10% and 25%, with the higher prevalence rates found among patients with intractable epilepsy. In one of the few population-based studies, Gaitatzis et al. found a prevalence of anxiety disorders of 11% among 5,834 PWE compared with 5.6% among 831,163 people without epilepsy.[53] The psychiatric diagnoses were obtained from primary care records. In a study of 174 consecutive PWE from five epilepsy centers, current anxiety disorders were identified in 53 patients and comprised 52.3% of all Axis I diagnoses established with the Mini International Neuropsychiatric Interview (MINI).[83] Agoraphobia (15.5%), GAD (13.2%), and social phobia (10.9%) were the most common diagnoses among the anxiety disorders. Among these 53 patients, 27 (50.9%) exhibited symptomatology that met criteria for two or more anxiety disorders.

Several studies have been carried out in refractory patients being evaluated for epilepsy surgery. For example, Wrench et al. found a prevalence of 23% among 43 patients being evaluated for an anterotemporal lobectomy and 18% among 17 patients with an extratemporal seizure focus (mostly frontal).[184] In the largest case series of patients who underwent an anterotemporal lobectomy (N = 322), Devinsky et al. found an anxiety disorder diagnosed before surgery with a structured interview in 18%.[48] In a study of 300 patients with refractory epilepsy (231 patients with a temporal lobe focus, 43 with a nontemporal lobe focus, and 26 with a generalized and multifocal seizure onset), Manchanda et al. found that 88 (29.3%) met criteria for a psychiatric syndrome and 54 (18.0%) for a personality disorder, with anxiety disorders being the most common psychiatric diagnosis (10.7%).[109]

Panic disorder is significantly more frequent among PWE than the general population. In a review of the literature, Beyenburg et al. estimated that PWE were six times more likely to suffer from PD than the general population, with point prevalence rates ranging between 5% and 30%,[15] compared with 3.5% in the general population.[96]

Karno et al. have analyzed the prevalence data of obsessive-compulsive disorder measured in five U. S. communities among more than 18,500 persons in residential settings as part of the National Institute of Mental Health–sponsored Epidemiologic Catchment Area program. Lifetime prevalence rates ranged from 1.9% to 3.3% across the five Epidemiologic Catchment Area sites for obsessive-compulsive disorder diagnosed without DSM-III exclusions and 1.2% to 2.4% with such exclusions.[95] On the other hand, the actual prevalence of OCD in PWE is yet to be established as there are no population-based studies in this group of patients and most of the available data are based on small studies carried out in tertiary care centers.

Several studies have evaluated anxiety in children with epilepsy. In one study of 100 children aged 5 to 16 years with complex partial seizures and similarly sized groups of both children with childhood absence epilepsy and normal children, those with complex partial seizures and childhood absence epilepsy were five times as likely to have an affective or anxiety disorder as normal controls; these disorders were identified in 33% of the epilepsy group.[26,27] Of note, anxiety disorder was the most frequent diagnosis among children with suicidal ideation. Within the epilepsy group, children with absence epilepsy were more likely to have an anxiety disorder alone than the children with complex partial seizures, who were more likely to have comorbid depression with anxiety and depression alone. One additional study confirmed the increased rate of anxiety disorders in children, as an anxiety disorder was present in 31% of 102 adolescents with epilepsy.[4]

CLINICAL MANIFESTATIONS

People with epilepsy can present the same clinical manifestations of the anxiety disorders included in the DSM-IV-TR classification,[6] though anxiety episodes/disorders with atypical semiology is not unusual. Such is the case when anxiety episodes are restricted to peri-ictal periods (see below). Thus, it is essential to establish the temporal relationship between the occurrence of psychiatric symptomatology and the seizures, as the duration, course, and response to treatment varies depending on whether an anxiety episode is ictal, postictal, or interictal.[90]

Comorbid mood disorders can be identified in a significant percentage of patients with primary anxiety disorders, and this is also the case in PWE. Thus, any investigation of anxiety symptoms/disorders must always be coupled with a search for mood disorders. This important point is discussed in greater detail below. For example, in a study of 199 PWE from five epilepsy centers, Kanner et al. found that 73% of patients with a history of depression met also DSM-IV criteria for an anxiety disorder.[91]

Interictal Anxiety Disorders

Generalized Anxiety Disorder

To meet diagnostic criteria of GAD, patients have to have experienced the following symptoms for a period of at least 6 months, occurring more days than not: (a) excessive worry and anxiety about a number of events or activities; (b) difficulty in controlling the worry; (c) the focus of the anxiety is not related to another psychiatric disorder (i.e., panic disorder, social phobia, etc.); (d) three or more of the following symptoms: restlessness or feeling on edge, being easily fatigued, difficulty concentrating, irritability, muscle tension, sleep disturbance manifested by either difficulty falling asleep and/or staying asleep and/or restless unsatisfying sleep; (e) symptoms cause clinically significant distress or impairment in the patients' social, occupational, or other areas of functioning; and (f) symptoms do not result from the use of medication or substances of abuse (including alcohol) or a general medical condition (i.e., hyperthyroidism) and do not occur exclusively during a mood or psychotic disorder.

Panic Disorder

PD consists of recurrent panic attacks with a frequency of at least one attack per week for a period of at least 1 month.[6] These attacks are characterized by a subjective sense of dread (feeling of impending doom), associated with a variety of autonomic symptoms including palpitations, sweating, subjective dyspnea, paresthesias, dizziness, nausea, feeling faint, and a sense of abdominal or central chest discomfort. Each attack may last between 5 and 30 minutes and may not have a clear precipitant. Anticipatory anxiety is the second feature of PD, so that the patients fear a recurrence of attacks and may enter a state of chronic lower-grade anxiety. Finally, the patients may show phobic avoidance of situations that they feel may provoke an attack, which may reach total avoidance of leaving the home or fear of being left alone (in which case patients are diagnosed with PD with agoraphobia). Comorbid depression is found in up to 70%, as is the development of secondary psychosocial problems, agoraphobia, and social phobias.[112] It is important to keep in mind that ictal fear can be often confused and misdiagnosed as panic attacks (see below).

Phobias

According to the DSM-IV-TR criteria, specific phobias are described as "marked and persistent fear that is excessive or unreasonable, cued by the presence or anticipation of a specific object or situation (i.e., flying, heights, animals, etc.)." Exposure to the phobic stimulus can trigger an anxiety reaction that may reach proportions of a panic attack.[6] In PWE, agoraphobia or social phobias are among the more frequent types, resulting from fear of injury or social embarrassment should a seizure occur in public. For example, in a study of postictal psychiatric symptoms carried out in 100 consecutive patients with pharmacoresistant partial epilepsy, Kanner et al. found postictal symptoms of agoraphobia in 29 patients; 18 of these patients (62%) attributed these symptoms to the fear of seizure recurrence, but none of these patients experienced seizures in clusters to explain the agoraphobic symptoms.[90] Nonetheless, none of these patients developed full-blown interictal agoraphobia.

Obsessive Compulsive Disorder

OCD consists of the presence of obsessions and/or compulsions causing marked distress, being time-consuming (occurring for at least 1 hour per day) and significantly interfering with the individual's normal routine, occupational functions, or social activities or relationships.[6] The DSM-IV-TR classification defines obsessions as recurrent and persistent thoughts, impulses, or images that are experienced at some time during the disturbance as intrusive and inappropriate and cause marked anxiety or distress. It defines compulsions as repetitive behaviors or mental acts that the person feels driven to perform in response to an obsession or according to rules that must be applied rigidly. These criteria call for the individual to recognize that the obsessions and compulsions are excessive or unreasonable.[6]

There have been several case reports of complete remission of OCD or marked improvement following epilepsy surgery that have spurned hypotheses suggesting common pathogenic mechanisms between OCD and epilepsy. For example, Barbieri et al. reported a patient who had developed obsessive-compulsive symptoms shortly after the onset of temporal lobe epilepsy and who exhibited almost complete symptom remission after being rendered seizure free after a temporal lobectomy.[11] Kanner et al. reported the case of a woman with OCD consisting primarily of obsessions that had been intractable to various pharmacologic and psychotherapeutic interventions prior to surgery and that remitted in toto after a right temporal lobectomy.[88] Remission of OCD has been restricted to TLE surgery. Guarnieri et al. reported two male patients with medically intractable frontal lobe epilepsy and OCD symptoms who experienced remission of obsessive-compulsive symptoms after anterior cingulate cortex ablation.[66]

Peri-ictal Symptoms of Anxiety

Few studies have investigated in a systematic manner the prevalence of peri-ictal anxiety symptoms or episodes, and those available have been limited to selected populations in tertiary centers. The lack of these data is not accidental as clinicians in general fail to inquire about such symptoms in their evaluations of PWE.

Pre-ictal Symptoms

Pre-ictal symptoms of anxiety can precede a seizure by several hours to several days. For example, Blanchet and Frommer identified symptoms of anxiety intermixed with symptoms of depression and irritability in a study of 27 patients who were asked to rate their mood on a daily bases for 1 month.[19] Thirteen patients experienced a variety of dysphoric symptoms, including symptoms of anxiety 3 days prior to the seizure occurrence that increased in severity as the time of the seizure got closer.

Ictal Symptoms of Anxiety

Ictal fear or ictal panic is the most frequent psychiatric symptom presenting as an expression of a simple partial seizure (or aura). It was identified in 60% of patients with auras consisting of psychiatric symptoms.[44,180] As stated above, ictal panic has been confused and misdiagnosed as a panic disorder. For example, in a series of 112 consecutive PWE, Sazgar et al. identified five patients with ictal fear as part of a partial seizure disorder of right mesial temporal origin who had been misdiagnosed with PD.[150] The difficulty in distinguishing the two disorders stems from the following: (a) an inaccurate and/or incomplete clinical history. (b) The absence of epileptiform activity in scalp interictal recordings in patients whose seizures originate from amygdala, a structure that generates epileptiform discharges with very narrow electric fields. In such patients, the use of video-electroencephalographic (V-EEG) monitoring studies may be necessary to record the actual seizure. Often, sphenoidal electrodes inserted under fluoroscopic guidance may be necessary to identify the electrographic ictal pattern of the aura.[89] (c) Ictal fear occurs often in the setting of a partial seizure disorder originating in the nondominant hemisphere. In such cases, patients may continue to respond during the ictus (including during a complex partial seizure) and neither witnesses to the seizure nor the patients may be able to identify a period of confusion or loss of awareness of their surroundings, lest a careful testing of the patient is conducted.

A detailed history can help distinguish a panic attack from ictal panic.[163] Indeed, ictal panic is typically brief (<30 seconds in duration), is stereotypical, occurs out of context to concurrent events, and may be followed by other ictal phenomena such as periods of confusion of variable duration and subtle or overt automatisms when and if the seizure evolves to a complex partial seizure. The intensity of the sensation of fear is mild to moderate and rarely reaches the intensity of a panic attack. On the other hand, panic attacks consist of episodes of 5 to 20 minutes' duration, which at times may persist for several hours, during which the feeling of fear or panic is very intense, often described as a feeling of impending doom and associated with a variety of autonomic symptoms, including tachycardia, diffuse diaphoresis, and shortness of breath. During a panic attack, patients may become completely absorbed by the panic experience to the point where they may not be able to report what is going on around them; nonetheless, there is no real confusion or loss of consciousness as in complex partial seizures. Finally, patients with panic attacks are more likely to develop agoraphobia, while this is rare among patients with ictal panic unless they suffer from interictal panic disorder as well.

Given the relatively high comorbidity of interictal panic disorder in PWE, the concurrent occurrence of ictal fear and interictal PD has to be investigated in all patients. For example, in a small study of 12 patients with temporal lobe epilepsy, Mintzer and Lopez found ictal fear and interictal panic disorder in four of these patients.[113] Two other patients had other forms of interictal anxiety disorder and eight patients had depressive disorder.

Finally, the presence of ictal fear can herald the development of postsurgical mood disorders. Thus, Kohler et al. studied the association of ictal fear with mood and anxiety disorders before and 1 year after temporal lobectomy.[99] They compared 22 patients with ictal fear with matched groups of patients with other types of auras and no auras at all. Mood and anxiety disorders declined in the control groups, but not in the ictal fear group after surgery.

Postictal Symptoms of Anxiety

Postictal symptoms of anxiety are relatively frequent among patients with refractory partial epilepsy. In a study of 100 consecutive patients with pharmacoresistant partial epilepsy cited above, Kanner et al. investigated in a systematic manner the occurrence of postictal psychiatric symptoms during a 3-month period.[90] The postictal period was defined as the 72 hours that followed a seizure. Only symptoms that occurred after more than 50% of seizures were recorded. A median of two postictal symptoms of anxiety (range: 1 to 5) were identified in 45 patients with a median duration of 24 hours (range: 0.5 to 148 hours). In 30 patients, at least 1 postictal symptom lasted 24 hours or longer (15 patients [33%] reported a cluster of 4 symptoms of at least 24 hours); 10 patients reported at least 1 symptom of 1 to 23 hours' duration; and 5 patients had anxiety symptoms lasting <1 hour. Thirty-two patients reported symptoms of generalized anxiety and/or panic; an additional ten patients also reported symptoms of compulsions and 29 patients experienced postictal symptoms of agoraphobia. In 37 of these 45 patients, postictal symptoms of depression were also identified. A prior history of anxiety disorder was identified in 15 patients (33%). There was an association between a history of anxiety disorder and the occurrence of two postictal symptoms of anxiety: Constant worrying and panicky feelings. In addition, there was a significant association between a history of anxiety and depressive disorders and a greater number of postictal anxiety symptoms.

Comorbid Occurrence of Anxiety and Depression Disorders

In patients with anxiety disorders with or without epilepsy, investigation of symptoms of anxiety is not complete without also screening for symptoms of depression or carrying out structured interviews looking for mood disorders (and vice versa). Thus, in a meta-analysis of studies that investigated comorbidity between *primary* depression and anxiety disorders, Dobson and Cheung concluded that among patients with a depressive disorder, a mean of 67% (range: 42% to 100%) also experienced anxiety disorders concurrently or in their lifetime.[49] Conversely, in patients with anxiety disorders, a mean of 40% (range: 17% to 65%) also suffered from depression. By the same token, comorbid occurrence of primary social phobia and both major depression and dysthymia of up to 70% have been reported,[112] while higher comorbidity is also identified in first-degree relatives.[135] Furthermore, improvement in one condition can be expected to have a positive impact on the other. For example, in a study carried out in a general medical clinic setting, 880 patients were screened for depression by using the Diagnostic Interview Schedule version of the DSM-III and the Zung Self-Rating Depression Scale, as well as the Zung Self-Rating Anxiety Scale[192]; 112 patients (13%) were found to have a depressive disorder. Comorbid symptoms of anxiety of moderate severity were identified in 67% of depressed patients. After a follow-up period of 1 year, during which symptoms of depression and anxiety were monitored at five time points, depressed patients who improved showed a significant decrease in severity of comorbid symptoms of anxiety, while depressed patients who worsened showed a significant increase in their anxiety index; the decrease in the anxiety index of patients in the no-change group was not statistically significant.

In PWE, the occurrence of comorbid anxiety and depressive disorders is also common. In a study of 199 patients with epilepsy from five epilepsy centers cited above, 73% of patients with a history of depression met also DSM-IV criteria for an anxiety disorder.[91] In that study the DSM-IV-TR diagnosis of a mood and/or anxiety disorder was established with the MINI and Structured Clinical Interview for Axis I Diagnosis (SCID). These patients completed a 46-item self-rating instrument, "The Mood and Anxiety Symptoms in Epilepsy" (MASE), that includes symptoms from eight domains (depression, anxiety, irritability, self-consciousness, physical symptoms, disturbances in socialization, suicidal ideation, and increased energy) on two occasions, 2 weeks apart. Sixty-seven patients met criteria for a DSM-IV Axis I diagnosis: Each of the 37 patients that met criteria for major depression reported symptoms of anxiety. Furthermore, several investigators dating back to Kraepelin, Bleuler, Gastaut, and more recently Blumer and Kanner have made a point of emphasizing the pleomorphic nature of the symptomatology of depressive disorders in PWE, in which symptoms of anxiety play a prominent role.[20,22,55,93,100]

Comorbid anxiety symptoms can also occur in subclinical or subsyndromic forms of depression. In the study of 199 consecutive PWE cited above,[91] 132 patients (64%) failed to meet any DSM-IV Axis I diagnosis according to the SCID and MINI; yet, using the self-rating instruments Beck Depression Inventory-II (BDI-II) or the Center for Epidemiologic Studies-Depression (CES-D), 32 patients (16% of the entire cohort) were also found to have been experiencing symptoms of depression of mild to moderate severity. Symptoms of anxiety were identified in 31 of these 32 patients with the MASE.

Screening of Anxiety Symptoms in the Clinic

Anxiety disorders in epilepsy *are not* homogeneous conditions, and often they occur in association with more than one type of anxiety and/or mood disorders. Thus, how can a neurologist identify an anxiety disorder in PWE? The use of self-rating *screening* instruments can be an *initial* step, but by themselves do not establish a diagnosis. Several instruments are available, but none has yet been validated in PWE. Self-rating screening instruments are obviously preferable to questionnaires that have to be administered by a health professional. In addition, instruments that also screen for symptoms of depression should be included for the reasons cited above. Among the multiple screening instruments available, the following can be considered:

1. Hospital Anxiety and Depression Scale[191]: This scale is specifically developed for use in patients with medical comorbidity, and consists of seven-item self-rated subscales for both depression and anxiety.
2. Beck Anxiety Inventory (BAI)[13]: The BAI is a 21-item self-report measure of anxiety severity. The scale consists of 21 items, each describing a common symptom of anxiety over the past week on a 4-point scale ranging from 0 (*Not at all*) to 3 (*Severely—I could barely stand it*). The items are summed to obtain a total score that can range from 0 to 63.
3. Goldberg's Depression and Anxiety Scales[62]: The instrument consists of nine questions assessing mood and anxiety over the previous month, and the full set of nine questions needs to be administered only if there are positive answers to the first four. The scales are devised specifically to be used by nonpsychiatrists in clinical investigations. Scores are from 0 to 9.
4. Hamilton Anxiety Rating Scale (HAM-A or HARS)[68]: This scale is a 14-item clinical interview scale (not self-reported) measuring somatic and psychic anxiety symptoms. The responses include five degrees of severity ranging from 0 (*None*) to 4 (*Frequent and severe symptomatology*). This instrument should be used with caution in PWE, given the large number of somatic symptoms included in this scale, which, in patients with epilepsy, can result from adverse effects of antiepileptic drugs (AEDs), potentially yielding false-positive suggestions of more severe anxiety symptomatology.

The Use of Screening Instruments in Research: A Cautionary Note!

One of the most frequent methodologic errors in research studies on psychiatric disorders and epilepsy is the sole reliance on *screening* instruments to establish a diagnosis. The argument for exclusively using screening instruments is that they have been "validated" to identify the condition at hand with acceptable levels of sensitivity and specificity and the severity of the depressive episodes. Yet, as stated above, patients may often experience more than one type of anxiety disorder at a given point in time and more often than not suffer from comorbid mood disorders. Accordingly, structured psychiatric evaluations are "a must," aimed at identifying the complexity of current and past psychiatric disorders. Short of that, the conclusions that can be derived from studies that assess any treatment modality or the course of symptomatology are limited.

For example, the course and response to treatment of GAD or PD in a patient with a comorbid history of bipolar disorder is different from that of a patient with major depressive disorder or without a comorbid mood disorder. In short, *screening* instruments identify "*symptoms*"; *structured interviews* establish the presence of a psychiatric disorder, according to classifications like the DSM-IV-TR. Thus, if the aim of a study is to identify the presence of an anxiety disorder, a psychiatric structured interview is necessary. Only once the presence of psychiatric disorders have been established in this manner should screening instruments be used to follow changes of symptom severity over time.

IMPACT OF ANXIETY DISORDERS ON QUALITY OF LIFE

Primary mood and anxiety disorders have a negative impact on the quality of life in the general population. In PWE, research on the effect of psychiatric disorders on health-related quality of life (HRQOL) has been focused on mood disorders (see also Chapter 205) and five studies carried out in patients with pharmacoresistant epilepsy have consistently demonstrated depression to be *the most* powerful predictor for each domain of health-related quality of life, even after controlling for seizure frequency, severity, and other psychosocial variables.[58,59,102,105,128] Cramer et al. also found that depression was significantly associated with poor quality of life scores on the Quality of Life in Epilepsy Inventory-89 (QOLIE-89) independently of the type of seizures; these investigators found, however, that seizure freedom for the last 3 months increased (i.e., improved) the quality-of-life ratings.[35]

Few studies have investigated the impact of anxiety symptoms and/or disorders on HRQOL of PWE. In a study of 87 patients with TLE, Johnson et al. found that symptoms of depression and anxiety were the strongest predictors of poor HRQOL.[82] These investigators found an independent effect of each class of symptoms on HRQOL, however. Furthermore, the psychiatric comorbidity explained more variance in HRQOL than did combined groups of clinical seizure or demographic variables. Furthermore, in a study of 154 outpatient adults with epilepsy carried out in South Korea, Choi-Kwon et al. found that the presence of anxiety symptoms was the most important variable mediating lower quality of life in patients with epilepsy.[32]

In the study of 199 patients described above, Kanner et al.[91] found that the scores of the QOLIE-89 were significantly lower (i.e., worse quality of life) among patients with anxiety disorders than those of asymptomatic patients. Furthermore, patients with comorbid anxiety and major depressive disorders had significantly lower scores in the QOLIE-89 than those with only major depressive episodes.

IMPACT OF ANXIETY ON SUICIDALITY

Suicidal ideation and attempts are significantly more frequent among PWE than in the general population.[84] Several studies have already established that anxiety disorders are risk factors for suicidal ideation and suicide attempts. For example, in a large population-based longitudinal study carried out in the Netherlands, Sareen et al. found that the presence of any anxiety disorder at the initial evaluation was significantly associated with suicidal ideation and suicide attempts in both the cross-sectional analysis (adjusted odds ratio [OR] for suicidal ideation, 2.29; 95% confidence interval [CI], 1.85 to 2.82; adjusted OR for suicidal attempts, 2.48; 95% CI, 1.70 to 3.62) and longitudinal analysis (adjusted OR for suicidal ideation, 2.32; 95% CI, 1.31 to 4.11; adjusted OR for suicide attempts, 3.64; 95% CI, 1.70 to 7.83).[149] Furthermore, the presence of any anxiety disorder in combination with a mood disorder was associated with a higher likelihood of suicide attempts in comparison with a mood disorder alone. Pilowsky et al. surveyed 2,043 patients attending a primary care clinic using the Primary Care Evaluation of Mental Disorders Patient Health Questionnaire, a screening instrument that yields provisional diagnoses of selected psychiatric disorders.[131] A provisional diagnosis of current panic disorder was identified in 127 patients (6.2%). After adjusting for potential confounders (age, gender, major depressive disorder, generalized anxiety disorder, and substance use disorders), patients with panic disorder were about twice as likely to present with current suicidal ideation, as compared to those without panic disorder (adjusted OR, 1.84; 95% CI, 1.06 to 3.18). After adjusting for panic disorder and the above-mentioned potential confounders, patients with major depressive disorder had a sevenfold increase in the odds of suicidal ideation, as compared to those without major depressive disorder (adjusted OR, 7.00; 95% CI, 4.42 to 11.08). Other studies have found that anxiety disorders may increase a suicidal risk only in the presence of comorbid mood disorders.[7]

The impact of anxiety disorders on suicidal ideation and suicide attempts has also been identified in children and adolescents but may not be as clear as in adults. For example, Strauss et al. carried out a study of 1,979 patients aged 5 to 19 years using the Schedule for Affective Disorders and Schizophrenia for School Aged Children–Present Episode at an outpatient mood and anxiety disorders clinic.[168] Subjects were stratified by age and categorized into mutually exclusive groups as being nonsuicidal (N = 817), having suicidal ideation (N = 768), or having attempted suicide (N = 394) in the current episode. After stratifying by age, the investigators found no differences among the ideators, attempters, and nonsuicidal youth in rates of an anxiety disorder in general or in specific rates of PD, agoraphobia, social phobia, simple phobia, and OCD. In older children (age >15 years), GAD was more prevalent in ideators (OR = 1.65; 95% CI, 1.03 to 2.66; $p = 0.03$) than in nonsuicidal patients. Whether similar findings would be identified in population-based studies is yet to be established.

The impact of anxiety disorders in suicidality of PWE has not been studied extensively. In one study by Jones et al. of 139 PWE, 17 met criteria for current suicidal ideation (12.2%), while a lifetime prevalence of suicidal attempts was found in 29 patients (20.8%).[84] Anxiety disorders were significantly more common among patients with current suicidal ideation (58.8%), while 41.2% of patients had comorbid anxiety and current major depressive disorders. On the other hand, lifetime major depressive disorder was the most frequent psychiatric disorder identified among patients with lifetime suicide attempt (51.7%).

PATHOGENIC MECHANISMS

There are several operant pathogenic mechanisms of anxiety in PWE, which can be classified into three groups: (a) psychosocial; (b) endogenous, which include neurochemical, neurophysiologic, neuroanatomic, and functional changes related to the seizure disorder per se; and (c) iatrogenic, including adverse effects of AEDs and complications of epilepsy surgery.

Psychosocial Factors

Patients with epilepsy face multiple psychosocial obstacles that can facilitate the development of symptoms of anxiety and/or (in patients with a predisposition) full-blown anxiety disorder. Stigma, to name one of such obstacles, accounts for the development of symptoms of anxiety. For example, in a study of more than 5,000 patients living in 15 countries in Europe, Baker et al. found that 51% reported feeling stigmatized, with 18% reporting feeling highly stigmatized.[9] High scores were correlated with worry, negative feelings about life, long-term health problems, injuries, and reported side effects of AEDs. Unfortunately, PWE's perception of being stigmatized is not only a function of their "insecurity" resulting from the epilepsy, but is also a real phenomenon illustrated in a study by Harden et al.[69] These investigators developed a survey consisting of three vignettes briefly describing a coworker with depression, multiple sclerosis, or epilepsy. Of note, the epilepsy vignette *did not describe a seizure*. Each vignette was followed by eight identical questions addressing the level of comfort during interactions with the vignette subject. The surveys were hand-distributed in two companies in New York City and returned anonymously by mail. Seventy-four of 200 distributed questionnaires were returned. Respondents reported more discomfort at the thought of interacting with a coworker with epilepsy than with depression or multiple sclerosis, but this difference did not reach significance. However, worry about sudden, unpredictable behavior for the coworker with epilepsy was significantly greater than that with multiple sclerosis. Responders had a significantly lower level of comfort providing first aid for the coworker with epilepsy than for the coworkers with depression and multiple sclerosis. Lower job level and lower income level correlated with more social discomfort for all three illnesses.

People with epilepsy have also been found to suffer from more frequent comorbid physical disorders, some of which are closely associated with stress and anxiety. For example, Téllez-Zenteno et al. analyzed epilepsy-specific and general population health data obtained through two previously validated, independently performed, door-to-door Canadian health surveys, the National Population Health Survey (N = 49,000) and the Community Health Survey (N = 130,882), which represent 98% of the Canadian population.[172] PWE were found to have higher comorbid stomach and intestinal ulcers, bowel disorders, migraine, and chronic fatigue. Likewise, Strine et al. analyzed data obtained from 30,445 adults aged 18 years or older who participated in the 2002 National Health Interview Survey in the United States.[169] They identified an estimated 1.4% subjects who were told by a health care professional that they had seizures; these subjects were significantly more likely than those without seizures to report lower levels of education, higher levels of unemployment, pain, hypersomnia and insomnia, and psychological distress (e. g., feelings of sadness, nervousness, hopelessness, and worthlessness). In addition, they were significantly more likely to report insufficient leisure time physical activity as well as physical comorbidities such as cancer, arthritis, heart disease, stroke, asthma, severe headaches, lower back pain, and neck pain. It is likely that the comorbid medical disorders play a significant role in the generation of symptoms of anxiety in PWE.

The Role of Seizure Frequency and Seizure Severity

As part of a large community-based study, Jacoby et al. investigated the variables associated with the clinical course of epilepsy and the development of anxiety and depression symptoms in an unselected population of people who had a recent history of seizures or were receiving AEDs.[76] Epilepsy data were collected from the medical records of the treating primary physicians and information about psychosocial functioning was obtained with questionnaires mailed to identified subjects, 71% of whom returned the questionnaire. Fifty-seven percent of the sample had had at least 2-year seizure-free periods and 46% were in a remission of at least 2 years' duration. There was a clear relationship between *current seizure frequency* and levels of anxiety and depression.

Smith et al. reported a study of 100 patients with medically refractory partial seizures who completed a quality-of-life questionnaire including measures of physical (seizure severity and frequency), social, and psychological well-being (anxiety, depression, self-esteem, locus of control, and happiness).[160] Multivariate analysis demonstrated that individual psychological variables were best predicted by other psychological variables. However, when these were removed from analysis, seizure severity, *but not seizure frequency,* was the most significant predictor of anxiety and self-esteem.

Similar findings have been reported in children with epilepsy, though data have been obtained from tertiary centers and not from population-based studies. For example, in a study of 35 children and adolescents aged 9 to 18 years and 35 healthy controls, Oguz et al. investigated the relationship between epilepsy-related factors and the development of symptoms of anxiety and depression.[123] Both study and control groups were divided into two age groups (9 to 11 and 12 to 18 years) to exclude the effect of puberty on anxiety and depression scores. Children and adolescents with epilepsy displayed higher scores on the measures of depression symptoms and suicidal ideation, and the mean trait anxiety score was significantly higher in the 9- to 11-year age group of epileptic patients than the corresponding control group, while the mean state, trait anxiety, and depression scores were significantly higher in the 12- to 18-year age group of epileptic children than in the control group. Duration of the epilepsy, seizure frequency, and polytherapy were the epilepsy-related factors associated with the development of anxiety and depression symptoms. Furthermore, in a study carried out in 102 adolescents aged between 12 and 18 from Nigeria, Abiodoun et al. identified an anxiety disorder in 32 (31.37%) of the adolescents with the Diagnostic Interview Schedule for Children Version IV (DISC-IV) and a depressive disorder in 29 (28.4%).[3] As in the above-cited studies, uncontrolled seizures, polytherapy, and felt stigma were identified as predictors of anxiety and depressive disorders by regression analysis. Family factors such as parents' psychopathology and family stress also played a moderately significant role. On the other hand, Williams et al. did not find a pathogenic role of seizure frequency in the development of anxiety symptoms. In a study of 101 children and adolescents between the ages of 6 and 16 years, mild to moderate symptoms of anxiety were reported by 23% of the patients.[183] The presence of comorbid learning or behavioral difficulties, ethnicity, and polytherapy were identified as the variables associated with increased anxiety scores.

Type of Seizure Disorder

The development of anxiety and mood disorders has been associated with seizure disorders involving limbic structures, such as seizures of temporal and frontal lobe origin. In fact, ictal fear can be identified in seizures originating in the amygdala, hippocampus, and cingulate gyrus.[28] Yet, anxiety symptoms can also be identified in primary generalized epilepsy. For example, among a group of 42 patients with idiopathic generalized epilepsy in adulthood, Cutting et al. found an anxiety disorder in nine patients (21%), seven of whom had GAD and two OCD.[40]

Endogenous Changes of Anxiety in Epilepsy

While it is tempting to conclude that anxiety in epilepsy is a simple reaction to having experienced the distress associated with seizures and living with the "Damocles sword" of future seizure risk, compelling evidence in the biologic realm would argue for a much higher degree of complexity to this association. While our understanding of the mechanisms underlying anxiety disorder is still in its infancy, knowledge of areas of potential commonality between anxiety and seizures has laid the foundation for better diagnosis and treatment of this distressing comorbidity. The common pathogenic mechanisms that may be operant in the development of anxiety disorders and epilepsy include (a) neurotransmitter abnormalities and (b) structural and functional abnormalities in common neuroanatomic structures, particularly the amygdala, hippocampus, and cingulate gyrus.

Neurotransmitter Abnormalities

Several neurotransmitters and neuropeptides have been found to play important pathogenic mechanisms in the development of anxiety disorders, including γ-aminobutyric acid (GABA), NE, serotonin (5-hydroxytryptamine, 5HT), and some of the hormones and neuropeptides involved in the hypothalamic-pituitary axis, particularly CRH. Interestingly enough, these neurotransmitters also play a significant pathogenic role in mood disorders and epilepsy and may explain the high comorbidity of these three disorders.

γ-Aminobutyric Acid One area of obvious neurochemical commonality involves the neurotransmitter GABA, which promotes inhibition of neuronal excitability by its effect upon chloride ion channels. The important role GABA plays in the pathogenesis of epilepsy is well known. For example, commonly utilized AEDs such as benzodiazepines, barbiturates, and tiagabine have anxiolytic properties through a potentiation and prolongation of GABA's synaptic inhibitory actions.[167] Barbiturates, for example, inhibit action potentials, neurotransmitter release, voltage-regulated calcium channels, and glutamate-mediated inhibitory synaptic activity.[134] By the same token, the effect of tiagabine and vigabatrin is mediated by an increase of GABA synaptic concentrations, through an inhibition of its reuptake or its metabolism, respectively. Some AEDs may indirectly enhance GABA through action upon sodium or calcium channels. For example, pregabalin, a pharmacologically active S-enantiomer of 3-aminomethyl-5-methylhexanoic acid, is a structural analog of GABA, although it is not active at GABA receptors, nor does it acutely alter GABA uptake or degradation. It binds with high affinity to the α^{54}–δ subunit protein of voltage-gated calcium channels in central nervous system (CNS) tissues and acts as a presynaptic modulator of the excessive release, in hyperexcited neurons, of various excitatory neurotransmitters. Binding of pregabalin to the α^{54}–δ subunit appears necessary for its demonstrable anxiolytic, analgesic, and anticonvulsant activities in animal models.[126]

The convulsant pentylenetetrazol (PTZ; a model for generalized seizures), which blocks $GABA_A$ receptor function, also promotes anxiety symptoms.[85] By the same token, anxiolytic effects of valproic acid identified in some animal models of anxiety are thought to be mediated through GABAergic processes as they can be reversed by the use of $GABA_A$ receptor antagonists.[159] Valproic acid has been reported to display antipanic efficacy and an anxiolytic effect in an open trial,[8] but no controlled studies have been carried out as of yet.

One theory posits that anxiety disorders may be due to defective neuroinhibitory processes, mediated in part through GABA, while abnormalities in the benzodiazepine receptors have also been suggested to play a pathogenic role in epilepsy.[29] The potential relationship between abnormalities in the benzodiazepine receptor system and anxiety disorder is suggested by the induction of panic symptoms in panic disorder patients, when the benzodiazepine antagonist flumazenil is administered.[121] It is further supported by the demonstration of widespread decreased binding of flumazenil to benzodiazepine receptors in panic disorder patients. Indeed, Malizia et al. compared fully quantitative, high-sensitivity positron emission tomography (PET) studies with flumazenil radiolabeled with carbon 11 between seven patients with panic disorder who had been off medication for at least 6 months and who had never abused alcohol and eight healthy controls.[108] Patients' PET studies displayed a global reduction in benzodiazepine site binding throughout the brain compared with controls. In addition, the areas with the largest regional decrease in binding (right orbitofrontal cortex and right insula) were areas thought to be essential in the central mediation of anxiety. The question is then raised whether down-regulation of these receptors is a consequence of exposure to stress or whether a preexisting low level of benzodiazepine receptor density may be a genetic risk factor for the development of stress-related anxiety disorders.

Noradrenergic Abnormalities

There are also very important links between the noradrenergic system and anxiety, since fear activates neurons of the locus coeruleus and increases NE secretion in the locus coeruleus; limbic structures such as the amygdala, hippocampus, and hypothalamus; and the cerebral cortex. With sustained stress in the learned helplessness animal model, depletion in norepinephrine can be demonstrated.[67] Furthermore, agents such as the norepinephrine reuptake inhibitor reboxetine are effective in the treatment of PD.[178] In fact, chronic symptoms experienced by anxiety disorder patients, such as panic attacks, insomnia, startle, and autonomic hyperarousal, are an expression of increased noradrenergic activity.[47] These symptoms can be alleviated with drugs that decrease the firing of neurons in the locus coeruleus, such as benzodiazepines, alcohol, and opiates, while drugs that increase its firing (i.e., cocaine) worsen these symptoms.[47]

Disturbances in the noradrenergic system have been found in epilepsy as well. For example, in animal models of epilepsy, the pathogenic role played by NE is illustrated in studies of two strains of genetic epilepsy-prone rats (GEPR), GEPR-3 and GEPR-9, which are characterized by predisposition to sound-induced generalized tonic–clonic seizures[34,79,81] and, particularly in GEPR-9 s, a marked acceleration of kindling.[78] Both strains of rats have innate noradrenergic pre- and postsynaptic transmission deficits. Noradrenergic deficiencies in GEPRs appear to result from deficient arborization of neurons arising from the locus coeruleus,[33,146] coupled with excessive presynaptic suppression of NE release in the terminal fields and lack of postsynaptic compensatory up-regulation.[78,187] GEPR-9 rats have a more pronounced NE transmission deficit and, in turn, exhibit more severe seizures than GEPR-3 rats.[80]

Increments of either NE transmission can prevent seizure occurrence, while reduction will have the opposite effect.[78,111] For example, drugs that interfere with the release or synthesis of NE exacerbate seizures in the GEPRs, including the NE storage vesicle inactivators reserpine or tetrabenazine and the NE false transmitter α-methyl-m-tryosine.

Another expression of the pathogenic role played by NE in epilepsy can be appreciated in the NE-mediated antiepileptic effect of the vagal nerve stimulator (VNS) in part through activation of the locus coeruleus.[117] Furthermore, a decrease in noradrenergic neurons reduces antiepileptic effects against electroshock or pentylenetetrazol-induced seizures.[25]

Serotonergic Abnormalities

An important pathogenic role has been identified in anxiety disorders and epilepsy. Serotonin's role in anxiety disorders is supported by the observation of potent anxiolytic effects of tricyclic antidepressants (TCAs) and selective serotonin reuptake inhibitors (SSRIs), which enhance 5-HT synaptic concentrations. Serotonin's anxiolytic effects may relate to an inhibition of noradrenergic activation through raphe nuclei projections to the locus coeruleus, periaqueductal gray inhibition of the freeze/flight responses, hypothalamic inhibition of corticotropin-releasing factor, and the amygdala inhibiting excitatory pathways from cortex and thalamus. PET studies with the selective $5\text{-}HT_{1A}$ radioligand[183] trans-4-fluoro-N-2-(4-(2-methoxyphenyl)piperazin-1-yl)ethyl)-N-(2-pyridyl)cyclohexanecarboxamide (FCWAY) permitting in vivo assessment of central $5\text{-}HT_{1A}$ binding have been instrumental in identifying abnormal 5-HT function in PD in a study of 16 unmedicated symptomatic outpatients with PD (seven of whom also suffered from a mood disorder of mild severity) and 15 matched healthy controls.[118] Neumeister et al. found lower distribution volume in the anterior cingulate, posterior cingulate, and raphe in patients compared to controls, indicating a reduction of $5\text{-}HT_{1A}$ receptors in these structures. Not surprisingly, agents that mediate their therapeutic effect through an increase of serotonergic activity in the brain such as TCAs and SSRIs have become the first line of therapy of PD and other anxiety disorders.[64]

The role of 5-HT in epilepsy has also been demonstrated in the GEPR animal model of epilepsy. The brain of this animal has deficits in serotonergic arborization and decreased postsynaptic $5\text{-}HT_{1A}$ receptor density in hippocampus. Conversely, drugs that enhance serotonergic transmission, such as the SSRI sertraline, resulted in a dose-dependent seizure frequency reduction in the GEPR that correlates to the extracellular thalamic serotonergic thalamic concentration.[186] The 5-HT precursor 5-hydroxy-L-tryptophan has anticonvulsant effects in GEPRs when combined with the SSRI fluoxetine.[185] SSRIs and monoamine oxidase inhibitors (MAOIs) can exert anticonvulsant effects in experimental animals, such as mice and baboons, that are genetically prone to epilepsy,[104,111] as well as nongenetically prone cats,[133] rabbits,[130] and rhesus monkeys.[189] In addition, an antiepileptic effect of $5\text{-}HT_{1A}$ receptors has been correlated to a membrane hyperpolarizing response, which is associated with increased potassium conductance in hippocampal kindled seizures in cats and in intrahippocampal kainic acid–induced seizures in freely moving rats.[12,124]

As mentioned, AEDs with established psychotropic effects (carbamazepine, valproic acid, and lamotrigine) can cause an increase in 5-HT.[41–43,162,182,188] In GEPRs, the anticonvulsant protection of carbamazepine can be blocked with 5-HT–depleting drugs.[111,116,187]

Dysfunction of the Hypothalamic-Pituitary-Adrenal Axis in Anxiety Disorders and Epilepsy

As mentioned in our introduction, the hypothalamic-pituitary axis (HPA) plays a fundamental pathogenic role in anxiety, mood disorders, and epilepsy.[143] Neurons in the paraventricular nucleus of the hypothalamus secrete CRH, which stimulates the secretion of ACTH from the pituitary gland. ACTH, in turn, releases glucocorticoids from the adrenal gland, which have an impact on various brain regions, and once in the circulation they exert an inhibitory effect on the HPA axis.[137] Under normal conditions, the hippocampus and amygdala play a role in the inhibition of the HPA axis as well.[70] High levels of CRH and glucocorticoids occur in acute and chronic stress as well as in anxiety disorders, particularly PTSD, depressive disorders, and epilepsy.[177] Intraventricular administration of CRH can mimic stress-induced phenomena. These include an increase in plasma norepinephrine, epinephrine, and glucose concentrations as well as an increase in heart rate and arterial blood pressure, large bowel transit, increase of locomotor activity in familiar environment, increased acoustic startle, grooming, and shock-induced freezing. These phenomena are not reversible by adrenalectomy or hypophysectomy but can be achieved with the use of CRH antagonists, which indicate a "direct" effect of CRH on the brain. Of note, CRH receptors are found in large numbers in the amygdala, which activate fear-related behaviors.[30] CRH receptors also are widely distributed in the cortex, and their function is believed to reduce reward expectation in animal models. Furthermore, CRH inhibits neurovegetative functions involving sexual activity and food intake as well as endocrine functions associated with reproduction and growth. Several studies have shown that early life stressors result in long-term increase of CRH activity in the CNS.

By the same token, an activation of the HPA axis demonstrated by an increase in the secretion of CRH, ACTH, and cortisol has been found in humans postictally following generalized tonic–clonic and complex partial seizures, as well as interictally. Furthermore, Wang et al. found significantly higher brain concentrations of CRH in postmortem brains from children with epilepsy compared to controls.[179] A direct pathogenic role of CRH was suggested by Baram et al. in studies of infants with infantile spasms who were found to have low cerebrospinal fluid ACTH and cortisol, which reflects a high brain CRH.[10]

Abnormalities of Neuroanatomic Structures

Similarities in the nature of symptoms of panic or other anxiety disorders and symptoms of some seizure types suggest that similar brain structures and pathways are involved in both conditions. For example, the intravenous administration of procaine in healthy volunteers produced diverse emotional symptoms of euphoria, anxiety, depression, fear, and derealization, all of which may be encountered in seizures, especially those involving limbic structures. PET scanning during this procedure reveals increased metabolic activity in anterior limbic and paralimbic areas.[157]

Abundant evidence demonstrates the central role of the amygdala in the fear conditioning model. For example, administering bilateral lesions to the lateral nucleus of the amygdala of the rat attenuates fear-induced freezing response to a conditioned auditory fear stimulus.[103] Bilateral lesions of the central nucleus of the rabbit amygdala result in loss of the fear-induced bradycardia response to a conditioned auditory fear stimulus.[94] Lesions of the central nucleus of the rat eliminate fear-potentiated startle.[73]

The amygdala is primarily responsible for mediating fear ("emotional reaction to aversive events") and anxiety ("the apprehension of an imminent aversive event"). The central nucleus is particularly crucial for this function. PET scan demonstrates increased perfusion to the amygdala when an individual is shown images of fearful as opposed to happy faces. Functional magnetic resonance imaging (MRI) can be used to show how individuals with social phobia exhibit increased amygdala activation in response to exposure to the stimulus of fearful faces, compared to healthy controls.[17]

The amygdala can be conceptually divided into three main groups of nuclei: The medial nucleus receives olfactory information and transmits excitatory signals to the hypothalamus. The lateral/basolateral nucleus receives diverse sensory information as well as information related to memories from the hippocampus. The central nucleus receives information from the lateral and basolateral nucleus of the amygdala and transmits excitatory signals to diverse regions that relate to arousal (e. g., hypothalamus, midbrain structures, pons, and medulla).[21,132]

There are numerous afferent and efferent connections to the basolateral nuclei. These connections may have important implications for response to fearful stimuli. Connections to the orbital frontal region play a role in the choice of behavioral responses to a fearful situation, providing an "emotional coloring" of events. Output to the dorsal and ventral striatum (structures believed to be integral to reward and motivation) is important for avoidance behavior and habitual behaviors. Connections to the central nucleus and/or lateral bed nucleus of the stria terminalis (BNST) lead to the "autonomic and somatic" manifestations of fear, and the individual's attention to specific stimuli.[30]

Efferent connections from the central nucleus of the amygdala may translate into many of the symptoms and signs commonly associated with anxiety. The role of the central nucleus in fear is further validated by the demonstration in animal studies of fearlike responses (freezing, shivering, and autonomic nervous system activation such as heart rate elevation and increase in blood pressure) in response to stimulation of this region.[30,60] This suggests that abnormal electrical activity, either experimental or spontaneous epileptiform in selective regions of the medial temporal lobe such as the amygdala, can produce intense sudden fear, reminiscent of the symptoms of panic disorder.[141]

Alternatively, lesions of amygdala nuclei reduce fearful behaviors. In a classic experiment in which the central nucleus is lesioned, the rat recurrently fails to react appropriately to the fearful stimulus of the ominous cat. In the face of danger, the rat no longer perceives sensory stimuli associated with the cat to be fearful and the normally expected autonomic nervous system activation is no longer produced.[18,86]

"Hyperexcitability" of fear circuits including the amygdala has been posited by some as a potential etiology for anxiety disorder. One might speculate then that seizures emanating from or involving the amygdala (as is commonly demonstrated on intracranial recordings in epilepsy surgery candidates) and its connections promote such a hyperexcitability, leading to heightened anxiety.[181]

Anxiety and the Hippocampus

Disturbances of structures other than the amygdala, such as the hippocampus, have been implicated in anxiety disorder.[129] High serum concentrations of corticosteroids, resulting from excessive CRH secretion, have been associated with damage to the hippocampal formation. Chronic exposure to high glucocorticoid serum levels has been blamed for hippocampal atrophy in patients with PTSD and major depressive disorders. Furthermore, in studies with rats and monkeys, prolonged increased concentrations of glucocorticoids have been found to damage hippocampal neurons, particularly CA3 pyramidal neurons, possibly by reduction of dendritic branching and loss of dendritic spines that are included in glutamatergic synaptic inputs.[147,153,158] Atrophy of CA3 pyramidal cells has been found following stress-induced secretion of glutamate in the hippocampus, which in turn resulted in high intracellular concentration of calcium, thus increasing the vulnerability of these cells and in that manner potentially increasing the risk of seizures; this effect was attenuated by *N*-methyl-D-aspartate (NMDA) antagonists. The deleterious effects of chronic glucocorticoid exposure was found to lead initially to a transient and reversible atrophy of the CA3 dendritic tree and an increased vulnerability to a variety of insults and finally to result in cell death under extreme and prolonged conditions.[147,148,153]

The interplay between the impact of high glucocorticoid levels and glutamate secretion in the hippocampus is of significant relevance in our attempts to understand the relationship between anxiety disorders such as PTSD, major depressive disorders, and epilepsy.[23,24,148,190] The role of excitatory neurotransmitters and the glutamate receptor NMDA site has been well established in epilepsy. Indeed, NMDA antagonists have been shown to have antiepileptogenic properties in the "kindling" animal model and to also display antiepileptic properties.[155]

Hypercortisolemia resulting from chronic stress or a depressive disorder has also been found to interfere with the development of new granule cell neurons in the adult hippocampal dentate gyrus. This effect is thought to be mediated by a decrease in the secretion of brain-derived neurotrophic factor (BDNF) in the dentate gyrus, pyramidal cell layer of hippocampus, amygdala. and neocortex.[161] These changes can be overturned with chronic (but not acute) antidepressant therapy, as chronic administration of antidepressant drugs increase BDNF expression and also prevent a stress-induced decrease in BDNF levels.[31,119] There is also evidence that antidepressant drugs can increase hippocampal BDNF levels in humans.[31,119] These data indicate that antidepressant-induced up-regulation of BDNF can hypothetically repair damage to hippocampal neurons and protect vulnerable neurons from additional damage. Recent studies have suggested, nonetheless, that BDNF increases cell survival by inhibition of cell cascades.

On the other hand, other studies suggest that it is those individuals with pre-existing hippocampal atrophy who are predisposed to develop anxiety disorders such as PTSD.[57,190] So similar to the controversial debate whether seizures induce or are a consequence of hippocampal atrophy, the directionality of hippocampal abnormalities and anxiety symptoms remains unclear.

Iatrogenic Mechanisms

Pharmacotherapy

Iatrogenic effects associated with AEDs can be caused by two mechanisms: (a) the introduction of AEDs with anxiogenic properties and (b) the discontinuation (often abruptly) of AEDs with positive psychotropic properties, primarily among patients with an underlying mood and/or anxiety disorder that had been "masked" or "controlled" by the discontinued AED.[92] The AEDs with known anxiolytic properties include the barbiturates, benzodiazepines, tiagabine, valproic acid, gabapentin, and pregabalin.[15,110]

The AEDs with anxiogenic properties include ethosuximide, felbamate, levetiracetam, phenytoin, topiramate, zonisamide, and vigabatrin. Paradoxically, these AEDs have a GABAergic effect, particularly and to a lesser degree topiramate, zonisamide, and felbamate.[15,110]

Abrupt discontinuation of benzodiazepines and barbiturates is known to cause severe "withdrawal" anxiety symptoms including severe panic attacks.[14] However, abrupt discontinuation of AEDs with positive psychotropic properties can also cause anxiety.[97] Such symptoms are often observed in the course of V-EEG monitoring studies in which AEDs are stopped abruptly to facilitate the occurrence of seizures.

Epilepsy Surgery

Postsurgical development of anxiety symptoms following anterotemporal lobectomy has been reported by several investigators. Fortunately, these symptoms are transitory and occur during the first 3 to 6 months after surgery. For example, in a study of 60 consecutive patients who underwent a temporal lobectomy for intractable epilepsy, Ring et al. found that half of those with no psychopathology preoperatively had developed symptoms of anxiety or depression at 6 weeks after surgery and 45% of all patients were noted to have increased emotional lability.[140] By 3 months after surgery emotional lability and anxiety symptoms had diminished, whereas depressive states tended to persist. Patients with a left hemispheric focus were more likely to experience persisting anxiety. Reuber et al. evaluated 76 patients with TLE for symptoms of depression and anxiety before and 12 months after surgery.[136] At baseline, depression and anxiety scores were high in patients with TLE, while after surgery, depression *but not anxiety* scores were significantly lower than at baseline.

Postsurgical OCD has also been reported. Chemali et al. described the case of a young woman with a simple motor tic disorder who after right temporal lobectomy for medically intractable epilepsy developed Tourette syndrome with complex motor and vocal tics, severe obsessive-compulsive disorder, and paranoia.[30a] Kulaksizoglu et al. published a case series of five patients with TLE with obsessive personality traits before surgery who underwent an anterotemporal lobectomy.[101] Within the first 2 postsurgical months two of these patients fulfilled OCD diagnostic criteria. These two patients did not differ from the other three patients with respect to age, age of onset of epilepsy, seizure types, and seizure frequency. All patients stopped having seizures postoperatively, but the OCD patients had worse quality of life postoperatively than preoperatively.

Treatment

The treatment options of anxiety disorders include pharmacotherapy, a variety of psychotherapeutic modalities (i.e., cognitive behavior therapy, desensitization behavioral therapy, supportive and psychodynamically oriented psychotherapies) and a combination of psychotherapy and pharmacotherapy. Before addressing the specific treatment strategies, it is important to review these basic principles:

1. Did the symptoms of the anxiety disorder appear following the introduction or increase in the dose of an AED known to cause psychiatric adverse events?
2. Did the anxiety symptoms follow the discontinuation of an AED with anxiolytic properties? In this case, the psychiatric symptoms may be the expression of recurrence of an anxiety disorder that had remitted with the AED that was discontinued.
3. Did the symptoms of the anxiety disorder occur after the introduction of an enzyme-inducing AED (carbamazepine, phenytoin, phenobarbital, primidone, high-dose topiramate, or oxcarbazepine) in a patient who was already taking a psychotropic drug for a previously recognized anxiety disorder? In such case, the symptom recurrence may have resulted from a pharmacokinetic interaction between the AED and the psychotropic drug on board that caused a drop in the psychotropic drug's serum concentration. Accordingly, a readjustment in the dose of the psychotropic drug may be sufficient to induce symptom remission.
4. Are the psychiatric symptoms temporally related to the seizure occurrence; that is, do they precede (pre-ictal), follow (postictal), or precede and follow; are they the expression of an ictal event; or do they occur interictally

with a peri-ictal exacerbation in severity? In the case of pre- or postictal without interictal symptoms, pharmacotherapy may fail to yield any benefit. Postictal breakthrough symptoms may occur in patients whose interictal symptoms had remitted with pharmacotherapy.

5. Is there a risk factor, other than epilepsy, for the development of the anxiety disorder, particularly a family history in first-degree relatives?
6. Is the anxiety disorder occurring in isolation or associated with other anxiety disorders (i.e., GAD and PD) and/or with a comorbid mood disorder?

Pharmacotherapy

Pharmacologic treatment of anxiety disorders in PWE follows the same drugs and dosages used in the treatment of primary anxiety disorders. Whether the anxiety disorder's response to pharmacotherapy differs between patients with and without epilepsy is yet to be established. Indeed, clinicians assume that primary anxiety disorders and those affecting patients with epilepsy are identical and hence should respond in the same manner, though such an assumption has yet to be proven. In short, pharmacotherapy of anxiety disorders in PWE remains empirical. We will therefore base our review on data from studies conducted in patients with primary anxiety disorders.

Pharmacologic treatment of anxiety disorders depends on the specific type of disorder. Five classes of drugs are typically used: (a) antidepressants, (b) benzodiazepines, (c) AEDs, (d) noradrenergic agents, and (e) buspirone. In the next section we will discuss the use of these drugs in the treatment of GAD, PD, social phobia, and OCD.

Antidepressant Drugs Today, antidepressants have become the first line of therapy in the management of the four anxiety disorders under consideration. In patients with epilepsy, clinicians have often been reluctant to use antidepressant drugs for fear of causing breakthrough seizures in seizure-free patients or worsening of seizures in patients with refractory epilepsy.[175] Data have shown, however, that with the exception of four agents (amoxapine, maprotiline, clomipramine, and bupropion), TCAs, SSRIs, and MAOIs can be safely used in PWE with the following caveats: If TCAs are prescribed, patients need to be started at a low dose and increments must be done in a stepwise manner to avoid toxic serum concentrations.[38,98,175] In fact, animal models of epilepsy have suggested that serotonergic and noradrenergic properties of antidepressant drugs have anticonvulsant properties.[171] A study by Khan et al. supported these observations; these investigators compared the incidence of seizures in depressed patients who were randomized to placebo or the SSRIs citalopram, escitalopram, fluoxetine, and fluvoxamine as well as the α_2 antagonist mirtazapine in Food and Drug Administration (FDA) regulatory studies. Patients randomized to placebo had a significant-higher frequency of seizures.[77]

Little data are available on the safety of the newer classes of antidepressants, such as the serotonin-noradrenaline reuptake inhibitors (SNRIs) venlafaxine (Effexor) and duloxetine (Cymbalta) and the α_2 antagonist mirtazapine (Remeron). Venlafaxine has been prescribed in more than 100 adults with pharmacoresistant epilepsy at the Rush Epilepsy Center without any evidence of worsening of seizure frequency or severity (unpublished data). A detailed discussion of the safety of antidepressant drugs in patients with epilepsy can be found in Chapter 205 and on the use of psychotropic drugs in epilepsy in Chapters 204 and 214. From a safety standpoint, other than seizure-related concerns, the antidepressant drugs of the SSRI family are considered to be the drugs of choice.

The most frequent adverse effects of SSRIs include gastrointestinal and sexual disturbances.[173] The latter may be of greater significance in PWE, as these patients have a significantly higher prevalence of sexual disorders resulting from an iatrogenic effect of AEDs and/or as a direct impact of the seizure disorder. The SSRI-related sexual adverse effects include decreased libido, anorgasmia, impotence, disturbances in ejaculation, and dyspareunia and have been reported in about 20% to 30% of patients.[173] Citalopram and its s-enantiomer escitalopram have the lowest incidence of sexual adverse events. Of note, mirtazapine also has a lower incidence of sexual adverse effects. Whether the adverse effects mediated by these drugs worsen already existing sexual disturbances in PWE is yet to be investigated. Tolerance may develop over time, and at times lowering of the dose or switching to another SSRI may improve these side effects.

By the same token, some SSRIs can cause weight gain (i.e., paroxetine, sertraline) that could potentially aggravate a weight gain problem triggered by AEDs like valproic acid, gabapentin, pregabalin, and carbamazepine. On the other hand, fluoxetine can cause weight loss in the first 3 months of therapy, but patients regain the weight lost thereafter.[173]

Pharmacokinetic interactions between antidepressants and AEDs have to be considered carefully in PWE, in particular: (a) the drop in serum concentration of antidepressants following the addition of enzyme-inducing AEDs, such as carbamazepine, phenytoin, phenobarbital, primidone, topiramate, and oxcarbazepine at high doses; and (b) the decrease in the clearance of certain AEDs with some of the SSRIs and SNRIs mediated by the inhibition of some of the hepatic cytochrome isoenzymes, which may lead to an increase in the serum concentrations of AEDs that are substrates for these isoenzymes.[52,65] For example, venlafaxine and paroxetine have the potential to inhibit hepatic cytochrome isoenzymes 2C19 and 3A4, which may lead to an increase in the serum concentrations of carbamazepine, tiagabine, and zonisamide via a moderate inhibition of 3A4. Venlafaxine is minimally inhibiting of 3A4 and of 2C19 as well, which could affect phenytoin and barbiturate levels. Likewise, fluoxetine is an inhibitor of 3A4 and 2C9/10, which can result in an increase in the serum concentrations of carbamazepine and phenytoin, while sertraline is a mild inhibitor of 3A4, leading to a potential increase in carbamazepine blood levels. On the other hand, citalopram and its enantiomer, escitalopram, have no interactions with the isoenzyme systems involved in antiseizure medicine metabolism.[176]

Other Precautions on the Use of Antidepressants

1. Patients with anxiety disorders may be extremely sensitive to adverse effects of antidepressant drugs. Accordingly, these drugs need to be started at low doses.
2. The high comorbidity between anxiety and mood disorders and the efficacy of antidepressants in anxiety disorders have made these agents an attractive option that would result in the remission of depressive and anxiety disorders with the use of a single agent. However, in the case of mood disorders, the use of antidepressants is indicated in major depressive episodes that are an expression of major depressive disorders, in dysthymic disorder, or in double depression. On the other hand, the use of antidepressants is not recommended in patients with bipolar disorders, lest they are administered in the presence of a mood-stabilizing agent, since they can worsen the course of bipolar disorders, facilitating the development of rapid cycling bipolar illness (defined as more than four manic and or major depressive episodes in a 12-month period), in which case symptom remission is less likely.[72] Accordingly, prior to the start of any antidepressant drug, it is necessary to take a careful history of manic or hypomanic episode and a family history of bipolar illness. Furthermore, a suspicion of potential bipolar illness increases in patients with a first major depressive episode before the age of 20. Indeed, Strober and Carlson

followed 60 adolescents hospitalized for major depressive episodes and followed them for a 3- to 4-year period. Twenty percent of these patients went on to develop bipolar illness.[170]

3. Discontinuation of TCAs, SSRIs, and SNRIs has to be carried out gradually through a tapering schedule to avert the development of discontinuation emergent symptoms.[152] These include somatic symptoms, such as nausea, vomiting, tremors, diaphoresis, ataxia, movement disorders, and sleep disturbances. SSRIs and SNRIs with the shorter half-lives are associated with a higher risk of developing these symptoms.

Efficacy of Antidepressants in Anxiety Disorders All of the SSRIs have shown efficacy in GAD, PD, and OCD.[166] Given the lack of pharmacokinetic interactions with AEDs and better tolerance, we recommend the use of escitalopram or citalopram first and sertraline as an alternative.[16,45,115,142] In the case of GAD and PD, absence of efficacy with an SSRI should be followed by a trial with the SNRI venlafaxine.[46,56,139] The anxiolytic effect of these drugs may not be apparent until the first 4 to 6 weeks after the start of therapy, for which a temporary use of a benzodiazepine is often an option.

Among the older antidepressant drugs, the TCA imipramine is the agent of choice in PD with a comparable efficacy to that of SSRIs, and has also been found to be as effective as benzodiazepines in the treatment of GAD.[151] MAOIs have been also found to be effective in the treatment of PD. Their use in PWE has been relegated to third place, however.

The SSRIs are the drugs of choice in the treatment of OCD, and all have been found to show comparable efficacy. In contrast to the treatment of GAD and PD, a therapeutic effect may not be noticed for 6 to 12 weeks, however.

Benzodiazepines Benzodiazepines occupied the first line of treatment of anxiety disorders before the antidepressants. Their efficacy has been demonstrated in GAD, PD, and anxiety secondary to life stressors or medical conditions.[39,51,122,138] The risk of physical dependence and development of tolerance after have limited their use to short-term trials. Typically, they are used in GAD and PD at the start of pharmacotherapy with antidepressants until the latter agents' therapeutic effect takes over. Alprazolam is the benzodiazepine preferred for PD, while clonazepam is used in GAD.

Noradrenergic Anxiolytics and Beta-Blockers The "overactivity" of noradrenergic neurons underlying anxiety states and evidenced by tachycardia, tremor, and excessive sweating has been the basis for the consideration of drugs that limit the secretion of norepinephrine through stimulation of α_2 autoreceptors and for which the α_2 agonist clonidine has been used. While it is effective in blocking the noradrenergic aspects of anxiety, it is not as effective in improving its subjective and emotional aspects. The use of beta-blockers can achieve this goal in a more effective manner, and they are often used in the treatment of social phobia.

Antiepileptic Drugs In addition to the benzodiazepines, tiagabine,[144,154,164] gabapentin,[165] pregabalin,[126] and valproic acid have been used by psychiatrists for anxiety disorders.[8,159] Tiagabine and pregabalin have been found to be effective in the treatment of GAD and gabapentin in social phobia in double-blind, placebo-controlled studies. Valproic acid, on the other hand, has been found to cause symptom remission in PD in a small study of 13 patients whose panic attacks failed to respond to antidepressant agents. These findings need to be confirmed in double-blind, controlled studies.[8] In PWE who suffer from seizures of frontal lobe origin, tiagabine should be used with caution as it can cause absence stupor.

Other Drugs Buspirone is a 5-HT_{1A} agonist agent that has been found to be effective for the treatment of GAD.[127] It is favored over the use of benzodiazepines because it does not cause drug dependence or withdrawal with long-term use and there is a lack of any significant pharmacokinetic interactions with other agents. Its onset of efficacy is delayed by several weeks, like that of antidepressant drugs.

Psychotherapies

Various types of psychotherapy have been used for a very long time for the treatment of anxiety disorders. In the last decade, however, cognitive behavior therapy (CBT) has gained much favor among health professionals as it has been recognized as an effective treatment for anxiety and depressive disorders. This therapy involves dismantling the patient's false or exaggerated beliefs that lead to anxiety and interfere with daily functioning. This alteration in cognitive outlook is then coupled with gradual desensitization to the anxiety-provoking stimuli, in order to improve the patient's ability to cope with anxiety. For example, in a pilot study by Goldstein et al., CBT was undertaken with six adults with chronic, poorly controlled seizures and coexisting psychiatric and/or psychosocial difficulties.[63] After 12 sessions of CBT from an experienced CBT nurse specialist, participants rated their initial epilepsy-related problem as having less impact on their daily lives, and at 1-month follow-up reported less deleterious impact on everyday life in terms of their psychological difficulties. In addition, participants demonstrated significant improvements in terms of their self-rated work and social adjustment and in their decreased use of escape-avoidance coping strategies.

The efficacy of CBT as monotherapy in GAD has been shown in a recent study of 36 patients randomized to CBT and 36 to no therapy for a 25-week period. Significant decreases in anxiety were found in the treatment group compared to the untreated group using both clinician-rated and subject-rated anxiety scales.[107] The efficacy of CBT has been found to be comparable to that of pharmacotherapy in the treatment of primary mood and anxiety disorders by several investigators, and there is a consensus that a combination of CBT and pharmacotherapy yields better results than either treatment modality given alone.[37,125,145] Given its proven efficacy in patients with primary psychiatric disorders, CBT should be tested in large studies with PWE. In theory, given its efficacy, short duration, and the fact that it can be administered by health professionals from multiple disciplines (i.e., psychologists, nurses and nurse practitioners, and social workers), CBT can be expected to play a major role in the treatment of anxiety and mood disorders in all epilepsy clinics. Furthermore, it may help alleviate the pervasive problem caused by the limited access to psychiatrists.

Therapeutic Effect of Epilepsy Surgery

While no one advocates the use of epilepsy surgery for the treatment of anxiety disorders in PWE, various studies have found a marked improvement in anxiety disorders/symptoms following epilepsy surgery, particularly temporal lobectomy. Such improvements have been associated with the achievement of seizure freedom. For example, Devinsky et al. compared the rate of anxiety disorders before an anterotemporal lobectomy (ATL) in 332 patients and 278 patients 2 years postsurgically and found a drop from 17.5% to 10.4%.[48] Furthermore, epilepsy surgery has resulted in remission of OCD in several cases, as indicated above.[11,66,88]

SUMMARY AND CONCLUSIONS

Anxiety disorders are frequent psychiatric comorbidities in PWE and together with mood disorders account to a great degree for the poor quality of life of these patients. Their early recognition and effective treatment should be part of the overall management of PWE. We have just begun to identify their multifactorial causes and multifaceted clinical expressions, but much research is needed to better understand their pathogenic mechanisms, identify the safest and most effective therapies, and establish the differences (if any) between anxiety disorders in epilepsy and primary anxiety disorders, as well as any difference in response to treatment.

References

1. Adamec R, Young B. Neuroplasticity in specific limbic system circuits may mediate specific kindling induced changes in animal affect-implications for understanding anxiety associated with epilepsy. *Neurosci Biobehav Rev.* 2000;24:705–723.
2. Adamec RE, Morgan HD. The effect of kindling of different nuclei in the left and right amygdala on anxiety in the rat. *Physiol Behav.* 1994;55:1–12.
3. Adewuya AO, Ola BA. Prevalence of and risk factors for anxiety and depressive disorders in Nigerian adolescents with epilepsy. *Epilepsy Behav.* 2005;6:342–347.
4. Adewuya AO, Ola BA Prevalence of and risk factors for anxiety and depressive disorders in Nigerian adolescents with epilepsy. *Epilepsy Behav.* 2005;6(3):342–347.
5. Alwash RH, Hussein MJ, Matloub FF. Symptoms of anxiety and depression among adolescents with seizures in Irbid, Northern Jordan. *Seizure.* 2000;9(6):412–416.
6. American Psychiatric Association. *Diagnostic and Statistical Manual of Mental Disorders IV-TR.* Washington, DC: American Psychiatric Press; 2000.
7. Arnold DH, Sanderson WC, Beck AT. Panic disorders and suicidal behavior. In: Asnis GM,van Praag HM, eds. *Panic Disorder. Clinical Biological and Treatment Aspects.* New York: John Wiley & Sons; 1995.
8. Baetz M, Bowen RC. Efficacy of divalproex sodium in patients with panic disorder and mood instability who have not responded to conventional therapy. *Can J Psychiatry.* 1998;43:73–77.
9. Baker GA, Brooks J, Buck D, et al. The stigma of epilepsy: a European perspective. *Epilepsia.* 2000;41:98.
10. Baram TZ, Mitchell WG, Brunson K, et al. Infantile spasms: hypothesis-driven therapy and pilot human infant experiments using corticotropin-releasing hormone receptor antagonists. *Dev Neurosci.* 1999;21(3–5):281–289.
11. Barbieri V, Lo Russo G, Francione S, et al. Association of temporal lobe epilepsy and obsessive-compulsive disorder in a patient successfully treated with right temporal lobectomy. *Epilepsy Behav.* 2005;6(4):617–619.
12. Beck SG, Choi KC. 5-Hydroxytryptamine hyperpolarizes CA3 hippocampal pyramidal cells through an increase in potassium conductance. *Neurosci Lett.* 1991;133:93–96.
13. Beck AT, Steer RA. *Manual for the Beck Anxiety Inventory.* San Antonio, TX: Psychological Corporation; 1990.
14. *Benzodiazepine Dependence, Toxicity, and Abuse: A Task Force Report of the American Psychiatric Association.* Washington, DC: American Psychiatric Association; 1990.
15. Beyenburg S, Mitchell AJ, Schmidt D, et al. Anxiety in patients with epilepsy: systematic review and suggestions for clinical management. *Epilepsy Behav.* 2005;7:161–171.
16. Bielski RJ, Bose A, Chang CC. A double-blind comparison of escitalopram and paroxetine in the long-term treatment of generalized anxiety disorder. *Ann Clin Psychiatry.* 2005;17(2):65–69.
17. Birbaumer N, Grodd W, Diedrich O, et al. fMRI reveals amygdala activation to human faces in social phobics. *NeuroReport.* 1998;9:1223–1226.
18. Blanchard DC, Blanchard RJ. Innate and conditioned reactions to threat in rats with amygdaloid lesions. *J Comp Physiol Psychol.* 1972;81:281–290.
19. Blanchet P, Frommer GP. Mood change preceding epileptic seizures. *J Nerv Ment Dis.* 1986;174:471–476.
20. Bleuler E. *Lehrbuch der Psychiatrie.* 8th ed. Berlin: Springer; 1949.
21. Blumenfeld H. *Neuroanatomy through Clinical Cases.* Sunderland, MA: Sinauer Associates; 2002.
22. Blumer D, Altshuler LL. Affective disorders. In: Engel J, Pedley TA, eds. *Epilepsy: A Comprehensive Textbook, vol. II,* Philadelphia: Lippincott-Raven; 1998:2083–2099.
23. Bremner JD, Randall P, Vermetten E, et al. Magnetic resonance imaging-based measurement of hippocampal volume in posttraumatic stress disorder related to childhood physical and sexual abuse: a preliminary report. *Biol Psychiatry.* 1997;40:23–32.
24. Bremner JD, Randall P, Scott TM, et al. MRI-based measurements of hippocampal volume in combat-related posttraumatic stress disorder. *Am J Psychiatry.* 1995;152:973–978.
25. Browning RA, Clark KB, Naritoku DK, et al. Loss of anticonvulsant effect of vagus nerve stimulation in the pentylenetetrazol seizure model following treatment with 6-hydroxydopamine or 5,7-dihyrdroxy-tryptamine. *Soc Neurosci.* 1997;23:2424.
26. Caplan R, Siddarth P, Gurbani S, et al. Psychopathology and pediatric complex partial seizures: seizure-related, cognitive, and linguistic variables. *Epilepsia.* 2004,45(10):1273–1281.
27. Caplan R, Siddarth P, Gurbani S, et al. Depression and anxiety disorders in pediatric epilepsy. *Epilepsia.* 2005;46(5):720–730.
28. Cendes F, Andermann F, Gloor P, et al. Relationship between atrophy of the amygdala and ictal fear in temporal lobe epilepsy. *Brain.* 1994;117:739–746.
29. Chang BS, Lowenstein DH. Epilepsy. *N Engl J Med.* 2003;349(13):1257–1266.
30. Charney DS, Bremner JD. The neurobiology of anxiety disorders. In: Charney DS, Nestler EJ, eds. *Neurobiology of Mental Illness.* 2nd ed.. New York: Oxford University Press; 2004:605–627.

30a. Chemali Z, Bromfield E. Tourette's syndrome following temporal lobectomy for seizure control. *Epilepsy Behav.* 2003;5:564–566.

31. Chen B, Dowlatshahi D, MacQueen GM, et al. Increased hippocampal BDNF immunoreactivity in subjects treated with antidepressant medication. *Biol Psychiatry.* 2001;50:260–265.
32. Choi-Kwon S, Chung C, Kim H, et al. Factors affecting the quality of life in patients with epilepsy in Seoul, South Korea. *Acta Neurol Scand.* 2003;108:428.
33. Clough RW, Peterson BR, Steenbergen JL, et al. Neurite extension of developing noradrenergic neurons is impaired in genetically epilepsy-prone rats (GEPR-3s): an in vitro study on locus coeruleus. *Epilepsy Res.* 1998;29:135–146.
34. Coffey LL, Reith MEA, Chen NH, et al. Amygdala kindling of forebrain seizures and the occurrence of brainstem seizures in genetically epilepsy-prone rats. *Epilepsia.* 1996;37:188–197.
35. Cramer JA, Blum M, Reed M, et al. , and Epilepsy Impact Project. The influence of comorbid depression on quality of life for people with epilepsy. *Epilepsy Behav.* 2003;4:515–521.
36. Cramer JA, Brandenburg N, Xu X. Differentiating anxiety and depression symptoms in patients with partial epilepsy. *Epilepsy Behav.* 2005;6(4):563–569.
37. Craske MG, Golinelli D, Stein MB, et al. Does the addition of cognitive behavioral therapy improve panic disorder treatment outcome relative to medication alone in the primary-care setting? *Psychol Med.* 2005;35(11):1645–1654.
38. Curran S, DePauw K. Selecting an antidepressant for use in a patient with epilepsy. Safety considerations. *Drug Saf.* 1998;18:125–133.
39. Cutler NR, Sramek JJ, Hesselink JMK, et al. A double-blind, placebo-controlled study comparing the efficacy and safety of ipsapirone versus lorazepam in patients with generalized anxiety disorder: a prospective multicenter trial. *J Clin Psychopharmacol.* 1993;13:429–437.
40. Cutting S, Lauchheimer A, Barr W, et al. Adult-onset idiopathic generalized epilepsy: clinical and behavioral features. *Epilepsia.* 2001;42:1395.
41. Dailey JW, Reith ME, Steidley KR, et al. Carbamazepine-induced release of serotonin from rat hippocampus in vitro. *Epilepsia.* 1998;39(10):1054–1063.
42. Dailey JW, Reith ME, Yan QS, et al. Carbamazepine increases extracellular serotonin concentration: lack of antagonism by tetrodotoxin or zero Ca2+. *Eur J Pharmacol.* 1997;328(2-3):153–162.
43. Dailey JW, Reith MEA, Yan QS, et al. Anticonvulsant doses of carbamazepine increase hippocampal extracellular serotonin in genetically epilepsy-prone rats: dose response relationships. *Neurosci Lett.* 1997;227(1):13–16.
44. Daly D. Ictal affect. *Am J Psychiatry.* 1958;115:97–108.
45. Davidson JR, Bose A, Wang Q. Safety and efficacy of escitalopram in the long-term treatment of generalized anxiety disorder. *J Clin Psychiatry.* 2005;66(11):1441–1446.
46. Davidson JRT, DuPont RL, Hedges D, et al. Efficacy, safety and tolerability of venlafaxine extended release and buspirone in outpatients with generalized anxiety disorder. *J Clin Psychiatry.* 1999;60:528–535.
47. Davis M. Functional neuroanatomy of anxiety and fear: a focus on the amygdala. In: Charney DS, Nestler EJ, Bunney BS, eds. *Neurobiology of Mental Illness.* New York: Oxford University Press; 1999:463–474.
48. Devinsky O, Barr WB, Vickrey BG, et al. Changes in depression and anxiety after resective surgery for epilepsy. *Neurology.* 2005;65(11):1744–1749.
49. Dobson KS, Cheung E. Relationship between anxiety and depression: conceptual and methodological issues. In: Maser JD, Cloninger CR, eds. *Comorbidity of Mood and Anxiety Disorders.* Washington, DC: American Psychiatric Press; 1990.
50. Ettinger A, Weisbrot DM, Nolan EE, et al. Symptoms of depression and anxiety in pediatric epilepsy patients. *Epilepsia.* 1998;39:595–599.
51. Fontaine R, Mercier P, Beaudry P, et al. Bromazepam and lorazepam in generalized anxiety: a placebo-controlled with measurement of drug plasma concentrations. *Acta Psychiatr Scand.* 1986;75:451–458.
52. Fritze J, Unsorg B, Lanczik M. Interaction between carbamazepine and fluvoxamine. *Acta Psych Scand.* 1991;84:583–584.
53. Gaitatzis A, Carroll K, Majeed A, et al. The epidemiology of the comorbidity of epilepsy in the general population. *Epilepsia.* 2004;45:1613.
54. Gaitatzis A, Trimble MR, Sander JW. The psychiatric comorbidity of epilepsy. *Acta Neurol Scand.* 2004;110:207.
55. Gastaut H, Roger J, Lesèvre N. Différenciation psychologique des épileptiques en fonction des formes électrocliniques de leur maladie. *Rev Psychol Appl.* 1953;3:237–249.

56. Gelenberg AJ, Lydiard RB, Rudolph RL, et al. Efficacy of venlafaxine extended-release capsules in nondepressed outpatients with generalized anxiety disorder: a 6-month randomized controlled trial. *JAMA.* 2000;282:3082–3088.
57. Gilbertson MW, Shenton ME, Ciszewski A, et al. Smaller hippocampal volume predicts pathologic vulnerability to psychological trauma. *Nat Neurosci.* 2002;5(11):1242–1247.
58. Gilliam F, Kuzniecky R, Faught E, et al. Patient-validated content of epilepsy-specific quality-of-life measurement. *Epilepsia.* 1997;38(2):233–236.
59. Gilliam F. Optimizing health outcomes in active epilepsy. *Neurology.* 2002;58(Suppl 5):S9–19.
60. Gloor P. Role of the amygdala in temporal lobe epilepsy. In: Aggleton JP, ed. *The Amygdala: Neurobiological Aspects of Emotion, Memory and Mental Dysfunction.* New York: Wiley-Liss; 1992:339–352.
61. Goddard GV, McIntyre DC, Leech CK. A permanent change in brain function resulting from daily electrical stimulation. *Exp Neurol.* 1969;25:295–330.
62. Goldberg D, Bridges K, Duncan-Jones P, et al. Detecting anxiety and depression in general medical settings. *BMJ.* 1988;297:897–899.
63. Goldstein LH, McAlpine M, Deale A, et al. Cognitive behaviour therapy with adults with intractable epilepsy and psychiatric co-morbidity: preliminary observations on changes in psychological state and seizure frequency. *Behav Res Ther.* 2003;41:447–460.
64. Gorman JM, Kent JM, Sullivan GM, et al. Neuroanatomical hypothesis of panic disorder, revised. *Am J Psychiatry.* 2000;157:493–505.
65. Grimsley S, Jann M, Carter J, et al. Increased carbamazepine plasma concentrations after fluoxetine coadministration. *Clin Pharmacol Ther.* 1991;50:10–15.
66. Guarnieri R, Araujo D, Carlotti CG Jr, et al. Suppression of obsessive-compulsive symptoms after epilepsy surgery. *Epilepsy Behav.* 2005;7(2):316–319.
67. Hales RE, Yudofsky SC. *Anxiety Disorders.* Washington, DC: American Psychiatric Publishing; 2003.
68. Hamilton M. The assessment of anxiety states by rating. *Br J Med Psychol.* 1959;32:50–55.
69. Harden CL, Kossoy A, Vera S, et al. Reaction to epilepsy in the workplace. *Epilepsia.* 2004;45:1134.
70. Herman JP, Cullinan WE. Neurocircuitry of stress: central control of the hypothalamo-pituitary-adrenocortical axis. *Trends Neurosci.* 1997;20:78–84.
71. Hermann BP, Whitman S, Wyler AR, et al. Psychosocial predictors of psychopathology in epilepsy. *Br J Psychiatry.* 1990;156:98–105.
72. Hirschfield RMA, Bowden CL, Gitlin MJ, et al. Practice guideline for the treatment of patients with bipolar disorder. *Am J Psychiatry.* 2002;159(Suppl 4):1–15.
73. Hitchcock JM, Davis M. Lesions of the amygdala, but not of the cerebellum or red nucleus, block conditioned fear as measured with the potentiated startle paradigm. *Behav Neurosci.* 1986;100:15.
74. Hoeppner TJ, Smith DC. Models of psychopathology in epilepsy. Lessons learned from animal studies. In: Ettinger AB, Kanner AM, eds. *Psychiatric Issues in Epilepsy; A Practical Guide to Diagnosis and Management.* New York: Lippincott Williams & Wilkins; 2001:273–287.
75. Isaacs KL, Philbeck JW, Barr WB, et al. Obsessive-compulsive symptoms in patients with temporal lobe epilepsy. *Epilepsy Behav.* 2004;5(4):569–574.
76. Jacoby A, Baker GA, Steen N, et al. The clinical course of epilepsy and its psychosocial correlates: findings from a U.K. community study. *Epilepsia.* 1996;37:148.
77. Jobe PC, Browning RA. The serotonergic and noradrenergic effects of antidepressant drugs are anticonvulsant, not proconvulsant. *Epilepsy Behav.* 2005;7(4):602–619.
78. Jobe PC, Dailey JW, Wernicke JF. A noradrenergic and serotonergic hypothesis of the linkage between epilepsy and affective disorders. *Crit Rev Neurobiol.* 1999;13:317–356.
79. Jobe PC, Dailey JW. Genetically epilepsy-prone rats (GEPRs) in drug research. *CNS Drug Rev.* 2000;6:241–260.
80. Jobe PC, Mishra PK, Adams-Curtis LE, et al. The genetically epilepsy-prone rat (GEPR). *Ital J Neurol Sci.* 1995;16:91.
81. Jobe PC, Mishra PK, Dailey JW, et al. Genetic predisposition to partial (focal) seizures and to generalized tonic/clonic seizures: interactions between seizure circuitry of the forebrain and brainstem. In: Berkovic SF, Genton P, Hirsch E, et al., eds. *Genetics of Focal Epilepsies.* Avignon, France: John Libbey & Company, Ltd.; 1999:251.
82. Johnson EK, Jones JE, Seidenberg M, et al. The relative impact of anxiety, depression, and clinical seizure features on health-related quality of life in epilepsy. *Epilepsia.* 2004;45(5):544–550.
83. Jones J, Hermann BP, Barry J, et al. Clinical assessment of axis I psychiatric morbidity in chronic epilepsy: a multicenter investigation. *J Neuropsychiatry Clin Neurosci.* 2005;17(2):172–179.
84. Jones JE, Hermann BP, Barry JJ, et al. Rates and risk factors for suicide, suicidal ideation, and suicide attempts in chronic epilepsy. *Epilepsy Behav.* 2003;4(Suppl 3):S31–38.
85. Jung ME, Lal H, Gatch MB. The discriminative stimulus effects of pentylenetetrazol as a model of anxiety: recent developments. *Neurosci Biobehav Rev.* 2002;26:429–439.
86. Kalin NH, Shelton SE, Davidson RJ. The role of the central nucleus of the amygdala in mediating fear and anxiety in the primate. *J Neurosci.* 2004;24(24):5506–5515.
87. Kalynchuk LE, Davis AC, Gregus A, et al. Hippocampal involvement in the expression of kindling-induced fear in rats. *Neurosci Biobehav Rev.* 2001;25:687–696.
88. Kanner AM, Morris HH, Stagno S, et al. Remission of an obsessive-compulsive disorder following a right temporal lobectomy. *Neuropsychiatry Neuropsychol Behav Neurol.* 1993;6:2:126–129.
89. Kanner AM, Ramirez L, Jones JC. The utility of placing sphenoidal electrodes under the foramen ovale with fluoroscopic guidance. *J Clin Neurophysiol.* 1995;12(1):72–81.
90. Kanner AM, Soto A, Gross-Kanner H. Prevalence and clinical characteristics of postictal psychiatric symptoms in partial epilepsy. *Neurology.* 2004;62:708–713.
91. Kanner AM, Wuu J, Barry J, et al. Atypical depressive episodes in epilepsy: a study of their clinical characteristics and impact on quality of life (abstract). *Neurology.* 2004;62(Suppl 5):A249.
92. Kanner AM. The complex epilepsy patient: intricacies of assessment and treatment. *Epilepsia.* 2003;44(Suppl 5):3–8.
93. Kanner AM, Kozak AM, Frey M. The use of sertraline in patients with epilepsy: is it safe? *Epilepsy Behav.* 2000;1(2):100–105.
94. Kapp BS, Frysinger RC, Gallgher M, et al. Amygdala central nucleus lesions: effects on heart rate conditioning in the rabbit. *Physiol Behav.* 1979;23:113.
95. Karno M, Golding JM, Sorenson SB, et al. The epidemiology of obsessive-compulsive disorder in five US communities. *Arch Gen Psychiatry.* 1988;45(12):1094–1099.
96. Kessler RC, McGonagle KA, Zhao S, et al. Life-time and 12 month prevalence of DSM-III-R psychiatric disorders in the United States: results from the National Comorbidity Survey. *Arch Gen Psychiatry.* 1994;51:8–18.
97. Ketter TA, Malow BA, Flamini R, et al. Anticonvulsant withdrawal-emergent psychopathology. *Neurology.* 1994;44:55–61.
98. Khan A, Alper K, Schwartz K, et al. Seizure risk among patients participating in psychopharmacology clinical trials. Poster Session I #148. American College of Neuropsychopharmacology (ACNP) 44th Annual Meeting, Waikoloa, Hawaii, 2005.
99. Kohler CG, Carran MA, Bilker W, et al. Association of fear auras with mood and anxiety disorders after temporal lobectomy. *Epilepsia.* 2001;42(5):674–681.
100. Kraepelin E. *Psychiatrie, vol 3.* Leipzig: Johann Ambrosius Barth; 1923.
101. Kulaksizoglu IB, Bebek N, Baykan B, et al. Obsessive–compulsive disorder after epilepsy surgery. *Epilepsy Behav.* 2004;5:113–118.
102. Boylan LS, Flint LA, Labovitz DL, et al. Depression but not seizure frequency predicts quality of life in treatment-resistant epilepsy. *Neurology.* 2004;62(2):258–261.
103. LeDoux JE, Cicchetti P, Xagoraris A, et al. The lateral amygdaloid nucleus: sensory interface of the amygdala in fear conditioning. *J Neurosci.* 1990;10:1062–1069.
104. Lehmann A. Audiogenic seizures data in mice supporting new theories of biogenic amines mechanisms in the central nervous system. *Life Sci.* 1967;6:1423.
105. Lehrner J, Kalchmayr R, Serles W, et al. Health-related quality of life (HRQOL), activity of daily living (ADL) and depressive mood disorder in temporal lobe epilepsy patients. *Seizure.* 1999;8(2):88–92.
106. Levine S. Stimulation in infancy. *Sci Am.* 1960;202:80–86.
107. Linden M, Zubraegel D, Baer T, et al. Efficacy of cognitive behaviour therapy in generalized anxiety disorders. Results of a controlled clinical trial (Berlin CBT-GAD Study). *Psychother Psychosom.* 2005;74(1):36–42.
108. Malizia AL, Cunningham VJ, Bell CJ, et al. Decreased brain GABA(A)-benzodiazepine receptor binding in panic disorder: preliminary results from a quantitative PET study. *Arch Gen Psychiatry.* 1998;55(8):715–720.
109. Manchanda R, Schaefer B, McLachlan RS, et al. Psychiatric disorders in candidates for surgery for epilepsy. *J Neurol Neurosurg Psychiatry.* 1996;61:82–89.
110. McConnell HW, Duncan D. Treatment of psychiatric comorbidity in epilepsy. In: McConnell HW, Snyder PJ, eds. *Psychiatric Comorbidity in Epilepsy.* Washington, DC: American Psychiatric Press; 1998:245–362.
111. Meldrum BS, Anlezark GM, Adam HK, et al. Anticonvulsant and proconvulsant properties of viloxazine hydrochloride: pharmacological and pharmacokinetic studies in rodents and epileptic baboon. *Psychopharmacology (Berlin).* 1982;76:212.
112. Merikangas KR, Angst J. Comorbidity and social phobia: evidence from clinical, epidemiologic and genetic studies. *Eur Arch Psychiatry Clin Neurosci.* 1995;244:297–303.
113. Mintzer S, Lopez F. Comorbidity of ictal fear and panic disorder. *Epilepsy Behav.* 2002;3(4):330–337.
114. Monaco F, Cavanna A, Magli E, et al. Obsessionality, obsessive-compulsive disorder, and temporal lobe epilepsy. *Epilepsy Behav.* 2005;7(3):491–496.
115. Montgomery SA, Nil R, Durr-Pal N, et al. A 24-week randomized, double-blind, placebo-controlled study of escitalopram for the prevention of generalized social anxiety disorder. *J Clin Psychiatry.* 2005;66(10):1270–1278.
116. Nadkarni S, Devinsky O. Psychotropic effects of antiepileptic drugs. *Epilepsy Curr.* 2005;5(5):176–181.
117. Naritoku DK, Terry WJ, Helfert RH. Regional induction of fos immunoreactivity in the brain by anticonvulsant stimulation of the vagus nerve. *Epilepsy Res.* 1995;22:53–62.

118. Neumeister A, Bain E, Nugent AC, et al. Reduced serotonin type 1A receptor binding in panic disorder. *J Neurosci*. 2004;24(3):589–591.
119. Nibuya M, Morinobu S, Duman RS. Regulation of BDNF and trkB mRNA in rat brain by chronic electroconvulsive seizure and antidepressant drug treatments. *J Neurosci*. 1995;15:7539–7547.
120. Nubukpo P, Preux PM, Houinato D, et al. Psychosocial issues in people with epilepsy in Togo and Benin (West Africa) I. Anxiety and depression measured using Goldberg's scale. *Epilepsy Behav*. 2004;5(5):722–727.
121. Nutt DJ, Glue P, Lawson CW, et al. Flumazenil provocation of panic attacks: evidence for altered benzodiazepine receptor sensitivity in panic disorders. *Arch Gen Psychiatry*. 1990;47:917–925.
122. Nutt DJ. Overview of diagnosis and drug treatments of anxiety disorders. *CNS Spectrum*. 2005;10(1):49–56.
123. Oguz A, Kurul S, Dirik E. Relationship of epilepsy-related factors to anxiety and depression scores in epileptic children. *J Child Neurol*. 2002;17(1):37–40.
124. Okuhara DY, Beck SG. 5HT1A receptor linked to inward-rectifying potassium current in in hippocampal CA# pyramidal cells. *J Neurophysiol*. 1994;71:2161–2167.
125. Otto MW, Bruce SE, Deckersbach T. Benzodiazepine use, cognitive impairment, and cognitive-behavioral therapy for anxiety disorders: issues in the treatment of a patient in need. *J Clin Psychiatry*. 2005;66(suppl 2):34–38.
126. Pande AC, Crockatt JG, Feltner DE, et al. Pregabalin in generalized anxiety disorder: a placebo-controlled trial. *Am J Psychiatry*. 2003;160:533–540.
127. Pande AC, Davidson JRT, Jefferson JW, et al. Treatment of social phobia with gabapentin: a placebo controlled study. *J Psychopharmacol*. 1999;19(4):341–348.
128. Perrine K, Hermann BP, Meador KJ, et al. The relationship of neuropsychological functioning to quality of life in epilepsy (see comments). *Arch Neurol*. 1995;52(10):997–1003.
129. Phillips RG, LeDoux JE. Differential contribution of amygdala and hippocampus to cued and contextual fear conditioning. *Behav Neurosci*. 1992;106:274–285.
130. Piette Y, Delaunois AL, De Shaepdryver AF, et al. Imipramine and electroshock threshold. *Arch Int Pharmacodyn Ther*. 1963;144:293.
131. Pilowsky DJ, Olfson M, Gameroff MJ, et al. Panic disorder and suicidal ideation in primary care. *Depress Anxiety*. 2006;23(1):11–16.
132. Pine DS. Development of the symptom of anxiety. In: Lewis M, ed. *Child and Adolescent Psychiatry. A Comprehensive Textbook*. 3rd ed. Philadelphia: Lippincott Williams & Wilkins; 2002:343–351.
133. Polc P, Schneeberger J, Haefely W. Effects of several centrally active drugs on the sleep wakefulness cycle of cats. *Neuropharmacology*. 1979;18:259.
134. Prichard JW, Ransom BR. Phenobarbital: mechanisms of action. In: Levy RH, Mattson RH, Meldrum BS, eds. *Antiepileptic Drugs*. 4th ed. New York: Raven Press; 1995:359–369.
135. Rende R, Weissman M, Rutter M. Psychiatric disorders in the probands of depressed probands II. Familial loading for comorbid non-depressive disorders based upon probands age of onset. *J Affect Disord*. 1997;42:23–28.
136. Reuber M, Andersen B, Elger CE, et al. Depression and anxiety before and after temporal lobe epilepsy surgery. *Seizure*. 2004;13(2):129–135.
137. Reul JM, Holsboer F. Corticotropin-releasing factor receptors 1 and 2 in anxiety and depression. *Curr Opin Pharmacol*. 2002;2:23–33.
138. Rickels K, Downing R, Schweizer E, et al. Antidepressants for the treatment of generalized anxiety disorder: a placebo-controlled comparison of imipramine, trazodone and diazepam. *Arch Gen Psychiatry*. 1993;50:884–895.
139. Rickels K, Pollack MH, Sheehan DV, et al. Efficacy of extended-release venlafaxine in nondepressed outpatients with generalized anxiety disorder. *Am J Psychiatry*. 2000;157:968–974.
140. Ring HA, Moriarty J, Trimble MR. A prospective study of the early post-surgical psychiatric associations of epilepsy surgery. *J Neurol Neurosurg Psychiatry*. 1998;64(5):601–604.
141. Ring HA, Nuri G-C. Epilepsy and panic disorder. In: Trimble MR, Schmitz B, eds. *The Neuropsychiatry of Epilepsy*. New York: Cambridge University Press; 2002:226–238.
142. Rocca P, Fonzo V, Scotta M, et al. Paroxetine efficacy in the treatment of generalized anxiety disorder. *Acta Psychiatr Scand*. 1997;95:444–450.
143. Romero LM, Sapolsky RM. Patterns of ACTH secretagog secretion in response to psychological stimuli. *J Neuroendocriol*. 1996;8:243–258.
144. Rosenthal M. Tiagabine for the treatment of generalized anxiety disorder: a randomized, open-label, clinical trial with paroxetine as a positive control. *J Clin Psychiatry*. 2003;64:1245–1249.
145. Roy-Byrne PP, Craske MG, Stein MB, et al. A randomized effectiveness trial of cognitive-behavioral therapy and medication for primary care panic disorder. *Arch Gen Psychiatry*. 2005;62(3):290–298.
146. Ryu JR, Jobe PC, Milbrandt JC, et al. Morphological deficits in noradrenergic neurons in GEPR-9s stem from abnormalities in both the locus coeruleus and its target tissues. *Exp Neurol*. 1999;156:84–91.
147. Sapolsky RM, Uno H, Rebert CS, et al. Hippocampal damage associated with prolonged glucocorticoid exposure in primates. *J Neurosci*. 1990;10:2897–2902.
148. Sapolsky RM. Glucocorticoids and hippocampal atrophy in neuropsychiatric disorders. *Arch Gen Psychiatry*. 2000;57:925–935.
149. Sareen J, Cox BJ, Afifi TO, et al. Anxiety disorders and risk for suicidal ideation and suicide attempts: a population-based longitudinal study of adults. *Arch Gen Psychiatry*. 2005;62(11):1249–1257.
150. Sazgar M, Carlen PL, Wennberg R. Panic attack semiology in right temporal lobe epilepsy. *Epileptic Disord*. 2003;5(2):93–100.
151. Schatzberg AF, Cole JO, DeBattista C. Antianxiety agents. In: *Manual of Clinical Psychopharmacology*. 5th ed. Washington, DC: American Psychiatric Association; 2005;313–330.
152. Schatzberg AF, Haddad P, Kaplan EM, et al. Serotonin reuptake discontinuation syndrome: a hypothetical definition (discontinuation consensus panel). *J Clin Psychiatry*. 1997;58(Suppl 7):5–10.
153. Schuff N, Marmar CR, Weiss DS, et al. Reduced hippocampal volume and n-acetyl aspartate in posttraumatic stress disorder. *Ann NY Acad Sci*. 1997;821:516–520.
154. Schwartz TL. The use of tiagabine augmentation for treatment-resistant anxiety disorders: a case series. *Psychopharmacol Bull*. 2002;36:53–57.
155. Scimemi A, Schorge S, Kullmann DM, et al. Epileptogenesis is associated with enhanced glutamatergic transmission in the perforant path. *J Neurophysiol*. 2006;95(2):1213–1220.
156. Selye H. *The Stress of Life*. New York: McGraw-Hill; 1978.
157. Servan-Schreiber D, Perlstein WM, Cohen JD, et al. Selective pharmacological activation of limbic structures in human volunteers: a positron emission tomography study. *J Neuropsychiatry Clin Neurosci*. 1998;10(2):148–159.
158. Sheline YI, Wnag PW, Gado MH, et al. Hippocampal atrophy in recurrent major depression. *Proc Natl Acad Sci USA*. 1996;93(9):3908–3913.
159. Silberstein S. Valproic acid: clinical efficacy in other neurologic disorders. In: Levy RH, Mattson RH, Meldrum BS, et al., eds. *Antiepileptic Drugs*. 5th ed. Philadelphia: Lippincott Williams & Wilkins; 2002:818–836.
160. Smith DF, Baker GA, Dewey D, et al. Seizure frequency, patient-perceived seizure severity and the psychosocial consequences of intractable epilepsy. *Epilepsy Res*. 1991;9:231–241.
161. Smith MA, Makino S, Kvetnansky R, et al. Effects of stress on neurotrophic factor expression in the rat brain. *Ann N Y Acad Sci*. 1995;771:234–239.
162. Southam E, Kirkby D, Higgins GA, et al. Lamotrigine inhibits monoamine uptake in vitro and modulates 5-hydroxytryptamine uptake in rats. *Eur J Pharmacol*. 1998;358(1):19–24.
163. Spitz MC. Panic disorder in seizure patients: a diagnostic pitfall. *Epilepsia*. 1991;32:33–38.
164. Sramek JJ, Tansman M, Suri A, et al. Efficacy of buspirone in generalized anxiety disorder with coexisting mild depressive symptoms. *J Clin Psychiatry*. 1996;57(7):287–291.
165. Stahl SM. Anticonvulsants as anxiolytics, part 1. Tiagabine and other anticonvulsants with actions on GABA. *J Clin Psychiatry*. 2004;65(3):292–293.
166. Stahl SM. Anxiolytics and sedative hypnotics. In: *Essential Psychopharmacology: Neuroscientific Basis and Practical Applications*. 2nd ed. Cambridge: Cambridge University Press; 2000:297–334.
167. Stahl SM. Psychopharmacology of anticonvulsants: do all anticonvulsants have the same mechanism of action? *J Clin Psychiatry*. 2004;65(2):149–150.
168. Strauss J, Birmaher B, Bridge J, et al. Anxiety disorders in suicidal youth. *Can J Psychiatry*. 2000;45(8):739–745.
169. Strine T, Kobau R, Chapman DP, et al. Psychological distress, comorbidities, and health behaviors among U.S. adults with seizures: results from the 2002 National Health Interview Survey. *Epilepsia*. 2005;46:1133.
170. Strober M, Carlson G. Bipolar illness in adolescents with major depression: clinical, genetic and psychopharmacologic predictors in a three to four year prospective follow-up investigation. *Arch Gen Psychiatry*. 1982;39:549–555.
171. Swinkels J, Jonghe F. Safety of antidepressants. *Int Clin Psychopharmacol*. 1995;9(Suppl 4):19–25.
172. Téllez-Zenteno JF, Matijevic S, Wiebe S. Somatic comorbidity of epilepsy in the general population in Canada. *Epilepsia*. 2005;46:1955.
173. Tollefson GD, Rosenbaum JF. Selective serotonin reuptake inhibitors. In: Schatzberg AF, Nemeroff CB, eds. *Textbook of Psychopharmacology*. 2nd ed. Washington, DC: American Psychiatric Association Press; 1998:219–237.
174. Torta R, Keller R. Behavioral, psychotic, and anxiety disorders in epilepsy: etiology, clinical features, and therapeutic implications. *Epilepsia*. 1999;40(Suppl 10):S2–20.
175. Tricyclic antidepressant induced seizures and plasma drug concentration. *J Clin Psychiatry*. 1992;53:160–162.
176. Trimble MR, Mula M. Antiepileptic drug interactions in patients requiring psychiatric drug treatment. In: Majkowski J, Bourgeois B, Patsalos P, et al., eds. *Antiepileptic Drugs: Combination Therapy and Interactions*. Cambridge: Cambridge University Press; 2006:350–368.
177. Van Praag HM, de Kloet R, van Os J. Stress the brain and depression. In: *Stress the Brain and Depression*. Cambridge: Cambridge University Press; 2004:225–259.
178. Versiani M, Cassano G, Perugi G, et al. Reboxetine, a selective norepinephrine reuptake inhibitor, is an effective and well-tolerated treatment for panic disorder. *J Clin Psychiatry*. 2002;63(1):31–37.
179. Wang W, Dow KE, Fraser DD. Elevated corticotropin releasing hormone/corticotropin releasing hormone-R1 expression in postmortem brain obtained from children with generalized epilepsy. *Ann Neurol*. 2001;50(3):404–409.

180. Weil A. Depressive reactions associated with temporal lobe uncinate seizures. *J Nerv Ment Dis*. 1955;121:505–510.
181. Wennberg R, Arruda F, Quesney LF, et al. Preeminence of extrahippocampal structures in the generation of mesial temporal seizures: evidence from human depth electrode recordings. *Epilepsia*. 2002;43(7):716–726.
182. Whitton PS, Fowler LJ. The effect of valproic acid on 5-hydroxytryptamine and 5- hydroxyindoleacetic acid concentration in hippocampal dialysates in vivo. *Eur J Pharmacol*. 1991;200:167–169.
183. Williams J, Steel C, Sharp GB, et al. Anxiety in children with epilepsy. *Epilepsy Behav*. 2003;4(6):729–732.
184. Wrench J, Wilson SJ, Bladin PF. Mood disturbance before and after seizure surgery: a comparison of temporal and extratemporal resections. *Epilepsia*. 2004;45:534–543.
185. Yan QS, Jobe PC, Dailey JW. Evidence that a serotonergic mechanism is involved in the anticonvulsant effect of fluoxetine in genetically epilepsy-prone rats. *Eur J Pharmacol*. 1993;252(1):105–112.
186. Yan QS, Jobe PC, Dailey JW. Further evidence of anticonvulsant role for 5-hydroxytryptamine in genetically epilepsy prone rats. *Br J Pharmacol*. 1995;115:1314–1318.
187. Yan QS, Jobe PC, Dailey JW. Thalamic deficiency in norepinephrine release detected via intracerebral microdialysis: a synaptic determinant of seizure predisposition in the genetically epilepsy-prone rat. *Epilepsy Res*. 1993;14:229–236.
188. Yan QS, Mishra PK, Burger RL, et al. Evidence that carbamazepine and antiepilepsirine may produce a component of their anticonvulsant effects by activating serotonergic neurons in genetically epilepsy-prone rats. *J Pharmacol Exp Ther*. 1992;261:652–659.
189. Yanagita T, Wakasa Y, Kiyohara H. Drug dependance potential of viloxazine hydrochloride tested in rhesus monkeys. *Pharmacol Biochem Behav*. 1980;12:155.
190. Yehuda R. Are glucocorticoids responsible for putative hippocampal damage in PTSD? How and when to decide. *Hippocampus*. 2001;11:85–89.
191. Zigmond AS, Snaith RP. The Hospital Anxiety and Depression Scale. *Acta Psychiatr Scand*. 1983;67:361–370.
192. Zung WWK, Magruder-Habib K, Velez R, et al. The comorbidity of anxiety and depression in general medical patients: a longitudinal study. *J Clin Psychiatry*. 1990;51(Suppl. 6):77–80.

CHAPTER 207 ■ PSYCHOGENIC NONEPILEPTIC SEIZURES AND EPILEPSY

W. CURT LAFRANCE, JR., ANDRES M. KANNER, AND TIM BETTS

INTRODUCTION

Psychogenic nonepileptic seizures (PNES) are similar to epileptic seizures (ES) in that they present as time-limited, paroxysmal alterations in behavior, sensation, motoric activity, autonomic signs, and/or consciousness. They differ from ES, however, in that they lack electroencephalographic ictal findings on EEG during the ictus. Treating the two disorders individually can present numerous challenges; the issues are multiplied in the 10% to 30% of patients with PNES who have comorbid ES. Much of the material on the diagnosis and treatment of patients with PNES is covered extensively in Chapter 282. In this chapter, we describe the epidemiology, diagnosis, and treatment of patients with mixed PNES/ES.

HOW FREQUENTLY IS IT A PROBLEM? EPIDEMIOLOGIC CONSIDERATIONS

Medical writings from the 19th century describe how to differentiate ES from PNES (then known as hystero-epilepsy). There is a great deal of interest in and controversy about whether people with PNES have an increased incidence of coexisting or previous epilepsy. Of the 1% of the U. S. population diagnosed with epilepsy, 5% to 20% have PNES.[29] It is estimated that 10% of those with PNES have mixed ES/PNES,[54] and estimates for the coexistence of ES and PNES vary from less than 10% to more than 40%.[69] The incidence of PNES has been estimated to be 3.03 per 100,000,[79] and the prevalence of PNES is estimated to be up to 33 per 100,000.[5] Patients with PNES are usually women (~80%) and are between 15 to 35 years old (~80%),[76] although children and the elderly can develop PNES. It is estimated that up to 50% of patients admitted to an intensive care unit from the emergency department in status epilepticus in fact have pseudostatus, as one manifestation of PNES.[72]

The literature on comorbid ES/PNES is confusing because different populations of patients have been studied by different investigators with diverse methodologies and because of the uncertainty about the diagnosis of PNES. In an attempt to clarify the available data, the following three questions must be addressed:

1. In a population of people with established epilepsy in whom the primary diagnosis is clear, how many might also have PNES?
2. In a population of people with PNES in whom the diagnosis is clear, how many have previously had a history of epilepsy, and could some of their seizures still be of epileptic origin so that, if anticonvulsant medication is withdrawn, epilepsy would re-emerge?
3. How often is a "misdiagnosis" of PNES made in some of the seizures of patients with an established diagnosis of epilepsy?

The following sections attempt to answer these questions.

How Often Does PNES Occur in Patients with an Established Diagnosis of Epilepsy?

The answer to this question is not known. If the cause of a particular patient's seizures is unclear, is it possible that two different types of seizure are present, one epileptic, the other not? The literature suggests that, in the assessment of a patient with an unknown attack disorder that has two different presentations, 5% to 30% of the time both with epilepsy and psychogenic PNES may be present.[69] The prevalence rates of concurrent ES and PNES may vary from one study to another according to whether a diagnosis of concurrent epilepsy was based on the capturing of actual seizures or on the recording of interictal epileptiform discharges only. For example, Devinsky et al. identified 20 patients with ES among a group of 99 PNES patients.[21] In contrast, in a study of 1,590 patients who underwent a video-electroencephalographic (V-EEG) study, Martin et al. found 514 (32.3%) diagnosed with PNES, of whom 29 (5.3%) were found to have both PNES and epilepsy.[55] Lesser et al. concluded that PNES and concurrent epilepsy occurred in about 10% of patients with PNES.[54] Using stringent criteria (as opposed to higher estimates in the past that based abnormalities—including slowing on EEG—as ictal evidence), Benbadis et al. identified three patients with interictal epileptiform activity among 32 patients (9.4%) with PNES.[4] These investigators did not record ES so it is not clear whether the seizure disorder was concurrent or the seizures had remitted with pharmacotherapy.

Studying the surgical population, Henry and Drury conducted a V-EEG in 145 patients who had temporal interictal EEG spikes, and they reported ictal semiology characteristic of temporal lobe seizures for presurgical evaluation of medically refractory seizures. PNES were unexpectedly identified in 12 (8%) of these patients.[37] A low prevalence was reported even in patient populations at greater risk. For example, Lelliott et al. found that, over a 5-year period, 7% of admissions to an epilepsy unit in a psychiatric hospital had PNES and concurrent epilepsy.[53]

An exception must be made among patients with cognitive developmental delay. Indeed, these are patients with epilepsy who may have found that their seizure activity can be reinforced or rewarded (i.e., having a seizure allows them to get out of unpleasant situations at school or workshop). As a result, they "learn to precipitate their epileptic seizures" at times when they try to avoid uncomfortable situations. These patients, therefore, are found to have higher prevalence rates of PNES and concurrent ES. For example, Neil and Alvarez evaluated 124 mentally retarded persons with behaviors suggestive of epilepsy.[57] Patients were monitored using an eight-channel radio-telemetered V-EEG recording system. Twenty patients (16%) were found to have only ES, 50 (40.5%) to have PNES, 11 to have both epileptic and PNES (9%), and 43 were classified as inconclusive. Among the patients with only PNES 15 had abnormal EEGs and four (37%) had epileptiform EEGs. Thus, in this study, among the 61 patients with PNES, 24.5% had a concurrent or past seizure disorder.

How Often Does PNES Develop in Patients with Prior History of Epileptic Seizures?

As for the previous question, no clear answer is obtained from the available literature. For example, in some studies it is also sometimes unclear, when the prevalence of the two conditions is compared, whether the investigator is referring to patients with PNES and concurrent ES or merely a history of past epilepsy. It is likely, as Ramsey et al. have concluded,[69] that if the history is one of past as opposed to present epilepsy, the proportion of patients with both epilepsy and nonepilepsy is likely to be higher, particularly in patients with cognitive developmental delay.[57]

A review of the literature[8,69] and the clinical studies[42,47,71] suggest that 10% to 40% of patients who appear to have established PNES also have a past history of ES. Sometimes the question can only be answered by withdrawing antiepileptic drugs (AEDs) in those patients whose interictal recordings reveal epileptiform activity or in whom a history of paroxysmal events with clinical manifestations is highly suggestive of ES (also see the next section). If epilepsy re-emerges upon discontinuation of AEDs, the possibility exists of a patient who has a seizure disorder that remitted with the use of AEDs, and who, at some point, went on to develop PNES. On the other hand, failure to record an ES upon discontinuation of AEDs does not rule out a seizure disorder that remitted with AEDs, above all in the presence of epileptiform activity in interictal recordings.

One example of patients with both PNES and a past history of epilepsy is found in those patients who have had successful temporal lobectomies and then went on to develop PNES, presumably because of an inability to adjust to a seizure-free life. Fortunately, this is not a common occurrence. In a study of 166 consecutive patients who underwent epilepsy surgery, Parra et al. found three patients (2%) who experienced postsurgical de novo PNES documented by V-EEG.[62] The interval between the date of surgery and the development of the symptoms was variable (8–47 months range). Two of the three patients had become seizure free after surgery, and one had significant improvement of her seizures. The clinical phenomena of PNES differed from those seen for the ES preceding surgery. The diagnosis of PNES had not been suspected before the diagnostic V-EEG. Following the diagnosis of PNES, spells stopped in two patients and recurred rarely in one. Davies et al. found de novo postsurgical PNES in eight (3.5%) of 228 patients who underwent epilepsy surgery.[14] PNES occurred between 6 weeks to 6 years (mean, 23 months) after surgery. Six had undergone a resection, and two had complete callosotomy. There was a significant excess of postoperative interictal dysphoric disorder (IDD) and operative complications (bone flap infections) in the PNES group. Ney et al. identified five patients (5%) with PNES among a group of 96 consecutive patients who underwent epilepsy surgery.[58] Two patients experienced operative complications. Compared with the surgical cohort, patients had a higher frequency of preoperative psychopathologic conditions, lower mean FSIQ, and a greater occurrence of operative complications. In a recent study completed at the Rush Epilepsy Center, Kanner et al. found that seven of 94 patients (7%) who underwent an anterotemporal lobectomy developed de novo PNES. As in other studies, most patients ($n = 6$) were women; six of the seven patients had a pre- and postsurgical psychiatric depression/anxiety disorder, whereas the seventh patient had a history of attention deficit disorder and personality disorder that was present before surgery and worsened after surgery. Three patients had gainful employment before and after surgery, whereas the remaining four did not seek or obtain work either before or after surgery. Given the small number of patients with de novo PNES, no statistical analyses were carried out (Kanner AM, unpublished data).

Glosser et al. tried to identify risk factors of postsurgical PNES by comparing the demographic, neurologic, and psychiatric variables of 22 medically refractory epilepsy patients in whom PNES was documented by electroencephalogram (EEG) after resective surgery to those of a larger series of epilepsy surgery patients.[33] Patients with PNES were significantly more likely to have a seizure onset later in life, to have undergone epilepsy surgery in the right hemisphere, and to be women, but these subjects failed to differ with respect to age, IQ, or preoperative psychiatric diagnoses. PNES tended to become apparent in the first few months after surgery.

How Often Does Epilepsy Lie Behind an Erroneous Diagnosis of PNES?

This question is difficult to answer, because it depends on the accuracy of the diagnosis of PNES, which is often impossible to determine in published series. In the literature, completely different methods have been used for diagnosing PNES, based sometimes on EEG criteria (but not necessarily EEGs recorded during the ictus itself), clinical criteria, or a mixture of both. For example, people with epilepsy often show emotional reactions to their auras, so that they may become afraid of them and develop hyperventilation or panic attacks or have an emotional reaction during the ES itself. When auras fail to evolve to complex partial seizures, and their scalp recordings fail to reveal an electrographic ictal pattern,[22] clinicians may be prone to misdiagnose these patients with simple partial seizures as having PNES. In fact, in 1885, Gowers suggested that minor seizures can elaborate into hysterical seizures.[34] A century later, Devinsky and Gordon reported the case of four patients in whom V-EEG–documented ES were temporally associated with PNES.[20] In one woman, the nonepileptic event followed an absence seizure, whereas in the other three patients, the seizures were partial and arose from right frontotemporal regions. Kapur et al. described three patients who convincingly elaborated simple partial seizures during EEG monitoring in order to ensure a result that would lead to surgery.[43] Clearly, one of the problems of assessing the cause of a seizure is that, during a simple partial seizure, some of what is observed may well be a behavioral manifestation of the patient's emotional reactions to an unpleasant epileptic experience. This understandable emotional reaction may be mistaken for a nonepileptic event.

Paradoxically, as clinicians have become increasingly aware of the existence of PNES, patients with certain types of seizure disorders are increasingly being erroneously diagnosed as having PNES. For example, Parra et al. studied 100 consecutive patients who were undergoing a diagnostic V-EEG.[61] Referring physicians correctly suspected a diagnosis of ES in only nine (43%) of 21 patients, whereas 12 (57%) patients were incorrectly thought to have PNES. This misdiagnosis was especially likely in patients with clinical seizures of mesial frontal or parietal lobe origin and stemmed from their "bizarre" or "atypical" manifestations or from the absence of any electrographic ictal activity concurrent with the event during the V-EEG.[41,56,84] Furthermore, it should be remembered that the electrographic ictal pattern on scalp recordings of simple partial seizures is identified in only 25% of these seizures.[22] The error rate in diagnosing PNES probably lies between 5% and 10% (i.e., in up to 10% of patients firmly diagnosed with PNES, the patient really has epilepsy).[69,85] This topic is reviewed in greater detail in Chapter 284.

STRATEGIES IN THE DIAGNOSIS OF PNES IN PATIENTS WITH EPILEPSY

Clinical History

Reaching a correct diagnosis of "only" PNES versus mixed PNES with concurrent or past ES is of the essence if a patient's AEDs are to be discontinued without placing her at risk of (epileptic) seizure recurrence. Clearly, a carefully obtained history and detailed description of all events witnessed by family members and the patient's own recollections are the first step in the diagnostic process and are of great importance when the existence of the two disorders in the same patient is suspected. The next step consists of a V-EEG to confirm the diagnosis. Unfortunately, few studies have investigated in a systematic manner the degree to which PNES and ES differ from one another in the same patient. The available data suggest that the two types of event differ clinically to a significant degree. In the Devinsky et al. study, analysis of PNES and ES on V-EEG revealed that the clinical features of PNES clearly differed from ES in 18 of 20 PNES cases.[21]

Although differentiating the two often is attempted by history, or even with observation of the ictal semiology, many epileptologists and neurologists know of cases in which a high suspicion for ES and V-EEG revealed PNES, or vice versa. Therefore, PNES is best diagnosed using the "gold standard" V-EEG, performed with the greatest humility because even the best have been fooled.

Differentiating PNES from ES Based on Ictal Semiology

This topic is reviewed in great detail in Chapter 282. We will therefore only refer to some of the salient clinical differences here. In many clinicians' minds, PNES presents as opisthotonic posturing with pelvic thrusting in a young female. Gates et al. showed that any presentation that epilepsy can have, PNES may have also,[30] but bedside examination reveals differences in the characteristics of the signs and movements.

During the ictus, some signs of PNES include geotropic eye movements, in which the eyes deviate downward to the side toward which the head is turned.[36] Eyelids are typically closed at the onset of PNES, and for a longer duration when as compared to temporal lobe epilepsy (TLE) or frontal lobe seizures (FLS) (20 seconds vs. ~2 seconds, respectively).[24] Along with ictal eye closure, weeping is associated with PNES.[7,27] Postictal nose rubbing and postictal cough are found in TLE, but not in PNES.[82] Pelvic thrusting has been reported to occur as commonly in FLS as it does in PNES. PNES and FLS differ, however, in that FLS are rarely associated with the overtly sexualized, often prolonged, display seen in some cases of PNES.[32]

It was once thought that absence of physical injury sustained during a seizure was a diagnostic indicator differentiating PNES from ES; however, more than half of all patients with PNES actually have a physical injury associated with their PNES.[40] PNES patients may have urinary incontinence and may injure themselves during the ictus. Tongue biting, self-injury, and incontinence are commonly associated with generalized seizures; however, two thirds of patients with PNES report one of these three signs, typically associated with ES.[15] Rug or floor burns on a patient's cheeks or body is viewed as being pathognomonic for PNES.[80]

Using Video-EEG

How Can the Video-EEG Monitoring Studies Help?

In ES, stereotyped ictal focal and generalized patterns appear on EEG. PNES, on the other hand, have a normal EEG background before, during, and after the events. EEG sensitivity and specificity increase with repeated tracings.[73] Although seizures associated with impaired consciousness (e. g., generalized convulsive and nonconvulsive seizures) are associated with typical, widespread ictal EEG abnormalities, some focal seizures may not show features of seizures with scalp electrodes.[69] The limitation of V-EEG is the same as that of routine EEG—that is, simple partial seizures and FLS may not show ictal patterns using scalp electrodes. Without V-EEG, a neurologists' ability to differentiate an ES from PNES by history has a specificity of 50%.[16]

The judicious use of neurophysiologic studies can help establish whether the patient experienced PNES with a concurrent or past seizure disorder that may have remitted with the administration of AEDs, surgical treatment, or spontaneously. When suspecting concurrent PNES and ES, patients should undergo a V-EEG study and not an ambulatory EEG without video, because capturing the events on video to distinguish the two types of paroxysmal episodes is of the essence. In our opinion, patients should be admitted to a V-EEG monitoring unit, and recordings should be obtained without modifying the AED dose for the first 48 hours. Indeed, as shown by several studies, PNES tend to occur within the first 2 days in more than 90% of patients.[63] The use of induction protocols with conventional activation procedures (hyperventilation and photic stimulation) can facilitate the recording of PNES without raising the ethical concerns of other induction procedures sometimes used.[6] Furthermore, no evidence suggests that the use of induction protocols based on "placebos" such as IV infusion of saline solution or the application of alcohol swabs over the carotid artery yielded a higher rate of event induction than the use of the maneuvers typically used in all EEGs to facilitate seizures[63] (see also Chapter 282).

Interictal Epileptiform Activity

The recording of interictal epileptiform activity (IEA) in the course of a V-EEG is the first clue of a potential comorbid (present or past) ES disorder in patients with PNES. Yet, the recording of IEA does not help to establish the timing of the patient's ES (i.e., remote versus present) or whether the patient's seizures may be in remission as long as the patient is on AEDs. Furthermore, IEA may be recorded in individuals who may have never experienced any ES, and who may have a first-degree relative with a history of epilepsy, above all primary generalized epilepsy. For example, in a review of the literature that looked at the prevalence of IEA in people without epilepsy, Pedley et al. identified six studies with prevalence rates ranging between 0.5% and 2.5%.[64] Of note, IEA were more common in children (1.9%–3.5%) than in adults (0.5%), and future seizures went on to occur in healthy children more often than in healthy adults. Among children, central midtemporal IEA and generalized spike-and-slow-wave discharges were among the most frequent types of IEA recorded, which is suggestive of epilepsy in siblings or other first-degree relatives or of asymptomatic manifestations of genetic traits.[64] Delgado-Escueta et al. reported the presence of IEA in nonsymptomatic siblings from 5 of 33 families (16%) with symptomatic probands.[17] Ultimately, the clinical significance of IEA may have to be resolved by discontinuation of AEDs.

Tapering of AEDs During V-EEG

A rapid taper of most AEDs is reasonable as long as the patient is undergoing an inpatient V-EEG. Abrupt discontinuation of AEDs, however, is known to precipitate ES. Therefore, abrupt discontinuation of AEDs in nonepileptic people should be avoided, because they may cause a false-positive diagnosis of ES. This includes primarily any of the benzodiazepines. Furthermore, abrupt discontinuation of these drugs can trigger withdrawal panic attacks and psychotic episodes, thus leading to further confusion with PNES and underlying psychiatric disorders.

Ictal Data

The recording of spontaneous seizures before tapering the AED dose clearly establishes the concurrent existence of ES and PNES. The occurrence of seizures only after discontinuation of AEDs does not rule out ES coexisting with PNES, but it raises the possibility that the ES may have remitted with AEDs. This question can be clarified by showing the video of the captured seizure to family members and inquiring about their occurrence in the present versus recent or remote past.

The issue of the specificity of EEG in the diagnosis of PNES has not been formally established. Ramsay et al. tested whether altered clinical behavior in the absence of EEG changes was diagnostic of PNES.[69] They evaluated 281 ictal recordings in 194 sequential patients who underwent V-EEG. In 46 (23.3%), the initial scalp EEG showed no epileptiform EEG changes during the clinical event. Subsequent monitoring revealed that, of the 46 with initial negative EEGs, 28 (61%) had PNES, 12 (26%) had epilepsy, and 6 (13%) had mixed PNES/ES. Of the patients with epilepsy, depth electrode recording revealed mesial temporal or inferior frontal areas of seizure onset that were not recorded with scalp electrodes.

Also, failure to record seizures even after discontinuation of AEDs does not rule out a concurrent or past ES disorder. In such cases, the patient's family is asked to make a video of the patient's events when they occur at home.

Ideally, clinicians should aim whenever possible to have V-EEG recordings of PNES and ES available to guide the pharmacologic treatment of ES. Patients, family members, and, when appropriate, friends and coworkers should be shown the two types of events so as to avoid an unnecessary hospitalization for PNES when the patient could be treated aggressively with parenteral AEDs. It is also advisable to give the patient and close family member a copy of the video demonstrating both PNES and ES events in case the patient is taken to an emergency room. The availability of such videos can help emergency-room physicians decide on the course of treatment in a more judicious manner.

Role of Neuroimaging Studies

Neuroimaging allows in vivo visualization of central nervous system (CNS) lesions causing alterations of consciousness. No static and no functional neuroimaging abnormalities have yet been found associated with cases of PNES. Abnormalities on structural neuroimaging neither confirm nor exclude ES or PNES. As shown in the data presented earlier, patients with PNES may have abnormal neurologic examinations, including abnormal MRI studies. However, in patients diagnosed with PNES, the identification of a structural lesion in mesial or orbitofrontal regions should lead the physician to seriously reconsider the diagnosis of PNES. The use of an ictal SPECT or SISCOM study can help clarify whether ES may have been misdiagnosed as PNES (see Chapter 282 as well). A lack of abnormality on scan SPECT studies report an average sensitivity of 72% for PNES and an average of 59% specificity for ES.[13] Case reports exist describing patients with other forms of sensory or motor impairments. Patients with astasia-abasia motor conversion disorder had left temporal hypoperfusion abnormalities on SPECT; however, this has not been seen in PNES.[87]

Role of Laboratory Tests

Serologic measures have been helpful in differentiating ES from PNES. Prolactin (PRL) is secreted from the anterior pituitary and is inhibited by tuberoinfundibular dopaminergic neurons in the arcuate nucleus of the hypothalamus.[31] Trimble found that elevated serum PRL in patients with generalized seizures helped distinguish ES from PNES.[81] A number of studies have since been conducted measuring prolactin in PNES and, with a lack of elevation of PRL, the average sensitivity to PNES was 89%.[13] Further, prolactin ES versus PNES studies have since shown that serum levels are elevated on average in 88% of generalized tonic–clonic (GTC) seizures, in 64% of temporal complex partial seizures (CPS), and in 12% of simple partial seizures. False positives for epilepsy include treatment with dopamine antagonists and some tricyclic antidepressants, breast stimulation, and syncope, and false negatives occur with use of a dopamine agonist or with status epilepticus, because PRL has a short half-life and may attenuate in postictal release.[2] PRL also does not rise after frontal seizures. The American Academy of Neurology's Therapeutics and Technology Assessment Subcommittee published their report on the use of serum PRL in differentiating ES from PNES. The authors reviewed the PRL seizure literature and concluded that a twice-normal relative or absolute serum PRL rise, drawn 10 to 20 minutes after the onset of the ictus, compared against a baseline nonictal PRL, is a useful adjunct in the differentiation of GTC or PCS from PNES.[12] Unfortunately, this test is not useful for differentiating those ES that are more likely to be confused with PNES (i.e., FLS) from PNES proper.

Other serum measure studies to differentiate GTC seizures from PNES have included the use of elevations in peripheral white blood count,[75] cortisol,[66] creatine kinase,[86] and neuron-specific enolase.[67] However, Willert et al. discussed the limited discriminative power of these serological tests in differentiating ES from PNES.[83] Ictal heart rate on EKG monitoring is higher, and a change in ictal heart rate is associated with ES, but not PNES.[25,59,60] Capillary oxygen saturation on pulse oximetry is lower for ES than for PNES.[38]

Role of Neuropsychometric Testing

A large number of studies exist describing the cognitive, emotional, personality, and psychomotor differences between the ES and PNES groups. Cragar et al. reviewed the literature on adjunctive tests for diagnosing PNES and reported sensitivity and specificity of the different measures.[13] A summary of their findings noted that PNES and ES patients did not differ on intelligence tests or on neuropsychological (NP) measures consistently. Both PNES and ES groups did have cognitive deficits when compared to normal controls, and patients with PNES tended to perform better than patients with ES on various NP tests. Studies examining intelligence, psychomotor function, motivational measures, and personality features in PNES suggest the following:

- Intelligence measures and cognitive testing. Comparing patients with PNES to those with ES, Binder et al. found no significant differences on tests of intelligence or learning and memory, including the Wechsler Adult

Intelligence Scale – Revised, Wisconsin Card Sort Test, or Rey Auditory Verbal Learning Test. Control subjects were significantly superior to both the PNES and ES groups.[9] Bortz et al. studied the California Verbal Learning Test results in PNES and ES patients, and the authors suggested that "failure to explicitly recognize words following repeated exposure" may be reflective of a negative response bias and psychological denial in patients with PNES.[11]

- Psychomotor measures. Kalogjera-Sackellares and Sackellares evaluated patients with PNES compared with matched normal controls and found reduced motor speed and grip strength in the PNES patients.[39] Some have interpreted this as a manifestation of motivation, which is discussed later. Dodrill and Holmes reported that patients with PNES performed better than those with ES on measures from the Halstead-Reitan Battery, with differences between Tactual Performance Test, Seashore Tonal Memory, and Trail-Making Part B.[23] Whereas finger tapping and grooved pegboard test results differed for controls compared with PNES and ES groups, Binder did not find differences between the ES and PNES groups on these measures.[9]
- Motivational measures. Motivational tests include the Portland Digit Recognition Test (PDRT), the Test of Memory Malingering (TOMM), and others; these tests are used to detect inadequate performance on NP testing. The presence of unconscious psychological stress is hypothesized as an explanation for variable effort in patients with PNES.[78] Binder et al. found that PNES patients performed more poorly when compared with patients with ES on the PDRT.[9,10] The authors noted that frank malingering occurs rarely in PNES, and the poorer performance in PNES may reflect a lack of psychological resources necessary to persist with a challenging NP battery.
- Personality testing. Results of the Minnesota Multiphasic Personality Inventory (MMPI/MMPI – 2) and Clinical Psychological Profiles and Family tests were reported. The majority of the MMPI studies in PNES report the "conversion V" profile, with elevations in Scales 1 (Hs, Hypochondriasis) and 3 (Hy, Hysteria), and depressions in Scale 2 (D, Depression).[13] Cragar et al. also reported an average sensitivity of 70% and specificity of 73% to PNES diagnosis using MMPI – 2 decision rules. The dramatic personality of patients with PNES was illustrated in a blinded pilot study of artwork drawn by patients with ES and PNES.[1] An 80% positive predictive value for PNES existed if subjects used 10 or more colors to draw their seizures. Galimberti et al. administered the Cognitive Behavioral Assessment (CBA) psychometric battery to patients with lone PNES, mixed ES/PNES, and ES controls. The CBA, which assesses personality characteristics and emotional adjustment, is comprised of scales rating introversion-extroversion, neuroticism, psychoticism, state-trait anxiety, psychophysiological distress, and depressive and other anxiety symptoms. These researchers found that the mean scores on the Psychophysiological Distress Scale for the PNES and the ES/PNES groups were higher than the mean scores of the ES control group.[28] The Rorschach test did not differentiate patients with PNES versus ES.[26] Krawetz et al. evaluated family functioning in patients with ES and PNES and their families.

They found that individuals with PNES view their families as being more dysfunctional, particularly in the area of communication, whereas family members of patients with PNES reported roles as being dysfunctional.[46]

In summary, compared with healthy controls, patients with ES and with PNES perform worse on a number of NP measures. However, few differences exist between ES and PNES groups on tests that would reliably differentiate ES from PNES. The impairments are thought to be due to at least three factors: (a) both the ES and the PNES patients were on AEDs, which may affect cognition; (b) structural lesions in ES patients and in some of the PNES patients with ES; and (c) emotional factors contributing to cognitive impairment in the PNES group.[78] Psychologically, patients with PNES appear to have personality characteristics of anxiety, cognitive dysfunction, and somatic distress, and they have difficulty in expressing and communicating that distress to family and others.

Role of Pharmaco-Diagnosis

Prior to the use of EEG, neurologists and psychiatrists frequently used sedatives or other pharmacologic agents to distinguish ES from PNES. One of the earliest pharmaco-diagnostic accounts from the late 1800s reads: "I administered a hypodermic injection of hyoscine hydrobromate, which caused the fits to cease and produced five hours' sleep. On awakening the patient was very emotional and far from well, but there were no return of the fits.

Hyoscine, we know, is most useful in cases of status epilepticus and in the convulsions associated with general paralysis of the insane; it appears to be of service also in this condition of hystero-epilepsy, and certainly it is much less tedious than the old chloroform method."[44]

Sodium Amytal and hypnosis were used in the mid-1900s to differentiate between ES and PNES.[52,65] Although these agents usually are not used diagnostically today, placebo saline injections and provocation techniques are used more frequently in some institutions.[3,18] The ethics of such procedures has been an issue of debate.[19,74,77] One acceptable technique incorporated at some epilepsy centers uses activation procedures (e.g., hyperventilation and photic stimulation) that are part of their routine EEG diagnostic protocol for PNES.[6]

TREATMENT STRATEGIES

We learn in medical school the physician's dictum, "Primum no nocere." But in the case of the PNES population, many times harm *is* done through inappropriate treatments and aggressive therapy to stop seizures. Although PNES are not responsive to treatment with AEDs, most patients with PNES receive unnecessary AEDs, and only half pursue recommended psychiatric follow-up.[45] Extensive observational data suggest that AEDs are ineffective or may worsen PNES.[48] In some cases, potentially dangerous invasive diagnostic studies, toxic parenteral medications, or emergent intubation are administered.[35,70] The patients, their families, and society bear an enormous cost if psychiatric care is not provided or if inappropriate neurologic therapy is instituted for PNES.

Pharmacotherapy Using AEDs Only Targeting Recognized Epileptic Seizures

We ask patients and their family members to give a detailed description of seizure events; many times, PNES and ES have markedly different phenomenology in the same patient.[20] Once documented historically, we give the patient a seizure calendar and ask patients and family members to chart events prospectively, noting the characteristics of the seizures and any particular triggers or precipitants. The frequency of ES and that of PNES are established and, in the following visit, the results are discussed. This process clarifies treatment targets not only for the patient, but also for the physician. We explain that, for one seizure type, we will use AEDs (e.g., "the seizure that occurs nocturnally, with lateral tongue biting, incontinence, and sore muscles upon regaining consciousness"). For the other type of seizure (e.g., "the one that occurs when watching a show on TV that reminds you of the past trauma of the assault, with 'zoning out' for a brief period of time and coming to just afterwards"), we will use a combination of medications for anxiety and psychotherapy. This method is a problem-oriented, practical approach that patients and their families understand and with which they can comply.

Psychiatric Treatment (Pharmacotherapy and Psychotherapeutic Interventions) for PNES

Intensive treatment using behavioral therapy, psychodynamic psychotherapy, occupational therapy, and education on an inpatient unit was the norm in earlier references to PNES treatment.[51,68] Success levels were higher than in the current outcomes reports, which incorporate a less intensive, outpatient treatment model, with up to 70% of patients with PNES continuing to have seizure events.[72]

Based on the clinical and research reports to date, we proposed the following assessment and treatment approach by a multispecialty neuropsychiatric team:[50]

- Proper diagnosis. Order a V-EEG for each patient with suspected PNES, or refractory or pharmacoresistant seizures.
- Presentation. Explain the PNES diagnosis in a clear, positive, nonpejorative manner. The patient may make the diagnosis presentation to the family members if cognitively and emotionally capable. This process helps reveal the level of understanding and initial acceptance of the diagnosis by the patient. Clarifications can be made by the physician, who is present. Communicate the diagnosis unambiguously to the referring physician and explain the need to eliminate unnecessary medications.
- Psychiatric treatment. Conduct a thorough psychiatric assessment to identify predisposing factors (including comorbid psychiatric disorders), seizure precipitants, and perpetuating factors. As diagnosis informs treatment, a dual-armed approach ensues using pharmacotherapy and/or psychotherapy, as indicated by the individual needs of the patient with PNES.

In patients with mixed ES/PNES, reduce high-dose or multiple AED therapy if possible based upon seizure calendar results. Use psychopharmacologic agents to treat mood, anxiety, or psychotic disorders. Enroll the patient in individual therapy with a psychiatrist or psychologist familiar with PNES and somatoform disorders, if a history of trauma, illness behavior, or specific interpersonal issues is identified in the assessment. Consider family therapy if the family functioning is found to be unhealthy, noting it to be a potential contributor to the symptoms.[49]

SUMMARY AND CONCLUSIONS

The majority of patients with PNES do not have epilepsy, and vice versa. In the 10% to 30% of patients who have mixed ES/PNES, diagnosis and treatment may present a significant challenge. A good history, documenting the various types of events the patient experiences, is an essential starting point. Long-term monitoring using V-EEG, to capture more than one of their typical events, aids in establishing the presence of mixed PNES and ES. Tapering AEDs during inpatient V-EEG greatly facilitates capturing the various seizure types. Provocation techniques using the routine activation procedures appear a safe and ethical procedure for seizure diagnosis.

Once the diagnosis of mixed ES/PNES is made, treatment entails addressing the patient and their family from a neuropsychiatric perspective. When ES coexists with PNES, this is most likely to occur in people with a previous history of epilepsy who have difficulty in adjusting to living without seizures and in patients who have coexisting psychiatric and physical disorders, which is not uncommon. Holistic assessment of the patient aids both diagnosis and management of coexisting epilepsy and nonepilepsy.

References

1. Anschel DJ, Dolce S, Schwartzman A, et al. A blinded pilot study of artwork in a comprehensive epilepsy center population. *Epilepsy Behav.* 2005;6(2):196–202.
2. Bauer J. Epilepsy and prolactin in adults: a clinical review. *Epilepsy Res.* 1996;24(1):1–7.
3. Bazil CW, Kothari M, Luciano D, et al. Provocation of nonepileptic seizures by suggestion in a general seizure population. *Epilepsia.* 1994;35(4):768–770.
4. Benbadis SR, Agrawal V, Tatum IV WO. How many patients with psychogenic nonepileptic seizures also have epilepsy? *Neurology.* 2001;57(5): 915–917.
5. Benbadis SR, Hauser WA. An estimate of the prevalence of psychogenic non-epileptic seizures. *Seizure.* 2000;9(4):280–281.
6. Benbadis SR, Johnson K, Anthony K, et al. Induction of psychogenic nonepileptic seizures without placebo. *Neurology.* 2000;55(12):1904–1905.
7. Bergen D, Ristanovic R. Weeping as a common element of pseudoseizures. *Arch Neurol.* 1993;50(10):1059–1060.
8. Betts T, Boden S. Diagnosis, management and prognosis of a group of 128 patients with non-epileptic attack disorder. Part I. *Seizure.* 1992;1(1):19–26.
9. Binder LM, Kindermann SS, Heaton RK, et al. Neuropsychologic impairment in patients with nonepileptic seizures. *Arch Clin Neuropsychology.* 1998;13(6):513–522.
10. Binder LM, Salinsky MC, Smith SP. Psychological correlates of psychogenic seizures. *J Clin Exp Neuropsychol.* 1994;16(4):524–530.
11. Bortz JJ, Prigatano GP, Blum D, et al. Differential response characteristics in nonepileptic and epileptic seizure patients on a test of verbal learning and memory. *Neurology.* 1995;45(11):2029–2034.
12. Chen DK, So YT, Fisher RS. Use of serum prolactin in diagnosing epileptic seizures: report of the Therapeutics and Technology Assessment Subcommittee of the American Academy of Neurology. *Neurology.* 2005;65(5):668–675.
13. Cragar DE, Berry DT, Fakhoury TA, et al. A review of diagnostic techniques in the differential diagnosis of epileptic and nonepileptic seizures. *Neuropsychol Rev.* 2002 Mar;12(1):31–64.
14. Davies KG, Blumer DP, Lobo S, et al. De novo nonepileptic seizures after cranial surgery for epilepsy: incidence and risk factors. *Epilepsy Behavior.* 2000;1:436–443.
15. de Timary P, Fouchet P, Sylin M, et al. Non-epileptic seizures: delayed diagnosis in patients presenting with electroencephalographic (EEG) or clinical signs of epileptic seizures. *Seizure.* 2002;11:193–197.
16. Deacon C, Wiebe S, Blume WT, et al. Seizure identification by clinical description in temporal lobe epilepsy: How accurate are we? *Neurology.* 2003;61(12):1686–1689.
17. Delgado-Escueta AV, Liu A, Serratosa J, et al. Juvenile Myoclonic Epilepsy: Is There Heterogeneity? In: Malafosse A, Genton P, Hirsch E, et al. *Idiopathic Generalized Epilepsies: Clinical, Experimental, and Genetic Aspects.* London: John Libbey; 1994:281–286.
18. Dericioglu N, Saygi S, Ciger A. The value of provocation methods in patients suspected of having non-epileptic seizures. *Seizure.* 1999;8(3):152–156.
19. Devinsky O, Fisher R. Ethical use of placebos and provocative testing in diagnosing nonepileptic seizures. *Neurology.* 1996;47(4):866–870.
20. Devinsky O, Gordon E. Epileptic seizures progressing into nonepileptic conversion seizures. *Neurology.* 1998;51(5):1293–1296.
21. Devinsky O, Sanchez-Villasenor F, Vazquez B, et al. Clinical profile of patients with epileptic and nonepileptic seizures. *Neurology.* 1996;46(6):1530–1533.
22. Devinsky O, Sato S, Kufta CV, et al. Electroencephalographic studies of simple partial seizures with subdural electrode recordings. *Neurology.* 1989;39(4):527–533.
23. Dodrill CB, Holmes MD. Chapter 13. Part Summary: Psychological and Neuropsychological Evaluation of the Patient with Non-Epileptic Seizures. In: Gates JR, Rowan AJ, eds. *Non-epileptic Seizures,* 2nd ed. Boston: Butterworth-Heinemann; 2000:169–181.
24. Donati F, Kollar M, Pihan H, et al. OPL145. Eyelids position—during epileptic versus psychogenic seizures. *J Neurologic Sci.* 2005;238(Suppl 1):S82–S83.

25. Donati F, Wilder-Smith A, Kollar M, et al. Abstract: epileptic versus psychogenic seizures: effect on heart rate. *Epilepsia*. 1996;37(Suppl 4):58.
26. Ferracuti S, Burla F, Lazzari R. Rorschach findings for patients with pseudoseizures. *Psychol Rep*. 1999;85(2):439–444.
27. Flügel D, Bauer J, Kaseborn U, et al. Closed eyes during a seizure indicate psychogenic etiology: a study with suggestive seizure provocation. *J Epilepsy*. 1996;9(3):165–169.
28. Galimberti CA, Ratti MT, Murelli R, et al. Patients with psychogenic nonepileptic seizures, alone or epilepsy-associated, share a psychological profile distinct from that of epilepsy patients. *J Neurol*. 2003;250(3):338–346.
29. Gates JR, Luciano D, Devinsky O. The Classification and Treatment of Nonepileptic Events. In: Devinsky O, Theodore WH, eds. *Epilepsy and Behavior*. New York: Wiley-Liss; 1991:251–263.
30. Gates JR, Ramani V, Whalen S, et al. Ictal characteristics of pseudoseizures. *Arch Neurol*. 1985;42(12):1183–1187.
31. Gerstik L, Poland RE. Chapter 6. Psychoneuroendocrinology. In: Schatzberg AF, Nemeroff CB, eds. *The American Psychiatric Publishing Textbook of Psychopharmacology*. 3rd ed. Washington, DC: American Psychiatric Publishing, Inc.; 2004:115–127.
32. Geyer JD, Payne TA, Drury I. The value of pelvic thrusting in the diagnosis of seizures and pseudoseizures. *Neurology*. 2000;54(1):227–229.
33. Glosser G, Roberts D, Glosser DS. Nonepileptic seizures after resective epilepsy surgery. *Epilepsia*. 1999;40(12):1750–1754.
34. Gowers WR. *Epilepsy and other chronic convulsive diseases: their causes, symptoms, and treatment,* 2nd ed. Brinklow, MD: Old Hickory Bookshop, 1963.
35. Gunatilake SB, De Silva HJ, Ranasinghe G. Twenty-seven venous cutdowns to treat pseudostatus epilepticus. *Seizure*. 1997;6(1):71–72.
36. Henry JA, Woodruff GHA. A diagnostic sign in states of apparent unconsciousness. *Lancet*. 1978;2(8096):920–921.
37. Henry TR, Drury I. Non-epileptic seizures in temporal lobectomy candidates with medically refractory seizures. *Neurology*. 1997;48(5):1374–1382.
38. James MR, Marshall H, Carew-McColl M. Pulse oximetry during apparent tonic-clonic seizures. *Lancet*. 1991;337(8738):394–395.
39. Kalogjera-Sackellares D, Sackellares JC. Impaired motor function in patients with psychogenic pseudoseizures. *Epilepsia*. 2001;42(12):1600–1606.
40. Kanner AM. Psychogenic nonepileptic seizures are bad for your health. *Epilepsy Curr*. 2003;3(5):181–182.
41. Kanner AM, Morris HH, Luders H, et al. Supplementary motor seizures mimicking pseudoseizures: some clinical differences. *Neurology*. 1990;40(9):1404–1407.
42. Kanner AM, Parra J, Frey M, et al. Psychiatric and neurologic predictors of psychogenic pseudoseizure outcome. *Neurology*. 1999;53(5):933–938.
43. Kapur J, Pillai A, Henry TR. Psychogenic elaboration of simple partial seizures. *Epilepsia*. 1995;36(11):1126–1130.
44. Kingdon WR. The diagnosis of hystero-epilepsy from status epilepticus. *Lancet*. 1898;152(3910):320–321.
45. Krahn LE, Reese MM, Rummans TA, et al. Health care utilization of patients with psychogenic nonepileptic seizures. *Psychosomatics*. 1997;38(6):535–542.
46. Krawetz P, Fleisher W, Pillay N, et al. Family functioning in subjects with pseudoseizures and epilepsy. *J Nerv Ment Dis*. 2001;189(1):38–43.
47. Krumholz A, Niedermeyer E. Psychogenic seizures: a clinical study with follow-up data. *Neurology*. 1983;33(4):498–502.
48. Krumholz A, Niedermeyer E, Alkaitis D, et al. Abstract: psychogenic seizures: a 5-year follow-up study. *Neurology*. 1980;30:392.
49. LaFrance WC, Jr., Barry JJ. Update on treatments of psychological nonepileptic seizures. *Epilepsy Behav*. 2005;7(3):364–374.
50. LaFrance WC, Jr. , Devinsky O. Treatment of nonepileptic seizures. *Epilepsy Behav*. 2002;3(5 Suppl 1):S19–S23.
51. LaFrance WC, Jr. , Devinsky O. The treatment of nonepileptic seizures: Historical perspectives and future directions. *Epilepsia*. 2004;45(Suppl 2):15–21.
52. Lambert C, Rees WL. Intravenous barbiturates in the treatment of hysteria. *BMJ*. 1944;2:70–73.
53. Lelliott PT, Fenwick P. Cerebral pathology in pseudoseizures. *Acta Neurol Scand*. 1991;83(2):129–132.
54. Lesser RP, Lueders H, Dinner DS. Evidence for epilepsy is rare in patients with psychogenic seizures. *Neurology*. 1983;33(4):502–504.
55. Martin R, Burneo JG, Prasad A, et al. Frequency of epilepsy in patients with psychogenic seizures monitored by video-EEG. *Neurology*. 2003;61(12):1791–1792.
56. Morris HH, 3rd, Dinner DS, Luders H, et al. Supplementary motor seizures: clinical and electroencephalographic findings. *Neurology*. 1988;38(7):1075–1082.
57. Neill JC, Alvarez N. Differential diagnosis of epileptic versus pseudoepileptic seizures in developmentally disabled persons. *Appl Res Ment Retard*. 1986;7(3):285–298.
58. Ney GC, Barr WB, Napolitano C, et al. New-onset psychogenic seizures after surgery for epilepsy. *Arch Neurol*. 1998;55(5):726–730.
59. Oliveira G, Gondim F, Hogan E. [P03.158] Movement-induced heart rate (HR) changes in epileptic and non-epileptic seizures. *Neurology*. 2004.
60. Opherk C, Hirsch LJ. Ictal heart rate differentiates epileptic from nonepileptic seizures. *Neurology*. 2002;58(4):636–638.
61. Parra J, Iriarte J, Kanner AM. Are we overusing the diagnosis of psychogenic non-epileptic events? *Seizure*. 1999;8(4):223–227.
62. Parra J, Iriarte J, Kanner AM, et al. De novo psychogenic nonepileptic seizures after epilepsy surgery. *Epilepsia*. 1998;39(5):474–477.
63. Parra J, Kanner AM, Iriarte J, et al. When should induction protocols be used in the diagnostic evaluation of patients with paroxysmal events? *Epilepsia*. 1998;39(8):863– 867.
64. Pedley TA, Mendriatta A, Walczak TS. Chapter 17. Seizures and Epilepsy. In: Ebersole JS, Pedley TA, eds. *Current Practice of Clinical Electroencephalography,* 3rd ed. Philadelphia: Lippincott Williams & Wilkins; 2003:506–587.
65. Peterson DB, Sumner JW, Jr. , Jones GA. Role of hypnosis in differentiation of epileptic from convulsive-like seizures. *Am J Psychiatry*. 1950;107:428–433.
66. Pritchard PB, 3rd, Wannamaker BB, Sagel J, et al. Serum prolactin and cortisol levels in evaluation of pseudoepileptic seizures. *Ann Neurol*. 1985;18(1):87–89.
67. Rabinowicz AL, Correale J, Boutros RB, et al. Neuron-specific enolase is increased after single seizures during inpatient video/EEG monitoring. *Epilepsia*. 1996;37(2):122–125.
68. Ramani V, Gumnit RJ. Management of hysterical seizures in epileptic patients. *Arch Neurol*. 1982;39(2):78–81.
69. Ramsay RE, Cohen A, Brown MC. Chapter 6. Coexisting Epilepsy and Non-Epileptic Seizures. In: Rowan AJ, Gates JR, eds. *Non-epileptic Seizures,* 1st ed. Stoneham, MA: Butterworth-Heinemann; 1993:47–54.
70. Reuber M, Baker GA, Gill R, et al. Failure to recognize psychogenic nonepileptic seizures may cause death. *Neurology*. 2004;62(5):834–835.
71. Reuber M, Fernandez G, Bauer J, et al. Interictal EEG abnormalities in patients with psychogenic nonepileptic seizures. *Epilepsia*. 2002;43(9):1013–1020.
72. Reuber M, Pukrop R, Bauer J, et al. Outcome in psychogenic nonepileptic seizures: 1 to 10-year follow-up in 164 patients. *Ann Neurol*. 2003;53(3):305–311.
73. Salinsky M, Kanter R, Dasheiff RM. Effectiveness of multiple EEGs in supporting the diagnosis of epilepsy: an operational curve. *Epilepsia*. 1987;28(4):331–334.
74. Schachter SC, Brown F, Rowan AJ. Provocative testing for nonepileptic seizures: attitudes and practices in the United States among American Epilepsy Society members. *J Epilepsy*. 1996;9(4):249–252.
75. Shah AK, Shein N, Fuerst D, et al. Peripheral WBC count and serum prolactin level in various seizure types and nonepileptic events. *Epilepsia*. 2001;42(11):1472–1475.
76. Shen W, Bowman ES, Markand ON. Presenting the diagnosis of pseudoseizure. *Neurology*. 1990;40(5):756–759.
77. Smith ML, Stagno SJ, Dolske M, et al. Induction procedures for psychogenic seizures: ethical and clinical considerations. *J Clin Ethics*. 1997;8(3):217–229.
78. Swanson SJ, Springer JA, Benbadis SR, et al. Chapter 9. Cognitive and Psychological Functioning in Patients with Non-Epileptic Seizures. In: Gates JR, Rowan AJ, eds. *Non-Epileptic Seizures,* 2nd ed. Boston: Butterworth-Heinemann; 2000:123–137.
79. Szaflarski JP, Ficker DM, Cahill WT, et al. Four-year incidence of psychogenic nonepileptic seizures in adults in Hamilton county, OH. *Neurology*. 2000;55(10):1561–1563.
80. Trimble MR. Chapter 10. Non-Epileptic Seizures. In: Halligan PW, Bass CM, Marshall JC, eds. *Contemporary Approaches to the Study of Hysteria: Clinical and Theoretical Perspectives*. Oxford, NY: Oxford University Press; 2001:143–154.
81. Trimble MR. Serum prolactin in epilepsy and hysteria. *Br Med J*. 1978;2(6153):1682.
82. Wennberg R. Postictal coughing and nose rubbing coexist in temporal lobe epilepsy. *Neurology*. 2001;56(1):133–134.
83. Willert C, Spitzer C, Kusserow S, et al. Serum neuron-specific enolase, prolactin, and creatine kinase after epileptic and psychogenic non-epileptic seizures. *Acta Neurol Scand*. 2004;109(5):318–323.
84. Williamson PD, Spencer DD, Spencer SS, et al. Complex partial seizures of frontal lobe origin. *Ann Neurol*. 1985;18(4):497–504.
85. Wyler AR, Hermann BP, Blumer D, et al. Chapter 8. Pseudo-Pseudoepileptic Seizures. In: Rowan AJ, Gates JR, eds. *Non-Epileptic Seizures,* 1st ed. Stoneham, MA: Butterworth-Heinemann; 1993:73–84.
86. Wyllie E, Lueders H, Pippenger C, et al. Postictal serum creatine kinase in the diagnosis of seizure disorders. *Arch Neurol*. 1985;42(2):123–126.
87. Yazici KM, Kostakoglu L. Cerebral blood flow changes in patients with conversion disorder. *Psychiatry Res*. 1998;83(3):163–168.

CHAPTER 208 ■ PSYCHIATRIC SIDE EFFECTS OF ANTIEPILEPTIC DRUGS

BETTINA SCHMITZ

INTRODUCTION

Central effects of antiepileptic drugs (AEDs) are not restricted to the modulation of cortical excitability. AEDs may also modify systems that regulate mood and behavior. Anticonvulsant and psychotropic effects are not independent. Effects on seizure control have indirect effects on the mental state. Patients who are seizure-free have no risk of developing seizure-related psychiatric complications. On the other hand, the sudden cessation of seizures may lead to an imbalance in the mental state, as in "forced normalization" (FN). Some AEDs have dose-related paradoxical proconvulsive properties that may cause behavioral disturbances through underlying nonconvulsive status epilepticus.

Psychotropic effects may be negative or beneficial in individual patients. These effects depend on the antiepileptic strength, the mode of action of the anticonvulsant, and the patient's biologic and psychological predisposition. With the increasing variety of AEDs available, behavioral drug profiles have become very important for optimal treatment choices in epilepsy. Recent quality-of-life studies have shown that measurements of depression and the tolerability of AEDs are more important to patients than seizure reduction.[16] Furthermore, the high psychiatric comorbidity in epilepsy often requires psychopharmacologic interventions, which may be avoided when those anticonvulsants used have positive psychotropic properties.

In clinical praxis, the adverse psychiatric effects of AEDs are often not recognized. Often patients don't complain about behavior or mood changes unless they are specifically interviewed. Many neurologists are not competent in the exploration of a mental state, or they don't have the additional time needed to evaluate a patient's mental state. Many depressed patients are not primarily troubled by obvious depressive symptoms such as sadness or feelings of guilt. Depression in epilepsy often presents with sleep disorders or somatoform complaints and memory problems, which makes the diagnosis difficult unless the full psychopathologic status is explored. If delayed adverse psychiatric effects occur after months or years of exposure, the causal relationship with drug treatment is often not considered and is in fact difficult to prove, unless drug withdrawal is followed by the remission of psychiatric symptoms.

The exact prevalence of psychiatric AED events is difficult to estimate. In a consecutive series of patients with epilepsy and significant depression, about 30% were considered to have AED-related symptoms.[21,39] With respect to psychoses, the percentage of episodes triggered by AEDs has been calculated to be 40% in one study.[30]

ADVERSE PSYCHIATRIC EFFECTS OF SPECIFIC AEDS

Conventional Drugs

Barbiturates

Several studies suggested a link between depression and treatment with barbiturates, both in adults and in children.[5,36.] Forty percent of school children treated with barbiturates were diagnosed with "major depression," as compared with only 4% of children treated with carbamazepine.[4] In children, a conduct disorder resembling attention deficit hyperactivity disorder may be provoked by many AEDs, the most frequently implicated drug being phenobarbitone. Irritability and aggressive behavior are side effects particularly often seen when barbiturates are used in mentally retarded patients. Withdrawal problems, which present with nervousness, dysphoria, and insomnia, may occur even when barbiturates are very slowly tapered down.

Phenytoin

Phenytoin may provoke schizophrenia-like psychoses at high serum levels.[32] These psychoses are dose related—and are thus toxic syndromes—but they are not associated with the cerebellar signs that are the most common central nervous system side effects of phenytoin. In a study of 45 patients with drug-related psychoses, 25 (56%) cases were attributed to treatment with phenytoin.[20] A chronic encephalopathy has also been described with phenytoin use, and has been referred to as "Dilantin dementia."[44]

Ethosuccimide

Psychoses typically following cessation of seizures and associated with a normalization of the electroencephalogram (EEG) occur in 2% of children treated with ethosuccimide. The risk of FN is higher (8%) in adolescents and adults treated with ethosuccimide for persisting absence seizures.[45]

Carbamazepine

Affective problems are rare complications of treatment with carbamazepine.[8] These complications present as either depressive disorders or mania, the latter being explained as a paradoxical effect due to the antidepressant properties of carbamazepine, which is chemically related to tricyclic antidepressants.[9]

TABLE 1

INCIDENCE RATES OF PSYCHOSES AND DEPRESSION IN CONTROLLED TRIALS (BESAG,[2] JANSSEN-CILAG,[18] AND LEVINSON AND DEVINSKY[28])

	Psychoses (%)	Depression (%)
Vigabatrin	2.5	12.1
Lamotrigine	0.2	–
Felbamate	0.02	–
Gabapentin	0.5	–
Topiramate	0.8	9–18
Tiagabine	0.8–2	5
Levetiracetam	0.3–0.7	0.5–2

Valproate

Rarely, valproate is associated with acute or chronic encephalopathies.[37,40,47] These encephalopathies are related to dose and perhaps polytherapy, and they are reversible with dose reduction.

Newer AEDs

Table 1 summarizes data from premarketing controlled trials suggesting a relatively high frequency of depressive reactions in vigabatrin, tiagabine, and topiramate, and relative low rates for lamotrigine, gabapentin, and levetiracetam. Obviously psychiatric risks of the newer AEDs are not the same for all compounds. Some of the drugs seem to have neutral effects, some have a relevant risk for negative effects, and some may have predominantely beneficial psychotropic effects. A general comment is that the overall psychiatric risks of newer AEDs are not lower than those of older AEDs.

Vigabatrin

The risk of psychiatric complications caused by vigabatrin has been analyzed in two meta-analyses. The overall incidence of psychoses and severe behavioral reactions leading to drug discontinuation in seven placebo-controlled European studies was 3.4% in the vigabatrin group and 0.6% in the placebo group.[13] Another meta-analysis on the psychiatric risks of vigabatrin[28] translated psychopathologic symptoms described in the investigator forms into standardized psychiatric terminology, which was then summarized into a syndromatic diagnosis. This analysis of U. S. and non-U. S. double-blind studies demonstrated a significantly increased risk for psychosis and particularly for depression. Psychoses occurred in 2.5% of patients treated with vigabatrin compared to an incidence of 0.3% in the placebo group ($p < 0.05$), and depression occurred in 12.1% of patients treated with vigabatrin in contrast to only 3.5% in the placebo group ($p < 0.001$).

Lamotrigine

Severe psychiatric complications are rare with lamotrigine, and psychosis and depression occurred only in very few cases in trials.[14] Insomnia, which may be associated with irritability, anxiety, or even hypomania, is the only significant psychiatric side effect, occurring in 6% of patients treated in monotherapy, compared with 2% in patients treated with carbamazepine and 3% in patients treated with phenytoin.[6]

When first reports surfaced of caregivers complaining that handicapped patients had become more alert and demanding, it was interpreted as reflecting inadequate rehabilitation facilities, rather than a negative side effect.[3] Besag refers to this as a "release phenomenon."[2] There are, however, a number of reports that children with learning difficulties and adults with mental handicaps develop behavioral problems such as aggression.[1,12] Reports have also noted the induction of a reversible Tourette syndrome, which in some cases was accompanied by obsessive compulsive symptoms.[29]

Felbamate

Felbamate is at present only used in a minority of patients, particularly those with Lennox-Gastaut syndrome, due to its hematologic and hepatic toxicity. Felbamate may lead to increased alertness, thus inducing sleep problems and behavioral problems related to agitation in some patients, particularly in children with learning disabilities.[31]

Gabapentin

Beyond somnolence, negative psychotropic effects have not been demonstrated in controlled studies of gabapentin. However, a number of studies suggest that gabapentin may induce behavioral problems such as aggression in children with learning disabilities and adults with mental handicap,[26,42,46] possibly related to rapid titration. In elderly people with reduced creatinine clearance, gabapentin may cause various neurotoxic symptoms due to its renal elimination.

Tiagabine

A specific problem with tiagabine is the paradoxical provocation of de novo nonconvulsive status epilepticus due to a relatively narrow therapeutic window.[38] Therefore, EEG registrations are necessary when behavioral problems arise, particularly when clinical signs such as mutism, qualitative change in consciousness, autisms, or myoclonia suggest status epilepticus.

In placebo-controlled add-on studies, nervousness and depressed mood were both increased in the tiagabine group[27] (12% vs. 3%, 5% vs. 1%). The incidence of serious adverse events presenting as psychosis was 2% versus 1% in the placebo group.

Topiramate

In premarketing studies, and possibly related to aggressive titration schemes, topiramate was associated with a relatively high rate of neurotoxic side effects. Psychotic reactions were, however, relatively infrequent, with a prevalence of 0.8%. In a postmarketing study comparing the psychiatric side effects of topiramate, lamotrigine, and gabapentin, psychotic episodes occurred in 12% of patients treated with topiramate compared with 0.7% of patients treated with lamotrigine and 0.5% of patients treated with gabapentin.[7] These data suggest an increased vulnerability in selected patient groups. A significant proportion of topiramate-associated psychoses are explained as alternative syndromes in patients who become seizure-free.[34]

The rate of affective symptoms is clearly dose-dependent, with an incidence of 9% and 19% with a daily dose of 200 mg and 1,000 mg, respectively, found in one premarketing study.[18] In an analysis of topiramate-related psychiatric complications, depression was significantly correlated with rapid titration and high dosages.[34] Two studies demonstrated a correlation between psychiatric adverse events and cognitive side effects, suggesting that neuropsychological and affective problems are closely interlinked.[22,34] The neuropsychological disorders caused by topiramate resemble a frontal lobe problem, and have been interpreted as regional behavioral toxicity. It would be interesting to investigate whether patients with epilepsies and frontal lobe dysfunction are more vulnerable to these effects.

TABLE 2

POSITIVE PSYCHOTROPIC EFFECTS OF ANTIEPILEPTIC DRUGS DEMONSTRATED IN CONTROLLED TRIALS

	Depression	Mania	Bipolar disorder	Anxiety
Carbamazepine	0	+	+	0
Oxcarbazepine	0	+	0	0
Valproate	0	+	+	0
Lamotrigine	0	0	+	0
Gabapentin	0	–	–	+/–
Topiramate	0	–	0	0
Tiagabine	0	–	0	0
Levetiracetam	0	0	0	–
Pregabaline	0	0	0	+
Zonisamide	0	0	0	0

+, positive results; –, negative results; 0, no published data.

Levetiracetam

Levetiracetam is not associated with a high risk for severe psychotic or depressive reactions. Significant affective episodes were reported in 2% and psychoses in 0.7% of patients treated in preclinical trials. Some of the levetiracetam-associated psychoses were explained as a manifestation of FN.

A clinically relevant psychiatric side effect of levetiracetam is the provocation of aggressive behavior and irritability, which occurs both in adults and children. In an English series of 517 adult patients treated with levetiracetam, 10% developed a psychiatric complication, most frequently presenting with aggressive behavior.[35] Aggression occurs particularly often, but not exclusively, in patients with preexisting irritability and dysphoria. Mesad and Devinsky[33] analyzed cases of severe aggressive behavior, defined by objective verbal or physical aggression, leading to withdrawal of levetiracetam. The prevalence was 18 out of 460 consecutive patients (3.9%). Seven patients had previous episodes of aggressive behavior.

Children may be at an even higher risk to develop aggression, including suicidal behavior, with prevalence rates up to 68%.[11] In children with preexisting neuropsychiatric symptomatology, levetiracetam may provoke an exacerbation of behavioral problems.[17] Kossoff[24] reported on four adolescents who developed a psychosis secondary to treatment with levetiracetam, which was reversible following withdrawal. All patients had preexisting behavioral problems, and two had become seizure-free, supporting the role of FN.

Zonisamide

Outside of Japan and the United States, there is still limited experience with this broad-spectrum AED. There are, however, indications of significant psychiatric adverse events, including affective problems and psychoses. In a Japanese series of patients with psychotic episodes, half of drug-related episodes were triggered by zonisamide.[30]

Pregabaline

Controlled trials of pregabaline show no evidence for significant psychiatric adverse events. However, clinical experience with this recently introduced drug is still limited.

POSITIVE PSYCHOTROPIC EFFECTS OF AEDS

Carbamazepine and valproate are established drugs for affective disorders, and all novel anticonvulsants have been tested in primary psychiatric disorders with respect to potential mood stabilizing properties. The advantages of anticonvulsants compared to classical mood stabilizers are the lack of proconvulsive risks, the lower potential to induce a switch from depression into mania, and a superior efficacy in atypical syndromes such as rapid-cycling bipolar disorder. So far, only lamotrigine has been approved for bipolar disorder. Pregabaline has shown efficacy in anxiety disorders and insomnia (Table 2).

The potentially positive psychotropic effects of AEDs have not been systematically studied in patients with epilepsy. This is unsatisfactory because the experience with primary psychiatric patients cannot easily be transferred to epilepsy. Many psychiatric disorders in epilepsy are different in their phenomenology and most likely also in their pathogenesis from "endogenous" disorders.

The evidence for the mood-stabilizing effects of carbamazepine and valproate when used in patients with epilepsy is based on few observations.[36,39,44] With respect to the newer AEDs, the only convincing evidence with respect to positive psychotropic effects relates to lamotrigine.[10,15,19,41]

RISK FACTORS FOR PSYCHIATRIC ADVERSE EVENTS

Patients with a biographic or genetic predisposition are presumably more at risk to develop AED-related psychiatric complications such as depression and psychosis (Table 3). Patients with previous depressive episodes are more likely to develop an affective disorder, whereas patients with previous schizophrenia-like psychoses are more likely to present with a psychotic reaction, suggesting that the clinical presentation of psychiatric adverse reactions depends on the individual psychopathologic predisposition. In patients with previous psychiatric problems, rapid titration should therefore be avoided, because aggressive titration schemes further increase the risk of behavioral toxicity.

Some studies have shown that patients with severe epilepsies are at a higher risk for psychiatric side effects. Mula[34] demonstrated that hippocampal sclerosis is more common in patients who develop depressive episodes secondary to treatment with topiramate, compared with patients without affective side effects, another indication for the close links between limbic dysfunction and affective disorders.

Children and adults with learning disability and multiple handicaps are particularly vulnerable to the behavioral adverse effects of AEDs. In these patients, the exact psychiatric

TABLE 3

RISK FACTORS FOR DEPRESSION AND PSYCHOSIS WITH VIGABATRIN, TOPIRAMATE, AND LEVETIRACETAM

	Vigabatrin* depression/psychoses $n = 22/28$	Topiramate** depression/psychoses $n = 46/16$	Levetiracetam*** depression/psychoses $n = 13/6$
Psychiatric history	+/+	+/+	+/+
Febrile seizures	?/?	+/?	+/?
Status epilepticus	?/?	?/?	+/?
Titration/dosage	+/–	+/–	–/–
Seizure freedom	–/+ (13 cases)	–/+ (10 cases)	–/+ (4 cases)
Severity of epilepsy	–/+	+/ ?	–/ ?
Cognitive side effects	?/?	+/–	–/–

*Thomas,[43] **Mula,[34] ***Mula[35]
+, significant relationship; –, no relationship; ?, not studied or too small numbers.

diagnosis may be difficult, and both depression and psychosis may manifest with aggressive behavior. Also, nonpsychiatric adverse events may lead to disturbed behavior because patients may have difficulties in otherwise expressing their discomfort. In these patients, drug changes should be monitored carefully, and it is recommended that the behavioral changes are carefully discussed with the health care/caregiver team. Occasionally, the interpretations of behavior changes are different within the team, particularly when patients become more alert and active because of positive psychotropic AED effects. These changes may be regarded as negative by some because they require attitude adjustments on the part of caregivers and make new treatment programs necessary.

MECHANISMS

Four major mechanisms explain behavioral effects of AEDs: (a) dosage-dependant toxicity, (b) dose-independent idiosyncratic drug effects, (c) withdrawal effects, and (d) indirect effects via anticonvulsive actions. Of these, the two most important mechanisms are pharmacodynamic side effects related to the drug's mode of action and effects that arise with seizure control—those alternative syndromes associated with the phenomenon of FN.

Trimble's hypothesis of a link between psychiatric complications and the γ-aminobutyric acid (GABA)-ergic mechanisms of AEDs was extended by Ketter,[23] who distinguished two categories of AEDs. The first category are GABAergic drugs with sedating, anxiolytic, and antimanic properties. This category includes barbiturates, benzodiazepines, valproate, vigabatrin, tiagabine, and gabapentin. The second category are the antiglutamatergic drugs, which are claimed to have activating, anxiogenic, and antidepressive effects: felbamate and lamotrigine. The authors suggest that anticonvulsant drugs have different psychiatric effects depending on the preexisting mental status of patients. They predict that patients who are primarily activated may benefit from drugs that belong to the "sedating" category and become worse with use of "activating" drugs. On the other hand, patients who are primarily sedated would benefit from a drug from the "activating" category, whereas the same patients would worsen with a "sedating" anticonvulsant. Taking the primary psychopathologic status of a patient into account explains the sometimes unexpected and seemingly paradoxical effects of some AEDs in individual patients. Based on clinical experiences, Table 4 suggests some "predictable" psychiatric AED risks that may depend on baseline psychopathology.

Forced Normalization

The concept of FN goes back to the publications of Landolt.[25] Cases of FN or alternative psychiatric syndromes have been reported with the use of all conventional and novel anticonvulsants, but seem to be particularly common with the more potent drugs such as vigabatrin, topiramate, and levetiracetam. FN has rarely been reported with tiagabine and lamotrigine, and is extremely rare with gabapentin. The best known manifestation of FN is a psychotic state. However, in a consecutive series by Wolf,[45] 50% of 36 consecutive patients presented with predominating affective symptomatology.

SUMMARY AND CONCLUSIONS

The risk of AED-related psychiatric complications is likely linked to the severity of epilepsy, polytherapy, rapid titration, and high dosages of drugs. Patients with previous psychiatric problems or a familial predisposition seem to be especially prone to behavioral side effects. Another risk group includes children and adults with learning disabilities, and perhaps elderly patients. It is important to recognize patients at risk, inform them and their families about the possibility

TABLE 4

PSYCHIATRIC RISKS OF ANTIEPILEPTIC DRUGS IN PATIENTS WITH PREEXISTING PSYCHIATRIC PROBLEMS

Patient	Possible contraindication	Possible side effect
Dysthymia	PHB, VGB, TPM, TGB	Major depression
Paranoia	DPH, VGB, TPM	Schizophrenic psychosis
Agitation	LTG	Insomnia, anxiety, hypomania
Hypermotor	LTG	Tourette-syndrome
Dysphoric	LEV	Aggression
Learning disability	All AEDs	Behavior disorders

PHB, phenobarbitone; LEV, levetiracetam; LTG, lamotrigine; TGB, tiagabine; TPM, topiramate; VGB, vigabatrin; DPH, phenytoin; AED, antiepileptic drug.

of psychiatric side effects, apply a careful titration scheme, and make sure that patients are seen frequently—and that the appropriate questions are asked. When recognized at an early stage, psychiatric AED complications are mild and reversible in most cases. Risk factors for psychiatric complications are not a strict contraindication for any particular drug, and it is not always necessary to completely withdraw the responsible drug. Depending on the pathophysiology and the severity of the syndrome, a dose reduction or comedication with an antipsychotic or antidepressive drug may be a good compromise.

Behavioral drug-effect profiles, both negative and positive psychotropic effects, ought to be considered in the choice of the optimal drug for an individual patient. More studies are needed specifically devoted to the psychiatric effects of AEDs in patients with epilepsy. We need these studies to better identify patients at risk of severe behavioral reactions with the use of specific drugs, and also to identify patients who have a good chance of benefiting from the potentially positive psychotropic effects of certain AEDs.

References

1. Beran RG, Gibson RJ. Aggressive behavior in intellectually challenged patients with epilepsy treated with lamotrigine. *Epilepsia.* 1998;39:280–282.
2. Besag FMC. Behavioral effects of the new anticonvulsants. *Drug Safety.* 2001;24:513–536.
3. Binnie DB. Lamotrigine. In: Engel J, Pedley TA, eds. *Epilepsy. A Comprehensive Textbook.* Philadelphia: Lippincott-Raven; 1997: 1531–1540.
4. Brent DA, Crumrine PK, Varma RR, et al. Phenobarbital treatment and major depressive disorder in children with epilepsy. *Pediatrics.* 1987;80:909–917.
5. Brent DA. Overrepresentation of epileptics in a consecutive series of suicide attempters seen at a children's hospital, 1978–1983. *J Am Acad Child Psychiatry.* 1986;25:242–246.
6. Brodie MJ, Richens A, Yuen AW. Double-blind comparison of lamotrigine and carbamazepine in newly diagnosed epilepsy. UK Lamotrigine/Carbamazepine Monotherapy Trial Group. *Lancet.* 1995;345:476–479.
7. Crawford P. An audit of topiramate use in a general neurology clinic. *Seizure.* 1998;7:207–211.
8. Dalby MA. Behavioral Effects of Carbamazepine. In: Penry JK, Daly DD, eds. *Complex Partial Seizures and Their Treatment. Advances in Neurology, Vol. 11.* New York: Raven Press; 1975: 331–343.
9. Drake ME, Peruzzi WT. Manic state with carbamazepine therapy of seizures. *J Natl Med Assoc.* 1986;78:1105–1107.
10. Edwards KR, Sackellares JC, Vuong A, et al. Lamotrigine monotherapy improves depressive symptoms in epilepsy: a double-blind comparison with valproate. *Epilepsy Behav.* 2001;2:28–36.
11. Estrada G, Wildrick D, Prantazelli M. Neuropsychiatric complications of levetiracetam in children with epilepsy. Abstract. *American Psychiatric Association,* 2002.
12. Ettinger AB, Weisbrot DM, Saracco J, et al. Positive and negative psychotropic effects of lamotrigine in patients with epilepsy and mental retardation. *Epilepsia.* 1998;39:874–877.
13. Ferrie CD, Robinson RO, Panaziotopoulos CP. Psychotic and severe behavioral reactions with vigabatrin: a review. *Acta Neurol Scand.* 1996;93:1–8.
14. Fitton A, Goa KL Lamotrigine. *Drugs.* 1995;50:691–713.
15. Gillham R, Kane K, Bryant-Comstock L, et al. A double-blind comparison of lamotrigine and carbamazepine in newly diagnosed epilepsy with health-related quality of life as an outcome measure. *Seizure.* 2000;9:375–379.
16. Gilliam F. Optimizing epilepsy management: seizure control, reduction, tolerability, and co-morbidities. Introduction. *Neurology.* 2002; 58(Suppl. 5):1.
17. Gustafson MC, Ritter FJ, Frost MD, et al. Behavioral and emotional effects of Levetiracetam in children with intractable epilepsy. Abstract. *Acad Psychiatry.* 2002.
18. Janssen-Cilag. *Topamax. Product monograph.* 1996.
19. Kalogjera-Sackellares D, Sackellares JC. Improvement in depression associated with partial epilepsy in patients treated with lamotrigine. *Epilepsy Behav.* 2002;3:510–516.
20. Kanemoto K, Tsuji T, Kawasaki J. Reexamination of interictal psychoses based on DSMIV psychosis classification and international epilepsy classification. *Epilepsia.* 2001;42:98–103.
21. Kanner AM, Kozak AM, Frey M. The use of sertraline in patients with epilepsy: is it safe? *Epilepsy Behav.* 2000;1:100–105.
22. Kanner AM, Wuu J, Faught E, et al. The PADS Investigators. A past psychiatric history may be a risk factor for topiramate-related psychiatric and cognitive adverse events. *Epilepsy Behav.* 2003;4(5):548–552.
23. Ketter TA, Post RM, Theodore WH. Positive and negative psychiatric effects of antiepileptic drugs in patients with seizure disorders. *Neurology.* 1999;53(Suppl. 2):53–67.
24. Kossoff EH, Bergey GK, Freeman JM, et al. Levetiracetam Psychosis in children with epilepsy. *Epilepsia.* 2001;42;1611–1613.
25. Landolt H. Serial Electroencephalographic Investigations During Psychotic Episodes in Epileptic Patients and During Schizophrenic Attacks. In: Lorentz de Haas AM, ed. *Lectures on epilepsy.* Amsterdam: Elsevier; 1958: 91–131.
26. Lee DO, Steingard RJ, Cesena M, et al. Behavioral side effects of gabapentin in children. *Epilepsia.* 1996;37:87–90.
27. Leppik E. Tiagabine: the safety landscape. *Epilepsia.* 1995;36(Suppl. 6):10–13.
28. Levinson DF, Devinsky O. Psychiatric adverse events during vigabatrin therapy. *Neurology.* 1999;53:1503–1511.
29. Lombroso CT. Lamotrigine-induced tourettism. *Neurology.* 1999;52:1191–1194.
30. Matsuura M. Epileptic psychoses and anticonvulsant drug treatment. *J Neurol Neurosurg Psychiatry.* 1999;67:231–233.
31. McConnell H, Snyder PJ, Duffy JD, et al. Neuropsychiatric side effects related to treatment with felbamate. *J Neuropsychiatry Clin Neurosci.* 1996;8:341–346.
32. McDanal CE, Bolman WM. Delayed idiosyncratic psychosis with diphenylhydantoin. *JAMA.* 1975;231:1063.
33. Mesad SM, Devinsky O. Levetiracetam related aggression. Abstract. *Acad Psychiatry.* 2002.
34. Mula M, Trimble MR, Lhatoo SD, Sander JW. Topiramate and psychiatric adverse events in patients with epilepsy. *Epilepsia.* 2003;44:659–663.
35. Mula M, Trimble MR, Yuen A, et al. Psychiatric adverse events during levetiracetam therapy. *Neurology.* 2003;61:704–706.
36. Robertson MM, Trimble MR, Townsend HRA. Phenomenology of depression in epilepsy. *Epilepsia.* 1987;28:364–372.
37. Sackellares JC, Lee SI, Dreifuss FE. Stupor following administration of valproic acid to patients receiving other convulsant drugs. *Epilepsia.* 1979;20:697–703.
38. Schapel G, Chadwick D. Tiagabine and non-convulsive status epilepticus. *Seizure.* 1996;5:153–156.
39. Schmitz B, Robertson M, Trimble MR. Depression and schizophrenia in epilepsy: social and biological risk factors. *Epilepsy Res.* 1999;35:59–68.
40. Schöndienst M, Wolf P. Zur Möglichkeit Neurotoxischer Spätwirkungen von Valproinsäure. In: Krämer G, Laub M, eds. *Valproinsäure.* Berlin: Springer; 1992: 259–265.
41. Smith D, Baker G, Davies G, et al. Outcomes of add on treatment with lamotrigine in partial epilepsy. *Epilepsia.* 1993;34:312–322.
42. Tallian KB, Nahata MC, Lo W, et al. Gabapentin associated with aggressive behavior in pediatric patients with seizures. *Epilepsia.* 1996;37:501–502.
43. Thomas L, Trimble MR, Schmitz B, et al. Vigabatrin and behavior disorders: a retrospective study. *Epilepsy Res.* 1996;25:21–27.
44. Trimble MR, Reynolds EH. Anticonvulsant drugs and mental symptoms: a review. *Psychol Med.* 1976;6:169–178.
45. Wolf P, Inoue Z, Röder-Wanner UU, et al. Psychiatric complications of absence therapy and their relation to alteration of sleep. *Epilepsia.* 1984;25:56–59.
46. Wolf SM, Shinnar S, Kang H, et al. Gabapentin toxicity in children manifesting as behavioral changes. *Epilepsia.* 1995;36:1203–1205.
47. Zaret BS, Cohen RA. Reversible valproic acid-induced dementia: a case report. *Epilepsia.* 1986;27:234–240.

CHAPTER 209 ■ PSYCHIATRY AND SURGICAL TREATMENT

STEFFI C. KOCH-STOECKER AND KOUSUKE KANEMOTO

INTRODUCTION

More than half a century after its development, epilepsy surgery has become a routine procedure, especially for resection of mesiotemporal sclerosis. Indications for epilepsy surgery are now well-established, and expected physical benefits following epilepsy surgery can be shown with some certainty. Nevertheless, the implicit hope of patients is that "favourable outcomes in social and psychological domains" will follow seizure relief.[82] In light of this background, any attempts at prognosis must include more than a prediction of favorable seizure outcome by epileptologic methods. A more comprehensive neuropsychiatric view of epilepsy surgery outcomes is necessary, the importance of which is also underlined by the results of numerous studies from different countries that show a high psychiatric comorbidity in candidates for epilepsy surgery (Table 1). In the last few years, an increasing number of studies support the notion that this comorbidity exists not merely as the parallel existence of two unrelated diseases, but as a common etiology for epilepsies and psychiatric disorders. Examples include the association of fear auras with postoperative mood and anxiety disorders following a temporal lobectomy,[46] the prediction of seizures in later life by a history of depression,[31] and the correlation between postoperative psychopathology and the extent of temporal resection.[4] As a result, the gap between "organic" and "psychiatric" topics has begun to shrink, forcing neurologists and psychiatrists to work together—and producing some encouraging effects, as seen in reports from epilepsy surgery centers.

THE IMPORTANCE OF PSYCHIATRIC EVALUATION IN THE CONTEXT OF EPILEPSY SURGERY

What do these promising developments mean for patients? The improvement in neuropsychiatric outcome prediction as a statistical piece of data is a helpful, although insufficient, frame in which to understand the complex situation of each individual patient. We know from psychiatric outcome studies[2,3] that mental instability may complicate the process of postoperative recovery. Following seizure cessation, affected patients may still suffer from their psychiatric disorders and may even acquire new ones. These patients face psychiatric disorder–related barriers that prevent them from making use of new opportunities in their seizure-free lives after surgery. Fortunately, individual outcome is not predicted by statistical data alone. We all know patients who transcend negative prognoses, profiting from the support and positive effects of relationships or internal strengths to make their way successfully through life post surgery. The best method for outcome prediction is a synthesis—a clinical psychiatric approach based on a balanced appreciation of the individual context and statistically evaluated group-predictors. The task of a neuropsychiatric assessment, beyond the evaluation of affiliation with special risk groups, is to understand the patient's motivations and aims within the frame of personal history, match them with realistic possibilities, communicate expected complications, treat actual disorders, and search for individual support strategies. Pre-, peri-, and postoperative psychiatric support during the process of surgery requires that the professional play the complex roles of physician, counselor, and container of hope simultaneously.

The majority of studies on this topic have focused on patients undergoing a temporal lobectomy or amygdalohippocampectomy because of the high proportion of temporal lobe epilepsies (TLEs) among epilepsy surgery candidates, but also of the prominence of psychiatric symptoms in patients with TLE. However, in the small number of reports that have mentioned the prevalence rate of psychiatric morbidities in temporal and extratemporal cases, no apparent difference has been found to exist when mental disorders are summed up as an entity.

This chapter does not cover the specific problems of epilepsy surgery in children, nor does it analyze in-depth psychosocial topics and questions concerning quality of life after surgery.

THE PREOPERATIVE PHASE: MENTAL CONDITIONS OF SURGICAL CANDIDATES

As shown in Table 1, the reported prevalence of psychiatric morbidities among surgical candidates varies so widely (27%–85%) that no representative figures can be presented. With few exceptions, the mean numbers of psychiatric cases in recent studies exceed 40%, which is lower than the very early data obtained during the 1970s, although still clearly higher than in normal and nonselected epilepsy populations. Recent changes in selection strategies for epilepsy surgery to more strict exclusion criteria for patients with severe psychiatric morbidities, as well as progress in the treatment of epileptic seizures and mental problems, may have decreased the total number of patients. On the other hand, the increasing attention paid to mental disorders in the context of surgery and changes in assessment strategies (such as the use of structured clinical interviews) may account for a more complete perception of the whole situation, at least in recent series that have been reported. However, there are still no generally recognized psychiatric assessment methods for use in surgical centers. Further, the insufficiency of diagnostic systems for use in epilepsy populations has complicated the problem, because it is becoming increasingly clear that some of the most common and disabling psychiatric problems in patients with epilepsy are atypical and cannot be

TABLE 1

PSYCHIATRIC MORBIDITIES PRE- AND POSTSURGERY

Author (Ref.)	Total *n*	Preoperation	Postoperation	Time of assessment
Temporal				
Taylor 1972[81]	100	87%	68%	1–10y
Jensen 1979[36]	74	85%	69%	?
Polkey 1983[67]	40	—	58%	?
Stevens 1990[80]	14	38%	36%	2–3y<
Naylor 1994[63]	37	35%	38%	?
Manchanda 1996[57]	231	45%	—	—
Ring 1998[72]	60	20%	57%	3m
Ring 1998[72]	60	20%	20%	6m
Blumer 1998[11]	44	57%*	39%	1–3y
Glosser 2000[26]	44	65%	65%	6m
Anhoury 2000[4]	109	44%	58%	12m
Kanemoto 2001[40]	52	42%	37%	2–12y
Inoue 2001[34]	226	27%	24%	>2y
Cankurtaran 2005	22	27%	27%	6m
Extratemporal				
Naylor 1994[63]	10	20%	10%	?
Manchanda 1996[57]	43	44.2%	—	—
Blumer 1998[11]	6	67%	83%	1–3y FLE

FLE, frontal lobe epilepsy.
Total *n* = number of subjects; m/y, months/years.
*Described as interictal dysphoric disorder.

classified easily within common psychiatric classification systems, such as the International Statistical Classification of Diseases and Health Related Problems (ICD) and the American Diagnostic and Statistical Manual of Mental Disorders (DSM).[11,89] Therefore, in the current situation, the variations of psychiatric morbidities among studies are due to the variety of selection methods used, improved treatment strategies, and investigation artifacts.

Although preoperative mental disorders may improve or even remit after surgery in some patients, a substantial portion of psychiatric morbidities emerge for the first time following surgical intervention, most within a few months after operation, with a limited timeframe of less than 1 year. As a net result, the prevalence rate of mental disorders after surgery tends to be close to that before surgery. Under the condition that epilepsy surgery is performed to cure epilepsy and not psychiatric disorders, practitioners should be content with these global outcome effects. However, the implicit expectations of patients, caregivers, and professionals transcend the expectation of mere freedom from seizures.

The Role of Surgical Expectations

Patients are subjected to a number of burdensome procedures during presurgical assessments. Strong motivation or a desire for surgery makes the stressful process more endurable for both patients and the doctors in charge. However, the beneficial effects of the strong desires seen prior to surgery often become a stumbling block after surgery, and might seriously undermine patient and caregiver satisfaction with a medically successful outcome, thus hindering social and psychological readaptation. Notably, Taylor et al.[84] designated such expectations as "desire beyond seizure freedom." Furthermore, in a series of insightful investigations, Wilson et al.[95] revealed that the major components of this desire beyond seizure freedom consist of various expectations of a social and psychological nature (e.g., getting married, increasing self-confidence), and that those who aimed at more "practical" benefits (e.g., driving, employment, travel) tended to be more satisfied with the results of surgery. In a similar study, Wheelock et al.[92] showed that those with realistic aims and satisfaction with postoperative results had solid family backgrounds and more stable affective situations prior to surgery. These results suggest that desire beyond seizure freedom and implicit agreements between surgeons and patients should be explored, made explicit, and clearly stated and weighted before surgery. All who are involved in surgical procedures for intractable epilepsy should be aware of the simple fact that a surgical procedure, even a successful one, does not automatically make life happier.

Anxiety and Depression

For surgical candidates, the majority of studies agree that, among psychiatric disorders, depression and anxiety prevail, although the reported prevalence rates vary greatly from 27%,[14] to 33%,[26] to 77%.[2] In this regard, it is noteworthy that the rate of preoperative depression may change substantially, depending on the classification criteria and assessment procedures used. The atypical mixed-mood disorder is commonly encountered in patients with longstanding, intractable temporal lobe epilepsy (TLE) and, when the criteria are strictly applied, this disorder does not fit easily into any single standard diagnostic categories based on ICD and DSM. Blumer and Montouris[10] revived Kraepelin's concept of "epileptische Verstimmung" and designated the pleomorphic, intermittent, rapid cycling presentation of mixed-mood disorder as "interictal dysphoric disorder." In addition to such a fundamental problem with diagnosis inevitably resulting from the insufficiency of the present standard diagnostic systems for neurobehavioral disorders, differences in assessment tools for affective symptoms as well as the observation period (whole life prior to the examination or a period at the time of examination) may well produce a profound effect on the results, which makes simple comparisons between studies virtually impossible.

It remains undetermined whether preoperative diagnoses of anxiety and depressive disorders are predisposed to postoperative anxiety and depressive disorders. Again, it seems plausible that a liability to depression or even a depressed personality structure will not automatically change following surgery for epilepsy, and contradicting data both for[2,68] and against[4,14,55] this argument have been provided. About one-third[26] to one-half[2] of all patients with presurgical depression experienced continuing relief from depression after surgery. In another report, virtually no overlapping was found between patients with depression prior to surgery and those after surgical intervention.[14]

As mentioned, in their study, Kohler at al.[46] added a special comment with regard to patients with ictal fear preceding temporal lobectomy. The authors observed that mood and anxiety disorders after a temporal lobectomy were more common in patients who had fear auras preoperatively, compared with patients with other auras or without auras, in particular if they were seizure-free. The role of the amygdala in fear conditioning, kindling, and the concept of forced normalization were suggested as a possible mechanism.

With regard to the laterality effect, some authors have postulated higher rates of depression in patients with left TLE at the time of the presurgical evaluation,[1,11,90] although more studies have suggested that serious affective dysfunction occurs predominantly in patients with right temporal lobe seizure focus.[22,24,26,47,81] There are also reports that deny any correlation between focus side and depression in surgical candidates.[2,55,57] However, a definitive trend is noted concerning postoperative depression, because right temporal surgery leads to a higher postoperative clinical depression index.[26,47,54,68,81]

Concerning the fate of patients with preoperative depression, the concept of "turning-in" proposed by Hill et al.[32] half a century ago is still worth noting. The authors found that some patients who had a reduction in outwardly turned aggressiveness that was apparent prior to surgery showed depressive mood swings that developed postoperatively, which recovered spontaneously in most cases within 18 months after surgery. Thereafter, a number of authors reported results supporting that tendency for aggression and irritability to ameliorate following a temporal lobectomy.[19,35,67,81,91]

At our center in Bethel, however, we have also observed changes in the opposite direction, as patients who were emotionally withdrawn preoperatively have gained after surgery impulsive energy that turned into irritable, polemic behavior. The case of a man who lost emotional responsiveness to his family members after surgery, presented by Lipson et al.,[53] points in a similar direction.

Psychosis

Stable interictal psychotic disorders are notably absent in recent surgical series, because such patients have obviously been screened out during presurgical assessment on the assumption that they are less likely to improve functionally[36,37,71,79] or even deteriorate after an anterior temporal lobectomy.[22,36,52,54,81,86] However, since Fenwick[21] advocated surgical treatment even for patients with chronic psychoses, using the argument that seizure freedom alone can be worthwhile for patients even if their psychoses persist, this policy of excluding interictal psychosis has slowly started to change.

Recently, two multiple case studies summarized sequels of temporal lobectomy in patients with chronic psychosis. In one of those studies, Reutens et al.[71] described five patients who had been diagnosed with schizoaffective disorder or schizophrenia based on DSM-IV criteria and rendered seizure-free after surgery, with a 2- to 8-year follow-up period. In two of those patients, activities associated with daily living improved visibly. In another two patients, mental as well as social status remained stable, but unchanged. However, in one patient, psychotic symptoms continued and were so crippling that the patient needed repeated admission. Marchetti et al.[58] reported six patients, five of whom achieved Engel class I seizure outcome and relative improvement in their mental condition. Of those, four patients had a left epileptogenic lesion and two received an initial diagnosis of postictal psychosis, which developed into persistent chronic psychosis later during the course of illness. Although the psychotic symptoms were ameliorated in all four patients with a left-sided lesion, only one of the two with a right-sided lesion improved mentally.

Table 2 lists the ratios of patients with a history of episodic interictal psychosis prior to surgery and the outcome of

TABLE 2

OUTCOME OF PREOPERATIVE PSYCHOSIS (TEMPORAL LOBECTOMY OR AMYGDALOHIPPOCAMPECTOMY)

		Outcome of psychosis		
Author (Ref.)	Total *n*	Preoperative psychosis	Unchanged/ aggravated	Improved/ remitted
Simmel 1958[78]	44	11 (25.0%)	11 (100%)	
Taylor 1972[81]	100	12 (12.0%)	9 (75%)	3 (25%)
Jensen 1979[36]	74	11 (14.9%)	5 (46%)	6 (54%)
Sherwin 1981[77]	63	7 (11.1%)	7 (100%)	
Walker 1984[91]	50	5 (10.0%)	5 (100%)	
Bruton 1988[13]	248	18 (7.3%)	12 (66.7%)	6 (33.3%)
Stevens 1990[80]	14	3 (21.4%)	2 (66.7%)	1 (33.3%)
Kanemoto 2001[40]	52	12 (23.1%)	8 (66.7%)	4 (33.3%)
Cankurtaran 2005[14]	22	0 (0%)		

Supplemented and modified from Matsuura's[59] review.
Patients with postictal psychosis were excluded, if recognized as such from descriptions.
Total *n* = number of subjects.

pre-existing psychotic symptoms after a temporal lobectomy reported in previous studies. The wide range (0%–25%) of rate of prevalence obtained at different surgical centers may well reflect different exclusion criteria for patients with intermittent (not persistent) psychotic episodes. Except for the Danish series, psychotic symptoms recurred in more than two-thirds of the patients after surgery. In our series, the average duration of postoperative psychotic disorders was far longer (7 months to 7 years; 50% longer than 2 years) than depression (2 to 17 months; 75% shorter than 6 months). It should be noted that a psychotic episode can recur even several years after surgery.[40,80]

In conclusion, treatment of interictal psychosis is not the aim of epilepsy surgery, and only seizure freedom (or improvement of seizure status) can be reasonably expected after surgical intervention. On this basis, patients should be informed that the postoperative development of their psychosis is unpredictable. However, with appropriate psychiatric support, patients can undergo epilepsy surgery and profit from seizure freedom in many respects.

In contrast to interictal psychosis, a number of studies suggest good outcomes for postictal psychotic episodes after a temporal lobectomy, thus rendering them as suitable surgical candidates.[19,22,40,74] The direct coupling of this type of psychosis to the occurrence of seizures predicts an excellent improvement under seizure-free postoperative conditions. In this regard, postictal psychosis has been described as a psychiatric indication for epilepsy surgery. However, in the postsurgical phase, those patients are especially liable to develop postoperative depression complicating their readaptation after surgery.[40] Two studies have reported frequencies of postictal psychoses in candidates for epilepsy surgery, which are rather high at 18%[87] and 13%.[40]

Other Psychiatric Disorders

In two case reports, rare associations of TLE and obsessive-compulsive disorder (OCD) were ameliorated after a right temporal lobectomy.[7,42] In contrast, Kulaksizoglu et al.[51] reported a worsening of preoperative obsessive-compulsive personality traits into a full-dressed OCD in two patients following an amygdalohippocampectomy. The authors hinted at the possible contribution of left-sided surgery to the development of OCDs.

Sexual behavior and function changes have also been listed as possible sequels after a temporal lobectomy. Postoperatively, both declines[12] and increases in sexual activity[5,6,9,12,65] have been reported, whereas abolition of aberrant sexual behaviors such as paraphilias[61] has also been noted. Postoperative sexual changes may persist several years after a temporal lobe resection and possibly more frequently after right-sided surgical intervention,[5,6] although the effect of laterality has been denied by others.[9]

Personality Disorders, Traumatic Stress, Nonepileptic Seizures

During the past decade, debate about the dubious character of the diagnostic category "personality disorder" (PD) has cooled down, possibly as a consequence of the descriptive, nonstigmatizing approach presented in the DSM classification system. Today, discussion tends toward a notion of PD as a result of maladaptive biographic developmental conditions, constitutional and/or experiential, which are expressed in behavior traits deviant from sociocultural norms. The capacity to cope with stressful life events is low in patients with a PD, and their liability to psychiatric decompensation is strengthened. It seems evident that, beyond other developmental risks, patients with chronic epilepsies are prone to additional personality problems due to their organic deficits, their epilepsy-specific social restrictions, and the side-effects of treatment. Candidates for epilepsy surgery with complex PDs could thus be expected to develop new psychiatric disorders. However, there are only a few studies on PDs in the context of epilepsy surgery. In 1957, Hill et al.[32] published a historical paper on personality changes after a temporal lobectomy. In that study, the authors investigated 27 patients both before and 2 to 5 years after temporal lobe surgery, of whom all but one had psychiatric disorders prior to surgery. Using a broad, not exactly specified definition of PD, the authors reported the following changes in personality: Loss of verbal learning abilities in dominant resections, reduction of aggressiveness by an increased tolerance of frustration, "turning-in" of aggressiveness with depressed mood (as mentioned earlier), changes in sexuality (mostly an increased sexual drive), and an increase of warmth in social relationships by a "lessening of egotism."

Two more early, but very instructive, studies with diligent case-descriptions were presented by Horowitz and Cohen in 1968[33] and Serafetinides in 1975,[75] which focused on the meaning of PDs in the context of epilepsy surgery. However, from that time, the topic more or less vanished as a research subject in regards to epilepsy surgery. Since then, most of the studies on presurgical psychiatric morbidity have only focused on DSM axis 1, namely clinical syndromes, and excluded personality diagnoses. One study found PDs in 18% of the candidates for epilepsy surgery.[57] In a group of 100 patients who underwent temporal lobe surgery at our Bethel epilepsy center, we found that 60% had PDs. A detailed analysis revealed that 15% had a severe PD due to epilepsy—that is, directly correlated to the disease—which was formerly called "organic PD." These patients, together with Cluster A patients (DSM-IV), showed a specific risk to develop new postoperative psychoses, whereas Cluster B patients were susceptible to dissociative disorders like depersonalization and nonepileptic seizures, but not to psychoses. The postoperative development of Cluster C patients was uncomplicated, except for those with additional cognitive deficits.[44] PDs also proved to predict severe postoperative psychiatric complications (defined by admittance to a psychiatric hospital during the first 2 years after surgery), because all psychiatrically hospitalized patients had suffered from PDs prior to surgery.[43]

As Ettinger[18] stressed in the editorial remarks to the recent re-edition of Hill's study, not only the topic of PDs but also Hill's scientific approach may need reactivation. The rigidity of the scientific community for only allowing the use of scales and scores as a basis for scientific publications too easily dismisses the detailed portrayals of patients' daily distress or missing skills, as well as analysis of their "essence."

Another topic that remains unexplored in the context of PDs in epilepsy patients is the role of psycho-traumatization in the genesis of epilepsy and during surgical procedures. Research in this field has shown that chronic complex trauma experienced during the phase of brain development may induce borderline PD as well as dissociative disorders, and may have a damaging effect on mesiotemporal structures. It is an open question if the origin of TLE in those patients is accidental or causally related to trauma history, the latter being subjective evidence of many affected patients. As mentioned earlier, in our Bethel group, the development of new dissociative symptoms after surgery has shown a strong link to the diagnosis of borderline PD with a trauma history. This concurs with the findings of Ney et al.,[64] who reported that new dissociative nonepileptic seizures after surgery were predicted (among other factors like low IQ and surgical complications) by serious preoperative psychopathologic conditions.

It is unclear whether nonepileptic seizures should be considered an independent disorder or a symptomatic expression of an underlying PD. To date, there is not much data on the percentage of patients with additional nonepileptic seizures in candidates for epilepsy surgery (ranging from 5%[64] to 10%[25]). Reuber et al.[70] followed-up 13 patients (out of 1,342 surgery candidates) with both seizure types and reported good postoperative outcomes in terms of epileptic seizure control with a good match to those without nonepileptic seizures. Similar to Henry and Drury,[27] who recommended that an operation should only be planned if nonepileptic attacks are well treated by psychotherapeutic interventions, Reuber et al. concluded that additional psychogenic seizures should not be considered an absolute contraindication for surgery.

POSTOPERATIVE PSYCHIATRIC DEVELOPMENT

De Novo Acquired Disorders and Their Treatment

In general, improvement in seizure frequency after a temporal lobectomy may increase the possibilities of participation in social life and contribute to a well-balanced psychosocial state. However, especially during the first 3 to 6 months after temporal lobe surgery, many studies indicate that even patients who experience seizure freedom should be prepared for at least transient psychiatric deterioration.[11,26,39,40,48,72] Some authors have pointed out that even over the long term, some exceptional patients continue to suffer from postoperative worsening of their mental condition.[40,80,81] Among psychiatric disorders, depression and anxiety are listed as the most frequently encountered conditions in many reports. Psychogenic seizures are not so common; however, these could become a serious problem for some individuals. Single cases of OCDs that developed following surgery have also been described. The majority of recent studies that have addressed psychotic symptoms agree that new psychosis after a temporal lobectomy is less frequent than assumed earlier.[26,60,63] However, the acquisition of a new psychosis is such a serious burden for patients that it is imperative to observe carefully if psychotic symptoms develop. These may be potentially reversed when appropriate therapy is provided.

Generally, the explanations for the occurrence of new psychiatric disorders suggested so far can be summarized as biologic and sociopsychological, a consequence of disrupted functioning within the temporal lobe structure, such as the amygdala, which is known to be involved in the modulation and expression of emotion,[72] forced normalization.[26,50,90] This system collapses under increased expectations for new role functions once seizures have been abolished or reduced.[9,23] However, these theories remain to be elucidated with further evidence.

Postoperative Depression, Anxiety, and Manic Disorders

It is widely accepted that patients are especially prone to develop depressive or anxious states during the first 3 months after surgical treatment.[9,11,17,72,89] Thus, the prevalence rate of postoperative depression in outcome studies is highly dependent on the time schedule of the psychiatric assessment (Table 3). Within 3 months after the operation, depression occurred in one-third of patients, a prevalence rate that amounted to approximately half of the patients when anxiety disorder was added in two studies.[11,72] In contrast, many studies agree that the prevalence drops to 5% to 14% at 6 months after surgery.[9,26,40,52,63] Except for the report of Anhoury et al.,[4] showing 17%, the prevalence rate of new depression ranges from 8% to 10% after 6 months. Further, Wrench et al.[96] found that temporal patients reported significantly higher rates of anxiety and depression than did extratemporal patients, stressing the pivotal role of temporal lobe involvement in the genesis of new depression.

Although the highest incidence of anxiety was achieved within 1 to 2 months after surgery, the highest morbidity of depression was found within 3 months.[55,72] Except for some exceptions,[45] many authors agree that anxiety disorders tend to have a shorter duration than do affective disorders.[14,55,72]

In extreme cases, significant levels of postoperative depression and anxiety can lead to attempted suicide, paradoxically even in patients who have been rendered seizure-free.[9,26,36] After the first alarming report of Taylor and Marsh of nine suicidal cases from Falconer's large series of 193 patients, suicide attempts have been reported (4.6%–8.1%), especially in earlier series.[36,83] Most authors agree that postoperative mood disorders are transitory, with a remission within the first year after surgery,[26,40] and that the occurrence of postoperative depression is independent of seizure outcome.[32,96]

In exceptional cases, mania can also occur de novo after a temporal lobectomy. Following the first case report,[38] a case control study[15] compared postoperative depression and mania

TABLE 3

POSTOPERATIVE DEPRESSION (TEMPORAL OR AMYGDALOHIPPOCAMPECTOMY)

Author (Ref)	Total *n*	Postop depression	New-onset only	Assessment time
Wrench 2005[96]	43		11 (26%)	1m
Ring 1998[72]	60	14 (24%)		1.5m
Ring 1998[72]	52	20 (38%)		3m
Glosser 2000[26]	39	3 (8%)		6m
Leinonen 1994[52]	57	5 (9%)		12m
Anhoury 2000[4]	109	35 (56%)	19 (17%)	12m
Naylor 1994[63]	37	5 (14%)	3 (8%)	23.5m*
Kanemoto 2001[40]	52		5 (10%)	24m–12y
Bladin 1992[9]	107	5 (5%)		4y*
Altshuler 1999[2]	49	14 (29%)	5 (10%)	9.6y*

Total *n* = number of subjects.
*Average follow-up duration at the last psychiatric assessment.
m/y, months/years.

groups, and indicated that postoperative mania patients were more likely to yield findings of additional brain dysfunction in the hemisphere contralateral to the side of surgery, particularly in the electroencephalogram (EEG). Episodes of mania, just as depression, were usually transient and remitted within 1 year after onset. The prevalence rates in previous studies were 1.8%,[52] 3.8%,[39] and 3.9%.[15] Right temporal lobectomy was more common in patients exhibiting mania.[15,39]

New Nonepileptic Seizures and Somatoform Disorders

Nonepileptic seizures occurred newly after a temporal lobectomy in 1.8% to 8.8% of patients.[4,25,62,66] Following the first report of Ferguson,[23] which emphasized psychological aspects, new-onset nonepileptic seizures following surgery have been neglected in studies. However, the recognition of postoperative new seizure events as nonepileptic seizures, both in patients following a successful operation and in those with persistent epileptic seizures, is mandatory to prevent a delay in finding the most effective coping strategy. Since those patients who develop nonepileptic seizures frequently suffer from complex biographic burdens, extensive psychotherapeutic interventions may be necessary.

Previous reports agree that female patients with a right-sided temporal lobectomy are more susceptible to developing new-onset nonepileptic seizures, which tend to appear within 6 months after surgical intervention.[25] Although some reports have stressed early epilepsy onset as a risk factor for the emergence of new-onset nonepileptic seizures,[23,49] others have reported the reverse.[25] Low intelligence has been also suggested to promote new-onset nonepileptic seizures,[64] although that has been denied by another report.[25] As an explanation for that discrepancy, Glosser suggested the heterogeneity of such patients. Further, Naga et al.[62] described rare cases of postoperative occurrence of somatoform disorders other than conversion, such as pain disorder and body dysmorphia. They found new-onset somatoform disorders exclusively in patients following a temporal lobectomy, especially after right-sided resections, and not in those with an extratemporal resection.

De Novo Psychoses

Over the years, special attention has been paid to the risk of development of de novo psychosis following epilepsy surgery, because psychotic symptoms, once emerged, may decisively damage the quality of postoperative life and can become the main obstacle to social and psychological adaptations following surgery.[11,36,54,56,57,73,80,81,86] Furthermore, a new development of postoperative psychosis can be observed even in the setting of complete relief of seizures. As a result, several earlier reports stressed the risk of a development of postoperative psychosis.[36,81] However, the majority of recent studies suggest that new psychotic symptoms are less common following epilepsy surgery than assumed earlier.[26,60,63] Despite this, because of the severity of the disorder and the clinical significance of early detection and effective treatment of even subtle psychotic complaints, the new occurrence of psychotic episodes deserves special attention.

The prevalence rates of postoperative new psychosis in available studies range from 3.8% to 12.1%, except for the very high rate of 35.7% reported by Stevens[80] (Table 4). In Stevens' series, three patients who had exhibited strong paranoid behavioral patterns even prior to surgery were also included as postoperative new psychosis. By excluding those patients from analysis, the prevalence rate for that report drops to 14.3%. Several clinical parameters have been listed as predictors for the postoperative occurrence of new psychosis, and some authors have postulated that patients with ganglioglioma are more susceptible.[3,73,81] In a recent case-control study of patients with new psychosis after a temporal lobectomy, more bilateral abnormalities in preoperative EEG findings were detected, as well as pathologies other than mesial temporal sclerosis in the excised lobe and a smaller amygdala on the unoperated side.[76]

As Trimble suggested,[85] an association between postoperative psychoses and right-sided temporal lobectomy is rather clear when previous studies are listed together (see Table 4). This is all the more conspicuous when considering that schizophrenic-like psychoses are more common in patients with left or language-dominant temporal lobe seizure focus before surgery.[24,81,86]

TABLE 4

DE NOVO PSYCHOSIS AFTER EPILEPSY SURGERY

Author (Ref.)	Total (R/L) n	New-onset psychosis	Side of lobectomy
Simmel 1958[78]	44	4 (9.0%)	(R = 1, L = 2)
Taylor 1972[81]	100	7 (7.0%)	?
Jensen 1979[36]	74	9 (12.1%)	?
Polkey 1983[67]	40	2 (5.0%)	(R = 2)
Walker 1984[91]	50	6 (12.0%)	?
Bruton 1988[13]	248 (121/127)	9 (3.6%)	(R = 5, L = 4)
Stevens 1990[80]	14* (10/4)	5 (35.7%)	(R = 4, L = 1)
Mace 1991[54]	—	6	(R = 6, L = 0)
Bladin 1992[9]	107	2 (1.9%)	?
Leinonen 1994[52]	57	3 (5.2%)	(R = 2, L = 1)
Naylor 1994[63]	37	0 (0%)	
Anhoury 2000[4]	109	0 (0%)	
Kanemoto 2001[40]	52 (22/30)	2 (3.8%)	(R = 2, L = 0)
Mayanagi 2001[60]	70	2 (2.9%)	(R = 2, L = 0)
Cankurtaran 2005[14]	22	1 (4.5%)	?

Supplemented and modified from Trimble.[85]
Total n = number of subjects.
R/L, right/left.

Some psychoses following surgery occur with postoperative freedom from seizures. They may be interpreted as "alternative psychosis" under the postoperative condition of forced normalization,[54] whereas others occur in patients with ongoing seizures, frequently as new "postictal psychosis," which has been reported to occur more often in male patients with right-sided surgery.[56] Recently, Christodoulou et al.[16] emphasized the significance of an emergence of new contralateral seizure foci after surgery, and suggested that new episodes of postictal psychosis were heralded by a new seizure type and originated from the side contralateral to the side of operation.

THE ROLE OF SEIZURE OUTCOME

Postoperative depression and psychosis can both occur with or without seizure freedom, and the relationship between seizure control and new psychiatric symptoms following surgery is still an open question. Glosser[26] noted a weak but noticeable trend that seizure-free patients may be at higher risk for the development of an early transient psychiatric worsening at 6 months after a temporal lobectomy. In contrast, seizure-free status is recognized to be the most powerful predictor of improved psychiatric and psychosocial adjustment outcome over the long term.[9,30,69,83,88,92]

On the other hand, several reports show weak but consistent evidence that the preoperative existence of a psychopathology is a negative predictor of seizure freedom. This supports the assumption of a common etiology between epileptic syndromes and psychiatric disorders.[4,63] At Bethel, we found seizure freedom in 89% of 100 patients without psychiatric comorbidities, whereas only 43% of patients with psychiatric disorders were seizure-free after temporal lobectomy.[44]

POSTOPERATIVE TREATMENT, ROLE CHANGES, AND LONG-TERM ADAPTATION

The first few postoperative weeks after epilepsy surgery are a vulnerable phase of irritability, anxiety, and the development of depression. One treatment strategy is to start early and broadly with antidepressants. Selective serotonin-reuptake inhibitors (SSRIs) are tolerated well and have been reported to be helpful, as have tricyclic antidepressants,[11] although control studies are missing.

If patients refuse to take antidepressants, it is necessary to instruct them to contact a neuropsychiatrist, at least when symptoms get stronger and indicate a manifest depressive episode. If patients, or more likely family members, should complain about withdrawal, delusions, and atypical suspiciousness, which are early symptoms of postoperative psychoses, an urgent outpatient contact is needed to plan careful treatment and convince the patient of the necessity of antipsychotic medication. Atypical substances, especially risperidone, in rather low doses are often sufficient, and instructions to the family along with clear advice about further treatment contacts are important. Generally, it is recommended to equip all patients with the phone number or e-mail address of a psychiatrist at the surgery center, which may also help to prevent suicide attempts during the first postoperative months. Although only a few patients make use of such contact offers, many report that the option to call or write is a substantial part of feeling secure during insecure times of change.

We concur with Wilson et al.,[94] in recommending a graduated return to work, starting no earlier than 6 to 8 weeks after surgery, to avoid the negative effects of early transient postoperative impairments (difficulties in word finding, memory, and concentration, distracted attention, affective lability) that may yield mistakes on the job and create a negative influence in the relationship between patients and employers.

Not only acute psychiatric complications bother patients and families after epilepsy surgery, but the complicated process of moving from chronically ill to normal and healthy. Since the early reports of Ferguson and Rayport,[23] who observed paradoxical worsening of behavior after successful surgery, and of Horowitz and Cohen,[33] who described that the loss of seizures may seem like the loss of "an old friend" during the process of readjusting to life without epilepsy, some papers have focused on the process of discarding roles associated with chronic epilepsy. Of special interest is the thoughtful application of the concept of "learned helplessness," a known trigger for depression, to chronic epilepsy patients.[28] Recurrent uncontrolled seizures support the development of a self-concept as being without personal resourcefulness and efficacy. This negative self-concept tends to persist after surgery and may lead to a poor postoperative psychosocial adjustment.[17] Ongoing feelings of helplessness, especially in the surroundings of growing external demands and the loss of being excused by the epilepsy are expressions of the "burden of normality."[9,93] Conversely, other patients have pushed themselves to their personal psychophysical limits before surgery to prove their normalcy. They may experience exhaustion after the cessation of seizures, instead of expected alleviation. Another hint that life remains complicated for patients who undergo surgery has been shown by Koch-Weser,[45] who found that the average burden of anxiety symptoms was higher in patients 2 to 7 years after surgery than in presurgical candidates. Over the long term, complete seizure relief is the best predictor of good psychosocial adaptation, and especially of an enduring remittance of depressive symptoms.[11,29]

PSYCHIATRIC CARE IN EPILEPSY SURGERY CENTERS: HISTORY, STATE, AND PERSPECTIVES

In the first Consensus Conference on epilepsy surgery at Palm Desert, Fenwick initiated a worldwide survey on psychiatric facilities in related centers.[20] At that time, 53 centers existed and 21 answered. The mean proportion of patients psychiatrically assessed before surgery was 31.7%, and after surgery the percentage was 41.5%. As a consequence, Fenwick advocated improvements in psychiatric facilities.

In their recommended standards, the International League Against Epilepsy (ILAE) commission on Neurosurgery (1993–1997) commented rather scantily on psychiatric necessities, saying that the preoperative workup should include "careful assessment of psychiatric state . . . using psychiatric rating scales when appropriate" and, with respect to the follow-up period, the recommendation was that "some form of psychiatric assessment should be used."[8]

Recently, Kanner[41] has advocated for more involvement of psychiatrists in epilepsy centers. He complains that "only a minority of (U.S. surgical) centers performs a psychiatric evaluation as part of their presurgical evaluation" and "in less than 25% of major epilepsy centers surveyed, the epilepsy team includes a psychiatrist who is available to evaluate every patient."

In the recent ILAE psychobiology commission (Trimble, Schmitz), a subcommission on epilepsy surgery (Koch-Stoecker, Krishnamoorthy, Kanemoto) has repeated a worldwide survey on psychiatric facilities in epilepsy surgery centers (unpublished data). The most important result is that 26 (43%) of the 60 responding centers stated that they perform both pre- and postoperative assessments for all patients, and another 40% at least have access to psychiatric crisis interventions. These results show substantial improvement; however, the survey did not cover the assessment strategies used, and it is probable that in many centers only standardized self-rating questionnaires are used which are no adequate substitute for a clinical diagnostic interview.

In times of economic pressure that lead to reductions in staff at most centers and no enhancement of psychiatric services, we recommend a psychiatric screening using rating scales for all patients, followed by an extensive interview with those who are screened out as belonging to a psychiatric risk group.

With respect to enhancement of psychiatric treatment options for epilepsy surgery patients, the development of specific psychiatric treatment manuals to be used in surgery centers as well as in local psychotherapies is desirable. These manuals should include topics such as a structured clearing of surgical expectations beyond seizure freedom; typical role-constellations and possible changes after surgery; education about symptoms of depression and psychosis; social skills training, along with instructions for the development of a reasonable self-concept; and education for coping with seizure recurrence.

Finally, psychiatric research in epilepsy surgery centers that stand at the interface between neurology and psychiatry must be promoted. In amplifying Ettinger's comments[18] on the rigidity of requirements for approval in peer reviews, more flexibility and creativity in study designs should be allowed to add new dimensions to our scientific knowledge. For example, individual case reports, in which psychosocial developments are extensively thought over and analyzed on the basis of the exchanges between patient and professional, or quality research strategies with expert discussion groups, are excellent and thoughtful means to supplement a statistically based understanding of mental disorders. Further, additional diversity in scientific exchange will inspire psychiatrists working in epilepsy surgery to participate in expanding the international network.

SUMMARY AND CONCLUSIONS

The close link between the epileptic condition and psychopathology, and the high frequencies of psychiatric disorders in epilepsy patients calls for psychiatric assessment and treatment in the context of epilepsy surgery. In addition, postoperative seizure freedom alone is no guarantee for an amelioration of quality of life, but mental stability and coping capacity are central preconditions in the challenging postoperative time of new role demands. Concerning depression, the most frequent disorder type, the predictive meaning of its preoperative existence is still equivocal, whereas postoperative depression is well-known as surgical complication during the first half year after surgery which occurs in about 10% of patients, especially after right sided resections.

Interictal psychoses are no longer seen as contraindications, because seizure relief can be of great value even if psychosis persists, and psychotic deteriorations after surgery are extremely infrequent. Postictal psychoses disappear together with seizures, but the probability of an episode of postoperative depression is high in this patient group. During the last decade the reports on new psychoses after surgery oscillate about a frequency of 2%. Despite this low incidence rate postoperative psychoses deserve special attention because of the severity of the disorder.

Personality disorders are very frequent in candidates for epilepsy surgery and complicate postoperative adaptation. The role of early traumatic experiences in the development of personality disorders, of the epilepsy causing lesion itself, and of non-epileptic dissociative attacks in epilepsy surgery candidates is not yet well understood.

In summary our knowledge about psychiatric disorders, their predictors and their treatment in the context of temporal lobe resections has grown during the last decade. Still there are many contradictory results, and conclusive etiological models are not available. Apart from future descriptive and controlled studies quality research and case studies could be helpful to create a more colourful picture of individual courses and to generate new hypotheses on psychobiological connections.

There is still too little presence of psychiatrists in epilepsy surgery units. Especially needed is more time for understanding patients' individual psychodynamics, the development of suitable assessment tools to meet the demands of atypical psychiatric disorders, and structured treatment instructions for special surgery related complications. If assessed and treated adequately mental disorders do not hinder patients on their way to a better quality of life after surgery in the long run.

References

1. Altshuler L, Devinsky O, Post RM, et al. Depression, anxiety, and temporal lobe epilepsy. *Arch Neurol.* 1990;47:284–288.
2. Altshuler L, Rausch R, Delrahim S, et al. Temporal lobe epilepsy, temporal lobectomy, and major depression. *J Neuropsychiatry Clin Neurosci.* 1999;11:436–443.
3. Andermann LF, Savard G, Meencke HJ, et al. Psychosis after resection of ganglioglioma or DNET: Evidence for an association. *Epilepsia.* 1999;40:83–87.
4. Anhoury S, Brown RJ, Krishnamoorthy ES, et al. Psychiatric outcome after temporal lobectomy: a predictive study. *Epilepsia.* 2000;41:1608–1615.
5. Baird AD, Wilson SJ, Bladin PF, et al. Hypersexuality after temporal lobe resection. *Epilepsy Behav.* 2002;3:173–181.
6. Baird AD, Wilson SJ, Bladin PF, et al. Sexual outcome after epilepsy surgery. *Epilepsy Behav.* 2003;4:268–278.
7. Barbieri V, Lo Russo G, Francione S, et al. Association of temporal lobe epilepsy and obsessive-compulsive disorder in a patient successfully treated with right temporal lobectomy. *Epilepsy Behav.* 2005;6:617–619.
8. Binnie CD, Polkey CE. Commission on Neurosurgery of the International League Against Epilepsy (ILAE) 1993–1997: Recommended standards. *Epilepsia.* 2000;41:1346–1349.
9. Bladin PF. Psychosocial difficulties and outcome after temporal lobectomy. *Epilepsia.* 1992;33:898–907.
10. Blumer D, Montouris G, Hermann BP. Psychiatric morbidity in seizure patients on a neurodiagnostic monitoring unit. *J Neuropsychiatr.* 1995;7:445–456.
11. Blumer D, Wakhlu S, Davies K, et al. Psychiatric outcome of temporal lobectomy for epilepsy: incidence and treatment of psychiatric complications. *Epilepsia.* 1998;39:478–486.
12. Blumer D, Walker AE. Sexual behaviour in temporal lobe epilepsy: A study of the effects of temporal lobectomy on sexual behaviour. *Arch Neurol.* 1967;16:37–43.
13. Bruton CJ. The neuropathology of temporal lobe epilepsy. Maudsley Monograph No. 31,Oxford: Oxford University Press; 1988.
14. Cankurtaran ES, Ulug B, Saygi S, et al. Psychiatric morbidity, quality of life, and disability in mesial temporal lobe epilepsy patients before and after anterior temporal lobectomy. *Epilepsy Behav.* 2005;7:116–122.
15. Carran MA, Kohler CG, O'Connor MJ, et al. Mania following temporal lobectomy. *Neurology.* 2003;61:770–774.
16. Chistodoulou C, Koutroumanidis M, Hennessy MJ, et al. Postictal psychosis after temporal lobectomy. *Neurology.* 2002;59:1432–1435.
17. Chovaz CJ, McLachlan RS, Derry PA, et al. Psychosocial function following temporal lobectomy: influence of seizure control and learned helplessness. *Seizure.* 1994;3:171–176.
18. Ettinger AB. Commentary on "Personality changes following temporal lobectomy for epilepsy." *Epilepsy Behav.* 2004;5:601–602.
19. Falconer MA. Reversibility by temporal lobe resection of the behavioural abnormalities of temporal lobe epilepsy. *N Engl J Med.* 1973;289:451–455.
20. Fenwick PB. Postscript: what should be Included in a Standard Psychiatric assessment? In: Engel J, ed. *Surgical Treatment of the Epilepsies.* New York: Raven Press; 1987:505–510.
21. Fenwick PB. Psychiatric assessment and temporal lobectomy. *Acta Neurol Scand.* 1988;78(Suppl 117):96–101.
22. Fenwick PB, Blumer D, Caplan R, et al. Presurgical Psychiatric Assessment. In: Engel J, ed. *Surgical Treatment of the Epilepsies,* 2nd ed. New York: Raven Press; 1993:273–290.
23. Ferguson SM, Rayport M. Living with epilepsy. *J Nerv Ment Dis.* 1965;140:26–37.

24. Flor-Henry P. Psychosis and temporal lobe epilepsy: A controlled investigation. *Epilepsia.* 1969;10:363–395.
25. Glosser G, Roberts D, Glosser DS. Nonepileptic seizures after resective epilepsy surgery. *Epilepsia.* 1999;40:1750–1754.
26. Glosser G, Zwil AS, Glosser DS, et al. Psychiatric aspects of temporal lobe epilepsy before and after anterior temporal lobectomy. *J Neurol Neurosurg Psychiatry.* 2000;68:53–58.
27. Henry TR, Drury I. Nonepileptic seizures in temporal lobectomy candidates with medically refractory seizures. *Neurology.* 1997;48:1374–1382.
28. Hermann BP, Trenerry MR, Colligan RC. Learned helplessness, attributional style, and depression in epilepsy. Bozeman Epilepsy Surgery Consortium. *Epilepsia.* 1996;37:680–686.
29. Hermann BP, Wyler AR. Depression, locus of control, and the effects of epilepsy surgery. *Epilepsia.* 1989;30:332–338.
30. Hermann BP, Wyler A, Somes G. Preoperative psychological adjustment and surgical outcome are determinants of psychosocial status after anterior temporal lobectomy. *J Neurol Neurosurg Psychiatry.* 1992;55:491–496.
31. Hesdorffer DC, Hauser WA, Annegers JF, et al. Major depression is a risk factor for seizures in older adults. *Ann Neurol.* 2000;47:246–249.
32. Hill D, Pond DW, Mitchell W, et al. Personality changes following temporal lobectomy for epilepsy. *J Ment Sci.* 1957;103,18–27.
33. Horowitz MJ, Cohen FM. Temporal lobe epilepsy—effect of lobectomy on psychosocial functioning. *Epilepsia.* 1968;9:23–41.
34. Inoue Y, Mihara T. Psychiatric disorders before and after surgery for epilepsy. *Epilepsia.* 2001;42(Suppl 6):13–18.
35. James IP. Temporal lobectomy for psychomotor epilepsy. *J Ment Sci.* 1960;106:543–558.
36. Jensen I, Larsen JK. Mental aspects of temporal lobe epilepsy. Follow-up of 74 patients after resection of a temporal lobe. *J Neurol Neurosurg Psychiatry.* 1979;42:256–265.
37. Jensen I, Larsen JK. Psychoses in drug-resistant temporal lobe epilepsy. *J Neurol Neurosurg Psychiatry.* 1979;42:948–954.
38. Kanemoto K. Hypomania after temporal lobectomy: A sequela to the increased excitability of the residual temporal lobe? *J Neurol Neurosurg Psychiatry.* 1995;59:448–449.
39. Kanemoto K, Kawasaki J, Mori E. Postictal psychosis as a risk factor for mood disorders following temporal lobectomy. *J Neurol Neurosurg Psychiatry.* 1998;65:587–589.
40. Kanemoto K, Kim Y, Miyamoto T, et al. Presurgical postictal and acute interictal psychoses are differentially associated with postoperative mood and psychotic disorders. *J Neuropsychiatry Clin Neurosci.* 2001;13:243–247.
41. Kanner AM. When did neurologists and psychiatrists stop talking to each other? *Epilepsy Behav.* 2003;4:597–601.
42. Kanner AM, Morris HH, Stagno S, et al. Remission of an obsessive-compulsive disorder following a right temporal lobotomy. *Neuropsychiatry Neuropsychol Behav Neurol.* 1993;6:126–129.
43. Koch-Stoecker S. Personality disorders as predictors of severe postsurgical psychiatric complications in epilepsy patients undergoing temporal lobe resections. *Epilepsy Behav.* 2002;3:526–531.
44. Koch-Stoecker S. Psychische Störungen im Kontext epilepsiechirurgischer Eingriffe bei Temporallappenepilepsien. Eine prospektive Pilotstudie bei 100 Patienten des Epilepsiezentrums Bethel. (Dissertation) Universitaet Luebeck; 2002.
45. Koch-Weser M, Garron DC, Gilley DW, et al. Prevalence of psychologic disorders after surgical treatment of seizures. *Arch Neurol.* 1988;45:1308–1311.
46. Kohler CG, Carran MA, Bilker W, et al. Association of fear auras with mood and anxiety disorders after temporal lobectomy. *Epilepsia.* 2001;42:674–681.
47. Kohler CG, Norstarnad JA, Baltuch G, et al. Depression in temporal lobe epilepsy before epilepsy surgery. *Epilepsia.* 1999;40:336–340.
48. Krahn LE, Rummans TA, Peterson GC. Psychiatric implications of surgical treatment of epilepsy. *Mayo Clin Proc.* 1996;71:1201–1204.
49. Krahn LE, Rummans TA, Sharbrough FW, et al. Pseudoseizures after epilepsy surgery. *Psychosomatics.* 1995;36:487–493.
50. Krishnamoorthy ES, Trimble MR, Sander JW, et al. Forced normalization at the interface between epilepsy and psychiatry. *Epilepsy Behav.* 2002;3:303–308.
51. Kulaksizoglu IB, Bebek N, Baykan B, et al. Obsessive-compulsive disorder after epilepsy surgery. *Epilepsy Behav.* 2004;5:113–118.
52. Leinonen E, Tuunainen A, Lepola U. Postoperative psychoses in epileptic patients after temporal lobectomy. *Acta Neurol Scand.* 1994;90:394–399.
53. Lipson SE, Sacks O, Devinsky O. Selective emotional detachment from family after right temporal lobectomy. *Epilepsy Behav.* 2003;4:449–450.
54. Mace CJ, Trimble MR. Psychosis following temporal lobe surgery: A report of six cases. *J Neurol Neurosurg Psychiatry.* 1991;54:639–644.
55. Malmgren K, Starmark JE, Ekstedt G, et al. Nonorganic and organic psychiatric disorders in patients after epilepsy surgery. *Epilepsy Behav.* 2002;3:67–75.
56. Manchanda R, Miller H, McLachlan RS. Post-ictal psychosis after right temporal lobectomy. *J Neurol Neurosurg Psychiatry.* 1993;56:277–279.
57. Manchanda R, Schaefer B, McLachlan RS, et al. Psychiatric disorders in candidates for surgery for epilepsy. *J Neurol Neurosurg Psychiatry.* 1996;61:82–89.
58. Marchetti RL, Fiore LA, Valente KD, et al. Surgical treatment of temporal lobe epilepsy with interictal psychosis: Results of six cases. *Epilepsy Behav.* 2003;4:146–152.
59. Matsuura M. Indication for anterior temporal lobectomy in patients with temporal lobe epilepsy and psychopathology. *Epilepsia.* 2000;41(Suppl 9):39–42.
60. Mayanagi Y, Watanabe E, Nagahori Y, et al. Psychiatric and neuropsychological problems in epilepsy surgery: Analysis of 100 cases that underwent surgery. *Epilepsia.* 2001;42(Suppl 6):19–23.
61. Mitchel W, Falconer MA, Hill D. Epilepsy with fetishism relieved by temporal lobectomy. *Lancet.* 1954;25:626–630.
62. Naga AA, Devinsky O, Barr WB. Somatoform disorders after temporal lobectomy. *Cogn Behav Neurol.* 2004;17:57–61.
63. Naylor AS, Rogvi-Hansen B, Kessing L, et al. Psychiatric morbidity after surgery for epilepsy: Short-term follow up of patients undergoing amygdalohippocampectomy. *J Neurol Neurosurg Psychiatry.* 1994;57:1375–1381.
64. Ney GC, Barr WB, Napolitano C, et al. New-onset psychogenic seizures after surgery for epilepsy. *Arch Neurol.* 1998;55:726–730.
65. Ozmen M, Erdogan A, Duvenci S, et al. Excessive masturbation after epilepsy surgery. *Epilepsy Behav.* 2004;5:133–136.
66. Parra J, Iriarte J, Kanner AM, et al. De novo psychogenic nonepileptic seizures after epilepsy surgery. *Epilepsia.* 1998;39:474–477.
67. Polkey CE. Effects of anterior temporal lobectomy apart from the relief of seizures. *J Roy Soc Med.* 1983;76,354–358.
68. Quigg M, Broshek DK, Heidal-Schiltz S, et al. Depression in intractable partial epilepsy varies by laterality of focus and surgery. *Epilepsia.* 2003;44:419–424.
69. Rausch R, Crandall PH. Psychological status related to surgical control of temporal lobe seizures. *Epilepsia.* 1982;23:191–202.
70. Reuber M, Kurthen M, Fernandez G, et al. Epilepsy surgery in patients with additional psychogenic seizures. *Arch Neurol.* 2002;59:82–86.
71. Reutens DC, Savard G, Andermann F, et al. Results of surgical treatment in temporal lobe epilepsy with chronic psychosis. *Brain.* 1997;120:1929–1936.
72. Ring HA, Moriarty J, Trimble MR. A prospective study of the early post-surgical psychiatric associations of epilepsy surgery. *J Neurol Neurosurg Psychiatry.* 1998;64:601–604.
73. Roberts GW, Done DJ, Bruton C, et al. A "Mock-up" of schizophrenia: Temporal lobe epilepsy and schizophrenia-like psychosis. *Biol Psychiatry.* 1990;28:127–143.
74. Savard G, Andermann F, Olivier A, et al. Postictal psychosis after partial complex seizures: A multiple case study. *Epilepsia.* 1991;32:225–231.
75. Serafetinides EA. Psychosocial aspects of neurosurgical management of epilepsy. In: Purpura DP, Penny JK, Walter RD, eds. *Advances in Neurology,* Vol. 8, New York: Raven Press; 1975:323–332.
76. Shaw P, Mellers J, Henderson M, et al. Schizophrenia-like psychosis arising de novo following a temporal lobectomy: Timing and risk factors. *J Neurol Neurosurg Psychiatry.* 2004;75:1003–1008.
77. Sherwin I. Psychosis associated with epilepsy: significance of the laterality of the epileptogenic lesion. *J Neurol Neurosurg Psychiatry.* 1981;44:83–85.
78. Simmel ML, Counts S. Clinical and Psychological Results of Anterior Temporal Lobectomy in Patients with Psychomotor Epilepsy. In: Baldwin M, Bailey P, eds. *Temporal Lobe Epilepsy.* Springfield, IL: Thomas; 1958:530–550.
79. Slater E, Beard AW. Schizophrenia-like psychoses of epilepsy. I. Psychiatric aspects. *Br J Psychiatry.* 1963;109:95–150.
80. Stevens JR. Psychiatric consequences of temporal lobectomy for intractable seizures: A 20–30-year follow-up of 14 cases. *Psychol Med.* 1990;20:529–545.
81. Taylor DC. Mental state and temporal lobe epilepsy: a correlative account of 100 patients treated surgically. *Epilepsia.* 1972;13:727–765.
82. Taylor DC, Hermann BP. Psychiatry and psychology in medical and surgical treatment. In: Engel J Jr, Pedley TA, eds. *Epilepsy: A Comprehensive Textbook.* Philadelphia: Lippincott-Raven; 1997:2117–2124.
83. Taylor DC, Marsh SM. Implication of long-term follow-up studies in epilepsy. In: Penry JK, ed. *Epilepsy: 8th International Symposium.* New York: Raven Press; 1977:27–34.
84. Taylor DC, McMacKin D, Staunton H, et al. Patients' aims for epilepsy surgery: Desires beyond seizure freedom. *Epilepsia.* 2001;42:629–633.
85. Trimble MR. *The Psychosis of Epilepsy.* New York: Raven Press; 1991:91–108.
86. Trimble MR. Behaviour change following temporal lobectomy, with special reference to psychosis. *J Neurol Neurosurg Psychiatry.* 1992;55:89–91.
87. Umbricht D, Degreef G, Barr WB, et al. Postictal and chronic psychoses in patients with temporal lobe epilepsy. *Am J Psychiatry.* 1995;152:224–231.
88. Vickrey BG, Hays RD, Engel J, et al. Outcome assessment for epilepsy surgery: The impact of measuring health-related quality of life. *Ann Neurol.* 1995;37:158–166.

89. Victoroff J. DSM-III-R psychiatric diagnosis in candidates for epilepsy surgery: Lifetime prevalence. *Neuropsychiatry Neuropsychol Behav Neurol.* 1994;7:87–97.
90. Victoroff J, Benson DF, Grafton ST, et al. Depression in complex partial seizures. *Arch Neurol.* 1994;511:155–163.
91. Walker AE, Blumer D. Behavioral effects of temporal lobectomy for temporal lobe epilepsy. In: Blumer D, ed. *Psychiatric Aspects of Epilepsy*. Washington DC: American Psychiatric Press; 1984:295–323.
92. Wheelock I, Peterson C, Buchtel HA. Presurgery expectations, postsurgery satisfaction and psychosocial adjustment after epilepsy surgery. *Epilepsia.* 1998;39:487–494.
93. Wilson SJ, Bladin PF, Saling MM. Paradoxical results in the cure of chronic illness: the "burden of normality" as exemplified following seizure surgery. *Epilepsy Behav.* 2004;5:13–21.
94. Wilson, SJ, Bladin PF, Saling MM, et al. Characterizing psychosocial outcome trajectories following seizure surgery. *Epilepsy Behav.* 2005;6:570–580.
95. Wilson SJ, Saling MM, Kincade P, et al. Patient expectations of temporal lobe surgery. *Epilepsia.* 1998;39:167–174.
96. Wrench J, Wilson SJ, Bladin PF. Mood disturbance before and after seizure surgery: A comparison of temporal and extratemporal resections. *Epilepsia.* 2004;45:534–543.

CHAPTER 210 ■ PSYCHIATRIC DISORDERS IN CHILDREN

ROCHELLE CAPLAN, CHRISTOPHER GILLBERG, DAVID W. DUNN, AND SARAH J. SPENCE

INTRODUCTION

The psychiatric and social aspects of epilepsy in childhood reflect the complex interaction of both general and specific illness-related factors on the child's life.[103] In terms of general factors, epilepsy is a chronic recurrent disorder and, like other chronic illnesses, this disorder affects the lives of the child and family. Among the specific illness-related factors, epilepsy involves brain function. In the developing child, chronic recurrent brief episodes of brain dysfunction might impact brain development, and, therefore, the development of behavior, cognition, and language. The maturation of these three areas of functioning has important implications for the psychiatric and social functioning of the child.

Two epidemiologic studies found a significantly higher rate of psychiatric disorders in children with neurologic disorders compared with children with chronic illnesses that do not involve the brain.[55,218] Furthermore, more specific seizure-related factors, such as type of seizure disorder, seizure control, the age of onset of seizures, and the number and type of antiepileptic drugs (AEDs) can impact the child's behavior.

This chapter summarizes the literature on these general and specific illness factors and how they are associated with psychopathology, cognition, and language in the child with epilepsy. It also presents the neurobehavioral aspects of selected early-onset epilepsy syndromes and how they affect children's behavior, cognition, language, and social skills.

The chapter then describes psychiatric disorders found in children with epilepsy. The chapter concludes by summarizing the most pertinent psychiatric and social issues of pediatric epilepsy. It also presents possible avenues for future research that would address the mental health needs of children with epilepsy.

DEFINITION AND PHENOMENOLOGY

Psychological Impact of a Chronic Illness on the Child and Family

A chronic illness like epilepsy is a stress factor for the child and his family. The child and family need to recruit coping or behavioral, emotional, and cognitive strategies to decrease the illness related "mismatch" with the environment.[98,218] Adaptive or maladaptive use of these coping strategies depends on the complex interaction of a "multivariate multiprocess system"[143] that involves the child and family, as well as the social, educational, and medical environments.

Several studies have demonstrated that maternal and family functioning are important predictor(s) of psychological functioning in children with a chronic illness, whereas illness severity merely mediates (moderates) the effects of psychosocial variables; the reader is directed to two reviews on this subject.[248,269] In pediatric epilepsy, maternal depression and family functioning primarily reflect the presence of comorbid behavioral problems in the child rather than illness severity.[164,232] Limited family mastery and lower levels of confidence in managing child problems also predicted behavior problems in children with epilepsy at baseline and 24 months later.[11]

From the psychodynamic perspective, a child with epilepsy is faced with several stresses. The first stress factor, unpredictability, is a hallmark of epilepsy because the child never knows when a seizure is going to happen.[276] From the child's perspective, this unpredictability can lead to a sense of lack of control, fear, anxiety, or need to be dependent and protected by significant adults.

During development, children acquire self-esteem as they begin to master their environment and can do more things by themselves. This sense of mastery fosters a feeling of competence and control while decreasing the child's need for dependence. In contrast, the need for dependence produces a sense of helplessness and lack of self-esteem that can lead to feelings of inadequacy, poor self-worth, and ultimately to depression.[144]

In addition to unpredictability, the lapse in consciousness during a seizure or the child's experience of having his limbs do things that he has no control over further increases the sense of lack of control. Similarly, the unpleasant sensation of epigastric distress during the aura of a complex partial seizure can exacerbate the sense of lack of control, fearfulness, and dependence. Furthermore, the manifestations of a seizure are often perceived by others as frightening and grotesque.[163] The child's peers might, therefore, react to a seizure in a negative manner.[163] This could increase the child's feelings of being different.

Several older studies have shown that children with epilepsy, particularly those with temporal lobe epilepsy (TLE), were more dependent than children with other chronic illnesses.[96,109,243] In these studies, dependence was related to the presence of psychiatric disturbances,[96,109,243] a sense of lack of control, and attribution of failures and successes (particularly those in the social realm) to external unknown sources.[163] More recent studies have shown that children with newly diagnosed epilepsy feel shame and guilt about having epilepsy[196] and that adolescents with epilepsy are aware of a stigma to this illness.[9] Caplin et al.[36] demonstrated a positive correlation of self-efficacy with positive self-concept and positive attitude toward illness in youth with epilepsy and a negative association of child self-efficacy with child worries and symptoms of depression. Austin et al.[11] have shown that greater worry, negative attitude, poor self-concept, and symptoms of depression were associated with an increased sense of stigma in a large sample of children with chronic epilepsy.

Furthermore, the child has to contend with the possible behavioral and cognitive side effects of AEDs. Young children and sometimes adolescents are often unaware of the connection between these effects and their medication. These side effects could, therefore, contribute to the child's feeling of not being in control. Finally, despite the previously described stressors, children with epilepsy, like their peers, need to function adequately in the academic and social environment. These are far from trivial stressors.

Three main factors affect the coping skills of children with a chronic illness: the marginality of the sick status, the episodic nature of the disease, and the age of onset of the disorder.[100,202] If a child has visible physical impairments, a disease that is not episodic, and onset of the disorder from the preschool period, she self-identifies as sick and others identify her as different. If the disease has no visible impairments, is episodic, and begins after kindergarten, the child does not feel different from other children. When ill, the child tries to regain and/or achieve normal status.

The emotional burden on the child increases the less visible the handicap and the more normal the child is expected to be.[100] The need to meet these expectations becomes increasingly taxing for the child with epilepsy with recurrent rather than well-controlled seizures.

From the conceptual perspective, children's understanding of the nature of their disorder is age-related and can impact how well they cope with the illness.[220] Thus, 5- to 7-year-old children are aware of the external aspects of their disorder.[23] For example, they take medication, have repeated blood tests, and visit the doctor. Older children with epilepsy are more aware of the brain's role in their disorder, and this knowledge sometimes becomes a source of concern for them.

Sanger et al.[220] found that 41% of epileptic children and adolescents between the ages of 5 and 16 years identify epilepsy as a disease that involves the brain. Some children[10] fear that they might die during a seizure, and this fear makes them more anxious and dependent. Many children have misconceptions about seizure disorders and lack disease-related information. Only 41% of the children identified epilepsy as a disease involving the brain.[220]

Compared with children with asthma and diabetes, those with epilepsy have more unanswered questions about their illness and feel excluded from discussions with doctors.[119] Supporting this finding, McNelis et al.[157] reported that more than half of children with new-onset seizures want more information on seizures, the cause of seizures, treatment, handling future seizures, and protection from injury 6 months after their first seizure. They want to talk to other people with seizures, and need help handling seizures at school. More than 30% have fears or concerns about having another seizure and how to tell others about their seizures.

The impact and ramifications of the unpredictability of seizures is as important for the parents as for the child. It causes a sense of anxiety and is confounded by fear that the child could get hurt[10] or die[277] during a seizure. This unpredictability results in the difficult task of having to tread the fine line between what might be perceived as an overanxious or overprotective parent versus a neglectful parent. Thus, mothers of children with epilepsy are more stressed than are parents of children with other chronic illnesses.[68]

Parents vacillate between the need to protect and make sure their child is safe at all times versus the need to allow the child autonomy. The way parents cope with this stress affects the child's sense of dependence/independence, competence, and self-esteem. The findings of studies on the relationship of maternal anxiety and maternal adjustment with child quality of life, severity of epilepsy, and child adaptation highlight the role psychosocial variables play in how families cope with having a child with epilepsy.

For example, a study conducted on a relatively small sample described mothers as more emotionally involved in the lives of their children with epilepsy compared with their children without epilepsy.[111] This study also found increased maternal criticism toward the children with epilepsy, and this finding was related to more antisocial behaviors and poorer self-esteem in the children with epilepsy compared with their siblings.

Williams et al.[266] found that a significantly higher rate of parents of children with epilepsy sleep with their children than do parents of children with diabetes. They suggested that anxious parents might be more likely to perceive more risks for their children and misinterpret information about their child's condition, such as the need to sleep with the child to monitor for seizures. In a later study, Williams and colleagues[268] demonstrated that families most vulnerable to reduced quality of life were those in which a child has poorly controlled epilepsy, comorbid disabilities, and increased parental anxiety. Similarly, Austin et al.[15] reported that maternal adjustment and attitude was significantly related to the severity of the child's seizures.

In a large sample of children with epilepsy, Shore et al.[231] used a conceptual model based on prior findings in the literature to investigate the associations among maternal and child characteristics, maternal beliefs, and maternal adaptation. They found that most mothers adapt relatively well to their children having epilepsy. However, more than one-third of mothers were depressed and felt inadequate at managing their child's seizure disorder and maintaining the family's usual leisure activities. Child behavior problems, maternal satisfaction with family, and maternal learned helplessness had the strongest associations with maternal outcomes. This study did not examine the relationship between maternal and child adaptation.

In terms of child functioning and adaptation, Lotham and Pianka[154] found that measures of child–mother interaction and child self-reliance were significantly related to adjustment measures in children with epilepsy. Chapieski et al.[48] reported that poor adaptive functioning, based on the Vineland Adaptive Behavior Scale[238] in children with epilepsy was significantly associated with maternal anxiety, as well as with an overprotective and overly directive parenting style.

The few studies that have included both mothers and fathers find similar concerns in both parents of children with new-onset epilepsy.[233] Although these concerns decrease over a 6–month period, mothers maintain a higher level of concern than do fathers. Fathers have also reported that mothers are more concerned than they are about their child's epilepsy.[66] These parental differences can influence what children feel about the impact of their illness on their parents and family functioning. Therefore, studies are needed to determine how differences in parental concerns, anxiety level, and attitude are reflected in child functioning and adaptation.

In addition to the previously reviewed child and parent psychological variables, sociodemographic variables, such as social class, current and previous family stresses, and the presence of other children might also contribute to both the child's psychosocial adjustment and the family's coping skills.[110] Within the family context, there is a debate in the literature on the impact of chronic illness on healthy siblings; this topic is reviewed by Sharpe.[228] Hoare[108] demonstrated that the siblings of children with new-onset epilepsy are not more maladapted than the siblings of children with new-onset diabetes. However, the siblings of children with chronic epilepsy were more maladapted than the siblings of children with chronic diabetes. These findings led Hoare to conclude that chronic epilepsy has a marked impact on the behavior of the affected child, the siblings, and the family.[108]

In terms of the external environment, both the child and parents must deal with the school system. From the psychodynamic perspective, the occurrence of seizures at school can increase the child's sense of lack of control and present the child with the difficulty of dealing with stigma from peers and teachers. The child is also often faced with repeated questions by peers after having a seizure at school and also with teachers' lack of knowledge and misconceptions about epilepsy.[24] Even though there is no medical indication, teachers sometimes send children home or to an emergency room when they have a seizure. As a result of repeated absences, the child has more work to catch up, and this may increase the already difficult work load.[202] Teachers also might underestimate the child's intellectual potential due to misconceptions about epilepsy.

From the parental perspective, their efforts to help the child deal with the school system might increase their stress and that of their child. Hoare and Kerley[110] have shown that families of children with epilepsy who attend special schools are under more stress than those of children in regular schools. Alternatively, Austin et al.[18] described a significant association between academic achievement and family mastery in children with epilepsy.

Regarding academic achievement, Fastenau et al.[72] demonstrated a moderating effect of family factors, particularly organized/supportive versus disorganized/unsupportive family structure, on the impact of neuropsychological deficits on the writing and reading skills of children with epilepsy. Supporting the importance of family functioning in the academic performance of children with epilepsy, Mitchell et al.[175] found that parental education rather than seizure variables plays an important role in the IQ of children with epilepsy. Taken together, these psychosocial factors could increase the demands facing the child and affect his academic functioning,[72] self-esteem,[162] and related social and school functioning.[42]

From the social perspective, the problems of adolescents with epilepsy deserve special mention. During adolescence, youth acquire more independence, yet vacillate between dependence and independence. Uncontrolled epilepsy could affect this process by increasing dependency. Alternatively, if adolescents experiment with the decision-making, they might make decisions that are potentially harmful for their illness.[33] For example, to conform to what they perceive as the expectations of peers, adolescents might be noncompliant with AEDs, go to sleep late, or use alcohol and drugs. These behaviors could lead to poor seizure control and possible denial of a driver's license. These circumstances can lead to a significant increase in family stress.[146]

In terms of coping skills, a study of a large sample of adolescents with epilepsy has shown increased negative attitude with increasing age and poor seizure control[99] using the Child Attitude Towards Illness Scale.[13] The authors of this study suggest that as youth get older, a better understanding of the restrictions and limitations of the illness might underlie the increased negative attitude. Despite seizure control, the mothers of adolescents with epilepsy report significantly more psychological, social, and school adjustment problems than do the mothers of adolescents with asthma.[14] Also, above and beyond the effects of seizure control, Sbarra et al.[224] found that adolescent perception of controlling maternal behavior was significantly associated with youth externalizing behaviors.

Dealing with the stigma of epilepsy during adolescence might also pose additional coping challenges, as reviewed by MacLeod.[157] Westbrook et al.[263] found that only one-third of 64 adolescents with epilepsy confirmed that they felt stigmatized, and this finding was associated with poor self-esteem. Similarly, using the Quality of Life in Epilepsy for Adolescents (QOLIE-AD-48), which includes a stigma scale, Devinsky et al.[57] found relatively low stigma and good quality of life in youth with epilepsy. In contrast, a 37-item questionnaire designed to measure familiarity with epilepsy, knowledge about epilepsy, and perceptions reflecting stigma filled out by 19,441 adolescents revealed lack of knowledge and misperceptions about epilepsy that suggest a high rate of stigma.[19] In addition, the finding that 70% of the epilepsy patients in the Westbrook et al.[263] study said that they do not talk with anyone about their epilepsy implies that they do not talk about their illness because of stigma.

Finally, the child and family also must interact with the medical system. Two studies, one conducted in the mid 1980s[50] and one in 2004 (Smith et al., in press) found a marked discrepancy between the concerns of parents of children with epilepsy regarding their children's needs compared to how the treating pediatric neurologists and pediatricians viewed the parents' concerns. Whereas the parents were mainly worried about their children's behavior and performance at school, physicians thought the parents were concerned primarily about the stigma of epilepsy and seizure control. This continued discrepancy, despite increasing evidence for behavioral, cognitive, linguistic, and quality-of-life difficulties experienced by children and adolescents with epilepsy, underscores the stresses faced by parents of children with epilepsy.

In summary, from the psychological perspective, the child's ability to cope with epilepsy is a function of his intrapsychic experiences, such as sense of mastery and understanding of the illness, how the child's parents and family deal with the illness, as well as how the school, peer group, and medical system respond to the illness.

THE EFFECT OF SEIZURE-RELATED FACTORS ON THE CHILD'S BEHAVIOR

This section reviews studies on the association among seizure-related factors, such as seizure type, seizure control, AEDs, and age of onset with behavior, cognition, and language of children with epilepsy.

Psychopathology by Seizure Type

The landmark Isle of Wight epidemiologic study on psychopathology in children found an increased rate in children with TLE.[218] However, very few children in that study met criteria for TLE. Subsequent studies, albeit nonepidemiologic, of psychopathology by seizure type in childhood inconsistently found a relationship between type of epilepsy and psychopathology.

These discrepancies reflect limitations inherent in including relatively small sample sizes of children with epilepsy, and, therefore, small numbers of children with different seizure types. This, in turn, reduces the power to examine possible confounding effects of other seizure variables (e.g., seizure control, age of onset, duration of illness, type and number of AEDs), as well as of comorbid cognitive and linguistic deficits, demographic variables, and premorbid behavior problems.

Moreover, studies differ in whether they classify children by epilepsy syndrome, type of epilepsy, or localization-related epilepsy, or include type of epilepsy as one of several seizure severity measures. In addition, they also vary in the technique used to collect behavioral information on the children (e.g., structured psychiatric interviews, questionnaires), the source of information (e.g., child, parent(s), teacher), and the measures (psychiatric diagnoses, scores).

With these limitations in mind, the findings of earlier studies suggested that a relationship exists between type of seizure disorder and behavioral problems. For example, Nuffield[190] described neurotic traits in childhood absence epilepsy. Several studies suggested that children with TLE have characteristic behavioral disturbances,[94,110,151,217,241,246] particularly if they have left-sided foci.[151,241] Their behavior problems, hyperactivity, aggression, and antisocial behavior were associated with male gender, poor seizure control, low IQ, and childhood rages.[94,110,151,217,241] However, other researchers were unable to identify differences in measures of psychopathology between children with temporal lobe and generalized epilepsy.[103,265]

Using structured psychiatric interviews, a recent study on a large sample of children with different types of seizure disorder has demonstrated similar rates of DSM-IV psychiatric diagnoses in 60% of the children with complex partial seizures and 58% of those with childhood absence epilepsy, compared with normal children.[198] Other than schizophrenia-like psychosis in 10% of children with complex partial seizures rather than childhood absence epilepsy,[41,150] children with complex partial seizures and childhood absence epilepsy have similar rates of disruptive, affective/anxiety, and both disruptive and affective/anxiety disorders. Controlling for seizure and demographic variables, IQ was the single predictor of a psychiatric diagnosis in children with complex partial and childhood absence groups.[198]

A long-term follow-up study of young adults with a history of childhood absence demonstrated that, compared with a control group of young adults with a juvenile rheumatoid arthritis history, they had a significantly higher rate of behavioral and school/academic problems.[270] This finding was unrelated to seizure variables. Thus, childhood absence epilepsy, considered by most neurologists to be completely benign, has both a high rate of psychopathology in childhood and poor outcome regarding behavior and academics by young adulthood.

In children with new-onset seizures, those with prior unrecognized seizures and subsequent development of partial or absence seizures have higher rates of behavior problems (based on Child Behavior Checklist [CBCL],[1] parent,[12] and teacher[65] total) internalizing, attention, thought, and somatic complaints scores than those with other types of seizures. Other studies on children with new-onset seizures, however, have not shown a relationship between severity of behavioral problems and type of epilepsy.[195] In fact, prior cognitive and behavioral problems, rather than seizure variables, predicted whether children with new-onset seizures continued to have behavior problems over time.[197]

A study on localization-related epilepsy describes parental reports of behavioral problems in 39% of 63 children with TLE.[97] However, this study did not include control groups of children with other types of epilepsy. A study comparing small samples of children with temporal, frontal, and absence epilepsy found increased attentional problems based on parent CBCL scores in those with frontal lobe epilepsy.[104]

Among the localization-related epilepsies, even the so-called "benign" epilepsies, benign epilepsy with centrotemporal spikes (BECTS) or benign occipital epilepsy (BOE) may be associated with psychopathology. In the last decade, more reports focus on the subtle behavioral alterations commonly seen with these syndromes. Nonspecific behavioral problems have been reported in 30% of children with centrotemporal spikes,[275] and these may be more prevalent in those with atypical features of BECTS.[260] Symptoms of attention-deficit hyperactivity disorder (ADHD) have also been reported and may be predicted by certain EEG characteristics.[161] Parents report more problems with attention, temper, and impulsiveness in children with BECTS compared with controls.[51] Of interest, centrotemporal spikes were found in 5% to 6% of a large sample of ADHD patients without a history of epilepsy,[117] and spike frequency appeared to be related to severity of symptoms.

In summary, irrespective of type of epilepsy, children with epilepsy, both new-onset and chronic epilepsy, have high rates of a wide range of behavioral disturbances. The small study sample sizes, wide age range, and different methods of assessing behavioral abnormalities in these studies highlights the importance of conducting prospective studies of large representative samples of children to demonstrate the consistency of the behavioral problems and their course, and whether type of epilepsy plays a role in the behavioral profile of children and adolescents with epilepsy.

Effects of Seizure Control on Behavior

Historically, Lindsay et al.'s[151] long-term outcome study of 100 pediatric TLE cases revealed that poor seizure control was associated with increased antisocial behavior in these children. Remission of seizures by age 12 years was associated with a better adult psychosocial outcome than remission after age 12.[150]

Hermann et al.[103] demonstrated that seizure control was the most robust predictor of total and externalizing CBCL scores in a large sample of children with epilepsy, controlling for the effects of demographic, biologic, and psychosocial variables. Numerous subsequent studies have examined this relationship using different behavioral instruments, control groups, informants, measures of seizure control, sample sizes, and youth cognitive ability. Some of these studies were cross-sectional and few were longitudinal. Only a few studies have controlled for possible confounding seizure variables to varying degrees. Retrospective and prospective treatment studies have also investigated the relationship between seizure control and behavioral outcome following intervention with AEDs and epilepsy surgery.

Due to space limitations, this section briefly summarizes the findings of the larger cross-sectional and longitudinal studies (including postsurgical intervention), conducted in children with epilepsy, that have examined the association with seizure control. It also indicates how these findings vary by type of behavioral instrument and informant.

In terms of cross-sectional studies there was no statistically significant relationship of seizure frequency with the presence and type of psychiatric disorders, as well as with CBCL scores in a large sample of children with complex partial seizures who have average IQ scores.[43] The DSM-IV psychiatric diagnoses of these children were based on information obtained on the child by a structured psychiatric interview administered separately to the child and to the parent.

In contrast to these findings, Schoenfeld et al.[225] reported significantly higher total and internalizing CBCL scores in children with complex partial seizures with the highest seizure frequency. However, they did not examine the possible effect of IQ on these findings.

Using CBCL scores, Austin et al.[16] also found significantly higher internalizing scores in children with epilepsy, aged 8 to 13 years, who had more severe seizures, a measure that includes seizure control. Follow-up of these children 4 years later revealed significantly higher internalizing CBCL scores in the girls with epilepsy who had more severe seizures both at baseline and follow-up.[9] These authors concluded that girls with more severe seizures might be more at risk for behavior problems as they moved through the teen years.

Children with new-onset seizures and subsequent recurrent seizures have significantly higher parent-[17] and teacher-based total and internalizing CBCL scores,[62] suggesting a relationship between seizure control and severity of behavioral problems. In contrast, Oostrom et al.[195] reported lack of persistence in behavior problems based on parent CBCL and teacher reports in their 3-, 12-, and 48-month follow-up study of children with new-onset epilepsy. Despite similar mean parent and teacher ratings, Oostrom et al.[195] found no agreement between parent and teacher ratings for individual children.

In terms of surgical studies, several older studies noted that some children with TLE become less aggressive, and their behavior improves once they attain seizure control after temporal lobectomy.[54,60,89,118,149] None of these studies, however, used standardized psychiatric instruments and control groups to follow the postoperative behavioral changes of a representative sample of children undergoing temporal lobectomy. In addition, these studies did not include a control group of medically treated children with epilepsy.

Using the CBCL,[1] Lendt et al.[145] found a significant decrease in the CBCL externalizing, internalizing, attention, and thought scores that had been within the clinical range 3 months after epilepsy surgery on 13 temporal and 11 extratemporal lobectomies, two hemispherectomies, and two callosotomies, compared with a control group of medically treated children with intractable epilepsy. Postsurgical seizure control rather than age, sex, onset, and duration of epilepsy; the site of the focus; and changes in AED regimen accounted for this finding.

In a 1-year follow-up study of a large sample of 30 children who underwent epilepsy surgery, Smith et al.[237] found no significant change in CBCL scores 1 year after surgery, compared with medically treated children with intractable epilepsy. Seizure control was unrelated to these findings.

In summary, the findings of cross-sectional and follow-up studies of children with new-onset and chronic epilepsy demonstrate an association of seizure frequency with the presence and severity of behavioral disturbances. However, recent evidence that verbal IQ predicts psychopathology, children with new-onset seizures have behavior problems prior to the onset of seizures, and children who undergo epilepsy surgery continue to have behavior problems irrespective of postsurgical seizure control suggest that psychopathology is a comorbid component of pediatric epilepsy irrespective of illness variables.

Effects of Antiepileptic Drugs on Behavior and Cognition

Although there are numerous reports on AED effects on behavior and cognition in children with epilepsy, no double-blind, randomized, controlled studies have examined these relationships in these children. For detailed information on extant studies and reports, the reader is referred to two reviews, one on the mechanisms of action of AEDs and the relevance to neurobehavioral adverse effects,[222] and the other on the cognitive side effects of AEDs in children with epilepsy (see also Chapter 201).[153]

This brief summary of the adverse effects of AEDs on cognition and behavior emphasizes the importance of controlling for these variables in neurobehavioral studies of children with epilepsy. In addition, different children appear to be vulnerable to these AED adverse effects. Thus, as described in adults with epilepsy,[138,181] increased risk for AED-related behavioral and cognitive side effects in children with epilepsy include AED polytherapy,[32,95,134,151,155] mental retardation or learning disabilities,[32,95] and a family history of psychiatric disorders.[28,30] Similarly, as shown in adults with epilepsy,[250] children with a past history of behavioral problems, as well as of prior adverse behavioral and cognitive effects to AEDs, might also be more vulnerable to these adverse effects.

It is important to note that children on high doses of combinations of AEDs might appear to be depressed because they are tired, apathetic, listless, and poorly motivated. Other children on polytherapy or high-dose monotherapy might respond with irritability, low frustration tolerance, poor impulse control, and hyperactivity.

However, AED polytherapy might also reflect the type or types of epilepsy, as well as comorbid cognitive and linguistic difficulties, all of which might increase the likelihood of behavioral problems. Therefore, clinicians should be aware that the functional impact of AED behavioral and cognitive side effects on the individual child's daily functioning and quality of life might be as severe as that of uncontrolled seizures.

In terms of specific behavioral side effects, AEDs that can trigger depression in children include phenobarbital,[28,30] primidone,[105] and valproic acid.[105] Adult studies also find depression associated with topiramate[182] and levetiracetam.[188] Manic behavior has been described in children with epilepsy treated with felbamate[45] and ethosuximide.

Case studies describe psychosis in children treated with topiramate,[206] levetiracetam,[134,274] vigabatrin,[35] and zonisamide.[177] Several case reports describe irritability, hyperactivity, and aggression in children with epilepsy on gabapentin,[129,172] phenobarbital,[34,261] vigabatrin,[3,230] and benzodiazepines.[81,249]

Slowing of cognitive processes and motor reaction time are attributed to the older AEDs, such as phenobarbital and benzodiazepines.[26,34,105,261] In adults with epilepsy, these effects are dose-related for carbamazepine, phenytoin, and valproic acid.[59] However, there have been no well designed studies on the new AEDs and cognition in children. The impaired word retrieval and cognitive slowing found in children treated with topiramate,[91,229] and the possible association with the speed of titration[221] must be studied in children.

To date, most clinicians have been impressed by the lack of adverse cognitive effects in children treated with lamotrigine.[221] The slow titration used in children with epilepsy to avoid the rash associated with lamotrigine treatment might contribute to this observation. However, well-designed studies are needed to examine the effects of the new AEDs on cognition.

In summary, double-blind, randomized studies using well-established behavioral and cognitive instruments sensitive to change are needed to determine which AEDs have behavioral and cognitive adverse effects and for which children with epilepsy. Studies of behavior and cognition in children with epilepsy, however, should include large samples of children to examine the possible role played by AEDs in the studies' findings. AED polytherapy and high therapeutic blood levels might be associated with more general behavioral problems, such as irritability, aggression, and hyperactivity, as well as slowing of cognitive processes in children. Children with epilepsy at risk for the adverse neurobehavioral effects of AEDs are those with mental retardation, learning disabilities, poor prior behavioral and cognitive responses to AEDs, psychiatric history of past behavioral and cognitive problems, and family history of psychiatric disorders.

Age of Onset and Duration of Illness

Increasing evidence suggests connectivity and structural changes caused by seizures in the brain of young animals despite the lack of cell loss (see review by Holmes[114]), an age-related effect on synaptic function,[141] and long-term cognitive and behavioral changes.[223] Maternal deprivation in the young animal has synergistic effects, with recurrent seizures in inducing long-term damage in the developing brain.[121] Although the impact of early seizures on brain development might reflect the underlying cause of the seizures rather than the effects of seizures,[113] the findings of animal studies support the previously reviewed clinical data suggesting that the child's immediate environment (i.e., home, school), rearing practices, recurrent ongoing seizures, and AEDs might impact the development of behavior and cognition.

The age of onset of epilepsy might be an indicator of the severity of the underlying pathology. Thus, early-onset epilepsy is often associated with mental retardation, and children with mental retardation have an earlier onset of epilepsy.[218] These age relationships imply that epilepsy and mental retardation in children with early onset are epiphenomena of underlying pathologic processes in the brain.

In terms of psychopathology, two epidemiologic studies have demonstrated significantly higher rates of psychopathology in children with epilepsy who have mental retardation[218] or complicated epilepsy, including learning disabilities[55] than those with normal intelligence or uncomplicated epilepsy. A population study of children with both mental retardation and epilepsy also revealed high rates of severe behavior problems.[239]

Nevertheless, it is still unclear how and to what degree recurrent seizures, both frequent and infrequent, and the need for high doses of AED polytherapy impair ongoing development of the brain and of emotional, social, cognitive, and linguistic skills in early childhood. It also remains to be determined through prospective studies if the behavioral, cognitive, and linguistic outcome in developmentally disabled children with earlier onset of epilepsy is worse than in children with later onset of their epilepsy. Whereas some studies suggest that epilepsy surgery and subsequent seizure control for early-onset intractable epilepsy changes the developmental course,[78] others do not.[44,133,135,237]

Regarding later onset of epilepsy, two of the most common types of pediatric epilepsy, complex partial seizure disorder and primary generalized epilepsy, typically begin in middle childhood. During middle childhood, acceleration occurs in the development of children's emotional, social, cognitive, and linguistic skills and continued maturation through adolescence. Ongoing seizures, high doses of multiple AEDs, and prolonged seizures might interrupt the functioning of the neural circuits involved in these maturational processes.

In children with onset of epilepsy in middle childhood, although the presence of psychopathology does not appear to be associated with age of onset,[43] earlier studies identify an association between early-onset and impaired cognitive functioning.[2,26,70,191] Yet, these findings might also reflect the confounding effects of poor seizure control, as well as AED polytherapy and high blood levels of treating drugs.[26]

More recent studies also find that cognition,[225] language,[225] verbal learning, and certain aspects of discourse skills[39,40] are associated with age of onset in children with complex partial seizures. For example, unrelated to lateralization of EEG findings, children with earlier onset of complex partial seizures have significantly lower scores on neuropsychological and linguistic tasks,[225] poor performance on long delay cued recall, and reduced monitoring and self-correction of errors in the organization of ideas during speech[39] than do those with later onset.

In summary, these findings suggest a dynamic interplay among brain development, age of onset, and maturation of cognition and language in children. They also highlight the importance of early treatment of seizures for optimal development of children's cognition, language, and discourse skills. Moreover, further studies are needed to determine if the higher rate of behavior problems found in studies of children with new-onset epilepsy[12] who had prior unrecognized seizures might represent the cumulative effects of early-onset seizures on the development of cognition, behavior, and language in these children.

EARLY-ONSET EPILEPSY SYNDROMES WITH SPECIFIC BEHAVIORAL, COGNITIVE, AND LINGUISTIC IMPAIRMENTS

Four early-onset epileptic syndromes, the West, Lennox-Gastaut, Landau-Kleffner, and continuous spike-and-slow wave syndromes and one disorder, tuberous sclerosis (TSC), are associated with behavioral social, cognitive, and linguistic impairments.

West Syndrome (Infantile Spasms)

The prototype for early-onset epilepsy syndromes is that of infantile spasms or West syndrome (Chapter 229). Seizure onset is usually by 4 to 6 months.[86] In the absence of seizure control, the developmental outcome for these children is usually poor both in the cognitive (see Caplan's review[38]) and behavioral domains, with varying degrees of impaired social relationships.[44,61,207]

Although the cause of the poor outcomes is still unknown, hypsarrhythmia, the severely epileptiform EEG found in this disorder, is present very early in development and has been implicated in the negative outcomes in these patients.[207] In fact, normalization of the EEG is thought to be the hallmark of successful treatment in this disorder.

Outcome studies in infantile spasms have mostly focused on cognitive rather than behavioral outcomes. Most studies show that a better cognitive profile at the onset (e.g., lack of significant regression), earlier treatment, and cryptogenic etiology are factors associated with improved cognitive outcome.[61,131,208]

More recently, early follow-up results from a large multicenter treatment trial[155] showed that the successfully treated subjects (those who showed cessation of spasms) had better scores on the Vineland Adaptive Behavior Scales than those who did not have cessation of spasms. Those with cryptogenic spasms also had better outcomes compared to those with symptomatic etiologies. But, in contrast to past results, there were no differences based on type of treatment, speed of normalization of the EEG, or time to treatment.

The behavioral or psychiatric abnormalities most strongly associated with infantile spasms are autism and autism spectrum disorders (ASD). According to a population study,[194] 6% of children with infantile autism had shown typical or atypical hypsarrhythmia with infantile spasms in the first year of life. Conversely, 13% of all children with infantile spasms were later diagnosed as suffering from infantile autism,[209] and several more showed severe degrees of autistic behavior. The autistic symptoms may be of a transient character in a large proportion of cases.[194,209] Another small prospective trial suggested that the etiology of the spasms was important in predicting later autistic behavior, with patients with symptomatic spasms showing a higher rate of autism.[8]

Given the high rate of infantile spasms in children with known genetic syndromes (e.g., TSC) and other brain abnormalities that are themselves associated with an increased rate of mental retardation and autism, this is undoubtedly a complex inter-relationship. The association with later autistic behavior in these patients, as well as the history of infantile spasms seen in ASD patients, points to the fact that epilepsy and, perhaps more importantly, epileptiform EEGs may play an important role in the development of autistic behaviors. Hyperactivity is another psychiatric disturbance seen in this syndrome. About two-thirds of those individuals with infantile spasms who have autism also meet criteria for hyperkinetic disorder. This is more than would be expected solely from the autism diagnosis.[209]

About 80% to 90% of children who had West syndrome in infancy will show cognitive delay either at the time of seizure onset or will be diagnosed with mental retardation later in childhood. Those with West syndrome, autism, and hyperkinetic disorders have mental retardation as often and of the same degree as children who do not. Thus, the well-known association of autism and hyperkinesis with cognitive impairment cannot in itself account for the link between these psychiatric disorders and West syndrome.

A meta-analysis of 67 studies showed that 17% of patients with infantile spasms developed Lennox-Gastaut syndrome (LGS).[120] The vast majority of these children will also appear severely withdrawn (autistic) and profoundly mentally retarded.

Lennox-Gastaut Syndrome

This syndrome is characterized by the early onset of intractable seizures (tonic, generalized tonic–clonic, atypical absence, atonic, and myoclonic) and bilateral slow spike-and-wave complexes on EEG (Chapter 241). Follow-up of children with LGS reveals that about half are retarded, in particular if they have minor motor seizures and multifocal independent spikes.[193] Treating clinicians all know that the behavioral aspects of this disorder are significantly impairing to the patient and family, but not much systematic study has been devoted to the area.[22] As in other cases of mental retardation, the children are sometimes irritable and hyperactive. These symptoms might decrease with seizure control or become exacerbated with some AEDs.

Landau-Kleffner Syndrome

Landau-Kleffner syndrome (LKS) is an acquired epileptic aphasia characterized by a gradual or rapid onset of aphasia that occurs in a previously normal child *plus* seizures and/or epileptiform changes on the EEG (Chapter 242).[142,257] The aphasia is often predominantly of a type referred to as "verbal auditory agnosia" (inability to understand spoken language).[205] All types of seizures have been reported in this syndrome, but nocturnal complex partial or simple motor may be most common.[21] The seizures are usually relatively infrequent and respond readily to AED treatment in most cases. EEG abnormalities frequently include focal or generalized spike-and-wave discharges that are activated during sleep.[161] At times, the patients meet criterion for electrical status epilepticus in sleep (ESES), with more than 80% to 85% of their sleep record consisting of spike-and-wave activity.[107]

The epidemiology of the disorder has not been properly studied. In clinical series, it appears to be about twice as common in boys as in girls. The etiology of LKS is unknown. There is a moderately increased rate of a family history of seizure disorder (10%–15%),[21] and the syndrome has been described in siblings. Taken together, these data suggest a genetic liability in some cases. However, it has also been described in conjunction with temporal lobe tumors,[186] cerebral arteritis,[199] and otitis media.[88] The possibility of electric dysregulation in several cortical areas as a pathophysiologic basis for this disorder has been emphasized by many authors, including Landau and Kleffner.[142]

The hallmark association is the language disturbance. This may fluctuate in severity, especially initially, when the impairment of verbal comprehension may first lead to suspicion of acquired deafness. Both receptive and expressive languages are affected.[236] Behavioral changes have also been reported. These include hyperactivity and inattentiveness,[107] psychosis and autistic behavior,[56] as well as oppositionalism, noncompliance, and frank aggression.[211,264]

LKS has been treated with traditional anticonvulsant medications,[56] corticosteroids,[147] intravenous immunoglobulin (IVIG),[173] and even epilepsy surgery[178] (see Tuchman[251] for review). Therapy that treats the EEG abnormalities has been associated with improved language[147,160] and behavior.[124,235] Robinson and colleagues reported that the duration of ESES was strongly correlated with language recovery, and that no child with prolonged ESES (>36 months) had a normal language outcome.[211] They also found that the severe behavioral disturbances in the acute phase were associated with frontal epileptiform activity during wakefulness.

On the other hand, the relationship between the seizures and/or the EEG abnormalities and the language and/or behavioral deficit is not completely clear. Many children do not begin to have seizures until after the period of regression, and some never have clinical seizures at all.[254] Some of the EEG abnormalities resolve spontaneously, and there are studies failing to demonstrate a correlation between EEG findings and the severity and course of the language impairment.[115,254,264] Van Hout[258] points out that, while the behavioral disturbances have been thought to be secondary to the severe language disturbance, there are cases where these disturbances precede the period of language regression. It has also been proposed that the epileptiform discharges are an epiphenomenon of the underlying brain abnormality rather than the actual cause of the language disturbance.[115]

Outcome in LKS is variable.[236] Seizure outcome is usually good, with resolution of seizures being the norm. But language and behavioral outcomes are more difficult to predict and range from muteness, persisting behavioral problems, and sometimes even intellectual impairment, to complete recovery in adult age. A considerable amount of variability of the clinical picture at the time of onset is supposedly a marker for relatively better outcome.

Continuous Spike-and-Wave Activity During Slow Sleep

Continuous spike-and-wave during sleep (CSWS) is the term most often used to describe a rare syndrome that strikes predominantly school-age males (Chapter 242). In 1971, Patry and colleagues[200] described the first patients, who presented with cognitive deterioration and the onset of epilepsy. The EEG showed a characteristic pattern of continuous spike-and-wave discharges during more than 85% of slow-wave sleep. The syndrome is now part of the epilepsy classification system as defined by the International League Against Epilepsy.[123] Individuals with the syndrome undergo severe language, behavioral, and global cognitive regression accompanied by epilepsy and the severely abnormal EEG pattern known as CSWS or ESES. Although the terminology is still not universal, most authors now use the term CSWS to refer to the clinical syndrome and ESES to refer to the EEG pattern.

As in LKS, this syndrome has its onset in childhood, shows a male predominance, and is associated with multiple seizure types. But unlike LKS, patients sometimes have preexisting developmental issues, the seizures are more frequent and harder to control,[236] the cognitive regression is significant and universal, and the behavioral difficulties are more prevalent.[79] Behavioral deficits include those similar to LKS (hyperactivity, inattentiveness, and aggression) but autism-like behavior has also been reported.[215] There are also motor impairments including weakness, dystonia, ataxia, and dyspraxia.[245] These more severe deficits in behavior, cognition, and motor function have been attributed to frontal and prefrontal dysfunction, perhaps as a result of the more frontal predominance of the EEG discharges.[33,215,236]

Outcomes are variable but overall are believed to be rather poor.[214] A recent study showed good behavioral outcome in all seven patients studied, but cognitive recovery (complete or partial) was seen in only three.[226] However, severe psychosis and lasting cognitive and motor impairment are also reported.[139,245]

Tuberous Sclerosis

TSC illustrates the complex relationship between brain malformations, epilepsy, behavior, and cognition. Epilepsy, both infantile spasms and partial epilepsy, and significant learning disability or mental retardation may be found in more than half the children with TSC.[52] Autistic disorder affects 25% to 50% of children with TSC.[25,94]

The severity of the neuropsychiatric problems associated with TSC seems dependent on the number and location of cortical tubers, although there are some inconsistencies in the literature. Bolton and Griffiths[25] found a strong association between temporal lobe tubers and autistic disorder. Positron emission tomography (PET) studies have shown decreased glucose metabolism in the temporal lobes, increased glucose metabolism in the cerebellar nuclei, and increased tryptophan uptake in the caudate nuclei.[7]

Age of seizure onset and seizure type also may be important. Both mental handicap and autistic disorder have been most consistently associated with infantile spasms and seizure onset before 2 years of age. Hunt and Dennis[122] found a history of infantile spasms in 40 of 45 children with TSC and autistic disorder.

The relative contribution of epileptiform discharges to autistic behavior remains a question. Tuchman and Rapin[255] found an association of autistic regression and epileptiform discharges in a population without TSC. Jambaqué et al.[125] treated seven children with TSC and infantile spasms with vigabatrin, with remission of the spasms in all the children. At follow-up, five of the six children with autistic symptoms showed improvement in behavior, and six of seven patients had improvements in developmental testing, thus suggesting some effect of epileptic discharges on cognitive function and behavior.

Thus, the brain areas that are dysfunctional in autism (and possibly certain variants of hyperkinetic disorder with cognitive impairment) may also be those that are affected in infantile spasms and in TSC with early symptom onset. According to one current theory for the development of autistic symptoms, dopaminergic (and other) nerve fibers arising in the brainstem and projecting onto structures in the striatum, medial temporal lobes, and prefrontal areas may be malfunctioning. Parts of these neural circuitries are also possibly involved in the pathogenic chain of events in infantile spasms. That they are often implicated in TSC has been known for a long time.[87]

CHILD PSYCHIATRIC DISORDERS ASSOCIATED WITH EPILEPSY

This section addresses the interface of behavior, cognition, language, social skills, and seizure variables as it pertains to psychiatric disorders commonly found in older children with epilepsy.

Autism, Asperger Syndrome, and Other Autism-Like Conditions

Autistic disorder, which occurs in about 1 to 2 children per 1,000, and about four times more often in boys than in girls,[77] is associated with a high rate of epilepsy, although reported rates have been extremely variable, with a range from 5% to 44%.[69,85,128,132,174,179,194,213,255,256,262,271] Seizure onset is usually either during the first 3 years of life,[194,262] or around the time of puberty.[80,82,218] New cases of epilepsy may also appear in early adult life.[53] The most common types of epilepsy encountered in autism are complex partial seizures, generalized tonic–clonic seizures, and combinations of seizures of various kinds.[53,194]

Autistic disorder is associated with mental retardation in approximately 70% of all cases.[76] Epilepsy is much more common in those individuals with autistic disorder who are also severely mentally retarded, but it is not a very rare phenomenon in those of low normal intelligence.[83,201,256]

The occurrence of epilepsy may also have a direct effect on language in ASD. The presence of a specific language profile (verbal auditory agnosia similar to that seen in LKS) predicts the presence of epilepsy and/or abnormal EEGs in autism.[256] Another, more controversial, association is that of language regression; conflicting reports exist regarding whether regression is or is not associated with a higher risk of epilepsy/EEG abnormalities.[128,132,148,152,156,183,184,213] For example, Tuchman and Rapin[255] found those with language regression had no increase in the frequency of clinical epilepsy, but did have significantly more isolated epileptiform EEG abnormalities compared with those without regression. Looking at this phenomenon in more detail, McVicar and colleagues[166,167] studied a sample with a high rate of ASD but that was ascertained for language regression; they showed that regression associated with pure language loss and occurring later was more frequently associated with epilepsy/EEG abnormalities than was more typical earlier autistic regression.

The variability in rates in the literature is likely due to sample heterogeneity. Factors such as differing ASD diagnostic classifications across the years,[58,210,256] variable epilepsy definitions,[85] differing age distributions in samples,[58,85,174,217,262,271] the inclusion of subjects with other specific genetic or neurologic disorders that are themselves associated with epilepsy,[201] as well as variability in the degree and type of associated cognitive or language deficits[20,253] could all influence rates of epilepsy in this population.

Asperger syndrome, which occurs in at least 3 to 4 out of every 1,000 children, and, again, much more often in boys than in girls,[67] may be associated with a slightly higher than expected rate of epilepsy,[47,81] but, to date, no large-scale epidemiologic study has been performed.

A group of autism-like conditions also exist that do not meet criteria for autism or Asperger syndrome. Some of these children are diagnosed as suffering from a "pervasive developmental disorder not otherwise specified" (PDD NOS). Others are never clinically diagnosed on the autism spectrum despite severe and typical problems, but receive diagnoses of "conduct disorder," "attention deficit hyperactivity disorder," or "hyperkinetic syndrome" instead, or have no other diagnosis than epilepsy (and possibly mental retardation). Just how frequently these autism-like conditions appear is not known. In a population study of all mentally retarded children with epilepsy, aged 8 to 12 years, several new cases of autism and autism-like conditions were found; these children had not been previously identified as suffering from a problem on the autism spectrum, and some had been missed in previous population studies of autism. Together they account for at least 1 in 1,000 children.[239] The gender ratio is almost equal in this group. It seems clear that the fact that they had early-onset epilepsy "deprived" them of recognition of the autistic symptoms. It is almost as though the specialists (often experienced child neurologists) treating these children for their epilepsy believed that the classical autistic symptoms evidenced were only to be expected in early-onset epilepsy and so required no additional diagnosis. The families, however, believed that, after the first year of diagnosis of the seizure disorder, they needed the most help with the autistic symptoms. However, no help was offered, because no diagnosis had been made. The children and their families were in a particularly difficult situation also because many of the AEDs (the benzodiazepines especially) tried appeared to contribute to enhancing the autistic symptomatology.

One of the many difficulties faced by the clinician caring for a family with a child affected by seizures and autistic behavior is to try to disentangle the effects of the neurologic from the psychiatric disorder. Many bizarre behaviors shown by children with autism are difficult to separate from clinical seizure activity. The empty, staring gaze might be mistaken for a "true" absence. Complex facial, hand, and arm mannerisms may suggest a complex partial seizure. Tics-like movements—very common in Asperger syndrome[67]—can be virtually impossible to separate from myoclonic jerks. The diagnostic problems are further enhanced by the fact that what is sometimes a symptom of epilepsy (for example, the upward turning of the eyes), may at other times be a stereotypic-catatonic phenomenon. An individual with an autism spectrum disorder may actually show the same—or a very similar—symptom as a consequence of epilepsy in one instance and of autism in another.

The EEG (including video monitoring) is sometimes very helpful in differential diagnosis, but this examination can be extremely difficult to accomplish in a child with severe behavior problems. A sleep EEG is sometimes all that can be obtained, but even the limited information one can get from this can be an essential part of the differential diagnostic work-up.

Literature also describes epileptiform discharges on EEGs in patients with autism without clinical seizure disorders. Tuchman and Rapin[255] reported 15% epileptiform sleep EEGs in patients without a history of epilepsy. Others report 20% to 30%[85,128,262] epileptiform EEG rates. Some evidence suggests that prolonged or overnight EEGs yield much higher rates of 46% to 60%.[49,252]

The exact association between the epileptiform discharges and the social, communication, and behavioral deficits seen in autism spectrum disorders is unknown. It is tempting to think there may be a causal relationship because that would have important implications for treatment. However, this has not been proven.

Pervasive Developmental Disorders Umbrella and the Spectrum Concept

The prevalence of epilepsy may be even higher in some of the other pervasive developmental disorders (PDD) umbrella disorders from the DSM. Rates in Rett syndrome range from 63% to 94%.[46,240] Patients also show an age-specific abnormal EEG pattern that may be related to the clinical disease progression.[86] Epilepsy rates of up to 77% are also seen in childhood disintegrative disorder.[179] Paroxysmal EEGs and ESES have been reported in higher numbers in CDD than in autism as well.[137,180,216]

These epilepsy and behavioral syndromes (e.g., autism with regression and epilepsy, other pervasive developmental disorders [Rett syndrome, CDD, developmental language disorder, LKS, CSWS, TSC]) all have in common characteristic seizures and/or epileptiform EEG patterns associated with specific behavioral, cognitive, and linguistic deficits. Thus, it has been the subject of much debate whether they could all exist along a single spectrum with a common underlying neuropathology and variable symptomatic presentation.[20,79,127,159,214,251,254,255] However, the exact role of the seizures and EEG abnormalities is still not understood. Given that the EEG pattern of ESES is seen in multiple epilepsy syndromes and not believed to be specific to the clinical syndrome of CSWS[259] it may be that the EEG pattern may affect behavioral, cognitive, and linguistic performance, regardless of the syndrome with which it is seen.

A better understanding of these phenomena is important both for elucidating pathophysiologic mechanisms underlying these disorders and for the development of proper treatment strategies. Indeed, some clinicians are adopting LKS and ESES treatment strategies, including drugs associated with significant side effects[251] and even epilepsy surgery,[185] for autistic patients with abnormal EEGs.

Attention-Deficit/Hyperactivity Disorder (ADHD)

Problems with attention and symptoms of attention deficit hyperactivity disorder (ADHD) are commonly reported in children with epilepsy. As previously described, children with TLE, particularly those with left-lobe TLE, were thought to demonstrate behaviors similar to ADHD (i.e., hyperactivity, distractibility, impulsivity) and conduct disorder (i.e., antisocial behaviors).[27,112,203,218,242] Using teacher and parent scales, Stores et al.[242] found that epileptic boys were more hyperactive and inattentive than nonepileptic boys. These two groups of subjects did not differ, however, on laboratory measures of attention, impulsivity, visual scanning, and distractibility.

Kinney et al.[130] concluded that epilepsy does not influence behavior adversely, because they did not find increased behavioral or learning disturbances in epileptic children with ADHD compared with nonepileptic children with ADHD. Hellgren et al.[101] found no increased rates of epilepsy in adolescents with a history of attentional deficits in preschool. However, the histories of these children indicated a significantly increased incidence of febrile seizures. Mitchell and colleagues[176] described decreased reaction time and inattention, but no impulsivity in children with epilepsy. These findings were unrelated to AEDs, IQ scores, duration of seizures, or seizure severity.

Reviewing ten recent studies of attention in children with epilepsy, Sánchez-Carpintero and Neville[219] found evidence of sustained attention deficits, particularly in children with complex partial seizures and BECTS. Deficits in divided attention were not found consistently. Studies using DSM criteria for the diagnosis of possible ADHD in children with epilepsy have reported prevalence rates of 30% to 40%.[63,102,227,247] There has been some suggestion that the inattentive type of ADHD may be more common than ADHD, combined type, in children with epilepsy.[63] As in the general population, children with epilepsy may have ADHD comorbid with other behavioral disorders. Caplan et al.,[43] in a study of children with complex partial epilepsy, found that 17% of children had disruptive behavior disorder (ADHD, oppositional defiant, or conduct disorders) and 23% had a disruptive disorder plus a mood or anxiety disorder.

Several risk factors are possible for attention problems in children with epilepsy. Neither gender nor seizure type have been consistent predictors. Early studies found more ADHD symptoms in boys with epilepsy, but in a recent study there was no difference by gender.[63] Similarly, although attention problems are often cited in children with partial complex seizures, some studies have found a higher rate in children with generalized seizures[102] or no effect by seizure type.[63] Seizure frequency may be important. Aldenkamp and Arends[4] found slowing of processing speed in children with frequent epileptiform discharges, and slow processing and attention problems in children with frequent nonconvulsive seizures. AEDs may be a factor. Attention problems have been reported with phenobarbital, benzodiazepines, and topiramate, but are less often found with newer AEDs.[26,153] ADHD may also be a risk factor for seizures. Hesdorffer et al.[106] found that ADHD, inattentive type, was a risk factor for subsequent unprovoked seizures, and Austin et al.[12] noted increased scores on the attention problem subscale of the CBCL at the time new-onset seizures were first recognized.

Treatment of attention problems in children with epilepsy is important. Williams et al.[267] have shown that problems with attention are better predictors of academic underachievement in children with epilepsy than are socioeconomic status, self-esteem, or measures of memory function. Although there have been concerns about the use of stimulants in children with seizures, the more recent recommendations and studies of stimulants in children with epilepsy have shown that methylphenidate is effective for symptoms of ADHD, is safe in children with well-controlled seizures, and is probably safe in children with uncontrolled seizures.[73,90,93,244]

Affective and Anxiety Disorders

Although epilepsy markedly impacts children's coping resources,[13,64] only a few mood and anxiety disorder studies have been conducted in children and adolescents with epilepsy. They demonstrate depression and anxiety in 16% to 23% of patients, with more anxiety disorders in younger patients[42,192] and depression in older youth.[64,71] Evidence for suicidal ideation in 20% of children with epilepsy, most of whom have both affective and disruptive disorders,[42] underscores the potential morbidity of these comorbid diagnoses in this population. Moreover, the higher rate of depression, anxiety, and suicidal acts, together with the poor quality of life in adult epilepsy patients,[84,126] highlight the need for early detection and treatment of depression and anxiety disorders in youth with epilepsy.

In a large epidemiologic study, Davies et al.[55] found emotional disorders (e.g., mood and anxiety disorders) in 16% of children with epilepsy, a prevalence of more than twice that found in children with diabetes (6.4%) and four times the rate found in the general population of youth (4.2%) using a structured psychiatric interview. Based on the Kiddie Schedule for Affective Disorders and Schizophrenia (K-SADS), Caplan et al.[42] found DSM-IV–based mood and anxiety disorder diagnoses in 33% of 171 children with epilepsy compared with 6% of 93 children without epilepsy. The most common diagnoses were anxiety (63%) and comorbid mood and disruptive disorders (26.1%), while only 5% had depression and 5% met criteria for both anxiety and depression.

Studies using the self-report Children's Depression Inventory[136] found depression in 25% of adolescents with epilepsy,[64] 26% of 7- to 18-year-old epilepsy youth,[71] as well as more depression in 12- to 18-year-old compared with 9- to 11-year-old children with epilepsy.[192] Although Ettinger et al.[71] reported anxiety in 16% of 7- to 18-year-old patients with epilepsy, both Caplan et al.[42] and Oguz et al.[192] found that anxiety, not depression, was more common in young children with epilepsy.

Inconsistent findings on the association of seizure variables with depression and anxiety disorders in youth with epilepsy could reflect methodological differences across studies, such as inclusion of different sample sizes and epilepsy variables, as well as use of different mood and anxiety instruments. Whereas several investigators report no association with seizure variables,[42,55,64] some find a relationship with duration of epilepsy and number of AEDs[192] and type of AED.[29,30] More children with complex partial seizures have depression than do those with absence epilepsy, who, in turn, have more anxiety disorders.[42]

Mood disorders also occur more frequently in children with epilepsy who have mental retardation[31,55] and lower average IQ scores.[42] Patients with comorbid psychopathology, depression and anxiety disorders, or disruptive and depression/anxiety disorders have significantly lower full scale and verbal IQ scores than do those with either depression or anxiety disorders alone.[42]

Finally, the association with demographic variables, such as gender and age, is similar to that described in the general population of youth with depression and anxiety disorders.[5,75] Thus, Dunn et al.[64] demonstrated more depression in adolescent girls with epilepsy. Younger children with epilepsy have more anxiety disorders, whereas adolescents have more depression.[41,192]

Psychosis

A recent epidemiologic study demonstrated a higher rate of a schizophrenia-like psychosis in epilepsy than in the general population.[204] They also found an association with both a family history of schizophrenia and a family history of psychosis. Unlike adults with epilepsy, postictal psychosis[189] has been rarely described in children. In contrast, about 10% of children with TLE[150] and complex partial seizures[37,41] have an interictal schizophrenia-like psychosis. These children present with hallucinations, delusions, and formal thought disorder, no negative signs, and poor seizure control.

Nonepileptic Seizures

Psychogenic nonepileptic seizures (PNES) can reflect a conversion disorder, a factitious disorder, malingering, or parental misinterpretation of the child's symptoms. The marked short- and long-term psychological morbidity associated with misdiagnosis of these disorders emphasizes the importance of recognizing these entities in youth with epilepsy.

Conversion Disorder (Pseudoseizures, Psychogenic Seizures, Nonepileptic Seizures)

In a conversion disorder,[8] the child's seizures or convulsions suggest that he has epilepsy and suffers significant distress or impairment from these attacks. Appropriate investigations do not confirm the epileptic basis for these episodes. Psychological factors, in the form of conflicts or stressors, however, initiate or exacerbate these attacks. The child with a conversion disorder does not intentionally produce or feign the seizures. This disorder is found in children and adolescents with normal IQ scores,[171] albeit varying degrees of learning difficulties, and in children with mild to moderate retardation.[116] Girls are affected more than boys,[74,92] and the incidence increases with age. The disorder is more common in children with a diagnosis of epilepsy and in those without epilepsy who have some exposure to epilepsy through a family member, a neighbor, or a friend.

The symptoms most commonly found in children and adolescents with PNES include: slow onset of seizures with a gradual build-up, prolonged duration, the absence of bodily injury or loss of continence, thrusting, jerking, or shaking motions rather than repeated fast flexion and extension, and the absence of a postictal period.[273]

These children often have difficulty expressing negative feelings, such as anger, or their expression of these feeling are unheard or minimized by family members. Social difficulties, strife with parents, learning difficulties,[234] or sexual abuse can give rise to the negative feelings associated with the primary conflict. The child's epileptic events increase the amount of attention the child gets and decreases demands, such as going to school. By reinforcing the child's symptoms, this secondary gain prevents the child from dealing with his problems in an adaptive manner. Although concerned about their seizures, these children minimize or deny any concern about the problems and difficulties in their lives even when these are significant.

Given the maladaptive nature of the symptoms of this disorder, a definitive diagnosis is needed as soon as possible. Wyllie et al.[273] reported a good outcome in 14 of 18 children and adolescents diagnosed with NES who had their symptoms for a mean duration of 7 months.

Factitious Disorders

Factitious disorders[8] involve intentional production or feigning of seizure symptoms specifically to assume the sick role. Unlike malingering, there are no external incentives for these behaviors, such as avoiding a legal responsibility like going to school. More commonly, the parent rather than the child has the factitious disorder and imposes a diagnosis of epilepsy on the child, as in Munchausen syndrome by proxy. Many of the reported Munchausen syndrome by proxy cases have presented with seizures.[140,165,212,272] In Meadow's series of 76 cases, 32 children had a primary diagnosis of epilepsy. In 21 cases, the mothers fabricated the symptoms of the illness.[168,170] In 11 cases, the mothers caused seizures by suffocation, carotid sinus pressure, or use of drugs. Sixteen of the children in Meadow's sample had medical symptoms other than seizures. In Rosenberg's series, 42% of the 117 cases presented with seizures.[212] It is important to note that Munchausen syndrome by proxy can also occur in a child with genuine epilepsy.[170]

Unlike other disorders, clinicians do not usually observe the seizures of children with epilepsy and need to rely on parental report for a description of the clinical manifestations of the child's seizure.[165] Because it is difficult to confirm parental reports, it is relatively easy for a parent to fabricate a history of seizures and a lack of response to AEDs in the child.[168]

These cases present with a history of uncontrolled seizures; an inconsistent description of the child's seizures; repeated normal EEG recordings; repeated consultation with different physicians, particularly if the physician determines that no evidence suggests that the child has epilepsy. Other than the parent, no medical or school personnel have observed the child have a seizure. The mothers of these children,[165] sometimes employed in the healthcare field, are often very knowledgeable about epilepsy, EEG findings, and the use of AEDs. They are concerned and devoted to the child, and appear at ease in the hospital, even forming close relationships with hospital staff. The fathers usually are absent or play no role in the sick process, so that they appear to be in "passive collusion"[170] with the mother. In some cases of Munchausen syndrome by proxy, the father has been described as the perpetrator.[158]

Misinterpretation of Children's Behavior

Misinterpretation of the child's behaviors as epileptic seizures can reflect parental anxiety.[169] Several investigators have shown that the primary reason for nonepileptic events in children, particularly those with impaired intellectual function, was misinterpretation of behavior by parents and caretakers.[60,171,187] These behaviors included staring episodes, abnormal reactions to environmental stimuli, and repetitive movements, such as rocking, shaking, or arm waving. Unusual movements based on abnormal muscle tone were also often misinterpreted as seizures.[187]

Unlike Munchausen syndrome by proxy, these cases usually present with fewer episodes. In addition, the parent's main concern is that their child recovers rather than need repeated medical examinations and procedures.

SUMMARY AND CONCLUSIONS

In summary, epilepsy is a chronic and episodic disease of the brain that can affect the child's emotional, cognitive, and linguistic functioning and, therefore, his intrapsychic and interpersonal functioning within the family, with peers, and in the academic and social environment of school. The response of the child's family to these stressors affects the way the child copes with the disorder. In addition to these psychodynamic and social factors, seizure-related (i.e., type of seizure disorder, seizure control, seizure duration, number and blood level of AEDs) and developmental factors (i.e., age of onset of seizures, level of cognitive and language function) affect the child's functioning and ability to cope with his illness.

The research of the past decade has demonstrated that epilepsy is a biopsychosocial disorder and that children with epilepsy have comorbid difficulties with behavior, cognition, and language. They have also shown that parents shoulder a heavy burden. Studies are sorely needed to determine optimal approaches for early identification and treatment of these comorbid problems, as well as how best to implement them.

ACKNOWLEDGMENTS

This work was supported by NINDs funded grants NS3270 (RC) and MH067187 (RC).

We wish to thank Anette Abeyta for her technical assistance in preparation of this manuscript.

References

1. Achenbach T. *Manual for the Child Behavior Checklist and Revised Child Behavior Profile*. Vermont: Department of Psychiatry, University of Vermont, 1991.
2. Addy DP. Cognitive function in children with epilepsy. *Dev Med Child Neurol*. 1987;29(3):394–397.
3. Aicardi J, Mumford JP, Dumas C, et al. Vigabatrin as initial therapy for infantile spasms: A European retrospective survey. Sabril IS Investigator and Peer Review Groups. *Epilepsia*. 1996;37(7):638–642.
4. Aldenkamp AP, Arends J. The relative influence of epileptic EEG discharges, short nonconvulsive seizures, and type of epilepsy on cognitive function. *Epilepsia*. 2004;45:54–63.
5. American Psychiatric Association. *Diagnostic and Statistical Manual of Mental Disorders,* 4th ed. (DSM-IV). Washington, DC: American Psychiatric Association, 1994.
6. Angold A, Costello E, Worthman C. Puberty and depression: The roles of age, pubertal status and pubertal timing. *Psychol Med*. 1988;28:51–61.
7. Asano E, Chugani DC, Muzik O, et al. Autism in tuberous sclerosis complex is related to both cortical and subcortical dysfunction. *Neurology*. 2001;57(7):1269–1277.
8. Askalan R, Mackay M, Brian J, et al. Prospective preliminary analysis of the development of autism and epilepsy in children with infantile spasms. *J Child Neurol*. 2003;18(3):165–170.
9. Austin J, Dunn D, Huster G. Childhood epilepsy and asthma: Changes in behavior problems related to gender and change in condition severity. *Epilepsia*. 2000;41:615–623.
10. Austin J, Dunn DW, Johnson CS. Behavioral issues involving children and adolescents with epilepsy and the impact of their families: Recent research data. *Epilepsy Behav*. 2004;5:S33–S41.
11. Austin J, Dunn D, Levstek D. First seizures: Concerns and needs of parents and children. *Epilepsia*. 1993;34(Suppl 6):24.
12. Austin J, Harezlak J, Dunn D, et al. Behavior problems in children before first recognized seizures. *Pediatrics*. 2001;107:115–122.
13. Austin J, Huberty T. Development of the Child Attitude Toward Illness Scale. *J Pediatr. Psychol*. 1993;18:467–480.
14. Austin J, Huster G, Dunn D. Adolescents with active or inactive epilepsy or asthma: A comparison of quality of life. *Epilepsia*. 1996;37:1228–1238.
15. Austin J, McBride A, Davis H. Parental attitude and adjustment to childhood epilepsy. *Nurs Res*. 1984;33:92–96.
16. Austin J, Risinger M, Beckett L. Correlates of behavioral problems in children with epilepsy. *Epilepsia*. 1992;33:1115–1122.
17. Austin JK, Dunn DW, Caffrey HM, et al. Recurrent seizures and behavior problems in children with first recognized seizures: A prospective study. *Epilepsia*. 2002;43:1564–1573.
18. Austin JK, Huberty TJ, Huster GA, et al. Academic achievement in children with epilepsy or asthma. *Dev Med Child Neurol*. 1998;40:248–255.
19. Austin JK, Shafer PO, Deering JB. Epilepsy familiarity, knowledge, and perceptions of stigma: Report from a survey of adolescents in the general population. *Epilepsy Behav*. 2002;3(4):368–375.
20. Ballaban-Gil K, Tuchman R. Epilepsy and epileptiform EEG: Association with autism and language disorders. *Ment Retard Dev Disabil Res Rev*. 2000;6(4):300–308.
21. Beaumanoir A. The Landau-Kleffner Syndrome. In: Dravet C, Bureau M, Dreifuss FE, Wolf P, eds. *Epileptic Syndromes in Infancy: Childhood and Adolescence*. London: John Libby, 1985.
22. Besag FM. Behavioral aspects of pediatric epilepsy syndromes. *Epilepsy Behav*. 2004;5(Suppl 1):S3–13.
23. Bibace R, Walsh ME. Development of children's concepts of illness. *Pediatrics*. 1980;66(6):912–917.
24. Bishop M, Slevin B. Teachers' attitudes toward students with epilepsy: Results of a survey of elementary and middle school teachers. *Epilepsy Behav*. 2004;5(3):308–315.
25. Bolton PF, Griffiths PD. Association of tuberous sclerosis of temporal lobes with autism and atypical autism [see comments]. *Lancet*. 1997;349(9049):392–395.

26. Bourgeois BF, Prensky AL, Palkes HS, et al. Intelligence in epilepsy: A prospective study in children. *Ann Neurol.* 1983;14(4):438–444.
27. Bradley C. Behavior disturbances in epileptic children. *JAMA.* 1951;146(5):436–441.
28. Brent D, Crumrine P, Varma R, et al. Phenobarbital treatment and major depressive disorder in children with epilepsy. *Pediatrics.* 1986;80:909–917.
29. Brent D, Crumrine P, Varma R, et al. Phenobarbital treatment and major depressive disorder in children with epilepsy. *Pediatrics.* 1987;80:909–917.
30. Brent D, Crumrine P, Varma R, et al. Phenobarbital treatment and major depressive disorder in children with epilepsy: A naturalistic follow up. *Pediatrics.* 1990;85:1086–1091.
31. Buelow J, Austin J, Perkins S, et al. Behavior and mental health problems in children with epilepsy and low IQ. *Dev Med Child Neurol.* 2003;45:683–692.
32. Bulteau C, Jambaque I, Viguier D, et al. Epileptic syndromes, cognitive assessment and school placement: A study of 251 children. *Dev Med Child Neurol.* 2000;42(5):319–327.
33. Bureau M. Continuous Spikes and Waves During Slow Sleep (CSWS): Definition of the Syndrome. In: Beaumanoir A, Bureau M, Deonna T, Mira L, Tassinari C, eds. *Continuous Spikes and Waves During Slow Sleep: Electrical Status Epilepticus During Slow Sleep.* London: John Libbey; 1995: 17–26.
34. Camfield CS, Chaplin S, Doyle AB, et al. Side effects of phenobarbital in toddlers; behavioral and cognitive aspects. *J Pediatr.* 1979;95(3):361–365.
35. Canovas Martinez A, Ordovas Baines JP, Beltran Marques M, et al. Vigabatrin-associated reversible acute psychosis in a child. *Ann Pharmacother.* 1995;29(11):1115–1117.
36. Caplin D, Austin JK, Dunn DW, et al. Development of a self-efficacy scale for children and adolescents with epilepsy. *Children Health Care.* 2002;31:295–309.
37. Caplan R, Arbelle S, Magharious W, et al. Psychopathology in pediatric complex partial and generalized epilepsy. *Dev Med Child Neurology.* 1998;40:805–811.
38. Caplan R, Austin JK. Behavioral aspects of epilepsy in children with mental retardation. *Ment Retard Dev Disabil Res Rev.* 2000;6(4):293–299.
39. Caplan R, Guthrie D, Komo S, et al. Conversational repair in pediatric complex partial seizure disorder. *Brain Language.* 2001;78:82–93.
40. Caplan R, Guthrie D, Komo S, et al. Social communication in children with epilepsy. *J Child Psychol Psychiatry.* 2002;43(2):245–253.
41. Caplan R, Shields WD, Mori L, et al. Middle childhood onset of interictal psychosis. *J Am Acad Child Adolesc Psychiatry.* 1991;30(6):893–896.
42. Caplan R, Siddarth P, Gurbani S, et al. Psychopathology and pediatric complex partial seizures: Seizure-related, cognitive, and linguistic variables. *Epilepsia.* 2004;45:1273–1286.
43. Caplan R, Siddarth P, Gurbani S, et al. Depression and anxiety disorders in pediatric epilepsy. *Epilepsia.* 2005;46(5):720–730.
44. Caplan R, Siddarth P, Mathern G, et al. Developmental outcome with and without successful intervention. *Int Rev Neurobiol.* 2002;49:269–284.
45. Carmant L, Holmes GL, Sawyer S, et al. Efficacy of felbamate in therapy for partial epilepsy in children. *J Pediatr.* 1994;125(3):481–486.
46. Cass H, Reilly S, Owen L, et al. Findings from a multidisciplinary clinical case series of females with Rett syndrome. *Dev Med Child Neurol.* 2003;45(5):325–337.
47. Cederlund M, Gillberg C. One hundred males with Asperger syndrome: A clinical study of background and associated factors. *Dev Med Child Neurol.* 2004;46(10):652–660.
48. Chapieski L, Brewer V, Evankovich K, et al. Adaptive functioning in children with seizures: Impact of maternal anxiety about epilepsy. *Epilepsy Behav.* 2005;7:246–252.
49. Chez MG, Chang M, Krasne V, et al. Frequency of epileptiform EEG abnormalities in a sequential screening of autistic patients with no known clinical epilepsy from 1996 to 2005. *Epilepsy Behav.* 2006;8(1):267–271.
50. Coulter DL, Koester BS. Information needs of parents of children with epilepsy. *J Dev Behav Pediatr.* 1985;6(6):334–338.
51. Croona C, Kihlgren M, Lundberg S, et al. Neuropsychological findings in children with benign childhood epilepsy with centrotemporal spikes. *Dev Med Child Neurol.* 1999;41(12):813–818.
52. Curatolo P. *Tuberous Sclerosis Complex: From Basic Science to Clinical Phenotypes.* London: MacKeith Press, 2003.
53. Danielsson S, Gillberg IC, Billstedt E, et al. Epilepsy in young adults with autism: A prospective population-based follow-up study of 120 individuals diagnosed in childhood. *Epilepsia.* 2005;46(6):918–923.
54. Davidson S, Falconer MA. Outcome of surgery in 40 children with temporal-lobe epilepsy. *Lancet.* 1975;1(7919):1260–1263.
55. Davies S, Heyman I, Goodman R. A population survey of mental health problems in children with epilepsy. *Dev Med Child Neurology.* 2003;45:292–295.
56. Deonna TW. Acquired epileptiform aphasia in children (Landau-Kleffner syndrome). *J Clin Neurophysiol.* 1991;8(3):288–298.
57. Devinsky O, Westbrook L, Cramer J, et al. Risk factors for poor health-related quality of life in adolescents with epilepsy. *Epilepsia.* 1999;40:1715–1720.
58. Deykin EY, MacMahon B. The incidence of seizures among children with autistic symptoms. *Am J Psychiatry.* 1979;136(10):1310–1312.
59. Dodrill CB, Temkin NR. Motor speed is a contaminating factor in evaluating the "cognitive" effects of phenytoin. *Epilepsia.* 1989;30(4):453–457.
60. Duchowny MS, Levin B JP, Resnick R, et al. Temporal lobectomy in early childhood. *Epilepsia.* 1992;33:298–303.
61. Dulac O, Plouin P, Jambaque I. Predicting favorable outcome in idiopathic West syndrome. *Epilepsia.* 1993;34(4):747–756.
62. Dunn D, Austin J, Caffrey H, et al. A prospective study of teachers' ratings of behavior problems in children with new-onset seizures. *Epilepsy Behav.* 2003;4:26–35.
63. Dunn DW, Austin JK, Harezlak J, et al. ADHD and epilepsy in childhood. *Dev Med Child Neurol.* 2003;45(1):50–54.
64. Dunn D, Austin J, Huster G. Symptoms of depression in adolescents with epilepsy. *J Am Acad Child Adolesc Psychiatry.* 1999;38:1132–1138.
65. Dunn DW, Harezlak J, Ambrosius WT, et al. Teacher assessment of behaviour in children with new-onset seizures. *Seizure.* 2002;11(3):169–175.
66. Eastman M, Ritter F, Risse G, et al. Impact of child's epilepsy on the parents. *Epilepsia.* 1999;40 (Suppl 7):129.
67. Ehlers S, Gillberg C. The epidemiology of Asperger syndrome. A total population study. *J Child Psychol Psychiatry.* 1993;34(8):1327–1350.
68. Eiser C, Havermans T, Pancer M, et al. Adjustment to chronic disease in relation to age and gender: Mothers' and fathers' reports of their childrens' behavior. *J Pediatr Psychol.* 1992;17(3):261–275.
69. Elia M, Musumeci SA, Ferri R, et al. Clinical and neurophysiological aspects of epilepsy in subjects with autism and mental retardation. *Am J Ment Retard.* 1995;100(1):6–16.
70. Ellenberg JH, Hirtz DG, Nelson KB. Age at onset of seizures in young children. *Ann Neurol.* 1984;15(2):127–134.
71. Ettinger AB, Weisbrot DM, Nolan EE, et al. Symptoms of depression and anxiety in pediatric epilepsy patients. *Epilepsia.* 1998;39:595–599.
72. Fastenau PS, Shen J, Dunn DW, et al. Neuropsychological predictors of academic underachievement in pediatric epilepsy: Moderating roles of demographic, seizure, and psychosocial variables. *Epilepsia.* 2004;45(10):1261–1272.
73. Feldman H, Crumrine P, Handen BL, et al. Methylphenidate in children with seizures and attention-deficit disorder. *Am J Dis Child.* 1989;143(9):1081–1086.
74. Finlayson RE, Lucas AR. Pseudoepileptic seizures in children and adolescents. *Mayo Clin Proc.* 1979;54(2):83–87.
75. Flemming J, Offord D. Epidemiology of childhood depressive disorders: A critical review. *J Am Acad Child Adolesc Psychiatry.* 1990;29:571–580.
76. Fombonne E. Epidemiological surveys of autism and other pervasive developmental disorders: An update. *J Autism Dev Disord.* 2003;33(4):365–382.
77. Fombonne E. Epidemiology of autistic disorder and other pervasive developmental disorders. *J Clin Psychiatry.* 2005;66(Suppl 10):3–8.
78. Freitag H, Tuxhorn I. Cognitive function in preschool children after epilepsy surgery: Rationale for early intervention. *Epilepsia.* 2005;46(4):561–567.
79. Galanopoulou A, Vidaurre J, McVicar KA, et al. Language and behavioral disturbances associated with epileptiform EEGs. *Am J End Technol.* 2002;42:181–209.
80. Gillberg C. Outcome and prognostic factors in infantile autism and similar conditions: A population-based study of 46 cases followed through puberty. *J Autism Dev Dis.* 1987;17:273–287.
81. Gillberg C. *Autism and Asperger Syndrome.* Cambridge: Cambridge University Press, 1991.
82. Gillberg C, Steffenburg S. Outcome and prognostic factors in infantile autism and similar conditions: A population-based study of 46 cases followed through puberty. *J Autism Dev Disord.* 1987;17(2):273–287.
83. Gillberg C, Steffenburg S, Jakobsson G. Neurobiological findings in 20 relatively gifted children with Kanner-type autism or Asperger syndrome. *Dev Med Child Neurol.* 1987;29(5):641–649.
84. Gilliam F. Diagnosis and treatment of mood disorders in persons with epilepsy. *Curr Opin Neurol.* 2005;18:129–133.
85. Giovanardi Rossi P, Posar A, et al. Epilepsy in adolescents and young adults with autistic disorder. *Brain Dev.* 2000;22(2):102–106.
86. Glaze DG. Neurophysiology of Rett syndrome. *Ment Retard Dev Disabil Res Rev.* 2002;8(2):66–71.
87. Gomez M. *Tuberous Sclerosis.* New York: Raven Press, 1988.
88. Gordon AG. Ear disease in Landau-Kleffner syndrome (LKS) and in adult psychiatry. *Can J Psychiatry.* 1989;34(1):77–78.
89. Green JR, Pootrakul A. Surgical aspects of the treatment of epilepsy during childhood and adolescence. *Ariz Med.* 1982;39(1):35–38.
90. Gross-Tsur V, Manor O, van der Meere J, et al. Epilepsy and attention deficit hyperactivity disorder: Is methylphenidate safe and effective? *J Pediatr.* 1997;130(4):670–674.
91. Gross-Tsur V, Shalev RS. Reversible language regression as an adverse effect of topiramate treatment in children. *Neurology.* 2004;62(2):299–300.
92. Gross M, Huerta E. Functional convulsions masked as epileptic disorders. *J Pediatr Psychol.* 1980;5(1):71–79.
93. Gucuyener K, Erdemoglu AK, Senol S, et al. Use of methylphenidate for attention-deficit hyperactivity disorder in patients with epilepsy or electroencephalographic abnormalities. *J Child Neurol.* 2003;18(2):109–112.
94. Gutierrez GC, Smalley SL, Tanguay PE. Autism in tuberous sclerosis complex. *J Autism Dev Disord.* 1998;28(2):97–103.
95. Harbord MG. Significant anticonvulsant side-effects in children and adolescents. *J Clin Neurosci.* 2000;7(3):213–216.
96. Hartlage LC, Green JB, Offutt L. Dependency in epileptic children. *Epilepsia.* 1972;13(1):27–30.

97. Harvey AS, Berkovic SF, Wrennall JA, et al. Temporal lobe epilepsy in childhood: Clinical, EEG, and neuroimaging findings and syndrome classification in a cohort with new-onset seizures. *Neurology.* 1997;49(4):960–968.
98. Hauser ST, DiPlacido J, Jacobson AM, et al. Family coping with an adolescent's chronic illness: An approach and three studies. *J Adolesc.* 1993;16(3):305–329.
99. Heimlich T, Westbrook L, Austin J, et al. Brief report: Adolescents' attitudes toward epilepsy: Further validation of the Child Attitude Toward Illness Scale (CATIS). *J Pediatr Psychol.* 2000;25:339–345.
100. Heisler AB, Friedman SB. Social and psychological considerations in chronic disease: With particular reference to the management of seizure disorders. *J Pediatr Psychol.* 1981;6(3):239–250.
101. Hellgren L, Gillberg IC, Bagenholm A, et al. Children with deficits in attention, motor control and perception (DAMP) almost grown up: Psychiatric and personality disorders at age 16 years. *J Child Psychol Psychiatry.* 1994;35(7):1255–1271.
102. Hempel A, Frost MD, Ritter FJ. Factors influencing the incidence of ADHD in pediatric epilepsy patients. *Epilepsia.* 1995;36(Suppl 4):122.
103. Hermann BP, Whitman S, Hughes JR, et al. Multietiological determinants of psychopathology and social competence in children with epilepsy. *Epilepsy Res.* 1988;2:51–60.
104. Hernandez M, Sauerwein HC J, Jambaque I, et al. Attention, memory, and behavioral adjustment in children with frontal lobe epilepsy. *Epilepsy Behav.* 2003;4:522–536.
105. Herranz J, Armijo JA, Arteaga R. Clinical side effects of phenobarbital, primidone, phenytoin, carbamazepine, and valproate during monotherapy in children. *Epilepsia.* 1988;29:794–804.
106. Hesdorffer DC, Ludvigsson P, Olafsson E, et al. ADHD as a risk factor for incident unprovoked seizures and epilepsy in children. *Arch Gen Psychiatry.* 2004;61(7):731–736.
107. Hirsch E, Marescaux C, Maquet P, et al. Landau-Kleffner syndrome: A clinical and EEG study of five cases. *Epilepsia.* 1990;31(6):756–767.
108. Hoare P. The development of psychiatric disorders among schoolchildren with epilepsy. *Dev Med Child Neurol.* 1984;26:3–13.
109. Hoare P. Does illness foster dependency? A study of epileptic and diabetic children. *Dev Med Child Neurol.* 1984;26(1):20–24.
110. Hoare P, Kerley S. Psychosocial adjustment of children with chronic epilepsy and their families. *Dev Med Child Neurol.* 1991;33(3):201–215.
111. Hodes M, Garralda ME, Rose G, et al. Maternal expressed emotion and adjustment in children with epilepsy. *J Child Psychol Psychiatry.* 1999;40:1083–1093.
112. Holdsworth L, Whitmore K. A study of children with epilepsy attending ordinary schools. II: Information and attitudes held by their teachers. *Dev Med Child Neurol.* 1974;16(6):759–765.
113. Holmes GL. Do seizures cause brain damage? *Epilepsia.* 1991;32(Suppl 5):S14–28.
114. Holmes GL. Effects of seizures on brain development: Lessons from the laboratory. *Pediatr Neurol.* 2005;33(1):1–11.
115. Holmes GL, McKeever M, Saunders Z. Epileptiform activity in aphasia of childhood: An epiphenomenon? *Epilepsia.* 1981;22(6):631–639.
116. Holmes GL, Sackellares JC, McKiernan J, et al. Evaluation of childhood pseudoseizures using EEG telemetry and video tape monitoring. *J Pediatr.* 1980;97(4):554–558.
117. Holtmann M, Schmidt MH. Behavior problems in nonepileptic children with rolandic epileptiform discharges. *Epilepsia.* 2003;44(6):875.
118. Hopkins IJ, Klug GL. Temporal lobectomy for the treatment of intractable complex partial seizures of temporal lobe origin in early childhood. *Dev Med Child Neurol.* 1991;33(1):26–31.
119. Houston EC, Cunningham CC, Metcalfe E, et al. The information needs and understanding of 5 10-year-old children with epilepsy, asthma or diabetes. *Seizure.* 2000;9(5):340–343.
120. Hrachovy RA, Frost JD, Jr. Infantile epileptic encephalopathy with hypsarrhythmia (infantile spasms/West syndrome). *J Clin Neurophysiol.* 2003;20(6):408–425.
121. Huang LT, Holmes GL, Lai MC, et al. Maternal deprivation stress exacerbates cognitive deficits in immature rats with recurrent seizures. *Epilepsia.* 2002;43(10):1141–1148.
122. Hunt A, Dennis J. Psychiatric disorder among children with tuberous sclerosis. *Dev Med Child Neurol.* 1987;29(2):190–198.
123. ILAE. Proposal for revised classification of epilepsies and epileptic syndromes. Commission on Classification and Terminology of the International League Against Epilepsy. *Epilepsia.* 1989;30(4):389–399.
124. Irwin K, Birch V, Lees J, et al. Multiple subpial transection in Landau-Kleffner syndrome. *Dev Med Child Neurol.* 2001;43(4):248–252.
125. Jambaque I, Chiron C, Dumas C, et al. Mental and behavioural outcome of infantile epilepsy treated by vigabatrin in tuberous sclerosis patients. *Epilepsy Res.* 2000;38(2–3):151–160.
126. Jones JE, Hermann BP, Barry JJ, et al. Rates and risk factors for suicide, suicidal ideation, and suicide attempts in chronic epilepsy. *Epilepsy Behav.* 2003;4(Suppl 3):S31–8.
127. Kanner AM. Commentary: The treatment of seizure disorders and EEG abnormalities in children with autistic spectrum disorders: Are we getting ahead of ourselves? *J Autism Dev Disord.* 2000;30(5):491–495.
128. Kawasaki Y, Yokota K, Shinomiya M, et al. Brief report: Electroencephalographic paroxysmal activities in the frontal area emerged in middle childhood and during adolescence in a follow-up study of autism. *J Autism Dev Disord.* 1997;27(5):605–620.
129. Khurana DS, Riviello J, Helmers S, et al. Efficacy of gabapentin therapy in children with refractory partial seizures. *J Pediatr.* 1996;128(6):829–833.
130. Kinney RO, Shaywitz BA, Shaywitz SE, et al. Epilepsy in children with attention deficit disorder: Cognitive, behavioral, and neuroanatomic indices. *Pediatr Neurol.* 1990;6(1):31–37.
131. Kivity S, Lerman P, Ariel R, et al. Long-term cognitive outcomes of a cohort of children with cryptogenic infantile spasms treated with high-dose adrenocorticotropic hormone. *Epilepsia.* 2004;45(3):255–262.
132. Kobayashi R, Murata T. Setback phenomenon in autism and long-term prognosis. *Acta Psychiatr Scand.* 1998;98(4):296–303.
133. Korkman M, Granstrom ML, Kantola-Sorsa E, et al. Two-year follow-up of intelligence after pediatric epilepsy surgery. *Pediatr Neurol.* 2005;33(3):173–178.
134. Kossoff EH, Bergey GK, Freeman JM, et al. Levetiracetam psychosis in children with epilepsy. *Epilepsia.* 2001;42(12):1611–1613.
135. Kossoff EH, Buck C, Freeman JM. Outcomes of 32 hemispherectomies for Sturge-Weber syndrome worldwide. *Neurology.* 2002;59(11):1735–1738.
136. Kovacs M. The Children's Depression Inventory (CDI). *Psychopharmacol Bull.* 1985;21:995–998.
137. Kurita H, Kita M, Miyake Y. A comparative study of development and symptoms among disintegrative psychosis and infantile autism with and without speech loss. *J Autism Dev Disord.* 1992;22(2):175–188.
138. Kwan P, Brodie MJ. Drug treatment of epilepsy: When does it fail and how to optimize its use? *CNS Spectr.* 2004;9:110–119.
139. Kyllerman M, Nyden A, Praquin N, et al. Transient psychosis in a girl with epilepsy and continuous spikes and waves during slow sleep (CSWS). *Eur Child Adolesc Psychiatry.* 1996;5(4):216–221.
140. Lacey SR, Cooper C, Runyan DK, et al. Munchausen syndrome by proxy: Patterns of presentation to pediatric surgeons. *J Pediatr Surg.* 1993;28(6):827–832.
141. Lado FA, Sankar R, Lowenstein D, et al. Age-dependent consequences of seizures: Relationship to seizure frequency, brain damage, and circuitry reorganization. *Ment Retard Dev Disabil Res Rev.* 2000;6(4):242–252.
142. Landau WM, Kleffner F. Syndrome of acquired aphasia with convulsive disorder in children. *Neurology.* 1957;7:523–530.
143. Lazarus R. *Stress, Appraisal, and Coping.* New York: Springer, 1984.
144. Lefkowitz MM, Tesiny EP, Gordon NH. Childhood depression, family income, and locus of control. *J Nerv Ment Dis.* 1980;168(12):732–735.
145. Lendt M, Helmstaedter C, Kuczaty S, et al. Behavioural disorders in children with epilepsy: Early improvement after surgery. *J Neurol Neurosurg Psychiatry.* 2000;69(6):739–744.
146. Leonard BJ. *The Adolescent with Epilepsy.* Orlando: Grune and Stratton; 1984.
147. Lerman P, Lerman-Sagie T, Kivity S. Effect of early corticosteroid therapy for Landau-Kleffner syndrome. *Dev Med Child Neurol.* 1991;33(3):257–260.
148. Lewine JD, Andrews R, Chez M, et al. Magnetoencephalographic patterns of epileptiform activity in children with regressive autism spectrum disorders. *Pediatrics.* 1999;104(3 Pt 1):405–418.
149. Lindsay J, Glaser G, Richards P, et al. Developmental aspects of focal epilepsies of childhood treated by neurosurgery. *Dev Med Child Neurol.* 1984;26(5):574–587.
150. Lindsay J, Ounsted C, Richards P. Long-term outcome in children with temporal lobe seizures I: Social outcome and childhood factors. *Dev Med Child Neurol.* 1979;21:285–298.
151. Lindsay J, Ounsted C, Richards P. Long-term outcome in children with temporal lobe seizures III: Psychiatric aspects in childhood and adult life. *Dev Med Child Neurol.* 1979;21:630–636.
152. Lord C, Shulman C, DiLavore P. Regression and word loss in autistic spectrum disorders. *J Child Psychol Psychiatry.* 2004;45(5):936–955.
153. Loring DW, Meador KJ. Cognitive side effects of antiepileptic drugs in children. *Neurology.* 2004;62(6):872–877.
154. Lothman D, Pianta R. Role of child-mother interaction in predicting competence of children with epilepsy. *Epilepsia.* 1993;34:658–669.
155. Lux AL, Edwards SW, Hancock E, et al. The United Kingdom Infantile Spasms Study (UKISS) comparing hormone treatment with vigabatrin on developmental and epilepsy outcomes to age 14 months: A multicentre randomised trial. *Lancet Neurol.* 2005;4(11):712–717.
156. Luyster R, Richler J, Risi S, et al. Early regression in social communication in autistic spectrum disorders: A CPEA study. *Dev Neuropsychol.* 2005;27(3):311–326.
157. MacLeod JS, Austin JK. Stigma in the lives of adolescents with epilepsy: A review of the literature. *Epilepsy Behav.* 2003;4(2):112–117.
158. Makar AF, Squier PJ. Munchausen syndrome by proxy: Father as a perpetrator. *Pediatrics.* 1990;85(3):370–373.
159. Mantovani JF. Autistic regression and Landau-Kleffner syndrome: Progress or confusion? *Dev Med Child Neurol.* 2000;42(5):349–353.
160. Marescaux C, Hirsch E, Finck S, et al. Landau-Kleffner syndrome: A pharmacologic study of five cases. *Epilepsia.* 1990;31(6):768–777.
161. Massa R, de Saint-Martin A, Hirsch E, et al. Landau-Kleffner syndrome: Sleep EEG characteristics at onset. *Clin Neurophysiol.* 2000;111(Suppl 2):S87–S93.
162. Matthews W, Barabas G, Ferrari M. Achievement and school behavior among children with epilepsy. *Psychol Sch.* 1983;20:10–12.

163. Matthews WS, Barabas G. *Perceptions of Control Among Children with Epilepsy*. New York: Oxford University Press, 1986.
164. McCusker C, Kennedy P, Anderson J, et al. Adjustment in children with intractable epilepsy: Importance of seizure duration and family factors. *Dev Med Child Neurology*. 2002;44(10):681–687.
165. McGuire TL, Feldman KW. Psychologic morbidity of children subjected to Munchausen syndrome by proxy. *Pediatrics*. 1989;83(2):289–292.
166. McVicar KA, Ballaban-Gil K, Raglin I, et al. Epileptiform EEG abnormalities in children with language regression. *Neurology*. 2005;65(1): 29–31.
167. McVicar KA, Shinnar S. Landau-Kleffner syndrome, electrical status epilepticus in slow wave sleep, and language regression in children. *Ment Retard Dev Disabil Res Rev*. 2004;10(2):144–149.
168. Meadow R. Fictitious epilepsy. *Lancet*. 1984;2(8393):25–28.
169. Meadow R. Munchausen syndrome by proxy. *Brit Med J*. 1989;299:248–250.
170. Meadow R. Neurological and developmental variants of Munchausen syndrome by proxy. *Dev Med Child Neurol*. 1991;33(3):270–272.
171. Metrick ME, Ritter FJ, Gates JR, et al. Nonepileptic events in childhood. *Epilepsia*. 1991;32(3):322–328.
172. Mikati MA, Choueri R, Khurana DS, et al. Gabapentin in the treatment of refractory partial epilepsy in children with intellectual disability. *J Intellect Disabil Res*. 1998;42(Suppl 1):57–62.
173. Mikati MA, Saab R. Successful use of intravenous immunoglobulin as initial monotherapy in Landau-Kleffner syndrome. *Epilepsia*. 2000;41(7):880–886.
174. Minshew N, Sweeney JA, Bauman ML. Neurologic Aspects of Autism. In: Cohen DJ, Volkmar FR, eds. *Handbook of Autism and Pervasive Developmental Disorders,* 2nd ed. New York: Wiley; 1997: 344–369.
175. Mitchell W, Chavez JM, Lee H, et al. Academic underachievement in children with epilepsy. *J Child Neurol*. 1991;6(1):65–72.
176. Mitchell WG, Zhou Y, Chavez JM, et al. Reaction time, attention, and impulsivity in epilepsy. *Pediatr Neurol*. 1992;8(1):19–24.
177. Miyamoto T, Kohsaka M, Koyama T. Psychotic episodes during zonisamide treatment. *Seizure*. 2000;9(1):65–70.
178. Morrell F, Whisler WW, Smith MC, et al. Landau-Kleffner syndrome. Treatment with subpial intracortical transection. *Brain*. 1995;118(Pt 6): 1529–1546.
179. Mouridsen SE, Rich B, Isager T. Epilepsy in disintegrative psychosis and infantile autism: A long-term validation study. *Dev Med Child Neurol*. 1999;41(2):110–114.
180. Mouridsen SE, Rich B, Isager T. A comparative study of genetic and neurobiological findings in disintegrative psychosis and infantile autism. *Psychiatry Clin Neurosci*. 2000;54(4):441–446.
181. Mula M, Trimble M. The importance of being seizure free: Topiramate and psychopathology in epilepsy. *Epilepsy Behav*. 2003;4:430–4.
182. Mula M, Trimble MR, Sander JW. The role of hippocampal sclerosis in topiramate-related depression and cognitive deficits in people with epilepsy. *Epilepsia*. 2003;44(12):1573–1577.
183. Nass R, Devinsky O. Autistic regression with rolandic spikes. *Neuropsychiatry Neuropsychol Behav Neurol*. 1999;12(3):193–197.
184. Nass R, Gross A, Devinsky O. Autism and autistic epileptiform regression with occipital spikes. *Dev Med Child Neurol*. 1998;40(7):453–458.
185. Nass R, Gross A, Wisoff J, et al. Outcome of multiple subpial transections for autistic epileptiform regression. *Pediatr Neurol*. 1999;21(1):464–470.
186. Nass R, Heier L, Walker R. Landau-Kleffner syndrome: Temporal lobe tumor resection results in good outcome. *Pediatr Neurol*. 1993;9(4):303–305.
187. Neil J, Alvarez N. Differential diagnosis of epileptic versus pseudoepileptic seizures in disabled persons. *Appl Res Ment Retard*. 1986;7:285–298.
188. Nicolson A, Lewis SA, Smith DF. A prospective analysis of the outcome of levetiracetam in clinical practice. *Neurology*. 2004;63(3):568–570.
189. Nissenkorn A, Moldavsky M, Lorberboym M, et al. Postictal psychosis in a child. *J Child Neurol*. 1999;14(12):818–819.
190. Nuffield EJ. Neuro-physiology and behaviour disorders in epileptic children. *J Ment Sci*. 1961;107:438–458.
191. O'Leary DS, Lovell MR, Sackellares JC, et al. Effects of age of onset of partial and generalized seizures on neuropsychological performance in children. *J Nerv Ment Dis*. 1983;171(10):624–629.
192. Oguz A, Kurul S, Dirik E. Relationship of epilepsy-related factors to anxiety and depression scores in epileptic children. *J Child Neurol*. 2002;17:37–40.
193. Ohtsuka Y, Amano R, Mizukawa M, et al. Long-term prognosis of the Lennox-Gastaut syndrome. *Jpn J Psychiatry Neurol*. 1990;44(2):257–264.
194. Olsson I, Steffenburg S, Gillberg C. Epilepsy in autism and autistic like conditions. A population-based study. *Arch Neurol*. 1988;45(6):666–668.
195. Oostrom KJ, Schouten A, Kruitwagen CL, et al. Behavioral problems in children with newly diagnosed idiopathic or cryptogenic epilepsy attending normal schools are in majority not persistent. *Epilepsia*. 2003;44(1):97–106.
196. Oostrom K, Schouten A, Olthof T, et al. Negative emotions in children with newly diagnosed epilepsy. *Epilepsia*. 2000;41:326–331.
197. Oostrom K, van Teeseling H, Smeets-Schouten A, et al. Dutch Study of Epilepsy in Childhood (DuSECh). Three to four years after diagnosis: Cognition and behaviour in children with "epilepsy only." A prospective, controlled study. *Brain*. 2005;128:1546–1544.
198. Ott D, Caplan R, Guthrie D, et al. Measures of psychopathology in children with complex partial seizures and primary generalized epilepsy with absence. *J Am Acad Child Adolesc Psychiatry*. 2001;40:907–914.
199. Pascual-Castroviejo I. Nicardipine in the treatment of acquired aphasia and epilepsy. *Dev Med Child Neurol*. 1990;32(10):930.
200. Patry G, Lyagoubi S, Tassinari CA. Subclinical "electrical status epilepticus" induced by sleep in children. A clinical and electroencephalographic study of six cases. *Arch Neurol*. 1971;24(3):242–252.
201. Pavone P, Incorpora G, Fiumara A, et al. Epilepsy is not a prominent feature of primary autism. *Neuropediatrics*. 2004;35(4):207–210.
202. Pless IB. Clinical assessment: Physical and psychological functioning. *Pediatr Clin North Am*. 1984;31(1):33–45.
203. Pond DA. Psychiatric aspects of epileptic and brain-damaged children. *Br Med J*. 1961;5265:1454–1459.
204. Qin P, Xu H, Laursen TM, et al. Risk for schizophrenia and schizophrenia-like psychosis among patients with epilepsy: Population based cohort study. *Br Med J*. 2005;331(7507):23.
205. Rapin I, Mattis S, Rowan AJ, et al. Verbal auditory agnosia in children. *Dev Med Child Neurol*. 1977;19(2):197–207.
206. Reith D, Burke C, Appleton DB, et al. Tolerability of topiramate in children and adolescents. *J Paediatr Child Health*. 2003;39(6):416–419.
207. Riikonen R. A long-term follow-up study of 214 children with the syndrome of infantile spasms. *Neuropediatrics*. 1982;13(1):14–23.
208. Riikonen R. Long-term outcome of patients with West syndrome. *Brain Dev*. 2001;23(7):683–687.
209. Riikonen R, Amnell G. Psychiatric disorders in children with earlier infantile spasms. *Dev Med Child Neurol*. 1981;23(6):747–760.
210. Rimland B. On the objective diagnosis of infantile autism. *Acta Paedopsychiatr*. 1968;35(4):146–161.
211. Robinson RO, Baird G, Robinson G, et al. Landau-Kleffner syndrome: Course and correlates with outcome. *Dev Med Child Neurol*. 2001;43(4):243–247.
212. Rosenberg D. Web of deceit: A literature review of Munchausen by proxy. *Child Abuse Negl*. 1987;11:547–563.
213. Rossi PG, Parmeggiani A, Bach V, et al. EEG features and epilepsy in patients with autism [see comments]. *Brain Dev*. 1995;17(3):169–174.
214. Rossi PG, Parmeggiani A, Posar A, et al. Landau-Kleffner syndrome (LKS): Long-term follow-up and links with electrical status epilepticus during sleep (ESES). *Brain Dev*. 1999;21(2):90–98.
215. Roulet Perez E, Davidoff V, Despland PA, et al. Mental and behavioural deterioration of children with epilepsy and CSWS: Acquired epileptic frontal syndrome. *Dev Med Child Neurol*. 1993;35(8):661–674.
216. Roulet Perez E, Seeck M, Mayer E, et al. Childhood epilepsy with neuropsychological regression and continuous spike waves during sleep: Epilepsy surgery in a young adult. *Eur J Paediatr Neurol*. 1998;2(6):303–311.
217. Rutter M. Autistic children: Infancy to adulthood. *Semin Psychiatry*. 1970;2(4):435–450.
218. Rutter M, Graham P, Yule W. *A Neuropsychiatric Study in Childhood*. London: S.I.M.P. William Heinemann Medical Books Ltd., 1970.
219. Sanchez-Carpintero R, Neville BG. Attentional ability in children with epilepsy. *Epilepsia*. 2003;44(10):1340–1349.
220. Sanger MS, Perrin EC, Sandler HM. Development in children's causal theories of their seizure disorders. *J Dev Behav Pediatr*. 1993;14(2):88–93.
221. Sankar R. Initial treatment of epilepsy with antiepileptic drugs: Pediatric issues. *Neurology*. 2004;63(10 Suppl 4):S30–S9.
222. Sankar R, Holmes GL. Mechanisms of action for the commonly used antiepileptic drugs: Relevance to antiepileptic drug-associated neurobehavioral adverse effects. *J Child Neurol*. 2004;19(Suppl 1):S6–S14.
223. Sayin U, Sutula TP, Stafstrom CE. Seizures in the developing brain cause adverse long-term effects on spatial learning and anxiety. *Epilepsia*. 2004;45(12):1539–1548.
224. Sbarra DA, Rimm-Kaufman SE, Pianta RC. The behavioral and emotional correlates of epilepsy in adolescence: A 7-year follow-up study. *Epilepsy Behav*. 2002;3(4):358–367.
225. Schoenfeld J, Seidenberg M, Woodard A, et al. Neuropsychological and behavioral status of children with complex partial seizures. *Dev Med Child Neurol*. 1999;41:724–731.
226. Scholtes FB, Hendriks MP, Renier WO. Cognitive deterioration and electrical status epilepticus during slow sleep. *Epilepsy Behav*. 2005;6(2):167–173.
227. Semrud-Clikeman M, Wical B. Components of attention in children with complex partial seizures with and without ADHD. *Epilepsia*. 1999;40(2):211–215.
228. Sharpe D, Rossiter L. Siblings of children with a chronic illness: A meta-analysis. *J Pediatr Psychol*. 2002;27:699–710.
229. Shechter T, Shorer Z, Kramer U, et al. Adverse reactions of topiramate and lamotrigine in children. *Pharmacoepidemiol Drug Saf*. 2005;14(3):187–192.
230. Sheth RD, Buckley D, Penney S, et al. Vigabatrin in childhood epilepsy: Comparable efficacy for generalized and partial seizures. *Clin Neuropharmacol*. 1996;19(4):297–304.
231. Shore C, Austin J, Dunn D. Maternal adaptation to a child's epilepsy. *Epilepsy Behav*. 2004;5:557–568.
232. Shore CP, Austin JK, Huster GA, et al. Identifying risk factors for maternal depression in families of adolescents with epilepsy. *J Spec Pediatr Nurs*. 2002;7(2):71–80.

233. Shore C, Austin J, Musick B, et al. Psychosocial care needs of parents of children with new-onset seizures. 3. *J Neurosci Nurs*. 1998;30(3):169–174.
234. Silver LB. Conversion disorder with pseudoseizures in adolescence: A stress reaction to unrecognized and untreated learning disabilities. *J Am Acad Child Psychiatry*. 1982;21(5):508–512.
235. Sinclair DB, Snyder TJ. Corticosteroids for the treatment of Landau-Kleffner syndrome and continuous spike-wave discharge during sleep. *Pediatr Neurol*. 2005;32(5):300–306.
236. Smith MC, Hoeppner TJ. Epileptic encephalopathy of late childhood: Landau-Kleffner syndrome and the syndrome of continuous spikes and waves during slow-wave sleep. *J Clin Neurophysiol*. 2003;20(6):462–472.
237. Smith ML, Elliott IM, Lach L. Cognitive, psychosocial, and family function one year after pediatric epilepsy surgery. *Epilepsia*. 2004;45(6):650–660.
238. Sparrow S, Balla D, Cicchetti D. *Vineland Adaptive Behavior Scales: Interview Edition survey form*. Circle Pines, MN: American Guidance Service, 1984.
239. Steffenburg S, Gillberg C, Steffenburg U. Psychiatric disorders in children and adolescents with mental retardation and active epilepsy. *Arch Neurol*. 1996;53(9):904–912.
240. Steffenburg U, Hagberg G, Hagberg B. Epilepsy in a representative series of Rett syndrome. *Acta Paediatr*. 2001;90(1):34–39.
241. Stores G. School-children with epilepsy at risk for learning and behaviour problems. *Dev Med Child Neurol*. 1978;20(4):502–508.
242. Stores G, Hart J, Piran N. Inattentiveness in schoolchildren with epilepsy. *Epilepsia*. 1978;19(2):169–175.
243. Stores G, Piran N. Dependency of different types in schoolchildren with epilepsy. *Psychol Med*. 1978;8(3):441–445.
244. Tan M, Appleton R. Attention deficit and hyperactivity disorder, methylphenidate, and epilepsy. *Arch Dis Child*. 2005;90(1):57–59.
245. Tassinari CA, Rubboli G, Volpi L, et al. Encephalopathy with electrical status epilepticus during slow sleep or ESES syndrome including the acquired aphasia. *Clin Neurophysiol*. 2000;111(Suppl 2):S94–S102.
246. Taylor DC. Aggression and epilepsy. *J Psychosom Res*. 1969;13(3):229–236.
247. Thome-Souza S, Kuczynski E, Assumpcao F, Jr, et al. Which factors may play a pivotal role on determining the type of psychiatric disorder in children and adolescents with epilepsy? *Epilepsy Behav*. 2004;5(6):988–994.
248. Thompson R Jr., Gustafson KE. *Adaptation to Chronic Childhood Illness*. Washington, DC: American Psychological Association Press, 1996.
249. Trimble M. *Benzodiazepines in Epilepsy*. London: John Wiley and Sons, 1983.
250. Trimble MR, Rusch N, Betts T, et al. Psychiatric symptoms after therapy with new antiepileptic drugs: Psychopathological and seizure related variables. *Seizure*. 2000;9(4):249–254.
251. Tuchman R. Treatment of seizure disorders and EEG abnormalities in children with autism spectrum disorders. *J Autism Dev Disord*. 2000;30(5):485–489.
252. Tuchman R, Jayakar P, Yaylali I, et al. Seizures and EEG findings in children with autism spectrum disorders. *CNS Spectrums*. 1997;3:61–70.
253. Tuchman R, Rapin I. Epilepsy in autism. *Lancet Neurol*. 2002;1(6):352–358.
254. Tuchman RF. Epilepsy, language, and behavior: Clinical models in childhood. *J Child Neurol*. 1994;9(1):95–102.
255. Tuchman RF, Rapin I. Regression in pervasive developmental disorders: Seizures and epileptiform electroencephalogram correlates. *Pediatrics*. 1997;99(4):560–566.
256. Tuchman RF, Rapin I, Shinnar S. Autistic and dysphasic children. II: Epilepsy [published erratum appears in *Pediatrics*. 1992 Aug;90(2 Pt 1):264]. *Pediatrics*. 1991;88(6):1219–1225.
257. van Dongen HR, De Wijngaert E, Wennekes MJ. The Landau-Kleffner Syndrome: Diagnostic Considerations. In: Martins IP, Castro-Caldas A, van Dongen HR,van Hout A, eds. *Acquired Aphasia in Children. Acquisition and Breakdown of Language in the Developing Brain*. London: Kluwer Academic Publishers; 1991.
258. van Hout A. Aphasia and Auditory Agnosia in Children with Landau-Kleffner Syndrome. In: Jambaque I, Lassonde M, Dulac O, eds. *Neuropsychology of Childhood Epilepsy*. New York: Kluwer Academic/Plenum; 2001: 191–198.
259. Veggiotti P, Beccaria F, Guerrini R, et al. Continuous spike-and-wave activity during slow-wave sleep: Syndrome or EEG pattern? *Epilepsia*. 1999;40(11):1593–1601.
260. Verrotti A, Latini G, Trotta D, et al. Typical and atypical rolandic epilepsy in childhood: A follow-up study. *Pediatr Neurol*. 2002;26(1):26–29.
261. Vining EP, Mellitis ED, Dorsen MM, et al. Psychologic and behavioral effects of antiepileptic drugs in children: A double-blind comparison between phenobarbital and valproic acid. *Pediatrics*. 1987;80(2):165–174.
262. Volkmar FR, Nelson DS. Seizure disorders in autism. *J Am Acad Child Adolesc Psychiatry*. 1990;29(1):127–129.
263. Westbrook L, Bauman L, Shinnar S. Applying stigma theory to epilepsy: A test of a conceptual model. *J Pediatr Psychol*. 1992;17:633–649.
264. White H, Sreenivasan U. Epilepsy-aphasia syndrome in children: An unusual presentation to psychiatry. *Can J Psychiatry*. 1987;32(7):599–601.
265. Whitman S, Hermann B, Black R, et al. Psychopathology and seizure type in children with epilepsy. *Psychol Med*. 1982;12:843–853.
266. Williams J, Lange B, Sharp G, et al. Altered sleeping arrangements in pediatric patients with epilepsy. *Clin Pediatr (Phila)*. 2000;39:635–642.
267. Williams J, Phillips T, Geiebel M, et al. Factors associated with achievement in children with controlled epilepsy. *Epilepsy Behav*. 2001;2:217–233.
268. Williams J, Steel C, Sharp GB, et al. Anxiety in children with epilepsy. *Epilepsy Behav*. 2003;4(6):729–732.
269. Williamson G, Walters A, Shaffer D. Caregiver models of self and others, coping, and depression: Predictors of depression in children with chronic pain. *Health Psychol*. 2002;21:405–410.
270. Wirrell EC, Camfield CS, Camfield PR, et al. Long-term psychosocial outcome in typical absence epilepsy. Sometimes a wolf in sheeps' clothing. *Arch Pediatr Adolesc Med*. 1997;151(2):152–158.
271. Wong V. Epilepsy in children with autistic spectrum disorder. *J Child Neurol*. 1993;8(4):316–322.
272. Woody RC, Jones JG. Neurologic Munchausen-by-proxy syndrome. *South Med J*. 1987;80(2):247–248.
273. Wyllie E, Friedman D, Rothner AD, et al. Psychogenic seizures in children and adolescents: Outcome after diagnosis by ictal video and electroencephalographic recording. *Pediatrics*. 1990;85(4):480–484.
274. Youroukos S, Lazopoulou D, Michelakou D, et al. Acute psychosis associated with levetiracetam. *Epileptic Disord*. 2003;5(2):117–119.
275. Yung AW, Park YD, Cohen MJ, et al. Cognitive and behavioral problems in children with centrotemporal spikes. *Pediatr Neurol*. 2000;23(5):391–395.
276. Ziegler RG. Impairments of control and competence in epileptic children and their families. *Epilepsia*. 1981;22(3):339–346.
277. Ziegler RG. Risk factors in childhood epilepsy. *Psychother Psychosom*. 1985;44(4):185–190.

CHAPTER 211 ■ SUICIDE: INCIDENCE, PSYCHOPATHOLOGY, PATHOGENESIS, AND PREVENTION

DIETRICH BLUMER

INTRODUCTION

Suicide among patients with epilepsy has been widely recognized as a serious problem. In modern times, its frequency appears to approach the frequency of death from seizures. However, the frequency of its incidence is still debated, its psychopathology and pathogenesis remains unclear, and no proper method of prevention has been established.

REVIEW OF LITERATURE

Frequency of Suicide

In a recent paper, Jallon[28] reviewed the significantly higher mortality of patients with epilepsy by status epilepticus, sudden unexplained death, and suicide, compared with the general population. He expressed concern that the reports on suicide were based on small samples from different populations and from highly selected groups of patients and used different methods of analysis. However, an analysis of the populations that differed in the numbers of suicide and an investigation (published in 2005) of the frequency of suicide in 29 cohorts of patients with epilepsy[44] provide answers to this concern.

Suicide is a rare event, occurring only slightly more than once among 10,000 persons annually in the United States.[41] In a review of completed suicide in manic-depressive patients, Goodwin and Jamison found a mean of 19% of deaths secondary to suicide in this population.[22] A similarly high suicide rate among patients with epilepsy has been documented: In a Danish study,[26] 164 of 2,763 patients with epilepsy suicided (an excess mortality rate of 273% compared with the number of deaths expected in Denmark); the case material included all adult patients discharged with the diagnosis of epilepsy at four neurologic clinics over 14 years, and any patient with a handicap other than epilepsy was excluded from the study. Although epilepsy was the immediate cause of death in 26%, suicide was the second leading cause of death in 20% (an excess mortality rate of 300%) at an average age at death of 32 years. According to eight reports, death by suicide occurs in 5% of patients with epilepsy, compared with 1.4% in the general population.[36] Based on a wider review of the literature, a fivefold increase in suicides among patients with epilepsy over the rate in the general population was found among those attending special clinics and was magnified to as much as 25-fold among patients with temporal lobe epilepsy (TLE).[1] A study by Hauser et al.,[24] on the other hand, included a general population of patients with epilepsy followed from the time of diagnosis, and not from the time of registration in a neurologic clinic; their patients were less severely affected, and they reported no suicides in excess of expected numbers. Suicide appears to represent a serious problem not in the general population of patients with epilepsy, but among those with more difficult epilepsy who require treatment in specialty clinics.

Since Jallon's review, Pompili et al.[44] investigated 29 studies of suicide in epilepsy, comprising 50,814 patients, of whom 187 committed suicide. Their meta-analysis showed that suicide in epilepsy is indeed more frequent than in the general population, but with significant exceptions. A study by Cockerell et al.[12] included patients with newly diagnosed or suspected epilepsy who were ascertained when attending a general practice, with a median follow-up of less than 7 years; a single suicide was registered among 792 patients. As in the study by Hauser et al.,[24] few severely affected patients were included. In contrast, the largest study cited by Pompili et al., 10,739 patients from our Epi-Care Center,[8] registered only five suicides (a rate lower than in the general population), not because of lack of severity of the epilepsy in the population, but because all patients with psychiatric complications were treated, at intake or as soon as needed, with proper psychotropic medication. This study will be fully reviewed, for a better understanding of suicide in epilepsy and to establish specific guidelines for its prevention.

Psychopathology Associated with Suicide in Epilepsy

The generally difficult psychosocial circumstances of patients with chronic epilepsy have often been considered the leading factor responsible for their elevated suicide rate, more important than the presence of psychiatric illness or the availability of drugs.[15] However, in general, psychiatric illness has been identified as the nearly universal antecedent of suicide, and psychosocial circumstances cannot be considered causes for suicide.[35,41] Very few reports have attempted to clarify the nature of the psychiatric disorder that may lead to suicide among patients with epilepsy.

Nilsson et al.[42] pointed out that studies are lacking in which persons with epilepsy who have committed suicide are compared with relevant controls to identify risk factors for suicide. In their case-control study of risk factors for suicide in epilepsy, they compared 26 cases of suicide and 23 cases of suspected suicide with 171 controls, within a cohort of 6,880 registered with a diagnosis of epilepsy in the Stockholm County Inpatient Register. They found a ninefold increase of suicide with mental illness and a tenfold increase in relative risk with the use of antipsychotic drugs. They arrived at a profile of the epilepsy patient who commits suicide as one with early onset, but not necessarily severe, epilepsy and with psychiatric illness (depression, psychosis, substance abuse).

Mendez et al.[40] studied the causative factors for suicide attempts by overdose in 22 patients with epilepsy (from 711 patients hospitalized for a suicide attempt) and concluded that interictal psychopathologic factors were of primary importance. A comparison of suicide attempts among patients with epilepsy and comparably handicapped controls with other chronic disabilities found that 30% of patients with epilepsy had attempted suicide, as compared with 7% of the controls.[38]

In 1992, Mendez and Doss[39] reported on the suicides in a substantial population of patients with epilepsy *and* included clinical details of all fatal outcomes. They documented the neuropsychiatric aspects of the four patients who died by suicide out of 1,611 patients with epilepsy followed in a neurology clinic over a period of 8 years: two male patients with chronic psychosis, depressive moods, and good seizure control; one male patient with brief psychotic episodes associated with confusion and increased bitemporal spikes and diffuse slowing on electroencephalogram (EEG) in the absence of seizures; and one female patient with episodes of profound ictal and postictal depression who suicided after three witnessed staring spells. The patient with brief psychotic episodes and one of the patients with chronic psychosis experienced voices commanding them to commit suicide. All four patients had suffered from complex partial seizures since childhood and committed suicide by medication overdose at a time when their seizures were controlled, except for the patient who suicided in a state of postictal depression.

Fukuchi et al.[17] reviewed the case records of all outpatients of two epilepsy centers who had died. Patients in one center were followed for 10 years and in the second center for 7 years. Those who had unclassified epilepsy or who died as the result of an underlying disease (such as neoplasm) were excluded. More than 4,000 subjects were reviewed, and the records of 43 deceased patients with well-classified epilepsy were analyzed. Suicide occurred in six patients (14% of the deaths), all with TLE, and three suicided by throwing themselves in front of an oncoming train in the midst of an episode of postictal psychosis. The authors noted the agreement of their findings with those of Mendez and Doss.[39] While providing fewer details, they concluded that most suicides in epilepsy were the result of an immediate causal relationship with ictal or interictal epileptic manifestations. The authors referred to reports of violent behavior directed outward following complex partial seizures, and proposed that this violence may eventually turn into a paroxysmal self-destructive impulse.[20,31]

Suicides After Successful Treatment of Seizures and After Surgical Treatment of the Epilepsy

For an understanding of the pathogenesis of suicide in epilepsy, evidence for the role of predominant inhibition ("forced normalization")[21,33,34,51] must be reviewed.

In 1969, Janz[29] stated that suicide does not occur among patients with severe epilepsy but does occur not infrequently among those patients who have just become free from seizures. With the guidance of Janz, Haltrich[23] studied the causes of death among 909 patients with epilepsy who had been treated at the neurology clinic of a German university during the preceding 8 years (1946–1953); his report includes a large number of suicides with highlights of their psychopathology. Of the 83 patients with symptomatic epilepsy, 51 died from brain tumors. The 11 recorded suicides all occurred among the 78 patients with cryptogenic epilepsy, and at 14.1% surpassed any other cause of death in this group; eight patients (10.3%) died from seizure status and six patients (7.7%) from single seizures. Among the 11 suicides, eight patients had complex partial seizures. Increased irritability was reported in six of the seven males (four with episodes of violence) and in one of the four females; four patients had a history of previous suicide attempts, and another three patients had experienced depressive moods with or without suicidal thoughts. Only one patient suicided during a psychotic state after three previous suicide attempts in psychotic or dysphoric states; he had been violence-prone and was the only patient requiring institutionalization among the 11 who suicided. Haltrich included three later cases of suicide when he reported that the 14 patients had responded well to treatment of their seizures; at the time of suicide, three had experienced only minor attacks, seven only very rare or no major seizures, and four had rare or no seizures of any type.

Taylor and Marsh[49] reported on the occurrence of suicide among 193 patients who had undergone temporal lobectomy and who were followed from 5 to 24 years. Of 37 deaths, nine were by suicide (24.3%). Including an additional six patients who died in unclear circumstances would have raised the suicide rate observed from 25-fold to 50-fold of that expected.[48] Five of the nine who definitely suicided had been rendered seizure-free by the surgery. The authors did not describe the mental state of the victims and merely documented the very high risk of suicide in their particular population.

In another series of surgically treated patients with epilepsy, Hennessy et al.[25] reported only one suicide among 20 deaths in their cohort of 305 consecutive patients who had TLE surgery over a 20-year period. A second patient ran onto a road and was killed by a passing car; both patients were seizure free. The authors suggested that the early series of Taylor and Marsh,[49] with its much higher postoperative suicide rate, had included many patients referred from the Maudsley psychiatric institution. However, the origin of the populations of patients surgically treated and with reports of postoperative mortality is usually not well defined. A large group surveyed from 1928 to 1973 by Jensen[30] includes 2,204 patients who had unilateral temporal lobectomy, with 164 postoperative deaths: due to epilepsy in 26%, suicide in 20%, and accidents in 11%; no details were provided about the suicides.

Of interest is the report by Bladin[2] who reported, with remarkable details of the psychosocial outcome, the results after temporal lobectomy of a series of 115 consecutive patients. They were followed as closely as possible for a mean of 4 years after temporal lobectomy. Five patients showed significant episodes of depression after the operation. In three of them, recognition and antidepressive therapy produced prompt improvement. Another patient, who was seizure-free, was rehabilitated by friends in a religious organization after two suicide attempts. The fifth patient, who lived at a distance and could not participate in the routine postoperative follow-up, was also free of seizures yet committed suicide following the unexpected death of mother and sibling. Three patients showed psychotic episodes more than 3 months after the operation and responded to appropriate therapy, including a neuroleptic. Postoperative anxiety was noted in about half the patients and responded to counseling, medication, or brief hospitalization. Increased sexual drive was reported only upon optimal seizure control. Bladin's report is unique in its report of the use of psychotropic medication for patients with epilepsy.

PSYCHOPATHOLOGY, PATHOGENESIS, AND PREVENTION OF SUICIDE: THE STUDY OF PATIENTS TREATED AT THE EPI-CARE CENTER

In Chapter 205 on affective disorders of epilepsy, we concluded that the pre-modern psychiatrists, who commonly observed patients with epilepsy on a daily basis, were correct when they recognized the interictal dysphoric disorder with its intermittent and pleomorphic symptomatology as the predominant specific psychiatric disorder of chronic epilepsy. The interictal dysphoric disorder includes episodes of anxiety, fear, elation, insomnia, anergia, pain, explosive irritability, and depressive moods that may be intense and associated with suicidality. The disorder, in its entirety, is well treated with low doses of antidepressant medication. Subsequent to the detailed report of our experience with suicide in a large population of patients attending our epilepsy center, the psychopathology, pathogenesis, and prevention of suicide in epilepsy will be discussed.

A total of 10,739 patients with epilepsy were treated at the Epi-Care Center in Memphis during a 12-year period (1987–1999). The population included a large number of referrals from the mid-South area and beyond. About 900 patients were surgically treated during this period. The comprehensive professional team of the Center consisted of a neurologist, neurosurgeon, electroencephalographer, neuropsychologist, and the same psychiatrist (D.B.) during the entire period. The tasks of the psychiatrist included evaluating all patients admitted for intensive neurodiagnostic monitoring (as candidates for surgical treatment of medically intractable epilepsy or for clarification of the differential diagnosis between epilepsy and nonepileptic seizures) and of every patient at the center who was judged by the team to have psychiatric difficulties. Every patient in need of psychiatric assistance was followed at the Center with the appropriate psychopharmacologic and supportive treatment regardless of geographic distance, as long as the patient and family were able to come for return visits. Patients who required psychiatric hospitalization were admitted under the care of the team psychiatrist in the same hospital where the team admitted its patients for evaluation and treatment of the epilepsy. The presence of a team psychiatrist at the Epi-Care Center and the effectiveness of the psychotropic treatment employed assured prompt referral of patients with psychiatric complications, who were not routinely evaluated by the psychiatrist, for early treatment beyond antiepileptic treatment. Neuropsychological testing of all patients admitted for intensive monitoring and of a large number of outpatients, as well as a weekly case conference, greatly facilitated the teamwork and the referrals to the psychiatrist for early treatment.

The gradual development of a standardized psychiatric evaluation by a comprehensive questionnaire for seizure patients using a semistructured interview of patients and next-of-kin and of an increasingly effective psychopharmacologic treatment has been reported elsewhere.[5,9–11] Initially, most patients with psychiatric complications of their epilepsy were treated by adding a modest dose of tricyclic antidepressant to the antiepileptic medication. With the development of treatment by double antidepressant medication (tricyclic plus serotonin-specific reuptake inhibitor) and the addition, if necessary, of a small dose of an atypical antipsychotic drug (risperidone), it became possible to treat successfully the vast majority of patients with any degree of psychopathology, including psychoses and suicidality.

The death of a patient with epilepsy at a treatment center is a memorable event. The number of patients who suicided was ascertained from medical records and the combined memories of the treatment team. The Epi-Care Center was the major center for treatment of epilepsy in the Mid-South and had a policy of careful follow-up of all patients. Thus, the death of one patient who had moved to a distant state about 1 year before her suicide (case 3) is included, as we had attempted to remain helpful.

Results

A total of five (four males, one female) of 10,739 patients attending the Center during the 12-year period committed suicide. The circumstances of these five treatment failures are reported here.

Case 1 (1989)

This male patient had had seizures since age 10. Following a 6-month marriage in late adolescence, he married two more times. His second wife had suicided following childbirth after 1 year of marriage; at that time, the patient became suicidal himself and required 2 months of psychiatric hospitalization. During the third marriage that lasted 4 years, he became suicidal when his wife left him with their child; he blamed his bad temper for the final breakup that had occurred 1 year prior to referral to the Center. His seizures became increasingly more frequent, occurring as often as three times daily. He was then treated by right temporal lobectomy at age 32.

After the operation, he experienced epileptic seizures on only two occasions after missing his medication. There had been a brief episode of feeling suicidal shortly after surgery, but soon he became enthusiastic about the success of the surgery, volunteered to talk to patients who were candidates for surgical treatment of their epilepsy, was active in the local chapter of the Epilepsy Foundation, and was working on a book about epilepsy. When he experienced an episode of dissociation with amnesia 12 months after his surgery, he was scheduled for psychiatric evaluation. Shortly thereafter, he developed frequent nonepileptic seizures.

He was first evaluated psychiatrically at age 33, 14 months after surgical treatment. He presented as an intensely emotional individual who felt he had a special mission in life and reported big mood shifts from very happy to very sad. He was at first treated with doxepin because of insomnia, then with the better-tolerated imipramine to 100 mg at bedtime, and he showed improvement. However, after 6 months of monthly visits, he felt accused of having "fake seizures," abruptly severed his relationship with the Center, moved to a neighboring state, and discontinued the antidepressant medication. On two occasions, at 7 and 11 months after he had discontinued his visits, he returned to the Center for only neurologic follow-up visits, stating that he had no seizures and was doing well. Six months after his last visit, he called the Center from out of state. He stated that his girlfriend had left him, he feared going off in a rage attack, and for the past 8 days he had been driving around with a rope in his car looking for a tree to hang himself. He refused any help and, 10 days later, 3 years after the operation, committed suicide by hanging.

Comment: This patient had a dysphoric disorder with marked depressive moods, irritability, and insomnia. The occurrence of nonepileptic seizures is not uncommon in patients who have become free of seizures after surgery.[13] We did not have the experience to deal with this predicament at that time; the patient became noncompliant and discontinued the antidepressant medication.

Case 2 (1990)

This male patient had had frequent seizures since the age of 6 weeks. He had three to five seizures per week, lived with his parents, and was active in church life. When he became unable to work because of back pain, he became depressed, with marked anergia and recurrent episodes of feeling suicidal, which required a brief psychiatric hospitalization.

Four months after onset of his pain, at age 34, he was evaluated at the Epi-Care Center. No pathology was found for his back pain, but a right temporal tumor was detected, and a right temporal lobectomy for a ganglioglioma was carried out.

Subsequent to the operation, he remained seizure free. At discharge, he was prescribed imipramine but discontinued the drug when it did not help his insomnia. He was referred for psychiatric follow-up near his home. Initially, he seemed improved but then continued to be depressed and preoccupied with his back pain. The psychiatric treatment consisted of counseling, fluoxetine, and a period of inpatient treatment 8 months after the operation. One year after the operation, he drowned himself. His family did not understand why this happened.

Comment: This patient had a dysphoric disorder with depressive moods, anergia, insomnia, and pain. He was treated psychiatrically near his home and, at that time, we did not have a more effective treatment to initiate or to recommend.

Case 3 (1991)

This female patient had had seizures since grammar school but was diagnosed only at age 18. After 18 years of education, she married but remained childless. She made one suicide attempt at age 38, and had several car accidents due to seizures.

She became a patient at the Epi-Care Center at the age of 43, initially for psychiatric treatment. Her main complaint was chronic pain with anergia and depressive moods of at least 5 years' duration; she also had insomnia and was hypochondriacal. Her primidone was phased out, and her pains and dysphoric symptoms vanished when the combination of carbamazepine and amitriptyline at 100 mg was prescribed. When her husband insisted on divorce, she regressed and had to be hospitalized for 1 month with a mixed manic and depressive state with recurrence of her pains. She again improved with the temporary addition of lithium.

Her seizures occurred perhaps every few weeks and, following finalization of the divorce, she had a right temporal lobectomy at age 45. The specimen showed hippocampal sclerosis, and she remained seizure-free. Six months after surgery, she felt great and decided to move to her far-away home state, where she did not find a supportive environment. Her pains and depression resumed, even though she maintained an antidepressant (trimipramine 100 mg daily). She returned to her original neurologist, who replaced the carbamazepine with primidone when she was found to have a low sodium level. At the age of 46, 18 months after surgery, she committed suicide by shooting herself.

Comment: This patient had a dysphoric disorder with depressive moods, anergia, insomnia, and pain. She did not seek local psychiatric help after her departure from the Center. The reintroduction of primidone possibly made her depressive moods worse.

Case 4 (1998)

This male patient began to have seizures at age 10, and was treated at the Epi-Care Center beginning at age 23. He underwent a left temporal lobectomy that showed hippocampal sclerosis, but he continued to have daily (although shorter) complex partial seizures. A further resection of the left hippocampus 6 months later was similarly ineffective. He was a serious and very religious young man, who admitted to some temper but showed no troublesome dysphoric symptoms at the time of his presurgical psychiatric evaluation at the Center, and he was not followed psychiatrically. He worked for 2 years after the operation and, after a failed marriage, resumed living with his parents. Over the subsequent 6 years, he was treated with all the latest antiepileptic drugs without any success until his seizures finally became controlled by the combination of zonisamide, gabapentin, and phenytoin. The subsequent follow-up was entirely by phone contact with the patient and his family. He resumed work and reported enjoying it. Following an unprecedented outburst of rage toward his parents 2 weeks after he had become seizure-free, he began to live in separate quarters on the family property. Antidepressant treatment suggested by our neurologist was not felt necessary by the family since he did well at work. Three months after becoming free of seizures, he was found dead, having inflicted a gunshot wound to the abdomen.

Comment: The first symptom of a dysphoric disorder in the form of an unexpected outburst of rage was reported after he had become seizure-free. There was no further warning or call for help.

Case 5 (1999)

This male patient suffered a head injury at age 6 and started to have seizures at age 17. He worked until age 35, and went to church faithfully. After age 41, he attended a family therapy center for a few years for depression and marital conflicts and took a drug overdose at the time of his divorce at age 45.

At age 48, he began treatment at the Epi-Care Center for complex partial seizures that tended to occur several times daily. On first evaluation, he was recognized as having a dysphoric disorder with intermittent depressive moods and occasional suicidal ideas, anergia, irritability, and anxiety. He refused antidepressant treatment. An anterior partial callosotomy early in his treatment at the Center did not improve the high daily frequency of his seizures.

At age 50, he married a domineering woman who had a history of skull fractures inflicted by her former husband and who had been treated for her own violent temper. Shortly thereafter, the couple elected treatment by vagal nerve stimulation (VNS) for his seizures, and he was reevaluated psychiatrically. Both the patient and his new wife admitted to being "hotheaded," but they adamantly refused to comply with advice given for the treatment of his dysphoric disorder. His seizure frequency gradually decreased over the initial 15 months of VNS until it diminished to only two complex partial seizures per day. At that point, the VNS was increased. Four months later, we learned from his local physician that he had become seizure-free for the first time since the onset of the epilepsy 35 years earlier and that he had killed his wife and then himself.

Comment: This patient had a dysphoric disorder with depressive moods, anergia, anxiety, and irritability. Whereas irritability to the point of paroxysmal outbursts of anger is a key symptom of the dysphoric disorder, dysphoric patients, like the majority of patients with epilepsy, tend to be very conscientious and often highly religious, and their outbursts are followed by genuine remorse. Their extreme rage tends to be turned against themselves, and homicide, as opposed to suicide, is an exceptionally rare occurrence in epilepsy.[6]

Discussion

The five suicides among the population of 10,739 patients seen at the Epi-Care Center over the period of 12 years share a surprisingly common pattern. All had a history of early onset (mean age 9.5 years) of long-standing complex partial seizures (mean duration 29 years) with very high (often daily) seizure frequency in all but one. Suicide occurred in all patients after a short interval (3 months to 3 years, mean 13 months) of having obtained full control of seizures for the first time by temporal lobectomy (three patients), medication, or VNS. All had symptoms of an interictal dysphoric disorder, and three of the four males had a significant problem with episodes of violent anger. All but one (case 4) had a history of previous suicidal moods or suicide attempts, but in three of the five, the suicidal act was precipitate and not anticipated at the time. All had experienced worse psychosocial predicaments in the past than were present at the time of completed suicide.

The four patients from the series of Mendez and Doss[39] likewise all had an onset of epilepsy in early life, with a mean duration of the seizure disorder of 25 years, and two of the three patients who committed suicide in a psychotic state were under good seizure control. The third patient suffered from unusual psychotic episodes that coincided with the presence of increased electroencephalographic epileptiform potentials in the absence of seizures; he will be discussed in the section on pathogenesis. The fourth patient suicided in a state of postictal depression. The patients from the series of Taylor and Marsh[49] who suicided after temporal lobectomy were reported without any details of their psychopathology, but five of the nine had been rendered seizure-free after surgical treatment.

Among the three series, 12 of 18 patients committed suicide after a long-standing seizure disorder was under control. This finding confirms the early reports by Janz[29] and Haltrich.[23] Janz was already well aware of the finding of forced normalization noted by Landolt[34]: Control of seizures may usher in dysphoric or psychotic disorders. Particularly notable is Haltrich's finding that six of the seven male patients had been markedly irritable, with a majority suffering from episodes of violent temper. The same finding is evident in three of our four male suicides.

Suicide among patients with epilepsy clearly is not the result of psychosocial difficulties caused by having seizures, but rather occurs in the presence of significant interictal and at times postictal psychopathology. Prior to reviewing the pathogenesis of suicide in epilepsy, the phenomenology of the interictal and peri-ictal psychopathology and their relationship to suicide must be clarified.

Psychopathology Associated with Suicide in Epilepsy

Premodern psychiatrists recognized an intermittent and pleomorphic disorder, termed the *dysphoric disorder*, as the most common psychiatric disorder of epilepsy. The interictal dysphoric disorder is a distinct disorder that had to be rediscovered.[6] One of its key symptoms—intermittent depressive mood—is associated with the episodic suicidal moods of patients with chronic epilepsy, primarily those with mesial TLE.[3,6,9,18,19,37] Kraepelin[32] precisely described the dysphoric disorder of patients with epilepsy: Dysphoric episodes present with depressive moods ("very frequently with utter disgust of life and suicidal bent"), irritability, anxiety, headaches, insomnia, but also with euphoric moods. The dysphoric episodes occur without external triggers, with rapid onset and termination, and recur fairly regularly in a uniform manner in the absence of clouding of consciousness. Dysphoric symptoms commonly can be observed as prodrome or aftermath of an attack but, most important, they appear as phenomena independent of the seizures, as interictal dysphoric episodes, with a frequency varying from every few days to every few months. As a rule, the dysphoric state lasts from 1 to 2 days but may dissipate after just a few hours.

Based on our own observations, we added anergia and phobic fears to Kraepelin's six key symptoms of the dysphoric disorder and have defined it by the presence of at least three of the eight key symptoms, each present to a troublesome degree.[9]

The risk of suicide in patients with epilepsy is primarily associated with the often sudden episodes of intense depressive mood of the interictal phase; therefore, suicide in epilepsy tends to occur in a precipitate manner. As noted by Haltrich[23] and in our own series, the occurrence of marked irritability with outbursts of violent behavior appears to represent a particular risk factor for suicide among male patients. As noted early by Kraepelin, the dysphoric symptoms also tend to occur peri-ictally, during the prodrome or aftermath of a seizure. The postictal phase in particular may be associated with marked depressive mood.[4] A high suicidal risk has been observed in patients who experience ictal depressive mood that extends into the postictal phase for a period of 1 hour to 3 days. Williams[52] reported 21 such cases among his 100 patients with ictal emotional experience, and five of the 21 patients had made suicide attempts during their postictal phase. The fourth case of Mendez and Doss represents a well-documented postictal suicide.[39]

As noted earlier by Kraepelin, interictal psychoses tend to develop as expansions of interictal dysphoric disorders.[32] The dysphoric disorder persists during the psychotic state, and suicidal depressive moods may occur in the course of an interictal psychosis when reasoning is impaired. Presence of the hallucination of voices commanding a patient to suicide represents a particular risk.

Pathogenesis of Suicide in Epilepsy

The treatment of seizures during the first four decades of the 20th century consisted chiefly of potassium bromide; phenobarbital, available since 1913, was widely shunned by psychiatrists because of its psychotoxic effects. In a modern era that considers epilepsy a neurologic disorder and has focused with growing success on the control of seizures with an expanding score of antiepileptic drugs and surgical procedures, dysphoric symptoms and psychotic episodes appear to have become more severe and chronic. Kraepelin[32] had noted a very brief duration of the dysphoric episodes, and stated that interictal psychotic episodes as a rule last only a few days and may persist for weeks or even months only in isolated cases; he noted a very frequent suicidal urge, but not completed suicide, associated with dysphoric episodes. The relative infrequency of suicide in the premodern era is documented by Prudhomme,[45] whose research included approximately 77,000 patients with epilepsy from the period of 1893 to 1940.

The emergence or worsening of psychopathology upon suppression of seizure activity has been widely reported. Since the early reports by Gibbs,[20] Hill,[27] and Landolt,[34] evidence has been increasing that the interictal psychopathology may emerge or worsen upon improvement of the epilepsy, as measured by seizure frequency and EEG abnormalities. Persuasive evidence suggests that the psychiatric disorders of epilepsy may result from the inhibitory activity that develops in reaction to the excessive excitatory activity of the chronic seizure disorder, as postulated by Stevens[47] and Engel.[16] The precise nature of the seizure-suppressing mechanisms is insufficiently understood, and the phenomenon of emergence of psychiatric disturbance with normalization of the EEG or with suppression of clinical seizures, has been usually referred to as *forced normalization* or *alternating psychosis*, respectively.[10,34,50] Landolt's early observations included dysphoric disorders upon normalization of the EEG,[34] but when the concept of the dysphoric disorder was forgotten, psychiatric observations began to focus on the psychotic disorders and to a lesser extent on isolated symptoms of the dysphoric disorder.[46] Early reports that suicide may occur as an alternating phenomenon when seizures are suppressed[29] were widely ignored.

The evidence of a linkage of the psychiatric changes to inhibitory mechanisms can be summarized as follows: (a) The development of interictal dysphoric and even more so of psychotic disorders is delayed following onset of epilepsy,[18,19] as inhibitory mechanisms become increasingly established; this predicament accords with the particular linkage of the psychiatric disorders of epilepsy with its most prominent chronic form (i.e., mesial TLE). (b) Upon decrease, and particularly upon full control of seizures, dysphoric symptoms and psychosis tend to be exacerbated or to emerge de novo.[6,10,21,27,34,50,51] (c) The same psychiatric changes emerge also at times when *acute* exacerbation of the seizure activity engages an enhanced inhibitory response, commonly in the prodromal and postictal phases, and rarely upon increased seizure activity as paraictal psychosis—a seeming opposite of forced normalization or alternating psychosis.[4,6,32,46] (d) After optimal surgical elimination of the epileptogenic zone, a delay of 6 to 18 months occurs before the psychiatric changes become phased out, presumably with only gradual fading of the inhibitory mechanisms.[10]

If predominance of inhibition results in persistent suppression of seizures in chronic epilepsy, some patients are at risk to develop the most severe psychiatric complications: A dysphoric disorder with suicidal depressive moods, psychosis, or a combination of both. On the other hand, the *acute* engagement of inhibitory mechanisms by the seizure event tends to result in peri-ictal dysphoric symptoms that may include postictal depressive mood with suicidality. The third case of Mendez and Doss[39] is exceptional: The patient's brief psychotic episodes would occur in the presence of *increased* epileptiform activity in the EEG in the *absence* of seizures, and the psychotic confusion was associated with voices commanding him to commit suicide. Demers-Desrosiers et al.[14] reported similar psychotic episodes in two patients who became psychotic shortly after discontinuing their antiepileptic medication, in association with *increased* epileptiform activity of the EEG in the *absence* of seizures; their psychotic state remitted upon resuming the antiepileptic medication. The authors correctly considered their findings as the antipode of forced normalization, since forced normalization is understood as the emergence of psychotic disturbance when the EEG is normalized. The three cases have in common that, in the presence of increased EEG abnormality, no seizures occurred, presumably as inhibitory mechanisms were acutely engaged, provoking psychotic episodes and suicidality as alternating phenomena.

A psychodynamic aspect in the pathogenesis of suicide is noteworthy. A core symptom of the dysphoric disorder, termed *irritability*, consists of the paroxysmal affect of anger that may be overcontrolled or range from short temper to the point of explosive rage; excessive anger conflicts with the notably conscientious and even hyper-religious personality of patients with epilepsy and may become intolerable,[6] prompting a precipitate and often unexpected act of suicide. Janz noted that a violent form of suicide (plunge from great height, throwing self under a train, drowning) occurred more frequently among patients with epilepsy than in the average population of suicides in Germany,[29] and similar reports came from Japan.[17]

Prevention of Suicide

If the hypothesis is correct that inhibition in chronic epilepsy may have a psychotoxic effect in many patients, then the treatment of psychopathology in epilepsy must aim to moderate the inhibitory mechanisms. Avoiding the antidepressant drugs that are most effective for this task for fear of lowering the seizure threshold of patients with epilepsy is ill-advised and carries the risk of fatal consequences.

The use of antidepressants for interictal psychiatric disorders was advocated as early as 1983.[43] We have successfully used antidepressants in modest doses for the psychiatric disorders of epilepsy for over 15 years in a large number of patients without increasing the seizure frequency, except in a rare patient with primary generalized seizures.[5,6,11] The proconvulsant antidepressant drugs at modest doses appear to serve as effective antagonists to the excessive inhibition and, in fact, are indispensable for successfully treating the interictal dysphoric and psychotic disorders. Gastaut et al.[19] pointed out that the interictal seizure threshold of patients with TLE (as measured by the response to Metrazol), in contrast to that of patients with primary generalized epilepsy, is higher than in nonepileptic individuals. The bias against the use of antidepressants for the psychiatric disorders of epilepsy, because they may lower the seizure threshold, is erroneous both on empirical and theoretical grounds. However, patients with primary generalized epilepsy who occasionally may experience dysphoric symptoms (presumably as a result of involvement of mesial temporal structures) still may have a lowered seizure threshold and need a more cautious dose of antidepressant medication.

In general, three of the eight key symptoms of the dysphoric disorder must be present before we initiate treatment with antidepressant medication. We add 100 mg (up to 150 mg) of imipramine at bedtime to the antiepileptic medication, making sure that the sleep disturbance is corrected; amitriptyline, doxepin, trimipramine, or nortriptyline may have to be substituted for that purpose. If the patient does not respond well, we add a serotonin-selective reuptake inhibitory antidepressant (SSRI) to the tricyclic, which is usually kept at a dose of 100 mg. Paroxetine has been our preferred SSRI, at 20 mg once to twice daily, but at times a different SSRI may be more effective. One may also proceed in the reverse order by starting with the SSRI and then adding a tricyclic drug if necessary. As a third step, for severe dysphoric disorders, risperidone at about 2 mg daily may have to be added. The response to this treatment extends to all the symptoms of the dysphoric disorder, including the depressive moods as well as the irritability, and occurs within days once a therapeutic dose is reached, allowing a rapid escalation of the prescription if necessary. If an interictal dysphoric disorder is associated with suicidality or with psychotic features, treatment should be started promptly with double antidepressant medication; a small dose of neuroleptic (risperidone 1 to 4 mg daily) may need to be added. Treating the interictal psychoses—dysphoric disorders with predominant psychotic features—should generally be carried out in identical fashion as for the severe dysphoric disorders and not simply by neuroleptic drugs.[10]

The number of suicides at the Epi-Care Center is a fraction of what is expected from previous surveys. When the three early patients (cases 1–3) from the Epi-Care Center suicided after successful epilepsy surgery, we had not yet learned to use the more effective augmented antidepressant treatment for severe dysphoric disorders. Mendez and Doss[39] reported the low rate of four suicides out of 1,611 patients (0.25%) followed for epilepsy in a neurology clinic over a period of 8 years. We had two suicides among the estimated 7,160 patients (0.03%) followed at the Epi-Care Center over the last 8 years of the study period, when we had the more effective psychotropic treatment in place; both patients had eluded this treatment (cases 4 and 5). Case histories of patients with the highest suicide risk but successfully treated at the Center have been previously reported.[5,7]

Suicide in epilepsy tends to be precipitate, but there may be recurrent warning from earlier dysphoric episodes with suicidal mood. All such patients require prompt and vigorous intervention with augmented antidepressant medication to stabilize their dysphoric disorder. However, a suicidal mood may emerge without a previous occurrence in a patient who had shown other symptoms of a dysphoric disorder (e.g., the outburst of rage in case 4). Prompt treatment of significant dysphoric symptoms assures not only an improved quality of life but prevents a suicidal outcome. Finally, patients with severe postictal depression, in our experience, can be protected from a suicidal impulse if they are maintained on antidepressant medication.

SUMMARY AND CONCLUSIONS

The increased risk of death by suicide among patients with epilepsy, while rarely disputed, has often been viewed as the unfortunate result of the psychosocial difficulties imposed by a chronic neurologic disease and has received scant psychiatric attention.

The study of suicides among 10,739 patients seen at the Epi-Care Center over 12 years confirms earlier findings[23,39] of suicide in epilepsy resulting from the specific neuropsychiatric disorders that are associated with epilepsy. These disorders include intermittent depressive moods with suicidal intensity among patients with interictal dysphoric disorder, psychotic episodes with concomitant dysphoric disorder and at times with command hallucinations, and severe postictal depressive states. The suicides may occur particularly in patients with long-standing TLE with high seizure frequency once seizures finally became controlled. Although a majority of patients with epilepsy will reach long-term remission, some patients with chronic epilepsy experience serious psychiatric complications when their seizures become controlled. Mendez and Doss implied that interictal depression may be relieved by having seizures, similar to the effect of electroconvulsive therapy.[39] The evidence suggests that a predominance of inhibitory mechanisms, interictally or postictally, may be psychotoxic, favoring the emergence of dysphoric and psychotic states and of a suicidal risk. The findings from the Epi-Care Center indicate that the early treatment of patients with epilepsy and dysphoric symptoms by the appropriate psychotropic medication can prevent suicides.

Suicide is only the most striking problem among the sizable number of patients with chronic epilepsy who suffer from dysphoric and psychotic disorders, and are well treatable by modern psychopharmacologic intervention. A much improved collaboration is required between neurologists who recognize the scope of the psychiatric complications of epilepsy and of psychiatrists who do not shun the field of epilepsy as alien to their specialty. The modern advances in suppressing seizures must become paired with the competence to treat the psychiatric consequences of improved seizure control in order to achieve optimal quality of life and to prevent fatal outcomes.

References

1. Barraclough BM. The suicide rate of epilepsy. *Acta Psychiatr Scand.* 1987; 76:339–345.
2. Bladin PF. Psychosocial difficulties and outcome after temporal lobectomy. *Epilepsia.* 1992;33:898–907.
3. Blumer D. *Psychiatric Aspects of Epilepsy.* Washington, D.C.: American Psychiatric Press; 1984.
4. Blumer D. Postictal depression: Significance for the treatment of the neurobehavioral disorder of epilepsy. *J Epilepsy.* 1992;5:214–219.
5. Blumer D. Antidepressant and double antidepressant treatment for the affective disorder of epilepsy. *J Clin Psychiatry.* 1997;58:3–11.
6. Blumer D. Dysphoric disorders and paroxysmal affects: recognition and treatment of epilepsy-related psychiatric disorders. *Harv Rev Psychiatry.* 2000;8:8–17.
7. Blumer D, Davies K. Psychiatric Issues in Epilepsy Surgery. In: Ettinger AB, Kanner AM, eds. *Psychiatric Issues in Epilepsy: A Practical Guide to Diagnosis and Treatment.* Philadelphia: Lippincott, Williams & Wilkins; 2001: 231–249.
8. Blumer D, Montouris G, Davies K, et al. Suicide in epilepsy: Psychopathology, pathogenesis, and prevention. *Epilepsy Behav.* 2002;3:232–241.
9. Blumer D, Montouris G, Hermann B. Psychiatric morbidity in seizure patients on a neurodiagnostic monitoring unit. *J Neuropsychiatry Clin Neurosci.* 1995;7:445–456.
10. Blumer D, Wakhlu S, Montouris G, Wyler A. Treatment of the interictal psychoses. *J Clin Psychiatry.* 2000;61:110–122.
11. Blumer D, Zielinski J. Pharmacologic treatment of psychiatric disorders associated with epilepsy. *J Epilepsy.* 1988;1:13–50.
12. Cockerell OC, Johnson AL, Sander JW, et al. Mortality from epilepsy: results from a prospective population-based study. *Lancet.* 1994;344:918–921.
13. Davies KG, Blumer DP, Lobo S, et al. *De novo* nonepileptic seizures after cranial surgery for epilepsy: Incidence and risk factors. *Epilepsy Behav.* 2000;1:436–443.
14. Demers-Desrosiers LA, Nestoros JN, Vaillancourt P. Acute psychosis precipitated by withdrawal of anticonvulsant medication. *Am J Psychiatry.* 1978;135:981–982.
15. Editorial. Suicide and epilepsy. *Br Med J.* 1980;281:530.
16. Engel J. *Seizures and Epilepsy.* Philadelphia: Davis; 1989.
17. Fukuchi T, Kanemoto K, Kato M, et al. Death in epilepsy with special attention to suicide cases. *Epilepsy Res.* 2002;51:233–236.
18. Gastaut H. État actuel des connaissances sur l'anatomie pathologique des épilepsies. *Acta Neurol Psychiatr Belg.* 1956;56:5–20.
19. Gastaut H, Morin G, Lesèvre N. Étude du comportement des épileptiques psychomoteurs dans l'intervalle de leurs crises: Les troubles de l'activité globale et de la sociabilité. *Ann Med Psychol (Paris). 1955;113:1–27.*
20. Gerard ME, Spitz MC, Towbin JA, et al. Subacute postictal aggression. *Neurology.* 1998;50:384–388.
21. Gibbs FA. Ictal and non-ictal psychiatric disorders in temporal lobe epilepsy. *J Nerv Ment Dis.* 1951;113:522–528.
22. Goodwin FK, Jamison KR. *Manic-Depressive Illness.* New York: Oxford University Press; 1990.
23. Haltrich E. *Todesursachen von Epilepsiekranken einer neurologischen Klinik und Poliklinik.* Heidelberg: Diss; 1960.
24. Hauser WA, Annegers JF, Elveback LR. Mortality in patients with epilepsy. *Epilepsia.* 1980;21:399–412.
25. Hennessy MJ, Langan Y, Binnie CD, et al. A study of mortality after temporal lobe epilepsy surgery. *Neurology.* 1999;53:1276–1283.
26. Henriksen B, Juul-Jensen PP, Lund M. The Mortality of Epileptics. In: Brackenridge RDC, ed. *Life Assurance Medicine.* London: Pitman; 1970:139–148.
27. Hill D. Psychiatric disorders of epilepsy. *Med Press.* 1953;229:473–475.
28. Jallon P. Mortality in patients with epilepsy. *Curr Opin Neurol.* 2004; 17:141–146.
29. Janz D. *Die Epilepsien. Spezielle Pathologie und Therapie.* Stuttgart: George Thieme; 1969.
30. Jensen I. Temporal lobe epilepsy: Late mortality in patients treated with unilateral temporal lobe resections. *Acta Neurol Scand.* 1975;52:374–380.
31. Kanemoto K, Kawasaki J, Mori E. Violence and epilepsy: A close relation between violence and postictal psychosis. *Epilepsia.* 1999;40:107–109.
32. Kraepelin E. *Psychiatrie,* 8th ed. Leipzig: Barth; 1923.
33. Landolt H. Serial Electroencephalographic Investigation during psychotic episodes in epileptic patients and during schizophrenic attacks. In: Lorentz de Haas AM, ed. *Lectures on Epilepsy.* Amsterdam: Elsevier; 1958:91–133.
34. Landolt H. Über Verstimmungen, Dämmerzustände and schizophrene Zustandsbilder bei Epilepsie: Ergebnisse klinischer und elektroenzephalographischer Untersuchungen. *Schweiz Arch Neurol Psychiatrie.* 1955;76:313–321.
35. Lönnqvist JK. Psychiatric aspects of suicidal behaviour: depression. In: Hawton K,van Heeringen K, eds. *Suicide and Attempted Suicide.* Chichester: Wiley; 2000:107–120.
36. Matthews WS, Barabas G. Suicide and epilepsy: a review of the literature. *Psychosomatics.* 1981;22:515–524.
37. Mendez MF. Disorders of Mood and Affect in Epilepsy. In: Sackellares JC, Berent S, eds. *Psychological Disturbances in Epilepsy.* Boston: Butterworth-Heinemann; 1996:125–141.
38. Mendez MF, Cummings JL, Benson DF. Depression in epilepsy. Significance and phenomenology. *Arch Neurol.* 1986;43:766–770.
39. Mendez MF, Doss RC. Ictal and psychiatric aspects of suicide in epileptic patients. *Int J Psychiatry Med.* 1992;22:231–237.
40. Mendez MF, Lanska DJ, Manon-Espaillat R, et al. Causative factors for suicide attempts by overdose in epileptics. *Arch Neurol.* 1989;46:1065–1068.
41. Murphy GE. Suicide and attempted suicide. In: Winokur G, Clayton PJ, eds. *The Medical Basis of Psychiatry.* Philadelphia: WB Saunders; 1994: 529–544.
42. Nilsson L, Ahlbom A, Farahmand BY, et al. Risk factors for suicide in epilepsy: A case control study. *Epilepsia.* 2002;43:644–651.
43. Ojemann LM, Friel PN, Trejo WJ, et al. Effect of doxepin on seizure frequency in depressed epileptic patients. *Neurology.* 1983;33:646–648.
44. Pompili M, Girardi P, Ruberto A, et al. Suicide in the epilepsies: A meta-analytic investigation of 29 cohorts. *Epilepsy Behav.* 2005;7:305–310.
45. Prudhomme C. Epilepsy and suicide. *J Nerv Ment Dis.* 1941;94:722–731.
46. Schmitz B, Wolf P. Psychoses in epilepsy. In: Devinsky O, Theodore WH, eds. *Epilepsy and Behavior.* New York: Wiley-Liss; 1991:97–128.
47. Stevens JR. Interictal clinical Manifestations of complex partial seizures. In: Penry JK, Daly DD, eds. *Advances in Neurology, Vol. 11: Complex Partial Seizures and Their Treatment.* New York: Raven; 1975:85–112.
48. Taylor DC. Psychiatric and social issues in measuring the input and outcome of epilepsy surgery. In: Engel J Jr., ed. *Surgical Treatment of the Epilepsies.* New York: Raven Press; 1987:485–503.
49. Taylor DC, Marsh SM. Implications of long-term follow-up studies in epilepsy: with a note on the cause of death. In: Penry JK, ed. *Epilepsy,*

the Eighth International Symposium. New York: Raven Press; 1977:27–35.
50. Tellenbach H. Epilepsy as a seizure disorder and as a psychosis: on alternative psychoses of a paranoid type with "Forced Normalization" (Landolt) of the electroencephalogram of Epileptics. In: Trimble MR, Schmitz B, eds. *Forced Normalization and Alternative Psychoses of Epilepsy*. Bristol, PA: Wrightson Biomedical Publishing; 1998 (English translation of the 1965 German paper).
51. Trimble MR, Schmitz B, eds. *Forced Normalization and Alternative Psychoses of Epilepsy*. Bristol, PA: Wrightson Biomedical Publishing; 1998.
52. Williams D. The structure of emotions reflected in epileptic experiences. *Brain*. 1956;79:29–67.

CHAPTER 212 ■ DISORDERS OF IMPULSE CONTROL

LUDGER TEBARTZ VAN ELST AND MICHAEL R. TRIMBLE

INTRODUCTION

Impulsivity in general is a frequent clinical problem that is related to many different primary psychiatric disorders as, for example, attention-deficit-hyperactivity disorder (ADHD), borderline personality disorder, bipolar disorder (in particular in hypomanic or manic states), and schizophrenia.[1,2] Furthermore, it is a common management problem in patients with mental retardation or organic brain disorders. Although the International Statistical Classification of Diseases and Health Related Problems (ICD-10) does not recognize specific independent disorders of impulse control,[1] the American Diagnostic and Statistical Manual of Mental Disorders (DSM-IV) defines the category of impulse-control disorders not elsewhere classified[2] and includes the entities of intermittent explosive disorder (IED; DSM-IV 312.34), kleptomania (DSM-IV 312.32), pyromania (DSM-IV 312.33), pathologic gambling (DSM-IV 312.31), and trichotillomania (DSM-IV 312.39).

Because impulsive aggression is the most clinically important and most troubling form of these impulse control disorders (see also Chapter 283 and the review by Tebartz van Elst[73]), in this chapter we will concentrate on the problem of aggression in the context of epilepsy. This issue has been the topic of other recent publications.[73] We discuss the putative relationship between epilepsy and the other aforementioned impulse control disorders briefly at the end of the chapter.

IMPULSIVE AGGRESSION IN EPILEPSY

The relationship between epilepsy and aggressive behavior is a particularly controversial issue.[33] In Chapter 283, we discussed the issue of episodic dyscontrol and IED in the context of the differential diagnosis of epilepsy, and also as an independent psychiatric entity. Here we want to dwell on the more general and less specific forms of impulsive aggression that do not fulfil the criteria of episodic dyscontrol, but still are seen in patients with epilepsy.

The precise prevalence of aggressive and violent behavior in the context of epilepsy is very difficult to assess and subsequently is still unknown. In patients with episodic affective aggression, a history of epilepsy is reported to be more common.[4] On the other hand,[22] most of the community-based studies did not find an increased prevalence of aggressive behavior in patients with epilepsy.[43,48] Different papers report wide-ranging prevalence figures of aggression in epilepsy in general, do not note the specific epileptic syndrome, and cite figures from as low as 4.8% [65] to as high as 50%.[31]

Currie et al. reported aggression in 7% of the patients in a large survey of 666 patients with temporal lobe epilepsy (TLE).[15] Falconer's group reviewed 100 patients from London's Maudsley Hospital referred for temporal lobectomy and found a prevalence of outbursts of aggressive behavior in as many as 27% of these patients.[24] However, like most of the other studies addressing this issue, these studies were hampered by selection bias, and thus the real prevalence of aggressive behavior in epilepsy remains controversial.[48]

In epilepsy, three different types of aggressive behaviors should be distinguished on the basis of their relationship to the seizures: ictal, postictal, and interictal aggression.[27,42,73,74]

Ictal Aggression

Ictal aggression is very rare.[36,66] Delgardo-Escueta et al. found an incidence of about 1 in 1,000 seizures with ictal aggression in a large survey of several thousand seizures documented by video-telemetry.[18] However, it can be argued that as such, looking for ictal aggression in the context of the tightly controlled arena of an electroencephalogram (EEG) suite is not going to provide a true view on the frequency of the problem. This is because patients with aggressive episodes are less likely to be accepted for evaluation, and such episodes of aggressive release are more likely to occur in a community rather than a laboratory setting. In ictal aggression, hostile and verbal or physical aggressive behavior is often directed toward nearby objects or persons and may or may not be provoked.[27] The patients are generally amnesic for these aggressive episodes and often express remorse or feelings of shame for their behavior after the event.[19,28]

Postictal Aggression

Postictal aggression is more common than ictal aggression and, although it is still believed to be rare, it may be underrecognized and unreported.[77] Postictal aggressive behavior usually follows a cluster of complex partial seizures or secondary generalized seizures in patients in whom such episodes are not the usually expression of their epilepsy. Some evidence points to ictal pain or dysphoria as predisposing factors for the later development of postictal aggressive behaviour.[32] If the episode occurs in the context of a postictal confusional state, poorly structured aggressive behavior is not that rare. This aggression is poorly directed, and the patient, rather than someone who is attacked, is most likely to come to harm. If postictal aggression is part of a postictal confusional state, the disruptive behavior immediately follows the seizure without a lucid interval intervening between the ictus and the outbreak of the disruptive behavior. In this state, patients are often resistive, but within their confusion can be very aroused, angry, and fearful.[41,46]

Postictal psychosis typically follows a cluster of complex partial or secondary generalized seizures in patients with long-standing chronic and often therapy-refractory epilepsy. Generally these states follow a lucid interval—the calm before the storm—which might last anywhere between hours and days up to 1 week. Observers may notice an insidious onset of affective symptoms with arousal, restlessness, agitation, and often anxiety, fear, and anger, although the behavioral state can erupt quite suddenly. Subsequently, overt psychotic symptoms with delusions and hallucinations might follow. The latter might be accompanied by aggressive behavior that sometimes is very dramatic and dangerous.[29,40,49,78] Although aggressive behavior in the context of a delusional state is often rather disorganized if there is some clouding of consciousness, this is not necessarily the case. Over 50% of patients with postictal psychotic states have minimal or no such associated confusion, and aggressive behavior can be well-structured and goal-directed. Patients often feel angry and aroused, although they may appear calm and concentrated to the observer.[41,72]

Kanemoto et al. make the important observation that well-directed and self-destructive behavior might even be a hallmark of postictal psychosis.[41] The psychosis may be missed, either because it is not probed for, or because the behavior is such that it is not possible to obtain a good mental state evaluation. The latter is the more problematic in those with learning disabilities. The aggressive behavior might then be structured and goal-directed, but without any obvious sign of delusions or hallucinations.[41,46,72] The awareness of the problem of postictal psychoses and associated aggressive behavior is of particular importance for epilepsy-monitoring centers because, in this context, many patients with chronic therapy-refractory epilepsy are seen and diagnosed following an acute reduction of their medication for diagnostic purposes. If a history of previous postictal events exists, doctors should be aware of the risk of postictal psychosis and aggression, and should closely monitor the behavior of these patients. Outbursts of aggression, especially with psychotic intensity, are dangerous not only for the patients but also the nurses and attending physicians themselves.

Interictal Aggression

Interictal aggressions are the most common, but generally less dramatic forms of aggressive behaviors in patients with epilepsy. These can be seen in the context of an antisocial personality disorder which, in turn, might be the consequence of the sometimes difficult psychosocial background and upbringing of patients with epilepsy, Or it might be part of a prolonged psychotic episode, an interictal affective disorder, or a psychosis of a paranoid- or schizophrenia-like type.[49,41]

In patients with epilepsy and mental handicap, interictal aggression is a common management problem. In these patients, the aggressive behavior is often the result of poor social and communication competence in expressing personal needs and rarely results in severe violence.[37]

An interictal syndrome of episodic affective aggression, independent of observable ictal activity, major psychiatric disorder, or antisocial personality disorder, is well described and has been referred to as *episodic dyscontrol* or *IED*.[4,23,47,52,64,71] Episodic dyscontrol is characterized by several discrete episodes of extreme arousal and rage that are out of proportion to any precipitating psychosocial stressor, but that result in severe aggressive and violent behavior. As mentioned earlier, this form of possible epilepsy-related aggression has been described and discussed in Chapter 283.

Irritability and impulsivity, in particular verbal aggression of mild to modest severity, might be a symptom of the dysphoric disorder of epilepsy (DDE). DDE is a specific form of epilepsy-related affective disorder characterized by symptoms like irritability, mood swings, anergia, diffuse pain, anxiety, fears, and disturbances of sleep. The paroxysmal affects, ranging from irritability through anger to rage, play a major role in DDE and make it an easy-to-recognize pattern of psychopathology for the experienced clinician.[10] Based on the relationship to the ictus, DDE can be subclassified as preictal, interictal, and postictal DDE.[44] In particular, in patients with learning disability, irritability and aggressive behavior might dominate the clinical picture of DDE and thereby obscure the diagnosis.

Finally, interictal aggression in the context of epilepsy can be a side effect of antiepileptic medication. Reports have been published, for example, for substances such as phenobarbital, several benzodiazepines, gabapentin (especially in adolescents), vigabatrin, topiramate, and levitiracetam.[3,8,16,20,30,54,57,67] This may be a part of a syndrome of forced normalization, an idiosyncratic reaction representing the precipitation of a nonconvulsive status epilepticus, or a manifestation of intoxication. However, from a different perspective, anticonvulsants may be quite helpful in treating impulsive aggression in patients with epilepsy, in whom aggression is postictal in nature or interictal as part of a mood instability syndrome, as they are in other aggressive patients without epilepsy.[5,6,39,58,59,68,69,75]

This complex constellation illustrates the need for a careful neuropsychiatric assessment of patients in whom impulsive aggression is a clinical problem, be it in the context of epilepsy or not.

TREATMENT OF AGGRESSION IN EPILEPSY

Establishing a correct diagnosis is the most important point in treating problems with aggression in the context of epilepsy (Fig. 1). A careful neurologic, psychiatric, and medical history and examination is a prerequisite to answer the following questions: Is there any medical condition that contributes to the aggressive behavior, such as an endocrinologic disease? Is there any medication that might contribute to the aggressive behavior—antiepileptic or otherwise? What is the correct neurologic diagnosis? Does the patient have epilepsy? Are there any other cerebral problems in addition to the epilepsy? Is there any specific epilepsy-related psychiatric disorder, either ictal or postictal, that might explain the aggressive behavior? Are any psychiatric diagnoses present, but possibly independent of the epilepsy, such as bipolar disorder or antisocial personality disorder?

With regards to the latter question, if the epilepsy started early in life, it is often impossible to establish if, for example, the clinical picture that fulfils the criteria for an antisocial personality disorder is or is not independent of the organic brain disease indicated by the epilepsy: Does the patient have an unassociated personality disorder or, alternatively, is the problem an organic personality disorder? A careful behavioral analysis, thorough anamnesis, and possibly video-telemetry should clarify if the aggressive behavior is ictal, postictal, or interictal and whether it occurs in the context of altered states of consciousness or psychosis.

Following syndromic and possibly nosologic diagnosis, treatment should be targeted to any treatable causes if possible, such as intervening medical problems like endocrinologic disorders. Neurological syndromes, such as the epilepsy itself, should be treated effectively, with as few medications as possible to avoid seizures, and with avoidance of medications most linked with alteration of mood and the release of aggressive behavior. Particular care should be taken to establish signs of depression, anxiety, or the common dysphoric disorder of epilepsy, because a close link exists between these psychopathologic states and affective aggression in epilepsy.[74] Affective symptoms should be treated medically and with psychotherapy at the same time.[34,50] In the medical treatment of depression in patients with epilepsy, selective serotonin reuptake inhibitors (SSRIs) or other new antidepressants such as

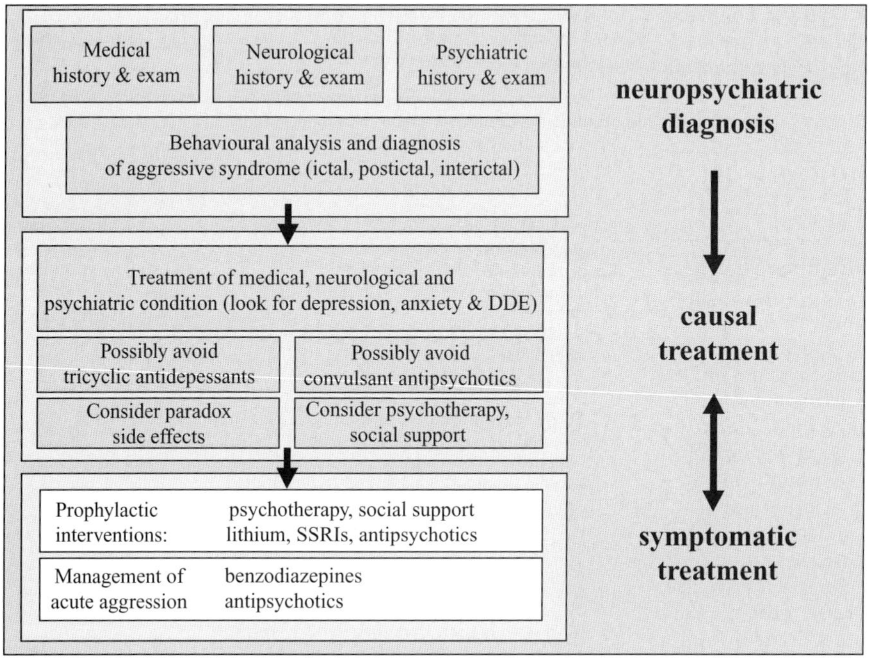

FIGURE 1. Therapeutic guidelines for the treatment of aggression in patients with epilepsy. (From Tebartz van Elst L. Aggression and epilepsy. In: Trimble M, Schmitz B, eds. *The Neuropsychiatry of Epilepsy*. Cambridge: Cambridge University Press; 2002: 81–106, with permission.)

venlafaxine should be preferred to the older tricyclic antidepressants (TCA) because the latter are more likely to provoke seizures.[9,45] The anticonvulsant effect of the SSRIs is well documented in animal models of epilepsy,[12,51,60,79] and is also described in humans.[26]

Following treatment of all medical, neurologic, and psychiatric conditions that may or may not contribute to the aggressive psychopathology, a symptomatic treatment of the aggression is mandatory. However, this depends on whether the aggression is an ictal, postictal, or interictal phenomenon.

Ictal aggression requires immediate attention to the seizures, and a nonconvulsive status epilepticus can be interrupted using, for example, benzodiazepines.[27] Apart from that, a patient who displays agitation and aggressive during a seizure should not be overly restricted, because defensive violence is more common in such situations, and the aggressive behavior is self-limited, as is the seizure.

The same is true for postictal confusional states: Even aggressive behavior in the context of postictal psychosis is self-limited. However, if the aggression is severe and disturbing or self-harming, medical treatment using benzodiazepines such as diazepam or clobazam and/or antipsychotics (usually one of the atypicals) should be started. Good seizure control that avoids clusters of complex partial or secondary generalized seizure is the best prophylactic intervention, because postictal confusional and psychotic states are more common after such episodes. If, after for example a cluster of attacks, the impending abnormal behavior can be predicted, the use of a benzodiazepine for about 48 hours may well be sufficient to abort the event. Patients or caregivers should have a supply of such medications and be given advice on how to use them judiciously.

In treating interictal aggression, one should again distinguish prophylactic and acute treatment. For the treatment of severe and etiologically unclear acute hyperarousal-dyscontrol syndromes, a combination of benzodiazepines, such as diazepam, and antipsychotics, such as haloperidol, is still the most effective and safest intervention. In cases of interictal psychoses, however, the antipsychotic medication should eventually be switched to one of the atypical antipsychotic agents with little proconvulsant potential, because these drugs are better tolerated. A good control of the psychosis is the best way to prevent aggression if it is part of the psychosis.

In cases of interictal aggressive syndromes like IED, no well-established medical prophylactic therapies are available. However, many anecdotal reports document the effective use of substances such as lithium, valproate, carbamazepine, phenytoin, antipsychotics, β-blockers, clonidine, and even psychostimulants (see Chapter 283 and several reviews[25,35,81]). However, because there are hardly any well-conducted systematic treatment studies at the moment, the medical treatment still is very experimental and single-case driven. Nevertheless, in the light of the very severe burden that is put on the patients, their relatives, and caregivers by the sometimes devastating behavioral episodes, a systematic trial of these agents seems justified.

If aggressive behavior is part of interictal DDE,[10] this should be treated with SSRIs in the first instance. Substances such as citalopram or escitalopram have few interaction problems with other antiepileptic drugs and have a minimal problem with lowering the seizure threshold. If these drugs are not effective in controlling dysphoric depression, one should consider others, such as venlafaxine, a TCA, or even a combination of the two. In some cases, additional treatment with a very low-dose atypical antipsychotic might also be helpful. However, one should always avoid high doses of these drug and be very careful with combination therapy, because this might lower the seizure threshold,[9] provoking further irritability or further postictal episodes.

Finally, as mentioned in Chapter 283 in the context of episodic dyscontrol, it must be stressed that anger management, contingency management, and psychotherapy all can be very helpful and successful in treating impulsive aggressive behavior. Particularly in the context of mental handicap and personality disorders, aggression and impulsivity might be part of attention seeking behavior and role testing. In these cases, feedback strategies and the reactions of relatives and caregivers are very important, and methods of contingency management may be a critical element of any successful treatment.[7,14] Behavioral therapy, in particular in patients with epilepsy and mental handicap, has been proven very effective.[17,38,63]

Different methods of anger management, cognitive behavior therapy, or skills training that have been developed irrespective of the context of impulsive behavior may be very helpful in the therapy of aggression.[17,70,76,80]

EPILEPSY AND OTHER DISORDERS OF IMPULSE CONTROL

To our knowledge, no papers in the literature address the question of a specific link between epilepsy and syndromes such as kleptomania and pathologic gambling. However, a few case reports discuss a putative link between very specific forms of epilepsy and trichotillomania and, in particular, pyromania or arson.[11,13,21,53,55,56,61,62] The latter has been discussed to be possibly triggered by a putative mechanism called the *limbic psychotic trigger reaction* (LPTR). This is believed to be a form of nonconvulsive behavioral seizure (NCBS); following this theory, seizure-like limbic pathomechanisms that are kindled by memory stimuli result in brief psychotic episodes in which the affected patients impulsively set fire.[61,62] However, it should be stressed that these hypotheses are purely based on a few case reports, and that no solid epidemiologic data support the theory that these forms of impulse control disorder are truly more common in epilepsy as compared to the general population.

SUMMARY AND CONCLUSIONS

Aggression in the context of epilepsy is not common but, when it occurs, it often imposes an immense burden on the patient, his relatives, and caregivers. The neurobiology and precise pathomechanisms of aggressive behavior, be it in the context of epilepsy or not, are most likely heterogeneous and very complex. Nevertheless, it is important to appreciate the interplay of social, psychological, and neurobiologic factors, all of which may contribute to aggression and violent behavior in any given case.

Clinically, it is crucial to first establish a correct diagnosis. Intervening medical, neurologic, and psychiatric disorders—in particular, depression, anxiety, and DDE—should be recognized and treated adequately. A correct syndromic diagnosis of the aggressive syndrome and its relation to the seizures should be made. Treatment should aim at possible underlying medical, neurologic, or psychiatric disorders. In symptomatic treatment of aggressive outbursts, the management of acute aggression and prophylactic treatment to prevent further episodes should be differentiated.

Pharmacologic treatment is often the mainstay of therapy, but psychological therapies in the form of anger management or other variations of cognitive behavior therapy are an integral part of management in many patients.

References

1. *International Klassifikation Psychischer Störungen*. Bern: Verlag Hans Huber; 2001.
2. American Psychiatric Association. *Diagnostic and Statistical Manual of Mental Disorders (DSM-IV)*. Washington, DC: American Psychiatric Association; 1994.
3. Armour DJ, Fidler C, Wright EC, et al. Vigabatrin in adults with poorly-controlled epilepsy and learning disabilities. *Seizure*. 1992;1:157–162.
4. Bach-Y-Rita G, Lion JR, Climent CE, et al. (1971) Episodic dyscontrol: A study of 130 violent patients. *Am J Psychiatry*. 1971;127:1473–1478.
5. Barratt ES, Kent TA, Bryant SG, et al. A controlled trial of phenytoin in impulsive aggression. *J Clin Psychopharmacol*. 1991;11:388–389.
6. Barratt ES, Stanford MS, Felthous AR, et al. The effects of phenytoin on impulsive and premeditated aggression: A controlled study. *J Clin Psychopharmacol*. 1997;17:341–349.
7. Berryman J, Evans IM, Kalbag A. The effects of training in nonaversive behavior management on the attitudes and understanding of direct care staff. *J Behav Ther Exp Psychiatry*. 1994;25:241–250.
8. Binder RL. Three case reports of behavioral disinhibition with clonazepam. *Gen Hosp Psychiatry*. 1987;9:151–153.
9. Blumer D. Antidepressant and double antidepressant treatment for the affective disorder of epilepsy. *J Clin Psychiatry*. 1997;58:3–11.
10. Blumer D. Dysphoric disorders and paroxysmal affects: Recognition and treatment of epilepsy-related psychiatric disorders. *Harv Rev Psychiatry*. 2000;8:8–17.
11. Brook R, Dolan M, Coorey P. Arson and epilepsy. *Med Sci Law*. 1996; 36:268–271.
12. Browning RA. Enhancement of the anticonvulsant effect of fluoxetine following blockade of 5-HT1A receptors. *Eur J Pharmacology*. 1997;336:1–6.
13. Carpenter PK, King AL. (1989) Epilepsy and arson. *Br J Psychiatry*. 1989;154:554–556.
14. Connor DF, Steingard RJ A clinical approach to the pharmacotherapy of aggression in children and adolescents. *Ann N Y Acad Sci*. 1996;794:290–307.
15. Currie S, Heathfield W, Henson R, et al. Clinical course and prognosis of temporal lobe epilepsy: A survey of 666 patients. *Brain*. 1974;94:173–190.
16. Daderman AM. Flunitrazepam (Rohypnol) abuse in combination with alcohol causes premeditated, grievous violence in male juvenile offenders. *J Am Acad Psychiatry Law*. 1999;27:83–99.
17. Davis GR, Armstrong HE Jr, Donovan DM, et al. Cognitive-behavioral treatment of depressed affect among epileptics: Preliminary findings. *J Clin Psychol*. 1984;40:930–935.
18. Delgado-Escueta AV, Mattson RH, King L, et al. Special report. The nature of aggression during epileptic seizures. *N Engl J Med*. 1981;305:711–716.
19. Devinsky O, Bear D. Varieties of aggressive behavior in temporal lobe epilepsy. *Am J Psychiatry*. 1984;141:651–656.
20. Dinkelacker V, Dietl T, Widman G, et al. Aggressive behavior of epilepsy patients in the course of levetiracetam add-on therapy: Report of 33 mild to severe cases. *Epilepsy Behav*. 2003;4:537–547.
21. Drogowski M, Orlicki B, Dawidowski E. [Pyromania as a symptom of a psycho-organic syndrome in the course of temporal lobe epilepsy]. *Neurol Neurochir Psychiatr Pol*. 1966;16:1433–1434.
22. Elliot FA. Neurological findings in adult minimal brain dysfunction and the dyscontrol syndrome. *J Nerv Ment Dis*. 1982;170:680–687.
23. Elliott FA. The episodic dyscontrol syndrome and aggression. *Neurologic Clin*. 1984;2:113–125.
24. Falconer MA. Reversibility by temporal-lobe resection of the behavioral abnormalities of temporal-lobe epilepsy. *N Engl J Med*. 1973;289:451–455.
25. Fava M. Psychopharmacologic treatment of pathologic aggression. [Review.] *Psychiatric Clin N Am*. 1997;20:427–451.
26. Favale E. Anticonvulsant effect of fluoxetine in humans [see comments]. *Neurology*. 1995;45:1926–1927.
27. Feddersen B, Bender A, Arnold S, et al. Aggressive confusional state as a clinical manifestation of status epilepticus in MELAS. *Neurology*. 2003;61:1149–1150.
28. Fenwick P. The nature and management of aggression in epilepsy. *J Neuropsychiatry Clin Neurosci*. 1989;1,418–425.
29. Fenwick PBC. Aggression and epilepsy. In: Trimble MR, Bolwig T, eds. *Epilepsy and Psychiatry*. Chichester: John Wiley and Sons; 1986:31–60.
30. File SE, Wilks LJ. Changes in seizure threshold and aggression during chronic treatment with three anticonvulsants and on drug withdrawal. *Psychopharmacology (Berl)*. 1990;100:237–242.
31. Gastaut H, Morrin G, Lesevre N. Etudes du compartment des epileptiques psychomoteur dans L'interval de leurs crises. *Ann Med Psychology*. 1955;113:1–29.
32. Gerard ME. Subacute postictal aggression [see comments]. *Neurology*. 1998;50:384–388.
33. Geschwind N. The clinical setting of aggression in temporal lobe epilepsy. In: Fields WS, Sweet WH, eds. *Neural Basis of Violence and Aggression*. St. Louis: Warren H. Green; 1975:273–281.
34. Goldstein LH. Effectiveness of psychological interventions for people with poorly controlled epilepsy. [Review.] *J Neurology, Neurosurg Psychiatry*. 1997;63:137–142.
35. Griffith JL. Treatment of episodic behavioral disorders with rapidly absorbed benzodiazepines. *J Nervous Ment Dis*. 1985;173:312–315.
36. Gunn J. Epilepsy, automatism, and crime. *Lancet*. 1971;1:1173–1176.
37. Gunn J. Criminal behavior and mental disorder. *Br J Psychiatry*. 1977; 130:317–329.
38. Holzapfel S. Behavioral psychophysiological intervention in a mentally retarded epileptic patient with brain lesion. *Appl Psychophysiol Biofeedback*. 1998;23:189–202.
39. Janowsky DS, Kraus JE, Barnhill J, et al. Effects of topiramate on aggressive, self-injurious, and disruptive/destructive behaviors in the intellectually disabled: An open-label retrospective study. *J Clin Psychopharmacol*. 2003;23:500–504.
40. Kanemoto K. Postictal psychosis: A comparison with acute interictal and chronic psychoses. *Epilepsia*. 1996;37:551–556.
41. Kanemoto K. Violence and epilepsy: A close relation between violence and postictal psychosis. *Epilepsia*. 1999;40:107–109.
42. Kanner AM. Recognition of the various expressions of anxiety, psychosis, and aggression in epilepsy. *Epilepsia*. 2004;45(Suppl 2):22–27.

43. Kligman D, Goldberg DA. Temporal lobe epilepsy and aggression. *J Nerv Ment Dis*. 1975;160:324–341.
44. Krishnamoorthy ES, Trimble MR, Blumer D. The classification of neuropsychiatric disorders in epilepsy: A proposal by the sub-commission on classification of the ILAE commission on epilepsy & psychobiology.
45. Lambert MV. Depression in epilepsy: Etiology, phenomenology, and treatment. [Review.] *Epilepsia*. 1999;40(Suppl 10):S21–S47.
46. Lancman M. Psychosis and peri-ictal confusional states. [Review.] *Neurology*. 1999;53:S33–S38.
47. Leicester J. Temper tantrums, epilepsy, and episodic dyscontrol. *Br J Psychiatry*. 1982;141:262–266.
48. Lishman WA. *Organic Psychiatry: The Psychological Consequences of Cerebral Disorder*. Boston: Blackwell Science; 1998.
49. Logsdail SJ, Toone BK. Post-ictal psychoses. A clinical and phenomenological description. *Brtish J Psychiatry*. 1988;152:246–252.
50. Lorenzen D. [Initial results of behavior therapy in Psychiatric Regional Hospital Weinsberg]. [German.] *Nervenarzt*. 1973;44:423–427.
51. Lu KT. Endogenous serotonin inhibits epileptiform activity in rat hippocampal CA1 neurons via 5-hydroxytryptamine1A receptor activation. *Neuroscience*. 1998;86:729–737.
52. Maletzky BM. The episodic dyscontrol syndrome. *Dis Nerv Syst*. 1973; 34:178–185.
53. Managoli S, Vilhekar KY. Tricotillomania as an ictal manifestation of partial seizure in a 4-year-old girl. *Indian J Pediatr*. 2003;70:843.
54. Marcus A. Benzodiazepine administration induces exogenic psychosis: A case of child abuse. *Child Abuse Neglect*. 1995;19:833–836.
55. Meinhard EA, Oozeer R, Cameron D. Photosensitive epilepsy in children who set fires. *Br Med J (Clin Res Ed)*. 1988;296:1773.
56. Milrod LM, Urion DK. Juvenile fire setting and the photoparoxysmal response. *Ann Neurol*. 1992;32:222–223.
57. Mula M, Trimble MR. The importance of being seizure free: Topiramate and psychopathology in epilepsy. *Epilepsy Behav*. 2003;4:430–434.
58. Nickel MK, Nickel C, Kaplan P, et al. Treatment of aggression with topiramate in male borderline patients: A double-blind, placebo-controlled study. *Biol Psychiatry*. 2005;57:495–499.
59. Nickel MK, Nickel C, Mitterlehner FO, et al. Topiramate treatment of aggression in female borderline personality disorder patients: A double-blind, placebo-controlled study. *J Clin Psychiatry*. 2004;65:1515–1519.
60. Pasini A. The anticonvulsant action of fluoxetine in substantia nigra is dependent upon endogenous serotonin. *Brain Res*. 1996;724:84–88.
61. Pontius AA. Motiveless firesetting: Implicating partial limbic seizure kindling by revived memories of fires in "limbic psychotic trigger reaction." *Percept Mot Skills*. 1999;88:970–982.
62. Pontius AA, Wieser HG. Can memories kindle nonconvulsive behavioral seizures in humans? Case report exemplifying the "limbic psychotic trigger reaction." *Epilepsy Behav*. 2004;5:775–783.
63. Rapport MD. Carbamazepine and behavior therapy for aggressive behavior. Treatment of a mentally retarded, postencephalitic adolescent with seizure disorder. *Behav Modif*. 1983;7:255–265.
64. Ratner RA, Shapiro D. The episodic dyscontrol syndrome and criminal responsibility. *Bull Am Acad Psychiatry Law*. 1979;7:422–431.
65. Rodin EA. Psychomotor epilepsy and aggressive behavior. *Arch Gen Psychiatry*. 1973;28:210–213.
66. Saver JL, Salloway SP, Devinsky O, et al. Neuropsychiatry of Aggression. In: Fogel BS, Schiffer RB, Rao SM, eds. *Neuropsychiatry*. Baltimore: Williams & Wilkins; 1996:523–548.
67. Sheth RD. Aggression in children treated with clobazam for epilepsy. *Clin Neuropharmacol*. 1994;17:332–337.
68. Stanford MS, Helfritz LE, Conklin SM, et al. A comparison of anticonvulsants in the treatment of impulsive aggression. *Exp Clin Psychopharmacol*. 2005;13:72–77.
69. Stanford MS, Houston RJ, Mathias CW, et al. A double-blind placebo-controlled crossover study of phenytoin in individuals with impulsive aggression. *Psychiatry Res*. 2001;103:193–203.
70. Stanley B, Bundy E, Beberman R. Skills training as an adjunctive treatment for personality disorders. *J Psychiatr Pract*. 2001;7:324–335.
71. Stone JL, McDaniel KD, Hughes JR, et al. Episodic dyscontrol disorder and paroxysmal EEG abnormalities: Successful treatment with carbamazepine. *Biol Psychiatry*. 1986;21:208–212.
72. Szabo CA, Lancman MSS. Postictal psychosis: A review. *Neuropsychiatry Neuropsychol Behav Neurol*. 1996;9:258–264.
73. Tebartz van Elst L. Aggression and Epilepsy. In: Trimble M, Schmitz B, eds. *The Neuropsychiatry of Epilepsy*. Cambridge: Cambridge University Press; 2002:81–106.
74. Tebartz van Elst L, Woermann FG, Lemieux L, et al. Affective aggression in patients with temporal lobe epilepsy: A quantitative MRI study of the amygdala. *Brain* 2000;123:234–243.
75. Thibaut F, Colonna L. [Carbamazepine and aggressive behavior: A review]. *Encephale*. 1993;19:651–656.
76. Thomas SP. Teaching healthy anger management. *Perspect Psychiatr Care*. 2001;37:41–48.
77. Treiman DM. *Psychobiology of Ictal Aggression*. New York: Raven Press; 1991:341–356.
78. Trimble MR. *The psychoses of epilepsy*. New York: Raven Press; 1991.
79. Wada Y. Prolonged but not acute fluoxetine administration produces its inhibitory effect on hippocampal seizures in rats. *Psychopharmacology*. 1995;118:305–309.
80. Willner P, Brace N, Phillips J. Assessment of anger coping skills in individuals with intellectual disabilities. *J Intellect Disabil Res*. 2005;49:329–339.
81. Yudofsky SC. Pharmacologic management of aggression in the elderly. [Review.] *J Clin Psychiatry*. 1990;51(Suppl):22–28.

CHAPTER 213 ■ PSYCHIATRY AND RESIDENTIAL CARE

STEPHEN W. BROWN AND FRANK M. C. BESAG

"Do poor Tom some charity, whom the foul fiend vexes."

—William Shakespeare, "King Lear," Act III, Scene IV

"What doubtless remained longer than leprosy, and would persist when the lazar houses had been empty for years, were the values and images attached to the figure of the leper as well as the meaning of his exclusion, the social importance of that insistent and fearful figure which was not driven off without first being inscribed within a sacred circle."

—Michel Foucault, *Madness and Civilization: A History of Insanity in the Age ofReason*[11]

INTRODUCTION

Historical Perspective on the Rise and Fall of Confinement

Development of Institutions

Hospitals, hostels, and hotels share functions that are reflected in the common Latin root of these words (*hospitalia*, "guest chambers"). It is possible that in Europe during the Middle Ages some cities kept hostels for local people who were not capable of looking after themselves. Also, some people with behavioral problems that would now be attributed to psychosis, brain damage, or other psychiatric conditions might congregate around certain religious shrines. Custodial institutions that were separate from prisons appeared in Europe from the late 17th century onward and, during the 18th century, there emerged specialized asylums for the insane. The reason for the growth in asylum building during that period of history has been a subject of speculation in this century. One argument has been that a real increase occurred in the population with psychosis.[12] Alternatively, sociologic explanations have been advanced, suggesting that the development of psychiatry was a self-perpetuating means of social control.[25] For example, Foucault, noting that leprosy had recently disappeared from Europe, postulated that the "formulas of exclusion" persisted, so that "... poor vagabonds, criminals, and 'deranged minds' would take the part played by the leper ...," and he refers to "... that major form of a rigorous division which is social exclusion but spiritual reintegration."[11] Houses of correction were established in England in 1575 by an act of Parliament for "the punishment of vagabonds and the relief of the poor," and in 1656 the Hôpital Général was founded in Paris to confine the poor. Foucault notes that this confinement included "the debauched, spendthrift fathers, prodigal sons, blasphemers, men who 'seek to undo themselves,' libertines, and, in about one-tenth of cases (Paris), the insane." There was, however, a gradual process of categorization whereby those in need of asylum were recognized as being respectively poor, insane, handicapped, or epileptic, and these groups in turn came to be regarded as separate from criminals. As asylums increased in number and became more concerned with mental illness, a more humane approach to care appeared. This was typified by the work of William Tuke (1732–1822) in York (who founded the York Retreat after the death of a fellow Quaker in the county asylum), and Philippe Pinel (1745–1826) in France. Both stressed moral aspects of treatment and advocated the avoidance of methods of physical constraint, such as chains. Pinel's pupil Maisonneuve studied epilepsy, and wrote that "... epilepsy, like all chronic diseases, can be studied well only in the hospitals; there alone is it possible to find all its varieties together, to see all its nuances, and to acquire in short time more experience of this disease than in the whole course of ordinary practice."[16] Another physician of Maisonneuve's generation, Jean Etienne Dominique Esquirol (1772–1840), advocated special facilities for people with epilepsy apart from the other asylum inmates. The reason for this, however, was not to protect those with epilepsy, but to protect the insane, for he believed "... that the sight of one epileptic attack might suffice to make a healthy person epileptic. Now if this held true of healthy people, how much greater was the danger for the mentally deranged, who were so much more impressionable."[27] Consequently, with the growth of provision for the insane there also came separate facilities within the asylums for people with epilepsy. It is not surprising that the next stage was the establishment of entirely separate institutions for people with epilepsy.

Epilepsy in Institutions and the Move Toward Colonies, Villages, and Schools

European writers of the 19th century became interested in the ways in which epilepsy might act on the mind and cause mental disorder. Morel[23] suggested that the disease could exist in a masked form (*epilepsie larvée*), in which the main features were of insanity, not seizures. Falret[10] attempted to classify the psychiatric disorders of epilepsy and, in addition to acknowledging the existence of interictal and peri-ictal phenomena, he followed Morel in proposing a category of epileptic insanity that was manifested as an alternative to seizures, the *folie épileptique*. Morel also offered the view that the behavioral disorders associated with epilepsy, in particular the "epileptic furore," might be a consequence of bad treatment, and that improvement of the patient's environment by segregation, recreation, and occupation would bring about improvement.[22] This debate added to the intellectual climate from which the argument for separate institutions for epilepsy was to emerge.

In 19th century Europe, the word *colony* did not carry a pejorative connotation. The notion of establishing separate living space for people with epilepsy was based on a belief that this would be therapeutic in itself. There was an understanding that the condition was perpetuated by restrictions placed on the activities of normal life, especially the opportunity to take part in work. This was the rationale for the colony movement, exemplified by the foundation in 1867 of Bethel, near Bielefeld in Germany, and by the foundation later in England of the Chalfont, Lingfield, and David Lewis colonies, and in the United States of the Craig colony. The emphasis was on social management, with early intervention by admission to the colony; discharge back to society was a possibility. Alan McDougall, the first medical director of the David Lewis colony, wrote, "Most of our colonists come to us too late to be cured of their fits. The children give brilliant results; one third of them become free from fits. Our ... experience seems to show that if all epileptic children, whatever their social position, were sent on the first appearance of epileptic symptoms to an epileptic colony, and kept there till the end of their school life, the benefits to themselves, to their relatives, and to the State would be enormous."[19] These epileptic colonies were sometimes, but not exclusively, situated in the countryside. They typically created a village-like atmosphere, and often included a residential school for children with epilepsy. Attention to lifestyle, as well as physical treatment, was considered important: "Most of the colonists take daily a 30-grain dose of Potassium Bromide. This appears in many cases to diminish the frequency of the fits, and the tendency to status. But other therapeutic means are even more important. Among these is the combined concert and dance that has been held without intermission every Saturday night of the year. Dancing (particularly the 'Lancers') is a valuable means of treatment, provided that it be practised frequently. On the first few occasions a fit may follow the dancing, but the patient soon becomes able to dance without unpleasant side effects. Classical treatment of Epilepsy follows the lines of forbidding the patient to do the things that might cause a fit; colony treatment attempts to rid the patient of fits while he is performing the acts of a normal person. The latter plan gives the better results."[17]

The development of colonies was the consequence of a philanthropic movement spearheaded by the social and religious conscience of the aristocracy and upper middle classes. Increasingly, the new wealthy class—the industrial bourgeoisie—undertook a scheme of building model villages for the working classes, exemplified by the work of the Cadburys in Bournville in the English Midlands, and in the building of Styal Village for the workers of Styal Mill in Cheshire. Also at this time, arts and crafts colonies developed, where a particular creative lifestyle could be followed, away from a society that Crichton-Browne described as "... a feverish and fidgety age in which an unappeasable restlessness pervades all ranks and classes."[7] This movement was not in any way the consequence of an overt desire to segregate or discriminate against elements of society regarded as difficult, dangerous, or undesirable. Thus, at this point, the history of the institutional management of epilepsy should diverge from that of institutional psychiatry. In particular, the epilepsy colonies (in Europe at least) were concerned from the beginning with destigmatization and normalization, with attaching value to people's social roles. The evidence is in stark contrast to that often offered by historians as explanations for the great confinement of the mentally ill in the 17th, 18th, and 19th centuries. Why is this? One explanation might be that some of the accepted historical cases in psychiatry have been overstated. Bynum wrote of Foucault, "... the power of his dark vision remains, although its empirical base has been questioned,"[3] and another modern historian noted, "... the view that the 17th and particularly the 18th centuries were a disaster for the insane in England has to be qualified...."[24] Alternatively, perhaps the epilepsy colony movement then was in opposition to social attitudes at the time. Indeed, the views of those advocating colony treatment are not congruent with ideas expressed by eminent psychiatrists much later in the 20th century. For example, in 1977, a leading English-language textbook of psychiatry contained the following passage describing personality deterioration in epilepsy: "There are also more constant and lasting affective changes. Most frequently these take the form of a mulish moroseness and rancour. Slights are felt to the quick, and malice is borne for months or years. In an epileptic ward gossip, lying or slander will all too easily reign.... Chronic epileptic patients are capable of actions of the most malicious and petty spite, and of combining them with self-justification and self-praise."[26]

Seven decades earlier, in 1909, Alan McDougall had noticed the opposite: "Each succeeding year, in spite of the constant increase in the population, there is less and less quarrelling among the colonists. Our experience leads us to believe that many of the unpleasant characteristics commonly ascribed to epileptics are due not so much to the disease as to the mishandling that the patient has received. When living with those who understand his special requirements, the epileptic is a very likeable person."[19] McDougall, however, did have a sanction that was not available to the alienist and, in the 1906 colony report, he noted, "Four have been discharged as unsuitable. Their persisting lack of consideration for their fellow colonists made it impossible to retain them. Yet had they entered a colony at an early stage of their illness, they would probably have been excellent colonists."[17]

COLONIES FOR PEOPLE WITH EPILEPSY: THEIR ROLE AND DEVELOPMENT

Special Schools, Centers, and Villages: Their Maximum Development and Subsequent Decline

The epilepsy colonies of Europe have not died; rather, their work has changed to keep pace with new developments in treatment and social expectations. Their achievements have been recognized and envied in other parts of the world: "Residential and treatment facilities must be built and improved to accommodate the unique problems of persons with epilepsy and associated disorders, perhaps on the model of the many splendid public epilepsy comprehensive treatment centers of western Europe, which have not a single counterpart anywhere in the United States."[28]

The demand for services has not diminished. For example, analysis of admission rates to the David Lewis Centre from 1920 to 1989 shows an almost exponential rise (Fig. 1). Although during this period there was some rise in the overall numbers of residents, most of this increase was matched by a corresponding rise in the rate of discharges, as the length of stay decreased. The founding fathers of the colonies had apparently believed that a return to the terrors of the outside world

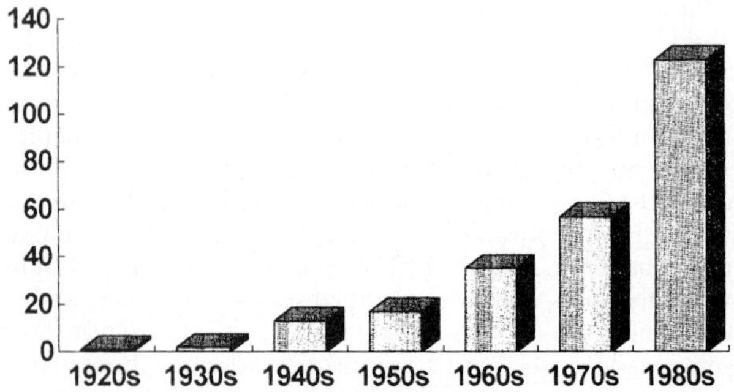

FIGURE 1. Admission rates to the Davis Lewis Centre for Epilepsy, 1920–1989.

was best avoided until cure was absolutely established: "It is very unwise to be hasty in removing from Colony conditions an improving patient; it is far wiser to wait till the improvement has become firmly established; otherwise there is great danger of relapse."[18] In these early days, however, probably the only effective medical treatment was bromide. Three factors developing during the 20th century were to influence the length of stay. These were treatment advances, secular social trends, and economics.

Treatment Advances

The introduction of barbiturates just before World War I, and of phenytoin just before World War II, made available a wider range of treatment options with potentially fewer side effects than bromides. Thus, an expectation of prolonged remission came to be part of the medical approach to epilepsy, with less medical objection to earlier return to the community. Those who still stayed behind would include a mixture of "good" colonists who had adapted well to colony life, so that neither the managers nor the clients themselves desired a change, together with those whose epilepsy or its associated problems failed to remit.

Secular Trends

The great confinement of the mentally ill began to end after World War II, probably mainly as a consequence of the introduction of phenothiazines in the 1950s, although the medicalization of psychiatry preceded this development by a century or so, with much of the intellectual impetus coming from the German-speaking world.[4] Similarly, the development of effective antituberculosis treatment at about the same time reduced the need for sanatoria. Thus, the concept of going away for long periods of time because of illness began to wither. It remained appropriate for sick people to spend time in the hospital for purposes of diagnosis and initiation of treatment, but after that the expectation was generally to return home. Although advances in epilepsy treatment were more modest, and despite the increased need for the services provided by epilepsy institutions as a consequence of increased numbers of cases of posttraumatic epilepsy resulting from two world wars, a view gradually began to emerge in parallel with these other developments, in which the emphasis shifted from fear of discharging too soon to fear of keeping patients too long.

Economics

Although most colonies were run as charitable institutions, and efforts were made to be as self-sufficient as possible in regard to providing food and services, residence always had to be paid for. Staffing and equipment costs increased along with the expectations of investigation, treatment, and care. Sponsors (families, insurance companies, national and local government agencies) were obliged to exert pressure to limit time spent during an admission.

Faced with these pressures, some establishments became smaller and a few closed, whereas others diversified their activities to meet the perceived needs of the changing market. During the 1960s, special short-stay assessment centers for epilepsy began to emerge within the colonies. Medical staff from epilepsy colonies became more involved in providing specialized epilepsy services in hospital settings. At about the turn of the decade, a significant change occurred; these venerable institutions faced the 1970s and beyond as "epilepsy centers," and the term *colony* was dropped forever. Since then, the larger centers have continued to provide more and more specialized facilities. The number of special residential schools declined, and those that remained came to include in their population an ever-larger proportion of children with severe learning disabilities. The charitable foundations responsible for the epilepsy centers began to become involved in wider issues, such as professional education and general public consciousness raising. In The Netherlands, the various epilepsy organizations, centers, and charities cooperated in producing an integrated epilepsy service for the nation that has remained a model of excellence. In the United Kingdom, the strength of the centers lay in their continuing independence from the state system in terms of business development, but their increasing reliance on statutory sources remained a weakness. In most parts of the world, an artificial distinction is made between health-related and social aspects of care, with different budgets available. A possibility arises for budget holders in health care or social services to attempt to shift the responsibility to the other area. No clearly accepted boundary exists at which social care takes over from "health." The situation is more complicated for children of school age in those areas where education authorities, faced with a bill for special education for a child with epilepsy, may be reluctant to fund aspects of care that are perceived as "medical" or "social." Thus, artificial difficulties may be put in the way of providing an integrated service. This is partly a consequence of social welfare and insurance systems that make no recognition of the particular issues in epilepsy. For example, the government of the United Kingdom, as part of a process of laying down minimum standards, sponsored a code of practice for residential care.[14] In this document, individual client groups are discussed, including the physically disabled, mentally ill, mentally handicapped, children and young people, the elderly, and people recovering from drug addiction and alcohol abuse. There is no mention of epilepsy. Therefore, there is no official "policy" for epilepsy—despite a number of expert reports, the recommendations of which have been largely ignored.[1,5,6,8] More recently, a further attempt at defining the scope of epilepsy services in the United Kingdom does seem to have had more impact, largely because of pressure from informed consumers.[2]

Current Residential Centers

At the beginning of the 21st century, the remaining residential epilepsy centers are the result of a heterogeneous evolution. The admission and discharge criteria and the range of services vary from country to country, and often from region to region, according to the prevailing social culture and the organization of health, education, and social services. Even so, some general themes are shared by most centers. The range of services includes (a) residential education for children, (b) residential assessment for children and adults, (c) long-stay provision and rehabilitation for adults, and (d) new areas of business.

Residential Education for Children

Some centers include a residential special school for children with epilepsy. There are, for example, currently three such schools in the United Kingdom, two of which are part of a larger center that also provides residential adult services. Admission criteria are the presence of a seizure disorder and educational failure. Many children arrive at residential special schools for epilepsy after a career of repeated failure in other settings. Frequently an additional psychiatric morbidity is present, manifested as a disorder of conduct, emotion, or both; however, in those cases where this has been studied, it seems that the rate of psychiatric disorders decreases with admission. This is probably a consequence of a mixture of efficient management of the seizure disorder, appropriate educational approach, and absence of stigmatization.[13] There is, therefore, a possibility of return to mainstream education after a period in a residential school, and this is achieved in some cases. Geographic separation from the home area may be beneficial in the initial stages but can restrict opportunities for reintegration.

Residential Assessment for Children and Adults

Since at least the 1960s, epilepsy centers have developed a role in short-term residential assessment. Access to high-quality neurophysiologic investigations is often available, which allows the possibility of electroencephalographic (EEG) monitoring in a homelike, nonhospital environment. Each case of epilepsy can be investigated, and the most appropriate medical treatment plan agreed. Such an admission is also an opportunity to assess living skills and determine the level of care and rehabilitation needs. The individual's and the family's knowledge (or lack of knowledge) of epilepsy can also be addressed. Admission criteria include the presence of a refractory seizure disorder with or without other problems of living, and the outcome might include rediagnosis, a medical treatment plan, and a personalized statement of care and rehabilitation needs. In some centers, short assessment admissions are also used as part of an evaluation for epilepsy surgery.

Where units for assessment of children exist, the relationships between epilepsy, interictal EEG activity, drug adverse effects, behavioral problems, speech and language development, and learning difficulties (both generalized and specific) can be studied in classroom and home-type situations, so that an optimal educational approach can be developed for each patient. This information can then be used to identify the most appropriate placement after the child leaves the assessment unit.

In the case of both children and adults, assessment units may offer specialized services for patients with epilepsy and learning disabilities or other coexisting psychiatric morbidity. Assessment units are therefore staffed by epileptologists, specialist nurses, educational and clinical psychologists and neuropsychologists, speech and language therapists, and social workers. Some centers also provide nonverbal approaches, such as art therapy and music therapy. Periods of admission for assessment vary from 2 to 12 weeks, and may depend on the reason for referral.

Long-stay Provision and Rehabilitation for Adults

Despite the trend toward deinstitutionalization in the last few decades, a long-stay residential population still remains in the epilepsy centers. It is slowly dwindling in size (Fig. 2), and comprises two groups of patients. First, there is an old long-stay group of patients who were admitted many years ago (and who would not have been admitted in modern times). These are people who have spent a large part of their lives in the epilepsy centers, are now growing old, and know no other home. Their numbers will continue to decrease, and this group will eventually disappear. Although their needs for care will increase with age, they do not make high demands on services compared with other groups in the epilepsy centers. Second, a new, small, but significant long-stay group of people is emerging who have particularly complex care needs as a result of refractory epilepsy, learning disability, challenging behavior, coexisting organic psychosyndromes, or any combination of these. Members of this group may eventually be able to return to the community as a clinical and social rehabilitation program achieves slow progress over a number of years. The final size of this group has yet to be determined.

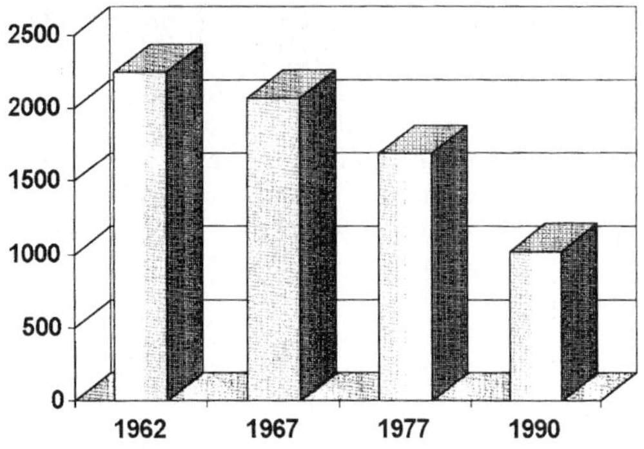

FIGURE 2. Numbers of patients living in epilepsy centers on a long-term basis. (From Duncan JS, Hart YM. Medical services. In: Laidlaw J, Richens A, Chadwick D, eds. *A Textbook of Epilepsy*. 4th ed. London: Churchill Livingstone; 1993:705–722, with permission.)

New Areas of Business

Keeping pace with secular trends in social care policy as well as advances in epilepsy management, the medical staff of epilepsy centers have developed working relationships with established neurology and psychiatry units, both academic and clinical. Epilepsy centers are now often involved in research and teaching in epileptology, and in the management of tertiary outpatient facilities. In some areas, epilepsy center staff members have started working directly with primary care physicians. Some residential epilepsy schools have developed links with mainstream education and send staff members to advise on educational approaches to children with epilepsy in mainstream schools, and they have also become involved in training teachers who will work in the educational mainstream. Finally, there is a trend to replace, wherever possible, the large, institutional-type housing of the long-stay clients with small, family-sized units that may be situated within the local community close to the facilities of the epilepsy center.

CURRENT TRENDS AND PURPOSES IN EPILEPSY INSTITUTIONS

Discharge of People with Epilepsy into the Community

Although actual discharge rates are difficult to determine on a large scale, the decline in total numbers of beds in the United Kingdom during the last years, set against the rise in overall admission rates mentioned previously, indicates a fairly marked process of deinstitutionalization (Fig. 2). The population remaining in residence does so for any of the following reasons: (a) A patient does not wish to be discharged; (b) there is no appropriate facility in the home area, even though the care needs are not excessively high; (c) care needs—whether social, medical, or both—are high, and the local services would be unable to provide the same level of support and, when appropriate, medical intervention.

Coassessment of Learning Disability (Mental Handicap)

Another problem arises in some cases for which service must provide guidance. Different professional groups may have varying views about a patient's primary problem; for example, neurologic services may see the main problem as psychiatric or social, and so on. This is why, in the United Kingdom, mental handicap (learning disability) services are increasingly taking on the management of learning disabled patients with complex epilepsy, although this currently identifies a need for training in staff working in this area. People with learning disability should have the same quality of investigation and treatment as the rest of the population. Epilepsy is very common among these individuals and, because of their special needs, intensive investigation may be necessary. The residential centers have the capacity to offer an integrated approach in which epilepsy and learning difficulties are assessed together. Medical assessment involves detailed observation of behavior and seizures in conditions that approximate those of everyday life. Education of both caregivers and clients can be achieved, and the needs of caregivers taken into account.[15] With children, the residential setting can provide a detailed multidisciplinary assessment for a prolonged period in a nonclinical environment, and then continued management with a true 24-hour curriculum. A detailed neuropsychiatric study of the children in one residential special school for epilepsy showed that, although nearly two-thirds had been referred because of behavioral problems, the rate of observed psychiatric disorder while they were at the school was only 42%. Given the overall disabilities of the sample population, (low IQ, brain damage, frequent seizures, poor family background), it was considered surprising that the prevalence of psychiatric disorder was not higher. The authors commented, "It may be that the stable environment of a residential school involves fewer stresses that might precipitate or maintain psychiatric disturbance.... Absence of stigma, efficient management of seizures and minimizing their effect on school attendance could also be beneficial in this respect."[13]

Outcome on Discharge from Special Schools, Centers, and Hospitals

Surprisingly little follow-up research has been done on the results of discharge from residential centers. Meyer and Gray[21] drew attention to the lack of community provision for people with epilepsy, which affected quality of life in their sample. Nearly a quarter of former residents were living independently, whereas half were in supported accommodation. Regular employment had been found only in 5% of cases. On the other hand, 50% reported a continuing decrease in seizure frequency, and 32% felt more alert. Medagoda and Brown[20] found that failures of successful rehabilitation were mainly related to inadequate medical follow-up or the inability of caregivers in the community to cope with behavioral problems or seizures. Breakdown of community placement after discharge was caused by a combination of inappropriate selection of placement by the receiving social services and a lack of appropriate medical services for epilepsy. It was possible, however, to readmit patients to the epilepsy center and achieve a successful, planned discharge later when these needs were met.

SUMMARY AND CONCLUSIONS

The former colonies remain repositories of expertise in the multifactorial assessment and management of epilepsy because they continue to carry a positive culture of destigmatization. The need for their services has not diminished, but the environment in which those services are provided is changing. On the site of the traditional countryside residential setting, services are being developed to provide residential assessment away from the clinical atmosphere of the hospital. People with epilepsy who also have challenging behavioral and learning disabilities can undergo specialized assessment and treatment in this setting. A special role in the future might be found for work in the field of forensic neuropsychiatry. Certainly the trend to shorter, focused admissions will continue, with the center at the same time reaching out into the community and offering preadmission services and postadmission follow-up. Some epilepsy centers in Europe are actively developing in-community care projects by establishing small living units that are closer to patients' friends and families. This last development, if successful, will further integrate the long-stay residential facility, which has the advantage of being able to provide prompt, appropriate medical and social care, in the tradition of the best colonies, into the mainstream of the community. Although residential schools are taking on the function of short-term assessment and rehabilitation, it is likely that at least some children with complex epilepsy and associated neuropsychiatric problems will receive a large part of their education in such places. Epilepsy centers will continue to be involved in teaching and research. The question remains whether truly integrated services comprising health, social work, and education can continue to thrive in a social market. Only time will tell.

References

1. Bennett-Morgan JD, Kurtz Z. *Special Services for People with Epilepsy in the 1970s*. London: HMSO; 1981.
2. Brown S, Betts T, Chadwick D, et al. An epilepsy needs document. *Seizure*. 1993;2:91–103.
3. Bynum WF. Biography and therapeutics. *Curr Opin Psychiatry*. 1988;1:598–601.
4. Bynum WF. Psychiatry in Its Historical Context. In: Shepherd M, Zangwill OL, eds. *General Psychopathology*. Cambridge, UK; Cambridge University Press; 1983:11–38 (*Handbook of Psychiatry*; vol 1).
5. Central Health Services Council. Report of the Sub-committee on the Medical Care of Epileptics (Chairman, H Cohen). London: HMSO; 1956.
6. Central Health Services Council. People with Epilepsy: Report of the Joint Sub-committee of the Standing Medical Advisory Committee and the Advisory Committee of the Health and Welfare of Handicapped persons (Chairman, J. A. Read). London: HMSO; 1969.
7. Crichton-Browne J. The cause of GPI 1871. Quoted in: Clare A. *Psychiatry in Dissent*. London: Tavistock; 1976:42.
8. DHSS Working Group. Report of the Working Group on Services for People with Epilepsy: a Report to the Department of Health and Social Security, Department of Education and Science and the Welsh Office. London: HMSO; 1986.
9. Duncan JS, Hart YM. Medical Services. In: Laidlaw J, Richens A, Chadwick D, eds. *A Textbook of Epilepsy*. 4th ed. London: Churchill Livingstone; 1993:705–722.
10. Falret J. De l'état mental des épileptiques. *Archives Générales de Médecine*, Ve série 16 (1860): 661–679; (1861): 461–491; 18 (1861): 423–443. Quoted in: Temkin O. *The Falling Sickness*. 2nd ed., revised. Baltimore: Johns Hopkins Press; 1971.
11. Foucault M. *Madness and Civilisation: a History of Insanity in the Age of Reason*. London: Tavistock; 1967.
12. Hare E. Was insanity on the increase? *Br J Psychiatry*. 1983;142:439–455.
13. Harvey I, Goodyer IM, Brown SW. The value of a neuropsychiatric examination of children with complex severe epilepsy. *Child Care Health Dev*. 1988;14:329–340.
14. *Home Life: a Code of Practice for Residential Care*. London: Centre for Policy on Ageing; 1984.
15. Jenkins LK, Brown SW. Some issues in the assessment of epilepsy occurring in the context of learning disability in adults. *Seizure*. 1992;1:49–55.

16. Maisonneuve JGF. Recherches et observations sur l'épilepsie, presentées à l'école de médecine de Paris. Quoted in: Temkin O. *The Falling Sickness*. 2nd ed., revised. Baltimore: Johns Hopkins Press; 1971.
17. McDougall A. Medical report. In: The David Lewis Manchester Epileptic Colony Report for the Year Ending August 31st 1906. Manchester: David Lewis Manchester Epileptic Colony; 1906.
18. McDougall A. Medical report. In: The David Lewis Manchester Epileptic Colony Report for the Year Ending August 31st 1908. Manchester: David Lewis Manchester Epileptic Colony; 1908.
19. McDougall A. Medical report. In: The David Lewis Manchester Epileptic Colony Report for the Year Ending August 31st 1909. Manchester: David Lewis Manchester Epileptic Colony; 1909.
20. Medagoda AS, Brown SW. Problems in implementing care in the community programme for people with chronic epilepsy. *Seizure*. 1992;1(Suppl A):P5/08.
21. Meyer J, Gray JMB. Discharges from the epilepsy centre 1987–1991. *Seizure*. 1992;1(Suppl A):P5/09.
22. Morel BA. Études cliniques. Traité théorétique et pratique des maladies mentales considérées dans leur nature, leur traitement, et dans leur rapport avec la médecine légale des aliénés. 2 vols. Nancy—Paris, 1852—1853. Quoted in: Temkin O. *The Falling Sickness*. 2nd ed., revised. Baltimore: Johns Hopkins Press; 1971.
23. Morel BA. D'une forme de délire, suite d'une surexcitation nerveuse se rattachant à une variété non encore décrite de l'épilepsie (épilepsie larvée). *Gazette Hebdomadaire de Médecine et de Chirurgie* 7 (1860): 773–775; 819–821; 836–841. Quoted in: Temkin O. *The Falling Sickness*. 2nd ed., revised. Baltimore: Johns Hopkins Press; 1971.
24. Schiller F. Pathographical history of psychiatry. *Curr Opin Psychiatry*. 1988;1:602–608.
25. Scull A. Was insanity increasing? A response to Edward Hare. *Br J Psychiatry*. 1984;144:432–436.
26. Slater E, Roth M. *Clinical Psychiatry,* 3rd ed., revised. London: Baillière Tindall; 1977.
27. Temkin O. *The Falling Sickness*. 2nd ed., revised. Baltimore: Johns Hopkins Press; 1971.
28. Wright GN. Rehabilitation and the Problem of Epilepsy. In: Wright GN, ed. *Epilepsy Rehabilitation*. Boston: Little, Brown; 1975:1–7.

CHAPTER 214 ■ PSYCHOPHARMACOLOGY OF PATIENTS WITH BEHAVIOR DISORDERS AND EPILEPSY

MICHAEL R. TRIMBLE AND MARCO MULA

INTRODUCTION

Psychiatric disorders are common in patients with epilepsy, and they encompass the spectrum of conditions from those that are a direct consequence of the epileptogenic activity to others that are simply comorbid.[45]

Therapy for behavioral disorders still remains unsatisfactory, and many patients with epilepsy receive psychotropic medications (Table 1) not always based on their psychiatric symptoms.[81] Effective therapy depends on a correct diagnosis and a combination of psychotropic drug treatments and behavioral interventions when other factors, such as emotional stressors, are present. In addition, antiepileptic drugs (AEDs) are important psychotropic agents with positive and negative psychotropic properties in their own right that should be taken into account when evaluating psychiatric symptoms in patients with epilepsy.

The present chapter focuses on the main problems that a clinician may encounter when treating psychiatric disorders in patients with epilepsy. We examine the effects of AEDs on mood and behavior, and we briefly review main factors that may affect choice of therapy, and patient's response and compliance, when prescribing antidepressants or antipsychotic drugs. In reviewing these agents, we concentrate specifically on drug interactions and any potential proconvulsive risk they may pose.

ANTIEPILEPTIC DRUGS AS PSYCHOTROPIC AGENTS

During the last 15 years, the number of AEDs available clinically has nearly trebled,[71] thus providing the possibility of providing better-tailored therapy according to patients' needs but also revealing a wide spectrum of adverse effects.

In some cases, emergent psychiatric symptoms may be side effects of the AED therapy,[5,42] the result of interactions between the drug and some biologic vulnerabilities of the patient. Subjects with more severe forms of epilepsy are generally more at risk to develop psychiatric adverse events (PAEs),[60,62] whereas specific lesions in the limbic system, such as hippocampal sclerosis, seem to be associated with the liability to develop depressive symptoms.[61] The *forced normalization phenomenon* is well known to be an idiosyncratic reaction to a sudden seizure cessation that may happen with different AEDs in predisposed patients, but whose characteristics are largely unknown.[59]

On the other hand, we have to take into account the fact that AEDs are extensively used in psychiatric practice for a broad spectrum of psychiatric disorders, especially bipolar disorders, and some are well known to stabilize mood. Since its introduction into the clinical management of epilepsy, carbamazepine has been reported to have psychotropic properties. Over time, several controlled studies have been carried out comparing the effects of carbamazepine in acute mania with placebo, lithium, or neuroleptics.[15] These studies have shown that carbamazepine is equivalent to lithium over a period of 8 weeks, and that the time course of the antimanic effect is a little slower than with neuroleptics but equivalent to lithium. This is relevant for those patients who are refractory to lithium and require an alternative to it. Carbamazepine has also been shown to be an effective treatment for the prophylaxis of bipolar disorder, with controlled studies suggesting that patients who are referred to as rapid cyclers (namely, patients with an unstable bipolar disorder with rapid fluctuations of more than four episodes a year), do best on carbamazepine or a combination of carbamazepine and lithium.[93] This approach has several advantages over the use of neuroleptics for such conditions, such as the avoidance of tardive extrapyramidal symptoms.

Valproate has been used in manic episodes, depressive episodes, and the maintenance therapy of bipolar disorder.[96] The strongest supporting evidence is for it use in acute mania, with somewhat less supporting evidence for the other conditions. Valproate may have an adverse effect on behaviors such as affective lability, aggression, and impulsivity across a range of different clinical contexts but, at the moment, controlled studies are available mainly for bipolar depression.

Among the new AEDs, some of them (e.g., tiagabine) have failed to show any efficacy in primary psychiatric disorders whereas others (e.g., topiramate) may have adjunctive uses, such as weight loss in the management of obesity. The data on the effects of oxcarbazepine on psychiatric disorders are limited and definitely less conclusive than those regarding carbamazepine. However, oxcarbazepine seems to be less effective than lithium but as effective as carbamazepine in acute mania; oxcarbazepine is probably better tolerated than carbamazepine.[94] The lack of efficacy of gabapentin in bipolar disorders has emerged from controlled studies have failed to detect such an effect.[29]

During clinical trials in the development of lamotrigine as an AED, it was observed that it had antidepressant properties. The cumulative results of the studies done so far provide evidence that lamotrigine is effective in the management of the depressed phase in bipolar disorder type II and in the long-term stabilization of mood in patients with rapid-cycling bipolar disorder.[36]

Among AEDs in development, pregabalin is probably the most interesting molecule. Controlled studies have demonstrated that it is better than placebo in anxiety disorders such as generalized anxiety disorder.[69]

Thus, data published to present suggest an important role for AEDs in psychiatric disorders. Unfortunately, it is difficult

TABLE 1

BRIEF CLASSIFICATION OF PSYCHOTROPIC DRUGS

ANTIDEPRESSANTS

- **Mono-Amino-Oxidase Inhibitors (IMAOs)**
  Moclobemide
- **Tricyclic antidepressant drugs (TCAs)**
  Amitriptyline, nortriptyline, clomipramine, imipramine, desipramine
- **Selective Serotonin Reuptake Inhibitors (SSRIs)**
  Fluoxetine, paroxetine, sertraline, fluvoxamine, citalopram, escitalopram
- **Noradrenergic uptake inhibitors (NARIs)**
  Reboxetine
- **Noradrenaline-Serotonin Uptake Inhibitors (NSRIs)**
  Venlafaxine, duloxetine
- **Noradrenaline-Selective Serotonin Antidepressants (NASSAs)**
  Mirtazapine
- **Serotonin Antagonist and Reuptake Inhibitors (SARIs)**
  Trazodone, nefazodone

ANTIPSYCHOTICS

- **Typical**
  - **Phenothiazines**
    Thioridazine, mesoridazine, chlorpromazine, prochlorperazine
  - **Butyrophenones**
    Haloperidol
- **Atypical**
  - **Benzisoxazoles and benzisothiazoles**
    Risperidone, ziprasidone, perospirone
  - **Thienobenzodiazepine, dibenzothiazepine, dibenzothiazepine derivatives**
    Clozapine, olanzapine, quetiapine

MINOR TRANQUILLIZERS – Barbiturates, Benzodiazepines, Others

MOOD STABILIZERS – Lithium

OTHERS – β-Blockers, buspirone

to extrapolate findings from these studies, performed with psychiatric patients, directly to patients with epilepsy. Obviously, it would be very useful to know whether AEDs have a positive influence on the psychic status of patients with epilepsy beyond their influence on seizure activity. However, there is little scientific evidence for this; most of the studies are uncontrolled and based on quality-of-life parameters rather than on a formal psychiatric evaluation. Because the simultaneous use of an AED as an anticonvulsant and antidepressant or mood stabilizer should be an important option for a rational pharmacotherapy in patients with uncontrolled epilepsy and comorbid psychiatric disorders, the need is great for further studies.

During the last few years, lamotrigine is the only AED investigated also as a psychotropic drug in patients with epilepsy. A randomized, placebo-controlled, double-blind, cross-over study of lamotrigine in 81 patients with refractory partial seizures showed some improvement in two subscales (happiness and alertness) in a health-related quality of life model but not on the other four scales specific for self-esteem, mood, anxiety, and depression.[82] Two double-blind studies of lamotrigine verus, respectively, carbamazepine[27] and valproate[16] demonstrated some improvement in quality of life outcomes. An open study[40] reported a significant antidepressant effect of lamotrigine in 13 patients with uncontrolled epilepsy and depression. Moreover, in two different studies, we have observed that lamotrigine significantly reduced the occurrence of PAEs during therapy with topiramate[60] or levetiracetam.[62] All these studies taken together suggest a possible role of lamotrigine as an antidepressant or mood stabilizer in those patients with uncontrolled epilepsy and depressive symptoms.

PHARMACOKINETIC INTERACTIONS BETWEEN ANTIEPILEPTIC DRUGS AND PSYCHOTROPIC DRUGS

Pharmacokinetic Interactions with Antidepressants

Several factors must be taken into account when predicting the outcome of a potential interaction: Patient-related (sex, age, ethnicity) and drug-related (the presence of active metabolites, the activity and potency at the enzyme site, the therapeutic window).[70] The role of the CYP450 enzyme system and glucuronosyltransferases (UGTs) in clinical psychopharmacology is increasingly recognized, and many papers have been published about pharmacokinetic interactions between AEDs and psychotropic drugs.[55,57,58]

Tricyclic antidepressants (TCAs) such as amitriptyline, clomipramine, and imipramine, are mainly metabolized by CYP1A2, -2D6, and -3A4 (Table 2). Nortriptyline and desipramine are, respectively, the active metabolites of amitriptyline and imipramine and are subsequently metabolized by CYP2D6.[80] Moclobemide is primarily metabolized by the CYP2 C subfamily, of which it is probably an inhibitor,[28] whereas the atypical antidepressants mianserin and trazodone are metabolized by CYP2D6.[11]

The selective serotonin reuptake inhibitors (SSRIs) fluoxetine and paroxetine are metabolized by CYP2D6, whereas sertraline, fluvoxamine, and citalopram are respectively metabolized by CYP3A4, -1A2, and -2 C.[64] Paroxetine and fluvoxamine are inhibitors of CYP2D6[74] and -1A2,[7] respectively (Table 3). Fluoxetine is a moderate inhibitor of CYP3A4, but, like paroxetine, is a potent inhibitor of CYP2D6. No clinically significant induction-inhibition properties have been demonstrated for sertraline and citalopram.[64]

Among the new generation of antidepressant drugs, venlafaxine is primarily metabolized by CYP2D6,[17] whereas CYP3A4 metabolizes nefazodone and reboxetine.[87] Nefazodone is a potent inhibitor of this enzymatic pathway.[87]

Generally, phenobarbital, carbamazepine, and phenytoin stimulate the metabolism of TCAs, whereas valproate can increase their plasma levels[55] (Table 4). An open-label study investigated the effect of valproate on amitriptyline and its active metabolite nortriptyline.[97] The mean area under curve (AUC) and the peak plasma concentration, for the sum of nortriptyline and amitriptyline, was 42% and 19% higher, respectively.

In a case series of 13 patients with major depression, the effects of carbamazepine on imipramine and desipramine serum concentrations have been investigated.[89] The authors demonstrated that carbamazepine affects not only the metabolism of both drugs but also their protein binding, thus leading to a significant increase in the free fraction.

Data about fluoxetine-carbamazepine interactions are contradictory and are still based on two old studies. The first one is a formal pharmacokinetic study using healthy male volunteers, in which the authors observed a slight increase in carbamazepine AUC levels and a decrease in 10,

TABLE 2

CYP ENZYMES INVOLVED IN PSYCHOTROPIC DRUG METABOLISM

CYP1A2	CYP2C9/10	CYP2C19	CYP2D6	CYP3A4
Antidepressants	**Antidepressants**	**Antidepressants**	**Antidepressants**	**Antidepressants**
TCAs	Sertraline	Citalopram	Fluoxetine	Nefazodone
Fluvoxamine	Fluoxetine	Escitalopram	Fluvoxamine	Sertraline
Mirtazapine	Amitriptyline	Sertraline	Citalopram	Venlafaxine
Duloxetine	Bupropion	Clomipramine	Escitalopram	Reboxetine
Antipsychotics	**Anticonvulsants**	Imipramine	Duloxetine	Escitalopram
Chlorpromazine	Phenytoin	Moclobemide	Paroxetine	Mirtazapine
Haloperidol	**Antipsychotics**	**Anticonvulsants**	Mianserin	Trazodone
Clozapine	Thioridazine	Phenytoin	Venlafaxine	TCAs
Olanzapine	Olanzapine	Mephenytoin	Trazodone	**Antipsychotics**
Ziprasidone		Esobarbital	Nefazodone	Haloperidol
		Mephobarbital	Maprotiline	Clozapine
		Phenobarbitone	Mirtazapine	Risperidone
		Primidone	TCAs	Ziprasidone
			Antipsychotics	Iloperidone
			Chlorpromazine	Quetiapine
			Thioridazine	Aripiprazole
			Haloperidol	**Anticonvulsants**
			Olanzapine	Carbamazepine
			Risperidone	Zonisamide
			Iloperidone	Tiagabine

11-carbamazepine epoxide AUC.[30] The second study is a small series of eight patients with epilepsy who showed no modifications in carbamazepine plasma levels before and after fluoxetine administration.[85] These two studies are not comparable mainly because the activity of CYP enzymes is influenced by different factors, namely age, sex (in the first study the authors used only male patients), ethnicity, and so on.

The inhibition properties of several SSRIs on phenytoin metabolism have been tested in an in vitro study with human liver microsomes.[86] The risk for a phenytoin-SSRI interaction seems to be higher with fluoxetine and less likely with the others (paroxetine and sertraline).

Possible kinetic interactions between paroxetine and carbamazepine, valproate, and phenytoin have been investigated in a single-blind, placebo-controlled, cross-over trial.[3]

TABLE 3

CYP ENZYMES INHIBITED OR INDUCED BY DIFFERENT PSYCHOTROPIC DRUGS

	Inhibitors		
CYP isoenzyme	**Antidepressants**	**Antipsychotics**	**Inducers**
CYP1A2	Fluvoxamine Fluoxetine Paroxetine Sertraline		St. John's wort
CYP2C9/10/19	Fluoxetine Sertraline Fluvoxamine	Thioridazine Clozapine	Phenobarbital Carbamazepine
CYP2D6	Fluoxetine Paroxetine Sertraline Bupropion Duloxetine Clomipramine	Thioridazine Haloperidol Clozapine Olanzapine Risperidone	
CYP3A4	Norfluoxetine Nefazodone Fluvoxamine	Chlorpromazine Thioridazine Haloperidol Risperidone	Carbamazepine Barbiturates Phenytoin St. John's wort

TABLE 4

PHARMACOKINETIC INTERACTIONS BETWEEN ANTICONVULSANT AND ANTIDEPRESSANT DRUGS

	Carbamazepine		Valproate		Phenytoin		Lamotrigine		Topiramate		Phenytoin		Gabapentin		Levetiracetam	
Fluoxetine		=↑		↓		↑									=*	=*
Paroxetine		=		=		=									=*	=*
Citalopram	↓	=	=*	=*	↓*	=*	=*	=*	=*	=*	↓*	=*	=*	=*	=*	=*
Escitalopram	=*	=*		=*		=*	=*	=*	=*	=*		=*	=*	=*	=*	=*
Sertraline	↓	=			↓	↑=					↓*		=*	=*	=*	=*
Fluvoxamine		=				↑							=*	=*	=*	=*
Venlafaxine		=		=*		=*		=*		=*		=*	=*	=*	=*	=*
Reboxetine	↓	=*		=*		=*		=*		=*		=*			=*	=*
Amitriptyline	↓		↑												=*	=*
Clomipramine	↓	↑	↑		↓						↓		=*	=*	=*	=*
Imipramine	↓°		↑		↓						↓		=*	=*	=*	=*
Desipramine	↓°		↑		↓						↓				=*	=*
Nortriptyline	↓		↑		↓						↓				=*	=*
Moclobemide		=													=*	=*
Mianserin	↓				↓						↓				=*	=*
Trazodone						↑									=*	=*
Mirtazapine	↓	=			↓	=					↓*				=*	=*
Nefazodone	↓	↑			↓*										=*	=*
Bupropion	↓			↑		↑		=							=*	=*
Viloxazine						↑		↑							=*	=*

Symbols on the left are referred to the antidepressant drug and on the right to the anticonvulsant drug, when prescribed in combination (in blank fields data are not available).

↑Increased plasma concentration, ↓ decreased plasma concentration, = unchanged plasma concentration.

*Theoretical data, no studies available.

°Dosage adjustments are not necessary.

Paroxetine caused no change in plasma concentrations and protein binding of the anticonvulsants. Studies of paroxetine plasma concentrations are lacking, but the major enzymatic pathway is a non-inducible enzyme (CYP2D6); therefore, modifications in plasma levels are unlikely when paroxetine is coadministered with AEDs with inducing properties.

Leinonen et al.[51] observed an increase in citalopram levels when carbamazepine was substituted with oxcarbazepine in two patients, demonstrating a significant induction effect of carbamazepine on citalopram metabolism. Steinacher et al. confirmed this observation in an open study of six patients, showing that a 4-week treatment with carbamazepine decreased the plasma concentration of S-citalopram and R-citalopram by 27% and 31%, respectively.[88]

The potential interaction between carbamazepine and fluvoxamine has been evaluated in a small open study of eight patients with epilepsy in steady-state for carbamazepine; no significant changes in carbamazepine and carbamazepine-10,11-epoxide occurred.[85] There are no studies of valproate-fluvoxamine interactions.

In the literature, two studies have investigated a possible effect of sertraline on phenytoin and carbamazepine metabolism. A double-blind, randomized, placebo-controlled study with 30 healthy volunteers showed no modifications in phenytoin pharmacokinetics.[77] The same authors, in a double-blind, randomized, placebo-controlled study on 14 healthy volunteers, observed no significant effects of sertraline on carbamazepine metabolism.[78] Conversely, Pihlsgard and Eliasson clearly showed that phenytoin and carbamazepine significantly reduced sertraline plasma concentrations.[72] Bonate et al.[6] demonstrated no drug interaction between clonazepam and sertraline in a randomized, double-blind, placebo-controlled, cross-over study with 13 subjects.

No clinical studies are available about potential interactions between venlafaxine and AEDs, whereas a randomized, cross-over study with 18 male subjects showed no pharmacokinetic interactions between venlafaxine and diazepam.[92]

Laroudie et al.[48] investigated kinetic interactions between nefazodone and carbamazepine in 12 healthy subjects. They observed a significant decrease in nefazodone AUC and an increase in carbamazepine AUC, demonstrating a potential inhibition property of nefazodone on carbamazepine metabolism.

An open-label, randomized, parallel group study in healthy male subjects investigated the possibility of pharmacokinetic interactions between mirtazapine and phenytoin. Coadministration of the antidepressant does not alter the steady-state pharmacokinetic of phenytoin, which, conversely, can decrease mirtazapine plasma levels by 46% on average.[83]

Ketter et al.[41] investigated the safety and efficacy of carbamazepine-moclobemide cotreatment in a double-blind study. The combination was well tolerated, with no modifications in carbamazepine kinetics, but they did not assess moclobemide plasma concentrations.

It has been well established that AEDs with induction properties determine a significant reduction in mianserin plasma concentrations.[58]

The use of bupropion is limited in patients with epilepsy because of a high seizure risk. Carbamazepine is a potent inducer of its metabolism, reducing the antidepressant plasma concentrations to undetectable levels.[75] On the other hand, bupropion has shown marked inhibition properties on valproate[75] and phenytoin metabolism.[90] In a randomized, open-label, crossover study with 12 healthy subjects, the kinetic parameters of a single 100-mg lamotrigine dose were not modified by steady-state, slow-release bupropion therapy.[65]

Pharmacokinetic Interactions with Antipsychotics

Neuroleptics, such as phenothiazines, are metabolized by intestinal sulfoxidases, although CYP2D6 plays an important role in chlorpromazine and thioridazine metabolism.[67] They are also partially metabolized by CYP1A2 and -2C, respectively, and partially inhibit CYP3A4.[12] Phenothiazines, in particular thioridazine, are potent inhibitors of CYP2D6.[67] Haloperidol is metabolized by CYP3A4 and -1A2, and only partially by -2D6.[46]

Among the atypical antipsychotics, clozapine undergoes extensive hepatic metabolism; multiple CYP enzymes are involved, however, the two most prominent are CYP1A2 and -3A4.[76,77]

The newer generation of antipsychotic drugs seem to have more favorable pharmacokinetic profiles. Risperidone is primarily metabolized by CYP2D6, although a correlation study using a panel of human microsomes suggested that CYP3A4 may also be involved.[22] Olanzapine undergoes extensive hepatic metabolism and shares some of its metabolic routes with the structurally and pharmacologically related clozapine, but UGTs appear to be a major metabolic pathway.[79] Quetiapine shares some pharmacologic and structural characteristics with clozapine and olanzapine, but CYP3A4 is most likely the main isoenzyme involved in its metabolism.[17]

Thioridazine is metabolized by intestinal sulfoxidases that are induced only partially by AEDs such as carbamazepine, phenytoin, and phenobarbital, but some authors have reported an increased clearance of thioridazine and a relevant decrease of mesoridazine (the active metabolite of thioridazine) levels in patients taking carbamazepine and or phenytoin.[70] On the other hand, thioridazine, as chlorpromazine and prochlorperazine, inhibits phenytoin, phenobarbital, and valproate metabolism[31] (Table 5).

Several studies have shown that haloperidol plasma levels decrease by 50% to 60% after carbamazepine coadministration, with concomitant worsening of the psychiatric clinical features.[37,38,43] In one study, therapeutic drug monitoring data from 231 schizophrenic inpatients demonstrated that haloperidol levels were 37% and 22% lower in patients comedicated with carbamazepine or phenobarbital, respectively.[35] Carbamazepine seems to decrease haloperidol concentrations in a dose- or concentration-dependent manner, even at subtherapeutic doses of the drug.[100] Interestingly, Iwahashi et al.[37] observed that serum carbamazepine concentrations in patients treated without haloperidol were significantly decreased (on average 40%), as compared with those treated with both carbamazepine and haloperidol. In a controlled clinical trial on the effects of carbamazepine and valproate cotreatment on the plasma levels of haloperidol and on the psychopathologic outcome in schizophrenic patients, valproate led to no significant effects on haloperidol plasma levels, and its use was associated with a better psychopathologic outcome.[34]

As far as new AEDs are concerned, the use of topiramate did not lead to clinically significant modifications on haloperidol pharmacokinetics in a formal pharmacokinetic study with healthy volunteers.[14]

Spina et al.[84] compared the risperidone total active moiety (risperidone plus its active metabolite, tamoxifen steady-state plasma concentrations in patients treated with risperidone alone and in patients comedicated with carbamazepine or valproate, matched for age, sex, body weight, and antipsychotic dosage. Although carbamazepine caused a significant decrease in active moiety concentrations, valproate (at dosages up to 1,200–1,500 mg/day) had minimal and clinically insignificant effects on plasma levels of risperidone-tamoxifen, suggesting

TABLE 5

PHARMACOKINETIC INTERACTIONS BETWEEN ANTICONVULSANT AND ANTIPSYCHOTIC DRUGS

	Carbamazepine		Phenobarbital		Phenytoin		Valproate		Lamotrigine		Topiramate		Gabapentin		Levetiracetam	
Chlorpromazine	↓	↑		↑		↑				=*					=*	=*
Thioridazine	↓		↓	↑	↓	↑		↑		=*					=*	=*
Mesoridazine	↓				↓										=*	=*
Haloperidol	↓	↑	↓		↓		=	=*	=*		=		=*	=*	=*	=*
Clozapine	↓		↓		↓		=↑						=*		=*	=*
Olanzapine	↓		↓*		↓*		↑*		=*		=*		=*	=*	=*	=*
Risperidone	↓	=↑	↓*		↓*		=				=*	=*	=*	=*	=*	=*
Ziprasidone	↓		↓*		↓*						=*		=*	=*	=*	=*
Iloperidone	↓*		↓*		↓*		=*				=*		=*		=*	=*
Quetiapine	↓		↓*	=*	↓	=*					=*		=*		=*	=*

Symbols on the left are referred to the antipsychotic drug and on the right to the anticonvulsant drug, when prescribed in combination (in blank fields data are not available).

↑ Increased plasma concentration, ↓ decreased plasma concentration, = unchanged plasma concentration.

*Theoretical data, no studies available.

that valproate could be added safely to an existing treatment with risperidone.

Recently, the relationship between CYP2D6 genotype and carbamazepine-risperidone interaction has been investigated, suggesting that the decrease in risperidone concentration is dependent on the CYP2D6 activity.[66] In an open study with eight patients with epilepsy, a mild increase in carbamazepine plasma levels has been described after the addition of risperidone 1 mg.[57] Although this interaction seems not to be clinically relevant, it may suggest that the antipsychotic, or more likely its metabolites, could modulate CYP3A4 activity and, interestingly, a different enantioselective 9-hydroxylation of risperidone by CYP2D6 and CYP3A4 has been shown in a separate study.[26]

Ziprasidone and perospirone are newly available antipsychotic drugs, and there are few clinical studies about their interactions. An open, randomized, parallel-group study using healthy volunteers showed a clinically insignificant reduction (<36%) in steady-state ziprasidone levels after carbamazepine prescription.[54]

Generally, phenytoin, phenobarbital, and carbamazepine[21,77] cause a decrease in clozapine plasma concentrations. However, carbamazepine is rarely used in combination with clozapine because of the high risk of hematologic side effects. Existing data on the effect of valproate coadministration are contradictory.[8,20] According to some authors, valproate may have a moderate inhibiting effect on the demethylation of clozapine (catalyzed by CYP1A2 and -3A4), but clozapine disposition is characterized by a large interindividual variability, being affected by age, gender, body weight, dose per kilogram, smoking habits, and ethnicity.[10]

Olanzapine plasma concentrations are decreased by carbamazepine,[53] but the authors of the study did not consider this interaction clinically relevant because of the wide therapeutic index of the antipsychotic. However, other authors have pointed that carbamazepine increases the metabolism of olanzapine, with a decrease in plasma concentrations of the latter by 38%.[52]

Quetiapine is a newly introduced atypical antipsychotic, and clinical data about pharmacokinetic interactions are lacking. Phenytoin seems to induce the metabolism of quetiapine, suggesting that dosage adjustment of quetiapine may be necessary when it is coprescribed with other AED enzyme inducers such as carbamazepine or phenobarbital.[98] Interestingly, Fitzgerald and Okos reported two patients who experienced markedly elevated levels of the carbamazepine active metabolite (carbamazepine-10,11-epoxide) with the occurrence of symptoms of neurotoxicity such as ataxia and agitation. The authors suggested that quetiapine may inhibit the epoxide hydrolase and/or glucuronidation of carbamazepine-10,11-trans-diol in the same way as valproate and lamotrigine possibly do.[23]

Pharmacokinetic Interactions with Anxiolytics

Generally, anxiolytics have a wide therapeutic index; therefore the clinical relevance of pharmacokinetic interactions is very limited. AEDs with enzyme-inducing properties may stimulate the biotransformation of many benzodiazepines. Carbamazepine has been reported to induce clobazam and diazepam metabolism,[86] and has also been demonstrated to enhance the clearance of clonazepam and alprazolam.[25,81] A clinically relevant interaction occurs between AEDs-inducers and midazolam and triazolam,[4] which are extensively metabolized by CYP3A4. Conversely, newer hypnosedatives such as zopiclone, zolpidem, and zaleplon are biotransformed by several CYP isoenzymes in addition to CYP3A4, resulting in CYP3A4 inducers having a lesser effect on their biotransformation.[33]

THE RISK OF SEIZURES WITH PSYCHOTROPIC DRUGS

Antidepressants

The association of antidepressants with the provocation of seizures is quite well known in medical literature. However, most of the data arise from studies using in vitro techniques, animal studies, and clinical observations; few specific clinical studies exist.[91] Within the therapeutic range for serum levels, the incidence of seizures is less than 0.5% for most antidepressants when other risk factors are excluded.

It has been known ever since their introduction that TCAs are proconvulsant and lead to seizures. This predilection, for example in overdose, is one method of fatality.[73] However, the mechanism responsible for inducing seizures with these heterocyclic antidepressants remains unclear. The most obvious explanation would be that the increase in serotonin and noradrenaline neurotransmission mediates this effect, because all antidepressants appear to display one or both of these properties. However, both these neurotransmitters have also been demonstrated to have some anticonvulsant effects in animal and human models. Such findings may explain those papers that suggest a possible therapeutic effect of antidepressants such as TCAs and newer antidepressants in low doses in the treatment of seizures.[99] Such observations have led to the suggestion of a biphasic effect, with lower levels being anticonvulsant and higher levels proconvulsant. Further, Leander[49] demonstrated, in an animal model of epilepsy, that the selective inhibition of serotonin uptake by fluoxetine can enhance the anticonvulsant potency of phenytoin and carbamazepine.

Antidepressants that pose a higher risk of seizures include mianserin, clomipramine, and maprotiline (Table 6). The risk associated with bupropion appears to be acceptably low when recommended prescribing practices are used. Of the newer generation of drugs, the SSRIs are considered to provoke less in the way of seizures than do TCAs.[32] Extensive clinical and research experience with all the SSRIs suggest that the epileptogenic potential of this class of drugs is quite low and not much different from placebo. However, a special caution

TABLE 6

SEIZURE RISK FOR SOME ANTIDEPRESSANT AND ANTIPSYCHOTIC DRUGS

High risk	Intermediate risk	Low risk
Antidepressants		
Bupropion	Mianserin	SSRIs
Clomipramine	Amitriptyline	Trazodone
Maprotiline	Imipramine	Venlafaxine
		IMAOs
		Mirtazapine
		Desipramine
		Nortriptyline
Antipsychotics		
Chlorpromazine (dose related)	Haloperidol	Risperidone
Clozapine (titration and dose related)	Quetiapine	Ziprasidone
	Olanzapine	

should be mentioned with regard to the risk of hyponatremia. This idiosyncratic phenomenon has been associated with all the SSRIs and represents an important variable that may precipitate seizures.

Antipsychotic Drugs

Traditional antipsychotics have long been recognized as a class of drugs that can increase the risk of seizures. To determine the risk for drug-induced seizures, different approaches have been adopted: Observational studies (case-control studies and case reports), drug-induced electroencephalographic (EEG) changes, animal models, and in vitro techniques in isolated tissue samples. One of the problems of the recent literature is that most of the studies have been performed on psychiatric patients, and it is not known whether drug related seizures in non–epileptic patients really predict risk in patients with epilepsy, and whether different epileptic syndromes have different risks for psychotropic-induced seizures.

Generally, chlorpromazine and clozapine are considered proconvulsant in epileptic patients, the former only at high doses (1,000 mg/daily) and the latter at medium and high doses (>600 mg/daily).[2] Clozapine frequently causes epileptiform EEG changes and seizures in 3% to 5% of patients treated, even at therapeutic doses. Devinsky et al.[13] observed a mean prevalence of seizures of 2.9% with clozapine and, considering different doses, the prevalence was respectively given at 1%, 2.7%, and 4.4% for doses of less than 300 mg, 300 to 600 mg, or 600 to 900 mg per day. Pacia and Devinsky[68] analyzed only patients without a previous history of seizures, and the prevalence of seizures was respectively 0.9%, 0.8%, and 1.5% for the same range of doses as in the previous study. Thus, with clozapine, the proconvulsant effect seems to be a dose-related phenomenon but the role of the titration time and rate of increase of dose probably is also important.[47] Although the incidence of seizures rises to about 5% at doses 600 mg and EEG changes may be recorded at lower doses, it should be noted that these results emerge from patients with schizophrenia, and not epilepsy.[2] The seizures are often myoclonic, but can be generalized tonic–clonic or partial, depending on the individual patient.

Although, olanzapine is structurally related to clozapine, it is in the thienobenzodiazepine class of atypical antipsychotics and, along with quetiapine, premarketing studies showed a seizure rate of 0.9%.[50] Risperidone seems to have a low risk of seizures (about 0.3%), but data are taken from premarketing and postmarketing studies[2,50] (Table 6).

THE USE OF LITHIUM IN PATIENTS WITH EPILEPSY

Lithium carbonate is frequently used for manic episodes in bipolar disorder, in association with valproate and carbamazepine. Carbamazepine also demonstrates antimanic properties, and a possibly favorable pharmacodynamic interaction could be suggested; however, carbamazepine can increase the incidence of lithium toxicity. Kramlinger and Post[44] studied the effects of this combination in 23 patients with affective disorders. They observed a significant increase in many hematologic parameters (mainly the mean white blood cell count; lithium likely counteracts the neutropenic properties of carbamazepine) and a significant modification in thyroid function, with decreases in T4 and free T4. The opposing effects of carbamazepine and lithium on electrolyte regulation are well-known, with the potential occurrence of severe hyponatremia when lithium alone is stopped.[95]

The combination of lithium and valproate is widely used in rapid-cycling, manic, depressive, and mixed episode in bipolar disorder. This combination has a higher tolerability than the coadministration with carbamazepine, and a pharmacodynamic synergistic interaction has been suggested.[32] However, the combination of lithium and valproate may induce additive side effects, such as weight gain, sedation, and tremor.[24]

Chen et al.[9] investigated lithium pharmacokinetics when coprescribed with lamotrigine in 20 healthy subjects. There were no significant differences in lithium pharmacokinetic parameters. Abraham and Owen described a single case of lithium toxicity associated with topiramate cotherapy.[1] The authors suggested that topiramate, as a carbonic anhydrase inhibitor, may reduce lithium clearance and lead to toxic plasma levels.

The neurotoxic and convulsant effects of lithium are well known, but seizures are most common when plasma levels exceed 3.0 mEq/L. At therapeutic levels, the effect of lithium on seizure frequency in individuals with epilepsy is inconsistent.[19,39] Thus, although reports are conflicting, it appears that lithium can be prescribed in patients with epilepsy when mood-stabilizing therapy is necessary and alternative agents either fail or are not tolerated. In these situations, vigilant monitoring of lithium blood levels and for clinical signs of neurotoxicity is warranted.

PRESCRIBING PSYCHOTROPIC DRUGS FOR PATIENTS WITH EPILEPSY

As noted earlier, most studies on the effects of AEDs on mood, or of psychotropic drug effects on seizures have been gathered from patients with psychiatric disorders and not from patients with epilepsy. However, some cross generalizations may be expected; for example, there is little reason to believe that a drug that is proconvulsant in psychiatric populations will not also be proconvulsant in people with epilepsy.

To minimize side effects and increase compliance, it is important to first of all discuss potential problems with the patient and, in particular, to settle any worries that the patient may have difficulty getting off the drugs because they may be addictive. Actually, the addictive potential of the antidepressant and the antipsychotic drugs is negligible, and some AEDs such as phenytoin are much more likely to be addictive and cause problems of abuse.

The psychotropic drugs should be introduced at low dosages, and the escalation rate should be slow (low and slow adage), but the patient's clinical progress must be carefully monitored. There is no point in prescribing the psychotropic and not seeing the patient again for several weeks.

Choice of drug is always difficult, especially because of so many newer agents from which to choose. The SSRIs are the favored antidepressants, and the atypical antipsychotics are best chosen for psychoses and in some settings for mood stabilization. If a patient has responded to a particular drug before, then it is sensible to opt for that prescription again.

The risk of an increase in seizures must always be mentioned, but this is not usually a problem in clinical practice, partly because patients are on AEDs, and partly because patients most susceptible to depression and psychoses are likely those with difficult-to-treat epilepsy, who have quite frequent seizures. In some patients who respond to the psychotropics but who do experience an exacerbation of seizures, a judicious increase in the AED therapy may be warranted.

A problem arises in the patient who has been seizure-free for a long time, but who develops a psychiatric disorder requiring treatment. Such patients are susceptible to the provocation of a seizure either on account of the proconvulsant potential of the drugs or because of a pharmacokinetic interaction. Careful discussion of the possibility of a seizure with the patient is mandatory.

Pharmacokinetic interaction possibilities are legion, as this chapter has demonstrated. Psychotropic drugs are not equivalent in their potential for drug interactions with AEDs. Each combination should be carefully considered, while taking into account all relevant variables related to the patient such as gender, age, ethnicity, smoking habits, body weight, and any associated renal or hepatic diseases.

Among antidepressants, the combination of nefazodone-carbamazepine is contraindicated because of the occurrence of toxic concentrations of the anticonvulsant. In other cases, from a clinical point of view, there are no particularly troublesome combinations. However, clinicians must be aware that fluoxetine has a long half-life, and the clearance of most antidepressants can be accelerated by enzyme-inducing AEDs.

As far as antipsychotic drugs are concerned, it must be kept in mind that the doses of neuroleptics should be always tailored on the patient's response. In almost all cases, enzyme inducers reduce the plasma levels of these drugs. The use of clozapine must be carefully monitored because its metabolism has high inter- and intraindividual variability and, especially in combination with valproate, interactions are difficult to predict. If there is concern about possible interactions, then serum AED levels should be taken before the administration of the psychotropic for later comparison.

Antidepressants must be given for at least 6 months to patients who have developed major depressive disorders, but variants, such as interictal dysphoric disorder (see Chapter 205), may resolve without therapy after a few days, or become repetitive and persistent, requiring longer-term mood stabilization. Antipsychotic drugs will be given at various schedules depending on the classification of the psychoses (see Chapter 204) and the severity. Stopping, as with starting these drugs, should be carried out slowly, and under adequate supervision.

Finally, the special role of clozapine in the psychoses should be noted. This drug may seem contraindicated in patients with epilepsy, especially on account of its proconvulsant liability. However, it has been used successfully in the management of the interictal psychoses of epilepsy, with certain provisions.[47] It is a remarkably useful antipsychotic in patients whose psychosis fails to respond to other atypical antipsychotics. The side effects of drooling and weight gain are further problems to its use, and it should not be used in patients who are on carbamazepine. However, a change of the latter to oxcarbazepine is an acceptable clinical maneuver. An EEG should be done before the administration of clozapine, in case of a deterioration of behavior, so that the development of a nonconvulsive status epilepticus can be identified and managed appropriately. The clozapine should be introduced slowly, white cell counts monitored, and increased in dose to between 300 and 600 mg if necessary, although some patients respond to lower doses.

The use of clozapine is most successful when given to a patient who has developed a psychosis and become seizure free, suggesting some variant of the theme of forced normalization and requiring perhaps a more proconvulsant antipsychotic for a clinical effect.

SUMMARY AND CONCLUSIONS

Although the mainstay of drug therapy in epilepsy relates to antiseizure medications, many patients have an associated psychopathology and receive psychotropic medications. In the past two decades the choice of such agents has increased considerably, and the introduction of new antidepressants such as the SSRIs and the atypical antipsychotics has allowed more patients to receive such drugs with a lessening of side effects. However, no psychotropic is free from treatment emergent effects, and they should only be prescribed when the clinical situation justifies it. It seems to be the case that many patients with epilepsy have unidentified psychiatric needs, and if anything psychotropic drugs are underprescribed.

Used judiciously, antidepressants and antipsychotic drugs can help bring resolution of psychopathology, but their use is always seen as part of a package of care which must also address social and psychotherapeutic needs.

References

1. Abraham G, Owen J. Topiramate can cause lithium toxicity. *J Clin Psychopharmacol.* 2004;24(5):565–567.
2. Alldredge BK. Seizure risk associated with psychotropic drugs: Clinical and pharmacokinetic considerations. *Neurology.* 1999;53(5 Suppl 2):S68–S75.
3. Andersen BB, Mikkelsen M, Vesterager A, et al. No influence of the antidepressant paroxetine on carbamazepine, valproate, and phenytoin. *Epilepsy Res.* 1991;10:201–204.
4. Backman TJ, Olkkola KT, Ojala M, et al. Concentrations and effects of oral midazolam are greatly reduced in patients on carbamazepine or phenytoin. *Epilepsia.* 1996;37:253–257.
5. Besag FM. Behavioural effects of the newer antiepileptic drugs: An update. *Expert Opin Drug Saf.* 2004;3(1):1–8.
6. Bonate PL, Kroboth PD, Smith RB, et al. Clonazepam and sertraline: Absence of drug interaction in a multiple-dose study. *J Clin Psychopharmacol.* 2000;20:19–27.
7. Brosen K, Skjelbo E, Rasmussen BB, et al. Fluvoxamine is a potent inhibitor of cytochrome P4501A2. *Biochem Pharmacol.* 1993;45:1211–1214.
8. Centorrino F, Baldessarini RJ, Kando J, et al. Serum concentrations of clozapine and its major metabolites: Effects of cotreatment with fluoxetine or valproate. *Am J Psychiatry.* 1994;151:123–125.
9. Chen C, Veronese L, Yin Y. The effects of lamotrigine on the pharmacokinetics of lithium. *Br J Clin Pharmacol.* 2000;50:193–195.
10. Chong SA, Remington G. Ethnicity and clozapine metabolism. *Br J Psychiatry.* 1998;172:97 [Letter].
11. Daniel W. Metabolism of psychotropic drugs: Pharmacological and chemical relevance. *Pol J Pharmacol.* 1995;47(5):367–379.
12. Daniel WA, Syrek M, Rylko Z, et al. Effects of phenothiazine neuroleptics on the rate of caffeine demethylation and hydroxylation in the rat liver. *Pol J Pharmacol.* 2001;53(6):615–621.
13. Devinsky O, Honigfeld G, Patin J. Clozapine-related seizures. *Neurology.* 1991;41 (3):369–371.
14. Doose DR, Kohl KA, Desai-Krieger D, et al. No clinically significant effect of topiramate on haloperidol plasma concentration. *Eur Neuropsychopharmacol.* 1999;9:S357 [Abstract].
15. Dunn RT, Frye MS, Kimbrell TA, et al. The efficacy and use of anticonvulsants in mood disorders. *Clin Neuropharmacol.* 1998;21(4):215–235.
16. Edwards KR, Sackellares JC, Vuong A, et al. Lamotrigine monotherapy improves depressive symptoms in epilepsy: A double-blind comparison with valproate. *Epilepsy Behav.* 2001;2(1):28–36.
17. Ereshefsky L. Pharmacokinetics and drug interactions: Update for new antipsychotics. *J Clin Psychiatry.* 1996;57(Suppl 11):12–25.
18. Ereshefsky L, Dugan D. Review of the pharmacokinetics, pharmacogenetics, and drug interaction potential of antidepressants: Focus on venlafaxine. *Depress Anxiety.* 2000;12 (Suppl 1):30–44.
19. Erwin CV, Gerber CJ, Morrison SD, et al. Lithium carbonate and convulsive disorders. *Arch Gen Psychiatry.* 1973;28(5):646–648.
20. Facciola G, Avenoso A, Scordo MG, et al. Small effects of valproic acid on the plasma concentrations of clozapine and its major metabolites in patients with schizophrenic or affective disorders. *Ther Drug Monit.* 1999;21:341–345.
21. Facciola G, Avenoso A, Spina E, et al. Inducing effect of phenobarbital on clozapine metabolism in patients with chronic schizophrenia. *Ther Drug Monit.* 1998;20:628–630.
22. Fang J, Bourin M, Baker GB. Metabolism of risperidone to 9-hydroxyrisperidone by human cytochromes P450 2D6 and 3A4. *Naunyn Schmiedebergs Arch Pharmacol.* 1999;359(2):147–151.
23. Fitzgerald BJ, Okos AJ. Elevation of carbamazepine-10,11-epoxide by quetiapine. *Pharmacotherapy.* 2002;22(11):1500–1503.
24. Freeman MP, Stool AL. Mood stabilizer combinations: A review of safety and efficacy. *Am J Psychiatry.* 1998;155(1):12–21.
25. Furukori H, Otani K, Yasui N, et al. Effect of carbamazepine on the single oral dose pharmacokinetics of alprazolam. *Neuropsychopharmacology.* 1998;18:364–369.

26. Furukory NY, Hidestrand M, Spina E, et al. Different enantioselective 9-hydroxylation of risperidone by the two human CYP2D6 and CYP3A4 enzymes. *Drug Metab Dispos*. 2001;29:1263–1268.
27. Gillham R, Kane K, Bryant-Comstock L, et al. A double-blind comparison of lamotrigine and carbamazepine in newly diagnosed epilepsy with health-related quality of life as an outcome measure. *Seizure*. 2000;9(6):375–379.
28. Gram LF, Guentert TW, Grange S, et al. Moclobemide, a substrate of CYP2C19 and an inhibitor of CYP2C19, CYP2D6, and CYP1A2: A panel study. *Clin Pharmacol Ther*. 1995;57(6):670–677.
29. Greist JH. Gabapentin. Clinical efficacy and use in psychiatric disorders. In: Levy RH, Mattson RH, Meldrum BS, Perucca E, eds. *Antiepileptic Drugs*, 5th ed. Philadelphia: Lippincott Williams & Wilkins; 2002:349–353.
30. Grimsley SR, Jann MW, Carter JG, et al. Increased carbamazepine plasma concentrations after fluoxetine coadministration. *Clin Pharmacol Ther*. 1991;50:10–15.
31. Guengerich FP. Role of cytochrome P450 enzymes in drug-drug interactions. *Adv Pharmacol*. 1997;43:7–35.
32. Hensiek A, Trimble MR. Relevance of new psychotropic drugs for the neurologist. *J Neurol Neurosurg Psychiatry*. 2002;72:281–285.
33. Hesse LM, von Moltke LL, Greenblatt DJ. Clinically important drug interactions with zopiclone, zolpidem and zaleplon. *CNS Drugs*. 2003;17(7):513–32.
34. Hesslinger B, Normann C, Langosch JM, et al. Effects of carbamazepine and valproate on haloperidol plasma levels and on psychopathologic outcome in schizophrenic patients. *J Clin Psychopharmacol*. 1999;19:310–315.
35. Hirokane G, Someya T, Takahashi S, et al. Interindividual variation of plasma haloperidol concentrations and the impact of concomitant medications: The analysis of therapeutic drug monitoring data. *Ther Drug Monit*. 1999;21:82–86.
36. Hurley SC. Lamotrigine update and its use in mood disorders. *Ann Pharmacother*. 2002;36:860–873.
37. Iwahashi K, Miyatake R, Suwaki H, et al. The drug-drug interaction effects of haloperidol on plasma carbamazepine levels. *Clin Neuropharmacol*. 1995;18:233–236.
38. Jann MW, Ereshefsky L, Saklad SR, et al. Effects of carbamazepine on plasma haloperidol levels. *J Clin Psychopharmacol*. 1985;5(2):106–109.
39. Jus A, Villenueve A, Gautier J, et al. Influence of lithium carbonate on patients with temporal epilepsy. *Can Psychiatr Assoc J*. 1973;18(1):77–78.
40. Kalogjera-Sackellares D, Sackellares JC. Improvement in depression associated with partial epilepsy in patients treated with lamotrigine. *Epilepsy Behav*. 2002;3(6):510–516.
41. Ketter TA, Post RM, Parekh PI, et al. Addition of monoamine oxidase inhibitors to carbamazepine: Preliminary evidence of safety and antidepressant efficacy in treatment-resistant depression. *J Clin Psychiatry*. 1995;56:471–475.
42. Ketter TA, Post RM, Theodore WH. Positive and negative psychiatric effects of antiepileptic drugs in patients with seizure disorders. *Neurology*. 1999;53(5 Suppl 2):S53–S67.
43. Kidron R, Averbuch I, Klein E, et al. Carbamazepine-induced reduction of blood levels of haloperidol in chronic schizophrenia. *Biol Psychiatry*. 1985;20(2):219–222.
44. Kramlinger KG, Post RM. Addition of lithium carbonate to carbamazepine: Haematological and thyroid effects. *Am J Psychiatry*. 1990;147:615–620.
45. Krishnamoorthy ES. Neuropsychiatric Disorders in Epilepsy—Epidemiology and Classification. In: Trimble MR, Schmitz B, eds. *The Neuropsychiatry of Epilepsy*. Cambridge, UK: Cambridge University Press; 2002:5–17.
46. Kudo S, Ishizaki T. Pharmacokinetics of haloperidol: An update. *Clin Pharmacokinet*. 1999;37(6):435–456.
47. Langosch JM, Trimble MR. Epilepsy, psychosis and clozapine. *Human Psychopharmacol Clin Exp*. 2002;17:115–119.
48. Laroudie C, Salazar DE, Cosson JP, et al. Carbamazepine-nefazodone interaction in healthy subjects. *J Clin Psychopharmacol*. 2000;20:46–53.
49. Leander JD. Fluoxetine, a selective serotonin-uptake inhibitor, enhances the anticonvulsant effects of phenytoin, carbamazepine and ameltolide (LY201116). *Epilepsia*. 1992;33:573–576.
50. Lee KC, Finley PR, Alldredge BK. Risk of seizures associated with psychotropic medications: Emphasis on new drugs and new findings. *Expert Opin Drug Saf*. 2003;2(3):233–247.
51. Leinonen E, Lepola U, Koponen H. Substituting carbamazepine with oxcarbazepine increases citalopram levels. A report on two cases. *Pharmacopsychiatry*. 1996;29:156.
52. Linnet K, Olesen OV. Free and glucuronidated olanzapine serum concentrations in psychiatric patients: Influence of carbamazepine comedication. *Ther Drug Monit*. 2002;24(4):512–517.
53. Lucas RA, Gilfillan DJ, Bergstrom RF. A pharmacokinetic interaction between carbamazepine and olanzapine: Observations on possible mechanism. *Eur J Clin Pharmacol*. 1998;54:639–643.
54. Miceli JJ, Anziano RJ, Robarge L, et al. The effect of carbamazepine on the steady-state pharmacokinetics of ziprasidone in healthy volunteers. *Br J Clin Pharmacol*. 2000;49(Suppl 1):S65–S70.
55. Monaco F, Cicolin A. Interaction between anticonvulsant and psychoactive drugs. *Epilepsia*. 1999;40 (Suppl 10):S71–S76.
56. Mula M, Monaco F. Antiepileptic-antipsychotic drug interactions. A critical review of the evidence. *Clin Neuropharmacol*. 2002;25(5):280–289.
57. Mula M, Monaco F. Carbamazepine-risperidone interactions in patients with epilepsy. *Clin Neuropharmacol*. 2002;25:97–100.
58. Mula M, Trimble MR. Pharmacokinetic interactions between antiepileptic and antidepressant drugs. *World J Biol Psychiatry*. 2003;4(1):21–24.
59. Mula M, Trimble MR. The importance of being seizure free: Topiramate and psychopathology in epilepsy. *Epilepsy Behav*. 2003;4(4):430–434.
60. Mula M, Trimble MR, Lhatoo SD, et al. Topiramate and psychiatric adverse events in patients with epilepsy. *Epilepsia*. 2003;44(5):659–663.
61. Mula M, Trimble MR, Sander JW. The role of hippocampal sclerosis in topiramate-related depression and cognitive deficits in people with epilepsy. *Epilepsia*. 2003;44(12):1573–1577.
62. Mula M, Trimble MR, Yuen A, et al. Psychiatric adverse events during levetiracetam therapy. *Neurology*. 2003;61(5):704–706.
63. Nelson MH, Birnbaum AK, Remmel RP. Inhibition of phenytoin hydroxylation in human liver microsomes by several selective serotonin re-uptake inhibitors. *Epilepsy Res*. 2001;44:71–82.
64. Nemeroff CB, De Vane CL, Pollock, BG. Newer antidepressants and cytochrome P450 system. *Am J Psychiatry*. 1996;153:311–320.
65. Odishaw J, Chen C. Effects of steady state bupropion on the pharmacokinetics of lamotrigine in healthy subjects. *Pharmacotherapy*. 2000;20:1448–1453.
66. Ono S, Mihara K, Suzuki A, et al. Significant pharmacokinetic interaction between risperidone and carbamazepine: Its relationship with CYP2D6 genotypes. *Psychopharmacology (Berl)*. 2002;162:50–54.
67. Otani K, Aoshima T. Pharmacogenetics of classical and new antipsychotic drugs. *Ther Drug Monit*. 2000;22(1):118–121.
68. Pacia SV, Devinsky O. Clozapine seizures: Experience with 5629 patients. *Neurology*. 1994;44:2247–2249.
69. Pande AC, Feltner DE, Jefferson JW, et al. Efficacy of the novel anxiolytic pregabalin in social anxiety disorder: A placebo-controlled, multicenter study. *J Clin Psychopharmacol*. 2004;24(2):141–149.
70. Patsalos PN, Perucca E. Clinically important drug interactions in epilepsy: Interactions between antiepileptic drugs and other drugs. *Lancet Neurol*. 2003;2(8):473–481.
71. Perucca E. NICE guidance on newer drugs for epilepsy in adults. *Br Med J*. 2004;328(7451):1273–1274.
72. Pihlsgard M, Eliasson E. Significant reduction of sertraline plasma levels by carbamazepine and phenytoin. *Eur J Clin Pharmacol*. 2002;57(12):915–916.
73. Pisani F, Oteri G, Costa C, et al. Effects of psychotropic drugs on seizure threshold. *Drug Saf*. 2002;25(2):91–110.
74. Pollock BG. Recent development in drug metabolism of relevance to psychiatrists. *Harvard Rev Psychiatry*. 1994;2:204–213.
75. Popli AP, Tanquary J, Lamparella V, et al. Bupropion and anticonvulsant drug interactions. *Ann Clin Psychiatry*. 1995;7:99–101.
76. Prior TI, Chue PS, Tibbo P, et al. Drug metabolism and atypical antipsychotics. *Eur Neuropsychopharmacol*. 1999;9(4):301–309.
77. Rapeport WG, Muirhead DC, Williams SA, et al. Absence of effect of sertraline on the pharmacokinetics and pharmacodynamics of phenytoin. *J Clin Psychiatry*. 1996;57(Suppl 1):24–28.
78. Rapeport WG, Williams SA, Muirhead DC, et al. Absence of sertraline-mediated effect on the pharmacokinetics and pharmacodynamics of carbamazepine. *J Clin Psychiatry*. 1996;57(Suppl 1):20–23.
79. Ring BJ, Catlow J, Lindsay TJ, et al. Identification of the human cytochromes P450 responsible for the in vitro formation of the major oxidative metabolites of the antipsychotic agent olanzapine. *J Pharmacol Exp Ther*. 1996;276(2):658–666.
80. Rudorfer MV, Potter WZ. Metabolism of tricyclic antidepressants. *Cell Mol Neurobiol*. 1999;19(3):373–409.
81. Shorvon SD, Tallis RC, Wallace HK. Antiepileptic drugs: Coprescription of proconvulsant drugs and oral contraceptives: A national study of antiepileptic drug prescribing practice. *J Neurol Neurosurg Psychiatry*. 2002;72(1):114–115.
82. Smith D, Baker G, Davies G, et al. Outcomes of add-on treatment with lamotrigine in partial epilepsy. *Epilepsia*. 1993;34(2):312–322.
83. Spaans E, van den Heuvel MW, Schnabel PG, et al. Concomitant use of mirtazapine and phenytoin: A drug-drug interaction study in healthy male subjects. *Eur J Clin Pharmacol*. 2002;58(6):423–429.
84. Spina E, Avenoso A, Facciolà G, et al. Plasma concentrations of risperidone and 9-hydroxyrisperidone: Effect of comedication with carbamazepine or valproate. *Ther Drug Monit*. 2000;22:481–485.
85. Spina E, Avenoso A, Pollicino AM, et al. Carbamazepine coadministration with fluoxetine or fluvoxamine. *Ther Drug Monit*. 1993;15:247–250.
86. Spina E, Perucca E. Clinical significance of pharmacokinetic interactions between antiepileptic and psychotropic drugs. *Epilepsia*. 2002;43(Suppl 2):37–44.
87. Spina E, Scordo MG, D'Arrigo C. Metabolic drug interactions with new psychotropic agents. *Fundam Clin Pharmacol*. 2003;17(5):517–538.
88. Steinacher L, Vandel P, Zullino DF, et al. Carbamazepine augmentation in depressive patients non-responding to citalopram: A pharmacokinetic and clinical pilot study. *Eur Neuropsychopharmacol*. 2002;12(3):255–260.
89. Szymura-Oleksiak J, Wyska E, Wasieczko A. pharmacokinetic interaction between imipramine and carbamazepine in patients with major depression. *Psychopharmacology (Berl)*. 2001;154:38–42.

90. Tekle A, al-Kamis KI. Phenytoin-bupropion interaction: Effect on plasma phenytoin concentration in the rat. *J Pharm Pharmacol.* 1990;42:799–801.
91. Torta R, Monaco F. Atypical antipsychotics and serotoninergic antidepressants in patients with epilepsy: Pharmacodynamic considerations. *Epilepsia.* 2002;43(Suppl 2):8–13.
92. Toy SM, Lucki I, Peirgies AA, et al. Pharmacokinetic and pharmacodynamic evaluation of the potential drug interaction between venlafaxine and diazepam. *J Clin Pharmacol.* 1995;35:410–419.
93. Trimble MR. Carbamazepine. Clinical efficacy and use in psychiatric disorders. In: Levy RH, Mattson RH, Meldrum BS, Perucca E, eds. *Antiepileptic Drugs,* 5th ed. Philadelphia: Lippincott Williams & Wilkins; 2002:278–284.
94. Trimble MR. Oxcarbazepine. Clinical efficacy and use in psychiatric disorders. In: Levy RH, Mattson RH, Meldrum BS, Perucca E, eds. *Antiepileptic Drugs,* 5th ed. Philadelphia: Lippincott Williams & Wilkins; 2002:476–478.
95. Vieweg V, Shutty M, Hundley P, et al. Combined treatment with lithium and carbamazepine. *Am J Psychiatry.* 1991;148:398–399.
96. Wang BPW, Ketter TA, Becker OV, et al. New anticonvulsant medication uses in bipolar disorder. *CNS Spectr.* 2003;8(21):930–932,941—947.
97. Wong SL, Cavanaugh J, Shi H, et al. Effects of divalproex sodium on amitriptyline and nortriptyline pharmacokinetics. *Clin Pharmacol Ther.* 1996;60:48–53.
98. Wong YW, Yeh C, Thyrum PT. The effects of concomitant phenytoin administration on the steady-state pharmacokinetics of quetiapine. *J Clin Psychopharmacol.* 2001;21:89–93.
99. Yan QS, Jobe PC, Dailey JW. Evidence that a serotonergic mechanism is involved in the anticonvulsant effect of fluoxetine in genetically epilepsy-prone rats. *Eur J Pharmacol.* 1994;252:105–112.
100. Yasui-Furukori N, Kondo T, Mihara K, et al. Significant dose effect of carbamazepine on reduction of steady-state plasma concentration of haloperidol in schizophrenic patients. *J Clin Psychopharmacol.* 2003;23(5):435–440.

CHAPTER 215 ■ OVERVIEW: SOCIAL ISSUES

ROBERT T. FRASER

INTRODUCTION

There has been longstanding concern in the field of epilepsy that, although progress continues to be made relative to medical management of the disability, including the development of new generations of antiepileptic medications, attention is less focused on the social adjustment of individuals with the disability. A survey of 420 individuals drawn from affiliates of the Epilepsy Foundation of America[17] suggests a number of ongoing concerns, including employment, marriage and money management, and diverse health-related concerns. An earlier study by Schacter et al.[16] indicates that 65% of the 150 respondents in an Epilepsy Association of Massachusetts study responded that they were psychosocially adversely affected by seizures and that this was true for even half of those with one seizure or less per year. A recent review by Theodore et al.[18] regarding epilepsy in North America describes poor quality of life, a high number of depression and anxiety days, marked unemployment and underemployment, continuing perceived stigma, and higher suicide rates. Although adults with well-controlled epilepsy[8] may not be as significantly affected as those with more active seizure conditions, this appears to be the minority of the epilepsy population.

The field of epilepsy is at a crossroads relative to addressing the psychosocial needs of people with this disability and their significant others. The impact of managed care, a lack of U.S. federal support for multidisciplinary centers, and other factors are reducing the emphasis on diverse aspects of social adjustment and needed psychosocial interventions. There is an increasing concern, however, about quality-of-life assessment related to medication or surgical intervention and diverse aspects of neuropsychological functioning, but a review of the presentations at the American Epilepsy Society's 2005 Annual Meeting in Washington, D.C., suggests less coverage and research investment in some of the areas discussed in this section of the book. There were almost no studies relating to psychosocial intervention. This underscores that clinical service demands and financial constraints are affecting the investment in psychosocial research and demonstration projects.

Overall, there are a number of areas in which the epilepsy population appears to be making some significant gains. In Chapter 216, Jacoby, Snape, and Baker make a helpful distinction between "felt" and "enacted" or actually experienced stigma. On an overview, attitudes toward people with epilepsy are continuing to become more positive. There are a number of mediators of attitudes toward epilepsy, including the educational levels of respondents and their perceptions of disability-related limitations. Jacoby et al. stress the importance of family support and clear intrafamily communication as being preventive of perceived stigma by offspring. They also endorse the importance of "target-specific change models," for example, geared to adolescent attitudes, involving multiple and multi-tiered strategies within each efforts.

Although employment continues to be an international concern, in Chapter 219, Thorbecke and Fraser highlight the various aspects of the vocational assessment process, workplace accommodation, different model programs, and relevant national legislation that affect employability for those with epilepsy. Employment rates through specialized programs have been recorded to be as high as 89% for referrals with "epilepsy only" as a disability.[6] There is no question, however, that associated cognitive deficits, behavioral difficulties, and so on, are making successful employment outcomes more challenging. Specialized epilepsy vocational programs, however, will continue to be more effective, particularly for individuals with more involved epilepsy and associated disabilities. Unfortunately, there has been a lessening of emphasis on provision of employment services by the national Epilepsy Foundation (EF) in the United States. Today in the United States, specialized epilepsy vocational programs exist only at the University of Washington-Seattle, the University of California-San Francisco, and some EF affiliate agencies. Germany and Holland are among the few other countries that have specialized programs of this nature.

As Beran and colleagues indicate in Chapter 221, a number of gains have been made in the areas of legislation, driver licenses, and access to insurance. The Americans with Disabilities Act (ADA), signed into law in 1990, not only forbids discrimination in employment, but also requires reasonable accommodation (e.g., job restructuring) if an individual cannot perform the essential functions of a job. This type of legislation, although not necessarily affecting initial hiring decisions, can assist people with epilepsy to maintain their job position within the context of discriminatory or whimsical employer decisions to terminate. Eligibility for coverage under ADA has been difficult to establish for persons with good seizure control, but advocacy efforts by the U.S. EF and collaborators are being made to rectify this situation.

In relation to driver licenses, there is a general trend toward shorter seizure-free periods and a review of favorable modifiers prior to categorical driver licensing suspensions. This is not to say that advocacy and targeted physician effort will not be necessary in different areas of the world or within some U.S. states. Some countries, such as Japan and Russia, preclude driving after one seizure.[4] There remains a delicate balance between patient benefit and acknowledging risk factors and general safety.

Within the area of legislation, however, there is a continuing international need for advocacy, specifically in relation to health care coverage and reform. A number of U.S. insurance companies have used outdated actuarial data and failed to note the advances in diagnosis and treatment of epilepsy in making their health care access and financial rate decisions. This issue is not unique to the United States. Beran et al. emphasize the need to advocate in other areas such as epilepsy research and development and services to families. They end their chapter with a helpful section on strategies for use with political representation.

Over the years there has been a growing recognition of the need for social support for individuals with epilepsy. In Chapter 217, Austin, de Boer, and Shafer review the plethora of issues affecting psychosocial adjustment in epilepsy and a range of issues that can be targeted for intervention. Of particular value are guidelines for dailing living both inside the home and within the community. They also draw attention to the need for more "self-management" education in relation to the disability and research into the value of group versus individual educational programs or programs combining education, counseling, and even recreation, among other isues.

Despite the fact that psychosocial gains are being made in a number of areas, certain issue areas deserve increasing attention. Although there is a dramatic increase in quality-of-life assessment and an effort to measure the impact of seizure severity on patients' lives, there is a continuing theme in the literature[1,2,7] that patients feel poorly educated not only about epilepsy, but also about medications and potential side effects. As Buck et al.[2] indicate, patients place a significant premium on physicians who are not only knowledgeable, but are also communicative and approachable. Within the current managed care context in a number of countries and given the institutional demands on the physicians' time, it can be very difficult for physicians to make the effort carefully to explain epilepsy and issues in medical management to a patient and family members. Somehow, however, this needs to be done because it directly relates to patient compliance, among other care variables, in the prevention of the disabling condition. Several studies[5,10] show sample noncompliance rates exceeding 50%. It appears that time spent educating each patient about epilepsy and medication is well spent.

In general, there is a need for more educational programs for individuals with epilepsy and their significant others. In Chapter 217, Austin et al. point out that although the literature supports the need for epilepsy education, few educational programs (exceptions are the Modular Service Package Epilepsy [MOSES] and Sepulveda Epilepsy Education [SEE] programs) have been presented and systematically evaluated. Internationally, only a few clinics have formal educational programs for their patients with regard to their epilepsy and medications, and only one program could be identified in the literature[11,12] for children with epilepsy and their parents. The SEE program[17] has shown some very beneficial results on quality of life and seizure management for adolescents with epilepsy and their parents.

Although the U.S. Epilepsy Foundation and other national epilepsy associations have quality educational materials available (e.g., on cognition and epilepsy), significant marketing efforts through the media might be needed to promote their utilization. An obvious role for epilepsy organizations internationally is the development of formal educational programs about epilepsy and associated issues that also help physicians to take the time required to discuss their patients' concerns. Medication noncompliance and continuing advances in medication management are areas that need to be attacked simultaneously.

Marriage and family concerns also deserve continued emphasis. Educational programs for both patients and the general public could be very helpful in improving the prognosis for marriage—particularly for men. As Thompson and Upton indicate,[19] levels of stress and dissatisfaction within families can be high because those with epilepsy often face difficulties in maintaining primary work careers or even receiving respite care for their children. Within the context of psychosocial research, interventions with families and their impact on medical and social adjustment have been largely overlooked.

In Chapter 218, Seidenberg and Clemmons discuss issues relating to school functioning and school-to-work transition. They present a comprehensive review of seizure and neuropsychological correlates of academic dysfunction and discuss subtypes of learning disabilities and a comprehensive perspective on educational and vocational assessment. They also offer approaches to working with parents, teachers, and state vocational rehabilitation representatives. Again, there is a paucity of recent research on school functioning or successful school-to-work transition.

Of particular interest in this section is Chapter 220 by Rubin, Wiebe, and Gilliam on health outcomes. The chapter underscores the importance of adverse medication effects and depression/anxiety on quality of life and the need to assess and intervene with regard to these issues. Although it is understood that other health-promoting behaviors such as sleep quality and exercise also can affect quality of life, we do not yet have an integrated model of effects on quality of life.

SUMMARY AND CONCLUSIONS

Although progress has been made relative to the social adjustment of people with epilepsy, there remains much to be done. Considerable challenges face those in less industrialized countries, in which some of the issues in discrimination, employment, and so on, are only recently becoming obvious and receiving media attention. As discussed by Collings,[3] we remain at the early stages of examining international differences in psychosocial well-being and quality of life for this population. The challenge remains not only to identify these differences, but also to find funds to mount education and other psychosocial intervention efforts that currently are lacking. Although it appears that intervention during childhood and particularly adolescence[15] is crucial within this population, most existing intervention efforts appear to be conducted within short-term summer camp structures.[5] Although these are valuable, they are insufficient. More comprehensive and sustained psychosocial interventions need to be pursued and evaluated.

ACKNOWLEDGMENT

I appreciate partial research review by the National Epilepsy Library at the Epilepsy Foundation (United States).

References

1. Brown SW. Quality of life: A view from the playground. *Seizure.* 1994; 3(Suppl 20A):11–15.
2. Buck D, Jacoby A, Baker GA, et al. Patients' experiences of and satisfaction with care for their epilepsy. *Epilepsia.* 1996;37:841–849.
3. Collings JA. International differences in psychosocial well-being: A comparative study of adults with epilepsy in three countries. *Seizure.* 1994;3:183–190.
4. Collings JA. Life fulfillment in an epilepsy sample from the United States. *Soc Sci Med.* 1995;40:1579–1584.
5. Cusher-Weinstein SM, Bethke-Pope L, Salpekar J, et al. *Camp designed for children with epilepsy.* Paper presented at the annual meeting of the American Epilepsy Society, Washington, D.C., December 3, 2005.
6. Dowse R, Futter WT. Outpatient compliance with theophylline and phenytoin therapy. *S Afr Med J.* 1991;80:550–553.
7. Fisher RS, Parsonage M, Beaussart M, et al. Epilepsy and driving: An international perspective. Joint Commission on Drivers' Licensing of the International Bureau for Epilepsy and the International League Against Epilepsy. *Epilepsia.* 1994;35:675–685.
8. Fraser RT, Clemmons DC, Koepnick D, et al. Evaluating seizure impact on employability [Abstract]. *Epilepsia.* 1996;37(Suppl 205):6.
9. Freeman GK, Richards SC. Personal continuity and the care of patients with epilepsy in general practice. *Br J Gen Pract.* 1994;44:395–399.
10. Jacoby A. Epilepsy and the quality of everyday life: Findings from a study of people with well controlled epilepsy. *Soc Sci Med.* 1992;6:657–666.
11. Jacoby A. Felt versus enacted stigma: A concept revisited. *Soc Sci Med.* 1994;38:269–274.
12. Krumholz A, Grufferman S, Orr ST. Seizures and seizure care in an emergency department. *Epilepsia.* 1989;30:175–181.
13. Lewis MA, Hatton CL, Salas I, et al. Impact of the children's epilepsy program on parents. *Epilepsia.* 1991;32:365–374.

14. Lewis MA, Salas L, de la Sota A, et al. Randomized trial of a program to enhance the competencies of children with epilepsy. *Epilepsia*. 1990;31:101–109.
15. Raty LK, Soderfeldt BA, Wilde Larson BM. *Psychosocial well being and quality of life in young adults with epilepsy*. Paper presented at the annual meeting of the American Epilepsy Society, Washington, D.C., December 3, 2005.
16. Schacter SC, Shafer PO, Murphy W. The personal impact of seizures: Correlation with seizure frequency, employment, cost of medical care, and satisfaction with physician care. *J Epilepsy*. 1993;6:224–227.
17. Shore CP, Perkins SM, Austen JK. *Efficacy of the SEE program on quality of life, seizure management and cost savings for adolescents with epilepsy and their parents*. Paper presented at the annual meeting of the American Epilepsy Society, Washington, D.C., December 3, 2005.
18. Theodore WH, Spencer SS, Wiebe S, et al. Epilepsy in North America: A report prepared by IBE, TLAE, and the WHO. *Epilepsia*. 2000;47:1700–1722.
19. Thompson FJ, Upton D. The impact of chronic epilepsy on the family. *Seizure*. 1992;1:43–48.

CHAPTER 216 ■ SOCIAL ASPECTS: EPILEPSY STIGMA AND QUALITY OF LIFE

ANN JACOBY, DEE SNAPE, AND GUS A. BAKER

INTRODUCTION

In this chapter, we turn from consideration of epilepsy as a biomedical condition and the province of health professionals to consideration of epilepsy as a negative social label and the concern of social theorists, social policy makers, and disability activists. Epilepsy has long been considered as "undesired differentness,"[44] and, as a consequence, it has involved the application of formal and informal rules and sanctions against those affected by it. Legal discrimination against people with epilepsy dates back centuries and operates still,[56] even though in many countries persons with epilepsy are now considered as having a prescribed disability and so are offered protections under the law. A significant literature traces the history of epilepsy as stigma and documents the role of stigma and discrimination in its present-day social reality. From this, it is clear that the social problems arising from a diagnosis of epilepsy and the repercussions for quality of life, especially for those in whom it proves to be clinically benign, can represent a greater challenge than its medical management. How these problems can be minimized thus represents an important aspect of the overall management of epilepsy.

EPILEPSY AS A SOCIAL LABEL

Although considered the "sacred disease" by the ancient Greeks, in many ancient and primitive societies epilepsy was believed to originate from malignant causes and to be associated with sin and demonic possession. Seizures were often considered bad omens. There are references in the New Testament to epilepsy as a form of madness, and the notion of people with epilepsy as "lunatic" held widespread currency throughout the mediaeval period. Theories of epilepsy as contagion can also be traced back to antiquity.[108] Temkin[108] saw epilepsy as representing the historical struggle between magical and scientific conceptions of disease, with its medicalization in the Western world a victory for the latter. It is apparent, however, from studies of lay attitudes and beliefs toward epilepsy (see later discussion) that remnants of the former attitude continue to inform popular concepts of the condition even through to the present day. What is more, even when biomedical explanations for epilepsy emerged as triumphant during the Enlightenment,[82] the evolution of epilepsy from "badness to sickness"[22] brought with it its own associations to stigma, with studies linking epilepsy to aggressive or even criminal behavior, abnormal sexual activity, hereditary degeneracy, and a specific "epileptic personality," all of which have had power to reinforce negative stereotypes and hence perpetuate stigma.

Although the biomedically driven concept of the epileptic personality may have been discounted in recent years, Scambler[97,98] proposed an alternative sociologic construct of "epileptic identity" resting firmly on the view of epilepsy as not just a clinical problem but also a social label. Scambler suggested that people with epilepsy react symbolically to having seizures and develop a special identity or "view of the world" underpinned by their expectations of stigma. This world view is not generally present in their lives, and is triggered by particular events; when it is triggered, however, it has the effect of predisposing them to try to cover up the signs of their condition and pass themselves off as "normal." Scambler found that almost everyone he interviewed was distressed by receiving a diagnosis of epilepsy because "they showed a more or less clearly defined awareness that a physician's diagnostic statement ... had transformed them from 'normal' persons to 'epileptics' and this was first and foremost a stigmatising condition." Their perceptions of epilepsy as stigmatizing were clearly anchored in what they believed to be the predominantly negative attitudes of others, which constituted a major source of anguish to them, but for which, Scambler argued, there was actually little empirical support.

Based on his analysis, he proposed a "hidden distress" model wherein the stigma of epilepsy and its repercussions for quality of life are best understood by making a distinction between "felt" and "enacted" stigma.[100] Felt stigma here refers to the shame of being epileptic and the fear of encountering epilepsy-linked enacted stigma, that is, enacted stigma to actual episodes of discrimination against people with epilepsy *solely* on the grounds of them having epilepsy. Scambler concluded that felt stigma was far more prevalent than enacted stigma, with almost everyone in his study appearing to suffer from it, even if only intermittently. It was also, in effect, a self-fulfilling prophecy inasmuch as their fear and shame about epilepsy led people to attempt to conceal their condition from others, denying themselves the opportunity to test whether the enacted stigma and discrimination they expected would, in fact, materialize.

The power of the social label of epilepsy is also illustrated in the work by Schneider and Conrad,[101] who reported that the people they interviewed with epilepsy saw it as a kind of "moral weight" they had to carry and so was far worse than simply having seizures. Some, described as "unadjusted" to their diagnosis, appeared to be overwhelmed by the shame of having epilepsy; they saw it as precluding or limiting their access to important personal and social resources, negatively affecting different aspects of their quality of life and preventing their happiness. For some people, referred to by Schneider and Conrad as "debilitated," it appeared that the label of epilepsy totally defined them, and their response was often to withdraw from contact with the nonepileptic world.

THEORIES OF STIGMA IN THE CONTEXT OF EPILEPSY

Goffman[44] defined stigma as "an undesired differentness." People are stigmatized because they possesses an attribute, such as epilepsy, that is undesired and deeply discrediting and by virtue of which they represent a discrepancy between the persons they might be and the persons they are—in Goffman's words, between their virtual and actual social identities. Goffman identifies three different types of stigma: (a) the tribal stigmas of race and religion, (b) blemishes of individual character, and (c) what he refers to as abominations of the body. Whichever of these prevails, Goffman argues that those who are stigmatized are seen by others as "not quite human" and the legitimate target for discrimination. Goffman notes that even though people who are stigmatized may attempt to rid themselves of their "contaminated" social identity, they cannot reacquire the status of normal, only that of someone who was once "contaminated." This problem is thrown into relief in the context of epilepsy by the fact that, in clinical terms, the condition may not be considered curable, only controllable, so that the threat of "contamination" can never be entirely eliminated. Because the possibility exists "that the offensive behaviour will recur,"[2] the stigma of epilepsy is irreversible and ineradicable.

Recent theoretical work on the concept of stigma has tended to emphasize two key dimensions, visibility/concealability and course/controllability,[29,65,66] both of which are highly relevant to epilepsy. Seizures, the "symptoms" of epilepsy, may be difficult to conceal and may become more salient over time depending on the clinical course of the condition and the degree to which it can be controlled. Four further dimensions, within each of which the stigma of epilepsy can be located, are disruptiveness, aesthetic aspects, origin, and peril (Table 1).[66] Seizures are clearly often highly disruptive to social interaction, causing those observing them to stand by powerlessly as "the terrified watcher."[116] Depending on their specific manifestations, they may also be aesthetically unpleasant to those observing them. The legacy of the old ideas about epilepsy as the product of malign forces or sinful behavior results in the issue of origin remaining ambiguous: It might be thought that people with epilepsy are somehow morally culpable for their condition. Moreover, although seizures present far greater dangers to those with epilepsy than to bystanders, the issue of peril is echoed in old ideas of epilepsy as contagion. Such ideas are still often dominant in resource-poor countries where the majority of those affected by epilepsy live, which commonly leads to their social ostracism.[21,64,83]

Even in resource-rich countries, the fact that often no definitive cause for epilepsy can be found creates the possibility for continuing misattributions. As shown in a recent study by Austin et al.,[5] 22% of American adolescents were uncertain whether epilepsy was a contagious condition.

TABLE 1

DIMENSIONS OF STIGMA ACCORDING TO JONES ET AL.[66]

Concealability	Extent to which the stigmatizing condition is visible to others
Course of the mark	Whether the condition becomes more salient over time
Disruptiveness	Degree to which it interferes with social interactions
Aesthetics	Subjective reactions of others to the unattractiveness of the stigmatizing condition
Origin	Whether seen as congenital, accidental, or intentional
Peril	Perceived danger of the condition to others

TABLE 2

COMPONENTS OF STIGMA ACCORDING TO LINK AND PHELAN[73]

Component 1	People distinguish and label *socially relevant* human differences
Component 2	Dominant cultural beliefs link labeled persons to *negative* stereotypes (e.g., "People with mental illness are a danger to others")
Component 3	Labeled persons are placed in distinct categories (e.g., "fat," "disabled," "epileptic") to separate them from others
Component 4	Labeled persons experience status loss and discrimination (and unequal health and socioeconomic outcomes)
Component 5	Social, economic, and political power allows components 1–4 to operate (those in positions of *low* power cannot impose labels, stereotypes, separation, status loss)

Social theorists have commented that a reason that conditions such as epilepsy are almost universally stigmatizing is that they represent some kind of tangible or symbolic danger either to individuals or entire cultures, including physical, moral, and health dangers.[32,104] With regard to epilepsy specifically, it has been argued[1,6,98,112] that seizures can be seen as uniquely dangerous to normal social interaction both by violating cultural norms or values and by representing human weakness and unpredictability and even "anomic terror." Recently, stigma theorists have also recognized the previously neglected role of power relations in the social construction of stigma.[73,99] Link and Phelan[73] commented, "it takes power to stigmatise." The social labeling, stereotyping, separation from others, and consequent status loss that are the key elements of stigma are only relevant in a power situation that allows them to unfold; in other words, they cannot be imposed by those in positions of low power (Table 2). How does this play out in epilepsy? Certainly within the current culture of biomedicine, clinicians hold power to impose a diagnosis of epilepsy on a set of often nebulous neurologic events or symptoms and, in so doing, to legitimize a historically based negative social label and its associated stereotypes. This then allows imposition of rules and sanctions that reinforce the differentness of having epilepsy.

Because it was developed in the context of epilepsy stigma specifically, it is worthwhile reevaluating Scambler's "hidden distress" theory in view of subsequent epilepsy-related research. Jacoby[54] revisited the concepts of felt and enacted stigma and found, like Scambler, that the former was far more commonly experienced than the latter, with few people able to recall any instances of enacted discrimination. Other research on epilepsy stigma in similar cultures supports this. It has been argued, however,[90] that much of the research reported has been concerned with identifying episodes at the hard end of enacted stigma only, for example, in relation to employment, while failing to document its more subtle expressions.

Furthermore, whereas felt stigma appears to be a much more pervasive element in North European cultures, it should not be assumed to be universally of greater relevance.[89] In some cultures, for example, sub-Saharan African ones,[87] enacted stigma may be of far greater concern, perhaps in part because the treatment gap increases the visibility of epilepsy. If we are to advance our understanding of the nature of epilepsy stigma, it will therefore be important to develop a shared theoretical framework and set of measurement tools that allow for cross-cultural and contextual adaptation.

VIEWS ABOUT EPILEPSY AS A SOCIAL LABEL

Views of People With Epilepsy

Labeling theorists maintain that the impact of a negative social label, for example, being "epileptic," can be quite profound inasmuch as the label overrides other aspects of a person's identity. In a sense, it becomes what has been termed the "master" status,[72] making it difficult for the affected person to continue to think of himself or herself as just "like everybody else."[30] Given that all illness can be defined negatively as a state of "deviance" from good health,[81] having epilepsy can be said to represent a state of double deviance,[55] its particular characteristics and social connotations ensuring that deviance also attaches to the condition per se. The process by which people with epilepsy come to acknowledge their deviant status and accept that they are not like everyone else has been the focus of attention of several authors.[98,101,118]

Parents emerge as key figures in these analyses because their reactions to a diagnosis of epilepsy in their child seem effectively to set the stage for the child's subsequent interpretation of its significance. When parental reactions are negative, their affected child learns to think of epilepsy as something shameful; when parental assumptions are that epilepsy will inevitably attract hostile reactions from others, their affected child learns to think of it as something to keep quiet about. Other key figures are likely to be teachers and health care professionals, both of which groups are known as sometimes having less-than-positive attitudes about the condition and limited knowledge about its implications (see later discussion).

It is not surprising, consequently, that people with epilepsy sometimes resort to trying to "renegotiate" the diagnosis into something more socially benign[98] or to taking active steps to conceal it from others.[74,98,101,120] Among the adult participants in the studies by Schneider, Conrad, and Scambler, concealment constituted a key management strategy. Similarly, in their study of adolescents with epilepsy, Westbrook et al.[119] found that more than half kept their condition a secret from others and almost three fourths said they rarely or never talked about it to others, even though denying that having epilepsy affected their friendships and perceived likeability among their peers.

Views of Other Groups

As noted, even today epilepsy remains shrouded in misinformation and misbeliefs.[78] Misattributions about the causes of epilepsy, for example, are common (Table 3). Historically, studies have presented a less-than-favorable picture for people with epilepsy. For example, Bagley[6] compared public attitudes toward people with epilepsy with those toward people with cerebral palsy and mental illness and found that people with epilepsy were much more often rejected than the other two groups. Both Vinson[115] and Harrison and West,[47] who interviewed people in two cities as part of the U.K. National Epilepsy Week, found that significant numbers of the people with whom they talked held images of people with epilepsy that were essentially negative. These included the views that people with epilepsy were violent, retarded, antisocial, and physically unattractive. Similarly negative traits were identified as peculiar to people with epilepsy in later street surveys carried out in the United Kingdom.[67,96]

TABLE 3

LAY UNDERSTANDING OF CAUSES OF EPILEPSY

Resource-rich countries	Resource-poor countries
■ Stress/pressure	■ Sorcery, witchcraft
■ Tiredness	■ Possession by devils, ancestral spirits
■ Heat	■ Infection, contagion
■ Mental illness	■ Saturation by foams
■ Brain/nervous system disorder	■ Insect/lizard in stomach/head
■ Congenital problem	
■ Old age	

In the United States, Baumann et al.[10] found that one fourth of respondents to a telephone survey believed there would be deterioration in the classroom environment were a child with epilepsy to join it. In the 1987 American Institute of Public Opinion survey,[70] 7% thought people with epilepsy were dangerous, 12% that they should not have children, and 33% that people think less of a person with epilepsy and their families. With regard to particular groups within the general population, research has also identified lack of knowledge and accompanying negative attitudes among employers,[40,50,91,94] coworkers,[46] health professionals,[11,109] and teachers.[13,31,42,75]

Rather more encouragingly, numerous surveys have documented improvements over time in attitudes to epilepsy,[19,20,33,39,51,52,61,63,79,80] indicating that its weight in some, if not all, "local moral worlds"[32] has lessened. For example, in the United States,[20] affirmative responses to questions asking people whether they would object to a child of theirs playing with one who had epilepsy and whether people with epilepsy should be barred from employment in the same jobs as others declined between 1949 and 1979 from 24% to 6% and from 35% to 9%, respectively. Jensen and Dam[63] reported that social acceptance of people with epilepsy was high in Denmark; Dawkins et al.[33] reported similarly in the United Kingdom. In a recent study carried out as part of the U.K. Omnibus Survey and involving >1,600 randomly selected members of the general public,[61] those questioned appeared generally well-informed about epilepsy, its causes, and its treatment, and most held highly favorable attitudes toward people with epilepsy, although one fifth thought people with epilepsy were more likely to have personality problems. Likewise, increasingly positive attitudes have been noted among key subgroups. For example, among primary and secondary level teachers surveyed in Greece,[68] most believed that children with epilepsy were as capable as others of achieving academically. Nonetheless, the continuing challenge of stigma is highlighted by a study published in the same year[95] documenting persistent widespread negative attitudes and bias toward epilepsy among teachers in Nigeria.

In a survey of 200 randomly selected U.K. employers, Jacoby et al.[60] found that although epilepsy continues to generate anxiety in the work context, the majority (and a larger proportion than in earlier surveys) reported that there were jobs in their companies suitable for people with epilepsy and were aware of the need and expressed clear willingness to comply with the principle of "reasonable adjustment." Overall such studies suggest significant improvements in public attitudes. It is interesting that, despite positive public attitude shifts, it has also been shown that epilepsy still sometimes evokes greater responses to rejection than other chronic conditions, even conditions such as AIDS/HIV infection and mental illness, which are recognized as deeply stigmatizing.[6,10,26,85] Reis[88] concluded that although the classic stereotypes of epilepsy may have less resonance today, they have tended to be replaced by new ones in which people with epilepsy are regarded as introverted, overanxious, and less open than others. Such present-day stereotypes, even if they are in any degree supported by available research, are inevitably disquieting to those against whom they are directed.

ROLE OF STIGMA IN QUALITY OF LIFE

Stigma has long been thought of as predisposing to psychopathology in people with epilepsy, although the relative lack of published studies involving formal and scientifically robust investigation of its role means that its supposed effects are less evidence based than a "taken for granted" assumption.[48] Studies that have attempted to examine the relationship between stigma and psychological health specifically, and quality of life more broadly, include those by Arnston et al.,[4] Hermann et al.,[49] Jacoby,[53,58] Baker et al.,[8] and Suurmeijer et al.[106] Jacoby[57] noted that consistent with sociologic theories about "the illness trajectory"[23] for people with epilepsy, the clinical course of their disease is important for their quality of life, including the degree of their stigma sense. She and her colleagues documented rates of stigma in persons starting to have seizures, experiencing seizures that prove to be intractable, and having seizures that go into remission. Among those newly diagnosed with epilepsy,[59] one-fourth reported feeling stigmatized despite the recency of application of the negative social label of "being epileptic." Two years later, only one tenth of those who had remained seizure free reported feeling stigmatized, compared with 45% of those experiencing continuing seizures. In contrast, among a separate cohort of persons with seizures in remission, only 14% reported feeling stigmatized, and this group also reported minimal impairments in other life domains.

The relationship between epilepsy stage or severity and stigma is also supported by Baker et al.'s study,[8] in which the percentage of people reporting feeling highly stigmatized rose from 10% of those who had been seizure free in the previous 12 months to 29% of those reporting ongoing seizures occurring more than once monthly. Competing evidence about the importance of factors other than these clinical ones is available, however; for example, the study by Ryan et al.[92] showed that the relationship between stigma perceptions and epilepsy severity was highly dependent on other mediating factors such as attained level of education and the perceived limitations imposed by epilepsy-related vulnerabilities. Such findings help to explain why a sense of stigma may persist for a small minority of people with apparently excellent seizure control and, conversely, are absent among some people with even very frequent seizures. They highlight the need for a psychosocial as well as a medical approach to the management of epilepsy.

Stigma was positively associated with impaired self-esteem, self-efficacy, sense of mastery, perceived helplessness, increased rates of anxiety and depression, increased somatic symptomatology, and reduced life satisfaction in studies by Arnston et al.,[4] Jacoby,[54,58] Westbrook et al.,[119] and Dilorio et al.[36] Baker et al.[7,8] also demonstrated a link between felt stigma and medication side effects, supporting Scambler's proposition about the potential for antiepileptic drugs to act as stigma cues. Both Baker et al.[7] and Youn and Hong[121] found that overall quality of life was poorer for persons reporting higher levels of stigma, either felt or enacted (Fig. 1). Suurmeijer et al.[106] used hierarchical regression analysis to demonstrate that perceived stigma was fourth in importance in predicting quality of life, after psychological distress, loneliness, and adjustment; it accounted for twice the amount of variance in quality-of-life scores as did clinical variables such as seizure frequency and antiepileptic drug side effects.

It is interesting that several hypotheses were not supported by the findings in the study by Westbrook et al.,[119] which focused on the link between stigma and self-esteem. For example, focal seizures, rather than tonic–clonic seizures, were predictive of lower self-esteem. In addition, contrary to the role proposed for it in stigma theory—namely, that the issue of disclosure management would be forced by the threat of frequent, visible symptoms—no relationship was shown between it and seizure type or frequency or epilepsy duration. These findings raise questions about the limitations of theory for lived experience and the need for more in-depth approaches to identify alternative and previously unrecognized mechanisms by which stigma exerts its effects.[74]

Stigma may also be implicated *indirectly* in quality of life by virtue of the fact that the quality of health and social care received by persons with stigmatizing health conditions may be suboptimal. Stigmatized conditions may fail to attract investment both for service provision and for research.[117]

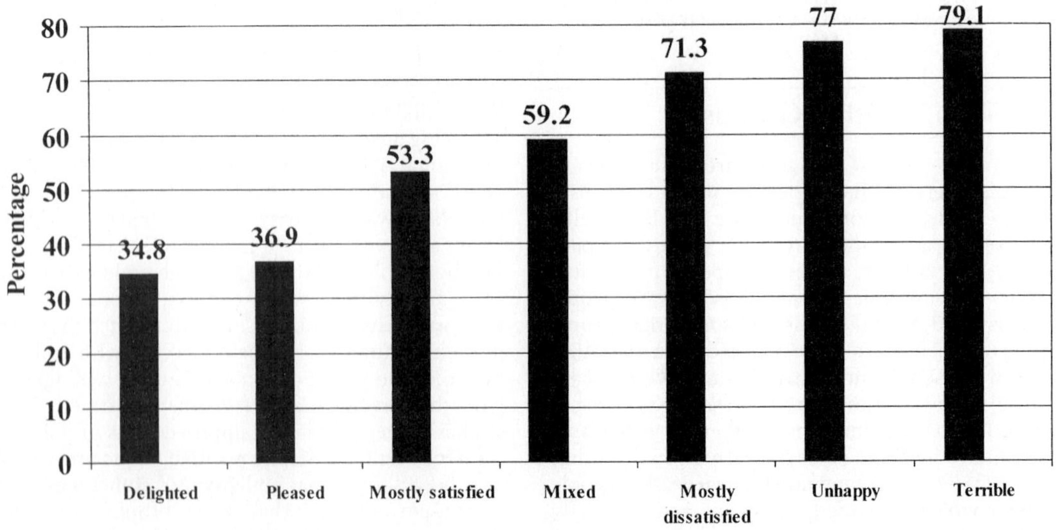

FIGURE 1. Stigma and overall quality of life. (From Baker GA, Brooks J, Buck D, et al. The stigma of epilepsy: a European perspective. *Epilepsia.* 2000;41:98–104, with permission.)

There is also some evidence to suggest that health and social care professionals, like other members of the general public, are susceptible to negative attitudes and beliefs about epilepsy. Recent surveys in the United Kingdom have suggested that health care for people with epilepsy is fragmented and underresourced, with many receiving care that is substandard in relation to published guidelines.[62,109,113] Significant levels of dissatisfaction with the quality of their medical, social, and educational care has been expressed by members of the United Kingdom's largest epilepsy support organization, Epilepsy Action.[15,16] The U.K. Clinical Standards Advisory Group[113] concluded that levels of disability and social exclusion for people with epilepsy would be considerably lessened by relatively simple and inexpensive changes in the delivery of their care. Among their suggestions were that formal mechanisms for eliciting the views of service users should be incorporated and that simple care protocols should be introduced for nonneurologic staff, for example, those working in accident and emergency departments.

Dilorio et al.[36] examined the relationship between felt stigma and perceptions of the quality of health care among adults with epilepsy living in the United States. They found that persons with higher levels of felt stigma reported lower levels of satisfaction with their care across a whole range of areas, including interpersonal, communication, technical competence, time spent with the doctor, and the accessibility of their care. They also experienced greater difficulty with managing their medication regime, reported less medication adherence, and reported less positive outcomes associated with taking medication. This lack of satisfaction may therefore reflect a combination of underresourcing and negative attitudes among care providers. As the authors acknowledge, however, the cross-sectional nature of their study precludes firm conclusions about the direction of effects.

MANAGING EPILEPSY STIGMA

Helping People With Epilepsy to Manage a Negative Social Label

Dell[35] noted that although identity politics is not "a comforting strategy" for those concerned, it does seek to establish society as the locus of stigma against people with epilepsy and force a reevaluation of their societal worth. Although people with epilepsy may have been slower than some other stigmatized groups to respond to the call, the epilepsy associations are moving rapidly from a view of their function as that of support and information to an increasingly political and campaigning role, agitating for better services and less discrimination for their members.[71]

Campaigns such as the Global Campaign Against Epilepsy[43] are raising its profile with governments and their health systems planners and providers worldwide.

At the individual level, there is evidence that whereas some people with epilepsy appear to admit to the permanence of epilepsy stigma, others show resourcefulness and resilience in putting it aside whatever the clinical prognosis.[92] Among factors identified as critical for developing such resilience are unconditional family support and clear intrafamilial communication.[1] Ablon[1] noted that living in such a positive environment helps to instill confidence and security in early life and encourages positive illness-coping behaviors in the affected person. Family members who openly discuss the practical and emotional issues associated with having a stigmatizing condition and who actively seek out high-quality health care for the affected person can do much to empower that person. Ablon commented that lack of knowledge on the part of other family members can seriously hamper the ability of persons with stigmatizing conditions to cope with them and make a positive adjustment, as can lack of knowledge on the part of affected persons themselves.[37] This suggests a need for targeted educational programs for people with epilepsy and their families; a number that have been formally evaluated are accessible for use.[76]

The importance of counseling as a means of helping people with epilepsy manage stigma had been stressed.[41] Although one-to-one counseling is expensive and therefore may be difficult to fund, Floyd-Richard and Gurung[38] studied the effect of group counseling for people with another chronic stigmatizing condition, leprosy, and concluded that this was a time-efficient and productive method of reducing the effects of stigma. They also argued, however, that counseling alone will not improve the self-image and acceptance of a stigmatized person, and other interventions, such as economic rehabilitation for the whole family and health education for the affected individual, their family, and the community, are also essential.

As shown earlier in this chapter, in the face of possible hostility and stigma, concealment appears to be a key management strategy adopted by people with epilepsy. Although this may make felt stigma "a self-fulfilling prophecy,"[98] disclosure is recognized as a potentially risky course of action[46,111] and is therefore a source of some considerable anxiety to people with epilepsy.[77] The advice from the epilepsy support organizations tends to be that people with epilepsy should approach the issue of disclosure carefully and thoughtfully.[12,17,86] Of course, people with epilepsy are often under a legal imposition to disclose their condition, for example, if they drive or are engaged in particular types of employment in which seizures would put them or others at risk. Ultimately, however, the decision of whether disclosure or nondisclosure is the wisest and least stressful course of action for managing possible stigma and discrimination must be made on an individual basis, although preferably with proper support.

Changing Negative Public Attitudes

With regard to improving public attitudes toward epilepsy, possible strategies include education and information provision, advocacy, inducing a greater degree of empathy toward epilepsy, and increasing the level of contact between people with epilepsy and people without epilepsy. The most frequently used strategy appears to be that of education, and findings from reviews[18,114] and single studies related both to epilepsy[5,14,64] and other health conditions[24,27,28,69,84,102,103,107] support it as an effective one. Evaluation, however, is often limited to fairly short-term assessments, and different kinds of educational interventions show mixed effects on patterns of attitude and behavioral change and stigma reduction. Interventions targeted at specific population subgroups appear more promising and cost-effective than broad-based public educational campaigns.[105] The overarching message appears to be that the type and content of educational interventions needs to be shaped within peoples' traditional way of thinking and must take account of the context in which stigma operates.

Advocacy focuses on provision of a supportive, enabling environment within which attempts can be made to influence legislative and policy change and is proposed as an important strategy for stigma reduction by several authors.[1,3,25] Given that attitude and behavior change initiatives appear to be more effective when targeted, Corrigan[25] proposed that advocacy groups should use a target-specific stigma-change model to ensure organization of diverse information into a coherent framework. The principle is to identify the group and stigmatizing attitudes that influence discriminatory behavior and the social context within which the group interacts with the stigmatized person(s). This, in turn, enables a specific change strategy to be identified. The success of the U.S. Epilepsy Foundation's "Entitled to Respect" campaign, targeted at young people, is a current example of advocacy at work.[110] Another good example is the U.K. group Epilepsy Bereaved, as a result of whose work the U.K. Department of Health commissioned the first U.K. audit into epilepsy-related death,[45] which led to a series of recommendations for the care of people with epilepsy.

Inducing empathy for a member of a stigmatized group can improve attitudes toward members of that group as a whole.[9] The assumption here is that by inducing others to see the world from the perspective of a stigmatized group member, they can be led to *feel* for this person and these empathetic feelings will generalize, resulting in a more positive attitude toward the group as a whole. Similarly, interventions based on increasing contact have been proposed as a means of reducing social distance toward affected persons. Such interventions can be targeted at individuals, groups, or the wider community; for example, the Horizon initiative in the Netherlands[34] involved placing people with epilepsy into employment and so exposing employers to them as employees directly. This initiative showed some degree of success despite findings from studies within other health contexts that increased contact in real-world settings, for example, job training, is largely ineffective. Brown et al.[18] argued that a contact strategy in conjunction with education is one of the most promising approaches to reducing negative attitudes.

Whatever strategy is adopted, the literature makes it clear that conducting stigma intervention programs requires diverse skills to engage and interact with targeted communities and community agencies. It also suggests that multistrategy, multilevel approaches are more effective in improving knowledge and reducing stigmatizing attitudes than are single interventions.[114] Furthermore, several studies report evidence of superficial changes in attitude based on improved knowledge but limited change in deep-seated fears, and little is known about what is required to bring about long-term attitude change. Within the field of epilepsy specifically, there is still limited evidence for the effectiveness of interventions to reduce stigma, despite the length of its history, but research suggests that stigma reduction must go hand in hand with improving access to health care and supporting treatment adherence.

SUMMARY AND CONCLUSIONS

In this chapter, we have focused largely on the literature relating to epilepsy stigma as played out in countries in the developed world. As we have tried to make clear, however, the implications of having epilepsy vary with time, geographic place, and sociocultural context, as do the ways in which people with epilepsy, their families, and their communities respond to the condition. What is without question is that for a significant proportion of those affected, stigma remains a real and present, if intangible, danger. Weiss and Ramakrishna[117] noted that a reformulation of the concept of stigma for health research would be that it is a process in which adverse social judgments are made that are medically unwarranted. This is a very relevant definition of stigma for the great majority of people with epilepsy whose condition can be easily and effectively controlled.[93] At a recent meeting on stigma and global health supported by the U.S. National Institutes of Health (available at www.stigmaconference.nih.gov), family, local community, health and social care systems, educational institutions, legal systems, employment, and insurance were all identified as areas in which people with epilepsy might encounter stigma. Continuing to challenge stigma in all these areas must remain a priority.

References

1. Ablon J. The nature of stigma and medical conditions. *Epilepsy Behav.* 2002;3:S2–S9.
2. Albrecht GL, Walker VG, Levy JA. Social distance from the stigmatised: A test of two theories. *Social Sci Med.* 1982;16:1319–1327.
3. Angermeyer MC, Matschinger H. Casual beliefs and attitudes to people with schizophrenia. *Br J Psychiatry.* 2005;186:331–334.
4. Arnston P, Drodge D, Norton R, et al. The perceived psychosocial consequences of having epilepsy. In: Whitman S, Herman B, eds. *Psychopathology in Epilepsy: Social Dimensions.* Oxford: Oxford University Press; 1986: 143–161.
5. Austin JK, Shafer PO, Deering JB. Epilepsy familiarity, knowledge and perceptions of stigma: Report from a survey of adolescents in the general population. *Epilepsy Behav.* 2002;3:368–375.
6. Bagley C. Social prejudice and the adjustment of people with epilepsy. *Epilepsia.* 1972;13:33–45.
7. Baker GA, Brooks J, Buck D, et al. The stigma of epilepsy: A European perspective. *Epilepsia.* 2000;41:98–104.
8. Baker GA, Jacoby A, Buck D, et al. Quality of life of people with epilepsy: A European study. *Epilepsia.* 1997;38:353–362.
9. Batson CD, Chang J, Orr R, et al. Empathy, attitudes, and action: Can feeling for a member of a stigmatized group motivate one to help the group? *Personal Soc Psychol Bull.* 2002;28:1656–1666.
10. Baumann RJ, Wilson JF, Weise HJ. Kentuckians' attitudes toward children with epilepsy. *Epilepsia.* 1995;36:1003–1008.
11. Beran RG, Jennings VR. Doctors' perspectives of epilepsy. *Epilepsia.* 1981;22:397–406.
12. Bishop M, Allen C. Employment concerns of people with epilepsy and the question of disclosure: Report of a survey of the Epilepsy Foundation. *Epilepsy Behav.* 2001;2:490–495.
13. Bishop M, Slevin B. Teachers' attitudes towards students with epilepsy: Results of a survey of elementary and middle school teachers. *Epilepsy Behav.* 2004;5:308–315.
14. Blake S, Coulson J. *Epilepsy: Stepping Out to Take Control. Findings of a Workshop for Young People with Epilepsy.* Leeds, UK: Epilepsy Action; 2003.
15. British Epilepsy Association. *Towards a New Understanding, a Charter for People with Epilepsy.* Leeds, UK: BEA; 1990.
16. British Epilepsy Association. *A Patient's Viewpoint.* Leeds, UK: BEA; 1996.
17. British Epilepsy Association. *Employment.* Leeds, UK: BEA; 2002.
18. Brown L, Trujillo L, Macintyre K. *Interventions to Reduce HIV/AIDS Stigma: What Have We Learned?* New Orleans, LA: Horizons Program/Tulane School of Public Health and Tropical Medicine; 2001.
19. Canger R, Cornaggia C. Public attitudes towards epilepsy in Italy: Results of a survey and comparison with USA and West German data. *Epilepsia.* 1985;26:221–226.
20. Caveness WF, Gallup GH. A survey of public attitudes towards epilepsy in 1979 with an indication of trends over the past thirty years. *Epilepsia.* 1980;21:509–518.
21. Conrad P. Epilepsy in Indonesia: Notes from development. *Central Issues Anthropol.* 1992;10:94–102.
22. Conrad P, Schneider JW. *Deviance and Medicalisation: From Badness to Sickness.* Philadelphia: Temple University Press; 1992.
23. Corbin J, Strauss AL. Accompaniments of chronic illness: Changes in body, self, biography and biographical time. In: Roth JA, Conrad P, eds. *The Sociology of Health Care.* Greenwich, CT: JAI Press; 1987.
24. Corrigan PW. Mental health stigma as social attribution: Implications for research methods and attitude change. *Clin Psychol Sci Pract.* 2000;7:48–67.
25. Corrigan PW. Target-specific stigma change: A strategy for impacting mental illness stigma. *Psychiatric Rehabil J* 2004;28:113–121.
26. Corrigan PW, Watson AC, Ottati V. From whence comes mental illness stigma? *Int J Soc Psychiatry.* 2003;49(2):142–157.
27. Crane SF, Carswell JW. A review and assessment of nongovernmental organization—based STD/AIDS education and prevention projects for marginalized groups. *Health Educ Res.* 1992;7:175–194.
28. Crisp A, Cowan L, Hart D. The College's anti-stigma campaign, 1998–2003. *Psychiatric Bull.* 2004;28:133–136.
29. Crocker J, Major B, Steele C. Social stigma. In: Gilbert DT, Fiske ST, Gardner L, eds. *The Handbook of Social Psychology.* Boston: McGraw-Hill; 1998:504–553.
30. Cuff EC, Sharrock WW, Francis DW. *Perspectives in Sociology,* 3rd ed. London: Routledge; 1992.
31. Dantas FG, Cariri GA, Ribeiro Filho AR. Knowledge and attitudes towards epilepsy among primary, secondary and tertiary level teachers. *Arq Neuro-Psiquiatria* 2001;59:712–716.
32. Das V. *Stigma, contagion, defect: Issues in the anthropology of public health.* Paper presented at U.S. NIH Conference on Stigma and Global Health: Developing a Research Agenda, Bethesda MD, 2001. Available at: http://www.stigmaconference.nih.gov.
33. Dawkins JL, Crawford PM, Stammers TG. Epilepsy: A general practice study of knowledge and attitudes among sufferers and non-sufferers. *Br J Gen Pract.* 1993;43:453–457.

34. de Boer H, Aldenkamp AP, Bullivant F, et al. Horizon: The trans-national epilepsy training project. *Int J Adolesc Med Health*. 1994;7:325–335.
35. Dell JL. Social dimensions of epilepsy: Stigma and response. In: *Psychopathology in Epilepsy: Social Dimensions*. Whitman S, Hermann B, eds. Oxford: Oxford University Press; 1986:185–210.
36. Dilorio C, Shafer PO, Letz R, et al. The association of stigma with self-management and perceptions of health care among adults with epilepsy. *Epilepsy Behav*. 2003;4:259–267.
37. Doughty J, Baker GA, Jacoby A, et al. Cross-cultural differences in levels of knowledge about epilepsy. *Epilepsia*. 2003;44:115–123.
38. Floyd-Richard M, Gurung S. Stigma reduction through group counselling of persons affected by leprosy—a pilot study. *Leprosy Rev*. 2000;71:499–504.
39. Fong CG, Hung A. Public awareness, attitude, and understanding of epilepsy in Hong Kong Special Administrative Region, China. *Epilepsia*. 2002;43:311–316.
40. Gade E, Toutges G. Employers' attitude hiring epileptics: Implications for job placement. *Rehabil Counsel Bull*. 1983:353–356.
41. Galletti F, Sturniolo MG. Counselling children and parents about epilepsy. *Patient Educ Counsel*. 2004;55:422–425.
42. Gallhofer B. Epilepsy and its prejudice: Teachers' knowledge and opinions—are they a response to psychopathological phenomena? *Psychopathology*. 1984;17:187–212.
43. Global Campaign Against Epilepsy. *Out of the Shadows: An Introduction to the Global Campaign and Its Demonstration Projects*. ILAE/IBE/WHO Global Campaign Against Epilepsy; 2001. Available at: http://www.who.int/mental˙health/media/en/37.pdf.
44. Goffman E. *Stigma: Notes on the Management of Spoiled Identity*. Englewood Cliffs, NJ: Prentice Hall; 1963.
45. Hanna NJ, Black M, Sander JW, et al. *The National Sentinel Audit of Epilepsy-Related Death*. London: The Stationery Office; 2002
46. Harden CL, Kossoy A, Vera S, et al. Reaction to epilepsy in the workplace. *Epilepsia*. 2004;45:1134–1140.
47. Harrison RM, West P. Images of a grand mal. *New Soc*. 1977;12(5):282.
48. Hermann BP, Whitman S. A multietiologic model. In Whitman S, Hermann BP, eds. *Psychopathology in Epilepsy, Social Dimensions*. New York: Oxford University Press; 1986:5–37.
49. Hermann BP, Whitman S, Wyler AR, et al. Psychosocial predictors of psychopathology in epilepsy. *Br J Psychiatry*. 1990;156:98–105.
50. Hicks RA, Hicks MJ. Attitudes of major employers towards the employment of people with epilepsy: A thirty year study. *Epilepsia*. 1991;32:86–88.
51. Hills MD, MacKenzie HC. New Zealand community attitudes toward people with epilepsy. *Epilepsia*. 2002;43:1583–1589.
52. Iivanainen M, Vutela A, Vilkkumaa I. Public awareness and attitudes towards epilepsy in Finland. *Epilepsia*. 1980;21:413–423.
53. Jacoby A. Epilepsy and the quality of everyday life. *Soc Sci Med*. 1992;38:261–274.
54. Jacoby A. Felt versus enacted stigma: A concept revisited. *Soc Sci Med*. 1994;38:269–274.
55. Jacoby A. *Psychosocial functioning in people with epilepsy in remission and the outcomes of antiepileptic drug withdrawal*. Ph.D. thesis, University of Newcastle upon Tyne, United Kingdom, 1995.
56. Jacoby A. Stigma, epilepsy and quality of life. *Epilepsy Behav*. 2002;3:S10–S20.
57. Jacoby A. *Course of quality of life for persons with epilepsy*. Invited presentation at 16th International Bethel-Cleveland Clinic Epilepsy Symposium, Beilefeld; 2005.
58. Jacoby A, Baker GA, Steen N, et al. The clinical course of epilepsy and its psychosocial correlates: Findings from a UK community study. *Epilepsia*. 1996;37:148–161.
59. Jacoby A, Gamble C, Doughty J, et al. Quality of life outcomes of immediate delayed AED treatment of early epilepsy and single seizures. *Neurology*. 2005;41:1978–1989.
60. Jacoby A, Gorry J, Baker GA. Employers' attitudes to employment of people with epilepsy: Still the same old story? *Epilepsia*. In press.
61. Jacoby A, Gorry J, Gamble C, et al. Public knowledge, private grief: A study of public attitudes to epilepsy in the UK and implications for stigma. *Epilepsia*. 2004;45:1405–1415.
62. Jacoby A, Graham-Jones S, Baker GA. et al. A General Practice Records Audit of the process of care for people with epilepsy. *Br J Gen Pract*. 1996;46:595–599.
63. Jensen R, Dam M. Public attitudes toward epilepsy in Denmark. *Epilepsia*. 1992;33:459–463.
64. JilekAall L, Jilek M, Kaaya J, et al. Psychosocial study of epilepsy in Africa. *Soc Sci Med*. 1997;45:783–795.
65. Jochim G, Acorn S. Living with chronic illness: The interface of stigma and normalisation. *Can J Nurs Res*. 2000;32:37–48.
66. Jones EE, Farina A, Hastorf AH, et al. *Social Stigma: The Psychology of Marked Relationships*. New York: Freeman; 1984.
67. Jordon S, Knight E, Vokins A. *Interpreting lay opinions on epilepsy*. Unpublished pre—clinical project, University of London, Middlesex Hospital Medical School; cited in Scambler G. Epilepsy. London: Tavistock Press; 1989.
68. Kaleyias J, Tzoufi M, Kotsalis C, et al. Knowledge and attitude of the Greek educational community toward epilepsy and the epileptic student. *Epilepsy Behav*. 2005;6:179–186.
69. Kemppainen JK, Dubbert PM, McWilliams P. Effects of group discussion and guided patient care experience on nurses' attitudes towards care of patients with AIDS. *J Adv Nurs*. 1996;24:296–302.
70. La Martina JM. Uncovering public misconceptions about epilepsy. *J Epilepsy*. 1989;2:45–48.
71. Lee P. Support groups for people with epilepsy. In: Baker GA, Jacoby A, eds. *Quality of Life in Epilepsy: Beyond Seizure Counts in Assessment and Treatment*. Amsterdam: Harwood Academic; 2000:273–281.
72. Lemert EM. *Social Pathology*. New York: McGraw-Hill; 1951.
73. Link BG, Phelan JC. Conceptualising stigma. *Annu Rev Sociol*. 2001;27:363–385.
74. MacLeod JS, Austin JK. Stigma in the lives of adolescents with epilepsy: A review of the literature. *Epilepsy Behav*. 2003;4:112–117.
75. Madsen LP. Danish primary school teachers' knowledge about epilepsy in children. *Ugsekrift Laeger*. 1996;158:1977–1980.
76. May TW, Pfafflin M. Psychoeducational programs for patients with epilepsy. *Disease Manage Health Outcomes*. 2005;13:185–199.
77. McEwan MJ, Espie CA, Metcalfe J, et al. Quality of life and psychosocial development in adolescents with epilepsy: A qualitative investigation using focus group methods. *Seizure*. 2004;13:15–31.
78. McLin WM, de Boer HM. Public perceptions about epilepsy. *Epilepsia*. 1995;36:957–959.
79. Mirnics Z, Czikora G, Zavecz T, et al. Changes in public attitudes toward epilepsy in Hungary: Results of surveys conducted in 1994 and 2000. *Epilepsia*. 2001;42:86–93.
80. Novotna I, Rektor I. The trend in public attitudes in the Czech Republic towards persons with epilepsy. *Eur J Neurol*. 2002;9:535–540.
81. Parsons T. *The Social System*. New York: Free Press; 1951.
82. Pasternak JL. An analysis of social perceptions of epilepsy: Increasing rationalisation as seen through the theories of Comte and Weber. *Soc Sci Med*. 1981;15E:223–229.
83. Peltzer K. Perceptions of epilepsy among black students at a university in South Africa. *Curationis*. 2001;24(2):62–67.
84. Pinfold V, Thornicroft G, Huxley P, et al. Active ingredients in anti-stigma programmes in mental health. *Int Rev Psychiatry*. 2005;17:123–131.
85. Pryor JB, Reeder GD, Landau S. A social-psychological analysis of HIV-related stigma: A two-factor theory. *Am Behav Sci*. 1999: 42(7):1193–1211.
86. Reid R. *To disclose or not: Can you afford to bring your epilepsy to work?* Epilepsy USA Newsletter, Epilepsy Foundation of America, 6 January 2004. Available at: http://www.epilepsyfoundation.org/epilepsyusa/disclosure.cfm.
87. Reis R. Explanatory concepts and stigmatisation: The case of epilepsy in Swaziland. *Behinderung Dritte Welf*. 2000;11:44–48.
88. Reis R. Epilepsy and self-identity among the Dutch. *Med Anthropol*. 2001: 19:355–382.
89. Reis R, Meinardi H. ILAE/WHO "Out of the Shadows Campaign" stigma: Does the flag identify the cargo? *Epilepsy Behav*. 2002;3:S33–S37.
90. Robson C. *Examining the social stigma of epilepsy: A qualitative analysis of attitudes, perceptions and understanding towards epilepsy and people with epilepsy among young adults in the undergraduate population*. M.Sci. thesis, University of York, Department of Health Sciences, UK; 2006.
91. Roessler RT, Sumner G. Employer opinions about accommodating employees with chronic illnesses. *J Appl Rehabil Counsel*. 1997;28:29–34.
92. Ryan R, Kempner K, Emlen AC. The stigma of epilepsy as a self-concept. *Epilepsia*. 1980;21:433–444.
93. Sander JWAS, Sillanpaa M. Natural history and prognosis. In: *Epilepsy: A Comprehensive Textbook*. Engel J, Pedley TA, eds.Philadelphia: Lippincott-Raven; 1997:69–86.
94. Sands H, Zalkind SS. Effects of an educational campaign to change employer attitudes toward hiring epileptics. *Epilepsia*. 1972;13: 87–96.
95. Sanya EO, Salami TAT, Goodman OO, et al. Perception and attitude to epilepsy among teachers in primary, secondary and tertiary educational institutions in middle belt Nigeria. *Tropical Doctor*. 2005;35: 153–156.
96. Scambler G. *Being epileptic: Sociology of a stigmatising condition*. Ph.D. thesis, University of London; 1983.
97. Scambler G. Perceiving and coping with stigmatizing illness. In: Fitzpatrick R, Hinton J, Newman S, et al., eds. *The Experience of Illness*. London: Tavistock; 1984:203–226.
98. Scambler G. *Epilepsy*. London: Tavistock; 1989.
99. Scambler G. Re-framing stigma: Felt and enacted stigma and challenges to the sociology of chronic and disabling conditions. *Soc Theory Health*. 2004;2:29–46.
100. Scambler G, Hopkins A. Being epileptic: Coming to terms with stigma. *Sociol Health Illness*. 1986;8:26–43.
101. Schneider JW, Conrad P. *Having Epilepsy: The Experience and Control of Illness*. Philadelphia: Temple University Press; 1983.
102. Schulze B, Richter-Werling M, Matschinger H, et al. Crazy? So what! Effects of a school project on students' attitudes towards people with schizophrenia. *Acta Psych Scand*. 2003;107:142–150.
103. Sharp LK. The short-term impact of a continuing medical education program on providers' attitudes toward treating diabetes. *Diabetes Care*. 1999;22:1929–1932.

104. Stangor C, Crandall CS. Threat and the social construction of stigma. In: Heatherton TF, Kleck RE, Hebl MR, et al., eds. *The Social Psychology of Stigma*. New York: Guilford Press; 2000:62–87.
105. Stuart H. Stigmatization. Lessons drawn from the programs aiming its reduction. *Mental Health Quebec*. 2003;28.
106. Suurmeijer TPBM, Reuvekamp MF, Aldenkamp BP. Social functioning, psychological functioning, and quality of life in epilepsy. *Epilepsia*. 2001: 42:1160–1168.
107. Tanaka G, Ogawa T, Inadomi H, et al. Effects of an educational program on public attitudes towards mental illness. *Psychiatry Clin Neurosci*. 2003;57:595–602.
108. Temkin O. *The Falling Sickness*. Baltimore: John Hopkins University Press; 1971.
109. Thapar AK, Stott NCH, Richens A, et al. Attitudes of GPs to the care of people with epilepsy. *Family Pract*. 1998;15:437–442.
110. The Epilepsy Foundation Editorial. *Epilepsy Behav*. 2004;5:276–276.
111. Troster H. Disclose or conceal? Strategies of information management in persons with epilepsy. *Epilepsia*. 1997;38:1227–1237.
112. Trostle JA. Social aspects: Stigma, beliefs and measurement. In: Engel J Jr, Pedley TA, eds. *Epilepsy: A Comprehensive Text Book*. Philadelphia: Lippincott—Raven; 1997:2183–2190.
113. UK Clinical Standards Advisory Group. *Services for Patients with Epilepsy*. London: HMSO; 2000.
114. Van der Meij S, Heijnders M. *The fight against stigma. Stigma reduction strategies and interventions*. A paper prepared for the International Stigma Workshop, Soesterberg, Netherlands, November 28 to December 2, 2004. Available at: http://www.kit.nl/smartsite.shtml?id=2542.
115. Vinson T. Towards de-mythologising epilepsy. *Med J Aust*. 1975;2:663–666.
116. Vizioli R. *An anthropo-phenomenological approach to the world of the epileptic*. Unpublished presentation, 1977, cited in Ziegler RG. Epilepsy: Individual illness, human predicament and family dilemma. *Family Relations* 1982;31:435–444.
117. Weiss MG, Ramakrishna J. *Interventions: Research on reducing stigma*. Paper presented at U.S. NIH Conference on Stigma and Global Health. Developing a Research Agenda. Bethesda, MD, 2001. Available at: http://www.stigmaconference.nih.gov.
118. West P. *Investigation into the social construction and consequences of the label 'epilepsy'*. Ph.D. thesis, University of Bristol, UK; 1979.
119. Westbrook LE, Bauman LJ, Shinnar S. Applying stigma theory to epilepsy: A test of a conceptual model. *J Pediatr Psychol*. 1992;17:633–649.
120. Wilde M, Haslam C. Living with epilepsy: A qualitative study investigating the experiences of young people attending outpatient clinics in Leicester. *Seizure*. 1996;5:63–72.
121. Youn SY, Hong SB. The relationship of stigma and quality of life in patients with epilepsy [Abstract]. In: *Sixth Conference of the Korean Epilepsy Society;* 2001:215.

CHAPTER 217 ■ DISRUPTIONS IN SOCIAL FUNCTIONING AND SERVICES FACILITATING ADJUSTMENT FOR THE CHILD AND THE ADULT

JOAN K. AUSTIN, HANNEKE M. DE BOER, AND PATRICIA O. SHAFER

INTRODUCTION

The impact of epilepsy on social functioning, or the ability to participate in a broad range of social activities and interpersonal relationships, can be quite varied. Although many people with epilepsy have few, if any, disruptions in social functioning, others have severe problems that prevent them from engaging in fully productive lives. The exact prevalence of social problems is difficult to establish because most studies have been carried out on clinic samples in which persons with more difficult-to-control epilepsy are served. Studies show that rates of social dysfunction are substantially higher in samples from clinics than in community samples.[104] Nevertheless, social problems are common in persons with epilepsy, and these problems need to be addressed by health care professionals.

In this chapter, we present an overview of the disruptions in social functioning that can be experienced by children and adults with epilepsy. We also describe factors associated with social problems and consider them within the context of tasks of normal psychosocial development. We conclude with guidelines for daily living, an overview of areas that need to be addressed in a comprehensive assessment, and the types of services that can facilitate social functioning in persons with epilepsy.

DISRUPTIONS IN SOCIAL FUNCTIONING

Social Problems

Persons with epilepsy have a higher prevalence of social problems than those from the general population. A longitudinal study of adults with childhood epilepsy indicated that epilepsy had a negative impact on social functioning.[97] Problems most commonly reported in persons with epilepsy include anxiety, poor self-esteem, social isolation, and symptoms of depression.[7,19,60,74,79,90,92,93]

Comparison studies show that children with epilepsy have poorer social functioning than children with other chronic physical conditions[89] such as asthma,[7,19] diabetes,[75] or learning disabilities.[74] In a recent study, adolescents with epilepsy showed greater social anxiety and interpersonal problems than adolescents without epilepsy.[20] Adults with epilepsy have also been found to have higher rates of social problems than the general population. Social problems include social isolation and problems with adaptation.[28,30,44,58] Problems in living with epilepsy related to social adjustment (e.g., driving and lack of employment opportunities) are also frequently reported in adults with epilepsy.[53,64] Long-distance travel can also be difficult for adults with epilepsy, especially for those with severe or frequent seizures. Social problems are important because they reduce quality of life and contribute to mental health problems such as depression, anxiety, and psychopathology in persons with epilepsy.[5,57]

Factors Associated With Social Problems

Empirical research carried out to identify factors associated with social dysfunction in persons with epilepsy identifies the following as risk factors:

- Severe and frequent seizures
- Presence of other chronic conditions or deficits
- Cognitive impairment and academic underachievement
- Negative attitudes toward epilepsy
- Inadequate knowledge about epilepsy
- Lack of a supportive family environment

Although social problems are more common in persons who have a chronic physical condition, youth with epilepsy have been found to have a poorer social functioning than youth with other chronic physical conditions.[4,19,88] Studies indicate that disruption in social functioning is greater for persons with severe epilepsy and other neurologic deficits or disabilities[29,56,100] than for those with epilepsy alone. Moreover, higher seizure frequency is generally found to be related to poorer social functioning.[6,17,20,59,60] Other seizure variables have not been found to be consistently associated with poorer social functioning. For example, Camfield et al.[25] did not find epilepsy-related variables (e.g., age at onset, seizure type, cause of seizures), neurologic deficits, and encephalographic data (e.g., focal slowing) to be strong predictors of social dysfunction in a sample of children and young adults with normal intelligence. Furthermore, even remission of epilepsy did not significantly predict social dysfunction. Only a learning disorder and >21 seizures before initiation of treatment were associated with at least one unfavorable social outcome in this population-based study.[25] In addition, poor cognitive functioning[26] and poor academic achievement[101] have also been found to be positively related to social problems in children with epilepsy.

Although most research identifying high rates of social problems are carried out on samples of persons with chronic epilepsy, studies of persons with new-onset epilepsy also indicate that social difficulties occur very early with the disorder. For example, Chaplin et al.[29] found that >10% of adults with recently diagnosed epilepsy rated four problems related to social functioning (fear of seizures, employment concerns, concerns about leisure, and decreased energy) as severe.

Negative attitudes toward having epilepsy have been found to be related to psychosocial problems in children with epilepsy.[13] Sometimes, negative perceptions about epilepsy are caused by excessive fears about seizures.[80] Austin and colleagues[8,16] found that children with new-onset epilepsy and their parents had many unfounded fears about seizures and their treatment, and greater concerns and fears have been associated with more-negative attitudes about having seizures.[11] Lack of accurate knowledge about epilepsy has been found to be associated with greater social anxiety and lower self-esteem in adolescents.[20]

The whole family is confronted with coping with the epilepsy. Studies exploring relationships between the family environment and social functioning in children indicate that family factors are related to social functioning in the child.[88] Austin et al.[17] found family stress, extended family social support, and family mastery and control to be related to psychosocial functioning. Lothman et al.[72] found praise in mother–child interactions to be related to child competence. What is not as well delineated is the nature of the relationship between the family environment and social functioning because most of the research is cross sectional. It is not known whether both the family and the child are reacting to the epilepsy, whether environment leads to social problems for the person with epilepsy, or whether the family is responding to the child's problems.

Few studies have been conducted on family environments of adults with epilepsy to identify whether there are factors that are associated with social problems. Thompson and Upton[103] found that caring for an adult with intractable epilepsy is quite stressful for the family. Approximately two thirds of the primary caregivers were dissatisfied with limitations on their social activities and intimate relationships. Caregivers identified the need for respite and increased social support.

In summary, although more research is needed to identify all the factors that lead to problems with social dysfunction, research has identified broad categories of variables that place persons at risk for social problems. It appears that a chronic, difficult-to-control condition and the presence of other deficits or disabilities are risk factors for social problems. Moreover, knowledge about epilepsy, how persons feel about having seizures, and characteristics of the family environment are related to social functioning in persons with epilepsy.

Developmental Tasks and Social Problems

Disruptions in social functioning in children need to be considered within the context of normal psychosocial development because epilepsy can interfere with the accomplishments of age-appropriate tasks. Furthermore, because epilepsy affects the whole family, it is important to consider how family factors influence the psychosocial adjustment to epilepsy.

Early and Middle Childhood

In early childhood, children need an environment in which they are able to become increasingly independent. They have daily routines and learn to master toilet training and other self-care activities, communicate with others, and become socialized.[22] For optimal psychosocial development, these children need an environment in which they can develop autonomy and initiative.[51] If parents are overly protective and concerned about the possibility of a seizure, they may overrestrict the child's activities and hinder the development of life skills. A recent study found increased levels of parental anxiety about their child's epilepsy was associated with poorer socialization in the child.[27] In middle childhood, children become more independent of parents. There is empirical evidence that children with epilepsy can have problems with completion of some of these developmental steps. For example, children with epilepsy have been found to be more dependent than children with tonsillectomies.[52]

Child social development has been found to be associated with parenting behaviors. Social maturity and social skills in children with epilepsy were found to be positively related to parental strictness. Lothman et al.[72] studied parenting behaviors in mother–child interactions and found praise to be related to child competence and child positive affect. Conversely, intrusive and overcontrolling parenting behaviors were related to decreased child autonomy and child confidence. In a recent longitudinal study, parent support of the child's autonomy predicted a better psychosocial adjustment.[10]

Adolescence

The primary developmental challenge of adolescence is identity formation.[22] Ideally, adolescents should begin adulthood with a strong sense of self and physical competence. Failure to develop a strong sense of self as competent can lead to problems with poor self-esteem and feelings of being different from others. Another important developmental task for adolescents is becoming independent and separating from the family of origin. Peer-group membership plays an important role in the social development of adolescents and in their becoming independent of their family. A recent study,[18] however, suggested that the social environment might not be supportive of the social development for the adolescent with epilepsy. In that study, adolescents in the general population were found to have a poor understanding of epilepsy. Almost three fourths believed that adolescents with epilepsy would be more likely to be bullied or "picked on" by others than other adolescents, and less than one third indicated that they would date an adolescent who had epilepsy.[18]

Young people with epilepsy can have problems meeting the developmental accomplishments of adolescence. The presence of a chronic condition such as epilepsy can interfere with the development of a strong sense of physical competence. Parental overprotection can deprive the child of experiencing the feelings of competence and, subsequently, affect later self-esteem.[76] The occurrence of seizures and the need to take medication can lead to a reduced sense of physical competence. The stigma associated with epilepsy can negatively impact how adolescents perceive themselves, socially and physically. A recent study indicated that adolescents with intractable epilepsy perceived that their having epilepsy set them apart from their peers.[47] Even adolescents with newly diagnosed epilepsy have been found to feel different from their peers and worry about being teased by them.[8] The episodic loss of control caused by seizures also can make it more difficult to become independent and separate from families. The inability to drive a car at an age-appropriate time can be a major problem for adolescents with epilepsy because it limits opportunities for developing independence and participation in social activities.[33]

A final way the presence of epilepsy might affect social functioning is poor academic performance. Success in school facilitates the development of initiative. School achievement also provides an opportunity for young people to receive recognition from others and to derive a sense of accomplishment. The school problems found in adolescents with epilepsy[19,79] reduce opportunities for the development of a sense of pride and accomplishment at school and also place these children at risk for later vocational problems.

Adulthood

Studies of psychosocial function of adults with epilepsy have many methodologic problems. Studies regarding these issues have mostly been clinic based, thus limiting generalization to the whole population of people with epilepsy. Recent research[102] was carried out in the north of the Netherlands concerning the quality of life reported by 210 adults with epilepsy and an average IQ of 101; 75% had a high school education or more. Of this group, 69.5% reported no social problems, 25.1% mentioned problems with adaptation, 5.5% reported feeling isolated or suffering from other problems in this area, and 89.7% mentioned no financial problems. Various subscales on health, self-confidence, coping, loneliness, stigma, life fulfillment, and psychological problems did not show many problems. It appeared as if early-onset epilepsy leads to adaptation and does not much influence the quality of life. The outcome of this study differed from those of many others probably because this was performed among a group of people with epilepsy living in the community rather than a clinic-based sample.

Being employed is an important predictor of quality of life of people with epilepsy. The World Health Organization also mentions the importance of employment for social health and, therefore, improved quality of life. It is widely recognized that a large number of people with epilepsy experience particular difficulties in gaining access to employment and vocational training on equal terms with other sections of the population, and it is also acknowledged that this situation is likely to get relatively worse, not better. Most figures concerning employment rates of people with epilepsy indicate that they do not perform as well on the labor market as others do. Although both research figures and research groups vary, unemployment rates generally are higher for people with epilepsy than for the general population.

Early employment studies showed that the situation for people with epilepsy was discouraging. Jacoby[64] found that 50% of people with epilepsy were unemployed, and Scambler and Hopkins[91] reported that 42% were unemployed. A research project set up among people with epilepsy in The Netherlands who were being treated at 10 special outpatient epilepsy clinics showed that compared to the general population, the study group tended to have a lower educational and a lower vocational level than the general Dutch population.[102] Of the study group, 44% were employed and 49% were unemployed (7% were in school).[34,86] A more recent study by Jacoby showed that when seizures are well controlled and there are no other handicaps, people with epilepsy do not experience employment problems.[65]

Young people with epilepsy especially are at a disadvantage when it comes to obtaining and retaining employment and may need special assistance and training to enable them to deal with difficulties they are likely to encounter. Even when the epilepsy is controlled, many find that their epilepsy is a barrier to employment.

Concerning marriage, Dutch research showed that 66.2% of patients were married and 14.8% were still living with parents.[102] This figure may be influenced by age, or there may be a regional (cultural) effect. Data from Montreal[32] showed that among study participants who developed seizures after the age of 20 years, 91.7% of women and 76.2% of men were married before the onset of seizures. These proportions were similar to those for the general population. However, if seizures occurred in the first decade, marriage were lower than expected for the general population. The rates were 32% for men and 58% for women. Ounsted and Lindsay[82] found that among their sample of 100 young people diagnosed as having temporal lobe epilepsy, the prognosis for marriage was good for girls (92% of them married), whereas only 41% of the boys married, even though they were not heavily handicapped. Pierzchala and Grudzinska[83] reported that of a group of 243 patients with epilepsy, 50.6% of men were married, which is a lower rate than both women with epilepsy and the general population.

Follow-up studies on people with epilepsy in the 1946 British birth cohort show very little difference concerning marriage between both uncomplicated and complicated cases and their controls at the age of 26 years.[23]

For many (young) people, marriage is one of the main goals in life. For a person with epilepsy, however, the chances of getting married can be particularly slim in the Third World. In some countries, a woman with epilepsy has virtually no chance of getting married at all, or when she does, epilepsy is a reason for an immediate divorce. In India, although the law forbidding people with epilepsy from getting married was repealed recently, such people still stand no chance of an arranged marriage, which is customary in that part of the world. Fundamentalist groups in many religious cultures, following ancient laws, still believe that epilepsy is inheritable, and of course these laws were originally intended to prevent the disease from spreading. Having epilepsy appears to affect the chances of marriage in the developing world as well as in the developed world, based on the erroneous idea that people with epilepsy are uneducable, unemployable, and a danger to the community; epilepsy is widely considered to be an inheritable disease requiring restriction of its spread. The severity of the epilepsy does not seem to make any difference in relation to marriage: Having seizures at all diminishes the chances.

There is a large literature on the medical aspects of pregnancy and epilepsy; however, the social aspects seem to be a neglected area. For the future mother with epilepsy, there are even more questions concerning having children than for other women. The questions include the following:

- Will my children also have epilepsy?
- What will happen to my seizures during pregnancy? Will they harm the baby?
- What is the effect of my medication on the baby?
- What happens if I have a seizure during delivery?
- Can I take care of a child safely?
- What changes do I need to make to take care of the child?

Up-to-date information concerning these often emotional questions is extremely important because the fear that they cause might not be verbalized. It is of the utmost importance that future mothers be able to discuss their desire for a child with the physician who treats their epilepsy. The importance of a good relationship between doctor and patient is vital.

Various practical measures for taking care of a baby may include sitting on the floor during feeding and washing and dressing the baby on the floor as well. Bathing should not be done when the mother is alone with the baby. When common sense and practical precautions as just described are applied, much of the fear of future mothers is in fact not necessary.

Epilepsy in a parent may have an impact on the family system. Few studies have explored the effects on child development of having a parent with epilepsy. Aldenkamp et al.[2] found acceptable patterns of communication about epilepsy between parent and child; 80% of the children were informed about their parents' seizure before witnessing one. This is contrary to the results from a study by Lechtenberg and Alkner,[68] which found little communication about the epilepsy. Information about epilepsy given before a child witnesses a seizure proved to be important for the adaptation of the child and prevention of serious personality disorders. The findings of the Aldenkamp study support the belief that children benefit from adequate information given in open and frank communication with their parents.

People with epilepsy sometimes state that it is very difficult, or even impossible, for them to make friends. This maybe caused, however, by their own attitude toward the disorder. Some people wear their epilepsy as a shield in front of them, thus creating a self-fulfilling prophecy, almost introducing themselves as a person with epilepsy. Friends probably should know about the epilepsy, but only when it is active. The following points to should be kept in mind:

- Do not scare the other person with your epilepsy.
- Only talk about your own epilepsy and your own seizures.
- Explain what happens when a seizure occurs.
- Explain what people can do to help.

When these rules are applied, neither the epilepsy nor the seizures should stand in the way of friendship.

GUIDELINES FOR DAILY LIVING

Risks at Home

Most accidents happen at home; this generalization applies to everyone, simply because we spend so much time there. Still, for people with epilepsy, there are extra risks, some of which can easily be avoided, as the following suggestions show:

Living Room
- An open fire or stove should be surrounded by a shield; sharp radiators should be covered (e.g., a wooden shield).
- Furniture should not have sharp edges.
- Unbreakable glass should be used in any windows below neck level.

Kitchen
- Gas or electric stoves can be protected with a low shield on top, as used for children.
- Microwave or induction cooking may be used.
- The hot water tap should be fitted with a temperature-control device.
- Electric tea- or coffeemakers are less risky than a hot water kettle.

Bathroom
- The door should be made to open from the outside.
- Baths should not be taken when the person is alone in the house.
- Showering is safer than bathing; any glass windows in the shower should be of unbreakable glass.
- The water taps must be fitted with a temperature-control device.

Bedroom
- If a person tends to fall out of the bed following seizures, a mattress may be placed on the floor. This is less restricting than a shield around the bed and it is quite safe.

Risks at School

Parents and teachers should avoid implementing rules for a regular and quiet life for children with epilepsy. Although fatigue and sleep deprivation may provoke seizures in some people with epilepsy, nothing should be left out of the lives of children with epilepsy unless it would be dangerous in that particular person. Education of parents, teachers, and children with epilepsy should decrease unsubstantiated fears about the condition and the implementation of unnecessary restrictions on their activities. Decisions must be made about participation in activities. The children should participate in this decision making about their participation in activities from a young age; otherwise, they might have difficulty in accepting real restriction or precautions. It is obvious that living a full, independent life between the seizures involves taking risks for everybody, and taking risks implies that, with statistical certainty, accidents will occur.

Risks at Work

The vast majority of jobs are suitable for people with epilepsy. When medical advice is sought about the suitability of particular jobs for people with epilepsy, the guidance given should take into account the requirements of the job, known facts about epilepsy, and the nature of the individual's seizures. More specifically, decisions should take into account information concerning the individual's epilepsy, such as the following:

- The diagnosis and prognosis of the individual's epilepsy
- Description of the seizures, including aura
- Seizure frequency
- Time pattern in which seizures occur (e.g., only during sleep)
- Recovery time
- Date of last seizure
- Any safety issues
- Medication

One area of misunderstanding is the prevalence of seizures caused by visual stimuli.[78] A recent comprehensive review of the empirical literature indicated that the chance of having a seizure caused by light or pattern is only 2% to 14% in people with epilepsy.[50] Children appear to be more vulnerable to visual stimuli than are adults. Therefore, blanket prohibitions should be avoided. Besides, often simple precautions can be taken to reduce the risks in the workplace, such as providing a chair with armrests to prevent the person from falling when having a seizure. In jobs known to carry a high degree of physical risk to the individual worker or to others, the organization of work practice should be examined to reduce this potential risk to an acceptable level. Only in those situations in which this cannot be achieved are restrictions on the employment of people with epilepsy justified.[63]

Traveling

Many people have the vague notion that persons with epilepsy are unfit to travel alone. Parents have nightmares of their children having a seizure in front of a train. In fact, traffic accidents caused by seizures are rare, and using public transport is possible for most people with active epilepsy. Traveling abroad is another issue of concern for many people with epilepsy and their caregivers. Having a seizure in a train or an airplane, however, is no more dangerous than having a seizure at home. An epilepsy "passport" assisting people with epilepsy when traveling abroad containing information on epilepsy in many languages may be very useful and is available in a number of countries. The International Bureau of Epilepsy (IBE) had developed such a passport, but this is now out of print. It would be useful to develop such passports either on a national or a regional basis. Holidays are organized by a number of IBE member organizations. All of these programs have one thing in common: They prove that epilepsy presents no constraint to traveling. Individuals who have frequent seizures, however, need to make sensible travel arrangements. Some general rules apply:

- Travelers need to take medication with them, preferably two sets, with one packed in the hand luggage and one in the checked bag.
- A letter from a doctor explaining the epilepsy and medication can be helpful (especially when dealing with customs).

- Travelers need to have appropriate travel insurance.
- Taking an epilepsy "passport" (as mentioned previously) is useful.
- Information issues concerning travel can be sought from a national epilepsy association or the IBE.

Cycling

In the literature, cycling is not considered more dangerous to people whose seizures are well controlled than to anybody else, and normal precautions should be taken, which may include wearing a helmet. If seizures are active, busy roads are best avoided, and cycling in the company of a supervisor may be advisable. All children will want to ride bicycles; in some countries, it is a regular part of growing up, and blanket restrictions may result in covert cycling in unsupervised situations, causing a greater danger than properly managed cycling. Furthermore, the use of tandem or properly fitted three-wheeler bikes can enable people who have frequent and severe seizures to ride a bike, thus offering them the feeling of freedom that comes with this activity.

Leisure Activities and Club Membership

Health professionals are often asked to give opinions about the risks for people with epilepsy engaging in leisure activities. Although this is an understandable question, there are no rules concerning risks for people with epilepsy in general, and no systematic study into such areas of ordinary daily activities has been made. It is, however, a well recognized that leisure activities such as going out and joining a club are highly desirable, especially for young persons when growing up and learning social skills, whether they have epilepsy or not. It also adds to the quality of life for adults. Going out may involve going to discotheques, which is a normal part of growing up and should not be avoided by young people with epilepsy who seek a full social life. Some people may find flashing or flickering lights unpleasant, but generally it is only bright white "strobe" lights operating at >5 flashes per second that may induce a seizure in some people with epilepsy.

Sports

Interest and active participation in sports is growing. Although studies do not indicate that people with epilepsy are at greater risk of developing seizures during various types of sports, it is assumed that fewer of them participate actively than might want to do so. Information on this or the advice given to people with epilepsy about active sports is not available. A survey in the Netherlands among patients and doctors showed that people with epilepsy are relatively interested in sports. Active participation is limited when either the doctor or the person with epilepsy sees epilepsy as a restricting factor. Clear advice from the professional is essential.[62] This advice should be based on the following rules:

- The risks following a seizure during sports depend on the type of seizure.
- When advising people with epilepsy concerning active participation, three categories of sports can be distinguished:
  - Sports with no restrictions.
  - Sports with some restrictions (safety precautions).
  - Sports that are prohibited.
- The risk of having a seizure during sports is usually smaller than during the relaxation period afterward.
- Sports, including contact sports (team sports) and fighting sports, generally do not provoke more, or more serious, seizures.
- Epilepsy is never a reason for not partaking in competitive sports at any level.
- Epilepsy is never a reason for denial of membership in a sports club.
- Besides to normal safety precautions, special guards need to be available with sports in or around water.
- Instructors and trainers need to know what to do when a seizure occurs.

(This list is the outcome of a symposium on epilepsy and sports organized by the Dutch League Against Epilepsy in 1989.)

Swimming

Most fatal accidents in epilepsy occur in the water (60%). However, very few people with epilepsy drown during swimming. Most accidents occur in the bath, while fishing, or from falling into water. As noted, research shows that very few seizures occur during active sports. They do occur, however, in the rest period afterward (e.g., when resting alongside the swimming pool). Still, certain precautions need to be taken in or around water when a person is not seizure free:

- Swimming in open waters is ill advised because first aid, in the case of a serious seizure, presents extra difficulties.
- Supervision is necessary.
- A person with epilepsy should never go into the water alone.
- When people have active seizures, they should have a person with lifesaving skills present.

SERVICES FOR FACILITATING SOCIAL ADJUSTMENT

The increased prevalence of social problems in people with epilepsy emphasizes the need for a comprehensive approach to treating people with this condition. Although seizure control is a critical factor affecting social function, managing the consequences of seizures on one's daily life is often the most challenging component of epilepsy care. Health care professionals must be aware of the multiple causes of social problems, how to screen for their occurrence, and how to provide appropriate referrals, education, and treatment. In addition, recent research highlighting the increased incidence of cognitive, mood, and behavior problems in children and adults with epilepsy stresses the need to identify and treat these problems early before the psychosocial consequences become intractable.

The ultimate goal of support services is to help persons with epilepsy and their families become as socially capable and competent as possible and live independent self-directed lives. Ideally, models of care and support systems will "foster empowerment and independence for people with epilepsy and support their efforts towards improved seizure control and a positive quality of life."[49] Critical elements that must be considered when making decisions about services include the following:

- Comprehensive assessments should be carried out on a regular basis.
- Early referral to services is recommended to prevent and treat social difficulties.
- Support services should be matched to specific needs of the persons with epilepsy and their families.

- Services should embrace the concepts of self-management and self-determination for persons with epilepsy and their families.

Comprehensive Assessment

Because a full explanation for the development of social problems is not available and persons with new-onset seizures have social concerns, it is important that the social functioning of all persons with seizures be assessed on a regular basis in the clinical setting. Moreover, persons with epilepsy can have different needs at different developmental stages. Therefore, it is important regularly to complete a comprehensive assessment of patient and family needs to obtain information critical to planning services to prevent and reduce social problems. A comprehensive assessment should provide the basis for designing intervention programs and services to enhance the quality of life of persons with epilepsy and their families. In the assessment, it is important to include both psychosocial functioning and the factors that are associated with social problems.

Assessments incorporating a functional status approach commonly used by nurses and rehabilitation specialists are easy to use in clinical settings and can help patients and families to identify target concerns, individualized goals, and treatment strategies. Assessments are generally carried out using structured interviews, rating scales, and self-report questionnaires. Some assessment instruments have norms, so results can be compared with general population norms or other populations. Areas of assessment and examples of scales to use in each area include the following:

Knowledge About Epilepsy and Its Treatment
- Fear of Seizures[80]
- Epilepsy Myths and Misunderstandings Questionnaire[48]
- Information Needs of Parents of Children with Epilepsy[31]
- Parent Need for Psychosocial Care Scale[9]
- Child Need for Psychosocial Care Scale[9]
- Learning Needs of People with Epilepsy[39]
- Knowledge of Women's Issues in Epilepsy[71]

Attitudes and Psychosocial Problems
- Rosenberg Self-Esteem Scale[90]
- Child Behavior Checklist[1]
- Child Depression Inventory[66]
- Washington Psychosocial Inventory (Adolescents)[21]
- Washington Psychosocial Inventory (Adult)[45]
- Child Attitude Toward Illness Scale (CATIS)[13]
- Quality of Life in Epilepsy[35]
- Child Stigma Scale[14]
- Parent Stigma Scale[14]
- Epilepsy Self-efficacy Scale[38]
- Epilepsy Self-management Scale[37,40]
- Epilepsy Regimen Specific Support Scale[40]

Family Environment
- Family Support Scale[46]
- Family Inventory of Resources for Management[77]
- Family APGAR[12,98]

Matching Services With Needs

Early referral to health care professionals, rehabilitation specialists, and educators is recommended for proper recognition and treatment of both seizures and their consequences. Because needs of patients and families may be assessed and prioritized differently by health care professionals and patients, incorporating the patient's perspective into the care planning is critical. Services and interventions can then be tailored to the individual and patient-centered goals established.

TYPES OF SERVICES

Programs and services for addressing social functioning may include various educational approaches, counseling, social skills training, cognitive rehabilitation, support networks, peer mentoring, vocational rehabilitation, and independent living programs. Many different health care providers and community-based rehabilitation and educational specialists may provide these services, depending on their areas of expertise and practice setting (i.e., nurses, social workers, psychologists, psychiatrists, educators, vocational rehabilitation therapists, recreation therapists, and resource specialists).

With the changing health care environment in many countries, care is increasingly being provided in outpatient settings. Residential programs, however, are still available in some countries. Specialized epilepsy centers offer the ability to provide education, counseling, and supportive services in both inpatient and outpatient settings and by professionals with expertise in epilepsy. Guidelines have been established by the National Association of Epilepsy Centers in the United States that incorporate the critical services that should be provided at level three and four epilepsy centers to provide education, counseling, neuropsychological evaluations, educational and vocational assessments, and rehabilitation services.[81]

Unfortunately, many people do not have access to specialty centers, lack insurance coverage, or are not referred to these services until secondary disabilities and social problems are difficult to treat. In these instances, a "shared control" concept of care between general neurologist and a specialized epilepsy program or between the person's health care providers and community-based agencies, support services, and rehabilitation specialists is often implemented.[95]

The Internet is increasingly becoming a major source of information, education, support, and resources. When used to supplement medical care, the Internet serves as a fascinating way to connect people with resources and support previously not accessible to many. Online support groups via community forums, information and education provided by reputable epilepsy organizations, academic distance learning, and job search programs hold the promise of overcoming major barriers for people with epilepsy such as the need to drive to be able to access needed services.

Self-management Education

Educating people with epilepsy and their families should be geared to more than just imparting information and should involve skill development and resource identification. Ideally, education should assist people in managing their epilepsy and its consequences. This process, often termed epilepsy self-management, can also be thought of as taking the steps necessary to manage seizures and their impact.[36]

Common components of self-management have focused on seizure, medication, and lifestyle management.[24,96] A psychosocial model of self-management has focused lifestyle management on stress and safety while adding the critical need to manage information and disclosure.[41,42] Other issues involving accessing care, managing health needs, and addressing social relationships and community living suggest that psychosocial concerns need to be addressed as an integral part of epilepsy education and care.[94]

Research into predictors and outcomes of self-management programs are sparse. Self-efficacy, or self-confidence in managing epilepsy, and patient satisfaction have been found to be important variables in epilepsy self-management, particularly medication management, and social support, stigma, depressive symptoms, and outcome expectancies influence self-efficacy.[43] Self-efficacy, together with locus of control and social support, has important influences on quality of life as well.[3]

Tailoring epilepsy education to individual needs is considered a critical element of program planning. Because responsibility for caring for children with chronic conditions rests primarily with the family,[61] the best way to enhance social functioning in children is to provide needed services to families. According to Dunst et al.,[46] addressing families' needs helps to empower them to successfully manage chronic conditions in family members. Interviews with families of children with new-onset epilepsy indicated that they had many learning needs, including the need for education about epilepsy, treatment issues, and strategies for managing the epilepsy.[16] Included in the strategies for management were parents' needs to handle the responses of others to their child's seizure disorder and to help their children to cope successfully. A recent psychoeducational intervention in which the information and support were tailored to the individual needs of the family members showed significant increases in knowledge about epilepsy for both children with epilepsy and their parents. In addition, after the intervention, these children had fewer worries and need for information, and their parents had significantly less need for information and support related to their child's epilepsy.[15]

Dilorio et al.,[39] in an assessment of learning needs, found that adults with epilepsy had a strong wish for information about the condition and how to manage it. Needs were identified in the following rank order: Information on medication, seizures, psychological factors, basic brain functioning and seizure causes, and general lifestyle factors.

Very few educational programs have been systematically evaluated for effectiveness and reported in the literature. Studies of psychoeducational groups for adults with epilepsy using the Sepulveda Epilepsy Education (SEE) and Modular Service Package Epilepsy (MOSES) programs have demonstrated positive outcomes (e.g., knowledge, coping, and seizure outcomes).[55,73] Study of 6-week structured program for adolescents with epilepsy and their parents using cognitive–behavioral strategies and support suggests a positive influence on quality of life; however, the sample size was quite small.[99] Finally, Lewis et al.[69,70] evaluated an intervention program for children with epilepsy and their parents and found that an educational program increased parents' knowledge about epilepsy, decreased parents' anxiety, and increased children's perceived social competence.

There are many other educational materials and programs that have been developed by specialized epilepsy centers or national organizations, such as the International Bureau for Epilepsy and country-specific organizations such as the Epilepsy Foundation in the United States. Most often programs are implemented on the community level and tailored to the needs of the learner for maximum effectiveness.

Unfortunately, research into the benefits of individual epilepsy education is sparse. A study of community-based specialty nurses demonstrated improved knowledge of people with newly diagnosed epilepsy, supporting the benefits of shared care in epilepsy between specialists and community-based professionals.[87] In addition, a recent nurse-led education intervention for adults with uncontrolled epilepsy showed a significant improvement in quality of life compared to a control group.[54] In this study, the areas of greatest improvement were physical limitations, health discouragement, and medication effects.

Recent advances in our understanding of self-management and health education have important implications for educational programming. In addition to giving information, improving the learner's self-efficacy or confidence and building social support networks also may be important strategies for managing social problems.

Counseling

Counseling approaches in epilepsy care are frequently used to address social problems, both individually and in group settings. Mental health counseling may help people to adjust to the challenges of living with epilepsy and treat comorbid conditions such as anxiety and symptoms of depression. Desired outcomes include improved attitudes related to the epilepsy and social functioning, as well as treatment and/or prevention of psychiatric complications. People who experience changes in seizures with emotional distress or stress may also use counseling to improve seizure control. Finally, group counseling can provide important opportunities for learning social skills and gaining support from others with similar problems.

Approaches may include psychotherapy, cognitive–behavioral techniques, and other stress management approaches. Combining or supplementing self-management education with counseling can help to build a person's self-efficacy or confidence in living with epilepsy. Because epilepsy affects more than just the individual with seizures, addressing family dynamics and problems is an important part of epilepsy care.

Counseling can also be provided by specialists in recreation therapy. Recreation therapy appears to be especially appropriate for persons with epilepsy because of their problems with social isolation and lack of satisfactory peer relationships. For example, Regan et al.[85] combined education and counseling with a recreational activity (a ski trip) and found improvement in self-concept.

Social Skills and Cognitive Rehabilitation

Some people with epilepsy have impaired social skills and cognitive problems that may be due in part to underlying brain dysfunction complicated by the effects of seizures and medications on their brain function. Rehabilitation professionals with expertise in brain injury and epilepsy can teach social awareness and help patients to learn social skills and develop specific strategies to compensate for cognitive problems such as memory deficits. These services can be provided within many specialized epilepsy centers, outpatient rehabilitation settings, and community-based programs.

Self-help and Support Groups

Self-help groups generally are groups of peers who have joined together to help each other with a common problem. Self-help groups can lead to improved social function by extending social networks, providing new opportunities for social learning, and changing cognitive perceptions about one's condition.[67] Courses have been organized to standardize methods for self-help groups in Italy.[84] In the United States, support groups can be found in many communities, established by individuals, health care facilities, or nonprofit agencies. The Epilepsy Foundation and affiliates offer support groups and networks that are often targeted to specific groups such as parents, teens, and women. Increasingly, varied ways of providing support are being tried, such as phone networks, online forums, and individual mentoring.

Vocational Rehabilitation

Because employment is a major problem for many people with epilepsy, all adolescents and adults should receive vocational counseling. Needs can include help in identifying medical and social factors that may affect employment, assisting people to become job-ready, educating potential employers about epilepsy, assisting with job searches, teaching people to develop new vocational skills that will build on strengths, and teaching people new vocational skills and how to find reasonable accommodations.

Independent Living Programs

Independent living programs aim at enhancing independence and self-determination for people with epilepsy. These programs may be provided in residential settings for people with significant difficulties living independently. Many people with less severe functional problems may still experience difficulties living on their own and can benefit from teaching and assistance in developing critical skills such as personal care, budgeting, home management, transportation, shopping, and other independent living skills. Funding for these services may be problematic, but some federal health or disability insurance or private agencies may help.

SUMMARY AND CONCLUSIONS

We have outlined some of the major social problems found in persons with epilepsy and placed them within the context of tasks of normal psychosocial development. We also have identified some of the risk factors for social dysfunction, provided some examples of instruments that might be used for a comprehensive assessment, and reviewed different types of services for facilitating social functioning. Although many persons with epilepsy function well socially, others experience difficulties. We propose that comprehensive assessments be carried out on a regular basis to facilitate early identification of social problems and referral for rehabilitation services. In addition, recent studies suggest that educational interventions can be helpful for persons with epilepsy.

ACKNOWLEDGMENT

This chapter was supported in part by grant NS22416 to Joan K. Austin from the National Institute of Neurological Disorders and Stroke.

References

1. Achenbach TM, Rescoria LA. *Manual for the ASEBA School-Age Forms & Profiles*. Burlington, VT: University of Vermont Research Center for Children, Youth & Families; 2001.
2. Aldenkamp AP, Bijvoet ME, Heisen TWM, et al. *The influence of Epilepsy in Parents on Psychosocial Functioning of Their Children. Advances in Epileptology*, Vol. 17. New York: Raven Press; 1989.
3. Amir M, Roziner I, Knoll A, et al. Self-efficacy and social support as mediators in the relation between disease severity and quality of life in patients with epilepsy. *Epilepsia*. 1999;40(2):216–224.
4. Apter A, Aviv A, Kaminer Y, et al. Behavioral profile and social competence in temporal lobe epilepsy of adolescence. *J Am Acad Child Adolesc Psychiatry*. 1991;30(6):887–892.
5. Arntson P, Droge D, Norton R, et al. The perceived psychosocial consequences of having epilepsy. In: Whitman S, Hermann BP, eds. *Psychopathology in Epilepsy. Social Dimensions*. New York: Oxford University Press; 1986:143–161.
6. Austin JK. Childhood epilepsy: Child adaptation and family resources. *J Child Adolesc Psychiatr Ment Health Nurs*. 1988;1:18–24.
7. Austin JK. Comparison of child adaptation to epilepsy and asthma. *J Child Adolesc Psychiatr Ment Health Nurs*. 1989;2:139–44.
8. Austin JK. Concerns and fears of children with seizures. *Clin Nurs Pract Epilepsy*. 1993;1(4):4–6.
9. Austin JK, Dunn D, Huster G, et al. Development of scales to measure psychosocial care needs of children with seizures and their parents. *J Neurosci Nurs*. 1998;30(3):155–160.
10. Austin JK, Dunn DW, Johnson CS, et al. Behavioral issues involving children and adolescents with epilepsy and the impact on their families: Recent research data. *Epilepsy Behav*. 2004;5:S33–S41.
11. Austin JK, Dunn DW, Perkins SM, et al. Youth with epilepsy: Development of a model of children's attitudes toward their condition. *Children's Health Care*. 2006;35(2):123–140.
12. Austin JK, Huberty TJ. Revision of the family Apgar for use by 8-year-olds. *Family Syst Med*. 1989;7(3):323–327.
13. Austin JK, Huberty TJ. Development of the Child Attitude Toward Illness Scale. *J Pediatr Psychol*. 1993;18(4):467–480.
14. Austin JK, MacLeod J, Dunn DW, et al. Measuring stigma in children with epilepsy and their parents: Instrument development and testing. *Epilepsy Behav*. 2004;5:472–482.
15. Austin JK, McNelis AM, Shore CP, et al. A feasibility study of a family seizure management program: Be Seizure Smart. *J Neurosci Nurs*. 2002;34(1):30–37.
16. Austin JK, Oruche UM, Dunn DW, et al. New-onset childhood seizures: Parents' concerns and needs. *Clin Nurs Pract Epilepsy*. 1995;2(2): 8–10.
17. Austin JK, Risinger MW, Beckett LA. Correlates of behavior problems in children with epilepsy. *Epilepsia*. 1992;33(6):1115–1122.
18. Austin JK, Shafer PO, Deering JB. Epilepsy familiarity, knowledge, and perceptions of stigma: Report from a survey of adolescents in the general population. *Epilepsy Behav*. 2002;3:368–375.
19. Austin JK, Smith MS, Risinger MW, et al. Childhood epilepsy and asthma: Comparison of quality of life. *Epilepsia*. 1994;35(3):608–615.
20. Baker GA, Spector S, McGrath Y, et al. Impact of epilepsy in adolescence: A UK controlled study. *Epilepsy Behav*. 2005;6:556–562.
21. Batzel LW, Dodrill CB, Dubinsky BL, et al. An objective method for the assessment of psychosocial problems in adolescents with epilepsy. *Epilepsia*. 1991;32(2):202–211.
22. Billingham KA. *Developmental Psychology for Health Care Professionals*. Boulder, CO: Westview Press; 1982.
23. Britten N, Morgan K, Fenwick PBC, et al. Epilepsy and handicap from birth to age 36. *Dev Med Child Neurol*. 1986;28:719–728.
24. Buelow JM. Epilepsy management issues and techniques. *J Neurosci Nurs*. 2001;33:260–269.
25. Camfield C, Camfield P, Smith B, et al. Biologic factors as predictors of social outcome of epilepsy in intellectually normal children: A population-based study. *J Pediatr*. 1993;122(6):869–873.
26. Caplan R, Sagun J, Siddarth P, et al. Social competence in pediatric epilepsy: Insights into underlying mechanisms. *Epilepsy Behav*. 2005;6: 218–228.
27. Chapieski L, Brewer V, Evankovich K, et al. Adaptive functioning in children with seizures: Impact of maternal anxiety about epilepsy. *Epilepsy Behav*. 2005;7:246–252.
28. Chaplin JE, Floyd M, Lasso RY. Early psychosocial adjustment and the experience of epilepsy: Findings from a general practice survey. *Int J Rehab Res*. 1993;16:316–318.
29. Chaplin JE, Lasso RY, Shorvon SD, et al. National general practice study of epilepsy: The social and psychological effects of a recent diagnosis of epilepsy. *Br Med J*. 1992;304:1416–1418.
30. Collins JA. Epilepsy and well-being. *Soc Sci Med*. 1990;31(2):165–170.
31. Coulter DL, Koester BS. Information needs of parents of children with epilepsy. *J Dev Behav Pediatr*. 1985;6(6):334–338.
32. Danksy LV, Andermann E, Andermann F. Marriage and fertility in epileptic patients. *Epilepsia*. 1980;21:261–271.
33. Dean P, Austin JK. Adolescent psychosocial adjustment issues in epilepsy. *Clin Nurs Pract Epilepsy*. 1996;3:4–6.
34. De Boer HM. Overview and perspectives of employment in people with epilepsy. *Epilepsia*. 2005;46(Suppl.1):52–54.
35. Devinsky O, Vickrey B, Hays R, et al. Quality of life in epilepsy: QOLIE-89 instrument development. *Neurology*. 1994;44(Suppl 2):A141.
36. DiIorio C. Epilepsy self-management. In: Gochman DS, ed. *Handbook of Health Behavior Research II: Provider Determinants*. New York: Plenum Press; 1997:213–230.
37. DiIorio C, Faherty B, Manteuffel B. The development and testing of an instrument to measure self-efficacy in persons with epilepsy. *J Neurosci Nurs*. 1992;24(1):9–13.
38. DiIorio C, Faherty B, Manteuffel B. The relationship of self-efficacy and social support in self management of epilepsy. *West J Nurs Res*. 1992;14(3):292–303.
39. DiIorio C, Faherty B, Manteuffel B. Learning needs of persons with epilepsy: A comparison of perceptions of persons with epilepsy, nurses and physicians. *J Neurosci Nurs*. 1993;25(1):22–29.
40. DiIorio C, Faherty B, Manteuffel B. Epilepsy self-management: Partial replication and extension. *Res Nurs Health*. 1994;17(3):167–74.
41. DiIorio C, Hennessey M, Manteuffel B. Epilepsy self-management: A test of a theoretical model. *Nurs Res*. 1996;45:211–217.

42. Dilorio C, Shafer P, Letz R, et al. The association of stigma with self-management and perceptions of health care among adults with epilepsy. *Epilepsy Behav.* 2003;4:259–267.
43. Dilorio C, Shafer PO, Letz R, et al., and Project EASE Study Group. Project EASE: A study to test a psychosocial model of epilepsy medication management. *Epilepsy Behav.* 2004;5(6):926–936.
44. Dodrill CB. Psychosocial characteristics of epileptic patients. In: Ward AA, Penry JK, Purpura D, eds. *Epilepsy.* New York: Raven Press; 1983:341–353.
45. Dodrill CB, Batzel LW, Queisser HR, et al. An objective method for the assessment of psychosocial problems among epileptics. *Epilepsia.* 1980;21:123–135.
46. Dunst CJ, Trivette CM, Deal AG. *Enabling and Empowering Families.* Cambridge, MA: Brookline Books; 1988.
47. Elliott IM, Lach L, Smith ML. I just want to be normal: A qualitative study exploring how children and adolescents view the impact of intractable epilepsy on their quality of life. *Epilepsy Behav.* 2005;7:664–678.
48. Epilepsy Foundation of America. *Epilepsy Myths and Misunderstandings Questionnaire. Issues and Answers: A Guide for Parents of Children with Seizures, Ages Six to Twelve.* Landover, MD: Epilepsy Foundation of America; 1993.
49. Epilepsy Foundation of America. *Report of the 2003 National Conference on Public Health and Epilepsy.* Landover, MD: Epilepsy Foundation of America; 2003.
50. Fisher RS, Harding G, Erba G, et al. Photic- and pattern-induced seizures: A review for the Epilepsy Foundation of America Working Group. *Epilepsia.* 2005;46:1426–1441.
51. Freiberg KL. *Human Development: A Life Span Approach,* 2nd ed. Monterey, CA: Wadsworth Health Sciences; 1983.
52. Hartlage LC, Green JB, Offutt L. Dependency in epileptic children. *Epilepsia.* 1972;13:27–30.
53. Hayden M, Penna C, Buchanan N. Epilepsy: Patient perceptions of their condition. *Seizure.* 1992;1(3):191–7.
54. Helde G, Bovim G, Brathen G, Brodtkorb E. A structured, nurse-led intervention program improves quality of life in patients with epilepsy: A randomized, controlled trial. *Epilepsy Behav.* 2005;7:451–457.
55. Helgeson DC, Mittan R, Tan SY, et al. Sepulveda Epilepsy Education: The efficacy of a psychoeducational treatment program in treating medical and psychosocial aspects of epilepsy. *Epilepsia.* 1990;31:75–82.
56. Hermann BP. Deficits in neuropsychological functioning and psychopathology in persons with epilepsy: A rejected hypothesis revisited. *Epilepsia.* 1981;22:161–167.
57. Hermann BP. The relevance of social factors to adjustment in epilepsy. In: Devinsky O, Theodore WH, eds. *Epilepsy and Behavior.* New York: Wiley-Liss; 1991:23–36.
58. Hermann BP, Whitman S. Behavioral personality correlates of epilepsy: A review, methodological critique, and conceptual model. *Psychol Bull.* 1984;95(3):451–497.
59. Hermann BP, Whitman S, Dell J. Correlates of behavior problems and social competence in children with epilepsy, aged 6–11. In: Hermann BP, Seidenberg M, eds. *Childhood Epilepsies: Neuropsychological, Psychosocial and Intervention Aspects.* New York: John Wiley; 1989:143–57.
60. Hoare P. The development of psychiatric disorder among school children with epilepsy. *Dev Med Child Neurol.* 1984;26:3–13.
61. Horner MM, Rawlins P, Giles K. How parents of children with chronic conditions perceive their own needs. *Am J Matern Child Nurs.* 1987;12(1):40–43.
62. Hupperts RMM, Habets JA. A written mail survey among 200 neurologists and 200 people with epilepsy. *Epilepsiebulletin.* 1989;2:14–17.
63. International Employment Commission of IBE. Principles of good practice for employers. *Epilepsia.* 1989;30(4):411–412.
64. Jacoby A. Epilepsy and the quality of everyday life. *Soc Sci Med.* 1992;34(6):657–666.
65. Jacoby A. Impact of epilepsy on employment status: Findings from a UK study of people with well-controlled epilepsy. *Epilepsy Res.* 1995;21:125–132.
66. Kovacs M. Rating scales to assess depression in school-aged children. *Acta Paedopsychiatr.* 1980/81;46:305–315.
67. Kurtz LF, Powell TJ. Three approaches to understanding self-help groups. *Soc Work Groups.* 1987;10(3):69–80.
68. Lechtenberg R, Alkner L. Psychological adaptation of children to epilepsy in a parent. *Epilepsia.* 1984;25(1):40–45.
69. Lewis MA, Hatton CL, Salas I, et al. Impact of the children's epilepsy program on parents. *Epilepsia.* 1991;32(3):365–374.
70. Lewis MA, Salas I, de la Sota A, et al. Randomized trial of a program to enhance the competencies of children with epilepsy. *Epilepsia.* 1990;31(1):101–109.
71. Long L, McAuley JW, Shneker B, et al. The validity and reliability of the Knowledge of Women's Issues and Epilepsy (KOWIE) questionnaires I and II. *J Neurosci Nurs.* 2005; 37(2):88–91.
72. Lothman DJ, Pianta RC, Clarson SM. Mother–child interaction in children with epilepsy: Relations with child competence. *J Epilepsy.* 1990;3:157–163.
73. May TW, Pfafflin M. The efficacy of an educational treatment program for patients with epilepsy (MOSES): Results of a controlled randomized study: Modular service package epilepsy. *Epilepsia.* 2002;43:539–549.
74. Margalit M, Heiman T. Anxiety and self-dissatisfaction in epileptic children. *Int J Soc Psychiatry.* 1983;29(3):220–24.
75. Matthews WS, Barabas G, Ferrari M. Emotional concomitants of childhood epilepsy. *Epilepsia.* 1982;23:671–681.
76. McCollum AT. *The Chronically Ill child: A Guide for Parents and Professionals.* New Haven, CT: Yale University Press; 1981.
77. McCubbin HI, Thompson AI. *Family Assessment Inventories for Research and Practice.* Madison, WI: Family Stress Coping and Health Project, University of Wisconsin-Madison; 1991.
78. Millett CJ, Fish DR, Thompson PJ. A survey of epilepsy-patient perceptions of video-game material/electronic screens and other factors as seizure precipitants. *Seizure.* 1997;6:457–459.
79. Mitchell WG, Chavez JM, Lee H, et al. Academic underachievement in children with epilepsy. *J Child Neurol.* 1991;6(1):65–72.
80. Mittan RJ. Fear of seizures. In: Whitman S, Hermann BP, eds. *Psychopathology in Epilepsy.* New York: Oxford University Press; 1986:90–121.
81. National Association of Epilepsy Centers. Report of the National Association of Epilepsy Centers: Guidelines for essential services, personnel, and facilities in specialized epilepsy centers in the United States. *Epilepsia.* 2001;42(6):804–814.
82. Ounsted C, Lindsay J. The long-term outcome of temporal lobe epilepsy in childhood. In: *Epilepsy & Psychiatry.* Edinburgh: Churchill Livingstone; 1981;185–215.
83. Pierzcha K, Grudzinska B. The number of children and marriage among men with epilepsy. *Neurol Neurochir Pol.* 1987;21:19–23.
84. Plazzini A, Moretti S. The first course on self-help groups in Italy. *Int Epilepsy News.* 1993:8–9.
85. Regan KJ, Banks GK, Beran RG. Therapeutic recreation programmes for children with epilepsy. *Seizure.* 1993;2:195–200.
86. Reuvekamp HF, de Boer HM, Bult I, et al. Employment of people with epilepsy, is there a problem? 23rd Epilepsy Congress. *Jansen-Cilag Med Sci News.* 1999;6:175–179.
87. Ridsdale L, Kwan I, Morgan M. How can a nurse intervention help people with newly diagnosed epilepsy? A qualitative study of patient views. *Seizure.* 2003;12:69–73.
88. Rodenburg R, Meijer AM, Dekovic M, et al. Family factors and psychopathology in children with epilepsy: A literature review. *Epilepsy Behav.* 2005;6:488–503.
89. Rodenburg R, Stams GJ, Meijer AM, et al. Psychopathology in children with epilepsy: A meta-analysis. *J Pediatr Psychiatry.* 2005;30(6):453–468.
90. Rosenberg M. *Society and the Adolescent Self-Image.* Princeton, NJ: Princeton University Press; 1965.
91. Scambler G, Hopkins A. Social class, epileptic activity and disadvantage at work. *J Epidemiol Commun Health.* 1980;34:129–133.
92. Scott DJ. Psychiatric aspects of epilepsy. *Br J Psychiatry.* 1978;132:417–430.
93. Seidenberg M. Academic achievement and school performance of children with epilepsy. In: Hermann BP, Seidenberg M, eds. *Childhood Epilepsies: Neuropsychological, Psychosocial and Intervention Aspects.* New York: John Wiley; 1989:105–118.
94. Shafer PO. Epilepsy and seizures: Advances in seizure assessment, treatment, and self-management: Neuroscience nursing for a new millennium. *Nurs Clin North Am.* 1999;34:743–759.
95. Shafer PO, Dilorio C. Managing life issues in epilepsy. Continuum—Lifelong Learning in Neurology. *Epilepsy.* 2004;(10)4:138–156.
96. Shope JT. Educating patients and families to manage a seizure disorder successfully. In: Santilli N, ed. *Managing Seizure Disorders: A Handbook for Health Care Professionals.* Philadelphia: Lippincott-Raven; 1996:123–134.
97. Sillanpaa M, Haataja L, Shinnar S. Perceived impact of childhood-onset epilepsy on quality of life as an adult. *Epilepsia.* 2004;45(8):971–977.
98. Smilkstein G. The family Apgar: A proposal for a family function test and its use by physicians. *J Family Pract.* 1978;6:1231–1239.
99. Snead K, Ackerson J, Bailey K, et al. Taking charge of epilepsy: The development of a structured psychoeducational group intervention for adolescents with epilepsy and their parents. *Epilepsy Behav.* 2004;5(4):547–556.
100. Steffenburg S, Gillberg C, Steffenburg U. Psychiatric disorders in children and adolescents with mental retardation and active epilepsy. *Arch Neurol.* 1996;53:904–912.
101. Sturniolo MG, Galletti F. Idiopathic epilepsy and school achievement. *Arch Dis Child.* 1994;70:424–428.
102. Suurmeijer TPBM, Reuvekamp MF, Aldenkamp AP. Social functioning, psychological functioning, and quality of life in epilepsy. *Epilepsia.* 2001;42:1160–1168.
103. Thompson PJ, Upton D. The impact of chronic epilepsy on the family. *Seizure.* 1992;1(1):43–48.
104. Trostle JA, Hauser WA, Sharbrough FW. Psychologic and social adjustment to epilepsy in Rochester, Minnesota. *Neurology.* 1989;39:633–637.

CHAPTER 218 ■ MAXIMIZING SCHOOL FUNCTIONING AND THE SCHOOL-TO-WORK TRANSITION

MICHAEL SEIDENBERG AND DAVID C. CLEMMONS

INTRODUCTION

Epilepsy is a common childhood neurologic disorder, affecting approximately 5 to 10 children in every 1,000. The vast majority of people with epilepsy begin having their seizures during the childhood years, and for many, the seizures persist for an extended period of time.[22] Thus, the view of epilepsy as a potentially chronic childhood disorder has important implications for long-term academic, social, and vocational adjustment.[38]

In this chapter, we discuss issues relevant to maximizing school and vocational adjustment in children and adolescents with epilepsy. A basic theme of this chapter is that a multidisciplinary assessment and intervention approach offers the most effective means to (a) identify children in need of educational or vocational services, (b) determine the nature and extent of services needed, and (c) develop effective intervention programs. The use of a multidisciplinary approach recognizes that multiple factors potentially influence academic and occupational development and requires the involvement of professionals from various disciplines (e.g., medicine, education, psychology, social service) as well as the participation of the family and the child. A major practical challenge for implementation of a multidisciplinary assessment and treatment approach is the establishment of the community linkages that enable the members of the various disciplines to interact effectively.

We begin with a review of the current data concerning the nature and extent of academic difficulties among children with epilepsy. Next, we discuss the factors that have been shown to be associated with academic vulnerability among children with epilepsy and their implications for evaluation and intervention. The final section provides the rationale for school-to-work transition programs along with a description of an integrated and comprehensive vocational intervention and training program.

Finally, although the specific condition of epilepsy is discussed here, the academic and vocations problems of many youth with epilepsy are often similar to those of persons with other neurologic conditions affecting the central nervous system (e.g., traumatic brain injury, stroke, multiple sclerosis, etc.). Thus, impairment of cognitive factors such as attention, memory, "multitasking," problem solving, and overall cognitive efficiency may be more important determinants of academic and vocational success than is their specific etiology. This is not always immediately apparent to many service providers, including many counselors and vocational advisors without specific training in this area.

SCHOOL PERFORMANCE OF CHILDREN WITH EPILEPSY

One can identify three basic questions in considering the school performance of children with epilepsy: (a) Is there increased risk of learning problems? (b) Why are there learning problems? (c) What can be done to help those children with learning problems?

Increased Risk of Learning Problems

A precise estimate of the incidence of academic difficulties among children with epilepsy is hampered by several important methodologic issues. First, most studies reported in the literature examined children seen at tertiary medical centers or specialized epilepsy centers. These children are unlikely to provide a representative sampling of children with epilepsy (e.g., seizure severity, seizure control), and this introduces a selection bias into the determination of the occurrence of academic dysfunction in this population. Second, many of the early studies did not employ objective and standardized measures of academic functioning and instead relied on teacher or parent ratings. Such ratings are potentially biased and invalid estimates of a child's functioning.

With these limitations in mind, and even though many children with epilepsy have minimal or no significant learning problems, there is considerable evidence of an increased risk for learning and academic problems in this population.[1,5,16,32,34,44] Although initial reports focused on reading skills, subsequent studies have shown that problems are often present in academic areas other than reading as well. Seidenberg et al.[36] reported that a substantial percentage of children with epilepsy being treated at a tertiary epilepsy center experienced significant levels of academic underachievement in four academic areas: (a) word recognition, (b) reading comprehension, (c) spelling, and (d) arithmetic.

Reasons for Learning Problems

The factors underlying academic vulnerability in children with epilepsy are multivariate, and one can anticipate the need to consider a variety of factors in attempts to establish a comprehensive evaluation and treatment program.[2,38] Seidenberg[35] identified four factors as important potential mechanisms linking epilepsy and academic difficulties: (a) seizure correlates,

(b) neuropsychological correlates, (c) medication effects, and (d) psychosocial correlates. Again, it is emphasized that an intervention that identifies the seizures themselves as the only or as the main focus of attention is likely to fall short of a student's needs.

Seizure Correlates of Academic Dysfunction

The determination of seizure-related correlates of academic dysfunction would be of potential use for early identification and screening of "at-risk" children. Clinical seizure correlates such as focal left-hemisphere spikes, early age of seizure onset, and seizure control have been implicated in some studies.[23,40] However, the findings have been inconsistent concerning the relationship of these variables to academic functioning.[10,24] Seidenberg et al.[36] found that the combined predictive significance of several clinical seizure characteristics (e.g., seizure type, age of seizure onset, seizure control, number of medications, laterality of electroencephalographic [EEG] abnormality) for academic achievement was moderate (between 6% and 17% of the variance). Thus, although knowledge of various aspects of seizure history and seizure characteristics is critical to the diagnosis and medical management of children with epilepsy, this information may be of more limited value in predicting academic outcome. Of interest for the current chapter, similar findings have been reported for predicting vocational adjustment and independent living of adolescents with epilepsy.[15]

Neuropsychological Correlates of Academic Dysfunction

In many instances, the academic difficulties do not reflect a generalized intellectual impairment, but instead are related to specific areas of cognitive deficit(s).[9] Impairments in attention and concentration have commonly been linked to academic dysfunction.[3,4,40,44] Seidenberg et al.[37] compared two groups of children with epilepsy—a group making adequate academic progress (AA) and a group making poor academic progress (UA)—on a battery of neuropsychological measures. Findings indicated that the UA group was distinctly impaired on measures of auditory perceptual skills, verbal memory, and attention and concentration relative to the AA group. The importance of these specific cognitive areas for academic functioning has been well documented in studies of learning-disabled children.[31,42]

Furthermore, similar to what is found in the broader learning disability literature, the nature of the underlying cognitive deficits associated with academic dysfunction is not similar for all children with epilepsy. Rather, there appear to be distinctive subtypes of learning deficits among children with epilepsy. A preliminary classification of "subtypes" of learning-disabled children with epilepsy was recently presented.[1] These workers proposed four distinct groups and possible seizure-related features that characterize them: (a) memory-deficit subtype, characterized by specific impairment in memory and learning (a relationship to temporal lobe dysfunction is suggested for these children); (b) attention-deficit type, characterized by global academic underachievement (this group was represented by a high frequency of children with generalized tonic–clonic seizures); (c) speed-factor type, which showed slower information processing and was found to be correlated with polytherapy and long-term treatment with phenytoin; and (d) problem-solving type, characterized by impairments in higher-order cognitive processes such as verbal reasoning and concept formation.

It is not surprising that cognitive deficits are an important mediating factor for school performance. These findings indicating cognitive subtypes serve to highlight the potential importance of detailed cognitive testing for identification and treatment planning for children at risk for academic dysfunction.

Medication Factors

The American Academy of Pediatrics Committee on Drugs[3] has called attention to the important effects that antiepileptic drugs (AEDs) can have on cognition and behavioral functioning of children with epilepsy. Several methodologic issues concerning the potential effects of AED on behavior remain open for study, including specific drug type effects, age at time of testing, and drug serum levels. Several investigators have documented the ill-advised use of polytherapy[43] and the adverse effects of phenobarbital on cognitive performance.[17] However, the cost–benefit analysis of seizure control versus side effects or direct negative effects of anticonvulsant medication on behavior is quite complicated. Once again, this issue emphasizes the need for data from multiple people involved in the treatment of the child to develop an effective treatment plan.

Psychosocial Factors

Taylor[41] described the "predicament of epilepsy," which extends beyond the medical neurologic aspects of the seizures themselves and touches on various parts of the person's life and interaction with the environment. Several investigators have reported an association between academic dysfunction and social environmental factors such as teacher attitudes, parental attitudes and expectations,[21,25] child self-esteem, and perceptions of reasons for school success and failure.[26] These environmental and behavioral or temperamental features are critical for the establishment of treatment programs to foster educational and vocational development. Freeman et al.[20] described a school-based program for children with epilepsy that included assessment and treatment of psychosocial problems (e.g., counseling, epilepsy education) as a critical component as well as vocational and more traditional academic programming. Findings indicated a decrease in school dropout rate and an increase in the numbers of students who later became employed or entered higher education programs or vocational training programs.

What Can Be Done?

For the individual child, one must be prepared to examine various potential sources of influence (seizure correlates, cognitive correlates, medications, psychosocial factors) and their interactions so that effective intervention programs can be developed. Thus, school planning for children with epilepsy requires the active involvement of parents, medical personnel, educators, and other specialists to ensure that these various factors are considered.[33] Early identification of the child who is at "high risk" for academic and learning difficulties is important. Parents are often the first to recognize that a child may have learning difficulties. Objective and standardized assessments provide a critical database for determining cognitive strengths and weaknesses and charting development in these areas. Medical input into the underlying seizure and neurologic characteristics and the medication regimen must be incorporated into the evaluation process. Parental and teacher observation of seizure activity and impressions about social adaptive development also form critical components of the assessment process.[8]

Unfortunately, the academic difficulties encountered during the early school years often continue into the high school years and ultimately translate into vocational and occupational limitations. Objective data concerning employment status for people with epilepsy are fraught with the same methodologic and selection bias issues described earlier for studies of academic and school performance. Nevertheless, it does appear that individuals with epilepsy have at least twice the rate of unemployment of the general population.[22]

Findings from a series of studies conducted at the University of Washington Regional Epilepsy Center provide information relevant to the issue of vocational and employment status among people with epilepsy.[11,12,15] Of 42 participants examined, 31% were dependent on government subsidy (supplemental security income) within 4 years of high school graduation. Only 29% of the sample was engaged in full-time employment within the same time period. Only 14% had obtained employment as a result of vocational services from the state rehabilitation agency. Although it can be argued that the study sample was not representative of the epilepsy population in general, the numbers are nevertheless disquieting. Fraser et al.[19] suggested that these findings are not isolated but instead represent a national trend. Emerging from these findings are three main concerns for providing rehabilitation services for youth with epilepsy: (a) the desirability of early vocational intervention programs, (b) the identification of "at-risk" youth based on assessment of neuropsychological status, and (c) the desirability of specialized rather than generic rehabilitation programs.

In the next section, we describe a specialized vocational intervention program for youth with epilepsy. The first part deals with assessment issues relevant to the development of a vocational rehabilitation plan, and the second part discusses strategies for implementation of the vocational treatment plan.

SCHOOL-TO-WORK TRANSITION: ASSESSMENT ISSUES

Similar to the area of academic achievement, the development of an individualized vocational rehabilitation plan involves multiple areas of assessment. Four general areas should be addressed: (a) neuropsychological functioning, (b) psychosocial functioning, (c) medical assessment, and (d) vocational assessment.

Neuropsychological Assessment

Neuropsychological assessment is frequently overlooked or deemphasized by those providing vocational services to youth with epilepsy. The following areas of brain function are frequent areas of concern for the vocational counselor working with persons with epilepsy: (a) sensory motor integrity, (b) attention and concentration, (c) memory (especially short-term memory and incidental memory), (d) verbal ability, (e) visuospatial ability, (f) cognitive efficiency, and (g) executive functions (i.e., the ability to plan, evaluate, implement, and monitor behavior).

It is important to realize that a neuropsychological test battery may be sensitive to difficulties that will not be observed with IQ tests or vocational aptitude batteries. It is also the case that many persons with subtle but vocationally significant neuropsychological problems may not present as "obviously" handicapped by their condition because of good adaptive skills, lack of expertise on the part of the observer, or other factors.

Not every youth with epilepsy who is referred for vocational services is an appropriate candidate for neuropsychological evaluation. Because epileptic seizures are a sign of an underlying pathology, however, it is important for the rehabilitation professional to ascertain whether the underlying cause of the seizures also presents cognitive difficulties that must be accounted for in a rehabilitation plan. Some of the most common signs of possible neuropsychological concerns include difficulty with short-term memory, problems doing multiple tasks or efficiently performing a task in the presence of distractors, and an unexplained discrepancy between apparent ability and performance. Other possible signs of neuropsychological difficulty include visual field cuts, "learning disability" symptoms, problems with attention and concentration, and unilateral weakness or clumsiness. None of the signs mentioned here is necessarily diagnostic of frank neuropsychological or cognitive difficulties, but they do serve as justification for referring a youth with epilepsy for more thorough screening.

Psychosocial Assessment

In carrying out a psychosocial assessment for youth with epilepsy, the following areas of concern should be addressed:

1. Adjustment within the family. Does the youth have a stable home situation with the appropriate balance of support and independence? Do the parents have realistic expectations of the youth? Is there sufficient education about epilepsy within the family group that there are no informational gaps that could cause difficulty within the family?
2. Does the youth have adequate information about epilepsy and seizures? Is the youth able to describe what happens during a seizure and discuss what first aid needs, if appropriate, may be necessary?
3. Is the youth satisfied with the medical care being provided?
4. Does the youth have an adequate peer group, circle of friends, and avenues of social support?
5. Are there any significant life goals that the youth feels are blocked by the presence of epilepsy?
6. Are there additional significant conditions (e.g., neuropsychological dysfunction, physical injury or impairment) that may interact with the condition of epilepsy? Although not all students with epilepsy manifest cognitive difficulties, the presence of the underlying conditions that propagate epileptic seizures places them at greater risk for cognitive concerns than individuals in the general population. The assignation of a student's academic or psychosocial difficulties to the presence of seizures may overlook less manifest, but more salient, variables.

In assessing psychosocial status, attention should be paid both to an individual's internal psychological adjustment and that individual's adjustment to his or her social network. Two useful instruments for overall psychosocial assessment are the Washington Psychosocial Seizure Inventory[15] developed at the University of Washington's Regional Epilepsy Center and its derivative, the Adolescent Psychosocial Seizure Inventory.[7] Each of these instruments has the advantage of being inexpensive, being easily administered and scored, and offering an indication of psychosocial status over a broad range of areas (e.g., adjustment to seizures, medical management, family background). These instruments are especially relevant because they were developed with and normed on an epilepsy population.

Medical Assessment

Medical assessment for vocational purposes goes beyond documenting the type of seizures and the medication involved. From a practical standpoint, and in keeping with federal regulation, access to or restriction from a given job because of epilepsy should be based on the individual's functional limitations. Blanket restrictions from certain types of occupations or duties (i.e., from "potentially dangerous" machinery, heights, driving, or meeting the public) should be avoided. The following checklist is useful in helping the counselor amass this information.

1. What happens during a seizure? For purposes of evaluation, the seizure should be operationally defined. Many persons think of seizures or epilepsy only in terms of the generalized tonic–clonic or "grand mal" seizure, which involves a complete loss of consciousness and a brief period of convulsive activity. Many other seizure types exist. It is important to know whether the client can walk about, whether consciousness is fully or partially lost, or whether the patient remains fully conscious.
2. Is a warning aura present? Many people with epilepsy have a dependable warning aura, which may precede a seizure by several minutes to several hours. Presence of a dependable aura frequently reduces functional limitations.
3. Temporal patterns. Many patients have seizures only when asleep. Others may have seizures only during certain times, such as early morning or later in the evening.
4. Ability of youth to attend to the medical regimen. Is the youth able to take medication on time and in the right amounts? One important question here is whether the youth's medical noncompliance is a vehicle for rebellion. This is an unfortunate, if not uncommon, complication for many youth with epilepsy, especially with individuals recently diagnosed. This is an important factor to assess not only because medical noncompliance is likely to increase the functional limitations of the person involved, but also because it may set the stage for potentially dangerous consequences, such as status epilepticus.

Advances in anticonvulsant medication and medical management are reviewed elsewhere in this book. Because significant progress in this area may occur within a short period of time, it is essential not only that youth with epilepsy have regular medical review, but that care should be taken to assure that the medical practitioner chosen has access to recent advances in epileptology.

Vocational Assessment

The vocational needs of many persons with epilepsy are sufficiently different from those of the general population that generalized approaches are often not helpful and may be damaging; the watchword here is individualized assessment. Generic assessment packages frequently confuse the issue by providing guidance that is inappropriate or irrelevant to the person with special needs related to a seizure condition. For example, an individual with any of a number of neurologic conditions, including epilepsy, may present with tested intellectual functioning well within or above normal limits while experiencing marked difficulties in areas of neuropsychological functioning, such as attention/concentration, memory, "multitasking," problem solving, and so on. This scenario is not uncommon, and it complicates counseling and planning efforts if it is not recognized and taken into consideration. Accordingly, standardized testing efforts should be supplemented by other information.

A student with apparent cognitive limitations should be offered a neuropsychological battery, as discussed earlier. Neuropsychological testing can be relatively expensive vis-à-vis vocational interest and aptitude or testing for intellectual functioning. This can sometimes present economic barriers to obtaining information about cognitive status, even though failing to do so may entail much higher long-term costs in terms of misdirected resources and poor vocational outcome. Neuropsychological testing for some specific purposes, such as vocational or educational planning, however, may have different aims than does testing for other purposes, such as medical or forensic investigation. A forensic or medical agenda may, for example, be concerned with such factors as pinpointing lesions sites and establishing liberalization or foci of dysfunction, in addition to a more general establishment of neuropsychological status. Vocational and educational uses of this testing are more likely to be more concerned with operational factors. Such considerations have led to an interest in the development and exploration of abbreviated batteries designed to target specific problems or populations. Among the benefits of such batteries would be reduction in cost, reduction in time expenditure, and more general availability of cognitive testing for special populations. Rao[29,30] has devoted much energy to this pursuit in the area of vocational and cognitive assessment in multiple sclerosis. Following this lead, Clemmons et al.[13] developed an abbreviated neuropsychological battery for use initially with a multiple sclerosis vocational rehabilitation population. Although research on ecological validity and on the utility of the battery with other neurologic populations is ongoing, the utility of this or quite similar batteries for use with neurologic populations, including epilepsy, appears warranted.

STRATEGIES FOR INTERVENTION

Working With Teachers and School Personnel

A key concern in working with teachers and school personnel is frequently the difference between a generalist and a specialist orientation. A useful tool for helping to bridge this gap is the individualized educational plan (IEP). The IEP is required by U.S. federal law for any student of public education who has educational needs that cannot be met via the general school curriculum.[6] The IEP is designed to identify and plan for special education needs and services. By U.S. law, parents may attend the IEP meeting and participate in its formulation. Because a school district may be obligated to provide services to a student qualifying for an IEP until the age of 21 years, care should be taken to avoid quick or expedient solutions. Both short-term and long-term goals need to be considered. For example, it may be desirable to avoid graduation or the attainment of a General Equivalency Diploma so as to offer the student a more intensive educational or pre-vocational experience. It should be noted that there may be considerable variation among individual school districts in developing and using IEPs. Much variation in expertise with neurologic conditions may also exist. If this is the case, parents may find that the use of an outside advocate or specialist in neurologic vocational habilitation is a desirable choice.

Parents or advocates should realize that an IEP can be modified to include goals that are not primarily academic but rather vocational and pre-vocational. Indeed, the point may be reached at which the inclusion of additional vocational training is more beneficial than specialized academic interventions. Experience at the Regional Epilepsy Center in Seattle, Washington, has shown that in some situations, the strategy of concentrating on work exploration and work experience issues is especially useful. Access to structured employment opportunities (such as job situations) through the IEP can be critical for development of employment skills and experience.

There are a number of strategies for providing a student with work experience. The most desirable is to develop part-time paid employment, with or without the ongoing support of a job coach or other supportive employment strategies. Frequently, however, the most viable option is the development of an unpaid work experience or job station in an area compatible with interests and abilities. In promoting unpaid work experience, it should be emphasized that these experiences may serve many desirable functions. These include an opportunity for vocational exploration, for assessing emotional and physical stamina in a job-like situation, work and social skills building, and adjustment or tolerance to a work-like situation (so-called "work hardening"). The unpaid work experience is also useful in providing a student with both work history and a positive work reference.

An unpaid work experience is successful to the extent that it mimics the working environment of a competitive job. To this end, an ideal goal is a situation that involves a minimum of 1 to 3 months of experience at 20 to 30 hours per week. Shorter time periods tend not to be useful for establishing a work history or for evaluating competitive status. Once the decision has been made to pursue the unpaid work experience as a training strategy, it may well become the focus of the rehabilitation plan. Many high schools recognize this fact and have developed strategies for awarding credits toward high school graduation for participation in specialized vocational programs.

Working With Parents and Family Members

The initial step in working with families should be the determination of their need for information about epilepsy and its vocational implications. Even families with relatively adequate general information about epilepsy may require more specific information with respect to their child's seizure disorder and its implications for educational and vocational planning. This may be particularly relevant for students with appreciable neuropsychological deficits. Conflicting perceptions or unrealistic expectations and objectives must be recognized and addressed.

A useful strategy is to present problematic issues with a general and neutral discussion of rehabilitation strategies, goals, barriers, and other issues. It is critical that the student, the parents, and the counselor meet early in the rehabilitation process to establish the goals of the intervention process. When the implicit assumption of the rehabilitation interaction is that the student has financial and social independence as long-term goals, this should be explored and made explicit. Not all students (or parents) see independence as a long-term goal. It is also important to attend to family time frames. Some families may see a set time frame, such as graduation from high school, the eighteenth birthday, or the twenty-first birthday as the appropriate time for the physical and financial separation of the child. Other families may have less specific time frames. The family's time frame may have significant impact on the motivation and investment of the rehabilitant. When rehabilitation or independence is not a particularly strong goal with the parent, the child also may have less urgent needs in this area.

Working With State Rehabilitation Agencies

At some point in the rehabilitation process, it is desirable to involve the state rehabilitation agency as an active participant in the rehabilitation plan. Various states have different age limits and policies determining when a juvenile may be referred formally for rehabilitation purposes, and these regulations may fluctuate both with time and with individual regions. Schools may have formal agreements with the state rehabilitation agency, or these may have to be developed on a specific basis. Although many state rehabilitation counselors have received specialized education and training with respect to epilepsy and allied concerns, many counselors are generalists and, as such, have very little specific knowledge with respect to working with persons with epilepsy. Fraser et al.[18] found that only a small percentage of persons with epilepsy referred to state vocational rehabilitation agencies actually entered competitive employment, whereas a much higher proportion from specific epilepsy rehabilitation programs did. This suggests the desirability of providing specialized information and resources to the state rehabilitation counselor.

Entry into a state rehabilitation system may be facilitated if the applicant has sufficient medical documentation to establish the presence of a vocationally handicapping condition. It may also be facilitated if the applicant has met with an epilepsy rehabilitation specialist and presents the state agency with at least the outline of a feasible rehabilitation plan proposal. In the absence of this groundwork, the state agency counselor may have to spend considerable time amassing the necessary medical documentation, scheduling testing and evaluative services, and developing a rehabilitation plan.

Once an individual has been accepted as a state rehabilitation agency client and a plan has been developed, it generally involves some support from the state agency in terms of counseling and guidance, tuition or training fees, provision of necessary clothes or equipment, and similar items. It should be noted that the availability of funds for any of these concerns may vary greatly, depending on the region, local economic concerns, and current policy. Funding is generally not available for such items as child support, counseling, or therapy not directly related to the vocational rehabilitation goal or for other items not specifically linked to the rehabilitation or employment process. In planning to approach a state rehabilitation agency, it is also important to realize that many agencies have "first-dollar" regulations. These regulations require that state money not be spent on the rehabilitation agenda (e.g., community college tuition) if other money is readily available.

Availability of funds for training and education may vary greatly from region to region, and the availability of first-dollar resources may have to be explored. Preemployment "work-hardening" experiences similar to those discussed earlier may be available through a state agency. Especially useful in some contexts are various economic incentives to employers. These may include an actual subsidization of a job for a limited period of time. This arrangement, ordinarily termed an "on-the-job training contract," is generally a good-faith agreement with an employer that, following a brief period of employment and training, the client will be hired as a permanent employee.

SUMMARY AND CONCLUSIONS

This chapter discussed issues relevant to school and vocational adjustment in children and adolescents with epilepsy. Several basic themes were highlighted, including the importance of early identification of children in need of additional educational and vocational services, the potential contribution of neuropsychological assessment, and the importance of a multidiscipline evaluation and intervention approach.

References

1. Aldenkamp AP, Alpherts WCJ, Dekker MJA, et al. Neuropsychological aspects of learning disabilities in epilepsy. *Epilepsia.* 1990;31(Suppl 4): S9–S20.
2. Aldenkamp AP, Dodson WE. Introduction. *Epilepsia.* 1990;31(Suppl 4): S1.
3. American Academy of Pediatrics Committee on Drugs. Behavioral and cognitive effects of anticonvulsant therapy. *Pediatrics.* 1985;76:644–647.
4. Baird HW, John ER, Ahn H, et al. Neurometric evaluation of epileptic children who do well and poorly in school. *Electroencephalogr Clin Neurophysiol.* 1980;48:683–693.
5. Bagley CR. The educational performance of children with epilepsy. *Br J Educ Psychol.* 1970;40:82–83.
6. Barbacovi DR, Clelland RW. Special education in transition. In: *Public Law.* Arlington, VA: American Association of School Administrators; 1978;94–142.
7. Batzel LW, Dodrill CB, Dubinsky BL, et al. An objective method for the assessment of psychosocial problems in adolescents with epilepsy. *Epilepsia.* 1991;32:202–211.

8. Berent S, Sackellares JC. Clinical monitoring of children with epilepsy: A neurologic and neuropsychological perspective. In: Hermann BP, Seidenberg M, eds. *Childhood Epilepsies: Neuropsychological, Psychosocial, Intervention Aspects*. London: John Wiley.
9. Binnie CD, Channon S, Marston D. Learning disabilities in epilepsy: Neurophysiological aspects. *Epilepsia*. 1990;31(Suppl 4):S2–S8.
10. Camfield PE, Gates R, Rosen G, et al. Comparison of cognitive ability, personality profile, and school success in epileptic children with pure right versus left temporal lobe EEG foci. *Ann Neurol*. 1984;15:122–126.
11. Clemmons DC, Dodrill CB. Vocational outcomes of high school students with epilepsy. *J Appl Rehab Counsel*. 1983;14:49–53.
12. Clemmons DC, Dodrill CB. Vocational outcomes of high school students with epilepsy and neuropsychological correlates with later vocational success. In Porter RJ, Mattson RH, Ward AA Jr, et al., eds. *Advances in Epileptology,* Vol. 15. New York: Raven Press; 1984: 611–614.
13. Clemmons DC, Fraser RT, Getter A, et al. An abbreviated neuropsychological battery in multiple sclerosis (MS) vocational rehabilitation. *Rehab Psychol*. 2004;4(2).
14. Dodrill CB. Neuropsychology of epilepsy. In: Filskov SB, Boll TJ, eds. *Handbook of Clinical Neuropsychology*. New York: John Wiley; 1981: 366–398.
15. Dodrill CB, Clemmons D. Use of neuropsychological tests to identify high school students with epilepsy who later demonstrate inadequate performances in life. *J Consult Clin Psychol*. 1984;52:520–527.
16. Farwell JR, Dodrill CB, Batzel LW. Neuropsychological abilities of children with epilepsy. *Epilepsia* 1985;26:395–400.
17. Farwell JR, Lee YJ, Hirtz DG, et al. Phenobarbital for febrile seizures: Effects on intelligence and seizure remission. *N Engl J Med*. 1990;322:364–369.
18. Fraser R, Trejo W, Blanchard W. Epilepsy rehabilitation evaluating specialized vs. general agency outcome. *Epilepsia*. 1984;26:332–337.
19. Fraser R, Trejo W, Temkin N, et al. Assessing the vocational interest of those with epilepsy. *Rehab Psychol*. 1985;30:29–33.
20. Freeman JM, Jacobs H, Vining E, et al. Epilepsy and the inner city schools: A school-based program that makes a difference. *Epilepsia*. 1984;25: 438–442.
21. Hartlage LC, Green JB. The relation of parental attitudes to academic and social achievement in epileptic children. *Epilepsia*. 1972;13:21–26.
22. Hauser WA, Hesdorffer DC. *Facts About Epilepsy*. Landover, MD: Epilepsy Foundation of America; 1990.
23. Holdsworth L, Whitmore K. A study of children with epilepsy attending ordinary schools. I. Their seizure patterns, progress and behavior in school. *Dev Med Child Neurol*. 1974;16:746–758.
24. Huberty TJ, Austin JK, Risinger MW, et al. Relationship of selected seizure variables in children with epilepsy to performance on school-administered achievement tests. *J Epilepsy*. 1992;5:10–16.
25. Long CG, Moore JR. Parental expectations for their epileptic children. *J Child Psychol Psychiatry*. 1979;20:299–312.
26. Matthews WS, Barabas G, Ferrari M. Emotional concomitants of childhood epilepsy. *Epilepsia*. 1982;23:671–681.
27. Mirsky A. Information processing in petit mal epilepsy. In: Hermann BP, Seidenberg M, eds. *Childhood Epilepsies: Neuropsychological, Psychosocial, Intervention Aspects*. London: John Wiley; 1989:51–70.
28. Pazzaglia P, Frank-Pazzaglia L. Record in grade school of pupils with epilepsy: An epidemiological study. *Epilepsia*. 1976;17:361–366.
29. Rao SM, Cognitive Function Study Group, National Multiple Sclerosis Society. *A Manual for the Brief Repeatable Battery of Neuropsychology Tests in Multiple Sclerosis*. New York: National Multiple Sclerosis Society; 1990.
30. Rao SM, Leo GJ, Ellington L, et al. Cognitive dysfunction in multiple sclerosis. II Impact on employment and social functioning. *Neurology*. 1991;41:692–696.
31. Rourke BP. Central processing deficiencies in children: Towards a developmental neuropsychological model. *J Clin Neuropsychol*. 1982; 4:1–18.
32. Rutter M, Graham P, Yule W. *A Neuropsychiatric Study in Childhood*. London: Spastics International; 1970.
33. Santilli N, Dodson WE, Walton AV. *Students with Seizures: A Manual for School Nurses*. Landover, MD: Epilepsy Foundation of America; 1991.
34. Seidenberg M. Academic achievement and school performance of children with epilepsy. In: Hermann BP, Seidenberg M, eds. *Childhood Epilepsies: Neuropsychological, Psychosocial, Intervention Aspects*. London: John Wiley; 1989:105–118.
35. Seidenberg M. Academic performance of children with epilepsy. In: Sackellares JC, Berent S, eds. *Psychological Disturbances in Epilepsy*. Newton, MA: Butterworth Heinemann; 1996:99–108.
36. Seidenberg M, Beck N, Geisser M, et al. Academic achievement of children with epilepsy. *Epilepsia*. 1986;27:753–759.
37. Seidenberg M, Beck N, Geisser M, et al. Neuropsychological correlates of academic achievement of children with epilepsy. *J Epilepsy*. 1987;1:23–30.
38. Seidenberg M, Berent S. Childhood epilepsy and the role of psychology. *Am Psychol*. 1992;47:1130–1133.
39. Stores G. Studies of attention and seizure disorders. *Dev Med Child Neurol*. 1973;15:376–382.
40. Stores G, Hart J. Reading skills of children with generalized or focal epilepsy attending ordinary school. *Dev Med Child Neurol*. 1976;18:705–716.
41. Taylor DC. Psychosocial components of childhood epilepsy. In: Hermann BP, Seidenberg M, eds. *Childhood Epilepsies: Neuropsychological, Psychosocial, Intervention Aspects*. London: John Wiley; 1989:119–142.
42. Townes BD, Trupin EW, Martin DC, et al. Neuropsychological correlates of academic success among elementary school children. *J Consult Clin Psychol*. 1980;48:675–684.
43. Trimble M. Antiepileptic drugs, cognitive function, and behavior in children: Evidence from recent studies. *Epilepsia*. 1990;31:S30–S34.
44. Yule W. Educational achievement. In Kulig BM, Meinardi H, Stores G, eds. *Epilepsy and Behavior*. Lisse, The Netherlands: Swets & Zerlinger; 1980: 162–168.

CHAPTER 219 ■ THE RANGE OF NEEDS AND SERVICES IN VOCATIONAL REHABILITATION

RUPPRECHT THORBECKE AND ROBERT T. FRASER

INTRODUCTION

The employment concerns for individuals with epilepsy have been repeatedly documented in the literature. The Epilepsy Foundation generally cites an unemployment rate of 13% to 25% for people with epilepsy in the U.S. labor force.[43] An earlier study by Emlen and Ryan[25] suggests that this statistic pertains to those who are maintaining an active job search. If persons who have been discouraged from seeking work were additionally included, the unemployment statistic would be closer to 34%. In the study of Emlen and Ryan, individuals having one or more generalized tonic–clonic or complex partial seizures a year had an even higher unemployment rate of 50%.

From an international perspective, the situation does not look appreciably different. A study from the United Kingdom[24] revealed an unemployment rate for vocationally active patients with epilepsy of 46%, compared with 19% in an appropriate age- and sex-matched group. A study from an Irish clinic[9] showed, for a period of 12 months, an unemployment rate of 34% in men, which compared poorly with the unemployment rate of 13% in the general population. A German study[7] found that 24% of a group of epileptic persons were unemployed, with unemployment in the general population being 8% to 10%. Mean duration of unemployment was 30 months, compared with 11.6 months in the general population. In an epidemiologic study in Germany in 1995, 29% of persons with epilepsy in the labor force were unemployed, with general unemployment being 10.4%, and 15% for persons with a disability certificate.[60] In a Finnish study, a cohort of 245 children younger than 16 years was recruited for a long-term follow-up. Thirty years later, of those with uncomplicated epilepsy 64% were seizure free for 5 years or more. In comparison to a matched control group 31% of those with epilepsy were unemployed, while 8% of the controls were unemployed. Further analysis gave hints that nonidiopathic etiology and learning disability might be relevant for these differences.[70,71] A caveat in understanding unemployment rates among this disabled group is that many studies have used populations from epilepsy clinics that are more severely impaired. For the United States, the Emlen and Ryan study,[25] which utilized a pharmacy register, and for Germany the Pfaefflin May study would be most representative.

Earlier studies have indicated that people with epilepsy can also be overrepresented in unskilled and semiskilled positions.[47,62] They may also drop out of the workforce prematurely.[59] In Germany in 2004, the mean age for early retirement because of illness or disability was 50.4 for men and 49.1 for women years, whereas for those with epilepsy it was 45.6 and 43.2 years, respectively. In addition, 12.1% of all men and 14.4% of all women with illness or disability retiring early were below 40 years of age, compared with 27.2% of men and 35.4% of women retiring because of epilepsy. These employment statistics are chiefly from industrialized countries, and the work difficulties experienced by persons with epilepsy in developing countries are not well documented.

It is of interest that in a German study up to 60% of employees with epilepsy had active seizures, but 70% had them outside work.[22] In an English study,[11] 51% of employees with epilepsy had a seizure at work, and this was even higher in a Tunisian study.[39] It is also of interest that risk of accident related to seizures in the workplace is either not higher than the nondisabled[52] or slightly higher and yet inconsequential as compared to impairing injury.[81,84] It is interesting to observe that in the European study 3% of persons with epilepsy (PWE), in contrast to 1% of controls, had an accident at the workplace in 24 months ($p < .01$); however, when seizure-related accidents were omitted the accident rate of PWE fell only to 2.5% ($p < .05$), indicating that medication side effects and neurologic deficits could be a more important factor.[81]

There is broad agreement in the literature that the employment problems of people with epilepsy cannot be reduced to one factor (i.e., seizure severity), but that they are rather the result of a bundle of adversive factors interacting with each other in a complex fashion. These factors include a lack of education and vocational training, neuropsychological deficits, lack of information, social isolation and resulting social skills deficits, and negative attitudes on the part of the family or employers. Unemployment appears to be minimally two to three times that of the general population (e.g., as shown in the 1979 Emlen and Ryan general pharmacy sample[25]) and still worse within the populations of specialized epilepsy clinics.

There appears to be two major issues. One is that of initial job access after secondary school. For example, at the University of Washington Epilepsy Center, vocational clients requesting services have approximately 13 years of education, which usually comprises high school and some additional community college course work. The common theme is that no specific vocational entry or transition plan exists, and youngsters with the disability simply "go on" to further community college training because it is considered "normative" despite often pronounced impairments. A second major issue is that people with epilepsy in the workforce often must deal with repeated and long periods of unemployment. It seems that these persons are a group with a specific cluster of problems and that their employment situation can be definitively improved by employment services addressing these problems as a whole rather than focusing on one simple concern, such as seizure status.

It is important to note that there is not one, but several profiles for job-seeking groups with epilepsy. Chaplin,[12] for purposes of understanding intervention needs, has proposed four categories of employment seekers with MS:

Group 1: Individuals with seizure control, a good work/educational background, and requiring minimal intervention other than some disclosure training.

Group 2: Those with acceptable seizure control, but unrealistic career goals based upon personal capacity. Vocational assessment (to include situational) can be very helpful.

Group 3: Those with unsatisfactory seizure control and interactive cognitive and emotional difficulties. They require comprehensive vocational and psychosocial intervention to achieve employment.

Group 4: Individuals who are typically not able to maintain competitive work due to seizure type, frequency, cognitive deficits, etc., and have typically required sheltered and supported work.

Traditionally, the latter group has been employed in sheltered workshops. There is now, however, a strong movement in bringing this group out of sheltered employment into the open labor market, and it is important to consider the implications of this movement for those currently in sheltered settings. It is beyond the scope of this chapter to review in detail vocational strategies for persons with epilepsy and associated disabilities—the associated disabilities can be a greater source of impairment than the epilepsy. New movements and legislation have brought about exciting developments in vocational rehabilitation for persons with epilepsy, but substantial challenges remain to include funding.

POSTSECONDARY SCHOOL VOCATIONAL ASSESSMENT

Unquestionably, a successful transition after secondary school into suitable employment or targeted vocational training is the best groundwork for stable employment in adult life. Nevertheless, studies or demonstration projects attempting to isolate the factors relevant for successful transition are surprisingly scarce.

Vocational Interests/Work Values

Some research is available that is specific to the vocational interests of individuals with epilepsy. Schultz and Thorbecke,[67] in a study of 116 people with epilepsy, including young adults, being assessed vocationally, found that initially 47% desired training for an occupation in the field of social sciences, for example, nurse or educator. As a result of the assessment, however, no one was recommended for training in this area. Fraser et al.[34] studied the vocational interests of 47 male and 24 female patients with epilepsy attending the University of Washington Regional Epilepsy Center using primarily the six major occupational scales and three special scales of the Strong-Campell Interest Inventory. Male patients with major motor seizures had lower Academic Orientation and Investigative scores than male normal controls ($p < .01$), and male patients with early-onset epilepsy had lower Investigative scores than normal controls ($p < .01$). Female vocational interests were not significantly different from those of the normal control group. The authors concluded that in line with previous research, male patients appear to be more greatly affected developmentally by epilepsy and that disability alone does not influence vocational orientation, but rather severity of the disability and age at disablement. The authors suggest supportive counseling, social experiences, and involvement in "hands on" and exploratory types of tasks for young men in the home and within the academic setting. Presently, there remains a need for further and more comprehensive studies of this type. It should be noted that work values or reinforcers ("things about the job") may be more important than interests in actual job choice. In one study,[29] securing a job close to home was significantly more important ($p < .01$) for those who found work than the unemployed. If this need couldn't be met, job outcome was less successful.

Pattern of Abilities

Studies of aptitudes or abilities present a number of other interesting issues. Clemmons[13] used the General Aptitude Test Battery (GATB), which has been in use throughout state employment and rehabilitation services in the United States. Fifty patients at the University of Washington Epilepsy Center were tested. Test scores did not discriminate between the successfully employed and unemployed. Furthermore, when the mean scores of the employed group were compared with the published GATB norms, all scores of the employed people with epilepsy were found to be significantly lower. The author emphasized that factors such as social support and appropriateness and psychosocial status might be more crucial job access variables than aptitudes.[13] Specialized vocational assistance and placement may also compensate for lesser abilities in highly motivated job seekers with epilepsy.

In a study by Clemmons and Dodrill,[16] the vocational outcome of 40 high school students with epilepsy 4.5 years after graduation was assessed. When looking for factors discriminating the unemployed from the employed, no influence of sex, age, or time since high school graduation could be detected. However, mean scores on the Wechsler Adult Intelligence Scale (WAIS) and the Halstead Impairment Index were significantly different across the groups ($p < .01$), with the strongest discriminator being the Aphasia Test ($p < .001$). The unemployed did significantly more poorly on these tests than those who were working. The working and nonworking groups were easily distinguished on the basis of neuropsychological and intelligence measures. The authors suggest identifying those at risk for unemployment based on these variables before they enter the workforce and offering them specialized and intensive vocational services.

Epilepsy-related Restrictions and Limitations

Scharfenstein and Thorbecke,[65] while performing a secondary analysis of vocational rehabilitation by the Department of Vocational Rehabilitation of the Berlin Labor Exchange, found severe epilepsy-related job restrictions in the records (Table 1). Only 11% of the records indicated the type of seizure and only 19% the seizure frequency. Such restrictions are in sharp contrast to the consistently reported low accident rates of people with epilepsy as noted previously. This holds true for persons known to the employer as having the disability and also for persons who do not disclose epilepsy.[77] Therefore, the development of approaches to assess the work-related risks of persons with epilepsy on an individual basis should be of high priority.

Behavioral Problems and Social Skills Deficits Associated with Epilepsy

In addition to some of the issues described above, there appear to be a number of variables affecting social and interpersonal

TABLE 1

WORK RESTRICTIONS FOR PEOPLE WITH EPILEPSY (DEPARTMENT OF VOCATIONAL REHABILITATION—BERLIN)

	Adults with epilepsy ($n = 32$)	Controls ($n = 32$)	Youths with epilepsy ($n = 32$)	Controls ($n = 32$)
No "dangerous tasks" (working with machinery, working in high places)	100%	22%	67%	11%
No "shift work"	94%	44%	60%	
No "piece work"	44%	22%	60%	
No "responsibility"	13%	9%	7%	11%
No "intellectually demanding tasks"	25%		27%	

behavior and competency for youth and adults coming into epilepsy rehabilitation programs. Work at the University of Washington Epilepsy Center[30] indicates that through several years (1988–1990) during which participants entered vocational services, additional disabilities were prevalent in 89% of this population. Mild to moderate neuropsychological impairment was salient; 37% to 54% (depending on the study group) had a specific documented brain insult, and 26% to 40% had an additional psychiatric diagnosis. The percentages of those with physical disability were minor. Wada et al. in a series of 278 patients in the unemployed found a significantly higher proportion with neuropsychiatric complications.[82]

Earlier work by Goldin et al.[38] suggests that children and adolescents with additional disabilities are more socially isolated and less involved in extracurricular and school social activities. Consequently, they have not had the exposure to social organizational activities through which social skills and competencies are developed. It would appear that youths with active seizures have increased dependency and are less involved in normal risk-taking and social activities, with a subgroup further restricted by additional emotional and cognitive limitations.

A lack of social skills development can be exacerbated by frequent seizure activity and side effects of drugs. As individuals with a seizure disorder mature, emotional and behavioral difficulties can become more pronounced as they react to isolation and failure in the social environment. Curly et al.[17] restricted their study of risk factors for psychosocial maladjustment to a sample of boys ($n = 60$) because they observed that boys seemed to have more adjustment difficulties than girls.[74] This has also been the experience of Fraser et al.[34] In the study by Curly et al., neuropsychological impairment, divisive parenting styles, and number of lifetime seizures accounted for approximately 50% of the variance related to the boys' behavioral disturbances—neuropsychologic impairment for 28% and the other two variables for 13%. Young boys in particular may be a subgroup having greater adjustment difficulty because of lack of support and greater expectations for performance within sports and the vocational areas.

SERVICES

Job access after school may vary between different countries because of different traditions. Therefore, the structure of some services will be outlined without a description of specific features.

Prevocational Intervention (Work Preparatory Courses, Social Rehabilitation)

Freeman and Gayle in 1978[36] initiated in Baltimore a school-based program to facilitate transition from school to employment. During the first 3 years of the program, 333 students with epilepsy were identified, with a mean age of 16 years (range, 12–21 years). The program provided counseling, epilepsy education, and work experience. Students in a first step participated in vocational training courses within their schools and then were offered job opportunities. When the employment outcome was evaluated 2 years after graduation, only 18% of the participating adolescents with epilepsy but 31% of the students without disabilities were identified as program dropouts (i.e., not holding a job or being in school or training).

The key factor to the success of this project was that it enabled the school system personnel to meet the requirements of the law (Public Law 94-142) in developing individualized programs for students with disabilities. In other words, the program assisted overworked and underfunded school personnel to complete required work activity.[35] It was "housed within the school system." Other projects, in Cleveland[80] and Seattle,[14] have encountered more significant difficulties in securing the cooperation of school personnel in obtaining access to youths with epilepsy for enrollment in school-to-work transition programs.

Similar programs were offered in the United Kingdom and in the Irish Republic. A work preparation course by the British Epilepsy Association[6] is conducted during 4 to 6 weeks and offers, in addition to epilepsy education, a comprehensive program of counseling, industrial visits, and work experience. Carroll[10] reported on a 6-month training program from Ireland, during which the trainees were assisted in developing social and communication skills and allowed to sample basic activities in art, drama, home management, and woodworking. On completion, 60% of the trainees with epilepsy versus 72% of the trainees without epilepsy were placed. One year later, 40% of the participants with epilepsy still were employed. When interviewed, participants with epilepsy found the program helpful in increasing their self-confidence and social skills.

At the Heemstede Center in Holland,[18] group training is provided in the following areas, considered vital to good vocational preparation: (a) Coping with seizures in work situations, (b) educating colleagues at work about epilepsy, (c) coping with colleagues' attitudes, and (d) interviewing techniques (role playing). As part of the group training, participants are given work experience during which they practice what has been learned. Similarly, in Germany, work preparatory courses lasting 1 or 2 years have been designed to integrate adolescents with disabilities into the general labor market as unskilled or semiskilled workers. In 2005 these courses were changed to a more open and flexible form including more practical work experience and allowing continuing with formal vocational training if the young adult shows sufficient capabilities.

Such courses are a valuable trajectory from school to employment for young adults with epilepsy for whom seizures are the main handicap. However, for those having additional physical or neuropsychological handicaps, vocational assessment and training are necessary to identify job goals more appropriately.

TABLE 2

EPILEPSY RISK CATEGORIES OF THE GERMAN TASK FORCE

"O"	No loss of consciousness; no loss of posture; control of own actions (seizures only with subjective symptoms)
"A"	No loss of consciousness; no loss of posture; impairment of ongoing activity
"B"	Impaired consciousness; interruption of ongoing activity; no loss of posture
"C"	No loss/loss of consciousness; loss of posture; interruption of ongoing activity
"D"	Impaired consciousness; no loss of posture; actions not in accordance with demands of the situation

Vocational Assessment and Its Components

Around the world in rehabilitation centers or epilepsy centers, assessment units have been set up for people with disabilities, including epilepsy. Vocational assessment typically involves the use of vocational interest inventories, work values inventories, academic achievement testing, intelligence assessment, assessment of emotional and personality functioning, and (depending on job goals) assessment of visual–spatial abilities, motor speed, and dexterity. For individuals with a known or suspected brain insult or impairment of functioning, a full neuropsychological evaluation is requested. For individuals more severely compromised by epilepsy and neuropsychological impairment, a number of commercially available or devised work samples may be utilized to identify a skill that might be transferable to repetitive work (e.g., filing by numbers). If an individual has no specific work goal that can be identified, time should be spent in identifying work-related values (e.g., aspects of work—an esthetically pleasing environment, working with a mixed group of young men and women) that might draw them into some type of work. At a number of the European rehabilitation or sheltered work facilities, a wide range of work activity that can be sampled is often available.

At the University of Washington Epilepsy Center Vocational Services, job tryouts are planned as they relate to a client's job goal, either in a volunteer setting within the hospital or within the private sector under a special 1993 U.S. Department of Labor waiver that allows unpaid work for up to 215 hours. In addition to a rehabilitation counselor monitoring this job tryout or community-based assessment, a job coach often is present to coach the client and take performance data. In the United States, sheltered work facilities are generally used for evaluation or training purposes only with the most impaired clients. Vocational assessment of people with epilepsy must always have two main components: (a) Evaluation of seizure-related restrictions and (b) Evaluation of abilities based on work samples and often neuropsychological testing (if there is a known brain insult).

A first step is always *a complete description of seizure variables* to assess vocational risks. Is there an aura or warning that allows the patient to prepare for a seizure? What is the state of consciousness during a seizure? Does the person with epilepsy fall, and what is the typical pattern of behavior during a seizure? How does the person behave after a seizure (e.g., confusion, disturbance of speech, paralysis of limbs, sleep)? How long does it take until the person is able to resume usual activity? At what time do seizures tend to occur (e.g., during sleep, after awakening), or are they completely unpredictable? Have seizure triggers been observed (e.g., sleep deprivation, alcohol intake, emotional issues)? Has the individual experienced other injuries secondary to a seizure incident? These are representative issues in assessing vocational concerns or risks.

A German group of epileptologists and professionals from rehabilitation centers, large companies, and state accident insurances recently suggested five categories of increasing risk that can be used to evaluate the occupational suitability of persons with epilepsy (Table 2).[1] Seizure frequency was grouped into four categories: More than one seizure per month, three to 11 per year, no more than two per year, and seizure free.

To demonstrate the practicality of these categories, vocations in electromechanics, metal work, health care, and pedagogics were assessed.[1]

Such guidelines facilitate assessment of suitability for certain "dangerous" vocations on an individual basis. However, before such an evaluation is performed, a person's drug regimen and compliance should be assessed to be sure that the person with epilepsy is grouped into the most appropriate category. In the United States, legislation requires consideration of workplace accommodations (adaptive procedures, physical modification of the job site, adaptive equipment that lowers risk). Nevertheless, there may remain situations in which the individual risk must be assessed using such a categorization.

Vocational planning traditionally has been done with the help of psychological testing. For people with epilepsy, however, such a strategy seems to be successful only if procedures are used that are sensitive to the specific abilities and deficits often found. As mentioned earlier, the GATB, which has been universally used in the United States, was not very predictive of the employment status of adolescents with epilepsy. On the other hand, neuropsychological tests predict job success at 1 year reasonably well[15] for those with epilepsy and known brain impairment.

In Germany, 46 rehabilitation centers now exist for young adults—all with a vocational assessment unit. Assessment is done both by evaluation of work samples from different occupational fields and by psychological testing. Finger[27] did an extended study within the assessment unit of the Bethel Epilepsy Rehabilitation Center. Seventy-eight young adults (mean age, 20.25 years; standard deviation [SD], 3.52) were given an extended battery of neuropsychological tests. In addition, epilepsy variables were documented carefully. The dependent variable was recommendation of formal training as a manual worker by the professional team (master educators or social workers) after evaluation of 3 months of work samples. The result was that none of the 10 persons with a history of status epilepticus was given a recommendation for training ($p < .05$).

The neuropsychological test battery, comprising Picture Arrangement, Digit Symbol Test, Concentration Endurance Test/d2, Stroop (Naming of Color Dots, Naming of Color Prints), Controlled Oral Word Association Test, Name Writing Preferred Hand, Trail Making Test Part B, and Purdue Pegboard Test (Preferred Hand and Both Hands Assembly), discriminated well between the trained and untrained groups. Stepwise discriminative function analysis correctly classified 73% of the persons without and 89% of those with training recommendation (81% and 60% in the cross-validation sample). These results underscore the importance of sensorimotor coordination, motor speed of the dominant side, speed of information processing of selective stimuli, cognitive flexibility, and mastery of abstract language concepts for vocational training.

It can be seen from these results that neuropsychological tests are a very effective tool for rehabilitation planning that includes special training considerations or appropriate job accommodations. It is important, however, not to ignore other capabilities of a client (e.g., compensatory capabilities or social skills). The final goal of vocational training is not successful training but successful placement, which can require additional abilities not measured through neuropsychological tests.

Vocational Training Courses for Young Adults with Epilepsy

Germany has a developed system of vocational training centers for young adults with disabilities. State legislation guarantees every young person with a disability vocational training that takes into account the limitations of the disability. To offer such training, 42 centers have been established, some with a focus on epilepsy and one (Bethel) specializing in assessing those with severe epilepsy or with epileptic and pseudoepileptic seizures. About 7% of the trainees in these centers (about 1,000 persons) have epilepsy.

Rehabilitation, as a rule, begins with an initial assessment by the Department of Vocational Rehabilitation (DVR). Skilled training in a rehabilitation center is proposed for about 60%, and a 3-month extended assessment for 40%. If the DVR counselor or the staff in the assessment unit concludes that it is still too early to enter formal training, a 1-year preparatory course may be offered through a rehabilitation center. During these courses, basic social and vocational skills are developed. Formal training as a rule takes 3 years. At the end, the trainees have to pass an examination in which they must solve the same tasks as an apprentice in a workshop or company elsewhere. The rate of success is high (see above), a consequence of careful selection during the different stages before formal training. Depending on the general unemployment rate between 1995 and 2003, between two-thirds and three fourths have been placed into competitive employment. There are, however, studies from the rehabilitation centers at Heidelberg and Bethel[83] showing that placement of young adults with epilepsy after successful training is more difficult than for trainees with other handicaps. This problem underscores the importance of specialized placement services being available.

School-to-work Transition

There remains a continuing need for developing and evaluating more integrated models of school-to-work transition in which the previously discussed issues are addressed at the same time (i.e., family education and family acceptance of new roles, vocational goal setting based an individual interests and work values, neuropsychological tests, and paid work experience with on-site support and assessment). At the end of such a sequence of activity, reassessment should be done with the aim of confirming or redesigning long-range employment goals.[68]

UNEMPLOYMENT, UNDEREMPLOYMENT, AND WORK-RELATED DIFFICULTIES OF THE EMPLOYED

It has long been understood that persons with epilepsy have much higher rates of unemployment than persons without epilepsy (see Introduction). Unemployment statistics, however, provide only one perspective. Another perspective relates to difficulties at work for those who are employed (e.g., being underemployed because of undue concern about a seizure disorder, or being "encouraged" toward early retirement because of disability).

Subgroups of the Unemployed and Underemployed

Chronically unemployed persons with epilepsy very often have additional handicaps, such as specific neurologic or neuropsychological deficits, physical handicaps, and emotional and behavioral difficulties. Fukoshima,[37] in a sample of 136 patients at Hirosaki University Hospital in Japan, found 100% of patients with controlled epilepsy and without additional handicaps in the regular workforce. On the other hand, 15% of those with uncontrolled seizures, 29% of those with an additional personality disorder, 36% of those with subnormal intelligence, and 41% of those with additional physical disability were unemployed. Dennerell et al.[19] analyzed in depth differences between 177 employed and unemployed adult patients with seizures. Utilizing verbal IQ, performance IQ, and education as predictors, they could correctly classify 67% of the patients as employed or unemployed. When scores from the Halstead-Reitan Neuropsychological Battery and the California Personality Inventory were included, 78% were correctly classified. It is likely that accurate employment classification would increase with additional information regarding disability or psychiatric status. It is the "epilepsy and additional disability" information that is generally unavailable relative to employment, but is available at the Michigan clinic.

Seizures and Unemployment

The influence of type and frequency of seizures as a risk for unemployment is controversial. Some studies[25,37,42,45,68] show a clear and consistent influence of type and frequency of seizures on rate of unemployment. In an epidemiologic study in Germany for a group of 660 persons between 15 and 60 years old, a consistent relation between seizure frequency and employment could be shown. Interestingly, unemployment of PWE aligned the general unemployment rate not before having become seizure free for 3 years or more.[60] Conversely, studies from epilepsy centers could not detect any significant influence of seizure frequency on unemployment, underscoring the larger role of psychiatric and neuropsychological factors in unemployment.[3,16] One explanation for this finding could be that specialized centers attract patients in whom psychiatric and neuropsychological difficulties are overrepresented. Another explanation could be that there has been a relative increase or identification of psychiatric difficulties in the last

30 years, as can be seen in the studies of Penin.[59] This author followed adults with epilepsy receiving early retirement between 1960 and 1979. In 1960, 75% of all early retirements were a consequence of high seizure frequency, whereas in 1979 this was true for only 25%. Instead of seizure frequency, psychiatric and neuropsychological variables were more in evidence. This is attributed by the author to better seizure control at the end of his study, in 1980, than at the beginning, in 1960.[59]

Some insight on the relationship between unemployment and seizure frequency comes from studies of the social outcome of surgical treatment. In a Norwegian study,[40] 156 surgically treated patients were followed for 17 years and then compared in regard to employment status with a group of nonsurgically treated patients. Treated patients who were employed at the time of surgery were significantly more involved in work at follow-up. On the other hand, those with epilepsy who were unemployed at the time of surgery were not better employed at follow-up than controls, although their seizure status was better than that of the controls and their self-reported "working ability" had improved highly significantly. A study from the Seattle group[28] showed similar results concerning the effects of surgery on employment. Furthermore, it was observed that those patients who remain employed after surgery gain a higher functional level—higher earnings, more working time, and wider responsibilities. In a U.S. study measuring long-term outcome after anterior temporal lobectomy, employment of the surgical group had significantly improved in comparison to the control group; there were, however, no differences between those having become seizure free and those with continuing seizures.[49]

A field of growing interest is changes in the psychosocial situation after a first epileptic seizure or with newly diagnosed epilepsy. There was one study on socioeconomic prognosis after a newly diagnosed unprovoked seizure. Unemployment was higher for those with continuing seizures.[53]

In sum, the relationship between seizure frequency and employment seems to be complex. Among the employed, some with severe epilepsy are not dismissed because of protective legislation in countries such as the United States and Germany. Seizure frequency may also be overshadowed by other factors—neuropsychological and psychiatric—important to employability. However, this does not mean that seizures can be neglected when the issue of unemployment is discussed. It would appear extremely important not to overlook seizure factors relevant for employment, such as the timing of seizure occurrence, potential warnings, provoking factors, falling, duration, and postictal confusion.[57]

Neuropsychological Deficits and Employability

Commonly used neuropsychological batteries include the Luria-Nebraska Neuropsychological Battery and the Halstead-Reitan Battery. Dodrill[21] established a comprehensive battery of 16 discriminative measures sensitive to brain impairment and epilepsy. This battery includes the Halstead Neuropsychological Battery for Adults; the Aphasia Screening Test; the Trail Making Test; the Logical Memory and Visual Reproduction parts of the Wechsler Memory Scale, Form 1; the Sensory-Perceptual Examination; the Stroop Test; and the Seashore Total Memory Test. This battery or others should enable an assessment of a broad range of capabilities, including motor performance, sensory-perceptual abilities, memory performance, attention span, language skills, visual-spatial abilities, problem-solving capacities, and general cognitive efficiency. For individuals referred to a regional or tertiary resource epilepsy center, it is these kinds of difficulties that will affect employability as much or more than seizures. It is common at the University of Washington Regional Epilepsy Center to refer an individual for a neuropsychological evaluation if there is a history of job losses and pronounced emotional difficulties. Sometimes individuals with both emotional problems and suspected cognitive deficits are also referred for assessment. Approximately 40% of the vocational program participants at the University of Washington Regional Epilepsy Center have experienced a head injury. In these cases, the importance of a neuropsychological assessment is further emphasized. Before neuropsychological information was utilized more carefully in vocational planning, it was very common for individuals to lose jobs because of memory difficulties, abstraction deficits, motor and visual-spatial problem-solving concerns, and general cognitive inefficiency.

In a cross-sectional validation study of 58 persons with epilepsy,[8] the neuropsychological scores of the Dodrill battery differentiated very well between the unemployed, the underemployed (working in sheltered employment settings or in competitive settings <20 hours per week), and the employed. The percentage of total test measures outside normal limits was 64% in the unemployed, 53% in the underemployed, and 22% in the employed ($p < .001$). When the subtests were inspected, the greatest differences could be found in tasks emphasizing motor performance and visual-spatial skills.[8] In another study from the University of Washington Epilepsy Center at Seattle,[32] 46 outpatients were followed prospectively in regard to employability. The best discriminators were the Digit Symbol Test from the WAISR Scale and the Name Writing Procedure. The neuropsychological battery for epilepsy correctly classified 70% of both employed and unemployed.[28] From this finding and general test data trends in the study, a picture emerged showing the unemployed having more difficulties with tasks requiring tactile, motor, perceptual, and spatial integration skills and having more neuropsychological deficits in general.

It is interesting to speculate on the development of such deficits in the course of epilepsy. Rodin[62] reported on 90 patients who were reassessed 6 years after their first evaluation at the Epilepsy Center of Michigan. Those who were unemployed at follow-up had several additional problems: Drug resistance, behavioral abnormalities, and neuropsychological deficits that had not been observed at the first examination 6 years earlier.[62] Dodrill,[20] in a very careful study assessing the association between number of generalized tonic–clonic seizures and neuropsychological functioning, reported a significant increase of neuropsychological deficits in comparing persons with two to 10, 11 to 100, and more than 100 generalized tonic–clonic seizures, and a history of status epilepticus. The sharpest loss of abilities was noted in the group of patients with a history of status epilepticus. It appears that neuropsychological variables are the most important predictors of employment stability or instability, and neuropsychological assessment tools are of immense practical value for rehabilitation planning.

Interactions with Employers and Colleagues

In one hypothesis for the high rate of unemployment among people with epilepsy, misinformation and the negative attitudes of employers are considered to be important causal factors. A study by Sands and Zalkind[63] of employment policies and attitudes toward persons with epilepsy showed that feelings about hiring people with epilepsy were more unfavorable than they were about hiring persons with heart disease, cancer, or diabetes. A similar result was found in a study from the United Kingdom,[48] in which the attitudes of 52 personnel officers toward employees with epilepsy were compared with their attitudes toward persons with heart conditions, loss of one eye or leg, diabetes, or chronic bronchitis. A recent study from the United Kingdom in which 240 employers were endorsed qualifies these findings.[46] About one fifth said that a prospective employee's epilepsy would be a major issue (mainly in respect to safety). When asked to consider a series of six conditions, epilepsy caused "the greatest overall concern" after depression or heart disease and the highest concern after depression with respect to absenteeism and accidents. About one fourth of the companies had experience employing PWE. In those companies the proportion of jobs deemed to be suitable for PWE and the willingness to make workplace accommodations were greater, and the belief that insurance costs could increase less likely. A higher proportion of jobs in larger businesses were regarded as suitable for PWE than in small ones.

It seems that the basis for negative employer attitudes is the lack of practical information about epilepsy. Holmes and McWilliams,[44] when surveying 116 employers in Tennessee, asking them, "If your company physician told you that an applicant with epilepsy was physically able to work, would you hire him?" got 72% positive answers and only a small proportion of negative responses; however, a relatively high proportion (24%) of employers expressed the view that they were unsure. From an earlier UK study,[48] it was also obvious that information deficits were one of the main barriers to employment; 43% of employers wrongly believed that insurance companies would not provide normal liability insurance rates.[48] The above findings suggest that employers could profit from basic educational to improve their hiring practices.

When looking at interactions with employers, there are also the emotional aspects that cannot be overseen. In all studies cited, there are prejudicial hints—high percentages of "unsure" answers or contradictions between positive and negative attitudes toward hiring in more specific questions. Sands and Zalkin,[63] in their demonstration project, undertook a rigorous education campaign over 1 year to change employer attitudes. The outcome was totally negative. There were no meaningful differences when the experimental (educational intervention) city was compared with the control city. From this the authors concluded the following:

> "Modification of employer attitudes toward hiring the epileptic may therefore require something more than the usual public education program. Employers must be actively involved in education campaigns by their actually seeking and providing jobs for qualified epileptics. As a result of such involvement in placement, the policy-level business executive will learn about epilepsy on an emotional level, which we postulate should result in an attitude change."[63]

It is just this approach that is often followed in modern vocational rehabilitation training and placement services. It would also be important to establish rules to prevent discriminatory hiring practices toward those with disabilities. A general framework for this is provided in the Americans with Disabilities Act, and specific guidelines are presented in the "principles for good practice" of the Employment Commission of the International Bureau for Epilepsy.[3]

There is now also a study in which the reactions of coworkers to PWE have been addressed.[41] When comparing the reactions to persons with depression, multiple sclerosis, and epilepsy, it seemed that coworkers are especially worried about sudden unpredictable behavior of PWE ($p < .013$) and feeling uncomfortable providing first aid to them ($p = .081$). This finding in accordance with the studies tapping employer attitudes suggests that educating people about epilepsy, especially about the concrete features of seizures and how to give first aid, could decrease worry and social avoidance.

Predictors of Long-term Employment Success

Prior sections of this chapter have dealt with seizures, neuropsychological deficits, behavioral abnormalities, additional handicaps, and employer attitudes as factors independently influencing the chances of persons with epilepsy to obtain or hold a job. From a broader perspective, it becomes obvious that these factors are interrelated. Frequent seizures may increase the likelihood of seizures occurring at work, which increases the risk for unemployment[76] and psychosocial problems.[20] Frequent seizures at the same time increase the risk for neuropsychological deficits,[20,62] and these in turn increase the risk for unemployment. It is also well known that unemployment increases the risk for psychiatric disorders and psychosocial problems, the latter being correlated with a bad seizure prognosis.[23]

Thus, it appears that services aimed at reducing the risk for unemployment will be effective only if they address joint factors at the same time and as early as possible. A second presupposition for long-term employment success is compensation for poor education and insufficient vocational training, which seem to be fundamental deficits in the unemployment status of people with epilepsy. Finally, it is insufficient simply to place these people in competitive, unsubsidized employment; they also need support to maintain steady employment and overcome periods of only cyclic employment.[33]

VOCATIONAL SERVICES

To address the employment problems of people with epilepsy, four types of services seem to be necessary:

1. Programs for assessment and short-term rehabilitation
2. Vocational retraining programs for those in occupations or trades unsuitable for anyone with a seizure disorder
3. Training and placement services for those who have completed vocational training or for those with poor work records
4. Services directed at keeping people with epilepsy employed (postplacement services)

It is obvious that such services in different countries may have different structures. For example, they may be separated or integrated, specialized for people with epilepsy, or specific for those with neurologic deficits or diverse disabilities.

Programs for Assessment and Short-term Rehabilitation

In 1983 in the United States, and then 15 years later in Germany, a type of service was launched that connected on the one hand high standard diagnosis and treatment approaches (including surgical treatment of the epilepsies) and on the other hand neuropsychological and psychiatric assessment and first steps of rehabilitation such as work experience, preparing structured vocational rehabilitation measures like retraining into a more suitable profession, or placement into competitive employment.

First data on the outcome of the U.S. program were given in 1983 by Fraser et al.[31]

From the German program, designed very similar to the American one, first data were given in 2004[73] comparing social and employment situations for a consecutive series of the first 96 patients before admission and 18 months after the 4- to 6-week enrollment in the program. Seventy-nine patients

(82%) had focal epilepsy. Physical comorbidity was found in 21%, and psychiatric comorbidity in 53% of the cohort. Compared with time point 1, seizure frequency and number of hospital admissions due to epilepsy were reduced at time point 2 ($p < 0.01$). Significant improvements were found in six out of seven quality-of-life domains (epilepsy-related fear, emotional adaptation, perceived restrictions, perceived stigma, mobility/independent living, and physical/emotional health) and in performance in daily life (e.g., going out alone, driving a car).

The employment situation also changed significantly: Unemployed, preadmission 48%, postenrollment 20%; employed, preadmission 33%, postenrollment 37%; sheltered employment, preadmission 6%, postenrollment 10%; vocational rehabilitation measures, preadmission 3%, postenrollment 11%; early disability pension, preadmission 2%, postenrollment 14%; homemaker, preadmission 8%, postenrollment 8%. Those who were employed preadmission and postenrollment reported significantly fewer problems at the workplace—time on sick leave, concentration and memory problems, and seizures at the workplace ($p = .014$).[72]

Retraining Centers for Adults

During the last 40 years in Germany, a network of centers has been developed; today, 28 centers have 14,500 retraining slots. They offer vocational retraining for a great number of occupations and trades. As a rule they have three components: (a) An assessment unit to assess interests and abilities over a 2- to 6-week period. At the end of the assessment, it is decided whether the client should be retrained, receive a disability pension, or be placed in unskilled or semiskilled employment without retraining. The decision to send a person to a retraining center is the responsibility of the local labor exchange's department of vocational rehabilitation or the rehabilitation department of the state pension insurance. (b) Retraining may begin with a 3-month preparatory course in which basic (school) abilities are retaught. (c) Two-year retraining follows. This is equivalent to 3 years of vocational training of young adults without disability after high school.

The proportion of people with epilepsy in these institutions is 1% to 3%. Some are specialized for persons with neurologic diseases, including epilepsy. Fifteen to 20% of the trainees drop out.

Schultz and Thorbecke[67] observed 73 people with epilepsy within the assessment unit of a Berlin retraining center for adults. Prognostic factors suggestive of training potential and level of retraining were age, number of additional handicaps, intellectual capacity, working pace, and drawing skills. Psychopathologic abnormalities sharply discriminated between those accepted versus not accepted for retraining.[67] No influence of seizure variables, which were carefully documented in the study, could be found.

In a study from the large retraining center at Heidelberg, Germany, Wöhrl[83] reported that 2 years after retraining, 68% of the persons with epilepsy ($n = 151$) were employed, whereas 79% of the persons with other disabilities ($n = 757$) were employed ($p < .01$), the level of vocational qualification being equivalent in both groups. This draws some attention to a need for specialized placement assistance for those with epilepsy.

Training and Placement Services

The most effective training and placement service for people with epilepsy worldwide has been the 20-year-old TAPS (training applicants for placement success) program of the Epilepsy Foundation of America (EFA). Over this time span, it grew continuously and became more specialized to the needs of special groups of people with epilepsy while simultaneously increasing the placement rate from about 55% at the beginning of the 1980s to nearly 70% at the beginning of the 1990s.

The background of the TAPS program was an EFA demonstration project in the 1960s in which group counseling was proved to be highly effective for the placement of job seekers with epilepsy and numerous other problems.[66] In 1976, with funding from the U.S. Department of Labor, the EFA started the TAPS program, which worked according to the same principles. The *client-oriented component* of TAPS is based on the principles of active peer support and shared responsibility. After intake and orientation sessions, participants received *training in job-seeking skills.* In the weekly meeting of the *job club,* they shared their actual job-seeking experiences and encouraged each other to continue the job search. During job club meetings, employers familiarized participants with their views of job applicants or did exercises with them to improve their job-seeking skills. Additionally, every participant received individual assistance as needed. *Placement* was achieved if an individual found part-time (15–29 hours) or full-time (30–40 hours) unsubsidized employment. *Follow-up services* were provided for 1 year following placement.

A second component of TAPS was aimed at *employer development and interagency collaboration.* Employer participation was to be found in all parts of the program. In *employer development,* staff gained information on current job opportunities and required qualifications through employer visits. Every regional TAPS had *a local advisory committee* composed of employers and representatives of relevant local agencies. Finally, staff provided *education and mediation services* for local employers regarding employment and epilepsy issues.

TAPS programs existed in 13 American cities, largely supported by the U.S. Department of Labor.[5] There were 1,351 persons with epilepsy enrolled in 1994, with 914 (68%) being placed in unsubsidized employment. Among these, 77% maintained employment 90 days after placement. Placement of women, however, reached only 39%, and placement of youth only 7%. Average cost per placement was approximately $750. Because of the great success of the TAPS methodology, EFA established further regional TAPS that were privately funded (e.g., by the Coelho Jobs Fund).

Troxell[79] reviewed a number of highlights from this large effort by the EFA and U.S. Department of Labor. It is of interest that seizures seemed to contribute little to employment outcome or retention. People receiving social funding assistance had more difficulty securing jobs and those unemployed for more than 1 year at intake had more difficulty keeping jobs. It is also important to note that although more than 65% achieved placement, only 70% of these maintained the job even at 90 days. Troxell ended his retrospective review of TAPS activities by calling for earlier vocational intervention, more comprehensive and intensive services for enrollees on social financial assistance programs, more in-depth assessment at intake, and the need for more intensive job-site support and follow-up postplacement.

Unfortunately, the U.S. Epilepsy Foundation is less involved in vocational programming today. Much of this relates to reduced available funding.

Fraser et al. conducted two studies[31,33] to evaluate the effectiveness of specialized training and placement services for people with epilepsy. In the first,[31] the vocational services program of the University of Washington Regional Epilepsy Center, which has nearly the same components as TAPS, was evaluated. Of 106 persons with epilepsy, 50 (47%) could be successfully placed. The strongest discriminators between the employed and dropouts were "months employed in the last 24 before entering the program" and treatment for psychiatric conditions or addictions before entering the program. The group achieving employment had an average of 12 months in employment of the prior 24, whereas dropouts approximated only 7 months. In later cross-validation, only months employed before entering the program proved to be a significant discriminator, the psychiatric and addiction category losing its influence because of program refinements targeting these issues.[31]

In the second study,[33] outcome from seven state placement agencies was compared with the outcome from the University of Washington placement program. State agencies had a placement rate ranging from 9% to 21%, except for one state with a 44% placement outcome. The University of Washington specialized program placement rate was about 50% (see above). There were no differences in client characteristics that could account for these differences. These authors provided some interesting explanations:

1. In state agencies, the client-to-rehabilitation counselor ratio is about 1:100, whereas in specialized TAPS programs it is between 1:30 and 1:40.
2. In the state agency with a placement rate as high as 44%, special efforts were made to increase placement of persons with epilepsy, such as hiring only counselors with a Master's degree and having a counselor with the disability provide detailed education on epilepsy for fellow counselors (also having an emotional impact).

From these experiences, the authors concluded that specialized agencies should be established in local epilepsy centers and associations. At the same time, specialized training should be developed for the state counselors so that they may better meet the needs of the job seeker with epilepsy. Through specialized training, counselors also acquire empathy for the cause.

Postplacement Services

After a person with epilepsy is assisted to placement, several problems may occur: Frequent sick leave, inadequate performance, conflicts with supervisors or colleagues, and uncertainty of supervisors and colleagues about an individual having epilepsy if this has not been previously disclosed. Different kinds of assistance may be needed: Medical treatment, accommodation of some type at the job site, transfer to another workplace, counseling of the person with epilepsy by supervisors or colleagues, medical leave, or early retirement. Support and counseling may be provided by different services. External services are affiliated with state agencies, epilepsy societies, or epilepsy clinics. Other services are situated at or near the work site, such as occupational health services. These services may be specialized for epilepsy or may accommodate persons with various disabilities.

As previously described, TAPS provided postplacement support until 1 year after placement. In Germany, external postplacement services for persons with mental illnesses and disabilities, which also support people with epilepsy, have been developed by the state. These services cooperate closely with psychiatric clinics, and in many cases support can begin before placement and be continued, if necessary, for years. These services seem to be effective in opening doors for unemployed persons, because the employer may rely on the service if there are difficulties after placement. It has also been observed that these services are effective if a chronic disorder develops in an employee. In this situation, an employer is generally in need of specific information concerning the disorder and is ready to accept suggestions from an external service (e.g., to look for specialized medical treatment or to retrain). If an employee with a chronic disorder, such as epilepsy, is employed for many years, support from the external postplacement services seems less applicable, because the company itself may have attempted many accommodations. Nevertheless, the external service can still give meaningful support, such as counseling, suggestions for transfer to another work site, or recommendations for specialized medical treatment.[54] These services seem to be highly effective for maintaining people with chronic illness on the job.

Postplacement support may also be given by occupational health services. Kleinsorge[50] reported on 65 persons with epilepsy in a large German chemical company. Only one of six had been known to have epilepsy when starting to work because of lack of disclosure. No one with epilepsy was dismissed when the epilepsy condition was disclosed; however, 25 of 65 had to be transferred to a more suitable workplace. Espir et al.[26] recently reported on 93 subjects with epilepsy who were referred to the British Civil Service Occupational Health Service during an 18-month period. Reasons for referral were prolonged or frequent sick leave, unsatisfactory work performance, and epilepsy starting during employment. After each case was inspected, it became evident that many referrals were not a consequence of epilepsy but of associated illness or handicaps. Twenty-six instances of prolonged sick leave were reported: Six caused by epilepsy, nine caused by side effects and disorders associated with epilepsy, and 11 caused by other disorders, such as internal medical problems, psychiatric problems, or alcohol abuse. Of 23 cases of unsatisfactory work performance, 14 were a consequence of epilepsy and nine were not.

It is interesting to review the results of the Occupational Health Service interventions. Of the six persons with epilepsy who had prolonged or frequent sick leave caused by epilepsy, only three continued to work. Of the 14 persons with epilepsy who had an unsatisfactory work performance caused by epilepsy, 12 continued to work. Among the 22 persons with epilepsy whose disability began during employment, 12 continued working. Of eight persons with undisclosed epilepsy, seven continued working, and of the 35 needing advice on working conditions, 28 continued. The authors emphasize the important role of the Occupational Health Service in solving these problems. However, the fact that only 12 of 22 persons with new-onset epilepsy occurring during employment continued to work engendered some criticism. This is not what would be expected for new-onset epilepsy, which has an excellent prognosis, and results could have been different with the advice of an experienced epileptologist.[26]

More research and demonstration project efforts with regard to specialized postplacement services are presently needed. It would be misleading to believe that only unemployed persons with epilepsy are a problem group. A second group, employed people with epilepsy, is at risk for dismissal or retirement, or these people are gradually losing their abilities because of lack of appropriate medical interventions. Postplacement services should be targeted at these groups.

WORKPLACE ACCOMMODATIONS

There are several categories of work-site accommodation, which include procedural accommodations, physical modifications to the workstation itself, and the use of adaptive or assistive technology (equipment that enables an individual to perform on the job). For most individuals with a seizure disorder, the primary issue falls within the first two categories.

Procedural changes can be easily implemented and are very helpful to an individual with a seizure disorder. Individuals with occasional loss of consciousness, particularly when there is no warning, may need to avoid certain physically hazardous work activities. Without consistent warning, there may be no way to ensure safety in a specific activity. For example, part of a job involving working in high places or driving might be reassigned to another worker. For some individuals with seizures, changing shifts can be detrimental to functioning. A regular day shift can at times be arranged so as not to disrupt sleep patterns or the manner in which drugs are absorbed. Individuals may also require work-site modifications specifically for safety purposes. This might involve some type of floor covering or matting, a machinery guard, or an automatic cutoff switch that would ensure safety if a seizure occurred. In sum, accommodation needs are primarily for those individuals with marginal seizure control and the potential for an accident or injury on the job. However, some individuals with new-onset epilepsy take some time (up to 1 year) to achieve reasonable control. During this period, procedural changes or work-site modification can help to keep them on the job.

Assistive equipment is primarily for individuals with epilepsy and neuropsychological impairment. Equipment can include electronic cueing devices and watches, telepagers, and other memory aids. For individuals with both memory and problem-solving deficits, computer software programs can be helpful in organizing work and improving cognitive efficiency. Other individuals may use palm-top computers to organize work and otherwise aid memory. Again, assistive equipment is not a typical work-site accommodation for an individual with a basic seizure disorder but is more commonly used for clients with additional cognitive or physical limitations.

Birgit's Case

Birgit S. came to the center at Bethel when she was 19 and in the third year of training as a lathe operator. Complex partial seizures preceded by an epigastric aura were diagnosed. Her aura, however, was too short to protect her from the seizures. Therefore, the foreman, the occupational physician, and the rehabilitation specialist decided to install a box of acrylic glass over the lathe to prevent the machine from starting without the box in the right position. Birgit completed her training as a lathe operator successfully and after several changes of drugs has achieved good seizure control.

Others who can profit from workplace accommodations are persons with epilepsy who have been employed for a long time in one company, persons with late-onset epilepsy, or those whose epilepsy status deteriorates. Such persons are often too old for retraining, cannot be dismissed because of seniority, and are often considered desirable by the employer for their long-term performance and contribution.

Christina's Case

Christina W. was employed as a production assistant. Her job was to take containers formed with synthetic material out of machinery, put away the metal-forming edges, and store the containers. When generalized tonic–clonic seizures developed and these tasks became too dangerous for her, the machinery was adapted. She is now using a new machine with an automatic starting button placed some distance away. The cost of this accommodation was paid by the Office for Handicapped People in the Work Force (Germany).

NATIONAL LEGISLATION AFFECTING JOB ACCESS

Germany

In 2001 the federal government bundled all rehabilitation laws and regulations in a complex rehabilitation act, which is based on the principles of the ICF (Sozialgestzbuch IX). The rehabilitation act also contained new forms of support (e.g., "work assistance"). An example for this would be that a person with epilepsy who sometimes to fulfill his or her professional tasks has to drive would get funded a driver. Persons who cannot reach their workplace because they are not able to use public transportation can ask for cost-free private transportation. Support of disabled persons at the workplace is organized by regional (state) offices for the disabled. These offices are also responsible for workplace accommodations and therefore provide technical services. They also have highly specialized outreach services to support persons with disabilities at the workplace. One shortcoming is that these institutions give only support to people who have the status as handicapped. One consequence of this is that persons after a first epileptic seizure cannot get support even though this is a group in high need of work-site accommodations or procedural changes for a limited time period.

Americans with Disabilities Act

The Americans with Disabilities Act, enacted between 1992 and 1994, is benchmark legislation in the United States extending the prohibition on disability-related discrimination to the private sector. Title 1 of the Act covers employment and companies with as few as 15 employees. A company cannot discriminate in employment practices against a person who has epilepsy (or even a record of experience with the disability). Persons with a seizure disorder cannot be discriminated against in employment if they can perform the *essential* functions of the job with or without *reasonable accommodation* (a change in procedure, physical modification to the work site, or some type of adaptive equipment). People with epilepsy do not have to disclose their disability in the interview unless it affects performance of the job's essential functions. A person with a seizure disorder no longer has to submit to a medical examination unless a job has been offered.

In a review of the claims[17] filed under the Act with the Equal Employment Opportunity Commission during the first year, McMahon et al.[58] determined that 86% of the complaints were related to individuals already on the job. The law seems to be helping people with disabilities to keep jobs, but not necessarily to be hired.

SHELTERED EMPLOYMENT VERSUS EMPLOYMENT OF PERSONS WITH EPILEPSY IN THE OPEN LABOR MARKET

Sheltered employment, or special work facilities for persons who are considered unemployable in the competitive labor market, exists in nearly all countries of the world. Typically, certain products or services are provided or subcontracted from a manufacturing company, but in recent years more sheltered workshops have developed their own products, such as toys. Although nearly universal, the types and extent of sheltered employment differ sharply between countries with comparable economic structures. In 1990, 5 of 1,000 workers in Germany, 14 of 1,000 in The Netherlands, and 1 in 1,000 in the United Kingdom and the United States were employees in sheltered workshops. The extent of sheltered employment seems to be more a reflection of national philosophies toward employing people with disabilities than an objective employment phenomenon.[75] In two sheltered facilities in Berlin, Thorbecke found that 5% to 10% of their employees had epilepsy, depending an each workshop's production structure. This result was congruent with findings in other countries.[2]

In a study on seizures and epilepsy within a mentally retarded population,[61] 26% of those with mental retardation, 6% of a borderline IQ group (IQ below 75), and 2% of the comparison group experienced two or more seizures. The authors have found not only persons with epilepsy and mental retardation in sheltered workshops, but also a second group who have epilepsy and other problems, such as learning disabilities, behavioral problems, and severe drug or cognitive side effects, or who have frequent uncontrolled seizures—a subgroup of persons with epilepsy who are chronically unemployed. Members of the first group as a rule enter sheltered workshops directly after school, whereas those in the second group come to them after integration efforts in the open labor market have failed, which may have serious consequences for their perception of the sheltered employment opportunity.

People with epilepsy in sheltered work are a minority. Therefore, their special needs can easily be neglected. For example, in Germany the responsible consulting physician in a sheltered workshop as a rule is neither an epileptologist nor a neurologist, and treatment status is assessed only on first entrance into sheltered employment, with no requirement for epilepsy education for supervisors. As a consequence, persons with epilepsy may be needlessly excluded from work at machinery that is highly valued and can pay better in the sheltered workshop setting. A further consequence may be that persons with epilepsy in sheltered employment who are not mentally retarded, after their epilepsy is well controlled, may not be sent for further vocational rehabilitation or placed in the open labor market, but rather remain in the sheltered workshop. These observations should, however, be grounded in more systematic studies (see also studies cited below).

NEW SERVICES

Models to Change Sheltered Employment

In the early 1970s, a U.S. movement arose for reducing sheltered employment and finding ways less conducive to segregation of employing those with severe disabilities. As a consequence, new forms of employment for this group in the open labor market, known as supported employment, were established. In the United States, supported employment emerged quickly because of amendments to the Developmental Disabilities Act in 1984. The concept of supported employment can be divided into four steps: (a) Placement, (b) training on the job by a job coach, (c) stabilization, and (d) maintenance. The time spent on job-site assistance decreases continuously from step one through step four.

Models of Supported Employment Placement

It should be noted that there is more than one model of supported employment:

1. Individual placement. Employer pays the client minimum federal wage or above while the client receives specific training with a job coach.
2. Enclave model. A group of individuals (usually fewer than eight) work together or at diverse work stations for one company and receive training or support from a job coach. Wages are usually at the minimum level. In some cases, individuals are integrated into the mainstream workforce on an individual basis.
3. Mobile crew model. In a single-purpose business, a general manager or trainer works with a group of four to five employees out of a mobile vehicle, such as a van. The work can involve activities such as landscaping or janitorial services, with wages at a minimum level or higher.
4. Entrepreneurial benchmark model. In a small, single-purpose business located in an integrated community setting, eight to 15 clients receive training or actively work. Wages are at a minimum level or higher and the workforce may be integrated, involving employees without disabilities.

Much work has been done to clarify supported employment program components: Community job analysis, job match and placement, job training with specific techniques of applied behavior analysis, and follow-up services and interagency coordination. (See special issues of the *Journal of Rehabilitation,* 1987;53[3]; the *American Journal of Applied Behavior Analysis,* 1989;Winter[4]; and the *American Journal on Mental Retardation,* 1989;94[1].)

A survey covering the years 1984 to 1985 and 1985 to 1986 in the United States showed that 17% to 19% of clients were transferred from sheltered into supported employment.[64] This trend within the United States has continued, so that the majority of clients are being served under a model of supported employment. Several benefit–cost analyses indicate positive results: The supported employee earns better pay and is more a part of mainstream life.[51,56,78] Three German federal states have large demonstration projects on ongoing supported employment: One aimed at direct transition from special school to employment in the open labor market, and the other two at transition from sheltered employment to competitive employment. In the Westfalian project including 141 persons, more than four/fifths of them had visited a special school for children with mild or severe learning disability and were placed in the general labor market. Twenty percent were in sheltered employment, the remaining unemployed or in work preparatory courses. Eighteen percent had epilepsy. Seven years later 125 could be revisited. Sixty-six percent still were employed in the general labor market, and 80% had been regularly employed for >50% of the follow-up time. No negative effects of epilepsy on the chances to keep employment could be detected; 93.6% got practical work experience before entering regular employment and got, if necessary, extensive support at the workplace organized by the integration service of the Westfalian office for the disabled. There was also an economic cost efficiency study showing that that there would be strong economic arguments for this approach, resulting in better funding of such services.[4]

Transition of People with Epilepsy from Sheltered Employment into the Open Labor Market

From the cited surveys, primarily persons with mild mental retardation or ratings of dull–normal on full-scale IQs (approximately the lower 70s) are served in supported employment. The proportion of persons with severe disabilities, such as traumatic brain injury, cerebral palsy, or autism, is low.[69] No specific data are available for persons with epilepsy. However, it is safe to assume that people with moderate or severe mental retardation as a primary disability who have epilepsy as an additional handicap are being served. It seems that issues concerning control of epilepsy in this group are the same as for persons without mental retardation, if treatment follows the principles of an effective anticonvulsant regimen.[55]

There is an urgent need for research to address the specific problems of those with epilepsy in sheltered employment who are truly candidates for supported employment in the open labor market.

SUMMARY AND CONCLUSIONS

In this chapter, the specific vocational needs of people with epilepsy and the services designed to meet them have been outlined. The background for this chapter has largely been experiences in vocational rehabilitation within the United States and in Germany. The service structure in these two countries is considerably different. In the United States, specific services exist for persons with epilepsy to a limited degree at certain affiliates of the national Epilepsy Foundation or at university epilepsy programs (e.g., University of Washington-Seattle or University of California-San Francisco).

In Germany, specific services are rare, while at the same time the "welfare state" makes intensive efforts to integrate all people with disabilities into the labor force. As a consequence, a network of labor-mediation agencies and integration services dealing with disability issues and rehabilitation centers for adolescents and adults has been developed. In Germany, the state agencies and training institutions try to remain sensitive to the specific needs of persons with epilepsy who are a minority, whereas in the United States, the vocational support such people receive depends more on the specialized vocational rehabilitation services that are available in their region. In some cases these services are exceptional, but in other cases within the United States, persons with epilepsy miss the benefits of a German type of integrated training or retraining system.

It is the authors' conviction that both approaches are needed: Specialized services for persons with epilepsy that are sufficiently flexible to accommodate their unique requirements and a network of integrated work access and training services for all people with disability with staff that knows and understands the special needs of those with epilepsy.

ACKNOWLEDGMENT

Appreciation is extended for partial research review by the National Epilepsy Library at the Epilepsy Foundation (United States).

References

1. Arbeitskreis zur Verbesserung der Eingliederungschancen von Personen mit Epilepsie: Empfehlungen zur Beurteilung beruflicher Möglichkeiten von Personen mit Epilepsie-Überarbeitung 1999. *Rehabilitation.* 2001;40:97–110.
2. The Commission for the Control of Epilepsy and Its Consequences. *Plan for Nationwide Action on Epilepsy* (Vol. IV). DHEW Publication No (NIH); 1978.
3. Employment Commission of the International Bureau for Epilepsy. Employing people with epilepsy: principles for good practice. *Epilepsia.* 1989;30:411–412.
4. *Monetäre Kosten-Nutzen-Analyse von Fachdiensten zur Integration von Menschen mit geistigen Beeinträchtigungen auf dem allgemeinen Arbeitsmarkt.* Münster: LWL; 1997.
5. *Training Applicants for Placement Success (TAPS).* Fourth-quarter report. Washington, D.C.: Epilepsy Foundation of America; 1994.
6. *Work Preparation Course for Young People with Epilepsy.* Northern Ireland: Association BE; 1981.
7. Bahrs O, in der Beek R. Epilepsie und Arbeitswelt - Zusammenfassende Darstellung einer empirischen Untersuchung unter besonderer Berücksichtigung von Wirklichkeit und Möglichkeit beruflicher Rehabilitation. *Rehabilitation.* 1990;29:100–111.
8. Batzel LW, Dodrill CB, Fraser RT. Further validation of the WPSI vocational scale: comparisons with other correlates of employment in epilepsy. *Epilepsia.* 1980;21:235–242.
9. Callaghan N, Crowley M, Goggin T. Epilepsy and employment, marital, education, and social status. *Irish Med J.* 1992;85:17–19.
10. Carroll D. Employment among young people with epilepsy. *Seizure.* 1992;1:127–131.
11. Chaplin JE. A Systems Analysis of the Employment Problems of People with Epilepsy, PhD thesis; 1993.
12. Chaplin JE. Vocational assessment and intervention for people with epilepsy. *Epilepsia.* 2005;46:55–56.
13. Clemmons D. Relationship of general aptitude test battery scores to successful employment for epileptics in a rehabilitation setting. *Epilepsia.* 1983;24:232–237.
14. Clemmons DC, Fraser RT, Dodrill CB, et al. *High School Prevocational Intervention Study.* National Institute of Neurological and Communicative Disorders and Stroke (NIH); 1983–1988.
15. Clemmons DC, Fraser RT, Dodrill CB, et al. Neuropsychological correlates of tested vocational aptitudes for adults with epilepsy in a rehabilitation setting. *J Appl Rehabil Counsel.* 1987;18:29–32.
16. Clemmons DC, Dodrill CB. Vocational outcomes of high school students with epilepsy. *J Appl Rehabil Counsel.* 1983;14(4):49–53.
17. Curly AD, Delaney RC, Mattson RH, et al. *Determinants of the behavioral disturbance in boys with seizures.* Annual Convention of the American Psychological Association, New York; 1987.
18. De Boer HM. Aspects of training for young adults as an entry to a working situation. *Int J Adolesc Med Health.* 1989;4/2:113–118.
19. Dennerll RD, Schwartz ML, Rodin EA. *Neurological, Psychological, and Social Factors Related to Employability of Persons with Epilepsy.* Final Report Project Number RD-1403-P. Detroit, MI; 1968.
20. Dodrill CB. Correlates of generalized tonic–clonic seizures with intellectual, neuropsychological, emotional, and social function in patients with epilepsy. *Epilepsia.* 1986;27(4):399–411.
21. Dodrill CB. A neuropsychological battery for epilepsy. *Epilepsia.* 1978; 19:611–623.
22. Elsner H, Thorbecke R. Anfallshäufigkeit und Verletzungsrisiko am Arbeitsplatz: Erfahrungen in metall- und textilverarbeitenden Berufen im BBW Bethel. In: Stefan H, Canger R, Spiel G, eds. *Epilepsie '93.* Berlin: Deutsche Sektion der Internationalen Liga gegen Epilepsie; 1993:28–138.
23. Elwes RDC, Johnson AL, Shorvon SDR, et al. The prognosis for seizure control in newly diagnosed epilepsy. *N Engl J Med.* 1984;11:944–947.
24. Elwes RDC, Marshall J, Beattie A, et al. Epilepsy and employment. A community based survey in an area of high unemployment. *J Neurol Neurosurg Psychiatry.* 1991;54:200–203.
25. Emlen AC, Ryan R. Analyzing Unemployment Rates among Men with Epilepsy. 30th Annual Western Institute on Epilepsy. Portland, OR; 1979.
26. Espir M, Floyd MC. Occupational aspects of epilepsy in the civil service. *Br J Indust Med.* 1991;48:665–669.
27. Finger M. *Prognostische Validität neuropsychologischer Tests in der beruflichen Rehabilitation von jungen Menschen mit Epilepsie.* Frankfurt: Peter Lang GmbH, Europäischer Verlag der Wissenschaften; 1996.
28. Fraser R, Dodrill CB, Clemmons DC. Vocational outcome following epilepsy surgery. *Epilepsia.* Submitted.
29. Fraser R, Koepnick D, Clemmons DC, et al. Poster Presentation: Work Values of Vocational Rehabilitation Clients With Epilepsy. American Epilepsy Society Meeting, Los Angeles, CA; 2000.
30. Fraser RT, Clemmons D, Andrechak D, et al. Paper: Pre-vocational Intervention in Epilepsy Rehabilitation: Outcome and Pre-/Post-Employability Correlates. Annual Meeting of the American Epilepsy Society. Seattle, WA; 1992.
31. Fraser RT, Clemmons D, Trejo W, et al. Program evaluation in epilepsy rehabilitation. *Epilepsia.* 1983;734–746.
32. Fraser RT, Clemmons DC, Dodrill CB, et al. The difficult-to-employ in epilepsy rehabilitation: predictions of response to an intensive intervention. *Epilepsia.* 1986;27:220–224.
33. Fraser RT, Trejo W, Blanchard W. Epilepsy rehabilitation: evaluating specialized versus general agency outcome. *Epilepsia.* 1984;25:332–337.
34. Fraser RT, Trejo WR, Temkin NR, et al. Assessing vocational interests of those with epilepsy. *Rehabil Psychol.* 1985;30(1):29–33.
35. Freeman J, Jacobs H, Vining ER, et al. Epilepsy and the inner city schools: a school-based program that makes a difference. *Epilepsia.* 1984;25(4):438–442.
36. Freeman JM, Gayle E. Rehabilitation and the clients with epilepsy: a survey of the client's view of the rehabilitation process and its results. *Epilepsia.* 1978;19:233–239.
37. Fukoshima Y. Occupation and epilepsy. *Fol Psychiatr Neurol Jpn.* 1978;32(3):449–450.
38. Goldin GJ, Perry SL, Margolin RJ, et al. *Rehabilitation of the Young Epileptic.* Lexington, MA: Lexington Books; 1997.
39. Gouider R, Fredj M, Mrabet A. Interaction between work and epilepsy in Tunisia. In: Chaplin JE, ed. *Epilepsy and Employment: Is There a Problem?* Heemstede: IBE; 1999:40–43.
40. Guldvog B, Loyning Y, Hauglie-Hanssen E, et al. Surgical versus medical treatment for epilepsy. II. Outcome related to social areas. *Epilepsia.* 1991;32:477–486.
41. Harden CL, Kossoy A, Vera S, et al. Reaction to epilepsy in the workplace. *Epilepsia.* 2004;45:1134–1140.
42. Hasegawa S, Sasagawa M, Tamura K. The ability to work and employment situation for people with epilepsy. *Jpn J Psychiatry Neurol.* 1988;42(3):578–579.
43. Hauser WA, Hesdorffer CC. *Epilepsy: Frequency, Causes, and Consequences.* New York: Demos; 1990.

44. Holmes DA, Williams JM. Employers attitudes towards hiring epileptics. *J Rehabil.* 1981;20–21.
45. Jacoby A, Baker GA, Steen N, et al. The clinical course of epilepsy and its psychosocial correlates: findings from a U.K. community study. *Epilepsia.* 1996;37:148–161.
46. Jacoby A, Gorry J, Baker GA. Employers' attitudes to employment of people with epilepsy: still the same old story? *Epilepsia.* 2005;46:1978–1987.
47. Janz D. Social prognosis in epilepsy, especially in regard to social status and the necessity for institutionalization. *Epilepsia.* 1972;13:141.
48. John C, McLellan DL. Employers' attitudes to epilepsy. *Br J Industr Med.* 1988;45:713–715.
49. Jones JE, Berven NL, Ramirez L, et al. Long-term psychosocial outcomes of anterior temporal lobectomy. *Epilepsia.* 2002;43:896–903.
50. Kleinsorge H. Anfallskranke Arbeiter der chemischen Industrie. *Zentralbl Arbeitsmed.* 1982;32:424–428.
51. Kregel J, Wehman PB, Banks PD. The effects of consumer characteristics and type of employment model on individual outcomes in supported employment. *J Appl Behav Anal.* 1989;22:407–415.
52. Lassouw G, Leffers P, de Krom M, et al. Epilepsy in a Dutch working population. Are employees diagnoses with epilepsy disadvantaged? *Seizure.* 1997;6:95–96.
53. Lindsten H, Stenlund H, Edlund C, et al. Socioeconomic prognosis after a newly diagnosed unprovoked epileptic seizure in adults: a population-based case-control study. *Epilepsia.* 2002;43:1239–1250.
54. Lohr-Wiegmann U. Betriebliche Rehabilitation psychisch Behinderter - Begleitende Hilfen im Arbeitsleben. *Rehabilitation.* 1988;27:14–17.
55. Marcus JC. Control of epilepsy in a mentally retarded population: lack of correlates with IQ, neurological status, and electroencephalogram. *Am J Ment Retard.* 1993;98:47–51.
56. McCaughrin WB, Ellis WK, Rusch FRH, et al. Cost-effectiveness of supported employment. *Ment Retard.* 1993;31(1):41–48.
57. McLellan DL. Epilepsy and employment. *J Soc Occup Med.* 1987;37:94–99.
58. McMahon BT, Shaw LR, Jaet DN. An empirical analysis: employment and disability from an ADA litigation perspective. *NARPPSJ.* 1995;10:3–14.
59. Penin H. Epilepsie und Berufsunfähigkeit. *Akt Neurol.* 1979;6:257–265.
60. Pfäfflin M, May T, Adelmeier U. Epilepsiebedingte Beeinträchtigungen im täglichen Leben und in der Erwerbstätigkeit - Querschnittstudie an Patienten niedergelassener Ärzte. *Neurol Rehabil.* 2000;6:140–148.
61. Richardson SA, Koller H, Katz M, et al. Seizures and epilepsy in a mentally retarded population over the first 22 years of life. *Appl Res Ment Retard.* 1980;1:123–138.
62. Rodin EA. *The Prognosis of Patients with Epilepsy.* Springfield, IL: Thomas; 1968.
63. Sands H, Zalkind SS. Effects of an educational campaign to change employer attitudes toward hiring epileptics. *Epilepsia.* 1972;13:87–96.
64. Schalock RL, McGaughey MJ, Kiernan WE. Placement into nonsheltered employment: findings from national employment surveys. *Am J Ment Retard.* 1989;94:80–87.
65. Scharfenstein J, Thorbecke R. Rehabilitation Epilepsiekranker in einem Arbeitsamtsbezirk. In: Remschmidt C, ed. *Epilepsie 1980.* Stuttgart: Thieme; 1981:22–28.
66. Schlesinger LE, Frank D. From demonstration to dissemination: gateways to employment for epileptics. *Rehabil Lit.* 1974;35:98–109.
67. Schultz U, Thorbecke R. Rehabilitationsprognose bei Epilepsiebeginn nach Eintritt ins Berufsleben. *Rehabilitation.* 1985;24:192–196.
68. Scrambler H, Hopkins A. Social class, epileptic activity and disadvantage at work. *J Epidemiol Commun Health.* 1980;34/2:129–133.
69. Shafer MS, Wehman P, Kregel J, et al. National supported employment initiative: a preliminary analysis. *Am J Ment Retard.* 1990;95:316–327.
70. Sillanpää M, Jalava M, Kaleva O, et al. Long-term prognosis of seizures with onset in childhood. *N Engl J Med.* 1998;338:1715–1722.
71. Sillanpää M, Shinnar S. Obtaining a driver's license and seizure relapse in patients with childhood-onset epilepsy. *Neurology.* 2005;64:680–686.
72. Specht U, Thorbecke R. In preparation. 2006.
73. Specht U, Thorbecke R, May T, et al. Comprehensive short term rehabilitation program for people with epilepsy: positive effects on quality-of-life and performance. *Epilepsia.* 2004;45:57.
74. Stores G. School children with epilepsy at risk for learning and behavior disorders. *Dev Med Child Neurol.* 1978;20:502–508.
75. Thorbecke R. Behindertenwerkstätten in der Bundesrepublik und in Europa. einfälle: Zeitschrift der Selbsthilfegruppen für und von Anfallkranken 1992;41:18–21.
76. Thorbecke R. Die Bedeutung von Anfallart und Anfallhäufigkeit für die Rehabilitation. In: Wolf P, ed *Epilepsie 88.* Reinbek: Einhorn-Presse Verlag GmbH; 1989:24–31.
77. Thorbecke R. Risks of accidents at work - personal comments. In: Cornaggia CM, ed. *Epilepsy and Risks: A First-step Evaluation.* Milano: Ghedini Editore; 1993:83–85.
78. Tines J, Rusch FR, McCaughrin W, et al. Benefit-cost analysis of supported employment in Illinois: a statewide evaluation. *Am J Ment Retard.* 1990;95:44–54.
79. Troxell J. The training and placement scheme (TAPS): a discussion of the Epilepsy Foundation of America's national employment project. In: *Epilepsy and Employment: Is There a Problem?* Prague: IBE; 2000:95–99.
80. Troxell J, Fraser R. *Epilepsy Rehabilitation: A Demonstration Project in School-to-Work Transition.* U.S. National Institute of Disability and Rehabilitation Research, Department of Education; 1993–1996.
81. van den Broek M, Beghi E. Accidents in patients with epilepsy: types, circumstances, and complications: a European cohort study. *Epilepsia.* 2004;45:667–672.
82. Wada K, Kawata Y, Murakami T, et al. Sociomedical aspects of epileptic patients: their employment and marital status. *Psychiatry Clin Neurosci.* 2001;55:141–146.
83. Wöhrl H-G. The integration into working life of persons with epilepsy after a vocational rehabilitation training in the Federal Republic of Germany. In: Canger R, Loeber JNC, F, eds. *Epilepsy and Society: Realities and Prospects.* Elsevier Science Publishers B.V. (Biomedical Division); 1988:139–147.
84. Zwerling CZ, Whitten PS, Davis CS, et al. Occupational injuries among workers with disabilities: the national interview survey. *JAMA.* 1997;278:2163–2167.

CHAPTER 220 ■ ISSUES IN HEALTH OUTCOMES ASSESSMENT

ZARYA A. RUBIN AND SAMUEL WIEBE

INTRODUCTION

Epilepsy is a multidimensional disorder with potential consequences for nearly every aspect of a patient's life, from physical effects, to social and vocational challenges, to personality and mood changes. In addition, total estimated health care costs are $12.5 billion in the United States annually.[12,46] Results of recent large clinical studies indicate that 25% to 40% of patients diagnosed with partial epilepsy will not be controlled with medication,[37,60,72–74,88] and a larger proportion experience adverse antiepileptic medication effects. Epilepsy patients are also more likely to suffer from comorbid depressive disorders than the general population or patients with other chronic illness, with prevalence rates of depression estimated to be 20% to 40%.[11,33,50,61,78,84] The comprehensive picture of the experience of epilepsy is more complex and detailed than is often assumed, reaching beyond the seizures themselves and extending into multiple domains of patients' overall health.

THE CONCEPT OF HEALTH-RELATED QUALITY OF LIFE IN EPILEPSY

Measures of success in treating medical illness have traditionally been characterized as freedom from disease or other intermediate quantifiable endpoints such as reduction in systolic blood pressure, serum glucose, or seizures.[21] Over the last decade, however, the emergence of health-related quality of life as a reliable, valid, and significant indicator of overall outcome in patients with epilepsy has begun to alter that perception.[28,41,49,95,101]

The concept of quality of life is not new, and dates back at least to the time of Aristotle, who attempted to define the attributes of happiness.[4] The Constitution of the World Health Organization defines health as "A state of complete physical, mental and social well-being and not merely the absence of disease or infirmity."[102] The current definition of quality of life encompasses both the concept of health and functional ability, as well as the patient's perceived satisfaction with this level of functioning. Thus, both objective and subjective measures are incorporated into the final assessment of overall quality of life.

As defined by Gotay et al.,[45]

> Quality of life is a state of well-being that is a composite of two components: (1) the ability to perform everyday activities that reflect physical, psychological and social well-being and (2) patient satisfaction with levels of functioning and the control of disease and/or treatment-related symptoms.

The initial formulation of an instrument designed to measure quality of life in health care occurred in 1948 with the development of the Karnofsky Performance Status Scale. The 100-point scale defined a patient's ability to perform various activities of daily living (where 100 is *capable of performing all normal activities* and 0 is *deceased*).[19,58] In 1992, Vickrey et al.[95] developed one of the first reliable and valid measure of quality of life in epilepsy, the Epilepsy Surgery Index-55. Baker et al.[9] concurrently constructed a model of assessment of physical, social, and psychological impairment related to refractory epilepsy. In 1995, Devinsky et al.[29] developed the Quality of Life in Epilepsy Inventory (QOLIE-89), an 89-item, disease-specific inventory to help characterize the impact of epilepsy on patients' global functioning. Since then, a QOLIE-10[25] has been developed in addition to other more specific inventories relating to aspects that contribute to overall quality of life in epilepsy such as medication side effects (Adverse Events Profile)[6] and the NDDI-E (Neurologic Disorders Depression Inventory for Epilepsy),[38] a newly developed tool for differentiating depression in epilepsy from antiepileptic drug (AED) and cognitive effects.

In a study of 81 consecutive epilepsy patients, Gilliam et al.[40] systematically assessed the specific concerns of patients with recurrent seizures. The most frequently cited concern was driving, at nearly 70%, whereas other significant factors listed by more than one third of patients included independence, work and education, social embarrassment, medication dependence, mood/stress, and safety (Table 1).

Although these patient-oriented outcome measures are not intended to replace traditional indicators of health status in epilepsy such as seizure frequency or severity, they may offer additional information that allows us to expand our knowledge of the experience of epilepsy and better treat our patients. This review examines the contributions of seizure status, outcomes of epilepsy surgery, mood effects, medication toxicity, and other comorbidities to overall health-related quality of life (HRQOL) in epilepsy.

SEIZURE FREQUENCY AND HEALTH-RELATED QUALITY OF LIFE

Although seizure frequency was previously believed to predict overall quality of life and seizure reduction continues to be a goal of therapeutic interventions for epilepsy, there in fact exists no clear gradient establishing a direct correlation between number of seizures and degree of HRQOL improvement or worsening. In fact, the only true amelioration in quality of life can be observed when patients are rendered entirely seizure free.[14,63,69,96]

In the multicenter study by Leidy et al.,[63] patients were classified according to seizure frequency and evaluated on the Medical Outcomes Short Study Form (SF-36), a "gold standard" measure of quality of life. Scores for seizure-free patients were similar to those of the general population, whereas

TABLE 1

QUALITY OF LIFE IN EPILEPSY-89 (QOLIE-89) TOTAL AND SUBSCALE SCORE DIFFERENCES BETWEEN GROUPS ACCORDING TO DEPRESSION DIAGNOSIS

	Difference between no and major	Difference between no and moderate	Difference between moderate and major
Total QOLIE-89	31	19	12
Health Perception	27	20	7
Overall Quality of Life	30	16	13
Physical Function	23	21	2
Role Physical	40	31	9
Role Emotional	54	24	29
Pain	29	18	11
Social Function	27	17	10
Energy-Fatigue	29	17	12
Emotional Well-Being	37	19	18
Attention-Concentration	32	17	15
Health Discouragement	38	20	17
Seizure Worry	24	15	8
Memory	27	18	9
Language	23	13	10
Medication Effect	21	8	13
Social Support	25	11	14
Social Isolation	37	21	16

Score difference >12 points are considered clinically significant. ANOVA, $p < .0001$, for all QOLIE-89 total and subscale raw scores by depression group.
Source: From Cramer JA, Blum D, Reed M, et al. The influence of comorbid depression on quality of life for people with epilepsy. *Epilepsy Behav.* 2003;4:515–521; with permission.

increasing frequency of seizures predicted a small but inverse shift in HRQOL across all domains.[63] Although some differences were observed between groups with differing seizure frequency, these differences were subtle, and the greatest discrepancy in quality-of-life scores was observed in the seizure-free group versus all seizure groups.[63] In a recent study by Birbeck et al.,[14] these results were confirmed using the QOLIE-31, QOLIE-89, and SF-36, with positive changes in HRQOL occurring only in the group that achieved seizure freedom and not in the groups that achieved seizure reduction. Thus, although many AED trials use a 50% reduction in seizure frequency as a desirable endpoint, it appears that the complete eradication of seizures provides the only definitive HRQOL benefits for patients with epilepsy.[14,63]

Vickrey et al.[95] compared the health status of patients who had undergone epilepsy surgery with those who suffered from other chronic illnesses such as hypertension, diabetes, and heart disease (Fig. 1). Although patients who were rendered completely seizure free scored higher on all measures than patients with chronic illness, patients who continued to have seizures, even without alteration in consciousness, scored similarly to patients with other chronic medical conditions in terms of social and emotional well-being; patients with residual complex partial or generalized tonic–clonic seizures scored significantly worse than patients with myocardial infarction or congestive heart failure on overall QOL and social and emotional well-being.[95]

These results further emphasize the importance of eliminating seizures to achieve adequate quality of life; even occasional auras impair quality of life to a degree similar to a chronic medical condition such as diabetes.[33] By achieving total cessation of seizures, through medical or surgical interventions, patients with epilepsy may attain of a level of quality of life that approaches or surpasses that of the general population.[14,63]

SURGERY AND HEALTH-RELATED QUALITY OF LIFE

In the first randomized, controlled trial comparing epilepsy surgery to conventional therapy, Wiebe et al.[100] demonstrated that surgery was far superior to medical treatment in terms of rendering patients free of disabling seizures (58% vs. 8%), with correlative improvements in quality of life. In a recent multicenter observational study with long-term follow-up by Spencer et al.,[90] 66% of patients experienced a 2-year remission. Success rates for temporal lobe epilepsy with corresponding mesial temporal sclerosis and supportive electroencephalographic (EEG) findings may be considerably higher.[39,83]

Despite compelling evidence in favor of epilepsy surgery, few patients who are possible candidates are being offered this potentially curative treatment, and those who are being considered for surgery may wait an average of 20 years from diagnosis.[42,61] The risks of delaying epilepsy surgery are not insignificant, given that the rate of epilepsy-related death may exceed 1%,[91] whereas the reported rate of mortality for epilepsy surgery is <0.2%.[13]

In addition to freedom from seizures, which is associated with significantly improved health outcomes, Gilliam et al.[42] looked at patient-oriented measures after temporal lobectomy for refractory epilepsy, using validated instruments for assessing HRQOL such as the Epilepsy Foundation of America's (EFA) Concerns Index, the Epilepsy Survey Inventory-55, the Adverse Events Profile, and the Profile of Mood States (POMS).[42] In a comparison of a presurgical group of 71 patients to 125 patients who had previously undergone anterior temporal lobectomy, 65% of postoperative patients were found to be seizure free (vs. 0%) and 60% (vs. 27%) were driving.[42] Multivariate regression analysis in the postoperative group

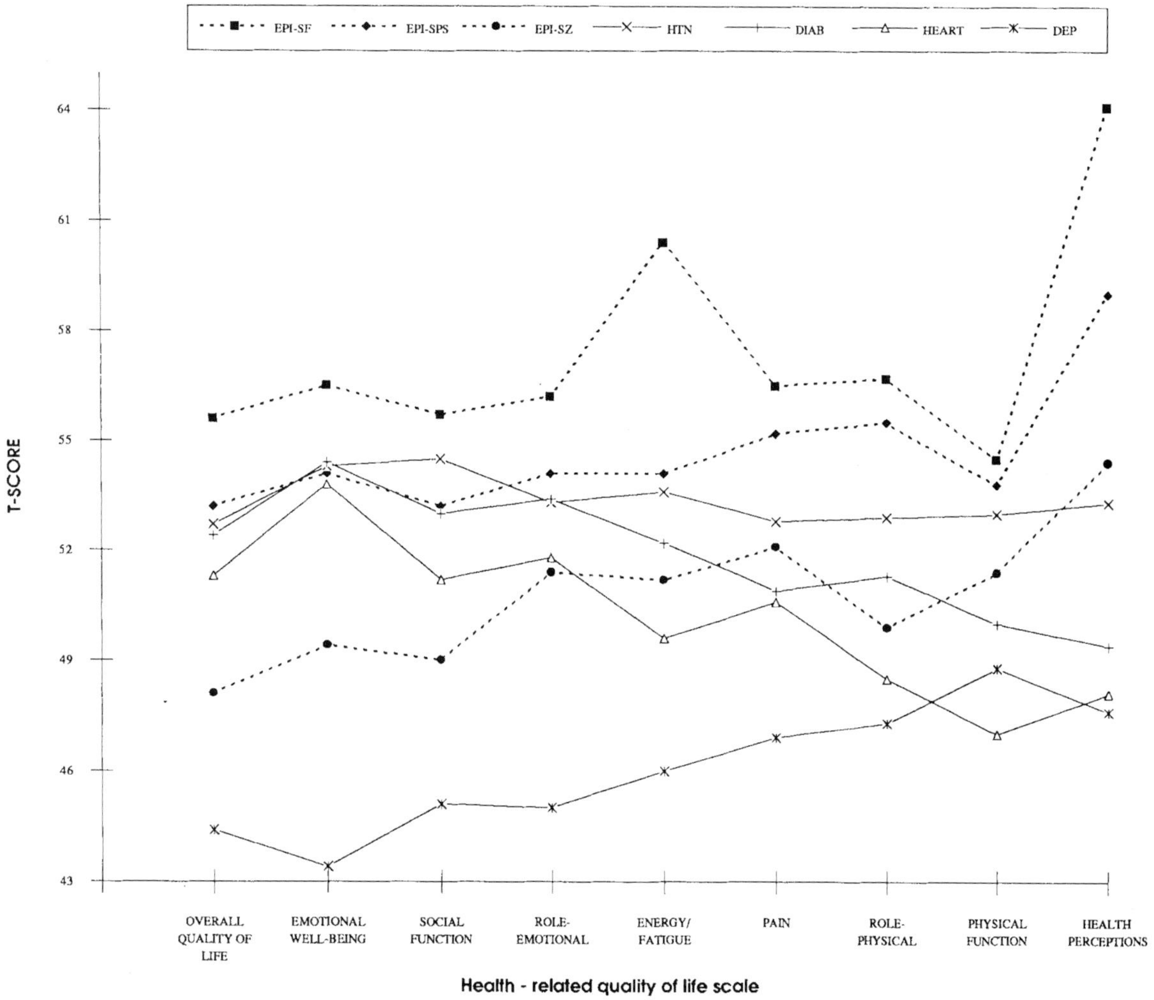

FIGURE 1. T-score distribution across nine health-related quality-of-life (QOL) domains in epilepsy surgery patients and Medical Outcomes Study Patients. EPI-SF, seizure free ($n = 55$, *solid squares*); EPI-SPS, simple partial seizures ($n = 44$, *solid diamonds*); EPI-SZ, one or more complex partial or generalized tonic–clonic GTC seizures or both ($n = 67$, *solid circles*); HTN, hypertension ($n = 1{,}224$, ×); DBT, diabetes ($n = 548$, +); DEP, depressive symptomatology ($n = 906$, *). (From Vickrey BG, Hays RD, Rausch R, et al. Quality of life of epilepsy surgery patients as compared with outpatients with hypertension, diabetes, heart disease, and/or depressive symptoms. *Epilepsia.* 1994;35:597–607; with permission.)

demonstrated that factors associated with improved quality of life included mood status, employment, driving, and AED cessation but did not include seizure freedom or IQ status.[42]

Markand et al.[69] found improvement in overall score and 10 of 17 scales of the QOLIE-89 in patients who had undergone temporal lobectomy versus those treated with conventional medical therapy. However, these improvements were dependent on achieving total seizure freedom.

These studies suggest a complex interaction among variables contributing to HRQOL in patients with epilepsy. By assuming that freedom from seizures, although a primary goal, is the only valuable postsurgical endpoint, we may be missing additional opportunities for intervention in the domains of transportation options, vocational counseling, and treatment of mood symptomatology with medication or psychotherapy. Through examination of the influence of patient-oriented outcomes on postoperative measures of success, we may better be able to characterize the impact of these factors on overall HRQOL in epilepsy and tailor therapeutic approaches accordingly.

MEDICATIONS AND HEALTH-RELATED QUALITY OF LIFE

Several recent studies have emphasized the importance of medication effects on overall HRQOL in epilepsy. Baker et al.[7] surveyed >5,000 European patients with epilepsy and found that 44% of respondents had changed their medications at least once in the last year due to unsatisfactory control. Only 12% of patients reported no side effects from medication; common side effects included tiredness (58%), memory problems (50%), difficulty concentrating (48%), sleepiness (45%), difficulty thinking clearly (40%), and nervousness or agitation (36%). Thirty-one percent of patients had changed their medication at least once in the last year due to side effects.[7] This study included patients' self-report of adverse effects from medication. Baker and colleagues also developed an instrument to systematically evaluate medication-related toxicity: The Adverse Events

Profile (AEP).[6] This 19-item instrument was tested and evaluated for internal consistency and was then administered to 200 consecutive epilepsy patients, 62 of whom met enrollment criteria. Patients were then randomized to receive usual care from a neurologist (no AEP) or to have the AEP provided to their neurologist at each visit. Baseline scores on the AEP correlated with scores on the QOLIE-89, and significant improvements in both the AEP and QOLIE-89 were observed in the group for which the neurologist had access to the AEP.[6,40] Availability of the AEP also resulted in a significant reduction in seizures as well as more adjustments in medication by their physician compared to patients for whom this additional information was not available.[6] These results emphasize the importance of measuring and evaluating medication toxicity as part of the overall care of the epilepsy patient, not only to control for side effects, but also to potentially reduce seizure frequency and improve overall quality of life.

Gilliam et al. specifically evaluated medication side effects and their association with HRQOL in a prospective study of 195 consecutive patients.[37] Patients were screened with the AEP, the QOLIE-89, and the Beck Depression Inventory (BDI). After controlling for age, gender, generalized tonic–clonic seizure frequency and depressive symptoms, adverse medication effects were the strongest predictor of HRQOL. Severity of depression was also found to be independently correlated with overall HRQOL; seizure frequency, however, was not.[37]

There has been equivocal evidence in the literature as to the relative superiority of monotherapy over "rational polypharmacy" in the treatment of medically refractory epilepsy.[82] Although monotherapy may be felt to be insufficient, polytherapy may not necessarily reduce seizure frequency but may incur a host of other, undesirable effects.

A recent study by Pirio Richardson et al.[82] looked at QOL and monotherapy in a group of patients with medically refractory epilepsy who had been converted to monotherapy and maintained on treatment for at least 12 months. Forty percent of patients became seizure free and experienced statistically significant improvements in quality of life in several domains, including memory loss, concern over medication long-term effects, difficulty in taking medications, trouble with leisure time activities, and overall state of health.[82] Despite methodologic issues in this small study, it suggests that further consideration be given to the notion of monotherapy in medically refractory epilepsy.

In a large study of 547 patients with partial-onset epilepsy and inadequate seizure control or intolerable side effects, conversion to monotherapy was achieved with lamotrigine. Patients were evaluated with the QOLIE-31 and showed significant improvement in multiple domains after conversion to monotherapy. This improvement was independent of seizure control.[24]

Baker et al.[7] conducted a cross-sectional community survey that compared 514 patients <60 years of age to 155 patients >60 years of age across various quality-of-life domains. Medication effects were assessed using the AEP, and results were significant for increased rates of dizziness, upset stomach, disturbed sleep, and memory problems among older patients. Older patients were also more likely to be taking older AED medications. Although senior adults (>60 years of age) represent the group with the highest age-specific rates of epilepsy and are likely to be the most vulnerable to drug interactions and AED-related side effects, few studies have specifically examined the effects of epilepsy treatment on HRQOL in this particular group.[70]

These studies emphasize the need methodically to approach the choice and monitoring of pharmacologic interventions for the treatment of epilepsy. By increasing our awareness of medication toxicity through careful, systematic screening and questioning of our patients at each office visit, we may be able significantly to improve health outcomes and overall quality of life. Instruments such as the AEP are ideally designed for such ends and should be employed routinely and without hesitation.

DEPRESSION AND HEALTH-RELATED QUALITY OF LIFE

Psychiatric comorbidities, particularly depression, have long been shown to negatively affect health outcomes and health-related quality of life in a variety of neurologic and nonneurologic conditions.[18,22,48,97–99] Epilepsy has extremely high rates of psychiatric illness, with depression being the most common comorbidity, with a prevalence of up to 55% among patients with refractory epilepsy.[43,50,61,78] Recent studies have consistently shown a negative correlation between mood status and overall quality of life in epilepsy, often with depression alone accounting the majority of variance in quality-of-life scores.[16,65,81]

In 1995, Perrine et al.[81] examined the relationship among neuropsychological functioning, mood, and quality of life in epilepsy patients at 25 centers across the United States. Results demonstrated that mood had the highest correlation and explained the greatest amount of variance (46.7%) in validated quality-of-life measures (QOLIE-89).

Lehrner et al.[62] studied patients with refractory epilepsy and measured degrees of depression and overall HRQOL using instruments validated for native German-speakers. Forty-five percent of patients were found to suffer from depression, and on multiple regression analysis, depression scores proved to be the major predictor on all six HRQOL scales. This was a linear correlation, with more severe depression scores predicting a lower quality of life. Seizure frequency was not found to predict either depressive mood or HRQOL score.[62]

Cramer et al.[23] studied the influence of comorbid depression on HRQOL for people with epilepsy using a postal survey and the QOLIE-89 and CES-D (Center for Epidemiologic Studies Depression Scale) (Fig. 2). Other variables, such as seizure frequency, medications, degree of disability, and economic factors, were also incorporated into the analysis. Depending on CES-D scores, patients were categorized into one of three groups: (a) no depression, (b) moderate depression, or (c) major depression. All QOLIE-89 subscales and total score were determined by degree of depression but were not significantly influenced by seizure type. Total scores decreased by 17 to 23 points between major and moderate depression, 8 to 13 points between moderate and no depression, and 30 to 32 points between major and no depression (Table 1).[23]

In a recent study, Loring et al.[65] examined the relative contribution of epilepsy-specific concerns, cognitive variables, and other clinical factors to overall HRQOL in patients undergoing evaluation for epilepsy surgery. Patients were evaluated with the QOLIE-89, Minnesota Multiphasic Personality Inventory-2, BDI, EFA Concerns Index, and various measures of general intelligence and cognitive function. Regression analysis revealed that the two most important factors associated with overall score on the QOLIE-89 were depressive symptomatology (accounting for 57% of the variance) and seizure worry (accounting for 42% of the variance) (Figs. 3 and 4).[65]

Until very recently there had been no specific diagnostic instrument for reliably and consistently diagnosing depression in patients with epilepsy, distinguishing mood status from other cognitive and medication-related effects. In a multicenter, multidisciplinary study by Gilliam et al.,[38] a six-item screening instrument, the NDDI-E (Neurological Disorders Depression

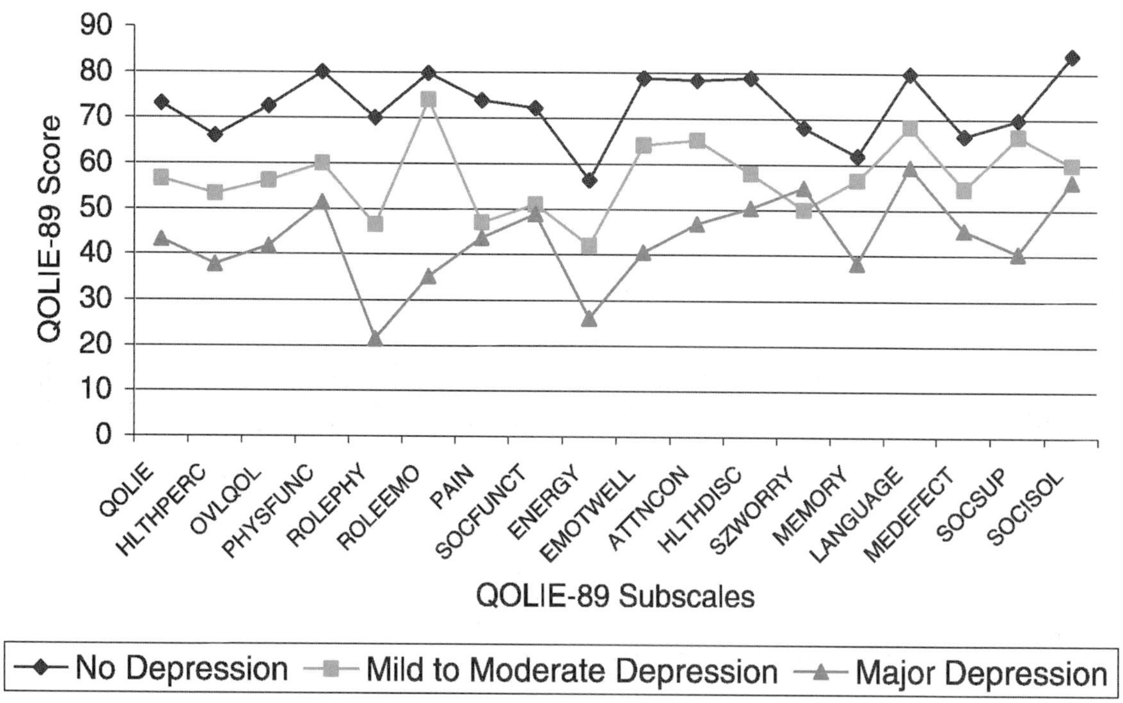

FIGURE 2. Quality of Life in Epilepsy Inventory-89 (QOLIE-89) total and subscale scores for patients with partial seizures by depression category. All scores significantly different by ANOVA across all groups. QOLIE, QOLIE-89 total; HLTHPERC, Health Perception; OVLQOL, Overall QOL; PHYSFUNC, Physical Function; ROLEPHY, Role Physical; ROLEEMO, Role Emotional; SOCFUNCT, Social Function; EMOTWELL, Emotional Well-Being; ATTCON, Attention-Concentration; HLTHDISC, Health Discouragement; SZWORRY, Seizure Worry; MEDEFECT, Medication Effect; SOCSUP, Social Support; SOCISOL, Social Isolation. (From Cramer JA, Blum D, Reed M, et al. The influence of comorbid depression on quality of life for people with epilepsy. *Epilepsy Behav.* 2003;4:515–521; with permission.)

Inventory for Epilepsy), was developed. Discriminant function analysis determined the items most likely to predict a diagnosis of depression based on *Diagnostic and Statistical Manual of Mental Disorders*, 4th edition[3] (DSM-IV)–based criteria and validated screening instruments (the Mini International Neuropsychiatric Interview [MINI] and the Structured Clinical Interview for DSM-IV [SCID]). The NDDI-E predicted major depression with a 90% specificity and 81% sensitivity, and together with drug toxicity, independently predicted 72% of the variance on the QOLIE-89 (adjusted $R^2 = 0.72$; $p < 0.0001$). Subjective health status as measured by the QOLIE-89 was independently predicted by total NDDI-E score (Fig. 5).[37]

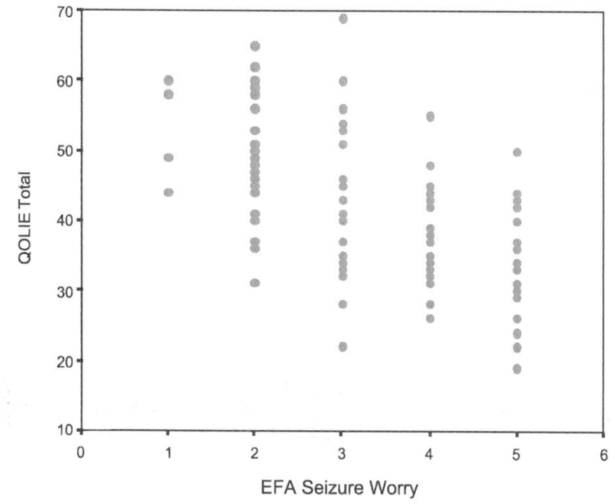

FIGURE 3. Correlation between Quality of Life in Epilepsy Inventory-89 (QOLIE-89) total score and the Epilepsy Foundation of America's Seizure Worry scale. (From Loring DW, Meador KJ, Lee GP. Determinants of quality of life in epilepsy. *Epilepsy Behav.* 2004;5:976–980; with permission.)

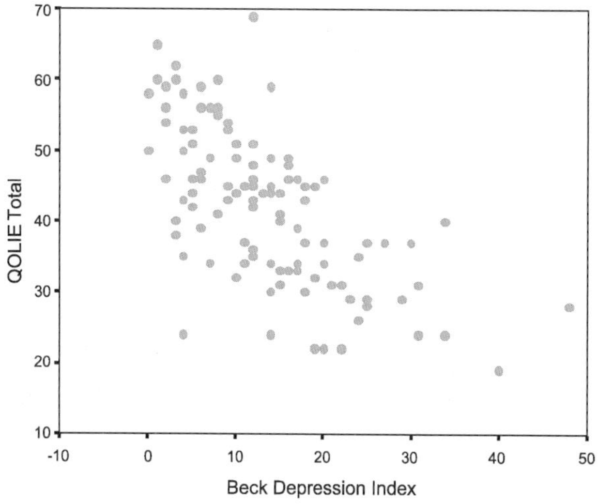

FIGURE 4. Correlation between Quality of Life in Epilepsy Inventory-89 (QOLIE-89) total score and Beck Depression Inventory score. (From Loring DW, Meador KJ, Lee GP. Determinants of quality of life in epilepsy. *Epilepsy Behav.* 2004;5:976–980; with permission.)

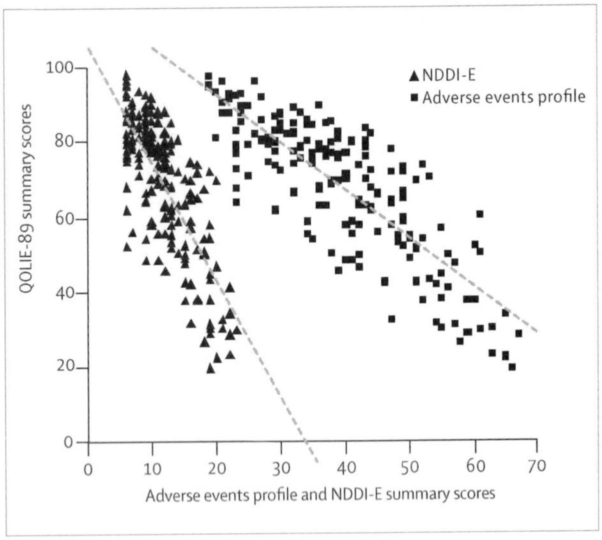

FIGURE 5. Correlation between Quality of Life in Epilepsy Inventory-89 (QOLIE-89) total score with Neurological Disorders Depression Inventory for Epilepsy (NDDI-E) score (partial $r = -0.39$, $p < 0.0001$) and Adverse Events Profile score (partial $r = -0.60$, $p < 0.0001$). Adjusted $R^2 = 0.72$ ($p < 0.0001$) on logistic regression with QOLIE-89 as the dependent variable. (From Gilliam F, Barry J, Hermann B, et al. Rapid detection of major depression in epilepsy: A multicentre study. *Lancet Neurol.* 2006:5;399–405, with permission.)

Although depression is the most common psychiatric comorbidity in epilepsy,[53] a recent multicenter study by Jones et al.[54] found a very high prevalence of DSM-IV anxiety disorders (52%) among patients attending tertiary care epilepsy clinics. Johnson et al.[52] looked at not only depression, but also the relative impact of anxiety and clinical seizure features on HRQOL in patients with temporal lobe epilepsy. Patients with temporal lobe epilepsy completed self-report measures of mood, anxiety, QOL, and seizure severity, including the Symptom Checklist-90 Revised, the BDI, the QOLIE-89, and the Liverpool Seizure Severity Scale. Significant inverse relationships were observed between depression and anxiety scores and overall HRQOL.

Although there is often considerable overlap of these two conditions, partial correlations demonstrated independent contributions by depression and anxiety symptoms to scores on the QOLIE-89. In addition, depression and anxiety independently accounted for the most variance in QOLIE-89 scores when compared to seizure variables and demographic characteristics.[53] These findings replicated the "dose-dependent" phenomenon of psychiatric illness on HRQOL measures seen previously for both depression and anxiety.[37,53]

Psychiatric illness is a highly prevalent, relatively underdiagnosed, and undertreated comorbidity in epilepsy that has the potential to significantly impact QOL.[43,56,57] There now exist highly specialized screening tools, such as the NDDI-E, that can rapidly and reliably detect depression in epilepsy patients, as well as differentiate symptoms of depression from those of medication toxicity and cognitive effects of epilepsy.[37] By recognizing the presence of this interictal phenomenon through systematic screening of epilepsy patients, we have the opportunity to intervene via psychotropic medications or psychotherapy and effect positive change in the overall HRQOL of patients with epilepsy.

OTHER COMORBIDITIES

In a recent population-based, nationwide Canadian study, Tellez-Zenteno et al.[93] found that people with epilepsy had a two- to fivefold higher risk of somatic comorbidities such as stroke, migraine, intestinal ulcers, and chronic fatigue than the general population. Although the reasons for these patterns were not directly explained in the study, this information further emphasizes the need to conceptualize epilepsy as a complex condition with diverse medical and psychiatric comorbidities, requiring a multidisciplinary, integrated approach.[93]

Sleep

A reciprocal relationship between sleep and epilepsy has been described over the last several centuries.[77] Circadian rhythms can affect the expression of epilepsy, and epilepsy itself has the potential to alter sleep patterns.[77] In addition, many antiepileptic drugs used to treat seizures have a disruptive effect on sleep architecture. There is a significant association between the presence of epilepsy and a comorbid sleep disorder, with rates of sleep apnea approaching 30% among patients with epilepsy.[34,51,66–68]

De Weerd et al.[26] examined the prevalence of various sleep disorders in patients with partial epilepsy and found significantly higher rates of disturbances such as insomnia, periodic leg movements, and excessive daytime sleepiness, with an overall twofold increase in sleep disorders compared to controls (38.6% vs. 18%; $p < 0.0001$). This study also examined the impact of sleep disturbances on overall quality of life in patients with epilepsy. The presence of epilepsy and a comorbid sleep disorder in the last 6 months was associated with the most substantial decrease in quality of life as measured by the SF-36, compared to patients with epilepsy alone and normal controls.[26]

In a large study of Mexican patients with epilepsy, patients were surveyed for factors contributing to quality-of-life scores as measured by the QOLIE-31.[1] On multiple regression analysis, the most significant factors predictive of lower QOLIE-31 scores were sleep disturbance and socioeconomic status. These factors were independent of seizure frequency, thus suggesting an independent association. Although this study was limited by the lack of screening instruments for detecting depression and medication toxicity, it further emphasizes the potential importance of comorbid sleep disturbances in determining quality of life in epilepsy.[1]

The increased prevalence of sleep disorders, particularly sleep apnea, among patients with epilepsy and their perceived impact on HRQOL should prompt increased awareness and screening by physicians who treat epilepsy.[44] Questioning regarding adequacy of sleep or excessive daytime somnolence may necessitate referral to a sleep specialist for polysomnography. General measures pertaining to proper sleep hygiene may also prove beneficial.[44] Because specific AEDs have the potential to both alter sleep architecture and increase daytime somnolence, judicious choice of medications favoring stimulating agents such as lamotrigine and felbamate, as well as the timing of medication with more-sedating agents used at bedtime, may also aid in restoring sleep.[10,44,51,77]

Exercise

Epilepsy patients have traditionally been counseled to avoid physical activity due to fear of physical injury or provocation of seizures, and as a result they tend to suffer from inactivity and general lack of physical fitness.[15,52,76,92] The issue of whether exercise exacerbates seizures is somewhat controversial, however; many studies point to a reduction in seizures in patients participating in regular exercise.[27,32,79] Several studies have examined fitness levels in epilepsy patients and results of exercise interventions on seizure control and overall health.

Steinhoff et al.[92] quantified objective measures of physical fitness such as body mass index, muscle strength endurance, and flexibility. Patients were also questioned about leisure time activities. Although leisure time activities did not differ considerably between epilepsy patients and normal controls, results based on the objective physical indicators reflected a significantly lower level of fitness in the epilepsy patients, including measures of aerobic endurance, muscle strength endurance, physical flexibility, and body mass index (BMI).[92]

Eriksen et al.[32] examined a small group of women with intractable epilepsy who were given an exercise regime of aerobic dance and strength training for 60 minutes, twice weekly, for 15 weeks. Seizure frequency was significantly reduced during the treatment phase, and a decrease in muscle pain, sleep disturbance, and fatigue was also observed.[32]

Roth et al.[85] studied associations among exercise levels, depression, and stressful life events in 133 adults with refractory epilepsy. Statistical analyses demonstrated lower levels of depression among the group who was more physically active, as well as an independent contribution of exercise and stressful life events on depression. This effect was separate from the influence of other predictor variables such as seizure frequency, age, and gender, suggesting that regular exercise and the avoidance of stress may lower depression in patients with epilepsy.[85]

In the first randomized, controlled trial of exercise in epilepsy, McAuley et al.[76] examined 23 patients with epilepsy who were randomized to either a 12-week, supervised, outpatient exercise program or to continue their current level of activity. Both clinical (seizure frequency, AED concentrations) and behavioral outcomes (QOLIE-89, POMS, Physical Self-Description Questionnaire, Self-Esteem) were measured. Results showed no appreciable difference in either seizure activity or AED levels; there were, however, significant improvements in overall score on the QOLIE-89 and significant decreases in mood disturbance among patients in the exercise group.[76]

These studies suggest a role for the implementation of an exercise program to promote overall HRQOL among patients with epilepsy without the risk of exacerbating seizures.

Migraine

Significant overlap between epilepsy and migraine is well known, in terms of both clinical presentation and prevalence of comorbid conditions in the same individual or family; having one disorder doubles a patient's risk of having the other disorder.[47,80]

Ottman and Lipton[80] investigated the comorbidity of migraine and epilepsy in a population-based study of >3,000 patients and found a greater-than-twofold increase in the rate of migraine among patients with epilepsy (24%) as well as their relatives with epilepsy (23%) compared to relatives without epilepsy (12%). Despite this increased association, no definitive causative factors, either genetic or environmental, have been identified, making this increased comorbidity likely the result of multiple contributory events.

Lipton et al.[64] examined the influence of migraine and depression on HRQOL in an international study involving patients in both the United States and the United Kingdom. Three hundred 89 migraine cases and 379 controls completed the SF-12, a generic measure of quality of life, and the Primary Care Evaluation of Mental Disorders, a mental health screening inventory. Patients with migraine had significantly lower scores on the SF-12 in both the physical and mental health domains. Depression was highly comorbid with migraine (adjusted prevalence ratio 2.7; 95% confidence interval 2.1–3.5), and both depression and migraine were independently correlated with lower HRQOL scores.[64]

A Turkish study by Velioglu et al.[94] specifically looked at the impact of migraine on epilepsy and prognosis. Cases with epilepsy and migraine and controls with epilepsy alone were followed prospectively over a 5- to 10-year period and assessed for medication use and seizure frequency. Despite similar initial baseline characteristics, the epilepsy-migraine group had a lower chance of becoming seizure free, a higher incidence of intractable seizures, a longer duration of illness, and a lower treatment response than did epilepsy controls. The reasons for poorer prognosis in the epilepsy-migraine group are not known; however, previous evidence suggesting neuronal hyperexcitability as the underlying pathophysiologic mechanism in migraine may explain the adverse outcomes in relation to seizure control.[5,47,59,94]

Given the increased prevalence of migraine and epilepsy, the adverse association with prognosis, quality of life, and depressed mood, and possible shared pathophysiology, it seems sensible to screen epilepsy patients for comorbid migraine headache and to prescribe pharmacologic treatments that target both disorders. Both topiramate[17,88] and valproate[35,87] have been shown to be effective in migraine prophylaxis and are approved by the U. S. Food and Drug Administration for this indication. Other antiepileptic drugs that may be useful in the treatment of migraine but lack evidence from large-scale trials include gabapentin,[71] levatiracetam,[33] tiagabine,[20] and zonisamide.[30] Very preliminary data in a small number of patients may show the efficacy of vagus nerve stimulation in refractory migraine.[75]

SUMMARY AND CONCLUSIONS

Traditionally, the study and treatment of epilepsy has considered the ictus itself to be of paramount importance. Whereas attempting to reduce or eliminate seizures is a worthy goal, the last decade of research in epilepsy, and particularly research relating to health outcomes, has begun to shift the focus from the ictal to the interictal period. By recognizing that pervasive and persistent interictal factors such as medication toxicity and comorbid psychiatric illness are responsible for the greatest amount of variance in overall HRQOL, we can see that the mere cessation of seizures may not be sufficient to positively affect HRQOL in patients with epilepsy.[16,37,65,81] The available instruments for measuring predictors of HRQOL should be employed routinely and frequently by neurologists and the epilepsy health care team at each outpatient encounter.

Numerous research-proven, validated instruments exist for measuring indicators of quality of life in epilepsy, including general measures such as the QOLIE-89 and instruments that target the most significant contributory subcategories, such as medication toxicity and mood status.[29,36,55,86] Current evidence from randomized, controlled trials suggests that instruments such as the Adverse Events Profile[5] for measuring medication toxicity and the newly developed Neurological Disorders Depression Inventory for Epilepsy[37] for screening for depression are relatively short, are easily completed in a busy neurologic practice, and may be the most valuable tools for improving the comprehensive care of patients with epilepsy.

References

1. Alanis-Guevara I, Pena E, Corona T, et al. Sleep disturbances, socioeconomic status, and seizure control as main predictors of quality of life in epilepsy. *Epilepsy Behav.* 2005;7:481–485.
2. Aldenkamp AP, Baker GA. The Neurotoxicity Scale—II. Results of a patient-based scale assessing neurotoxicity in patients with epilepsy. *Epilepsy Res.* 1997;27:165–173.
3. American Psychiatric Association. *Diagnostic and Statistical Manual of Mental Disorders,* 4th ed. Washington, DC: American Psychiatric Association; 1994.

4. Aristotle. De Anima. In: McKeon R, ed. *Introduction to Aristotle.* New York: Modern Library; 1947: 148–153.
5. Aurora SK, Cao Y, Bowyer SM, et al. The occipital cortex is hyperexcitable in migraine: Experimental evidence. *Headache.* 1999;39:469–476.
6. Baker GA, Frances P, Middleton E. Initial development, reliability, and validity of a patient-based adverse events scale. *Epilepsia.* 1994;80.
7. Baker GA, Jacoby A, Buck D, et al. Quality of life of people with epilepsy: A European study. *Epilepsia.* 1997;38:353–362.
8. Baker GA, Jacoby A, Buck D, et al. The quality of life of older people with epilepsy: Findings from a UK community study. *Seizure.* 2001;10: 92–99.
9. Baker GA, Smith DF, Dewey M, et al. The initial development of a health-related quality of life model as an outcome measure in epilepsy. *Epilepsy Res.* 1993;16:65–81.
10. Bazil CW. Sleep, sleep apnea, and epilepsy. *Curr Treat Options Neurol.* 2004;6:339–345.
11. Beghi E, Spagnoli P, Airoldi L, et al. Emotional and affective disturbances in patients with epilepsy. *Epilepsy Behav.* 2002;3:255–261.
12. Begley CE, Famulari M, Annegers JF, et al. The cost of epilepsy in the United States: An estimate from population-based clinical and survey data. *Epilepsia.* 2000;41:342–351.
13. Behrens E, Schramm J, Zentner J, et al. Surgical and neurological complications in a series of 708 epilepsy surgery procedures. *Neurosurgery.* 1997;41:1–9; discussion, 9—10.
14. Birbeck GL, Hays RD, Cui X, et al. Seizure reduction and quality of life improvements in people with epilepsy. *Epilepsia.* 2002;43:535–538.
15. Bjorholt PG, Nakken KO, Rohme K, et al. Leisure time habits and physical fitness in adults with epilepsy. *Epilepsia.* 1990;31:83–87.
16. Boylan LS, Flint LA, Labovitz DL, et al. Depression but not seizure frequency predicts quality of life in treatment-resistant epilepsy. *Neurology.* 2004;62:258–261.
17. Brandes JL, Saper JR, Diamond M, et al. Topiramate for migraine prevention: A randomized controlled trial. *JAMA.* 2004;291:965–973.
18. Broadhead WE, Blazer DG, George LK, et al. Depression, disability days, and days lost from work in a prospective epidemiologic survey. *JAMA.* 1990;264:2524–2528.
19. Buelow J,Estwing Ferrans C. Quality of life in epilepsy. In: Ettinger A, Kanner A, eds. *Psychiatric Issues in Epilepsy: A Practical Guide to Diagnosis and Treatment.* Philadelphia: Lippincott Williams & Wilkins; 2001: 307–319.
20. Capuano A, Vollono C, Mei D, et al. Antiepileptic drugs in migraine prophylaxis: State of the art. *Clin Ther.* 2004;155:79–87.
21. Clancy CM, Eisenberg JM. Outcomes research: Measuring the end results of health care. *Science.* 1998;282:245–246.
22. Covinsky KE, Fortinsky RH, Palmer RM, et al. Relation between symptoms of depression and health status outcomes in acutely ill hospitalized older persons. *Ann Intern Med.* 1997;126:417–425.
23. Cramer JA, Blum D, Reed M, et al. The influence of comorbid depression on quality of life for people with epilepsy. *Epilepsy Behav.* 2003;4:515–521.
24. Cramer JA, Hammer AE, Kustra RP. Quality of life improvement with conversion to lamotrigine monotherapy. *Epilepsy Behav.* 2004;5:224–230.
25. Cramer JA, Perrine K, Devinsky O, et al. A brief questionnaire to screen for quality of life in epilepsy: The QOLIE-10. *Epilepsia.* 1996;37:577–582.
26. de Weerd A, de Haas S, Otte A, et al. Subjective sleep disturbance in patients with partial epilepsy: A questionnaire-based study on prevalence and impact on quality of life. *Epilepsia.* 2004;45:1397–1404.
27. Denio LS, Drake ME Jr, Pakalnis A. The effect of exercise on seizure frequency. *J Med.* 1989;20:171–176.
28. Devinsky O, Penry JK. Quality of life in epilepsy: The clinician's view. *Epilepsia.* 1993;34(Suppl 4):S4–S7.
29. Devinsky O, Vickrey BG, Cramer J, et al. Development of the quality of life in epilepsy inventory. *Epilepsia.* 1995;36:1089–1104.
30. Drake ME Jr, Greathouse NI, Renner JB, et al. Open-label zonisamide for refractory migraine. *Clin Neuropharmacol.* 2004;27(6):278–280.
31. Drake ME, Greathouse N, Armentbright AD, et al. Levetiracetam for preventive treatment of migraine. *Cephalalgia.* 2001;21:373.
32. Eriksen HR, Ellertsen B, Gronningsaeter H, et al. Physical exercise in women with intractable epilepsy. *Epilepsia.* 1994;35:1256–1264.
33. Ettinger A, Reed M, Cramer J. Depression and comorbidity in community-based patients with epilepsy or asthma. *Neurology.* 2004;63:1008–1014.
34. Foldvary-Schaefer N. Obstructive sleep apnea in patients with epilepsy: Does treatment affect seizure control? *Sleep Med.* 2003;4:483–484.
35. Freitag FG, Collins SD, Carlson HA, et al. A randomized trial of divalproex sodium extended-release tablets in migraine prophylaxis. *Neurology.* 2002;58:1652–1659.
36. Gillham R, Bryant-Comstock L, Kane K. Validation of the Side Effect and Life Satisfaction (SEALS) inventory. *Seizure.* 2000;9:458–463.
37. Gilliam F. Optimizing health outcomes in active epilepsy. *Neurology.* 2002;58:S9–S20.
38. Gilliam F, Barry J, Hermann B, et al. Rapid detection of major depression in epilepsy: A multicentre study. *Lancet Neurol.* 2006;5:399–405.
39. Gilliam F, Bowling S, Bilir E, et al. Association of combined MRI, interictal EEG, and ictal EEG results with outcome and pathology after temporal lobectomy. *Epilepsia.* 1997;38:1315–1320.
40. Gilliam F, Carter J, Vahle V. Tolerability of antiseizure medications: Implications for health outcomes. *Neurology.* 2004;63:S9–S12.
41. Gilliam F, Kuzniecky R, Faught E, et al. Patient-validated content of epilepsy-specific quality-of-life measurement. *Epilepsia.* 1997;38: 233–236.
42. Gilliam F, Kuzniecky R, Meador K, et al. Patient-oriented outcome assessment after temporal lobectomy for refractory epilepsy. *Neurology.* 1999;53:687–694.
43. Gilliam FG. Diagnosis and treatment of mood disorders in persons with epilepsy. *Curr Opin Neurol.* 2005;18:129–133.
44. Gilliam FG, Mendiratta A, Pack AM, et al. Epilepsy and common comorbidities: Improving the outpatient epilepsy encounter. *Epileptic Disord.* 2005;7(Suppl 1):27–33.
45. Gotay CC, Korn EL, McCabe MS, et al. Quality-of-life assessment in cancer treatment protocols: Research issues in protocol development. *J Natl Cancer Inst.* 1992;84:575–579.
46. Hauser WA, Annegers JF, Kurland LT. Incidence of epilepsy and unprovoked seizures in Rochester, Minnesota: 1935—1984. *Epilepsia.* 1993;34:453–468.
47. Haut SR, Bigal ME, Lipton RB. Chronic disorders with episodic manifestations: Focus on epilepsy and migraine. *Lancet Neurol.* 2006;5: 148–157.
48. Hays RD, Wells KB, Sherbourne CD, et al. Functioning and well-being outcomes of patients with depression compared with chronic general medical illnesses. *Arch Gen Psychiatry.* 1995;52:11–19.
49. Hermann BP. Developing a model of quality of life in epilepsy: The contribution of neuropsychology. *Epilepsia.* 1993;34(Suppl 4):S14–S21.
50. Hermann BP, Seidenberg M, Bell B. Psychiatric comorbidity in chronic epilepsy: Identification, consequences, and treatment of major depression. *Epilepsia.* 2000;41(Suppl 2):S31–S41.
51. Hollinger P, Khatami R, Gugger M, et al. Epilepsy and obstructive sleep apnea. *Eur Neurol.* 2006;55:74–79.
52. Jalava M, Sillanpaa M. Physical activity, health-related fitness, and health experience in adults with childhood-onset epilepsy: A controlled study. *Epilepsia.* 1997;38:424–429.
53. Johnson EK, Jones JE, Seidenberg M, et al. The relative impact of anxiety, depression, and clinical seizure features on health-related quality of life in epilepsy. *Epilepsia.* 2004;45:544–550.
54. Jones JE, Hermann BP, Barry JJ, et al. Clinical assessment of Axis I psychiatric morbidity in chronic epilepsy: A multicenter investigation. *J Neuropsychiatry Clin Neurosci.* 2005;17:172–179.
55. Jones JE, Hermann BP, Woodard JL, et al. Screening for major depression in epilepsy with common self-report depression inventories. *Epilepsia.* 2005;46:731–735.
56. Kanner AM. Depression in epilepsy: A frequently neglected multifaceted disorder. *Epilepsy Behav.* 2003;4(Suppl 4):11–19.
57. Kanner AM, Palac S. Depression in epilepsy: A common but often unrecognized comorbid malady. *Epilepsy Behav.* 2000;1:37–51.
58. Karnofsky D, Abelmann W, Craver L. The use of nitrogen mustards in the palliative treatment of carcinoma. *Cancer.* 1948;4:634–656.
59. Koch UR, Musshoff U, Pannek HW, et al. Intrinsic excitability, synaptic potentials, and short-term plasticity in human epileptic neocortex. *J Neurosci Res.* 2005;80:715–726.
60. Kwan P, Brodie MJ. Early identification of refractory epilepsy. *N Engl J Med.* 2000;342:314–319.
61. Lambert MV, Robertson MM. Depression in epilepsy: Etiology, phenomenology, and treatment. *Epilepsia.* 1999;40(Suppl 10):S21–S47.
62. Lehrner J, Kalchmayr R, Serles W, et al. Health-related quality of life (HRQOL), activity of daily living (ADL) and depressive mood disorder in temporal lobe epilepsy patients. *Seizure.* 1999;8:88–92.
63. Leidy NK, Elixhauser A, Vickrey B, et al. Seizure frequency and the health-related quality of life of adults with epilepsy. *Neurology.* 1999;53: 162–166.
64. Lipton RB, Hamelsky SW, Kolodner KB, et al. Migraine, quality of life, and depression: A population-based case—control study. *Neurology.* 2000;55:629–635.
65. Loring DW, Meador KJ, Lee GP. Determinants of quality of life in epilepsy. *Epilepsy Behav.* 2004;5:976–980.
66. Malow BA, Levy K, Maturen K, et al. Obstructive sleep apnea is common in medically refractory epilepsy patients. *Neurology.* 2000;55:1002–1007.
67. Manni R, Tartara A. Evaluation of sleepiness in epilepsy. *Clin Neurophysiol.* 2000;111(Suppl 2):S111–S114.
68. Manni R, Terzaghi M, Arbasino C, et al. Obstructive sleep apnea in a clinical series of adult epilepsy patients: Frequency and features of the comorbidity. *Epilepsia.* 2003;44:836–840.
69. Markand ON, Salanova V, Whelihan E, et al. Health-related quality of life outcome in medically refractory epilepsy treated with anterior temporal lobectomy. *Epilepsia.* 2000;41:749–759.
70. Martin R, Vogtle L, Gilliam F, et al. Health-related quality of life in senior adults with epilepsy: What we know from randomized clinical trials and suggestions for future research. *Epilepsy Behav.* 2003;4:626–634.
71. Mathew NT, Rapoport A, Saper J, et al. Efficacy of gabapentin in migraine prophylaxis. *Headache.* 2001;41:119–128.
72. Mattson RH, Cramer JA, Collins JF. A comparison of valproate with carbamazepine for the treatment of complex partial seizures and secondarily generalized tonic—clonic seizures in adults. The Department of Veterans Affairs Epilepsy Cooperative Study No. 264 Group. *N Engl J Med.* 1992;327:765–771.

73. Mattson RH, Cramer JA, Collins JF. Prognosis for total control of complex partial and secondarily generalized tonic clonic seizures. Department of Veterans Affairs Epilepsy Cooperative Studies No. 118 and No. 264 Group. *Neurology*. 1996;47:68–76.
74. Mattson RH, Cramer JA, Collins JF, et al. Comparison of carbamazepine, phenobarbital, phenytoin, and primidone in partial and secondarily generalized tonic-clonic seizures. *N Engl J Med*. 1985;313:145–151.
75. Mauskop A. Vagus nerve stimulation relieves chronic refractory migraine and cluster headaches. *Cephalalgia*. 2005;25(2):82–86.
76. McAuley JW, Long L, Heise J, et al. A prospective evaluation of the effects of a 12-week outpatient exercise program on clinical and behavioral outcomes in patients with epilepsy. *Epilepsy Behav*. 2001;2:592–600.
77. Mendez M, Radtke RA. Interactions between sleep and epilepsy. *J Clin Neurophysiol*. 2001;18:106–127.
78. Mendez MF, Cummings JL, Benson DF. Depression in epilepsy. Significance and phenomenology. *Arch Neurol*. 1986;43:766–770.
79. Nakken KO, Bjorholt PG, Johannessen SI, et al. Effect of physical training on aerobic capacity, seizure occurrence, and serum level of antiepileptic drugs in adults with epilepsy. *Epilepsia*. 1990;31:88–94.
80. Ottman R, Lipton RB. Comorbidity of migraine and epilepsy. *Neurology*. 1994;44:2105–2110.
81. Perrine K, Hermann BP, Meador KJ, et al. The relationship of neuropsychological functioning to quality of life in epilepsy. *Arch Neurol*. 1995;52:997–1003.
82. Pirio Richardson S, Farias ST, Lima AR 3rd, et al. Improvement in seizure control and quality of life in medically refractory epilepsy patients converted from polypharmacy to monotherapy. *Epilepsy Behav*. 2004;5:343–347.
83. Radhakrishnan K, So EL, Silbert PL, et al. Predictors of outcome of anterior temporal lobectomy for intractable epilepsy: A multivariate study. *Neurology*. 1998;51:465–471.
84. Robertson MM, Trimble MR. Depressive illness in patients with epilepsy: A review. *Epilepsia*. 1983;24(Suppl 2):S109–S116.
85. Roth DL, Goode KT, Williams VL, et al. Physical exercise, stressful life experience, and depression in adults with epilepsy. *Epilepsia*. 1994;35:1248–1255.
86. Salinsky MC, Storzbach D. The Portland Neurotoxicity Scale: Validation of a brief self-report measure of antiepileptic-drug—related neurotoxicity. *Assessment*. 2005;12:107–117.
87. Silberstein SD, Collins SD. Safety of divalproex sodium in migraine prophylaxis: An open-label, long-term study. Long-term Safety of Depakote in Headache Prophylaxis Study Group. *Headache*. 1999;39:633–643.
88. Silberstein SD, Neto W, Schmitt J, et al. Topiramate in migraine prevention: Results of a large controlled trial. *Arch Neurol*. 2004;61:490–495.
89. Sillanpaa M, Haataja L, Shinnar S. Perceived impact of childhood-onset epilepsy on quality of life as an adult. *Epilepsia*. 2004;45:971–977.
90. Spencer SS, Berg AT, Vickrey BG, et al. Predicting long-term seizure outcome after resective epilepsy surgery: The multicenter study. *Neurology*. 2005;65:912–918.
91. Sperling MR, Feldman H, Kinman J, et al. Seizure control and mortality in epilepsy. *Ann Neurol*. 1999;46:45–50.
92. Steinhoff BJ, Neususs K, Thegeder H, et al. Leisure time activity and physical fitness in patients with epilepsy. *Epilepsia*. 1996;37:1221–1227.
93. Tellez-Zenteno JF, Matijevic S, Wiebe S. Somatic comorbidity of epilepsy in the general population in Canada. *Epilepsia*. 2005;46:1955–1962.
94. Velioglu SK, Boz C, Ozmenoglu M. The impact of migraine on epilepsy: A prospective prognosis study. *Cephalalgia*. 2005;25:528–535.
95. Vickrey BG, Hays RD, Graber J, et al. A health-related quality of life instrument for patients evaluated for epilepsy surgery. *Med Care*. 1992;30:299–319.
96. Vickrey BG, Hays RD, Rausch R, et al. Quality of life of epilepsy surgery patients as compared with outpatients with hypertension, diabetes, heart disease, and/or depressive symptoms. *Epilepsia*. 1994;35:597–607.
97. Wells KB, Stewart A, Hays RD, et al. The functioning and well-being of depressed patients. Results from the Medical Outcomes Study. *JAMA*. 1989;262:914–919.
98. Whooley MA, Browner WS. Association between depressive symptoms and mortality in older women. Study of Osteoporotic Fractures Research Group. *Arch Intern Med*. 1998;158:2129–2135.
99. Whooley MA, Simon GE. Managing depression in medical outpatients. *N Engl J Med*. 2000;343:1942–1950.
100. Wiebe S, Blume WT, Girvin JP, et al. A randomized, controlled trial of surgery for temporal-lobe epilepsy. *N Engl J Med*. 2001;345:311–318.
101. Wiebe S, Derry PA. Measuring quality of life in epilepsy surgery patients. *Can J Neurol Sci*. 2000;27(Suppl 1):S111–S115; discussion, S121–S115.
102. World Health Organization. The constitution of the World Health Organization. *WHO Chron*. 1947;1:29.

CHAPTER 221 ■ LEGAL CONCERNS AND EFFECTIVE ADVOCACY STRATEGIES

ROY G. BERAN, JOHN DEVEREUX, WILLIAM MCLIN, CYNTHIA LEHMAN, JOHAN FALK-PEDERSEN, HANNEKE M. DE BOER, AND ALEXANDRA FINUCANE

INTRODUCTION

For too many years, people with disabilities—particularly people with epilepsy—were a voiceless minority. These individuals had many unmet needs in the areas of civil rights, education, employment, residential and community services, and provision of appropriate health care. Many lived at home, rarely venturing out. Too many were segregated from society and they were forced to live in large state residential institutions for the intellectually disabled or mentally ill. Until recent decades, laws, even in countries whose citizens pride themselves on liberal views about such matters, such as the United States, restricted the rights of people with epilepsy to marry and provided for their involuntary sterilization.[3] The prevailing belief was that people with epilepsy could not be employed because they might have a seizure on the job and hurt themselves or others.

Over the years, these beliefs and conditions have been challenged in various countries by advocacy efforts led by citizens with disabilities, family members, professionals, policy makers, and the courts. Gradually, society is coming to recognize that many of the problems faced by those with disabilities are not inevitable but are rather the result of discriminatory policies based on unfounded, outmoded stereotypes and perceptions deeply grounded in irrational fears and prejudices toward such people.

In recent decades, some countries have enacted laws specifically prohibiting discrimination on the basis of disability. One example of a broad-reaching antidiscrimination law is the Americans with Disabilities Act (ADA), enacted in 1990, which prohibits discrimination on the basis of disability in employment, in the programs and services of state and local governments, by places of public accommodation, in public and private transportation services, and in communications. The ADA grants all individuals with disabilities uniform protection, regardless of the state in which they live.[2]

Even with the passage of laws like the ADA and its international equivalents, epilepsy raises a variety of legal concerns, including employment discrimination, driver licensing requirements, access to appropriate educational services, access to insurance, and even possible arrest for seizure-related behavior. This chapter summarizes some of the legal issues that patients with epilepsy face, some of the legal remedies, the issues physicians may face as they advocate for their patients, continuing areas of legislative advocacy, and effective advocacy strategies for those wishing to change current laws.

This chapter emphasizes U.S. law because space does not permit a full discussion of legal issues from the perspective of each country and because insufficient recent information exists about legal issues from an international perspective, except in the area of driver licensing. Additional publications on legal or psychosocial issues in various countries may be of interest.[1,4,6,9–12,15,16,19,21,23–25]

THE AMERICANS WITH DISABILITIES ACT—EMPLOYMENT PROVISIONS

Although laws do not eliminate discriminatory attitudes, antidiscrimination statutes such as the ADA have forced many employers to reevaluate and subsequently change their employment practices and have given employees important legal tools with which to seek redress from unfair employment practices.

The concept of disability under the ADA encompasses three parts: (a) does the individual have, does the individual have a record of, or is the individual regarded as having, a physical or mental impairment? If so, does the physical or mental impairment the individual has, has a record of, or is regarded as having (b) substantially limit (c) one or more of that individual's major life activities?

Under the ADA, employers with 15 or more employees are prohibited from discriminating on the basis of disability against individuals who can do the essential functions of the job or who could do so with reasonable accommodation. Reasonable accommodation is a flexible concept. Examples of accommodations that might be appropriate for individuals with epilepsy include job restructuring (e.g., if driving is a marginal duty, driving tasks could be reassigned to another employee); permitting part-time or modified work schedules; allowing time off for doctor's visits and to recover from seizures; installing a safety device around a piece of machinery; padding a concrete floor at the employee's work site; and allowing the individual to work at a job site close to home or, in some cases, at home.

Employers are not required to provide an accommodation under the ADA if it would be an "undue hardship" on the employer, that is, if it would cause the employer significant difficulty or expense. This is evaluated in light of the employer's overall business. If a particular accommodation would impose an undue hardship on an employer, the employer may be required to provide other reasonable accommodations. The ADA does not require employers to accommodate the needs of employees who miss work to care for family members with medical problems. However, in the United States, employees who need to miss a significant amount of work because of their serious health problems or those of family members may benefit from the Family and Medical Leave Act (FMLA), which requires employers with 50 or more employees to provide up to 12 weeks of unpaid leave to eligible employees and to retain the employee's benefits. It is recognized that this may be a uniquely U.S. situation, but it highlights the way in which the rights of individuals are becoming protected by law. Further information about FMLA can be obtained from the Wage and Hour Division of the U.S. Department of Labor.

Safety Issues

For most jobs, simply having occasional seizures will not significantly affect the person's ability to do the job's essential functions. Having seizures does not render a person unqualified under the ADA simply because seizures require occasional use of sick time, do not look good, or may result in injury or possible use of worker's compensation. In the U.S. example, employers do not have to offer a job or retain an individual in a job because of a disability if the individual poses a "direct threat" to safety. Direct threat is defined as "a significant risk of substantial harm which cannot be lessened by reasonable accommodation."

Except in very limited circumstances (e.g., commercial airline pilots), a mere diagnosis of epilepsy will not mean that an individual poses a direct threat. Similarly, a possibility or even a probability that an individual will experience a seizure at work is usually not enough to make that person a direct threat without showing that the individual's workplace or essential job duties pose a particular risk of harm. An evaluation must also be made as to whether the factors causing the increased risk can be reduced through a reasonable accommodation. Using laws similar to the ADA, people with epilepsy have successfully obtained and retained such high-risk jobs as firefighter, police officer, and butcher (see, e.g., the case of *Jansen v Food Circus Supermarkets*[13]).

Unsubstantiated fears about risks from the employment environment may not be used by an employer to disqualify a person with epilepsy. Under the ADA, employers must evaluate the individual and the specific situation using reasonable medical judgment that relies on the most current knowledge and best objective evidence. If the specific job tasks suggest possible safety concerns, the treating physician may be asked by the employer or employee for advice about whether the employee should avoid certain tasks. In evaluating a person with epilepsy for a position that might pose safety concerns, it is important to consider the type of job, the essential job duties, the degree of seizure control, the types of seizures (whether the person has simple partial onset to warn of possible evolution), the person's reliability in taking prescribed seizure medication, any side effects of medication, and any accommodations that might lessen the risk.[17]

The ADA's focus on individual capabilities is especially important for the individual with epilepsy because the term epilepsy refers to a broad range of symptoms and underlying causes. Depending on their individual circumstances, some people with active seizures should avoid certain job tasks, such as driving, or certain environmental conditions, such as exposure to open fire, hot substances, dangerous moving objects, mechanical and electrical hazards, and situations in which a danger of falling exists. If an employee is no longer able to do the job for which he or she was hired, even with reasonable accommodations, an employer may be required to reassign that employee to another position, if one is available, for which the employee is qualified. The position should be equivalent in terms of pay and other job status. Within this scheme, an employer is permitted to reassign an individual to a lower-grade position if that is the only position available for which the individual is qualified.

Medical Inquiries by Employers

Employers who are covered by the ADA are prohibited from asking any questions about whether an applicant has a medical condition or about the nature and severity of the condition until after they have extended the applicant a job offer. This is particularly important for individuals with epilepsy, who historically have been denied interviews and refused employment solely because an employer learned of their epilepsy. Again focusing on the U.S. situation, once a job offer has been made, an employer may ask medical questions or request that an individual have a medical examination, so long as all employees selected for that job classification are required to do so. Once an individual has been employed and is on the job, medical inquiries must be job related and consistent with business necessity. In other words, the need for the examination must be triggered by some evidence of problems related to job performance or safety, or an examination may be necessary to determine whether individuals in physically demanding jobs continue to be suitable for duty. In addition, a request for reasonable accommodation by an employee may trigger medical inquiries to verify the need and scope of accommodation. All medical information must be kept separate from an employee's personnel file, and the information must be kept confidential.

Many countries have enacted privacy laws, and transgression of these may provide an alternate source of remedy if the person with epilepsy has been exposed against his or her will.

Complaint Process Under the Americans with Disabilities Act

Individuals may file employment discrimination complaints under the ADA with the U.S. Equal Employment Opportunity Commission (EEOC) or, in many cases, with their state Human Rights Commission. If an employer is not covered by the ADA, because the business does not have 15 or more employees, one should investigate whether there is a state law that applies. Further information about state antidiscrimination laws should be available from the state Human Rights Commission (HRC), and most industrialized countries now have local equivalents of the EEOC and HRC. These bodies have international legitimacy because their host nation is usually a signature nation of the International Parent Body run under the auspices of the United Nations. The U.S. example is far from unique, and was merely provided as a focus on which local proceedings can be examined and used to protect the rights of people with epilepsy.

The Supreme Court's Interpretation of the Americans with Disabilities Act—Important Limitations

It is important to note that, despite the apparently clear nature of protection against discrimination afforded by the ADA, its recent interpretation by the Supreme Court of the United States has limited the protection provided by the Act. In a trilogy of cases (*Sutton v United Airlines, Inc*; *Murphy v United Parcel Service, Inc*; and *Albertson's Inc v Kirkinberg*), the Court held that, in determining whether a person was suffering from a disability, mitigating factors (such a medication) must be taken into account. Thus, in *Sutton*, although the applicants had poor eyesight (20/200 in the right eye and 20/400 in the left eye), when corrected with glasses or contact lenses, their vision was 20/20. The applicants were not disabled. Similarly, the applicant in *Murphy* had chronic hypertension, which, without medication, was extremely high. With medication, it was within acceptable ranges. A recent reaffirmation of these cases is *Cutrera v Board of Supervisors of Louisiana State University* (429 F.3 d 108, 2005).

The effect of these cases on people suffering from epilepsy is obvious. A person whose epilepsy is controlled by medication will not be regarded as having a disability, and thus will not be afforded the protections of the ADA.

DRIVER LICENSING

Driver licensing laws and policies vary significantly from country to country. There is, however, a consensus among experts worldwide that driving should be permitted when seizures are adequately controlled. There is less consistency among different countries as to the length of time considered to be adequate following seizure activity.

Most countries require a seizure-free period of 1 to 3 years.[20] In the United States, most states use a firm seizure-free period of 1 year, 6 months, or 3 months. Many states also provide for exceptions to the usual seizure-free requirement, for example, when an individual has a breakthrough seizure due to medication change or withdrawal and is back on the original medication.[14]

Experts in the international community and in the United States have recently developed separate reports on driving and epilepsy.[18,20] In general, these experts recommend that licenses should be granted after a short prescribed period of freedom from seizures, the decision should be based on an assessment of the medical history of the individual and there should be room for exceptions to the prescribed period of seizure freedom. This assessment should be done either by an independent neurologic specialist or by a Medical Advisory Board on which a neurologic specialist serves. Variations in determining whether to license an individual come from differences in the seizure history, type of seizure, and causative factors. Reassessments should occur periodically or when the individual reports changes in seizure experience.

Current practice in the United States is that, whereas the ultimate licensing decision lies with the state Department of Motor Vehicles (DMV), the agency looks to the treating physician for a variety of information ranging from details about the patient's seizure disorder to the physician's opinion about the patient's ability to drive safely. Most states also require periodic medical updates, at least for several years.

There has been a general trend in recent years to move toward shorter seizure-free periods and exceptions to the general rule. Those U.S. physicians who want to influence DMV policies may want to join their state DMV's medical advisory board, if one exists. In states where the criteria for licensing people with epilepsy was enacted by the legislature, any major changes would be made on the legislative level, but in many places the rules are controlled by regulations pertaining to the act; thus, alteration is far simpler. Physicians may want to contact a local epilepsy organization about state-wide legislative initiatives. A model driver licensing law developed by the Epilepsy Foundation of American (EFA), the American Academy of Neurology (AAN), and the American Epilepsy Society (AES) is available from the EFA.[18] The EFA, AAN, and AES support the use of a 3-month seizure-free interval in driver licensing with consideration of the following favorable and unfavorable factors that may modify that interval:

Favorable modifiers

- Seizures during medically directed medication changes
- Simple partial seizures that do not interfere with consciousness or motor control
- Seizures with consistent and prolonged auras
- Established pattern of pure nocturnal seizures
- Seizures secondary to acute metabolic or toxic states not likely to recur
- Sleep-deprived seizures
- Seizures related to reversible acute illness

Unfavorable modifiers

- Noncompliance or lack of credibility
- Alcohol or drug abuse within last 3 months
- Increased number of seizures in the last year
- Prior bad driving record
- Structural brain lesion
- Noncorrectable brain functional or metabolic condition
- Frequent seizures after seizure-free interval
- Prior crashes due to seizures in the last 5 years

According to their report on driving and epilepsy, international experts from the International Bureau for Epilepsy (IBE) and the International League Against Epilepsy (ILAE) have not recommended a specific seizure-free period but generally describe a range from 3 months to 2 years as appropriate, depending on various factors.[20] The medical issues critical to licensing, and which they recommend should be assessed, are generally similar to the criteria described here. For example, the report on driving suggests that no restrictions on driving may be necessary if the seizure follows an acute cerebral illness from which there has been full recovery or in cases of sensory-evoked seizures. Only a short period of seizure freedom may be necessary prior to licensure if a seizure is the result of physician-supervised medication changes. Whether to license individuals who have seizures due to metabolic disorders depends on the nature of the underlying condition or disease. The report thus clearly emphasizes an individualized assessment based on various factors.

Some people who suffer from seizures have incurred civil or criminal liability as the result of seizure-related accidents. In the United States, such liability has occurred when individuals have driven against medical advice, without a valid license, without the state DMV being aware of their medical condition, or with the knowledge that there was a particular reason that they should not be driving at that time.

In a disturbing trend that is yet to show up in the United States, a court in New South Wales, Australia, in deciding the unreported case of *R v Gillett*, disregarded physician- and state-endorsed guidelines established to determine fitness to drive in assessing the liability of a man with epilepsy who had a motor vehicle accident causing death to others.

In the United States, few reported cases exist on the issue of physician liability to third parties for certifying a patient to drive. Those cases that have been brought in the area of certifying fitness to drive suggest that the risk of liability is minimal. In the United States and internationally, experts recommend that physicians should not be liable for recommendations to the state driver licensing agency as long as those recommendations were arrived at in a reasonable manner and consistent with the prevailing standard of care.[18,20]

Some cases brought by third parties against physicians have been based on the theory that the physician did not use due care in the diagnosis or treatment of the patient. Most courts that have considered these cases in the United States have recognized that physicians cannot "control" their patients; thus, they do not have a duty to prevent them from driving. They may, however, have a duty to warn their patients not to drive due to recent seizures or side effects of medication, and they may be liable to third parties if they fail to give such instructions. Physicians should provide the warnings and advice that are required under prevailing standards of care. Patients who should not be driving, or who should be driving only under certain circumstances, should be so advised in writing. Similarly, confirmation of having given such advice should be written in the patient's medical records as an added protection, should the physician be faced with litigation.

As long as the physician is using reasonable medical judgment and proper documentation, a third-party suit should not result in liability. If a physician has specific concerns, however (such as a patient who is driving against medical advice), he or she may want to consult with an attorney.

The EFA, the IBE, and the ILAE oppose laws requiring physicians to report their patients with epilepsy to the state. In the United States, states currently having such laws include California, Delaware, Nevada, New Jersey, Oregon, and Pennsylvania. Instead, the EFA, the IBE, and the ILAE support laws that give physicians "good faith" immunity for participating in the driver licensing process and for voluntarily reporting those patients who pose an imminent threat to public safety because they are driving against medical advice. In Australia, physicians are not required to report (except in South Australia and the Northern Territory) and are protected against invasion of privacy, except in Western Australia.[5]

EDUCATION

The educational process can pose significant obstacles to children with epilepsy. Obstacles include the physical and psychosocial effects of seizures, the effects of antiepileptic medications, underlying cognitive difficulties, and an educational system that, all too often, does not provide the necessary support or understanding.[22]

In 1975, in response to pressure from organized groups, the U.S. Congress passed the Education of All Handicapped Children Act (PL. 94–142), which guarantees that all children shall receive a free, appropriate public education in the "least restrictive environment." The underlying notion was that children with disabilities were to be educated alongside their nondisabled peers whenever possible. This law was yet another step in the evolution of a public policy goal of total integration of people with disabilities into U.S. society. In 1990, this law was renamed the Individuals with Disabilities Education Act (IDEA).

The Individuals with Disabilities Education Act is the central vehicle through which the U.S. federal government maintains a partnership with the states and localities to provide an appropriate education for children with disabilities requiring special education and related services. To receive funds, state and local education agencies must follow the law's requirements for identifying, evaluating, and providing services to eligible children aged 3 to 21 years. Children with epilepsy are eligible for services if their epilepsy adversely affects their educational performance. Infants and toddlers who have developmental disabilities or who are at risk of having a disability may be eligible for early intervention services.[8] Treating physicians play an important role in establishing a child's need for services.

ARREST FOR SEIZURE-RELATED BEHAVIOR

Some seizure-related behaviors, particularly those associated with complex partial seizures, may result in the individual with epilepsy being arrested and charged with such offenses as public intoxication, trespassing, breaking and entering, shoplifting, resisting arrest, and assault. Assault charges sometimes result when an individual having a seizure is restrained and reacts reflexively. Whether the behavior in question was consistent with the individual's seizures is an issue best addressed by the treating neurologist. Sometimes, intervention by a medical professional will result in charges being dropped. If charges are brought, the individual should seek the advice of a criminal defense lawyer. The type of defense that is appropriate varies from country to country. Some countries and some U.S. states recognize an "automatism" defense for individuals who were not aware of their actions at the time of the alleged criminal behavior. Expert opinion at trial will be crucial in proving a defense. In some countries, one must be careful of the concept of "sane" versus "insane" automatism, and legal judgment is mandatory.

To reduce the number of inappropriate arrests of those with epilepsy, the EFA, in conjunction with the Police Executive Research Forum, has developed training materials for police officers. The materials encourage police to consider the possibility that certain types of behaviors stem from seizures. Police should consider information from bystanders or family members or from observation at the scene that give clues that a person's confusion or unusual behavior was seizure related. Other national bodies, such as the National Epilepsy Association of Australia (NEAA), as it was then called, have also developed police training materials.

In a number of cases, individuals have sought to use epilepsy as a defense against charges of serious violent crimes. The circumstances under which violent or aggressive behaviors occur, as the result of epileptic seizures, is controversial, and the types of legal defense that would be used vary from country to country and from state to state.[26] In a text such as this, it is not possible to fully debate such defense strategies, but it is vital that the rights of both the individual with epilepsy and the public at large be protected and that the defense provided by "epilepsy" be correctly applied and not abused.

CONTINUING AREAS OF ADVOCACY

Health Care Reform

Issues of access to health care services are central to ethical concerns regarding quality of life for people with epilepsy in all countries. Decisions about access and adequacy of services made at executive and legislative levels, as well as in the private sector, affect the choices that are available to clinicians and patients. A major public policy priority for the epilepsy community in the United States is comprehensive reform of the health care system. The existing mix of public and private insurance in the United States has failed to provide insurance to an estimated 39 million Americans, including many individuals with chronic health conditions such as epilepsy. Private health insurance is increasingly priced beyond the reach of individuals and businesses. Benefits for individual consumers are being trimmed in an attempt to control costs, yet the costs of health care continue to skyrocket. The greatest flaw in the existing health care delivery system in the United States is the fact that those individuals who most need access to health care, namely people with chronic health conditions or disabilities, are the most likely to be denied health insurance.

In 1989, the EFA commissioned a study of insurance industry practices toward people with epilepsy. This study found that most, if not all, companies base their underwriting decisions on medical outcome data that are seriously outdated. The report concluded that existing underwriting guidelines used by U.S. insurance companies fail to reflect the major advances in the diagnosis and treatment of epilepsy. Clearly, the question that lies at the heart of today's U.S. health care debate is, "How do we ensure access to appropriate health care for everyone?" Many options have been considered by the U.S. Congress, including mandating health insurance coverage at the workplace and significantly restructuring the health care system in a comprehensive way. Some have advocated for a single-payer national health plan patterned on the Canadian system. Clearly, passage of legislation ensuring universal access to health insurance would have a profound effect on the lives of thousands of people with epilepsy who currently are unable to obtain coverage. Although Congress has failed to pass appropriate health care reform legislation, disability rights advocates will continue to press for comprehensive reform.

Epilepsy Research and Drug Development

Enormous advances in our understanding of epilepsy have occurred in the last 20 years that have already affected, or will affect, the care of patients with epilepsy and their quality of life. Particularly in the 1990s, dubbed the "decade of the brain," there was enormous enhancement of tools available with which to treat epilepsy, such as vigabatrin, lamotrigine, gabapentin, felbamate, and topiramate.

Concurrent with these developments has emerged a need to examine commitment to research and a review of ethical questions and indemnification of those, namely researchers, ethics committees, and people who take part as volunteers, within such research programs. Each of the antiepileptic medications mentioned encountered problems in development (addressed elsewhere in this text), but, coupled with these difficulties, the issues of legal standing, for all concerned, emerge. This is highlighted by the case of felbamate, the development of which has been arrested on a worldwide scale, even though there are still 150,000 people in the United States who depend on this medicine to achieve better seizure control. A similar, though quite different, situation existed with zonisamide, an agent whose U.S. development was initially stopped while the drug was still in use in Japan, before it reemerged in the United States.

The epilepsy movement, through its international parent bodies of the ILAE and the IBE, and local agencies such as the EFA and the AES, has long been committed to supporting research at all levels of society with its own programs and those of national bodies such as the National Health Scheme (United Kingdom), the National Institutes of Health (United States), and the National Health and Medical Research Council (Australia).

Where problems arise as a result of federal (national) government regulation or intrusion into the availability of or access to existing or new agents, the local chapters of the ILAE and the IBE have proven highly persuasive. This is evidenced by the Australian experience in which the government restricted access to valproate to authority-only prescription, which made it difficult to get the drug. The combined efforts of the NEAA (as it was then called) and the Epilepsy Society of Australia (ESA) reversed this decision and ensured ongoing easy access to this effective treatment. Similarly, the EFA interacts with the U.S. Food and Drug Administration on a frequent basis to improve the regulatory function of evaluating the safety and efficacy of medications, including the standards used to determine the therapeutic bioavailability of generic antiepileptic drugs.

The international epilepsy movement has also demonstrated its commitment to the exchange of ideas within the scientific community at all levels with the sponsorship of international meetings that provide a forum to consider not only the pure science of epileptology, but also advocacy and legal ramifications, as evidenced by the 1987 and 1995 meetings, during which the main themes examined were epilepsy and the law.

Family Support Services

The literature on the psychosocial adaptation of children with epilepsy indicates that the adjustment of the child to his or her disability is significantly affected by the attitudes of the adults in the family, community, and educational environment.[27] Families of children with disabilities experience enormous stress on a day-to-day basis. Lack of family support often renders even the strongest family unable to cope effectively. In the face of complicated medical, social, and educational issues, families in this situation may not be able to provide the support and nurturing a child with epilepsy needs to reach his or her full potential. In addition, families often do not have a clear understanding of the right of their children to an appropriate education in the least restrictive environment and how to advocate effectively for these services. For these reasons, the epilepsy community is actively advocating for greater family support services in the following areas: information, respite care, counseling support and communication, evaluation, and coordination of services.

In the United States, efforts are underway in several states to establish programs providing families of people with disabilities with financial support, the specific uses of which are to be determined by the family, not the government. At the federal level, legislation has been passed that would provide eligible families with assistance. Efforts are underway to secure funding for the initiative. The epilepsy community and other disability organizations have been working very hard on these types of initiatives at the state and federal levels.

EFFECTIVE STRATEGIES WITH POLITICAL REPRESENTATIVES

In an era of diminishing public resources and increasingly complex public policy debates, it is especially important for the epilepsy community to expand on its current advocacy activities and relationships with public policy makers. The following strategies have proven effective in building such relationships:

- Write letters and make phone calls to policy makers on issues of concern. Similarly, write or call to thank legislators for supporting an issue.
- Conduct meetings on a regular basis with legislators in their home district offices.
- Invite elected representatives to local activities, such as board meetings, support group meetings, fund-raising events, and medical conferences.
- Include articles about public policy issues and legislators in organizational newsletters.
- Get involved in local political campaigns; however, these activities must be conducted only on personal time and cannot include contributions or expenditures by tax-exempt organizations.
- Develop or join coalitions of groups with coinciding interests or positions.
- Develop local grass-roots letter-writing and telephone networks that can be activated to influence decision makers when issues arise.
- Add legislators to mailing lists for newsletters and special event announcements.
- Write letters to the editors of local newspapers on issues of importance to the epilepsy community.
- Organize rallies and events when important issues are being considered by your state or federal legislators and invite the press to attend.

A strong advocacy network, at national and local levels, is needed to protect the rights of people with epilepsy and to ensure that their specific concerns will be fully considered as new policies are developed. To accomplish this, continuing contacts and interactions with legislators and other policy makers are essential.

SUMMARY AND CONCLUSIONS

Although one can point to significant gains in the areas of legal rights, education, employment and training, and development of safer, more effective therapies, much remains to be done if people with epilepsy truly are to be given the opportunity to reach their full potential in our society. An area of particular need in some countries continues to be access to appropriate health care services. No longer should those with epilepsy be routinely denied the benefits of timely and quality health care services. The epilepsy community will continue to advocate strongly in this and other areas, with the goal of further reducing the burden of this serious disorder.

References

1. Aldenkamp AD, Das Gupta A, Saxena VS, eds. *Epilepsy and Education*. London: International Bureau for Epilepsy; 1989.
2. Americans with Disabilities Act. 42 U.S.C. 12101 et seq 1990.
3. Barrow RL, Fabing HD. *Epilepsy and the Law,* 2nd ed. New York: Harper & Row; 1966.
4. Beaussart-Defaye J. Is the legal rehabilitation of epileptics possible? In: Porter RJ, Mattson RH, Ward AA, et al., eds. *Advances in Epileptology, Vol. 15*. New York: Raven Press; 1984: 619–624.
5. Beran RG. An analysis and overview of the guidelines for assessing fitness to drive for commercial and private vehicle drivers. *Int Med J*. 2005;35: 364–368.
6. Castellano F, Canger R. Governmental influence on public attitude. In: Porter RJ, Mattson RH, Ward AA, et al., eds. *Advances in Epileptology, Vol. 15*. New York: Raven Press; 1984: 663–655.
7. Dodrill CB, Beier R. Kasparick M. Psychosocial problems in adults with epilepsy: comparison of findings from four countries. *Epilepsia*. 1984: 25(2):176–183.
8. *Epilepsy Foundation of America. School Plum nm*. Landover, MD: Epilepsy Foundation of America; 1994.
9. Fenwick P. Epilepsy and the law. In Hopkins A, ed. *Epilepsy*. New York: Demos; 1987: 553–562.
10. Fraser RT, de Boer H, Oxley J, et al. Epilepsy and employment: an international survey. In: Manelis J, Bental F, Loeber JN, et al., eds. *Advances in Epileptology, Vol. 17*. New York: Raven Press; 1989: 474–478.
11. Gerstle de Pasquet F, Avondet M, Castelli Y, et al. Employment and employability among epileptic patients of Uruguay. In Porter RI, Mattson RH, Ward AA, et al., eds. *Advances in Epileptology, Vol. 15*. New York: Raven Press; 1984:615–618.
12. Gorsky D. Epilepsy and human rights legislation in Canada: an assessment of the Ontario Human Rights Code. In: Manelis J, Bental E, Locher JN, et al., eds. *Advances in Epileptology, Vol. 17*. New York: Raven Press; 1989: 413–420.
13. *Jansen v Food Circus Supermarkets, Inc.,* 541 A.2d 682 (NJ 1988).
14. Krumholz A, Fisher RS, Lesser RP, et al. Driving and epilepsy. A review and reappraisal. *JAMA*. 1991;265:622–626.
15. Lai CW, Huang X, Lai YH. Survey of public awareness, understanding, and attitudes toward epilepsy in Henan Province, China. *Epilepsia*. 1990;31(4):182–187.
16. Laidlaw J, Richens A, Oxley J, eds. *A Textbook of Epilepsy,* 3rd ed. New York: Churchill Livingstone; 1988.
17. Lehman C, Marder K. *The Legal Rights of Persons with Epilepsy,* 6th ed. Landover, MD: Epilepsy Foundation of America; 1992.
18. Lipman IJ. Consensus Conference on Driver Licensing and Epilepsy: American Academy of Neurology, American Epilepsy Society, and Epilepsy Foundation of America. *Epilepsia*. 1994;35(3):662–664.
19. Mani KS, Hedge NS. Epilepsy and the law: position in India. In: Manelis J, Bental E, Loeber IN, et al., eds. *Advances in Epileptology, Vol. 17*. New York: Raven Press; 1989: 428–431.
20. Parsonage M, Beaussart M, Bladin PF, et al. *Epilepsy and Driving License Regulations: Report by the ILAE/IBE Commission on Driver's Licensing*. Heemstede, Netherlands: International Bureau for Epilepsy; 1992.
21. Peper C. The practice of statutory regulations with regard to epilepsy. In: Manelis J, Bental E, Loeber IN, et al., eds. *Advances in Epileptology, Vol. 17*. New York: Raven Press; 1989;421–424.
22. Santilli N, Dodson WE, Walton AV. *Students with Seizures, A Manual for School Nurses*. Cedar Grove, NJ: HealthScan; 1991.
23. Shorvon SD, Farmer PJ. Epilepsy in developing countries: a review of epidemiological, sociocultural, and treatment aspects. In: Trimble MR, ed. *Chronic Epilepsy: Its Prognosis and Management*. New York: Wiley; 1989: 209–241.
24. Steinmeyer HD, Werner C. *Rechtsfiagen bei Epilepsie,* 3rd ed. Bonn, Germany: Stiftung Michael; 1992.
25. Strauss SA. The legal rights of the person with epilepsy: an introduction. In: Manelis J, Bental E, Loeber JN, et al., eds. *Advances in Epileptology, Vol. 17*. New York: Raven Press; 1989: 425–427.
26. Treiman DM. Epilepsy and the law. In: Laidlaw J, Richens A, Chadwick C, eds. *A Textbook of Epilepsy,* 4th ed. New York: Churchill Livingstone; 1993: 645–659.
27. Whitman S, Hermann BP, eds. *Psychopathology in Epilepsy, Social Dimensions*. New York: Oxford University Press; 1986.

CHAPTER 222 ■ OVERVIEW: NEONATAL SYNDROMES

JEAN AICARDI

INTRODUCTION

The neonatal period is conventionally limited to the first 28 days of life. However, some seizures with onset in the first 2 to 3 months of life display similar features and will be considered here. The vast majority of neonatal seizures, however, occur during the first 10 days of life. Most neonatal seizures are short-lived events, lasting only a few days, and usually do not herald a chronic convulsive disorder unless structural damage is present whether due to malformations or acquired disease. Therefore, the term *epilepsy,* meaning a chronic, recurrent disorder with unprovoked paroxysmal events, is only rarely adequate, and the noncommittal term of *neonatal seizures* or *convulsions* is more appropriate. Seizures are one of the most common neurologic problems in the first days of life. Their real frequency is not known because it is becoming clear that all abnormal, stereotyped, and periodically recurring movements may not be epileptic seizures in the sense of excessive discharges of the gray matter, but they can be due to other mechanisms, such as release of brainstem tonic mechanisms from cortical control as a result of lesions or dysfunction of the cortex.[5] The clinical features of neonatal seizures are often relatively unimpressive (see Chapter 56). Generalized seizures are rare, although occasionally cases of infantile spasms or massive myoclonias may occur.[1,3] Focal or multifocal seizures are the rule and several types are recognized. Focal clonic seizures may remain in a fixed location or may involve several focal areas at the same time or in succession (migratory seizures). Clonic seizures are usually associated with typical rhythmic electroencephalographic (EEG) discharges, although these may also occur with tonic or subtle seizures. Tonic seizures may be localized to a single segment; when generalized, they are more often the result of nonepileptic tonic liberation than truly epileptic. *Subtle seizures,*[30] sometimes referred to as *motor automatisms,*[19] are frequent and may include random and roving eye movements, sucking, chewing motions, tongue protrusion, rowing or swimming or boxing movements of the arms, and pedaling or bicycling movement of the lower limbs. Apneic seizures are relatively common.[31] Although some subtle seizures are associated with rhythmic ictal EEG discharges and are clearly epileptic, ictal EEG often does not show typical epileptic activity, and the nature of the clinical events is difficult to determine. In some cases, such ictal phenomena can be provoked by external stimuli that can demonstrate temporal and spatial summation, or they can be inhibited by restraint or repositioning of the involved part. Such features may be more suggestive of brainstem release phenomena, and these events are mainly interpreted as nonepileptic. The absence of an EEG discharge, however, does not completely rule out the possibility of an epileptic phenomenon, thus raising a difficult diagnostic problem.

Ictal EEG discharges in neonates may be highly polymorphic. The two main components, which may be associated with one another, are repetitive sharp waves or spikes and abnormal paroxysmal rhythms including beta, alpha, theta, or delta rhythms that usually remain focal or involve only one hemisphere.[13,16,21] Almost all paroxysmal EEG activity in the neonate begins focally. Ictal discharges are extremely variable in appearance, voltage, frequency, and polarity, and their aspect can change suddenly. Unrelated discharges of various shapes and rhythms frequently occur independently at different locations in both hemispheres. Bilateral symmetric discharges are rare and are associated specifically with unusual ictal phenomena such as myoclonias or spasms. In benign familial neonatal convulsions, they may consist of generalized flattening of the tracing, followed by high-amplitude, slow theta waves,[12,26] but these events follow a focal onset.

Although such differences between neonatal epileptic versus nonepileptic seizures can be of practical value because the use of anticonvulsant drugs that depress cortical activity might be contraindicated in nonepileptic release phenomena,[5] a firm differentiation of epileptic from nonepileptic seizures in neonates may be impossible.

From a clinical viewpoint, seizures must be differentiated from jittering or tremulations, shuddering, and benign neonatal sleep myoclonus.

Ictal EEG recording is helpful when showing clear paroxysmal activity. Ictal EEG events may not be easily differentiated from other patterns that are not infrequently seen in the neonatal EEG. These include brief intermittent repetitive discharges (BIRDS). Most investigators, therefore, require discharges of at least 10 seconds to accept their ictal nature.[28,29] Isolated interictal sharp waves should not be regarded as pointing necessarily to a diagnosis of seizures. However, some seizures with all the clinical features of classical epileptic seizures are not accompanied by typical discharges on the scalp.[8] Conversely, many characteristic EEG discharges are not associated with any clinical manifestation,[13] and such electroclinical dissociation seems to occur especially following long series of seizures. It is not currently possible to decide whether such purely electrical seizures have the same significance as electroclinical attacks, carry the same risk of brain damage, and require the same treatment.

Neonatal seizures rarely occur as isolated events. In most cases, the seizures are frequently repeated over a period of a few days and may result in status epilepticus.[28] They then subside, irrespective of whether the cause is a major brain lesion—as in hypoxic-ischemic encephalopathy—or a benign, purely functional disturbance—as in benign familial neonatal convulsions. The duration of individual seizures is usually brief, even in cases of status. An average duration of 137 ± 11 sec was found in one study.[7] This brief duration may be one reason for the absence of residual damage in such cases as hypocalcemic seizures that leave no residua even if they are repeated over several days.

The causes of neonatal seizures differ considerably from those of seizures in older children. A majority are due to organic brain damage of prenatal or perinatal origin or to acute metabolic disturbances. The role of neonatal hypoxic-ischemic encephalopathy is probably less than formerly thought because of improvements in prenatal and obstetric care. Moreover, a significant proportion of seizures attributed to anoxia are of the subtle type and may not be epileptic. A relatively poor correlation has been found between such variables as Apgar scores, cord pH, and abnormalities of cardiac rhythms and the occurrence of convulsions.[20] Conversely, emphasis has been put more recently on the etiologic role of brain damage of prenatal origin[27] and congenital brain anomalies.

Other significant lesional causes include intracranial hemorrhage and neonatal and fetal infections such as bacterial meningitis and sepsis that require emergency treatment. Strokes due to arterial thrombosis or embolism of undetermined origin have proved to be a frequent cause of focal seizures of fixed location occurring in the first few days of life. These are usually of clonic type and are often repeated in long series or status epilepticus. A persisting hemiplegia is observed in about half of the cases, but the neurodevelopmental outcome is relatively favorable.[30] Strokes of venous origin may also be observed.[9]

Acute metabolic disturbances are relatively uncommon with the virtual disappearance of late hypocalcemia and the decrease in frequency of electrolytic derangements and of hypoglycemia. Hypoglycemia remains an important cause, however, because it is a treatable condition that is observed mainly in post-term infants often following prolonged labor and difficult birth. It may rarely reveal pancreatic disease or may result from other metabolic errors. An abnormality of the transport of glucose[10] usually becomes manifest later in the neonatal period and is responsible for hypoglycorrhachia without hypoglycemia, thus requiring CSF level of glucose study for diagnosis.[10]

There are a number of chronic metabolic diseases with neonatal manifestations. Disorders of organic acids and amino acid metabolism most often manifest in the neonatal period with subtle seizures or abnormal movements that, in most cases, do not seem to be of a true epileptic nature. True epileptic attacks can be observed perhaps more commonly in urea cycle disorders.[2] They are also a feature of glycine encephalopathy in which erratic myoclonus is frequent. Rare disorders of neurotransmitters and sulfite oxidase and manganese cofactor occur. Pyridoxine dependency is another treatable cause and occurs selectively in the first days of life.[11] Convulsions responding to pyridoxal-phosphate but resistant to pyridoxine, which are also treatable, have been recently described.[15] These causes individually, in rare cases collectively, form a sizable group and are important because treatment is possible in some situations, or at least diagnosis is possible for counseling purposes. Other nonlesional causes include drug withdrawal and inadvertent injection of local anesthetics in the fetus during peridural anesthesia.[14]

Benign syndromes of infantile seizures have emerged during the last two decades and their recognition is important because, in contrast with most neonatal convulsions, their outcome is favorable and families should not be given the poor prognosis that is applicable to many neonatal seizures (see Chapter 227). They include two groups. *Benign familial neonatal seizures* have recently attracted considerable attention (see Chapter 223). Such cases are dominantly transmitted and in some families have been shown to result from ion channel dysfunction affecting usually K^{2+},[18] but also Na channels.[4] Whether these cases form one or several clinical syndromes is not clear. Genetically, they are heterogeneous, with at least three different loci, and responsible genes have been located most commonly on chromosome 20 and, rarely, on chromosome 8, although many cases do not demonstrate any of these linkages.[18,24] However, in most families no gene is currently known. They are dominantly inherited. The seizures have some special characteristics[12,26] and disappear, usually in a few days or weeks, although some 15% of affected children may have other types of seizures in later life.

Despite their rarity, these cases are of great significance because they represent the first known disease of pure epilepsy of monogenic origin and may be significant for the understanding of the mechanisms of more common forms of epilepsy. They are also of theoretical interest as demonstrating the role of ion channels, in this case K channels. *Benign nonfamilial seizures*, sometimes termed fifth-day fits[24,25] because their most common occurrence consists of episodes of repeated brief seizures of clonic and apneic types in the normal newborn between days 3 and 7, recur for 24 to 48 hours and disappear without leaving apparent sequelae. Their features do not differ from those of the familial seizures. No cause has been consistently found, and the frequency of the syndrome may be fluctuating with time, suggesting the possibility of environmental causes. The definition of the syndrome, however, is loose, and this may account for the discrepant frequencies reported.[17] Nonetheless, its existence underlines the fact that some syndromes in neonates are benign.

The outlook of neonatal convulsions varies with their cause. Seizures due to brain damage are of unfavorable significance when associated with structural brain defects. Predictors of poor prognosis include the persistence of abnormal neurologic signs at the end of the first week of life[17] and the presence of marked interictal EEG anomalies, such as inactive or depressed tracings and periodic bursts of paroxysmal activity on a generally inactive background (paroxysmal tracings). The major problem is the development of mental retardation or cerebral palsy rather than the persistence of seizures. The frequency of later epilepsy varies between 18% and 26% following convulsions of hypoxic-ischemic origin. In many cases, late seizures develop after a free interval and are often infantile spasms.[3] The persistence of partial seizures is the rule with brain malformations.[19] In rare cases, infantile spasms may begin in the neonatal period.[3] They are a part of Ohtahara syndrome, in association with a burst-suppression EEG (see Chapter 225). The syndrome is often due to extensive brain malformations and has a very poor outlook.[21] The same sort of burst-suppression tracing may be associated with erratic myoclonus and partial seizures in the syndrome of neonatal (or early) myoclonic encephalopathy.[21] The two syndromes may be related, although the latter seems to be more often of genetic, perhaps metabolic, origin. This is definitely the case of glycine encephalopathy, a common cause of neonatal myoclonic encephalopathy.

Treatment of neonatal seizures hinges mainly on etiology (see Chapter 123). Many uncertainties persist concerning the significance of the seizures themselves as a cause of possible additional brain damage[17,30] and, consequently, concerning how important it is to control seizures (with the additional unsolved problem of purely EEG discharges, as discussed earlier). Therefore, a rapid but complete assessment of the infant with special attention to infections and possible metabolic disturbances such as hypoglycemia, hypocalcemia, and electrolyte disturbances is essential and should lead to appropriate correction treatment. More severe metabolic diseases should be vigorously treated. There is no agreement on the anticonvulsant drugs to be used.[16] Many investigators[22] favor phenobarbital or phenytoin in large doses, with initial loading, followed by maintenance therapy for variable periods. In general, short-term treatment is advised, but actual duration may be a few days to a few months. Recently doubt has been raised concerning the innocuousness and effectiveness of large doses of phenobarbital.[23] An alternative method is to use diazepam or lorazepam by intravenous route as the first anticonvulsant agent.

SUMMARY AND CONCLUSIONS

The clinical significance of neonatal seizures is more of an indicator of underlying serious brain damage or dysfunction than a predictor of chronic seizure persistence despite the recent realization that benign "idiopathic" cases do exist. Much remains to be learned about the basic mechanisms of neonatal seizures such as answers to such fundamental issues as the ability of the seizures to produce brain damage and the role of brain maturation in their electroclinical expression and response to therapy. In any case, their significance is more of an indication of brain damage than in terms of etiology. Pending the answers, empirical therapy and supportive treatment will remain essential.

References

1. Aicardi J. *Epilepsy in Children,* 2nd ed. New York: Raven Press; 1994.
2. Aicardi J. Epilepsy in inborn errors of metabolism. In: Roger J, Bureau M, Dravet C, et al., eds. *Epileptic Syndromes in Infancy Childhood and Adolescence,* 2nd ed. London: John Libbey; 1992: 12–23.
3. Arzimanogmou A, Guerrini R, Aicardi J. Neonatal seizures. In: *Aicardi's Epilepsy in Children,* 3rd ed. Philadelphia: Lippincott Williams & Wilkins; 2004: 188–209.
4. Berkovic ZF, Heron SE, Giordano L, et al. Benign familial neonatal-infantile seizures: further characterization of a new sodium channelopathy. *Ann Neurol.* 2004;55:550–557.
5. Camfield PR, Camfield CS. Neonatal seizures: a commentary on selected aspects. *J Child Neurol.* 1987;2:244–251.
6. Caraballo R, Cersosimo R, Espeche A, et al. Benign familial and non-familial infantile seizures: a study of 64 patients. *J Child Neurol.* 2002;17:695–699.
7. Clancy RR, Legido A. The exact ictal and interictal duration of electroencephalographic neonatal seizures. *Epilepsia.* 1987;28:537–541.
8. Clancy RR, Legido A, Lewis D. Occult neonatal seizures. *Epilepsia.* 1988;29:256–261.
9. DeVeber G, Andrew M, Adams C, et al. Cerebral sinovenous thrombosis in children. *N Engl J Med.* 2001;345:417–423.
10. De Vivo DC, Trifiletti RR, Jacobson RI, et al. Defective glucose transport across the blood–brain barrier as a cause of persistent hypoglycorrhachia, seizures and developmental delay. *N Engl J Med.* 1991;325:703–709.
11. Haenggeli CA, Girardin E, Pannier L. Pyridoxine dependent seizures, clinical and therapeutic aspects. *Eur J Pediatr.* 1991;120:452–455.
12. Hirsch E, Velez A, Sellal F, et al. Electroclinical signs of benign neonatal familial convulsions. *Ann Neurol.* 1993;34:835–841.
13. Kellaway PM, Mizrahi EM. Clinical, electroencephalographic, therapeutic and pathophysiologic studies of neonatal seizures. In: Wasterlain CG, Vert P, eds. *Neonatal Seizures.* New York: Raven Press; 1990: 1–13.
14. Kim WY, Pomerance JJ, Miller AA. Lidocaine intoxication in a newborn following local anesthesia for episiotomy. *Pediatrics.* 1979;64:643–645.
15. Kuo MF, Wang HS. Pyridoxal-responsive epilepsy with resistance to pyridoxine. *Pediatr Neurol.* 2002;26:146–147.
16. Lombroso CT. Neonatal seizures. In: Resor SR, Kutt H, eds. *The Medical Treatment of Epilepsy.* New York: Marcel Dekker; 1992: 115–125.
17. Lombroso CT. Neonatal seizures: a clinician's overview. *Brain Dev.* 1996;18:1–28.
18. Malafosse A, Leboyer M, Dulac O, et al. Confirmation of linkage of benign familial neonatal convulsions to D20S19 and D20S20. *Hum Genet.* 1992;89:54–58.
19. Mizrahi EM, Kellaway PM. Characterization and classification of neonatal seizures. *Neurology.* 1987;37:1837–1844.
20. Nelson KB, Ellenberg JH. Apgar scores as predictors of chronic neurologic disability. *Pediatrics.* 1981;68:36–44.
21. Otani K, Abe J, Futagi Y, et al. Clinical and electroencephalographic follow-up study of early myoclonic encephalopathy. *Brain Dev.* 1989;11:332–337.
22. Painter J, Bergman I, Crumrine P. Neonatal seizures. *Pediatr Clin North Am.* 1986;33:91–109.
23. Painter MJ, Scher MS, Paneth NS, et al. Randomized trial of phenobarbital as phenytoin treatment of neonatal seizures. *Pediatr Res.* 1994;35:384A.
24. Plouin P. Benign idiopathic neonatal convulsions (familial and non-familial). In: Roger J, Bureau M, Dravet C, et al., eds. *Epileptic Syndromes in Infancy, Childhood and Adolescence.* London: John Libbey; 1992: 3–11.
25. Plouin P. Benign idiopathic neonatal convulsions (familial and non-familial): open questions about these syndromes. In: Wolf P, ed. *Epileptic Syndromes and Seizures.* London: John Libbey; 1994: 193–201.
26. Ronen GM, Rosales TO, Connelly M, et al. Seizure characteristics in chromosome 20 benign partial convulsions. *Neurology.* 1993;43:1355–1360.
27. Scher MS. Prenatal neonatal neurologic consultations: identifying brain disorders in the context of feto-maternal placental disorders. *Semin Pediatr Neurol.* 2001;8:55–73.
28. Scher MS, Hamid MY, Steppe DA, et al. Ictal and interictal electrographic seizure durations in preterm and term neonates. *Epilepsia.* 1993;34:284–288.
29. Scher MS, Hamid MY, Steppe DA, et al. Ictal and interictal electrographic seizure durations in preterm and term neonates. *Epilepsia.* 1993;34:284–288.
30. Volpe JJ. Neonatal seizures: current concepts and classification. *Pediatrics.* 1989;84:422–428.
31. Watanabe K, Hara K, Miyazaki S, et al. Apneic seizures in the newborn. *Am J Dis Child* 1982;15:584–596.

CHAPTER 223 ■ BENIGN FAMILIAL NEONATAL SEIZURES AND BENIGN IDIOPATHIC NEONATAL SEIZURES

PERRINE PLOUIN

INTRODUCTION

In 1989, the International Classification of Epilepsies, Epileptic Syndromes and Related Disorders[15] included two neonatal syndromes among idiopathic conditions in the section on generalized epilepsies and syndromes: *benign familial neonatal convulsions* and *benign neonatal convulsions*. At that time, no video-electroencephalogram (EEG) recording of seizures had been reported, and newborn infants were considered as presenting more generalized than focal seizures. Nevertheless, since 2001, it has been proposed to consider at least benign familial neonatal convulsions as a focal clonic or adversive epilepsy. Plouin[47] proposed that the appellation *benign neonatal convulsions* was not sufficiently precise: Some symptomatic cases such as hypocalcemia may also be benign, and it would be more accurate if the word *idiopathic* was added: *benign idiopathic neonatal convulsions*. Since then, the word "convulsions" has been replaced by the word "seizures" because "convulsions" refer only to the motor components of seizures, excluding the autonomic components. These two syndromes are now called benign familial neonatal seizures (BFNS) and benign idiopathic neonatal seizures (BINS). Only the first remains in the proposed classification because it seems that no new cases of BINS have been reported in the last 15 years.

These two syndromes do not strictly fulfill the criteria for idiopathic generalized epilepsies; the typical trait of generalized spike-and-wave discharge is not present. It can be argued that the immaturity of the central nervous system is responsible for this absence. Nevertheless, since 2001, it has been proposed that at least BFNS be considered a focal clonic or adversive epilepsy.

Benign neonatal seizures are defined by a favorable outcome, that is, normal psychomotor development and the absence of secondary epilepsy. Benign familial neonatal seizures and benign idiopathic neonatal seizures fulfill these criteria, even if some questions remain open.

Recognition of these syndromes allows the prediction of a favorable outcome from the neonatal period, and long-term antiepileptic treatment is not indicated.

BENIGN FAMILIAL NEONATAL SEIZURES

Historical Perspectives

In 1964, Rett and Teubel[51] reported the first BFNS family, with eight cases over three generations. On the third day of life, the male proband developed an initial tonic phase with cyanosis followed by clonic movements of the whole body including the face and eye muscles, and he had 15 to 20 seizure events on the following day. A brother born 16 months later had a similar experience. Several interictal EEGs were reported for these two boys and single EEGs for three other affected relatives. No ictal EEG was recorded. The authors noted the familial history, the normality of the interictal EEG, and the favorable outcome.

In a second family, 14 members in five generations had similar clinical histories.[9] After a normal delivery, seizures (sometimes with cyanosis) usually started on the third day of life but stopped within 1 month. A few seizures were observed up to 7 months in three children and up to 10 years in two others.

In 1979, Quattlebaum[50] reported a family in which 11 individuals had seizures that started on or before 3 days of age, 1 at 3 weeks, and 3 at 3 months. Most had seizures until 6 or 8 months, but all were otherwise normal.

Between 1964 and 1989, 26 families were reported, with all authors agreeing on a probable autosomal-dominant inheritance.

In 1989, Leppert et al.[32] studied 48 individuals in four generations of a family (Quattelbaum's family), 19 of them having the characteristics of BFNS. They localized the gene on the long arm of chromosome 20, possibly to 20q13.2, the first linkage to be reported for an epilepsy syndrome. This was soon confirmed in a Newfoundland, Canada, family with 69 affected invividuals,[53] in a northern European family,[55] and in six French families.[38] The BFNS syndrome that maps to chromosome 20q has been designated EBN1. Since then, >25 families have been genetically studied in different countries. For 20 of them, the same genetic localization on the long arm of chromosome 20 has been proved.

In 1991, however, Ryan et al.[55] studied two families with BFNS that did not link to chromosome 20 and concluded that the syndrome of BFNS was genetically heterogeneous. Further study of that family[34] demonstrated tight linkage to a locus on 8q, thus verifying heterogeneity (the BFNS syndrome on 8q is designated EBN2). In other families, no linkage could be found on either 20q or 8q.[35]

In 1995, Anderson et al.[1] characterized a candidate gene for BFNS: the human alpha 4 subunit of the nicotine acetylcholine receptor (hCHRNA4). In 1998, the sequencing of genes that are mutated in EBN1 and EBN2 was reported.[58] The new gene was named *KCNQ2*, and analysis of five other ENB1 families yielded two transmembrane missense mutations, two frameshifts, and one splice-site mutation.

A search of the human genome databases for sequences homologous to *KCNQ2* detected one in the chromosome 8q24 region.[14] The new gene was named *KCNQ3*, and a mutant DNA fragment from it was found to segregate perfectly with the EBN2 phenotype in a *Mexican-American family*.[58]

New EBN1 kindreds have been reported with variations in seizure history or in types of mutation. A wide range of clinical manifestations has been observed, including partial seizures in later life with corresponding focal neurologic deficits. Thus far, however, there is little evidence for a correlation between type of mutation and seizure history.[8,33]

The condition of benign familial neonatal seizures is a rare, dominantly inherited epileptic syndrome with a penetrance as high as 85%.

For more details about the genetics of this syndrome see Chapter 18.

Definitions

The diagnosis of BFNS can be considered as a diagnosis by exclusion if every other etiology has been excluded and if there is a family history of neonatal seizures without any severe epilepsy in family members.

Epidemiology

No epidemiologic study of infant or childhood epilepsy has determined the prevalence of BFNS. Among a population of 76 newborns with seizures referred to the neuropediatric unit of Saint Vincent de Paul Hospital between 1994 and 2002 and with video-EEG–recorded seizures, we had only 2 cases of BFNS. The best estimate thus far of the population rate for BFNS comes from a recent prospective, population-based study that involved all obstetric and neonatal units across the province of Newfoundland.[52] Five cases of BFNS (none of whom were part of the kinship reported by Ronen et al.[53]) were observed among 34,615 live births from 1 January 1990 to 31 December 1994. Thus the incidence of BFNS was reported as 14.4 per 100,000 live births.

All reported families represent isolated cases. It is probable that families with BFNS are more numerous than would appear from the medical literature; families with this syndrome often know that the outcome is favorable and do not always report the occurrence of seizures to their physician.

Three hundred and fifty-five cases have been reported in the medical literature since the first article by Rett and Teubel.[51] These neonates belong to 44 families. The number of affected generations varies from one to five (Table 1).

TABLE 1

BENIGN FAMILIAL NEONATAL SEIZURES

Study	Cases per family	Generations per family
Rett and Teubel 1964[51]	8	3
Bjerre and Corelius 1968[9]	14	5
Steejohnsen 1968	8	?
Rose and Lombroso 1970[54]	3	3
Goutières 1977[26]	8	3
	2	1
Carton 1978[13]	9	4
Quattelbaum 1979[50]	15[a]	4
Pettit and Fenichel 1980[45]	5	3
Tibbles 1980[59]	2	2
	6	2
	3	2
Pavone et al. 1982[44]	7	2
Giacoia 1982[23]	7	4
Plouin 1984[46]	2	2
	2	1
Kaplan and Lacey 1983[31]	12	4
Palencia and Berjon 1985[43]	4	2
Shevell et al. 1986[57]	5	3
	4	3
Nieto Barrera et al. 1986[41]	14	3
Calero Garcia et al. 1988[11]	17	4
Cunniff et al. 1988[17]	8	2
Giroud et al. 1989[24]	2	2
	2	2
	2	1
Malafosse et al. 1990[37]	6[a]	3
	4[a]	3
	4[a]	2
Webb and Bobele 1990[63]	9	5
Camfield et al. 1991[12]	5	2
Ryan et al. 1991[55]	14[a]	3
	15[b]	3
Schiffmann et al. 1991[56]	4	1
Wakai et al. 1991[61]	5	2
Aso and Watanabe 1992[4]	3	2
Malafosse et al. 1992[38]	9[a]	4
	3[a]	2
	9[a]	4
Mami et al. 1993[39]	4	2
Ronen et al. 1993[53]	69[a]	5
Hirsch et al. 1993[30]	6[a]	2
Bye 1994[10]	5	3
Berkovic et al. 1994[6]	10[a]	4
Total 1964–1995: 355 cases, 44 families		

[a]Families mapped to chromosome 20 (linkage analysis of Quattelbaum's family by Leppert et al.[32]).
[b]Family mapped to chromosome 8 (linkage analysis of Lewis et al.[34]).

Etiology and Basic Mechanisms

By definition, an idiopathic syndrome does not have a specific underlying etiology. This is the case for BFNS.

Basic mechanisms in this syndrome are probably close to those involved in other types of neonatal convulsions. Immature brain is more likely to respond to any kind of injury with epileptic seizures. In this syndrome, genetic susceptibility during the first week of life in full-term neonates is responsible for the appearance of seizures; the cause is a deficit of a specific channelopathy, but the precise mechanism is unknown. The fact that seizures occur in premature infants when they reach 39 to 41 weeks of gestational age means that a step in maturation has to be reached for the channelopathy to be expressed.

Clinical Presentation

One can consider the diagnosis of BFNS as a diagnosis by exclusion reinforced by the familial history of neonatal seizures.

The clinical data come from the 44 families reported between 1964 and 1996, including 355 cases (Table 1). Since 1996, more isolated families have been reported, but mostly by geneticists, and few details appear in these papers about the electroclinical presentation of seizures.

In documented cases, birth was always at full term (except for three cases of Ronen et al.[53]), with a normal birth weight and an Apgar score >7 at the first minute of life. None of these neonates was in an intensive care unit. There was always a seizure-free interval between birth and occurrence of seizures.

The gender ratio shows an equal distribution between boys and girls.

In 80% of cases, seizures start on the second or third day of life, but some infants start having seizures later, during the first or even up to the third month of life. Ronen et al.,[53] in their large family, report that two of the individuals in whom seizures started at 1 month of age were premature. Premature infants would not be able to have seizures before reaching full-term neurologic state; this point is important, given the strict age dependence of the syndrome.

The neurologic state of the infants remains normal in most cases, and they can nurse or drink from a bottle between seizures; a mild transitory hypotonia can be noticed in some cases. None of these infants was transferred to neonatal intensive care units.

In the first reported families, before the use of video-EEG monitoring, seizures were described as a clonic type, sometimes with apneic spells. Tonic seizures were reported in two cases. Clonic or tonic seizures were short (lasting from 1 to 3 minutes) and frequently repeated within a period of 7 days, whereas isolated seizures could occur in some cases during the following weeks.

Seizures had already been described in previous reports,[12,16,23,57] but there was no evidence in these cases for a homogeneous presentation. More recently, Ronen et al.[53] listed all the clinical components of the 70 seizures they could analyze in their large family. They concluded that most of the time, seizures started with tonic, autonomic, or oculofacial features, being of a mixed type. Hirsch et al.[30] recorded 14 seizures in three neonates with video-EEG monitoring. All seizures started with a tonic phase, with a right or left maximum. Seizures varied from one to the next in a given infant and were always accompanied by tachycardia and a short period of apnea. The clonic phase (partial or generalized) was introduced by vocalization or chewing. We had the opportunity to record seizures in five cases with video-EEG monitoring (unreported families): Seizures were stereotyped, starting with a diffuse hypertonia and a short apnea, followed by autonomic or oculofacial features and symmetric or asymmetric clonic movements of the limbs. In 1994, Bye[10] reported a new case of BFNC, with two seizures recorded and videotaped. Both seizures started with an arousal, but in one, groping and clonic movements of the limbs remained localized to the left side, whereas in the second, these movements were generalized. From these different video recordings, it appears that in most cases, seizures start with a diffuse tonic component, followed by various autonomic and motor changes, which can be unilateral or bilateral, symmetric or not. The only cases without an initial tonic component are those of Bye.[10] No myoclonic seizures or spasms have been reported nor in fact true generalized tonic–clonic seizures.

When described, interictal EEG was normal, discontinuous, or included focal or multifocal abnormalities or a *théta pointu alternant* pattern (Figs. 1 and 2). Patterns suggesting a poor prognosis, such as a paroxysmal, inactive, or suppression-burst pattern, were never reported.

In first reports, some seizures were recorded, but the EEGs were not published or were incomplete. In the cases we recorded, the ictal pattern was very similar to the one published by Ronen et al.[53] and to the cases of Hirsch et al.[30] On the EEG, seizures started with a generalized flattening of the background activity followed by focalized or generalized spikes or slow waves lasting as long as the clinical manifestations. A prolonged flattening of the EEG could follow the seizures. Hirsch et al.[30] studied the ictal EEG very carefully and found that the length of the flattening could vary from 5 to 19 seconds and the complete seizure from 59 to 155 seconds. All of these individuals had BFNS mapped to chromosome 20. The electro-clinical presentation of these seizures suggests that they are of

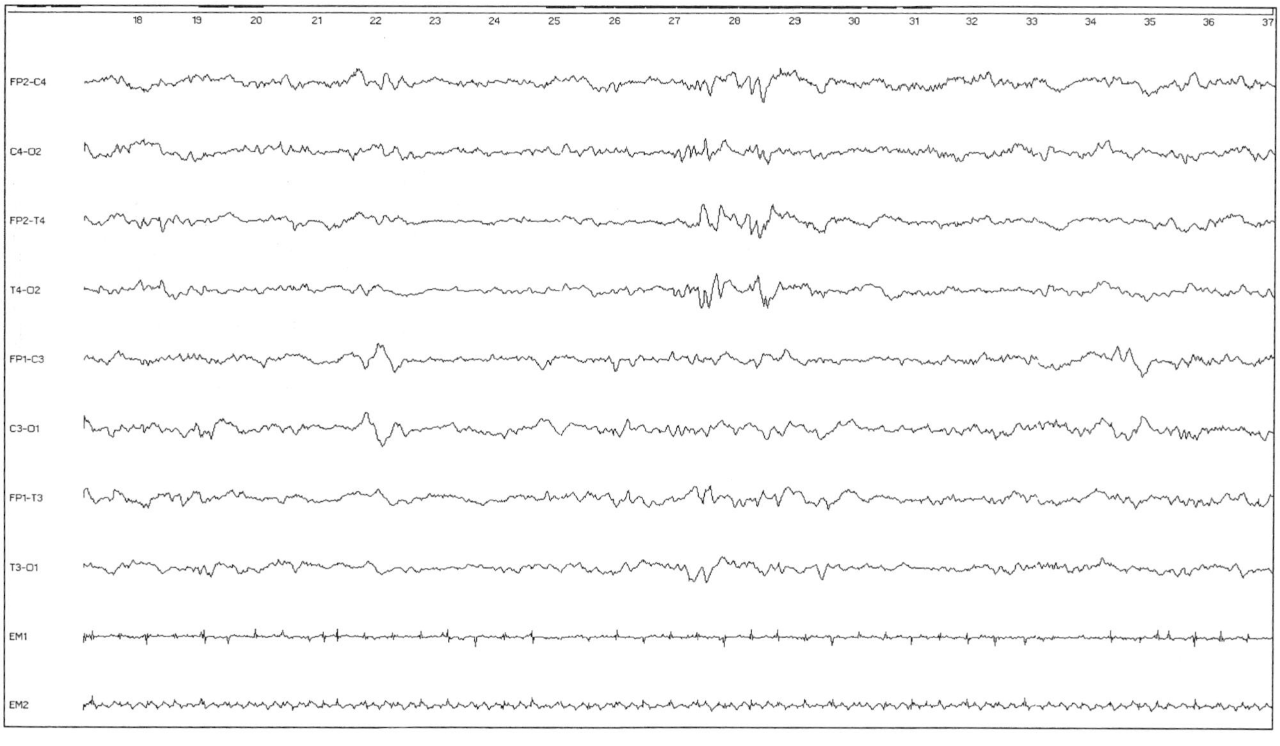

FIGURE 1. Interictal waking electroencephalogram (EEG) in a 5-day-old full-term neonate with benign idiopathic neonatal seizures (BFNS); short bursts of theta rhythms are more marked on the right hemisphere.

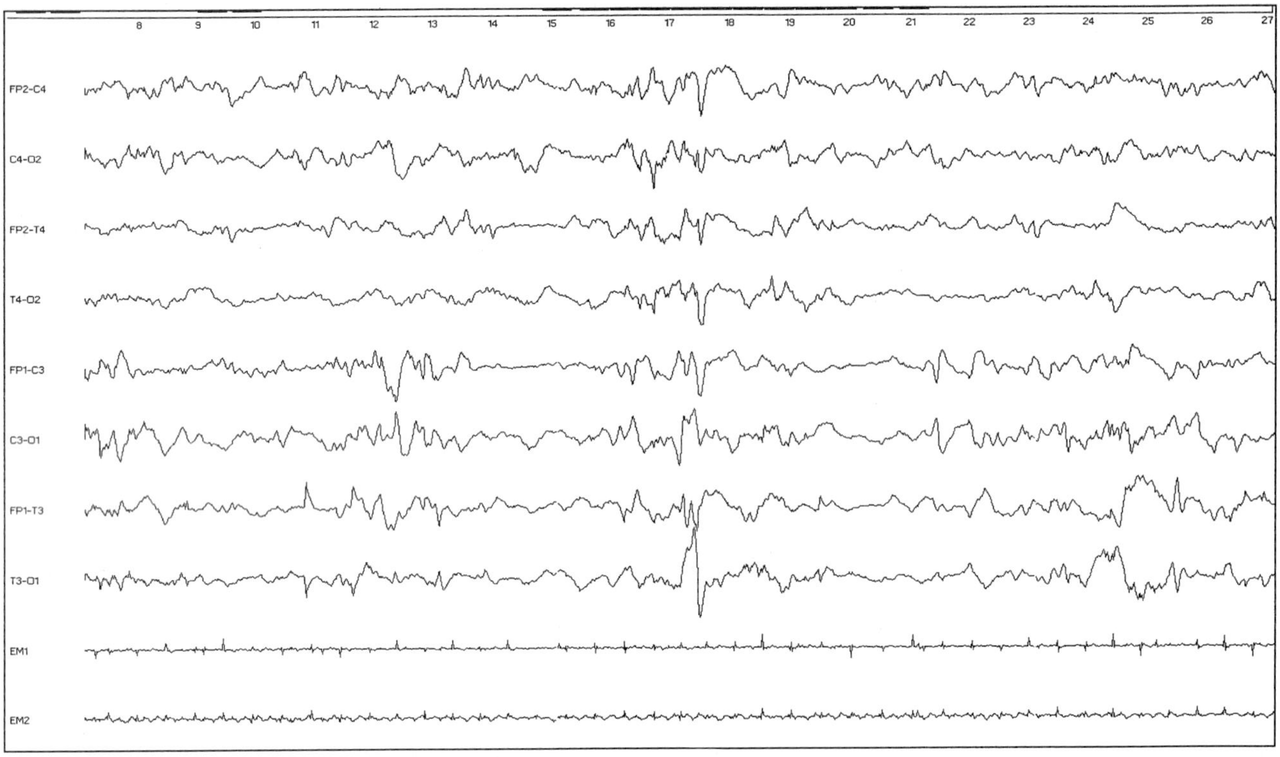

FIGURE 2. Interictal sleep electroencephalogram (EEG) in the same neonate with benign idiopathic neonatal seizures (BFNS); short bursts of bilateral asynchronous theta rhythms are more marked on the left hemisphere.

a generalized type. Aso and Watanabe[4] discussed this point because they recorded a unilateral seizure in a 3-month-old infant having had BFNS.

The publication of Hirsch et al.[30] emphasized that the initial flattening of the EEG is generalized from the start and that the successive symptoms occurring during a seizure (tonic, apnea, clonic phases) are identical to those reported in generalized tonic clonic seizures in children and adults. The same authors suggested that the asymmetric character of some clinical and EEG signs during the tonic or the clonic phase could be related to the absence of maturation of the corpus callosum during the first weeks of life.[5] In all of our recorded seizures we noticed a unilateral predominance of the EEG pattern, even if the initial flattening seemed to be generalized, and at the end of the seizures, we noticed a focal temporal discharge, the same side as the frontal initial spikes and slow waves (Fig. 3). Bye[10] and Hirsch et al.[29] discussed the place of BFNS among idiopathic generalized epilepsies: At the time the classification was adopted (1989), no videotape of BFNS existed, whereas it now appears that some partial seizures may be present, but most of them are of a generalized type.

We suggest nonetheless that this syndrome not be included among the generalized ones: The electroclinical presentation is closer to partial epilepsies such as benign infantile familial seizures or epilepsy with centrotemporal spikes, both benign age-dependent focal epilepsy syndromes. This opinion is shared by Watanabe et al.[62] and Engel.[22]

Diagnostic Evaluation

The diagnosis of BFNS is based on the clinical presentation and the familial history. Cases of BFNS will be found in the family history, but whereas only cases of BFNS are seen in some families, in other families, cases of BFNS are found along with other types of seizures, mostly belonging to the idiopathic generalized epilepsies. The EEG is normal or mildly abnormal. If recordings are made, the electroclinical presentation of seizures is relatively stereotyped.

Nevertheless it seems necessary to exclude any other etiology—metabolic or infectious—and for that purpose a clinical workup and a lumbar puncture should be done. Computed tomography (CT) is not indicated as long as the neurologic state of the infant remains normal.

Differential Diagnosis

Benign familial neonatal seizures must be differentiated from nonepileptic paroxysmal phenomena of neonates (see Chapter 273) and from other types of neonatal convulsions (see Chapter 56).

Among nonepileptic phenomena in neonates, tremulousness and benign sleep myoclonus should be eliminated. Tremulousness occurs in normal neonates during waking and sleep; it can be very intense, and its main characteristic is that it can be stopped by restraining the involved limb and the EEG is normal. Benign neonatal sleep myoclonus occurs only during quiet sleep. The EEG is strictly normal between and during the fits. This phenomenon disappears spontaneously within days to weeks, and the child develops normally.[20]

Symptomatic neonatal convulsions are the most frequent, occurring secondary to hypoxo-ischemic encephalopathy, metabolic disturbances, or infectious processes. These etiologies can be assessed with different diagnostic tools, and the convulsions do not have the typical clinical presentation of BFNC, differing in regard to day of onset, clinical type of seizures, duration and repetition of seizures, and neurologic

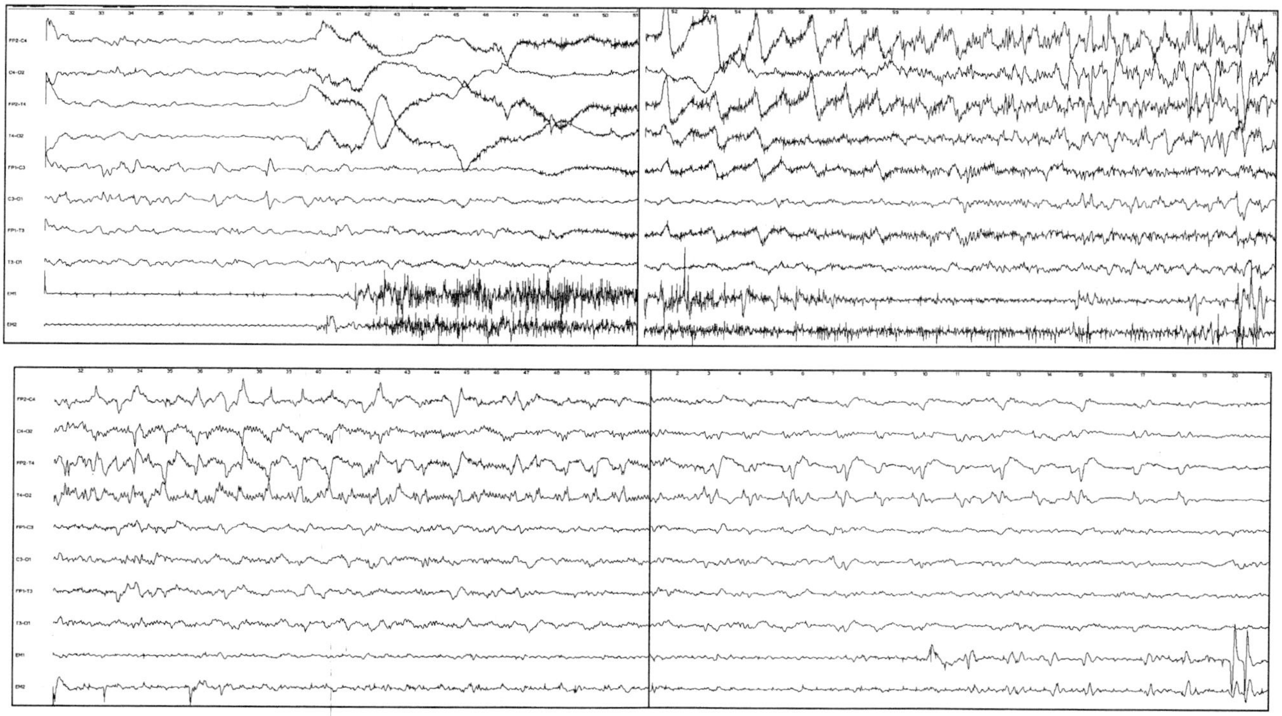

FIGURE 3. Polygraphic recording of a focal seizure in the same neonate. Initial flattening is more marked on the right hemisphere, followed by frontal delta waves; notice the right temporal spikes at the end of the seizures; the duration of the seizures is 80 seconds.

state. Interictal and ictal EEGs also show different patterns according to etiology and severity of the pathology, from normal to very abnormal tracings.

A new sodium channelopathy was reported in 2002[27] in a family with benign neonatal-infantile seizures, the phenotype being described later by Berkovic et al.[6] In this situation, the members of a given family may have neonatal or infantile seizures, with a favorable outcome in all cases. This could be considered an intermediate situation between BFNS and benign familial infantile seizures.[60]

Treatment and Outcome

No guideline has been proposed concerning the treatment of BFNC. In the past, probably no treatment was given. In some families, mostly coming from around the Mediterranean Sea, the best reported treatment was to put a cold key in the neck of the infant. Different authors give their own experience in the treatment of these infants. The drug used depends on country, continent, and year of publication.

Most infants were given phenobarbital for 2 to 6 months, rarely longer. In our experience, sodium valproate is effective, leading to a rapid cessation of seizures. Some authors have also used diphenylhydantoin. The question remains open about the usefulness of an antiepileptic drug treatment: Grandparents of these infants were not treated and did well. If a treatment is initiated at the time of the seizures, it seems reasonable to interrupt it by the third or sixth month.

Long-Term Prognosis

No longitudinal study has been published of BFNC. When we reviewed the literature,[47] we found that infants with BFNS have a 5% risk for febrile convulsions, which is not very different from the general population risk. Concerning secondary epilepsy, the mean risk is around 11% among these infants, higher than in the general population. However, no case of severe epilepsy was noticed in this population. In 1999 Maihara et al.[36] reported two siblings with BFNS who later developed epilepsy with centrotemporal spikes: Both stopped having seizures with carbamazepine and had a normal psychomotor development. No case of psychomotor retardation or mental impairment has been reported among this population of BFNS.

BENIGN IDIOPATHIC NEONATAL SEIZURES

Historical Perspectives

The first report about BINS was by Dehan et al. in 1977.[19] They described 20 neonates with convulsions occurring around the fifth day of life, no specific underlying etiology, and a favorable neurologic outcome in an article entitled "Les convulsions du cinquième jour: un nouveau syndrome?" ("Fifth day's fits: a new syndrome?"). Other French authors reported similar cases.[2,3,21,40,48] The first non-French study was by Pryor et al.[49] from Australia, followed by that of North et al.[42]

During the 1980s, the only reports were French and Australian. In 1992, however, Herrmann et al. from Germany reported 21 recent cases.[28] No study of this syndrome came from the United States.

Table 2 summarizes the 299 published cases.

Definitions

The diagnosis of BINS is made in full-term infants who are neurologically normal and have no familial history of neonatal

TABLE 2

BENIGN IDIOPATHIC NEONATAL SEIZURES

Study	Collection period	Cases
Dehan et al. 1977[19]	1973–1976	20
André et al. 1978[3]	1972–1976	4
Pryor et al. 1981[49]	1973–1977	90
Dreyfus-Brisac et al. 1981[21]	1974–1979	11
Plouin et al. 1981[48]	1966–1980	39
Navelet et al. 1981[40]	1976–1980	18
North et al. 1989[42]	1972–1985	94
André et al. 1990[2]	1980–1981	2
Herrmann et al. 1993[28]	1989–1991	21
Total	1966–1991	299

convulsions, negative findings on workup, and a favorable outcome with respect to both psychomotor development and the absence of secondary epilepsy. Again, this diagnosis is made by exclusion of any specific underlying etiology.

Epidemiology

The incidence of BINS is not clearly apparent in epidemiologic studies dealing with childhood epilepsy. This condition is quite well known among neonatologists and neuropediatricians but not among epileptologists.

Plouin[46] tried to determine the prevalence of BINS among neonatal convulsions. Studies of neonatal convulsions or neonatal status epilepticus published between 1959 and 1982 were analyzed to identify those that could be defined as BINS. Among these studies, special attention was paid to the description by Dehan et al.[18] of neonatal convulsions with unknown etiology occurring around the fifth day of life.

The 15 published studies exhibited a great disparity regarding material and methods. Among the 2,042 cases reported in these 15 studies, a majority of the cases of neonatal convulsions of unknown etiology had a good outcome (120 of 195 documented cases; mean, 62%; range, 28%–93%), and cases with unknown etiology and favorable outcome account for 6.6% of all neonatal convulsions (range, 0%–28%).

This suggests that cases of BINS were already present in the literature before their formal description by Dehan et al. in 1977.[18] Their prevalence can be estimated to be about 7% of neonatal convulsions; this percentage decreases to 2% if only the cases for which the date of occurrence of seizures and the interictal EEG patterns are reported are taken into account. In reported series of BINS, the prevalence varies from 4% to 38% of neonatal convulsions, and this large scatter probably reflects differences in patients' referral and recruitment—intensive care units, maternity clinics, and departments of neonatology or pediatric neurology. The true prevalence of BINS is in good agreement with the range of 2% to 7% cited previously.

Finally, North et al.[42] insisted on the fact that no case of BINS has been observed in their department since 1982. Moreover, the incidence of neonatal convulsions, which was very high during the 1970s, has decreased since the beginning of the 1980s. Others in Australia noted the same facts, leading to the hypothesis of an epidemic phenomenon of BINS, with the etiology undetermined.

In 1990, Dehan, Navelet, and D'Allest carried out a retrospective study to determine the number of cases of BINS referred to neonatology and pediatric department intensive care units as well as maternity units each year between 1979 and 1989. The results were presented at the first Réunion d'Actualités en Epileptologie in Geneva in 1991. The authors concluded that sporadic cases existed among all departments (0.5 to 1.5 cases per year per department), with an important peak in 1981 (comparable with the one of 1975 that led to the first report of BINS).

Herrmann et al.[28] also reported the epidemic occurrence of BINS, with 21 cases referred between 1989 and 1991. The fact that they found a rotavirus infection associated with 95% of their cases reinforces the hypothesis of an epidemic phenomenon but does not explain the relationship to the convulsions.

Etiology and Basic Mechanisms

Metabolic, viral, other infectious, and toxic etiologies have been looked for in this syndrome.

Goldberg and Sheehy proposed one etiologic hypothesis.[25] After a 3-year prospective study, they found an acute zinc deficiency in the cerebrospinal fluid of infants with BINS when compared with a group of infants in whom a cause of convulsions had been identified and with another group of infants without convulsions but with other health problems. This hypothesis has not been confirmed. Moreover, in Australia and France, very complete metabolic, toxic, and viral inquiries have been performed, without any significant results.

More recently, Herrmann et al.[28] reported 21 cases of BINS referred between 1989 and 1991 among 1,917 neonates hospitalized during the same period. They tested for rotavirus in the feces of 19 infants with BINS, 30 healthy controls (age, 4–6 days), and 202 sick neonates without convulsions. They found rotavirus in the feces of 18 of the 19 infants with BINS (95%), whereas only 40% of the healthy controls ($p < 0.001$) and 48% of the sick neonates without convulsions ($p < 0.001$) had positive findings. The authors suggested a causal relationship between BINS and rotavirus infection, although rotavirus was not present in the cerebrospinal fluid of 6 rotavirus-positive infants with BINS. They concluded that pathogenic mechanisms remain unclear. This syndrome remains idiopathic.

Clinical Presentation

The gender distribution reveals a majority of boys (62%). Only full-term infants have been reported. Pregnancy and delivery were normal, and seizures started after a seizure-free interval. In all cases, seizures occurred between days 1 and 7; 90% occurred between days 4 and 6, and 97% between days 3 and 7. No videotape recording has been reported for any of these cases.

When described, the seizures were always of the clonic type, mostly partial, with or without apnea, but never tonic. North et al.[42] reported apneic seizures in 31% of their cases. Clonic seizures were often lateralized, starting on one side and then affecting the other side, and rarely of a generalized type. They lasted from 1 to 3 minutes. They were frequently repeated, leading to status epilepticus. The mean duration of status epilepticus was about 20 hours, but it could be shorter (2 hours) or longer (up to 3 days).

The neurologic state of the infants is usually normal at onset of convulsions. Infants then become drowsy and hypotonic, the various antiepileptic drugs given to stop the convulsions being partly responsible for this evolution. Drowsiness and hypotonia may last for several days after the end of status epilepticus, but the infants soon recover to a normal neurologic state.

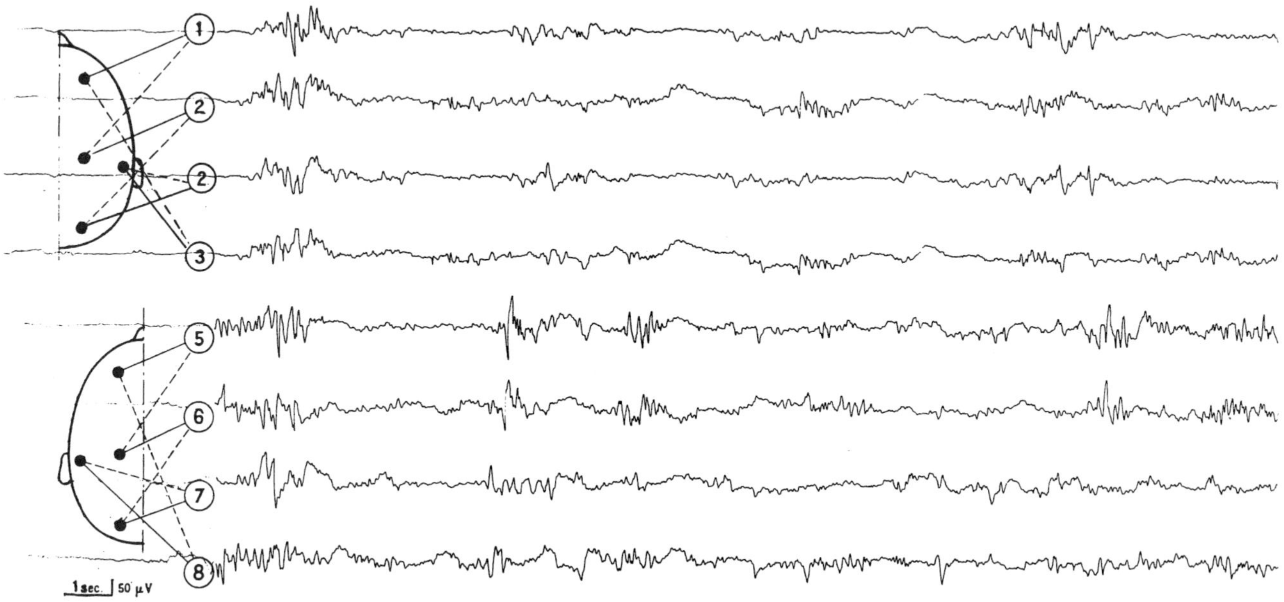

FIGURE 4. Interictal electroencephalogram (EEG) of a *théta pointu alternant* pattern in an infant with benign idiopathic neonatal seizures (BINS).

Interictal EEG patterns were described in 101 of the 299 published cases. The interictal EEG was normal in 10 infants, discontinuous in 6, and showed "focal or multifocal abnormalities" in 25. The *théta pointu alternant* pattern was present in the remaining 60 infants. This pattern was first described by Dehan et al.[18] as a dominant theta activity, alternating or discontinuous, unreactive, with sharp waves and frequent interhemispheric asynchrony. The *théta pointu alternant* pattern may be present in cases of status epilepticus of different etiologies (hypocalcemia, neonatal meningitis, subarachnoidal hemorrhage) and cannot be considered as specific for BINS.[40,46] Nevertheless, it is associated with a favorable neurologic prognosis (Fig. 4).

Seizures have been recorded in most of the 101 cases. They last from 1 to 3 minutes and have no remarkable EEG features—mostly rhythmic spikes or rhythmic slow waves. They can be localized to any area but are more frequently present in the rolandic areas. They can be strictly unilateral, immediately generalized, or first localized and then generalized. Electroclinical seizures or subclinical discharges (so-called electroencephalographic seizures) can be recorded; clinical seizures without EEG modifications have also been reported.

Diagnostic Evaluation

The diagnosis of BINS is based on the clinical presentation, the ictal and interictal EEG, and the elimination of any specific underlying etiology, such as metabolic disturbances, neonatal meningitis, viral infections, or malformations of the central nervous system.

Differential Diagnosis

The differential diagnosis of BINS is not different from that of BFNS. The familial convulsions are different from the idiopathic convulsions in several ways: BFNS is a familial disease having an autosomal mode of inheritance linked to genetic markers localized to the long arm of chromosome 20, at least in the majority of cases; conversely, a family history is very rare in BINS (0.2%). Seizures start earlier in BFNS (days 2–3) and persist longer than in BINS (starting on days 4–5, and lasting no more than 20 hours). Occurrence of secondary epilepsy is more frequent in BFNS (11%) than in BINS (0.5%). Minor neurologic impairment is more frequent in cases of BINS.

Treatment and Outcome

Many antiepileptic drugs have been used for BINS (phenobarbitone, phenytoin, diazepam, paraldehyde, chloral hydrate, clomethiazole), often in combination, without a consistent effect on the duration of seizures. The seizures usually stop without treatment, but occasionally the end seems to be related to administration of diazepam or phenytoin. Dehan et al.[19] suggested that these infants not be treated if alternative diagnoses have been eliminated.

Long-Term Prognosis

The long-term favorable outcome must be confirmed by more numerous and more extensive studies. The 90 cases reported by Pryor et al.[49] have not been followed beyond the neonatal period. The 92 cases reported by French authors were followed from 6 months to 6 years. In five cases, a transitory psychomotor retardation was noted until the age of 1 year; one child had a simple febrile convulsion, and another had a convulsion without fever at the age of 3 years.[18]

Among the 94 cases reported by North et al.,[42] 33 (38%) were followed between the ages of 6 months and 2 years. In roughly half of these 33 infants, the authors found abnormalities. Although there is no control group, the percentage of abnormalities seems excessive in this study. One can consider that children with medical problems were exposed to more frequent consultations than were children without any problems. These authors concluded that their results do not allow assessment of the benignity of this syndrome.

SUMMARY AND CONCLUSIONS

Benign Familial Neonatal Seizures

Recognizing the phenotype of BFNS is important, first because of the prediction of a favorable neurologic outcome, and second for the contribution to genetic studies, which comprise a dynamic area of epilepsy research, especially for the idiopathic epilepsies.

The classic phenotype of BFNS comprises the following features: (a) normal pregnancy and delivery; (b) seizure-free interval before onset of seizures (mostly on days 2 and 3); (c) neurologically normal state between seizures; (d) normal interictal EEG; (e) tonic–clonic seizures, symmetric or not; and (f) familial history of BFNS or other types of epilepsy (mostly idiopathic epilepsies). The families of such infants should be considered appropriate for genetic studies.

Benign Idiopathic Neonatal Seizures

Benign idiopathic neonatal seizures can be recognized by the clinical and paraclinical characteristics that comprise the syndrome. Diagnosis allows one to predict a favorable neurologic outcome. However, the *théta pointu alternant* EEG pattern is present in only 60% of cases and is not specific. Further reports with a longer follow-up period will perhaps lead to a better understanding of this syndrome and more precise determination of the outcome. The "episodic character" of this syndrome and the nonspecific EEG pattern as well as the type of seizures make it questionable to maintain it in the International Classification of Epilepsies and Epilepsy Syndromes.

References

1. Anderson VE, Stauffer D, Peiffer A, et al. Testing the hCHRNA4 gene as a candidate for benign familial neonatal convulsions. *Epilepsia.* 1995;36 (Suppl 3):S7.
2. André M, Matisse N, Vert P. Prognosis of neonatal seizures. In: Wasterlain CG, Vert P, eds. *Neonatal Seizures.* New York: Raven Press; 1990: 61–67.
3. André M, Vert P, Bouchez T. Ápropos des convulsions du cinquième jour. *Arch Fr Pediatr.* 1978;35:922–923.
4. Aso K, Watanabe K. Benign familial neonatal convulsions: generalized epilepsy? *Pediatr Neurol.* 1992;8:226–228.
5. Bardovick AJ, Kjos BO. Normal post natal development of the corpus callosum as demonstrated by MR imaging. *AJNR Am J Neuroradiol.* 1988;3:487–491.
6. Berkovic SF, Heron SE, Giordano L, et al. Benign familial neonatal-infantile seizures: characterization of a new sodium channelopathy. *Ann Neurol.* 2004;55:550–755
7. Berkovic SF, Kennerson ML, Howell RA, et al. Phenotypic expression of benign familial neonatal convulsions linked to chromosome 20. *Arch Neurol.* 1994;51:1125–1128.
8. Biervert C, Steinlein OK. Structural and mutational analysis of *KCNQ2* the major gene locus for benign neonatal familial convulsions. *Hum Genet.* 1999;104:234–240.
9. Bjerre I, Corelius E. Benign neonatal familial convulsions. *Acta Paediatr Scand.* 1968;57:557–561.
10. Bye AME. Neonate with benign familial neonatal convulsions: recorded generalized and focal seizures. *Pediatr Neurol.* 1994;10:164–165.
11. Calero Garcia JL, Nieto Barrera M, Moruno Tirado A, et al. Convulsiones neonatales familiares benignas. Aportacion de una nueva familia. *Rev Esp Epilepsia.* 1988;4:32–35.
12. Camfield PR, Dooley J, Gordon K, et al. Benign familial neonatal convulsions are epileptic. *J Child Neurol.* 1991;6:340–342.
13. Carton D. Benign neonatal familial convulsions. *Neuropädiatrie.* 1978;9:167–171.
14. Charlier C, Singh NA, Ryan SG, et al. A pore mutation in a novel KQT-like potassium channel gene in an idiopathic epilepsy family. *Nature Genet.* 1998;18:53–55.
15. Commission on Classification and Terminology of the International League Against Epilepsy. Proposal for revised classification of epilepsies and epileptic syndromes. *Epilepsia.* 1989;30:389–399.
16. Crispen C, Kelly T. Benign familial neonatal convulsions. *Iowa Med.* 1985;75:397–401.
17. Cunniff C, Wieldlin N, Lyons Jones K. Autosomal dominant benign neonatal seizures. *Am J Med Genet.* 1988;30:963–966.
18. Dehan M, Navelet Y, D'Allest AM, et al. Quelques précisions sur le syndrome des convulsions du cinquième jour de vie. *Arch Fr Pediatr.* 1982;39:405–407.
19. Dehan M, Quilleron D, Navelet Y, et al. Les convulsions du cinquième jour de vie: un nouveau syndrome? *Arch Fr Pediatr.* 1977;34:730–742.
20. Di Capua G, Vigevano F. Benign neonatal sleep myoclonus. *Mov Disord.* 1993;812:191–194.
21. Dreyfus-Brisac C, Peschanski N, Radvanyi MF, et al. Convulsions du nouveau-né. Aspects cliniques, électroencéphalographiques, étiopathogéniques et pronostiques. *Rev EEG Neurophysiol.* 1981;11:367–378.
22. Engel J Jr; International League Against Epilepsy (ILAE). A proposed diagnostic scheme for people with epileptic seizures and with epilepsy: report of the ILAE Task Force on Classification and Terminology. *Epilepsia.* 2001;42:796–803.
23. Giacoia GP. Benign familial neonatal convulsions. *South Med J.* 1982;75:629–630.
24. Giroud M, Soichot P, Nivelon-Chevalier A, et al. Les convulsions néo-natales familiales: leurs aspects électrocliniques et génétiques. *Neurophysiol Clin.* 1989;19:47–54.
25. Goldberg HJ, Sheehy EM. Fifth day fits: an acute zinc deficiency syndrome? *Arch Dis Child.* 1983;57:633–635.
26. Goutières F. Convulsions néonatales familiales bénignes. In: *Congrès de la Société de Neurologie Infantile.* Marseilles: Diffusion Générale de Librairie; 1977: 281–286.
27. Heron SE, Crossland KM, Andermann E, et al. Sodium-channel defects in benign familial neonatal-infantile seizures. *Lancet.* 2002;360:851–852.
28. Herrmann B, Lawrenz-Wolf B, Seewald C, et al. 5-Tages-Krämpfe des Neugeborenen bei Rotavirusinfektionen. *Monatsschr Kinderheilkd.* 1993;141:120–123.
29. Hirsch E, de Saint Martin A, Marescaux C. Convulsions néonatales familiales bénignes: un modèle d'épilepsie idiopathique. *Rev Neurol.* 1999;155:463–467.
30. Hirsch E, Velez A, Sellal F, et al. Electroclinical signs of benign neonatal familial convulsions. *Ann Neurol.* 1993;34:835–841.
31. Kaplan RE, Lacey DJ. Benign familial neonatal-infantile seizures. *Am J Med Genet.* 1983;16:595–599.
32. Leppert M, Anderson VE, Quattlebaum T, et al. Benign familial neonatal convulsions linked to genetic markers on chromosome 20. *Nature.* 1989;337:647–648.
33. Leppert M, Singh N. Benign familial neonatal epilepsy with mutations in two potassium channel genes. *Curr Opin Neurol.* 1999;12:143–147.
34. Lewis TB, Leach RJ, Ward K, et al. Genetic heterogeneity in benign familial neonatal convulsions: identification of a new locus on chromosome-8q. *Am J Hum Genet.* 1993;53:670–675.
35. Lewis TB, Shevell MI, Andermann E, et al. Evidence of a third locus for benign familial convulsions. *J Child Neurol.* 1996;11:211–214.
36. Maihara T, Tsuji M, Higuchi Y, et al. Benign familial neonatal convulsions followed by benign epilepsy with centro-temporal spikes in two siblings. *Epilepsia.* 1999;40:110–113.
37. Malafosse A, Leboyer M, Dulac O, et al. Convulsions néonatales familiales bénignes: un modèle d'étude des bases moléculaires des facteurs génétiques des épilepsies. *Epilepsies.* 1990;2:64–71.
38. Malafosse A, Leboyer M, Dulac O, et al. Confirmation of linkage of benign familial neonatal convulsions to D20S19 and D20S20. *Hum Genet.* 1992;89:54–58.
39. Mami C, Tortorella R, Manganaro R, et al. Les convulsions néonatales familiales bénignes. *Arch Fr Pediatr.* 1993;50:31–33.
40. Navelet Y, D'Allest AM, Dehan M, et al. Ápropos du syndrome des convulsions néonatales du cinquième jour. *Rev EEG Neurophysiol.* 1981;11:390–396.
41. Nieto Barrera M, Borrego S, Aguilar Quero F. Convulsiones neonatales familiares benignas y crises asociadas. *Rev Esp Epilepsia.* 1986;2:66–70.
42. North KN, Storey GNB, Handerson-Smart DJ. Fifth day fits in the newborn. *Aust Paediatr J.* 1989;25:284–287.
43. Palencia R, Berjon MC. Convulsiones neonatales familiares benignas, crises febriles y epilepsia. Su coincidencia en una familia. *An Esp Pediatr.* 1985;23:65–67.
44. Pavone L, Mazzone D, La Rosa M, et al. Le convulsioni familiari benigne. Studio di una famiglia. *Ped Oggi.* 1982;11:375–378.
45. Pettit RE, Fenichel GM. Benign familial neonatal seizures. *Arch Neurol.* 1980;37:47–48.
46. Plouin P. Benign idiopathic neonatal convulsions (familial and non-familial). In: Roger J, Bureau M, Dravet C, Dreifuss FE, et al., eds. *Epileptic Syndromes in Infancy, Childhood and Adolescence.* London: John Libbey; 1984: 3–11.
47. Plouin P. Benign idiopathic neonatal convulsions (familial and non-familial). In: Roger J, Bureau M, Dravet C, et al., eds. *Epileptic Syndromes in Infancy, Childhood and Adolescence.* London: John Libbey; 1992: 3–11.
48. Plouin P, Sternberg B, Bour F, et al. États de mal néonataux d'étiologie indéterminée. *Rev EEG Neurophysiol.* 1981;11:385–389.

49. Pryor DS, Don N, Macourt DC. Fifth day fits: a syndrome of neonatal convulsions. *Arch Dis Child*. 1981;56:753–758.
50. Quattelbaum TG. Benign familial convulsions in the neonatal period and early infancy. *J Pediatr*. 1979;95:257–259.
51. Rett A, Teubel R. Neugeborenen Krampfe im Rahmen einer epileptisch belasten Familie. *Wien Klin Wochenschr*. 1964;76:609–613.
52. Ronen GM, Penney S, Andrews W. The epidemiology of clinical neonatal seizures in Newfoundland: A population-based study. *J Pediat*. 1999;134:71–75.
53. Ronen GM, Rosales TO, Connolly MED, et al. Seizure characteristics in chromosome 20 benign familial neonatal convulsions. *Neurology*. 1993;43:1355–1360.
54. Rose AL, Lombroso CT. Neonatal seizure states. A study of clinical pathology and EEG features in 137 full-term babies with a long-term follow-up. *Pediatrics*. 1970;45:405–425.
55. Ryan SG, Wiznitzer M, Hollman C, et al. Benign familial neonatal convulsions: evidence for clinical and genetic heterogeneity. *Ann Neurol*. 1991;29:469–473.
56. Schiffmann R, Shapira Y, Ryan G. An autosomal recessive form of benign familial neonatal seizures. *Clin Genet*. 1991;40:467–470.
57. Shevell MI, Sinclair DB, Metrakos K. Benign familial neonatal seizures: clinical and electroencephalographic characteristics. *Pediatr Neurol*. 1986;2:272–275.
58. Singh NA, Charlier C, Stauffer D, et al. A novel potassium channel gene, KCNQ2, is mutated in an inherited epilepsy of newborns. *Nature Genet*. 1998;18:23–29.
59. Tibbles JAR. Dominant benign neonatal seizures. *Dev Med Child Neurol*. 1980;22:664–667.
60. Vigevano F. Benign familial infantile seizures. *Brain Dev*. 2005;27(3):172–177.
61. Wakai S, Tachi N, Chiba S, et al. Benign familial neonatal convulsions: clinical features of the propositus and comparison with the previously reported cases. *Acta Paediatr Jpn*. 1991;33:77–82.
62. Watanabe K, Miura K, Natsume J, et al. Epilepsies of neonatal onset: seizure type and evolution. *Dev Med Child Neurol*. 1999;41:318–322.
63. Webb R, Bobele G. "Benign" familial neonatal convulsions. *J Child Neurol*. 1990;5:295–298.

CHAPTER 224 ■ EARLY MYOCLONIC ENCEPHALOPATHY (NEONATAL MYOCLONIC ENCEPHALOPATHY)

ALEKSANDRA DJUKIC, FEDERICO VIGEVANO, PERRINE PLOUIN, AND SOLOMON L. MOSHÉ

INTRODUCTION

In 1978, Aicardi and Goutieres described a group of five patients with "neonatal myoclonic encephalopathy" commencing in the hours immediately after birth and consisting of erratic, asynchronous, nonperiodic myoclonus associated with generalized jerks and a distinctive electroencephalogram (EEG).[3] Since then, the syndrome has been referred to as early myoclonic encephalopathy and also as myoclonic encephalopathy with neonatal onset,[8] neonatal epileptic encephalopathy with periodic EEG bursts, and early myoclonic epileptic encephalopathy[9] and neonatal myoclonic encephalopathy.[3,39]

In 1989, the ILAE Commission of Classification and Terminology recognized the syndrome as "early myoclonic encephalopathy (EME)" and classified it as generalized symptomatic epilepsies of nonspecific etiology.[16] In 2001 the entity was finally recognized as one of the "epileptic encephalopathies" together with early infantile epileptic encephalopathy with suppression-bursts (EIEE, Ohtahara syndrome), West syndrome, and Lennox-Gastaut syndrome. Since 1978, there have been published reports on 50 patients with the characteristic clinical picture—onset of symptoms during the first month of life consisting of erratic, fragmentary myoclonus, massive myoclonus, partial seizures, suppression-burst EEG pattern, and, later, tonic spasms; the prognosis is grave.[4] Some controversial issues on differential diagnosis from EIEE and physiopathology remain; there are several cases of early encephalopathy with seizures and a suppression-burst pattern that do not fulfill the criteria for either EIEE or EME.[4,10,18,33]

EPIDEMIOLOGY

The syndrome is rare. An epidemiologic study of childhood epilepsy in Japan detected 4 cases of EME (0.168%) among 2,378 children with epilepsy >10 years of age.[6,28] In a study of 75 infants with epilepsy of neonatal onset, Watanabe et al.[42] observed 2 cases (2.7%) of EME. A gender difference, with female-to-male ratio of 1:1.3, is seen in the 30 cases published in the English literature.[10]

ETIOLOGY

In most cases, the etiology of EME is unknown. Although EME is assumed to be associated with inborn errors of metabolism, even the most frequently reported diagnosis—nonketotic hyperglycinemia—is rarely documented.[2,5,9,13,27,33,38,39] Other identified inborn errors of metabolism are D-glyceric acidemia, propionic acidemia, molybdenum cofactor deficiency, methylmalonic acidemia, mitochondrial dysfunction, and abnormal urinary oligosaccharides.

Structural brain malformations (cerebellar hypoplasia, migrational disorder with cortical dysgenesis) have also been reported.[11,23]

Wang and colleagues reported a patient with a clinical picture of early myoclonic encephalopathy and an atypical suppression-burst pattern, with full recovery after administration of pyridoxine.[40] The syndromes of retinal pigmentary degeneration and nephronophthisis, congenital nephrotic syndrome, and Zellweger disease have all also presented with EME.[2,5,9,13,15,19,21,23,27,33,39–40]

Familial occurrence has been reported,[2,9,33,40] reflecting the genetic nature of the underlying diseases. Because the gene locations for these metabolic errors vary widely, however, it is more likely that EME does not develop due to a specific genetic abnormality but rather due to extensive cortico-subcortical dysfunction as a consequence of a severe metabolic disorder.[27]

CLINICAL PRESENTATION

Seizure Characteristics

In this condition, a child usually born without dysmorphic features and after an uneventful delivery undergoes a regression as the seizures emerge and becomes less alert and irritable and with poor interactions.[9] The distinctive clinical characteristic of EME is myoclonias, which are the first presenting symptom, starting usually within the first week of life. The majority of the patients present within the first month of life. Onset during the prenatal period and during the second or third month of life has been reported but is rare.[9,11,40]

Myoclonus is fragmentary and erratic and shifts from one to another body part in a random, asynchronous fashion; it can become massive and generalized in some cases.[4] Initially, it involves eyelids, face, and limbs in the form of twitches of small to moderate amplitude. Sometimes, twitches are restricted to a very small territory (eyebrow, corner of the mouth). The frequency of myoclonic jerks also varies from occasional to almost continuous from the onset. It may persist during sleep.[9]

Shortly after the onset, partial seizures occur and can be subtle, consisting of only eye deviations or autonomic phenomena according to Dalla Bernardina et al.[9] Tonic seizures are observed later, usually around 3 to 4 months of age.[2,4]

Diagnostic Evaluations

Electroencephalographic Features

There is no normal background activity during wakefulness or sleep.[2] There is a burst-suppression EEG pattern characterized

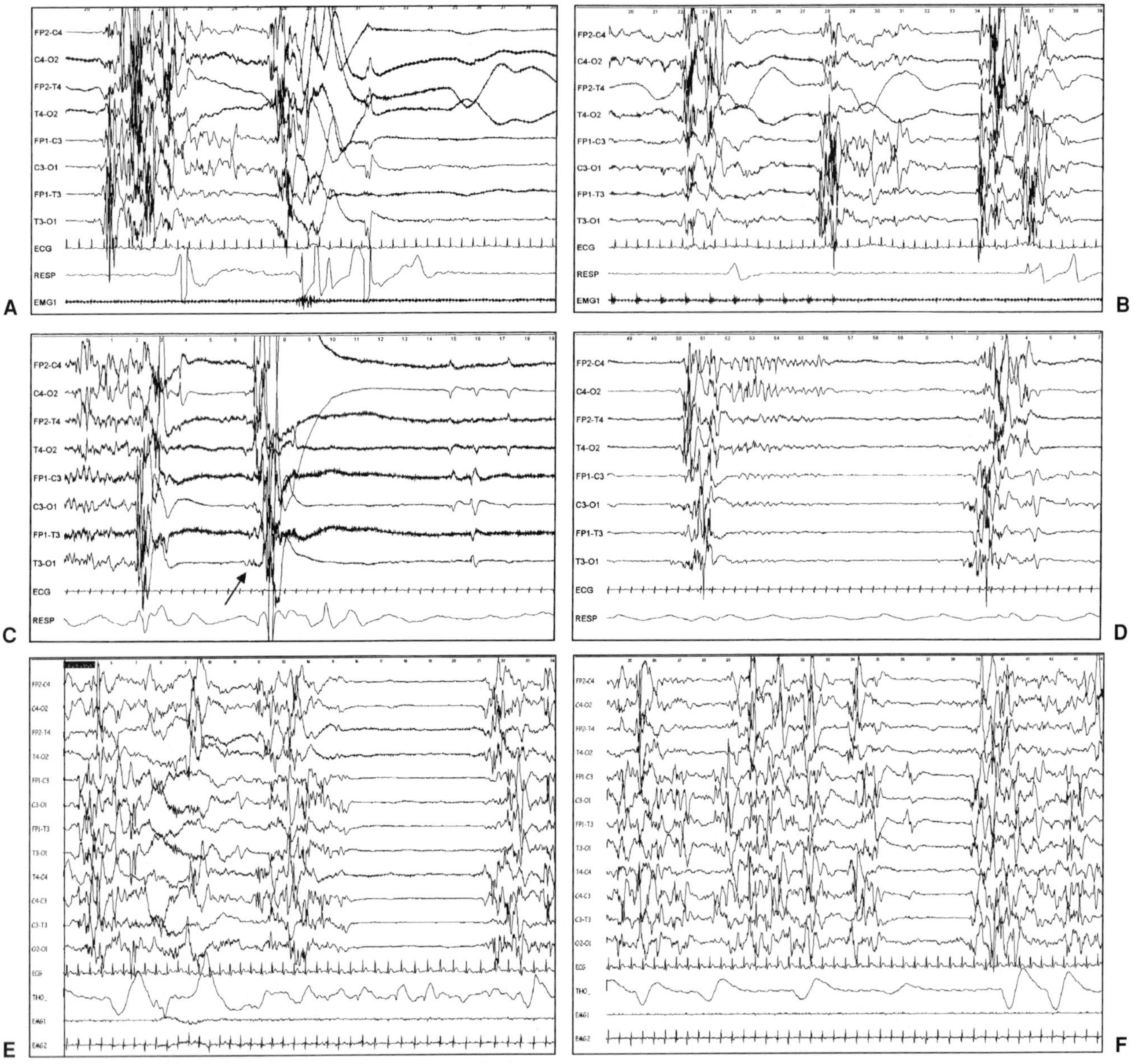

FIGURE 1. Electroencephalograms (EEGs) from an infant with early myoclonic encephalopathy. Panels A to D were obtained when the infant was 1 month old. **A, B:** Awake state. **C:** The occurrence of a myoclonic jerk (*arrow*). **D:** Asleep. Panels E and F were obtained when the infant was 3 month old **E:** Awake. **F:** Asleep. Notice that the burst-suppression pattern is present during wakefulness and sleep. Time scale is 15 mm/s; sensitivity is 100 μV/cm.

by bursts of spikes, sharp waves, and slow waves irregularly intermingled and separated by periods of electrical silence. The duration of the bursts is usually 1 to 5 seconds, and the duration of the silent periods is 3 to 10 seconds (Fig. 1A–D). The EEG paroxysms may be either synchronous or asynchronous over both hemispheres. This pattern is often more marked during sleep. Usually after a few months, it evolves into hypsarrhythmia (more or less typical) or into multifocal paroxysmal discharges without normal patterns. In some cases the burst-suppression pattern may persist for a few months (Fig. 1E, F).

Erratic myoclonus generally may not have an ictal EEG correlate. Axial myoclonias that can be recorded with surface electromyography (EMG) on both deltoid muscles are immediately preceded by a burst of bilateral polyspikes.[3] They occur more frequently during wakefulness and may occur in clusters (Fig. 1). These myoclonias can be differentiated from epileptic spasms: The clinical manifestation is a short tonic contraction, and the EEG pattern consists of a complex of slow waves associated with fast rhythms. Later, multifocal seizures may emerge and the interictal EEG pattern evolves to hypsarrhythmia.[29]

Imaging Findings

Computed tomography (CT) and magnetic resonance imaging (MRI) in most cases are initially normal. In some cases, serial brain imaging shows development of diffuse brain atrophy even in those children with normal imaging findings at onset. Malformations have been reported as a cause of EME. The imaging may show the different pattern of brain malformation cited in the section on etiology.

Other Laboratory Investigations

Because the inborn errors of metabolism are the major cause of EME, a metabolic workup (amino acids, organic acids, lactate, and pyruvate) should be considered in all patients in the blood and in the cerebrospinal fluid (CSF). A pyridoxine challenge should be performed because the association of massive and erratic myoclonias leading to a very hyperexcitable infant with a suppression-burst EEG pattern can be the expression of B6 dependency. In these cases myoclonic jerks stop as soon as the B6 is administered intravenously. To confirm this diagnosis, the specific treatment should be stopped later; if the myoclonic seizures recur, the diagnosis is definite.

DEVELOPMENTAL COURSE

Psychomotor development becomes arrested. The prognosis is grave. In 91% of the patients described in sufficient detail, the outcome is poor: Death occurs during the first years of life in at least 50%; those surviving have severe psychomotor retardation or remain in a persistent vegetative state.[2,10] In rare cases, signs of peripheral neuropathy were reported.[2] Normal developmental outcome has been limited to one case with pyridoxine dependency.[40] The progressive nature and the high fatality of EME cases can be attributed to the progressive nature and systemic influences of conditions with inborn errors of metabolism that remain undetected or untreated in addition to an electroencephalographic abnormality.

Seizure control is poor. The erratic myoclonus usually disappears after a few weeks or months,[4] and partial seizures become intractable. Tonic seizures develop at age 3 to 4 months. Once tonic seizures occur, the overall poor prognosis becomes even graver. In review of 30 patients from the literature, Djukic et al.[10] found that of 22 patients with EME and tonic seizures, 11 died, whereas none of the patients without tonic seizures did. The burst-suppression EEG pattern evolves into hypsarrhythmia in one third of patients. Focal or multifocal abnormalities develop in the remaining patients.

PATHOPHYSIOLOGIC BASIS

Neither the occurrence of the constellation of symptoms and findings in EME nor the pathophysiologic basis of the changing clinical picture that follows the progression of the disease have been well explained.

Ohtahara et al.[25] approached the problem from the standpoint of the characteristic EEG findings. They drew an analogy to the pathophysiologic basis of the other, more common conditions with suppression-burst EEG (deep anesthesia, normal premature infants <30–32 weeks of gestation, severe hypoxic ischemic encephalopathy). They pointed to a theory of abnormal "neuronal connectivity, suggesting that a disconnection in brain circuits may be involved in the genesis of EEG" and emphasized the "indispensable role of brain lesions both at the subcortical and cortical level."[27]

An alternative hypothesis is more symptom oriented, based on evidence from experimental studies and analysis of the clinical stages in the evolution of EME; it proposes that EME and EIEE may represent a continuum based on the burden of disease at the onset of symptoms.[10] Rodin's animal studies[31,32] clearly showed the brainstem structures associated with the onset of generalized seizures, such as tonic seizures, with the earliest sustained discharges appearing in the pons. During clonic seizures, the cortical discharges lead. Thus, there it has been suggested that clonic seizures originate in the forebrain, whereas tonic seizures originate in the brainstem.[36] This conclusion is supported by studies using precollicular transections: Tonic seizures also occurred when seizures were induced in animals with transections, whereas clonic seizures required forebrain connections.[1,7,12] Other studies show that repeated generalized seizures in experimental animals can kindle secondary seizure foci.[43] These secondary epileptic foci may persist even after the bilateral or generalized seizures abated, because descending inhibition from the hemispheres increases with maturation.[22]

Thus, it is tempting to speculate that in EME, there is initially involvement of cortical structures. The repeated myoclonic seizures may "kindle" the development of focal seizures, and with time there may be a spread to the brainstem (in some cases). Tonic seizures develop once the brainstem lesion burden exceeds the threshold for seizures. Patients with EIEE may have already exceeded this threshold at birth and present with tonic seizures early. In EME, brainstem involvement may be less severe, and tonic seizures are not the presenting symptom. Over time, the brainstem alterations may allow the emergence of tonic seizures possibly as a result of a kindling process increasing seizure susceptibility or as a release of the brainstem from cortical inhibitory control as the metabolic disease progresses.

The pathologic data are consistent with this view. Autopsies were performed in five patients with EME.[11,14,15,17,20,24,30,34,35] All patients had tonic seizures, and clinical signs of brainstem anomalies were present in all of them.

Genetic mapping of an autosomal-recessive form of EME to chromosome 11p15.5 led to the identification of a missense mutation (p.Pro206Leu) in the gene encoding GCI, a protein in the mitochondrial inner membrane that cotransports glutamate with H^+.[21] Expression of this protein has an age-specific distribution: At 20 weeks of gestation, the highest gene expression is identified in the cortex, brainstem, and cerebellum. A moderate to high level of expression is observed within the brainstem in the red nuclei, the substantia nigra, and the olivary complexes and the dentate nucleus in the cerebellum. It is interesting that many of these structures, especially the substantia nigra pars reticulata and its output circuits, play a prominent role in the control of seizures as a function of age and gender.[37] The observation that EME results from a defect in GC1 suggests a role for either glutamate metabolism, mitochondrial pathology, or both in EME.

DIFFERENTIAL DIAGNOSIS

Early myoclonic encephalopathy and Ohtahara syndrome share many common clinical and EEG characteristics such as onset in the first few months of life, suppression-burst pattern on EEG, and grave prognosis. The boundary between the two syndromes unfortunately is not always clear,[18,33,40] and the classification is sometimes questionable even among the published cases.[4] Once tonic seizures occur in patients with EME, the differential diagnosis becomes even more difficult, perhaps implying common pathogenetic mechanisms as discussed earlier. Perhaps the term *neonatal epileptic encephalopathy* is more appropriate to encompass both conditions.

The critical difference between EME and EIEE appears to be in the presumed etiologies and the prevailing seizure type at the onset of the clinical seizures. EIEE typically manifests with tonic seizures at onset, whereas EME is most associated with myoclonic seizures. However, erratic myoclonus may be absent even in the most frequently identified cause of EME: glycine encephalopathy (J. Aicardi, personal communication). In its classification, the International League Against Epilepsy emphasizes the symptomatic nature and nonspecific etiology of both syndromes.[16] The majority of cases of EIEE are associated with structural brain anomalies, whereas the majority of EME cases are associated with metabolic disorders.[4,9,19,26,38,40] There is an overlap, however, and often the underlying etiology remains unclear.[42] The observation that under some circumstances multiple etiologies can produce either syndrome suggests that EIEE and EME may represent a continuum.

The initial differentiation of EIEE and EME based on the presence or absence of myoclonic or tonic seizures at onset may better indicate the stage of the progression of the brainstem pathology/dysfunction than a phenotype specific to one syndrome or another. A major differentiating point is the absence of myoclonias in EIEE. A common unifying feature is the eventual appearance of tonic seizures. As the brainstem disease burden approaches the threshold for tonic seizures, EME patients become less distinguishable clinically from patients with EIEE.

The EEG pattern and persistence of "burst-suppression" distinguishes EME and EIEE from other conditions that produce neonatal burst-suppression, such as hypoxic–ischemic encephalopathy and neonatal convulsions.

TREATMENT

With the exception of cases with pyridoxine dependency, there is no effective management for EME. Neither the conventional antiepileptic medications nor adrenocorticotropic hormone or corticosteroids alter the progressive nature of the disease and improve the poor outcome. Treatments directed at correcting the underlying metabolic deficit may improve the outcome. A trial of treatment with pyridoxine is justified in all cases with EME because it is still the only efficient treatment for the small subgroup of patients in whom it is effective.

SUMMARY AND CONCLUSIONS

EME is a malignant epileptic syndrome with typical onset during the neonatal period. The main seizure type at onset is erratic myoclonus, but as the disease progresses, other seizure types develop, including tonic seizures at 3 to 4 months of age. The EEG is characterized by a suppression-burst pattern and often evolves into hypsarrhythmia. The etiology of EME is diverse: Congenital errors of metabolism are the most frequently identified, followed by cryptogenic and cases with structural brain malformations. Except in rare cases responsive to treatment with pyridoxine, control of seizures is poor. Prognosis is grave, with high early mortality and severe neurologic handicap in survivors.

It is possible that EME presents a continuum with EIEE and the phenotypic differences reflect the severity of the underlying pathologic process. In the future, a systematic approach including comprehensive evaluations (morphometric and functional imaging studies, neurophysiologic evaluations with multimodal evoked potentials, and possibly CSF neurotransmitter studies) performed during different stages of the diseases and especially during periods of clinical transitions could help to provide a better understanding of the underlying pathophysiologic processes. Shifting the goal of the diagnostic evaluation from detecting a specific abnormality to detecting a progressive pathologic change might permit the identification of more subtle changes before they become significant and allow the introduction of new treatments.

References

1. Ackermann RF, Engel J Jr, Baxter L. Positron emission tomography and autoradiographic studies of glucose utilization following electroconvulsive seizures in humans and rats. *Ann N Y Acad Sci.* 1986;462:263–269.
2. Aicardi J. Early myoclonic encephalopathy (neonatal myoclonic encephalopathy). In: Roger J, Bureau M, Dravet C, et al., eds. *Epileptic Syndromes in Infancy, Childhood and Adolescence,* 2nd ed. London: John Libbey; 1992:13–23.
3. Aicardi J, Goutieres F. Encephalopathie myoclonique neonatale. *Rev Electroencephalogr Neurophysiol Clin.* 1978;8(1):99–101.
4. Aicardi J, Ohtahara S. Severe neonatal epilepsies with suppression-burst pattern. In: Roger J, Bureau M, Dravet C, et al., eds. *Epilepsy Syndromes in Infancy, Childhood and Adolescence,* 3rd ed. London: John Libbey; 2002: 33–44.
5. Aukett A, Bennett M, Hosking GP. Molybdenum co-factor deficiency: an easily missed inborn error of metabolism. *Dev Med Child Neurol.* 1988;30(4):531–535.
6. Bartschwinkler S. Cycle of earthquake-induced aggradation and related tidal channel shifting, Upper Turnagain Arm, Alaska, USA. *Sedimentology.* 2000;35(4):621.
7. Browning RA, Nelson DK. Modification of electroshock and pentylenetetrazol seizure patterns in rats after precollicular transections. *Exp Neurol.* 1986;93(3):546–556.
8. Cavazzuti G, Nalin A, Ferrari F, et al. Encephalopatia epilettica ad insorgenza neonatale. *Clin Pediatr.* 1978(60):239–246.
9. Dalla Bernardina B, Dulac O, Fejerman N, et al. Early myoclonic epileptic encephalopathy (E.M.E.E.). *Eur J Pediatr.* 1983;140(3):248–252.
10. Djukic A, Lado FA, Shinnar S, et al. Are early myoclonic encephalopathy (EME) and the Ohtahara syndrome (EIEE) independent of each other? *Epilepsy Res.* 2006;70(Suppl 1)S68–S76.
11. Du Plessis AJ, Kaufmann WE, Kupsky WJ. Intrauterine-onset myoclonic encephalopathy associated with cerebral cortical dysgenesis. *J Child Neurol.* 1993;8(2):164–170.
12. Engel J Jr, Wolfson L, Brown L. Anatomical correlates of electrical and behavioral events related to amygdaloid kindling. *Ann Neurol.* 1978;3(6):538–544.
13. Grandgeorge D, Favier A, Bost M, et al. L'acidemie D-glycerique. A propos d'une nouvelle observation anatomo-clinique. *Arch Fr Pediatr.* 1980;(37):577–584.
14. Harding BN, Boyd SG. Intractable seizures from infancy can be associated with dentato-olivary dysplasia. *J Neurol Sci.* 1991;104(2):157–65.
15. Hirabayashi S, Shigematsu H, Iai M, et al. A neurodegenerative disorder with early myoclonic encephalopathy, retinal pigmentary degeneration and nephronophthisis. *Brain Dev.* 2000;22(1):24–30.
16. ILAE. Proposal for revised classification of epilepsies and epileptic syndromes. Commission on Classification and Terminology of the International League Against Epilepsy. *Epilepsia.* 1989;30(4):389–399.
17. Itoh M, Hanaoka S, Sasaki M, et al. Neuropathology of early-infantile epileptic encephalopathy with suppression-bursts; comparison with those of early myoclonic encephalopathy and West syndrome. *Brain Dev.* 2001;23(7):721–726.
18. Kelley KR, Shinnar S, Moshe SL. A 5-month-old with intractable epilepsy. *Semin Pediatr Neurol.* 1999;6(3):138–144; discussion, 144–145.
19. Lombroso CT. Early myoclonic encephalopathy, early infantile epileptic encephalopathy, and benign and severe infantile myoclonic epilepsies: a critical review and personal contributions. *J Clin Neurophysiol.* 1990;7(3):380–408.
20. Miller SP, Dilenge ME, Meagher-Villemure K, et al. Infantile epileptic encephalopathy (Ohtahara syndrome) and migrational disorder. *Pediatr Neurol.* 1998;19(1):50–54.
21. Molinari F, Raas-Rothschild A, Rio M, et al. Impaired mitochondrial glutamate transport in autosomal recessive neonatal myoclonic epilepsy. *Am J Hum Genet.* 2005;76(2):334–339.
22. Moshe SL, Albala BJ. Maturational changes in postictal refractoriness and seizure susceptibility in developing rats. *Ann Neurol.* 1983;13(5):552–557.
23. Nishikawa M, Ichiyama T, Hayashi T, et al. A case of early myoclonic encephalopathy with the congenital nephrotic syndrome. *Brain Dev.* 1997; 19(2):144–147.
24. Ogihara M, Kinoue K, Takamiya H, et al. A case of early infantile epileptic encephalopathy (EIEE) with anatomical cerebral asymmetry and myoclonus. *Brain Dev.* 1993;15(2):133–139.
25. Ohtahara S, Ohtsuka Y, Erba G. *Epilepsy: A Comprehensive Textbook.* Philadelphia: Lippincott-Raven; 1998.
26. Ohtahara S, Ohtsuka Y, Yamatogi Y, et al. The early-infantile epileptic encephalopathy with suppression-burst: developmental aspects. *Brain Dev.* 1987;9(4):371–376.
27. Ohtahara S, Yamatogi Y. Epileptic encephalopathies in early infancy with suppression-burst. *J Clin Neurophysiol.* 2003;20:398–407.
28. Oka E, Ishida S, Ohtsuka Y, et al. Neuroepidemiological study of childhood epilepsy by application of international classification of epilepsies and epileptic syndromes (ILAE 1989). *Epilepsia.* 1995;36:658–661.
29. Otani K, Abe J, Futagi Y, et al. Clinical and electroencephalographical follow-up study of early myoclonic encephalopathy. *Brain Dev.* 1989;11:332–337.
30. Robain O, Dulac O. Early epileptic encephalopathy with suppression bursts and olivary-dentate dysplasia. *Neuropediatrics.* 1992;23(3):162–164.
31. Rodin E, Onuma T, Wasson S, et al. Neurophysiological mechanisms involved in grand mal seizures induced by Metrazol and Megimide. *Electroencephalogr Clin Neurophysiol.* 1971;30:62–72.
32. Rodin EA. Some relationships of induced seizure patterns to clinical findings in epileptic patients. *Epilepsia.* 1964;23:21–32.
33. Schlumberger E, Dulac O, Plouin P. Early infantile epileptic syndrome(s) with suppression burst: nosological considerations. In: Roger J, Bureau M, Dravet

C, et al., eds. *Epileptic Syndromes in Infancy, Childhood and Adolescence.* London: John Libbey; 1992:35–44.
34. Spreafico R, Angelini L, Binelli S, et al. Burst suppression and impairment of neocortical ontogenesis: electroclinical and neuropathologic findings in two infants with early myoclonic encephalopathy. *Epilepsia.* 1993;34(5):800–808.
35. Trinka E, Rauscher C, Nagler M, et al. A case of Ohtahara syndrome with olivary-dentate dysplasia and agenesis of mamillary bodies. *Epilepsia.* 2001;42(7):950–953.
36. Veliskova J. Behavioral characterization of seizures in rats. In: Pitkanen A, Schwartzkroin P, Moshe S, eds. *Animal Models of Epilepsy.* San Diego, CA: Elsevier; 2005:601–611.
37. Veliskova J, Caludio OI, Galanopoulou AS, et al. Developmental aspects of the basal ganglia and therapeutic perspectives. *Epileptic Disord.* 2002;4(Suppl 3):S73–S82.
38. Vigevano F, Bartuli A. Infantile epileptic syndromes and metabolic etiologies. *J Child Neurol.* 2002;17(Suppl 3):3S9–3S13; discussion, 3S14.
39. Vigevano F, Cincinnati P, Bertini E, et al. Neonatal myoclonic encephalopathy. Contribution of a case with suspected dysmetabolic etiology [in Italian]. *Riv Neurobiol.* 1981;27(34):458–466.
40. Wang PJ, Lee WT, Hwu WL, et al. The controversy regarding diagnostic criteria for early myoclonic encephalopathy. *Brain Dev.* 1998;20(7):530–535.
41. Watanabe K, Miura, K, Natsume J, et al. Epilepsies of neonatal onset: seizure type and evolution. *Dev Med Child Neurol.* 1999;41:318–322.
42. Williams AN, Gray RG, Poulton K, et al. A case of Ohtahara syndrome with cytochrome oxidase deficiency. *Dev Med Child Neurol.* 1998;40(8):568–570.
43. Wong BY, Moshe SL. Mutual interactions between repeated flurothyl convulsions and electrical kindling. *Epilepsy Res.* 1987;1(3):159–164.

CHAPTER 225 ■ OHTAHARA SYNDROME

SHUNSUKE OHTAHARA, YASUKO YAMATOGI, AND YOKO OHTSUKA

INTRODUCTION

Epileptic or chronic seizures occurring during the neonatal and early infantile periods are rarely observed compared with those occurring during other stages of childhood, because of the morphologic and biochemical immaturity of the central nervous system. Only a few epileptic syndromes begin in these periods, most of them refractory and catastrophic epilepsies.[3,7,21] Of these, this chapter describes the Ohtahara syndrome (OS): Early infantile epileptic encephalopathy with suppression-burst.

This syndrome, which has not only characteristic clinical and electroencephalographic (EEG) features, but also a distinct age dependence and evolution of epileptic syndromes with age, is considered the youngest form of the age-dependent epileptic encephalopathy.

HISTORICAL PERSPECTIVE

In 1976, Ohtahara et al.[27] first described OS as an independent epileptic syndrome. It is the earliest form of the age-dependent epileptic encephalopathies, which include OS, West syndrome, and Lennox-Gastaut syndrome. Although each of these is an independent clinicoelectrical entity with individual clinical and EEG features, they have the following characteristics in common: (a) predominance in a certain age group (age dependence); (b) a peculiar type of frequent, minor, generalized seizure; (c) a severe and continuous epileptic EEG abnormality; (d) heterogeneous etiology; (e) frequent association with a mental defect; and (f) poor response to treatment and grave prognosis.[25,26,29] Furthermore, these syndromes often evolve with age. During their clinical course, a considerable number of cases of OS evolve into West syndrome and then from West syndrome into Lennox-Gastaut syndrome.[25,28,49] Because of their common characteristics and their transitions with age, Ohtahara applied the inclusive term *age-dependent epileptic encephalopathy* to this group of three syndromes.[25,26,29]

We adopt the term "epileptic encephalopathy" instead of "epilepsy" based on the following characteristics: (a) the presence of serious underlying disorders, (b) extremely frequent seizures, (c) continuously appearing marked epileptic EEG abnormality, and (d) mental stagnation or deterioration often manifesting with the persistence of seizures.

Although the etiologies of these syndromes are heterogeneous, each syndrome occurs predominantly within a certain age range and is associated with specific clinical and EEG traits. Because the clinical and electrical characteristics of each syndrome are based on a diverse group of etiologies, age should be considered the common factor underlying the manifestation of specific features. Thus, these syndromes may represent an age-specific epileptic reaction to various nonspecific exogenous insults to the brain occurring at an age-specific developmental stage.

DEFINITIONS

Ohtahara syndrome is characterized by very early onset, within a few months of birth, frequent tonic spasms, and a suppression-burst pattern in the EEG.[27,29,31,32] This periodic EEG pattern is consistently observed in both awake and sleep states. The main seizure pattern is tonic spasms but not myoclonic seizures. Tonic spasms appear often in clusters but sometimes sporadically. Partial motor seizures may occur. Although the etiologies are heterogeneous, neuroimaging usually discloses gross structural abnormalities due to mainly prenatal cerebral dysgenesis. The prognosis is serious: For example, early death or marked psychomotor retardation and intractable seizures with frequent evolution to West syndrome and still further to Lennox-Gastaut syndrome in some cases[28,29,49] or to severe epilepsy with multiple independent spike foci.[51] The Commission on Classification and Terminology of the International League Against Epilepsy (ILAE)[7] placed this syndrome among "symptomatic generalized epilepsies and syndromes with nonspecific etiology," and the proposed diagnostic scheme of the ILAE[10] categorized it as "epileptic encephalopathy."

EPIDEMIOLOGY

Several dozen cases of OS have been reported, but occurrence has been rare in comparison with West syndrome (WS) and Lennox-Gastaut syndrome. An epidemiologic study of childhood epilepsy carried out in Okayama Prefecture, Japan, detected 1 case of OS (0.04%) among 2,378 epileptic children <10 years of age.[36] The prevalence of this syndrome was much lower than that of West syndrome (40 cases, or 1.68%). Similarly, Kramer et al.[18] described 1 case of OS (0.2%) and 40 cases of WS (9.1%) in a cohort of 440 consecutive children <15 years of age with epilepsy in Tel Aviv, Israel. Thus, the relative prevalence of OS to WS may be 1:40 or less. On the other hand, in a study of 75 infants with epilepsy of neonatal onset who were monitored intensively, Watanabe et al. observed 8 cases (10.7%) of OS and no case of WS.[46]

No obvious racial differences have been observed in the respective incidences. No significant gender difference was confirmed, but male slightly exceeded female cases by 9:7 in our series.[50]

ETIOLOGY AND BASIC MECHANISMS

Although the etiologies of OS are heterogeneous, the majority are static gross brain pathologies such as cerebral dysgenesis, although some are cryptogenic. Development of neuroimaging techniques, particularly magnetic resonance imaging (MRI), has disclosed that various types of cerebral dysgenesis are the greatest underlying pathologies of this syndrome.[40,50] It is also important that asymmetry is often observed in structural abnormalities of the brain. Porencephaly, Aicardi syndrome,[34,50] cerebral dysgenesis, olivary-dentate dysplasia,[13,39,44] hemimegalencephaly,[12,33,50] linear sebaceous nevus,[15] Leigh encephalopathy,[42] and subacute diffuse encephalopathy[29] have been reported.

Of 16 cases in our series, 5 (31.3%) were cryptogenic.[50] With regard to genetic factors, no sibling case was reported except for Leigh encephalopathy.

With regard to metabolic disorders, although they are very rare, Williams et al.[14,48] first reported a case with cytochrome oxidase deficiency. This case, however, had only transient reversible deficiency that may have caused impaired neuronal migration or demyelination due to energy depletion during a critical period. Miller et al.[20] reported the absence of γ-aminobutyric acid (GABA) in cerebrospinal fluid (CSF) in a case with diffuse cerebral migration disorder. Fusco et al.[11] described one case each with pyridoxine dependency and carnitine palmitoyltransferase deficiency.

Fundamentally, the age factor should be emphasized, on the basis of polyetiology.

The pathophysiologic mechanisms underlying suppression-bursts are not fully elucidated. Aso et al.[4] found that the suppression-burst pattern correlated with multifocal severe brain damage, although no one structure was consistently affected. Any of these anomalies can prevent the establishment of normal neuronal connectivity necessary for the EEG ontogeny. This hypothesis is corroborated by the observation that a normal EEG pattern at any age can revert to a suppression-burst pattern after catastrophic events that cause laminal necrosis of the cortex, as in severe hypoxic-ischemic encephalopathy.[47] Similar but less readily identifiable cortical and subcortical abnormalities must be invoked to explain cryptogenic cases of OS and those with olivary-dentate dysplasia. Spreafico et al.[41] suggested that in OS and early myoclonic encephalopathy (EME) the suppression-burst (SB) pattern primarily reflects a diffuse structural or junctional disturbance of gray matter connectivity.

Its similarity to tracé alternant in neonatal quiet sleep and to burst-suppression in brain-damaged neonates may suggest an excessive subcortical neuronal discharge modified by subcorticocortical dysregulation or disconnection and by cortical lesions.[27,29] Trinka et al.[44] also considered that in olivary dentate dysplasia or focal cortical dysplasia, mild additional supratentorial/cortical anomalies or infratentorial anomalies contribute to the SB pattern in OS.

The markedly asymmetric and sometimes unilateral SB pattern reported in hemimegalencephaly further suggests the indispensable role of brain lesions at both the subcortical and cortical levels in generating the SB pattern.[23,33,35]

Two types of mechanisms have been suggested in the pathogenesis of SB, as mentioned later.

CLINICAL PRESENTATION

The onset of the initial seizures or tonic spasms is early, within the first 3 months after birth, mainly within 1 month. Du Plessis et al.[9] extended the earliest age of onset into the intrauterine period. Clarke et al.[6] also suspected an intrauterine onset in four of their eight cryptogenic cases based on observations of violent fetal movement.

The main seizure type is tonic spasms with or without clustering. These occur not only during the waking state, but also during sleep in most cases. In 6 of our 16 patients (37.5%), hemiconvulsions, tonic seizures, or clonic seizures preceded one to several weeks before the onset of tonic spasms.[50] Myoclonic seizures are rare.[29,50]

An evolutionary pattern is characteristic: From OS to West syndrome in the middle period of infancy (between 3 and 6 months of age in many cases) and from West syndrome to Lennox-Gastaut syndrome in early childhood.[28–30,45,50]

DIAGNOSTIC EVALUATION

Electroencephalographic Findings

The most characteristic feature of EEG in OS is the suppression-burst pattern, which is consistently seen during both awake and sleep states (Fig. 1). The suppression-burst pattern is characterized by high-voltage bursts alternating with nearly flat periods at an approximately regular rate. Bursts last 1 to 3 seconds and comprise high-voltage (150–350 μV) slow waves intermixed with spikes. Duration of the suppression phase is 3 to 5 seconds. The interval measured from beginning to beginning of bursts ranges from 5 to 10 seconds. The suppression-burst pattern shows some asymmetry in approximately two thirds of cases, presumably reflecting the underlying brain lesions. There is no awake/sleep differentiation. The suppression-burst pattern evolves to hypsarrhythmia in many cases, and then from hypsarrhythmia to diffuse slow spike-waves in some cases.[28,30]

The EEG pattern of OS needs to be differentiated from (a) the periodic type of hypsarrhythmia, in which periodicity becomes remarkable in the sleeping state and sleep spindles may be observed in the interburst phase, and (b) the burst-suppression pattern in severely abnormal neonates, which is characterized by a longer depressed phase with irregular and atypical appearance of bursts including fewer spike components.

The ictal EEG during tonic spasms shows desynchronization with or without fast activity. Tonic spasms in OS often appear concomitant with burst, but the SB pattern often disappears during a cluster of spasms. Partial seizures show focal repetitive or rhythmic discharges, which are often followed by a series of tonic spasms.

NEUROIMAGING AND OTHER LABORATORY EXAMINATIONS

Computed tomography (CT) and MRI reveal structural abnormalities that are often asymmetric, even at an early stage of the disorder. Single-photon emission computed tomography and positron emission tomography often show corresponding abnormalities.

No abnormalities are found in serum and urine amino acids, cerebrospinal fluid, bone marrow, enzyme assay of white blood cells, serum pyruvate and lactate, ammonia, liver function, serum immunoglobulin, or TORCH (antibodies of *Toxoplasma*, rubella virus, cytomegalovirus, and herpes simplex virus).[29]

With evoked potentials, abnormalities are often found in auditory brainstem responses and visual responses in OS.[29]

DIFFERENTIAL DIAGNOSIS

Ohtahara Syndrome and West Syndrome

The age of onset is different in the two syndromes. It is between the neonatal and early infantile periods in OS and between middle and late infancy in West syndrome (see Chapter 229). Lombroso[19] claimed that OS might be regarded as an early form of West syndrome. There is a close relationship between OS and West syndrome, and in a considerable number of cases OS evolves to West syndrome. However, OS is certainly a different epileptic syndrome than West syndrome. Although

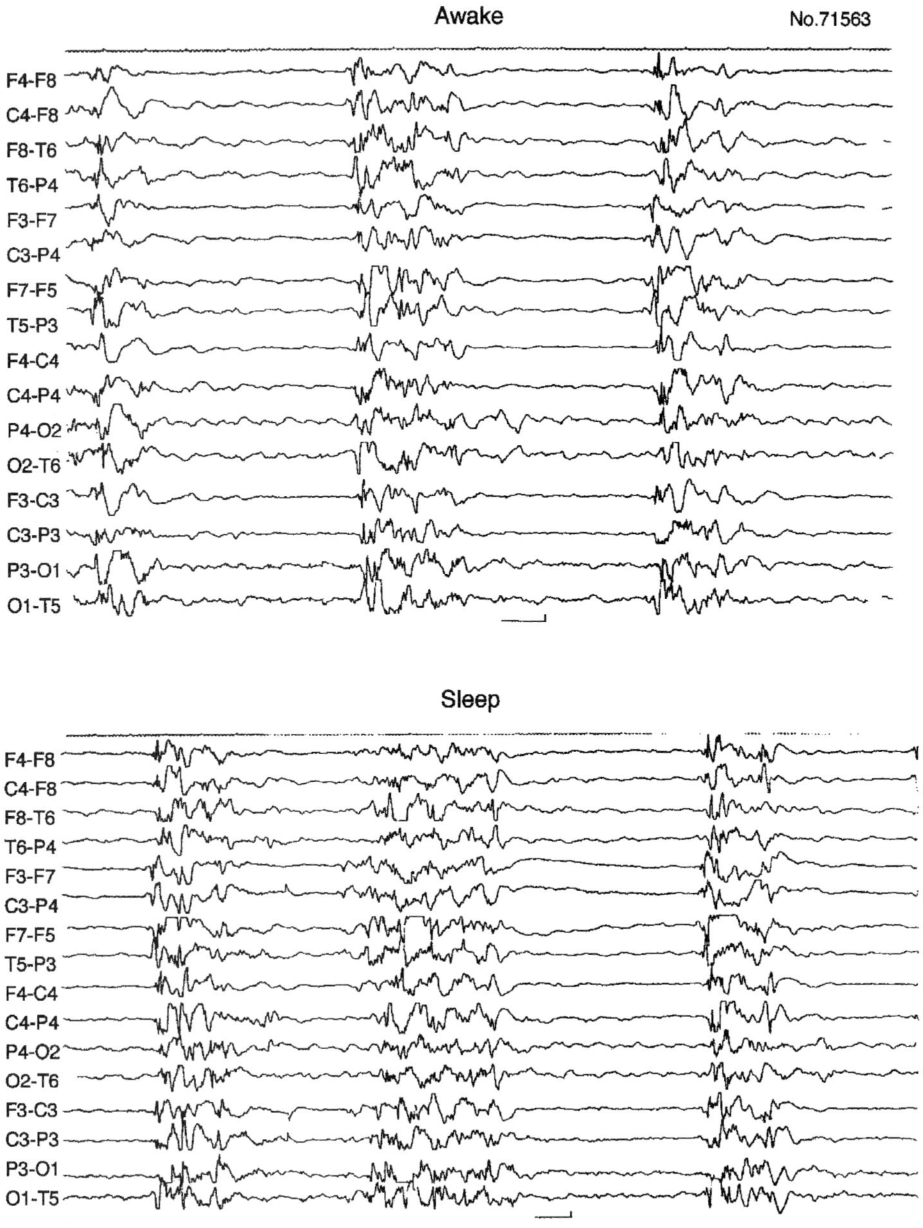

FIGURE 1. Interictal electroencephalogram. Suppression-burst pattern in a 2-month-old boy with Ohtahara syndrome. **Top:** Awake. **Bottom:** Natural sleep. The horizontal calibration mark denotes 1 second, the vertical one, 50 μV.

the main seizure type is tonic spasms in both syndromes, tonic spasms in OS appear during both awake and sleep states, and also with and without clustering in many cases. Partial seizures are also more often observed in some OS cases. Most cases with OS show severe cortical pathology, often with asymmetric lesions displayed on neuroimaging.

With regard to EEG findings, the suppression-burst pattern is seen in OS, in contrast to hypsarrhythmia in West syndrome. The suppression-burst pattern differs from the periodic type of hypsarrhythmia, in which periodicity becomes distinct only during sleep. Seizures are more intractable in OS, and adrenocorticotropic hormone (ACTH) is poorly effective in most cases. Prognosis is far less favorable in OS than in West syndrome.

Ohtahara Syndrome and Early Myoclonic Encephalopathy

Because OS and EME[1–3,8] have both clinical and electrical characteristics in common, such as onset during the neonatal and early infantile periods and the EEG suppression-burst pattern, differential diagnosis of these syndromes warrants discussion (see also Chapter 224).[31,32]

Clinical Features

Tonic spasms are the main seizure type in OS, whereas EME is characterized by myoclonia, especially erratic myoclonia, and very frequent partial seizures. In contrast, episodes of myoclonia are rarely seen in OS.

Electroencephalographic Findings

The suppression-burst pattern is a common feature of both syndromes, although its form and the mode of its appearance and its period of persistence differ considerably between the two. With regard to mode of appearance, the suppression-burst pattern in OS appears consistently and unchangingly during both the awake and sleep states; in EME, the suppression-burst pattern is enhanced during sleep and often is not apparent in the awake state.[32] Regarding the period of its persistence, the suppression-burst pattern appears at the onset of disease and disappears within the first 6 months of life in OS, whereas in EME, the suppression-burst pattern appears at 1 to 5 months of age in some cases and characteristically persists for a prolonged period.[22,31,32]

Evolution During the Clinical Course

Evolution of the EEG pattern during the clinical course is a characteristic feature of OS: From the suppression-burst pattern to hypsarrhythmia in many cases, and then from hypsarrhythmia to diffuse slow spike-waves in some cases.[29,31,32,45,50] In contrast, the suppression-burst pattern in EME reappears and persists for a prolonged period after a transient appearance of atypical hypsarrhythmia that may be observed during the clinical course in some cases.[22,32] Thus, the patterns of EEG evolution with age differ considerably between the two syndromes.

As already mentioned, considering the evolution of disorder type with age and the mode of appearance in relation to the wake-and-sleep cycle, the existence of two types of SB, those observed in OS and EME, is a very interesting and important finding, one that might contribute to the understanding of the mechanism of SB.

With regard to the evolution of epileptic syndromes, OS shows a specific pattern of evolution into other forms of the age-dependent epileptic encephalopathies, whereas EME has no such age-related evolution. Furthermore, it is also significant that no transition is observed between OS and EME.

Etiology

In OS, obvious brain lesions, such as malformations, are often seen, and CT and MRI abnormalities are usually detected even at an early stage. No familial cases of OS have been reported. In contrast, the frequent occurrence of familial cases of EME suggests some congenital metabolic disorders as the etiology.[3,40,43]

These findings strongly suggest that OS and EME are separate clinicoelectrical entities. Schlumberger et al.[40] found definite clinical and symptomatologic differences between these two syndromes and no overlap. However, there are cases that are truly difficult to separate because they have cerebral malformation and metabolic/genetic disorders.

TREATMENT AND OUTCOME

Seizures are intractable. Synthetic ACTH exerted a limited efficacy in some cases.[50] Phenobarbital,[37] pyridoxal phosphate or vitamin B6, valproate, benzodiazepines, and a ketogenic diet were poorly effective in general.

There are recent reports of cases responsive to zonisamide[24,50] and vigabatrin.[5] Successful resection has been reported in patients with focal cortical dysplasia and has been associated with relatively improved neurologic development after surgery.[16,17,38]

Although they are intractable, seizures come under control by school age in approximately half of the patients. Prognosis for psychomotor development remains very poor; all survivors have severe disabilities, both mental and physical. Many such patients died, especially in the early stage of the disease.[50] One fourth of our patients died before 2 years of age.

LONG-TERM PROGNOSIS

In 8 survivors of 16 OS cases in our series, the age at follow-up ranged from 5 years and 0 months to 28 years and 0 months.[50] All but 2 were >10 years of age. All survivors had severe mental retardation. Six were bedridden with quadriplegia; only 2, with hemiplegia, were ambulant. Seizures persisted in 2 of the survivors: Tonic spasms in 1 and focal motor seizures in the other.

With EEG follow-up, only 2 of 8 survivors were spike-free. Focal spikes were detected in 6 others: Multiple independent spike foci were found in 4 and other cortical foci in 2; 3 of them showed diffuse generalization.

SUMMARY AND CONCLUSIONS

OS is a peculiar epileptic syndrome with strong age dependence in the neonatal period and very early infancy, and it is the earliest form of the age-dependent epileptic encephalopathies. In describing the clinicoelectrical characteristics of this syndrome and its evolution with age, we stressed the importance of taking a developmental approach in epilepsy research. This approach is very effective for establishing new syndromes and differentiating them from related disorders/syndromes as well as clarifying prognoses. In discussion differential diagnosis focused particular attention on early myoclonic encephalopathy.

References

1. Aicardi J. Early myoclonic encephalopathy (neonatal myoclonic encephalopathy). In: Roger J, Bureau M, Dravet C, et al., eds. *Epileptic Syndromes in Infancy, Childhood and Adolescence,* 2nd ed. London: John Libbey; 1992: 13–23.
2. Aicardi J, Goutieres F. Encéphalpathie myoclonique néonatale. *Rev EEG Neurophysiol.* 1978;8:99–101.
3. Aicardi J, Ohtahara S. Severe neonatal epilepsies with suppression-burst pattern. In: Roger J, Bureau M, Dravet C, et al., eds. *Epileptic Syndromes in Infancy, Childhood and Adolescence,* 4th ed. Montrouge: John Libbey Eurotext; 2005:39–50.
4. Aso K, Scher MS, Barmada MA. Neonatal electroencephalography and neuropathy. *J Clin Neurophysiol.* 1989;6:103–123.
5. Baxter PS, Gardnerr-Medwin D, Barwick DD, et al. Vigabatrin monotherapy in resistant neonatal seizures. *Seizure.* 1995;4:57–59.
6. Clarke M, Gill J, Noronha M, et al. Early infantile epileptic encephalopathy with suppression burst: Ohtahara syndrome. *Dev Med Child Neurol.* 1987;29:520–528.
7. Commission on Classification and Terminology of the International League Against Epilepsy. Proposal for revised classification of epilepsies and epileptic syndromes. *Epilepsia.* 1989;30:389–399.
8. Dalla Bernardina B, Dulac O, Fejerman N, et al. Early myoclonic epileptic encephalopathy (EMEE). *Eur J Pediatr.* 1983;140:248–252.
9. Du Plessis AJ, Kaufmann WE, Kupsky WJ. Intrauterine-onset myoclonic encephalopathy associated with cerebral cortical dysplasia. *J Child Neurol.* 1993;8:164–170.
10. Engel J Jr. ILAE Commission report. A proposed diagnostic scheme for people with epileptic seizures and with epilepsy: report of the ILAE Task Force on Classification and Terminology. *Epilepsia.* 2001;42:796–803.
11. Fusco L, Pachatz C, Di Capua M, et al. Video/EEG aspects of early-infantile epileptic encephalopathy with suppression–bursts (Ohtahara syndrome). *Brain Dev.* 2001;23:708–714.
12. Guzzetta F, Battaglia D, Lettori D, et al. Epileptic negative myoclonus in a newborn with hemimegalencephaly. *Epilepsia.* 2002;43:1106–1109.
13. Harding BN, Boyd SG. Intractable seizures from infancy can be associated with dentato–olivary dysplasia. *J Neurol Sci.* 1991;104:157–165.
14. Higgins C, Gray G, Ramani P, et al. Transient cytochrome oxidase deficiency with Ohtahara syndrome. *Dev Med Child Neurol.* 2000;42:785–786.
15. Hirata Y, Ishikawa A, Somiya K. A case of linear nevus sebaceous syndrome associated with early infantile epileptic encephalopathy with suppression burst (EIEE). *No To Hattatsu.* 1985;17:577–582.
16. Hmaimess G, Raftopoulos G, Kadhim H, et al. Impact of early hemispherotomy in a case of Ohtahara syndrome with left parieto-occipital megalencephaly. *Seizure.* 2005;14:439–442.
17. Komaki H, Sugai K, Maehara T, et al. Surgical treatment of early-infantile epileptic encephalopathy with suppression-burst associated with focal cortical dysplasia. *Brain Dev.* 2001;23:727–731.
18. Kramer U, Nevo Y, Neufeld MY, et al. Epidemiology of epilepsy in childhood: a cohort of 440 consecutive patients. *Pediatr Neurol.* 1998;18:46–50.
19. Lombroso CT. Early myoclonic encephalopathy, early infantile epileptic encephalopathy, and benign and severe infantile myoclonic epilepsies: a critical review and personal contributions. *J Clin Neurophysiol.* 1990;7:380–408.
20. Miller SP, Dilenge ME, Meagher-Villemure K, et al. Infantile epileptic encephalopathy (Ohtahara syndrome) and migrational disorder. *Pediatr Neurol.* 1998;19:50–54.

21. Mizrahi EM, Clancy RR. Neonatal seizures: early-onset seizure syndromes and their consequences for development. *Ment Retard Dev Disabil Res Rev.* 2000;6:229–241.
22. Murakami N, Ohtsuka Y, Ohtahara S. Early infantile epileptic syndromes with suppression-bursts: early myoclonic encephalopathy vs. Ohtahara syndrome. *Jpn J Psychiatry Neurol.* 1993;47:197–200.
23. Ogihara M, Kinoue K, Takamiya H, et al. A case of early infantile epileptic encephalopathy with anatomical cerebral asymmetry and myoclonus. *Brain Dev.* 1993;15:133–139.
24. Ohno M, Simotsuji Y, Abe J, et al. Zonisamide treatment of early infantile epileptic encephalopathy (EIEE). *Pediatr Neurol.* 2000;23:341–344.
25. Ohtahara S. A study on the age-dependent epileptic encephalopathy. *No To Hattatsu.* 1977;9:2–21.
26. Ohtahara S. Clinico-electrical delineation of epileptic encephalopathies in childhood. *Asian Med J.* 1978;21:499–509.
27. Ohtahara S, Ishida T, Oka E, et al. On the specific age-dependent epileptic syndrome: the early-infantile epileptic encephalopathy with suppression-burst. *No To Hattatsu.* 1976;8:270–280.
28. Ohtahara S, Ohtsuka Y, Yamatogi Y, et al. The early-infantile epileptic encephalopathy with suppression-burst: developmental aspects. *Brain Dev.* 1987;9:371–376.
29. Ohtahara S, Ohtsuka Y, Yamatogi Y, et al. Early-infantile epileptic encephalopathy with suppression-bursts. In: Roger J, Bureau M, Dravet C, et al., eds. *Epileptic Syndromes in Infancy, Childhood and Adolescence,* 2nd ed. London: John Libbey; 1992:25–34.
30. Ohtahara S, Yamatogi Y. Evolution of seizures and EEG abnormalities in childhood onset epilepsy. In: Wada JA, Ellingson RJ, eds. *Clinical Neurophysiology of Epilepsy.* Amsterdam: Elsevier; 1990:457–477.
31. Ohtahara S, Yamatogi Y. Epileptic encephalopathies in early infancy with suppression-burst. *J Clin Neurophysiol.* 2003;20:398–407.
32. Ohtahara S, Yamatogi, Y. Ohtahara syndrome: with special reference to its developmental aspects for differentiating from early myoclonic encephalopathy. *Epilepsy Res.* 2006;70 (Suppl):S58–S67.
33. Ohtsuka Y, Ohno S, Oka E. Electroclinical characteristics of hemimegalencephaly. *Pediatr Neurol.* 1999;20:390–393.
34. Ohtsuka Y, Oka E, Terasaki T, et al. Aicardi syndrome: a longitudinal clinical and electroencephalographic study. *Epilepsia.* 1993;34:627–634.
35. Ohtsuka Y, Sato M, Sanada S, et al. Suppression-burst patterns in intractable epilepsy with focal cortical dysplasia. *Brain Dev.* 2000;22:135–138.
36. Oka E, Ishida S, Ohtsuka Y, et al. Neuroepidemiological study of childhood epilepsy by application of international classification of epilepsies and epileptic syndromes (ILAE 1989). *Epilepsia.* 1995;36:658–661.
37. Ozawa H, Kawada Y, Noma S, et al. Oral high-dose phenobarbital therapy for early infantile epileptic encephalopathy. *Pediatr Neurol.* 2002;26:222–224.
38. Pedespan JM, Loiseau H, Vital A, et al. Surgical treatment of an early epileptic encephalpathy with suppression-bursts and focal cortical dysplasia. *Epilepsia.* 1995;36:37–40.
39. Robain O, Dulac O. Early epileptic encephalopathy with suppression bursts and olivary-dentate dysplasia. *Neuropediatrics.* 1992;23:162–164.
40. Schlumberger E, Dulac O, Plouin P. Early infantile epileptic syndrome(s) with suppression-burst: nosological considerations. In: Roger J, Bureau M, Dravet C, et al., eds. *Epileptic Syndromes in Infancy, Childhood and Adolescence,* 2nd ed. London: John Libbey; 1992:35–42.
41. Spreafico R, Angelini L, Binelli S, et al. Burst suppression and impairment of neocortical ontogenesis: electroclinical and neuropathologic findings in 2 infants with early myoclonic encephalopathy. *Epilepsia.* 1993;34:800–808.
42. Tatsuno M, Hayashi M, Iwamoto H, et al. Leigh's encephalopathy with wide lesions and early infantile epileptic encephalopathy with burst-suppression: an autopsy case. *No To Hattatsu.* 1984;16:68–75.
43. Terasaki T, Yamatogi Y, Ohtahara S, et al. A long-term follow-up study on a case with glycine encephalopathy. *No To Hattatsu.* 1988;20:15–22.
44. Trinka E., Rauscher C, Nagler M, et al. A case of Ohtahara syndrome with olivary-dentate dysplasia and agenesis of mamillary bodies. *Epilepsia.* 2001;42:950–953.
45. Verrotti A, Domizio S, Sabatino G, et al. Early infantile epileptic encephalopathy: a long-term follow-up study. *Child's Nerv Syst.* 1996;12:530–533.
46. Watanabe K, Miura K, Natsume J, et al. Epilepsies of neonatal onset: seizure type and evolution. *Dev Med Child Neurol.* 1999;41:318–322.
47. Widaicks EP, Parisi JE, Sharbrough FW. Prognostic value of myoclonus status in comatose survivors of cardiac arrest. *Ann Neurol.* 1994;35:239–243.
48. Williams AN, Gray RG, Poulton K, et al. A case of Ohtahara syndrome with cytochrome oxidase deficiency. *Dev Med Child Neurol.* 1998;40:568–570.
49. Yamatogi Y, Ohtahara S. Age-dependent epileptic encephalopathy: a longitudinal study. *Folia Psychiatr Neurol Jpn.* 1981;35:321–331.
50. Yamatogi Y, Ohtahara S. Early-infantile epileptic encephalopathy with suppression-bursts, Ohtahara syndrome; its overview referring to our 16 cases. *Brain Dev.* 2002;24:13–23.
51. Yamatogi Y, Ohtahara S. Severe epilepsy with multiple independent spike foci. *J Clin Neurophysiol.* 2003;20:442–448.

CHAPTER 226 ■ OVERVIEW: SYNDROMES OF INFANCY AND EARLY CHILDHOOD

JEAN AICARDI

INTRODUCTION

The incidence of epilepsy is very high in the first years of life, reaching a peak in the first year and remaining at high levels throughout infancy and early childhood. The epilepsies with onset in infancy, although a heterogeneous group, share some special characteristics, and this applies up to the age of approximately 3 to 4 years. The following chapters, therefore, are concerned with all epilepsies that begin before the age of 4 years.

The special features of the epilepsies of early onset are the result of several etiologic, anatomic, and neurophysiologic factors. One major factor is the immaturity of the infant's brain. At this period, dendritic development is actively proceeding, and myelin formation and deposition are far from complete, which may be responsible for imperfect synchronization of the hemispheres. Brain circuitry is different from that in later life. In particular, the number of synapses increases rapidly during the first years of life and far exceeds the ultimate number.[16] A high proportion of these synapses is eliminated before 8 to 10 years of age, and this pruning process depends on activity and, therefore, on environmental stimuli. There is evidence that functional synapses become stabilized, whereas unused ones disappear; this is probably one of the mechanisms of brain plasticity. Development and maturation of the brain are associated with changes in neurotransmitters and receptors and their effects. For example, some γ-aminobutyric acid (GABA) receptors have been shown to be excitatory during fetal life and the early postnatal period,[19] and glutamate receptors may not be sufficient to produce brain damage through activation of the glutamate cascade. Such changes are likely profoundly to modify the excitability of the infant's brain. The conjunction of these factors undoubtedly accounts for some of the features of early seizures, such as the generally imperfect organization of seizure discharges, the rarity of full-fledged tonic–clonic attacks, and the higher frequency of unilateral or predominantly unilateral seizures in response to diffuse systemic disturbances such as fever or metabolic imbalances. However, the infant's brain is capable of occasionally producing 3-Hz spike-wave discharges and massive myoclonias and even, although rarely, absence attacks.[2] Seizures of focal origin are the most common seizures in this age range. They may be associated with focal clinical manifestations and electroencephalogram (EEG) discharges of several forms with different degrees of propagation. Many focal seizures are associated with extensive brain lesions, indicating that the infant brain may be unable to organize complete seizure sequences as observed at a later age. The atypical clinical expression of many seizures in the infantile range probably results from the neurophysiologic factors already mentioned, from the late maturation of some areas of the brain such as the frontal lobe, as well as from the inability of infants to experience or express some of the more complex features of seizures and the difficulty or impossibility for observers to detect such symptoms as loss or impairment of consciousness.[20] Conversely, focal brain lesions or abnormalities may be associated with diffuse clinical symptoms and with extensive EEG paroxysms, one common type being infantile spasms with the so-called hypsarrhytmic pattern of high-amplitude disorganized tracing, suggesting that focal origin of seizures may be expressed in generalized attacks and is probably even more common in young children than previously thought.[13]

The etiology of early-onset epilepsies is also responsible for many of their clinical and evolutive characteristics. As in older patients, the two main factors are a propensity to fitting (mostly genetically determined) and the presence of brain lesions; however, both have age-specific peculiarities.

The *epileptogenic lesions* are often extensive, even when they give rise to partial seizures. Some are destructive and may be related to mechanical or hypoxic-ischemic injuries. A majority, however, are of developmental origin, the most common being abnormalities of cortical development. These include heterotopias, diffuse pachygyria-lissencephaly, hemimegalencephaly, and focal cortical dysplasias, the latter being the most common cause of epilepsy at this age.[15] It is of interest that the nature, location, and extent of organic brain damage—and not only the age of the child—are responsible, at least in part, for the ictal symptomatology. Thus, tuberous sclerosis often determines infantile spasms, and Aicardi syndrome determines a mixture of focal seizures and spasms.

The propensity to seizures of infants is mainly expressed by febrile convulsions (see Chapter 227) and less often in the form of other benign epilepsy syndromes. Febrile convulsions (FCs) are by far the most common frequent manifestation of a genetic predisposition to seizures. Although febrile seizures are not termed *epilepsy* because they do not fulfill the definition of a chronic unprovoked condition but are classified as *occasional seizures* or *situation-related seizures*,[1,14] they have undoubted physiopathologic and genetic relationships with the epilepsies and may be regarded as a benign expression of the main basic phenomenon. This genetic relationship is best illustrated by the occurrence of afebrile convulsions following FC, which, although rare, are much more common than in the general population and in rare instances by the syndrome of generalized epilepsy with febrile seizures plus (GEFS+).

The importance of age in the expression of infantile epilepsy is clearly shown by the age dependence of several types of seizures. West syndrome rarely begins after 1 year of age and has a well-defined modal age of onset at 5 to 6 months (Chapter 229). Several types of seizures may occur in succession in the same patient with an unchanged pathologic basis; for example, Ohtahara syndrome can precede infantile spasms, followed by the development of the Lennox-Gastaut syndrome; focal or unilateral seizures may precede the development of West or Lennox-Gastaut syndrome. Such changes may reflect not only the maturation of the brain, but perhaps also the plasticity of the central nervous system. Some of the changes could result from the capacity for reorganization of the infant's brain following an insult or even a prolonged dysfunction without any lesion. It is conceivable that unusual regulation and development of receptors or preferential stabilization of certain synapses as a result of prolonged abnormal epileptic activity in certain pathways may lead to altered connectivity, with corresponding clinical changes. Such a mechanism could account for some of the characteristics of epileptic deterioration, such as its spontaneous arrest after disappearance or improvement of epileptic activity and incomplete recovery in spite of apparent cure of epilepsy. Deterioration associated with, and possibly resulting from, intense epileptic activity, whether marked by seizures or only by EEG alterations, is a remarkable feature of some early epilepsies,[3,5,11] sometimes termed *epileptic encephalopathies* or *catastrophic epilepsies* (see Chapter 230). Although epileptic deterioration is not limited to young children, as shown by its occurrence in such syndromes as the Landau-Kleffner syndrome or that of continuous spike-waves of slow sleep,[5] it is clearly prominent in this age bracket (see Chapter 242). Other factors possibly responsible for deterioration include evolution of the underlying lesions, frequency and consequences of seizures, psychological problems, side effects of drugs, and other environmental influences.

Finally, epilepsy in infants is often associated with other neurologic problems, such as cerebral palsy or mental retardation, and seizures not only add to children's difficulties, but also multiply the total impairment so that attempts at control are particularly important.

The seizures of early-onset epilepsies often differ from those in older patients (see Chapter 56). Some types of seizures observed in later life are sometimes seen in children <3 years of age. These include generalized—especially myoclonic—seizures that may have their onset from a few months of age.

Tonic–clonic seizures tend to be less well organized and less symmetric and to feature a longer tonic phase than in older children. Atypical absences often feature changes in tone, and their EEG manifestations (slow spike-wave complexes or fast rhythms) are completely different from those of typical absences, which are very rare in the first 2 to 3 years.[3] Partial seizures are probably more common, but they often have unusual clinical features with predominance of head deviation and unilateral or asymmetric tonic phenomena over clonic jerks.[12] More precise classification of partial seizures is difficult because of the difficulties of assessing awareness and the limited register of motor manifestations, even though some investigators have reported on "complex" focal seizures in infants.[26,27] Some types of seizures are particularly characteristic of young children, although none is completely restricted to them. These include infantile spasms, tonic and atonic seizures, atypical absences, and episodes of nonconvulsive status epilepticus often with myotonic manifestations. Such seizures are major components of the catastrophic epilepsies or epileptic encephalopathies.[3,11] Other seizures have a very limited clinical expression, such as simple arrest of activity, subtle changes in tone (hypertonia or hypotonia), simple staring, pallor, perioral cyanosis, blinking of eyelids, or isolated eye deviation.[22] Such atypical attacks often evolve into more characteristic partial seizures when the children grow older.

The frequency of the various types of seizures is not well known. In two large series of epilepsy in infants <1 year of age,[7,8] infantile spasms were the most frequent type (230 of 437 and 183 of 387, respectively), followed by other generalized seizures (99 and 87, respectively) and partial seizures (57 and 51, respectively). In a large group of 504 children <3 years old, Dalla Bernardina et al.[10] ascribed 163 patients to the group of the epileptic encephalopathies, 189 to the partial epilepsies, and 80 to the generalized epilepsies (34 with myoclonic seizures). These figures were drawn from specialized referral centers, so the proportion of severe seizures is likely to be less in the general population.

As in other age groups, epilepsy syndromes, that is, clusters of signs and symptoms occurring customarily together,[11,14] are recognizable among infantile epilepsies. However, syndromic classification is more difficult than in older patients because of the uncharacteristic features of many cases and the fact that the clinical and EEG manifestations are rapidly changing in many cases, so that several syndromes may evolve in succession in the same child. For example, partial seizures may precede infantile spasms, and these frequently herald the development of the Lennox-Gastaut syndrome. The most common epilepsy syndromes in infants are described in the following chapters. The best characterized are West syndrome (Chapter 229), severe myoclonic epilepsy (Chapter 230), and the Lennox-Gastaut syndrome (Chapter 241) (although its onset is often slightly later in life). These syndromes usually have a poor prognosis. West syndrome and the Lennox-Gastaut syndrome are of lesional origin in most cases, and abnormalities of cortical development are a major etiologic factor, especially in the case of infantile spasms.[13] Despite their generalized clinical and EEG features, seizures in these two syndromes are probably due in a significant proportion of cases to localized lesions, some of which may be amenable to surgical treatment. Severe myoclonic epilepsy (renamed Dravet syndrome because myoclonic seizures may be absent in some cases) is a clinically well defined syndrome with onset in the first year of life with febrile convulsions, often prolonged and frequently recurrent, followed in the second or third year by myoclonic attacks and multiple seizure types. It is due in most cases to a new sodium channelopathy.[21] Other tentative syndromes have been proposed. One is the syndrome of partial migrating infantile seizures,[9] whose specificity has been debated.[17]

More-benign syndromes of infantile seizures have been recognized more recently, indicating that the outcome of infantile seizures is not always poor and this has to be taken into account when giving a prognosis. Their frequency is much lower than that of the more severe types but may be greater than shown by statistics coming from referral centers and may be higher in some Asian countries[18] (Chapters 236 and 238). Clinical manifestations are brief partial seizures occurring in clusters in the first 2 years of life and disappearing before the age of 2 years. In some cases, a benign movement disorder may supervene after several years.[23] Benign partial infantile seizures are often genetically determined.[24,25] Some have been mapped to different loci on chromosomes 16, and the mutant gene has been isolated in one family.[6] Nongenetic benign syndromes have also been described.[12]

SUMMARY AND CONCLUSIONS

Infantile epilepsies have distinctive clinical characteristics due in large part to neurophysiologic features related to age. Their treatment is often unsatisfactory as a result of the lesional nature of many cases, the extent of responsible brain damage, and the consequences of epilepsy for cognitive and behavioral development. The respective indications of conventional and new drug treatment and of agents such as adrenotropic hormone or steroids are not yet clear. Surgical treatment has been shown to be possible and to give results on seizures similar to those obtained in older patients. However, its effects on neurodevelopment are yet to be assessed.

The important point is that experience with the catastrophic epilepsies of this age shows that epilepsy is more than simply having seizures and may have pervasive effects on development, even when paroxysmal manifestations are absent or mild.

References

1. Aicardi J. Syndromic classification in the management of childhood epilepsy. *J Child Neurol.* 1994;9(Suppl):2514–2518.
2. Aicardi J. Typical absences in the first two years of life. In: Ducan JS, Panayiotopoulos CP, eds. *Typical Absences and Related Epileptic Syndromes.* London: Churchill Communication Europe; 1995.
3. Aicardi J. Epilepsy: the hidden part of the iceberg. *Eur J Paediatr Neurol.* 1999;443–448.
4. Arzimanoglore A, Guerrini R, Acardi J. *Aicard's Epilepsy in Children*, 3rd ed. Philadelphia: Lippincott Williams & Wilkins; 2004.
5. Beaumanoir A, Burea N, Deonna T, et al. Continuous Spikes and Waves during Slow Sleep. London: John Libbey; 1995.
6. Berkovic SF, Heron SE, Giordano L, et al. Benign familial neonatal-infantile seizures: characterization of a new sodium channelopathies. *Ann Neurol.* 2004;55:550–557.
7. Cavazzuti GB, Ferrari P, Lalla M. Follow-up of 482 cases with convulsive disorders in the first year of life. *Dev Med Child Neurol.* 1984;26:425–437.
8. Chevrie JJ, Aicardi J. Convulsive disorders in the first year of life. Neurologic and mental outcome and mortality. *Epilepsia.* 1978;19:67–74.
9. Coppola G, Plouin P, Chiron C, et al. Migrating partial seizures in infancy: a malignant disorder with developmental arrest. *Epilepsia.* 1995;36:1017–1024.
10. Dalla Bernardina B, Colamaria V, Capovilla G, et al. Nosological classification of epilepsies in the first three years of life. In: *An Update on Research and Therapy.* New York: Alan Liss: 1983;165–183.
11. Donat JF. The age-dependent epileptic encephalopathies. *J Child Neurol.* 1992;7:7–21.
12. Duchowny MS. Complex partial seizures of infancy. *Arch Neurol.* 1987;44:911–914.
13. Dulac O, Tuxhorn I. Infantile spasms and West syndrome. In: Roger J, Bureau M, Dravet C, et al., eds. *Epileptic Syndromes in Infancy, Childhood and Adolescence.* London, John Libbey; 2002:53–72.
14. Engel J Jr. A proposed diagnostic scheme for people with epileptic seizures and epilepsy: report of the ILAE Task Force for Classification and Terminology, International League Against Epilepsy (ILAE). *Epilepsia.* 2001;42:796–803.
15. Guerrini R, Sicca F, Parmeginni L. Genetic malformations of the cerebral cortex and epilepsy. *Epilepsia.* 2005;46(Suppl 1):32–37.
16. Huttenlocher P. Synaptic density in human frontal cortex. Developmental changes and effect of aging. *Brain Res.* 1979;163:195–205.
17. Ishii K, Oguni H, Hayashi K, et al. Clinical study of catastrophic infantile epilepsy with focal seizures. *Pediatr Neurol.* 2002;27:366–377.
18. Lee WL, Low PS, Rajan U. Benign familial infantile epilepsy. *J Pediatr.* 1993;123:588–590.
19. Moshé SL, Holmes GL, Mares P. Epileptogenesis and the immature brain subcortical mechanisms. In: Klee MR, Lux HD, Speckmann EJ, eds. *Physiology, Pharmacology and Development of Epileptic Phenomena.* Berlin: Springer; 1991: 147–149.
20. Nordli DR Jr, Bazil CW, Scheuer ML, et al. Recognition and classification of seizures in infants. *Epilepsia.* 1997;38:553–558.
21. Oguni H, Hayashi K, Osawa M, et al. Severe myoclonic epilepsy in infants. Typical and borderline groups in relation to *SCN1A* mutations. In: Delgado-Escueta V, Guerrini R, Medina MT, et al., eds. *Myoclonic Epilepsies.* Philadelphia: Lippincott Williams & Wilkins; 2004:103–117.
22. Okumura A, Hayakawa F, Kato T, et al. Early recognition of benign partial epilepsy in infancy. *Epilepsia.* 2000;41:714–717.
23. Szepetowski P, Rochette E, Berquin P, et al. Familial infantile convulsions and paroxyxmal choreoathetosis: a new neurological syndrome linked to the pericentric region of human chromosome 16. *Am J Hum Genet.* 1997;61:889–898.
24. Vigevano F, Fusco L, Di Capua M, et al. Benign infantile familial convulsions. *Eur J Pediatr.* 1992;151:608–612.
25. Vigevano F, Fusco L, Ricci S, et al. Dysplasias. In: Dulac O, Chugani H, Dalla Bernardina, eds. *Infantile Spasms and West Syndrome.* London: Saunders; 178–191.
26. Watanabe K, Negoro T, Aso K. Benign partial epilepsy with secondary generalized seizures in infancy. *Epilepsia.* 1993;34:635–638.
27. Watanabe K, Yamamoto N, Negoro T, et al. Benign infantile epilepsy with complex partial seizures. *J Clin Neurophysiol.* 1990;7:409–416.

CHAPTER 227 ■ BENIGN FAMILIAL AND NONFAMILIAL SEIZURES

FEDERICO VIGEVANO, NICOLA SPECCHIO, ROBERTO CARABALLO, AND KAZUYOSHI WATANABE

INTRODUCTION

Benign familial and nonfamilial forms of infantile seizure and partial epilepsies of infancy are significant categories of pediatric epilepsies. In the past, seizures with onset during the first months of life were considered to have a bad prognosis and a symptomatic etiology. Since the first description by Fukuyama, the existence of infantile seizures with a benign evolution has been defined and accepted.

The international classification of epilepsies and epileptic syndromes[17] includes benign infantile seizures, which are divided into familial and nonfamilial forms. In recent years, variants of these two forms and similar entities have been described.

HISTORICAL PERSPECTIVE

In 1963, Fukuyama was the first to report cases with onset within the first 2 years of life that were characterized by generalized convulsions, absence of etiologic factors, and benign outcome.[18] This type of infantile convulsion was the subject of many subsequent studies, but only after 20 years were the true clinical entities clarified. Reports have specified the localization and semiology of seizures, which have been defined as being of partial type[69,71,72] and in terms of the presence or absence of familial occurrence.[6–8]

Vigevano and coworkers focused on cases exhibiting a family history of convulsions with benign outcome during infancy and autosomal-dominant inheritance, and they proposed the term *benign infantile familial convulsions* (BIFC).[67] Later, other such cases were reported in many different parts of the world,[16,21,35,40,45] thus confirming them as new epileptic syndromes. When these entities were included in the list of epileptic syndromes by the International League Against Epilepsy (ILAE) Task Force on Classification and Terminology, it was suggested that the term "seizure" should be used rather than the term "convulsion."[17] Just like benign seizures with neonatal onset, benign infantile seizures are divided into familial and nonfamilial forms.[17] These two forms, however, can have overlapping features.[39] Genetic studies of familial forms led to the identification of a chromosome marker on chromosomes 19,[23] 16,[11] and 2.[42]

An association between *benign familial infantile seizures* (BFIS) and variably expressed paroxysmal choreoathetosis was reported in 1997 by Szepetowski et al.[61] A specific marker on chromosome 16 has been identified in this familial variant, called *infantile convulsions and choreoathetosis* (ICCA).

Heron et al.[25] in 2002 and later Berkovic et al.[3] proposed a new entity and coined the term *benign familial neonatal-infantile seizures* (BFNIS) to describe families with onset at an intermediate age between neonatal and infantile forms.

Considering that convulsive manifestations are limited to a short period of time, some authors hypothesized the existence of particular etiologic factors in some sporadic cases such as cases of benign infantile convulsions associated with episodes of diarrhea caused by rotavirus infections.[12,28,30] Finally, Capovilla et al. described a peculiar form of benign epilepsy occurring within the second year of life and with a typical sleep electroencephalographic (EEG) pattern.[5,6]

DEFINITION

Benign partial seizures in infancy are a group of diseases characterized by onset during the first 2 years in otherwise normal children. They could be familial, with a characteristic autosomal-dominant trait of inheritance and a typical onset around 6 months, or nonfamilial, which usually occur later. Seizures are partial with or without secondarily generalization and are typically grouped in clusters of many per day. In most cases, interictal EEGs are normal, except for the midline spikes during slow sleep described by Capovilla, but this form of epilepsy is under discussion. Outcome is always excellent, with a normal psychomotor development after seizures.

EPIDEMIOLOGY

Several cases with this syndrome have been described from all over the world. Data on prevalence and incidence are not available. In a series described by Caraballo et al.,[9] benign infantile seizures were listed as the third-most-common type of epilepsy in the first 2 years of life.

ETIOLOGY AND BASIC MECHANISMS

Autosomal-dominant transmission is evident in BFIS. Due to the close similarity to *benign familial neonatal seizures* (BFNS), researchers first tried to find the chromosome markers described in this latter syndrome.[37,55,57] In 1994, Malafosse et al.[43] demonstrated that BFIS is not an allelic form of BFNS, excluding the marker on chromosome 20.

In 1997, linkage analysis was carried out in five Italian BFIS families, and a locus was mapped on chromosome 19q12–13.1 between markers D19S49 and D19245.[23] Gennaro et al.[20] later conducted a linkage analysis of seven families of Italian origin and demonstrated the presence of linkage to chromosome 19q in a single family, suggesting genetic heterogeneity within the examined families. Studies of familial cases with ICCA are particularly interesting. Szepetowski et al.[61] demonstrated linkage to the pericentromeric region of chromosome 16 in the families with this syndrome. This finding was then confirmed by Lee et al.[36] in a family of Chinese origin. In 2001, Caraballo et al.[11] found linkage on chromosome 16p12-q12, the same region as for ICCA, in seven families with only benign familial infantile seizures. There was a previous report describing a large family affected by paroxysmal kinesigenic dyskinesia without infantile convulsions with linkage to the ICCA region.[33] Therefore, Caraballo et al. hypothesized that chromosome 16p12-q12 is a major genetic locus underlying both benign familial infantile seizures and paroxysmal dyskinesias.[11] Weber reported similar results in 14 families with benign familial infantile seizures without paroxysmal choreoathetosis.[73]

In 2001, Malacarne et al.[42] mapped a novel locus to chromosome 2q24 in eight Italian families, thus demonstrating a genetic heterogeneity, as in other autosomal-dominant idiopathic epilepsies.

In cases described as having *benign familial neonatal-infantile seizures*—an intermediate form between BFIS and benign familial neonatal seizures—a missense mutation in the *SCN2A* gene has been found, leading to the hypothesis of the existence of a third form,[20] although recently a similar mutation of the same gene has been described in a family with clinical features typical of BFIS.[58]

A particular etiologic factor has been recognized in some infantile seizures associated with mild gastroenteritis, with positivity to the rotavirus antigen. In the other nonfamilial forms, no clear etiologic factors have been described.

CLINICAL PRESENTATION

Benign Nonfamilial Infantile Seizures

Watanabe et al.[3] described a series of infants having focal seizures with benign evolution. The majority of the cases were not familial. They described nine infants with benign complex partial seizures as diagnosed by simultaneous electroencephalogram and video recording. At ages of 3 to 10 months, most of these infants presented with clusters of seizures consisting of motion arrest, decreased responsiveness, staring, or blank eyes, mostly with simple automatisms and mild convulsive movements associated with focal paroxysmal discharges, most frequently in the temporal area. Carbamazepine or phenobarbital was used to control the seizures, and all patients were seizure free for >3 years. All patients showed normal interictal electroencephalogram and psychomotor development.

Later, the same authors described the cases of 7 infants with benign idiopathic partial epilepsy presenting with apparently generalized tonic–clonic seizures (GTCs), which turned out to be partial seizures evolving to secondarily generalized seizures (SGS).[69] In subsequent years, other reports confirmed this syndrome, for example, Berger et al.[2] and Capovilla et al.,[7] who reported the cases of 12 children with complex partial seizures having similar electroclinical features.

The term *benign partial epilepsy in infancy* (BPEI) was proposed to combine the two previously described entities.[2,69] Clinical characteristics of benign partial epilepsy in infancy, which is now classified as benign nonfamilial infantile seizures, are summarized in Table 1.

TABLE 1

CLINICAL CHARACTERISTICS OF BENIGN NONFAMILIAL INFANTILE SEIZURE, WHICH COMPRISES BENIGN PARTIAL EPILEPSY OF INFANCY WITH COMPLEX PARTIAL SEIZURES AND BENIGN PARTIAL EPILEPSY WITH SECONDARILY GENERALIZED SEIZURES IN INFANCY

Benign Partial Epilepsy of Infancy With Complex Partial Seizures	Benign Partial Epilepsy With Secondarily Generalized Seizures in Infancy
• Normal development before onset	• Normal development before onset
• No underlying disorders or neurologic abnormalities	• No underlying disorders or neurologic abnormalities
• Onset mostly within the first year of life	• Onset mostly within the first year of life (3–20 mo)
• Complex partial seizures, often occurring in clusters	• Partial seizures (stare, blank eyes, or crying)
• Normal interictal EEG	• With secondary generalization, often occurring in clusters
• Ictal EEG most often showing temporal focus	• Normal interictal EEG
• Excellent response to treatment	• Ictal EEG most often showing a centroparietal origin
• Normal developmental outcome	• Excellent response to treatment
	• Normal developmental outcome

EEG, electroencephalogram.

Benign Familial Infantile Seizures

Vigevano and coworkers described cases with benign epilepsy in infancy and a family history of convulsions.[69] All of them had a benign outcome and autosomal-dominant inheritance, and the authors suggested the term *benign infantile familial convulsions*.[67] In subsequent years, autosomal-dominant familial cases have been reported by other authors, confirming the existence of this syndrome.[10,21,35,40,46,65]

The first series described by *Vigevano et al.*[67] consisted of five infants—three girls and two boys. All of them had one or more paternal relatives with a history of benign seizures occurring at the same age. It was found that 13 of their relatives had analogous seizures. Age at onset ranged from 4 to 7 months in the probands, whereas in their relatives it was 4 to 8 months, and peaked around 6 months. Onset was never in the neonatal period or after the eighth month of life.

This syndrome is included in the most recent classification and terminology proposed by the ILAE under the term *benign familial infantile seizures.*

Clinical characteristics are summarized in Table 2. Psychomotor development of all children before the onset of seizures is absolutely normal. A common characteristic to almost all cases is the occurrence of seizures in a cluster—mostly brief and successive seizures, a maximum of 8 to 10 per day, which do not reach a true status epilepticus. Interictal clinical condition is normal, with occasional stupor, most probably caused by drugs. Seizures are usually longer in the beginning, lasting 2 to 5 minutes, and become shorter as treatment takes effect. The cluster can last 1 to 3 days.

Vigevano's patients presented with seizures that were clinically characterized by psychomotor arrest, slow deviation of the head and eyes to one side, diffuse hypertonia, cyanosis, and unilateral limb jerks, which became bilateral and synchronous or asynchronous. Although the seizures were highly stereotyped, the direction of the head and eye deviation sometimes changed from seizure to seizure in the same patient.

TABLE 2

CLINICAL AND ELECTROENCEPHALOGRAPHIC CHARACTERISTICS OF BENIGN FAMILIAL INFANTILE SEIZURES

- Family history of seizures (similar age at onset, autosomal-dominant trait)
- Normal development before onset
- No underlying disorders or neurologic abnormalities
- Onset between 4 and 8 mo of age
- Seizures in clusters
- Partial seizures localized in the occipitoparietal areas
- Semiology: psychomotor arrest, cyanosis, head/eye deviation to one side (variable), tonic contraction, bilateral clonic jerks
- Normal interictal electroencephalogram
- Ictal electroencephalogram: fast activity originating in the occipitoparietal area
- Postictal electroencephalogram: lateralized occipitoparietal delta waves and spikes
- Normal developmental outcome
- Benign course

Benign Familial Infantile Seizures Associated With Other Neurologic Symptoms

In 1997, Szepetowski et al.[61] identified and described in four French families an association of BFIS with paroxysmal choreoathetosis appearing later in life, and they proposed a new syndrome called *familial infantile convulsion and choreoathetosis* (ICCA). Linkage to chromosome 16 and dominant transmission were also clearly defined.[61] This entity has been confirmed by other authors.[1,4,6,8,60,63]

Familial hemiplegic migraine (FHM) is a rare, severe autosomal-dominant subtype of migraine with aura associated with hemiparesis.[29] Most of the families that have been reported were linked to chromosome 19p13 and had missense mutations in the *CACNA1A* gene.[16] In two families with FHM linked to 1q23, two missense mutations in the *ATP1A2* gene were identified.[65] Two novel mutations in the *ATP1A2* gene were also found. In particular, one mutation was detected in a Dutch-Canadian family in which FHM was associated with BFIS.[45,62] In this family, BFIS were followed at an older age by FHM and cosegregated to chromosome 1q23.[65] This finding suggests that BFIS may have a wider association with other neurologic diseases.

Benign Familial Neonatal-Infantile Seizures

A seizure onset occurring between neonatal and infantile ages was reported by Kaplan and Lacey in 1983.[32] The onset of seizures varied from 2 days to 3.5 months.[32] The authors used the term *benign familial neonatal-infantile seizure* (BFNIS). In 2002, Heron et al.[25] described two families with afebrile, secondarily generalized partial seizures occurring between 1.9 and 3.8 months of life and having an autosomal-dominant mode of inheritance, and they described a missense mutation in *SCN2A*, the gene coding for the $\alpha 2$ subunit of the voltage-gated sodium channel. In 2004,[3] a novel missense mutation in *SCN2A* gene was found in five similar families in addition to the first family described by Kaplan and Lacey: a new sodium channelopathy was identified. Clinical characteristics are summarized in Table 3. The semiology of the seizures was characterized by a predominant focal motor manifestation, with head and eye deviation followed by tonic and clonic movements. Most of the seizures were relatively long, lasting up to 4 minutes, and were of variable frequency, with some patients having few seizures per day and others having clusters of seizures. Interictal EEGs were normal or showed some epileptiform discharges in the posterior areas. When ictal EEGs were recorded, they showed a focal posterior onset of discharges. All patients had a normal development before and after the seizure occurrence. The authors concluded that this mutation represents a new sodium channelopathy, despite the possible overlap with the previously described cases of BFIS.

TABLE 3

CLINICAL CHARACTERISTICS OF BENIGN FAMILIAL NEONATAL-INFANTILE SEIZURE

- Family history of seizures (autosomal-dominant trait)
- Normal development before onset
- No underlying disorders or neurologic abnormalities
- Onset between 2 d and 7 mo of age
- Frequency ranging from few attacks to clusters
- Afebrile secondarily generalized partial seizures
- Ictal electroencephalogram: onset in the posterior areas
- Remission within 12 mo
- Benign course

Recently, Striano et al.[58] reported a novel heterozygous mutation c3003 T→A in the *SCN2A* gene in a family with three affected individuals over three generations. All individuals experienced clusters of partial seizures with or without secondary generalization and onset between 4 and 12 months of life. They have been diagnosed with BFIS. No patients developed other seizures later in life, and all of them had a normal development outcome. This report provides new evidence that BFNIS and BFIS may show some overlapping clinical and genetic characteristics.

Benign Infantile Seizures Associated With Mild Gastroenteritis

Morooka[46] was the first to describe this entity (BIS with MG) in Japan in 1982. It is characterized by nonfebrile generalized seizures associated with symptoms of gastroenteritis in previously healthy patients between 6 months and 3 years of age. Seizures often occurred in clusters, and laboratory examination results, including blood and cerebrospinal fluid (CSF) glucose, were normal. Interictal EEG was normal in all patients, and all of them had an excellent outcome.

After the first report by Morooka, numerous (>60) reports have been published in Japan[30,31,33,36,49,53,56,64,67] but only nine from other countries.[20,22,27,38,42,54,61,68,76] Cases of BIS with MG are likely to fall within the category of situation-related seizures, although they are not described in the proposed ILAE classification and seizure terminology.[17] Seizure recurrence, also without prophylactic antiepileptic treatment, has not been reported in BIS with MG, although it can occur in a few cases when an infant has repeated episodes of gastroenteritis.[19] In a recent study by Okumura et al.[51] on the efficacy of antiepileptic drugs during a cluster, lidocaine was reported as the most effective drug for seizure cessation.

BIS with MG are characterized by mostly brief and partial seizures evolving to secondary generalization, often occurring in clusters, in infants and children aged 1 to 2 years. Seizures occurred within the first 5 days of the gastroenteritis episode,

TABLE 4

CLINICAL CHARACTERISTICS OF BENIGN INFANTILE SEIZURES ASSOCIATED WITH MILD GASTROENTERITIS

- Healthy patients
- Age between 1 and 2 yr
- Brief partial seizures evolving to secondary generalization
- Symptoms of gastroenteritis
- Seizures in clusters
- Seizures within the first 5 days of gastroenteritis
- More than 50% positive to rotavirus antigen
- Seizure recurrences rare, only during recurrence of mild gastroenteritis
- Benign course

TABLE 5

CLINICAL AND ELECTROENCEPHALOGRAPHIC CHARACTERISTICS OF BENIGN INFANTILE FOCAL EPILEPSY WITH MIDLINE SPIKES AND WAVES DURING SLEEP

- Normal psychomotor development
- Family history (half of patients)
- Age between 4 and 30 mo
- Semiology: cyanosis, staring, rare lateralizing signs, automatisms
- Electroencephalographic marker: spike followed by bell-shaped slow wave (midline region) during sleep
- Sporadic seizures
- Favorable outcome
- Majority of patients not treated
- Benign course

and the proportion of positive rotavirus antigen was greater than half.[64] Table 4 summarizes the clinical characteristics of this condition.

Benign Infantile Focal Epilepsy With Midline Spikes and Waves During Sleep

First Bureau and Maton[4] and later Capovilla and Beccaria[5] and Capovilla et al.[6] described a form of epilepsy in children with homogeneous electroclinical features and a benign course that they hypothesized to be a new form of benign focal epilepsy. A distinctive aspect of this condition was that all of the described children presented particular interictal EEG abnormalities that were detectable during sleep and characterized by isolated or grouped spikes and waves from the midline region to the central regions. The authors pointed out that these abnormalities could be an EEG marker that is clearly distinct from other typical EEG markers at an older age. They highlighted, however, that it could not be only an EEG marker because it was found in a group of infants presenting with homogeneous clinical features, thus suggesting a possible new epileptic syndrome. Capovilla had previously described this syndrome with the term *benign partial epilepsy in infancy and early childhood with vertex spikes and waves during sleep*.[5] He later[6] proposed to replace *vertex spikes* with *midline spikes* in order not to confuse them with physiologic sleep vertex spikes.

The general features of this condition (Table 5) are neurologic and neuroradiologic normality, a normal psychomotor development, a positive family history, and a benign evolution in all cases. With regard to clinical features, age at onset is between 4 and 30 months, with a peak between 13 and 19 months (more than two thirds of cases are within this age range). The frequency of seizures is low; some children have a single episode, and others have multiple episodes per year. The seizure length is between 1 and 5 minutes. The episodes usually occur during wakefulness; in one fourth of cases, they occur during sleep. The age of the last seizure is between 24 and 43 months. The semiology of seizures is characterized by loss of contact—staring as a rule—and cyanosis. Perioral cyanosis and motion arrest are among the main clinical symptoms. Instead, lateralizing signs and automatisms are rarely observed. EEG is normal when awake, with typical sleep EEG abnormalities, well differentiated from the typical high-voltage diphasic spikes followed by a slow wave found in benign epilepsy with centrotemporal spikes.[13] All of the children reported had a normal development during the follow-up period.

DIAGNOSTIC EVALUATION

As a general rule, it is not necessary to perform many diagnostic evaluations in these forms of epilepsy except for prolonged wake and sleep EEGs. All of these children have a normal psychomotor development and in some cases a clear familial recurrence: this history since onset can help to bring the clinician to a diagnosis of idiopathic epilepsy. The follow-up and the EEG evaluations of these patients confirm the diagnosis of benign forms. Magnetic resonance imaging (MRI) is always normal, as are all other diagnostic evaluations. In cases in which mild gastroenteritis is suspected as an etiologic factor, it is necessary to look for rotavirus antigen, which has been found in half of the cases.

Electroencephalographic Findings

Interictal EEG is normal or fails to show any diagnostic elements in all forms except for the midline spikes during sleep reported by Capovilla, who hypothesized the existence of this peculiar and rare form.[6]

The EEG characteristics are well defined in BFIS as described by Vigevano et al.[67]; during a cluster of seizures, interictal EEGs showed lateralized slow waves and spikes in the occipitoparietal areas, whereas outside the cluster of seizures, the interictal EEG is normal. Ictal EEG disclosed a focal discharge characterized by a recruiting rhythm of increasing amplitude with onset in the occipitoparietal regions, spreading over the hemisphere and involving the entire brain. Recordings in the same patient of seizures with onset sometimes on the right hemisphere (Fig. 1) and sometimes on the left (Fig. 2) confirmed the alternating clinical pattern. The site of seizure origin seems to be a characteristic distinguishing this form from that described by Watanabe. The temporal area is the site of origin in cases described as BPEI with CPS,[71] whereas in cases described as BPEI with SGS, the site of origin is centroparietal.[69] In familial cases, the seizures originate mostly in the parieto-occipital area, with the side varying from one seizure to another.[66]

The distinctive aspect of benign infantile focal epilepsy with midline spikes and waves during sleep is that all of the described children presented particular interictal EEG abnormalities that

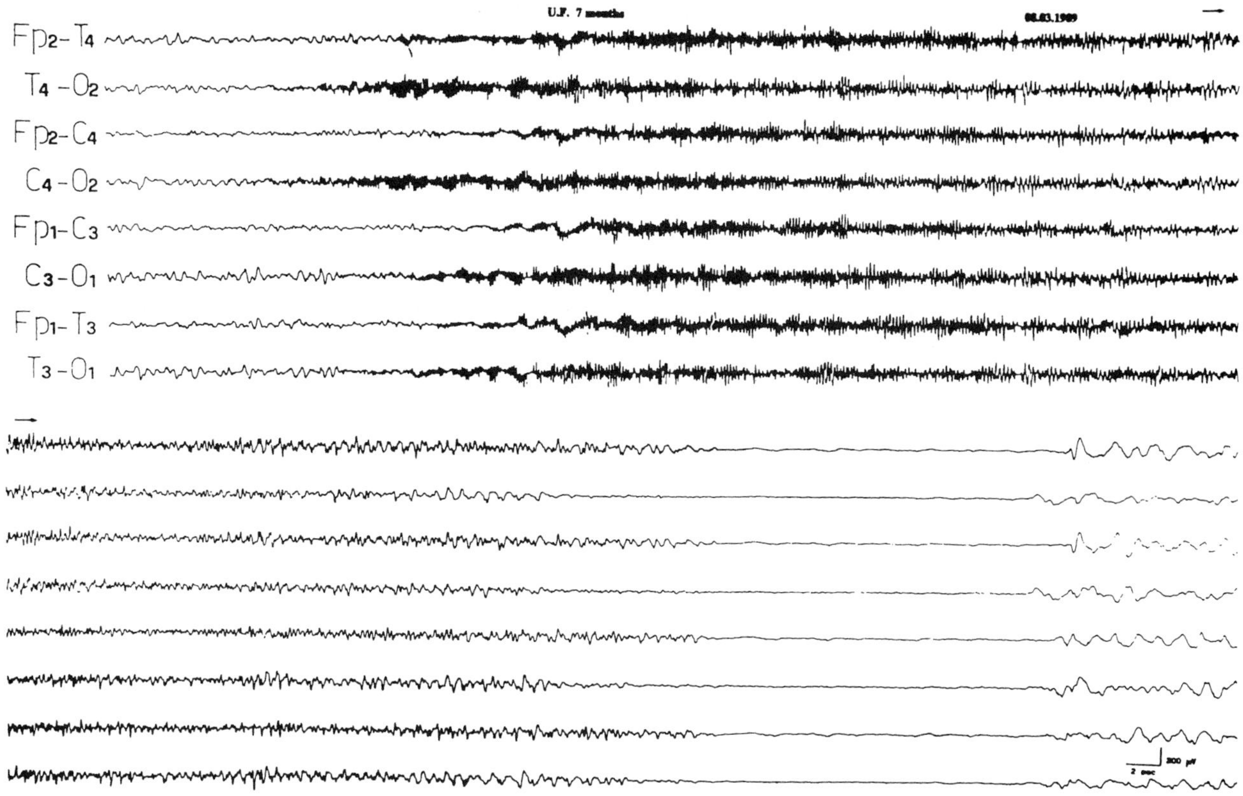

FIGURE 1. A 5-month-old boy affected by a familial form of benign infantile seizure. The seizure starts over the right parieto-occipital region.

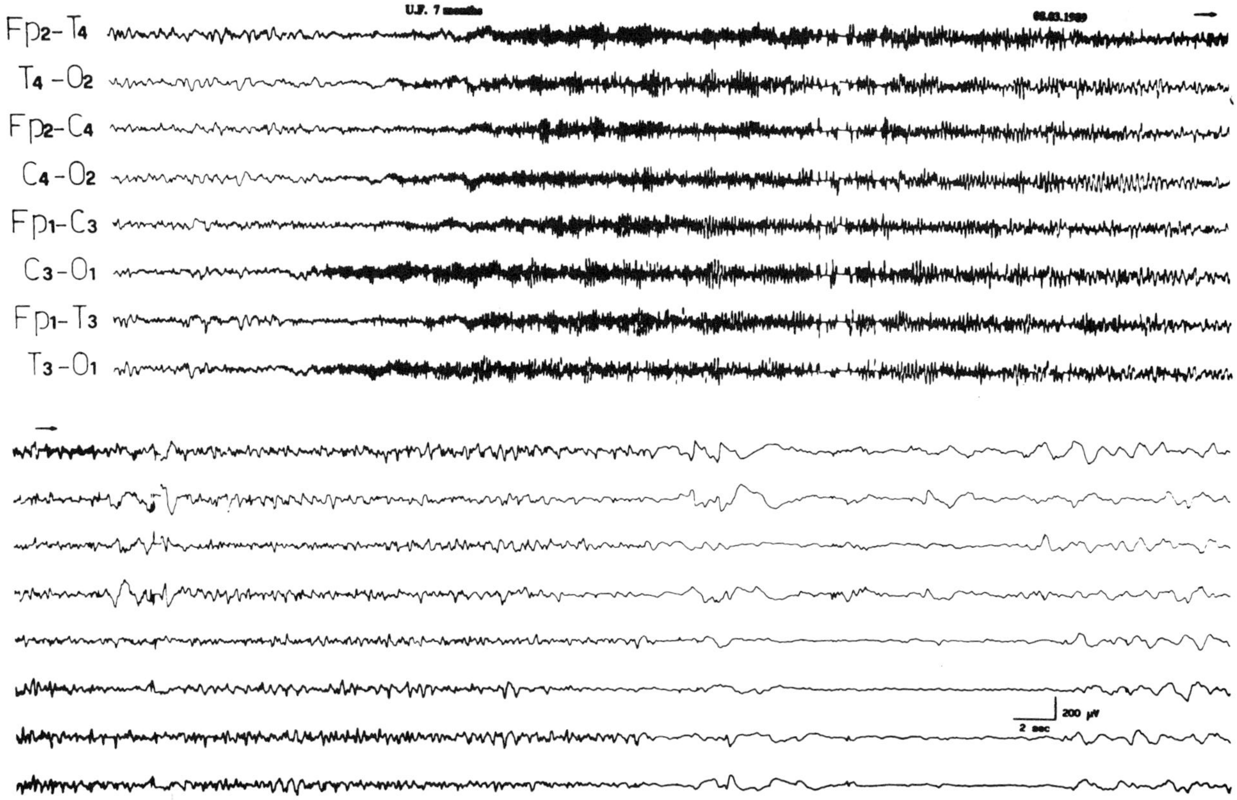

FIGURE 2. The same patient after 2 hours, experiencing a second seizure, which in this case starts over the left parieto-occipital region, thus demonstrating the alternating clinical and electroencephalographic pattern.

are detectable during sleep and characterized by isolated or grouped spikes and waves from the midline region to the central regions; Capovilla described these abnormalities as fast spikes, followed by a slow wave, in the midline region. They tend to spread to both central regions and are followed by a higher, bell-shaped slow wave.

Neuroimaging and Laboratory Assessment

Brain MRI is normal in all patients. The need to perform such examinations is based on the difficulty of diagnosing these epilepsies as benign from the onset. In cases with a clear autosomal-dominant pattern of inheritance and clear clinical features of benignity, it is possible to postpone the brain MRI. There are no particular indications for the laboratory assessment: Cardiovascular and respiratory function parameters have to be carefully monitored in children with BFIS or BNFIS during the cluster. A determination of glycemia could be useful at the onset and during the cluster of seizures.

In cases with BIS and MG, it is necessary to monitor the patient's hydration and general clinical conditions and investigate the presence of rotavirus antigen.

It is useful to collect such familial cases for linkage studies. The aim of genetic studies is to confirm the mutations that have been identified and provide genetic counseling. The possibility of new genetic mutations responsible for benign infantile seizures is sufficiently important to justify proposing a genetic study of these families.

DIFFERENTIAL DIAGNOSIS

The different forms of benign epilepsy in infancy recently have been examined by the ILAE in a proposed classification,[17] although their nosologic definition presents some difficulties.

The first report on the possible existence of benign forms of epilepsy in infancy dates back to 1963. In that year, Fukuyama[18] described a series of infants having apparently generalized seizures and benign course, as confirmed by Sugiura et al.[59]

On the other hand, partial epilepsies in infancy had long been considered as epilepsies with an unfavorable prognosis and as an expression of brain injury. Some authors also doubted the existence of partial idiopathic epilepsy in early infancy.[15] With the work of Watanabe et al.,[69,71,72] who reported cases of infants with complex partial seizures and seizures evolving to secondarily generalized seizures, a form of benign epilepsy was identified with partial seizures and onset in infancy. Afterward, Vigevano et al. focused on cases with similar features but also having a clear familial origin. They identified a specific form of benign epilepsy with onset within the first year of life and autosomal-dominant inheritance.[67] After the first study by Vigevano et al.,[67] a number of other reports confirmed the existence of such a benign epileptic syndrome. Furthermore, inheritance patterns have been confirmed with the identification, through linkage analysis of numerous families, of gene loci on chromosomes 19, 16, and 2.[11,23,42,58]

In this regard, other clinical entities with similar features to that described by Vigevano et al. but associated with other neurologic symptoms have been mapped to the same chromosomes where the syndrome described by Vigevano et al. was mapped.

ICCA, in which BIS are associated with paroxystic choreoathetosis,[61] has been mapped in various families on chromosome 16 in a region very close to that identified in families with BFIS.

The distinction between BFIS and other forms of benign epilepsy with neonatal onset (BFNS) appeared to be clear due to both the tight correlation with age and the difference in linkage analysis showing the existence of two genes, *KCNQ2* and *KCNQ3*, on chromosomes 20 and 8 responsible for BNFS.[37,55] Genetic studies failed to demonstrate the same gene defect in families with BFIS, thus dispelling all doubts about a possible overlap between BFIS and BFNS,[43] which are now also clearly distinct in the latest classification proposed by the ILAE.[17]

In 2004, a form of benign epilepsy with an intermediate onset between the neonatal and infantile forms was identified as BFNIS.[3] For this syndrome, a mutation of the gene *SCN2A* has been demonstrated. The onset of seizures in families affected by BFNIS is reported to occur between 7 days and 4 months of age. Although the mutation of the gene *SCN2A* appears to be distinctive to these families, age of onset and seizure semiology seem to overlap with BFNS and BFIS. We believe that it is of crucial importance to study new families with the described clinical picture to confirm the actual existence of a third form of benign familial epilepsy. To this purpose, we recently reported a new mutation of the gene *SCN2A* in a family with clinical features of BFIS, demonstrating a clinical and genetic overlap between BFNS and BFIS.[58]

From the clinical point of view, benign epilepsies of infancy are entities for which it is not easy to make a diagnosis. Clinical criteria described for BNFS and BFIS are not indicative for the diagnosis, although the presence of familiality may be helpful information. Sporadic forms may be even more difficult to diagnose. As reported by Okumura et al.,[50] recognition of BPEI is possible, to some extent, at the first presentation, but a confirmation can actually be obtained only by following these children over time to verify whether other seizures occur and other EEG abnormalities are found. These concepts are also relevant to pharmacologic treatment: It is difficult not to treat these epilepsies at the onset because these infants present with clusters of seizures. After the acute phase, many infants continue to follow a chronic therapy. In familial forms, the tendency is to interrupt the therapy as early as possible. In nonfamilial forms, instead, the indication is to wait and follow the evolution; should the benign diagnosis be confirmed, it is possible to stop the treatment within 18 months after the last seizure.

The phenotype of familial and nonfamilial forms is likely to be very similar. There may be some differences in the seizure semiology and in the site of the seizure onset (more anterior in the sporadic forms and more parieto-occipital in the familial forms).

It is certain, however, that there are familial forms with an autosomal-dominant trait as well as sporadic forms. Therefore, in our opinion, the major criterion for distinguishing these forms of benign epilepsy should be the presence or absence of familiality, as proposed in the most recent classification.[17]

All of the aforementioned entities do not present any interictal EEG abnormality and are characterized by seizures occurring exclusively in a short period of infancy. For all of these reasons, we agree with the proposal of the ILAE Task Force on Classification and Terminology that these conditions be defined with the term *seizures* and not *epilepsy*.[17]

Benign infantile focal epilepsy with midline spikes and waves during sleep (BIMSE) can be distinguished from other infantile benign forms because infants with this syndrome, as reported by Bureau and Maton[4] and later by Capovilla et al.,[5,6] have a slightly later onset, with no seizures in clusters, and with characteristic sleep EEG abnormalities. This syndrome is more similar to other benign epilepsies with partial seizures generally occurring at older ages, such as early-onset benign occipital seizure susceptibility syndrome (EBOSS) and benign epilepsy of childhood with centrotemporal spikes (BECTS), in which the interictal EEG shows particular epileptiform abnormalities.

TABLE 6

BENIGN NON FAMILIAL INFANTILE SEIZURES

	BNFIS	BFIS	BFNIS	BIS AND MG	BIMSE
Genetic	Sporadic	AD	AD	Sporadic	Sporadic
Onset					
Typical		5–6 mo	Within 3rd mo	?	17 mo
Range		3–9 mo	2 d –7th mo	5–36 mo	4–30 mo
Type of seizure	Focal sometimes with SGS	Focal with SGS	Focal with SGS	Focal	Focal
Occurrence	Cluster	Cluster	Cluster	Repetitive	Rare
Other type of seizure	—	—	—	—	—
Other clinical features	—	Paroxysmal choreoathetosis migraine	—	—	—
Interictal EEG	NS	NS	NS	NS	Midline spikes during sleep
Chromosomal loci	—	16,19,2	2	—	—
Gene	—	*SCN2A*	*SCN2A*	—	—

AD, autosomal dominant; BFIS, benign familial infantile seizures, BNFIS, benign non familial infantile seizures, BIS and MG, benign infantile seizures and mild gastroenteritis; BIMSE, benign infantile focal epilepsy with midline spikes and waves during sleep; EEG, electroencephalogram; NS, not significative; SGS, secondarily generalized seizures.

Although in BIMSE, as in the other epilepsies described, there seems to be a characteristic EEG pattern, a wider number of patients should be studied to confirm the actual existence of this new form of benign epilepsy. At present, this entity is being studied and is not included in the international classification of epilepsies.

In contrast to the previously discussed entities, benign infantile seizures associated with mild gastroenteritis (BIS with MG) are more likely to be considered as situation-related seizures than as epilepsy. This syndrome can be misdiagnosed as epilepsy because seizures are nonfebrile and may occur in clusters. It is important further to study and understand this entity.

In conclusion, benign epilepsies of infancy encompass a wide spectrum of entities with differences in age at onset, genetic aspects, seizure semiology, and EEG characteristics (when available). Table 6 summarizes the main features of benign epilepsies. Follow-up of these infants is important because it allows us to confirm the benign outcome over time.

TREATMENT AND OUTCOME

Although, as in other benign forms of infant epilepsy, seizures in these forms should not be treated, in clinical practice it is difficult to not treat these patients. At the very beginning these children present seizures in clusters (seizure every 2–3 hours), which sometimes require a rapid intervention with drugs. Patients not treated after the first cluster can have other seizures or clusters. When such children arrive at the emergency department, the etiology of their seizures may appear clearly only after EEG monitoring and with a normal neurologic evaluation. For these reasons, the majority of children receive antiepileptic treatment. In cases that exhibit a familial recurrence, it is possible to withhold the treatment because the diagnosis is simpler. In anecdotal reports, all drugs have demonstrated efficacy in benign infantile seizures (valproate, carbamazepine, phenobarbital, and phenytoin), with apparently no differences. Recently, Japanese authors[44] reported the efficacy of low doses of carbamazepine in a series of patients with benign infantile seizures. In this study, carbamazepine was administered at a once-daily dose of 5 mg/kg; seizures did not recur in any patient. The treatment can be withdrawn 1 year after onset.

LONG-TERM PROGNOSIS

Unpublished data from the Division of Neurology, Bambino Gesù Children's Hospital, of a 14 year-follow-up period confirm that any patients have had seizure recurrence without treatment. Neuropsychological development appears to be normal in all of them, except for one patient, who has mild mental retardation, which was evident before the seizure onset. Most of the patients have had several follow-up EEGs that failed to show any abnormalities. Some data have been published that confirm the benign prognosis for these patients.[49,52]

SUMMARY AND CONCLUSIONS

Benign epilepsies during infancy are a large topic needing both clinical and nosologic clarification. In 1963, Fukuyama reported patients with seizures during infancy with a benign outcome. In the late 1980s and early 1990s, Watanabe reported series of infants with complex partial seizures or partial seizures with secondary generalization, with a normal development before onset and a benign outcome. In the same years, Vigevano focused on familial cases: He described several families with seizures with onset around 6 months of age and an autosomal-dominant mode of inheritance. To define this condition, he coined the term *benign familial infantile seizures* (BFIS). Later studies of families with this phenotype detected loci on chromosomes 19, 16, and 2 responsible for it. Similar loci were found in families affected by BFIS and subsequent choreoathetosis and BFIS associated with familial hemiplegic migraine. More recently, a new form of benign epilepsy has been proposed with an intermediate onset between the neonatal and infantile ages, *benign familial neonatal-infantile seizures* (BFNIS). This condition might have some clinical and genetic features overlapping with BFIS. Seizures with a benign outcome also have been reported in infants during episodes of mild gastroenteritis (BIS with MG), frequently with positive rotavirus antigen. Finally, Capovilla et al. reported sleep EEG abnormalities in children with a peculiar form of epilepsy that they defined as *benign infantile focal epilepsy with midline spikes and waves during sleep* (BIMSE). Some of these entities have been included in the most recent classification proposed by the ILAE and have been differentiated into familial and nonfamilial forms.

We believe that there is a series of clinical entities with seizures in clusters that are limited to a short period of life. All of these entities are idiopathic, without EEG interictal abnormalities, and benign, and we define them as "seizures" and not "epilepsies."

Benign infantile focal epilepsy with midline spikes and waves during sleep should be placed at the upper border of this age range. Infants with this syndrome have a later onset, and it has more similarities with benign focal epilepsies appearing later in life such as early-onset benign occipital seizure susceptibility syndrome (EBOSS) and benign epilepsy of childhood with centrotemporal spikes (BECTS).

References

1. Bennett LB, Roach ES, Bowcock AM. A locus for paroxysmal kinesigenic dyskinesia maps to human chromosome 16. *Neurology.* 2000;54:125–130.
2. Berger A, Diener W, Stephani E, et al. Benigne fruekindliche partialepilepsie nach Watanabe. *Epilepsie Blaetter.* 1997;10:76–81.
3. Berkovic SF, Heron SE, Giordano L, et al. Benign familial neonatal-infantile seizures: characterization of a new sodium channelopathy. *Ann Neurol.* 2004;55:550–557.
4. Bureau M, Maton B. Valeur de l'EEG dans le prognostic précoce des epilepsies partielles non-idiopathiques de l'enfant. In: Bureau M, Kahane P, Munari C, eds. *Epilepsies Partielles Graves Pharmacorésistantes de L'énfant: Strategies Diagnostiques et Traitements Chirurgicaux.* Montrouge, France: John Libbey; 1998: 67–78.
5. Capovilla G, Beccaria F. Benign partial epilepsy in infancy and early childhood with vertex spikes and waves during sleep: a new epileptic form. *Brain Dev.* 2000;22:93–99.
6. Capovilla G, Beccaria F, Montanini A. "Benign focal epilepsy in infancy with vertex spikes and waves during sleep." Delineation of the syndrome and recalling as "benign infantile focal epilepsy with midline spikes and waves during sleep" (BIMSE). *Brain Dev.* 2006;28:85–91.
7. Capovilla G, Giordano L, Tiberti S, et al. Benign partial epilepsy in infancy with complex partial seizures (Watanabe's syndrome): 12 non-Japanese new cases. *Brain Dev.* 1998;20:105–111.
8. Caraballo R, Cersosimo R, Amartino H, et al. Benign familial infantile seizures: further delineation of the syndrome. *J Child Neurol.* 2002;17:696–699.
9. Caraballo R, Cersosimo R, Espeche A, et al. Benign familial and non-familial infantile seizures: a study of 64 patients. *Epileptic Disord.* 2003;5:45–49.
10. Caraballo R, Cersosimo R, Galicchio S, et al. Convulsiones familiares benignas de la infancia. *Rev Neurol (Barcelona).* 1997;25:682–684.
11. Caraballo R, Pavek S, Lemainque A, et al. Linkage of benign familial infantile convulsions to chromosome 16p12–q12 suggests allelism to the infantile convulsions and choreoathetosis syndrome. *Am J Hum Genet.* 2001;68,788–794.
12. Contino MF, Lebby T, Arcinue EL. Rotaviral gastrointestinal infection causing afebrile seizures in infancy and childhood. *Am J Emerg Med.* 1994;12:94–95.
13. Dalla Bernardina B, Sgrò V, Fejerman N. Epilepsy with centro-temporal spikes and related syndromes. In: Roger J, Bureau M, Dravet C, et al., eds. *Epileptic Syndromes in Infancy, Childhood and Adolescence,* 4th ed. Eastleigh, UK: John Libbey; 2005: 203–225.
14. Ducros A, Denier C, Joutel A, et al. The clinical spectrum of familial hemiplegic migraine associated with mutations in a neuronal calcium channel. *N Engl J Med.* 2001;341:7–24.
15. Dulac O, Cusmai R, de Oliveira K. Is there a partial benign epilepsy in infancy? *Epilepsia.* 1989;30:798–801.
16. Echenne B, Humbertclaude V, Rivier F, et al. Benign infantile epilepsy with autosomal dominant inheritance. *Brain Dev.* 1994;16:108–111.
17. Engel J Jr. A proposed diagnostic scheme for people with epileptic seizures and with epilepsy: report of the ILAE Task Force on Classification and Terminology. *Epilepsia.* 2001;42:796–803.
18. Fukuyama Y. Borderland of epilepsy with special reference to febrile convulsions and so-called infantile convulsions. *Seishin-Igaku (Clin Psychiatry).* 1963;5:211–223.
19. Fukuyama Y, Sakauchi M. Benign infantile seizure syndromes complex. From classic to recent advances. *Epilepsies.* 2006;18:8–23.
20. Gennaro E, Malacarne M, Carbone I, et al. No evidence of a major locus for benign familial infantile convulsions on chromosome 19q12–q13.1. *Epilepsia.* 1999;40:1799–1803.
21. Giordano L, Accorsi P, Valseriati D, et al. Benign infantile familial convulsions: natural history of a case and clinical characteristics of a large Italian family. *Neuropediatrics.* 1999;30:99–101.
22. Gomez-Lado C, Garcia-Reboredo M, Monasterio-Corral L, et al. Benign seizures associated with mild gastroenteritis: Apropos of two cases. *An Pediatr.* 2005;63:558–560.
23. Guipponi M, Rivier F, Vigevano F, et al. Linkage mapping of benign familial infantile convulsions (BFIC) to chromosome 19. *Hum Mol Genet.* 1997;6:473–477.
24. Hattori H, Fujii T, Nigami H, et al. Co-segregation of benign infantile convulsions and paroxysmal kinesigenic choreoathetosis. *Brain Dev.* 2000;22:432–435.
25. Heron SE, Crossland KM, Andermann E, et al. Sodium-channel defects in benign familial neonatal infantile seizures. *Lancet.* 2002;360:851–852.
26. Hung JJ, Wen HY, Yen MH, et al. Rotavirus gastroenteritis associated with a febrile convulsion in children: clinical analysis of 40 cases.*Chang Gung Med J.* 2003;26:654–659.
27. Iglesias Escalera G, Usano Carrasco AI, Cueto Calvo E, et al. Benign afebrile convulsion due to rotavirus gastroenteritis. *An Pediatr.* 2005;63:82–83.
28. Imai K, Otani K, Yanagihara K, et al. Ictal video-EEG recording of three partial seizures in a patient with the benign infantile convulsions associated with mild gastroenteritis. *Epilepsia.* 1999;40:1455–1458.
29. International Headache Society. Classification and diagnostic criteria for headache disorders, cranial neuralgias and facial pain. Headache Classification Committee of the International Headache Society. *Cephalalgia.* 1988;8:1–96.
30. Itou J, Takahashi Y, Kusunoki Y, et al. Convulsions associated with mild acute diarrhea. *Shonika Rinsho (Jpn J Pediatr).* 1988;41:2011–2015.
31. Kajiyama M, Fukuyama Y. Infantile convulsions associated with mild diarrhea [in Japanese]. *Nihon Shonika Gakkai Zasshi.* 1984;88:883–889.
32. Kaplan RE, Lacey DJ. Benign familial neonatal-infantile seizures. *Am J Med Genet.* 1983;16:595–599.
33. Kobayashi K, Araki K, Kobayashi S, et al. Infantile afebrile clustered convulsions associated small round structured virus infection [in Japanese]. *Shonika Rinsho.* 1999;52:56–62.
34. Komori H, Wada M, Eto M, et al. Benign convulsions with mild gastroenteritis: a report of 10 recent cases detailing clinical varieties. *Brain Dev.* 1995;17:334–337.
35. Lee WL, Low PS, Rajan U. Benign familial infantile epilepsy. *J Pediatr.* 1993;123:588–590.
36. Lee WL, Tay A, Ong HT, et al. Association of infantile convulsions with paroxysmal dyskinesias (ICCA syndrome): confirmation of linkage to human chromosome 16p12–q12 in a Chinese family. *Hum Genet.* 1998;103:608–612.
37. Leppert M, Anderson VE, Quattlebaum T, et al. Benign familial neonatal convulsions linked to genetic markers on chromosome 20. *Nature.* 1989;337:647–648.
38. Lionetti P, Salvestrini C, Trapani S, et al. An 18-month-old child with seizures and bloody diarrhea. *Inflamm Bowel Dis.* 2005;11:209–210.
39. Lispi ML, Cusmai R, Vigevano F. Benign partial epilepsy in infancy: sporadic versus familial forms. *Ann Neurol.* 2001(Suppl 1):102.
40. Luovigsson P, Olafsson E, Rich SS, et al. Benign infantile familial epilepsy: three families with multiple affected members in three generations. *Epilepsia.* 1993;34:18.
41. Lynch M, Lee B, Azimi P, et al. Rotavirus and central nervous system symptoms: cause or concomitant? Case reports and review. *Clin Infect Dis.* 2001;33:932–938.
42. Malacarne M, Gennaro E, Madia F, et al. Benign familial infantile convulsions: mapping of a novel locus on chromosome 2q24 and evidence for genetic heterogeneity. *Am J Hum Genet.* 2001;68:1521–1526.
43. Malafosse A, Beck C, Bellet H, et al. Benign infantile familial convulsions are not an allelic form of the benign familial neonatal convulsions gene. *Ann Neurol* 1994;35:479–482.
44. Matsufuji H, Ichiyama T, Isumi H, et al. Low-dose carbamazepine therapy for benign infantile convulsions. *Brain Dev.* 2005;27:554–557.
45. McCallenbach P, De Coo RFM, Vein AA, et al. Benign familial infantile convulsions: a clinical study of seven Dutch families. *Eur J Paediatr Neurol* 2002;6:269–283.
46. Morooka K. Convulsions and mild diarrhea [in Japanese]. *Shonika.* 1982;23:131–137.
47. Nakai M, Soda M. Benign convulsions with mild diarrhea [in Japanese]. *Shonika Rinsho.* 1982;35:2855–2859.
48. Narchi H. Benign afebrile cluster convulsion with gastroenteritis: an observational study. *BMC Pediatr.* 2004;4:2.
49. Nelson GB, Olson DM, Hahn JS. Short duration of benign partial epilepsy in infancy. *J Child Neurol.* 2002;17:440–445.
50. Okumura A, Hayakawa F, Kato T, et al. Early recognition of benign partial epilepsy in infancy. *Epilepsia.* 2000;41:714–717.
51. Okumura A, Uemura N, Negoro T, et al. Efficacy of antiepileptic drugs in patients with benign convulsions with mild gastroenteritis. *Brain Dev.* 2004;26:164–167.
52. Okumura A, Watanabe K, Negoro T, et al. Long-term follow-up of patients with benign partial epilepsy in infancy. *Epilepsia.* 2006;47:181–185.
53. Omata T, Tamai K, Kurosaki T, et al. Clinical study of convulsions with mild gastroenteritis [in Japanese]. *Nihon Shonika Gakkai Zasshi.* 2002;106:368–371.

54. Posner E. "Benign convulsion with mild gastroenteritis" a worldwide clinical entity. *Brain Dev*. 2003;25:529.
55. Ryan SG, Wiznitger M, Hollman C, et al. Benign familial neonatal convulsions: evidence for clinical and genetic heterogeneity. *Ann Neurol*. 1991;29:469–473.
56. Shikano T, Kikukawa H, Kato M, et al. Clinical findings of infants with afebrile seizures associated with mild diarrhea [in Japanese]. *Shonika Rinsho*. 1998;51:1074–1078.
57. Singh NA, Charlier C, Stauffer D, et al. A novel potassium channel gene, KCNQ2, is mutated in an inherited epilepsy of newborns. *Nat Genet*. 1998;18:25–29.
58. Striano P, Bordo L, Lispi ML, et al. A novel SCN2A mutation in family with benign familial infantile seizures. *Epilepsia*. 2006;47:218–220.
59. Sugiura M, Matsumoto A, Watanabe K, et al. Long-term prognosis of generalized convulsions in the first year of life, with special reference to benign infantile convulsions. *Jpn J Epil Soc*. 1983;1:116–121.
60. Swoboda KJ, Soong BW, McKenna C, et al. Paroxysmal kinesigenic dyskinesia and infantile convulsions. Clinical and linkage studies. *Neurology*. 2000;55:224–230.
61. Szepetowski P, Rochette J, Berquin P, et al. Familial infantile convulsions and paroxysmal choreoathetosis: a new neurological syndrome linked to the pericentromeric region of human chromosome 16. *Am J Hum Genet*. 1997;61:889–898.
62. Terwindt GM, Ophoff RA, Lindhout D, et al. Partial cosegregation of familial hemiplegic migraine and a benign familial infantile epileptic syndrome. *Epilepsia*. 1997;38:915–921.
63. Tomita H, Nagamitsu S, Wakui K, et al. Paroxysmal kinesigenic choreoathetosis locus maps to chromosome 16p11.2–q12.1. *Am J Hum Genet*. 1999;65:1688–1697.
64. Uemura N, Okumura A, Negoro T, et al. Clinical features of benign convulsions with mild gastroenteritis. *Brain Dev*. 2002;24:745–749.
65. Vanmolkot KR, Kors EE, Hottenga JJ, et al. Novel mutations in the Na+, K+-ATPase pump gene ATP1A2 associated with familial hemiplegic migraine and benign familial infantile convulsions. *Ann Neurol*. 2003;54:360–366.
66. Vigevano F. Benign familial infantile seizures. *Brain Dev*. 2005;27:172–177.
67. Vigevano F, Fusco L, Di Capua M, et al. Benign infantile familial convulsions. *Eur J Pediatr*. 1992;151:608–612.
68. Vigevano F, Sebastianelli R, Fusco L, et al. Benign infantile familial convulsions. In: Malafosse A, Genton P, Hirsch E, et al., eds. *Idiopathic Generalized Epilepsies: Clinical, Experimental and Genetic Aspects*. London: John Libbey; 1994: 45–49.
69. Watanabe K, Negoro T, Aso K. Benign partial epilepsy with secondarily generalized seizures in infancy. *Epilepsia*. 1993;34:635–638.
70. Watanabe K, Okumura A. Benign partial epilepsies in infancy. *Brain Dev*. 2000;22:296–300.
71. Watanabe K, Yamamoto N, Negoro T, et al. Benign complex partial epilepsies in infancy. *Pediatr Neurol*. 1987;3:208–211.
72. Watanabe K, Yamamoto N, Negoro T, et al. Benign infantile epilepsy with complex partial seizures. *J Clin Neurophysiol*. 1990;7:409–416.
73. Weber YG, Berger A, Bebek N, et al. Benign familial infantile convulsions: linkage to chromosome 16p12–q12 in 14 families. *Epilepsia*. 2004;45:601–609.
74. Wong V. Acute gastroenteritis-related encephalopathy. *J Child Neurol*. 2001;16:906–910.

CHAPTER 228 ■ MIGRATING PARTIAL SEIZURES IN INFANCY

MARIA ROBERTA CILIO, OLIVIER DULAC, RENZO GUERRINI, AND FEDERICO VIGEVANO

INTRODUCTION

Epileptic syndromes with onset in the neonatal period or infancy with very poor prognosis have been recognized or better defined in recent years due to developments in diagnostic techniques, including video-electroencephalography, brain imaging, and cytogenetics. Migrating partial seizures in infancy (MPSI) is a rare, newly recognized, age-specific epileptic syndrome first described in 1995 by Coppola et al.[3] In the proposed revision of the International League Against Epilepsy (ILAE) diagnostic scheme for people with epileptic seizures and with epilepsy, MPSI was labeled as a syndrome in development and included among symptomatic and probably symptomatic focal epilepsies.[7] It is characterized by onset in the first 6 months of age, after a normal early development, of nearly continuous multifocal partial seizures arising independently and sequentially from both hemispheres, progression through a period of intractable seizures, subsequent neurologic deterioration or arrest with complete loss of both cognitive and motor abilities and, in most children, progressive decline of head circumference percentile.

HISTORICAL PERSPECTIVES

MPSI was first reported in 1995 by Coppola et al.,[3] who described 14 infants with a severe epileptic disorder characterized by seizure onset in the first year of life; nearly continuous multifocal seizures involving both hemispheres; no identifiable immediate or remote cause; normal neuroimaging studies at onset; and intractability to conventional antiepileptic drugs (AEDs), including phenobarbital, phenytoin, carbamazepine, valproate, vigabatrin, clobazam, nitrazepam, biotin, vitamin B_6, and corticosteroids. In this first description, the outcome was very poor with regard to both the seizure disorder and psychomotor development. Only 2 of 14 patients stopped having seizures with a combination of stiripentol and clonazepam and showed some neurologic improvement. Eleven patients developed microcephaly during the first year of life, and three patients died. After this original report, additional cases from Australia, Europe, Japan, and the United States were published.[4,10,11,13,15,17,22] Thirty-three cases have now been reported. In particular, two cases have been reported from Australia[22] that fulfill the diagnostic criteria proposed by Coppola et al.[3] Both infants presented with intractable partial seizures arising independently from multiple regions of both hemispheres, with interictal electroencephalograms (EEGs) revealing multifocal epileptiform activity. There was no response to AEDs, pyridoxine, and corticosteroids, and developmental arrest followed seizure onset. Extensive investigations failed to identify an underlying cause. Both infants died. One of them underwent postmortem examination, which was normal.

Veneselli et al. reported three infants in whom seizure onset occurred before 3 months of age and was characterized by focal motor manifestations with a gradually increasing frequency.[17] Either hemibody was alternatively and randomly involved, and secondary generalization was evident only during the evolution of the disease. Conventional AEDs were uneffective. No etiologic factors have been identified. Neurologic status and evolution were highly unfavorable, resulting in death in one case and severe neurodevelopmental morbidities in the others. The same malignant course, with regard to both seizure disorder and ultimate outcome, was described by Gross-Tsur et al. in two additional cases.[10] One infant, microcephalic at birth, developed at age 4 months clusters of nearly continuous multifocal seizures with secondary generalization, refractory to antiepileptic drugs. By the age of 4.5 years she was seizure free but remained without any cognitive or motor function. The other, born with a normal head circumference, began seizures at the age of 3 months, never became seizure free, and died at age 18 months. Neuroimaging findings showed progressive subcortical atrophy. In both cases, extensive evaluation including skin and muscle biopsy did not clarify the etiology. However, more recently, Marsh et al.[13] reported six new patients with the same clinical and electroencephalographic characteristics as those described by Coppola et al.[3] but with the prospect of a more optimistic developmental outcome, raising the difficult distinction at onset with benign infantile or neonatal-infantile seizures. Each patient underwent comprehensive brain imaging and neurometabolic evaluations, which were unrevealing. Five patients had a long-term follow-up. Whereas all had some degree of neurodevelopmental sequelae, a few of them appeared to be less severely affected: One was able to walk, one developed some degree of spoken language, two showed developmental quotients between 50% and 100%, and only one was profoundly impaired. In terms of seizure outcome, one was still having intractable seizures when lost to follow-up. For five of six patients, six or more AEDs failed. Two patients received adrenocorticotropic hormone (ACTH); two were treated with folinic acid, and two were placed on ketogenic diet. None of them was more successful than the others. In contrast, successful seizure control was obtained with potassium bromide by Okuda et al. in two patients with a diagnosis of MPSI and refractory to conventional AEDs.[15] Moreover, once seizures were controlled, both patients showed some degree of neurologic recovery. A recently published case report by Hmaimess et al. in 2006 described the first neonatal case of MPSI and documented a positive response to levetiracetam.[11] Unfortunately, despite the dramatic decrease in seizure activity, which paralleled a positive clinical evolution in terms of psychomotor development, the child died unexpectedly at 14 months of age. The most recent three cases at the time of this review have been reported by Coppola et al., who performed a mutational scanning of potassium, sodium, and chloride ion channels (KCNQ2, KCNQ3, SCN1A, SCN2A, and MECP2) but failed to find any mutations.[4] Finally, it is important to consider that studies on drug-resistant seizures with early onset classified as "catastrophic infantile epilepsy" may include cases of MPSI. Ishii et al.[12] investigated clinicoelectrical and etiologic characteristics of 15 patients with catastrophic infantile epilepsy. Although some of these patients did not belong to MPSI, a number of them, mainly those without a clear etiology, clinically and electroencephalographically resemble this syndrome.

DEFINITIONS

MPSI is a severe, probably symptomatic, age-dependent focal epilepsy defined by the following diagnostic criteria: (a) normal development before seizure onset; (b) seizures beginning before age 6 months; (c) migrating focal motor seizures at onset; (d) multifocal seizures becoming nearly continuous; (f) intractability to conventional AEDs; (e) lack of demonstrable etiology; and (g) severe psychomotor delay on follow-up. The clinical features and EEG pattern suggest that MPSI may rank among the catastrophic epilepsies of infancy. Moreover, due to the high frequency of seizures and the intense epileptiform activity that contribute to the progressive disturbance of cerebral function, MPSI could also be included in the epileptic encephalopathies.

EPIDEMIOLOGY

Its prevalence is unknown because only small series of patients have been published.[4,10,11,13,15,17,22] Both sexes are equally affected.

ETIOLOGY AND BASIC MECHANISMS

The etiology is not known, but a functional or metabolic disorder is suspected. All reported patients had normal magnetic resonance imaging (MRI) and computed tomography (CT) scans at the onset of seizures. There is no evidence of familiarity because no familial recurrence of migrating seizures has been reported, and there is no consanguinity. In the series reported by Coppola et al., three patients had family history of febrile seizures and four of epilepsy.[3] Veneselli et al. reported one patient with a family history of first-degree seizures.[17] Neurometabolic evaluations performed in all cases have excluded inborn errors of metabolism. In those cases that were examined with postmortem, neuropathology failed to demonstrate cortical dysplasia, neuronal migration defects, or cortical vacuolation.[3,22] Preliminary genetic studies excluded any abnormality in the coding region of several relevant sodium, potassium, and chloride ion channel gene involved in other epileptic syndromes of the first year of life, suggesting lack of any molecular link between benign familial neonatal or neonatal-infantile seizures or Dravet syndrome and MPSI.[4]

CLINICAL PRESENTATION

The first seizure occurs before 6 months of age (1 day to 6 months; mean 25 days) in normal infants, who have no antecedent risk factors. Seizures begins with focal motor movements that can alternate from one side of the body to another with lateral deviation of the head and eyes and eye jerks, twitching of the eyelids, limb myoclonic jerks, and increased tone of one or both limbs.[3,4,10,11,13,15,17,22] At the beginning, many of the motor manifestations are relatively subtle and easily overlooked both by parents and the nursing staff, such as fixed sight, psychomotor arrest, lateral deviation of the eyes, and chewing-like movements. Sometimes, electrical seizures are not associated with any clinical manifestations, although they may spread and involve both hemispheres.[13,22] It is also worth mentioning that in very young patients motor and autonomic signs are often the only clinically relevant symptoms of seizures. Focal motor components are often accompanied by autonomic signs including flushing of the face, salivation, and apnea.[3,13,15,17] Epileptic spasms have been described in only one patient, appearing during the course of the disease and associated with a focal discharge.[3] Truly generalized tonic–clonic seizures are very rare.[22] The combination of these various manifestations produces a wide range of ictal semiology that may vary in a given infant from one seizure to another, although there are predominant focal motor components. Prolonged observation soon shows that both sides are alternatively affected, which demonstrates the involvement of the whole brain cortex. Seizures are relatively brief, but often last several minutes, and thus are longer than observed in patients with benign seizures in infancy. In addition, they tend to recur in series of 5 to 30 seizures during drowsiness and/or at awakening, several times a day. Such clusters may last up to 2 to 5 days. Initially seizures are rare, occurring roughly once a week. Nevertheless, two patients presented with status epilepticus.[3] Soon after, seizure frequency tend to increase and, at an age ranging from 24 days to 10 months, become almost continuous in most of the reported cases. These consecutive seizures can overlap, with one seizure beginning before the end of the previous one (Fig. 1).[3,11] At this stage, seizures tend to cluster, and clusters of seizures may last up to 2 to 5 days. Between seizures during these clusters, infants are floppy, drooling, often somnolent, and unable to drink and swallow. Between clusters, the infant may recover partially. As patients recover slightly, however, the next cluster occurs and patients regress. Moreover, with time, seizures tend to generalize more frequently.

Psychomotor development before seizure onset has been normal in most cases.[3,4,10,13,17,22] One patient presented with microcephaly at birth,[10] and two patients had evidence of mild psychomotor delay before onset of seizures.[3] However, in some cases the first symptoms appear as early as the first days of life, making developmental evaluation prior to the seizure onset more difficult. There is progressive neurologic deterioration with the development of major axial and limb hypotonia, loss of visual contact, inability to grasp, and complete loss of other motor and social skills in most children. Most patients show progressive loss of head circumference percentiles over time and development. In most cases, the condition is progressive, and patients lose all skills within a few months of onset of the illness. However, in a few cases,[3,11,13,15] seizures were eventually controlled, and these children partly recovered motor and cognitive abilities. In all series, developmental outcome is better when seizures are controlled compared to those with continued intractable seizures. Some patients die.[3,10,11,17,22] Although death can be a consequence of very frequent seizures complicated by respiratory distress and[17] intercurrent infections,[3,22] the cause of death often remains unclear and is largely undocumented.[10,11] Marsh et al. published a series of infants with MPSI and a slightly better outcome than previously reported, underscoring the difficult distinction with benign conditions at onset.[13] In particular, although all of their patients had a period of intractable seizures and developmental plateau or regression, the developmental outcome was borderline mild mental retardation in one patient and mild to moderate retardation in another. Three patients had developmental quotients between 50% and 100%, and only one was profoundly impaired. These findings are not dissimilar to those of other types of early-onset epileptic encephalopathies, such as West syndrome, in which a few children may recover without severe adverse sequelae.[6]

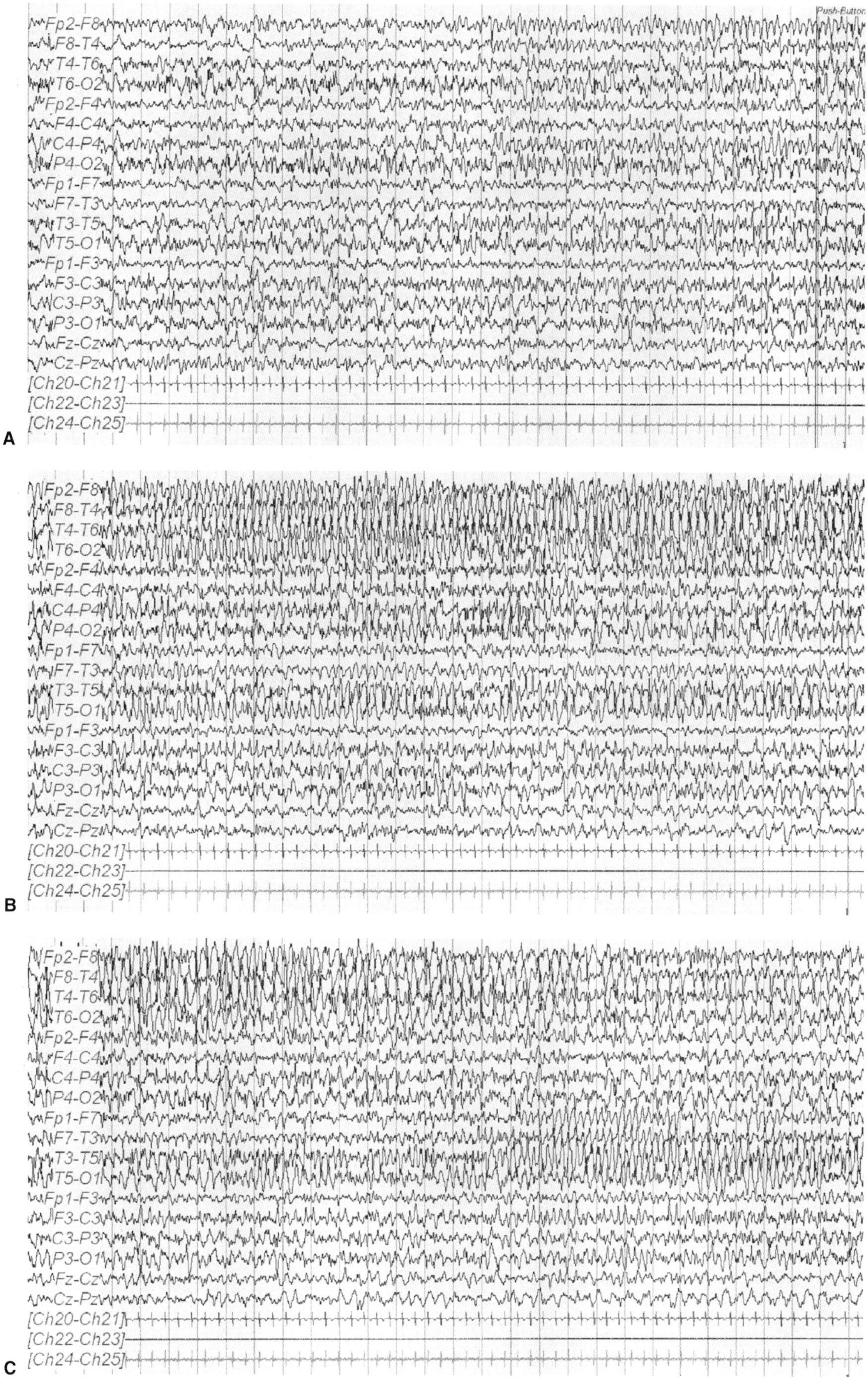

FIGURE 1. Ictal recording of a 6-month-old girl affected by migrating partial seizures in infancy showing apparently random onset of electroencephalographic discharges. **A:** A seizure starts over the right frontotemporal region. **B:** Another seizure starts in the left frontotemporal region, before the end of the first event. **C:** Simultaneous discharges involve two different areas, the right frontotemporal region and the left temporal region. *(Continued)*

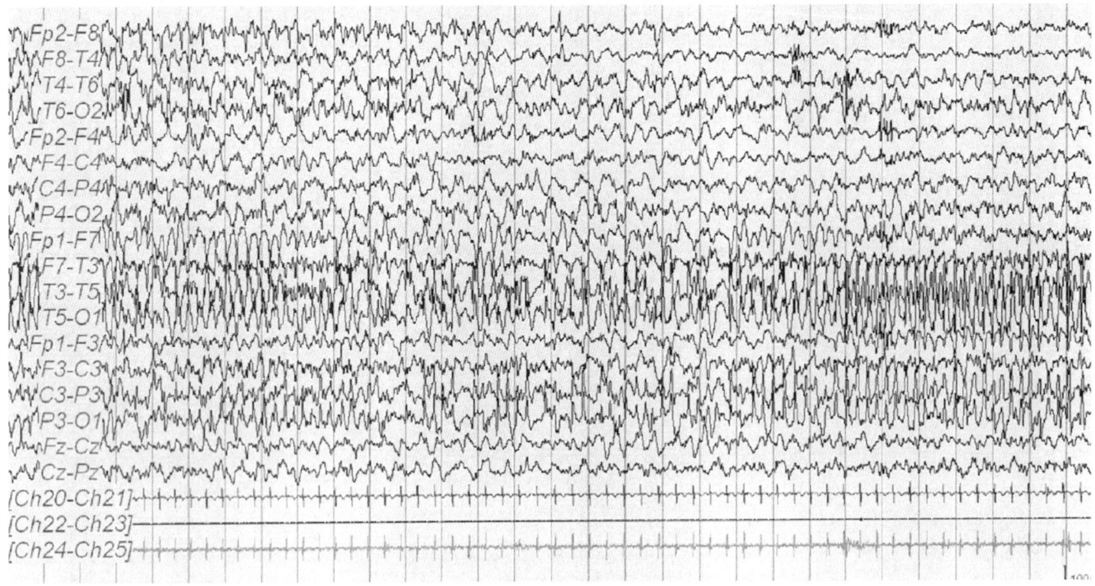

D

FIGURE 1. *(Continued)* D: The seizure over the right hemisphere ends, whereas the seizure over the left hemisphere persists.

DIAGNOSTIC EVALUATION

Electroencephalographic Findings

At onset, interictal EEG background varies from normal to diffuse slowing,[3,13] and epileptiform discharges may be rare, with unifocal or multifocal interictal patterns. Initial EEGs and video-EEGs may indicate a localized onset of seizures if only few seizures are recorded. The multifocal character of the seizures becomes evident only with prolonged video-EEG monitoring,[22] suggesting that long-term monitoring has an important role in the diagnosis of this disease. EEGs reflect the escalation of seizure activity, because no infant continues to have a normal EEG. Soon, the EEG background activity becomes slow with fluctuating asymmetry, one hemisphere exhibiting slow activity on one recording, the other one on the next recording. Multifocal spikes are present in all instances. When seizures become very frequent, an interictal state can no longer be identified. All patients have electrographic seizures with a monomorphic pattern that is identical from seizure to seizure in each patient. It consists of focal rhythmic theta or alpha activity beginning in one region and progressively involving the adjacent areas. The location of the ictal onset varies not only from side to side, but also within a hemisphere. Electrographically, the single ictal event can shift from one region to another and from one hemisphere to the other, and additional seizures beginning in other areas in either hemisphere could start before the end of the first event or immediately follow it (Fig. 1).[3,11] The centrotemporal region seems to be the most common site of seizure onset,[10,13] although posterior temporal, frontal, and occipital onsets are also observed. Most seizures are electroclinical, but frequent subclinical discharges also occur.[3,13] Although in some studies video-EEG makes it possible to define the correlation between the topography of the EEG ictal discharge and the clinical manifestations,[2,3] in others the clinical features did not correlate with the hemisphere involved.[10] When there is a good clinical/EEG correlation,[2,3] occipital EEG seizures correlate with lateral deviation of head and eyes and lateral eye jerks; rolandic discharges correspond to contralateral limb clonus; temporal discharges are associated with chewing movements and staring; and frontal seizures are related to limb hypertonia of either side. In older children, the amplitude of ictal discharge tends to increase, more seizures generalize, and the frontal areas are more frequently affected. In children EEG documented the disappearance of spikes and sharp waves and the reappearance of sleep/wake differentiation.[11,15] In contrast, if seizures continue, stopping only when they "burn out," EEG is characterized by low-voltage, slow activity, as described by Gross-Tsur et al.[10]

Neuroimaging and Laboratory Examinations

CT and MRI performed at the beginning of the illness are normal, as are single photon emission computed tomography (SPECT),[15] fluoro-2-deoxyglucose/positron emission tomography (PET) scan,[11] and MRI with spectroscopy.[13] On follow-up, CT and MRI, when abnormal, show progressive atrophy of both the cortex and subcortical white matter with enlargement of subarachnoid and ventricular spaces.[3,10] MRI spectroscopy discloses decreased *N*-acetyl aspartate in the frontal cortex and basal ganglia.[10]

Laboratory findings, including karyotype, cerebrospinal fluid (CSF) biochemistry and neurotransmitters, liver function tests, extensive metabolic evaluation with ammonia, serum lactate and pyruvate, serum amino acids, urine organic acids, CSF amino acids, CSF lactate/pyruvate, serum folate, sulfocystein, succinylpurine screening, serum copper level, ceruloplasmin, chromatography purine and pyrimidine, uricemia, β-galactosidase, β-hexosaminidase A and B, as well as respiratory chain enzymes, are unrevealing. Skin, muscle, and liver biopsies are normal. In most cases, brainstem auditory-evoked responses (BAERs), electroretinogram, visual- and somatosensory-evoked potentials (VEPs and SEPs), as well as nerve conduction velocities are also normal. In one case, SEP showed a mild increase in central conduction time,[17] and in another, BAERs had absent waves I and II in the left side, right interpeak latency prolonged, and decreased amplitude of wave V bilaterally.[15] Autopsy was performed in three cases.[3,22] Although neuropathologic examination manifested no evidence of hippocampal sclerosis, cortical dysplasia, or neuronal migration defects in one case,[22] there was revealed severe hippocampal neuronal loss and accompanying gliosis in the two others.[3] In particular, in those cases, there was almost complete neuronal loss, with reactive gliosis of the CA1 sector of the pyramidal layer of the Ammon horn in the hippocampus and also a mild neuronal loss and gliosis in the hilus of the dentate gyrus. The neocortex exhibited only minimal lesions, consisting of microvacuolization and gliosis in discrete areas of the molecular layer in one case, whereas it was normal in the other. The cerebellum was normal in both.

DIFFERENTIAL DIAGNOSIS

The spectrum of neonatal and early infantile epilepsy syndromes is broad and ranges from relatively mild to severe.[1,6,16] In addition, there are symptomatic and cryptogenic focal epilepsies beginning in the neonatal period. MPSI may be misdiagnosed as refractory focal epilepsy, which could lead to inappropriate surgical procedures.[8] Indeed, initial EEGs and video-EEG monitoring may initially suggest a localized onset for the seizures, and their multifocal character becomes evident only later, and when prolonged video-EEG monitoring. Whereas in symptomatic or probably symptomatic focal epilepsies seizures alway arise from the same cortical area, indicating a localized pathologic process, seizures in MPSI, originate from multiple focal areas, demonstrating the involvement of the whole cortex. Given the unique clinical and EEG features exhibited by children with MPSI, it is extremely unlikely that this condition could be mistaken for one of the severe epileptic syndromes of neonatal or infantile periods, such as early myoclonic encephalopathy (EME),[1] early infantile epileptic encephalopathy (EIEE),[1] or West syndrome.[6] All of these entities have typical interictal EEG patterns, such as burst-suppression in EME and EIEE and hypsarrhythmia in West syndrome. In contrast to EIEE and West syndrome, spasms are lacking in MPSI.

Multifocal electrographic seizures in the neonate are a common nonspecific feature following various types of brain insults, such as infections, metabolic disorders, or hypoxia-ischemia.[20] However, in these conditions, frequent seizures tend to be confined to the acute phase of the illness. Cerebral damage from hypoxic-ischemic encephalopathy or infection is readily demonstrated with neuroimaging, which is normal in MPSI.

Pyridoxine and pyridoxal phosphate dependencies should be considered, especially in those cases with onset of multifocal seizures within the first hours or days of life and no apparent cause. The differential diagnosis is made by a therapeutic trial of intravenous pyridoxine with simultaneous EEG monitoring or oral pyridoxal phosphate, the lack of response excluding these hypotheses.

Alpers disease is a rare autosomal recessive hepatocerebral syndrome of early onset characterized by progressive neuronal degeneration with liver involvement. This entity has been recently associated with mitochondrial DNA depletion and mutations.[5,14] Neurologic symptoms of Alpers disease include loss of previously learned skills and intractable myoclonic seizures. Progressive liver failure is considered an important hallmark of Alpers disease, and in the reported patients with MPSI, liver function tests and/or liver biopsy were normal. However, none of them underwent mitochondrial DNA testing.

The normal development before onset of seizures, absence of an identifiable cause, time of onset, tendency of seizures to occur in clusters, as well as the clinical and EEG features of the seizures may overlap similiar features in the benign partial epilepsies in neonates or infants, such as benign partial epilepsy in infancy,[21] benign familial and nonfamilial neonatal seizures,[16] and benign infantile familial seizures.[9,18,19] Even in the most benign conditions, such as benign neonatal seizures and benign infantile familial seizures, seizures can occur in clusters involving various areas of the cortex. The ictal manifestations in these benign syndromes show many similarities to those of MPSI, including eye deviation, head rotation, clonic movements of the face and limbs, tonic stiffening, and secondary generalization. However, although intense, the period of seizure activity is usually brief and there is a marked difference in outcome. Giordano et al.[9] described a large family with benign familial infantile seizures in which seizures began at 3 to 4 months of age and stopped by 11 months in every infant with no treatment. All were seizure free with normal psychomotor development at follow-up, in contrast to MPSI, in which seizures are almost continuous for several months, there is developmental regression, and interictal EEG becomes progressively more abnormal with both multifocal epileptiform activity and slowing.

TREATMENT AND OUTCOME

Conventional AED treatments, including phenobarbital, phenytoin, carbamazepine, valproate, vigabatrin, clonazepam, nitrazepam, midazolam, lamotrigine, steroids, and ACTH, have proved ineffective. Vigabatrin and carbamazepine may worsen seizures. These data should help in avoiding overtreatment with conventional AEDs that are consistently ineffective. Trials with various vitamins, including pyridoxine, biotin, and folinic acid, have been done without success. Four patients have been placed on the ketogenic diet with little or no improvement.[13,15] Among the new antiepileptic drugs, zonisamide and topiramate (C. Chiron, personal communication) have been tried and found to be ineffective. Successful control of seizures was reported with a combination of clonazepam and stiripentol in two patients[3] and with potassium bromide in two others[15] but was not confirmed in another.[11] The first use of levetiracetam was recently reported in a newborn with MPSI[11] and proved to be well tolerated and effective in reducing the seizure frequency even if complete seizure control was never achieved. Among the 33 cases with MPSI, death has been reported in 8 patients (25%), mostly before the age of 1 year.[3,10,11,17,22] The majority of these patients failed to respond favorably to various AED combinations. Nevertheless, one of them died unexpectedly despite a positive evolution over several months in terms of seizure control and clinical improvement.[11] The cause of death in this syndrome remains unclear and largely undocumented. In many cases, the parent's denial of postmortem examination precluded a proper investigation into the causes of death.

LONG-TERM PROGNOSIS

In most cases, the prognosis has been poor. Seizures remained severely intractable, patients develop microcephaly and hypotonia during the first year of life, and all skills are typically lost within a few months of onset of the illness. There is a trend toward progressively diminishing head-circumference percentiles, hypotonia, and developmental delay, but a few patients are occasionally less severely affected, with only mild to moderate mental retardation. These findings of a slightly better outcome are not dissimilar to those of other types of early-onset catastrophic epilepsies such as West syndrome, in which a few children may escape the expected sever outcomes.

SUMMARY AND CONCLUSIONS

Various epileptic syndromes with onset in the neonatal period or infancy have been identified by age of onset, seizure types, and interictal clinical and EEG characteristics.[7] MPSI is a newly recognized epileptic syndrome, unusual but often overlooked, that begins in the first 6 months of life in apparently normal infants, and in which very frequent seizures involve multiple independent areas of both hemispheres with arrest of psychomotor development. No causes have been identified, and no familial cases have been reported. Clinical, EEG, and follow-up data suggest that MPSI may rank among the catastrophic seizure syndromes of infancy. It is unclear whether the progression of the disease is the cause of the intractable seizures or its consequence. In our opinion, the high frequency of seizures and epileptiform abnormalities is a major cause of the psychomotor deterioration observed in these infants in coincidence with the onset of seizures. For this reason, we believe that MPSI should be included among the epileptic encephalopathies as defined by the ILAE in 2001.[7]

References

1. Aicardi J, Ohtahara S. Severe neonatal epilepsies with suppression-burst pattern. In: Roger J, Bureau M, Dravet C, et al., eds. *Epileptic Syndromes in Infancy, Childhood and Adolescence,* 4th ed. Eastleigh, UK: John Libbey; 2005:39–50.
2. Chiron C, Soufflet C, Pollack C, et al. Semiology of cryptogenic multifocal partial seizures in infancy. *Clin Neurophysiol.* 1988;70:9P–16P.
3. Coppola G, Plouin P, Chiron C, et al. Migrating partial seizures in infancy: a malignant disorder with developmental arrest. *Epilepsia.* 1995;36:1017–1024.
4. Coppola G, Veggiotti P, Miraglia del Giudice E, et al. Mutational scanning of potassium, sodium and chloride ion channels in malignant migrating partial seizures in infancy. *Brain Dev.* 2006;28:76–79.
5. Davidzon G, Mancuso M, Ferraris S, et al. POLG mutations and Alpers syndrome. *Ann Neurol.* 2005;57:921–923.
6. Dulac O, Tuxhorn I. Infantile spasms and West syndrome. In: Roger J, Bureau M, Dravet C, et al., eds. *Epileptic Syndromes in Infancy, Childhood and Adolescence,* 4th ed. Eastleigh, UK: John Libbey; 2005:53–72.
7. Engel JJ. International League Against Epilepsy. A proposed diagnostic scheme for people with epileptic seizures and with epilepsy: report of the ILAE Task Force on Classification and Terminology. *Epilepsia.* 2001;42:796–803.
8. Gérard F, Kaminska A, Plouin P, et al. Focal seizures versus focal epilepsy in infancy: a challenge distinction. *Epileptic Disorders.* 1999;1:135–139.
9. Giordano L, Accorsi P, Valseriati D, et al. Benign infantile familial convulsions: natural history of a case and clinical characteristics of a large Italian family. *Neuropediatrics.* 1999;30:99–101.
10. Gross-Tsur V, Ben-Zeev B, Shalev RS. Malignant migrating partial seizures in infancy. *Pediatr Neurol.* 2004;31:287–290.
11. Hmaimess G, Kadhim H, Nassogne MC, et al. Levetiracetam in a neonate with malignant migrating partial seizures. *Pediatr Neurol.* 2006;34:55–59.
12. Ishii K, Oguni H, Hayashi K, et al. Clinical study of catastrophic infantile epilepsy with focal seizures. *Pediatr Neurol.* 2002;27:369–377.
13. Marsh E, Melamed SE, Barron T, et al. Migrating partial seizures in infancy: expanding the phenotype of a rare seizure syndrome. *Epilepsia.* 2005;46:568–572.
14. Naviaux RK, Nguyen KV. POLG mutations associated with Alpers' syndrome and mitochondrial DNA depletion. *Ann Neurol.* 2004;55:706–712.
15. Okuda K, Yasuhara A, Kamei A, et al. Successful control with bromide of two patients with malignant migrating partial seizures in infancy. *Brain Dev.* 2000;22:56–59.
16. Plouin P, Anderson VE. Benign familial and non-familial neonatal seizures. In: Roger J, Bureau M, Dravet C, et al., eds. *Epileptic Syndromes in Infancy, Childhood and Adolescence,* 4th ed. Eastleigh, UK: John Libbey; 2005:3–15.
17. Veneselli E, Perrone MV, Di Rocco M, et al. Malignant migrating partial seizures in infancy. *Epilepsy Res.* 2001;46:27–32.
18. Vigevano F. Benign familial infantile seizures. *Brain Dev.* 2005;27:172–177.
19. Vigevano F, Fusco L, Di Capua M, et al. Benign infantile familial convulsions. *Eur J Pediatr.* 1992;151:608–612.
20. Volpe JJ. *Neurology of the Newborn.* 4th ed. Philadelphia: WB Saunders; 2001.
21. Watanabe K, Okumura A. Benign partial epilepsies in infancy. *Brain Dev.* 2000;22:296–300.
22. Wilmshurst JM, Appleton BD, Grattan-Smith PJ. Migrating partial seizures in infancy: two new cases. *J Child Neurol.* 1999;15:717–722.

CHAPTER 229 ■ WEST SYNDROME

OLIVIER DULAC, BERNARDO DALLA BERNARDINA, AND CATHERINE CHIRON

INTRODUCTION

The occurrence of clusters of axial movements in the first year of life, combined with major and subcontinuous electroencephalographic (EEG) paroxysmal activity called hypsarrhythmia, is the most frequent cause of psychomotor deterioration in infancy. This condition, usually termed either infantile spasms (IS) or West syndrome (WS), is a model for the study of epilepsy, because although the etiology, clinical and EEG expression, and outcome vary greatly from one patient to another, there is growing evidence that the etiology determines both expression and outcome in each given patient. The term *IS* denotes a specific age of onset and is therefore a syndromic concept. Because the concept of *West syndrome* usually includes hypsarrhythmia, this term should be considered more restrictive than the term *IS*. The clinical and EEG pattern is described in Chapter 54 (Spasms). This chapter concentrates on recent findings concerning correlation with etiology and the contribution of these findings to the understanding of pathophysiology.

HISTORICAL PERSPECTIVES

Over 160 years ago, West reported a condition that is probably the first epilepsy syndrome ever described. It was characterized by spasms as a particular seizure type not reported earlier and also by occurrence in infancy and mental deterioration. The condition did not become widely recognized as an epilepsy syndrome until 100 years later, however, when the particular EEG pattern was defined. Nevertheless, epileptic spasms were not recognized as a particular type of seizure and were therefore not included in the international classification,[80] although it is clear that their occurrence is not restricted to West syndrome, and they may occur beyond infancy.

BASIC MECHANISMS

A large variety of cerebral lesions may cause IS. Classic concepts of basic mechanisms suggest that IS are generated in subcortical structures, with ascending activity producing hypsarrhythmia and descending activity producing the seizures, a concept very similar to that of so-called centrencephalic epilepsy.[39,43] This view fails to take in account the predominantly cortical lesions determined radiologically and by neuropathologic studies. According to a newer concept, based on the potential recovery following removal of cortical lesions, the subcortical structures supposedly producing hypsarrhythmia and spasms are triggered by discharges in the cortical lesion.[10,15] During an ictal event, electrocorticography recording detects a focal spike triggering the fast-wave burst[2] and near-infrared spectroscopy multiple cortical areas activated simultaneously or sequentially.[70] However, this hypothesis does not clarify the age relationship, the variability of outcome, and especially the correlation of clinical and EEG pattern with etiology. The neurobiologic characteristics of the developing brain cortex, including age-dependent hyperexcitability and anteroposterior gradient of maturation, are the features most likely to contribute to the clinical and EEG pattern, including variations in outcome of epilepsy and cognitive disorders.[26] According to this hypothesis, continuous paroxysmal activity in the cortex, resulting from cortical damage, age-related functional instability, or both, produces nonconvulsive status epilepticus, accounting for the psychomotor deterioration, and determines the disinhibition of subcortical structures that generate the spasms. A model based on an unbalanced maturational pattern in brain structures leading to developmental desynchronization has recently been proposed for IS.[38] A transient developmental particularity is also the key of Baram's hypothesis at the origin of IS: The excessive secretion by hypothalamus of a highly convulsant peptide in immature brain, cortico-releasing factor, would be reduced by feedback using adrenocorticotropic hormone (ACTH) as treatment of IS.[4]

CLINICAL CHARACTERISTICS OF THE SYNDROME

For these, see also Chapter 54.

Seizures

Epileptic spasms consist of axial contractions that may occur in flexion, extension, or both, and that may be symmetric or asymmetric. Asymmetry may involve the upper limbs, head, or eyes, and video recording is often required for detailed analysis. The contractions are usually brief and differ from myoclonic and tonic fits. They occur in clusters, occasionally combined with a focal discharge. Between spasms of a cluster, the interictal EEG pattern may or may not recur, which distinguishes "independent" from "nonindependent" spasms. Other types of seizures—myoclonic, tonic, or partial—may occur before, in combination with, or after the cluster of spasms.

Psychomotor Development

Psychomotor development can be been normal or abnormal before the first spasms. Deterioration at onset of spasms is a usual feature. However, some patients do not deteriorate and may even make further progress in development after onset of the disorder.

Interictal Electroencephalogram

The interictal EEG pattern is quite variable. Hypsarrhythmia as defined by Gibbs and Gibbs,[40] consisting of more or less continuous activity of high-amplitude, asynchronous spikes-and-slow-waves without any physiologic activity, involves only a small proportion of cases. Other patterns consist of asymmetric hypsarrhythmia, focal or multifocal spikes with secondary generalization during sleep, and patterns that are more specific to particular causes of the disorder, including suppression bursts.

Age of Onset

Onset of IS usually occurs in the middle of the first year of life. Onset is rare before 3 months and after 1 year of age, which is considered to be the upper limit of occurrence of the syndrome in the classification of epilepsy syndromes.[80] In one series, however, >2% of patients with IS had their first seizure after the age of 12 months, and cases with onset in the fourth year of life are on record.[5]

Outcome

The range of outcomes is wide; spontaneous recovery may occur in 6% to 16% of patients. Others still have spasms after the end of the first decade of life. Different types of seizure disorders may occur, including partial epilepsy with one or more foci, Lennox-Gastaut syndrome, and other types of symptomatic generalized epilepsy. Mental retardation and various types of specific cognitive disorders are involved.

Thus, the pattern of IS is extremely variable from patient to patient in terms of clinical and EEG features and outcome. Etiology seems to be the major factor determining the characteristics of each component. Whatever the cause, age of onset and seizure type are similar among patients. The syndrome can therefore either be subdivided according to specific patterns or considered as a single disorder. The following discussion will show that both approaches are productive in terms of understanding clinical expression and outcome.

PATTERN OF INFANTILE SPASMS ACCORDING TO ETIOLOGY

Malformations

Aicardi Syndrome

Aicardi syndrome is characterized by IS, chorioretinal lacunae, and callosal agenesis. Although often overlooked, the presence of widespread polymicrogyria probably contributes to the severe epilepsy; paraventricular heterotopia and occasional plexus papilloma are also frequently observed.

Initial seizures occur before 3 months of age in 68% of patients and before 1 month in 23%. Partial seizures usually precede epileptic spasms by 1 to 6 weeks, and spasms most often are characterized by asymmetry of contraction of the upper limbs and lateral deviation of the head and eyes.

Interictal EEG is characterized by asymmetry or asynchrony of both hemispheres with unilateral hypsarrhythmia, a pattern called *split brain*[34]; it is now clear, however, that the pattern does not result from callosal agenesis, because patients with callosal agenesis and IS of other etiology do not exhibit a similar pattern. At disease onset, patients often have a diffuse, asymmetric, or unilateral suppression-burst pattern. Focal discharges may arise from the smaller or more malformed hemisphere.[21] Electroencephalographic recordings of ictal events demonstrate that in many instances the cluster of spasms is combined with a focal discharge.[9,10] Spasms prove to be extremely resistant to treatment, and they often persist after the end of the first decade. Most patients exhibit severe mental retardation and remain bedridden, and the mortality rate is high. However, some patients acquire the ability to walk.[65]

Agyria, Pachygyria, and Laminar Heterotopia

Various forms of diffuse disorders of cortical development, ranging from the four-layered cortex of agyria to laminar heterotopia, may produce IS. Agyria with microcephaly resulting from chromosomal deletion of 17p13 and agyria-pachygyria with no obvious chromosomal deletion produce IS in most cases.[8,24] Laminar heterotopia mainly involves female infants and rarely produces IS.[74,75] A few families have been reported with girls exhibiting laminar heterotopia and boys agyria, with X-linked dominant transmission.[22,78]

In cases of agyria and pachygyria, epilepsy may be manifested by early partial seizures before epileptic spasms occur. Interictal EEG demonstrates diffuse, high-amplitude rhythmic activity in the theta or alpha range that becomes discontinuous during sleep.[32] A similar pattern is occasionally seen in laminar heterotopia. Polygraphic recording shows the disappearance of high-amplitude interictal activity between spasms of a cluster. A functional imaging study with single-photon emission computed tomography (SPECT) showed no anteroposterior gradient of cerebral blood flow and no modification with age, in contrast with the maturation observed in normal infants, thus demonstrating the lack of normal maturation of the cortex.[14] This is correlated with the persistence of spasms, which may last beyond the end of the first decade.

Hemimegalencephaly, Focal Cortical Dysplasia, and Hamartoma

In hemimegalencephaly, one hemisphere and the corresponding lateral ventricle are larger than the other, and the cortex on the affected side is thick with giant neurons and abnormal lamination.[83] In focal cortical dysplasia, similar but less extensive histologic abnormalities are observed.

Epileptic spasms occur in half of cases of hemimegalencephaly.[104] During a spasm, contraction of the upper limbs is asymmetric. The period of IS is usually preceded and followed by partial seizures. A similar pattern may be produced by focal cortical dysplasia, particularly when it is located in the occipital lobe[58] or recently individualized as hemi-hemimegalencephaly if extended to the posterior quadrant.[20] Here, the asymmetry involves eye deviation rather than the upper limbs. Electroencephalographic findings may include triphasic spikes in the first week of life. During the period of IS, EEG usually demonstrates an asymmetric suppression-burst pattern.[73] Detection of focal cortical dysplasia may be difficult, even on new-generation magnetic resonance imaging (MRI machines). Functional imaging is helpful,[16] but IS are often associated with transient cortical, especially occipital, hypometabolic foci that are not necessarily associated with structural lesions and do not indicate a poor prognosis.

Several cases of prepeduncular hamartoma have been reported with IS.[37]

Bilateral Perisylvian Microgyria

Bilateral perisylvian microgyria appears to result from some ischemic event related to rapid growth of the perisylvian area in the second trimester of gestation. A small proportion of patients are affected with IS.[56] The EEG pattern consists of asymmetric hypsarrhythmia.

Neurocutaneous Syndromes

Tuberous Sclerosis

Half of all patients with tuberous sclerosis have IS, and tuberous sclerosis is the major cause of IS,[49] accounting for 7% to 25% of cases. The IS are often asymmetric or are preceded by or combined with partial seizures. Most patients with partial seizures in the first month of life progress to IS. This pattern is rare when partial seizures begin after 6 months of age.[27] Interictal EEG demonstrates diffuse spike-and-slow-wave activity that is rarely of the typical hypsarrhythmic pattern type. Waking traces usually show one or several spike-and-slow-wave foci with generalization during sleep. During drowsiness, spikes associated with physiologic hypnagogic hypersynchrony simulate the hypsarrhythmic pattern.[27] Even patients who exhibit true hypsarrhythmia have focal spikes or slow waves in a significantly higher proportion than do patients with cryptogenic West syndrome, particularly after administration of diazepam. Polygraphic recordings show that clusters of spasms may be initiated by a tonic or a focal discharge. The tracing between spasms does not return to the pattern seen before the onset of the cluster. Few spasms are isolated. Video recording shows that during the spasm the eyes or head may turn to the side opposite the interictal focus.

In 75% of patients, epileptic foci are correlated with the topography of large cortical tubers, suggesting that these malformations are the main epileptogenic cause.[17] The correlation is stronger for occipital than for frontal foci[96] because frontal foci are rare before the age of 2 years and because bilateral synchrony predominates in the frontal regions.[16] A functional imaging study in 25 patients used SPECT and MRI and showed that cortical tubers are hypoperfused, even before the first seizure occurs.[11] In active epilepsy, the area of hypoperfusion may be wider than that of the corresponding tuber. Patients with intractable epilepsy exhibit hypoperfused areas without corresponding cortical tubers, localized mostly in the temporal regions. This suggests that secondary epileptogenic foci contribute to intractability.

In the past, more than two thirds of patients with tuberous sclerosis and IS were left with mental retardation and behavioral disorders, and more than half exhibited autistic traits,[45] a rate twice that for all patients with IS. Mental retardation is linked to the number of tubers together with IS.[71] Intellectual outcome is significantly improved by the control of spasms and subsequent seizures.[41,48] Early treatment with vigabatrin, which controls spasms in >90% of cases,[13] prevents the development of autistic features in most instances, even in patients who still have intractable partial seizures.[47] Topography of tubers also plays a major role. Autistic traits with TS were linked to bilateral and combined anterior and posterior tubers,[49] whereas mental retardation is associated more with other generalized seizures in patients with bilateral anterior tubers. Patients with selective cognitive defects had had either transient IS rapidly controlled by therapy or infrequent partial seizures, and they had a single detectable cortical tuber.

Neurofibromatosis

The combination of neurofibromatosis and West syndrome is not coincidental.[69] Spasms are usually symmetric, with a typical hypsarrhythmic EEG, "independent" spasms on ictal EEG and no focal features. This is the only symptomatic condition having the clinical and EEG characteristics of "idiopathic West syndrome" in most patients. A single case of hemimegalencephaly with neurofibromatosis has been reported.[18]

Perinatal Hypoxia-Ischemia

Severe hypoxia-ischemia in full-term newborns producing convulsions in the neonatal period and IS in infancy has become a rare condition in developed countries. Electroencephalographic features are a markedly depressed tracing followed by a progressive return to normal or near normal before focal or multifocal spikes or sharp waves appear and foretell hypsarrhythmia.[107] The outcome of the spasms is rarely favorable,[103] and partial epilepsy with multiple foci or generalized epilepsy may occur in more than half of patients.

In premature infants, numerous positive rolandic spikes lasting several weeks indicate a high risk for periventricular leukomalacia. In two of nine patients, the spikes were followed by development of West syndrome.[72] Outcome of the epilepsy is favorable in most patients following steroid treatment, although they are left with spastic diplegia.[88] Regarding patients with periventricular leukomalacia, the occurrence of paroxysmal discharges as irregular spikes-and-waves and polyspikes-and-waves, mainly in bilateral parietooccipital areas, is predictive of the development of WS.[93] The timing of brain insult in premature infants who develop WS is determined by maturation, not by the term of delivery.[72]

Porencephaly

Among 173 patients with IS investigated by computed tomography (CT), Cusmai et al. found 10% to have focal lesions, mainly porencephaly.[19] Most patients had spasms as the first seizure type, although occasionally partial seizures preceded them.[1] Epileptic spasms are asymmetric in one third of cases, and the EEG shows asymmetric hypsarrhythmia with striking focal features.[19] Outcome is favorable, but partial epilepsy may occur by 2 to 3 years of age, mainly in patients with frontal porencephaly.

Chromosome Disorders

Down Syndrome

WS involves 1% to 3% of patients with Down syndrome. WS may result from ischemic brain lesions produced during delivery or may be caused by congenital heart disease. Nonetheless, the combination of Down syndrome and WS is not coincidental. In a series of 14 patients with Down syndrome who were followed from their first spasms,[89] spasms had begun at a mean age of 8 months, spasms were symmetric and associated with no other type of seizure, and mental deterioration involved tone and eye contact. Hypsarrhythmia was typical in 13 cases, asymmetric in 1. The spasms of 8 patients were recorded; these were "independent," and intravenous diazepam failed to show any focal feature. Therefore, the neurophysiologic features were those of idiopathic WS. However, unlike idiopathic WS, this condition is particularly resistant to treatment when its onset is delayed by >2 months, with significantly increased risk of autistic features and pharmacoresistance.[33,81] During the following years, patients often exhibited other types of seizures—myoclonic, tonic–clonic, or absences—that were usually easy to control. Thus, in contrast to brain malformations and tuberous sclerosis, and despite the fact that the gyral pattern in the temporal lobe is abnormal, Down syndrome does not exhibit the features of focal or diffuse brain malformations; rather, the characteristics are mainly those of a functional phenomenon, as in idiopathic epilepsies. However, functional consequences may be severe, possibly related to diagnostic delay with postural delay and the development of autistic features.

Deletions and Mutations

Sex-linked dominant inheritance involves incontinentia pigmenti; other families had Xp11.4-Xter, Xp11.4-Xp22.11[92] chromosomal translocation, and others had Williams[68] syndrome. Dysmorphia, hypotonia, and pyramidal signs are combined with inversion duplication[6] and partial hexasomy[44] of chromosome 15q. The 1p36 deletion with characteristic craniofacial abnormalities and mental retardation includes epilepsy, which often consists of severe IS when there is loss of the potassium channel beta-subunit gene, KCNAB2. Various familial dysmorphias are combined with IS, including broad thumbs,[98] cleft lip, and exophthalmos.[101] Familial IS with microcephaly and nephrotic syndrome[84] has been reported. Monogenic conditions are being recognized. Various abnormalities of Aristaless-related homeobox gene, ARX, produce IS in 12.5%[76] to 34% of the cases.[91] However, IS are not the only type of seizures, and myoclonic epilepsy does occur,[100] with some apparent genotype–phenotype correlation.[53] Missense mutations,[97] frameshift deletions,[87] and de novo balanced X autosome translocations[52] in the X-linked cyclin-dependent kinase–like 5 (CDKL5/STK9) gene produce early-onset severe IS. Mutation of the ATPase-sensitive potassium channel Kir6.2 is associated with IS.

Inborn Errors of Metabolism

They are rare and comprise a wide variety in which IS are but one expression of infantile convulsions. However, Menkes disease,[94] phenylketonuria and biopterin deficiency, and mitochondrial disease due to NARP mutation[62] comprise a high proportion of patients who develop IS. In Menkes disease, West syndrome is constant following the first occurrence of status.[4a] In phenylketonuria, WS affects 1 patient of 6, and the phenylalanine-free diet can only prevent its occurrence when started before the age of 3 months.[108] In biopterin deficiency with WS, the diet does not permit solution of the epilepsy, which needs steroid therapy.[66] The NARP mutation produces pharmacosensitive WS.[23] Complexes I, III, and IV and combined I and IV have also been reported in combination with WS.[7] Spasticity, nystagmus, apnea, and cardiac problems are usually combined in these cases.[99] The latter is easily recognized based on T2 hypersignal in the basal ganglia. Blood lactate is usually normal in patients with IS.[86] Schinzel-Giedion syndrome, which comprises several facial dysmorphisms, midface hypoplasia, and multiple skeletal anomalies, produces IS in one fourth of the cases.[42] In some families, hypsarrhythmia was combined with congenital encephalopathy, edema, and optic atrophy (PEHO) and was inherited as an autosomal recessive trait.[36,55,102]

Cryptogenic/Idiopathic West Syndrome

Of patients with IS, 15% to 32% have a normal development before the onset of spasms and exhibit no evidence of brain lesion.[54,63] These cases are classically designated as cryptogenic[39] or idiopathic.[50] According to the 1989 classification of epilepsies and epileptic syndromes, the terms are not synonymous; *cryptogenic* indicates that the origin is hidden, whereas *idiopathic* means that there is no cause other than the disease itself. In addition, according to this classification,[80] West syndrome may be either symptomatic or cryptogenic, but not idiopathic. However, a number of patients with West syndrome exhibit spontaneous disappearance of epilepsy and complete recovery of mental development.[3] The proportion of cryptogenic/idiopathic cases varies in the reported series from 15% to 53%, probably as a result of varying definitions of the condition. For idiopathic cases, the figures are 26% and 6% in the only two available series.[28,105] The latter series also show that based on clinical and neurophysiologic characteristics, it is often possible to differentiate cryptogenic from idiopathic cases.

Cases are considered to be *cryptogenic* when indirect evidence of focal or multifocal cortical involvement exists. Focal ictal discharges may be recorded between clusters of spasms by 24-hour ambulatory EEG.[79] During a cluster, a focal discharge may occur, and hypsarrhythmia does not usually recur between consecutive spasms.[25] In most instances, however, no focal discharge is recorded during a cluster, but again hypsarrhythmia does not recur between spasms, thus showing that the whole cluster is a single seizure. Parents often notice that the child's behavior changes before the first spasm, as an "aura" easily overlooked by the medical staff. Focal interictal abnormalities can be evidenced by reducing the amplitude of the recording or by the intravenous administration of diazepam. Neuropsychologic investigation at the onset of the disease may demonstrate loss of eye tracking or babbling, or asymmetry of grasping.[29] Focal dysplasia may be overlooked by MRI until myelination shows the blurred border between gray and white matter by the end of the second year of life. Inversion recovery or thin slices may be helpful. Functional imaging by SPECT[12] and positron emission tomography (PET)[15] may detect single or multiple abnormal cortical areas. Cases with demonstrated abnormalities should then be considered as symptomatic and treated as such. A majority of the remaining patients later exhibit partial or generalized epilepsy, including Lennox-Gastaut syndrome, associated with development of mental retardation, autistic features, speech delay with hyperkinesia, and visual disorders. The latter disorders are correlated with the topography of EEG and functional imaging foci, and a correlation could be found between subscores of the Brunet-Lézine test battery at onset of West syndrome and on follow-up.[46] Very few neuropathologic investigations have been reported. In patients with focal abnormalities, cortical dysplasia is usually observed. The pathologic significance of more widespread heterotopic neurons remains to be demonstrated.[64]

The term *idiopathic West syndrome* is used to designate the condition of patients who are considered to have no brain lesion and for whom epilepsy is a purely functional phenomenon. Identification of these patients at onset of the disease is based on lack of indirect signs of brain lesion. Normal development before spasms is extremely difficult to determine. In a prospective study, 12 of 14 patients had acquired the ability to grasp objects and all had acquired smiling and eye tracking; loss of milestones was mild, with only 1 patient having lost eye tracking.[31] Hypsarrhythmia is symmetric, with no spike-and-slow-wave focus after intravenous diazepam. Recorded clusters show reappearance of hypsarrhythmia between spasms and no focal discharge. In a later article, it was shown that significant diagnostic features include no loss of eye tracking and smiling. In regard to ictal EEG, it was shown that 12- to 14-hour ambulatory recording is necessary to analyze the characteristics of the cluster of spasms.[79]

"Lumping" Versus "Splitting"

It has become clear that the clinical and EEG features of IS mainly depend on its cause. Asymmetric spasms indicate a cortical brain lesion, thus demonstrating the cortical contribution to the genesis of the spasms. The EEG pattern may be specific for a given brain malformation, thus showing that it is determined by the cortical abnormality, not by the epilepsy. Secondary generalization may result from single focal or multifocal epileptogenic brain lesions, such as tuberous sclerotic lesions or anoxoischemic lesions after term delivery.

Hypsarrhythmia is an age-related dysfunction of the brain cortex occurring around a focal lesion or without any evidence of structural lesion.[26]

This correlation of clinical and EEG expression with etiology has three implications: (a) The diagnosis may be suspected based on clinical and EEG characteristics, which may contribute to an improved imaging workup; (b) evaluation of the prognosis may be improved, particularly when the characteristics of idiopathic West syndrome are present; and (c) therapeutic decisions may be made more specifically, according to etiology. For instance, vigabatrin has been shown to be better than steroids in tuberous sclerosis in a randomized, prospective trial.[13]

TREATMENT

The major drugs that have been shown to be effective in IS are steroids and vigabatrin. Considering an evidence-based approach, ACTH is "probably" effective in the short-term treatment and vigabatrin (VGB) "possibly" effective.[61] They both have side effects, although different in potential severity: Vigabatrin may induce bilateral restriction of the peripheral visual field in around 20% of cases, whereas steroid therapy carries a mortality rate from 2.3%[57] to 4.9%.[82] Most conventional antiepileptic compounds are ineffective, but some patients respond to valproic acid, lamotrigine, high doses of pyridoxine, topiramate, sulthiame, and zonisamide. Carbamazepine may even worsen the condition, which is an important finding in view of the possible combination of IS with focal seizures.[95] Very little has been reported with ketogenic diet in WS. In our hands, it proved occasionally but rarely effective in patients who had not responded to VGB and steroids. The evidence for an effect as first-line treatment remains to be evaluated.[85]

It has been advocated not to give aggressive treatment, that is, steroids, to patients with IS symptomatic of brain injury because the side effects would exceed the mild benefits. However, this assertion mainly results from the major dispersion of mental functions before the first spasms, of psychomotor regression at the onset of the disorder, and of the ability of treatment to control seizures and interictal paroxysmal activity. When focusing on a single etiology, it appears that treatment schedules are not equal. For instance, vigabatrin as initial therapy proved to be more efficient than steroids in tuberous sclerosis[13] but less in other etiologies[59] at 2-week treatment. Developmental and socialization outcomes are favorably influenced by early and rapid control of spasms with vigabatrin in tuberous sclerosis[47] but with steroids in cryptogenic cases.[35,60] On the other hand, up to 10% of patients seem to recover spontaneously.[3,30] Therefore, early, tailored and sometimes aggressive treatment is required to achieve total control of seizures and paroxysmal EEG abnormalities.

Treatment strategy mainly depends on drug availability in different countries. In most countries, VGB is considered the drug of choice as first-line monotherapy, the major remaining question being for how long. In cryptogenic cases, 6 months seems reasonable. For tuberous sclerosis, the risk of a severe and intractable relapse persists until the age of 5 years. Adding steroids to VGB seems to be more effective than steroids alone, but, again, whether VGB should be continued for a long period needs to be clarified. In a prospective population study, it could be shown that tailored choices are useful for steroid treatment, using hydrocortisone for 2 weeks and then switching to ACTH in case of failure. Recovery is only considered when both the spasms and EEG paroxysmal activities have ceased.[106]

Surgical removal of an epileptogenic cortical brain lesion can be effective, provided it is the only lesion. Patients with tumors, focal dysplasia or hemimegalencephaly, and porencephaly have all benefited from removal or disconnection of the lesion, with cessation of epilepsy and improvement in psychomotor development.[67,90] The earlier the surgery, the better is the developmental outcome.[51] Identifying the lesion by imaging may be an issue before the age of 18 months, when myelin has become mature, thus showing properly the white/gray border. Total callosotomy was useful in 80% of children who underwent this procedure after having acquired walking. However, if the child is able to speak, it should be performed before the age of 10 years to avoid the risk of deterioration of this ability. Both anterior and posterior sections proved to be ineffective.[77]

SUMMARY AND CONCLUSIONS

Although each of the various causes of IS is associated with quite specific features, the age of onset, main seizure type, and occurrence of generalized paroxysmal activity are similar for all patients. The similarity of these three characteristics among patients is sufficient to delineate a syndrome, although other characteristics vary widely according to underlying cause.

References

1. Alvarez LA, Shinnar S, Moshe SL. Infantile spasms due to unilateral cerebral infarcts. *Pediatrics.* 1987;79(6):1024–1026.
2. Asano E, Juhasz C, Shah A, et al. Origin and propagation of epileptic spasms delineated on electrocorticography. *Epilepsia.* 2005;46(7):1086–1097.
3. Bachman DS. Spontaneous remission of infantile spasms with hypsarhythmia. *Arch Neurol.* 1981;38(12):785.
4. Baram TZ, Mitchell WG, Brunson K, et al. Infantile spasms: hypothesis-driven therapy and pilot human infant experiments using corticotropin-releasing hormone receptor antagonists. *Dev Neurosci.* 1999;21(3–5):281–289.
5. Bednarek N, Motte J, Soufflet C, et al. Evidence of late-onset infantile spasms. *Epilepsia.* 1998;39(1):55–60.
6. Bingham PM, Spinner NB, Sovinsky L, et al. Infantile spasms associated with proximal duplication of chromosome 15q. *Pediatr Neurol.* 1996;15(2):163–165.
7. Blanco-Barca O, Pintos-Martinez E, Alonso-Martin A, et al. Mitochondrial encephalomyopathies and West's syndrome: a frequently underdiagnosed association [in Spanish]. *Rev Neurol.* 2004;39(7):618–623.
8. Bordarier C, Robain O, Rethore MO, et al. Inverted neurons in agyria. A Golgi study of a case with abnormal chromosome 17. *Hum Genet.* 1986;73(4):374–378.
9. Bour F, Chiron C, Dulac O, et al. Electroclinical characteristics of seizures in the Aicardi syndrome [in French]. *Rev Electroencephalogr Neurophysiol Clin.* 1986;16(4):341–353.
10. Carrazana EJ, Lombroso CT, Mikati M, et al. Facilitation of infantile spasms by partial seizures. *Epilepsia.* 1993;34(1):97–109.
11. Chiron C, Dulac O. Brain function imaging in epileptic children [in French]. *Arch Fr Pediatr.* 1990;47(9):629–632.
12. Chiron C, Dulac O, Bulteau C, et al. Study of regional cerebral blood flow in West syndrome. *Epilepsia.* 1993;34(4):707–715.
13. Chiron C, Dumas C, Jambaque I, et al. Randomized trial comparing vigabatrin and hydrocortisone in infantile spasms due to tuberous sclerosis. *Epilepsy Res.* 1997;26(2):389–395.
14. Chiron C, Nabbout R, Pinton F, et al. Brain functional imaging SPECT in agyria-pachygyria. *Epilepsy Res.* 1996;24(2):109–117.
15. Chugani HT, Shields WD, Shewmon DA, et al. Infantile spasms: I. PET identifies focal cortical dysgenesis in cryptogenic cases for surgical treatment. *Ann Neurol.* 1990;27(4):406–413.
16. Curatolo P, Seri S, Verdecchia M, et al. Infantile spasms in tuberous sclerosis complex. *Brain Dev.* 2001;23(7):502–507.
17. Cusmai R, Chiron C, Curatolo P, et al. Topographic comparative study of magnetic resonance imaging and electroencephalography in 34 children with tuberous sclerosis. *Epilepsia.* 1990;31(6):747–755.
18. Cusmai R, Curatolo P, Mangano S, et al. Hemimegalencephaly and neurofibromatosis. *Neuropediatrics.* 1990;21(4):179–182.
19. Cusmai R, Ricci S, Pinard JM, et al. West syndrome due to perinatal insults. *Epilepsia.* 1993;34(4):738–742.
20. D'Agostino MD, Bastos A, Piras C, et al. Posterior quadrantic dysplasia or hemi-hemimegalencephaly: a characteristic brain malformation. *Neurology.* 2004;62(12):2214–2220.
21. de Jong JG, Delleman JW, Houben M, et al. Agenesis of the corpus callosum, infantile spasms, ocular anomalies (Aicardi's syndrome). Clinical and pathologic findings. *Neurology.* 1976;26(12):1152–1158.

22. des Portes V, Pinard JM, Billuart P, et al. A novel CNS gene required for neuronal migration and involved in X-linked subcortical laminar heterotopia and lissencephaly syndrome. *Cell.* 1998;92(1):51–61.
23. Desguerre I, Pinton F, Nabbout R, et al. Infantile spasms with basal ganglia MRI hypersignal may reveal mitochondrial disorder due to T8993G MT DNA mutation. *Neuropediatrics.* 2003;34(5):265–269.
24. Dobyns WB, Stratton RF, Greenberg F. Syndromes with lissencephaly. I: Miller-Dieker and Norman-Roberts syndromes and isolated lissencephaly. *Am J Med Genet.* 1984;18(3):509–526.
25. Donat JF. The age-dependent epileptic encephalopathies. *J Child Neurol.* 1992;7(1):7–21.
26. Dulac O, Chiron C, Robain O, et al. Infantile spasms: a pathophysiological hypothesis. *Semin Pediatr Neurol.* 1994;1(2):83–89.
27. Dulac O, Lemaitre A, Plouin P. Maladie de Bourneville: aspects cliniques et électroencéphalographiques de l'épilepsie dans la première année. *Boll Lega Ital Epil.* 1984: 39–42.
28. Dulac O, Plouin P, Jambaque I. Predicting favorable outcome in idiopathic West syndrome. *Epilepsia.* 1993;34(4):747–756.
29. Dulac O, Plouin P, Jambaque I. Predicting favorable outcome in idiopathic West syndrome. *Epilepsia.* 1993;34(4):747–756.
30. Dulac O, Plouin P, Jambaque I, et al. Benign epileptic infantile spasms [in French]. *Rev Electroencephalogr Neurophysiol Clin* 1986;16(4):371–382.
31. Dulac O, Plouin P, Jambaque I, et al. Benign epileptic infantile spasms [in French]. *Rev Electroencephalogr Neurophysiol Clin.* 1986 Dec;16(4):371–382.
32. Dulac O, Plouin P, Perulli L, et al. Electroencephalographic aspects of classic agyria-pachygyria [in French]. *Rev Electroencephalogr Neurophysiol Clin.* 1983;13(3):232–239.
33. Eisermann MM, DeLaRaillere A, Dellatolas G, et al. Infantile spasms in Down syndrome—effects of delayed anticonvulsive treatment. *Epilepsy Res.* 2003;55(1–2):21–27.
34. Fariello RG, Chun RW, Doro JM, et al. EEG recognition of Aicardi's syndrome. *Arch Neurol.* 1977;34(9):563–566.
35. Ferrie CD, Beaumanoir A, Guerrini R, et al. Early-onset benign occipital seizure susceptibility syndrome. *Epilepsia.* 1997;38(3):285–293.
36. Field MJ, Grattan-Smith P, Piper SM, et al. PEHO and PEHO-like syndromes: report of five Australian cases. *Am J Med Genet A.* 2003;122(1): 6–12.
37. Fohlen M, Lellouch A, Delalande O. Hypothalamic hamartoma with refractory epilepsy: surgical procedures and results in 18 patients. *Epileptic Disord.* 2003;5(4):267–273.
38. Frost JD Jr, Hrachovy RA. Pathogenesis of infantile spasms: a model based on developmental desynchronization. *J Clin Neurophysiol.* 2005;22(1): 25–36.
39. Gastaut H, Roger J, Soulayrol R, et al. *L'encephalopathie myoclonique infantile avec hypsarythmie (syndrome de West).* Paris: Masson; 1964.
40. Gibbs FA, Gibbs EL. *Atlas of electroencephalography.* Reading, MA: Addison-Wesley; 1952.
41. Goh S, Kwiatkowski DJ, Dorer DJ, et al. Infantile spasms and intellectual outcomes in children with tuberous sclerosis complex. *Neurology.* 2005;65(2):235–238.
42. Grosso S, Pagano C, Cioni M, et al. Schinzel-Giedion syndrome: a further cause of West syndrome. *Brain Dev.* 2003;25(4):294–298.
43. Hrachovy RA, Frost JD Jr, Kellaway P. Sleep characteristics in infantile spasms. *Neurology.* 1981;31(6):688–693.
44. Huang B, Bartley J. Partial hexasomy of chromosome 15. *Am J Med Genet A.* 2003;121(3):277–280.
45. Hunt A, Dennis J. Psychiatric disorder among children with tuberous sclerosis. *Dev Med Child Neurol.* 1987;29(2):190–198.
46. Jambaque I, Chiron C, Dulac O, et al. Visual inattention in West syndrome: a neuropsychological and neurofunctional imaging study. *Epilepsia.* 1993;34(4):692–700.
47. Jambaque I, Chiron C, Dumas C, et al. Mental and behavioural outcome of infantile epilepsy treated by vigabatrin in tuberous sclerosis patients. *Epilepsy Res.* 2000;38(2–3):151–160.
48. Jambaque I, Cusmai R, Curatolo P, et al. Neuropsychological aspects of tuberous sclerosis in relation to epilepsy and MRI findings. *Dev Med Child Neurol.* 1991;33(8):698–705.
49. Jeavons PM, Bower BD. *Infantile Spasms: A Review of the Literature and a Study of 112 Cases.* London: Heinemann Medical; 1964.
50. Jeavons PM, Bower BD, Dimitrakoudi M. Long-term prognosis of 150 cases of "West syndrome." *Epilepsia.* 1973;14(2):153–164.
51. Jonas R, Asarnow RF, LoPresti C, et al. Surgery for symptomatic infant-onset epileptic encephalopathy with and without infantile spasms. *Neurology.* 2005;64(4):746–750.
52. Kalscheuer VM, Tao J, Donnelly A, et al. Disruption of the serine/threonine kinase 9 gene causes severe X-linked infantile spasms and mental retardation. *Am J Hum Genet.* 2003;72(6):1401–1411.
53. Kato M, Das S, Petras K, et al. Polyalanine expansion of ARX associated with cryptogenic West syndrome. *Neurology.* 2003;61(2):267–276.
54. Kellaway P, Hrachovy RA, Frost JD, et al. Precise characterization and quantification of infantile spasms. *Ann Neurol.* 1979;6(3):214–218.
55. Klein A, Schmitt B, Boltshauser E. Progressive encephalopathy with edema, hypsarrhythmia and optic atrophy (PEHO) syndrome in a Swiss child. *Eur J Paediatr Neurol.* 2004;8(6):317–321.
56. Kuzniecky R, Andermann F, Guerrini R. Infantile spasms: an early epileptic manifestation in some patients with the congenital bilateral perisylvian syndrome. *J Child Neurol.* 1994;9(4):420–423.
57. Lombroso CT. A prospective study of infantile spasms: clinical and therapeutic correlations. *Epilepsia.* 1983;24(2):135–158.
58. Lortie A, Plouin P, Chiron C, et al. Characteristics of epilepsy in focal cortical dysplasia in infancy. *Epilepsy Res.* 2002;51:133–145.
59. Lux AL, Edwards SW, Hancock E, et al. The United Kingdom Infantile Spasms Study comparing vigabatrin with prednisolone or tetracosactide at 14 days: a multicentre, randomised controlled trial. *Lancet.* 2004;364(9447):1773–1778.
60. Lux AL, Edwards SW, Hancock E, et al. The United Kingdom Infantile Spasms Study (UKISS) comparing hormone treatment with vigabatrin on developmental and epilepsy outcomes to age 14 months: a multicentre randomised trial. *Lancet Neurol.* 2005;4(11):712–717.
61. Mackay M, Weiss S, Snead OC III. Treatment of infantile spasms: an evidence-based approach. *Int Rev Neurobiol.* 2002;49:157–184.
62. Makela-Bengs P, Suomalainen A, Majander A, et al. Correlation between the clinical symptoms and the proportion of mitochondrial DNA carrying the 8993 point mutation in the NARP syndrome. *Pediatr Res.* 1995;37(5):634–639.
63. Matsumoto A, Watanabe K, Negoro T, et al. Infantile spasms: etiological factors, clinical aspects, and long term prognosis in 200 cases. *Eur J Pediatr.* 1981;135(3):239–244.
64. Meencke HJ, Janz D. The significance of microdysgenesia in primary generalized epilepsy: an answer to the considerations of Lyon and Gastaut. *Epilepsia.* 1985;26(4):368–371.
65. Menezes AV, MacGregor DL, Buncic JR. Aicardi syndrome: natural history and possible predictors of severity. *Pediatr Neurol.* 1994;11(4):313–318.
66. Mikaeloff Y, Pinton F, Sevin C, et al. Progressive convulsive encephalopathy: considering an abnormality of biopterin metabolism [in French]. *Arch Pediatr.* 1999;6(7):759–761.
67. Mimaki T, Ono J, Yabuuchi H. Temporal lobe astrocytoma with infantile spasms. *Ann Neurol.* 1983;14(6):695–696.
68. Mizugishi K, Yamanaka K, Kuwajima K, et al. Interstitial deletion of chromosome 7q in a patient with Williams syndrome and infantile spasms. *J Hum Genet.* 1998;43(3):178–181.
69. Motte J, Billard C, Fejerman N, et al. Neurofibromatosis type one and West syndrome: a relatively benign association. *Epilepsia.* 1993;34(4):723–736.
70. Munakata M, Haginoya K, Ishitobi M, et al. Dynamic cortical activity during spasms in three patients with West syndrome: a multichannel near-infrared spectroscopic topography study. *Epilepsia.* 2004;45(10):1248–1257.
71. O'Callaghan FJ, Harris T, Joinson C, et al. The relation of infantile spasms, tubers, and intelligence in tuberous sclerosis complex. *Arch Dis Child.* 2004;89(6):530–533.
72. Okumura A, Watanabe K, Hayakawa F, et al. The timing of brain insults in preterm infants who later developed West syndrome. *Neuropediatrics.* 2001;32(5):245–249.
73. Paladin F, Chiron C, Dulac O, et al. Electroencephalographic aspects of hemimegalencephaly. *Dev Med Child Neurol.* 1989;31(3):377–383.
74. Palmini A, Andermann F, Aicardi J, et al. Diffuse cortical dysplasia, or the 'double cortex' syndrome: the clinical and epileptic spectrum in 10 patients. *Neurology.* 1991;41(10):1656–1662.
75. Palmini A, Andermann F, Olivier A, et al. Focal neuronal migration disorders and intractable partial epilepsy: a study of 30 patients. *Ann Neurol.* 1991;30(6):741–749.
76. Partington MW, Turner G, Boyle J, et al. Three new families with X-linked mental retardation caused by the 428–451dup(24bp) mutation in ARX. *Clin Genet.* 2004;66(1):39–45.
77. Pinard JM, Delalande O, Chiron C, et al. Callosotomy for epilepsy after West syndrome. *Epilepsia* 1999;40(12):1727–1734.
78. Pinard JM, Motte J, Chiron C, et al. Subcortical laminar heterotopia and lissencephaly in two families: a single X linked dominant gene. *J Neurol Neurosurg Psychiatry.* 1994;57(8):914–920.
79. Plouin P, Dulac O, Jalin C, et al. Twenty-four-hour ambulatory EEG monitoring in infantile spasms. *Epilepsia.* 1993;34(4):686–691.
80. Proposal for revised classification of epilepsies and epileptic syndromes. Commission on Classification and Terminology of the International League Against Epilepsy. *Epilepsia.* 1989;30(4):389–399.
81. Rasmussen P, Borjesson O, Wentz E, et al. Autistic disorders in Down syndrome: background factors and clinical correlates. *Dev Med Child Neurol.* 2001;43(11):750–754.
82. Riikonen R, Donner M. ACTH therapy in infantile spasms: side effects. *Arch Dis Child.* 1980;55(9):664–672.
83. Robain O, Floquet C, Heldt N, et al. Hemimegalencephaly: a clinicopathological study of four cases. *Neuropathol Appl Neurobiol.* 1988;14(2):125–135.
84. Roos RA, Maaswinkel-Mooy PD, vd Loo EM, et al. Congenital microcephaly, infantile spasms, psychomotor retardation, and nephrotic syndrome in two sibs. *Eur J Pediatr.* 1987;146(5):532–526.
85. Rubenstein JE, Kossoff EH, Pyzik PL, et al. Experience in the use of the ketogenic diet as early therapy. *J Child Neurol.* 2005;20(1):31–34.
86. Sadleir LG, Connolly MB, Applegarth D, et al. Spasms in children with definite and probable mitochondrial disease. *Eur J Neurol.* 2004;11(2):103–110.

87. Scala E, Ariani F, Mari F, et al. CDKL5/STK9 is mutated in Rett syndrome variant with infantile spasms. *J Med Genet.* 2005;42(2):103–107.
88. Schlumberger E, Dulac O. A simple, effective and well-tolerated treatment regime for West syndrome. *Dev Med Child Neurol.* 1994;36(10):863–872.
89. Silva ML, Cieuta C, Guerrini R, et al. Early clinical and EEG features of infantile spasms in Down syndrome. *Epilepsia.* 1996;37(10):977–982.
90. Soufflet C, Bulteau C, Delalande O, et al. The nonmalformed hemisphere is secondarily impaired in young children with hemimegalencephaly: a pre- and postsurgery study with SPECT and EEG. *Epilepsia.* 2004;45(11):1375–1382.
91. Stromme P, Mangelsdorf ME, Scheffer IE, et al. Infantile spasms, dystonia, and other X-linked phenotypes caused by mutations in Aristaless related homeobox gene, ARX. *Brain Dev.* 2002;24(5):266–268.
92. Stromme P, Sundet K, Mork C, et al. X linked mental retardation and infantile spasms in a family: new clinical data and linkage to Xp11.4–Xp22.11. *J Med Genet.* 1999;36(5):374–378.
93. Suzuki M, Okumura A, Watanabe K, et al. The predictive value of electroencephalogram during early infancy for later development of West syndrome in infants with cystic periventricular leukomalacia. *Epilepsia.* 2003;44(3):443–446.
94. Sztriha L, Janaky M, Kiss J, et al. Electrophysiological and 99mTc-HMPAO-SPECT studies in Menkes disease. *Brain Dev.* 1994;16(3):224–228.
95. Talwar D, Arora MS, Sher PK. EEG changes and seizure exacerbation in young children treated with carbamazepine. *Epilepsia.* 1994;35(6):1154–1159.
96. Tamaki K, Okuno T, Ito M, et al. Magnetic resonance imaging in relation to EEG epileptic foci in tuberous sclerosis. *Brain Dev.* 1990;12(3):316–320.
97. Tao J, Van EH, Hagedorn-Greiwe M, et al. Mutations in the X-linked cyclin-dependent kinase–like 5 (CDKL5/STK9) gene are associated with severe neurodevelopmental retardation. *Am J Hum Genet.* 2004;75(6):1149–1154.
98. Tsao CY, Ellingson RJ. Infantile spasms in two brothers with broad thumbs syndrome. *Clin Electroencephalogr.* 1990;21(2):93–95.
99. Tsuji M, Kuroki S, Maeda H, et al. Leigh syndrome associated with West syndrome. *Brain Dev.* 2003;25(4):245–250.
100. Turner G, Partington M, Kerr B, et al. Variable expression of mental retardation, autism, seizures, and dystonic hand movements in two families with an identical ARX gene mutation. *Am J Med Genet.* 2002;112(4):405–411.
101. Tutuncuoglu S, Ozkinay F, Genel F, et al. A case report: corpus callosum dysgenesis, microcephaly, infantile spasm, cleft lip-palate, exophthalmos and psychomotor retardation. *Clin Genet.* 1996;49(4):220–222.
102. Vanhatalo S, Somer M, Barth PG. Dutch patients with progressive encephalopathy with edema, hypsarrhythmia, and optic atrophy (PEHO) syndrome. *Neuropediatrics.* 2002;33(2):100–104.
103. Velez A, Dulac O, Plouin P. Prognosis for seizure control in infantile spasms preceded by other seizures. *Brain Dev.* 1990;12(3):306–309.
104. Vigevano F, Bertini E, Boldrini R, et al. Hemimegalencephaly and intractable epilepsy: benefits of hemispherectomy. *Epilepsia.* 1989;30(6):833–843.
105. Vigevano F, Fusco L, Cusmai R, et al. The idiopathic form of West syndrome. *Epilepsia.* 1993;34(4):743–746.
106. Villeneuve N, Soufflet C, Plouin P, et al. Treatment of infantile spasms with vigabatrin as first-line therapy and in monotherapy: apropos of 70 infants [in French]. *Arch Pediatr.* 1998;5(7):731–738.
107. Watanabe K, Takeuchi T, Hakamada S, et al. Neurophysiological and neuroradiological features preceding infantile spasms. *Brain Dev.* 1987;9(4):391–398.
108. Zhongshu Z, Weiming Y, Yukio F, et al. Clinical analysis of West syndrome associated with phenylketonuria. *Brain Dev.* 2001;23(7):552–557.

CHAPTER 230 ■ SEVERE MYOCLONIC EPILEPSY IN INFANCY (DRAVET SYNDROME)

CHARLOTTE DRAVET AND MICHELLE BUREAU

INTRODUCTION

Severe myoclonic epilepsy in infancy is one of the most severe epilepsies affecting the infants and deserves to be recognized as soon as possible in order to manage it appropriately. However, the diagnosis is not easy and every infant who presents with long and repeated febrile convulsions before the end of the first year of life must be carefully followed because he is at risk for this epilepsy. Up to now, no antiepileptic drug has allowed controlling the seizures completely and almost all the childern have an abnormal psychomotor development and cognitive impairment at the adult age. In the last years, the genetic origin of this epilepsy has been demonstrated, most of the patients being carriers of a *de novo* mutation in the SCN1A gene, but not all. Currently, many studies aim to discover either the other mutations that could be responsible or the function of the known mutations.

HISTORICAL PERSPECTIVES

Severe myoclonic epilepsy in infants (SMEI) was first defined in 1982[14] and recognized as a syndrome in the most recent international classification of the epilepsies.[9] Since 1982, about 445 cases have been published in the literature. Most cases are reported from Southern Europe and Japan, but descriptions also come from other regions.[3,26,30] The name of the syndrome was used in the first description to underscore the ictal and interictal, myoclonic component, which allowed differentiating this syndrome from the Lennox-Gastaut syndrome. In the latter, the ictal hallmarks are occurring by generalized tonic seizures, mainly during sleep, and atypical absences. Later, it appeared that myoclonus could be absent in some patients. Seizures were polymorphic, and it was more difficult to find an appropriate semiologic designation.[1] For this reason the Commission on International Classification has proposed using the eponym "Dravet syndrome."[9] Since 2000, because of the discovery of a mutation in the sodium channel gene *SCN1A* in some patients,[8] this syndrome has been the target of a number of genetic studies that have given new insights to its pathophysiology.

DEFINITION

Severe myoclonic epilepsy in infants is characterized by febrile and afebrile, generalized and unilateral clonic or tonic–clonic seizures that occur in the first year of life in an otherwise normal infant. Later there is with myoclonus, atypical absences, and partial seizures. All seizure types are resistant to antiepileptic drugs. Developmental delay becomes apparent within the second year of life and is followed by definite cognitive impairment and personality changes. The disorder has been categorized among "epilepsies and syndromes undetermined as to whether they are focal or generalized" because the syndrome shows both generalized and localized seizure types and electroencephalographic (EEG) paroxysms.[9] In the most recent proposal it is placed among the "epileptogenic encephalopathies."[15]

Many children have been reported with a similar picture but without myclonus, and this condition has been designated as "borderline SMEI" (SMEIB).[33] These patients can have different EEG features but have the same course and outcome as patients with myclonus, and they can be included in the same syndrome. Recent genetic studies have demonstrated of *SCN1A* mutations in SMEIB patients but with differences in the type and the site of these mutations.

EPIDEMIOLOGY

SMEI is a rare condition. In the patient population of the Centre Saint-Paul, SMEI was diagnosed in 63 of 6,300 patients (1%) between 1970 and 1990. Hurst[26] estimated an incidence of at least 1 case in 40,000 children <7 years of age in the general population, and Yakoub et al.[50] gave a slightly higher figure (1/20,000 or 1/30,000). In children with seizure onset in the first year of life, the proportion varies from 3%[2] to 5%.[50] These findings show that this syndrome deserves to be recognized in infants with early convulsions. Mild male predominance has been reported.[13]

ETIOLOGY AND BASIC MECHANISMS

SMEI shares some characteristics with the idiopathic epilepsies (genetic predisposition, photosensitivity, generalized seizures, and generalized spikes-and-waves on EEG), but they are also associated with features of localization-related epilepsies (focal seizures, focal EEG anomalies, cognitive impairment). Moreover, the course of the disease—progressive during the first stage and always severe—could suggest a metabolic disease. However, none has been identified.

Until recently, magnetic resonance imaging (MRI) was said to be normal, even when repeated some years after the onset. However, in 2005, new data were published by Siegler et al.,[40] who performed the first systematic neuroimaging study with repeated MRI at different ages. They found hippocampal sclerosis (HS) in 10 of 14 patients with SMEI. In 6 of them, HS was not present on the first MRI, performed during the first 2 years in 5 patients and at 11 years in 1 patient, but developed later, between 14 months and 16 years. In the other 4 children, the first examination was not performed before the age of 4 years. In the last 4 children, MRI, performed between 6 and 17 years, remained normal. Because all the patients had a history of numerous hemiconvulsions and generalized tonic–clonic seizures (GTCS) during the first year, these results support the hypothesis that HS is a consequence of prolonged febrile seizures, even if it is unclear why 4 of the patients did not show HS.

Neuropathologic findings reported by Renier and Renkawek[37] from an autopsied case included cerebellar microdysgenesis, irregular lamination of cerebral cortex, and threefold spinal cord canals. There are no other neuropathologic studies.

A mitochondrial cytopathy was suspected in three patients who presented with an extremely severe picture.[5,6,16] However, according to Dravet et al.[13] and Giovanardi-Rossi et al.[20] no structural or histochemical abnormality was present in the biopsy samples from muscles in respectively five and nine patients.

A family history of epilepsy or febrile seizures is often present, ranging from 25% to 71%.[13] Five families have been reported with two affected siblings in each.[13,33,47]

Monozygotic twins have been reported by Fujiwara et al.,[17] Musumeci et al.,[31] and Ohki et al.[35] Recently, several publications described SMEI cases in the syndrome of generalized epilepsy with febrile seizures plus (GEFS+).[41,42,47] Thus, a genetic etiology could be suspected and was confirmed by the recent discovery of a de novo mutation in the sodium channel gene *SCN1A*.[8] Several publications have reported analogous findings in a high proportion of patients with SMEI but not in all. The percentage varies from 35% among 93 patients,[32] to 62% among 76 patients[19] (in part already published in the Nabbout et al. study[32]), to 71.4% among 12 patients,[44] to 82.7% among 29 patients.[36] Only two studies reported a *GABRG2* mutation,[25,28] which was not found by Madia et al.,[29] in 53 patients without the *SCN1A* mutation. Different mutation types were reported (truncating, missense, nonsense) in different sites of the gene. Correlations of phenotypes to genotypes were variable in different studies. Mutations were observed also in SMEIB,[18] but truncating mutations were largely predominant in the typical form.

CLINICAL PRESENTATION

Initially, prolonged, generalized, or unilateral clonic seizures are typically but not always triggered by fever. In some patients, isolated episodes of focal myoclonic jerking are noted by parents. Shortly thereafter, seizures also appear without fever. These convulsive seizures tend to be long (>20 minutes), recur in clusters in the same day, and evolve to status epilepticus. Their lateralization is variable, from one side to the other, either in different episodes or even in the same episode (alternating seizures). Generalized or erratic myoclonus, or both, appear between the ages of 1 and 4 years in typical cases. Jerks are usually mild, and falling is infrequent.

Other seizure types are observed during the course of the disease. Atypical absences accompanied by myoclonus occur in 40% of patients, often as absence status associated with convulsive seizures. The status consists of impaired consciousness, variable in intensity, with fragmentary and segmental, erratic myoclonias of low amplitude involving the limbs and the face, sometimes associated with a slight increase in muscular tone. According to the degree of altered consciousness, patients can or cannot react to stimuli, and have simple activities interrupted by short episodes of complete loss of contact and staring. Convulsive seizures can either initiate, occur during, or terminate the status. The EEG is characterized by diffuse slowing, intermixed with focal and diffuse spikes, sharp waves, and spike-wave discharge, of higher voltage in the frontal areas and the vertex, with random correspondence between spikes and myoclonias. Simple partial motor seizures or complex partial seizures, with prominent vegetative symptoms, occur in 46% of children observed as a complex partial status in one case.[48] Without EEG video recordings it is often difficult to differentiate between atypical absences and complex partial seizures. Generalized tonic seizures are exceptional but can be observed in the later stage of the disease. Other clinical paroxysmal events are described by parents, but we do not know if they are epileptic seizures.

Psychomotor delay becomes progressively evident. After children have started walking and producing first words at a normal age, they develop an unsteady gait for an unusually long time, and language skills are delayed, if acquired at all. After the age of 2 years, children become hyperkinetic, with recalcitrant behavior and major learning problems. About 60% of children have an ataxic gait, and 20% show mild pyramidal signs. Interictal EEGs are usually normal at the beginning. However, postictal recordings show asymmetry after unilateral seizures, and a photoparoxysmal response is evident before the age of 2 years in 20% of patients (Fig. 1). Interictal generalized spike-and-wave (SW) complexes appear within the second year of life in most children and can be frequent or infrequent, and only slightly activated by sleep. They are associated with focal and multifocal abnormalities in the majority of cases. Background activity is also usually normal at the beginning. Myoclonus is easily demonstrated by polygraphic recordings, accompanied by generalized SW or polySW when generalized, and without detectable EEG changes if erratic (Figs. 1 and 2).

Neuroimaging does not show any definite abnormality at the onset.[13]

TREATMENT AND OUTCOME

Typically, the course of SMEI is characterized by three phases, as emphasized by Lambarri San Martin et al.[27] The first phase ("febrile phase" according to these authors) covers the first year, with onset of seizures in a normal infant, often febrile or related to infectious episodes and vaccinations. The second phase ("catastrophic phase") extends from the second to the fourth year, with explosion of frequent and various types of seizures, myoclonus, status epilepticus, psychomotor delay, behavioral disturbances, neurologic signs, and EEG worsening. After 4 years ("sequelae phase"), progressive improvement is observed with decreased seizures and EEG discharges, slow cognitive improvement, and attenuation of the neurologic signs.

However, other periods of worsening are not actually excluded. Although results of medical treatment are in general disappointing, valproic acid (VPA) and benzodiazepines are preferable to other drugs at the very beginning. The first seizures should be treated vigorously, whether, febrile or not, to avoid development of status with its deleterious consequences. Rectal diazepam is the drug of choice and can be used by parents and caretakers. Phenobarbital (PB) can be necessary in case of status. Phenytoin does not offer any advantage and may produce more severe side effects than PB. Continuous oral treatment by VPA should be given when febrile seizures are long and repeated, and when afebrile seizures and myoclonic jerks occur.[38] Among the newer antiepileptic drugs, topiramate is the most promising and should be used as soon as VPA resistance appears.[10] In case of repeated status, stiripentol is the best choice, combined with VPA and clobazam.[7,46] Other options are possible, such as bromides[13] and ketogenic diet.[2,3] Ethosuximide may be helpful in reducing myoclonus and atypical absences. In older patients (third phase), vigabatrin has given promising results, reducing convulsive seizures in patients in whom myoclonus was not a prominent symptom.[23] Conversely, severe worsening of convulsive seizures and myoclonus has been observed with add-on carbamazepine and

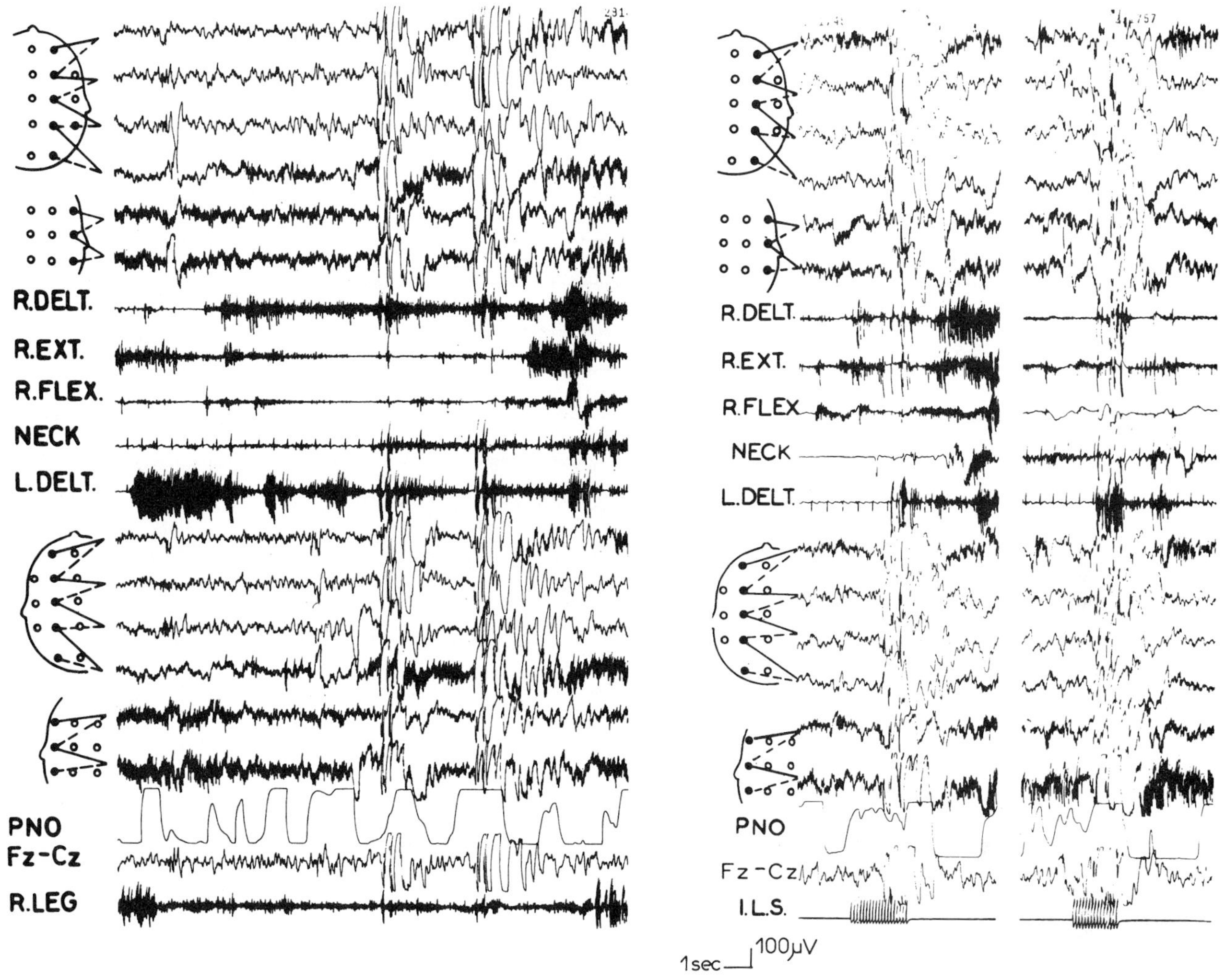

FIGURE 1. Boy, age 1 year, 8 months. **Left:** Polygraphic recording of spontaneous myoclonic attacks is accompanied by generalized spike-and-wave complexes. **Right:** Electroclinical findings of intermittent light stimulation (ILS)–induced generalized myoclonus are similar to those of the spontaneous attacks. L. DELT., left deltoid; R. LEG, extensor of the right leg; R. DELT., right deltoid; R. EXT., extensors of the right wrist; R. FLEX., flexors of the right wrist; PNO, pneumogram.

lamotrigine, and these should be avoided.[21,48] Particular attention should be given to avoiding intercurrent infections and to prevent the occurrence of status epilepticus because any febrile episode may be complicated by convulsive status.

Peculiar features are remarkable temperature, sensitivity and photosensitivity. Seizures can be triggered by slight variations in the body temperature of only few degrees (e. g., going from 36.5 °C to 37.5 °C) without associated infection, sometimes related to external temperature or physical efforts. In Japan, hot baths are a frequent triggering factor.[45] Other triggering factors are variations in the environmental light, eye closure, and pattern fixation leading to self-stimulation.

LONG-TERM PROGNOSIS

Follow-up in the series by Dravet et al.[13] varied from 2 years, 6 months to 33 years, 8 months (median, 11 years, 6 months). Long-term outcome was always unfavorable. Convulsive seizures persist, with a tendency to be localized at night. They are described as generalized but often have a localized onset, proved by ictal video-EEG recordings. The course of myoclonus is variable. It may persist, more or less attenuated, disappears, or occur only just before a convulsive seizure. Complex partial seizures usually no longer occur after the first years but the age of disappearance is not homogeneous.[13,35] Atypical absences and absence status also tend to cease. Electroencephalographic findings may vary by age from one patient to another. Generalized SWs tend to disappear. Focal abnormalities, often localized in the central areas, are activated during sleep. Background activity can deteriorate during the course of the disease, mainly when convulsive seizures are frequent, especially between the ages of 5 to 10 years, and then return almost to normal. Temperature sensitivity decreases. Photosensitivity and pattern sensitivity can be constant during the course or occur inconsistently. All patients are cognitively impaired, with 50% of those 10 years and older having severe retardation. The mental impairment constitutes itself progressively during the first 4 to 6 years and then remains more or less equal without further deterioration. A single neuropsychological study was conducted in Marseille, France,[4,49] on 20 patients aged from 11 months to 16 years, with a follow-up of >3 years in 10 cases. Cognitive and behavioral difficulties were always present at varying degrees. Neuropsychological deficits involved all skills, with motor, linguistic and visual abilities being most affected. Behavior was

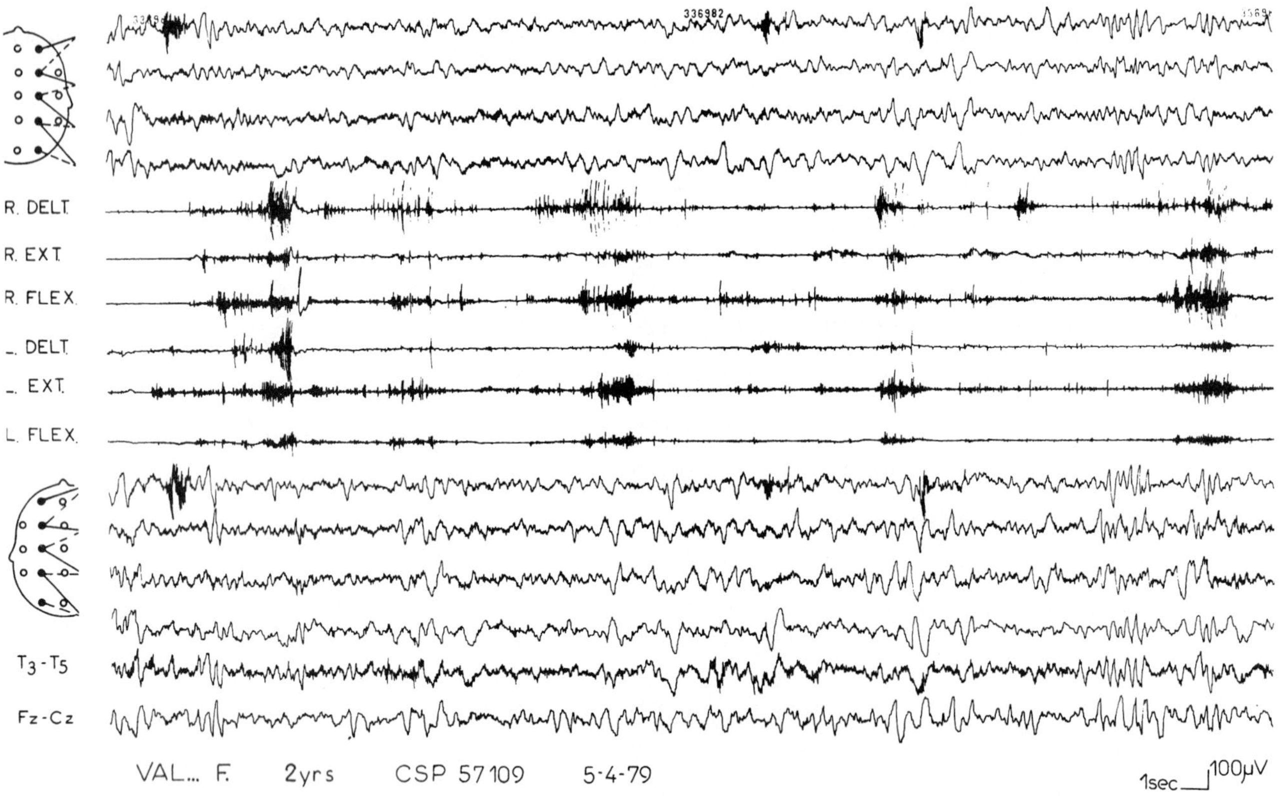

FIGURE 2. Girl, age 2 years. Polygraphic recording of segmental myoclonus at rest and during muscular contraction. Myoclonic potentials are not accompanied by time-locked paroxysmal electroencephalographic abnormalities. L. DELT., left deltoid; L. EXT., extensor of the left wrist; L. FLEX., flexor of the left wrist; R. DELT., right deltoid; R.. EXT., extensors of the right wrist; R. FLEX., flexors of the right wrist.

marked by hyperactivity, psychotic type of relationships, and some autistic traits. The appearance of neuropsychological disorders seemed to be related to the severity of epilepsy during the first 2 years of life.

The mortality rate is very high, around 15% in our most recent series.[13] Several other authors have also reported this high incidence of early deaths.[11,33,34] Causes of death are various, and include drowning, accident, status epilepticus with hepatic or multiorgan failure, severe infection, and sudden unexpected death.

In adulthood, these patients present as dependent persons with mental disabilities, with poor language, poor fine motor function, generalized slowness, sometimes autistic features, and rarely aggressiveness or other psychiatric features. They have few or no school skills, are unable to work, and live in specialized institutions or with their family. However, we underline that therapeutic possibilities have strongly increased with the use of new and more efficacious drugs and strategies. We can hope to see a better outcome for these patients due to these improvements.

DIFFERENTIAL DIAGNOSIS

The first seizures must be differentiated from febrile convulsions. Long duration and clustering of attacks despite treatment should lead one to suspect SMEI. Appearance of myoclonus, established by EEG and electromyographic recordings, and photosensitivity are typical. However, in some children with a similar outcome, myoclonus is a minor feature or is absent.[43] Differentiation from benign myoclonic epilepsy is quite easy and is based on three major features: (a) onset with brief generalized myoclonic attacks, (b) which represent the only ictal manifestation in a normal child, (c) with generalized SWs on the EEG.[12] In the rare patients having benign myoclonic epilepsy with febrile seizures, these seizures are always simple and infrequent. The differences between SMEI and Lennox-Gastaut syndrome are clear enough (see Chapter 241). On the contrary, more difficulty arises in differentiating SMEI from myoclonic-astatic epilepsy (MAE),[22,24] a syndrome category in which some children are first seen with early-onset generalized convulsive seizures triggered by fever.

Although this onset is very similar to that of SMEI, it is not the most common in MAE, and the course is different, with myoclonic-astatic seizures (drop attacks) becoming a major feature with absence of any focal clinical or EEG manifestation. The long-term outcome is variable. Some of the affected children remain intractable and have a severe cognitive impairment, but others improve and become seizure free. Another condition that must be ruled out is a progressive myoclonic epilepsy resulting from metabolic disorders, mainly the neuronal ceroid lipofuscinoses. The absence of visual disturbances and of abnormalities of the fundus coupled with negative results of relevant laboratory investigations eliminate this diagnosis. The last differential diagnosis is with a cryptogenic focal epilepsy, which may have the same onset, with febrile seizures rapidly associated with focal seizures. However, these patients do not present atypical absences and myoclonic jerks in the later course, and their EEG shows focal abnormalities that remain localized in the same area. Moreover, this diagnostic is very improbable when the hemiclonic seizures are alternating.[39]

SUMMARY AND CONCLUSIONS

Severe myoclonic epilepsy in infants is characterized by febrile and afebrile generalized and unilateral clonic or tonic-clonic seizures that occur in the first year of life in an otherwise normal infant and are later associated with myoclonus, atypical absences, and partial seizures. All seizure types are resistant to antiepileptic drugs. Developmental delay becomes apparent within the second year of life and is followed by definite cognitive impairment and personality disorders. Some cases do not present with all the features and are described as borderline or atypical forms. In the most recent proposal it is placed among the "epileptogenic encephalopathies."

In more than 60% of patients in the most recent studies, mutations in the sodium channel gene SCN1A have been found. In more than 60% of patients in the most recent studies, different mutations types were reported in different sites of the gene. Correlations of phenotypes to genotypes are not well established.

Initial prolonged, generalized, or unilateral clonic seizures are typically but not always triggered by fever, and seizures also appear without fever. They tend to evolve into status epilepticus. They are generalized or lateralized (alternating seizures). Later on, myoclonic seizures, atypical absences, absence status, simple partial motor seizures or complex partial seizures, with prominent vegetative symptoms, are observed. Interictal erratic myoclonus also appears between the ages of 1 and 4 years in typical cases. Psychomotor delay and behavioral disturbances become progressively evident, often associated with ataxia and pyramidal signs. Interictal EEGs are usually normal at the beginning. Later on, generalized spike-and-wave discharges associated with focal and multifocal abnormalities appear in the majority of cases, and photosensitivity is frequently observed. Neuroimaging does not show any definite abnormality at onset.

Typically, three phases characterize the course of the disease: the "febrile phase" (first year), the "catastrophic phase" (from the second to the fourth year), and the "sequelae phase" (after 4 years) with decrease in seizures and EEG discharges, slow cognitive acquisitions, and attenuation of the neurologic signs, other periods of worsening being not actually excluded. Triggering seizure effect of temperature variations persists all over the life, whereas photosensitivity is fluctuating.

Treatment is disappointing. Valproate, benzodiazepines, topiramate and stiripentol are the most useful antiepileptic drugs. Carbamazepine and lamotrigine should be avoided during the first phases. Particular attention must be given to avoiding intercurrent infections and to vigorously treating the febrile seizures to prevent the occurrence of status epilepticus (rectal and intravenous diazepam).

In published series, long-term prognosis was always unfavorable, and no adult patient became seizure free. All patients were cognitively impaired, with 50% of those 10 years and older having severe retardation. The mental impairment remained more or less static without further deterioration after the age of four. Mortality rates are very high, around 15%, ofen due to sudden unexpected death. Differential diagnosis mainly includes febrile seizures, myoclonic astatic epilepsy, progressive myoclonus epilepsies, cryptogenic focal epilepsies.

Dravet syndrome should be recognized in infants with early convulsions because it affects 3% to 5% of children seizures in the first year of life. Early diagnosis could allow improved management and, perhaps, a less severe prognosis.

References

1. Arzimanoglou A, Guerrini R, Aicardi J. *Epilepsy in Children,* 3rd ed. Philadelphia: Lippincott Williams and Wilkins; 2004:51–57.
2. Caraballo R, Tripoli J, Escobal L, et al. Ketogenic diet: efficacy and tolerability in childhood intractable epilepsy [in Spanish]. *Rev Neurol.* 1998;26:61–64.
3. Caraballo RH, Cersosimo RO, Sakr D, et al. Ketogenic diet in patients with Dravet syndrome. *Epilepsia.* 2005;46:1539–1544.
4. Cassé-Perrot C, Wolff M, Dravet C. Neuropsychological aspects of severe myoclonic epilepsy in infancy. In: Jambaqué I, Lassonde M, Dulac O, eds. *The neuropsychology of childhood epilepsy.* New York: Plenum Press/Kluwer Academic; 2001:131–140.
5. Castro-Gago M, Eiris J, Fernandez-Bustillo J, et al. Severe myoclonic epilepsy associated with mitochondrial cytopathy. *Child's Nerv Syst.* 1995;11:630–633.
6. Castro-Gago M, Martinon Sanchez JM, Rodriguez-Nunez A, et al. Severe myoclonic epilepsy and mitochondrial cytopathy. *Child's Nerv Syst.* 1997;(11–12):570–571.
7. Chiron C, Marchand MC, Tran A, et al. Stiripentol in severe myoclonic epilepsy in infancy: a randomised placebo-controlled syndrome-dedicated trial. STICLO study group. *Lancet.* 2000;356(9242):1638–1642.
8. Claes L, Del-Favero J, Ceulemans B, et al. De novo mutations in the sodium-channel gene *SCN1A* cause severe myoclonic epilepsy of infancy. *Am J Hum Genet.* 2001;68:1327–1332.
9. Commission on Classification and Terminology of the International League Against Epilepsy. Proposal for revised classification of epilepsies and epileptic syndromes. *Epilepsia.* 1989;30:389–399.
10. Coppola G, Capovilla G, Montagnini A, et al. Topiramate as add-on drug in severe myoclonic epilepsy in infancy: an Italian multicenter open trial. *Epilepsy Res.* 2002;49:45–48.
11. Dooley J, Camfield P, Gordon K. Severe polymorphic epilepsy of infancy. *J Child Neurol.* 1995;10:339–340.
12. Dravet C, Bureau M. Benign myoclonic epilepsy in infancy. In: Roger J, Bureau M, Dravet C, et al., eds. *Epileptic Syndromes in Infancy, Childhood and Adolescence,* 4th ed. London: John Libbey; 2005:77–88.
13. Dravet C, Bureau M, Oguni H, et al. Severe myoclonic epilepsy in infancy (Dravet syndrome). In: Roger J, Bureau M, Dravet C, et al., eds. *Epileptic Syndromes in Infancy, Childhood and Adolescence,* 4th ed. London: John Libbey; 2005:89–113.
14. Dravet C, Roger J, Bureau M, Dalla Bernardina B. Myoclonic epilepsies in childhood. In: Akimoto H, Kazamatsu M, Seino M, et al., eds. *Advances in Epileptology: The XIIIth Epilepsy International Symposium.* New York: Raven Press; 1982:135–140.
15. Engel J Jr. A proposed diagnostic scheme for people with epileptic seizures and with epilepsy: report of the ILAE Task Force on Classification and Terminology. International League Against Epilepsy (ILAE). *Epilepsia.* 2001;42:796–803.
16. Fernàndez-Jaén A, Leon MC, Martinez-Granero MA, et al. Diagnostico en la epilessia mioclonica severa de la infancia: estudio de 13 casos. *Rev neurol.* 1998;26:759–762.
17. Fujiwara T, Nakamura H, Watanabe M, et al. Clinicoelectrographic concordance between monozygotic twins with severe myoclonic epilepsy in infancy. *Epilepsia.* 1990;31:281–286.
18. Fukuma G, Oguni H, Shirasaka Y, et al. Mutations of neuronal voltage-gated Na+ channel $\alpha 1$ subunit gene *SCN1A* in core severe myoclonic epilepsy in infancy (SMEI) and in borderline SMEI (SMEB). *Epilepsia.* 2004;45:140–148.
19. Gaggero R, Mancardi M, Striano P, et al. Genetic predisposition to severe myoclonic epilepsy of infancy (Dravet syndrome): analysis of cases with and without *SCN1A* mutations [Abstract]. *Epilepsia.* 2005;46(Suppl 6):50.
20. Giovanardi-Rossi P, Pini M, Santucci M, et al. Studio istologico, istochimico e biochimico muscolare nella epilessia mioclonica severa. In: Scarcella M, Perniola T, eds. *Atti XV Congresso Nazionale, S.I.N.P.I, Bari, 14–17 ottobre 1992.* Bologna: Monduzzi; 1992:279–284.
21. Guerrini R, Dravet C, Genton P, et al. Lamotrigine and seizure aggravation in severe myoclonic epilepsy. *Epilepsia* 1988;39:508–512.
22. Guerrini R, Dravet C, Gobbi G, et al. Idiopathic generalized epilepsies with myoclonus in infancy and childhood. In: Malafosse A, Genton P, Hirsch E, et al., eds. *Idiopathic Generalized Epilepsies: Clinical, Experimental and Genetic Aspects.* London: John Libbey; 1994:267–280.
23. Guerrini R, Paglia G, Dravet C, et al. Efficacy of vigabatrin as add-on therapy in relation to type of epilepsy or epileptic syndrome: retrospective study of 120 patients. *Epilepsia.* 1994;35(Suppl 7):S65.
24. Guerrini R, Parmeggiani L, Bonanni P, et al. Myoclonic astatic epilepsy. In: Roger J, Bureau M, Dravet C, et al., eds. *Epileptic Syndromes in Infancy, Childhood and Adolescence,* 4th ed. London: John Libbey; 2005:115–124.
25. Harkin LA, Bowser DN, Dibbens LM, et al. Truncation of the $GABA_A$-receptor $\gamma 2$ subunit in a family with generalized epilepsy with febrile seizures plus. *Am J Hum Genet.* 2002;70:530–536.
26. Hurst DL. Epidemiology of severe myoclonic epilepsy of infancy. *Epilepsia.* 1990;31:397–400.
27. Lambarri San Martin I, Garaizar Axpe C, Zuazo Zamalloa E, et al. Epilepsia polimorfa de la infancia: revision de 12 casos. *An Esp Pediatr.* 1997;46:571–575.
28. Lerche H. Idiopathic generalized epilepsies and GEFS+ [Abstract]. *Epilepsia.* 2004;45(Suppl 3):45.
29. Madia F, Gennaro E, Cecconi M, et al. No evidence of *GABRG2* mutations in severe myoclonic epilepsy of infancy. *Epilepsy Res.* 2003;53:196–200.

30. Mukhin Kiu, Nikanorova Miu, Temin PA, et al. Severe myoclonic epilepsy in infancy. *Zh Nevrol Psikhiatr Im S S Korsakova*. 1997;97:61–64.
31. Musumeci SA, Elia M, Ferri R, et al. Epilessia mioclonica grave in due gemelli monozigoti con sindrome di Rud. *Boll Lega Ital Epil*. 1992;79/80: 81–82.
32. Nabbout R, Gennaro E, Dalla Bernardina B, et al. Spectrum of *SCN1A* mutations in severe myoclonic epilepsy of infancy. *Neurology*. 2003;60:1961–1967.
33. Ogino T, Ohtsuka Y, Yamatogi Y, et al. The epileptic syndrome sharing common characteristics during early childhood with severe myoclonic epilepsy of infancy. *Jpn J Psychiatr Neurol*. 1989;43:479–481.
34. Oguni H, Hayashi K, Awaya Y, et al. Severe myoclonic epilepsy in infants—a review based on the Tokyo Women's Medical University series of 84 cases. *Brain Dev*. 2001;23:736–748.
35. Ohki T, Watanabe K, Negoro K, et al. Severe myoclonic epilepsy in infancy: evolution of seizures. *Seizure*. 1997;6:219–224.
36. Ohmori I, Ouchida M, Ohtsuka Y, et al. Significant correlation of the *SCN1A* mutations and severe myoclonic epilepsy in infancy. *Biochem Biophys Res Commun*. 2002;295:17–23.
37. Renier WO, Renkawek K. Clinical and neuropathological findings in a case of severe myoclonic epilepsy of infancy. *Epilepsia*. 1990;31:287–291.
38. Sankar R, Wheless JW, Dravet C, et al. Treatment of myoclonic epilepsies in infancy and early childhood. In: Delgado-Escueta AV, Guerrini R, Medina MT, et al. *Advances in Neurology, Vol. 95. Myoclonic Epilepsies*. Philadelphia: Lippincott Williams & Wilkins; 2005:289–298.
39. Sarisjulis N, Gamboni B, Plouin P, et al. Diagnosing idiopathic/cryptogenic epilepsy syndromes in infancy. *Arch Dis Child*. 2000;82:226–230.
40. Siegler Z, Barsi P, Neuwirth M, et al. Hippocampal sclerosis in severe myoclonic epilepsy in infancy: a retrospective MRI study. *Epilepsia*. 2005;46: 704–708.
41. Singh R, Andermann E, Whitehouse WP, et al. Severe myoclonic epilepsy of infancy: extended spectrum of GEFS+? *Epilepsia*. 2001;42:837–844.
42. Singh R, Scheffer IE, Whitehouse W, et al. Severe myoclonic epilepsy of infancy is part of the spectrum of generalized epilepsy with febrile seizures plus (GEFS+) [Abstract]. *Epilepsia*. 1999;40(Suppl 2):175.
43. Sugama M, Oguni H, Fukuyama Y. Clinical and electroencephalographic study of severe myoclonic epilepsy in infancy (Dravet). *Jpn J Psychiatry Neurol*. 1987;41:463–465.
44. Sugawara T, Mazaki-Miyazaki E, Fukushima K, et al. Frequent mutations of *SCN1A* in severe myoclonic epilepsy in infancy. *Neurology*. 2002;58:1122–1124.
45. Sumi K, Nagaura T, Nagai T, et al. A clinical study of seizures induced by hot bathing. *Jpn J Psychiatry Neurol*. 1993;47:350–351.
46. Thanh TN, Chiron C, Dellatolas G, et al. Efficacité et tolérance à long terme du Stiripentol dans le traitement de l'épilepsie myoclonique sévère du nourrisson (syndrome de Dravet). *Arch Pediatr*. 2002;11:1120–1127.
47. Veggiotti P, Cardinali S, Montalenti E, et al. Generalized epilepsy with febrile seizures plus and severe myoclonic epilepsy in infancy: a case report of two Italian families. *Epileptic Disord*. 2001;3:29–32.
48. Wakai S, Ikehata M, Nihira H, et al. "Obtundation status (Dravet)" caused by complex partial status epilepticus in a patient with severe myoclonic epilepsy in infancy. *Epilepsia*. 1996;37:1020–1022.
49. Wolff M, Cassé-Perrot C, Dravet C. Neuropsychological disorders in children with severe myoclonic epilepsy [Abstract]. *Epilepsia*. 2001;42(Suppl 2):61.
50. Yakoub M, Dulac O, Jambaque I, et al. Early diagnosis of severe myoclonic epilepsy in infancy. *Brain Dev*. 1992;14:299–303.

CHAPTER 231 ■ IDIOPATHIC MYOCLONIC EPILEPSY IN INFANCY

CHARLOTTE DRAVET AND FEDERICO VIGEVANO

INTRODUCTION

The syndrome of benign myoclonic epilepsy in infancy (BMEI) was not clearly identified before its first description in seven infants in 1981.[10] These authors defined it as the occurrence of myoclonic seizures (MS) without other seizure types, except rare simple febrile seizures (FS), in the first 3 years of life in otherwise normal infants. These myoclonic seizures were easily controlled and remitted during childhood. Psychomotor development remained normal, and no severe psychological consequences were observed. Many other cases have been published since. BMEI was classified among the generalized idiopathic epilepsies in the 1989 international classification.[4] Some authors have described cases with reflex myoclonic seizures, triggered by noise or contact, and have proposed to distinguish two separate entities, the second one being named "reflex myoclonic epilepsy in infancy."[24] We do not think this distinction is necessary,[11] and we will describe all cases as BMEI.

As of 2006, there were 155 cases published in the literature, of which 123 corresponded to the classical description and 32 were reported as "reflex BMEI" (for a review, see Auvin et al.[2] and Dravet and Bureau[11]). The 22 cases reported by Darra et al.[6] are not counted because it is not known how many were already included in other reports. In the first description, onset was before 3 years of age, whereas in subsequent reports, some cases had a later onset, up to 4 years 8 months.[17] This means that the same type of epilepsy may appear at different ages but tends to be more frequent in some periods.[18] The adjective "benign" is considered problematic, because some patients do not have an actually benign evolution, particularly from the neuropsychological point of view.[2,22] For this reason, the name "myoclonic epilepsy in infancy" has been proposed, but it is ambiguous. This BMEI is idiopathic, and to distinguish this syndrome from other myoclonic epilepsies, we propose replacing the *benign* by *idiopathic*. Thus, the condition should be termed "idiopathic myoclonic epilepsy in infancy (IMEI)," but, in this chapter, we continue to use BMEI, which is the designation best known to epileptologists.

In this chapter, the numbers reported without reference citation are taken from the extensive review of the literature by Dravet and Bureau,[11] supplemented by the paper of Auvin et al.[2]

GENERAL CONSIDERATIONS

Epidemiology

According to the few available epidemiologic data, BMEI seems to represent <1% of all epilepsies[20] (unpublished data from the Centre Saint-Paul, 1999), 2% of all idiopathic generalized epilepsies (unpublished data from the Centre Saint-Paul, 1997), and around 2% of epilepsies that begin in the first 3 years of life.[5]

Gender Distribution

There is a prevalence of male patients, with a male-to-female ratio of 2:1.

Genetics

The genetics of BMEI are unknown. Cases are rare, and no family cases of BMEI have been described. A family history of epilepsy or FS is present in 50.5% of cases. Epilepsy types found in relatives are difficult to assess. In one case, the mother presented with juvenile myoclonic epilepsy (JME).[6] In another case, the mother had a myoclonic-astatic epilepsy (EMAS). In the case described by Arzimanoglou et al.,[1] the proband was the second of two brothers, and the oldest was affected by typical EMAS. A similar situation was reported in 2006 by Darra et al.[6]

Personal History

Most patients do not have any relevant history prior to the onset of the myoclonic seizures. Only two (1.9%) had an associated disease: Down syndrome[13] and hyperinsulinic diabetes.[3] However, the occurrence of FS is not uncommon (28%). They are always simple, usually rare (one or two), and are observed before the onset of myclonus and before initiation of treatment. In one patient, two isolated nocturnal orofacial seizures occurred 6 months before appearance of myoclonic seizures.[6]

CLINICAL AND ELECTROENCEPHALOGRAPHIC MANIFESTATIONS

The age at onset is usually between 4 months and 3 years; earlier onset is uncommon. Rarely, later onset, between 3 and 5 years, is reported.[17,18]

Initially, the myoclonic seizures are brief, often rare, and involve the upper limbs and the head, rarely the lower limbs. In infants, they may be barely noticeable, and the parents sometimes have difficulty determining their exact onset and their frequency. They often speak of "spasms" or "head nodding." Later, the frequency increases.

Video-electroencephalographic (EEG) and polygraphic recordings have facilitated precise analysis of these seizures. They are more or less massive myoclonic jerks, involving the axis of the body and the limbs, provoking a head drop and an upward-outward movement of the upper limbs, with flexion of the lower limbs, and sometimes a rolling of the eyes. Their intensity varies from one child to another and from one attack to another in the same child. The most severe forms cause a sudden projection of objects held in the hands and sometimes a fall. The mildest forms provoke only brief forward movement of the head or even a simple closure of the eyes. As a rule, seizures are very brief (1–3 seconds), although they may be longer, especially in older children, consisting of pseudo-rhythmically repeated jerks lasting no more than 5 to 10 seconds. They occur several times a day at irregular and unpredictable times. Unlike infantile spasms, they do not occur in long series. They are not activated by awakening, but rather by drowsiness, except in some cases. In some patients, they can be triggered by intermittent photic stimulation (IPS). In patients with the reflex BMEI, myclonus is triggered by a sudden noise, more often by a sudden contact. The state of consciousness is difficult to assess in isolated seizures. Only when seizures are repeated is there slight impairment of consciousness without interruption of activity. In reflex myoclonic seizures, the myoclonus is elicitable both in wakefulness and in sleep, with a threshold lower in stage I and increasing gradually during the slower stages.[24] No rapid eye movement (REM) sleep has been recorded and tested in patient with reflex myoclonic seizures.

As development continues normally, parents and pediatricians tend not to consider these movements as pathologic events.

When an EEG is performed, it can be normal during the awake state if no myoclonic fits are recorded.

However, myoclonias are always associated with an EEG discharge. Polygraphic recordings demonstrate that myclonic are accompanied by a discharge of fast generalized spike-waves (SW) or polyspike-waves (PSW) at >3 Hz, lasting for the same time as the myoclonia (Figs. 1 and 2). This discharge is more or less regular and can start in the two frontal areas and the vertex. Myoclonias are brief (1–3 seconds) and usually isolated. Each myoclonic jerk may be followed by a brief loss of time. Sometimes, after the attack, there is a voluntary movement, visible as a normal muscular contraction. In only one patient did we observe the association of myclonus in the deltoid muscle with pure atonia in the neck muscles. During drowsiness, there is enhancement of the myclonic jerks; they usually, but not always, disappear during slow sleep. The myoclonic seizures triggered by tactile and acoustic stimuli have the same characteristics (Fig. 2). Ricci et al.[24] noted that the initial manifestation generally, but not always, consisted of a blink, followed 40 to 80 msec later by the first myoclonic arm jerk. After a myoclonic attack, there was a refractory period, lasting 20 to 30 seconds to 1 to 2 minutes, during which sudden stimuli did not provoke attacks, even when the startle reaction was easily elicitable. IPS can also provoke myoclonic seizures.

The interictal EEG is normal. Spontaneous SW discharges are rare; some slow waves may be found over the central areas. Darra et al.[6] described rhythmic, 4- to 5-Hz theta activity over the rolandic regions and the vertex in 4 of 22 children. IPS does not provoke SW without concomitant myclonus at the onset. Nap sleep recordings have shown a normal organization of sleep; generalized SW discharges may occur during REM sleep.

EVOLUTION AND TREATMENT

No other type of seizure is observed in children with BMEI, even if they are left untreated (for up to 8.5 years in one of our patients). In particular absence or tonic seizures do not

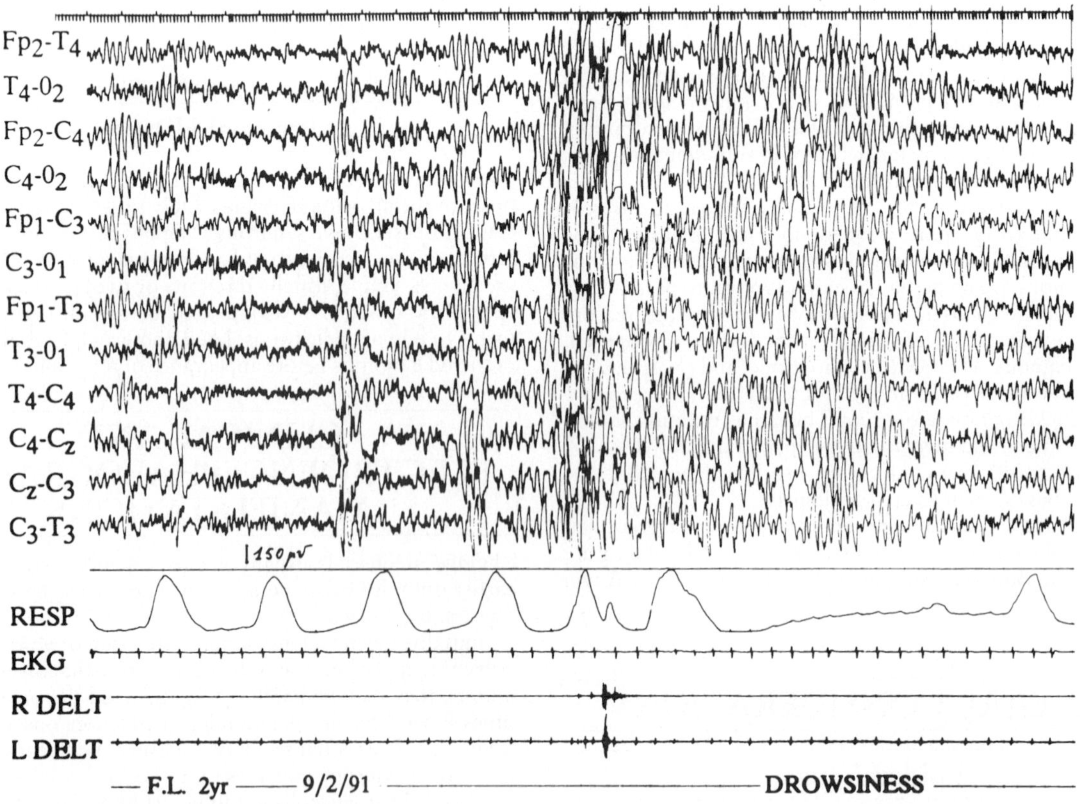

FIGURE 1. Infant with benign myoclonic epilepsy. A spontaneous massive myoclonic jerk was recorded during drowsiness. The ictal EEG shows a brief discharge of generalized spike-wave and polyspike-wave complexes. EKG, electrocardiogram; L DELT, left deltoid; R DELT, right deltoid; RESP, respiration.

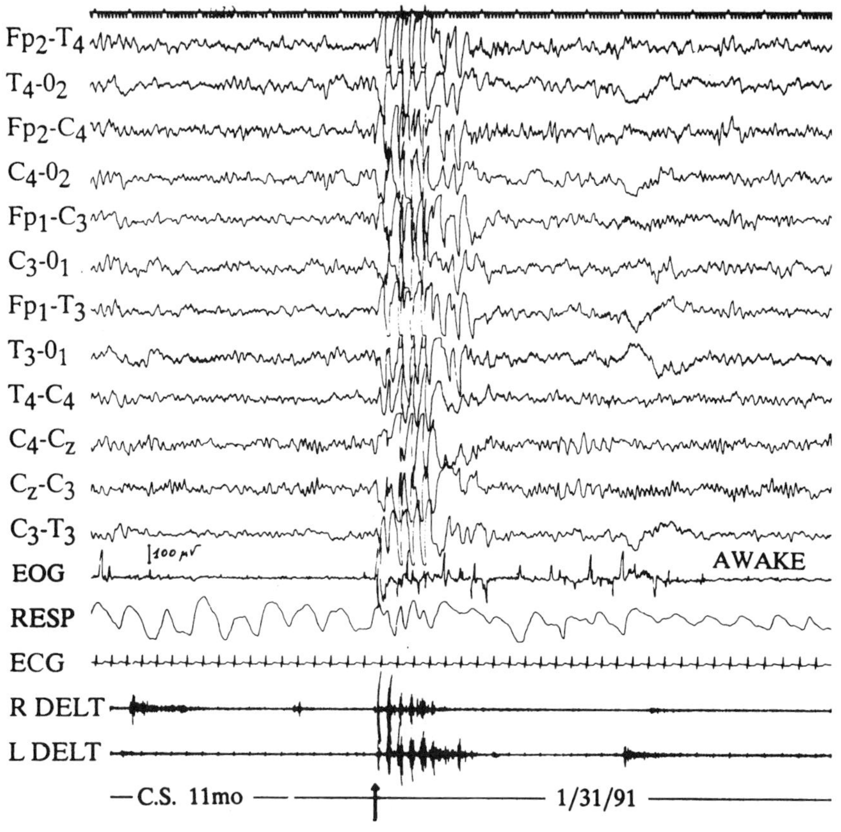

FIGURE 2. Patient affected by reflex benign myoclonic epilepsy in infancy. A sudden noise (*arrow*) triggers a brief cluster of myoclonic jerks; ictal electroencephalogram consists of generalized spike-and-wave complexes. ECG, electrocardiogram; L DELT, left deltoid; R DELT, right deltoid; RESP, respiration.

occur. Clinical examination is normal. Interictal myoclonus was described only by Giovanardi-Rossi et al.,[17] in 6 patients. In reviewing our patients, we found mild interictal myoclonus in 2 patients, revealed by polygraphic recordings. Many patients were not investigated, but when computed tomography (CT) scan and magnetic resonance imaging (MRI) were performed, they were normal (46 patients).

The outcome seems to depend on an early diagnosis and treatment. Myoclonic jerks are easily controlled by valproate (VPA), and the child may then develop normally. If left untreated, patients continues to experience myoclonic attacks, and this may lead to impaired psychomotor development and behavioral disturbances.

The therapeutic modalities have been reported in 131 patients. Monotherapy was used in 109 patients (104 with VPA), polytherapy in 15, and no therapy in 7. Ninety-nine (95.2%) became seizure free on monotherapy. All of the others became seizure free using, usually including VPA and one benzodiazepine, rarely phenobarbital (PB), ethosuximide (ESM), or lamotrigine (LTG). Only in 1 patient did myoclonic seizures persist in spite of various drug combinations and even one ketogenic diet.[23] Finally, 7 patients, 4 of whom presented with reflex seizures, did not receive any treatment and became seizure free spontaneously. On the whole, 125 (95.4%) became seizure free. The study of Darra et al.[6] confirmed these findings, the control of myoclonic seizures having been achieved in all 22 patients.

These data support the VPA as the drug of first choice in BMEI. Treatment must be monitored using plasma drug levels, because irregular intake can lead to relapse and falsely mimic drug-resistant epilepsy. Lin et al.[19] gave a well-detailed account of treatment in their patients. They also underscored the necessity of monitoring and of using high doses at the onset (30–40 mg/kg) to obtain levels >100 mg/L at 3 hours after the morning intake in some patients. The daily dose was reduced to usual therapeutic plasma levels (50–100 mg/L) after seizures were controlled.

LONG-TERM OUTCOME AND PROGNOSIS

The length of follow-up is known in 112 cases, from 9 months to 27 years, and ≥5 years in 85.

In all these cases, myoclonic seizures disappeared. Their duration is known in 69 cases. In most patients they lasted <1 year. The longest duration (6 years 4 months) was observed only in the first publication, before recognition of the syndrome and its treatment.[13] When duration of follow-up is longer, the number of patients who have other seizure types after the end of the myoclonic seizures increases. Excluding FS, there were 17 reported among the 112 cases with known follow-up (15.2%). They were rare generalized tonic–clonic seizures (GTCS) in 12 patients, without associated myoclonic seizures. It is interesting that only 2 patients with BMEI evolved to juvenile myoclonic epilepsy (JME) at 9 and 12 years, respectively, with seizures well controlled by VPA.[2] Two other patients presented absences, respectively, at 10 and 11 years.[23] They were described as "petit mal" in the first patient and as absences with marked eyelid myoclonia in the second. The last patient, with reflex BMEI, had complex partial motor seizures from 6 years on, with normal EEG, with good response to the combination of carbamazepine and PB.[2] In a series of 22 patients,[6] 4 presented occasional isolated seizures after the age of 5 years: 1 spontaneous GTCS, 1 IPS-induced massive myoclonic seizures, 1 IPS-induced GTCS, and 1 television-induced GTCS.

The EEG outcome is known for 88 patients. EEGs remained abnormal after myoclonic seizures have disappeared, with generalized SW, sometimes focal without clinical correlate (frontal, frontocentral, frontoparietal, frontotemporal), but they became normal later in the majority of patients. It is interesting to note that photosensitivity can appear after the disappearance of myoclonic seizures, as reported by several authors, and can persist for many years after cessation of myoclonic seizures even to adult ages. In once older patients, photo sensitivity is only an EEG response without clinical correlate. Darra et al.[6] confirmed the persistence of photosensitivity. They reported one case with association of generalized SW and typical rolandic spikes, the latter persisting at 9 years, several years after seizure remission and withdrawal of treatment.

These findings affirm the usual good prognosis of BMEI. Attacks provoked by noise or contact were more easily controlled than spontaneous ones. Conversely, photosensitivity was more difficult to control and persisted several years after cessation of seizures.

On the whole, psychological outcome is favorable, and most patients are normal. Outcome is known in 96 cases. Seventy-nine (82.3%) were normal, of whom 56 were age 5 years or older. Twelve (12.5%) presented with mild retardation and attended specialized schools, but none was institutionalized. Five patients (5.2%) had cognitive deficits and personality disturbances. One of them had Down syndrome and strong photosensitivity, and another had myoclonic seizures until age 5 years, with sensitivity to IPS and eye closure. The psychological outcome of cases reported by Darra et al.[12] was also favorable, and 77% had normal cognitive skills at follow-up.

One recent study[22] analyzed of the neuropsychological and behavioral outcomes in seven patients affected by BMEI, with an average follow-up of 6 years 9 months (range: 4 years 9 months–9 years 2 months). The mean full-scale intelligence quotient of the group was 74, with a significantly higher verbal IQ score in all but one patient. Five were within normal limits, one had slight mental retardation, and one had moderate retardation. All but one also had attention-deficit disorder. The authors underlined the young age at onset of the disease in the patients who had neuropsychological deficits.

In our opinion, the psychological outcome partly depends on an early diagnosis, allowing appropriate treatment and reassurance of the family for the future. The early occurrence of epilepsy often generates great anxiety and leads to wrong educational attitudes. There are, however, also other factors related either to an associated pathology or to an abnormal family structure and a disturbed mother/infant relationship. Finally, it cannot be excluded that the biologic process that causes the myoclonic attacks also interferes with the development of cognitive functions when it occurs in a very immature brain.

DIFFERENTIAL DIAGNOSIS

Differential diagnosis must be made with respect to the other epileptic and nonepileptic manifestations that appear in the first years of life. These include *benign nonepileptic myoclonus* described by Lombroso and Fejerman.[21] In this condition, both ictal and interictal EEG patterns are always normal, and the ictal manifestation is not a true myoclonus, but rather a movement similar to a shiver.

When myoclonic seizures start in the first year of life, the other diagnosis that comes to mind is that of *cryptogenic infantile spasms* (IS). IS are clinically different from benign myoclonias: They are more intense, and they involve a strong flexion (or extension) of the whole body, which is never observed in BMEI. In addition isolated, sporadic spasms are always associated with serial spasms in the same infant, and long serial spasms are more likely with awakening. Polygraphic recordings of IS show a typical pattern of a brief tonic contraction, well described by Fusco and Vigevano,[15] only rarely a prolonged myoclonia. The ictal EEG is not a fast, generalized PSW. It is variable, accompanied by a sudden flattening with or without superimposed fast rhythms, or a large slow wave followed by a flattening, or even no visible change. The occurrence of IS is associated with behavioral changes, poor quality of contact, and psychomotor delay leading to arrest and regression. Interictal EEGs are always abnormal, demonstrating either hypsarrhythmia or modified hypsarrhythmia, or focal abnormalities; they never show the isolated or brief bursts of bilateral synchronous SW as in BMEI.

In the first year of life, *severe myoclonic epilepsy of infancy* (see Chapter 230) might be considered, but it always starts with long and repeated febrile and afebrile convulsive seizures. Exceptionally, they can be immediately preceded by myoclonic attacks, more often focal.[12] They are drug resistant and associated with other seizure types. Psychomotor development becomes delayed during the second year of life with behavioral disturbances.

When myoclonic seizures begin after the end of the first year of life, the diagnosis of a *cryptogenic Lennox-Gastaut syndrome* (LGS) may come to mind. In LGS (see Chapter 241), seizures are typically tonic, leading to sudden falls and injuries, and atypical absences, sometimes associated with atonic seizures. Myoclonic seizures are rare. The ictal EEG shows either a recruiting rhythm, a flattening, or a high slow wave followed by runs of low-voltage rapid rhythms. Interictal awake EEGs are characterized by bursts of diffuse slow SW, and sleep EEGs by PSW and diffuse, high-voltage, rapid rhythms. When these EEG features are not present at the very beginning, the diagnosis is based on the rapid association of different types of seizures such as atypical absences and axial tonic seizures, constant impairment of behavior and learning, and lack of efficacy of antiepileptic drugs.

If myoclonic seizures remain isolated or are associated with GTCS, the diagnosis *of epilepsy with myoclonic astatic seizures* (EMAS) (see Chapter 232) must be entertained, although the onset of myoclonic astatic seizures in this syndrome is rare before the age of 3 years.[8] There are two essential differences. The first one is the clinical aspect of the seizures, which associate myoclonic jerks without fall and myoclonic-atonic or pure atonic seizures leading to violent drop attacks. In BMEI, only rarely do the myoclonic seizures provoke falls on the ground. In EMAS, the myoclonic seizures are combined with other seizure types, such as repeated GTCS, atypical absences, and minor epileptic status with stupor, which are never observed in BMEI. The second difference lies in EEG features. SW and PSW are more numerous, often interictal, and grouped in long bursts with an irregular frequency. They are activated by sleep where polyspikes can predominate. The typical theta rhythm over the centroparietal areas described in the seminal Doose's study[8] is not always present. Other differential criteria appear during the following months, including pharmacoresistance and slowing down of psychomotor delay. Some cases included by Doose,[8] however, should probably be classified as BMEI. In the same way, the group studied by Delgado-Escueta et al.[7] under the name of early childhood myoclonic epilepsy (ECME) seems to include cases of both EMAS and BMEI. On the other hand, some relationship between the two syndromes is strongly suspected (see later discussion).

A recent study[23] emphasized the relationship between BMEI and the syndrome of *eyelid myoclonias with absence* because the authors observed eyelid myoclonias with myoclonic seizures in three children. One of them later, at 10 years of age, had this seizure type. Other authors have not observed this evolution.

Finally, one should consider other epilepsies beginning in the first 3 years of life in which myoclonias are the main seizure type and which have a variable prognosis. They are heterogeneous: There is a combination of other types of seizures, constant presence of EEG focal abnormalities, previous delayed psychomotor development, poor response to drugs, and uncertain prognosis.[9,11] Most probably those are cases of symptomatic myoclonic epilepsies. We also mention the *autosomal-recessive benign myoclonic epilepsy of infancy* described in a single family,[27,28] in which myoclonic seizures were associated with GTCS persisting in adulthood. The locus was mapped to chromosome 16p13 in this family.

DIAGNOSTIC EVALUATION

The diagnostic workup is simple. It requires a good clinical description and repeated polygraphic video-EEG recordings to demonstrate the presence of myoclonic seizures with generalized SW discharges, either spontaneous or facilitated by drowsiness, noise, contact, or IPS. A sleep recording shows slight activation of discharges without change in morphology, without appearance of rapid rhythms and focal abnormalities. Neuroimaging can be useful to confirm the absence of brain lesions but is not mandatory when the symptomatology is typical. Neuropsychological assessment is more useful to check psychomotor development and follow its evolution. Biologic investigations may be necessary in cases where associated symptoms suggest another disease.

MANAGEMENT

Treatment of choice is VPA monotherapy, which must be prescribed as soon as possible. The use of solution is preferable to that of syrup because it is better tolerated by the infant. Plasma levels must be monitored carefully. A dose of 30 mg/kg divided three times a day is usually sufficient, but higher doses are necessary in some patients.[18] VPA is also effective against possible febrile seizures. If myoclonias are not completely controlled by VPA, the addition of either a benzodiazepine (clobazam or nitrazepam) or ESM can be considered, and the diagnosis must be reviewed. Treatment should be continued for 3 to 4 years if it is well tolerated. In cases of purely reflex seizures, drug therapy may be avoided. When used, seizures can usually be stopped early, except in cases of photosensitivity. The occurrence of a GTCS at adolescence can require another brief period of treatment. The medical treatment must be associated with psychological help to the family, who may be extremely anxious and need to be reassured concerning the good prognosis of this epilepsy.

In practice, the diagnosis of BMEI should be restricted to patients fulfilling the following criteria:

- Brief myoclonic seizures, spontaneous or provoked by noise or contact
- Onset between 4 months and 3 years
- Previously normal infant, often with a family history of epilepsy or FS
- Not associated with other seizure types, except rare simple FS
- In the EEG:
    - Generalized fast SW and PSW during myoclonic seizures
    - Rare interictal SW when awake
    - SW enhanced by drowsiness and slow sleep, sometimes by IPS
    - Normal background
    - Absence of focal discharges
- Good response to VPA monotherapy

In patients with this typical picture, treatment given without delay leads to a good clinical outcome in terms of seizures and cognitive function. In cases with less typical features, particularly in the presence of focal EEG discharges, the diagnosis remains uncertain until a long remission is observed.[26] When the onset is later than 3 years, the diagnosis may be the same.[18]

NOSOLOGY

This syndrome belongs to the group of idiopathic generalized epilepsies.[4] It seems to be the infantile equivalent of JME. Auvin et al.[2] reported the first two cases in whom the two syndromes were observed successively, and Darra et al.[6] reported a single case of a mother affected by JME. Delgado-Escueta et al.[7] did not find cases of JME in their study of 24 affected family members with ECME, although they found 76% with other types of idiopathic generalized epilepsies. The relationship with EMAS should be investigated as suggested by the case reported by Arzimanoglou et al.[1] and Darra et al.[6] Moreover, Doose[8] mentioned the case of a patient with EMAS who had two children. The first was affected by EMAS and the second by BMEI.

The last problem is that of the terminology this syndrome. In 1981, it was legitimate to name it "benign" because of the constant disappearance of seizures and the usually good psychological outcome. Today, how benign it is questionable, in light of the definition given by the ILAE Commission report[14] "a benign epilepsy syndrome is a syndrome characterized by epileptic seizures that are easily treated, or require no treatment, and remit without sequelae." It is now established that a small proportion of patients with BMEI have other seizures later (15.2%) or are not psychologically normal (17.7%) after remission of epilepsy. Whether the cognitive and personality disorders described in rare patients are the sequelae of their epilepsy is difficult to establish, however, given the early age of onset. In some patients, the syndrome can be associated with another conditions, as is accepted in other idiopathic and benign epilepsies, such as the benign epilepsy with centrotemporal spikes.[16,25]

We had the opportunity to read the paper by Zuberi et al.[29] only after the end of our work and have not included their six cases in our analysis.

SUMMARY AND CONCLUSIONS

In this chapter we have used the name "benign myoclonic epilepsy in infancy" (BMEI), and the terminology is discussed because it has recently been proposed as a substitute for "idiopathic myoclonic epilepsy in infancy."

BMEI epilepsy is defined as the occurrence of myoclonic seizures (MS) without other seizure types, except rare simple febrile seizures (FS), in the first 3 years of life in otherwise normal infants. These myoclonic seizures are easily controlled by a simple treatment and remit during childhood. The psychomotor development remains normal, and no severe psychological consequences are observed. Some patients present with a reflex form, in which the myoclonic seizures are usually triggered by noise or contact.

BMEI was classified among the generalized idiopathic epilepsies in the 1989 international classification. It seems to represent <1% of all epilepsies and around 2% of epilepsies that begin in the first 3 years of life. Genetics is unknown. A family history of epilepsy or FS is present in 50.5% of cases. Juvenile myoclonic epilepsy (JME) and epilepsy with myoclonic astatic seizures (EMAS) were reported in four families.

Age at onset is usually between 4 months and 3 years, exceptionally between 3 and 5 years.

The myoclonic seizures consist of very brief shock-like seizures, affecting mainly the upper limbs and the head, isolated or grouped in short clusters, accompanied by a generalized spike-wave discharge of the same duration in the EEG.

Interictal EEG discharges are rare, more often during drowsiness and sleep. An extensive clinical and EEG description of the myoclonic seizures is given.

The outcome seems to depend on early diagnosis and treatment. Myoclonic seizures are easily controlled by valproate (VPA) alone, and the child may then develop normally. If left untreated, the patient continues to experience myoclonic attacks, and this may lead to impaired psychomotor development and behavioral disturbances. On the whole, 95.4% of the patients reported in the literature became seizure free. However, the use of high doses of VPA and the monitoring of the plasma levels are necesssary at the onset. After seizures are controlled, the dosage can be reduced. In the reflex form, pharmacological treatment can be avoided .

Other types of idiopathic generalized seizures can occur after the disappearance of the myoclonic seizures (15.2% of the published patients) and these respond well to treatment. In two patients BMEI evolved to JME, well controlled by VPA. One patient, after a reflex BMEI, had complex partial motor seizures with a normal EEG.

On the whole, psychological outcome is favorable, and about 80% of the patients are normal. The others have slight to moderate mental retardation. Attention-deficit disorders are also described.

Differential diagnosis includes non-epileptic benign myoclonus of infancy, infantile spasms, severe myoclonic epilepsy in infancy (Dravet syndrome), and epilepsy with myoclonic astatic seizures.

References

1. Arzimanoglou A, Prudent M, Salefranque F. Epilepsie myoclono-astatique et épilepsie myoclonique bénigne du nourrisson dans une même famille: quelques réflexions sur la classification des épilepsies. *Epilepsies.* 1996;8:307–315.
2. Auvin S, Pandit F, De Bellecize J, et al. , and the Epilepsy Study Group of the French Pediatric Neurology Society. Benign myoclonic epilepsy in infants: electroclinical features and long-term follow-up of 34 patients. *Epilepsia.* 2006;47:1–7.
3. Colamaria V, Andrighetto G, Pinelli L, et al. Iperinsulinismo, ipoglicemia ed epilessia mioclonica benigna del lattante. *Boll Lega It Epil.* 1987;58–59:231–233.
4. Commission on Classification and Terminology of the International League Against Epilepsy: proposal for revised classification of epilepsies and epileptic syndromes. *Epilepsia.* 1989;30:389–399.
5. Dalla Bernardina B, Colamaria V, Capovilla G, et al. Nosological classification of epilepsies in the first three years of life. In: Nistico G, Di Perri R, Meinardi H, eds. *Epilepsy: An Update on Research and Therapy.* New York: Alan Liss; 1983: 165–183.
6. Darra F, Fiorini E, Zoccante L, et al. Benign myoclonic epilepsy in infancy (BMEI): a longitudinal electroclinical study of 22 cases. *Epilepsia.* 2006;47(Suppl 5):S31–S35.
7. Delgado-Escueta AV, Greenberg D, Weissbecker A, et al. Gene mapping in the idiopathic generalized epilepsies: juvenile myoclonic epilepsy, childhood absence epilepsy, epilepsy with grand mal seizures, and early childhood myoclonic epilepsy. *Epilepsia.* 1990;31(Suppl 3):S19–S29.
8. Doose H. Myoclonic astatic epilepsy of early childhood. In: Roger J, Bureau M, Dravet C, et al., eds. *Epileptic Syndromes in Infancy, Childhood and Adolescence,* 2nd ed. London: John Libbey; 1992: 103–114.
9. Dravet C. Les épilepsies myocloniques bénignes du nourrisson. *Epilepsies.* 1990;2:95–101.
10. Dravet C, Bureau M. L'épilepsie myoclonique bénigne du nourrisson. *Rev EEG Neurophysiol.* 1981;11:438–444.
11. Dravet C, Bureau M. Benign myoclonic epilepsy in infancy. In: Roger J, Bureau M, Dravet C, et al., eds. *Epileptic Syndromes in Infancy, Childhood and Adolescence,* 4th ed. London: John Libbey; 2005: 77–88.
12. Dravet C, Bureau M, Oguni H, et al. Severe myoclonic epilepsy in infancy (Dravet syndrome). In: Roger J, Bureau M, Dravet C, et al., eds. *Epileptic Syndromes in Infancy, Childhood and Adolescence,* 4th ed. London: John Libbey; 2005: 89–113.
13. Dravet C, Bureau M, Roger J. Benign myoclonic epilepsy in infants. In: Roger J, Bureau M, Dravet C, et al., eds. *Epileptic Syndromes in Infancy, Childhood and Adolescence,* 2nd ed. London: John Libbey; 1992: 67–74.
14. Engel J Jr. A proposed diagnostic scheme for people with epileptic seizures and with epilepsy: report of the ILAE Task Force on Classification and Terminology. *Epilepsia.* 2001;42:1–8.
15. Fusco L, Vigevano F. Ictal clinical and electroencephalographic findings of spasms in West syndrome. *Epilepsia.* 1993;34:671–678.
16. Gelisse P, Genton P, Raybaud C, et al. Benign childhood epilepsy with centro-temporal spikes and hippocampal atrophy. *Epilepsia.* 1999;40:1312–1315.
17. Giovanardi Rossi P, Parmeggiani A, Posar A, et al. Benign myoclonic epilepsy: long-term follow-up of 11 new cases. *Brain Dev.* 1997;19:473–479.
18. Guerrini R, Dravet C, Gobbi G, et al. Idiopathic generalized epilepsies with myoclonus in infancy and childhood. In: Malafosse A, Genton P, Hirsch E, et al., eds. *Idiopathic Generalized Epilepsies: Clinical, Experimental, and Genetic Aspects.* London: John Libbey; 1994: 267–280.
19. Lin YP, Itomi K, Takada H, et al. Benign myoclonic epilepsy in infants: video-EEG features and long-term follow-up. *Neuropediatrics.* 1998;29:268–271.
20. Loiseau P, Duché B, Loiseau J. Classification of epilepsies and epileptic syndromes in two different samples of patients. *Epilepsia.* 1991;32: 303–309.
21. Lombroso CT, Fejerman N. Benign myoclonus of early infancy. *Ann Neurol.* 1977;1:138–143.
22. Mangano S, Fontana A, Cusumano L. Benign myoclonic epilepsy in infancy: neuropsychological and behavioural outcome. *Brain Dev.* 2005;27:218–223.
23. Prats-Vinas JM, Garaizar C, Ruiz-Espinosa C. Benign myoclonic epilepsy in infants [in Spanish]. *Rev Neurol.* 2002;34:201–204.
24. Ricci S, Cusmai R, Fusco L, et al. Reflex myoclonic epilepsy: a new age-dependent idiopathic epileptic syndrome related to startle reaction. *Epilepsia.* 1995;36:342–348.
25. Santanelli P, Bureau M, Magaudda A, et al. Benign partial epilepsy with centro-temporal (or rolandic) spikes and brain lesion. *Epilepsia.* 1989;30:182–188.
26. Sarisjulis N, Gamboni B, Plouin P, et al. Diagnosing idiopathic/cryptogenic epilepsy syndromes in infancy. *Arch Dis Child.* 2000;82:226–230.
27. Zara F, De Falco FA. Autosomal recessive benign myoclonic epilepsy of infancy. In: Delgado-Escueta V, Guerrini R, Medina MT, et al., eds. *Advances in Neurology, Vol. 95. Myoclonic Epilepsies.* Philadelphia: Lippincott Williams & Wilkins; 2005: 139–145.
28. Zara F, Gennaro E, Stabile M, et al. Mapping of a locus for a familial autosomal recessive idiopathic myoclonic epilepsy of infancy to chromosome 16p13. *Am J Hum Genet.* 2000;66:1552–1557.
29. Zuberi SM, O'Regan ME. Developmental outcome in benign myoclonic epilepsy in infancy and reflex myoclonic epilepsy in infancy: a literature review and six new cases. *Epilepsy Res* 2006;70S:S110–S115.

CHAPTER 232 ■ EPILEPSY WITH MYOCLONIC ASTATIC SEIZURES

OLIVIER DULAC AND ANNA KAMINSKA

INTRODUCTION

Epilepsy with myoclonic–astatic seizures (EMAS) is a recently identified type of idiopathic, potentially severe epilepsy. It is characterized by a combination of seizures, including drop attacks, and psychomotor deterioration beginning in early childhood. These features are similar to those of Lennox-Gastaut syndrome, and the syndrome's nosologic limits, particularly with regard to the Lennox-Gastaut syndrome, are still not clearly determined. A "myoclonic variant of Lennox-Gastaut syndrome" has even been reported that most likely corresponds to one subtype of EMAS. Epilepsy with myoclonic–astatic seizures was identified on the basis of two distinct approaches by two different schools of epileptology: German researchers in Kiel identified genetic predisposition as an etiologic factor in severe pediatric epilepsy at the same time that researchers in Marseille were developing the concept of epilepsy syndromes.[5] A clear definition therefore needs to be established distinguishing EMAS from both the Lennox-Gastaut syndrome and other kinds of myoclonic epilepsy occurring in childhood.[8]

In this chapter, we describe the development of EMAS as a syndrome, delineate it nosologically, describe the specific pattern of cognitive and motor dysfunction, define the therapeutic strategy, and describe the present pathophysiologic hypotheses.

HISTORICAL PERSPECTIVES

To understand the apparent contradictions that have paved the way for the identification of EMAS, one has to consider two major schools of epileptology following parallel pathways. The German school—Janz and Christian for adults[9] and Doose and coworkers for children—was making considerable effort to clarify the genetic basis of epilepsy.[7] Careful neurophysiologic analysis played a major role, particularly for children. Doose established a correlations between several electroencephalographic (EEG) patterns and familial antecedents of epilepsy, namely theta rhythms, generalized spike waves, spontaneous or triggered by hyperventilation, and photosensitivity (for a review, see Doose[6]). This allowed him to identify epilepsy conditions affecting early childhood that were thought to be due to genetic predisposition with polygenic inheritance. He called this group, in which myoclonic seizures causing drop attacks were a predominating feature, "centrencephalic myoclonic–astatic petit mal."[7] The main practical interest in the recognition of this group was to show that children with severe epilepsy involving the whole brain and producing drop attacks and cognitive deterioration did not all have Lennox-Gastaut syndrome, and thus some kind of brain lesion, but they could have genetically inherited epilepsy in an undamaged brain.

Patients within "centrencephalic myoclonic–astatic petit mal (CMAPM)" exhibited a range of different types of seizures: tonic–clonic, myoclonic, myoclonic–astatic, tonic, absence, and various types of epilepsy status, mainly myoclonic and absence. However, within this group, Doose distinguished various patterns correlated with different courses[5]:

- Patients who exhibit only generalized myoclonic seizures as the sole seizure type usually have good outcome.
- Patients with clonic seizures from the first year of life experience a severe course and the occurrence of long-lasting clonic status epilepticus contrasting with very few or even no spike waves on EEG.
- Poor outcome is also the case for patients who develop frequent tonic seizures in sleep and for those who have episodes of myoclonic status and develop dementia. Such cases usually begin after the second year of life.
- However, other patients, beginning after 2 years of age, may completely recover, even if they have experienced tonic seizures and daily drop attacks for weeks and their EEG shows a very active spike and wave pattern.

Therefore, although CMAPM features myoclonic seizures and generalized spike-waves, which are assumed to express genetic predisposition, it is completely heterogeneous in terms of clinical presentation, EEG characteristics, and outcome. It is thus not a syndrome, but an etiologic concept of difficult-to-treat generalized epilepsies resulting from genetic predisposition.

In the meantime, the Marseille school developed the concept of epilepsy syndromes following the observation that patients with epilepsy have a variable course ranging from full recovery to pharmacoresistance with major impact on cognitive and motor functions, and that this variability is not related solely to age of onset, seizure type, interictal EEG, or etiology. Indeed, etiology is identified in only one fourth of patients, and the variability also affects both patients without identifiable etiology and those with a given etiology. The type of seizure is not linked to etiology or the course because a given seizure type may occur in epilepsies with the most benign as well as those with the most severe outcome. Children with epilepsy usually exhibit several types of epileptic seizures, and therefore it is not possible to distinguish the various types of epilepsy according to seizure types only. In addition, the neurologic condition prior to onset of seizures, the age of onset, and the interictal clinical and EEG phenomena also vary greatly. However, there are groups of patients that have similar age of onset, seizure types, interictal EEG pattern, and course. These characteristics form the basics of epilepsy syndromes. This concept appeared soon after the clinical introduction of EEG. It became possible to distinguish between two major EEG patterns of generalized spike waves, respectively "petit mal" and "petit mal variant" patterns, which were correlated with different seizure types and distinct courses. In addition, the "hypsarrhythmic" EEG pattern was linked to infantile spasms. This approach to the separation of various epilepsy patterns with distinct courses was then systematized in Marseille. In Lennox-Gastaut syndrome, drop attacks result from tonic seizures or atypical absences, whereas myoclonic seizures are rare. Therefore, it differs from conditions that include mainly myoclonic seizures. When myoclonic epilepsy has begun in infancy without any identifiable cause, two groups with respectively severe (Dravet syndrome) and benign courses could be distinguished. In the last decade of the twentieth century, it became clear that these two conditions were included in Doose's "centrencephalic myoclonic–astatic petit mal."

In addition, in some patients, "centrencephalic myoclonic–astatic petit mal" starts later in life, after the age of 2 years, in which severe myoclonic seizures cause the patient to fall, as in Lennox-Gastaut syndrome. Indeed, that can be difficult to distinguish this from Lennox-Gastaut syndrome. Patients with Lennox-Gastaut syndrome and EMAS share age of onset (early school age, various kinds of seizures including absences and drop attacks), generalized spike waves, and a major impact on cognitive functions. Thus, the usual understanding, expressed by Aicardi, was that there is a range from Lennox-Gastaut syndrome to myoclonic epilepsy, with myoclonic–astatic epilepsy between these two extremes.[1] This concept of a continuum was similar to that of the Montreal school regarding idiopathic generalized epilepsy (e. g., Berkovic et al.[3]). However, the concept of a continuum was inconsistent with the idea that one condition was genetically determined, whereas the other resulted from a brain lesion. Some difference should therefore exist. The difficulty in making reliable and reproducible distinctions lies to in the fact that the number of characteristics to be taken in account challenges our ability to identify possible differences. By applying a special mathematical method called "multiple correspondence analysis,"[10] it proved possible to recognize reproducible differences. This method can identify within a group of items belonging to a population those clusters of individuals that differ from the rest of the population for specific items and identify these items.[2] This method was applied to patients with various types of generalized seizures and various patterns of generalized spike waves, including either 3-Hz spike waves (SW) or slow spike waves (SSW), negative brain imaging, and first seizures between 1 and 10 years of age; two groups could be distinguished:

One group had onset between 5 and 7 years of age had mainly tonic and absence seizures together with SSW, and the course was unfavorable. There was an excess of focal EEG abnormalities. The sex ratio in this group was equal. This is the usual pattern of the Lennox-Gastaut syndrome.

The other group began slightly earlier, between 2 and 5 years of age, with tonic–clonic seizures before the occurrence of myoclonic–astatic seizures and 3-Hz SW. There was an excess of boys. The course was favorable in a majority after 2 or 3 years, although one third had recorded tonic seizures, a feature previously not mentioned in patients who recover. However, in a sizeable proportion, vibratory tonic and absence seizures and long-lasting myoclonic status occurred and the course was unfavorable: Following the disappearance of myoclonic status, clusters of vibratory tonic seizures at the end of night sleep and slow spike waves persisted for years together with major cognitive impact.

DEFINITIONS

Epilepsy with myoclonic–astatic seizures is defined by the combination of myoclonic–astatic seizures and other kinds of generalized seizures, including tonic–clonic, myoclonic, and eventually tonic seizures, absences and erratic myoclonus, and generalized spike-waves beginning in early childhood, between 2 and 5 years of age. The outcome ranges from complete recovery to intractable epilepsy persisting after the end of the second decade and consisting of tonic seizures in sleep with dramatic deterioration of cognitive and motor functions. This syndrome is not related to any brain lesion, but rather to genetic predisposition combined with brain maturational features.

EPIDEMIOLOGY

The epidemiology is not known because this condition has long been confused with Lennox-Gastaut syndrome. It is likely that the incidence is at least in the same range as that of Lennox-Gastaut syndrome if not higher.

ETIOLOGY AND BASIC MECHANISMS

Although the etiology is unknown, familial studies suggest that some genetic predisposition is at work. However, the variable course has no explanation, and the search for gene mutations has been negative.[13] The only differences between favorable and unfavorable cases have been with regard to gender, with a poorer prognosis for boys than girls, and the age of onset, with poorer prognosis in case of late onset.[10]

Mechanism of Intractability and Cognitive Difficulties

The clinical presentation and course mentioned earlier are characteristic and result from the combination of two groups of factors:

- Generalized tonic–clonic seizures, myoclonus, and bursts of 3-Hz generalized SW seem to be determined mainly by genetic predisposition to idiopathic generalized epilepsy thought to involve the thalamocortical circuits. The rhythmicity in this model is generated by the thalamic reticular nuclei and the cortical contribution mainly involving the rolandic strip, generating myoclonus.
- Tonic seizures, atypical absences, and slow spike-waves suggest epileptogenicity-related and age-related hyperexcitability, and therefore a relation to brain maturation, which involves mainly both frontal lobes at that age. Irregular and slow spike-waves probably result from secondary bilateral synchrony involving both frontal lobes through the corpus callosum.

The pattern in patients with early onset but unfavorable course is consistent at onset with the pattern of the first group (genetic). In terms of the course of the disorder, it is consistent with the second group (maturation of frontal lobes) in the course of the disorder.

The relative contribution of these two factors determines the severity of the condition: The combination of both epileptogenic factors could explain the long-lasting episodes of myoclonic status with drowsiness. The interaction of two distinct paroxysmal activities, respectively rhythmic at 3 Hz and irregular and slow at 2 Hz, could generate the apparently chaotic, irregular, and asynchronous spike and slow-wave activity and replace massive myoclonus by erratic myoclonus. The predominance of the latter in the perioral and tongue areas and in distal parts of the upper limbs is consistent with involvement of pyramidal pathways, because these areas are those mainly represented in the rolandic strip. In addition, the combination of two epileptogenic factors could also generate pharmacoresistance.

This formulation also clarifies similarities with Lennox-Gastaut syndrome, because in the latter, there is a combination of some cortical lesion with the same age-related hyperexcitability involving frontal maturation, ensuring pharmacoresistance. Therefore, in Lennox-Gastaut syndrome, pharmacoresistance would result from the combination of two etiologic factors—focal cortical lesion and maturation—whereas in unfavorable cases of EMAS, it would result from the combination of genetic predisposition with maturation. Because one factor is shared by Lennox-Gastaut syndrome and EMAS, the clinical and EEG patterns have similarities that have generated long-lasting confusion. Finally, in favorable cases of EMAS, the contribution of maturation factors would be milder, explaining the neater clinical pattern and lack of pharmacoresistance.

Neuropsychological findings are also consistent with this understanding of pathophysiology: Major features are dysarthria and apraxia, in addition to the ataxia that is often linked to myoclonus. Dysarthria and apraxia both involve areas of the cortex that are adjacent to the rolandic strip. Cases with unfavorable outcome exhibit in addition slowness and attention deficit, which are eventually additional features of frontal lobe dysfunction. The latter is shared with Lennox-Gastaut syndrome.

What Is the Precise Nature of the Genetic Predisposition?

The identification of a specific genetic predisposition to Dravet syndrome may open another way to understand the difference between favorable and unfavorable cases because a specific monogenic predisposition might apply only to unfavorable cases of EMAS.[4] The slightly lower incidence of familial antecedents of epilepsy in unfavorable cases would be consistent with this hypothesis. However, it is also consistent with the hypothesis previously mentioned of a combination of genetic and maturational features. In the case of Dravet syndrome, the characteristic pattern in patients with the mutation in *SCNA1* can be recognized from the beginning of the disorder because they exhibit unilateral clonic seizures. The only way to answer the questions thus opened on the neurobiologic basis of the various aspects of EMAS is through extensive search of the molecular predisposition in this disorder combined with very precise phenotyping. To date, however, such search has been negative.[13]

CLINICAL PRESENTATION

Seizures

Myoclonic–astatic epilepsy begins between 2 and 5 years of age in a previously healthy child, usually with repeat tonic–clonic seizures that may repeat on the same day. Febrile seizures may have occurred, but this is not the rule.

Within a few days or weeks, the patient starts to have falling episodes due to myoclonic seizures. These drop attacks may be very severe, causing face injuries.

At this point, the child exhibits tonic–clonic, clonic, absence, myoclonic flexor, and atonic, and myoclonic–astatic seizures. The child becomes hyperkinetic and inattentive.

Pattern of Cognitive and Motor Dysfunction

The main findings in patients who are mildly affected are ataxia together with abnormal fine movements due to dyspraxia, and speech difficulties. Many patients suffer from attention deficit disorder with hyperkinesia that may persist for many months after the last seizure has occurred. Patients who undergo prolonged episodes of myoclonic status develop dementia.[11]

DIAGNOSTIC EVALUATION

Electroencephalographic Findings

At onset, the interictal EEG shows slowing of the background activity, and generalized spike-waves increase when the patient is falling asleep (Fig. 1). When drop attacks have occurred, videopolygraphic recording shows different mechanisms underlying the falling: myoclonic flexor seizures, atonic seizures, and particularly myoclonic–atonic seizures, which are very particular because they combine myoclonic and atonic components (Fig. 1).[14]

Therefore, the combination of video-EEG and simultaneous recording of the surface EMG is most useful in this situation. It makes it possible to show that the drop attacks are due to the

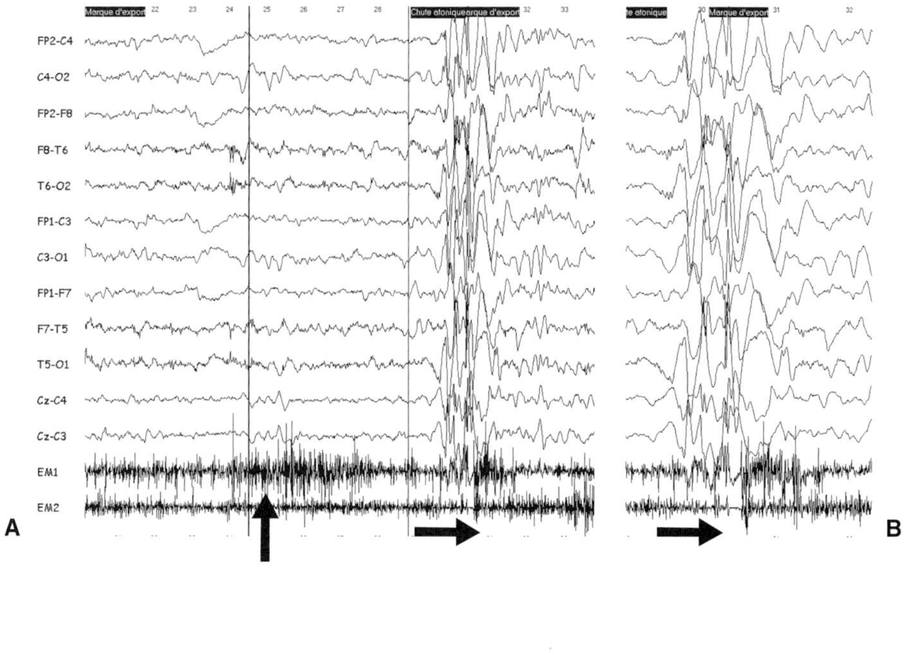

FIGURE 1. Polygraphy in a 3-year-old boy with drop attacks due to epilepsy with myoclonic–astatic seizures (EMAS). Notice that the jerk indicated by the arrow coincides with the spike and precedes the disappearance of muscle tone that coincides with the slow wave, which explains why the child is unable to protect his face from the injury. **A:** 15 mm/s; **B:** 30 mm/s.

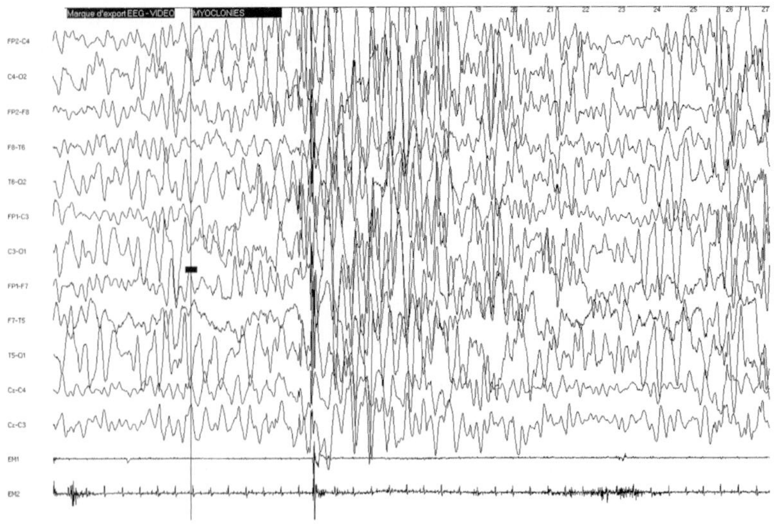

FIGURE 2. Myoclonic status. 1 cm = 100 μV, 15 mm/s; lack of physiologic rhythms, high-amplitude slow waves, and spike waves. Segmentary myoclonus.

patient being thrown forward and losing the ability to protect himself or herself with the upper limbs. This is the cause of severe injury to the face.

Neuroimaging and Other Laboratory Examinations

Neuroimaging is by definition negative, including in those cases with unfavorable outcome. Other laboratory investigations are also negative.

DIFFERENTIAL DIAGNOSIS

At this early stage, there are a few diagnostic issues. Some patients exhibit occasional partial seizures in addition to the generalized tonic–clonic seizures. They are distinct from partial seizures of focal epilepsy because they do not appear as repeated and stereotyped with an interictal EEG focus, as would be the case in focal epilepsy. The distinction is of major importance for the choice of medication. At onset of the disease, it is more dangerous to miss EMAS than to miss partial epilepsy, because the risk of iatrogenic worsening mainly concerns EMAS. On the other hand, the EEG may exhibit major slowing of the background activity, suggesting acute brain damage instead of epilepsy. Again, the physician treating a 2- to 5-year old child who starts having generalized tonic–clonic seizures should always consider the possibility of EMAS because it is highly treatable and, if overlooked, may destroy brain functions.

TREATMENT AND OUTCOME

The Risk for Worsening

One characteristic of this disorder is drug-induced worsening, which has been reported by a number of research groups, including situations before the nosologic characteristics were identified (for review, see Perucca et al.[16]). Carbamazepine was long considered as the drug of first choice for children with epilepsy. It is now clearly established that this drug aggravates EMAS. It is difficult to give the incidence of aggravation due to the lack of controlled data, but Kaminska et al. found in their series that this occurred in more than half of the cases.[10]

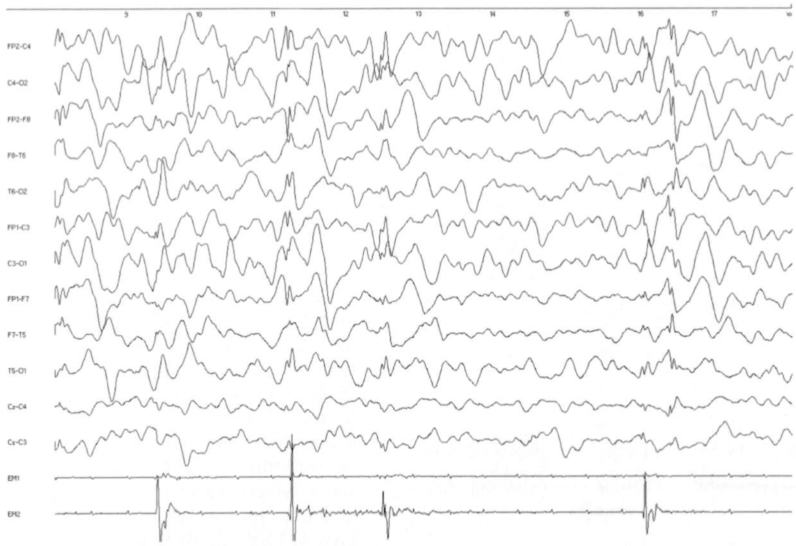

FIGURE 3. Myoclonic status. 1 cm = 200 μV, 1 cm = 30 mm; slow waves with multifocal spikes correlated with erratic myoclonus. Note that the spike activity is very mild.

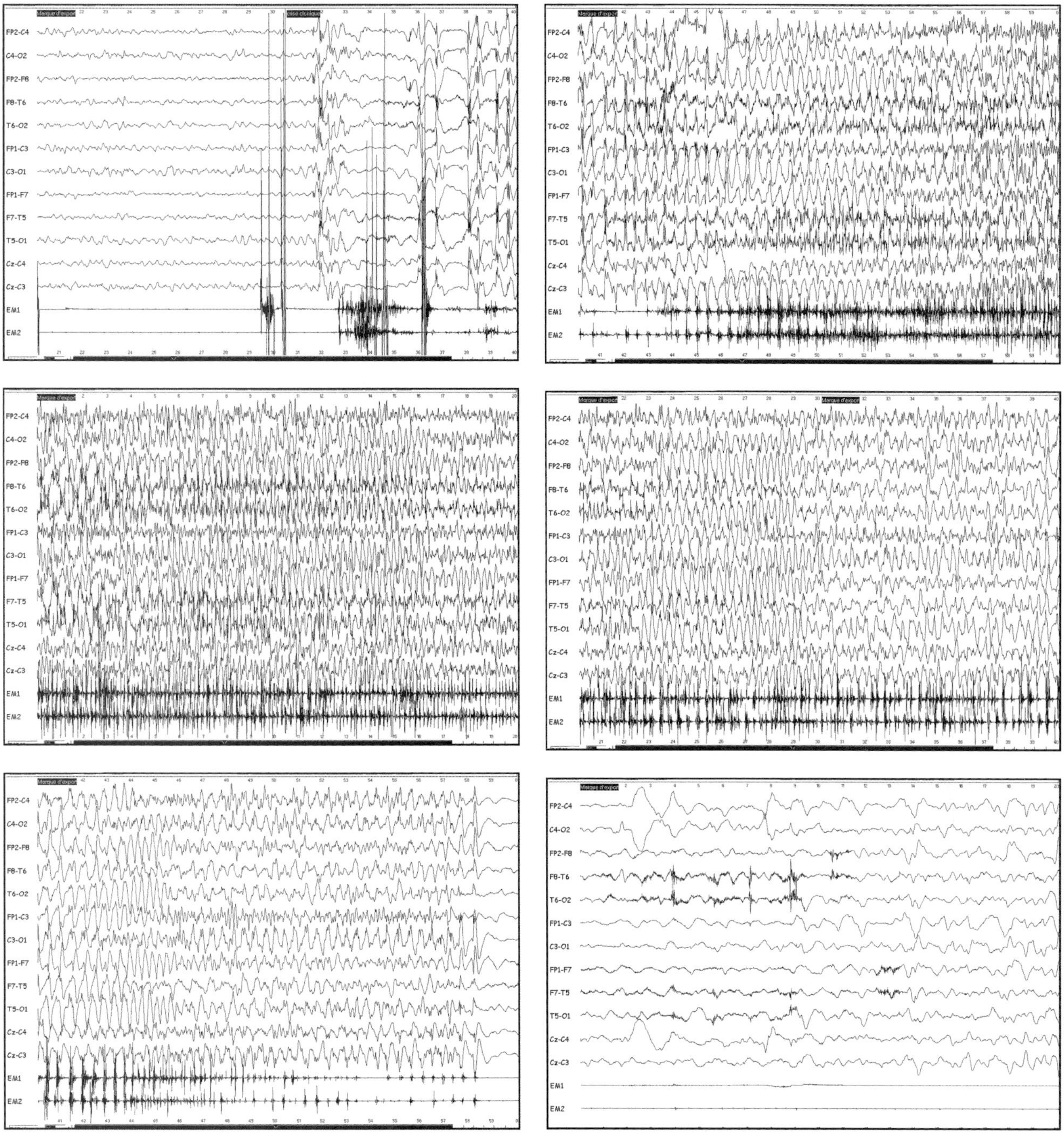

FIGURE 4. Myoclonic–tonic–clonic seizure. 1 cm = 200 μV, 1 cm = 30 mm. Note the complexity of the pattern compared to a classic tonic–clonic seizure observed in adolescence or adulthood, and the major postictal slowing.

The same applies to phenytoin, although this is less often administered to children. It is, however, an excellent drug for the treatment of status epilepticus, and it is then tempting to switch from the intravenous to the oral formulation.

Vigabatrin is also likely to worsen the condition.[12] Although the use of this drug has been restricted due to its potential retinal toxicity, it is very helpful for infants and children with pharmacoresistant epilepsies.

The risk related to the administration of phenobarbital is not as clear. However, given the high incidence of absence seizures in this type of epilepsy and the ability of phenobarbital to precipitate nonconvulsive status epilepticus, this compound clearly represents a theoretical risk for aggravation.

Benefits From Therapy

Valproate has some effect on tonic–clonic, absence, and myoclonic seizures. Ethosuximide is helpful for absences and myoclonic seizures. Benzodiazepines are indicated for the treatment of status epilepticus, but the benefit of long-term everyday administration is less clear for two reasons: These compounds may increase the incidence of tonic seizures or even precipitate tonic status epilepticus, and the chronic administration of the compound may reduce the potential of these compounds to interrupt status epilepticus. In addition, withdrawing benzodiazepines following chronic administration may be challenging because of progressive dependence; it needs to be done over several months. The introduction of lamotrigine has led to a revolution in the treatment of EMAS, with more than three fourths of patients experiencing >75% decrease in seizure frequency and many stopping seizures altogether.[10] Topiramate was effective, reducing seizure frequency by half in more than half of the cases.[18] Levetiracetam seems promising, provided moderate doses are administered at onset, but wider experience is required before it can be advised early in the course of the disorder.

In practice, the occurrence of a first tonic–clonic seizure in a 2- to 5-year-old child requires an EEG, in contrast to later age ranges. Slow basic activity, and even more so the presence of spike waves, indicates the need for administration of valproate. The occurrence of further seizures indicates the addition of lamotrigine. Although the epilepsy may prove intractable for months and could encourage dropping this therapy in favor of less appropriate compounds, seizure frequency tends to decrease progressively. The ketogenic diet is useful in this context, particularly in cases of recent worsening of seizure frequency.[15] Steroids may be useful in cases of frequent absence seizures or myoclonic status.

LONG-TERM PROGNOSIS

The course is variable, with total recovery within a few months to 3 years in most cases, although behavioral abnormalities improve only slowly. A number of patients develop myoclonic status in which the child is drowsy with erratic myoclonus involving the mouth and tongue, the hands, and eventually the rest of the body. The EEG shows high-amplitude polymorphic delta slow waves, with rare and erratic spikes. Other kinds of motor seizures appear mainly at the end of the night, between 5 AM and 7 AM, in clusters consisting of axial hypertonia with a rapid clonic, vibratory component (Figs. 2–4). When unrecognized this status may last several weeks. The term status itself may not be appropriate because the long duration of this kind of seizure activity is also seen in epileptic encephalopathy. Following this episode of epileptic encephalopathy, erratic myoclonus disappears and consciousness improves, but the patient has lost cognitive abilities and become very slow in thoughts and behavior. The long-term unfavorable course is characterized by the persistence of clusters of vibratory tonic seizures at the end of night sleep many years later, even by the beginning of the third decade.

Mental retardation and persisting seizures are the two major features that prevent the patients from normal social integration ($p < 0.001$).[10] The major factors for developing mental retardation are lack of familial antecedents and presence of short 3-Hz SW bursts, as shown with univariate analysis of electroclinical variables. Logistic regression analysis added the presence of tonic and absence seizures at onset as major risk factors ($p = 0.01$). On follow-up, univariate analysis showed that the main factors were duration of epilepsy >3 years ($p < 0.001$), presence of vibratory tonic seizures ($p < 0.001$), and myoclonic status epilepticus ($p = 0.02$). Factors relating to poor school performance in children with epilepsy were shown to include behavior problems, early onset, and polytherapy.[17] Although these children have onset of epilepsy after age 2 years, they have the two other risk factors.

SUMMARY AND CONCLUSIONS

Severe, generalized cryptogenic epilepsies comprise a particularly important model for understanding the respective roles of the three major categories of factors predisposing to epilepsy in childhood: (a) cortical lesions, (b) genetic predisposition, and (c) maturation of the brain. They also contribute to the understanding of factors of intractability in this age range. In addition, they make it possible to apply a mathematical method—multiple correspondence analysis—that is particularly useful in distinguishing discrete groups of patients with epilepsy that may appear as a continuum to the clinician, even though they result from distinct etiologic factors and thus from distinct neurobiologic mechanisms. This has made it possible to confirm mathematically the existence of EMAS as an epilepsy syndrome distinct from Lennox-Gastaut syndrome. The impression of a continuum is given by the combination of several factors in some patients. In addition, recent findings concerning the genetic predisposition to epilepsy suggest that genetic predisposition is heterogeneous due to several monogenic conditions, and thus this heterogeneity also contributes to the impression of a continuum. In addition, modulating genetic factors yet to be identified could also increase the clinical variability and thus the impression of a continuum.

References

1. Aicardi J. *Epilepsy in Children.* New York: Raven Press; 1986.
2. Benzecri J. *Handbook of Correspondance Analysis.* New York: Dekker; 1992.
3. Berkovic SF, Andermann F, Andermann E, et al. Concepts of absence epilepsies: discrete syndromes or biological continuum? *Neurology.* 1987;37:993–1000.
4. Claes L, Del Favero J, Ceulemans B, et al. De novo mutations in the sodium-channel gene *SCN1A* cause severe myoclonic epilepsy of infancy. *Am J Hum Genet.* 2001;68(6):1327–1332.
5. Doose H. Myoclonic astatic epilepsy of early childhood. In: Roger J, Bureau M, Dravet C, et al., eds. *Epileptic Syndromes in Infancy, Childhood and Adolescence.* London: John Libbey; 1992: 103–114.
6. Doose H. *Epilepsien im Kindes- und Jugendalter,* 11th ed. Flensburg, Germany: Desitin Arzneimittel; 1998.
7. Doose D, Gerken H, Morstmann T, et al. Centrencephalic myoclonic-astatic petit mal. *Neuropediatrics.* 1970; 2:59–78.
8. Dulac O, Plouin P, Shewmon A. Myoclonus and epilepsy in childhood: 1996 Royaumont Meeting. *Epilepsy Res.* 1998;30(2):91–106.
9. Janz D, Christian W. Impulsive-Petit mal. *Dtsch Z Nervenheilk.* 1957;176:346.
10. Kaminska A, Ickowicz A, Plouin P, et al. Delineation of cryptogenic Lennox-Gastaut syndrome and myoclonic astatic epilepsy using multiple correspondence analysis. *Epilepsy Res.* 1999;36(1):15–29.
11. Kieffer-Renaux V. Cognitive deterioration in Lennox-Gastaut syndrome and Doose epilepsy. In: Kaminska A, Dulac O, eds. *Neuropsychology of Childhood Epilepsy.* New York: Kluwer; 2001: 185–190.
12. Lortie A, Chiron C, Mumford J, et al. The potential for increasing seizure frequency, relapse, and appearance of new seizure types with vigabatrin. *Neurology.* 1993;43(11 Suppl 5):S24–S27.
13. Nabbout R, Kozlovski A, Gennaro E, et al. Absence of mutations in major GEFS+ genes in myoclonic astatic epilepsy. *Epilepsy Res.* 2003;56(2–3):127–133.
14. Oguni H, Fukuyama Y, Imaizumi Y, et al. Video-EEG analysis of drop seizures in myoclonic astatic epilepsy of early childhood (Doose syndrome). *Epilepsia.* 1992;33(5):805–813.
15. Oguni H, Tanaka T, Hayashi K et al. Treatment and long-term prognosis of myoclonic–astatic epilepsy of early childhood. *Neuropediatrics* 2002;33(3):122–132.
16. Perucca E, Gram L, Avanzini G, et al. Antiepileptic drugs as a cause of worsening seizures. *Epilepsia.* 1998;39(1):5–17.
17. Sabbagh SE, Soria C, Escolano S, et al. Impact of epilepsy characteristics and behavioral problems on school placement in children. *Epilepsy Behav.* 2006;9(4):573–578.
18. Wheless JW. Use of topiramate in childhood generalized seizure disorders. *J Child Neurol.* 2000;15(Suppl 1):S7–S13.

CHAPTER 233 ■ HEMICONVULSION-HEMIPLEGIA-EPILEPSY SYNDROME

ALEXIS ARZIMANOGLOU, CHARLOTTE DRAVET, AND PATRICK CHAUVEL

INTRODUCTION

Hemiconvulsion-hemiplegia-epilepsy (HHE), described by Gastaut et al.[17] in 1957, was not considered as a syndromic entity in the 1989 International League Against Epilepsy (ILAE) classification of epilepsies and epilepsy syndromes. Indeed, one could argue that the initial episode of a prolonged unilateral convulsion can be classified as a unique episode of a motor partial status, with hemiplegia as the main sequela. The later development of focal seizures can be considered, and consequently classified, as a form of partial symptomatic epilepsy. In 2001, HHE was introduced as a syndrome in the published report of the ILAE Task Force on Classification and Terminology.[12] In fact, it is *the stereotyped sequence of events* (hemiconvulsions followed by hemiplegia and leading to a focal epilepsy) that makes HHE "a complex of signs and symptoms that defines a unique epilepsy condition," that is, a syndrome.

As mentioned, taken separately each of its components cannot be considered as an identifiable syndrome because they can be classified into other categories. However, as for progressive myoclonic epilepsies, maintaining HHE as a syndrome is still useful because of the unique characteristics of the condition and their importance when dealing with complex issues and concepts such as secondary epileptogenesis, role of febrile convulsions, and neuroprotection.

HISTORICAL PERSPECTIVES AND DEFINITIONS

The sequence of prolonged hemiconvulsions (the term *unilateral status* could be used to differentiate them from focal status restricted to a body segment) immediately followed by hemiplegia and, secondarily, focal epileptic seizures was identified by Pierre Marie[26] in 1885 within the setting of infantile infectious disorders and described by Gowers in 1886 as "posthemiplegic epilepsy."[18] Similar descriptions advocated a vascular[13] or "acute encephalitic"[7] etiology.

In 1957, Gastaut et al.[17] grouped cases of hemiplegia in childhood following convulsions due to various causes (excluding cases of preexisting brain damage) and were the first to use the term HHE. In their series of 150 patients, they found that >80% of cases of chronic epilepsy occurred after a free interval of <1 year and 50% of cases of "psychomotor" epilepsy after >3 years. Partial seizures were considered to be of temporal origin. Further studies[8,9,33,34] have demonstrated that the initial episode may be observed in various situations and that the subsequent partial epilepsy can be temporal, extratemporal, or multifocal.

The term hemiconvulsion-hemiplegia (HH) is often used to describe the initial stage of the syndrome. It is considered as appearing in a child without antecedents, usually before the age of 4 years. Using current ILAE classification criteria for the definition of syndromes, one cannot consider HH as an epilepsy syndrome, because it corresponds to a unique paroxysmal episode.

The incidence of HHE has declined considerably over the last 20 years. Between 1967 and 1978 the number of HHE cases in the district of Geneva decreased from 7.7 to 1.64 per 10,000 children (Beaumanoir, cited by Roger et al.[35]). A *PubMed* search reveals that the most recent publication of a series on HHE dates back in 1988[21]; it reported on computed tomography (CT) and electroencephalogram (EEG) abnormalities in 25 children with post-hemiconvulsive hemiplegia hospitalized between 1968 and 1980. Since 1995 not more than ten small series or isolated case reports have been published. It is expected that it would be difficult for isolated cases to be accepted for publication. The lack of published large series, however, probably reflects the dramatic improvement in the acute treatment of prolonged seizures in young children. As a consequence, some children who experienced HH avoid motor sequelae and late-onset epilepsy, whereas others do not develop the full HHE clinical picture and are considered as focal epilepsies with antecedents of an acute, usually febrile, convulsive episode.

AGE AT ONSET

The HH initial episode has its peak of incidence during the first 2 years of life; 60% to 85% of the cases occur between 5 months and 2 years of age, with only few patients who are 4 years or older.[3,36] In approximately three fourths of patients, the HH episode evolves to the secondary appearance of partial epilepsy. The average interval from the prolonged initial convulsion to chronic epilepsy was 1 to 2 years, with 85% of the epilepsies having started within 3 years in one study.[3] However, this series was biased in favor of the early onset of complex partial seizures, and these often occur 5 to 10 years after the initial episode.

CLINICAL PRESENTATION AND DIAGNOSTIC EVALUATION

The first stage of the syndrome, *hemiconvulsion*, constitutes a particular form of status epilepticus corresponding to the *unilateral seizures* described by Gastaut et al.[15] As stated in the previous edition of this book and by Arzimanoglou et al.,[6] this type of seizure deserves to be distinguished because it occurs frequently in infants and young children, diffuses to the whole of the affected side and can last 30 minutes or more (up >24 hours if untreated). In children, most of the long-lasting hemiconvulsions, particularly in the presence of fever, are the initial epileptic manifestations,[2,3,30] which explains the impossibility of prevention. Recognition of this type of seizure by general practitioners, pediatricians, and nurses is of primary importance because in most of the cases the outcome is favorable,[27,39] provided treatment is administered early in the course of the seizure. The seizure is predominantly of the clonic type, with saccadic adversion of head and eyes to one side and unilateral, more or less rhythmic jerks of the limb muscles (with contralateral involvement), variable degree of impairment of consciousness, and autonomic symptoms (cyanosis, hyersalivation, respiratory dysfunction) of variable severity.

The ictal discharge consists of rhythmic (2–3/s) bilateral slow waves, with higher amplitude on the hemisphere contralateral to the clinical seizure. On this side they are intermingled with recruiting rhythms of 10 cycles/s, which predominate posteriorly (Fig. 1). Ictal EEG is variable because of changes in shape, frequency, and topography of the slow and fast components. Pseudorhythmic Spike-waves (SWs) contralateral to the clinical seizure, periodically interrupted by electrodecremental events of 1 to 2 seconds' duration, also may occur. Polygraphic recordings do not demonstrate any consistent relationship between muscle jerks and spikes. Spontaneous seizure termination is brisk, with a brief extinction of all rhythms followed by delta waves of higher amplitude on the ictally engaged hemisphere alternating with short periods of suppression. On the opposite side, physiologic rhythms progressively reappear. At this time the hemiplegia is noted. When the seizure is stopped by intravenous diazepam, arrest of muscle jerks is immediate. The ictal discharge progressively vanishes, persisting longer on the ictally engaged hemisphere. Postictal asymmetry is obvious, with abundant drug-induced rapid rhythms invading the contralateral hemisphere.[8]

The second stage of the syndrome, *hemiplegia*, immediately follows the prolonged convulsive episode. It is initially flaccid and fairly massive but tends to become spastic and less marked as time passes. The minimum duration of the hemiplegia is arbitrarily set at <7 days, to separate it from the more common postictal or Todd paralysis. In 20% of the cases of Gastaut et al., the hemiplegia was not permanent and disappeared within 1 to 12 months. In our experience,[6] some degree of spasticity, increased deep tendon reflexes, and pyramidal tract signs persist, even when the paralysis clears. The hemiplegia is usually predominant in the arm, but the face is constantly involved, an important sign that differentiates an acquired hemiplegia from a congenital one in cases of early onset.

The third component of HHE is *focal epilepsy*. The average interval from initial convulsions to chronic epilepsy is 1 to 4 years,[17] with 85% of the epilepsies having started within 3 years of the first hemiconvulsive episode in one study.[3] Vivaldi,[43] in his series of 45 cases, reported a range of 1 month to 9 years after the acute episode. Approximately two thirds of the late seizures are focal seizures with alteration of consciousness.[36,43] Focal seizures without alteration of consciousness, mainly clonic motor seizures, occur in approximately 30% of the patients; secondarily generalized seizures are reported in 20% and other episodes of status in approximately 10%.[36] Gastaut et al. considered that the epilepsy is always made of focal seizures originating from the temporal lobe (previously called "psychomotor seizures").

In an attempt to further characterize the types of epilepsy within the setting of HHE syndrome, Chauvel and Dravet[8] analyzed a series of 37 adult patients investigated in Sainte-Anne Hospital in Paris for surgical therapy. They were selected based on having a history of convulsions in infancy or early childhood, immediately followed by a hemideficit, and after a free interval (ranging from 1 month to 19 years; mean 5.6 years), having developed epilepsy. They had all underwent a stereotactic neuroradiologic investigation as part of the epilepsy surgery evaluation. The age of HH syndrome ranged from 1 month to 9 years. Only 19% presented the initial episode after the age of 3 years. The majority of the patients had several seizure types, whereas only 9 (24%) had one type of seizure. All the patients presented focal seizures, but 3 of them also had "absences" and seizures generalized at onset. The epileptogenic zone was considered unifocal in 29 and multifocal in 8. In the unifocal group, a striking predominance of suprasylvian localizations was found as compared to the pure temporal lobe epilepsies (5 patients). In 14 of those 29 (nearly 50%) the epileptogenic zone included the frontocentral and parietocentral regions; prefrontal epilepsies were rare, and no pure occipital epilepsy was reported. In the multifocal group, a predominant involvement of the parietal lobe was noticed (7 of 8 patients). These results clearly show that epilepsy in HHE is not always of temporal origin, as initially suggested by some authors.

Diagnostic evaluation following the initial acute episode mainly consists in identifying the cause or triggering event responsible (see the later section on the etiology of HHE). Immediately after the HH episode, CT scan may evidence swelling and edema of the hemisphere involved in the epileptic discharge. Later, a rather characteristic uniform hemiatrophy with midline displacement is observed. This evolution was initially reported using pneumoencephalography[2,17,20] or CT scan.[16,21] Case reports including magnetic resonance imaging (MRI) investigation confirmed this pattern.[14] Morimoto et al.'s case[29] showed a unilateral swelling and damaged cortex and subcortical white matter with a high-intensity signal in T2-weighted images at day 17 from status, followed, on day 25 and day 36 neuroimaging, by a severe hemispheric atrophy. Kawada et al.[22] reported a similar evolution, with atrophy being detected from day 15. Follow-up reports on the evolution of hemiatrophy are lacking, but in our experience it remains relatively stable (Fig. 2).

To our knowledge, the longitudinal evolution of interictal EEG abnormalities during the free interval period has not been studied in detail. In the Sainte-Anne series,[8] when the patients were seen for intractable epilepsy, interictal EEG showed multifocal spikes and sharp waves, as well as generalized and bilateral slow waves, in 56% of 37 patients. Widespread interictal abnormalities were more frequently encountered in the symptomatic category (see later discussion) of HHE patients. Even when radiologic studies suggested a strictly unilateral pathology, the distribution of EEG slow waves frequently suggested a more extended lesion (especially in the contralateral hemisphere), and interictal spiking frequently suggested multiple epileptogenic zones.[8]

ETIOLOGY

Prolonged clonic convulsions with a marked unilateral predominance usually occur in the course of a febrile disease. A number of acute cerebral disorders have been occasionally related to the occurrence of the syndrome (meningitis, subdural effusions, head trauma, etc.). In many cases no cause is obvious (*idiopathic hemiconvulsion-hemiplegia* according to Roger et al.[33]), and such cases may represent only prolonged (complicated) febrile convulsions that do not otherwise differ from common febrile convulsions. In such cases the seizure activity itself could be responsible for the appearance of new lesions occurring in a previously normal brain. As Aicardi and Chevrie[3,4] pointed out, "febrile, cryptogenic status epilepticus is only the most severe expression of idiopathic febrile convulsions and differs from the common brief, benign seizures in severity, not in nature." They proposed that "epilepsy and neurological sequelae might be the direct consequence of seizures *per se*." In the same way, Lennox-Buchtal[25] insisted that in cases in which febrile convulsions were focal and prolonged there was a definite risk for mental and neurologic sequelae as well as for subsequent development of epilepsy. The two preceding

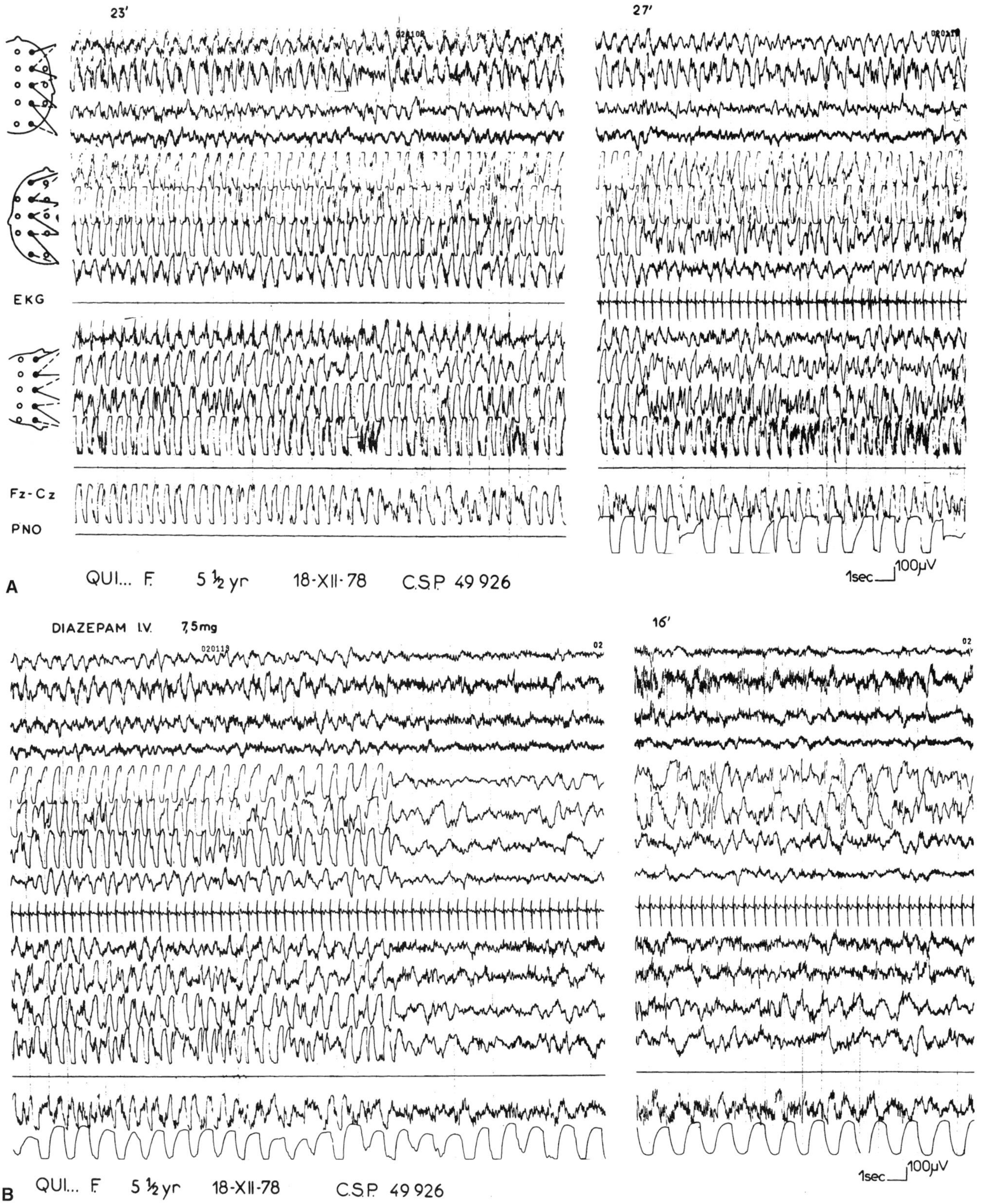

FIGURE 1. Right hemiclonic seizure in course in a 5-year-old boy afflicted with this type of seizure since the age of 3 years. **A:** Recordings 23 and 27 minutes after seizure onset. On the left hemisphere, high-amplitude rhythmic slow waves with superimposed small spikes; on the right hemisphere, rhythmic slow waves over the frontocentral area, with superimposed myoclonic jerks recorded from scalp electrodes. Tachycardia and slight irregularities in respiration. **B:** End of the seizure following intravenous injection of 7.5 mg of diazepam. On the left hemisphere, rhythmic slow waves stop abruptly; 16 minutes later, SW appear over the frontal area. On the right hemisphere, slow waves are replaced at the end of the seizure by fast rhythms caused by diazepam. Respiration becomes more regular. EKG, electrocardiogram; PNO, pneumogram.

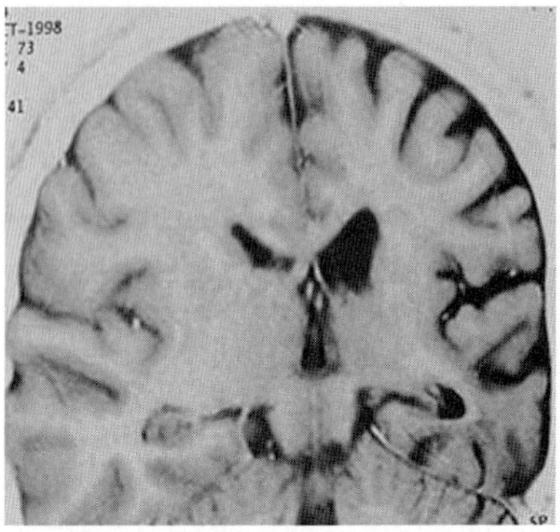

FIGURE 2. Magnetic resonance imaging (MRI) scan of a patient with hemiconvulsion-hemiplegia syndrome. The left hemisphere is diffusely atrophic with ventricular dilation and cortical atrophy. The MRI picture corresponds to the neuropathologic aspect known as hemiatrophia cerebri. It differs from the localized atrophy observed in congenital hemiplegias resulting from arterial occlusion, and it is seen only with acquired post-convulsive hemiplegia. (Reproduced from Arzimanoglou A, Guerrini R, Aicardi J. Epilepsies characterized by partial seizures. In: *Aicardi's Epilepsy in Children*, 3rd ed. Philadelphia: Lippincott Williams & Wilkins; 2004, with permission.)

studies stressed the importance of prompt treatment of febrile convulsions to prevent their sequelae. Furthermore, they stressed the importance of prevention with prophylactic treatment of febrile status in children at risk.

Alternatively, the presence of a preexisting asymptomatic lesion, of perinatal or prenatal origin, may be responsible in a number of cases (*symptomatic hemiconvulsion-hemiplegia* according to Roger et al.[33]) for the initiation or localization of the seizure. The prolonged seizure would then produce or contribute to the development of irreversible brain damage with resultant partial epilepsy.[3–5,25,35,37]

The difference between "idiopathic" and "symptomatic" forms is not always easy to establish. As for "probably symptomatic" focal epilepsies, one could expect that showing some of the related lesions (particularly those due to a migration disorder) depends on the quality and capacity of the means of investigation. Particularly for cases investigated only by pneumoencephalography, CT scan, or early-generation MRI machines, a minor lesion would be difficult to detect. The combination of an "idiopathic" febrile seizure and a potentially epileptogenic lesion would then favor the prolonged character of the convulsive episode and the development of a "symptomatic" HHE syndrome.

The role of long-lasting febrile convulsions, as part of a hemiconvulsion-hemiplegia episode, in the genesis of hippocampal sclerosis and consequent mesial temporal lobe epilepsy also remains disputed. A statistical association is well demonstrated,[32] and there are strong arguments in favor of an etiologic relationship,[19] although the presence or absence of other contributing factors is not clearly established.[5,38,41]

PATHOPHYSIOLOGY

The pathophysiologic mechanisms involved are not clearly elucidated. They most probably involve issues related to the pathophysiology of complicated febrile seizures (genetic factors, the triggering or predisposing role of a preexisting lesion, etc.), the duration of the initial event, the cortical structures involved in the propagation of the initial seizure, and the epileptogenicity of the brain lesions resulting from the initial event.

Chauvel and Dravet[8] recently reviewed the hypotheses on the pathogenesis of the syndrome. They underscored that radiologic studies appear to establish a sequential relation between early repetitive seizures, brain edema, cortical and subcortical atrophy. and, in a good proportion of the cases, chronic epilepsy. For that reason, pathogenesis of the HHE syndrome is of special interest, relating directly to major controversies in the pathogenesis of brain damage in human epilepsy. The principal arguments in this controversy center around two extreme positions: On one hand, it is argued that hypoxic damage (diffuse or selective) would be the result of deficient blood supply (directly by mechanical distortion of the brain at birth, or vascular thrombosis; indirectly by arterial or venous thrombosis of infectious origin[42] or secondary to brain edema); on the other hand, as emphasized by Meldrum and Corsellis,[28]

> insults such as a severe infection or a head injury may well be important factors in some cases, but the most sinister event commonly found to have occurred in epileptic patients with "hypoxic" brain damage is the onset of fits in infancy or in childhood.

The existence of a predisposing genetic factor has been discussed.[31] A high incidence of family history of febrile convulsions is frequently present. Tanaka and colleagues reported ictal and postictal single photon emission computed tomography (SPECT) findings in a 5-month-old boy.[41] When the SPECT was realized during left-sided hemiconvulsions and during the third day after partial status, diffuse hyperperfusion was revealed in the right hemisphere. On the seventh and tenth days after status, diffuse hypoperfusion was exhibited in the right hemisphere. Striking neuroimaging findings suggestive of diffuse cytotoxic edema confined to one hemisphere, including extensive diffusion-weighted imaging abnormalities, were reported by Freeman et al.[14] following early MRI screening. Japanese authors discussed the possible role played by hypercytokinemia[44] and elevated level of interleukin-6 in the cerebrospinal fluid,[23] whereas Scantlebury et al.[37] reported two patients for whom the HHE syndrome could be attributed to the factor V Leiden mutation.

MANAGEMENT

The incidence of hemiconvulsion-hemiplegia-epilepsy syndrome has declined considerably in countries in which emergency care is highly developed.[5,8,35]

Most cases of fever and prolonged convulsions occur during the first 18 months of life. The most important factor is the prompt recognition and early vigorous treatment of prolonged infantile seizures of whatever origin, especially of febrile convulsions. This seems to be the only way to reduce the incidence of postconvulsive hemiplegia and late-onset partial epilepsy. Symptomatic therapy of the acute convulsive episode uses mainly benzodiazepines, particularly diazepam. It can be easily administered by either venous or rectal route. The usual dose is 0.5 to 1 mg/kg given as a single dose. The dose may be repeated after 10 to 20 minutes. Clonazepam, midazolam, or lorazepam may also be used. Antithermic drugs are used in combination. According to the eventual causal agent, additional anti-infectious therapy is required. Prophylactic treatment of febrile convulsions is necessary after HH, but it does not prevent later epilepsy. The outcome of the HH syndrome has become less severe, and subsequent epilepsy seems to be less frequent in idiopathic cases.

In the complete form of the syndrome, partial seizures of temporal or extratemporal origin should be treated like any other type of focal symptomatic epilepsy, using antiepileptic drugs. Surgical treatment is an alternative. However, epilepsies due to extended brain damage may prove difficult to handle surgically. The possibility for a limited cortectomy will usually need an invasive presurgical evaluation performed by a group specialized in epilepsy surgery. Of the 37 patients explored in Sainte-Anne,[8] it was estimated that surgery was possible in only 20. Following surgery, 9 patients (45%) became seizure free or experienced <1 seizure per year; three patients (15%)

showed a significant reduction (40%) in seizure frequency, and no change was obtained in 7 patients (35%). One patient died during a postoperative status.

Hemispherectomy (total, subtotal, or "functional") may be another surgical alternative, particularly when limited cortectomy is not feasible. Delalande et al.[10] included 7 children with HHE syndrome in a series of 53 patients submitted to hemispherotomy. Indications and clinical outcomes of hemispherectomy for epilepsy of various etiologies have been recently reviewed.[11]

Kwan et al.[24] reported on 4-year follow-up in three children who underwent callosotomy. All patients experienced a significant reduction of "generalized tonic seizures," whereas partial seizures of the sensory type were unchanged.

SUMMARY AND CONCLUSIONS

Hemiconvulsion-hemiplegia-epilepsy syndrome can be considered as a unique epilepsy condition because of the stereotyped sequence of events that characterize it. Onset is in the form of an isolated episode of motor partial status (unilateral status) followed by hemiplegia. The seizure is predominantly of the clonic type, with saccadic adversion of head and eyes to one side and unilateral, more or less rhythmic jerks of the limb muscles (with contralateral involvement), variable degree of impairment of consciousness, and autonomic symptoms (cyanosis, hyersalivation, respiratory dysfunction) of variable severity. Hemiplegia, immediately follows the prolonged convulsive episode. It is initially flaccid and fairly massive but tends to become spastic and less marked as time passes. After a free interval the patient will develop focal seizures and neuroimaging will evidence a rather characteristic cerebral hemiatrophy. The complete sequence of event defines HHE. The HH initial episode has its peak of incidence during the first two years of life. The average interval from the prolonged initial convulsion to chronic epilepsy is one to three years. Diagnostic evaluation, following the initial acute episode, mainly consists in identifying the cause or triggering event responsible. The pathophysiological mechanisms involved are not clearly elucidated.

The most important factor that can influence long-term outcome is the prompt recognition and early vigorous treatment of prolonged infantile seizures of whatever origin, especially of febrile convulsions. This seems to be the only way to reduce the incidence of post convulsive hemiplegia and late onset partial epilepsy. In the complete form of the syndrome, partial seizures of temporal or extratemporal origin should be treated as any other type of focal symptomatic epilepsy.

Hemiconvulsion-hemiplegia-epilepsy syndrome is a form of focal epilepsy, more often symptomatic. It is the stereotyped sequence of events that justifies its recognition as a syndromic entity. The HH initial prolonged episode has its peak during the first two years of life and may or may not be related to fever. After a free interval of usually not more than 2 to 3 years approximately three fourths of the children will develop a focal epilepsy, temporal, extratemporal or multifocal.

Vigorous and early treatment of the initial episode, usually with rectal administration of a benzodiazepine, is the most appropriate way to reduce neurological sequelae. The incidence of HHE syndrome has declined considerably in countries in which emergency care is highly developed.

References

1. Aicardi J. Febrile convulsions and other occasional seizures. In: Aicardi J, ed. *Diseases of the Nervous System in Childhood,* 2nd ed. Cambridge: Cambridge University Press; 1998:605–607.
2. Aicardi J, Baraton J. A pneumo-encephalographic demonstration of brain atrophy following status epilepticus. *Dev Med Child Neurol.* 1971;13:660–667.
3. Aicardi J, Chevrie JJ. Convulsive status epilepticus in infants and children: a study of 239 cases. *Epilepsia.* 1970;11:187–197.
4. Aicardi J, Chevrie JJ. Febrile convulsions: neurological sequelae and mental retardation. In: Brazier MA, Coceani F, eds. *Brain Dysfunction in Infantile Febrile Convulsions.* New York: Raven Press; 1976:247–257.
5. Arzimanoglou A, Dravet C. Hemiconvulsion-hemiplegia-epilepsy syndrome. *Medlink Neurology,* 2002. Available: http://www.medlink.com.
6. Arzimanoglou A, Guerrini R, Aicardi J. *Aicardi's Epilepsy in Children,* 3rd ed. Philadelphia: Lippincott Williams & Wilkins; 2003.
7. Bernheim M, Girard P, Larbre F. Le rôle des phlébites cérébrales dans les "encéphalites aiguës de l'enfant." *Sem Hop Paris.* 1955;31:1–14.
8. Chauvel P, Dravet C. The HHE syndrome. In: Roger J, Bureau M, Dravet C, et al., eds. *Epileptic Syndromes in Infancy, Childhood, and Adolescence.* Eastleigh, UK: John Libbey; 2005:277–293.
9. Chauvel P, Dravet C, Di Leo M, et al. The HHE syndrome. In: Lüders H, ed. *Epilepsy Surgery.* New York: Raven Press; 1991:183–196.
10. Delalande O, Fohlen M, Jalin C, et al. From hemispherectomy to hemispherotomy. In: Lüders HO, Comair YG, eds. *Epilepsy Surgery,* 2nd ed. Philadelphia: Lippincott-Raven; 2001:741–746.
11. Devlin AM, Cross JH, Harkness W, et al. Clinical outcomes of hemispherectomy for epilepsy in childhood and adolescence. *Brain.* 2003;126:556–566.
12. Engel J Jr. A proposed diagnostic scheme for people with epileptic seizures and with epilepsy. Report of the ILAE Task Force on Classification and Terminology. *Epilepsia.* 2001;42:796–803.
13. Ford FR, Schaffer AJ. The etiology of infantile acquired hemiplegia. *Arch Neurol Psychiatry.* 1927;18:323.
14. Freeman JL, Coleman LT, Smith LJ, et al. Hemiconvulsion-hemiplegia-epilepsy syndrome: characteristic early magnetic resonance imaging findings. *J Child Neurol.* 2002;17:10–16.
15. Gastaut H, Broughton R, Roger J, et al. Unilateral epileptic seizures. In: Vinken PJ, Gruyn GW, eds. *The Epilepsies. Handbook of Clinical Neurology,* Vol. 15. Amsterdam: Elsevier; 1974:235–245.
16. Gastaut H, Pinsard N, Gastaut JL, et al. Etude tomodensitométrique des accidents cérébraux responsables des hémiplégies aiguës de l'enfant. *Rev Neurol.* 1977;133:595–607.
17. Gastaut H, Vigouroux M, Trevisan C, et al. Le syndrome "hémiconvulsion-hémiplégie-epilepsie" (syndrome HHE). *Rev Neurol.* 1957;97:37–52.
18. Gowers WR. *Epilepsy and Other Chronic Convulsive Diseases: Their Causes, Symptoms and Treatment.* London: Churchill; 1886.
19. Holthausen H. Febrile convulsions, mesial temporal sclerosis and temporal lobe epilepsy. In: Wolf P, ed. *Epileptic Seizures and Syndromes.* London: John Libbey; 1994:449–467.
20. Isler W. Acute hemiplegias and hemisyndromes in childhood. In: *Clinics in Developmental Medicine.* London: Heinemann; 1971:131–140.
21. Kataoka K, Okuno T, Mikawa H, et al. Cranial computed tomographic and electroencephalographic abnormalities in children with post-hemiconvulsive hemiplegia. *Eur Neurol.* 1988;28:279–284.
22. Kawada J, Kimura H, Yoshikawa T, et al. Hemiconvulsion-hemiplegia syndrome and primary human herpes virus 7 infection. *Brain Dev.* 2004;26:412–414.
23. Kimura M, Tasaka M, Sejima H, et al. Hemiconvulsion-hemiplegia syndrome and elevated interleukin-6: case report. *J Child Neurol.* 2002;17:705–707.
24. Kwan SY, Wong TT, Chang KP, et al. Postcallosotomy seizure outcome in hemiconvulsion-hemiatrophy-epilepsy syndrome. *Zhonghua Yi Xue Za Zhi (Taipei).* 2000;63:503–511.
25. Lennox-Buchtal MA. Febrile convulsions. A reappraisal. *Electroencephalogr Clin Neurophysiol.* 1973;32:1–132.
26. Marie P. Hémiplégie cérébrale infantile et maladies infectieuses. *Prog Med.* 1885;2:167.
27. Maytal J, Shinnar S. Febrile status epilepticus. *Pediatrics.* 1990;86:611–616.
28. Meldrum BS, Corsellis JAN. Epilepsy. In: Hume Adams J, Corsellis JAN, Duchen LW, eds. *Greenfield's Neuropathology.* New York: Wiley; 1984: 921–950.
29. Morimoto T, Fukuda M, Suzuli Y, et al. Sequential changes of brain CT and MRI after febrile status epilepticus in a 6-year-old girl. *Brain Dev.* 2002;24(3):190–193.
30. Nelson KB, Ellenberg JH. Prognosis in children with febrile seizures. *Pediatrics.* 1978;61:720–727.
31. Ounsted C, Lindsay J, Norman R. *Biological Factors in Temporal Lobe Epilepsy. Clinics in Developmental Medicine,* No. 2. London: Spastics Society and Heinemann Medical; 1996.
32. Rocca WA, Sharbrough FW, Hauser WA, et al. Risk factors for complex partial seizures: a population-based case-control study. *Ann Neurol.* 1987;21:22–31.
33. Roger J, Bureau M, Dravet C, et al. Les données EEG et les manifestations épileptiques en relation avec l'hémiplégie cérébrale infantile. *Rev EEG Neurophysiol.* 1972;2:5–28.
34. Roger J, Dravet C, Bureau M. Unilateral seizures (hemiconvulsion-hemiplegia syndrome and hemiconvulsion-hemiplegia-epilepsy syndrome). *Electroencephalogr Clin Neurophysiol.* 1982;35(Suppl):211–221.
35. Roger J, Dravet C, Bureau M. Unilateral seizures: hemiconvulsions-hemiplegia syndrome (HH) and hemiconvulsions-hemiplegia-epilepsy syndrome (HHE). In: Broughton RJ, ed. *Henri Gastaut and the Marseilles School's Contribution to the Neurosciences.* Amsterdam: Elsevier Biomedical Press; 1982:203–219.

36. Roger J, Lob H, Tassinari CA. Status epilepticus. In: Vinken PJ, Bruyn GW, eds. *Handbook of Neurology,* Vol. 15, *The Epilepsies*. Amsterdam: North-Holland; 1974:145–188.
37. Scantlebury MH, David M, Carmant L. Association between factor V Leiden mutation and the hemiconvulsion, hemiplegia, and epilepsy syndrome: report of two cases. *J Child Neurol*. 2002;17:713–717.
38. Scott RC, Gardian DG, King MD, et al. Magnetic resonance imaging findings within 5 days of status epilepticus in childhood. *Brain*. 2002;125:1951–159.
39. Shinnar S, Pellock JM, Berg AT, et al. Short-term outcomes of children with febrile status epilepticus. *Epilepsia*. 2001;42:47–53.
40. Shinnar S, Maytal J, Krasnoff L, et al. Recurrent status epilepticus in children. *Ann Neurol*. 1992;31:598–604.
41. Tanaka Y, Nakanishi Y, Hamano S, et al. Brain perfusion in acute infantile hemiplegia studied with single photon emission computed tomography [in Japanese]. *No To Hattatsu*. 1994;26:68–73.
42. Veith G, Spittler JF. Früherworbene Hemiparesen und chronische Epilepsie, eine Klinisch-Pathologische Studien um 64 Fällen. *Fortschr Neurol Psychiatr*. 1981;49:77–87.
43. Vivaldi J. *Les crises hémicloniques de l'enfant: modalités évolutives*. Thèse, Marseille; 1976.
44. Wakamoto H, Ohta M, Nakano N. Hypercytokinemia in hemiconvulsions-hemiplegia syndrome associated with dual infection with varicella zoster and Epstein-Barr viruses. *Neuropediatrics*. 2002;33:262–265.

CHAPTER 234 ■ MYOCLONIC STATUS IN NONPROGRESSIVE ENCEPHALOPATHY

BERNARDO DALLA BERNARDINA

INTRODUCTION

Despite the existence in the literature of proof of the possible occurrence in infants and young children of an absence status with myoclonias of variable severity and duration called by various names, such as "minor epileptic status," "minor motor status," "myoclonic status," "obtundation with myoclonias," "nonconvulsive states with ataxia," "myoclonic state with impaired consciousness," "myoclonic status in symptomatic cases of myoclonic astatic epilepsy," and so on,[1–3,6,9,10,24,27,28,32,36,38,42] reports documenting the existence of an epileptic syndrome characterized by the recurrence of long-lasting or subcontinuous myoclonic status in children with a nonprogressive encephalopathy are relatively rare.[7,11,13,15,16,18–21,25,33] In fact a very similar electroclinical picture has been described in children with Angelman syndrome,[8,25,33–35,37,39,41,43,45,47,52] in some children with 4p- syndrome,[44,46,53] and in some children with Rett syndrome,[17] but very few authors have stressed how, in these cases, the electroclinical picture was typically that of "myoclonic status in nonprogressive encephalopathy,"[15–19,22,40,44] a syndromic entity recently proposed by the ILAE Task Force on Classification and Terminology[41] in its category "syndromes in development."

DEFINITIONS

The syndrome is characterized by the recurrence of long-lasting myoclonic status, that is often difficult to recognize and frequently refractory to different treatments, in children with a nonprogressive encephalopathy of variable etiology.

EPIDEMIOLOGY

The prevalence of this condition is unknown; it seems to be rare because the only three series available[7,11,17] account for a total of 96 cases. The true prevalence is probably higher than reported, considering that many similar cases can remain misdiagnosed particularly in the absence of polygraphic recordings. There appears to be a female predominance, with a male:female ratio of 1:2. Familial antecedents for epilepsy are present in about 15% of cases.

ETIOLOGY AND BASIC MECHANISMS

A genetic disorder (4p- syndrome, Rett syndrome, and especially Angelman syndrome) is present in nearly half of the reported cases. In such cases, nonsignificant abnormalities are neuroradiologically detectable.

A history of prenatal anoxic injury is well documented in about 15% of the cases. In about half of these cases, the neuroradiologic investigation shows cortical atrophy of variable degree that maximally affects the frontal regions.

In about one third of cases, neuroradiologic investigations reveal brain developmental malformations such as unilateral or bilateral micropolygyria, complete or partial callosal agenesis, vermis hypoplasia, or bilateral hippocampal dysgenesis, in most cases probably genetically determined.[7,17]

In the remaining 10% of cases, the etiology is unknown, with normal neuroradiologic and other laboratory investigations.

In some of the genetic cases, as in Angelman syndrome and 4p- syndrome, hyperexcitability of the motor cortex might be related to reduced GABAergic inhibition. In pre and perinatal anoxic cases, a similar "localized" hyperexcitability could be induced by a circulatory disturbance in late pregnancy causing selective dysfunction in the motor cortex.[11]

ELECTROCLINICAL PRESENTATION

Neurological impairment, which may be severe, has been observed at onset in almost three fourths of the cases. There is axial hypotonia of variable degree associated with abnormal movements, presenting a picture of "ataxic" cerebral palsy of a dystonic dyskinetic syndrome, severe mental retardation and, in some cases, microcephaly with dysmorphisms.

In one fourth of the cases, the neurologic impairment at onset is less obvious, characterized only by delayed postural acquisitions and language skills.

Age at first seizure ranges between 1 month and 5 years, with a mean age of 10 months.

Onset of epilepsy in several cases has been characterized by a myoclonic status with very frequent daily or subcontinuous "absences" accompanied by periorbital and perioral myoclonias and rhythmic and arrhythmic jerks of distal muscles in nearly half of the cases. In other childern, the initial seizures are mostly partial motor, brief myoclonic absences, massive myoclonias, and, more rarely, generalized or unilateral clonic seizures. Massive startles frequently occur at rest and during drowsiness.

The average age at which myoclonic status is recognized is 14 months (range: 3 months–5 years). Because of severe mental retardation and continuous abnormal movements, both the paroxysmal attention disturbances ("absences") and the myoclonias can remain unrecognized for several months. Considering its insidious appearance, it is probable that the age of onset of the status, in many cases, may be significantly earlier than when it is recognized.

In many cases, the myoclonias are subcontinuous but asynchronous in different muscles, and their relationship to the paroxysmal electroencephalographic (EEG) activity is difficult to appreciate because they are arrhythmic and subtle and also because the paroxysmal nature of the EEG pattern is often difficult to recognize.

In some cases the myoclonias are more obvious, involving rhythmic contractions of both arms and orofacial muscles. In other cases, the myoclonias are followed by a brief silent period constituting a mixture of positive and negative phenomena. In others, negative myoclonus is predominant, continuously fragmenting the voluntary movements and inhibiting the maintenance of any fixed antigravitary postures.

Even when the child is awake, the EEG is characterized by slow and poorly reactive activity with paroxysmal abnormalities. These consist of relatively monomorphic subcontinuous delta-theta activity (3–6 c/s) that varies in amplitude and occurs asynchronously over the frontocentral regions. In addition, there are brief sequences of rhythmic delta waves with superimposed spikes constituting unusual spike and wave complexes.

When the myoclonias are rhythmic, synchronous on the two sides, and strictly related to the diffuse paroxysmal bursts, they constitute an ictal pattern similar to that of a brief myoclonic absence.

The myoclonias become easier to recognize when there is motor arrest, such as during absence or drowsiness when all other abnormal movements disappear.

During drowsiness and slow wave sleep, spikes and waves become continuous to the point that sleep spindles are not recognizable. During stages II and III of the following nocturnal cycles, the paroxysmal activation ceases and spindles are clearly represented. During slow wave sleep, the myoclonias vanish, reappearing briefly at arousal. During rapid eye movement (REM) sleep when the diffuse discharges disappear, there is continuous rhythmic theta activity involving mainly the vertex and rolandic regions. The same theta activity strictly related to myoclonias is transitorily observed during alerting.

Based on the electroclinical picture, three main subgroups can be recognized.

The *first group* consists of patients who show a mixed pattern of brief myoclonic absences and subcontinuous rhythmic positive jerks, eventually followed by a brief silent period related to subcontinuous delta-theta activity involving the central areas accompanied by brief sequences of rhythmic delta waves with superimposed spikes mainly involving the parieto-occipital regions and often elicited by eye closure.

In this group, the status can be recognized during the first year of life. These are events of variable duration recurring sporadically in about half of the cases, whereas they are more "chronic" (lasting for years) in about one fourth of the cases. No other types of seizures are observed except for rare unilateral or generalized seizures that often occur in the setting of a febrile illness.

This electroclinical picture has been observed mainly in children with Angelman syndrome and with 4p- syndrome.

As we have described previously,[16–19,22,23] and as confirmed by other authors,[7,25,33,40] we consider this electroclinical picture to be the earliest diagnostic indicator of Angelman syndrome. Many authors have, in fact, described a very similar status in cases of Angelman syndrome, but they didn't recognize the preeminent myoclonic character.[5,30,37,39,41,43,45,47,48]

The *second subgroup* is made up of patients showing a pattern characterized by the marked predominance of inhibitory phenomena mixed with a severe fragmented dystonic component and sudden irregular, fast, lightning-like jerks. In these cases, the status is often difficult to recognize because of the very severe mental impairment, which is present from onset, and the abundance of continuous polymorphic and coarse abnormal movements. The jerks are mostly erratic and are therefore difficult to distinguish from violent dyskinetic movements. Moreover, the EEG paroxysmal abnormalities consist of subcontinuous multifocal slow spike waves that predominate in the frontocentral regions but fluctuate in amplitude and extent, making it very difficult to correlate with the positive and negative myoclonias. The result is an epileptic status characterized by a complex dysregulated motor pattern inducing a peculiar "hyperkinetic complete motor inhibition."

Except for brief generalized tonic-clonic seizures sometimes in clusters, other types of seizures are very rare.

Patients showing this electroclinical picture are females affected by a nonprogressive encephalopathy of unknown etiology or by associated with a cortical malformation.[7,17]

The *third subgroup* is made up of children who have only mild neurologic impairment at onset. Initially they have partial motor seizures or brief myoclonic absences. More or less rapidly and more or less subtly, a progressive myoclonic status begins, characterized initially by a subcontinuous sequence of generalized spike-wave paroxysms related to the rhythmic myoclonias of face and limbs. With time, there is progressive deterioration of the electrical activity and a morphologic modification of the paroxysms to sharp theta wave type with very slow pseudorhythmic continuous spikes in the central regions and vertex. At the same time, motor function is progressively compromised and pyramidal signs and intention tremors appear. In addition, continuous myoclonic inhibitory phenomenon appears that sometimes can be recognized clinically and polygraphically only when postural tone is increased. Complete motor inhibition is invariably the result.

In one fourth of the cases, magnetic resonance imaging (MRI) shows a probable disturbance, in gyration such as focal bilateral micropolygyria. Some children have Rett syndrome.[7,17]

Partial motor seizures, predominantly tonic and only sometimes followed by generalization, are frequent even at long follow-up intervals, whereas other types of seizures are absent.

DIFFERENTIAL DIAGNOSIS

Because of the significant progressive increase of both neurological impairment and EEG paroxysmal abnormalities as well as worsening polymorphic myoclonic manifestations, the first and often most complex step is the need to exclude a progressive disease, particularly the late infantile form of neuronal ceroid-lipofuscinosis.[4,49,50] The absence of progressive visual impairment with persistence of normal visual evolved potentials (VEP) even when, as frequently observed, the somatosensory evoked potentials (SEP) are abnormal, there is an absence of a paroxysmal response to photic stimulation and there is persistence of recognizable spindles can help to suggest a correct diagnosis.

Neuropathologic and molecular genetic analyses are required to rule out a progressive disease, particularly neuronal ceroid-lipofuscinosis.

Another somewhat difficult differential diagnosis can be with the cases reported in the literature as having a "newborn continuous partial epilepsy,"[14] "early-onset progressive encephalopathy with migrant continuous myoclonus,"[29] or "migrating partial seizures of early infancy"[12,31,51] because many of these can present, soon after onset, long-lasting status characterized by continuous discharges of diffuse spikes and waves accompanied by bilateral asynchronous myoclonias with obtundation and drooling.

TREATMENT AND OUTCOME

In children showing the first electroclinical picture, the status frequently lasts for years refractory to treatment, and even benzodiazepines and adrenocorticotropic hormone generally have only a transitory effect. Nevertheless, in many cases ethosuximide plus valproic acid and levetiracetam leads to a significant improvement, and as the status resolves the clinical picture improves dramatically. Continuous disabling jerks are reduced and some children become able to walk. In about one third of cases, even if the status disappears, intention myoclonus becomes predominant, constituting the picture described by Guerrini et al.[33,35,36] as cortical myoclonus.

In children with the second electroclinical picture, the long-term prognosis is always unfavorable. The status is refractory to different therapies and permanent in evolution, with definitive aposturality and severe mental deficit. Some patients die in long-lasting motor status.

The third electroclinical pattern is a pharmacoresistant progressive epilepsy not associated with a progressive disease. The neurologic impairment increases dramatically over a few years: In one third of the cases, cortical-subcortical and cerebellar atrophy becomes recognizable on MRI.

SUMMARY AND CONCLUSIONS

This particular type of symptomatic myoclonic epilepsy, characterized essentially by the recurrence of long-lasting atypical status associated with an impaired attention and continuous polymorphic jerks mixed with other complex abnormal movements in infants suffering from a nonprogressive encephalopathy, constitutes a unique syndromic entity.

Although this condition is difficult to diagnose clinically, it can be easily recognized by polygraphic recordings, which show rhythmic discharges of diffuse slow spike-waves accompanied by more or less rhythmic asynchronous myoclonias that are continuous during wakefulness and, in many cases, persist during sleep.

It is probable that becuase it is not routine to perform polygraphic recordings in clinical practice, the frequency of this condition has been underestimated.

This status is invariably accompanied by concomitant worsening of the child's neurological condition. The etiology can be varied, and is probably mainly malformative and genetic.

Electroclinical analysis makes it possible to distinguish three subsets of the disorder that have important diagnostic and prognostic significance. The first is characterized by the association of absences, subcontinuous jerks, at times rhythmic or arrhythmic and mainly positive, brief myoclonic absences, and hypnagogic startles. These suggest a diagnosis of Angelman syndrome or the up-syndrome.

The second affects mainly females and is characterized by the association of absence status and continuous rhythmic myoclonus, mainly negative, mixed with sudden, uncontrolled continuous dyskinetic movements leading to a clinical picture of hyperkinetic aposturality, generally sustained by a cortical malformation.

The third is characterized by continuous spike activity over the rolandic regions that persists throughout life accompanied by bilateral rhythmic myoclonias followed by an inhibitory phenomenon leading to a progressive neuromotor deterioration. This presents as a form of myoclonic progressive epilepsy in the absence of a progressive disease. In these cases, cortical dysplasia involving the motor area is frequently recognized.

References

1. Aicardi J, Chevrie JJ. Myoclonic epilepsies of childhood. *Neuropaediatrie.* 1971;3:177–190.
2. Arzimanoglou A, Guerrini R, Aicardi J. Epilepsies with predominantly myoclonic seizures. In: Arzimanoglou A, Guerrini R, Aicardi J, eds. *Aicardi's Epilepsy in Children.* Philadelphia: Lippincott Williams & Wilkins; 2004: 58–80.
3. Bennett HS, Selman JE, Rapin I, et al. Non convulsive epileptiform activity appearing as ataxia. *Am J Dis Child.* 1982;136:30–32.
4. Binelli S, Canafoglia L, Panzica F, et al. Electroencephalographic features in a series of patients with neuronal ceroid lipofuscinoses. *Neurol Sci.* 2000;21(3 Suppl):S83–S87.
5. Boyd SG, Harden A, Patton MA. The EEG in early diagnosis of the Angelman (Happy Puppet) syndrome. *Eur J Pediatr.* 1988;147:508.
6. Brett EM. Minor epileptic status. *J Neurol Sci.* 1966;3:52–75.
7. Caraballo et al. Myoclonic status in Non-progressive encephalopathies. In preparation.
8. Casara GL, Vecchi M, Boniver C, et al. Electroclinical diagnosis of Angelman syndrome: A study of 7 cases. *Brain Dev.* 1995;17:64–68.
9. Cavazzuti GB, Nalin A, Ferrari F, et al. Encefalopatie miocloniche nel primo anno di vita. *Riv Ital EEG Neurofisiol Clin.* 1979;2:253–261.
10. Chevrie JJ, Aicardi J. Childhood encephalopathy with slow spike wave. A statistical study of 80 cases. *Epilepsia.* 1972;13:259–271.
11. Chiron C, Plouin P, Dulac O, et al. Epilepsies myocloniques des encephalopathies non progressives avec etats de mal myoclonique. *Neurophysiol Clin.* 1988;18:513–524.
12. Coppola G, Plouin P, Chiron C, et al. Migrating partial seizures in infancy: A malignant disorder with developmental arrest. *Epilepsia.* 1995;36(10):1017–1024.
13. Dalla Bernardina B, Colamaria V, Capovilla G, et al. Nosological classification of epilepsies in the first 3 years of life. In: Nisticò G, Di Perri R, Meinardi H, eds. *Epilepsy: An Update on Research and Therapy.* New York: Alan R. Liss; 1983: 165–183.
14. Dalla Bernardina B, Colamaria V, Capovilla V, et al. Epilessia parziale continua del lattante. *Boll Lega It Epil.* 1987;58/59:101–102.
15. Dalla Bernardina B, Fontana E, Darra F. Myoclonic status in non-progressive encephalopathies. In: Roger J, Bureau M, Dravet C, et al., eds. *Epileptic Syndromes in Infancy, Childhood and Adolescence,* 3rd ed. London: John Libbey; 2002: 137–144.
16. Dalla Bernardina B, Fontana E, Darra F. Myoclonic status in non–progressive encephalopathies. In: Roger J, Bureau M, Dravet C, et al., eds. *Epileptic Syndromes in Infancy, Childhood and Adolescence,* 4th ed. London: John Libbey; 2005: 149–157.
17. Dalla Bernardina B, Fontana E, Darra F. Myoclonic status in nonprogressive encephalopathies. In: Gilman S, Goldstein GW, Waxman SG, eds. *Neurobase.* San Diego, CA: Arbor Publishing; 2001.
18. Dalla Bernardina B, Fontana E, Sgrò V, et al. Myoclonic epilepsy ('myoclonic status') in non-progressive encephalopathies. In: Roger J, Dravet C, Bureau M, et al., eds. *Epileptic Syndromes in Infancy, Childhood and Adolescence,* 2nd ed. London: John Libbey; 1992: 89–96.
19. Dalla Bernardina B, Fontana E, Zullini E, et al. Angelman syndrome: Electroclinical features of ten personal cases. *Gaslini.* 1995;27:75–78.
20. Dalla Bernardina B, Trevisan C, Bondavalli S, et al. Une forme particulière d'épilepsies myoclonique chez des enfants porteurs d'encéphalopathie fixée. *Boll Lega It Epil.* 1980;29–30:183–187.
21. Dalla Bernardina B, Trevisan E, Colamaria V, et al. Myoclonic epilepsy ('myoclonic status') in non-progressive encephalopathies. In: Roger J, Dravet C, Bureau M, et al., eds. *Epileptic Syndromes in Infancy, Childhood and Adolescence.* London: John Libbey; 1985:68–72.
22. Dalla Bernardina B, Zullini E, Fontana E, et al. Electroclinical longitudinal study of ten cases of Angelman's syndrome. *Epilepsia.* 1993;34(Suppl 2): 71.
23. Dalla Bernardina B, Zullini E, Fontana E, et al. Sindrome di Angelman: Studio EEG-poligrafico di 8 casi. *Boll Lega It Epil.* 1992;79/80: 257–259.
24. Doose H. Myoclonic astatic epilepsy of early childhood. In: Roger J, Bureau M, Dravet C, et al., eds. *Epileptic Syndromes in Infancy, Childhood and Adolescence.* London: John Libbey; 1992: 103–114.
25. Dulac O, Plouin P, Shewmon A, Contributors to the Royaumont Workshop. Myoclonus and epilepsy in childhood. 1996 Royaumount Meeting. *Epilepsy Res.* 1998;30:91–106.
26. Engel J. A proposed diagnostic scheme for people with epileptic seizures and with epilepsy: Report of the ILAE Task Force on Classification and Terminology. *Epilepsia.* 2001;42(6):796–803.
27. Erba G, Lombroso CT. Angelman's (Happy Puppet) syndrome: Clinical, CT scan and serial electroencephalographic study. *Clin Electroencephalogr.* 1973;20:128–140.
28. Fejerman N. Myoclonus and epilepsies in children. *Rev Neurol.* 1991;147(12):782–797.
29. Gaggero R, Baglietto MP, Curia R, et al. Early-onset progressive encephalopathy with migrant, continuous myoclonus. *Child's Nerv Syst.* 1996;12(5):254–261.
30. Ganji S, Duncan MC. Angelman's (Happy Puppet) syndrome: Clinical, CT scan and serial electroencephalographic study. *Clin Electroencephalogr.* 1989;20:128–140.
31. Gérard F, Kaminska A, Plouin P, et al. Focal seizures versus focal epilepsy in infancy: A challenging distinction. *Epileptic Disord.* 1999;1(2): 135–139.
32. Giovanardi Rossi P, Pazzaglia P, Cirignotta F, et al. Le epilessie miocloniche dell'infanzia. *Riv Ital EEG Neurofisiol Clin.* 1979;2:321–328.
33. Guerrini R, Bonanni P, Rothwell J, et al. Myoclonus and epilepsy. In: Guerrini R, Aicardi J, Andermann F, et al, eds. *Epilepsy and Movement Disorders.* Cambridge: Cambridge University Press; 2002: 165–210.
34. Guerrini R, Carrozzo R, Rinaldi R, et al. Angelman syndrome: Etiology, clinical features, diagnosis, and management of symptoms. *Pediatr Drugs.* 2003;5(10):647–661.

35. Guerrini R, De Lorey TM, Bonanni P. Cortical myoclonus in Angelman syndrome. *Ann Neurol.* 1996;40:39–48.
36. Guerrini R, Parmeggiani L, Volzone A, et al. Cortical myoclonus in early childhood epilepsy. In: Majkowski J, Owczarek K, Zwolinski P, eds. *3rd European Congress of Epileptology.* Bologna: Monduzzi Editore; 1998: 99–105.
37. Laan LA, Renier WO, Arts WF, et al. Evolution of epilepsy and EEG findings in Angelman syndrome. *Epilepsia.* 1997;38(2):195–199.
38. Lombroso C, Erba G. Myoclonic seizures: Considerations in taxonomy. In: Akimoto H, Kazamatsuri H, Seino M, et al., eds. *Advances in Epileptology: The XIIIth Epilepsy International Symposium.* New York: Raven Press; 1982: 129–134.
39. Matsumoto A, Kumagai T, Miura K. Epilepsy in Angelman syndrome associated with chromosome 15q deletion. *Epilepsia.* 1992;33:1083.
40. Mizuguchi M, Tsukamoto K, Suzuki Y, et al. Myoclonic epilepsy and a maternally derived deletion of 15pter (r) q13. *Clin Genet.* 1994;45: 44–47.
41. Moncia A, Malzac P, Livet MO, et al. Angelman syndrome resulting from UBE3A mutations in 14 patients from eight families: Clinical manifestations and genetic counseling. *J Med Genet.* 1999;36:554–560
42. Pazzaglia P, Giovanardi Rossi P, Cirignotta F, et al. Nosografia delle epilessie miocloniche. *Riv Ital EEG Neurofisiol Clin.* 1979;2:245–252.
43. Rubin DI, Patterson MC, Westmoreland BF, et al. Angelman's syndrome: Clinical and electroencephalographic findings. *EEG Clin Neurophysiol.* 1997;102:299–302.
44. Sgrò V, Riva E, Canevini MP, et al. 4p- syndrome: A chromosomal disorder associated with a particular EEG pattern. *Epilepsia.* 1995;36(12): 1206–1214.
45. Sugimoto T, Yasuhara A, Ohta T, et al. Angelman syndrome in three siblings: Characteristic epileptic seizures and EEG abnormalities. *Epilepsia.* 1992;33:1078.
46. Valente KD, Freitas A, Fiore LA, et al. A study of EEG and epilepsy profile in Wolf-Hirshhorn syndrome and considerations regarding its correlation with other chromosomal disorders. *Brain Dev.* 2003;25:283–287.
47. Valente KD, Koiffmann CP, Fridman C, et al. Epilepsy in patients with Angelman Syndrome caused by deletion of the chromosome 15q11–13. *Arch Neurol.* 2006;63(1):122–128.
48. Van Lierde A, Atza MG, Giardino D, et al. Angelman's syndrome in the first year of life. *Dev Med Child Neurol.* 1990;32:1011–1021.
49. Veneselli E, Biancheri R, Buoni S, et al. Clinical and EEG findings in 18 cases of late infantile neuronal ceroid lipofuscinosis. *Brain Dev.* 2001;23(5):306–311.
50. Veneselli E, Biancheri R, Perrone MV, et al. Neuronal ceroid lipofuscinoses: Clinical and EEG findings in a large study of Italian cases. *Neurol Sci.* 2000;21(Suppl 3):S75–S81.
51. Veneselli E, Perrone MV, Di Rocco M, et al. Malignant migrating partial seizures in infancy. *Epilepsy Res.* 2001;46(1):27–22.
52. Viani F, Romeo A, Viri M, et al. Seizure and EEG patterns in Angelman's syndrome. *J Child Neurol.* 1995;10(6):461–71.
53. Zankl A, Addor MC, Maeder-Ingvar M, et al. A characteristic EEG pattern in 4p- syndrome: Case report and review of the literature. *Eur J Pediatr.* 2001;160:123–127.

CHAPTER 235 ■ OVERVIEW: SYNDROMES OF LATE CHILDHOOD AND ADOLESCENCE

JEAN AICARDI

INTRODUCTION

The incidence of epilepsy declines after the first few years of life but remains higher than in adults.[21] Greater maturity of the brain is associated with an increasing frequency of the classic types of seizures, such as generalized tonic–clonic, absence, and simple or complex partial seizures, and with a decreased incidence of the seizure types characteristic of infancy, such as infantile spasms, atypical absences, and febrile convulsions. Although lesional epilepsies of various causes can begin in this age range, a remarkable feature of many of the epilepsies of late childhood and adolescence is their occurrence in a previously normal child without neurologic or neurodevelopmental defects. Even more remarkable is the fact that a significant proportion of the epilepsies of late childhood and preadolescence tend to be self-limited and disappear after a few years without any detectable sequelae, and several such epilepsy syndromes with variable degree of benignity are described in the following chapters.

Such benign or favorable courses reflect the nonlesional nature of many of the epilepsies of this age, which are mainly determined by genetic factors.[14,16,32] Familial grouping of cases is well recognized, but there is still considerable uncertainty regarding the modes of inheritance of various types and the identification and localization of the responsible genes. Several monogenic syndromes have been described, but in most epilepsies of childhood and adolescence, only a few loci or genes have been characterized, and multigenic determination is considered probable. Even clinically homogeneous syndromes such as juvenile myoclonic epilepsy are genetically heterogeneous, and the current trend is to think in terms of susceptibility genes rather than of direct causation. This applies, for instance, to juvenile myoclonic epilepsy[23] and even more clearly to the syndrome of generalized epilepsy with febrile seizures plus (GEFS+), for which at least three genes have been identified,[17] and probably to other epilepsies.[32]

Two major groups of nonlesional, probably genetically determined, epilepsies are recognized: (a) the idiopathic generalized and (b) the benign partial epilepsies. The first group includes epilepsies with primary generalized tonic–clonic convulsions and several forms of myoclonic and absence epilepsies. The most common types in childhood and adolescence are childhood absence epilepsy (Chapter 239) and juvenile myoclonic epilepsy (Chapter 244). Absence epilepsy appears to be a clinically heterogeneous syndrome, and several distinct syndromes of absence epilepsy exist, whose recognition is probably important for prognostic purposes.[27] Childhood absence epilepsy has an excellent outcome, whereas juvenile absence epilepsy[34] and absences associated with juvenile myoclonic epilepsy are likely to persist into adult life. The exact nosologic place of some rare syndromes, such as eyelid myoclonia with absences[4] and absences with prominent perioral myoclonus between absence and myoclonic epilepsies, is not definitely determined. Juvenile myoclonic epilepsy is a common and well-defined syndrome in adolescents. The characteristic myoclonus on awakening easily goes unrecognized, and the diagnosis is often missed, so that the correct prognosis and treatment might not be given.[9,23] Juvenile myoclonic epilepsy, idiopathic grand mal epilepsies, and juvenile absence epilepsy may represent a spectrum of related syndromes (sometimes termed primary generalized epilepsies) with some types presenting only tonic–clonic seizures (awakening grand mal) and others with associated juvenile absences. It is not clear whether these different clinical presentations form different electroclinical and/or genetic entities or more likely belong to what is basically a single condition due to a common predisposition with specific factors determining the seizure expression, so that the group might be better termed primary generalized epilepsy.[30] Despite these different clinical aspects, the epilepsies in this group are benign in terms of neurodevelopment but tend to be persistent and not to remit for many years. They may even be lifelong, thus requiring continuous treatment.

The second group of partial idiopathic epilepsies has proved to be one of the most common types of epilepsy in older children. *Benign rolandic epilepsy* (Chapter 236), first described in the 1960s,[24] has been extensively studied.[5] The charactristic nocturnal sensorimotor facial seizures of short duration occurring in healthy children has now become familiar to neurologists and is easily recognized, even though the paroxysmal electroencephalogram (EEG) abnormalities may be more variable than initially thought.[34] The virtually complete benign nature of the syndrome has been repeatedly confirmed, although exceptional cases of an identical clinical syndrome in association with focal opercular lesions are on record.[3] However, recent studies have shown that disturbances of language and of other cognitive and behavioral functions may often be found, usually to a mild degree.[11,12] Long- term follow-up studies are necessary to assess the significance of these findings.

Cases closely related to benign rolandic epilepsy but with unusual features have received recent attention, and different aspects have been described. Opercular status epilepticus applies to rare cases with dysarthria, drooling, and pseudobulbar features lasting days to weeks, which might be considered as status of benign rolandic epilepsy, as confirmed by EEG recording.[8,11] Atypical benign partial epilepsy[1,20] is marked by the appearance of atonic seizures following a period of typical facial seizures, associated with intense spike-wave activity in slow sleep, and may wrongly suggest the diagnosis of Lennox-Gastaut syndrome. Electrical status epilepticus of slow sleep (ESES) is defined mainly by the EEG features and clinically by cognitive and behavioral deterioration. It is a heterogeneous group of patients, with approximately half of the cases having lesional causes.[18,19] The Landau-Kleffner syndrome (Chapter 242) often shares the EEG features of ESES and is clinically characterized by prominent language disturbances.[7,10] The very delineation of these syndromes is not entirely clear, and their relationship to benign rolandic epilepsy, which is suggested by the interictal EEG findings and the ultimate remission of epilepsy, is not straightforward because some cases may be due to brain lesions and the reasons for the different clinical expression and course are obscure. The mechanism of epileptic encephalopathy outlined here is probably an important causal factor.

Benign childhood epilepsy with occipital paroxysms (Chapters 237 and 238) is a second form of idiopathic focal epilepsy. Its clinical presentation is variable. Most commonly it presents in young children with infrequent nocturnal seizures, vomiting, loss of consciousness, and eye deviation. Most seizures are brief, but some may last several hours,with prominent autonomic manifestations, and they may simulate abdominal emergencies.[26] Visual symptoms are more common in older children, mainly in the form of transient loss of vision. Striking EEG abnormalities include continuous spike-wave complexes arrested by eye opening. Less typical abnormalities may be more common, however, in the form of spikes over the posterior part of the head. The course is consistently benign. Similarities and sometimes coexistence between rolandic and occipital epilepsy have suggested the concept of benign seizure susceptibility syndrome. Other syndromes, such as epilepsy with evoked parietal spikes and benign psychomotor epilepsy, have not been validated.

New syndromes of partial nonlesional epilepsies have been recently reported. Nocturnal frontal lobe epilepsy[2] presents with nocturnal seizures and is often misdiagnosed as sleep disorder (Chapter 249). It is transmitted as an autosomal-dominant trait and, in some families, has been shown to be due to mutations in the gene for α- and β-nicotinic cholinergic receptors or of the γ-aminobutyric acid (GABA) receptor GABRG2.[17] No linkage to these loci was present in other families, however, indicating further genetic heterogeneity. Several distinct syndromes of dominant partial epilepsy are now recognized. They include benign multifocal partial epilepsy,[2] benign rolandic epilepsy with pseudobulbar features,[31] and benign dominant mesial and lateral temporal lobe epilepsies,[6] which may not be rare but have not been recognized before adolescence (Chapter 248).

The benign couse and even the nonlesional nature of some of the newly described partial epilepsy syndromes are difficult to establish because similar cases can be of lesional origin. In general, the use of the term *benign* should be reserved for those cases in which a favorable outcome of the epilepsy and normal neurodevelopment have been consistently found. The term is not synonymous with *idiopathic* or *genetic* because cases belonging to the latter categories may have a severe outcome.

Seizures of lesional origin in children and adolescents may have quite variable manifestations. Late cases of the Lennox-Gastaut syndrome (Chapter 241) and even of epileptic spasms may appear. Well-defined complex partial seizures tend to become increasingly frequent as the patients grow older. The causes of lesional seizures in this age range differ from those found in adults. Developmental brain abnormalities are still common.[18] Cases of mesial temporal lobe epilepsy (Chapter 247) with typical temporal lobe seizures and evidence of hippocampal sclerosis on neuroimaging begin to appear in the latter part of the period. In younger children, cortical dysplasia and related migration abnormalities tend to predominate. They can involve any part of the brain, which explains the greater frequency of extratemporal epilepsies in children than in adults. Frontal lobe seizures are especially common and may be difficult to distinguish both from temporal lobe seizures and from pseudoseizures. In many frontal lobe seizures, consciousness is preserved despite unresponsiveness of the child and complex movements and attitudes.[5] Tumors are rare as a cause of seizures in children and adolescents. A majority are developmental tumors, commonly associated with neighboring dysplasias (developmental neuroepithelial tumors and gangliogliomas). Their diagnosis by neuroimaging has been reviewed.[29] A rare but important form of partial lesional epilepsy is Rasmussen syndrome (Chapter 243), a progressive inflammatory brain disorder of unknown origin that often causes epilepsia partialis continua and a progressive neurologic deficit requiring surgical therapy.

SUMMARY AND CONCLUSIONS

An important proportion of the epilepsies of childhood and adolescence are of idiopathic origin and relatively benign. Overtreatment should be avoided in these cases, and some epileptologists believe that drug treatment is unnecessary when the outcome can be firmly predicted. Intractable lesional epilepsies may be medically intractable and amenable to surgical therapy. However, the majority of the epilepsies with onset in late childhood and adolescence respond well to antiepileptic agents and are compatible with a reasonably normal quality of life in the cases in which no definitive remission is to be expected.

References

1. Aicardi J, Chevrie JJ. Atypical benign partial epilepsy in childhood. *Dev Med Child Neurol.* 1982;24:281–292.
2. Andermann F, Kobayashi E, Andermann E. Genetic focal epilepsies: state of the art and paths to the future. *Epilepsia.* 2005;46:61–67.
3. Ambrosetto G. Unilateral opercular macrogyria and benign epilepsy with centrotemporal (rolandic) spikes: report of a case. *Epilepsia.* 1992;33:499–503.
4. Appleton RE, Panayiotopoulos CP, Acamb BA, et al. Eyelid myoclonia with typical absences: an epilepsy syndrome. *J Neurol Neurosurg Psychiatry.* 1993;56:1312–1316.
5. Arzimanoglou A, Guerrini R, Aicardi J. *Aicardi's Epilepsy in Children,* 3rd ed. Philadelphia: Lippincott Williams & Wilkins; 2003.
6. Berkovic SF, Howell A, Hopper JL. Familial temporal lobe epilepsy: a new syndrome with adolescent/adult onset and a benign course. In: Wolf P, ed. *Epileptic Seizures and Syndromes.* London: John Libbey; 1994: 257–263.
7. Bureau M. Continuous spikes and waves during slow sleep (CSWS): definition of the syndrome. In: Beaumanoir MBA, Deonna T, Mira L, et al., eds. *Continuous Spikes Waves During Slow Sleep. Electrical Status Epilepticus During Slow Sleep: Acquired Epileptic Aphasia and Related Conditions.* London: John Libbey; 1992: 17–26.
8. Colamaria V, Sgro V, Caraballo R, et al. Status epilepticus in benign rolandic epilepsy manifesting as anterior operculum syndrome. *Epilepsia.* 1991;32:329–334.
9. Delgado-Escueta AV, Liu A, Serratosa J, et al. Juvenile myoclonic epilepsy: is there heterogeneity? In: Malafosse A, Genton P, Hirsch E, et al., eds. *Idiopathic Generalized Epilepsies.* London: John Libbey; 1995: 281–286.
10. Deonna T, Beaumanoir A, Gaillard F, et al. Acquired aphasia in childhood with seizure disorder: a heterogeneous syndrome. *Neuropaediatrie.* 1977;8:263–273.
11. Deonna T, Roulet E, Fontan D, et al. Speech and oromotor deficits of epileptic origin in benign partial epilepsies of childhood with rolandic spikes (BECRS). *Neuropediatrics.* 1993;24:83–87.
12. Deonna T, Zesinger P, Davidoff V, et al. Benign partial epilepsy of childhood: a longitudinal neuropsychological and EEG study of cognitive functions. *Dev Med Child Neurol.* 2000;42:595–603.
13. Doose H. Symptomatology of children with focal sharps of genetic origin. *Eur J Pediatr.* 1989;149:210–215.
14. Doose H, Baier W. Genetic aspects of childhood epilepsy. *Cleve Clin J Med.* 1989;56(Suppl):S105–S110.
15. Fejermann N, Caraballo R, Tenenbaum SN. Atypical evolutions of benign localization-related epilepsies in children: are they predictable?
16. Gardiner M. Genetics of idiopathic generalized epilepsies. *Epilepsia.* 2005;46(Suppl 9):15–20.
17. Gerard F, Pereira S, Robaglia-Schlupp A, et al. Clinical and genetic analysis of a new multigenerational pedigree with GEFS+ (generalized epilepsy with febrile seizures plus). *Epilepsia.* 2002;43:581–586.
18. Guerrini R, Andermann F, Canapicchi R, et al., eds. *Dysplasias of Cerebral Cortex and Epilepsy.* New York: Lippincott-Raven; 1996.
19. Guerrini R, Genton P, Bureau M, et al. Multiple polymicrogyria, intractable drop attacks seizures, and sleep-related status electrical epilepticus. *Neurology.* 2000;51:504–512.
20. Hahn A, Pistohl J, Neubauer BA, et al. Atypical "benign" partial epilepsy or pseudo-Lennox syndrome. Part I: Symptomatology and long-term prognosis. *Neuropediatrics.* 2001;32:1–8.

21. Hauser WA. The prevalence and incidence of convulsive disorders in children. *Epilepsia*. 1993;35(Suppl 2):S1–S6.
22. Hirose S, Mitsudome A, Okada M, et al. Genetics of idiopathic epilepsies. *Epilepsia*. 2005(Suppl 1):38–43.
23. Janz D. Juvenile myoclonic epilepsy: epilepsy with impulsive petit mal. *Cleve Clin J Med*. 1989;56(Suppl):S23–S33.
24. Lombroso CT. Sylvian seizures and midtemporal spike foci in children. *Arch Neurol*. 1967;17:52–59.
25. Nordli DR Jr. Idiopathic generalized epilepsies recognized by the International League Against Epilepsy. *Epilepsia*. 2005;46(Suppl 9):48–56.
26. Panayiotopoulos CP. Early-onset benign childhood occipital seizures/a syndrome to recognize. *Epilepsia*. 1999;40:621–630.
27. Panayiotopoulos CP, Obeid T, Waheed G. Absences in juvenile myoclonic epilepsy: a clinical and video-electroencephalographic study. *Ann Neurol*. 1989;25:391–397.
28. Panayiotopoulos CP, Obeid T, Waheed G. Differentiation of typical absence seizures in epileptic syndromes. A video EEG study of 224 seizures in 20 patients. *Brain*. 1989;112:1039–1056.
29. Raymond AA, Halpin SFS, Alsanjari N, et al. Dysembryoplastic neuroepithelial tumour: features in 16 patients. *Brain*. 1994;117:461–475.
30. Sander T, Schultz H, Saar K, et al. Genome search for susceptibility loci of common idiopathic generalized epilepsies. *Hum Mol Genet*. 2000;9:1465–1473.
31. Scheffer IE, Bhatia KP, Lopes-Cendes I, et al. Autosomal dominant rolandic epilepsy and speech dyspraxia: a new syndrome with anticipation. *Ann Neurol*. 1995;38:633–642.
32. Tassinari CA, Bureau M, Dravet C, et al. Epilepsy with continuous spikes and waves during slow sleep-otherwise described as ESES (epilepsy with status epilepticus during slow sleep). In: Roger J, Bureau M, Dravet C, et al., eds. *Epileptic Syndromes in Infancy, Childhood and Adolescence*. London: John Libbey; 1992:245–256.
33. Wirrel EC, Camfield PR, Gordon KE, et al. Benign rolandic epilepsy: atypical features are very common. *J Child Neurol*. 1995;10:455–458.
34. Wolf P. Juvenile absence epilepsy. In: Duncan JS, Panayiotopoulos CP, eds. *Typical Absences and Related Epileptic Syndromes*. London: Churchill Communication Europe; 1995:161–167.

CHAPTER 236 ■ BENIGN CHILDHOOD EPILEPSY WITH CENTROTEMPORAL SPIKES

NATALIO FEJERMAN

INTRODUCTION

The recognition that some epilepsies in children have focal clinical manifestations and unilateral electroencephalographic (EEG) discharges with benign evolution has been one of the most interesting contributions to pediatric epileptology in the last 50 years.

The concept of idiopathic and benign focal epilepsies of childhood is relevant not only from the theoretical point of view, but also as a practical tool, because the term implies both absence of structural brain lesions and a genetic predisposition associated with age-dependent seizures. Benign childhood epilepsy with centrotemporal spikes (BCECTS) is the most frequent of the benign focal epilepsies of childhood and represents 15% to 25% of epilepsy syndromes in children <15 years of age. In addition, it is the most frequent epilepsy syndrome in school-age children.[25,101,125]

HISTORICAL PERSPECTIVES

Yvette Gastaut was the first to state, in 1952, that "pre-rolandic spikes" could be "functional" instead of an indicator of a cortical lesion.[48] In 1958, Bancaud et al.[6] and Nayrac and Beaussart[91] reported the first series of patients, emphasizing that rolandic or pre-rolandic spikes or spike-waves constituted EEG features that were typical of childhood, and that should not induce "neurosurgical behaviors," although they did not describe a clear electroclinical correlation. In 1960, Gibbs and Gibbs[51] stated that prognosis was much better in children with centrotemporal spikes than in those with spikes in the anterior temporal regions. In the same year Faure and Loiseau[39] wrote of "Rolandic spike-waves without focal significance," referring to age of onset and sleep as a trigger of seizures, and to spontaneous electroclinical normalization in puberty. Clinical features of seizures were not defined, however, because they found generalized seizures in 13 of their 15 cases. In 1966, Trojaborg[114] published a longitudinal study in a cohort of 519 children with focal spike discharges. Two hundred and eighty of these patients had cerebral palsy. The main purpose of this work was a detailed analysis of the significance of acute sharp waves in the EEG and their correlation with brain lesions. The author recognized that one prognosis was good in children with centrotemporal spikes, but did not determine their clinical correlates. Also in 1966 the most important series of children with temporal lobe epilepsy was published.[97] Among the 100 children followed, 33 constituted a subgroup without pathologic history and with mean age of onset of seizures between 7 and 8 years. It is now easy to imagine that a significant proportion of these 33 children might have had the diagnosis of BCECTS.

One year later, two independent groups reported their series of patients with a peculiar form of epilepsy to be differentiated from other focal epilepsies, mainly from temporal lobe epilepsy. Loiseau et al.[78] presented 122 cases with onset of seizures at school age and rolandic sharp waves in the EEG. In 80% of their patients, seizures occurred during sleep and were frequently motor with predominant involvement of the face. Lombroso[81] provided a clear description of the seizures, emphasizing somatosensitive symptoms in tongue, oral mucosa, and gums, along with speech arrest, and proposed the term "sylvian seizures," recognizing also the particular focal EEG features. Both Loisseau et al. and Lombroso stressed the benign character of the condition in terms of the evolution of seizures and normalization of the EEG. In 1972, Blom et al.[13] reported a prevalence and follow-up study and proposed that the condition be named "benign epilepsy of children with centrotemporal EEG foci." Several long-term follow-up studies confirmed the good prognosis.[8,9,72,80] Atypical and not-so-benign evolutions have been reported in some patients.[1,40,43,44,46,54] This form of epilepsy is now called benign childhood epilepsy with centrotemporal spikes and is placed in the group of idiopathic localization-related (focal, local, partial) epilepsies in the International Classification of Epilepsies and Epileptic Syndromes.[21,36]

DEFINITIONS

The most common name besides BCECTS appearing in the literature referring to this condition is "benign rolandic epilepsy." The term "benign" has been questioned for other epilepsy syndromes because some epileptologists believe that benign implies a natural evolution to remission of seizures and EEG abnormalities even without treatment. In this sense, BCECTS conforms to the aforementioned concept, even if we must accept that there are exceptions to the rule.

Onset during childhood with hemifacial motor, seizures, speech arrest, and sialorrhea, occurring mostly during sleep, along with distinctive centrotemporal spikes in the EEG are well-defined features that allow a prompt diagnosis and assure a good prognosis, although subsets of atypical cases with slight compromise of neurological functions are increasingly being reported.[102,120,122]

EPIDEMIOLOGY

Benign childhood epilepsy with centrotemporal spikes accounts for between 15% and 25% of all epileptic syndromes in children between the ages 4 and 12 years.[19,25,101,121] Its annual incidence has been reported to be between 7.1 and 21 per 100,000 in children <15 years of age.[56] Because nocturnal seizures can be overlooked in diagnosis, this disorder may be even more common than generally suspected. There is a slight male predominance.[82]

The prevalence of epilepsy is much higher among close relatives of children with BCECTS than in a matched control group.[17] In one study, 15% of siblings had seizures and rolandic spikes, 19% of siblings had rolandic spikes without attacks, and 11% of the parents had had childhood seizures that had disappeared by adulthood.[57]

In an epidemiologic study of epilepsy in a cohort of 440 consecutive children, benign rolandic epilepsy of childhood accounted for 8% of patients (neonatal seizures were excluded from the analysis).[67]

ETIOLOGY AND BASIC MECHANISMS

The high incidence of a positive family history for epilepsy and focal EEG abnormalities indicates the importance of genetic factors in the etiology of BCECTS.[13,17,27,82] Most authors speak of an autosomal-dominant trait with variable penetrance.[17,57] This type of inheritance was also suggested by studies of monozygotic twins with rolandic discharges[64] and of HLA antigens and their haplotypes.[34] However, in another study of clinical and genetic aspects in children with benign focal sharp waves, including 134 probands with seizures (24% of which had typical rolandic seizures), the findings agreed with a multifactorial pathogenesis with "benign" focal epileptiform sharp waves.[32] Epileptic seizures appear in only 25% or less of individuals with this EEG trait.[82] Expression of the gene may be influenced by other genetic and environmental factors.[79] Linkage to chromosome 15q14 was found in 54 patients of 22 families with benign childhood epilepsy with centrotemporal spikes.[92] However, in a study of 70 families with BCECTS in Italy, the same linkage could not be found.[104] Approximately 10% of patients have a history of febrile seizures, and this also supports a genetic predisposition for febrile seizures expressed at earlier ages in children with BCECTS.[63,71]

A family with nine affected individuals in three generations was reported showing the features of rolandic epilepsy associated with oral and speech dyspraxia and cognitive impairment.[109] Similar seizures and the EEG phenotype of BCECTS were found in three children with de novo terminal deletions of the long arm of chromosome 1q, and the authors suggested that it could be a potential site for a candidate gene.[118]

Although the pathophysiology of BCECTS is unknown, and there is no associated structural lesion, the typical ictal clinical behavior and EEG discharge indicate a disturbance in the sylvian and rolandic areas.[37] Electrophysiologic studies, however, fail to demonstrate a discrete generator, and a large, shifting area of regional cortical dysfunction may be present. In some patients with BCECTS, the occurrence of generalized spike-wave EEG discharges, as well as focal spikes in other areas, suggests a relationship between BCECTS and the idiopathic generalized epilepsies, as well as with other idiopathic localization-related partial epilepsies.[73,82] Between 10% and 20% of patients with centrotemporal spikes may also have sharp slow wave complexes in other cortical locations.[100]

Combined recording of interictal spikes and somatosensory-evoked potentials led to the conclusion that in some patients multiple simultaneous neuronal populations are active within the central region.[7]

Magnetoencephalographic (MEG) analysis of generator sources and propagation of rolandic discharges in BCECTS using three-dimensional dipole localization suggested that rolandic discharges are generated through a mechanism similar to that of somatosensory-evoked responses.[86] A localization analysis of spontaneous magnetic brain activities also suggested the value of MEG for pathophysiologic studies.[65] Six children with bilateral centrotemporal synchronous discharges were studied using MEG and EEG with equivalent current dipole modeling. Results implied cortical epileptogenicity in bilateral perirolandic areas.[75] Interictal spikes were recorded in seven children during functional magnetic resonance imaging (fMRI) acquisition using a MR-compatible digital EEG system. Spike-related activation in the perisylvian central region was found in three of them.[14] High-resolution EEG and MEG and a realistic volume conductor model were used to study the spatiotemporal aspects of the sources of spikes in children with benign rolandic epilepsy. Results for EEG and MEG were different. Both high-resolution EEG and MEG revealed that in some cases there were multiple sources for spikes that were well separated in space and time, whereas in other cases only single-source activity was present.[61]

Recent papers considered BCECTS, Landau-Kleffner syndrome, and electrical status epilepticus in sleep as a spectrum of disorders with a common transient, age-dependent, nonlesional, genetically based epileptogenic abnormality, involving a perisylvian epileptic network. Halasz et al. refer to "mild to severe epileptic encephalopathy limited to the perisylvian network, where the cognitive impairment is caused by epileptic discharges interfering with cognitive development."[55]

CLINICAL PRESENTATION

We discuss the main clinical features of BCECTS, assuming that this is an idiopathic focal epilepsy that appears in children with normal neurological development, although this syndrome has also been reported in patients with nonevolutive brain lesions.[108]

1. BCECTS begins between 4 and 10 years of age in 90% of patients, and the median age of onset is approximately 7 years. There are no reports of BCECTS occurring during the first year of life or after age 15 years, and cases with seizure onset before the age of 2 years are extremely rare.[25,42]
2. BCECTS is seen more frequently in males, with a male-to-female ratio of 3:2.
3. Seizures are clearly related to sleep, whether during the night or the day. This is seen in 80% to 90% of patients. Seizures during waking hours are more likely to occur shortly after awakening,[82] although on many occasions, during the early morning the child wakes up with a seizure that really started during sleep. Seizure frequency is usually low, and around 10% of cases have only one seizure. In about 20% of the children, however, seizures are frequent and may even occur several times per day.[25] Most patients have a single type of seizure, but 20% to 25% of children experience more than one type.[79] Loiseau and Beaussart[77] described 35 signs or components of 275 seizures analyzed in 190 children with BCECTS. We can reduce this number to a small group of characteristic manifestations of seizures:
   a. *Orofacial motor signs*, especially tonic or clonic contractions of one side of the face, with predilection for the labial commissure (contralateral to the centrotemporal spikes). There are also contractions of the tongue or jaw, guttural sounds, and drooling from hypersalivation and swallowing disturbance.
   b. *Speech arrest,* most probably due to tonic contractions of pharyngeal and buccal muscles, constituting anarthric seizures. In fact, the patient cannot speak during the seizure because either he or she wakes up with hemifacial contractions or while awake opens his or her mouth with the intention to speak but stays blocked in that position.
   c. *Somatosensory symptoms*, namely unilateral numbness or paresthesia of the tongue, lips, gums, and

cheek, are frequent, but sometimes have to be looked for in the context of recalling previous events.

d. The three mentioned groups of manifestations are related to an epileptic activation of lower rolandic motor and somatosensory areas. In terms of sialorrhea, it is not clear whether it corresponds to increased salivation, a swallowing disturbance, or both. In general, these seizures only last a few minutes. Although partial seizures are characteristic of this disorder, generalized seizures are not infrequently observed, particularly in younger children.[71,82] The initial event is often a nocturnal hemifacial convulsion, which may spread to the arm and the leg or may become secondarily generalized. It is highly probable that in these cases a focal seizure begins during sleep with a rapid generalization and loss of consciousness, which makes it difficult for the child to remember what happened. This is in line with the fact that almost all seizures that start while the person is awake are focal.

4. Behavioral and learning problems are less frequent than in other forms of childhood epilepsy.[58] It is often mentioned that children with BCECTS are free of neurological and psychological impairments.[45,46,71] In recent years, however, several reports based on meta-analyses of published series, retrospective analysis of patients, or prospective cohort studies have reported a higher incidence of learning and/or language difficulties in these children. In a study of 40 children with centrotemporal spikes with and without seizures compared with 40 healthy controls, patients were significantly impaired in IQ, visual perception, short-term memory, and psychiatric status. The deficits in IQ correlated more with frequency of EEG spikes than with the frequency of seizures.[122] Similar findings were reported in 19 children with this syndrome.[29] An increased frequency of rolandic spikes has been reported in children with attention deficit hyperactivity disorder.[59] One study found a consistent pattern of language dysfunction in 13 of 20 children with BCECTS, suggesting interictal dysfunction of the perisylvian language areas.[113] A longitudinal study of one boy with acquired epileptic dysgraphia was reported. Most probably, in this case, the acquired regression of graphomotor skills was associated with an increase in spike frequency as happens in cases with atypical evolution of this syndrome.[33] In a more recent report, written language skills were compared in 32 children with typical BCECTS with 36 controls. As a group, the patients with BCECTS performed significantly worse than controls in spelling, reading aloud, and reading comprehension, presented dyslexic-type errors, and frequently had below-average school performance.[102] Language assessment in 16 children with BCECTS also showed that the domains of expressive grammar and literacy skills were affected in a significant proportion of the cases.[89] A comprehensive study of neuropsychological and language profiles of 42 children with BCECTS selected using strict clinical and EEG criteria showed that the patients have normal intelligence and language ability, although a specific pattern of difficulties in memory and phonologic awareness was found. No correlation between EEG features and the aforementioned impairments was demonstrated.[94]

Atypical features in benign childhood epilepsy with centrotemporal spikes can be seen both clinically (daytime-only seizures, postictal Todd paresis, prolonged seizures, or even status epilepticus) and in EEG features (atypical spike morphology, unusual location, or abnormal background). In a retrospective case series, atypical clinical features were seen in 50% of patients and atypical electrographic features in 31%.[123] In a follow-up study of 74 children with typical rolandic epilepsy and 14 with atypical features, a significantly higher percentage of learning and behavioral disabilities was found in the second group.[120]

Several cases of partial status epilepticus have been reported. The manifestations include hemifacial seizures, dysarthria or anarthria, and persistent drooling.[20,43,44,52,66,106,107]

DIAGNOSTIC EVALUATION

Electroencephalographic Findings

After recognition of typical clinical features, the cornerstone of the diagnosis of BCECTS lies in the characteristic interictal EEG pattern, which include the following features:

1. Background EEG activity is symmetric, well organized, and normally reactive during wakefulness, and the physiologic patterns of sleep are also normal.[25,26]
2. Interictal epileptic discharges and location of spikes are characterized as follows:
   a. *Characteristics of spikes*: Typical centrotemporal spikes (CTS) are located in centrotemporal or rolandic areas (Fig. 1). They are broad, diphasic, high-voltage (100–300 μV) sharp waves, with a transverse dipole, and they are often followed by a slow wave. The spikes may occur isolated or in clusters, with a rhythm of about 1.5 to 3 Hz.[79] Focal rhythmic slow activity is occasionally observed in the region in which the spikes are seen, especially when spikes are frequent.[87] They may be seen in only one hemisphere or independently on both sides of the head (Fig. 2).[37] The CTS tend to spread to adjacent regions. Several authors emphasized the characteristic dipole orientation in the EEG.[53,76,115] Two groups of patients have been found based on EEG findings (maximal negativity was registered in high- and low-central regions, but never in midtemporal regions): (a) a high-central-region group with more frequent hand involvement and (b) a low-central group with common orofacial symptoms.[70] The source distribution of benign rolandic spikes along and across the central sulcus was examined in 15 patients between 7 and 15 years of age. The equivalent current dipoles of the spikes measured by whole-head MEG were compared to the spike distributions detected by simultaneous scalp EEG. Rolandic spikes are consistent with by a precentral origin, assuming that the surface negative potential is continuous from the gyral to fissural cortices.[62]
   b. *Enhancement of discharges*: The centrotemporal spikes are not enhanced by eye opening or closure, hyperventilation, or photic stimulation. Moreover, hyperventilation sometimes reduces the frequency of rolandic spikes.[45,121] The discharge rate is increased in drowsiness and in all stages of sleep, and in about one third of children, the spikes appear only in sleep.[81] Sleep EEG organization is preserved.[23] In spite of their increasing frequency during sleep, the CTS show the same morphology as during wakefulness. A change in morphology, particularly the appearance of fast spikes or polyspikes, a marked increase in the slow component, or a brief depression of voltage, suggests an organic etiology even when the ictal features are suggestive of BCECTS.[25] There is no correlation between intensity of spike discharges in the EEG and

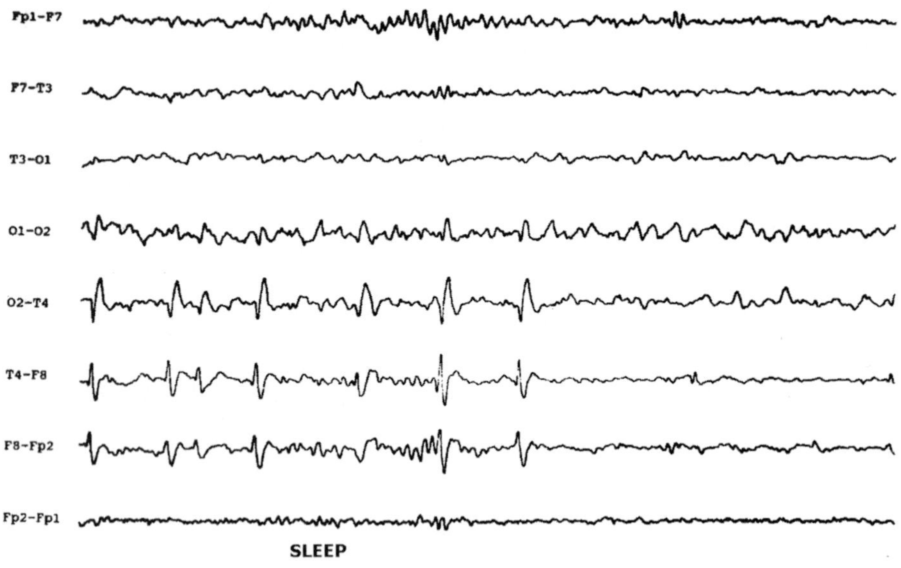

FIGURE 1. Sleep electroencephalogram (EEG) in a 6-year-old girl with typical seizures and right centrotemporal spikes.

frequency, length, or duration of clinical seizures.[72] In fact, extreme discrepancies between the rarity of seizures and the activity of the EEG foci are not uncommon, and clinical experience indicates that the EEG is often relatively unchanged, even with effective treatment.[5]

c. *Spikes in other areas and spike-wave discharges*: Spike foci may coexist in other areas independent of their clinical correlation.[71,100] Generalized spike-wave discharges are rarely seen in the waking state but are not infrequent during drowsiness and sleep.[11,45] The real incidence of spike-wave discharges in children with BCECTS is not established; numbers vary between 7% and 65%.[25,27] One must be cautious in interpreting this because bursts of slow waves with spikes in drowsiness are seen in up to 20% of children between 3 and 6 years of age, especially those with history of febrile seizures.[2] We will see later that the coexistence of BCECTS with the Panayiotopoulos type of benign occipital epilepsy is not rare, whereas its association with absence epilepsy is exceptional.

3. With regard to the frequency of discharges and the correlation with cognitive deficits, the association of more frequent discharges or multifocal paroxysms with complicated evolution in BCECTS is a debated subject.[25,85] It is clear, however, that the appearance of bilateral synchronies leading to continuous spikes and waves during sleep are frequently associated with severe cognitive and language impairment.[43] In a recent study of 20 children with benign partial epilepsies who were studied by combined EEG, MEG, and MRI, location of spikes was determined by dipole source estimates. There was a cor-

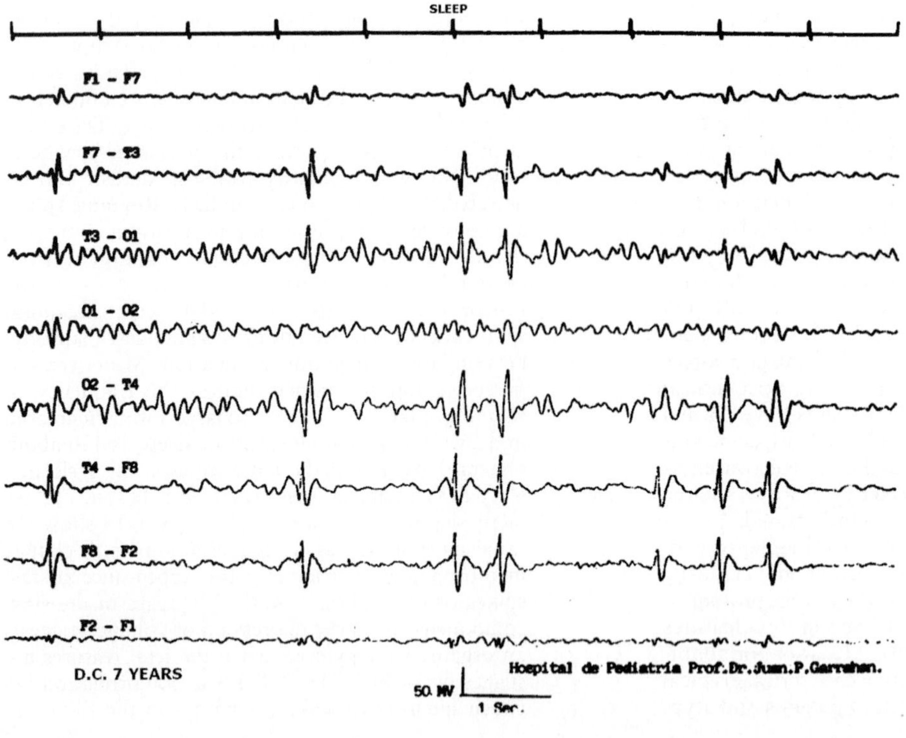

FIGURE 2. Sleep electroencephalogram (EEG) in a 7-year-old boy with typical seizures and bilateral centrotemporal spikes.

relation between location of spikes and selective cognitive deficits, with left perisylvian spikes associated with poorer language test results in 11 cases, whereas 6 children with right perisylvian location performed within normal ranges in all parts of the tests.[124] In a small group of patients with status epilepticus in BCECTS, the finding of independent right and left seizures was considered a risk factor.[52]

4. EEG studies in large numbers of healthy children revealed centrotemporal spikes in 2.1% of 533 children between 6 and 15 years of age;[35] in 2.4% of 3,726 children between 6 and 13 years of age;[19] and in 3.5% of 1,057 children between 6 and 12 years of age.[95] Considering that in many of the cases the EEGs were performed in the waking state, we may assume that the actual figures should be higher. The fact is that in a vast majority of children with CTS, a genetically determined cortical excitability produces the EEG abnormalities, which in a few patients are associated with clinical seizures. It has been estimated that <25% of children with CTS have seizures.[82] The presence of CTS was also reported in children with Rett syndrome and fragile X syndrome and even in children with brain tumors.[69,90,93]
5. Reports in the literature on ictal EEGs in children with BCECTS are scarce and only deal with isolated cases.[3,26] The ictal pattern is generally characterized by a sequence of rhythmic spikes remaining quite monomorphic throughout the discharge. Lerman described a diurnal seizure with local decremental activity followed by dense spikes confined to the centrotemporal area during the tonic phase and with spike-waves during the clonic phase.[71]

Neuroimaging and Other Laboratory Examinations

When the clinical and EEG features are typical, the diagnosis is certain, and therefore neuroimaging in BCECTS has been regarded as superfluous by many authors.[5,71] However, several reports called attention to a higher percentage of brain abnormalities in children with typical BCECTS. Gelisse et al.[50] presented the case of a 10-year-old-boy with marked right hippocampal atrophy, although they concluded that the seizure disorder could not be ascribed to this abnormality. The same group reported computed tomography (CT) or MRI abnormalities in 10 of 71 consecutive patients with BCECTS, but the sample was most probably biased because 2 of the 5 children showing enlargement of the lateral ventricle had shunted hydrocephalus.[49] Hippocampal asymmetries and white matter abnormalities in MRI have been reported in 33% of 18 children with BCECTS, but the relationship was considered unclear.[83,84] On the other hand, because of a few cases that have presented the clinical and EEG phenotype of BCECTS in whom cortical dysplasia[3,40,110] and even brain tumors[111] were found, one might question whether an MRI study is indicated. Based on these findings and the evaluation of what happens in everyday practice, it is legitimate to obtain an MRI study to avoid the possibility of ignoring existing abnormalities.

Very few studies using positron emission tomography (PET) have been performed in children with BCECTS. De Saint-Martin et al.[30] reported a longitudinal study of a child with BCECTS using F-fluorodeoxyglucose (FDG) PET. They found a bilateral increase of glucose metabolism in the temporal opercular regions interictally during the "active" phase of the epilepsy. In 11 children with BCECTS studied with FDG-PET, no interictal side differences in glucose metabolism were demonstrated.[117]

DIFFERENTIAL DIAGNOSIS

Several series of children with BCECTS have included some patients with cerebral palsy.[13,72,82] Distinction between benign childhood epilepsy with centrotemporal spikes and more serious nonidiopathic epileptic conditions, such as mesial temporal lobe epilepsy, can usually be made easily on the basis of history and the unique dipole pattern of the centrotemporal spike. However, benign focal epileptiform discharges were found in 2 of 17 preadolescent children who eventually underwent anteromesial temporal resection for refractory temporal lobe epilepsy due to hippocampal sclerosis, and the authors suggested that it might not have been an incidental finding.[98] Because of their prevalence, fortuitous associations may be found between benign childhood epilepsy with centrotemporal spikes and nonprogressive brain lesions.[108] Isolated cases of children with BCECTS and unilateral opercular neuronal migration disorders have been published.[3,40,110] Cerebral tumors presenting as pseudo-benign partial epilepsy in childhood with centrotemporal spikes were reported in five patients.[111] Five children with a so-called "malignant rolandic-sylvian epilepsy" secondary to neuronal migration disorders and gliosis were reported as presenting similar clinical and EEG features of benign childhood epilepsy with centrotemporal spikes. The authors emphasized the role of MEG in the differential diagnosis.[96]

The pathophysiologic relationships that may exist between benign childhood epilepsy with centrotemporal spikes and other benign partial nonrolandic epilepsies can make differential diagnosis difficult. The coexistence of two types of benign partial epilepsies in children, namely Panayiotopoulos type of benign occipital epilepsy and BCECTS, has been reported, presenting either in sequence one after the other or at the same time,[18,22,99] although treatment and prognosis are the same.[73]

TREATMENT AND OUTCOME

In considering outcome in children with BCECTS, it is necessary to consider control of seizures on one hand and the incidence of neurological impairments, either transitory or persistent, on the other. Antiepileptic drug treatment is usually effective, although many authors believe that drug treatment is not necessary in the benign focal epilepsies of childhood.[25,47,100] Therefore, continuous treatment should be considered only in patients with frequent seizures and when the ictal events are disruptive to the patient or family. Carbamazepine was always the drug of choice. However, the use of benzodiazepines at night may be considered in those children who have seizures only during sleep. Benzodiazepine treatment for several weeks was also recommended.[28] In comparison with valproate and carbamazepine, clonazepam was found to be more effective in suppressing rolandic discharges after 4 weeks of treatment.[88] Sulthiame has been recommended in several reports.[31,71,74] In a double-blind, placebo-controlled study of 66 children with BCECTS, sulthiame was found to be remarkably effective in preventing seizures and was well tolerated.[105] A more recent report also showed the benefits of sulthiame.[38] Among new drugs, oxcarbazepine and levetiracetam showed good results.[10,116] Curiously enough, an ictal clinical and EEG study in one child suggested that voluntary protrusion of the tongue could stop seizures and EEG discharges.[119]

A meta-analysis of outcome in 794 patients in 13 cohorts, concluded that early prediction of seizure outcome in a new patient cannot be given with certainty.[15] It was stated that the only predictor for a disease course in children with multiple seizures is onset before 3 years of age.[68]

In a prospective study of treatment in childhood epilepsy, it was concluded that 1 year of treatment can be recommended in children with benign childhood epilepsy with centrotemporal spikes.[16] In fact, once the decision to treat is made, it is not possible to make a firm recommendation regarding duration, but there is no need to wait for normalization of the EEG to stop medication. Relapse of seizures, however, may occur after premature withdrawal.[79]

If it is considered that there is risk of an atypical evolution due to worsening of the EEG, an increase in the number of seizures, the presence of inhibitory seizures, or evidence of neuropsychologic abnormalities, the following steps should be taken: First, stop the medication if it is carbamazepine, oxcarbazepine, phenytoin, or valproic acid, and then switch to a benzodiazepine, ethosuximide, or sulthiame. Two of our cases of BCECTS status only responded to treatment with steroids.[44] Sulthiame seems to be the drug of choice in patients presenting atypical evolution associated with secondary bilateral synchrony in the EEG.[41,43]

LONG-TERM PROGNOSIS

In general, benign childhood epilepsy with centrotemporal spikes is associated with an excellent prognosis. Seizures are difficult to control in only a small number of cases.[9,12] The prognosis is favorable even in patients whose seizures are difficult to control as seizures almost always remit spontaneously in adolescence. In their investigation of 168 patients 7 to 30 years after cessation of epilepsy with centrotemporal spikes, Loiseau et al. reported that seizures persisted in only 3 cases after adulthood.[80] The seizures were all generalized tonic–clonic seizures. Two of the 3 had obviously isolated incidences. This incidence of generalized seizures in adults with a history of epilepsy with centrotemporal spikes in childhood is nevertheless higher than that of seizures in the general population.[80] Cognitive functions were evaluated in 23 adolescents and young adults in complete remission from BCECTS and showed no significant differences from controls. However, qualitative analysis suggested a different organizational pattern for cerebral language in adolescents and young adults in remission.[60]

The presence of atypical interictal epileptiform EEG patterns does not appear to alter prognosis.[11] However, atypical evolutions may cause doubt about the prognosis. For example, in the cases of benign atypical partial epilepsy described by Aicardi and Chevrie,[1] affected children showed partial or generalized atonic fits leading to multiple daily falls. These inhibitory attacks appeared in clusters that lasted for weeks, and the EEG showed continuous spikes-and-waves during slow wave sleep (Fig. 3). Status lasting days or weeks including motor facial seizures and anarthria with persistent drooling constitute other complications of this syndrome.[43,44] Both complications were still associated ultimately with a good prognosis. However, acquired epileptic aphasia and the syndrome of continuous spikes-and-waves during slow sleep have also been associated with BCECTS, and in these cases the risk of permanent language dysfunction or neurological abnormalities is clearly present.[40,43] EEG activity in these atypical evolutions seems to be a kind of secondary bilateral synchrony, but it is not understood why some children develop this EEG pattern. In some cases, certain antiepileptic drugs seemed to be responsible.[18,103,112]

SUMMARY AND CONCLUSIONS

Benign childhood epilepsy with centrotemporal spikes is an idiopathic childhood epilepsy characterized by well-defined

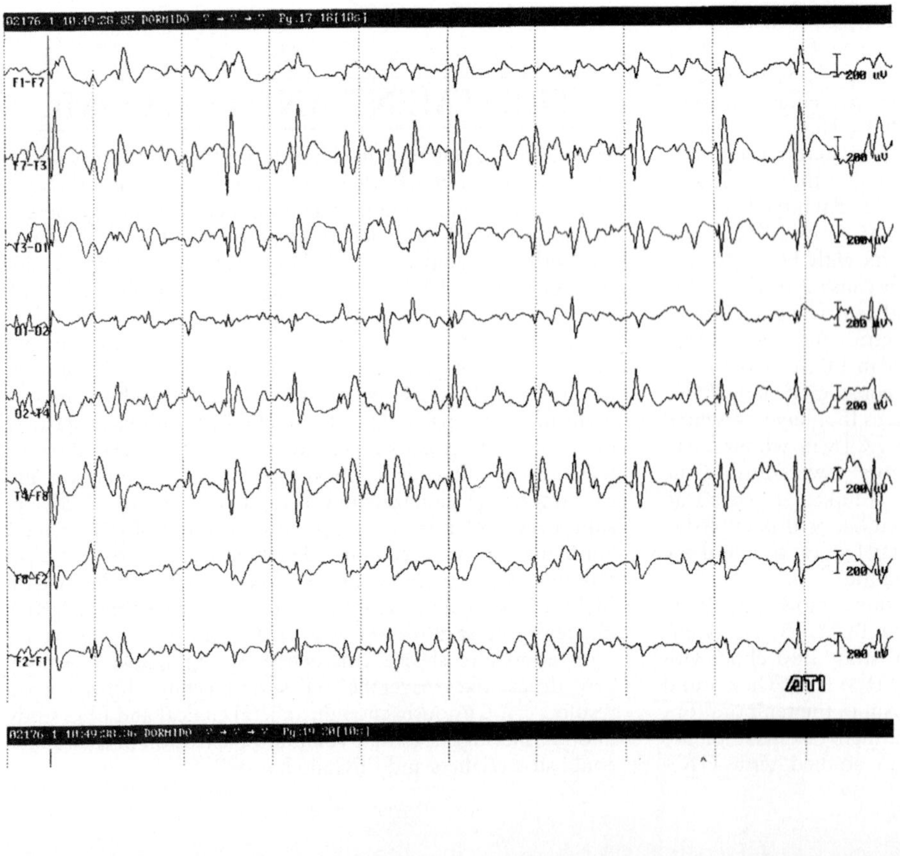

FIGURE 3. Sleep electroencephalogram (EEG) in a 7-year-old boy with a history of typical benign childhood epilepsy with centrotemporal spikes and onset of inhibitory seizures. Bilateral, almost continuous spike-wave discharges are seen.

electroclinical features, including brief hemifacial motor seizures, with sialorrhea and speech arrest, occurring more frequently during sleep, associated with centrotemporal spikes in the interictal EEG. It is the most frequent epilepsy syndrome in children between 4 and 12 years of age.

In general, BCECTS is associated with very good prognosis, with electroclinical normalization in puberty. There are rare cases (approximately 2%) with atypical evolutions leading to significant neuropsychologic impairments. This event should be recognized as early as possible.

Treatment is not always necessary. Common antiepileptic drugs can be used, but in the presence of atypical features such as increase in the number of seizures, onset of inhibitory seizures, continuous spike and waves during slow sleep in the EEG, and language or behavioral involvement, the best choice is benzodiazepines or sulthiame.

References

1. Aicardi J, Chevrie JJ. Atypical benign partial epilepsy of childhood. *Dev Med Child Neurol.* 1982;24:281–292.
2. Alvarez N, Lombroso CT, Medina C, et al. Paroxysmal spike and wave activity in drowsiness in young children: its relationship to febrile convulsions. *Electroencephalogr Clin Neurophysiol.* 1983;56:406–413.
3. Ambrosetto G. Unilateral opercular macrogyria and benign childhood epilepsy with centrotemporal (rolandic) spikes. *Epilepsia.* 1992;33:499–503.
4. Ambrosetto G, Gobbi G. Benign epilepsy of childhood with rolandic spikes or a lesion? EEG during a seizure. *Epilepsia.* 1975;16:793–796.
5. Arzimanoglou A, Guerrini R, Aicardi J. Epilepsies characterized by partial seizures. In: Arzimanoglou A, Guerrini R, Aicardi J, eds. *Aicardi's Epilepsy in Children,* 3rd ed. Philadelphia: Lippincott Williams & Wilkins; 2004: 114–175.
6. Bancaud J, Colomb D, Dell MB. Les pointes rolandiques: un symtôme EEG prope à l'enfant. *Rev Neurol (Paris).* 1958;99:206–209.
7. Baumgartner C, Graf M, Doppelbauer A, et al. The functional organization of the interictal spike complex in benign rolandic epilepsy. *Epilepsia.* 1996;37:12:1164–1174.
8. Beaussart M. Benign epilepsy of children with rolandic (centrotemporal) paroxysmal foci. *Epilepsia.* 1972;13:795–811.
9. Beaussart M, Faou R. Evolution of epilepsy with rolandic paroxysmal foci: a study of 324 cases. *Epilepsia.* 1978;19:337–342.
10. Bello-Espinosa LE, Roberts SL. Levetiracetam for benign epilepsy of childhood with centrotemporal spikes—three cases. *Seizure.* 2003;12: 157–159.
11. Beydoun A, Garofalo EA, Drury I. Generalized spike-waves, multiple loci, and clinical course in children with EEG features of benign epilepsy of childhood with centrotemporal spikes. *Epilepsia.* 1992;33:1091–1096.
12. Blom S, Heijbel J. Benign epilepsy of children with centrotemporal EEG foci: a follow-up study in adulthood of patients initially studied as children. *Epilepsia.* 1982;23:629–631.
13. Blom S, Heijbel J, Bergfors PG. Benign epilepsy of children with centrotemporal foci: prevalence and follow-up study of 40 patients. *Epilepsia.* 1972;13:609–619.
14. Boor S, Vucurevic G, Pfleiderer C, et al. EEG-related functional MRI in benign childhood epilepsy with centrotemporal spikes. *Epilepsia.* 2003;44(5):688–692.
15. Bouma PA, Bovenkerk AC, Westendorp RG, et al. The course of benign partial epilepsy of childhood with centrotemporal spikes: a meta-analysis. *Neurology.* 1997;48:2:430–437.
16. Braathen G, Andersson T, Gylje H, et al. Comparison between one and three years of treatment in uncomplicated childhood epilepsy: a prospective study. I. Outcome in different seizure types. *Epilepsia.* 1996;37(9):822–832.
17. Bray PF, Wiser WC. Evidence for a genetic etiology of temporal central abnormalities in focal epilepsy. *N Engl J Med.* 1964;271:926–933.
18. Caraballo R, Cersosimo R, Fejerman N. Idiopathic partial epilepsies with rolandic and occipital spikes appearing in the same children. *J Epilepsy.* 1998;11:261–264.
19. Cavazzuti GB. Epidemiology of different types of epilepsy in school age children of Modena, Italy. *Epilepsia.* 1980;21:57–62.
20. Colamaria V, Sgro V, Caraballo R, et al. Status epileptics in benign rolandic epilepsy manifesting as anterior operculum syndrome. *Epilepsia.* 1991;32:329–334.
21. Commission on Classification and Terminology of the International League Against Epilepsy. Proposal for revised classification of epilepsies and epileptic syndromes. *Epilepsia.* 1989;30:389–399.
22. Covanis A, Lada C, Skiadas K. Children with rolandic spikes and ictal vomiting: rolandic epilepsy or Panayiotopoulos syndrome?. *Epileptic Disord.* 2003;5(3):139–143.
23. Dalla Bernardina B, Beghini G. Rolandic spikes in children with and without epilepsy. *Epilepsia.* 1976;17:161–167.
24. Dalla Bernardina B, Sgro V, Caraballo R, et al. Sleep and benign partial epilepsies of childhood: EEG and evoked potential study. In: Degen R, Rodin EA, eds. *Epilepsy, Sleep and Sleep Deprivation.* Amsterdam: Elsevier; 1991: 83–96.
25. Dalla Bernardina B, Sgro V, Fejerman N. Epilepsy with centrotemporal spikes and related syndromes. In: Roger J, Bureau M, Dravet C, et al., eds. *Epileptic Syndromes in Infancy, Childhood and Adolescence,* 3rd ed. Montrouge, France: John Libbey; 2005: 203–225.
26. Dalla Bernardina B, Tassinari CA. EEG of a nocturnal seizure in a patient with benign epilepsy of childhood with rolandic spikes. *Epilepsia.* 1975;16:497–501.
27. Degen R, Degen HE. Some genetic aspects of rolandic epilepsy: waking and sleep EEGs in siblings. *Epilepsia.* 1990;31:795–801.
28. De Negri M, Baglietto MG, Gaggero R. Benzodiazepine (BDZ) treatment of benign childhood epilepsy with centrotemporal spikes. *Brain Dev.* 1997;19(7):506.
29. Deonna T, Zesiger P, Davidoff V, et al. Benign partial epilepsy of childhood: a longitudinal neuropsychological and EEG study of cognitive function. *Dev Med Child Neurol.* 2000;42(9):595–603.
30. De Saint-Martin A, Petiau C, Massa R, et al. Idiopathic rolandic epilepsy with "interictal" facial myoclonia and oromotor deficit: a longitudinal EEG and PET study. *Epilepsia.* 1999;40:614–620.
31. Doose H, Baier WK, Ernst JP, et al. Benign partial epilepsy: treatment with sulthiame. *Dev Med Child Neurol.* 1988;30:683–684.
32. Doose H, Brigger-Heuer B, Neubauer B. Children with focal sharp waves: clinical and genetic aspects. *Epilepsia.* 1997;38(7):788–796.
33. Dubois CM, Zesiger P, Perez ER, et al. Acquired epileptic dysgraphia: a longitudinal study. *Dev Med Child Neurol.* 2003;45(12):807–812.
34. Eeg-Olofsson O. Further genetic aspects in benign localized epilepsies in early childhood. In: Degen R, Dreifuss FE, eds. *Benign Localized and Generalized Epilepsies of Early Childhood.* Amsterdam: Elsevier; 1992: 117–119.
35. Eeg-Olofsson O, Petersen I, Selden U. The development of the electroencephalogram in normal children from the age of 1 through 15 years. *Neuropediatrie.* 1971;2:375–404.
36. Engel J Jr. A proposed diagnostic scheme for people with epileptic seizures and with epilepsy: report of the ILAE Task Force on Classification and Terminology. *Epilepsia.* 2001;42(6):796–803.
37. Engel J, Fejerman, N. Benign childhood epilepsy with centrotemporal spikes. In: Engel J, Fejerman N, eds. *MedLink Neurology (Section of Epilepsy).* San Diego, CA: MedLink; 1999–2005. Available: www.medlink.com.
38. Engler F, Maeder-Ingvar M, Roulet E, et al. Treatment with sulthiame (Ospolot) in benign partial epilepsy of childhood and related syndromes: an open clinical and EEG study. *Neuropediatrics.* 2003;34(2):105–109.
39. Faure J, Loiseau P. Une corrélation clinique particulière des pointes-ondes sans signification focale. *Rev Neurol.* 1960;102:399–406.
40. Fejerman N. Atypical evolutions of benign partial epilepsies in children. *Int Pediatr.* 1996;11(6):351–356.
41. Fejerman N. Benign focal epilepsies in infancy, childhood and adolescence. *Rev Neurol.* 2002;34(1):7–18.
42. Fejerman N, Caraballo R, Tenembaum S. Epilepsias parciais idiopaticas. In: Costa da Costa J, Palmini A, Yacubian EMT, et al., eds. *Benign Childhood Epilepsy with Centrotemporal Spikes.* Sao Paulo, Brazil: Lemos; 1998.
43. Fejerman N, Caraballo R, Tenembaum SN. Atypical evolutions of benign localization-related epilepsies in children: are they predictable?. *Epilepsia.* 2000;41(4):380–390.
44. Fejerman N, Di Blasi AM. Status epilepticus of benign partial epilepsies in children: report of two cases. *Epilepsia.* 1987;28:351–355.
45. Fejerman N, Medina CS. *Convulsiones en la infancia.* Buenos Aires: El Ateneo; 1986: 166–178.
46. Fejerman N, Medina CS, Caraballo R. Síndromes epilepticos en la infancia y adolescencia. In: Fejerman N, Fernadez-Alvarez E, eds. *Neurologia Pediátrica,* 2nd ed. Buenos Aires: Panamericana; 1997: 536–538.
47. Galanopoulou A, Bojko A, Lado F, et al. The spectrum of neuropsychiatric abnormalities associated with electrical status epilepticus in sleep. *Brain Dev.* 2000;22:279–295.
48. Gastaut Y. Un element deroutant de la semeiologie electroencephalographique: les pointes prerolandiques sans signification focale. *Rev Neurol (Paris).* 1952;87:488–490.
49. Gelisse P, Corda D, Raybaud C, et al. Abnormal neuroimaging in patients with benign epilepsy with centrotemporal spikes. *Epilepsia.* 2003;44(3):372–378.
50. Gelisse P, Genton P, Raybaud C, et al. Benign childhood epilepsy with centrotemporal spikes and hippocampal atrophy. *Epilepsia.* 1999;40:1312–1315.
51. Gibbs EL, Gibbs FA. Good prognosis of mid-temporal epilepsy. *Epilepsia.* 1960;1:448–453.
52. Gregory DL, Farrell K, Wong PK. Partial status epilepticus in benign childhood epilepsy with centrotemporal spikes: are independent right and left seizures a risk factor?. *Epilepsia.* 2002;43(8):936–940.
53. Gregory DL, Wong PK. Topographical analysis of the centrotemporal discharges in benign rolandic epilepsy of childhood. *Epilepsia.* 1984;25:705–711.

54. Hahn A, Pistohl J, Neubauer BA, et al. Atypical "benign" partial epilepsy or pseudo-Lennox syndrome. Part I: Symptomatology and long-term prognosis. *Neuropediatrics*. 2001;32(1):1–8.
55. Halasz P, Kelemen A, Clemens B, et al. The perisylvian epileptic network. A unifying concept. *Ideggyogy Sz*. 2005;58(3–4):104.
56. Heijbel J, Blom S, Bergfors PG. Benign epilepsy of children with centrotemporal EEG foci. Study of incidence rate in outpatient care. *Epilepsia*. 1975;16:657–664.
57. Heijbel J, Blom S, Rasmuson M. Benign epilepsy of childhood with centrotemporal EEG foci: a genetic study. *Epilepsia*. 1975;16:285–293.
58. Heijbel J, Bohman M. Benign epilepsy of children with centrotemporal EEG foci: intelligence, behavior and school adjustment. *Epilepsia*. 1975;16:679–687.
59. Holtmann M, Becker K, Kentner-Figura B, et al. Increased frequency of rolandic spikes in ADHD children. *Epilepsia*. 2003;44(9):1241–1244.
60. Hommet C, Billard C, Motte J, et al. Cognitive function in adolescents and young adults in complete remission from benign childhood epilepsy with centro-temporal spikes. *Epileptic Disord*. 2001;3(4):207–216.
61. Huiskamp G, van Der Meij W, van Huffelen A, et al. High resolution spatio-temporal EEG-MEG analysis of rolandic spikes. *J Clin Neurophysiol*. 2004;21(2):84–95.
62. Ishitobi M, Nakasato N, Yamamoto K, et al. Opercular to interhemispheric source distribution of benign rolandic spikes of childhood. *Neuroimage*. 2004;25(2):417–423.
63. Kajitani T, Kimura T, Sumita M, et al. Relationship between benign epilepsy of children with centrotemporal EEG foci and febrile convulsions. *Brain Dev*. 1992;14:230–234.
64. Kajitani T, Nakamura M, Ueoka K, et al. Three pairs of monozygotic twins with rolandic discharges. In: Wada J, Penny J, eds. *Advances in Epileptology. The Tenth International Symposium*. New York: Raven Press; 1980: 171–175.
65. Kamada K, Moller M, Saguer M, et al. Localization analysis of neuronal activities in benign rolandic epilepsy using magnetoencephalography. *J Neurol Sci*. 1998;154(2):164–172.
66. Kramer U, Ben-Zeev B, Harel S, et al. Transient oromotor deficits in children with benign childhood epilepsy with central temporal spikes. *Epilepsia*. 2001;42(5):616–620.
67. Kramer U, Nevo Y, Neufeld MY, et al. Epidemiology of epilepsy in childhood: a cohort of 440 consecutive patients. *Pediatr Neurol*. 1998;18(1):46–50.
68. Kramer U, Zelnik N, Lerman-Sagie T, et al. Benign childhood epilepsy with centrotemporal spikes: clinical characteristics and identification of patients at risk of multiple seizures. *J Child Neurol*. 2002;17(1):17–19.
69. Kraschnitz W, Scheer P, Korner K, et al. Rolandic spikes as an EEG manifestation of an oligodendro-glioma. *Pediatr Pathol*. 1988;23:313–319.
70. Legarda S, Jayakar P, Duchowny M, et al. Benign rolandic epilepsy: high central and low central subgroups. *Epilepsia*. 1994;35:1125–1129.
71. Lerman P. Benign childhood epilepsy with centrotemporal spikes. In: Engel J, Pedly TA, eds. *Epilepsy: A Comprehensive Textbook*. Philadelphia: Lippincott-Raven; 1998: 2307–2314.
72. Lerman P, Kivity S. Benign focal epilepsy of childhood. A follow-up study of 100 recovered patients. *Arch Neurol*. 1975;32:261–264.
73. Lerman P, Kivity S. The benign partial nonrolandic epilepsies. *J Clin Neurophysiol*. 1991;8:275–287.
74. Lerman P, Lerman-Sagie T. Sulthiame revisited. *J Child Neurol*. 1995;10:241–242.
75. Lin YY, Chang KP, Hsieh JC, et al. Magnetoencephalographic analysis of bilaterally synchronous discharges in benign rolandic epilepsy of childhood. *Seizure*. 2003;12(7):448–455.
76. Lischka A, Graf M. Benign rolandic epilepsy of childhood: topographic EEG analysis. *Epilepsy Res Suppl*. 1992;6:53–58.
77. Loiseau P, Beaussart M. The seizures of benign childhood epilepsy with rolandic paroxysmal discharges. *Epilepsia*. 1972;14:381–389.
78. Loiseau P, Cohadon F, Mortureux Y. A propos d'une forme singulière d'epilepsie de l'enfant. *Rev Neurol (Paris)*. 1967;116:244–248.
79. Loiseau P, Duche B. Benign childhood epilepsy with centrotemporal spikes. *Cleve Clin J Med*. 1989;56:S17–S22.
80. Loiseau P, Duche B, Cordova S, et al. Prognosis of benign childhood epilepsy with centrotemporal spikes. A follow-up study of 168 patients. *Epilepsia*. 1988;29:229–235.
81. Lombroso CT. Sylvian seizures and midtemporal spike foci in children. *Arch Neurol*. 1967;17:52–59.
82. Luders H, Lesser RP, Dinner DS, et al. Benign focal epilepsy of childhood. In: Luders H, Lesser RP, eds. *Epilepsy: Electroclinical Syndrome*. Berlin: Springer-Verlag; 1987: 303–346.
83. Lundberg S. *Rolandic epilepsy*. Thesis, University of Uppsala; 2004.
84. Lundberg S, Eeg-Olofsson O, Raininko R, et al. Hippocampal asymmetries and white matter abnormalities on MRI in benign childhood epilepsy with centrotemporal spikes. *Epilepsia*. 1999;40(12):1808–1815.
85. Massa R, de Saint-Martin A, Carcangiu R, et al. EEG criteria predictive of complicated evolution in idiopathic rolandic epilepsy. *Neurology*. 2001;57:1071–1079.
86. Minami T, Gondo K, Yamamoto T, et al. Magnetoencephalographic analysis of rolandic discharges in benign childhood epilepsy. *Ann Neurol*. 1996;39(3):326–334.
87. Mitsudome A, Ohu M, Yasumoto S, et al. Rhythmic slow activity in benign childhood epilepsy with centrotemporal spikes. *Clin Electroencephalogr*. 1997;28(1):44–48.
88. Mitsudome A, Ohfu M, Yasumoto S, et al. The effectiveness of clonazepam on the rolandic discharges. *Brain Dev*. 1997;19(4):274–278.
89. Monjauze C, Tuller L, Hommet C, et al. Language in benign childhood epilepsy with centro-temporal spikes abbreviated form: Rolandic epilepsy and language. *Brain Lang*. 2005;92(3):300–308.
90. Musumeci SA, Colognola RM, Ferri R, et al. Fragile-X syndrome: a particular epileptogenic EEG pattern. *Epilepsia*. 1988;29:41–47.
91. Nayrac P, Beaussart M. Les pointes-ondes prerolandiques: expression EEG tres particuliere. Etude electroclinique de 21 cas. *Rev Neurol (Paris)*. 1958;99:201–206.
92. Neubauer BA, Fiedler B, Himmelein B, et al. Centrotemporal spikes in families with rolandic epilepsy: linkage to chromosome 15q14. *Neurology*. 1998;51(6):1608–1612.
93. Niedermeyer E, Naidu S. Further EEG observations in children with the Rett syndrome. *Brain Dev*. 1990;12:53–54.
94. Northcott E, Connolly AM, Berroya A, et al. The neuropsychological and language profile of children with benign rolandic epilepsy. *Epilepsia*. 2005;46(6):924–930.
95. Okubo Y, Matsuura M, Asai T, et al. Epileptiform EEG discharges in healthy children: prevalence, emotional and behavioural correlates, and genetic influences. *Epilepsia*. 1994;35:832–841.
96. Otsubo H, Chitoku S, Ochi A, et al. Malignant rolandic-sylvian epilepsy in children: diagnosis, treatment, and outcomes. *Neurology*. 2001;57(4):590–596.
97. Ounsted C, Lindsay J, Norman R. *Biological Factors in Temporal Lobe Epilepsy. Clinics in Developmental Medicine, No. 22*. London: Heinemann Medical; 1966.
98. Pan A, Gupta A, Wyllie, E, et al. Benign focal epileptiform discharges of childhood and hippocampal sclerosis. *Epilepsia*. 2004;45(3):284–288.
99. Panayiotopoulos CP. Benign childhood partial epilepsies: benign childhood seizure susceptibility syndrome. *J Neurol Neurosurg Psychiatry*. 1993;56:2–5.
100. Panayiotopoulos CP. *Benign Childhood Partial Seizures and Related Epileptic Syndromes*. London: John Libbey; 1999.
101. Panayiotopoulos CP. *The Epilepsies*. Oxford: Bladon; 2005.
102. Papavasiliou A, Mattheou D, Bazigou H, et al. Written language skills in children with benign childhood epilepsy with centrotemporal spikes. *Epilepsy Behav*. 2005;6(1):50–58.
103. Prats JM, Garaizar C, Garcia-Nieto ML, et al. Antiepileptic drugs and atypical evolution of idiopathic partial epilepsy. *Pediatr Neurol*. 1998;18(5):402–406.
104. Pruna D, Persico I, Serra D, et al. Lack of association with the 15q14 candidate region for benign epilepsy of childhood with centro-temporal spikes in a Sardinian population. *Epilepsia*. 2000;41:164.
105. Rating D, Wolf C, Bast T. Sulthiame as monotherapy in children with benign childhood epilepsy with centrotemporal spikes: a 6-month randomized, double-blind, placebo-controlled study. Sulthiame Study Group. *Epilepsia*. 2000;41(10):1284–1288.
106. Roulet E, Deonna T, Despland PA. Prolonged intermittent drooling and oromotor dyspraxia in benign childhood epilepsy with centrotemporal spikes. *Epilepsia*. 1989;30:564–568.
107. Salas-Puig J, Perez-Jimenez A, Thomas P, et al. Opercular epilepsies with oromotor dysfunction. In: Guerrini R, Aicardi J, Andermann F, et al., eds. *Epilepsy and Movement Disorders*. London: Cambridge University Press; 2002: 251–268.
108. Santanelli P, Bureau M, Magaudda A, et al. Benign partial epilepsy with centrotemporal (or rolandic) spikes and brain lesion. *Epilepsia*. 1989;30(2):182–188.
109. Scheffer IE, Jones L, Pozzebon M, et al. Autosomal dominant rolandic epilepsy and speech dyspraxia: a new syndrome with anticipation. *Ann Neurol*. 1995;38(4):633–642.
110. Sheth RD, Gutierrez AR, Riggs JE. Rolandic epilepsy and cortical dysplasia: MRI correlation of epileptiform discharges. *Pediatr Neurol*. 1997;17(2):177–179.
111. Shevell MI, Rosenblatt B, Watters GV, et al. "Pseudo-BECRS": intracranial focal lesions suggestive of a primary partial epilepsy syndrome. *Pediatr Neurol*. 1996;14(1):31–35.
112. Shields WD, Saslow E. Myoclonic, atonic, and absence seizures following institution of carbamazepine therapy in children. *Neurology*. 1983;33(11):1487–1489.
113. Staden U, Isaacs E, Boyd SG, et al. Language disfunction in children with rolandic epilepsy. *Neuropediatrics*. 1998;29:242–248.
114. Trojaborg W. Focal spike discharges in children: a longitudinal study. *Acta Paediatr Scand*. 1966(Suppl):168.
115. Tsai ML, Hung KL. Topographic mapping and clinical analysis of BCECS. *Brain Dev*. 1998;20(1):27–32.
116. Tzitiridou M, Panou T, Ramantani G, et al. Oxcarbazepine monotherapy in benign childhood epilepsy with centrotemporal spikes: a clinical and cognitive evaluation. *Epilepsy Behav*. 2005;7(3):458–467.
117. Van Bogaert P, Wikler D, Damhaut P, et al. Cerebral glucose metabolism and centrotemporal spikes. *Epilepsy Res*. 1998;29(2):123–127.
118. Vaughn BV, Greenwood RS, Aylsworth AS, et al. Similarities of EEG and seizures in del(1q) and benign rolandic epilepsy. *Pediatr Neurol*. 1996;15(3):261–264.

119. Veggiotti P, Beccaria F, Gatti A, et al. Can protrusion of the tongue stop seizures in rolandic epilepsy?. *Epileptic Disord.* 1999;1(4):217–220.
120. Verrotti A, Latini G, Trotta D, et al. Typical and atypical rolandic epilepsy in childhood: a follow-up study. *Pediatr Neurol.* 2002;26(1):26–29.
121. Watanabe K. Benign partial epilepsies. In: Wallace SJ, Farrell K, eds. *Epilepsy in Children,* 2nd ed. London: Arnold 2004:199–220.
122. Weglage J, Demsky A, Pietsch M, et al. Neuropsychological, intellectual, and behavioral findings in patients with centrotemporal spikes with and without seizures. *Dev Med Child Neurol.* 1997;39(10):646–651.
123. Wirrell EC, Camfield PR, Gordon KE, et al. Benign rolandic epilepsy: atypical features are very common. *J Child Neurol.* 1995;10(6):455–458.
124. Wolff M, Weiskopf N, Serra E, et al. Benign partial epilepsy in childhood: selective cognitive deficits are related to the location of local spikes determined by combined EEG/MEG. *Epilepsia.* 2005;46(10):1661–1667.

CHAPTER 237 ■ EARLY-ONSET BENIGN CHILDHOOD OCCIPITAL EPILEPSY (PANAYIOTOPOULOS TYPE)

NATALIO FEJERMAN

INTRODUCTION

In the first edition of this book, only a few lines mentioned this condition under the heading of Childhood Epilepsy With Occipital Spikes and Other Benign Localization-Related Epilepsies.[33] At present, early-onset benign childhood occipital epilepsy (Panayiotopoulos type) (EOCOE) is not only a clearly recognized syndrome, but it also represents the second-most-frequent benign focal epilepsy syndrome in childhood after benign childhood epilepsy with centrotemporal spikes (BCECTS). The characteristic clinical features of this syndrome should be known not only by epileptologists and neurologists, but also by pediatricians. An early diagnosis would avoid undue interventions and concerns on account of its really benign outcome.

HISTORICAL PERSPECTIVES

In the International League Against Epilepsy (ILAE) classification of Epilepsy syndromes,[11] besides the well-known BCECTS, only childhood epilepsy with occipital paroxysms (CEOP), as described by Gastaut, is recognized.[29] In comparison with BCECTS, which has a prevalence of approximately 15% among children with epilepsy,[15,18,52] the Gastaut type of CEOP is rare, of uncertain boundaries, and often of unpredictable prognosis.[8] This condition is characterized by brief seizures with mainly visual symptoms such as elementary visual hallucinations, illusions, or amaurosis, followed by hemiclonic convulsions. Postictal migraine headaches occur in half of the patients. Age at onset is approximately 8 to 9 years. The electroencephalogram (EEG) shows occipital spike-wave paroxysms that attenuate or disappear when the eyes are open.[11,29,30,47]

In 1989, two significant papers of Panayiotopoulos based on an already long follow-up of his patients called attention to the particular cluster of symptoms present in what he called "benign nocturnal childhood occipital epilepsy."[49,50] He had already emphasized vomiting as an ictal symptom in epileptic seizures in children 1 year earlier.[48] Another peculiar clinical feature of EOCOE was the "cerebral insult–like" partial status epilepticus including autonomic symptoms.[38,57,64] To stress the variable phenotypes of benign focal epileptic syndromes in childhood, Panayiotopoulos and coworkers used the term "benign childhood seizure susceptibility syndromes."[51,52] After 1996, Fejerman and coworkers proposed naming this syndrome early-onset benign childhood occipital epilepsy (Panayiotopoulos type) as opposed to late-onset childhood occipital epilepsy (Gastaut type).[7,8,19–22] Three important series of children with this syndrome were published about this time.[25,37,45] Retrospective analysis of the clinical histories allowed the authors to study the variants of childhood epilepsies with occipital paroxysms and to recognize this early-onset variant. In the same year, the first prospective study of 66 children with EOCOE was published.[8] In 2001, the task force on Classification and Terminology of the ILAE published a proposed diagnostic scheme for people with epilepsy.[17] It adopted the names proposed by Fejerman including eponymic designations to emphasize the differences between the Gastaut type and the Panayiotopoulos type of childhood epilepsy with occipital paroxysms, keeping intentionally the term "benign" only for this early-onset form.[19,20] Thereafter, several authors preferred the eponymic term "Panayiotopoulos syndrome" (PS) to include patients with and without occipital spikes or occipital ictal origins.[3,8,13,14,16,26–28,36,42,54,56,59] Considering the emphasis given in recent years to the presence of autonomic seizures and autonomic status epilepticus in this condition, that occipital EEG abnormalities are not found in a certain proportion of the cases, and that there is no clear documentation of an occipital origin of seizures, we agree that the name PS might be more appropriate. As a practical measure, we will continue to refer to EOCOE as PS in this chapter.

DEFINITIONS

Types of seizures, age of onset, normal neurologic status of patients, and spontaneous evolution allow us to define the PS as a benign, age-related focal epilepsy syndrome occurring in early and mid-childhood. The analysis of several large series of published cases and our own present series clearly demonstrates the significant frequency of PS, which is seen about one third as often as BCECTS.

EPIDEMIOLOGY

PS is seen only in children, with a peak incidence between 4 and 5 years of age. Given that the official recognition of EOCOE or PS took place only in 2001, it is very difficult to find epidemiologic studies in a childhood population that include PS among the diagnoses. Additionally, most studies are based more on seizure types than syndromes. One study included a mix of seizures and syndromes for the recognition of epilepsies in 440 consecutive pediatric patients. Thirty-six (8%) of the cases were diagnosed as benign rolandic epilepsy of childhood and 8 cases (2%) as benign occipital epilepsy of childhood. We may assume that this last group was underevaluated, and we do not know how many of the cases corresponded to PS.[39] A cohort of 407 children with their first unprovoked seizure was followed for a mean of 9.4 years, and distribution of epilepsy syndromes was reported: Of 114 children with localization-related epilepsy syndromes, 26 were idiopathic, 24 were rolandic, and only 2 were occipital.[60] Another study of a population-based, active-prevalence cohort in children <16 years of age was able to classify syndromes in 235 (96%) of the 245 patients followed for many years. However, no specific data about PS were included in any of these three studies because they were based on the 1989 ILAE Classification.[61] Therefore, one has to credit the everyday experience of active epileptologists caring for children, who have become aware of this condition in the last few years:[3]

- Oguni et al. 1999: Among 649 children with localization-related epilepsy selected from their database, 62 met the criteria for diagnosis of PS.
- Kivity et al. 2000: A file review of patients with occipital EEG paroxysms disclosed 72 children with typical PS.
- Caraballo et al. 2000: A prospective study selected 66 patients with PS with strict criteria for inclusion.
- Lada et al. 2003: A retrospective analysis of clinical and EEG records included 1,340 children with focal seizures; 43 who had PS and >2 years since they were seizure free were followed-up.
- Caraballo and Fejerman 2005: The addition of new cases after the 66 reported in 2000 provided a total of 156 children with typical PS who were followed prospectively.
- Panayiotopoulos 2005: In an ongoing hospital-based, prospective study at the end of 3 years, 228 children aged 1 through 14 years with one or more seizures had one or more EEGs. Fourteen of them (6.1%) had Panayiotopoulos syndrome.[54]

ETIOLOGY AND BASIC MECHANISMS

As an idiopathic epilepsy syndrome, PS is by definition not associated with remote symptomatic or acute symptomatic etiology. Most likely, it is genetically determined, although neither a gene nor a chromosomal locus has been found in PS. Linkage with chromosome 15 has been reported in BCECTS,[43] although in another study this locus was not found.[58] One affected sibling with PS was reported in one series,[25] and two pairs of affected siblings were seen in each of two other series.[8,42] Three siblings were reported in 1987 as having benign occipital epilepsy as described by Gastaut, although the paper indicates that the three siblings showed seizures starting at ages 4 and 5 years, and the clinical features were quite compatible with PS.[40]

There is a high prevalence of febrile seizures in children with PS, ranging from 16% to 45%.[8,13,14,25,45,64] A family history of epilepsy was found in 30.3% of the cases.[8] The finding of several children with PS who at the same time or later had rolandic seizures and centrotemporal spikes typical of BCECTS as well as siblings who had either rolandic epilepsy or PS speaks in favor of a genetic linkage of these two syndromes, perhaps expressed as a reversible functional derangement of the brains cortical maturation.[6,8,13,14,24,50,52,54,56] Basic mechanisms and pathophysiology of PS are largely unknown. Clinical findings indicate that there is a diffuse cortical hyperexcitability, which is related to maturation.[14,26,54] Even when the majority of cases show occipital spikes, a significant number of patients have spikes in other areas, and according to the mentioned reference of PS and BCECTS in the same children, spikes may appear in two areas at the same time or over the course of time.[6,13] In addition, the high frequency of ictal vomiting indicates that epileptic discharges are generated at various cortical locations. The same concept is valid for other autonomic manifestations. As we will see later, different cortical locations in patients with PS were also documented with magnetoencephalography.[36]

CLINICAL PRESENTATION

Panayiotopoulos syndrome occurs in children who are otherwise normal; it is not associated with neurodevelopmental problems. Although it has been described as starting as early as 1 year of age and as late as 14 years of age, the large majority of patients have their first seizure around the age of 4 to 5 years. Three fourths of patients have their first seizure between the ages of 3 and 6 years. It affects boys and girls almost equally. Seizures occur predominantly during sleep, and only in sleep in two thirds of patients. In seizures occurring while the patient is awake, onset may be inconspicuous with pallor, agitation, feeling sick, and vomiting. At this stage, the epileptic nature of the event can hardly be suspected in the absence of motor convulsive symptoms that, if present, may be rightly considered as secondary to an ongoing serious brain insult. It is only the normal postictal state of the child that should be reassuring.

The duration of the seizures is usually long, commonly >5 minutes, and in approximately 40% of the cases, >30 minutes, constituting then a focal or secondarily generalized status epilepticus. Three groups of symptoms are recognized, as shown in Table 1.

Core Clinical Features

Ictal Emetic Symptoms and Other Autonomic Manifestations

Ictal vomiting, which is considered to be exceptional in other epilepsies, occurs in approximately 80% of the cases with PS.[8,13,25,42,45,48–50,54,55] In one prospective study, vomiting was considered a criterion for inclusion, although we now know that vomiting is not present in 100% of the cases.[8] In nocturnal seizures, it is usually the first apparent symptom, whereas in seizures occurring while the patient is awake, other symptoms of the emetic spectrum such as nausea or retching may appear along with or before vomiting.[13]

TABLE 1

FREQUENCY OF SEIZURE TYPES IN CHILDREN WITH PANAYIOTOPOULOS SYNDROME

Core clinical features
- Ictal emetic symptoms and other autonomic manifestations
- Deviation of the eyes
- Impairment of consciousness

Frequent types of seizures
- Unilateral clonic or tonic–clonic seizures
- Secondary generalized tonic–clonic seizures
- Encephalopathy-like status epilepticus (focal motor—unilateral or generalized—and autonomic)

Less frequent but not rare symptoms and signs
- Visual symptoms
- Migraine-like headaches
- Incontinence of urine and feces
- Syncope-like symptoms
- Other

Vomiting may occur repetitively or only once during the seizure.

Pallor is the most frequent autonomic manifestation. It occurs mainly at onset and commonly together with vomiting. In seizures starting while the patient is awake, pallor, nausea, and "feeling sick" are frequent symptoms.

Deviation of the Eyes

Unilateral deviation of the eyes is as common as vomiting and also occurs in approximately 80% of the patients.[8,25,45,48,49,54,56] The eye deviation may be brief or prolonged and is frequently accompanied by head deviation. It may be continuous or, less often, intermittent. Consciousness is often but not invariably impaired at this stage. It should be noted that exact details of this symptom are rarely witnessed because seizures occur mostly at night.

Impairment of Consciousness

Consciousness is usually intact at seizure onset but becomes impaired in 80% to 90% of cases as the seizure evolves. Impairment of consciousness may be mild or moderate, with the child retaining some ability to respond to verbal commands but often talking out of context. In seizures with motor components occurring during sleep, complete loss of consciousness may be seen, especially in all those that are prolonged into status. In diurnal seizures, clouding of consciousness usually starts after the appearance of autonomic and behavioral symptoms. Awareness may be preserved throughout the ictal state in 10% to 20% of the seizures.[25,45,46,50,54,56]

Frequent Features of Seizures

Unilateral Clonic or Tonic–Clonic Seizures

Unilateral clonic convulsions in face and extremities at onset or following vomiting and eye deviation are seen in 25% to 30% of the cases.[8,54,55]

Secondarily Generalized Tonic–Clonic Seizures

This type of seizure rarely appears at onset and usually follows seizures starting with focal motor manifestation. In one series of patients, this course was seen in nearly 40% of the cases.[8]

Status Epilepticus

This is usually nonconvulsive, lasts >30 minutes, and occurs in approximately 30% of cases in all series.[8,25,45,49,54–56] This "encephalopathy-like" form of status epilepticus may progress to hemiconvulsions. We will show under the heading of differential diagnosis how important it is to recognize PS when it may mimic other pathologies caused by true cerebral insult.

Less Frequent, but Not Rare, Symptoms

Visual Symptoms

Visual symptoms are typical of the Gastaut type of CEOP. However, in patients with PS, elementary visual hallucinations, illusions, and blindness were registered in <10% of children who were able to describe them.

Migraine-Like Headaches

These are rarely present, and in older children may sometimes cast doubt on a differential diagnosis with the Gastaut type of CEOP.

Incontinence of Urine and Feces

This may occur when consciousness is impaired.

The occurrence of syncope-like symptoms is another autonomic manifestation that has been emphasized more recently. Children becoming completely irresponsive and flaccid, often without convulsions, are not considered rare by many authors.[13,14,26,54,56]

DIAGNOSTIC EVALUATION

Neuroimaging and Other Laboratory Examinations

By definition of an idiopathic epilepsy syndrome, neurologic and neuropsychological evaluations of children with PS are normal. Some of the initial symptoms may mislead the pediatrician regarding the nature of the condition, mainly when vomiting and other autonomic symptoms are present. Excessive laboratory examinations might then be undertaken. When syncope-like manifestations occur, cardiology consultation is required.

Brain imaging studies are normal. However, the spectacular nature of ictal features, and especially the frequency of status epilepticus, makes magnetic resonance imaging (MRI) necessary to rule out conditions that can provoke focal, unilateral, or generalized seizures.

Electroencephalographic Findings

The most useful laboratory test is EEG. Ictal EEG reports are rare because seizures are infrequent. The ictal discharge in PS is characterized by rhythmic monomorphic decelerating theta or delta activity that is markedly different from the episodic fast activity of visual seizures of the Gastaut type CEOP and starts either from the posterior[2,16,45,64,65] or frontal regions.[14,45] We recently registered an ictal EEG in a 4-year-old girl with a seizure consisting of vomiting, pallor, and loss of consciousness; rhythmic spike discharges could be seen starting in the right occipital region and propagating to frontal areas (Fig. 1).[4]

Because most patients with PS are first seen between ages 3 and 6 years, many of these EEGs are obtained during sleep. Sleep activates the appearance of occipital spikes in these children (Fig. 2).[8] Occipital spikes are bilateral and synchronous, often with voltage asymmetry, or unilateral. In awake EEGs, occipital paroxysms of high amplitude with sharp and slow-wave complexes that occur immediately after closing the eyes are often registered. These paroxysms are eliminated, or markedly attenuated, when the eyes are opened, a phenomenon due to fixation of sensitivity.[47,54,55] This phenomenon, which should be sought in every EEG laboratory, was considered pathognomonic of the Gastaut type of CEOP, but it is not. It has been reported not only in patients with PS, but also in patients with other conditions.[12,44]

Even when occipital spikes and spike-wave paroxysms are the main EEG feature, their absence does exclude the diagnosis of PS. It has been emphasized that extraoccipital spikes (centrotemporal, frontal, parietal) may also be found in children with PS.[14,45,52] Generalized spike and wave discharges are not seen in children with PS as frequently as they are in children

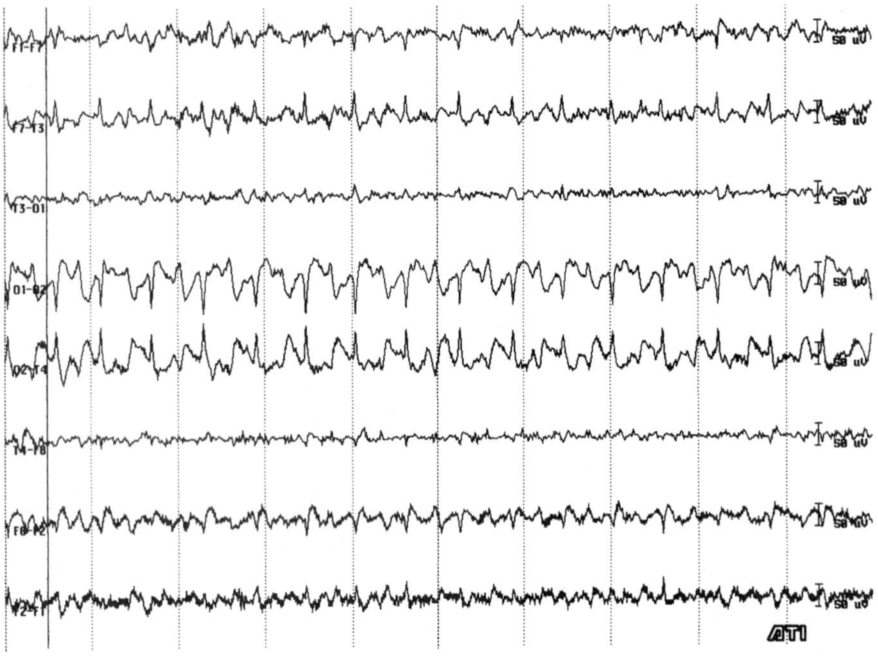

FIGURE 1. A 4-year-old girl. Ictal EEG: The seizure started 5 seconds before the discharges seen in this sample, with rhythmic spikes in the right occipital area and propagated to frontal areas.

with BCECTS.[18] Normal EEGs during sleep are exceptional according to a recent consensus report.[26]

The evolution of EEG discharges in 76 children with PS was followed with repeated sleep EEG examinations. These showed that the occipital spike pattern was prevalent in the first few years of the diagnosis and later became associated with frontal or centrotemporal spikes.[46]

An interesting recent paper related to EEG in PS showed that a group of EEG technicians trained on the clinical features of PS were able to diagnose the condition in 14 children, and in 9 of the cases their information was crucial to achieving a diagnosis.[59]

In a recent study of eight children with PS, dipole analysis of the interictal spike discharges was performed. The various types of spikes observed in PS had similar and stable dipole locations. The dipoles showing high stability were located in the mesial occipital area and were accompanied by dipoles located in the rolandic area, suggesting a possible pathogenetic link between PS and BCECTS.[66]

Other Neurophysiologic Studies

In 13 children with PS who ranged in age from 3 to 14 years, the localizations of equivalent current dipoles (ECDs) of spike discharges by magnetoencephalography were examined. Eleven patients (84.6%) showed clustered ECDs in areas alongside the parietooccipital sulcus and/or the calcarine sulcus. Five of

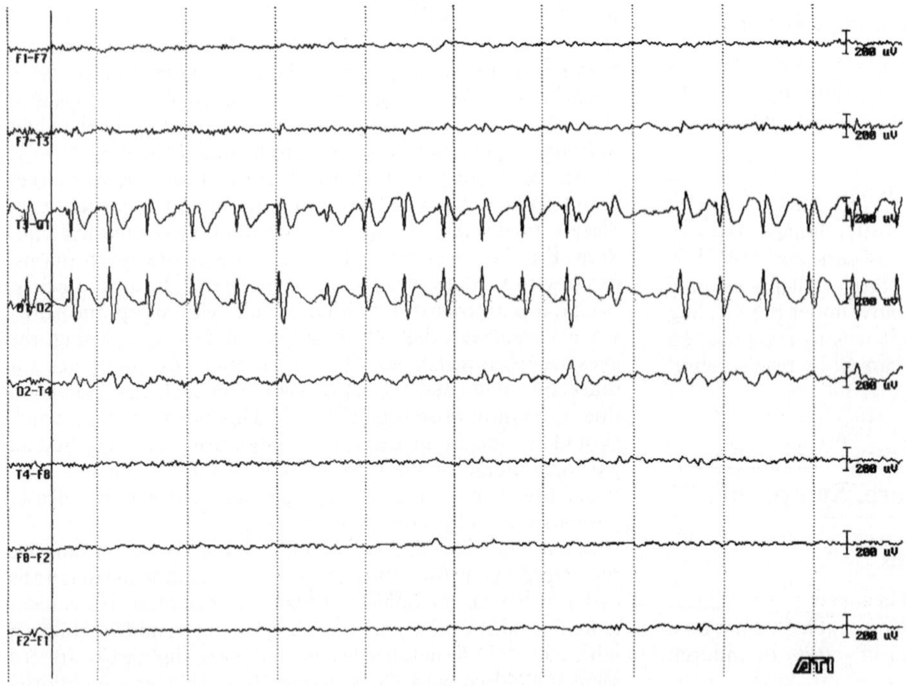

FIGURE 2. A 7-year-old boy. Left occipital spikes activated by sleep.

the children who also presented rolandic seizures showed in addition clustered ECDs in rolandic areas.[36]

Studies of visual-evoked potentials (VEPs) were performed in 9 children with PS and 10 children with the Gastaut type of CEOP. High-amplitude VEP responses attributed to hyperexcitability of the occipital cortical structures were present in all 19 patients.[34]

DIFFERENTIAL DIAGNOSIS

Despite sound clinical-EEG manifestations, for many years Panayiotopoulos syndrome escaped recognition, for many reasons. Ictal vomiting is rarely considered as an ictal event. When this is associated with deteriorating level of consciousness followed by convulsions, encephalitis or other acute cerebral insults are the prevailing diagnoses at the acute stage. If the seizures are hemigeneralized, a more focal cerebral insult is always looked for. If the child is seen after complete recovery, atypical migraine, gastroenteritis, or a first seizure is a likely diagnosis. Table 2 lists the main differential diagnoses of PS. The presence of prolonged seizures in a previously healthy child inevitably leads to consideration of acute cerebral insults due to encephalitis; intoxication; acute disseminated encephalomyelitis; mitochondrial encephalopathy, lactic acidosis, and stroke-like episodes (MELAS); or acute cerebrovascular event. Complete recovery after $\geq$1 hours of seizures makes these diagnoses improbable, although, as stated before, brain imaging studies are usually obtained. Basilar or other infrequent forms of atypical migraine are among the main differential diagnoses in cases with prolonged or repeated vomiting with other autonomic symptoms. Both conditions may appear abruptly, and in both, full recovery is seen. Impaired consciousness does not rule out the diagnosis of migraine.[53] However, it is extremely rare for migraine to start with vomiting interrupting sleep in young children.

Syncope-like episodes with pallor, irresponsiveness, and flaccidity may lead to consideration of real syncopal attacks and to ask for cardiology examination. Of course, common syncope in children does not appear during sleep, but nausea, pallor, and sick feeling in an awake child can be the first symptoms of a syncopal attack.

Table 3 shows the differential diagnosis between PS and the Gastaut type of CEOP.

The mean age of onset of BCECTS is approximately 7 to 8 years of age, and its typical features differ clearly from those of PS. However, we will note later that it is not rare to see children presenting at the same time ictal symptoms of both syndromes. As for the idiopathic photosensitive occipital lobe epilepsy, its mean age of onset is around 11 years, and all ictal events are preceded by the exposure to photic stimulation, either intermittent lights or TV or computer game screens.[35] This condition is quite rare and less frequent than other reflex epilepsies secondary to visual stimuli.

Symptomatic occipital epilepsies may present clinical features similar to those of the idiopathic occipital epilepsies. The EEG may even show the occipital spike-and-wave discharges disappearing after eye opening that is so typical of the Gastaut type of CEOP but may also be seen in PS.[12,44] There are two particular conditions to consider in children with seizures manifested by visual symptomatology and occipital spikes or spike-waves. One is celiac disease with occipital calcifications and epilepsy. The majority of patients with this condition do not have overt symptoms of celiac disease. That is why, in the presence of occipital discharges and seizures, posterior cerebral calcifications have to be discarded. If they are present, specific studies for celiac disease are mandatory because in these children their epilepsy improves with a gluten-free diet.[1,32] Silent celiac disease was investigated in a study of 72 patients observed consecutively over a 5-year period with an initial diagnosis of idiopathic partial epilepsy. In the 47 children with BCECTS, specific antibodies were not found, but in 2 of the 25 cases with childhood partial epilepsy with occipital paroxysms (CEOP), the results were positive and later confirmed by jejunal biopsy.[41] This study did not attempt to distinguish between the Gastaut type and the Panayiotopoulos type of CEOP.

In a recent series of 12 patients, we showed a clear association between history of neonatal hypoglycemia and posterior cerebral lesions provoking seizures. Epileptic seizures in these children were usually well controlled by antiepileptic drugs (AEDs), but most of the cases presented intellectual impairment.[8]

TABLE 2

DIFFERENTIAL DIAGNOSIS OF PANAYIOTOPOULOS SYNDROME

With other neurologic conditions
- Encephalitis
- Acute toxic encephalopathy
- Acute disseminated encephalomyelitis (ADEM)
- Mitochondrial encephalopathy with lactic acidosis and stroke (MELAS)
- Acute cerebrovascular event
- Migraine (basilar artery migraine)
- Diseases of the autonomic nervous system

With other epilepsy syndromes
- With other idiopathic epilepsy syndromes
  - Childhood epilepsy with occipital paroxysms (Gastaut type)
  - Benign childhood epilepsy with centrotemporal spikes
  - Idiopathic photosensitive occipital epilepsy
- With symptomatic occipital epilepsies
  - Celiac disease, occipital calcifications, and epilepsy
  - Occipital epilepsy after neonatal hypoglycemia
  - Other symptomatic occipital epilepsies

Association of Panayiotopoulos Syndrome With Other Idiopathic Epilepsy Syndromes

Isolated cases with electroclinical features of BCECTS are occasionally found in children with idiopathic occipital epilepsies.[24,38,49,54] In 1998, idiopathic partial epilepsies with both rolandic and occipital spikes appearing were reported in ten patients. Five of them had first PS and after $\geq$2 years presented hemifacial motor seizures with anarthria typical of BCECTS. The other five patients presented anarthria and hemifacial contractions with sialorrhea and ictal vomiting with head deviation as typical seizures of PS and BCECTS in the same epoch and even in the same episodes.[6] This finding was later confirmed by another group of authors.[13]

Another small series of cases reporting the presence of two idiopathic epilepsy syndromes in the same children showed that absence epilepsy was associated with the Gastaut type of CEOP in five patients and with PS in one child.[10]

TREATMENT AND OUTCOME

There is no consensus about treatment in PS. Because approximately one third of the patients only have one seizure, either

TABLE 3

DIFFERENTIAL DIAGNOSIS BETWEEN PANAYIOTOPOULOS SYNDROME AND GASTAUT-TYPE CHILDHOOD OCCIPITAL EPILEPSY

	Panayiotopoulos syndrome	Gastaut-type childhood occipital epilepsy
Prevalence among benign focal epilepsies in childhood (%)	27	3
Age at onset (yr)	1–14 (mean: 4–5)	3–16 (mean; 8–9)
Duration of seizures		
• <2 min	Exceptional	As a rule
• >5 min	As a rule	Rare
High seizure frequency	Rare	As a rule
Seizures during sleep	>2/3 of cases	<1/3 of cases
Features of seizures		
• Ictal vomiting	Frequent	Exceptional
• Deviation of the eyes	Frequent	Rare
• Impairment of consciousness	Frequent	Rare
• Visual hallucinations	Rare	As a rule
• Loss of vision	Exceptional	Frequent
• Autonomic disturbances	Not rare	Rare
• Postictal headache	Rare	Frequent
Seizures evolving into status	Frequent	Exceptional
Interictal electroencephalogram	Frequent occipital spikes; less frequent spikes in other areas.	Spike-wave occipital paroxysms reactive to eye opening
Prognosis		
• Remission within 1–3 yr from first seizure	As a rule	Rare
• Evolution into Continuous spike and waves during slow sleep	Rare (3 cases reported)	Rare (2 cases reported)
• Overall prognosis	Excellent	Uncertain

brief or prolonged, many authors recommend not starting AED treatment.[14,56] However, it is not so easy for pediatric neurologists to advise parents after their child has had a prolonged seizure that there is no need to try to prevent further events using medication. Even when both authors of this chapter agree about the good outcome in patients without medication, one of us prefers to medicate after the first seizure when it was prolonged. Carbamazepine and valproic acid are the drugs of choice, and the latter is preferred when the EEG shows spike-and-wave discharges instead of spikes. At any rate, clear instructions should be given to parents on how to use rectal diazepam immediately after onset of a new seizure.

LONG-TERM PROGNOSIS

Despite the high incidence of seizures evolving into status epilepticus, PS is a remarkably benign epilepsy syndrome.[8,14,54,56,62] One third of the patients have only a single seizure, and most of the cases present no more than two to five seizures. Remission usually occurs 1 or 2 years after the first seizure, and there are no comparable data on whether there is a significant difference in cases treated with AEDs.

Regarding the risk of persistence of seizures or of developing other types of epilepsy in adult life, except for the personal experience of Dr. Panayiotopoulos, no series has reached a sufficient long-term follow-up to provide information.

A need for caution in reference to neuropsychological findings has recently been raised. A study of 22 children with PS showed that intellectual quotients were within normal limits, but selective dysfunctions were found relating to verbal and visual-spatial memory, visual-motor integration global abilities, reading and writing, and arithmetic ability.[31]

Atypical Evolutions in Patients with Panayiotopoulos Syndrome

As stated before, a number of cases presenting BCECTS after the onset of PS are well documented, and even one case with typical absence epilepsy following PS was recently reported. The concept is that even when these associations occur, long-term prognosis is almost always benign. We say "almost" because nothing is absolute in medicine. We showed three cases with typical features of PS that presented atypical evolutions quite like those described in BCECTS.[23] The three children started with inhibitory seizures and drops, atypical absences, and language and behavioral impairment associated with continuous spike-and-waves discharges in the sleep EEG (Fig. 3). They were well managed with appropriate changes in AEDs, but we do not know what the natural evolution of this complication would have been.[5,28] Moreover, ictal cardiorespiratory

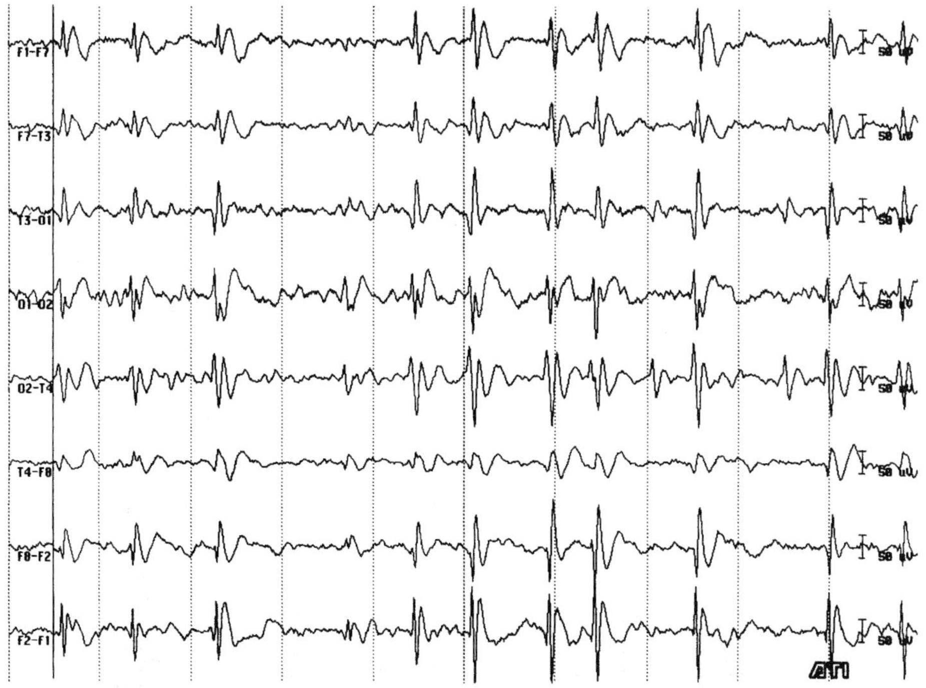

FIGURE 3. A 5.5-year-old boy. Atypical evolution of Panayiotopoulos syndrome with frequent bilateral spike-wave discharges in sleep.

arrest was recently reported in a patient with PS,[63] an exception confirming the rule of very good long-term prognosis.

SUMMARY AND CONCLUSIONS

- Early-onset benign childhood occipital epilepsy (Panayiotopoulos type), or Panayiotopoulos syndrome, is a clearly identifiable epilepsy syndrome that is second in frequency to benign childhood epilepsy with centrotemporal spikes among idiopathic focal epilepsies with onset in childhood.
- Vomiting and other autonomic ictal manifestations are very frequent and should call attention to the possibility of PS. The other frequent seizure features are eye deviation and impairment of consciousness.
- Approximately one third of patients present prolonged seizures evolving into status; one third of children have only one seizure.
- Sleep EEG shows occipital spikes in a majority of patients, although spikes in other areas can also be seen in more than one third of patients.
- There is no clear understanding of the mechanisms of vomiting and other autonomic ictal features and their association with interictal epileptiform discharges in the EEGs of these children.
- Prognosis is excellent despite prolonged seizures or the rare event of atypical evolutions with continuous spike-and-waves during slow sleep and its clinical correlations.
- Future research should clarify the not rare association between PS and BCECTS, perhaps based on a finding of genetic linkage explaining the different phenotypic expressions within a wider group of benign focal epilepsies in infancy and childhood.

References

1. Arroyo HA, De Rosa S, Fejerman N. Epilepsy, cerebral calcifications and coeliac disease: Argentine multicentre experience. In: Gobbi G, Andermann F, Naccarato S, et al., eds. *Epilepsy and Other Neurological Disorders in Coeliac Disease*. London: John Libbey; 1997:93–101.
2. Beaumanoir A. Semiology of occipital seizures in infants and children. In: Andermann F, Beaumanoir A, Mira L, et al., eds. *Occipital Seizures and Epilepsies in Children*. London: John Libbey; 1993:71–86.
3. Berg AT, Panayiotopoulos CP. Diversity in epilepsy and a newly recognized benign childhood syndrome [Editorial]. *Neurology*. 2000;55:1073–1074.
4. Caraballo R. Personal communication; 2005.
5. Caraballo RH, Astorino F, Cersosimo R, et al. Atypical evolution in childhood epilepsy with occipital paroxysms (Panayiotopoulos type). *Epileptic Disord*. 2001;3:157–162.
6. Caraballo RH, Cersosimo R, Fejerman N. Idiopathic partial epilepsies with rolandic and occipital spikes appearing in the same children. *J Epilepsy*. 1998;11:261–264.
7. Caraballo RH, Cersosimo RO, Medina CS, et al. Epilepsias parciales idiopáticas con paroxismos occipitales. *Rev Neurol*. 1997;25:1052–1058.
8. Caraballo R, Cersosimo R, Medina C, et al. Panayiotopoulos-type benign childhood occipital epilepsy: a prospective study. *Neurology*. 2000;55:1096–1100.
9. Caraballo RH, Sakr D, Mozzi M, et al. Symptomatic occipital lobe epilepsy following neonatal hypoglycemia. *Pediatr Neurol*. 2004;31(1):24–29.
10. Caraballo RH, Sologuestua A, Grañana N, et al. Idiopathic occipital and absence epilepsies appearing in the same children. *Pediatr Neurol*. 2004;30(1):24–28.
11. Commission on Classification and Terminology of the International League Against Epilepsy. Proposal for revised classification of epilepsies and epileptic syndromes. *Epilepsia*. 1989;30:389–399.
12. Cooper GW, Lee SI. Reactive occipital epileptiform activity: is it benign? *Epilepsia*. 1991;32:63–68.
13. Covanis A, Lada C, Skiadas K. Children with rolandic spikes and ictus emeticus: rolandic epilepsy or Panayiotopoulos syndrome? *Epileptic Disord*. 2003;5:139–143.
14. Covanis A, Ferrie CD, Koutroumanidis M, et al. Panayiotopoulos syndrome and Gastaut type idiopathic childhood occipital epilepsy. In: Roger J, Bureau M, Dravet CH, et al., eds. *Epileptic Syndromes in Infancy, Childhood and Adolescence,* 4th ed. Montrouge, France: John Libbey; 2005:227–253.
15. Dalla Bernardina B, Sgrò V, Fejerman N. Epilepsy with centro-temporal spikes and related syndromes. In: Roger J, Bureau M, Dravet CH, et al., eds. *Epileptic Syndromes in Infancy, Childhood and Adolescence,* 4th ed. Montrouge, France: John Libbey; 2005:203–225.
16. Demirbilek V, Dervent A. Panayiotopoulos syndrome: video-EEG illustration of a typical seizure. *Epileptic Disord*. 2004;6:121–124.
17. Engel J Jr. A proposed diagnostic scheme for people with epileptic seizures and with epilepsy: report of the ILAE Task Force on Classification and Terminology. *Epilepsia*. 2001;42:796–803.
18. Engel J, Fejerman N. Benign childhood epilepsy with centrotemporal spikes. In: Engel J, Fejerman N, eds. *MedLink Neurology (Section of Epilepsy)*. San Diego, CA: MedLink; 1999/2005. Available: www.medlink.com.
19. Fejerman N. Atypical evolutions of benign partial epilepsies in children. *Int Pediatrics*. 1996;11:351–356.
20. Fejerman N. New idiopathic partial epilepsies. *Epilepsia*. 1997;38 (Suppl 7):26.

21. Fejerman N. Benign focal epilepsies in infancy, childhood and adolescence. *Rev Neurol.* 2002;34:7–18.
22. Fejerman N. Epileptic syndromes and diseases. In: Aminoff M, Daroff RB, eds. *Encyclopedia of the Neurological Sciences.* San Diego, CA: Academic Press; 2003:264–288.
23. Fejerman N, Caraballo RH, Tenembaum S. Atypical evolutions of benign localization-related epilepsies in children. Are they predictable? *Epilepsia.* 2000;41:380–390.
24. Ferraro SM, Daraio MC, Mazzola ME, et al. Coexistence of two forms of benign childhood partial epilepsies. *Epilepsia.* 1997;38 (Suppl 7):38.
25. Ferrie CD, Beaumanoir A, Guerrini R, et al. Early-onset benign occipital seizure susceptibility syndrome. *Epilepsia.* 1997;38:285–293.
26. Ferrie CD, Caraballo RH, Covanis A, et al. Panayiotopoulos syndrome: a consensus view. *Dev Med Child Neurol.* 2006;48(3):236–240.
27. Ferrie CD, Grunewald RA. Panayiotopoulos syndrome: a common and benign childhood epilepsy [Commentary]. *Lancet.* 2001;357:821–823.
28. Ferrie CD, Koutroumanidis M, Rowlinson S, et al. Atypical evolution of Panayiotopoulos syndrome: a case report (published with video-sequences). *Epileptic Disord.* 2002;4:35–42.
29. Gastaut H. A new type of epilepsy: benign partial epilepsy of childhood with occipital spike-waves. *Clin Electroencephalogr.* 1982;13:13–22.
30. Gastaut H, Roger J, Bureau M. Benign epilepsy of childhood with occipital paroxysms. Up-date. In: Roger J, Bureau M, Dravet C, et al., eds. *Epileptic Syndromes in Infancy, Childhood and Adolescence.* London: John Libbey; 1992:201–217.
31. Germano E, Gagliano A, Magazu A, et al. Benign childhood epilepsy with occipital paroxysms: neuropsychological findings. *Epilepsy Res.* 2005;64(3):137–150.
32. Gobbi G, Bertani G, and the Italian Working Group on Coeliac Disease and Epilepsy. Coeliac disease and epilepsy. In: Gobbi G, Andermann F, Naccarato S, et al., eds. *Epilepsy and Other Neurological Disorders in Coeliac Disease.* London: John Libbey; 1997:65–80.
33. Gobbi G, Guerrini R. Childhood epilepsy with occipital spikes and other benign localization-related epilepsies. In: Engel J, Pedley TA, eds. Epilepsy. A Comprehensive Textbook. Philadelphia: Lippincott-Raven; 1998:2315–2326.
34. Gokcay A, Celebisoy N, Gokcay F, et al. Visual evoked potentials in children with occipital epilepsies. *Brain Dev.* 2003;25(4):268–271.
35. Guerrini R, Dravet C, Genton P, et al. Idiopathic photosensitive occipital lobe epilepsy. *Epilepsia.* 1995;36:883–891.
36. Kanazawa O, Tohyama J, Akasaka N, et al. A magnetoencephalographic study of patients with Panayiotopoulos syndrome. *Epilepsia.* 2005;46(7):1106–1113.
37. Kivity S, Ephraim T, Weitz R, et al. Childhood epilepsy with occipital paroxysms: clinical variants in 134 patients. *Epilepsia.* 2000;41:1522–1523.
38. Kivity S, Lerman P. Stormy onset with prolonged loss of consciousness in benign childhood epilepsy with occipital paroxysms. *J Neurol Neurosurg Psychiatr.* 1992;55:45–48.
39. Kramer U, Nevo Y, Neufeld Y, et al. Epidemiology of epilepsy in childhood: a cohort of 440 consecutive patients. *Pediatric Neurol.* 1998;18(1):46–50.
40. Kuzniecky R, Rosenblatt B. Benign occipital epilepsy: a family study. *Epilepsia.* 1987;28:346–350.
41. Labate A, Gambardella A, Messina D, et al. Silent celiac disease in patients with childhood localization related epilepsies. *Epilepsia.* 2001;42(9):1153–1155.
42. Lada C, Skiadas K, Theodorou V, et al. A study of 43 patients with Panayiotopoulos syndrome: a common and benign childhood seizure susceptibility. *Epilepsia.* 2003;44:81–88.
43. Neubauer BA, Fiedler B, Himmelein B, et al. Centro-temporal spikes in families with Rolandic epilepsy: linkage to chromosome 15q14. *Neurology.* 1998;51:1608–1612.
44. Newton R, Aicardi J. Clinical findings in children with occipital spike-wave complexes suppressed by eye-opening. *Neurology.* 1983;33:1526–1529.
45. Oguni H, Hayashi K, Imai K, et al. Study on the early-onset variant of benign childhood epilepsy with occipital paroxysms otherwise described as early-onset benign occipital seizure susceptibility syndrome. *Epilepsia.* 1999;40:1020–1030.
46. Ohtsu M, Oguni H, Hayashi K, et al. EEG in Children with early-onset benign occipital seizure susceptibility syndrome: Panayiotopoulos syndrome. *Epilepsia.* 2003;44:435–442.
47. Panayiotopoulos CP. Inhibitory effect of central vision on occipital lobe seizures. *Neurology.* 1981;31:1330–1333.
48. Panayiotopoulos CP. Vomiting as an ictal manifestation of epileptic seizures and syndromes. *J Neurol Neurosurg Psychiatr.* 1988;51:1448–1451.
49. Panayiotopoulos CP. Benign childhood epilepsy with occipital paroxysms: a 15-year prospective study. *Ann Neurol.* 1989;26:51–56.
50. Panayiotopoulos CP. Benign nocturnal childhood occipital epilepsy: a new syndrome with nocturnal seizures, tonic deviation of the eyes, and vomiting. *J Child Neurol.* 1989;4:43–49.
51. Panayiotopoulos CP. Benign childhood epilepsy with occipital paroxysms. In: Andermann F, Beaumanoir A, Mira L, et al. *Occipital Seizures and Epilepsies in Children.* London: John Libbey; 1993:151–164.
52. Panayiotopoulos CP. *Benign Childhood Partial Seizures and Related Epileptic Syndromes.* London: John Libbey; 1999.
53. Panayiotopoulos CP. Elementary visual hallucinations, blindness, and headache in idiopathic occipital epilepsy: differentiation from migraine. *J Neurol Neurosurg Psychiatry.* 1999;66:536–540
54. Panayiotopoulos CP. Panayiotopoulos syndrome: a common and benign childhood epileptic syndrome. London: John Libbey; 2002.
55. Panayiotopoulos CP. Early onset benign childhood occipital epilepsy (Panayiotopoulos syndrome). In: Engel J, Fejerman N, eds. *MedLink Neurology (Section of Epilepsy).* San Diego, CA: MedLink; 1999/2005. Available: www.medlink.com.
56. Panayiotopoulos CP. Benign childhood focal seizures and related epileptic syndromes. In: Panayiotopoulos CP, ed. *The Epilepsies: Seizures, Syndromes and Management.* Oxford: Bladon; 2005:223–269.
57. Panayiotopoulos CP, Igoe DM. Cerebral insult–like partial status epilepticus in the early-onset variant of benign childhood epilepsy with occipital paroxysms. *Seizure.* 1992;1:99–102.
58. Pruna D, Persico I, Serra D, et al. Lack of association with the 15q14 candidate region for benign epilepsy of childhood with centro-temporal spikes in a Sardinian population. *Epilepsia.* 2000(Suppl Florence):164.
59. Sanders S, Rowlinson S, Manidakis I, et al. The contribution of the EEG technologists in the diagnosis of Panayiotopoulos syndrome (susceptibility to early onset benign childhood autonomic seizures). *Seizure.* 2004;13:565–573.
60. Shinnar S, O'Dell C, Berg AT. Distribution of epilepsy syndromes in a cohort of children prospectively monitored from the time of their first unprovoked seizure. *Epilepsia.* 1999;40(10):1378–1383.
61. Sillanpaa M, Jalava M, Shinnar S. Epilepsy syndromes in patients with childhood-onset seizures in Finland. *Pediatr Neurol.* 1999;21(2):533–537.
62. Verrotti A, Domizio S, Guerra M, et al. Childhood epilepsy with occipital paroxysms and benign nocturnal childhood occipital epilepsy. *J Child Neurol.* 2000;15:218–221.
63. Verrotti A, Salladini C, Trotta D, et al. Ictal cardiorespiratory arrest in Panayiotopoulos syndrome: a case report. *Neurology.* 2005;64:1816–1817.
64. Vigevano F, Lispi ML, Ricci S. Early onset benign occipital susceptibility syndrome: video-EEG documentation of an illustrative case. *Clin Neurophysiol.* 2000;111(Suppl 2):S81–S86.
65. Vigevano F, Ricci S. Benign occipital epilepsy of childhood with prolonged seizures and autonomic symptoms. In: Andermann F, Beaumanoir A, Mira L, et al., eds. *Occipital Seizures and Epilepsies in Children.* London: John Libbey; 1993:133–140.
66. Yoshinaga H, Koutroumanidis M, Shirasawa A, et al. Dipole analysis in Panayiotopoulos syndrome. *Brain Dev.* 2005;27:46–52.

CHAPTER 238 ■ LATE-ONSET CHILDHOOD OCCIPITAL EPILEPSY (GASTAUT TYPE)

GIUSEPPE GOBBI, RENZO GUERRINI, AND SALVATORE GROSSO

INTRODUCTION

Occipital epilepsies commonly start in childhood or adolescence and include two etiologic groups: Symptomatic and idiopathic epilepsies. Symptomatic occipital epilepsies may be caused by brain malformations (focal cortical dysplasia, polymicrogyria, subcortical band heterotopia, periventricular heterotopia), metabolic disorders (Lafora disease, juvenile neuronal ceroid lipofuscinosis, mitochondrial disorders such as MERRF [syndrome of myoclonus epilepsy and ragged red fibers] and MELAS [syndrome of mitochondrial encephalopathy, lactic acidosis, and strokelike episodes]), and occipital bilateral calcifications (often associated with celiac disease).[95] Among the idiopathic group, the new classification system of the International League Against Epilepsy (ILAE) Task Force[30] recognizes three epilepsy syndromes: (a) the early-onset benign childhood occipital epilepsy (Panayiotopoulos type), (b) the late-onset childhood occipital epilepsy (Gastaut type), and (c) the idiopathic photosensitive occipital lobe epilepsy. The latter is included among the reflex epilepsies.

The late-onset childhood occipital epilepsy–Gastaut type (LOCOE-Gastaut type) is the topic of this chapter, while the early-onset benign childhood occipital epilepsy (Panayiotopoulos type) and the idiopathic photosensitive occipital lobe epilepsy are described in Chapters 237 and 257.

HISTORICAL PERSPECTIVES

Benign occipital epilepsy was first described by Gastaut.[35] It was considered an epilepsy syndrome with a typical clinical history and interictal electroencephalographic (EEG) pattern. The existence of an idiopathic/cryptogenic benign childhood occipital epilepsy was already evident in the first reports of Gastaut in 1950[34] and Gibbs and Gibbs in 1952.[42] Further observations corroborated the identification of "benign occipital epilepsy,"[10,25,68,93] but discussions about a new "benign migraine-epilepsy syndrome" developed among authors.[1,16,71,78,90,94] The controversy regarding whether the origin of this syndrome was epileptic or migrainous was resolved by Gastaut,[35,36] who critically reviewed the four children reported by Camfield et al.[16] and concluded that their benign occipital epilepsy constituted "a primary and independent epileptic disorder." Gastaut[36] and Gastaut and Zifkin[39] considered both visual ictal symptoms and the interictal occipital spikes and waves that appeared upon closing the eyes as the main clinical and EEG signs of the benign childhood epilepsy with occipital paroxysms (CEOP). However, it was already known that occipital foci in young children might also be a sign of a "maturational" factor in a variety of cerebral dysfunctions.[63] In fact, occipital lobe epileptogenesis with occipital spikes may occur in genetically predisposed children with visual defects at a critical stage of development.[67,73] Reactive occipital spikes have been reported in children without epileptic seizures[2,11,60,76] as well as in patients having cryptogenic or symptomatic occipital epilepsies[2,23,27,36,41,51,76,98] and those having occipital epilepsies associated with progressive disorders.[29,49,50,74,89,91] Finally, visual symptoms and reactive occipital paroxysms may be absent in CEOP.[41,54] These data cast some doubt on the existence of a true benign and idiopathic occipital epilepsy as defined, using the clinical and EEG criteria proposed by Gastaut.[35] Among patients with occipital epilepsy and occipital EEG abnormalities suppressed by eye opening, a series emerged with "nonlesional" epilepsy, remarkable age-dependent seizure onset, familial predisposition, and benign evolution.[6,23,98] According to these criteria, CEOP was included in the ILAE classification[21] as an idiopathic form having the clinical and EEG findings suggested by Gastaut,[35,36] but with an uncertain long-term prognosis. More recently, Panayiotopoulos[80,81] described a form of CEOP characterized by early onset, nocturnal seizures with tonic deviation of the eyes, and vomiting,[80,81] which has an excellent prognosis with seizure remission occurring within 1 to 2 years. On that basis, Caraballo et al.[17] proposed designating this early-onset CEOP as "Panayiotopoulos-type benign childhood occipital epilepsy," and "Gastaut type of benign childhood occipital epilepsy" the occipital epilepsy described by Gastaut.

Finally, the latest diagnostic scheme for people with epilepsy proposed by the ILAE Task Force on Classification and Terminology[30] recognized this syndrome as "late-onset childhood occipital epilepsy–Gastaut type."

DEFINITION

LOCOE-Gastaut type is an age-related, possibly genetically determined, epilepsy syndrome, with onset ranging from 4 to 13.2 years, and with a peak of incidence at 8 years. Girls and boys are equally affected.[85]

Epileptic seizures are characterized by brief, frequent, diurnal visual hallucinations; blindness; or both. Although commonly preserved, the consciousness is mainly impaired when seizure progresses toward a hemiclonic or generalized convulsion or automatism. In 25% to 50% of cases, visual seizures are followed by pulsating headache, associated with nausea and vomiting in about 10% of patients.

Interictal EEG features consist of high-voltage spikes-and-wave complexes or sharp waves recurring rhythmically in the occipital and posterior temporal areas of one or both hemispheres, but only when the patient's eyes are closed. Fixation-off sensitivity is typical. Ictal EEG is characterized by the sudden appearance of an occipital discharge consisting of fast activity and/or spikes, which may spread to the central or temporal regions.[85]

Since both clinical and EEG findings do not exclude a symptomatic epilepsy, neurophysiologic, neuropsychological, neuroimaging, and laboratory assessment are always indicated. At present, no definite statement on prognosis is possible,[21] even though it seems to be relatively benign, especially using rigid criteria of selection.[99]

EPIDEMIOLOGY

LOCOE-Gastaut type is a rare condition with a probable prevalence of 0.2% to 0.9% of all epilepsies, and 2% to 7% of benign childhood partial seizures. On average, LOCOE-Gastaut type is considered five times less frequent than Panayiotopoulos type.[85] Higher figures have been reported by Gokcay et al.,[52] who observed ten patients with LOCOE-Gastaut type among 29 cases presenting with idiopathic occipital epilepsies. A slightly higher frequency of LOCOE-Gastaut type than the Panayiotopoulos type has also been found by Tsai et al.,[99] which was attributed to the inclusion of patients with migrainous headache with focal occipital paroxysms and the exclusion of patients with adversive seizure and EEG foci beyond the occipital area.

ETIOLOGY AND PATHOPHYSIOLOGY

Gastaut[36,37] stressed the presence of genetic or functional factors, such as a predisposition to epilepsy and febrile convulsions, in 36.6% to 47% of the cases. However, patients with lesional epilepsy related to premature birth, mild perinatal distress, and HHE (hemiconvulsion-hemiplegia-epilepsy) syndrome were also included in LOCOE-Gastaut type.[36,37,41] A thalamocortical mechanism, similar to the reticulocortical mechanism of idiopathic generalized epilepsies[46] but limited to a localized thalamocortical area, was hypothesized.[34] According to the concept of "idiopathic" epilepsy, symptomatic cases are no longer included in this group of patients.

A role of genetic factors as part of the etiology is still presumed, and the recognition of familial cases strongly suggests this hypothesis. A family history of epilepsy varying from 33% to 43% in patients with occipital epilepsy has been reported by several authors.[6,60,98] Kuzniecky and Rosenblatt[65] suggested "an autosomal dominant pattern for the EEG abnormalities with age-dependent expression and variable penetrance of the seizure disorder." Nagendran et al.[75] reported a family in which two siblings had visual seizures and occipital paroxysms, and another presented with centrotemporal spikes on the EEG. Moreover, there may be an association between idiopathic generalized epilepsies and LOCOE-Gastaut type. In fact, generalized spike-wave discharges in addition to occipital epileptiform activity were noted in this group of patients.[36] In turn, in idiopathic generalized epilepsies there may be focal activity, which is typically frontal but may also occur in posterior areas.[77] Caraballo et al.[18] reported the occurrence of childhood absence epilepsy in 5 out of 35 children with LOCOE-Gastaut type. Patients with both types of epilepsy have also been reported by Sofue et al.[92] and by Grosso et al.,[53] respectively. Typical absences have mainly been found in patients with LOCOE-Gastaut type (14% of patients) rather than in the much larger group with the Panayiotopoulos type (0.6%). Therefore, it has been suggested that childhood absence epilepsy may have a closer genetic relationship to LOCOE-Gastaut type than to the Panayiotopoulos type.[18]

From a pathogenetic point of view, mechanisms underlying LOCOE-Gastaut type remain to be established. The primary visual cortex (VI or Brodmann area 17) represents the site where elementary visual hallucinations are generated. Simple visual symptoms can also be evoked by stimulation of extra-striate and prestriate (Brodmann areas 18 and 19) cortical regions. The stimulation of the latter areas can also provoke visual illusions. Recently, it has been confirmed that both the mesial and lateral occipital lobe may be involved in generating elementary visual phenomena, and that there is a wide semiologic overlapping of visual symptoms between seizures originating from these occipital areas.[15] In fact, mesial foci rapidly spread to the lateral occipital region and vice versa.[20] Occipital epileptogenic activity spreads extensively to the adjacent neocortex and to limbic structures through the projections from the occipital cortex to lateral and mesial temporal areas.[15]

In particular, reciprocal connections between temporal neocortex and the primary visual cortex have recently been confirmed.[3,62] Complex visual seizures have been considered to represent seizure spread to the temporal lobe. Blume et al.[15] suggested that structured visual phenomena require the involvement of both neocortical and limbic regions. This is consistent with the clinical occurrence of initial occipital symptoms followed by structured visual hallucinations and other temporal lobe findings.[5,102] Actually, the role of the temporal lobe in determining visual symptoms appears to be more complex. Indeed, it should be remembered that simple visual phenomena have also occasionally been reported in temporal (lateral or medial) epilepsy. Motor phenomena of both lateral and mesial occipital epileptogenesis may be explained by their access to supra-Sylvian or to brainstem motor regions.[15]

The pathophysiologic mechanisms leading to postictal headache remain also to be clarified. Migraine is considered a paroxysmal and unique neurovascular disorder.[101] According to Goadsby,[47] migraine is a disorder of sensory dysmodulation that involves the trigeminovascular system and central nervous system modulation of the pain-producing structures of the cranial structures. A multitude of factors able to increase neuronal and network hyperexcitability may trigger migraine attack. Thus, it is possible that an occipital ictal discharge triggers a genuine migraine headache through trigeminovascular or brainstem mechanisms.[84] It has been pointed out that postictal migraine headache occurs in predisposed children with impaired or labile cerebrovascular autoregulation. On that basis, occipital ictal activity may result in a persistence of vasodilation in the posterior territory of cerebral and basilar arteries with subsequent plasma extravasation and neuropeptide release.[101]

CLINICAL PRESENTATION

The mean age at onset ranges from 3 to 4 to 13 to 16 years.[85,99] Gastaut and Zifkin[41] reported an upper age at onset of 19 years.

The main clinical findings of LOCOE are represented by *visual seizures*. Usually, they occur in the daytime, but are not invariably present. In some instances, triggering or facilitation stimuli have been reported: Extinction of light,[69,79] passage from light to darkness or vice versa,[8,37] and darkness.[86] In some teenage girls, seizures seem to occur with menstruation.[37,41] *Elementary visual hallucinations* are brief (5 to 20 seconds, rarely more than 3 minutes or even 15 to 20 minutes) seizures, which usually occur as an initial ictal symptom, and may represent the only seizure type (30% of the patients)[64,84] or be associated with other occipital symptoms such as illusions of ocular movements, tonic deviation of the eyes, and eyelid fluttering. This type of seizure may also be prolonged, especially when visual symptoms are followed by autonomic-migrainous postictal symptoms, and may progress to hemiconvulsions or generalized tonic–clonic seizures. *Positive elementary visual hallucinations* may consist of perception of white flashes or colored (bright red, yellow, blue, and green are prominent) unformed or formed phenomena, usually circular, commonly appearing in the periphery of a hemifield, evolving into multicolored circular patterns that multiply and enlarge during seizure progression, flashing or static, with a possible horizontal movement toward the other side.[84] Sometimes the patient may turn his or her head and eyes to look at them.[64] In each patient elementary visual hallucinations have a stereotypic appearance regarding morphology, colors, location, and movement. *Negative elementary visual seizures*[6,36,37] are the second most common seizure type. They consist of a sudden ictal blurred vision or amaurosis, lasting up to 5 minutes. Ictal amaurosis may be the sole event in a patient who, during other seizures, has visual hallucinations without blindness. Blindness may involve the whole visual field or be confined to a part of it (quadrantanopia, hemianopia). Hemianopia may be both ictal and postictal. The elementary visual seizures in nontreated patients may be frequent, up to several per day or week. Responsiveness is commonly preserved. Loss of consciousness usually occurs at the onset of other ictal manifestations following visual hallucinations or amaurosis, such as eye deviation or convulsions.[85]

Complex visual hallucinations and visual illusions are rare in LOCOE-Gastaut type patients, occurring in <10% of the patients. *Complex visual hallucinations* represent the progress of elementary visual seizures, and consist of hallucinations of animals, people, or scenes, or of numerals or letters, stationary or moving. In complex hallucinations an evident emotional component, such as elements from memory, unfulfilled wishes, or intense affects related to them, which is lacking in simple hallucinations, is experienced by the patient. *Ictal visual illusions* may be simple with alteration in perception of objects, such as micropsia/macropsia (dysmegalopsia), dyschromatopsia, achromatopsia, metamorphopsia, plagiopsia, kinetopsia, and teichopsia, or may be complex, such as palinopsia, teleopsia, macroproxiopia, and microtlepsia.[6,36–39,41,78,81] *Sensory hallucinations of ocular movements and pain* without detectable motion usually occur with progression of ictal elementary visual hallucinations

Nonvisual ictal seizures with occipital lobe origin may also be present in the context of the clinical picture. *Adversive seizures with contralateral eye deviation*, often associated with head turning, is the most common nonvisual symptom. Kivity et al.[64] reported that 79% of patients with visual symptoms experienced adversive manifestations, either independently, as a separate entity that preceded or followed the visual symptoms by weeks or months or even years, or as a part of the same event. In the latter, usually they start after visual hallucinations or occur while hallucinations persist. More often these events are severe with impairment of consciousness and may evolve into secondary generalizations or hemiconvulsions with or without secondary generalization. *Forced eyelid closure and eyelid blinking* occur in approximately 10% of LOCOE patients.[84,85] They may precede by months the onset of elementary visual hallucinations (personal observations). Other nonvisual seizures may occur as a result of seizure propagation. Visual symptoms may be followed by *hemiclonic* (44%), *complex partial* (19%), or *generalized tonic–clonic seizures* (8%).[34–41] *Partial status epilepticus* is rare.[64] Contrary to what occurs in symptomatic occipital epilepsies, progression to hemiclonic seizures is more frequent than to complex partial seizures,[24,98] and symptoms related to the temporal lobe are more evocative of a symptomatic cause.[85] *Ictal vomiting* is rare in LOCOE-Gastaut type.[32]

Rarely, *migraine-type headache* with photophobia, nausea, and vomiting with or without impairment of consciousness preceded the seizures,[2] sometimes by several hours.[41,69] Some patients may have headache during their seizures at the same time as visual symptoms.[66] It is unclear whether these were migraine-triggered seizures or migrainelike ictal symptoms. Undoubtedly, headache as an ictal event is rare.[85] By contrast, *postictal headache* is common and observed in 30% to 50% of LOCOE-Gastaut type patients. Headache is bilateral, throbbing, and often associated with nausea and vomiting, photophobia and phonophobia, and sometimes obfuscation of consciousness.[36,37,78,98] Postictal headache may be indistinguishable from migraine, especially when it follows a simple visual seizure, which may be considered as the presenting visual event of migraine with aura attack.[41] Duration ranges from 30 minutes to several hours, and appears to be proportional to the duration and severity of the preceding seizures. Postictal headache may also be present in the cases of symptomatic occipital seizures.[85]

Finally, an association between LOCOE-Gastaut type and *typical absences* has been reported. In these patients typical absences appeared at the same time as visual seizures or after 1 year. All patients had typical occipital paroxysms and a 3-Hz generalized spike-wave on the EEG.[18,53,92] *Febrile convulsions* have been reported in 14% of the patients as well.[85]

DIAGNOSTIC EVALUATION

Interictal EEG

EEG shows normal background activity[6] and typical occipital dysphasic spike-and-wave complexes, spikes, or sharp-wave paroxysms of high voltage (200 to 300 μV) with a strong negative peak followed by a small-amplitude positive peak and a negative slow wave.[35–39] The occipital spike component has been found to be usually higher in amplitude than the negative slow waves, often exceeding 100 μV, with a duration <70 msec.[96] Occipital paroxysms are rhythmic at a frequency of 1 to 4 Hz in bursts or sequences.[36,37,81] In 5% of cases, occipital paroxysms consist of rhythmic posterior slow waves.[41] Distribution of paroxysmal abnormalities is over the occipital and posterior temporal regions of one hemisphere or over both hemispheres, synchronously or independently. When bilateral, the spikes are frequently asymmetric.[81] Topographic mapping may show the focus mainly at the occipital area mostly spreading to the parietal or temporal area. No superficial dipole field was noted by the voltage mapping of scalp EEG.[99] Other independent epileptiform discharges may be found, in addition to occipital spikes.[99] Photic stimulation does not usually affect occipital paroxysms[36,37,82] but may occasionally have an inhibitory effect.[66,82] Activation during hyperventilation has occasionally been reported.[60,66,98] Discharges are usually, but not invariably, increased during non–rapid eye movement (REM) sleep.[6,41] In some patients, discharges appear only during sleep.[66] Usually, occipital spikes disappear upon eye opening and reappear 1 to 20 seconds after eye closure.[35–37] Panayiotopoulos[79] and Lugaresi et al.[69] found that occipital spikes are also activated by darkness, and that in darkness they were suppressed by fixation on a very small light source (fixation-off sensitive spikes). This would indicate that the abolition of central vision (macular vision) is responsible for the appearance of occipital paroxysms.[79] The absence of the typical EEG paroxysms does not exclude the diagnosis[41,55,81,96] if the other clinical and EEG criteria are present. Moreover, occipital spikes may often occur only between the ages of 3 and 5 years.[61] Occipital paroxysms may remain in the same location during follow-up or may shift from side to side, and they sometimes may be replaced by, or associated with, bilateral rolandic spikes.[43,45,54,55,82,98] Spikes and seizures usually disappear simultaneously,[6] but epileptiform EEG abnormalities may outlast seizures.[37,54,80,96]

Although the normal background and the suppression of occipital paroxysmal discharges operated by eye opening were considered to be distinctive and characteristic of LOCOE-Gastaut type,[40,60,95] further studies showed that these features were not very specific, since they may also be observed in symptomatic epilepsies[49,50,56] and in epilepsies with undefined complex partial seizures.[70]

Ictal EEG

Electroencephalographic seizure patterns do not differ from those of other occipital epilepsies.[6] In general, in the case of brief seizures there are ictal discharges localized in one or both occipital areas and characterized by rapid spikes that slow progressively.[6,36,37] Panayiotopoulos[81,84,85] observed that in complex visual seizures the discharges are slower than in simple ones, and that ictal EEG anomalies during amaurosis are represented by pseudoperiodic slow waves and spikes, which are different from those observed during visual hallucinations. Brief seizures recorded during sleep show disappearance of interictal occipital discharges, followed by repetitive spikes of about 10 Hz that sometimes spread to the parietal region.

Other Neurophysiologic Investigations

Visual-evoked potentials (VEPs) and somatosensory-evoked potentials (SEPs) had a higher amplitude in the involved hemisphere.[41,87] Gokcay et al.[52] also reported that P100 potential amplitude values of LOCOE-Gastaut type patients were significantly higher than those recorded in healthy subjects and mostly attributed to hyperexcitability of the occipital cortical structures.

Neuroimaging and Other Laboratory Examinations

Neuroimaging is normal by definition. However, since both clinical and EEG findings do not exclude a symptomatic epilepsy[2] with unfavorable outcome, especially at the onset of the disorder,[48,51] further diagnostic investigation is needed, including neuroimaging, especially with high resolution, visual field assessment, and full laboratory evaluation (see Differential Diagnosis section).

Neuropsychological Assessment

Neuropsychological assessment could be important in children for diagnostic purposes, as well as early detection of possible cognitive disturbances accompanying nonidiopathic forms. However, to our knowledge, apart three reported cases with evolution to continuous spike-wave during sleep (CSWS) and cognitive deterioration,[31,97] any data available are on the neuropsychological profile in patients with LOCOE-Gastaut type. The few studies addressing that topic included patients presenting with both early- and late-onset childhood occipital epilepsy.[19] Since the occipital lobes are mainly involved in both low-level and high-level visual processing, including object identification and localization and face recognition, it is possible that any interictal dysfunction of occipital circuitries may have visuoperceptual difficulties as a clinical counterpart. In fact, lower performance in visuoperceptual tasks, attention, memory, and verbal functions were reported in idiopathic childhood occipital epilepsy,[58] even though studies that compared the neuropsychological outcome of patients with idiopathic childhood epilepsy with occipital paroxysms with normal controls revealed no significant differences in basic neuropsychological functions. However, a cognitive profile with relatively better verbal than performance abilities, a high incidence of scholastic disabilities, and the presence of psychiatric disturbances in the form of anxiety and depressive disorders was found in a cohort of patients with idiopathic occipital epilepsy.[19]

DIFFERENTIAL DIAGNOSIS

LOCOE-Gastaut type has to be differentiated from the Panayiotopoulos-type childhood-onset epilepsy, photosensitive idiopathic occipital epilepsy, symptomatic occipital epilepsies (including malformations of cortical development), temporal epilepsies, idiopathic generalized epilepsy, and migraine.

Concerning the Panayiotopoulos-type childhood-onset epilepsy, cardinal differences are age at onset of seizures, higher frequency, shorter duration, and daily occurrence of seizures. Ictal vomiting is commonly lacking, even though it may sometimes occur after visual symptoms.[33,99]

In the case of photosensitive idiopathic occipital epilepsy, age at onset is around the fourth year of life with visual symptoms consisting of either blurred vision or ictal amaurosis followed by secondary tonic–clonic generalization. Seizures are typically triggered by televisions or less often by video games. Interictal EEG shows occipital paroxysms activated by intermittent photic stimulation. Ictal EEG is characterized by spike-and-wave occipital paroxysms spreading to the temporal areas.[57,82–85]

Symptomatic occipital epilepsies often imitate LOCOE-Gastaut type. In fact, although Gastaut and Zifkin[41] stated that the ictal symptoms are different in idiopathic and in symptomatic occipital lobe epilepsy, seizure semiology analysis cannot invariably help to distinguish between different forms of occipital lobe epilepsy.[84,85,100] Therefore, clinical examination; neurophysiologic investigations; neuroimaging studies, including high-resolution magnetic resonance imaging (MRI) for the detection of subtle lesions; and neuropsychological assessment are needed for a correct etiologic diagnosis. Interictal EEG in symptomatic forms may show focal or diffuse abnormal background activity,[98] occipital polymorphous delta activity,[41] and prolonged bursts of sharp waves in temporo-occipital regions,[23] frequently associated with secondary generalization, occipital bursts of fast activity,[48] or multifocal spikes that are semiologically different from those of benign childhood epilepsy with centrotemporal spikes. The interictal abnormalities are enhanced during sleep and often show morphologic modification into rapid rhythms or polyspikes and waves.[51] Sleep interictal EEG is especially useful in the differential diagnosis of some symptomatic cases in whom the clinical and waking EEG features resemble those of a LOCOE-Gastaut type at the beginning of disease[44,51,76] but in whom progressive severity becomes apparent after a benign onset (Fig. 1). In this "malignant variant," occipital polyspikes or rapid rhythms during sleep are the only early warning sign.[48,51] Brain mapping of the occipital spikes in LOCOE-Gastaut type shows the spike maximum in the occipital area, while in symptomatic occipital lobe epilepsy it is located away from the occipital pole, often in the temporo-occipital or the parieto-occipital areas.[72] Clinical and EEG findings in the different forms of occipital epilepsy are summarized in Table 1.

Finally, among the symptomatic occipital epilepsy causes should be considered celiac disease[49,50] Lafora disease[89]; neuroaxonal dystrophy with myoclonus epilepsy; mitochondrial diseases, such as MELAS and MERRF[4,29,91]; and metabolic disorders such as hyperglycemia,[59] in which occipital lobe seizures and EEG abnormalities may be present in the early stages, before other clinical features are present; and hypercalcemia, nonketotic hyperglycinemia, hypoglycemia (in neonatal age), and glycogenosis.

Childhood epilepsies with posterior temporal seizure onset[28,41,66] and complex partial seizures accompanied by

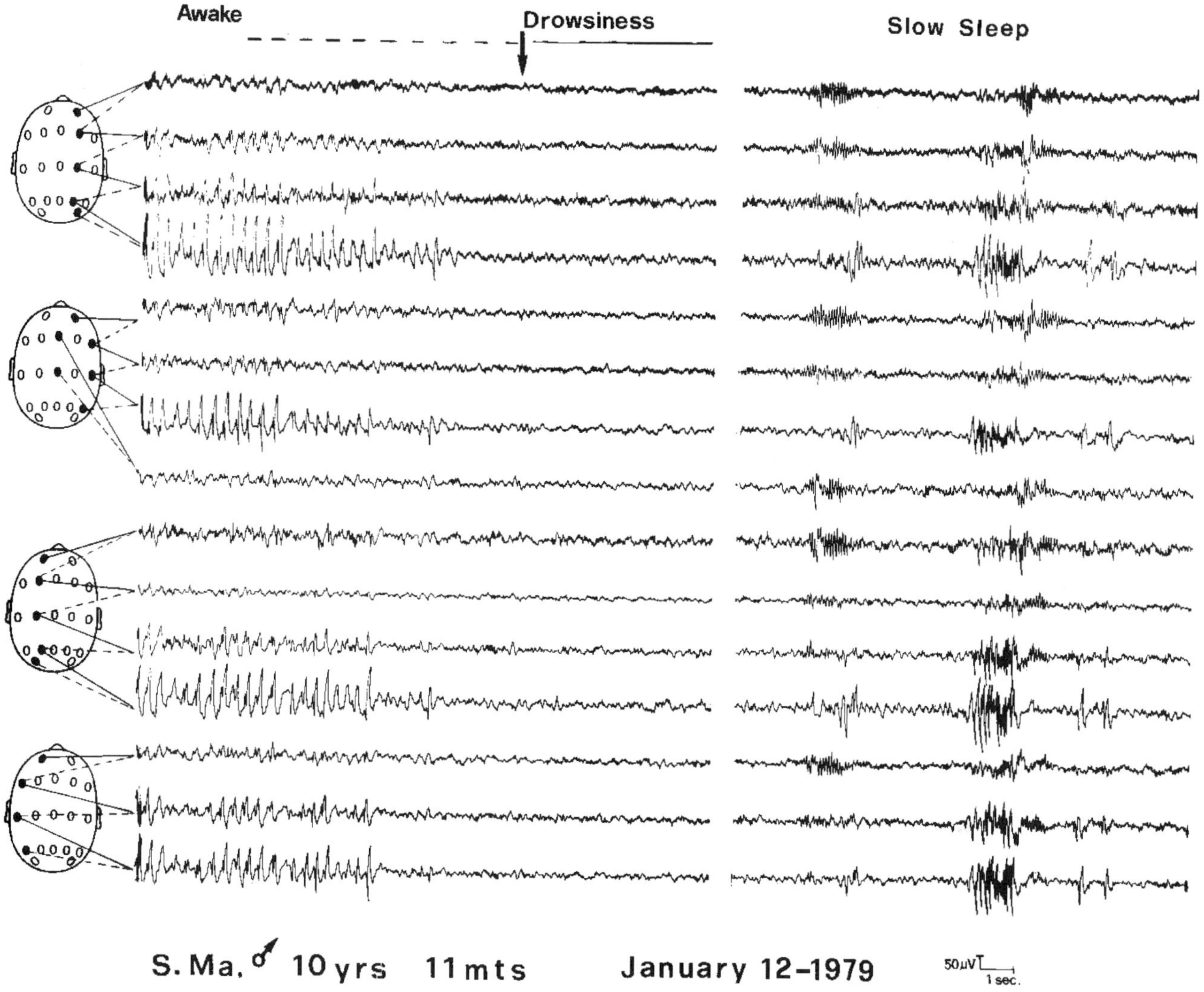

FIGURE 1. Patient with cryptogenic occipital epilepsy and severe evolution, 5 months after the epilepsy onset. **Left** (awake to drowsiness): Rhythmic bilateral occipital spikes and waves disappear in drowsiness. **Right:** Bilateral occipital polyspikes and rapid rhythms appear during slow sleep instead of occipital spikes and waves.

illusions or hallucinations, followed by motor ictal phenomena, also have to be assessed. The so-called "concentric changes of visual field" seizures, which consist of continuous progressive restriction of the visual field, referred to as "tunnel vision" by patients and often associated with emotional distress, are strictly related to either the hippocampus or the temporolateral neocortex.[12] In these cases ictal and interictal EEG abnormalities are usually localized over the temporal, central, and posterior frontal region.

There may be diagnostic confusion between idiopathic occipital epilepsy and idiopathic generalized epilepsy. In fact, in idiopathic occipital epilepsies of childhood there may be generalized spike-wave discharges, and, conversely, EEG of idiopathic generalized epilepsies may show focal activity, which typically occurs in the frontal regions but may also occur in posterior areas. Moreover, patients with absences or even myoclonus may report brief "blacking out" of vision, mimicking a simple visual seizure. Distinction is possible through careful electroclinical analysis.[96]

Differential diagnosis between migraine with aura, basilar migraine, and LOCOE-Gastaut type should not be difficult if all of their components are present and properly evaluated.[85] In general, the age at onset of basilar migraine is during adolescence.[7,9,13] The persistent occipital abnormalities of LOCOE-Gastaut type have rarely been reported in cases of basilar migraine.[16,78,90,94] However, elementary visual seizures followed by headache and vomiting may be especially confusing. In fact, classic distinctive criteria, suggesting that in migraine the prodrome is usually longer than 5 minutes, as opposed to the very brief epileptic aura,[26] have proved to be unreliable.[14,56,57] On the other hand, visual auras, when of epileptic origin, are multicolored with circular or spherical patterns, as opposed to the predominantly black-and-white linear pattern of migraine attacks,[83] and are followed by eye deviation and lateralized or generalized convulsions, and there are no brainstem or cerebellar symptoms.[98] Eventually, postictal EEG commonly return quickly to the pre-ictal state, in contrast to the prolonged postcritical EEG abnormalities of migrainous attacks.[6]

TREATMENT AND OUTCOME

Unlike other benign childhood partial epilepsies that may not need treatment, LOCOE-Gastaut type should be treated because seizures, although brief and mild, are frequent with

TABLE 1

CLINICAL AND EEG FINDINGS DIFFERENTIATING THE IDIOPATHIC AND SYMPTOMATIC OCCIPITAL EPILEPSIES

Occipital epilepsies	Age at onset of occipital seizures, y	Main seizure patterns	Photoparoxysmal response	Photically induced occipital seizures	Interictal EEG findings	Outcome	References
EOBCOE-Panayiotopoulos type	2–14, peaks 4–5	Sleep-related—tonic eye deviation, unresponsiveness, vomiting	Never reported	Never reported	Normal background, occipital S or SW reactive to eye	Remission within 1–2y, before 12 y	90,91
LOCOE-Gastaut type	3–16, mean 8	Diurnal visual seizures, followed by postictal headache and often by CPS or hemiclonic seizures	Never reported	Never reported	Normal background, occipital S or SW reactive to eye	Seizures persisting into late adolescence	40,41
Idiopathic photosensitive occipital lobe epilepsy	5–17, peak at about 15	Visual symptoms, epigastric discomfort, headache, version, vomiting	Constant posterior, generalized, or both	Constant	Normal background, occipital S or SW reactive to eye opening	Good in most patients; seizures may persist with wide photosensitivity range	50,79
Symptomatic/cryptogenic epilepsy (unspecific etiology)	Variable	Varies with suprasylvian/ intrasylvian spread	Not infrequent: posterior	Sporadic	Usually abnormal background, S or SW reactive or not to eye opening evolving in to rapid rhythm or pSW during sleep	Variable, with progressive occipital lobe severity (malignant variant)	56,60
Special conditions that may be associated with recurrent occipital seizures:							
Occipital lobe epilepsy (with and without occipital calcifications) and occipital lobe epilepsy with occipital calcifications (without celiac disease)	2–14	Visual and versive first; tonic, atypical/atonic absences if worsening	Not infrequent: posterior	Not infrequent	Normal or abnormal background, occipital S or SW reactive or not to eye opening, in celiac disease	Variable: favorable, or steady orprogressive severity	5,54,55
Lafora disease	6–19, peak at about 11	Visual, clonic, GTC, myoclonus	Almost constant: occipital, generalized, or both	Sporadic	Normal or abnormal background, occipital and generalized S and pSW	Progressive myoclonus, epilepsy, and mental deterioration	106
Hyperglycemia	Adulthood	Visual and versive	Never reported	Never reported	Normal or abnormal background, occipital slow waves	Drug-resistant if glucose levels abnormal	61

EOBCOE, early onset benign childhood occipital epilepsy; LOCOE, late onset childhood occipital epilepsy; S, spikes; SW, spikes-and-waves; CPS, complex partial seizures; GTC, generalized tonic–clonic; pSW, polyspikes-and-waves.

possible secondary generalization, and the active period is variable. Most of the available data on treatment are based on studies performed when the distinction between early- and late-onset variants had not yet been defined, and the results reported could therefore be biased. In prospective studies of patients with strictly defined diagnoses, carbamazepine was able to control visual seizures.[84,85,100] It may be possible that delaying appropriate medication may adversely affect prognosis. Antiepileptic drugs do not necessarily normalize EEGs, and the epileptiform abnormalities may persist for a few years after the cessation of seizures and withdrawal of drugs.[36,54] Clusters of seizures do not seem to be influenced by antiepileptic drugs. Clobazam seems to control the seizures and spikes and waves after a few days in some difficult cases.[41,66]

Among patients who had been treated, drugs were successfully withdrawn before the age of 16 in 33% of cases. According to Panayiotopoulos,[85] slow reduction of medication 2 to 3 years after the last visual or other minor or major seizure may be advisable, but if visual seizures reappear, treatment should be restored. However, a relapse at drug withdrawal is possible even after a 2-year seizure-free period,[54] and long-lasting spontaneous remission is not guaranteed. The duration of the active phase may be difficult to predict, and consequently optimal duration of treatment is hard to assess.

LONG-TERM PROGNOSIS

Prognosis of LOCOE is not firmly established. Prognosis variability may depend on the selection criteria of the patients. In the early series of Gastaut, seizures were completely controlled by medication in only 60% of cases.[36,41] Beaumanoir reported seizure control before the age of 13 years, whereas Gastaut found 19 years to be the upper limit.[10] Patients initially classified as having idiopathic epilepsy but with a less favorable course turned out to have minor lesions on high-resolution MRI, which had not been detected in earlier neuroimaging studies.[72] When strict inclusion criteria such as normal neurologic examination and normal imaging studies are fulfilled, most patients have a favorable outcome.[99] Brain mapping seems to be valuable predictor of seizure outcome.[72]

SUMMARY AND CONCLUSIONS

In general, occipital epilepsies constitute a rare condition, but it is common opinion that they are probably underestimated because, especially at the onset, they may emulate other epilepsies since the visual hallucinations, which are the most important symptom for diagnosis, may lack or may be difficult to elicit on history, especially from younger children. The typical EEG abnormalities may also be absent, and if the no-visual seizures are the predominating ictal event, a different localization-related epilepsy may be supposed.

The usual clinical picture of LOCOE-Gastaut type is a normal child within the typical age range having either short visual seizures or eye-adversive seizures accompanied by visual ictal phenomena, which may be followed by hemi- or generalized convulsions. Elementary visual seizures are frequent, up to more than one per day. In about 50% of the patients, ictal hallucinations are followed by unilateral and pulsating headache, and in 10% of the cases they are associated with nausea and vomiting, making visual seizures indistinguishable from migraine with aura or basilar migraine attacks. Even though specific studies are needed to draw definite conclusions, these patients might be at risk for lower intellectual performance, scholastic disabilities, and psychiatric disorders. In particular, specific deficits in the visuoperceptual domain might occur.

LOCOE-Gastaut type has to be differentiated from the Panayiotopoulos-type childhood-onset epilepsy, photosensitive idiopathic occipital epilepsy, symptomatic occipital epilepsies, temporal epilepsies, idiopathic generalized epilepsy, and migraine. Especially important differential diagnoses are symptomatic occipital epilepsies. The following features should be considered as indications of a symptomatic or cryptogenic origin: Neuropsychological and neuroradiologic abnormalities, brief (>30 minutes) and persistent frequent partial seizures that may be associated with an alteration of consciousness, polymorphous seizures, abnormal background EEG activity, focal slowing, multiple spike foci, secondary generalization, and a change in the morphology of paroxysmal abnormalities during sleep.[6,22,51,61,88,98] A full neurophysiologic, neuropsychological, neuroimaging, and laboratory assessment is invariably mandatory in all patients with occipital epilepsy.

Prognosis and outcome of LOCOE-Gastaut type is not more firmly established than in other benign idiopathic epilepsies. This variability may depend on the selection criteria of the patients. When strict inclusion criteria are fulfilled, most patients have a favorable outcome. Because of prognosis uncertainty; seizures, though brief and mild, are frequent with possible secondary generalization; and the active period is variable, LOCOE-Gastaut type should be early treated. It may also be possible that delaying appropriate medication may adversely affect prognosis. Carbamazepine seems able to control visual seizures.

References

1. Aicardi J, Chevrie JJ. Epilepsie partielle avec foyer rolandique de la seconde enfance. *Journ Paris Pédiatr.* 1969;4:125–142.
2. Aicardi J, Newton R. Clinical findings in children with occipital spike-wave complexes suppressed by eye opening. In: Andermann F, Lugaresi E, eds. *Migraine and Epilepsy.* London: Butterworth; 1987:111–124.
3. Albright TD, Stoner GR. Contextual influences on visual processing. *Annu Rev Neurosci.* 2002;25:339–379.
4. Andermann F. Occipital epileptic abnormalities in mitochondrial disorders—preferential involvement, illustrations of clinical patterns, current progress in neurobiology, and a hypothesis. In: Andermann F, Beaumanoir A, Mira L, et al., eds. *Occipital Seizures and Epilepsies in Children.* London: John Libbey; 1993:111–120.
5. Aykut-Bingol C, Bronen RA, Kim JH, et al. Surgical outcome in occipital lobe epilepsy: implications for pathophysiology. *Ann Neurol.* 1998;44:60–69.
6. Beaumanoir A. Infantile epilepsy with occipital focus and good prognosis. *Eur Neurol.* 1983;22:43–52.
7. Beaumanoir A. An EEG contribution to the study of migraine and of the association between migraine and epilepsy in childhood. In: Andermann F, Beaumanoir A, Mira L, et al., eds. *Occipital Seizures and Epilepsies in Children.* London: John Libbey; 1993:101–110.
8. Beaumanoir A, Capizzi G, Nahory A, et al. Scotogenic seizures. In: Beaumanoir A, Gastaut H, Naquet R, eds. *Reflex Seizures and Reflex Epilepsies.* Geneve: ditions Médecine et Hygiène; 1989:219–223.
9. Beaumanoir A, Grandjean E. Occipital spikes, migraine and epilepsy. In: Andermann F, Lugaresi E, eds. *Migraine and Epilepsy.* London: Butterworth; 1987:97–110.
10. Beaumanoir A, Premet I, Safran AB. Concerning the association amblyopia-epilepsy. *Electrencephalogr Clin Neurophysiol.* 1977;42:435.
11. Bickerstaff ER. Basilar artery migraine. *Lancet.* 1961;1:15–17.
12. Bien CG, Benninger FO, Urbach H, et al. Localizing value of epileptic visual auras. *Brain.* 2000;123:244–253.
13. Bille B. Migraine in school children. *Acta Paediatr Scand Suppl.* 1962;51:1–151.
14. Bladin PF. The association of benign rolandic epilepsy with migraine. In: Andermann F, Lugaresi E, eds. *Migraine and Epilepsy.* London: Butterworth; 1987:145–152.
15. Blume WT, Wiebe S, Tapsell LM. Occipital epilepsy: lateral versus mesial. *Brain.* 2005;128:1209–1225.
16. Camfield PR, Metrakos KK, Andermann F. Basilar migraine, seizure and severe epileptiform EEG abnormalities: a relatively benign syndrome in adolescents. *Neurology.* 1978;28:584–588.
17. Caraballo R, Cersosimo R, Medina C, et al. Panayiotopoulos-type benign childhood occipital epilepsy: a prospective study. *Neurology.* 2000;55:1096–1100.

18. Caraballo RH, Sologuestua A, Granana N, et al. Idiopathic occipital and absence epilepsies appearing in the same children. *Pediatr Neurol.* 2004;30:24–28.
19. Chilosi AM, Brovedani P, Moscatelli M, et al. Neuropsychological findings in idiopathic occipital lobe epilepsies. *Epilepsia.* 2006;47:76–78.
20. Collins RC, Caston TV. Functional anatomy of occipital lobe seizures: an experimental study in rats. *Neurology.* 1979;29:705–716.
21. Commission on Classification and Terminology of the International League Against Epilepsy. Proposal for classification of epilepsies and epileptic syndromes. *Epilepsia.* 1989;30:389–399.
22. Cooper GW, Lee SI. Reactive occipital epileptiform activity: is it benign? *Epilepsia.* 1991;32:63–68.
23. Dalla Bernardina B, Fontana E, Cappellaro O, et al. The partial occipital epilepsies in childhood. In: Andermann F, Beaumanoir A, Mira L, et al., eds. *Occipital Seizures and Epilepsies in Children.* London: John Libbey; 1993:173–181.
24. Dalla Bernardina B, Sgro V, Fontana E, et al. Les épilepsies partielles idiopathiques de l'enfant. In: Roger J, Bureau M, Dravet C, et al., eds. *Les Syndromes pileptiques de l'Enfant et de l'Adolescent.* London: John Libbey; 1992:173–188.
25. Delwaide PJ, Barragan M, Gastaut H. Remarques sur l'épilepsie partielle occipitale. *Acta Neurol Belg.* 1971;71:383–391.
26. Deonna T. Paroxysmal disorders which may be migraine or may be confused with it. In: Hockaday JM, ed. *Migraine in Childhood.* London: Butterworth; 1988:55–87.
27. Deonna T, Ziegler HL, Despland PA. Paroxysmal visual disturbance of epileptic origin and occipital epilepsy in children. *Neuropediatrics.* 1984;15:131–135.
28. Duchowny M, Jayakar P, Resnick T, et al. Posterior temporal epilepsy electroclinical features. *Ann Neurol.* 1994;35:427–431.
29. Dvorkin GS, Andermann F, Carpenter S, et al. Classical migraine, intractable epilepsy and multiple strokes: a syndrome related to mitochondrial encephalopathy. In: Andermann F, Lugaresi E, eds. *Migraine and Epilepsy.* London: Butterworth; 1987:203–231.
30. Engel J Jr, International League Against Epilepsy (ILAE). A proposed diagnostic scheme for people with epileptic seizures and with epilepsy: report of the ILAE Task Force on Classification and Terminology. *Epilepsia.* 2001;42:796–803.
31. Fejerman N. Atypical evolution of benign partial epilepsies in children. *Int Pediatr.* 1996;11:351–356.
32. Ferrie CD, Beaumanoir A, Guerrini R, et al. Early-onset benign occipital seizure susceptibility syndrome. *Epilepsia.* 1997;38:285–293.
33. Ferrie C, Caraballo R, Covanis A, et al. Panayiotopoulos syndrome: a consensus view. *Dev Med Child Neurol.* 2006;48:236–240.
34. Gastaut H. vidence électrographique d'un mécanisme sous-cortical dans certaines épilepsies partielles—la signification clinique des "secteurs eréo-thalamiques." *Rev Neurol.* 1950;83:396–401.
35. Gastaut H. L'épilepsie bénigne de l'enfant à pointes-ondes occipitales. *Bull Acad R Méd Belg.* 1981;136:540–555.
36. Gastaut H. A new type of epilepsy: benign partial epilepsy of childhood with occipital spike-waves. *Clin Electroencephalogr.* 1982;13:13–22.
37. Gastaut H. Épilepsie bénigne de l'enfance avec paroxysmes occipitaux. In: Roger J, Bureau M, Dravet C, et al., eds. *Les Syndromes Épileptiques de l'Enfant et de l'Adolescent.* London: John Libbey; 1992:201–217.
38. Gastaut H, Aguglia U, Tinuper P. Benign versive or cycling epilepsy with bilateral 3-cps spike-and-wave discharges in late childhood. *Ann Neurol.* 1986;19:301–303.
39. Gastaut H, Zifkin BG. Ictal visual hallucinations of numerals. *Neurology.* 1984;34:950–953.
40. Gastaut H, Zifkin BG. Classification of epilepsies. *J Clin Neurophysiol.* 1985;2:313–326.
41. Gastaut H, Zifkin BG. Benign epilepsy of childhood with occipital spike-and-wave complexes. In: Andermann F, Lugaresi E, eds. *Migraine and Epilepsy.* London: Butterworth; 1987:47–81.
42. Gibbs FA, Gibbs EL. *Atlas of Electroencephalography.* Cambridge, MA: Addison-Wesley; 1952:222–224.
43. Gibbs EL, Gillen HV, Gibbs FA. Disappearance and migration of epileptic foci in children. *Am J Dis Child.* 1954;88:596–603.
44. Giroud M, Borsotti JP, Michiels R, et al. Épilepsie et calcifications occipitales bilatérales: 3 cas. *Rev Neurol.* 1990;4:288–292.
45. Giroud M, Soichot P, Weyl M, et al. L'épilepsie à pointe-ondes occipitales. Sa place parmi les épilepsies bénignes. *Ann Pediatr.* 1986;33:131–135.
46. Gloor P, Metrakos J, Metrakos K, et al. Neurophysiological, genetic, and biochemical nature of epileptic diathesis. *Electroencephalogr Clin Neurophysiol.* 1982;35:45–56.
47. Goadsby PJ. Migraine pathophysiology. *Headache.* 2005;45(Suppl 1):14–24.
48. Gobbi G, Ambrosetto G, Parmeggiani A, et al. The malignant variant of partial epilepsy with occipital spikes in childhood. *Epilepsia.* 1991;32(Suppl 1):16–17.
49. Gobbi G, Ambrosetto P, Zaniboni MG, et al. Coeliac disease, posterior cerebral calcifications and epilepsy. *Brain Dev.* 1992;14:23–29.
50. Gobbi G, Bouquet F, Greco L, et al. Coeliac disease, epilepsy and cerebral calcifications. *Lancet.* 1992;340:439–443.
51. Gobbi G, Sorrenti G, Santucci M, et al. Epilepsy with bilateral occipital calcifications: a benign onset with progressive severity. *Neurology.* 1988;38:913–920.
52. Gokcay A, Gokcay F, Ekmekci O, et al. Occipital epilepsies in children. *Eur J Paediatr Neurol.* 2002;6:261–268.
53. Grosso S, Galimberti D, Gobbi G, et al. Typical absence seizures associated with localization-related epilepsy: a clinical and electroencephalographic characterization. *Epilepsy Res.* 2005;66:13–21.
54. Guerrini R, Battaglia A, Dravet C, et al. Outcome of idiopathic childhood epilepsy with occipital paroxysms. In: Andermann F, Beaumanoir A, Mira L, et al., eds. *Occipital Seizures and Epilepsies in Children.* London: John Libbey; 1993:165–171.
55. Guerrini G, Bonanni P, Ferrari AR, et al. Épilepsie occipitale idiopathique de l'enfant: limites et incertitudes du diagnostic EEG. *Epilepsies.* 1995;7:153–166.
56. Guerrini G, Dravet A, Genton P, et al. Idiopathic photosensitive occipital lobe epilepsy. *Epilepsia.* 1995;36:883–891.
57. Guerrini R, Ferrari AR, Battaglia A, et al. Occipitotemporal seizures with ictus emeticus induced by intermittent photic stimulation. *Neurology.* 1994;44:253–259.
58. Gulgonen S, Demirbilek V, Korkmaz B, et al. Neuropsychological functions in idiopathic occipital lobe epilepsy. *Epilepsia.* 2000;41:405–411.
59. Harden CL, Rosenbaum DH, Daras M. Hyperglycemia presenting with occipital seizures. *Epilepsia.* 1991;32:215–220.
60. Herranz Tanarro FJ, Saenz Lope E, Christobal Sassot S. La pointe-onde occipitale avec et sans épilepsie bénigne de l'enfant. *Rev EEG Neurophysiol.* 1984;14:1–7.
61. Holmes GL. Benign focal epilepsies of childhood. *Epilepsia.* 1993;34(Suppl 3):49–61.
62. Kastner S, Ungerleider LG. Mechanisms of visual attention in the human cortex. *Annu Rev Neurosci.* 2000;23:315–341.
63. Kellaway P. The incidence, significance and natural history of spike foci in children. In: Henry CE, ed. *Current Clinical Neurophysiology.* New York: Elsevier/North-Holland; 1980:151–175.
64. Kivity S, Ephrain T, Weitz R, et al. Childhood epilepsy with occipital paroxysms: clinical variants in 134 patients. *Epilepsia.* 2000;41:1522–1533.
65. Kuzniecky P, Rosenblatt B. Benign occipital epilepsy: a family study. *Epilepsia.* 1987;28:346–350.
66. Lerman P, Kivity S. The benign partial non-rolandic epilepsies. *J Clin Neurophysiol.* 1991;8:275–287.
67. Levinson JD, Stillerman ML. The correlation between electroencephalographic findings and eye disorders in children. *Electroencephalogr Clin Neurophysiol.* 1950;2:226.
68. Ludwig BI, Ajmone-Marsan C. Clinical ictal pattern in epileptic patients with occipital electroencephalographic foci. *Neurology.* 1975;25:463–471.
69. Lugaresi E, Cirignotta F, Montagna P. Occipital lobe epilepsy with scotosensitive seizures: the role of central vision. *Epilepsia.* 1984;25:115–120.
70. Maher J, Ronen GM, Ogunyemi AO, et al. Occipital paroxysmal discharges suppressed by eye opening: variability in clinical and seizure manifestations in childhood. *Epilepsia.* 1995;36:52–57.
71. Manzoni GC, Terzano MG, Mancia D. Possible interference between migrainous and epileptic mechanisms in intercalated attacks. *Eur Neurol.* 1979;18:124–128.
72. Mennink S, van Nieuwenhuizen O, Jennekens-Schinkel A, et al. Early prediction of seizure remission in children with occipital lobe epilepsy. *Eur J Paediatr Neurol.* 2003;7:161–165.
73. Mira L, Van Lierde A. EEG in children with visual pathways damage. In: Andermann F, Beaumanoir A, Mira L, et al., eds. *Occipital Seizures and Epilepsies in Children.* London: John Libbey; 1993:65–70.
74. Montagna P, Sacquegna T, Cortelli P, et al. Mitochondrial abnormalities in migraine. Preliminary findings. *Headache.* 1988;28:477–480.
75. Nagendran K, Prior PF, Rossiter MA. Benign occipital epilepsy of childhood: a family study. *J R Soc Med.* 1990;83:804–805.
76. Nalin A, Ruggerini C, Ferrari E, et al. Clinique, diagnostique différentielle et évolution des crises épileptiques visuelles de l'enfant. *Neurophysiol Clin.* 1989;19:25–36.
77. Niedermeyer E. Primary (idiopathic) generalized epilepsy and underlying mechanisms. *Clin Electroecephalogr.* 1996;27:1–21.
78. Panayiotopoulos CP. Basilar migraine? Seizure and severe epileptiform EEG abnormalities. *Neurology.* 1980;30:1122–1125.
79. Panayiotopoulos CP. Inhibitory effect of central vision on occipital lobe seizures. *Neurology.* 1981;31:1331–1333.
80. Panayiotopoulos CP. Benign nocturnal childhood epilepsy: a new syndrome with nocturnal seizures, tonic deviation of eyes, and vomiting. *J Child Neurol.* 1989;4:43–48.
81. Panayiotopoulos CP. Benign childhood epilepsy with occipital paroxysms: a 15-year prospective study. *Ann Neurol.* 1989;26:51–56.
82. Panayiotopoulos CP. Benign childhood epilepsy with occipital paroxysms. In: Andermann F, Beaumanoir A, Mira L, et al, eds. *Occipital Seizures and Epilepsies in Children.* London: John Libbey; 1993:151–164.
83. Panayiotopoulos CP. Elementary visual hallucinations in migraine and epilepsy. *J Neurol Neurosurg Psychiatry.* 1994;57:1371–1374.
84. Panayiotopoulos CP. Elementary visual hallucinations, blindness, and headache in idiopathic occipital epilepsy: differentiation from migraine. *J Neurol Neurosurg Psychiatry.* 1999;66:536–540.

85. Panayiotopoulos CP. Idiopathic childhood occipital epilepsies. In: Roger J, Bureau M, Dravet CH, et al., eds. *Epileptic Syndromes in Infancy, Childhood, and Adolescence*. Eastleight: John Libbey; 2002:203–227.
86. Pazzaglia P, Sabatini L, Lugaresi E. Crisi occipitali precipitate dal buio. *Rev Neurol*. 1970;40:184–192.
87. Plasmati R, Blanco R, Michelucci R, et al. SEP study in idiopathic infantile epilepsies. In: Beaumanoir A, Gastaut H, Naquet R, eds. *Reflex Seizures and Reflex Epilepsies*. Geneve: ditions Médecine et Hygiène; 1989:75–81.
88. Roger J, Bureau M. Postface: épilepsie bénigne de l'enfance avec paroxysmes occipitaux. In: Roger J, Bureau M, Dravet C, et al., eds. *Les Syndromes Épileptiques de l'Enfant et de l'Adolescent*. London: John Libbey; 1992:205–215.
89. Roger J, Pellissier JF, Bureau M, et al. Le diagnostic précoce de la maladie de Lafora. Importance des manifestations paroxystiques visuelle et intérêt de la biopsie cutanée. *Rev Neurol*. 1983;139:115–124.
90. Slatter KH. Some clinical and EEG findings in patients with migraine. *Brain*. 1968;91:85–98.
91. So N, Berkovic SF, Andermann F, et al. Myoclonus epilepsy and ragged red fibers (MERRF). Electrophysiological studies and comparison with the other progressive myoclonus epilepsies. *Brain*. 1989;112:1261–1276.
92. Sofue A, Okumura A, Negoro T, et al. Absence seizures in patients with localization-related epilepsy. *Brain Dev*. 2003;25:422–426.
93. Sorel L, Rucquoy-Ponsar M. Lépilepsie fonctionelle de maturation. *Rev Neurol*. 1969;121:288–297.
94. Swanson JW, Vick NA. Basilar artery migraine: 12 patients with an attack recorded electroencephalographically. *Neurology*. 1978;28:782–786.
95. Talwar D, Rask CA, Torres F. Clinical manifestations in children with occipital spike-wave paroxysms. *Epilepsia*. 1992;33:667–674.
96. Taylor I, Scheffer IE, Berkovic S. Occipital epilepsies: identification of specific and newly recognized syndromes. *Brain*. 2003;126:753–769.
97. Tenembaum S, Deonna T, Fejerman N, et al. Continuos spike-waves and dementia in childhood epilepsy with occipital paroxysms. *J Epilepsy*. 1997;10:139–145.
98. Terasaki T, Yamatogi Y, Ohtahara S. Electroclinical delineation of occipital lobe epilepsy in childhood. In: Andermann F, Lugaresi E, eds. *Migraine and Epilepsy*. London: Butterworth; 1987:125–137.
99. Tsai ML, Lo HY, Chaou WT. Clinical and electroencephalographic findings in early and late onset benign childhood epilepsy with occipital paroxysms. *Brain Dev*. 2001;23:401–405.
100. Van den Hout BM, Van der Meij W, Wieneke GH, et al. Seizure semiology of occipital lobe epilepsy in children. *Epilepsia*. 1997;38:1188–1191.
101. White HS. Molecular pharmacology of topiramate: managing seizures and preventing migraine. *Headache*. 2005;45(Suppl 1):48–56.
102. Williamson PD, Thadani VM, Darcey TM, et al. Occipital lobe epilepsy: clinical characteristics, seizure spread patterns, and results of surgery. *Ann Neurol*. 1992;31:3–13.

CHAPTER 239 ■ CHILDHOOD AND JUVENILE ABSENCE EPILEPSIES

EDOUARD HIRSCH, PIERRE THOMAS, AND CHRYSOSTOMOS P. PANAYIOTOPOULOS

INTRODUCTION

Typical Absences: The Symptoms

Typical absences (TAs) are epileptic seizures manifested by impairment of consciousness and 2.5- to 4-Hz generalized spike-and-slow-wave discharges[47,85,187] (see Chapter 49). Impairment of consciousness may be mild (requiring special testing)[1,7,27,112,122,161,162,199,205,206,208] or severe and may be associated with other clinical manifestations, such as automatisms,[184] regional or widespread myoclonia (rhythmic or random), and autonomic disturbances.[46] Furthermore, the electroencephalographic (EEG) discharge may be brief or long, continuous or fragmented, with multiple or single spikes that are consistently associated or not associated with the slow wave. The intradischarge frequency may be relatively constant or vary.[161]

Thus, the term *typical absences* does not refer to a stereotyped symptom, but to a cluster of clinico-EEG manifestations that may be syndrome related. It should be appreciated that like any other physical symptoms in medicine, a detailed study of the manifestations of TAs is a prerequisite for a meaningful syndrome-related diagnosis. The clinico-EEG manifestations of absences have been best described in the eminent video-EEG studies by Penry et al.[185] and Stefan et al.,[211] but it is only recently that an attempt has been made for their syndrome-related characterization with video-EEG analysis.[108,109,158–161,170–172] It has been shown that some of the manifestations of TA may be more specifically related to an epileptic syndrome than others, but no single symptom is sufficient to define an epileptic syndrome.[173]

Epileptic Syndromes with Typical Absences

An epileptic syndrome, by definition, requires the nonfortuitous clustering of many symptoms and signs.[48]

Four epileptic syndromes with TAs have been recognized by the International League Against Epilepsy (ILAE)[48]: Childhood absence epilepsy (CAE), juvenile absence epilepsy (JAE), juvenile myoclonic epilepsy (JME), and myoclonic absence epilepsy (MAE). The first three (CAE, JAE, JME) are considered as part of idiopathic generalized epilepsies (IGEs), whereas the fourth (MAE) is categorized among the symptomatic or cryptogenic generalized epilepsies.

There may be more epileptic syndromes with TAs, such as eyelid myoclonia with absences (EMA), perioral myoclonia with absences, and others awaiting further studies and confirmation.[166,168,171,177,178] Furthermore, idiopathic generalized tonic–clonic seizures on awakening are often associated with mild absences.[175] Many of these syndromes are different in presentation, severity, and prognosis. Children with CAE in their majority will remit, those with MAE are affected by or may develop mental and behavioral problems, and those with JME in their midteens may develop lifelong myoclonic jerks and generalized tonic–clonic seizures (GTCSs). Other patients may have subtle clinical manifestations during the typical 3-Hz spike-and-wave discharges of which they are not aware (phantom absences); often they seek medical consultation only after a generalized tonic–clonic seizure develops, probably a long time after the onset of absences.

Some investigators[11,21,23–26,117,192,193] have proposed that all these disorders, not only idiopathic (for which some theoretical justification may exist) but also those whereby the seizures arise from known brain damage, constitute a neurobiologic continuum.

HISTORICAL PERSPECTIVES

This topic has been discussed in detail elsewhere.[66,67,116,125,127,134,135,139,194] According to Temkin,[216] the first description of absences was made in 1705 by Poupart. Tissot in 1770[217] described a girl with absences "*avec un très léger mouvement dans les yeux*" associated with frequent GTCSs. The term *epileptic absences* was first used by Calmeil[35] in his doctoral thesis of 1824. The term of *petit mal* was introduced by Esquirol in 1815.[73] Gowers in 1881[97] gave the most accurate description of absence seizures "without conspicuous convulsions," and Hughlings Jackson in 1879[115] discussed the differences between absences and complex partial seizures. Absences also have been described on clinical grounds, without EEG, by Friedmann.[83] Although he believed that these absences were not epileptic, he gave an excellent description of the attacks and a long-term favorable prognosis. Sauer[204] originated the term *pyknolepsy* (from the Greek *pyknos* indicating closely packed, dense, aggregated). Adie.[2] based on his own observations but mainly, as he admitted, on those of Friedmann,[83] Heilbronner,[106] and Stier,[212] defined pyknolepsy in the most admirable way as follows:

> "A disease with an explosive onset between the ages of 4 and 12 years, of frequent short, very slight, monotonous minor epileptiform seizures of uniform severity, which recur almost daily for weeks, months or years, and which are uninfluenced by anti-epileptic remedies, do not impede normal and psychical development, and ultimately cease spontaneously never to return. At most the eyeballs may roll upwards, the lids may flicker and the arms may be raised by a feeble tonic spasm. Clonic movements, however slight, obvious vasomotor disturbances, palpitations and lassitude or confusion after the attacks, are equivocal symptoms strongly suggestive of oncoming grave epilepsy, and for the present they should be considered as foreign to the more favourable disease."

The electroclinical characteristics of absences were described by Gibbs.[94,95] The petit mal triad of Lennox,[126,127] which was misused and misunderstood, was finally clarified by the ILAE[47] with the differentiation of typical and atypical absences.

The present ILAE distinction[48] between CAE and JAE is mainly based on the pioneer work of Doose et al.[61] and Janz.[116] Doose et al.,[61] in a study of 149 children with absences, found three different groups with emphasis at the age of onset: (a) an absence epilepsy of early onset from birth to 4 years of age, (b) CAE (pyknolepsy) with onset at 4 to 8 years of age, and (c) JAE with onset before puberty and with absences occurring in clusters (cycloleptic) or sporadically (spanioleptic). Janz[116] emphasized the significance of the frequency of the absences in a comparative study of 505 pyknoleptic and 197 nonpyknoleptic cases and confirmed Doose's conclusions regarding differences of age at onset and sex.[116,118,119]

Tassinari et al.,[215] by describing myoclonic absences, and Jeavons,[121] by describing eyelid myoclonia with absences, were probably the first authors to report absences starting in childhood but having different characteristics and prognoses than in CAE.

DEFINITIONS

Childhood Absence Epilepsy

According to the international classification of epilepsies,[48] CAE represents an idiopathic generalized epilepsy defined as follows: Pyknolepsy occurs in children of school age (peak manifestation age 6 to 7 years), with a strong genetic predisposition in otherwise normal children. It appears more frequently in girls than in boys. It is characterized by very frequent (several to many per day) absences. The EEG reveals bilateral, synchronous symmetric spike-waves, usually 3 Hz, on a normal background activity (Fig. 1). During adolescence, generalized tonic–clonic seizures often develop. Otherwise, absences may remit or, more rarely, persist as the only seizure type.

This brief definition of the ILAE Commission[48] mainly based on retrospective studies was a source of confusion. Thus, many authors make the arbitrary interpretation that CAE is any type of epilepsy with onset of absences in childhood. Therefore, epidemiology, genetics, age at onset, clinical manifestations, other types of seizures, long-term prognosis, and treatment do not accurately reflect the syndrome of CAE. A more precise definition of childhood absence epilepsy has been recently proposed by the ILAE Task Force on Classification defining inclusion and exclusion criteria.[140] It takes into account several important diagnostic points, such as the degree of impairment of consciousness, the morphology of spike-wave discharges, and the place of generalized tonic–clonic seizures. Clear exclusion criteria were also proposed[140]: Eyelid myoclonia (which is predominantly myoclonic and has minimal consciousness impairment) and TAs consistently provoked by specific stimuli. The same applies for multiple spikes (more than three spikes per wave) that also indicate a bad prognosis and coexistent myoclonic jerks or GTCSs.[160]

The following definition may better represent CAE (Table 1):

> Childhood absence epilepsy is an age-related idiopathic generalized epilepsy, which occurs in otherwise normal children, more frequently girls, with a strong genetic predisposition. Age of onset is between 4 and 10 years of age, with a peak at 5 to 7 years. Absences are frequent, tens to hundreds per day. Their duration varies from 4 to 20 seconds, though most of them last around 10 seconds. Clinically, there is abrupt and severe impairment (loss) of consciousness, with cessation of voluntary activity, which is not restored during the ictus. The eyes spontaneously open; overbreathing, speech, and other voluntary activity stop within the first 3 seconds from the onset of the discharge. Automatisms are frequent but have no significance in the diagnosis. The eyes stare or move slowly, and random eyelid blinking (usually not sustained) may occur.
>
> Persistent eyelid myoclonia, rhythmic massive limb jerking, and single or arrhythmic myoclonic jerks of the head, trunk, or limbs are probably not compatible with childhood absence epilepsy. However, milder myoclonic elements, particularly at the onset of the seizure discharge, may be a feature of childhood absence epilepsy. Generalized tonic–clonic seizures and other types of seizures like myoclonic jerks should not be featured in childhood absence epilepsy. Visual (photic) and other sensory precipitation are most likely against a diagnosis of childhood absence epilepsy. Mild or no impairment of consciousness is not compatible with childhood absence epilepsy.
>
> The EEG has a normal background, with sometimes rhythmic posterior delta activity. Ictal discharges consist of generalized high-amplitude spike- and double (maximum occasional three spikes are allowed)-spike-and-slow-wave complexes. They are rhythmic at around 3 to 4 Hz (>2.5 Hz) with a gradual and regular (0.5 to 1 Hz) slowdown from the initial to the terminal phase of the discharge. The first 1 to 2 seconds of the onset of the discharge is usually fast and unreliable for these measurements. There are no marked variations in the relation of spike to the slow wave, no fluctuations in the intradischarge frequency, and certainly no fragmentations of the ictal discharges.
>
> Remission usually occurs before the age of 12 years but infrequent GTCSs may develop in adolescence.

Juvenile Absence Epilepsy

According to the Revised International Classification of Epilepsies and Epileptic Syndromes,[48] JAE is one of the age-related idiopathic generalized epilepsies. The following description is given:

> The absences of JAE are the same as in pyknolepsy, but absences with retropulsive movements are less common. Manifestation occurs around puberty. Seizure frequency is lower than in pyknolepsy, with absences occurring less frequently than every day, mostly sporadically. Association with GTCS is frequent, and GTCSs precede the absence manifestations more often than in childhood absence epilepsy, often occurring on awakening. Not infrequently, the patients also have myoclonic seizures. Response to therapy is excellent.

A similar but slightly more restrictive definition has been proposed by Panayiotopoulos.[166]

EPIDEMIOLOGY

Childhood Absence Epilepsy

The annual incidence of CAE is low and may vary from 1.9 to 8 per 100,000 children below the age of 16 years, and the prevalence is probably in the range of 2% to 10% of children with epileptic disorders.[23,30,133,200,201] A twofold preponderance in girls than boys may be a realistic estimate, although some studies have reported that boys and girls are equally affected.

Juvenile Absence Epilepsy

There are no population-based epidemiologic data on this syndrome. According to Janz,[118] JAE represented 10% of the age-related epilepsies with petit mal seizures.

ETIOLOGY AND BASIC MECHANISMS

According to Tissot,[217] "To produce epilepsy, two things are necessary: (i) a tendency for the brain to fall into spasm more readily than during health; (ii) a source of irritation that can precipitate this tendency." These two factors (genetic factor

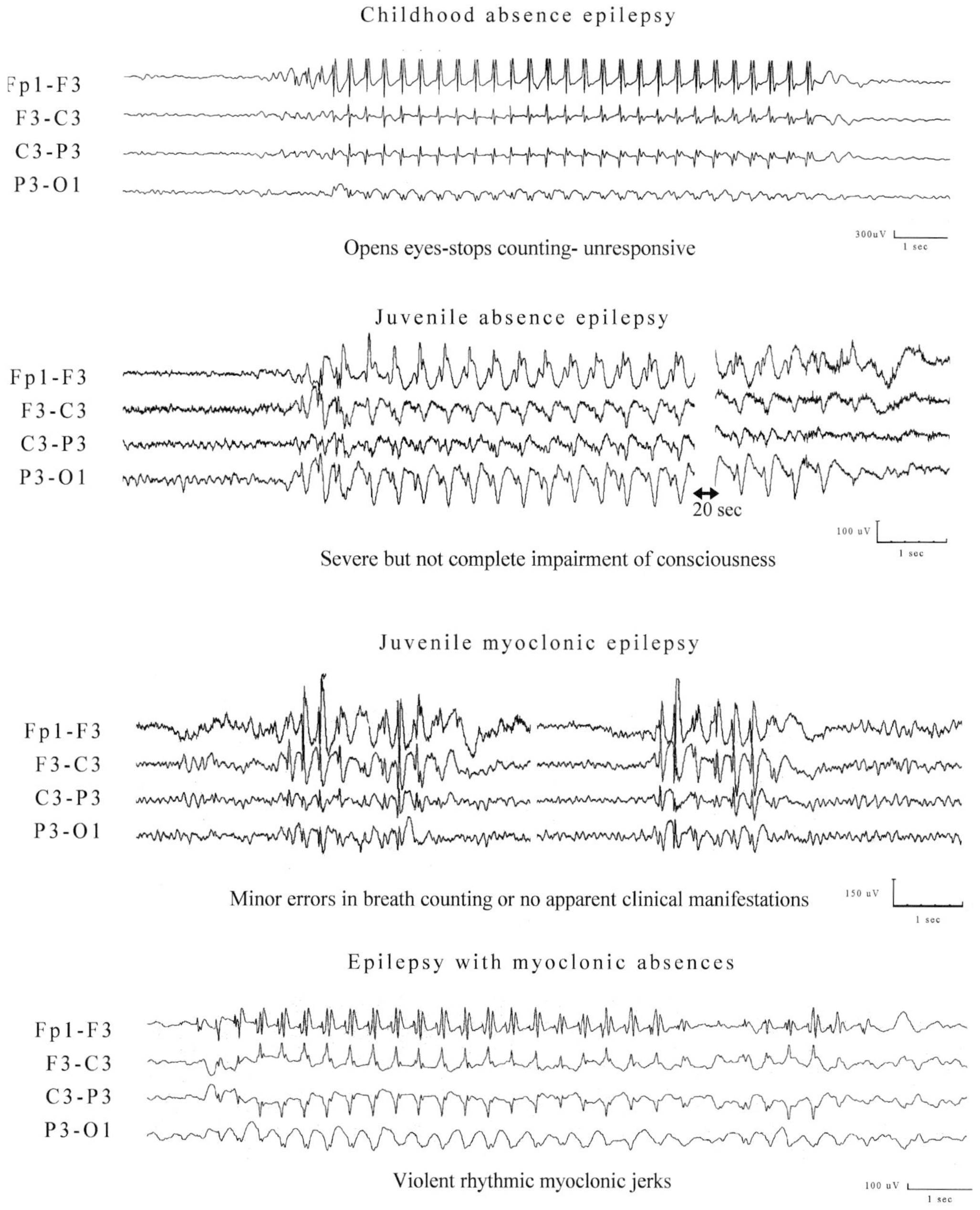

FIGURE 1. Video-electroencephalographic (EEG) recordings. **Upper:** This trace is from a 7-year-old girl with frequent daily typical absences (TAs). She stops overbreathing and counting within the first 3 seconds after onset of the EEG 3-Hz spike-and-slow-wave discharge, she is unresponsive, and she demonstrates features described in the text for CAE. Automatisms are seen in some of her seizures, but there is no eyelid or perioral or limb myoclonia. She is not photosensitive. Note the regularity and rhythmicity of the ictal paroxysm. **Upper middle:** This trace is from a 33-year-old woman who has experienced frequent daily absences that were highly resistant to treatment since 8 years of age. Ten long spontaneous absences were recorded during the 3-hour video-EEG session, but they were mainly provoked by overbreathing. She experiences severe impairment of consciousness, but she may recall events occurring toward the end of the ictus, usually keeps her eyes closed, and may restore counting during the discharge. The long ictal EEG is as rhythmic and regular as that of CAE. **Lower middle:** This image is from a 38-year-old woman with juvenile myoclonic epilepsy (JME). Note the brief fragmented discharges with "W"s. Impairment of consciousness may be detected with breath counting (annotated with numbers) where there is a significant delay in pronouncing the next number after a discharge. **Lower:** This trace is from an 11-month-old boy with mild developmental delay and a 1-month history of absences. In video-EEG these were manifested with 3-Hz rhythmic multiple spike-and-slow-waves with rhythmic myoclonic jerking of the head, body, and shoulders.

TABLE 1

INCLUSION AND EXCLUSION CRITERIA FOR CHILDHOOD ABSENCE EPILEPSY

INCLUSION CRITERIA FOR CHILDHOOD ABSENCE EPILEPSY

(1) Age at onset between 4 and 10 years and a peak at 5–7 years
(2) Normal neurologic state and development
(3) Brief (4–20 seconds, exceptionally longer) and frequent (tens per day) absence seizures with abrupt and severe impairment (loss) of consciousness. Automatisms are frequent but have no significance in the diagnosis.
(4) EEG ictal discharges of generalized high-amplitude spike- and double (maximum occasional three spikes are allowed) spike-and-slow-wave complexes. They are rhythmic at around 3 Hz with a gradual and regular slowdown from the initial to the terminal phase of the discharge. Their duration varies from 4 to 20 seconds.

EXCLUSION CRITERIA FOR CHILDHOOD ABSENCE EPILEPSY

The following may be incompatible with childhood absence epilepsy:

(1) Other than typical absence seizures such as generalized tonic–clonics seizures or myoclonic jerks prior to or during the active stage of absences
(2) Eyelid myoclonia, perioral myoclonia, rhythmic massive limb jerking, and single or arrhythmic myoclonic jerks of the head, trunk, or limbs. However, mild myoclonic elements of the eyes, eyebrows, and eyelids may be featured—particularly in the first 3 seconds of the absence seizure.
(3) Mild or no impairment of consciousness during the 3- to 4-Hz discharges
(4) Brief EEG 3- to 4-Hz spike-wave paroxysms of <4 seconds, multiple spikes (more than three), or ictal discharge fragmentations
(5) Visual (photic) and other sensory precipitation of clinical seizures

From Loiseau P, Panayiotopoulos CP. Childhood absence epilepsy. In: Gilham S, ed. *Neurobase*. San Diego, CA: Arbor Publishing Corp.; 2000, with permission.

and acquired factor) exist with a very unequal significance in absences epilepsies.

Genetic Factors

Childhood Absences

Although CAE is genetically determined, the precise mode of inheritance and the genes involved remain largely unidentified.[9,10,84,154] A positive family history of epilepsy was found in 15% to 44% of cases.[20,53,59,62,63,108,127,205] Ascertainment of family history of epilepsy has to be considered: When keeping only epilepsy in parents and siblings, the frequency decreases from 42.6% to 20.7%.[111] In two series, epilepsy in first-degree relatives was found in 17% of CAE.[36,137] These seizures are TAs and GTCSs. In studies on twins, 84% of monozygotic twins had 3-Hz spike-waves, and TA developed in 75% of pairs and dizygotic twins 16 times less often.[127] An Australian study of epilepsy in twins confirmed that in concordant pairs, twins developed a similar syndrome.[26] Bianchi et al.[28] found that in 24 families with a CAE proband, there was a high concordance (33.3%) for the same clinical form in first-degrees relatives, while febrile convulsions (46.7%) and GTCSs (30%) were more common in distant relatives. Epilepsy risk in children of patients with CAE would be 6.8%.[17]

Currently, various chromosomal loci have been identified in families with absences of childhood onset (not necessarily equated with CAE). Linkage to chromosome 1 was found in families with absences starting in childhood and the later development of myoclonic jerks and GTCSs, as in JME.[58] Linkage analysis in five generations of a family in which affected patients had childhood absences and GTCSs provided evidence of a locus on chromosome 8q24.[58,81] The candidate region for this locus, designated ECA 1, has been refined, but a gene remains to be identified. According to the criteria proposed in this chapter, neither of these groups is CAE. There are also reports implicating chromosome 5q31.1 and 19p13.2.[52] Furthermore, there is now evidence available to suggest that mutations in genes encoding GABA receptors[145] or brain-expressed voltage-dependent calcium channels[44] may underlie CAE. Marini et al.[145] found $GABA_A$ receptor γ-2 subunit gene mutations on chromosome 5 in a large family with CAE and febrile seizures (including febrile seizures plus and other seizure phenotypes). This gene mutation segregated with febrile seizures and CAE, and also occurred in individuals with the other phenotypes. The clinical and molecular data suggested that the $GABA_A$ receptor subunit mutation alone could account for the febrile seizure phenotype, but an interaction of this gene with another gene or genes was required for the childhood absence phenotype in this family. Linkage analysis for a putative second gene contributing to the childhood absence phenotype suggested possible loci on chromosomes 10, 13, 14, and 15. Chen et al.[44] found 68 variations, including 12 missense mutations in the calcium channel *CACNA1H* gene in CAE patients. The identified missense mutations occurred in the highly conserved residues of the T-type calcium channel gene.

Juvenile Absences

A family history of epilepsy is frequent, and identical twins who both have the syndrome have been reported.[26] Obeid[156] reported that in a Saudi Arabian population where consanguineous marriages are frequent and can be found in 47% of the families of patients with JME,[152] this was only true for 1 out of 14 JAE families. This could indicate that a recessive gene is important in JME but not JAE. In the clinical genetic study of families with idiopathic generalized epilepsy,[146] phenotypic concordance within families of JAE was 10%, which was low compared to families of other IGE syndromes. Because 31% of JAE relatives had CAE but only 2.5% had JME, the authors suggested that CAE and JAE share a close genetic relation, whereas JME may be a more distinct entity. There are several reports of mutation of the CACNA1 A α-1 subunit of the CaV2.1 Ca2+ channel, or the CACNB4 β-4 subunit, with the phenotype of absence seizures with ataxia,[72,114] which does not fit in any of the known absence epilepsies. The paper of Escayg et al.[72] comprises an observation of a mutation in a family with an identical locus in CACNB4 as in the *lethargic* mouse mutant but which resulted in a quite different human phenotype. Findings with the genetically well-defined series of mouse mutants with absences can probably not be easily transferred to human epilepsies.

Acquired Factors

As concordance in monozygotic twins is not 100%, nongenetic factors are likely.[26] Perinatal complications, postnatal head trauma, and cerebral inflammatory disease were found in the case histories of 7% to 30% of patients,[146,225] and only 3.9% in the Janz series.[118] However, these cerebral aggressions are very common in children and were not risk factors in a population-based case-control study.[196] A history of febrile convulsions is frequent: 20% to 23% of cases.[196,205] More than a risk factor, febrile convulsions are probably the first manifestation of an epileptic diathesis.[196] This is in accordance with results of studies on the phenotype of families with "febrile convulsions plus" related or not to mutations of voltage-dependant sodium channel gene mutations (SCN1A or SCN1B). In such families, tonic–clonic, tonic, and absence seizures have been reported.[14,128]

Pathology and Structural Brain Imaging

Autopsy[147,148] and magnetic resonance imaging (MRI)[225] studies found microdysgenesis and other cerebral structural changes in some patients with CAE. Meencke and Janz[148] reviewed autopsy findings in CAE and confirmed their previous reports on microdysgenesis[147] with the frontal lobe more severely affected. Using quantitative MRI, Woermann et al.[225] found that patients with idiopathic generalized epilepsy had significantly larger cortical gray matter volumes than control subjects. Abnormalities of the regional distribution of cerebral gray and subcortical matter were frequent in other patients with IGE but only in 1 out of 10 patients with childhood absence epilepsy. However, all cases of Meenke[149] had frequent absences from childhood to adulthood and GTCSs, which would not conform to a strict diagnosis of the syndrome of CAE. Similar may be the single patient with abnormal MRI of Woermann et al.[225] Recently, thalamic atrophy was demonstrated, using optimized voxel-based morphometry in a series of absence epilepsy patients. Bilateral thalamic atrophy may be either a result of damage from seizures (as in hippocampal sclerosis) in this group of patients with difficult to treat absences or a reflection of a primary underlying pathology as the cause of absence seizures.[41]

Basic Mechanisms

Current thinking about the pathogenesis of absence seizures dates to the landmark experiments of Jasper and Droogleever-Fortuyn.[120] They demonstrated that 3 c/s stimulation of the midline and intralaminar nuclei of the thalamus in cats could produce bilaterally synchronous spike-wave discharges in the cortical EEG of those animals. Over the next 50 years, a debate ensued in the literature as to which was pre-eminent in controlling synchronous spike-wave discharge that characterized absence seizures: The cortex, the thalamus, or both. With the advent of number of animal models of generalized absence seizures, this controversy has been at least partially resolved.[210] Moreover, the availability of these models has advanced our understanding of the basic mechanisms of absence seizures. The unifying hypothesis coming from animal data and in vitro neurophysiologic data will be briefly summarized in this chapter.

Animal Models of Generalized Absence Seizures

A valid animal model of generalized absence seizures should reflect the clinical and pharmacologic characteristics of this disorder.[42,113,144,155] The criteria for animal models of absence seizures are EEG findings and behavior analogous to human absence epilepsy; reproducibility; predictability; ability to standardize and quantitate; attenuation or blockage by ethosuximide, trimethadione, valproic acid, and benzodiazepines; appropriate ontogeny; exacerbation by γ-aminobutyric acid (GABA)-ergic drugs; blockage by $GABA_B$ antagonists; spike-wave discharges that originate in the thalamus, cortex, or both; and hippocampus silent during seizure activity. There are two main genetic models of absence seizures in rats: WAG/Rij[46] and GAERS (genetic absence epilepsy rats from Strasbourg).[56] A number of other well-characterized genetic mouse models of absence seizures are reported. However, these models manifest a variety of neurologic abnormalities and in some cases other seizures types besides absence epilepsy. Several pharmacologic models of generalized absence seizures are described (γ-hydroxybutyrate [GHB], pentylenetetrazol, penicillin, etc.). These pharmacologic models are all electrographic models because bilaterally synchronous spike-wave discharges are observed.

Unifying Hypothesis

The animal data suggest that three interacting neuropharmacologic forces within the context of the thalamocortical circuitry are involved in the pathogenesis of absence seizures: (a) postsynaptic events required for the occurrence of generalized absence seizures are glutamate-mediated excitatory postsynaptic potentials (EPSPs) followed by $GABA_A$- and $GABA_B$-mediated inhibition that triggers a low-threshold calcium current in nuclear reticularis thalamus neurons; (b) the overall setpoint of thalamic and cortical excitability is modulated by means of ascending cholinergic pathways that project to the thalamus and noradrenergic and dopaminergic neurons projecting to the cortical end of the thalamocortical loop; and (c) presynaptic $GABA_B$ and GHB receptors may contribute to the regulation of thalamocortical rhythmicity by means of precise control of excitation and inhibition through modulation of GABA and glutamate release within the involved thalamocortical circuitry.

Genetic Identifiers of Animal Models of Absence Epilepsy

Studies have uncovered the causative genes for absencelike mice models. Tottering and leaner mice have defects in the calcium channel α subunit, lethargic mouse in the calcium channel β-4 gene, and stargazer and waggler mice in the calcium channel γ subunit gene. These mice mutants show some characteristics of absence epilepsy; however, all affected mice show some degree of cerebellar degeneration, which is quite different from human absence epilepsy.[110] Attempts to identify the genetic defects in calcium channel genes that underlie human absence epilepsy have so far failed.[201] Similar mutations of P/Q-type voltage-gated calcium channel CaV2.1 have been reported in a family with autosomal dominant transmission of absences and episodic ataxia.[114] Genetic studies in GAERS suggest a polygenic mode of inheritance of the EEG phenotype with at least three gene loci on chromosomes 4, 7, and 8.[197]

CLINICAL PRESENTATION

Childhood Absences

The age at onset of CAE is classically between 4 and 8 years, with a peak at 6 to 7 years, although some investigators have suggested a much wider range reflecting differences in definition criteria. For example, Janz et al.,[118] using frequency of absences as a selection criterion, found that pyknoleptic absences first occur at 3 to 16 years of age, with a peak at 7.5 years. Girls are affected twice as frequently as boys.

The description of Gowers[97] probably best describes the clinical manifestations of TA in CAE:

> "Transient loss of consciousness without conspicuous convulsions. A patient stops for a moment whatever he or she is doing, very often turns pale, may drop what ever is in the hand.... There may be a slight stoop forward, or a slight quivering of the eyelids.... The attack usually lasts only a few seconds. The return of the consciousness may be sudden and the patient after the momentary lapse, may

be in just the same state as before the attack, may even continue a sentence or action which was commenced before it came on, and suspended during the occurrence."

The absences of CAE are easily precipitated by hyperventilation,[34] which may be used during clinical examination for observation. They are easily studied with EEG because untreated children with CAE invariably manifest clinical absences with 3-Hz generalized spike and slow waves during well-performed overbreathing.

A typical case of CAE is of a girl with normal intelligence and development who at the age of 6 years started having absences with severe impairment of consciousness. They were brief, lasting around 8 seconds, and occurred many times (tens or hundred) per day. The EEG, as nearly always with CAE, demonstrated 3-Hz regular spike-and-slow-wave generalized discharges that were mainly provoked by hyperventilation.[33] Video-EEG confirmed exclusion and inclusion criteria for CAE. There was no evidence of photosensitivity. Cessation of seizures was achieved by administration of sodium valproate, but because of body weight increase this was changed to ethosuximide, which also successfully controlled her absences. Two years later, ethosuximide was gradually withdrawn. At 21 years of age, she is well, attends college, and plans to start a family.

Juvenile Absence Epilepsy

Age of onset is mostly in the range of 7 to 17 years with a peak at 10 to 12 years.[69,174,227,228] The seizure frequency is lower than in pyknolepsy, with clinical absences occurring less frequently than every day, mostly sporadically. The same types of absence occur as in CAE, but absences with retropulsive movements are less common. In one video-based study,[160,161] language functions in JAE absences were less rapidly abolished, consciousness was less severely impaired, and hyperventilation stopped later than in CAE. Spontaneous eye opening was rare, and simple absences were more common. However, this study is based on only three cases of JAE and is therefore not necessarily representative.

The majority of patients also have GTCSs, but it may be that the diagnosis is often missed if absences are the only seizure type. If the patients also have GTCSs, their manifestation precedes that of the absences more often than in CAE. Most frequently, they belong to the awakening type. Association with myoclonic seizures of the type seen in JME is more common than in CAE, probably in the order of 15% to 20%.

DIAGNOSTIC EVALUATION

Electroencephalographic Findings

Childhood Absence Epilepsy

Video-EEG studies showed that CAE demonstrates the following ictal symptoms[108]:

1. The impairment of consciousness is severe. There is no verbal or other response to commands, and recollection of verbal ictal events is lost.
2. The eyes are open, overbreathing stops, and speech discontinues within 3 seconds after the onset of the discharge.
3. Automatisms occur in two thirds of the seizures but are not stereotyped. The same patient may have simple and complex absences. Automatisms may be evoked by passive movements. Automatisms in absences indicate severe impairment of consciousness and do not occur in patients with mild impairment of cognition, even if the discharges last for more than 8 seconds.
4. Rhythmic blinking at 3 Hz is an infrequent, unsustained feature. The eyes may stare, but they also may move during the ictus, particularly if the child is loudly called by name.
5. Retropulsive movements of the eyes and head, which characterize eyelid myoclonia with absences, are not a usual clinical feature of CAE but may occur at the onset of the absence.
6. The duration of absences in CAE is shorter than in JAE (mean 12.4 and 16.3 seconds, respectively).

The clinical manifestations of CAE are associated with the following EEG features:

1. The interictal EEG is normal or shows rhythmic posterior delta activity. Occasionally, centrotemporal or occipital spikes may be seen.
2. The ictal EEG shows generalized, spike- or double-spike (no more than three spikes are seen)-and-slow-wave complexes at 3 Hz (no less than 2.7 Hz and no more than 4 Hz at the initial phase of the discharge with gradual and smooth decline in frequency from the initial to the terminal phase). The discharge is regular, with well-formed spikes that retain a constant relationship with the slow waves. The duration is usually around 10 to 12 seconds, no less than 4 seconds, and no more than 20 seconds (Fig. 1).

Partial seizures, myoclonic jerks, GTCSs, and other more bizarre fits have been described with absences starting in childhood (not necessarily CAE).[14,75] GTCSs occurring before the onset of TAs should not be accepted in CAE.

Juvenile Absence Epilepsy

In the EEG, the background activity is usually normal. The characteristic feature of the interictal and ictal EEG is generalized symmetric spike-and-waves discharge with frontal accentuation. The spike-and-waves frequency is usually faster than 3 Hz (3.5 to 4 Hz), the first complex of a group sometimes being even faster.[220] Often, the slow wave is preceded by two or three spikes. The above-mentioned preliminary study of Panayiotopoulos et al.[160] indicated that the ictal discharges may be longer in JAE (16.3 $\pm$ 7.1 seconds) than in CAE (12.4 $\pm$ 2.1 seconds) and in JME (6.6 $\pm$ 4.2 seconds). They were more regular than in JME but could show fragmentation unlike in CAE. In one study,[226] photosensitivity was less common than in other idiopathic generalized epilepsies, but this was not confirmed in the only other study.[220,229]

Neuroimaging

Functional imaging with positron emission tomography demonstrates normal cerebral glucose metabolism and benzodiazepine receptor density in absence epilepsies with diffuse hypermetabolism during 3-Hz spike-and-wave discharges.[71,188,198] There is no evidence of any interictal overall abnormality of opioid receptors, though typical absences have been found to displace 11 C-diprenorphine from the association areas of the neocortex. In contrast, binding of 11 C-flumazenil to cBZRs has been shown not to be affected by serial absences.[71] Functional MRI-EEG study of absences seizures in adult patients with JAE demonstrated bilateral activation of the thalamus and widespread deactivation of the cortex maximal in frontal regions.[6,124,199] Substraction interictal-ictal single photon emission computed tomography (SPECT) coregistered to MRI (SISCOM) was used to evaluate cerebral blood flow changes during the ictal and immediate postictal phase in four children with CAE.[153] The authors reported a widespread decrease of cerebral blood flow during ictal phase and an increase during post ictal phase. Those studies confirm in humans data observed in animal models, which suggest a crucial role of the thalamo-cortical loop and specific metabolic modifications during absence seizures.

DIFFERENTIAL DIAGNOSIS

The diagnosis of CAE may be difficult, even by specialists. Three child neurologists independently classified epilepsy syndromes in a cohort of children with newly diagnosed epilepsy and 7 of 74 CAEs were not diagnosed as such by one of the three.[18] In practical terms, a child suspected of typical absences should be asked to overbreathe for 3 minutes counting his or her breaths. Hyperventilation will provoke an absence in nearly all untreated children with CAE.[224] This procedure should preferably be videotaped for documentation of the clinical features.

CAE and JAE are epileptic syndromes that have to be distinguished from a variety of conditions such as nonepileptic manifestation (attention disturbance and daydreaming)[80] or focal epilepsies. Differential diagnosis of absence epilepsies from focal epilepsies should be easy, though alteration of consciousness and automatisms may be common in both. Temporomesial seizures could be characterized by staring and automatisms, reasons that in the past it was improperly called "pseudoabsences" or "temporal lobe absences." However, in temporal mesial seizures, loss of consciousness is preceded by vegetative aura; seizure ending could be characterized by postictal signs (asthenia, aphasia). A main problem is "typical absence seizures" from frontopolar lobe origin that may also have concomitant more or less regular bilateral 3-Hz spike-wave discharges.[75,77,219] Focal motor components, asymmetric ictal discharges, or stable interictal frontal foci in the EEG may help in their differentiation. MRI may demonstrate frontal abnormalities[77] or subependymal gray matter heterotopia.[190] However, rare focal EEG abnormalities are possible in CAE.[16,141,231] Loss of consciousness of milder intensity is observed during atypical absences in Lennox-Gastaut syndrome. Lennox-Gastaut syndrome is characterized by the association of atypical absences with tonic and atonic seizures, runs of rapid spikes in non-REM sleep, and status epilepticus. Resistance to therapy and persistence of epilepsy are among the most frequent features. Mental retardation is a leading symptom, occurring on average in 90% of cases.

Other Epilepsies with Typical Absence Seizures Starting in Childhood or Early Adolescence

The differentiation of CAE from other IGEs with absences may be difficult without video-EEG comparisons (Fig. 2). Eyelid myoclonia with absences is the easiest of all to differentiate from CAE because of brief, mainly eyelid myoclonia; minor impairment of consciousness; EEG generalized discharges of predominantly polyspikes; and photosensitivity. Myoclonic absence epilepsy and absences with perioral myoclonia have clinically apparent myoclonic jerks, and EEG discharges usually show polyspikes. The major problem is with JAE and JME that may start with typical absence seizures long before the appearance of myoclonic jerks and GTCSs.

Juvenile Myoclonic Epilepsy (Janz Syndrome)

Absence seizures occur in one third of JME patients, but these are usually very mild, are often inconspicuous, and have different EEG patterns.[100,160,165,167] The main seizure type of JME is myoclonic jerks upon awakening, and these do not occur in CAE. The problem is when JME starts with absences prior to the onset of myoclonic jerks, but again, there are a number of clinico-EEG differences such as milder impairment of consciousness, frequent polyspikes, and fragmentations of the EEG discharges in JME.[160,207] Some authors consider these cases as CAE evolving or progressing to JME.[58,223] In our opinion, this is JME starting with absences in childhood. In the majority of these patients with JME starting with TAs in childhood, video-EEG studies would clearly differentiate them from the TAs of CAE.[160] However, there may be cases where their differentiation is difficult and JME will not be diagnosed until many years after with the appearance of myoclonic jerks and GTCSs.

Absence Epilepsy of Early Childhood

A syndrome of absence epilepsy of early childhood was proposed in the 1960s[61] and later,[8,29,38,40,55,57,65] that included a heterogenous group of patients, some of whom had CAE. It was characterized by an onset before the age of 5 years; possible occurrence, at the onset or later, of GTCSs and/or myoclonic-astatic seizures; irregular 2- to 3-Hz spike-and-waves discharges on the EEG; and often an unfavorable prognosis. Later, its heterogeneity was admitted.[64] Age at onset artificially covers various idiopathic generalized epilepsies with a polygenic inheritance. Absence epilepsies of early childhood include early-onset CAE and other absence epilepsies in which more important environmental factors explain the frequency of GTCSs and a less favorable outcome. The "intermediate petit mal" described by the Bologna school[142] probably corresponds to similar situations.

Myoclonic Absence Epilepsy

This syndrome described by Tassinari et al.[214,215] is also incorporated in the ILAE Classification[48] as a rare generalized cryptogenic/symptomatic absence epilepsy. Severe bilateral rhythmic clonic jerks, often associated with a tonic contraction, occur during the absence.[143] Awareness of the jerks may be maintained. Seizures occur many times a day. Other types of seizures are rare. Age of onset is around 7 years, and there is a male preponderance. Prognosis is not good because of resistance to therapy, mental deterioration, and possible evolution to other types of epilepsy such as Lennox-Gastaut syndrome.[215]

Eyelid Myoclonia with Absences (Jeavons Syndrome)

The syndrome of eyelid myoclonia with absences was first described by Jeavons in 1977 as a form of photosensitive epilepsy[70,121] and was confirmed by other investigators.[12,13,15,55,79,90,91,96,99,103] Eyelid myoclonia with absences is frequently familial.[182] It is considered more a myoclonic than an absence syndrome.[177,213] The following definition was proposed by Panayiotopoulos[181]: Jeavons syndrome (eyelid myoclonia with absences) is an idiopathic epileptic syndrome manifested by frequent (pyknoleptic) seizures, consisting of eyelid myoclonia often associated with absences. Onset is usually in early childhood. The seizures are brief (3 to 6 seconds) and occur mainly after eye closure.[169,176,222] They consist of eyelid myoclonia, which persists throughout the attack with or without absences. Absences without eyelid myoclonia do not occur. The eyelid myoclonia consists of marked, rhythmic, and fast jerks of the eyelids, often associated with jerky upward deviation of the eyeballs and retropulsion of the head. There is probably an associated tonic component of the involved muscles. If the seizure is prolonged, impairment of consciousness occurs. The latter is mild or moderately severe

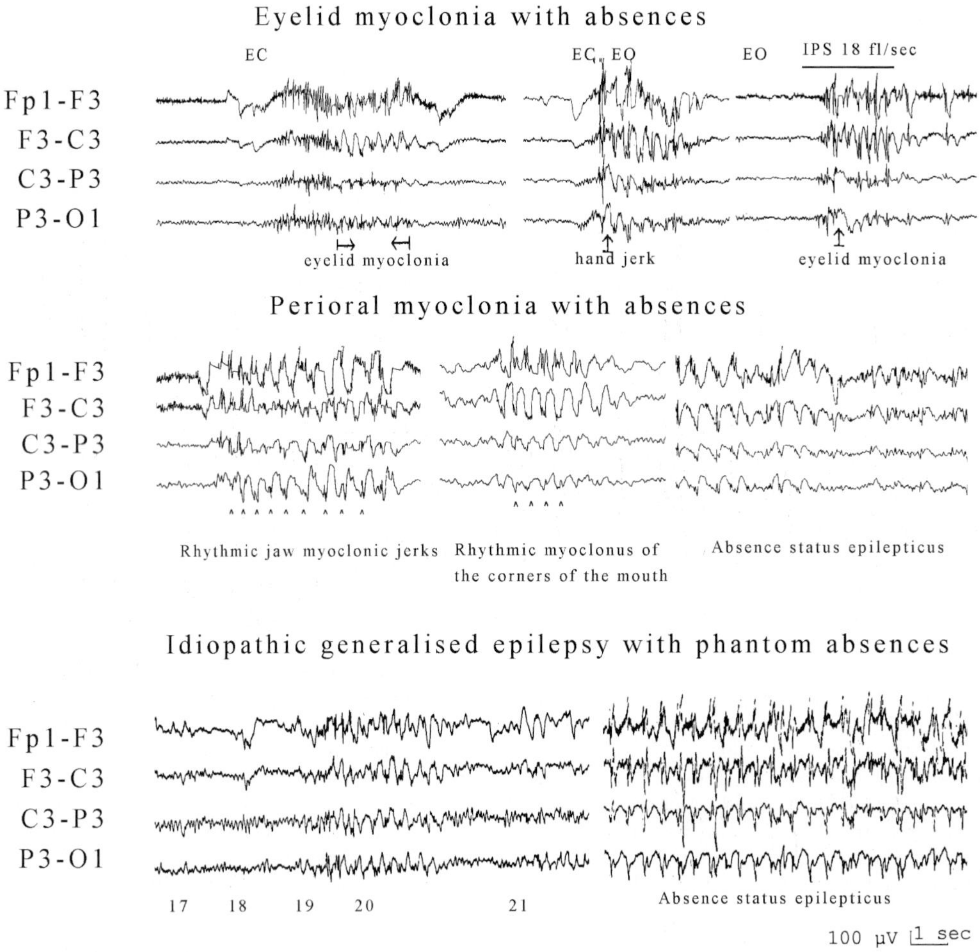

FIGURE 2. Video-electroencephalographic (EEG) recordings. **Upper left:** Brief ictal discharges consisting mainly of polyspikes and slow waves are induced after eye closure in a 32-year-old woman with eyelid myoclonia with absences (EMA). They are associated with eyelid myoclonus and occasionally mild impairment of consciousness. Similar abnormalities are seen in a 17-year-old girl on eye closure (**middle**) and intermittent photic stimulation (**right**). In the latter case, mild myoclonic jerks of the hands also were seen. Details of these patients have been reported by Giannakodimos and Panayiotopoulos.[50] **Middle left:** Rhythmic jaw jerking (annotated with *arrows*) with mild impairment of consciousness were the characteristic clinical features during these brief discharges in an 18-year-old woman with intractable absences, generalized tonic–clonic seizures (GTCSs), jerks, and possible absence status. Similar EEG abnormalities associated with rhythmic contractions of the depressor anguli oris were recorded in a 37-year-old man with infrequent absence status followed by GTCSs (**middle**). An episode of absence status with perioral myoclonia and cloudiness of consciousness ending in a GTCS was recorded via EEG in a 29-year-old woman with frequent absences and absence status with GTCSs (**right**). Details of these patients have been reported by Panayiotopoulos et al.[102,103] **Lower right:** Phantom absences manifested with delays in counting during overbreathing (numbers) in a 17-year-old girl with a single GTCS at 17 years of age (**left**). Similar brief and mild absences were recorded in another 56-year-old woman who also had two episodes of de novo absence status of late onset (**right**). Details for these patients have been reported by Panayiotopoulos et al.[106]

without associated automatisms. Milder seizures of eyelid myoclonia without absences are common, particularly in adults and treated patients, and may occur without EEG accompaniments. All patients are highly photosensitive in childhood, but this declines with age. Infrequent GTCSs, either induced by lights or spontaneous, are probably inevitable in the long term and are likely to occur after sleep deprivation, fatigue, and alcohol indulgence. Myoclonic jerks of the limbs may occur, but are infrequent and random. The eyelid myoclonia of Jeavons syndrome is resistant to treatment and may be lifelong. However, clinical absences may become less frequent with age.

The EEG ictal manifestations consist mainly of generalized polyspike-waves at 3 to 6 Hz, which are more likely to occur after eye closure in an illuminated room. Total darkness abolishes the abnormalities related to eye closure. Photoparoxysmal responses are recorded from all untreated young patients.

Perioral Myoclonia with Absences

Panayiotopoulos et al.[168] reported that TAs associated with marked perioral myoclonia may constitute a new epilepsy syndrome defined as follows:

> Perioral myoclonus with absences is a syndrome of idiopathic generalized epilepsy with onset in childhood or adolescence, characterized by frequent typical absences with variable severity of impairment of consciousness and ictal localized rhythmic myoclonus of

the perioral facial muscles (lip myoclonus) or occasionally of the masticatory muscles (jaw myoclonus). TA duration is usually brief, ranging from 2 to 10 seconds. Ictal EEG shows generalized discharges of spikes, more often irregular polyspikes and slow waves at 3 to 5 Hz. They are not associated with eye closure and photosensitivity. Perioral myoclonia with absences often associates with absence status.[5] GTCSs always occur either early or several years after the onset of TA; they are usually heralded by clusters of TAs or absence status and may be infrequent. The syndrome is lifelong and often resistant to medication. A family history of epilepsy is common.[181]

Lips and chin myoclonia are by themselves insufficient symptoms to justify a syndromic individualization, because of a possible moderate myoclonic component in CAE and JAE.[37,108] However, a unique combination of characteristic clinico-EEG features is likely in perioral myoclonia with absences.

Phantom Absences and Generalized Tonic–Clonic Seizures

Phantom absences is the term we have coined to denote TAs that are so mild that they are inconspicuous to the patient and imperceptible to the observer.[76,88,180] They have been known for many years as "subclinical or larval absences."[1] The absences are simple, occasionally with eyelid blinking. They are common in patients with idiopathic generalized epilepsies but are often unrecognized. Based on patient information, the absences often start after patients' teen years. The absences were shown on video-EEG recordings with breath counting and consisted of brief (3 to 4 seconds) generalized discharges of 3- to 4-Hz spikes or multiple spike-and-slow-wave discharges, during which mild impairment of cognition manifested with consistent errors and discontinuation of breath counting. Absence status occurred, either in isolation or terminating in GTCSs.[209] In these patients GTCSs were consistently preceded by absence status. After recognition of this sequence, GTCSs were often preventable with rectal benzodiazepine, self-administered while in absence status. Long-term prognosis may be the same as in other syndromes of IGE with TAs and GTCSs. In view of the high incidence of absence status, patients should be advised to use rectal diazepam.

Symptomatic Absence Seizures

In genetically predisposed individuals, brain damage may precipitate TA occurrence, most often associated with neurologic signs and/or mental retardation. This category comprised 10% of patients with TA in a Swedish population-based study.[158] Ferrie et al.[77] made a list of diffuse and focal cerebral pathologies in which TAs have been reported. They are as follows, in alphabetic order: Arteriovenous malformations, autism, biochemical disturbances, brain tumors, cerebral abscess, congenital microcephaly, craniostenosis, Down syndrome, drugs/drug withdrawal, encephalitides, endocrine disturbances, head injury, hemiplegia, hydrocephalus, hypothalamic lesions,[152] juvenile Batten disease, mitochondrial encephalopathies, neonatal intracranial hemorrhage, precocious puberty, progressive myoclonic epilepsy, Sturge-Weber syndrome, subacute sclerosing panencephalitis, tuberculous meningitis, and tuberous sclerosis. Most of these reports are old and, hence, poorly documented, and one may wonder how many patients fitted with CAE characteristics. Subtentorial lesions[189,191] are noteworthy, because they may disturb the corticothalamic oscillatory networks. Prognosis is that of the underlying pathology. In most cases, the association is probably coincidental. However, cerebral pathology may modify the expression of genetic seizure susceptibility.[77] In these cases, the correct diagnosis is not CAE, but symptomatic absence epilepsy, with a less favorable outcome.

TREATMENT AND OUTCOME

Childhood Absence Epilepsy

Childhood absence epilepsy needs treatment because absences are very frequent throughout the day and may adversely affect cognitive functioning.[32,68] However, clinicians should avoid overtreatment with antiepileptic drugs (AEDs), which may induce cognitive side effects. First-line drugs are ethosuximide, sodium valproate, and lamotrigine, alone or in combination.[78,164,195] Clonazepam, clobazam, and acetazolamide are second-line drugs for CAE, sharing a similar risk of tolerance and adverse effects.[98,179] Amantadine could be effective in association as a third-line drug in pharmacoresistent absence epilepsies with few adverse events. Despite this clear-cut evidence of antiabsence drug efficacy, many children with typical absence seizures would still be treated with inappropriate drugs.[183] Sodium valproate controls absences in 75% of patients[22] and has the advantage also of controlling generalized tonic–clonic seizures (70%) and myoclonic jerks (75%), but may be undesirable for women. Rare cases of paradoxical aggravation in CAE with valproate have been reported; this might be related to a genetic heterogeneity of CAE.[129] Similarly, lamotrigine may control absences in possibly 50% to 60% and GTCSs in 50% to 60%, but may worsen myoclonic jerks; hypersensitivity immune reaction are possible.[49,50,82,89] Ethosuximide controls 70% of absences, but it is undesirable as monotherapy if other generalized seizures are at risk. Combination of any of these three drugs may be needed for resistant cases. Minute doses of lamotrigine added to sodium valproate may have a dramatic beneficial effect. Clonazepam, particularly in absences with myoclonic components, acetazolamide, and amantadine may be useful adjunctive drugs. Diones are no longer used.[186] Conversely, carbamazepine, vigabatrin, gabapentin, and tiagabine are contraindicated because of their proabsence effect.[39] Phenytoin and phenobarbital are contraindicated because of their usual inefficacy.[179,181] The place of topiramate, levetiracetam, and vagal nerve stimulation is still unknown.

Monotherapy with sodium valproate, ethosuximide, or lamotrigine should be the choice and should not be abandoned before making sure that the maximum tolerated dose has been achieved if smaller doses have failed. There are anecdotal reports whereby children may not respond to syrup of sodium valproate despite adequate levels, but seizures stop if this is replaced by tablets or microspheres of sodium valproate. If monotherapy fails or unacceptable adverse reactions appear, then replacement of one by the other is the alternative. The best possible combination is adding small, minute doses of lamotrigine to adequate doses of sodium valproate. Gradual withdrawal of medication is recommended in patients with CAE who are seizure free for 1 to 2 years and have a normalized EEG. EEG confirmation of the seizure-free state is needed during this withdrawal period.

Juvenile Absence Epilepsy

First-line drugs are sodium valproate and lamotrigine, alone or in combination. When there is concern about teratogenicity, lamotrigine can be given as first-line monotherapy,[82] although onset of action is much slower compared to valproate.[49] There is at present no study specifically investigating the newer AEDs such as topiramate and levetiracetam in JAE. Carbamazepine and oxcarbazepine may aggravate the seizures of JAE.[87]

LONG-TERM PROGNOSIS

Childhood Absence Epilepsy

Most of the available evidence is inconclusive regarding evolution and prognosis of CAE. This is because of markedly different classification criteria in the relevant reports or of too-short follow-up periods. Most authors include in CAE any child with absences before the age of 10 years, which may not be CAE.[19,31,140,181] Retrospective studies in adults may lack accurate initial data. Patients must be followed beyond 18 or 20 years of age.[132,136,138] Our view is that CAE, if properly defined, has an excellent prognosis.

Prognosis of Typical Absence Seizures

At a time when no antiabsence drug existed, Adie[2] concluded that even if absence seizures in pyknolepsy persisted for a long time, they ultimately ceased, never to return. This is consistent with recent findings that absences of CAE, even if they may persist several years, finally disappear with age in more than 90% of cases.[132,136,138,202,203] In a Swedish population-based study, a 91% remission rate was found when patients with absence epilepsy had only absences.[105]

Typical absence seizures persist for a mean time of 6.6 years[53] and disappear between age 3 and 19 years, with a mean age of 10.5[107] or 14 years.[53] "The tendency for petit mal to cease is present at all ages and not just at puberty. In about a quarter of patients the attacks cease before the age of 15 and by the age of 30 years petit mal had ceased in about three quarters of the patients."[92,93] In this study, with a follow-up of about 5 years, only 3% of patients experienced TAs beyond 50 years of age. In another study,[130] of the 92 controlled patients, 89 were aged 20 or younger at the time of cessation of absence seizures.

Thus, TA persistence is rare, reported to occur in about 6% of patients.[157] In adults, attacks tend to be infrequent and milder, and occur with precipitating factors such as fatigue, sleep deprivation, and menstruation,[53,86,161,181] though in some cases absences may be very severe.[5]

Two favorable prognostic signs are age at onset of TAs and medication efficacy. In patients diagnosed early and followed beyond 20 years of age, TAs had disappeared in 95% and 90% of cases according to an age at onset of 8 or 10 years, respectively.[135,136] Their cessation soon after prescription of a convenient antiepileptic drug is considered as a favorable sign.[53,131]

Generalized Tonic–Clonic Seizures

However, cessation of absence seizures may not mean remission. This again depends on diagnostic inclusion and exclusion criteria. Considering all absences with onset in childhood as CAE, prognosis is uncertain and with great variations.[31,181] GTCSs may appear and patients may develop juvenile myoclonic epilepsy.[223] Absence seizures in these patients may persist, improve, or disappear.

It has been estimated that GTCSs occurs in 36% to 60% of patients with onset of TAs in childhood.[53,130] Most often, GTCSs occur 5 to 10 years after onset of TAs,[132] that is, mainly between 8 and 15 years of age,[43,60,130] and sometimes beyond 20 and even 30 years of age.[86] They have been considered as infrequent and easily controlled.

Different risk factors have been suggested, as follows:

- Age at onset of TAs: The later the onset of TAs, the higher the risk is for subsequent convulsive seizures.[20,43,51,54,102,127,130]
- Absence status, especially when absences occur late in the course of epilepsy,[60] but this may not be childhood absence epilepsy.[3,4,5,104]
- Sex: TAs are more frequent in girls and TAs + GTCSs are more frequent in boys.[157]
- EEG: Usually, clinical/EEG correlation is fair. However, the predictive value of the EEG is not absolute; spike-wave discharges may persist after clinical recovery, and conversely GTCSs may occur in spite of a normalized EEG.[105] When initial tracings show posterior delta rhythms, GTCSs rarely occur.[45,105,157] An abnormal background activity, multiple spikes,[74] and focal abnormalities are considered as unfavorable signs, but are likely to correspond to erroneous diagnoses.
- Therapy: With an early institution of effective therapy, GTCSs occurred in 30% of cases, and 68% after incorrect therapy.[20] GTCSs manifested in 85% of incorrectly treated patients.[60]

A change of CAE into epilepsy with focal seizures has been reported. It probably corresponds to erroneous diagnosis: Either TAs with automatisms or absence epilepsy other than CAE such as in febrile seizures plus.[123]

Complete Remission

A wide range of remission rates has been given: 78% to 33%. The reasons for this are as follows: (a) patients with absence epilepsies other than CAE were included; (b) patients' age at last clinic visit, with, for instance, inclusion of 82% of patients when beyond 18 years of age but only 65% in those beyond 20[60]; (c) follow-up duration, with relapse in 19% of patients who had been seizure free for 2 years or more; and (d) therapy[60]: With early and adequate therapy, 70% of patients were included, whereas 18% with an incorrect therapy were included.[20]

Social Prognosis

Social adaptation of patients having had CAE would be poor in one third of patients, even when in remission.[60,102,107,142] In childhood absence epilepsy, TAs are very frequent and the EEG shows brief discharges of bilateral spike-waves without apparent clinical impairment. Neuropsychological studies have documented cognitive dysfunctioning (reaction time tasks and sustained attention tests) during these discharges. "The transitory bursts of spike-wave activity represent the tip of an iceberg. Below the surface there may be a more or less continuously active pathophysiological process, which is reflected in impaired performance on tests of attention and in alterations in event-related brain potentials."[150,151] Therefore, long-term sequelae of scholastic difficulties are not surprising. Furthermore, a psychomotor slowing beginning late in follow-up has been found in some patients with TAs persisting after the age of 30 to 61 years.[86] It was supposed to be multifactorial in origin.

Juvenile Absence Epilepsy

The response to therapy is good in spite of the frequent combination with GTCSs. Wolf and Inoue,[230] in their cross-sectional study of 229 adolescents and adults who had a diagnosis of absences and still were in treatment, reported that all were seizure free if they had only had absences (n = 21), and 87% were seizure free if there had not been more than ten GTCSs. If there were more GTCSs (which was the case in 123 patients), the response was still very good, but 24% were not seizure free. The response was better in JAE (85% seizure free) than in CAE (80%, $p < 0.02$), and combination with myoclonic seizures did not affect the therapy prognosis. In these patients, the absences were mostly treated with ethosuximide, valproate, or both—and in some cases with mesuximide—and if necessary the doses were increased to the maximum the patients could tolerate. If GTCSs were present, these were often treated with an additional drug, especially with succinimide treatment for absences. In the study of Trinka et al.,[218] 40 (62%) of 64 JAE patients were seizure free for at least 2 years, which was almost similar to the seizure-free rate of CAE patients (56%).

SUMMARY AND CONCLUSIONS

Childhood absence epilepsy is an idiopathic generalized epilepsy that should not be equated with any type of absences first appearing in childhood. It may be as benign as the benign childhood partial seizures,[163] but further prospective studies must be conducted with strict clinico-EEG criteria of the classification. A better definition of CAE and related syndromes allows a better classification of patients with idiopathic absence epilepsies. However, 33% of patients are still difficult to classify.[101] This syndromic approach is necessary for the improvement of genetic and pharmacologic studies. Juvenile absence epilepsy is an idiopathic form of epilepsy that is probably lifelong. It is characterized by frequent absences with severe impairment of consciousness (imitating CAE) associated with GTCSs and occasionally with myoclonic jerks (imitating JME). Thus, the phenotypic manifestations of JAE are intermediate between CAE and JME. Whether this is also the case for their genotypes remains to be seen. Incidence, prevalence, long-term prognosis, genetics, and what is the most realistic treatment (which may be lifelong) need to be studied.

References

1. Aarts HR, Binnie CD, Smit AM, et al. Selective cognitive impairment during focal and generalised epileptiform EEG activity. *Brain*. 1984;107:293–308.
2. Adie WJ. Pyknolepsy: a form of epilepsy occurring in children with a good prognosis. *Brain*. 1924;47:96–102.
3. Agathonikou A, Giannakodimos S, Koutroumanidis M, et al. Idiopathic generalised epilepsies in adults with onset of typical absences before the age of 10 years. *Epilepsia*. 1997;38(Suppl 3):213.
4. Agathonikou A, Koutroumanidis M, Panayiotopoulos CP. Fixation-off sensitive epilepsy with absences and absence status: video EEG documentation. *Neurology*. 1997;48:231–234.
5. Agathonikou A, Panayiotopoulos CP, Giannakodimos S, et al. Typical absence status in adults: diagnostic and syndromic considerations. *Epilepsia*. 1998;39:1265–1276.
6. Aghakhani Y, Bagshaw AP, Benar CG, et al. fMRI activation during spike and wave discharges in idiopathic generalized epilepsy. *Brain*. 2004;127:1127–1144.
7. Aicardi J. Epilepsies with typical absence seizures. In: Aicardi J, ed. *Epilepsy in Children*. New York: Raven Press; 1994:94–117.
8. Aicardi J. Typical absences in the first two years of life. In: Duncan JS, Panayiotopoulos CP, eds. *Typical Absences and Related Epileptic Syndromes*. London: Churchill Livingstone; 1995:284–288.
9. Andermann E. Genetic aspects of epilepsy. In: Robb P, ed. *Epilepsy Updated: Causes and Treatment*. New York: Year Book Medical Publisher; 1980:11–24.
10. Andermann E. The genetics of typical absences-future directions-consensus statement. In: Duncan JS, Panayiotopoulos CP, eds. *Typical Absences and Related Epileptic Syndromes*. London: Churchill Livingstone; 1995:338–343.
11. Andermann F. Typical absences are all part of the same disease. In: Duncan JS, Panayiotopoulos CP, eds. *Typical Absences and Related Epileptic Syndromes*. London: Churchill Livingstone; 1995:300–304.
12. Appleton RE, Panayiotopoulos CP, Acomb BA, et al. Eyelid myoclonia with typical absences: an epilepsy syndrome. *J Neurol Neurosurg Psychiatry*. 1993;56:1312–1316.
13. Appleton RE. Eyelid myoclonia with absences. In: Duncan JS, Panayiotopoulos CP, eds. *Typical Absences and Related Epileptic Syndromes*. London: Churchill Livingstone; 1995:213–220.
14. Audic-Gerard F, Szepetowski P, Genton P. GEFS + syndrome: phenotypic variations from the newborn to the adult in a large French pedigree. *Rev Neurol (Paris)*. 2003;159:189–195.
15. Barclay CL, Murphy WF, Lee MA, et al. Unusual form of seizures induced by eye closure. *Epilepsia*. 1993;34:289–290.
16. Beaumanoir A, Ballis T, Varfis G, et al. Benign epilepsy of childhood with rolandic spikes. *Epilepsia*. 1974;15:301–315.
17. Beck-Mannagetta G, Janz D, Hoffmeister U, et al. Morbidity risk for seizures and epilepsy in offsprings of patients with epilepsy. In: Beck-Mannagetta G, Anderson WE, Doose H, et al., eds. *Genetics of the Epilepsies*. Berlin Heidelberg: Springer-Verlag; 1989:119–126.
18. Berg AT, Levy SR, Testa FM, et al. Classification of childhood epilepsy syndromes in newly diagnosed epilepsy: interrated agreement and reasons for disagreement. *Epilepsia*. 1999;40:439–444.
19. Berg AT, Shinnar S, Levy SR, et al. How well can epilepsy syndromes be identified at diagnosis? A reassessment two years after initial diagnosis. *Epilepsia*. 2000;41:1267–1275.
20. Bergamini L, Bram S, Broglia S, et al. L'insorgenza tardiva di crisi Grande Male nel Piccolo Male puro. Studio catamnestico di 78 casi. *Arch Suisses Neurol Neurochir Psychiatr*. 1965;96:306–317.
21. Berkovic SF, Andermann F, Andermann E, et al. Concepts of absence epilepsies: discrete syndromes or biological continuum? *Neurology*. 1987;37:993–1000.
22. Berkovic SF, Andermann F, Gubbermann A, et al. Valproate prevents the recurrence of absence status epilepticus. *Neurology*. 1989;39:1294–1297.
23. Berkovic SF. Generalised absence seizures. In: Wyllie E, ed. *The Treatment of Epilepsy: Principles and Practice*. Philadelphia: Lea & Febiger; 1993:401–410.
24. Berkovic S. Lessons from twin studies. In: Wolf P, ed. *Epileptic Seizures and Syndromes*. London: John Libbey; 1994:155–164.
25. Berkovic S, Reutens DC, Andermann E, et al. The epilepsies: specific syndromes or a neurobiological continuum? In: Wolf P, ed. *Epileptic Seizures and Syndromes*. London: John Libbey; 1994:25–37.
26. Berkovic SF, Howell RA, Hay DA, et al. Epilepsy in twins. In: Wolf P, ed. *Epileptic Seizures and Syndromes*. London: John Libbey and Co; 1994:157–164.
27. Berkovic SF. Childhood absence epilepsy and juvenile absence epilepsy. In: Wyllie E, ed. *The Treatment of Epilepsy: Principles and Practice*. Baltimore: Williams & Wilkins; 1996:461–466.
28. Bianchi A, the Italian League Against Epilepsy Collaborative Group. Study of concordance of symptoms in families with absence epilepsies. In: Duncan JS, Panayiotopoulos CP, eds. *Typical Absences and Related Epileptic Syndromes*. London: Churchill Livingstone; 1995:328–337.
29. Binnie CD, Jeavons PM. Photosensitive epilepsies. In: Roger J, Bureau M, Dravet C, et al., eds. *Epileptic Syndromes in Infancy, Childhood and Adolescence*. London: John Libbey; 1992:299–305.
30. Blom S, Heijbel J, Bergfors PG. Incidence of epilepsy in children: a follow-up study three years after the first seizure. *Epilepsia*. 1978;19:343–350.
31. Bouma PA, Westendorp RG, van Dijk JG, et al. The outcome of absence epilepsy: a meta-analysis. *Neurology*. 1996;47:802–808.
32. Brodie MJ. The treatment of typical absences and related epileptic syndromes-consensus statement. In: Duncan JS, Panayiotopoulos CP, eds. *Typical Absences and Related Epileptic Syndromes*. London: Churchill Livingstone; 1995:381–383.
33. Browne TR, Dreifuss FE, Penry JK, et al. Clinical and EEG estimates of absence seizure frequency. *Arch Neurol*. 1983;40:469–472.
34. Bureau M, Guey J, Dravet C, et al. Etude de la répartition des absences chez l'enfant en fonction de ses activités. *Rev Neurol (Paris)*. 1968;118: 493–494.
35. Calmeil LF. *De l'épilepsie etudiée sous le rapport de son siège et de son influence sur la production de l'aliénation mentale*. Paris: Thèse; 1924.
36. Callenbach PMC, Geerts AT, Arts WFM, et al. Familial occurrence of epilepsy in children with newly diagnosed multiple seizures: Dutch study of epilepsy in childhood. *Epilepsia*. 1998;39:331–336.
37. Capovilla G, Rubboli G, Beccaria F, et al. A clinical spectrum of the myoclonic manifestations associated with typical absences in childhood absence epilepsy. A video-polygraphic study. *Epileptic Disord*. 2001;3: 57–62.
38. Cavazzuti GB, Ferrari F, Galli V, et al. Epilepsy with typical absences with onset during the first year of life. *Epilepsia*. 1989;30:802–806.
39. Chadwick D. Gabapentin and felbamate. In: Duncan JS, Panayiotopoulos CP, eds. *Typical Absences and Related Epileptic Syndromes*. London: Churchill Livingstone; 1995:376–380.
40. Chaix Y, Daquin G, Monteiro F, et al. Absence epilepsy with onset before age three years: a heterogeneous and often severe condition. *Epilepsia*. 2003;44:944–949.
41. Chan CH, Briellmann R, Pell GS, et al. Thalamic atrophy in childhood absence epilepsy. *Epilepsia*. 2006;47:399–405.
42. Chapman AG. Anti-epileptic drugs in animal models-consensus statement. In: Duncan JS, Panayiotopoulos CP, eds. *Typical Absences and Related Epileptic Syndromes*. London: Churchill Livingstone; 1995:69–73.
43. Charlton MH, Yahr MD. Long term follow-up of patients with petit mal. *Arch Neurol*. 1967;16:595–598.

44. Chen Y, Lu J, Pan H, et al. Association between genetic variation of CACNA1H and childhood absence epilepsy. *Ann Neurol.* 2003;54:239–243.
45. Cobb WA, Gordon N, Matthews SC, et al. The occipital delta rhythm in petit mal. *Electroencephalogr Clin Neurophysiol.* 1961;13:142–143.
46. Coenen AM, Van Luijtelaar EL. Genetic animal models for absence epilepsy: a review of the WAG/Rij strain of rats. *Behav Genet.* 2003;33:635–655.
47. Commission on Classification and Terminology of the International League Against Epilepsy. Proposal for revised clinical and electroencephalographic classification of epileptic seizures. *Epilepsia.* 1981;22:489–501.
48. Commission on Classification and Terminology of the International League Against Epilepsy. Proposal for revised classification of epilepsies and epileptic syndromes. *Epilepsia.* 1989;3:389–399.
49. Coppola G, Auricchio G, Federico F, et al. Lamotrigine versus valproic acid as first-line monotherapy in newly diagnosed typical absence seizures: an open-label, randomized, parallel-group study. *Epilepsia.* 2004;45:1049–1053.
50. Coppola G, Licciardi F, Sciscio N, et al. Lamotrigine as first-line drug in childhood absence epilepsy: a clinical and neurophysiological study. *Brain Dev.* 2004;26:26–29.
51. Covanis A, Skiadas K, Loli N, et al. Absence epilepsy: early prognostic signs. *Seizure.* 1992;1:281–289.
52. Crunelli V, Leresche N. Childhood absence epilepsy: genes, channels, neurons and networks. *Nat Rev Neurosci.* 2002;3:371–382.
53. Currier RD, Kooi KA, Saidman J. Prognosis of pure petit mal: a follow-up study. *Neurology.* 1963;13:959–967.
54. Dalby MA. Epilepsy and 3 per second spike and wave rhythms. A clinical, electroencephalographic and prognostic analysis of 346 patients. *Acta Neurol Scand Suppl.* 1969;40:181–183.
55. Dalla Bernardina B, Sgro V, Fontana F, et al. Eyelid myoclonias with absences. In: Beaumanoir A, Gastaut H, Naquet R, eds. *Reflex Seizures and Reflex Epilepsies.* Geneva, Switzerland: Medecine et Hygiene; 1989:193–200.
56. Danober L, Deransart C, Depaulis A, et al. Pathophysiological mechanisms of genetic absence epilepsy in the rat. *Prog Neurobiol.* 1998;55:27–57.
57. Darra F, Fontana E, Scaramuzzi V, et al. Typical absence seizures in the first three years of life: electroclinical study of 31 cases. *Epilepsia.* 1996;37(Suppl 4):95.
58. Delgado-Escueta AV, Medina MT, Serratosa JM, et al. Mapping and positional cloning of common idiopathic generalized epilepsies: juvenile myoclonus epilepsy and childhood absence epilepsy. *Adv Neurol.* 1999;79:351–374.
59. De Marco P. Eyelid myoclonia with absences in two monovular twins. *Clin Electroencephalogr.* 1989;20:193–195.
60. Dieterich E, Baier WK, Doose H, et al. Long term follow-up of childhood epilepsy with absences. I. Epilepsy with absences at onset. *Neuropediatrics.* 1985;16:149–154.
61. Doose H, Volzke E, Scheffner D. Verlaufsformen kindlicher epilepsien mit spike wave-absencen. *Arch Psychiatr Nervenkr.* 1965;207:394–415.
62. Doose H, Gerken H, Horstmann T, et al. Genetic factors in spike-wave absences. *Epilepsia.* 1973;14:57–75.
63. Doose H, Baier WK. Generalized spikes and waves. In: Beck-Managetta G, Andewn VE, Doose H, et al., eds. *Genetics of the Epilepsies.* Berlin: Springer; 1989:95–103.
64. Doose H. Absence epilepsy of early childhood—genetic aspects. *Eur J Pediatr.* 1994;153:372–377.
65. Doose H. Discussion: absence epilepsy of early childhood. In: Wolf P, ed. *Epileptic Seizures and Syndromes.* London: John Libbey; 1994:133–135.
66. Dreifuss FE. Absence epilepsies. In: Dam M, Gram L, eds. *Comprehensive Epileptology.* New York: Raven Press; 1991:145–153.
67. Dreifuss FE. Historical aspects of typical absences and related epileptic syndromes. In: Duncan JS, Panayiotopoulos CP, eds. *Typical Absences and Related Epileptic Syndromes.* London: Churchill Livingstone; 1995: 1–7.
68. Duncan JS. Treatment strategies for typical absences and related epileptic syndromes. In: Duncan JS, Panayiotopoulos CP, eds. *Typical Absences and Related Epileptic Syndromes.* London: Churchill Livingstone; 1995:354–360.
69. Duncan JS, Panayiotopoulos CP. Juvenile absence epilepsy: an alternative view. In: Duncan JS, Panayiotopoulos CP, eds. *Typical Absences and Related Epileptic Syndromes.* London: Churchill Livingstone; 1995:167–173.
70. Duncan JS, Panayiotopoulos CP. The differentiation of 'eye-closure' from 'eyes-closed' EEG abnormalities and their relation to photo- and fixation-off sensitivity. In: Duncan JS, Panayiotopoulos CP, eds. *Eyelid Myoclonia with Absences.* London: John Libbey & Company Ltd.; 1996: 77–87.
71. Duncan JS. Positron emission tomography receptor studies. *Adv Neurol.* 1999;79:893–899.
72. Escayg A, De Waard M, Lee D, et al. Coding and noncoding variation of the human calcium-channel beta4-subunit gene CACNB4 in patient with idiopathic generalized epilepsy and episodic ataxia. *Am J Hum Genet.* 2000;66:1531–1539.
73. Esquirol J. De l'épilepsie. In: *Traité des maladies mentales.* Vol. I. Paris: Baillière Publishers; 1838:274–355.
74. Fakhoury T, Abou-Khalil B. Generalized absence seizures with 10–15 Hz fast discharges. *Clin Neurophysiol.* 1999;110:1029–1035.
75. Fegersten L, Roger J. Frontal epileptogenic foci and their clinical correlations. *Electroencephalogr Clin Neurophysiol.* 1961;13:905–913.
76. Ferner R, Panayiotopoulos CP. "Phantom" typical absences, absence status and experiential phenomena. *Seizure.* 1993;2:253–256.
77. Ferrie CD, Giannakodimos S, Robinson RO, et al. Symptomatic typical absence seizures. In: Duncan JS, Panayiotopoulos CP, eds. *Typical Absences and Related Epileptic Syndromes.* London: Churchill Livingstone; 1995:241–252.
78. Ferrie CD, Robinson RO, Knott C, et al. Lamotrigine as an add-on drug in typical absence seizures. *Acta Neurol Scand.* 1995;91:200–202.
79. Ferrie CD, Agathonikou A, Parker A, et al. The spectrum of childhood epilepsies with eyelid myoclonia with absences. In: Duncan JS, Panayiotopoulos CP, eds. *Eyelid Myoclonia with Absences.* London: John Libbey & Company Ltd.; 1996:39–48.
80. Fish DR. Blank spells that are not typical absences. In: Duncan JS, Panayiotopoulos CP, eds. *Typical Absences and Related Epileptic Syndromes.* London: Churchill Livingstone; 1995:253–262.
81. Fong GC, Shah PU, Gee MN, et al. Childhood absence epilepsy with tonic-clonic seizures and electroencephalogram 3–4-Hz spike and multispike-slow wave complexes: linkage to chromosome 8q24. *Am J Hum Genet.* 1998;63:1117–1129.
82. Frank LM, Enlow T, Holmes GL, et al. Lamictal (lamotrigine) monotherapy for typical absence seizures in children. *Epilepsia.* 1999;40:973–979.
83. Friedmann M. Uber die nichtepileptischen Absencen oder kurzen narkoleptischen Anfalle. *Dtsch Z Nervenheilkd.* 1906;30:462–492.
84. Gardiner M. Genetics of human typical absence syndromes. In: Duncan JS, Panayiotopoulos CP, eds. *Typical Absences and Related Epileptic Syndromes.* London: Churchill Livingstone; 1995:320–327.
85. Gastaut H. Clinical and EEG classification of epileptic seizures. *Epilepsia.* 1970;17:102–113.
86. Gastaut H, Zifkin BG, Mariani E, et al. The long-term course of primary generalized epilepsy with persisting absences. *Neurology.* 1986;36:1021–1028.
87. Gelisse P, Genton P, Kuate C, et al. Worsening of seizures by oxcarbazepine in juvenile idiopathic generalized epilepsies. *Epilepsia.* 2004;45:1282–1286.
88. Genton P. Epilepsy with 3-Hz spike-and-waves without clinically evident absences. In: Duncan JS, Panayiotopoulos CP, eds. *Typical Absences and Related Epileptic Syndromes.* London: Churchill Livingstone; 1995:231–238.
89. Gericke CA, Picard F, de Saint-Martin A, et al. Efficacy of lamotrigine in idiopathic generalized epilepsy syndromes: a video-EEG-controlled, open study. *Epileptic Disord.* 1999;1:159–165.
90. Giannakodimos S, Panayiotopoulos CP. Eyelid myoclonia with absences in adults: a clinical and video-EEG study in adults. *Epilepsia.* 1996;37:36–44.
91. Giannakodimos S, Panayiotopoulos CP. Eyelid myoclonia with absences in adults. In: Duncan JS, Panayiotopoulos CP, eds. *Eyelid Myoclonia with Absences.* London: John Libbey & Company Ltd.; 1996:57–68.
92. Gibberd FB. The prognosis of petit mal. *Brain.* 1966;89:531–538.
93. Gibberd FB. The prognosis of petit mal in adults. *Epilepsia.* 1972;3:171–175.
94. Gibbs FA, Davis H, Lennox WG. The electroencephalogram in epilepsy and in conditions of impaired consciousness. *Arch Neurol Psychiatry.* 1935;34:1133–1148.
95. Gibbs FA, Gibbs EL, Lennox WG. Electrographic classification of epileptic patients and control subjects. *Arch Neurol Psychiatry.* 1943;50: 111–128.
96. Gobbi G, Bruno L, Mainetti A, et al. Eye-closure seizures. In: Beaumanoir A, Gastaut H, Naquet R, eds. *Reflex Seizures and Reflex Epilepsies.* Geneva, Switzerland: Medecine et Hygiene; 1989:181–191.
97. Gowers WR. *Epilepsies and Other Chronic Convulsive Diseases. Their Causes, Symptoms and Treatment.* London: JA Churchill; 1881.
98. Gram L. Acetazolamide, benzodiazepines and lamotrigine. In: Duncan JS, Panayiotopoulos CP, eds. *Typical Absences and Related Epileptic Syndromes.* London: Churchill Livingstone; 1995:368–375.
99. Grinspan A, Hirsch E, Malafosse A, et al. Epilepsie absences photosensible familiale: un nouveau syndrome? *Epilepsies.* 1992;4:245–250.
100. Grunewald RA, Panayiotopoulos CP. Juvenile myoclonic epilepsy: a review. *Arch Neurol.* 1993;50:594–598.
101. Guilhoto LM, Manreza ML, Yacubian EM. Syndromic classification of patients with typical absence seizures. *Arq Neuropsiquiatr.* 2003;61:580–587.
102. Guiwer J, Valenti MP, De Saint-Martin A, et al. Pronostic des épilepsies idiopathiques avec absences. *Epilepsies.* 2004;2:67–74.
103. Gumnit RJ, Niedermeyer E, Spreen O. Seizure activity uniquely inhibited by patterned vision. *Arch Neurol.* 1965;13:363–368.
104. Guye M, Bartolomei F, Gastaut JL, et al. Absence epilepsy with fast rhythmic discharges during sleep: an intermediary form of generalized epilepsy? *Epilepsia.* 2001;42:351–356.
105. Hedström A, Olsson I. Epidemiology of absence epilepsy: EEG findings and their predictive value. *Pediatr Neurol.* 1991;7:100–104.

106. Heilbronner. Gehaufte Kleine Anfalle. *Deut Zeitschr f Nervenheilk.* 1907;31:472(cited by Addie).
107. Hertoft P. The clinical, electroencephalographic and social prognosis in petit mal epilepsy. *Epilepsia.* 1963;4:298–314.
108. Hirsch E, Blanc-Platier A, Marescaux C. What are the relevant criteria for a better classification of epileptic syndromes with typical absences? In: Malafosse A, Genton P, Hirsch E, et al, eds. *Idiopathic Generalized Epilepsies: Clinical, Experimental and Genetic Aspects.* London: John Libbey; 1994:87–93.
109. Hirsch E, Marescaux C. Should absence epilepsies be classified according to the age of onset? In: Duncan JS, Panayiotopoulos CP, eds. *Typical Absences and Related Epileptic Syndromes.* London: Churchill Livingstone; 1995:310–314.
110. Hirose S, Okada M, Kanedo S, et al. Are some idiopathic epilepsies disorders of ion channels?: A working hypothesis. *Epilepsy Res.* 2000;41:191–204.
111. Hollowack J, Thurston DL, O'Leary JL. Petit mal epilepsy. *Pediatrics.* 1962;60:893–901.
112. Holmes GH, MacKeever M, Adamson M. Absence seizures in children: clinical and electroencephalographic features. *Ann Neurol.* 1987;21:268–273.
113. Hosford DA, Lin F, Cao Z, et al. Action of anti-epileptic drugs in animal models: mechanistic frame-work of absence seizures with a focus on the lethargic (1h/1h) mouse model. In: Duncan JS, Panayiotopoulos CP, eds. *Typical Absences and Related Epileptic Syndromes.* London: Churchill Livingstone; 1995:41–50.
114. Imbrici P, Jaffe SL, Eunson LH, et al. Dysfunction of the brain calcium channel CaV2.1 in absence epilepsy and episodic ataxia. *Brain.* 2004;127:2682–2692.
115. Jackson HJ. On temporary mental disorders after epilepsy paroxysms. In: Taylor J, ed. *Selected Writings of John Hughlings Jackson.* Vol 1. London: Hodder and Stoughton; 1981:119–134.
116. Janz D. Die Epilepsien. *Spezielle Pathologie und Therapie.* Stuttgart: Georg Thieme; 1969.
117. Janz D, Beck-Mannagetta G, Waltz S. Do idiopathic generalised epilepsies share a common susceptibility gene? *Neurology.* 1992;42(Suppl 5): 48–55.
118. Janz D, Beck-Mannagetta G, Sproder B, et al. Childhood absence epilepsy (pyknolepsy) and juvenile absence epilepsy: one or two syndromes? In: Wolf P, ed. *Epileptic Seizures and Syndromes.* London: John Libbey; 1994:115–126.
119. Janz D, Waltz S. Juvenile myoclonic epilepsy with absences. In: Duncan JS, Panayiotopoulos CP, eds. *Typical Absences and Related Epileptic Syndromes.* London: Churchill Livingstone; 1995:174–183.
120. Jasper HH, Drooglever-Fortuyn J. Experimental studies on the functional anatomy of petit mal epilepsy. *Res Publ Assoc Nerv Ment Dis.* 1947;26:272–298.
121. Jeavons PM. Nosological problems of myoclonic epilepsies of childhood and adolescence. *Dev Med Child Neurol.* 1977;19:3–8.
122. Jus A, Jus K. Retrograde amnesia in petit mal. *Arch Gen Psychiatry.* 1962;6:163–167.
123. Kobayashi K, Ohtsuka Y, Ohmori I, et al. Clinical and electroencephalographic characteristics of children with febrile seizures plus. *Brain Dev.* 2004;26:262–268.
124. Labate A, Brielmann RS, Abott DF, et al. Typical childhood absence seizures are associated with thalamic activation. *Epileptic Disord.* 2005;7: 373–377.
125. Lennox WG. The petit mal epilepsies. *JAMA.* 1945;129:1069–1073.
126. Lennox WG, Davis JP. Clinical correlates of the fast and slow spike-wave electroencephalogram. *Pediatrics.* 1950;5:626–644.
127. Lennox WG, Lennox MA. *Epilepsy and Related Disorders.* Boston: Little, Brown and Co.; 1960:546–574.
128. Lerche H, Weber YG, Baier H, et al. Generalized epilepsy with febrile seizures plus: further heterogeneity in a large family. *Neurology.* 2001;57:1191–1198.
129. Lerman-Sagie T, Watemberg N, Kramer U, et al. Absence seizures aggravated by valproic acid. *Epilepsia.* 2001;42:941–943.
130. Livingston S, Torres I, Pauli LL, et al. Petit mal epilepsy. Results of a prolonged follow-up study of 117 patients. *JAMA.* 1965;194: 227–232.
131. Loiseau P, Cohadon F, Cohadon S. Le petit mal qui guérit, guérit rapidement. *J Med Lyon.* 1966;1108:1557–1565.
132. Loiseau P, Pestre M, Dartigues JF, et al. Long term prognosis in two forms of childhood epilepsy: typical absence seizures and epilepsy with rolandic (centrotemporal) EEG foci. *Ann Neurol.* 1983;13:642–648.
133. Loiseau J, Loiseau P, Guyot M, et al. Survey of seizure disorders in the French Southwest. I. Incidence of epileptic syndromes. *Epilepsia.* 1990;31:391–396.
134. Loiseau P. Childhood absence epilepsy. In: Roger J, Bureau M, Dravet C, et al., eds. *Epileptic Syndromes in Infancy, Childhood and Adolescence.* London: John Libbey; 1992:135–150.
135. Loiseau P, Duche B. Childhood absence epilepsy. In: Duncan JS, Panayiotopoulos CP, eds. *Typical Absences and Related Epileptic Syndromes.* London: Churchill Livingstone; 1995:152–160.
136. Loiseau P, Duche B, Pedespan JM. Absence epilepsies. *Epilepsia.* 1995;36:1182–1186.
137. Loiseau P, Duché B, Pédespan JM. Splitting or lumping absence epilepsies. *Epilepsia.* 1995;36:116.
138. Loiseau P, Duché B. Childhood absence epilepsy. In: Duncan JS, Panayiotopoulos CP. eds, *Typical Absences and Related Epileptic Syndromes.* Edinburgh: Churchill Livingstone; 1995:152–160.
139. Loiseau P, Panayiotopoulos CP. Childhood absence epilepsy. In: Gilman S, ed. *Neurobase.* San Diego, CA: Arbor Publishing Corp.; 2000.
140. Loiseau P, Panayiotopoulos CP. Childhood absence epilepsy. In: Gilman S, ed. *Medlink Neurology.* San Diego, CA: Arbor Publishing Corp.; 2005.
141. Lombroso CT. Consistent EEG focalities detected in subjects with primary generalized epilepsies monitored for two decades. *Epilepsia.* 1997;38:797–812.
142. Lugaresi E, Pazzaglia PP, Franck L, et al. Evolution and prognosis of primary generalised epilepsy of the petit mal absence type. In: Lugaresi E, Pazzaglia PP, Tassinari CA, eds. *Evolution and Prognosis of Epilepsy.* Bologna, Italy: Auto Gaggi; 1973:3–22.
143. Manonmani V, Wallace SJ. Epilepsy with myoclonic absences. *Arch Dis Child.* 1994;70:288–290.
144. Marescaux C, Vergnes M. Animal models of absence seizures and absence epilepsies. In: Duncan JS, Panayiotopoulos CP, eds. *Typical Absences and Related Epileptic Syndromes.* London: Churchill Livingstone; 1995: 8–18.
145. Marini C, Harkin LD, Wallace RH, et al. Childhood absence epilepsy and febrile seizures: a family with GABA(A) receptor mutation. *Brain.* 2003; 126:230–240.
146. Marini C, Scheffer IE, Crossland KM, et al. Genetic architecture of idiopathic generalized epilepsy: clinical genetic analysis of 55 multiplex families. *Epilepsia.* 2004;45:467–478.
147. Meencke HJ, Janz D. Neuropathological findings in primary generalised epilepsy: a study of eight cases. *Epilepsia.* 1984;25:8–21.
148. Meencke HJ, Janz D. The significance of microdysgenesia in primary generalized epilepsy: an answer to the considerations of Lyon and Gastaut. *Epilepsia.* 1985;26:368–371.
149. Meencke HJ. Pathological findings in childhood absence epilepsy. In: Duncan JS, Panayiotopoulos CP, eds. *Typical Absences and Related Epileptic Syndromes.* London: Churchill Livingstone; 1995:122–132.
150. Mirsky AF, Duncan CC, Myslobodsky MS. Petit mal epilepsy: a review and integration of recent information. *J Clin Neurophysiol.* 1986;3: 179–208.
151. Mirsky AF, Duncan CC, Levav ML. Neuropsychological and psychophysiological aspects of absence epilepsy. In: Duncan JS, Panayiotopoulos CP, eds. *Typical Absences and Related Epileptic Syndromes.* Edinburgh: Churchill Livingstone; 1995:112–121.
152. Mullatti N, Selway R, Nashef L, et al. The clinical spectrum of epilepsy in children and adults with hypothalamic hamartoma. *Epilepsia.* 2003;44:1310–1319.
153. Nehlig A, Valenti MP, Thiriaux A, et al. Ictal and interictal perfusion variations measured by SISCOM analysis in typical childhood absence seizures. *Epileptic Disord.* 2004;6:247–253.
154. Noebels JL. Genetic and phenotypic heterogeneity of inherited spike-and-wave epilepsies. In: Malafosse A, Genton P, Hirsch E, et al., eds. *Idiopathic Generalized Epilepsies: Clinical, Experimental and Genetic Aspects.* London: John Libbey; 1994:215–225.
155. Noebels JL. Genetic mechanisms of spike wave epilepsies in mouse mutants. In: Duncan JS, Panayiotopoulos CP, eds. *Typical Absences and Related Epileptic Syndromes.* London: Churchill Livingstone; 1995:29–38.
156. Obeid T. Some clinical and genetic aspects of juvenile absence epilepsy. *J Neurol.* 1994;241:487–491.
157. Oller-Daurella L, Sanchez ME. Evolucion de las ausencias tipicas. *Rev Neurol.* 1981;9:81–102.
158. Olsson I. Absence epilepsy in Swedish children. Clinical epidemiology—psychosocial adjustment [MD Thesis]. University of Goteborg, Sweden; 1990.
159. Panayiotopoulos CP. Fixation-off-sensitive epilepsy in eyelid myoclonia with absence seizures. *Ann Neurol.* 1987;22:87–89.
160. Panayiotopoulos CP, Obeid T, Waheed G. Absences in juvenile myoclonic epilepsy: a clinical and video-electroencephalographic study. *Ann Neurol.* 1989;25:391–397.
161. Panayiotopoulos CP, Chroni E, Daskalopoulos C, et al. Typical absence seizures in adults: clinical, EEG, video-EEG findings and diagnostic/syndromic considerations. *J Neurol Neurosurg Psychiatry.* 1992;55:1002–1008.
162. Panayiotopoulos CP, Baker A, Grunewald R, et al. Breath counting during 3 Hz generalised spike and wave discharges. *J Electrophysiol Technol.* 1993;19:15–23.
163. Panayiotopoulos CP. Benign childhood partial epilepsies: benign childhood seizure susceptibility syndromes. *J Neurol Neurosurg Psychiatry.* 1993;56:2–5.
164. Panayiotopoulos CP, Ferrie CD, Knott C, et al. Interaction of lamotrigine with sodium valproate. *Lancet.* 1993;1:445.
165. Panayiotopoulos CP, Obeid T, Tahan A. Juvenile myoclonic epilepsy: a 5-year prospective study. *Epilepsia.* 1994;35:285–296.
166. Panayiotopoulos CP. The clinical spectrum of typical absence seizures and absence epilepsies. In: Malafosse A, Genton P, Hirsch E, et al., eds. *Idiopathic Generalized Epilepsies: Clinical, Experimental and Genetic Aspects.* London: John Libbey; 1994:75–85.

167. Panayiotopoulos CP. Juvenile myoclonic epilepsy: an underdiagnosed syndrome. In: Wolf P, ed. *Epileptic Seizures and Syndromes*. London: John Libbey; 1994:221–230.
168. Panayiotopoulos CP, Ferrie CD, Giannakodimos S, et al. Perioral myoclonia with absences: a new syndrome? In: Wolf P, ed. *Epileptic Seizures and Syndromes*. London: John Libbey; 1994:143–153.
169. Panayiotopoulos CP. Fixation-off sensitive epilepsies: clinical and EEG characteristics. In: Wolf P, ed. *Epileptic Seizures and Syndromes*. London: John Libbey; 1994:55–66.
170. Panayiotopoulos CP, Giannakodimos S. A comprehensive clinical and video-EEG study of idiopathic generalised epilepsies with typical absences in adults [Abstract]. *J Neurol Neurosurg Psychiatry*. 1995;59: 203(abst).
171. Panayiotopoulos CP, Ferrie CD, Giannakodimos S, et al. Perioral myoclonia with absences. In: Duncan JS, Panayiotopoulos CP, eds. *Typical Absences and Related Epileptic Syndromes*. London: Churchill Livingstone; 1995:221–230.
172. Panayiotopoulos CP, Giannakodimos S, Chroni E. Typical absences in adults. In: Duncan JS, Panayiotopoulos CP, eds. *Typical Absences and Related Epileptic Syndromes*. London: Churchill Livingstone; 1995:289–299.
173. Panayiotopoulos CP. Typical absences are syndrome-related. In: Duncan JS, Panayiotopoulos CP, eds. *Typical Absences and Related Epileptic Syndromes*. London: Churchill Livingstone; 1995:304–314.
174. Panayiotopoulos CP. Juvenile absence epilepsy. In: Wallace S, ed. *Childhood Epilepsy*. London: Chapman & Hall; 1996:325–332.
175. Panayiotopoulos CP. Epilepsy with generalised tonic-clonic seizures on awakening. In: Wallace S, ed. *Childhood Epilepsy*. London: Chapman & Hall; 1996:349–353.
176. Panayiotopoulos CP. Epilepsies characterised by seizures with specific modes of precipitation (reflex epilepsies). In: Wallace S, ed. *Childhood Epilepsy*. London: Chapman & Hall; 1996:355–375.
177. Panayiotopoulos CP, Agathonikou A, Koutroumanidis M, et al. Eyelid myoclonia with absences: the symptom. In: Duncan JS, Panayiotopoulos CP, eds. *Eyelid Myoclonia with Absences*. London: John Libbey & Company Ltd.; 1996:17–26.
178. Panayiotopoulos CP, Giannakodimos S, Agathonikou A, et al. Eyelid myoclonia is not a maneouvre for self-induced seizures in eyelid myoclonia with absences. In: Duncan JS, Panayiotopoulos CP, eds. *Eyelid Myoclonia with Absences*. London: John Libbey & Company Ltd.; 1996: 93–106.
179. Panayiotopoulos CP. The treatment of typical absence seizures and related epileptic syndromes. *Paediatr Drugs*. 2001;3:379–403.
180. Panayiotopoulos CP, Ferrie CD, Koutroumanidis M, et al. Idiopathic generalised epilepsy with phantom absences and absence status in a child. *Epileptic Disord*. 2001;3:63–66.
181. Panayiotopoulos CP. Idiopathic generalised epilepsies. In: Panayiotopoulos CP, ed. *The Epilepsies: Seizures, Syndromes and Management*. Oxford: Bladon Med; 2005:271–348.
182. Parker A, Gardiner M, Ferrie CD, et al. Genetics and family observations in eyelid myoclonia with absences. In: Duncan JS, Panayiotopoulos CP, eds. *Eyelid Myoclonia with Absences*. London: John Libbey & Company Ltd.; 1996:107–114.
183. Parker APJ, Agathonikou A, Robinson RO, et al. Inappropriate use of carbamazepine and vigabatrin in typical absence seizures. *Dev Med Child Neurol*. 1998;40:517–519.
184. Penry JK, Dreifuss FE. Automatisms associated with the absence of petit mal epilepsy. *Arch Neurol*. 1969;21:1942–1949.
185. Penry JK, Porter RJ, Dreifuss FE. Simultaneous recording of absence seizures with video tape and electroencephalography: a study of 374 seizures in 48 patients. *Brain*. 1975;98:427.
186. Peterman MG. Abstract of discussion on "The petit mal epilepsies: their treatment with tridione." *JAMA*. 1945;129:1074.
187. Porter RJ. The absence epilepsies. *Epilepsia*. 1993;34(Suppl 3):S42–S48.
188. Prevett MC, Duncan JS. Functional imaging in humans. In: Duncan JS, Panayiotopoulos CP, eds. *Typical Absences and Related Epileptic Syndromes*. London: Churchill Livingstone; 1995:83–91.
189. Raymond AA, Sisodiya S, Fish DR, et al. Subependymal heterotopia: a distinct neuronal migration disorder associated with epilepsy. *J Neurol Neurosurg Psychiatry*. 1994;57:1195–1202.
190. Raymond AA, Fish DR, Sidodiya A, et al. Abnormalities of gyration, heterotopias, tuberous sclerosis, focal cortical dysplasia, microdysgenesis, dysembryoplastic neuroepithelial tumour and dysgenesis of the archicortex in epilepsy. Clinical, EEG and neuroimaging features in 100 adult patients. *Brain*. 1995;118:629–660.
191. Raymond AA, Fish DR. EEG features of focal malformations of cortical development. *J Clin Neurophysiol*. 1996;13:495–506.
192. Reutens DC. Aspects of the nosology and pathophysiology of the idiopathic generalised epilepsies of adolescence [PhD Thesis]. University of Melbourne, Australia; 1992.
193. Reutens DC, Berkovic SF. Idiopathic generalized epilepsy of adolescence: are the syndromes clinically distinct? [see comments]. *Neurology*. 1995;45:1469–1476.
194. Reynolds JR. Epilepsy, Its Symptoms, Treatment. London: Churchill; 1861.
195. Richens A. Ethosuximide and valproate. In: Duncan JS, Panayiotopoulos CP, eds. *Typical Absences and Related Epileptic Syndromes*. London: Churchill Livingstone; 1995:361–367.
196. Rocca WA, Sharbmugh FW, Hauser WA, et al. Risk factors for absence seizures: a population-based case-control study in Rochester, Minnesota. *Neurology*. 1987;37:1309–1314.
197. Rudolf G, Therese Bihoreau M, F Godfrey R, et al. Polygenic control of idiopathic generalized epilepsy phenotypes in the genetic absence epilepsy rats from Strasbourg (GAERS). *Epilepsia*. 2004;45:301–308.
198. Ryvlin P, Mauguière F. Imagerie fonctionnelle dans les épilepsies généraliées idiopathiques. *Rev Neurol (Paris)*. 1998;154:691–696.
199. Salek-Haddadi A, Lemieux L, Merschhemke M, et al. Functional magnetic resonance imaging of human absence seizures. *Ann Neurol*. 2003;53:663–667.
200. Sander JWAS. The epidemiology and prognosis of typical absence seizures. In: Duncan JS, Panayiotopoulos CP, eds. *Typical Absences and Related Epileptic Syndromes*. London: Churchill Livingstone; 1995: 135–144.
201. Sander T, Peters G, Jaliz D, et al. The gene encoding the 1A-voltage-dependant calcium channel (CACN1A4) is not a candidate for causing common subtypes of idiopathic generalized epilepsy. *Epilepsy Res*. 1998;29:115–122.
202. Sato S, Dreifuss FE, Penry JK. Prognostic factors in absence seizures. *Neurology*. 1976;28:788–796.
203. Sato S, Dreifuss FE, Penry JK, et al. Long term follow-up of absence seizures. *Neurology*. 1983;33:1590–1595.
204. Sauer H. Uber Gehaufte Kleine Anfalle by Kindern (pyknolepsie). *Mschr Psychiatr Neurol*. 1916;40:276–300.
205. Sgro V, Paola M, Canevini M, et al. Absence epilepsy: electroclinical study of 37 cases. *Epilepsia*. 1996;37(Suppl 4):106.
206. Schwab RS. Method of measuring consciousness in attacks of petit mal epilepsy. *Arch Neurol Psychiatry*. 1939;41:215–217.
207. Serratosa JM, Delgado-Escueta AV. Generalized myoclonic seizures. In: Wyllie E, ed. *The Treatment of Epilepsy: Principles and Practice*. Philadelphia: Lea & Febiger; 1993:411–424.
208. Shimazono Y, Hirai T, Okura T, et al. Disturbance of consciousness in petit mal epilepsy. *Epilepsia*. 1953;2:49–55.
209. Shorvon S. Absence status epilepticus. In: Duncan JS, Panayiotopoulos CP, eds. *Typical Absences and Related Epileptic Syndromes*. London: Churchill Livingstone; 1995:263–274.
210. Snead OC III, Depaulis A, Vergnes M, et al. Absence epilepsy: advances in experimental animal models. In: Delgado-Escueta AV, Wilson WA, Olsen RW, et al., eds. *Jasper's Basic Mechanisms of the Epilepsies, Third Edition: Advances in Neurology.* Vol. 79. Philadelphia: Lippincott Williams & Wilkins; 1999:253–278.
211. Stefan H. *Epileptische Absencen*. Stutgard, Germany: Georg Thieme; 1982:1–269.
212. Stier E. Zeitschr f d ges. *Neur u Psych, Orig*. 1922–23;80:143 (cited by Addie).
213. Striano S, Striano P, Nocerino C, et al. Eyelid myoclonia with absences: an overlooked epileptic syndrome? *Neurophysiol Clin*. 2002;32: 287–296.
214. Tassinari CA, Lyagoubi S, Santos V, et al. Etude des decharges des pointes ondes chez l'homme. II. Les aspects cliniques et EEG des absences myocloniques. *Rev Neurol*. 1969;121:379–383.
215. Tassinari CA, Michelucci R, Rubboli G, et al. Myoclonic absence epilepsy. In: Duncan JS, Panayiotopoulos CP, eds. *Typical Absences and Related Epileptic Syndromes*. London: Churchill Livingstone; 1995:187–195.
216. Temkin C. *The Falling Sickness. A History of Epilepsy from the Greeks to the Beginning of Modern Neurology* 2nd ed. Baltimore: Johns Hopkins Press; 1971.
217. Tissot SA. *Traite de l'epilepsie, faisant le tome troisieme du traite des nerfs et de leurs maladies*. Paris: Didot le jeune; 1770.
218. Trinka E, Baumgartner S, Unterberger I, et al. Long-term prognosis for childhood and juvenile absence epilepsy. *J Neurol*. 2004;251:1235–1241.
219. Tukel K, Jasper H. The EEG in parasagittal lesions. *Electroencephalogr Clin Neurophysiol*. 1952;4:284–290.
220. Waltz S. Electroenzephalographische befunde bei der epilepsie mit pyknoleptischen absencen und der juvenilen absnecen-epilepsie [Inaugural Dissertation]. Frei University, Berlin; 1993.
221. Weir B. The morphology of the spike-wave complex. *Electroencephalogr Clin Neurophysiol*. 1965;19:284–290.
222. Wilkins A. Towards an understanding of reflex epilepsy and the absence. In: Duncan JS, Panayiotopoulos CP, eds. *Typical Absences and Related Epileptic Syndromes*. London: Churchill Livingstone; 1995:196–205.
223. Wirrell EC, Camfield CS, Camfield PR, et al. Long-term prognosis of typical childhood absence epilepsy: remission or progression to juvenile myoclonic epilepsy. *Neurology*. 1996;47:912–918.
224. Wirrell EC, Camfield PR, Gordon KE, et al. Will a critical level of hyperventilation-induced hypocapnia always induce an absence seizure? *Epilepsia*. 1996;37:459–462.
225. Woermann FG, Sisodiya SM, Free SL, et al. Quantitative MRI in patients with idiopathic generalized epilepsy. Evidence of widespread cerebral structural changes. *Brain*. 1998;121:1661–1667.
226. Wolf P, Goosses R. Relation of photosensitivity to epileptic syndromes. *J Neurol Neurosurg Psychiatry*. 1986;49:1386–1391.

227. Wolf P. Juvenile absence epilepsy. In: Roger J, Bureau M, Dravet C, et al., eds. *Epileptic Syndromes in Infancy, Childhood and Adolescence*. London: John Libbey; 1992:307–312.
228. Wolf P. Juvenile absence epilepsy. In: Duncan JS, Panayiotopoulos CP, eds. *Typical Absences and Related Epileptic Syndromes*. London: Churchill Livingstone; 1995:161–167.
229. Wolf P, Goosses R. Relation of photosensitivity to epileptic syndromes. *J Neurol Neurosurg Psychiatry*. 1986;49:1386–1390.
230. Wolf P, Inoue Y. Therapeutic response of absence seizures in patients of an epilepsy clinic for adolescents. *J Neurol*. 1984;231:225–229.
231. Yoshinaga H, Ohtsuka Y, Tamai K, et al. EEG in childhood absence epilepsy. *Seizure*. 2004;13:296–302.

CHAPTER 240 ■ EPILEPSY WITH MYOCLONIC ABSENCES

CARLO ALBERTO TASSINARI, ROBERTO MICHELUCCI, ELENA GARDELLA, AND GUIDO RUBBOLI

INTRODUCTION

Epilepsy with myoclonic absences (MAs) is an epileptic syndrome characterized clinically by absence seizures associated with rhythmic, bilateral myoclonic jerks of severe intensity. The diagnosis is based on clinical observation and ictal video-polygraphic recordings. Indeed, in video-polygraphic investigations (recording an electroencephalogram [EEG] and electromyogram [EMG] from upper limb muscles, such as deltoids), MAs are characterized by rhythmic, bilateral, synchronous, symmetric 3-Hz spike-wave (SW) discharge, as in typical absences, associated with EMG myoclonic bursts at 3 Hz, superimposed to a progressively increasing tonic contraction.

Demonstration of MA seizures is essential for the diagnosis; thus, epilepsy with MAs belongs to the group of epilepsy syndromes that is defined by a specific seizure type (as, for example, juvenile myoclonic epilepsy or myoclonic astatic epilepsy [Doose syndrome]). Indeed, since the early description of MAs,[13,15,16] it has been believed that this seizure type could characterize a distinct epileptic condition that could be identified and separated from other forms of generalized epilepsy, such as childhood absence epilepsy. The Commission on Classification and Terminology of the International League Against Epilepsy (ILAE) accepted this view, recognizing epilepsy with MAs as an autonomous syndromic entity that was included, in the 1989 ILAE Proposal for Revised Classification of Epilepsies and Epileptic Syndromes,[6] in the group of cryptogenic or symptomatic generalized epilepsies, due to an overall dismal and heterogeneous prognosis. On the other hand, in the more recent Proposed Diagnostic Scheme for People with Epileptic Seizures and with Epilepsy produced by the ILAE Task Force on Classification and Terminology,[9] it has been tentatively placed among idiopathic generalized epilepsies. Recent reviews on this epileptic condition by Bureau and Tassinari[2,3] and Tassinari et al.[21] acknowledged the existence of at least two forms of epilepsy with MAs: one with a more benign course, and eventually disappearance of seizures, in which MAs are the sole, or predominant, seizure type; and the other with MAs associated with other seizure types (particularly, frequent generalized tonic–clonic seizures) that bears a more severe prognosis, as compared to other idiopathic generalized epilepsies. Furthermore, cases with "atypical" features in which MAs were part of a clinical picture characterized by some degree of mental retardation, neurologic deficits (e.g., congenital hemiparesis), and chromosomopathy[7,8,11] have been reported.

CLINICAL DATA

General Remarks

Epilepsy with MAs is a rare condition; in a selected population of epileptic patients attending the Centre St. Paul in Marseilles, it accounts for 0.5% to 1% of all epilepsies. There is a male preponderance (69%), at variance with childhood absence epilepsy in which females are more frequently affected. Etiologic factors reported in about 35% of cases are prematurity, perinatal damage, consanguinity, congenital hemiparesis, and chromosomopathy.[2,3] The evidence in some cases of associated chromosomal dysfunction has led to the hypothesis that abnormal expression of genes located in the affected chromosome segments may play a role in the pathogenesis of myoclonic absence epilepsy.[7,8] A genetic susceptibility, as demonstrated by a positive family history of epilepsies, has been observed in about 20% of cases.

The mean age of onset of MAs is 7 years, with a range between 11 months and 12.2 years. Reports describing cases with onset of MAs in the first year of life have been published in the last years.[1,14,19,22]

Myoclonic Absences

MAs are characterized by the following:

Impairment of consciousness, which can vary in intensity, ranging from a mild disruption of contact to a complete loss of consciousness. Sometimes the patients are aware of the jerks and may recall the words pronounced by the examiner during the seizures.

Motor manifestations, which consist of bilateral myoclonic jerks, often associated with a discrete tonic contraction that has been clearly documented in proximal upper limb muscles. The myoclonias mainly involve the muscles of the shoulders, arms, and legs; facial myoclonias, when present, are more evident around the chin and the mouth, whereas eyelid twitching is typically absent or rare. Due to concomitant tonic contraction, the jerking of the arms is accompanied by a progressive elevation of the upper extremities, giving rise to a quite constant and recognizable pattern. When the patient is standing, falling is uncommon. In some patients, asymmetric features, such as head and trunk deviation, may occur.

Autonomic manifestations, which consist of an arrest of respiration and inconstant loss of urine.

MAs last for 10 to 60 seconds, and recur at a high frequency (many seizures per day), being often precipitated by hyperventilation or awakening. MAs may also be observed during the early stages of sleep. Episodes of MA status are distinctly rare.

Seizures Other Than Myoclonic Absences

MAs represent the only seizure type in about one third of patients. The remaining cases can suffer from other seizure types, which can appear before the onset of MAs or occur in association with MAs. They consist of generalized tonic–clonic seizures, absences, or epileptic falls.

Neurologic and Neuropsychologic Examination

Neurologic examination is normal, except in those cases with congenital hemiparesis. Mental retardation is present in about 45% of cases before the onset of MAs. During the course of MAs, mental retardation may worsen, or even appear, in patients previously normal, particularly in those patients with frequent tonic–clonic seizures associated with MAs. These data constitute a very significant difference for this subgroup of patients when compared with the cognitive status observed in childhood absence epilepsy.

NEUROPHYSIOLOGIC DATA

Interictal EEG

The interictal EEG shows a normal background activity in all cases. In one third of cases, bursts of generalized SWs or, more rarely, focal or multifocal SWs are present. It is noteworthy to point out that the sinusoidal posterior slow rhythm has never been observed, as reported in childhood absence epilepsy.

Ictal EEG

The ictal EEG consists of rhythmic SW discharges at 3 Hz, which are bilateral, synchronous, and symmetric, as observed in typical absences. The onset and the end of SWs are abrupt. Polygraphic (EEG-EMG) recording discloses the appearance of bilateral myoclonias, at the same frequency as the SW, which begin around 1 second after the onset of EEG paroxysmal discharges and are followed by a tonic contraction, maximal

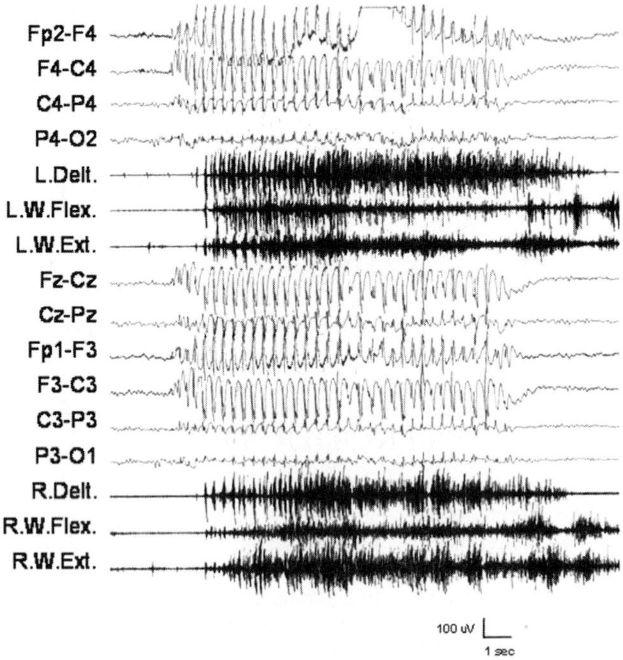

FIGURE 1. Spontaneous myoclonic absence. Electroencephalogram (EEG): Rhythmic spike-wave (SW) discharge at 3 Hz, bilateral, synchronous, and symmetric, as observed in typical absences. Electromyogram (EMG): Rhythmic myoclonia, at the same frequency of the SW, involving the upper extremities, and starting about 1.5 seconds after the onset of the EEG paroxysmal discharge, associated with a tonic contraction with progressively increasing intensity. Delt., deltoid; W.Flex., wrist flexor; W.Ext., wrist extensor; R., right; L., left.

in the shoulder and deltoid muscles (Fig. 1). Original investigations by Tassinari et al.[16,17] by means of high-speed oscilloscopic analysis provided a detailed description of the relationships between the EEG SW and motor events, showing a strict and constant relation between the spike of the SW discharge and the myoclonia (Fig. 2). These studies emphasized the relationships between the positive transient encompassed in the SW complex,[24] which in MAs is of high amplitude and is followed on the EMG by a myoclonia with a latency of 15 to 40 msec for the more proximal muscles and of 50 to 70 msec for the more distal muscles. This myoclonia is itself followed by a brief silent period (60 to 120 msec), which breaks the tonic contraction. Recently, Gardella et al.[10] demonstrated that the first myoclonic jerks were restricted to the facial musculature, then spreading to the neck and upper limbs muscles. Back-average of the EEG activity triggered from the onset of the first myoclonia confirmed the correlation of the

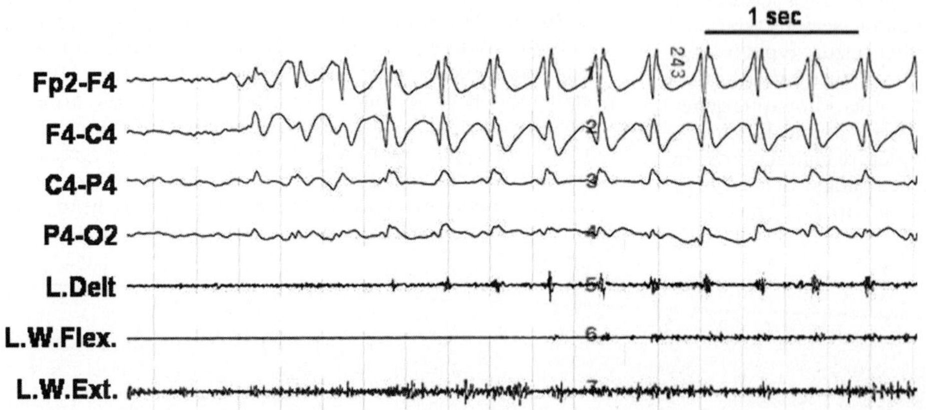

FIGURE 2. High-speed polygraphic recording of a myoclonic absence (MA) seizure, showing the relationship between the spike of the spike-wave (SW) complex and the myoclonic potential. The first three SW complexes are not associated with any evident myoclonic activity. Delt., deltoid; W.Flex., wrist flexor; W.Ext., wrist extensor; L., left.

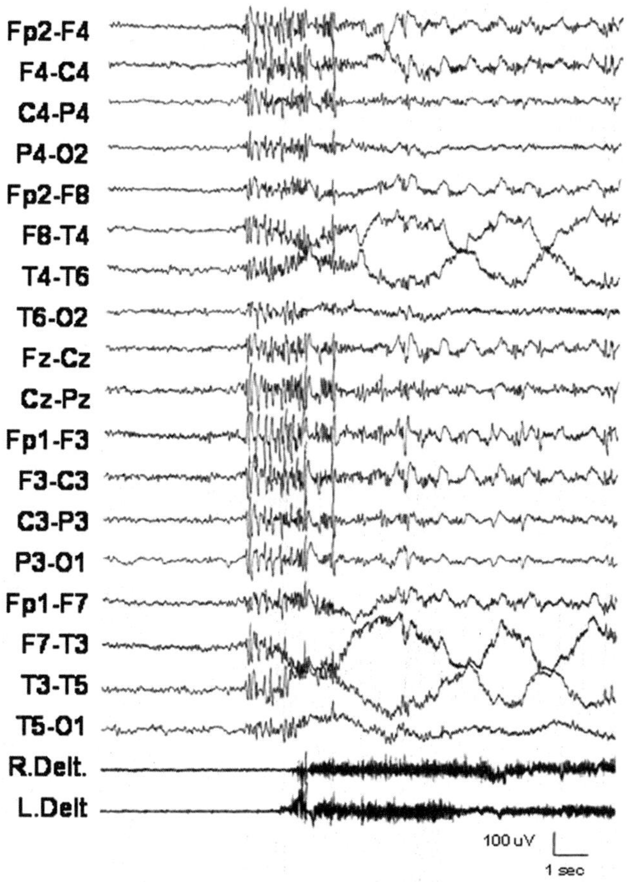

FIGURE 3. Tonic seizure during light sleep in a 45-year-old patient who started to suffer from myoclonic absences when she was 11 years old. Tonic muscular activity appears about 1 second after the onset of a rhythmic polyspike discharge. Delt., deltoid; R., right; L., left.

myoclonic phenomenon with the positive transient of the SW complex.

Physiopathogenetic hypotheses on the peculiar muscular pattern that characterizes MA seizures admit that the tonic muscular contraction component that is superimposed on the myoclonic activity might be related to the involvement of secondary motor areas,[3] possibly in the frontomesial cortex.[12] Indeed, tonic contractions occur always in MAs, but after the appearance of few SW complexes, possibly suggesting a spread of paroxysmal activity to frontomesial areas. During the evolution, some cases may evolve to a "Lennox-Gastaut–like syndrome" with tonic seizures, particularly during wakefulness or light sleep, associated in the EEG with rhythmic polyspike waves (Fig. 3). In these patients, the disappearance of SW complexes might be observed, replaced by focal frontal spikes; although infrequently, a frontal partial status may occur that can be controlled by phenytoin administration.

Sleep EEG

Sleep organization is constantly normal and physiologic patterns are symmetrically present. During sleep the evolution of the SW discharges is similar, on the whole, to that observed in childhood absence epilepsy.[18] MAs may occur during stage I of sleep, awakening the subject. During stage II, SW discharges, of brief or long duration, are also observed, sometimes associated with bursts of myoclonias.

EVOLUTION

Classical data on the evolution of MAs indicate that these are still present in about two thirds of the cases followed up for a mean period of 10 years, whereas they disappear in the remaining patients after a mean period of 5.5 years from the onset.[2,3,21] The two groups of patients differ in the frequency and type of associated seizures: in fact, patients with "refractory" MAs have a high incidence (80%) of associated seizures, mainly of generalized tonic–clonic and atonic types. On the contrary, patients with remitting MAs have a lower incidence (40%) of associated seizures, mainly of the absence type. The long duration of MAs is likely to be an important factor for the appearance of mental retardation, since intellectual functions are always preserved in children with rapid remission of MAs. In rare cases, the disappearance of MAs has been followed by the onset of other seizure types, namely absences with atypical SW discharges and clinical and subclinical tonic seizures, giving rise to a clinical picture similar to the Lennox-Gastaut syndrome.[19,20]

DIAGNOSIS

The diagnosis of MAs mainly rests on the polygraphic demonstration of SW discharges at 3 Hz (as in typical absences) accompanied by rhythmic myoclonias. Therefore, polygraphic recording is mandatory when the clinical suspicion of MAs is raised. Since the anamnestic data may sometimes be misleading (asymmetric MAs may be misdiagnosed as partial motor seizures, MAs with mild myoclonias may be misdiagnosed as typical petit mal absences, etc.), we suggest that polygraphic recording should be performed also in patients with "drug-resistant" absence seizures and in cases with refractory "myoclonic" or "partial motor seizures."

Capovilla et al.[4] reported a group of patients with childhood absence epilepsy exhibiting absence seizures associated with mild myoclonic jerks, involving mainly the facial and neck muscles (eyebrows, nostrils, perioral region, chin, sternocleidomastoideus). Indeed, the electroclinical characteristics (particularly, benign course with excellent response to treatment, and possible drug withdrawal in the evolution, and mild myoclonia without a background of tonic contraction) differentiate this clinical picture from epilepsy with MAs. Moreover, myoclonic phenomena have also been described in children with early-onset typical absences (before age 2 to 3 years).[5]

Finally, MAs must be differentiated from absence seizures with more or less rhythmic myoclonias associated with 2.5–3 Hz irregular SWs observed in nonspecific diffuse epileptic encephalopathies.[20]

TREATMENT

Data on outcome suggest that the correct medical therapy for MAs consists of the associated use of valproic acid and ethosuximide at high doses, with serum plasma levels ranging from 80 to 130 μg/mL and 70 to 110 μg/mL, respectively. Recent studies found lamotrigine, particularly in combination with valproate, or in one case ethosuximide, to be useful when other measures had failed.[14,23] In individual cases, good seizure control was achieved by using a combination of phenobarbitone, valproic acid, and benzodiazepines. It must be pointed out that since epilepsy with MAs is a relatively rare condition, no comparative or controlled clinical trials have ever been performed; therefore, the only available data are of retrospective nature. In particular, the efficacy of more recent antiepileptic drugs that are currently used in the treatment of refractory absences or in myoclonic epilepsies, such as levetiracetam, topiramate, and zonisamide, has not been adequately investigated in epilepsy with MAs. Finally, it should be mentioned that drugs such as carbamazepine or phenytoin (and possibly vigabatrin, gabapentin, tiagabine, and oxcarbazepine) might theoretically worsen MAs; however, as above mentioned, in patients who present with partial status, phenytoin may be useful to stop seizure activity.

SUMMARY AND CONCLUSIONS

The syndrome of epilepsy with MAs is a distinct form of childhood epilepsy characterized by a peculiar seizure type that identifies this epileptic condition. Recognition of MAs relies on direct clinical observation and polygraphic recording; in particular, the EEG-EMG ictal pattern bears specific features that allow differential diagnosis with other generalized seizure types. It can be stated that the demonstration of MAs is sufficient for the diagnosis. Regarding the natural history and prognosis of epilepsy with MAs, two forms may be identified: a form in which MAs are the sole or predominant seizure type and a form in which MAs are associated with other seizure types and particularly with numerous generalized tonic–clonic seizures; this latter form bears a poor prognosis in terms of seizure control and neuropsychological deterioration.

ACKNOWLEDGMENTS

We thank Prof. G. Avanzini and Prof. S. Franceschetti from the Neurological Institute "C. Besta" in Milan for providing the case illustrated in Figure 1, and Mrs. C. Giardini for her help in the preparation of the manuscript.

References

1. Aicardi J. Typical absences in the first two years of life. In: Duncan JS, Panayiotopoulos CP, eds. *Typical Absences and Related Syndromes*. London: Churchill Livingstone; 1995:284–288.
2. Bureau M, Tassinari CA. The syndrome of myoclonic absences. In: Roger J, Bureau M, Dravet C, et al., eds. *Epileptic Syndromes in Infancy, Childhood and Adolescence*. 3rd ed. Moutroupe: John Libbey & Co. Ltd.; 2002:305–312.
3. Bureau M, Tassinari CA. The syndrome of myoclonic absence. In: Roger J, Bureau M, Dravet CH, et al., eds. *Epileptic Syndromes in Infancy, Childhood, and Adolescence*. 4th ed. Moutroupe: John Libbey Eurotext Ltd.; 2005: 337–344.
4. Capovilla G, Rubboli G, Beccaria F, et al. A clinical spectrum of the myoclonic manifestations associated with typical absences in childhood absence epilepsy. A video-polygraphic study. *Epileptic Disord*. 2001;3:57–61.
5. Chaix Y, Daquin G, Monteriro F, et al. Absence epilepsy with onset before age three years: a heterogeneous and often severe condition. *Epilepsia*. 2003;44:944–949.
6. Commission on Classification and Terminology of the International League Against Epilepsy. Proposal for revised classification of epilepsies and epileptic syndromes. *Epilepsia*. 1989;30:389–399.
7. Elia M, Musumeci SA, Ferri R, et al. Trisomy 12p and epilepsy with myoclonic absences. *Brain Dev*. 1998;20:127–130.
8. Elia M, Guerrini R, Musumeci SA, et al. Myoclonic absence-like seizures and chromosome abnormality syndrome. *Epilepsia*. 1998;39:660–663.
9. Engel JJ. A proposed diagnostic scheme for people with epileptic seizures and with epilepsy: report of the ILAE Task Force on classification and terminology. *Epilepsia*. 2001;42:796–803.
10. Gardella E, Rubboli G, Meletti S, et al. Polygraphic study of muscular activation pattern in myoclonic absence seizures. *Epilepsia*. 2002;43(Suppl 8):98–99.
11. Guerrini R, Bureau M, Mattei MG, et al. Trisomy 12p syndrome: a chromosomal disorder associated with generalized 3 Hz spike-and-wave discharges. *Epilepsia*. 1990;31:557–566.
12. Ikeda A, Nagamine T, Kunieda T, et al. Clonic convulsions caused by epileptic discharges arising from the human supplementary motor area as studied by subdural recording. *Epileptic Disord*. 1999;1:21–26.
13. Lugaresi E, Pazzaglia P, Franck L, et al. Evolution and prognosis of primary generalized of the petit mal absence type. In: Lugaresi E, Pazzaglia P, Tassinari CA, eds. *Evolution and Prognosis of Epilepsy*. Bologna: Aulo Gaggi; 1973:2–22.
14. Manonmani V, Wallace SJ. Epilepsy with myoclonic absences. *Arch Dis Child*. 1994;70:288–290.
15. Tassinari CA, Bureau M. Epilepsy with myoclonic absences. In: Roger J, Dravet C, Bureau M, et al., eds. *Epileptic Syndromes in Infancy, Childhood, and Adolescence*. London: John Libbey; 1985:123–131.
16. Tassinari CA, Lyagoubi S, Santos V, et al. Etude des décharges de pointes ondes chez l'homme. Il. Les aspects cliniques et electroencephalographiques des absences myocloniques. *Rev Neurol*. 1969;121:379–383.
17. Tassinari CA, Lyagoubi S, Gambarelli F, et al. Relationships between EEC discharge and neuromuscular phenomena. *Electroencephalogr Clin Neurophysiol*. 1971;31:176.
18. Tassinari CA, Bureau-Paillas M, Dalla Bernardina B, et al. Generalized epilepsies and seizures during sleep: a polygraphic study. In: Van Praag HM, Meinardi H, eds. *Brain and Sleep*. Amsterdam: De Erven Bhon; 1974:154–166.
19. Tassinari CA, Bureau M, Thomas P. Epilepsy with myoclonic absences. In: Roger J, Bureau M, Dravet C, et al., eds. *Epileptic Syndromes in Infancy, Childhood, and Adolescence*. 2nd ed. London: John Libbey; 1992:151–160.
20. Tassinari CA, Michelucci R, Rubboli G, et al. Myoclonic absence epilepsy. In: Duncan JS, Panayiotopoulos CP, eds. *Typical Absences and Related Syndromes*. London: Churchill Livingstone; 1995:187–195.
21. Tassinari CA, Rubboli G, Gardella E, et al. Epilepsy with myoclonic absences. In: Wallace SJ, Farrell K, eds. *Epilepsy in Children*. 2nd ed. London: Arnold; 2004:189–194.
22. Verrotti A, Greco R, Chiarelli F, et al. Epilepsy with myoclonic absences with early onset: a follow-up study. *J Child Neurol*. 1999;14:746–749.
23. Wallace SJ. Myoclonus and epilepsy in childhood: a review of treatment with valproate, ethosuximide, lamotrigine, and zonisamide. *Epilepsy Res*. 1998;29:147–154.
24. Weir B. The morphology of the spike-wave complex. *Electroencephalogr Clin Neurophysiol*. 1965;19:284–290.

CHAPTER 241 ■ LENNOX-GASTAUT SYNDROME

PIERRE GENTON AND CHARLOTTE DRAVET

INTRODUCTION

Among childhood epilepsies, Lennox-Gastaut syndrome (LGS) is one of the most severe. It is characterized clinically by frequent seizures, including sudden falls, marked resistance to therapy, and progressive mental and behavioral disturbances. The syndrome is difficult to treat, even with the most recent antiepileptic drugs. Although the physiologic and pathogenic mechanisms of LGS are not fully understood, it has precise, well-defined clinical and neurophysiologic characteristics that restrict the diagnosis to a fairly homogenous, albeit rather uncommon entity. Historically, its main trait (i.e., the presence of diffuse slow spike-wave discharges), has led to overdiagnoses and confusion with other encephalopathic epilepsies; not all diffuse slow spikes-and-waves, not all epileptic drop attacks, and not all severe, polymorphic encephalopathic childhood-onset epilepsies are caused by LGS. Indeed, some cases previously diagnosed as LGS would nowadays be reclassified into other categories, like myoclonic astatic epilepsy or the Dravet syndrome.

LGS has many possible causes, and modern concepts have stressed the major part played in the genesis of LGS by secondary bilateral synchrony originating from the frontal cortex. In spite of its relative rarity, LGS has in recent years been the object of specific clinical trials evaluating the efficacy of newer antiepileptic agents, probably because it still represents the archetype of a recognizable, yet severe, intractable childhood epileptic encephalopathy.

HISTORICAL PERSPECTIVE

Early authors had already noticed the poor prognosis of some types of childhood seizures (i.e., atypical absences, tonic seizures, and astatic seizures), when Gibbs in 1938[38] and then Gibbs et al.[39] in 1939 identified an electroencephalographic (EEG) pattern characterized by slow (about 2-Hz) spikes-and-waves. They called this the *petit mal variant* as opposed to the less severe *petit mal absence*, characterized by 3-Hz spikes-and-waves. Lennox in 1945[57] and Lennox and Davis in 1950[59] established the clinical correlates of this pattern and described a symptomatic triad comprising slow diffuse spikes-and-waves, mental deficiency, and three seizure types: Myoclonic jerks, atypical absences, and head drops or falls, the latter successively described as *akinetic seizures*, *astatic seizures*, and finally *drop attacks*.

The further studies by Sorel[80] and Doose et al.,[25] and the MD dissertation of Dravet, published by Gastaut et al.,[33] allowed precise characterization of the electroclinical features of the syndrome. Different denominations were used over the years (including such complex ones as *childhood epileptic encephalopathy with diffuse slow spike-waves*) until the consensual denomination of *Lennox-Gastaut syndrome* was proposed by Margaret Buchtal-Lennox in 1966, in tribute to both the initial work of Lennox[57,58] and the thorough clinical description performed by the Marseille school. Further investigations included the long-term studies of large series reported by Oller Daurella,[69] Gastaut et al.,[34] Loubier,[60] Ohtahara et al.,[68] Beaumanoir,[11] and Chevrie and Aicardi.[18] Of particular interest from a clinical, genetic, and therapeutic perspective is the progressive delineation of LGS from other encephalopathic epilepsies like myoclonic astatic epilepsy (the Doose syndrome), severe myoclonic epilepsy of infancy (the Dravet syndrome), the syndrome of continuous spikes-and-waves during slow-wave sleep, and specific encephalopathies like the Angelman syndrome.

DEFINITIONS

In the International Classification of Epilepsies and Epileptic Syndromes,[20] LGS is classified among the symptomatic or cryptogenic generalized epilepsies. It is defined by several criteria:

a. Onset during childhood
b. Coexistence of several seizure types, with mainly atypical absence, axial tonic, and atonic seizures; the presence of tonic seizures during sleep is a constant feature; other seizures (myoclonic, generalized tonic–clonic, focal) can occur
c. Diffuse slow spikes-and-waves and bursts of fast rhythms at 10 to 12 Hz during sleep
d. Permanent psychologic disturbances with psychomotor delay, personality disorders, or both

The seizure frequency is high, and episodes of status are not uncommon. In the EEG, focal and multifocal abnormalities can be associated with the diffuse slow spikes-and-waves. These electroclinical features may occur in a previously normal child, without pathologic antecedents and without signs of brain lesion, usually between the ages of 1 and 8 years, and constitute the cryptogenic form of LGS. They also can occur in a child with prior signs of brain damage, sometimes in the wake of another type of epilepsy, such as infantile spasms or focal epilepsy, and constitute the symptomatic forms of LGS. In the latter cases, the range of ages at onset may be wider (between 1 and 15 years, rarely more).

In the 2001 proposal of the ILAE,[29] LGS was classified among epileptic encephalopathies, a category of epilepsies *in which the epileptiform abnormalities may contribute to progressive dysfunction.*

EPIDEMIOLOGY

Epidemiologic data on LGS vary greatly. Different criteria were used in selecting cases. Some studies have included all forms of severe childhood epilepsies associated with slow spikes-and-waves on the EEG. Others have restricted the criteria to those defined above. Its frequency has thus been estimated to range from 3% to 10.7% of all cases of childhood epilepsies.[4,11,34] In the population observed in the Centre St. Paul, which specializes in the treatment of severe epilepsies, the figure is 3.7% in the whole population (children and adults) and 6.6% in patients with onset before age 10 (personal data from a prospective registry of all newly referred epilepsy cases seen between 1986 and 1996). A study performed in metropolitan Atlanta, GA, found a prevalence of 4% among children aged <10.[84] Another study performed in Finland found a yearly incidence of 2 per 100,000 of "broadly defined" LGS among children aged 1 to 14 years.[47]

There is no particular geographic or ethnic distribution. Boys are slightly more often affected than girls.[60,61,68] A closer look at patient registries would probably show that the incidence has declined in recent years, due to stricter diagnostic criteria, leading to other specific diagnoses and to changes in the early treatment of severe childhood epilepsies that may have avoided the progression of symptomatic cases into the full-blown LGS. In our recent experience, the incidence of LGS has been comparable to that of myoclonic astatic epilepsy and the Dravet syndrome.

ETIOLOGY AND BASIC MECHANISMS

LGS can be symptomatic or cryptogenic. Numerous etiologies can be found in the symptomatic forms[12]: Perinatal anoxic ischemia; antenatal or perinatal vascular accident; antenatal, perinatal, or postnatal cerebral and cerebromeningeal infection; HHE (hemiconvulsion-hemiplegia-epilepsy) syndrome; both diffuse and lateralized or even focal brain malformation and migration disorders; tuberous sclerosis, Down syndrome, hydrocephalus, head trauma, brain tumor and radiotherapy for brain tumor, and many others. There are numerous publications on uncommon etiologies, and a sample may be quoted here to underline the etiologic heterogeneity of this syndrome. LGS may, for instance, occur following chemo- and whole-brain radiotherapy for acute lymphocytic leukemia[63]; in an encephalitic form of neurocysticercosis[1]; or in common variable immunodeficiency with acute disseminated encephalomyelitis.[53]

In some cases, despite psychomotor retardation before the onset of seizures or of mild to moderate, nonspecific cerebral atrophy demonstrated by computed tomography (CT) and magnetic resonance imaging (MRI), there is no recognizable etiology. When epilepsy starts in the first year of life, it is often in the form of infantile spasms, followed by LGS. Otherwise, LGS can be preceded by focal seizures, or all the features of LGS may be manifesting at onset or soon thereafter. It must also be stressed that the typical features of LGS can be observed only transiently in some patients.[11] In the cryptogenic forms, there is no etiology by definition. However, "cryptogenicity" may depend on the amount of investigation, and this category may have shrunk since the availability of MRI. Some authors have been enticed to subdivide LGS patients in three categories: Symptomatic, noncryptogenic, and cryptogenic, the latter category referring to individuals with strict criteria of normal development, lack of dysmorphism, and normal MRI[41]: Using such criteria, these authors found no difference in seizure outcome between these etiologic categories.

The mechanisms underlying LGS are not well understood. In 1987, Theodore et al.[82] used positron emission tomography (PET) to investigate the cerebral metabolism of ten patients, and Chugani et al.[19] that of five, without considering the various etiologies. Their results appear too heterogeneous to be significant. Microscopic studies of samples obtained at autopsy and brain biopsy from 15 patients were reported by Roger and Gambarelli-Dubois.[75] Selective neuronal necrosis was observed in the neocortex, hippocampus, thalamus, and cerebellum, but in eight cases the necrosis was restricted to the cerebellum. Electron microscopic examination of biopsy material from eight patients showed that neuronal loss occurred mainly at postsynaptic sites. Quantitative analysis confirmed the rarefaction of cortical dendrites and synaptic contacts. In two cases studied by Renier,[73] there were a few swollen astrocytes around the neurons in the deeper cortical layers, poor dendritic arborization, and disturbed synaptic development of the pyramidal cells restricted to the inner cortical layers. He hypothesized that these findings were the origin and not the consequence of LGS, and were perhaps related to an autoimmune process. A virologic and immunologic approach was adopted by Smeraldi et al.,[79] but the results of their studies were not significant. Eeg-Olofsson[28] discussed the relationships between a genetic defective immune mechanism and the occurrence of LGS.

Genetic factors do not seem to play a major part in LGS, and no multiplex families with LGS have been reported. The frequency of cases with a family history of epilepsy ranges from 2.5%[18] to 28%.[60] Boniver et al.[16] noted that 48% of patients with cryptogenic LGS had a family history of either epilepsy or febrile convulsions, but their series may have included patients with myoclonic astatic epilepsy. Interestingly, no case of LGS has been reported in large generalized epilepsy with febrile seizures plus (GEFS+) families, which include patients with Dravet syndrome or myoclonic astatic epilepsy. Among genetically determined cortical brain malformations, LGS may occur in patients with micropolygyria and in those with the XLIS mutation, which causes subcortical band heterotopia in females and pachygyria in males. In the latter example, the occurrence of LGS seems to be correlated with the thickness of the band or severity of pachygyria.[42]

The neurophysiologic processes leading to the production of interictal EEG changes and seizures in LGS have received some attention. Processes related to those occurring in idiopathic generalized epilepsies play a limited part, since abnormal sleep patterns found in patients with cryptogenic LGS seem to originate outside the usual thalamocortical circuit.[88] Secondary bilateral synchrony (SBS), which is of cortical origin, appears to be at the origin of the apparently generalized EEG changes: In their study comparing myoclonic seizures found in LGS and in (truly idiopathic) myoclonic astatic epilepsy, Bonnani et al.[15] convincingly demonstrated propagation from a lateralized origin in LGS. There is no satisfactory explanation for the genesis of this abnormal tendency to SBS and related inhibition of function, but this phenomenon clearly plays a major part in the genesis of both seizures and cognitive impairment. The occurrence of the LGS at a crucial stage of neurodevelopment is of course a major factor of the learning difficulties and progressive retardation, and Blume[14] has hypothesized that the intensity of interictal and ictal discharges diverts the brain from normal developmental processes toward seizure control mechanisms.

In the light of recent data, LGS appears to be an acquired, nonspecific, age-dependent diffuse encephalopathy, occurring without specific familial predisposition, and the reason why it appears in either normal or brain-damaged patients is not known.[12] There is evidence of major focal factors, related to the frontal lobes, but these coexist with a predisposition to bilateral synchrony, which accounts for most of the clinical features. Until we know more, this epileptic encephalopathy should thus still be ranked among the "generalized" syndromes.

CLINICAL PRESENTATION

The onset is before the age of 8, with a peak between 3 and 5 years. Onset after age 10 is unusual. In cryptogenic cases,[16] the first seizures can be myoclonic, atypical absences, or falls, sometimes repeated in status. Sometimes, an isolated seizure—tonic, clonic, tonic–clonic, or even a unilateral seizure—has preceded the typical seizures by several months. Nocturnal tonic attacks are usually not observed at the very onset. Psychological and cognitive disturbances can be concomitant with the first seizures or can develop later, insidiously. Thus, it is not easy to make the diagnosis of LGS very quickly. The EEG features at onset can consist of either diffuse slow spikes-and-waves or only more or less diffuse slow waves. A single case study of nocturnal sleep at this stage has been published,[21] demonstrating the presence of bursts of low-voltage rapid rhythms evoking subclinical tonic seizures. When LGS follows infantile spasms, there are two possible modalities: Either infantile spasms are replaced by tonic seizures without a free interval, or infantile spasms disappear and both the EEG and the psychomotor development improve for some time before falls, atypical absences, and diffuse slow spikes-and-waves appear, accompanied by a new slowing of development. When LGS complicates other types of epilepsy, the diagnosis is marked by the onset of falls and behavioral/cognitive changes. Several authors have reported the occurrence of LGS in adolescents and young adults who previously had an idiopathic type of generalized epilepsy.[59,68,74]

Interictal Symptomatology

The neuropsychological and psychiatric symptoms consist of arrest or slowing of psychomotor development, apparent deterioration of cognitive abilities, and appearance of psychiatric conditions, the expression of which depends on age. The youngest children are seen with physical and intellectual instability, mood lability, inability to acquire new skills, and progressive disharmony. Older children exhibit slowness of ideation and expression; language deterioration resulting from motor dysfunction, particularly changes in muscular tone of the orolaryngopharyngeal area[10]; aggression; irritability; loss of social relationships; tendency to isolation; and sometimes psychotic outcome. Personality disorders are always present in the cryptogenic forms.[89] There are no neurologic signs that can be considered specific to LGS, apart from transient cerebellar, pyramidal, or extrapyramidal signs during prolonged status. However, in some patients the recurrent episodes of status are so long and so frequent that this semiology can become permanent after more than 10 years of evolution. Iatrogenic factors may contribute to neurologic deterioration.

On the EEG, the background can be disorganized, with diffuse slow waves, poor reactivity, and lack of topographic differentiation. Such disorganization can be permanent (67% of patients) or transient, appearing only during periods of worsening of seizures. Constant disorganization is a sign of poor prognosis. Hyperventilation can elicit slow spike-and-wave discharges with or without clinical correlates (atypical absences), whereas intermittent photic stimulation has no effect. Paroxysmal changes are frequent, with discharges of diffuse slow spikes-and-waves and slow polyspikes-and-waves. In 75% of children, they are associated with focal and multifocal changes (spikes, slow spikes, slow spikes-and-waves), with constant or variable focalization, frequently frontal or temporal. They are increased during slow sleep, when the diffuse slow spikes-and-waves become more synchronous and rhythmic, with prominent polyspikes. During sleep, specific bursts of fast rhythms appear (see below). The differentiation of sleep stages can be preserved or can be blurred[7] (Fig. 1).

Ictal Symptomatology

In order of decreasing specificity, LGS, a disorder associated with multiple seizure types, includes tonic seizures, atypical absences, atonic seizures, and other types. Both tonic and atonic seizures may cause falls.

Tonic seizures are the main feature of the syndrome and are reported in 74%[11,34] to 90%[60] of patients. They can be axial, axorhizomelic, or complete, and symmetric or markedly unilateral. They can occur while patients are awake or asleep. The neck and body are suddenly flexed, the shoulders and arms are raised in a semiflexed or extended position, the legs are extended, the facial muscles (sometimes only of the lower lip) contract, and the eyes roll up. Apnea and facial flushing are apparent. The victim may fall suddenly. Loss of consciousness does not always occur and is rarely the initial symptom. Return to normal consciousness always coincides with the end of the EEG discharge. Enuresis can occur. The pupils are usually dilated. When these seizures are short and involve only rolling of the eyes and respiratory changes (which is usually the case during sleep), they may remain unnoticed. When they last for more than 10 seconds, they can culminate in a tremor that affects the whole body (resulting in a "vibratory" seizure). In tonic–automatic seizures, described by Oller Daurella[70] in 72% of late-onset cases, there is a final phase of gestural, sometimes ambulatory automatisms. Slow-wave sleep facilitates the occurrence of tonic seizures. The EEG during tonic seizures (Fig. 2) consists of either a bilateral discharge of fast rhythms, predominantly in the anterior areas and at the vertex, or a flattening of the background, or a combination of these two patterns, sometimes preceded by generalized spikes-and-waves, followed by diffuse slow waves and slow spikes-and-waves, that last longer in patients with "tonic–automatic" seizures. There is no postictal silence. The fast discharges are particularly common during slow-wave sleep, when they can be nearly subclinical. Gibbs[38] inappropriately described this ictal pattern recorded during sleep as the *grand mal pattern*.

Atypical absences are observed in a vast majority of patients. Clinically, they are often difficult to diagnose: The onset and end are gradual, contact is impaired but not completely lost, a simple activity can be continued, eyelid myoclonus is not rhythmic, perioral myoclonus is frequent, and slow forward motion of the head caused by loss of tone, as well as drooling, is also frequent. In the EEG, atypical absences are associated with often irregular, more or less symmetric discharge of diffuse slow spikes-and-waves at 2 to 2.5 Hz (Fig. 3), or with a burst of rapid rhythms, or with a mixed pattern.

Atonic, myoclonic–atonic, and myoclonic seizures are not easy to differentiate by clinical observation alone. Most authors group these seizures with falls under the name of *akinetic* or *astatic* seizures,[32] or *drop attacks*. They may provoke a sudden fall, either of the head only or of the whole body, which may cause injuries. This is followed by an immediate recovery (there may, however, be loss of consciousness and progressive recovery in case of significant head concussion). The EEG correlates are polymorphous: Slow spikes-and-waves, slow polyspike-and-waves, and decremental events. The simultaneous video-EEG and polygraphic recordings allow an accurate characterization of the seizure type. They occur together in the same patient in 95% of cases.

Other seizure types, not specific for LGS, can be observed: Generalized tonic–clonic, generalized clonic, and focal seizures. Reflex seizures may be seen in some cases, like seizures provoked by eating[56] or, more commonly, in Down syndrome patients with LGS, in whom a "startle" reaction may trigger tonic seizures or atypical absences.[43]

All the seizure types occur as status in a majority of patients (54%,[60] 75%[11]). Status consists of periods of more or less profound obtundation/stupor, intermixed with serial tonic attacks, sometimes with myoclonic–atonic falls. When tonic attacks are predominant, they constitute a tonic status. The main characteristics of status episodes are their long duration

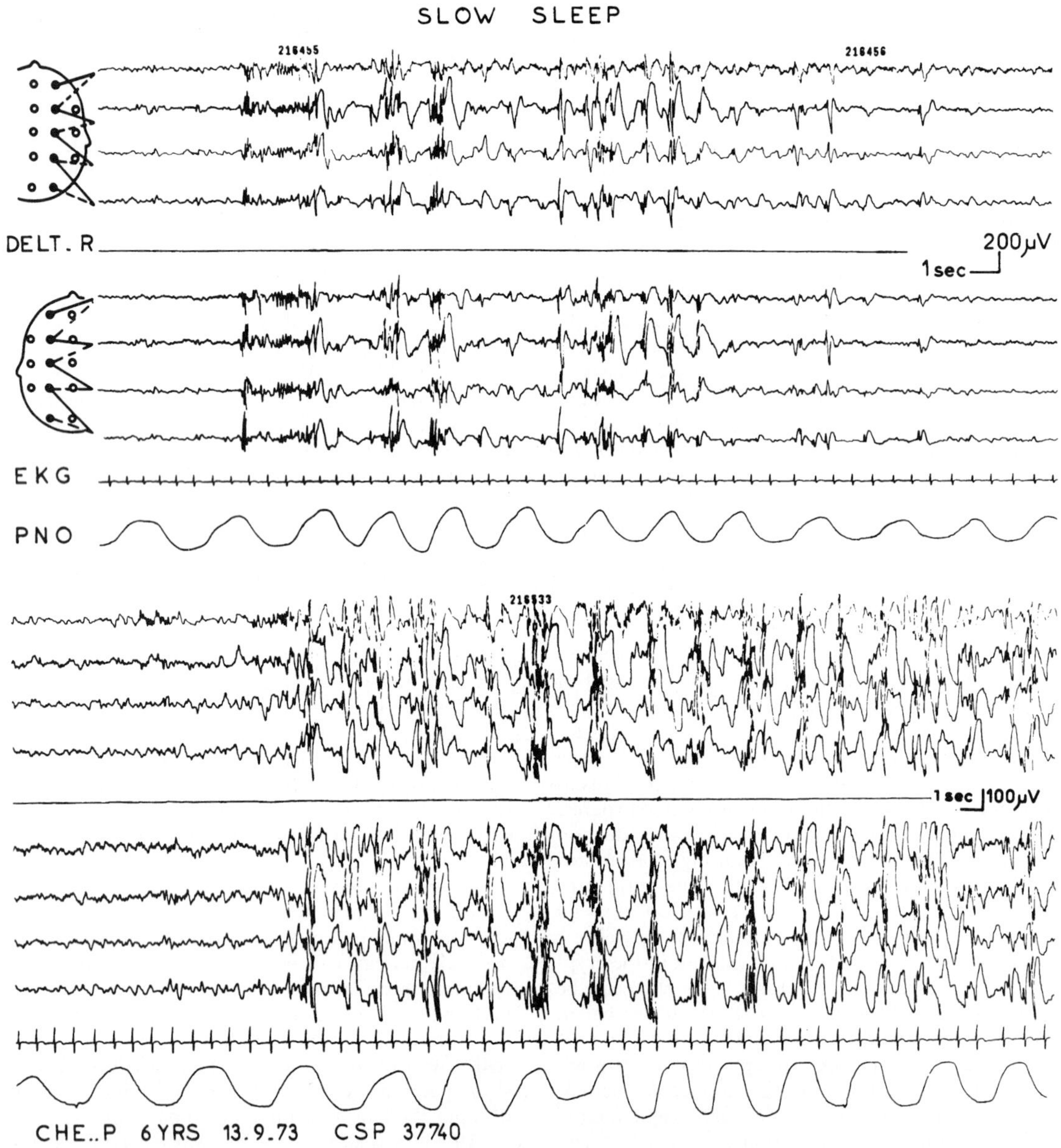

FIGURE 1. Electroencephalographic recording during sleep in cryptogenic Lennox-Gastaut syndrome. **Top:** Typical bursts of subclinical rapid rhythms, variable in amplitude and duration, recorded with decreased amplification. **Bottom:** Other runs of rapid rhythms recorded with the normal gain, accompanied by a slight change in respiration. DELT R, right deltoid; PNO, pneumogram.

(days to weeks), resistance to treatment, and tendency to occur repeatedly. During status, the EEG becomes almost hypsarrhythmic. It has been suggested that this represents only a temporary worsening of the usual interictal symptomatology.[11,26] The occurrence and frequency of nonconvulsive status is considered to contribute to the poor cognitive outcome of LGS.[48]

Clinical Variants

In the myoclonic variant of LGS, which represents 18% of the cases of Chevrie and Aicardi,[18] massive myoclonus and myoclonic–atonic attacks are the prominent seizure types. Tonic seizures are mainly nocturnal, and epileptic status is characterized by stupor and myoclonus. The awake EEG is not different from the typical form, but there are fewer runs of rapid rhythms during sleep. This myoclonic variant is cryptogenic in 64% of cases, and its mental prognosis is more favorable. Probably some of the patients reported to have "myoclonic LGS" in the literature actually had myoclonic astatic epilepsy.[24]

Late-onset LGS has been studied by Oller Daurella,[69] Bauer et al.,[9] and Roger et al.[74] These authors have distinguished between LGS following idiopathic generalized epilepsy, LGS following partial epilepsy, and LGS appearing initially as the typical cryptogenic syndrome. The age of onset is usually between 10 and 20 years but in some cases was between 20 and 30 years. Patients with Down syndrome will usually initiate LGS with reflex seizures, between the ages of 8 and 12 years.[43] The clinical characteristics of late-onset LGS are the presence of tonic–automatic and generalized tonic–clonic seizures in addition to drop attacks and atypical absences. The psychologic features are mainly ideomotor slowness and psychotic change of personality. In the EEG, slow spikes-and-waves are often associated with fast spikes-and-waves.

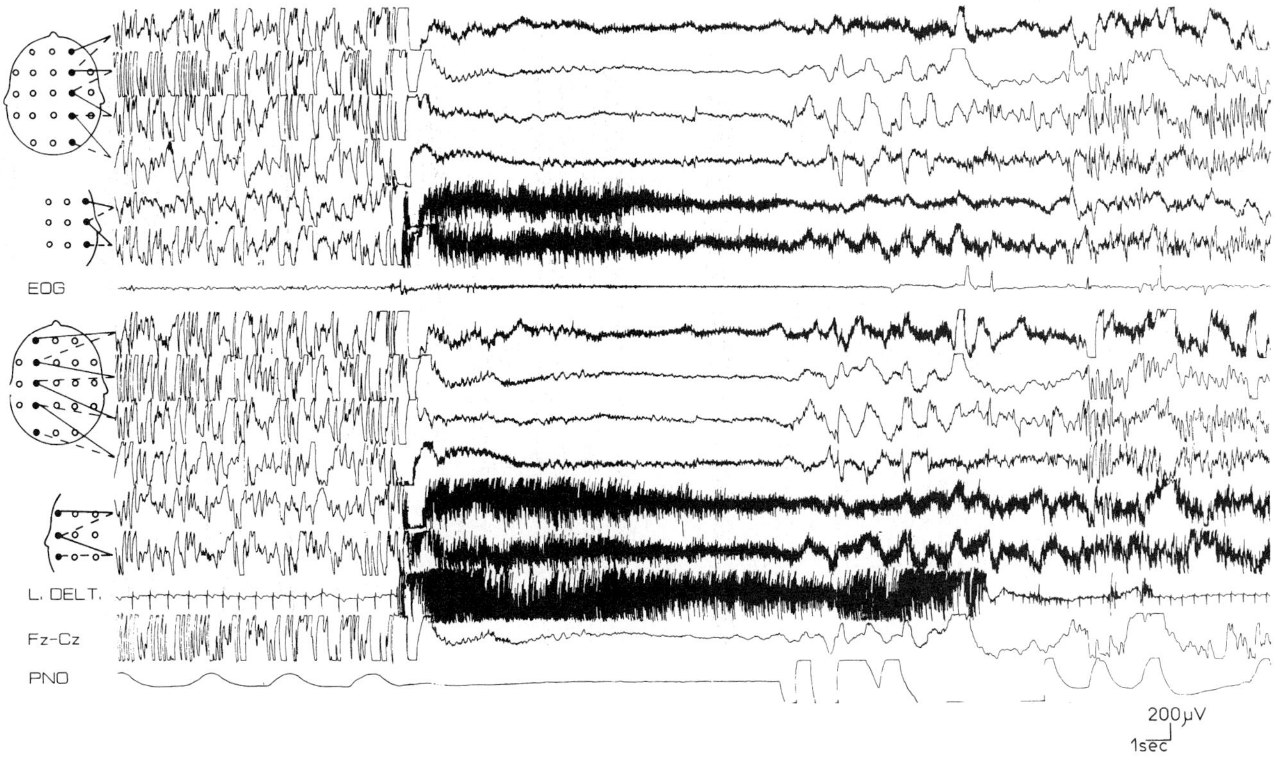

FIGURE 2. Awake recording of a tonic seizure in a boy with symptomatic Lennox-Gastaut syndrome. Interictal slow spikes-and-waves are abruptly interrupted by flattening, with superimposed rapid rhythms and muscular artifacts, for 15 seconds, followed by diffuse slow waves and then a burst of sharp waves. Polygraphy shows intense tonic contraction of the deltoid and apnea. (Note the decreased recording amplification used here.) EOG, oculogram; L DELT, left deltoid; PNO, pneumogram.

DIAGNOSTIC EVALUATION

The diagnosis of LGS is based on electroclinical findings, which must be carefully collected. A precise description of seizures must be obtained so that atypical absences and nocturnal tonic seizures can be detected. A sleep EEG must be performed, and an afternoon sleep recording after partial sleep deprivation is usually sufficient. If the results are not informative, the EEG must be repeated, as the whole clinical and EEG picture can establish itself progressively over time. Given the subtle nature of atypical absences and sometimes of the atonic or tonic seizures, polygraphic recording with axial EMG leads is compulsory, and the importance of video-EEG monitoring has been stressed.[8] Simultaneous etiologic investigations (neurocognitive, fundus, MRI, biology) help distinguish symptomatic from cryptogenic cases.

Criteria for an early diagnosis were proposed by Boniver et al.[16] Existence of one or several seizures typical for the syndrome, presence of diffuse slow spikes-and-waves in the EEG, and cognitive impairment were considered major criteria; high frequency of seizures, drug resistance, and atypical seizures were considered minor criteria. The presence of at least two major criteria during the first 6 months of the epilepsy was strongly predictive of the diagnosis.

During the course of the disorder, the diagnosis rests on the demonstration of tonic seizures or subclinical runs of fast rhythms at 10 to 12 Hz during sleep, not on the presence of diffuse slow spikes-and-waves alone. Thus, at least one EEG must be recorded during sleep. The best way to confirm the diagnosis is to make a long video and polygraphic EEG recording with the patient awake and engaged in some activities, and again with the patient asleep (recording during an afternoon nap may be sufficient), so that interictal and ictal patterns can be studied. It is also necessary to follow the psychomotor and cognitive development of the child by the appropriate psychometric testing in order to react quickly to special educational needs.

DIFFERENTIAL DIAGNOSIS

Diffuse slow spikes-and-waves do not constitute a sufficient criterion for the diagnosis of LGS; they can appear secondarily during the course of other types of epilepsy,[59] as reported by Beaumanoir[11] in 38 of 103 patients seen with severe epilepsy resembling LGS. They can also be observed in cases of idiopathic generalized epilepsies modified by iatrogenic factors, and in other specific settings like the Angelman syndrome, which should be easily recognizable. A multiple seizure-type disorder with cognitive decline like the Dravet syndrome (severe myoclonic epilepsy in infancy) should not be confused with LGS, due to its own many specific diagnostic features. The main characteristics of encephalopathic epilepsies of childhood are summarized in Table 1.

The main nosologic and clinical problems involved in the differential diagnosis of LGS are different in cryptogenic and symptomatic forms, and depend partly on age at onset.

For cryptogenic LGS, the main differential diagnosis is myoclonic astatic epilepsy of early childhood (MAE, Doose syndrome), which has often been poorly separated from LGS, especially in patients with MAE and an unfavorable course, which may be associated with tonic seizures during sleep.[24] Contrary to LGS, MAE is a truly idiopathic type of epilepsy, with a strong genetic component. An in-depth clinical evaluation[52] has stressed the differential features of MAE, all of which are apparent within 1 year from seizure onset: A family history

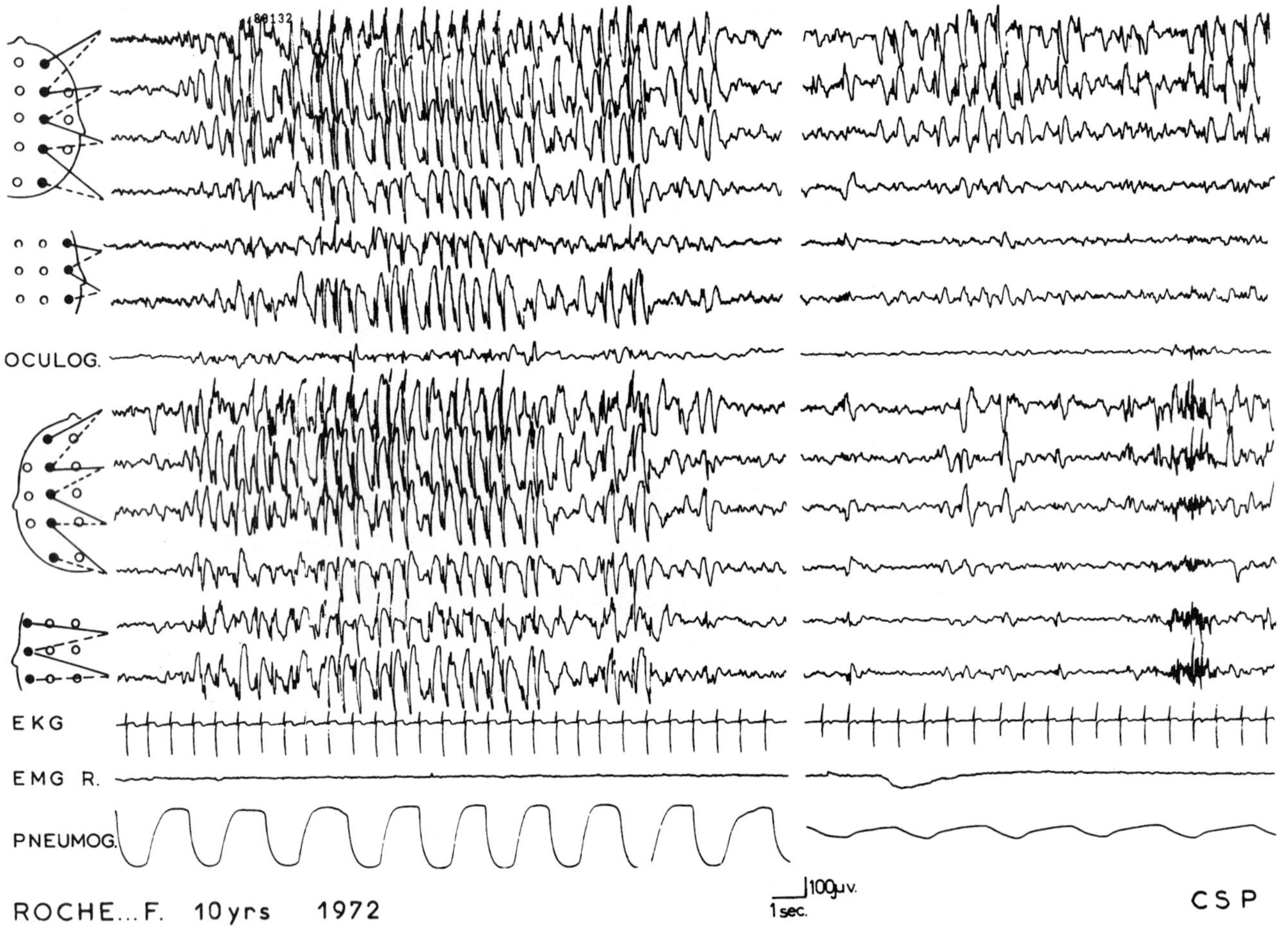

FIGURE 3. **Left:** Atypical absence with asymmetric, irregular, slow spikes-and-waves. **Right:** During slow sleep, one burst of frontal slow spikes-and-waves in the right hemisphere and a burst of rapid rhythms in the left hemisphere. In this girl, Lennox-Gastaut syndrome was preceded by partial seizures. EMG R, electromyogram of right deltoid.

of idiopathic epilepsy, earlier onset, fast spike-and-waves, and myoclonic and generalized tonic–clonic seizures are markers of a benign type of MAE with good outcome. Additionally, children with MAE may exhibit myoclonic status, vibratory tonic seizures, and marked slow components on the EEG, and may have a less favorable outcome. In this series, patients with a final diagnosis of LGS had atypical absences, no vibratory tonic seizures, no myoclonus, and a later age at onset, and all experienced mental degradation. Neurophysiology may also help in this differential diagnosis, with the evidence, on back-averaging studies of the EEG correlates of myoclonus, of SBS in the LGS versus a truly generalized aspect in MAE.[15]

Another condition has long been confused with LGS: Epilepsy with continuous spikes-and-waves during slow sleep (CSWS). Like LGS, CSWS, first described by Patry et al.,[71] can occur in children who were previously normal or already retarded, and in children with brain lesions or with normal MRI. It can succeed to partial or generalized epilepsy. It is characterized by atypical absences, drop attacks, mental deterioration, and diffuse slow spikes-and-waves in the EEG, especially pronounced during sleep. However, children with CSWS never have tonic seizures, either awake or during sleep, nor are runs of rapid rhythms or subclinical tonic seizures apparent in their sleep EEG. The typical sleep EEG pattern is one of continuous diffuse slow spikes-and-waves, which occupy at least 85% of slow sleep and are fragmented during rapid eye movement (REM) sleep. This pattern also occurs in children with acquired aphasia with auditory agnosia (Landau-Kleffner syndrome), which is not observed in patients with LGS. In CSWS, the epileptic seizures and EEG changes are strictly age related and always disappear at the latest during puberty.

Atypical benign partial epilepsy, described by Aicardi and Chevrie,[2] is difficult to diagnose at first, because it differs from CSWS only by its outcome and the absence of mental deterioration. It can be confused with LGS when electroclinical symptomatology worsens. At this stage, it is essential to look for factors that might explain these changes, such as inappropriate treatment or intercurrent disease, and to perform sleep EEG recordings to demonstrate the absence of tonic seizures and fast activities. This type of childhood epilepsy clearly overlaps with benign epilepsy with centrotemporal spikes and with CSWS. In the German-speaking area, the term of "pseudo-Lennox" syndrome is often used, even recommended, to describe such patients.[45]

There are severe focal epilepsies, usually of frontal lobe origin, in which seizures consist of sudden falls that resemble the drop attacks observed in the generalized epilepsies. However, in these disorders the electroclinical symptoms do not mimic those of LGS. In some cases, however, the diagnosis of focal epilepsy with SBS must be considered, to the point that the diagnosis may fluctuate between focal epilepsy with SBS and LGS at various moments during follow-up, as some age-dependent traits of LGS may disappear with maturation or may become less prominent due to medication.

TABLE 1

DISTINCTIVE FEATURES OF ENCEPHALOPATHIC CHILDHOOD EPILEPSIES

	Age at onset	First seizure	Other seizures	EEG changes	Mental outcome
LGS	2–8 yr	Variable	Falls Tonic, atonic Atypical absence Other (GTC, focal) Frequent status	Abnormal BA Slow SW 10–12 activities during sleep Multifocal changes	Abnormal
MAE	1–5 yr	Myoclonic, myoclonic astatic	Falls, GTC Myoclonic Atonic Obtundation state	Normal BA Centroparietal theta Generalized SW	Normal or abnormal
SME	<1 yr	Febrile clonic	Clonic, GTC, unilateral, Pseudogeneralized Myoclonic, absence, other	Normal BA at onset Multifocal Photosensitivity	Abnormal
ABPE	3–8 yr	Partial	Falls, focal Atypical absence neg. myoclonus	Normal BA Focal and diffuse	Normal

ABPE, atypical benign partial epilepsy; BA, background activity; GTC, generalized tonic–clonic; LGS, Lennox-Gastaut syndrome; MAE, myoclonic-astatic epilepsy; SME, severe myoclonic epilepsy; SW, spike-and-wave.

The concept of SBS was introduced by Jasper[51] and Tükel and Jasper.[85] SBS was described as bursts of high-amplitude, synchronous, slow spike-and-wave complexes, more or less symmetric over both hemispheres, caused by a unilateral epileptogenic lesion of the mesial surface of the frontal or temporal lobe. SBS is contrasted with *primary* bilateral synchrony, which is manifested by more rapid symmetric and synchronous spike-and-wave discharges over both hemispheres and is caused by a generalized epileptic process independent of any focal hemispheric lesion. Many authors have discussed this concept. Gastaut and Zifkin[35] and Blume[13] tried to establish the differences between epilepsy with SBS and LGS. According to the former, epilepsy with SBS begins later (mean age of onset, 10 years and 9 months); focal neurologic signs are much more frequent (hemiplegia in 30% vs. in 9% of those with LGS); obvious mental retardation is less frequent (35% vs. 87%); seizure frequency is lower; multiple seizure types are less often present in the same patient; partial seizures are more frequent; astatic seizures are less frequent; atypical absences are not observed; bursts of slow spikes-and-waves are more often asymmetric (50% vs. 23%); a constant, localized epileptic focus is seen in all cases of epilepsy with SBS versus a rather variable localized predominance of slow spikes-and-waves in LGS; and runs of rapid recruiting rhythms in slow sleep are less frequent (15% vs. 79%). The same EEG aspects were described by Niedermeyer et al.[65] in cases of severe head trauma associated with generalized tonic–clonic and complex partial seizures. Lesions are mainly frontal and temporal, and SBS can be the significant mechanism in such posttraumatic epilepsies. Epilepsy with SBS can be as severe as LGS. It is, however, important to recognize this situation, because surgery may be the treatment of choice in epilepsy with SBS—with either removal of the primary lesion when possible or callosotomy. Thorough functional imaging investigations can help determine the diagnosis and indication for surgery. Indeed, a study using ^{18}F-fluorodeoxyglucose (FDG)-PET in children with epileptic encephalopathies showed the absence of abnormal focal findings in five children with cryptogenic LGS, while focal changes were present in three fourths with an atypical LGS, and five sixths in LGS following infantile spasms.[30] It is clear that there is no tight border between LGS and epilepsy with SBS, especially in symptomatic, lesional cases.

TREATMENT

LGS is highly drug resistant. Classic antiepileptic drugs (AEDs) usually do not bring total seizure control, and the "gold standard" of monotherapy can seldom be applied.[12] Polytherapy, with a combination of drugs respectively active against the main seizure types, is the rule. A mixed seizure disorder with frequent attacks that requires polytherapy, like LGS, is a likely candidate for paradoxic aggravation of seizures,[37] and this phenomenon may escape attention due to the subtle character of seizures, to the unlikelihood of self-reporting, and to the spontaneously fluctuating course of the condition. Drugs that may aggravate typical absences are likely to increase atypical absences as well as myoclonic or astatic seizures. Specific aggravation has been described in LGS following the use of IV clonazepam, which may induce tonic status,[81] and following the use of gabapentin,[90] but these reports concern only the tip of the iceberg. Clinicians should thus remain acutely aware of the possibility of drug-induced aggravation in patients with LGS. Moreover, unwanted side effects of AED are more likely to occur in LGS, due to polytherapy and use of high daily doses, and they may be overlooked because of the spontaneous severity of the condition and the lack of adequate communication with the patient. Clinicians should also be aware of this. Recent considerations about treatment attitudes have stressed that individual risk–benefit considerations should apply.[77] Overtreatment is probably common, and may contribute in part to the unfavorable long-term evolution. Treatments used in LGS include classic MAE, recent MAE, and nonpharmacologic treatments like the ketogenic diet, vagus nerve stimulation, and surgery.

Among the classic AEDs, carbamazepine, valproate, and benzodiazepines are often used, mostly in combination. Despite their metabolic interactions, carbamazepine and valproate give interesting results when given in combination. Carbamazepine (like phenytoin) is effective against tonic seizures, but may increase absences, while valproate (like ethosuximide) is effective against atypical absences and myoclonic or atonic seizures, but has little effect on tonic seizures. Clobazam and nitrazepam have fewer side effects than clonazepam and may need to be prescribed alternatively because tolerance may occur. Nitrazepam, which has been recommended by the Marseille school in the treatment of LGS nearly 40 years ago, is seeming to enjoy a revival, with estimated responder rates above 50% and few side effects besides sedation and drooling.[49] Phenytoin can be used in adolescents and adults for the vibratory tonic and tonic–clonic attacks, and is often initiated during a tonic status. Ethosuximide can also help control the atypical absences.

Among the newer AEDs, vigabatrin has not proved very useful. However, it is worth trying, and some good results have been reported in LGS associated with cortical dysplasia.[44] Lamotrigine has proven efficacy in open studies[23,83] and in controlled trials,[64] apparently mostly when used in combination with valproate, which matches our own experience. Felbamate retains selective indications in LGS, with proven efficacy,[6] and a favorable effect on cognitive function and behavior[36]; its efficacy may be due in part to its combination with valproate.[78] Topiramate has been proven efficacious, especially against drop attacks, both in open-label, long-term studies[40] and in shorter controlled trials.[76] However, its efficacy is less prominent in LGS than in other epileptic encephalopathies like the Dravet syndrome.[62] There is a single study alluding to a possible positive effect of levetiracetam in LGS, especially against myoclonic and generalized tonic–clonic seizures, without effect, however, on tonic seizures.[22] Zonisamide has been used for more than 15 years in Japan, and is considered appropriate for use in LGS.[67] Among AEDs still in development, rufinamide has received an orphan drug designation in Europe for patients with LGS.[5]

The course of the disease is characterized by a succession of bad and better periods. During the better periods, only nocturnal seizures are observed, and patients are less handicapped in their daily life. But series of tonic seizures can occur suddenly, without obvious reason, particularly in the early morning. Even when epilepsy has improved, cognitive impairment and behavioral disturbances persist, requiring educational and psychological support. The degree of mental deficit is variable, from slight to profound. In cryptogenic cases, it increases with age and repetition of seizures, but it is less marked than in symptomatic cases.

One of the aims of treatment is to avoid episodes of status. Sometimes they are provoked by triggering factors, such as intercurrent illness, changes in drug regimen, and psychological stress.[26] In case of impending status, it is better not to change the treatment dramatically and not to hospitalize the patient in a nonspecialized unit. Rectal injections of diazepam or oral intake of a high dose of clobazam (30 to 40 mg) can stop serial attacks and avoid hospital admission. Overt status can be treated with IV benzodiazepines and/or phenytoin, sometimes with concomitant steroids, and with respiratory assistance if necessary. It must be noted that status is much less life threatening in LGS than in other types of epilepsies. Recovery is relatively swift. Steroids may be tried in children early in the course of the disease, as in infantile spasms.

Other treatments have been used in LGS, without controlled trials. IV γ-globulins have been proposed,[17] as has thyrotropin-releasing hormone.[54] The ketogenic diet has been used, but not in controlled trials.

Surgical procedures are not often considered as treatment options. Callosotomy brought significant seizure relief to 31 of 48 (64.6%) patients with LGS,[55] but is reputedly less efficacious than in focal epilepsies with SBS. There are only isolated reports on successful lesional surgery in patients with focal brain pathology and LGS.[27] Conversely, vagal nerve stimulation (VNS) has been used quite extensively in LGS, and is considered well tolerated. A Dutch study showed marked cognitive improvement, which did not correlate with the modest effect on seizures (26.9% average seizure reduction).[3] This contrasts with the 52.2% seizure reduction observed in a U.S. study,[50] in which 3 of 13 patients reached a 90% reduction in seizure frequency. Indeed, the response may increase over time, with seizure reduction of 42% at 1 month, 58.2% at 3 months, and 57.9% at 6 months.[31] Stimulation procedures differing from VNS, especially deep brain stimulation, have been tried in selected patients,[88] apparently with some positive results against atypical absences and tonic seizures.[86,87] Modern recommendations are that the baseline treatment for LGS should rely on valproate, benzodiazepines, and either lamotrigine or topiramate as second-line add-ons,[77] with the valproate + lamotrigine or valproate + topiramate probably representing the most logical, synergistic combinations. They carry their own risks, cumulating the potential side effects of either drug with the specific side effects of these combinations. According to a recent Cochrane review, none of the recent AED has shown spectacular power against LGS, and each case should be considered individually.[46] Indications for nonpharmacologic treatments should also be assessed individually. The multiplicity of therapeutic proposals does not really mask—and indeed, rather underlines—the relative impotency of medical intervention in LGS. Practical management is also a matter of common sense and restraint.

LONG-TERM PROGNOSIS

As stressed by all authors who have studied this syndrome, its long-term prognosis is unfavorable, and it is too soon to know whether it will be improved by recent advances in epilepsy treatment. Unfortunately, the availability of many new treatment options has not changed the global outlook for patients with LGS, in contrast with the apparently improved prognosis of MAE and Dravet syndrome.

Complete seizure-free recovery is rare: 13.7% of patients for Ohtahara et al.,[68] 6.7% for Gastaut et al.,[34] and none of the cryptogenic cases followed up for more than 15 years by Beaumanoir.[11] Among 72 patients followed over more than 10 years, 33% of the cryptogenic and 55% of the symptomatic cases had lost the characteristics of LGS, turning into nonspecific generalized symptomatic epilepsies, severe epilepsy with multiple independent spike foci, or localization-related epilepsies.[66] In another long-term study, with an average follow-up of 16 years, only 33% of 102 patients retained LGS.[91] Few studies have considered the epilepsy outcome in adulthood. Roger et al.[74] reported that only 47% of patients maintained a complete LGS profile in adulthood. Most had cryptogenic LGS with an onset before the age of 4 years. In 16%, generally those with symptomatic LGS, the syndrome as such disappeared, but an often severe, mostly unifocal epilepsy persisted, together with symptoms of frontal lobe dysfunctions. In 20%, seizures were rare, probably partial, but gross psychological disturbances were present. In 17%, epilepsy seemed to be nearly completely cured, with a normal or subnormal mental state. Rai et al.[72] reported on 17 patients institutionalized in an epilepsy center for a period of 16 years. The severity of epilepsy decreased even though the seizure types remained more or less unchanged. However, an attempt to reduce polytherapy failed, and a global improvement was observed only in three patients who had a relatively late onset of LGS between ages 5 and 10.

Mental deficiency is observed in 85% to 92% of patients. Major changes in behavior may occur at adolescence, with onset of violence, often directed against close family members. Frequently, but not consistently, patients become psychotic. Many patients are finally institutionalized, either in centers for epileptic patients or in homes for mentally handicapped people. Some children who are absolutely normal before the onset of cryptogenic LGS have a relatively good social outcome, with normal or near-normal schooling, and reach employment (often in a sheltered context) despite persisting seizures. The EEG features often attenuate with age, but some patients will retain

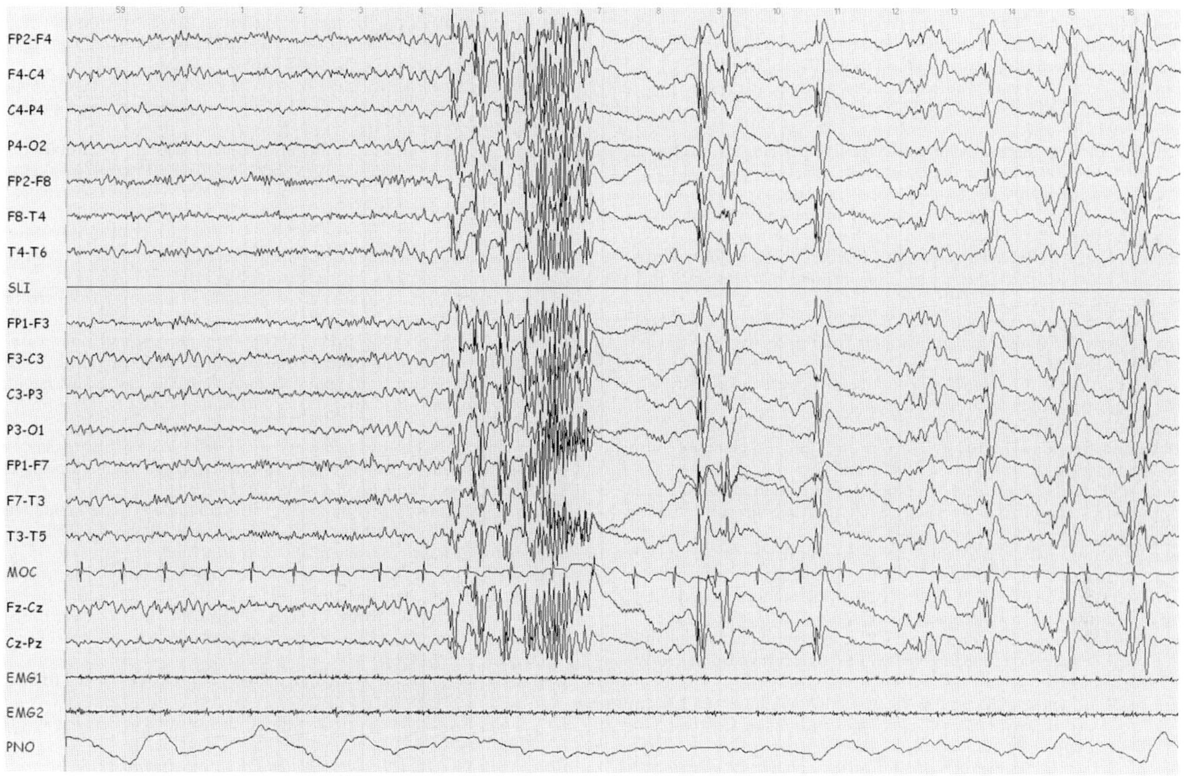

FIGURE 4. Sleep electroencephalogram (EEG) in a 48-year-old patient with cryptogenic Lennox-Gastaut syndrome since the age of 5. She lives in a home for the handicapped and has part-time sheltered employment. She still has several falls per month, atypical absences, and frequent nocturnal tonic seizures (usually several per night), with rare generalized tonic–clonic seizures. She receives a combination of valproate, felbamate, phenobarbital, and clobazam. Her waking EEG shows normal background α activity and is devoid of paroxysmal changes (not shown). During an afternoon sleep recording, there were few physiologic sleep transients and numerous high-amplitude bursts of fast activities, as well as suppressions and isolated spike-waves.

the full-blown LGS symptomatology, including the typical EEG traits, especially during sleep (Fig. 4), while awake EEGs may show only a slow background without slow spike-and-wave discharges.

Death is caused by intercurrent disease or accident, rarely by epilepsy itself. The mortality rate is difficult to assess: About 3% in the series of Gastaut et al.[34] with a mean follow-up of 8 years and 7 months, and 7% in that of Loubier[60] with a mean follow-up of 9 years and 9 months.

The main factors for a poor prognosis are the symptomatic nature of the syndrome, particularly after infantile spasms; early age at onset, before 3 years; high frequency of seizures; long duration of worsening periods; frequent status; and the presence of constantly slow background activity and multifocal localized abnormalities on the EEG.

SUMMARY AND CONCLUSIONS

Lennox-Gastaut syndrome is a well-defined epilepsy syndrome that can be easily recognized using a careful clinical and EEG approach and applying consensual diagnostic criteria. It is still overdiagnosed due to the prevalent concept that slow spike-waves and mental handicap is synonymous with LGS. It may be difficult to distinguish from myoclonic astatic epilepsy, and from epilepsies with secondary bilateral synchrony. It stands out among epileptic encephalopathies as a true syndrome, with multiple etiologies and a fairly homogenous presentation and prognosis. The multiplicity of therapeutic proposals does not really mask—and indeed, rather underlines—the relative impotency of medical intervention in LGS. Practical management is a matter of common sense and restraint. Here, as in other difficult-to-treat epilepsies, one shouldn't do anything just because not much can be done.

References

1. Agapejev S, Padula NA, Morales NM, et al. Neurocysticercosis and Lennox-Gastaut syndrome: case report. *Arq Neuropsiquiatr.* 2000;58:538–547.
2. Aicardi J, Chevrie JJ. Atypical benign partial epilepsy of childhood. *Dev Med Child Neurol.* 1982;24:281–292.
3. Aldenkamp AP, Van de Veerdonk SH, Majoie HJ, et al. Effects of 6 months of treatment with vagus nerve stimulation on behavior in children with Lennox-Gastaut Syndrome in an open clinical and nonrandomized study. *Epilepsy Behav.* 2001;2:343–350.
4. Alving J. Classification of the epilepsies and investigation of 402 children. *Acta Neurol Scand.* 1979;60:157–163.
5. Anonymous. Rufinamide: CGP 33101, E 2080, RUF 331, Xilep. *Drug R D.* 2005;6:249–252.
6. Avanzini G, Canger R, Dalla Bernardina B, et al. Felbamate in therapy-resistant epilepsy: an Italian experience. Felbamate Italian Study Group. *Epilepsy Res.* 1996;25:249–255.
7. Baldy-Moulinier M, Touchon J, Billiard M, et al. Nocturnal sleep studies in the Lennox-Gastaut syndrome. In: Niedermeyer E, Degen R, eds. *The Lennox-Gastaut Syndrome.* New York: Alan R. Liss; 1988:243–260.
8. Bare MA, Glauser TA, Strawsburg RH. Need for electroencephalogram video confirmation of atypical absence seizures in children with Lennox-Gastaut syndrome. *J Child Neurol.* 1998;13:498–500.
9. Bauer G, Aichner F, Saltuari L. Epilepsies with diffuse slow spikes and waves of late onset. *Eur Neurol.* 1983;22:344–350.
10. Beaumanoir A, Martin F, Panagopoulos M, et al. Le syndrome de Lennox. *Schweiz Arch Neurol Neurochir Psychiatr.* 1968;102:31–62.
11. Beaumanoir A. The Lennox-Gastaut syndrome. A personal study. *Electroencephalogr Clin Neurophysiol Suppl.* 1982;35:85–99.

12. Beaumanoir A, Blume WT. The Lennox-Gastaut syndrome. In: Roger J, Bureau M, Dravet C, et al., eds. *Epileptic Syndromes in Infancy, Childhood and Adolescence*. 4th ed. London: John Libbey; 2005:125–148.
13. Blume WT. Lennox-Gastaut syndrome and secondary bilateral synchrony: a comparison. In: Wolf P, ed. *Epileptic Seizures and Syndromes*. London: John Libbey; 1994:285–297.
14. Blume WT. Lennox-Gastaut syndrome: potential mechanisms of cognitive regression. *Ment Retard Dev Disabil Res Rev*. 2004;10:150–153.
15. Bonanni P, Parmeggiani L, Guerrini R. Different neurophysiologic patterns of myoclonus characterize Lennox-Gastaut syndrome and myoclonic astatic epilepsy. *Epilepsia*. 2002;43:609–615.
16. Boniver C, Dravet C, Bureau M, et al. Idiopathic Lennox-Gastaut syndrome. In: Wolf P, Dam M, Janz D, et al., eds. *Advances in Epileptology*. Vol. 16. New York: Raven Press; 1987:195–200.
17. Brett EM. The Lennox-Gastaut syndrome: therapeutic aspects. In: Niedermeyer E, Degen R, eds. *The Lennox-Gastaut Syndrome*. New York: Alan R. Liss; 1988:329–339.
18. Chevrie JJ, Aicardi J. Childhood epileptic encephalopathy with slow spike-wave. A statistical study of 80 cases. *Epilepsia*. 1972;13:259–271.
19. Chugani HT, Mazziotta JC, Engel J, et al. The Lennox-Gastaut syndrome. Metabolic subtypes determined by 2-deoxy-2-(18F)fluoro-glucose positron emission tomography. *Ann Neurol*. 1987;231:4–13.
20. Commission on Classification and Terminology of the International League Against Epilepsy. Proposal for a revised classification of epilepsies and epileptic syndromes. *Epilepsia*. 1985;26:268–278.
21. Costa P, Beaumanoir A. Modalités de début du syndrome de Lennox-Gastaut: à propos d'un cas. *Epilepsies*. 1992;4:221–228.
22. De Los Reyes EC, Sharp GB, Williams JP, et al. Levetiracetam in the treatment of Lennox-Gastaut syndrome. *Pediatr Neurol*. 2004;30:254–256.
23. Donaldson JA, Glauser TA, Olberding LS. Lamotrigine adjunctive therapy in childhood epileptic encephalopathy (the Lennox-Gastaut syndrome). *Epilepsia*. 1997;38:68–73.
24. Doose H. Myoclonic-astatic epilepsy of early childhood. In: Roger J, Bureau M, Dravet C, et al., eds. *Epileptic Syndromes in Infancy, Childhood and Adolescence*. London: John Libbey; 1992:103–114.
25. Doose H, Gerken H, Leonhardt R, et al. Centrencephalic myoclonic-astatic petit mal. *Neuropädiatrie*. 1970;2:59–78.
26. Dravet C, Natale O, Magaudda A, et al. Les états de mal dans le syndrome de Lennox-Gastaut. *Rev Neurophysiol Clin*. 1985;15:361–368.
27. Dravet C. Lennox-Gastaut syndrome: a surgically remediable epilepsy. In: Lüders HO, Comair YG, eds. *Epilepsy Surgery*. Philadelphia: Lippincott Williams & Wilkins; 2001:165–175.
28. Eeg-Olofsson O. Genetic factors. In: Niedermeyer E, Degen R, eds. *The Lennox-Gastaut Syndrome*. New York: Alan R. Liss; 1988:65–71.
29. Engel J. A proposed diagnostic scheme for people with epileptic seizures and with epilepsy: report of the ILAE Task Force on Classification and Terminology. *Epilepsia*. 2001;42:796–803.
30. Ferrie CD, Maisey M, Cox T, et al. Focal abnormalities detected by 18FDG PET in epileptic encephalopathies. *Arch Dis Child*. 1996;75:102–107.
31. Frost M, Gates J, Helmers SL, et al. Vagus nerve stimulation in children with refractory seizures associated with Lennox-Gastaut syndrome. *Epilepsia*. 2001;42:1148–1152.
32. Gastaut H. The Lennox-Gastaut syndrome: comments on the syndrome's terminology and nosological position amongst the secondary generalized epilepsies in childhood. *Electroencephalogr Clin Neurophysiol Suppl*. 1982;35:71–84.
33. Gastaut H, Roger J, Soulayrol R, et al. Childhood epileptic encephalopathy with diffuse slow spike-waves (otherwise known as "petit mal variant") or Lennox syndrome. *Epilepsia*. 1966;7:139–179.
34. Gastaut H, Dravet C, Loubier D, et al. Évolution clinique et prognostic du syndrome de Lennox-Gastaut. In: Lugaresi E, Pazzaglia P, Tassinari C, eds. *Evolution and Prognosis of Epilepsies*. Bologna: Aulo Gaggi; 1973:133–154.
35. Gastaut H, Zifkin B. Secondary bilateral synchrony and Lennox-Gastaut syndrome. In: Niedermeyer E, Degen R, eds. *The Lennox-Gastaut Syndrome*. New York: Alan R. Liss; 1988:221–242.
36. Gay PE, Mecham GF, Coskey JS, et al. Behavioral effects of felbamate in childhood epileptic encephalopathy (Lennox-Gastaut syndrome). *Psychol Rep*. 1995;77:1208–1210.
37. Genton P. When antiepileptic drugs aggravate epilepsy. *Brain Dev*. 2000;22:75–80.
38. Gibbs FA. The electroencephalogram in epileptic seizures. *Tabul Biol ('s-Grav)*. 1938;16:128.
39. Gibbs FA, Gibbs EL, Lennox WG. The influence of the blood sugar level on the wave and spike formation in petit mal epilepsy. *Arch Neurol Psychiatry*. 1939;41:1111–1116.
40. Glauser TA, Levisohn PM, Ritter F, et al. Topiramate in Lennox-Gastaut syndrome: open-label treatment of patients completing a randomized controlled trial. Topiramate YL Study Group. *Epilepsia*. 2000;41(Suppl 1):S86–90.
41. Goldsmith IL, Zupanc ML, Buchhalter JR. Long-term seizure outcome in 74 patients with Lennox-Gastaut syndrome: effects of incorporating MRI head imaging in defining the cryptogenic subgroup. *Epilepsia*. 2000;41: 395–399.
42. Guerrini R. Genetic malformations of the cerebral cortex and epilepsy. *Epilepsia*. 2005;46(Suppl 1):32–37.
43. Guerrini R, Genton P, Bureau M, et al. Reflex seizures are frequent in patients with Down syndrome and epilepsy. *Epilepsia*. 1990;31:406–417.
44. Guerrini R, Paglia G, Dravet C, et al. Efficacy of vigabatrin as add-on therapy in relation to type of epilepsy or epileptic syndrome: retrospective study of 120 patients. *Epilepsia*. 1994;35(Suppl 7):65.
45. Hahn A, Pistohl J, Neubauer BA, et al. Atypical "benign" partial epilepsy or pseudo-Lennox syndrome. Part I: symptomatology and long-term prognosis. *Neuropediatrics*. 2001;32:1–8.
46. Hancock E, Cross H. Treatment of Lennox-Gastaut syndrome. *Cochrane Database Syst Rev*. 2003;3:CD003277.
47. Heiskala H. Community-based study of Lennox-Gastaut syndrome. *Epilepsia*. 1997;38:526–531.
48. Hoffmann-Riem M, Diener W, Benninger C, et al. Nonconvulsive status epilepticus–a possible cause of mental retardation in patients with Lennox-Gastaut syndrome. *Neuropediatrics*. 2000;31:169–174.
49. Hosain SA, Green NS, Solomon GE, et al. Nitrazepam for the treatment of Lennox-Gastaut syndrome. *Pediatr Neurol*. 2003;28:16–19.
50. Hosain S, Nikalov B, Harden C, et al. Vagus nerve stimulation treatment for Lennox-Gastaut syndrome. *J Child Neurol*. 2000;15:509–512.
51. Jasper H. Étude anatomo-physiologique des épilepsies. In: Fischgold H, ed. *Compte-rendus du 2ème Congrès International d'EEG, Paris, 1949*. Paris: Masson; 1949:99–111.
52. Kaminska A, Ickowicz A, Plouin P, et al. Delineation of cryptogenic Lennox-Gastaut syndrome and myoclonic astatic epilepsy using multiple correspondence analysis. *Epilepsy Res*. 1999;36:15–29.
53. Kondo M, Fukao T, Teramoto T, et al. A common variable immunodeficient patient who developed acute disseminated encephalomyelitis followed by the Lennox-Gastaut syndrome. *Pediatr Allergy Immunol*. 2005;16:357–360.
54. Kubek MJ, Garg BP. Thyrotropin-releasing hormone in the treatment of intractable epilepsy. *Pediatr Neurol*. 2002;1:9–17.
55. Kwan SY, Lin JH, Wong TT, et al. Prognostic value of electrocorticography findings during callosotomy in children with Lennox-Gastaut syndrome. *Seizure*. 2005;14:470–475.
56. Lee IH, Kwan SY, Su MS. Eating seizures in Lennox-Gastaut syndrome. *Eur Neurol*. 2001;45(2):123–125.
57. Lennox WG. The petit mal epilepsies; their treatment with tridione. *JAMA*. 1945;129:1069–1074.
58. Lennox WG. *Epilepsy and Related Disorders*. Boston: Little Brown; 1960.
59. Lennox WG, Davis JP. Clinical correlates of the fast and the slow spike-wave electroencephalogram. *Pediatrics*. 1950;5:626–644.
60. Loubier D. *Le syndrome de Lennox-Gastaut: modalités évolutives (Thèse Médecine)*. Marseille: 1974.
61. Markand O. Slow wave activity in EEG and associated clinical features: often called "Lennox" or "Lennox-Gastaut" syndrome. *Neurology*. 1977;27:746–757.
62. Mikaeloff Y, de Saint-Martin A, Mancini J, et al. Topiramate: efficacy and tolerability in children according to epilepsy syndromes. *Epilepsy Res*. 2003;53:225–232.
63. Mitsufuji N, Ikuta H, Yoshioka H, et al. Lennox-Gastaut syndrome associated with leukoencephalopathy. *Pediatr Neurol*. 1996;15:63–65.
64. Motte J, Trevathan E, Arvidsson JF, et al. Lamotrigine for generalized seizures associated with the Lennox-Gastaut syndrome. Lamictal Lennox-Gastaut Study Group. *N Engl J Med*. 1998;339:851–852.
65. Niedermeyer E, Walker AE, Burton C. The slow spike-wave complex as a correlate of frontal and fronto-temporal post-traumatic epilepsy. *Eur Neurol*. 1970;3:330–346.
66. Oguni H, Hayashi K, Osawa M. Long-term prognosis of Lennox-Gastaut syndrome. *Epilepsia*. 1996;37(Suppl 3):44–47.
67. Ohtahara S. Zonisamide in the management of epilepsy-Japanese experience. *Epilepsy Res*. 2006;68(Suppl 2):25–33.
68. Ohtahara S, Yamatogi Y, Ohtsuka Y. Prognosis of the Lennox syndrome. Long-term clinical and electroencephalographic follow-up study, especially with special reference to relationship with the West syndrome. *Folia Psychiatr Neurol Jpn*. 1976;30:275–287.
69. Oller Daurella L. *"El Sindrome de Lennox."* Barcelona: Espaxs; 1967.
70. Oller Daurella L. Un type spécial de crises observées dans le syndrome de Lennox-Gastaut d'apparition tardive. *Rev Neurol (Paris)*. 1970;122:459–462.
71. Patry G, Lyagoubi S, Tassinari CA. Subclinical electrical status epilepticus induced by sleep. An electroencephalographical study of six cases. *Arch Neurol*. 1971;24:242–252.
72. Rai PV,Fülöp T, Erçal S. Clinical course of Lennox-Gastaut syndrome in institutionalized adult patients. In: Niedermeyer E, Degen R, eds. *The Lennox-Gastaut Syndrome*. New York: Alan R. Liss; 1988:409–418.
73. Renier WO. Neuromorphological and biochemical analysis of a brain biopsy in a second case of idiopathic Lennox-Gastaut syndrome. In: Niedermeyer E, Degen R, eds. *The Lennox-Gastaut Syndrome*. New York: Alan R. Liss; 1988:427–432.
74. Roger J, Remy C, Bureau M, et al. Le syndrome de Lennox-Gastaut de l'adulte. *Rev Neurol (Paris)*. 1987;143:401–405.
75. Roger J, Gambarelli-Dubois D. Neuropathological studies of the Lennox-Gastaut syndrome. In: Niedermeyer E, Degen R, eds. *The Lennox-Gastaut Syndrome*. New York: Alan R. Liss; 1988:73–93.
76. Sachdeo RC, Glauser TA, Ritter F, et al. A double-blind, randomized trial of topiramate in Lennox-Gastaut syndrome. Topiramate YL Study Group. *Neurology*. 1999;52:1882–1887.
77. Schmidt D, Bourgeois B. A risk-benefit assessment of therapies for Lennox-Gastaut syndrome. *Drug Saf*. 2000;22:467–477.

78. Siegel H, Kelley K, Stertz B, et al. The efficacy of felbamate as add-on therapy to valproic acid in the Lennox-Gastaut syndrome. *Epilepsy Res*. 1999;34:91–97.
79. Smeraldi E, Smeraldi RS, Cazzullo CL, et al. Immunogenetics of the Lennox-Gastaut syndrome: frequency of HL-A antigens and haplotypes in patients and first degree relatives. *Epilepsia*. 1975;16:699–703.
80. Sorel L. L'épilepsie myokinétique grave de la première enfance avec pointe-onde lente et son traitement. *Rev Neurol* (*Paris*). 1964;110:215–223.
81. Tassinari CA, Dravet C, Roger J, et al. Tonic status epilepticus precipitated by intravenous benzodiazepines in five patients with the Lennox-Gastaut syndrome. *Epilepsia*. 1972;13:421–435.
82. Theodore WH, Rose D, Patronas N, et al. Cerebral glucose metabolism in the Lennox-Gastaut syndrome. *Ann Neurol*. 1987;21:14–21.
83. Timmings PL, Richens A. Lamotrigine as add-on drug in the management of Lennox-Gastaut syndrome. *Eur Neurol*. 1992;32:305–307.
84. Trevathan E, Murphy CC, Yeargin-Allsopp M. Prevalence and descriptive epidemiology of Lennox-Gastaut syndrome among Atlanta children. *Epilepsia*. 1997;38:1283–1288.
85. Tükel K, Jasper H. The electroencephalogram in parasagittal lesions. *Electroencephalogr Clin Neurophysiol*. 1952;4:481–494.
86. Velasco M, Velasco F, Velasco AL. Centromedian-thalamic and hippocampal electrical stimulation for the control of intractable epileptic seizures. *J Clin Neurophysiol*. 2001;18:495–513.
87. Velasco F, Velasco M, Jimenez F, et al. Stimulation of the central median thalamic nucleus for epilepsy. *Stereotact Funct Neurosurg*. 2001;77:228–232.
88. Velasco M, Eugenia-Diaz-de Leon A, Marquez I, et al. Temporo-spatial correlations between scalp and centromedian thalamic EEG activities of stage II slow wave sleep in patients with generalized seizures of the cryptogenic Lennox-Gastaut syndrome. *Clin Neurophysiol*. 2002;113:25–32.
89. Viani F. Le syndrome de Lennox-Gastaut. Problèmes actuels et perspectives de recherche. *Epilepsies*. 1991;3:2–3.
90. Vossler DG. Exacerbation of seizures in Lennox-Gastaut syndrome by gabapentin. *Neurology*. 1996;46:852–853.
91. Yagi K. Evolution of Lennox-Gastaut syndrome: a long-term longitudinal study. *Epilepsia*. 1996;37(Suppl 3):48–51.

CHAPTER 242 ■ LANDAU-KLEFFNER SYNDROME AND CSWS

MICHAEL C. SMITH AND CHARLES E. POLKEY

INTRODUCTION

Landau-Kleffner syndrome (LKS) and the syndrome of continuous spikes-and-waves during slow sleep (CSWS) were described independently and have been considered separate disorders. Both have been given distinct recognition by the Commission on Classification and Terminology of the International League Against Epilepsy[13] and by the World Health Organization in the International Classification of Diseases.[74] More recently, however, emphasis has been placed on the possibility that there may be common features in the pathophysiology of these two syndromes[15,25,27,28,41,43,62,71] and that LKS may actually be a subtype of CSWS.[25,43,46,62] A major symposium on this subject was held in Venice in 1993 and published in 1995.[8]

LKS and CSWS appear to represent points on a spectrum of functional age-related epilepsies ranging from the "benign" idiopathic localization-related childhood syndromes, such as benign childhood epilepsy with centrotemporal spikes (BECT), to full-blown continuous spikes-and-waves in slow sleep associated with behavioral disturbances.[62] They differ from the secondary generalized epilepsies, such as Lennox-Gastaut syndrome (LGS), in being a truly functional disturbance induced by age-related, self-limited paroxysmal activity.

HISTORICAL PERSPECTIVES

In 1957 Landau and Kleffner[37] reported six children with a syndrome of "acquired aphasia with a convulsive disorder." One of the children became aphasic and hemiplegic after a head injury, but the other five children's developmental aphasia was related to their convulsive disorder. These five children were presented in detail, with one added as an addendum. Landau and Kleffner described an aphasia that developed over days to months that then persisted from 2 weeks to several years. The associated seizures included grand mal, petit mal, and myoclonic seizures, and the paroxysmal abnormality was usually bilateral, most prominent over the temporal lobes.

They felt that although the relationship was not perfect, the severity of the paroxysmal disturbance on the electroencephalogram (EEG) did correspond to the severity of language disturbance. Landau and Kleffner noted that the seizures were easily controlled and the prognosis was generally good. They hypothesized that persistent convulsive discharge in brain tissue responsible for linguistic communication results in the functional ablation of these areas for normal language behavior. Their thesis was supported by the fact that these children did not have clouded consciousness like patients in petit mal status and had good performance on nonverbal intelligence tests.[37]

Since that time there have been over 350 published cases of acquired aphasia associated with a paroxysmal EEG.[4] The EEG abnormality is a predominantly bilateral posterior temporal spike or spike-and-wave discharge that is activated by slow-wave sleep. Most observers agree that the ultimate language outcome correlates with the age of onset of this epileptic disturbance, as well as its severity, bilateral anatomic location, and duration of the active phase.[15,28,41,62]

In 1971 Patry et al.[52] described "subclinical electrical status epilepticus" induced by sleep in children. They reported on six children who displayed seizures; cognitive decline, including language dysfunction; and severe paroxysmal EEG disturbance. The patients ranged in age from 7 to 12, four boys and two girls. There was a history of birth trauma in three, consanguinity in two, and epilepsy in the family of one. All displayed continuous spikes-and-waves in 85% of the non–rapid eye movement (REM) sleep record for an extended period of time. Seizures were described as atonic, generalized tonic–clonic, convulsive, clonic, and atypical absence. Five of the six children were mentally retarded and two failed to acquire language. The authors noted that the degree of mental retardation was related to the age of onset of the seizures and hypothesized that this syndrome represented a form of encephalopathy secondary to a focal or multifocal brain lesion. The activation of the paroxysmal activity during sleep, especially slow-wave sleep, was due to a particularly active synchronizing system during slow sleep.[52]

Tassinari et al. later retitled this syndrome electrical status epilepsy during sleep (ESES)[69] and then CSWS,[67] as a result of the criticism that clinical seizures were not seen during the spike-and-wave discharges. Tassinari et al. concluded that the persistent continuous spike-and-wave discharges over years were responsible for the complex and severe neurologic impairment.[67]

DEFINITIONS

LKS is a functional disorder of childhood usually described as having the following features: Acquired aphasia, paroxysmal EEG that is usually bitemporal, seizures that are easily treatable and self-limited, no demonstrable brain pathology that is sufficient to explain the behavioral symptomatology, and some degree of improvement when the epileptic condition resolves.[17,25,36,46,49,53,57]

Although these features are commonly cited in the literature, there are exceptions. The language disturbance is described as an acquired aphasia, but both these terms have been challenged. Rapin et al. argued that it is not an aphasia, but a verbal agnosia.[56] In fact, recent evidence suggests that it is an auditory agnosia.[49] Acquired aphasia implies a demonstrable age-appropriate language prior to onset of the CSWS. Early onset of the same process could prevent language function before any language is clearly demonstrable; however, a diagnosis of LKS would be impossible in this situation unless the aphasia is reversed by stopping the epileptic activity.

The paroxysmal EEG is commonly described as predominantly bitemporal and activated by sleep, especially slow-wave sleep. It usually becomes continuous in slow-wave sleep and persists for an extended period.[46] However, the paroxysmal disturbance may be interrupted by normal sleep EEG patterns, and eventually the epileptiform EEG disturbances disappear completely.[29] Furthermore, as will be discussed later, there is evidence to suggest that the primary epileptogenic region is unilateral.[46,49] Awake EEGs may be normal, even in the active phase of spike-and-wave during sleep. Seizures are not always seen, and when present may be quite subtle and not reported.[17,27,49]

Although there is no demonstrable brain pathology sufficient to explain the language dysfunction, multiple nonspecific structural abnormalities have been associated with LKS,[63] which presumably accounts for the epileptiform disturbances.

There is improvement in language function in all patients with the resolution of the active phase of spike-and-wave discharges; however, permanent sequelae in language function are usually seen, especially when there has been early onset of epileptic EEG activity[8,25,53,62] and when the epileptic activity is not eliminated before the critical period for language development is over.[44,49,57,58] LKS therefore represents an age-dependent functional disruption of language induced by a localized paroxysmal EEG disturbance.

CSWS is a functional disorder of childhood with the following features: Severe paroxysmal EEG disturbance, occupying at least 85% of sleep (sleep index 85%); seizures that may be severe but self-limited; behavioral deterioration, with or without premorbid developmental disturbances; no demonstrable brain pathology sufficient to explain the behavioral deterioration; and stabilization or improvement of behavior once the epileptiform EEG abnormalities resolve.[9,68]

These features are not invariably agreed upon. Although Tassinari et al.[68] have maintained that a sleep index of 85% is a necessary component of the diagnosis, the ILAE definition did not require it (ILAE 1989). There may be fluctuations, fragmentation, and variability in the continuity of the spike-and-wave discharges over time. Seizures are usually seen, but they may be subtle and go unreported.[9,68] Traditional antiepileptic drugs usually prevent the expression of the seizures but do not eliminate the paroxysmal EEG abnormality. Although behavioral deterioration is seen in all patients, it may not be as marked in those with previously abnormal development.[68]

Prior abnormal neurologic development is not uncommon in CSWS. Demonstrable brain pathology is seen, but it is insufficient to explain the deterioration of function. There is spontaneous resolution of the epileptiform discharges by the midteenage years with stabilization and often improvement of the neuropsychological and behavioral deterioration. However, significant permanent sequelae are seen in the majority of patients that appear to be related to the duration of the active phase of spike-and-wave activity.[9,53,73] CSWS, therefore, also appears to be an age-dependent disturbance of brain function, induced by a severe paroxysmal disturbance that resolves over time.

EPIDEMIOLOGY

The frequency of Landau-Kleffner syndrome cannot be accurately ascertained. Using the strict diagnostic criteria discussed earlier, LKS is a rare disorder. There have been over 350 published cases since 1957. There were 81 cases reported between 1957 and 1980, but 117 cases were reported between 1980 and 1990.[3] Dugas et al.[21] observed one new case per year in a Parisian psychiatric clinic. Males are affected more commonly than females, with a peak onset between 5 and 7 years of age.[10]

The frequency of CSWS is also unknown. Using the strict criteria of continuous spike-and-wave discharge during 85% of sleep associated with cognitive and behavioral decline, CSWS is a rare disorder. Between 1971 and 1984, Tassinari et al. reported 19 personal cases from the Centre St. Paul in Marseille and an additional 25 from the literature.[67] Since 1984, ten new cases have been seen at the Centre St. Paul, a rate of one to two per year.[68] Males are affected more commonly than females, with a peak onset between 5 and 7 years of age.[10]

ETIOLOGY AND BASIC MECHANISMS

A convergence of evidence suggests that LKS and CSWS are due to a common pathophysiologic mechanism,[14,25,27,29,41,43,46,62,71] and a specific hypothesis has been proposed for LKS.[46,49] Both disorders develop during a period of cortical synaptogenesis when the basic functional circuitry is being established (age 1 to 8). Synaptogenesis involves an overabundant growth of axonal processes and synaptic contacts thought to be twice the number found in mature adults.[31,32,54,55] Neuronal activity or synaptic use is the major factor that determines which synapses will be strengthened and which will be pruned.[31,54] The environment, more than genetic programming, plays the crucial role in the establishment of permanent synaptic contacts. If a significant paroxysmal EEG disturbance is present during this age-dependent synaptogenesis, it acts to strengthen synaptic contacts that should have degenerated in order for the neuronal aggregates to mediate normal behavior.[49] In the case of LKS, the paroxysmal activity reinforces inappropriate contacts in the developing temporoparietal cortex, thus producing a permanent language dysfunction.[49] In addition, the disturbance must have a bilateral effect to prevent transfer of function to the contralateral homotopic cortex. In CSWS, the most prominent paroxysmal activity appears to be in the frontal area, which would disrupt higher cognitive and executive function and attention before producing language dysfunction. Because the functional disruptions induced by paroxysmal EEG activity can spread to involve a larger cortical area, the symptom complexes of LKS and CSWS tend to merge as the disease goes on, producing severe cognitive, behavioral, and social dysfunction, much like the child with severe autism.

This proposed underlying mechanism predicts that, if unsuccessfully treated, those children affected earlier in this period of synaptogenesis will suffer the most serious neuropsychological sequelae after the epileptiform disturbances remit. Several authors have reported this in their series.[8,23,57,58,70] The importance of overactive inhibition as well as overactive excitation in these syndromes has been recently highlighted. This combination results in coexistence of a lack of overt seizures at the same time as severe cognitive/language dysfunction—a hallmark of the epileptic encephalopathies.[27]

Multiple nonspecific pathologic abnormalities can be associated with these syndromes and, although insufficient to explain the behavioral deterioration, may be responsible for the epileptic disturbances. Common etiologies in CSWS include congenital hydrocephalus, periventricular, and diffuse atrophy.[7,20] The pathologic findings associated with LKS in the literature are similar to those seen in other partial epilepsies; they include encephalitis, vasculitis, subpial gliosis, cysticercosis, and neuronal migration disorders.[12] The biopsy material taken from the temporal pole, at a distance from the primary epileptic site, in one surgical series of 14 patients with LKS revealed a variety of pathologic abnormalities in 13.[63]

The mechanistic hypothesis presented here raises the question of whether other epilepsies might also induce progressive behavioral dysfunction. BECT and other idiopathic localization-related epilepsies involving frontal, temporal, parietal, and occipital lobes all could have deleterious effects on cortical development and function where the abnormality is maximal. It may be that we cannot clinically detect the permanent sequelae because of the poor sensitivity of our testing.

CLINICAL PRESENTATION

Landau-Kleffner Syndrome

LKS is an acquired epileptic aphasia or auditory agnosia, occurring in a previously normal child, in language function, in association with paroxysmal EEG abnormalities with or without clinically apparent seizures, and without a structural substrate sufficient to account for the behavioral deterioration. The disorder begins most commonly between the ages of 3 and 8 in children who have already developed age-appropriate speech. The onset may be subacute or stuttering and initially consists of a loss of verbal understanding (i.e., receptive disturbances predominate). Soon, however, speech output is affected and paraphasias and phonologic errors appear. In the most severe cases, the child becomes entirely mute and will fail to respond to even nonverbal sounds—such as the ring of a telephone, a knock on the door, or a dog barking—that were previously well attended to. Behavioral disorders such as hyperactivity and attention deficit are common. Rarely, there is progression to severe disinhibition and psychosis.[3,46,49]

Seizures vary in type, but most commonly are associated with eye blinking or brief ocular deviation, head drop, and minor automatisms with occasional secondary generalization. They bear a variable relationship to the language deficit, and, indeed, from 20% to 30% of patients do not exhibit behavioral seizures.[4] The seizures have a benign course, are readily responsive to antiepileptic drugs, and generally subside by the age of 15 years. The language disturbance, as a rule, has a much less satisfactory prognosis, although early on the symptoms may show marked fluctuation, and even complete recovery, within weeks or months of onset.[15] However, if the aphasia persists for more than 2 to 3 years, complete recovery is most unusual; such patients may expect a lifelong linguistic defect.[8,36,46,49,53,57]

A critical component of LKS is the presence of continuous 1.5- to 5-Hz spike-and-wave EEG discharges in slow sleep that fragment or disappear during REM sleep[29,41,42,46,49] (Fig. 1). It is this latter feature that links the two conditions under discussion and provides the impetus to seek clinical similarities. A distinctive feature of LKS, however, is that the spike-and-wave discharges predominate in the posterior temporal regions. Most patients do not show spike-and-wave activity for 85% or more of slow sleep at the time of study, and some may not show continuous spike-and-wave during sleep at all; however, it has been assumed that this condition was met at some point during the course of the disorder.[46] During the active phase, brief posterior temporal epileptiform discharges can also be seen during wakefulness on the routine EEG, which can be localized to one posterior temporal region. With the use of the methohexital suppression test,[47,64] intracarotid amobarbital, EEG dipole mapping, and magnetoencephalogram (MEG), it can be shown that most, if not all, children have a unilateral primary epileptogenic region.[39,46,49,51,65] This can involve either side, since the contralateral propagation of paroxysmal discharges creates bilateral dysfunction that disrupts normal language development, regardless of the side of origin.

Continuous Spikes-and-Waves during Slow Sleep

The EEG pattern of CSWS consists of bilateral generalized, 1.5- to 5-Hz spike-and-wave discharges strongly activated by sleep, being present for 85% to 90% of slow-wave sleep and interrupted during REM episodes or in the waking state. REM and wakefulness are characterized by focal or multifocal paroxysmal EEG activity, or by brief bursts of bilateral spike-and-wave discharges.[52] Focal spikes tend to be frontal.

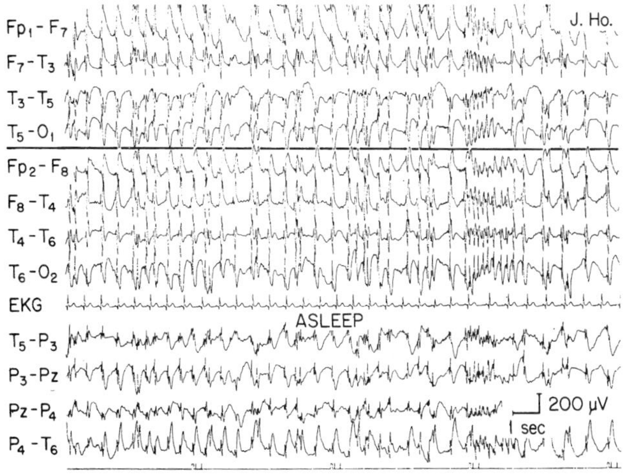

FIGURE 1. Electroencephalogram tracing taken during sleep in a patient with Landau-Kleffner syndrome prior to treatment. Such patterns may occupy 80% to 90% of the hours normally given to slow-wave sleep. The first four channels derive from the left hemisphere, the second four from the homotopic regions on the right. The lowest four channels show a transverse array, left to right, across the parietal region. Electrode designations are those of the standard "10 to 20" international system. (From Morrell F, Whisler WW, Smith MC, et al. Landau-Kleffner syndrome: treatment with subpial intracortical transection. *Brain.* 1995;118:1529–1546.)

Generally, the seizures associated with CSWS are focal motor or hemiclonic, partial motor, complex partial, absence, or secondarily generalized tonic–clonic. Tonic seizures do not occur. Although the seizures may be frequent, they are usually responsive to medical management and disappear entirely in the middle teens.[10,68]

Much more serious are the cognitive disturbances. These may include aphasias and apraxias, but generally embody widespread multisystem cognitive decline leading to substantial retardation and dementia.[9,68] Although the cognitive symptoms are highly correlated in time with the onset of CSWS, antiepileptic drugs do not improve them.

Tassinari et al.[68] have distinguished three groups of patients with CSWS based on clinical seizures. The first group suffers rare orofacial, generalized tonic–clonic, and myoclonic seizures in sleep. These patients resemble children with BECT. The second group suffers unilateral partial, generalized tonic–clonic, and absence seizures. The frequency of seizures in this group is greater, and seizures occur in wakefulness. The third group has unilateral partial and generalized tonic–clonic seizures in sleep and absence, absence status, and atonic seizures with falls in wakefulness.[68]

When reviewing the psychomotor development and neuropsychological disturbances, Tassinari et al.[68] distinguished two groups. The first has a normal development prior to the CSWS. During the active phase of epileptic discharge, there is a severe decrease in IQ, marked reduction in language function in the majority, severe disturbance of temporospatial orientation, and a marked behavioral disturbance in all. The behavioral disturbance includes reduced attention span, hyperactivity, aggressiveness, disinhibition, and difficulty in contact with the environment. The second group has pre-existing abnormalities of psychomotor development. These patients suffer deterioration of function and worsening of behavior, but this condition

TABLE 1

COMPARISON OF LKS VERSUS CSWS[a]

	LKS	CSWS
Sex	(Sex) 68% male	(Sex) 63% male
Antecedent history	3% encephalopathy	31%; 36% cerebral palsy; 36% encephalopathy
FH epilepsy	3%	10%
Age of onset	Peak, 5–7; 5% after 9 years of age	Peak, 5–7; 20% after 9 years of age
First symptom	Seizure, 60%	Seizure, 80%
Second symptom	Neuropsychological, 40%	Neuropsychological, 40%
Seizure types	GTC seizure, 35%; unilateral, 26%; unilateral status, 6%	Unilateral, 50%; unilateral status, 6%; absence, GTC, CPS
During active phase of spike-and-wave	(−) atonic seizure, not significant ↑ seizure, clonic/unilateral, CPS	+ atonic seizure/with fall, significant ↑ in seizures, ↑ absence, ↑ atonic seizure, ↑ atypical absence
After active phase of spike-and-wave	19% rare seizure: 81% seizure free	16% rare seizure; 84% seizure free
Neuroimaging	13% abnormal	33% abnormal
Meet criteria for 85% spike-and-wave in sleep	<50%	78%
Frequency of spike-and-wave	2 Hz	2 Hz
Ictal discharge awake	26%	67%
Focal discharges	Centrotemporal/parietal, 60%	Frontal, 60%
Regional predominance of continuous spike-and-wave during sleep	Posterior	Anterior

[a] N = 103. CSWS = 71; LKS = 31. FH, = family history; GTC, generalized tonic-clonic convulsions; CPS complex partial seizures.
Adapted from Refs. 3 and 10.

is not as marked from pre-existing baseline as that of the first group. Long-term outcome in a CSWS patient is generally poor, with significant mental retardation common and frontal lobe syndrome and frontal lobe epilepsy described.[53,73]

OVERLAP BETWEEN THE SYNDROMES

A major problem in our understanding of this spectrum of age-related functional cognitive disorders induced by paroxysmal activity has been the low frequency of reported cases in a given institution. At the Venice colloquium,[6] case reports from an international group were analyzed, yielding 103 patients. Of this group, 71 best fit the syndrome of CSWS and 31 best fit that of LKS. One could not be classified. This substantial body of information allows a direct comparison of these two syndromes.[10] Not all the cases could be used in each reported analysis because of the insufficient or poorly described information. Nonetheless, these data confirm the significant overlap between these proposed separate syndromes (Table 1). The reported differences in clinical presentation, seizure type, and neurologic and behavioral sequelae appear to be due to the primary cortical area involved; the age of onset of epileptiform EEG abnormalities in relation to age-dependent synaptogenesis; severity of the continuous spikes-and-waves during sleep, as measured by the sleep index; and length of time the EEG abnormality persisted.[66] Because of the commonality of features and the more specific localization of the epileptogenic region in LKS, it might be considered a subtype of CSWS.[46]

DIAGNOSTIC EVALUATION

In the evaluation of children with suspected LKS or CSWS, a careful developmental history is taken and physical and neurologic examinations are done. Documentation of premorbid language and of cognitive and behavioral performance is sought, including school testing and intelligence testing.[49]

All children with suspected LKS or CSWS should undergo careful neuropsychological testing by a specialist team experienced in both linguistic and nonlinguistic capacity. This testing allows one to judge whether there are specific deficits in cognitive function, as expected in LKS in the language domain, or whether there is frontal dysfunction, as expected in CSWS.

Laboratory testing includes structural and functional neuroimaging. Routine EEG is essential, and either closed-circuit television (CCTV)-EEG monitoring or ambulatory monitoring can be helpful.[3,46,49] More sophisticated investigations, which are of value for LKS when surgical treatment is considered, can include MEG,[39,51,65] computerized amplitude mapping of EEG, and intracranial EEG recordings, as reviewed by Morrell et al.[49]

In general, structural neuroimaging is usually normal in LKS but abnormal in CSWS, reflecting the prior neurologic insult.[49,68] The structural abnormalities reported in CSWS include unilateral atrophy, focal porencephaly, focal pachygyria, diffuse atrophy, congenital hydrocephalus, and minor white matter abnormalities. The abnormalities reported in LKS include focal pachygyria and mild diffuse atrophy.[7,10,20]

Functional neuroimaging has been reported in only a minority of patients with LKS and CSWS. An important point in interpreting these results is to know whether radionucleotide injection and scan was performed during the active phase of spike-and-wave and whether it was performed in the wake or asleep state. In general, if scans are performed in the wake state or after the period of active spike-and-wave activity, both single photon emission computed tomography (SPECT) and positron emission tomography with ^{18}F-fluorodeoxyglucose (FDG-PET) show an area of decreased blood flow or glucose utilization, whereas if they are done in sedated patients with induced continuous spikes-and-waves, they show a focal area of increased blood flow or glucose utilization.[41,49] Hirsch et al. reported increased glucose metabolism during the active phase of spike-and-wave during both the asleep and wake states in both disorders, though the area of increased metabolism was greater in sleep.[28] It is not noted whether the paroxysmal activity was present during the wake scan. The hypermetabolism was restricted to focal or regional cortical association areas and the type of neuropsychological impairment was in good agreement with the topography of this disturbance.[28,41] The pattern seen in both LKS and CSWS combined features of immature brain with superimposed focal abnormalities. The metabolic abnormalities of these two syndromes displayed significant overlap, suggesting that they represent two parts of the same spectrum of functional disorders of childhood.[28,41] Some patients who underwent FDG-PET scans after the active phase of spike-and-wave discharges had resolved showed persistent regions of hypometabolism in areas that previously showed hypermetabolism, documenting enduring metabolic change.[41]

EEG recordings in slow sleep are important in the diagnosis of LKS and CSWS, but, because of the short recording time, routine studies rarely record slow-wave sleep. Amitriptyline at a dose of 1 to 2 mg/kg and a prolonged recording of 3 hours significantly improves the chance of observing slow sleep. The Venice colloquium provided direct comparison of EEG data in LKS and CSWS[6] (see Table 1). During the active phase of spike-and-wave discharges, more patients with CSWS met the criteria of a sleep index of 85% than those with LKS. The average frequency of the spikes-and-waves was 2 Hz in each disorder. Sleep spindles were absent in 10% of patients, more commonly in the CSWS group than in the LKS group. If a patient had a frontal EEG spike focus, he or she was more likely to have a sleep index of 85% or greater, suggesting that intrinsic circuitry and dense callosal connections of the frontal lobe predispose to generalization during sleep. Patients could be divided into two groups, depending on the severity of the EEG abnormality. The first group had a sleep index of 85% or greater, frequently disrupted sleep spindles, only rare focal discharges during sleep, and bursts of spikes-and-waves in wakefulness. This EEG pattern was seen in 70% of patients with CSWS and in 40% of those with LKS. The second, less severely affected group, showed a sleep index between 50% and 80%, often recognizable sleep spindles, more frequent focal spiking during sleep, and absent or rare spike-and-wave discharges during wakefulness. This set of EEG findings was seen in 30% of the CSWS group and in 60% of the LKS group. These data support the significant overlap in EEG findings, although those with CSWS are more likely to have a severely affected EEG.[6] In addition, focal spikes tend to be frontal in CSWS and are temporoparietal in LKS.

Magnetoencephalography on a number of patients with LKS revealed a focus of slow waves and epileptiform activity in the posterior temporal area adjacent to the sylvian fissure, supporting an origin in the dorsal surface of the superior temporal gyrus[24,39,49,53,65] (Fig. 2). Computerized amplitude and polarity mapping has also been performed in a few patients with LKS and CSWS. In LKS, isolated unilateral spikes during the methohexital suppression test or the first spike in a burst of spikes-and-waves displays a tangential dipole with suprasylvian negativity and infrasylvian positivity, also indicating the origin to be in the dorsal surface of the superior temporal gyrus.[30,41] Amplitude mapping of spikes during wakefulness in three cases of CSWS showed two to be predominantly left frontal with temporal spread and one right frontal with frontal and temporal spread. The sleep spikes tended to have a more diffuse distribution.[24,62] Although the number of cases studied is small, they support differences in maximal cortical areas involved in these syndromes.

A few children with LKS have undergone chronic intracranial electrode and intraoperative recordings in the course of surgical treatment.[33,49,59] These studies confirmed that the common paroxysmal abnormality is in the area of the posterior temporal lobe, often maximal on the superior temporal gyrus (Fig. 3). At times the epileptogenic region is confined within the sylvian fissure near the Heschl gyrus (Fig. 4).

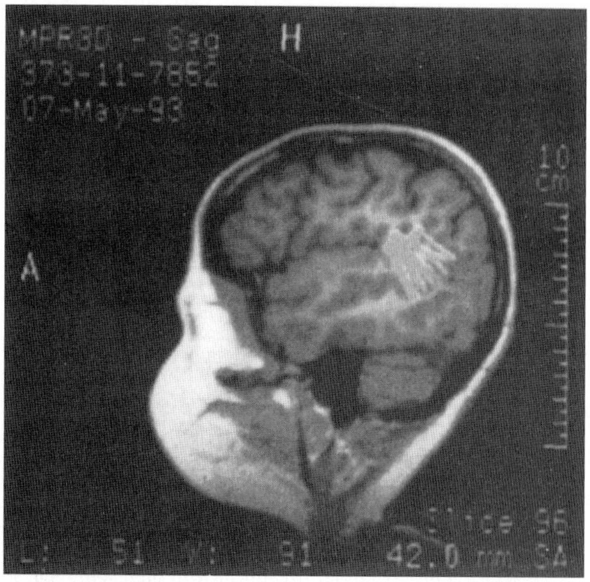

FIGURE 2. Magnetic resonance image (MRI) of another patient with Landau-Kleffner syndrome. In this example, the entire dipole, including its orientation, is displayed on the MRI. In (A) a sagittal section of the left sylvian region is shown. The dipolar orientation is perpendicular to the sylvian fissure and is angled in the anterior–posterior dimension, the suprasylvian projection being anterior to the intrasylvian one.

DIFFERENTIAL DIAGNOSIS

The differential diagnosis between LKS and CSWS, whether or not the former is considered to be a subtype of the latter, is difficult (see Table 1). LKS tends to affect a slightly younger population, presenting first with language dysfunction and only later with other cognitive and behavioral deterioration. In CSWS the children affected tend to be slightly older, presenting with more global neuropsychological and behavioral deterioration before language dysfunction appears.[9] The severity of the seizures and

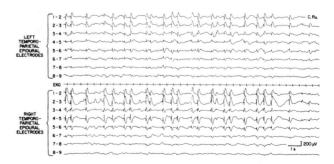

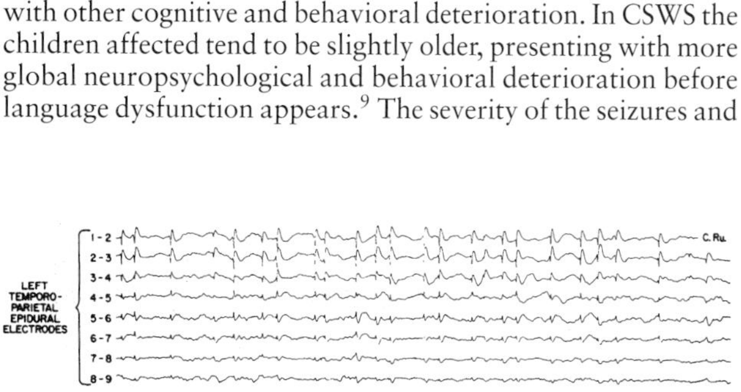

FIGURE 3. Electroencephalogram derived from implanted epidural electrodes in a 5-year-old child. The bilateral spike and spike-wave pattern is well seen. Electrodes were placed symmetrically over the sylvian fissure in each hemisphere. (From Morrell F, Whisler WW, Smith MC, et al. Landau-Kleffner syndrome: treatment with subpial intracortical transection. *Brain.* 1995;118:1529–1546.)

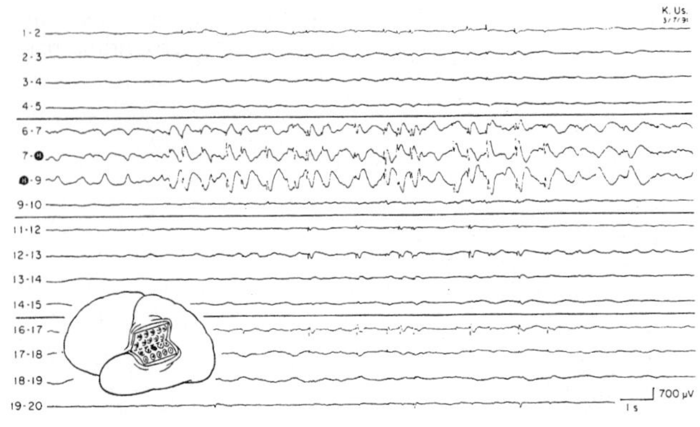

FIGURE 4. Electrocorticographic recordings derived from a pad of electrodes inserted between the lips of the surgically opened sylvian fissure. A vigorous epileptiform discharge was encountered at electrode number 8, whereas highly attenuated spikes were detected in adjacent electrodes of the pad. Electrode 8 lay directly on the dorsal surface of the superior temporal gyrus immediately posterior to the transverse gyrus of Heschl. (From Morrell F, Whisler WW, Smith MC, et al. Landau-Kleffner syndrome: treatment with subpial intracortical transection. *Brain.* 1995;118:1529–1546.)

EEG abnormality is not as pronounced in LKS as in CSWS. The spike-and-wave discharges are maximal in the centrotemporal and posterior head region in LKS and in the frontal head region in CSWS.[6]

The disorders most commonly confused with LKS and CSWS are pervasive developmental delay (PDD) and autism.[25,62,71] The most important distinguishing feature is the loss of previously achieved developmental milestones with LKS and CSWS. In contrast to LKS, children with PDD and autism display abnormal, nonverbal intelligence as well as language dysfunction. Children with early-onset and persistent CSWS may deteriorate more globally and begin to mimic autism. However, although PDD and autism may be associated with paroxysmal EEG abnormalities, they do not have the continuous spike-and-wave discharges during slow sleep of CSWS.

Mental retardation from a wide variety of causes can occasionally be misdiagnosed as LKS or CSWS. A careful history will usually document that motor developmental milestones were not met and suggest the child was affected from birth. The neurologic examination is often abnormal, demonstrating abnormalities in the motor and other systems. These children may also display EEG abnormalities reflecting the underlying cortical pathology; however, these abnormalities rarely meet criteria for continuous spikes-and-waves.[17]

Developmental dysphasia is another disorder that may mimic LKS. Children with this condition do not develop language skills in the usual time frame. They often have a normal neurologic examination and nonverbal intelligence. EEG abnormalities are uncommon, and a continuous spike-and-wave abnormality has not been described.[17] If a child presented with continuous spikes-and-waves in sleep and developmental dysphasia, early-onset LKS is possible.

Once seizures and EEG recordings have indicated the presence of an epileptic disorder, other epileptic syndromes must be considered. These include BECT; other idiopathic, localization-related epilepsies; and Lennox-Gastaut syndrome.[9] Although clear features distinguish LKS and CSWS from Lennox-Gastaut syndrome, there is an overlap with BECT and related disorders.

Classic CSWS and Lennox-Gastaut syndrome (see Chapter 241) share some common features. These include the presence of atypical absence and atonic seizures. The EEG of Lennox-Gastaut syndrome typically shows slow spikes-and-waves that may activate with sleep, but not to the extent of CSWS. In addition, the EEG of Lennox-Gastaut syndrome, but not CSWS or LKS, typically includes polyspikes-and-waves as well as bursts of rhythmic fast activity.[9,25,62,68] Finally, children with Lennox-Gastaut syndrome, but not with CSWS or LKS, display tonic seizures as a prominent component of their disorder.[25,62,68]

Although there are clear clinical differences in these syndromes, a common feature may be that severe epileptiform activity is responsible for progressive cognitive dysfunction. In CSWS and LKS, the paroxysmal abnormality is more restricted and time dependent, whereas in Lennox-Gastaut syndrome the epileptiform activity is multifocal, persistent, and secondary to central nervous system (CNS) injury that also contributes to cognitive disturbance that is not time dependent; this results in a chronic seizure disorder and permanent cognitive dysfunction.[9,68]

The idiopathic localization-related epilepsies (see Chapters 236, 237, and 238) are more difficult to distinguish pathophysiologically from LKS and CSWS but are readily separated clinically.[9,25,43,62,71] These disorders may have less of an effect on cognitive function because the active spike-and-wave activity is less severe, or because it involves different, more "silent" cortical areas. Aicardi and Chevrie[1] reported a syndrome that displayed active spike-and-wave discharges that became continuous with sleep. These children had no detectable cognitive or intellectual deterioration. However, the sleep index and the duration of the active phase of spike-and-wave were not documented.[7] Deonna et al.[19] had six similar cases, but documented increasing neuropsychological dysfunction at the time of EEG deterioration. Polypharmacy may have worsened the clinical status, and all of Deonna's cases improved with antiepileptic drug (AED) taper. It is probable that this syndrome is a subset of CSWS with an older onset and a shorter course of the active phase of continuous spikes-and-waves. It may also be that more careful neuropsychological testing would be able to detect cognitive deficits.[10]

Benign childhood epilepsy with centrotemporal spikes is easily distinguished from LKS by the absence of acquired aphasia; however, BECT may also be a subset of CSWS.[25,62] In Tassinari's clinical division into various subsets of CSWS, one type with orofacial and generalized tonic–clonic seizures in sleep mimics BECT. Absence seizures have been reported with BECT.[68] There are differences, however, in EEG manifestations. In CSWS, focal abnormalities predominate in the frontal areas, whereas in BECT they are maximal in the centrotemporal areas. There is a clear activation of epileptiform activity in BECT during sleep, at times becoming continuous spikes-and-waves; however, the sleep index never reaches 85%.[9,11,25,62] There was one reported case of BECT that worsened with the introduction of carbamazepine and reached a sleep index of 85%; clinical deterioration with atypical absence and falls resolved with withdrawal of the carbamazepine.[11] Mental retardation and a history of prior neurologic insult are commonly seen in CSWS but not in BECT. Family history of epilepsy is reported in 40% with BECT but in only 10% with CSWS.[9] Despite these clinical differences, it is probable that a child with early-onset and persistent BECT with a high sleep index would display cognitive or motoric deficits if carefully tested.

TREATMENT AND OUTCOME

As previously noted, the clinical seizures in LKS and CSWS, as with the other idiopathic localization-related epilepsies, are, for the most part, not severe and are easy to control.[10,25,41,46,49,62]

The one important exception to this is in the subgroup of CSWS with daily atypical absences and drop attacks.[68] In this group, clinical seizures are severe and at times difficult to treat. The clinical seizures in both groups are self-limited, with only rare seizures in about 20% of both groups once the active phase of spike-and-wave has resolved.[10] All available AEDs have been used individually and in combination for the treatment of LKS and CSWS. The Venice colloquium confirmed this and listed the medications used by participating investigators.[72] During the active phase of spike-and-wave, polytherapy was the rule, with only 9% of patients treated with monotherapy. Efficacy was difficult to judge, because in general, all AEDs were effective in treating the clinical seizures, but there was poor response of the paroxysmal EEG. There have been reports of carbamazepine causing a worsening of seizures, especially atypical absence and atonic falls.[11] In reviewing which AEDs, if any, were being used at the time of resolution of the CSWS, there were data on 88 patients. Seven of these patients were not on any medication at the time of resolution of CSWS, documenting its self-limited nature. Of the other 81 patients, 55 were taking valproate, 19 as monotherapy. Thirty-nine of the patients were on a benzodiazepine, mostly clobazam. A small number were on phenobarbital, vigabatrin, ethosuximide, and carbamazepine. These data indicate that valproate alone or in combination with a benzodiazepine has been the treatment of choice.

Corticosteroid therapy, either with adrenocorticotropic hormone (ACTH) or prednisone, appears to have favorable and long-lasting effects.[61,72] Although there were too few cases and insufficient follow-up time to permit a definitive conclusion on their effectiveness, some authors suggest that ACTH or corticosteroids should be the treatment of choice, especially in new-onset disease in a young patient.[18,29,38] Lerman et al.[38] reviewed the literature and reported on four cases with LKS that they treated with either ACTH or corticosteroids. They tended to use a high dose for a prolonged period of time (ACTH 80 IU/day with a 3-month taper; prednisone 60 mg/day with a 3-month taper). They noted, and this was confirmed in the Venice colloquium,[72] that there may be relapses with steroid reduction and some children may need to be on steroids for months to years. A commonly accepted dose is 3 to 5 mg/kg/day of prednisone for at least 3 months. It appears that the earlier treatment is initiated, the shorter the duration of steroids required, and the better is the ultimate outcome.[38] With steroid wean, most of these children were on additional AEDs, most commonly valproate or benzodiazepines. Lower-dose protocols with fewer adverse effects have been reported to be helpful.[61]

The long-term use of corticosteroids is fraught with side effects, including weight gain, cushingoid appearance, hypertension, glucose intolerance, electrolyte abnormalities, sleep disturbance, mood changes, and more serious conditions, including cataract formation, proximal myopathy, pathologic fracture, and immune dysfunction (see Chapter 144). The risks versus benefits must be clearly thought out and explained to all concerned parties, including patients, parents, and primary care physicians. Side effects of steroids may be acceptable in patients with an early onset of the active phase of spike-and-wave discharges and a severe and persistent epileptic disturbance because this group is at highest risk for significant residual neuropsychological sequelae.

Current practice is to treat initially with valproate with or without a benzodiazepine. If epileptiform EEG abnormalities and cognitive dysfunction persist despite high therapeutic AED levels, a course of prednisone 3 to 5 mg/kg/day[1] with careful laboratory and physical examination follow-up is usually offered. It is important to obtain serial EEGs that include slow-wave sleep in order to judge the efficacy of therapy. An attempt can be made to convert to every-other-day dosing in the second month of therapy, if there is therapeutic success. A slow wean during the third month is performed, although relapses are not uncommon.[18,38,46]

Morrell et al. originally reported on the surgical treatment by multiple subpial transection (MST) of 14 children suffering from LKS.[49] All children had been unable to use language meaningfully for more than 2 years and displayed continuous spike-and-wave discharges that were demonstrated to arise unilaterally in the superior temporal gyrus and surrounding perisylvian cortex. After MST resolved the paroxysmal EEG abnormality, there was dramatic improvement in language function over time, with 50% recovering age-appropriate language and returning to regular classroom school and 29% showing a marked improvement in language function but still undergoing speech therapy. They concluded that success in restitution of language function depended on proper selection of patients and resolution of the severe epileptiform EEG abnormality.[49] Presurgical evaluation requires delineation of an epileptogenic region involving one posterior temporal lobe, which is usually accomplished not only by standard imaging and electrophysiologic investigations, but also by the methohexital suppression test, and occasionally intracarotid amobarbital, electrical dipole mapping, and magnetic resonance imaging.[49]

Longer-term follow-up on the original 14 patients found that 11 of 14 demonstrated significant postoperative improvement in receptive-expressive language and that gains in language function are most likely to be seen years rather than months after surgery.[26] These results indicate that early accurate diagnosis and effective treatment optimizes outcome. This series has been recently extended to 24 children treated with MST to treat severe persistent language disturbance of more than 18 months' duration. MST resulted in recovery of functional language (speaking in complex sentences) in two thirds of children treated.[35]

Other investigators have confirmed these original findings that MST is an effective treatment in children with active CSWS and acquired aphasia despite treatment.[33,59]

The clinical response to MST in atypical LKS or autistic regression with epileptiform EEG, at times CSWS, had been reported, but long-term functional language improvement had not been demonstrated,[39,50] making accurate diagnosis critical in patient selection for MST.[62]

There is now a better understanding of treatment options in LKS and CSWS. It is necessary to eliminate the severe paroxysmal EEG disturbance to prevent serious neuropsychological sequelae in some patients.[41,46,66] Aggressive treatment is indicated in those with early onset of the active phase of spike-and-wave discharges who have a severe and persistent paroxysmal disturbance affecting neocortex that is critical to language and other higher cognitive function. In these children, high doses of traditional AEDs, corticosteroids, and occasionally surgery are justified because of the risk of serious and permanent cognitive dysfunction that will affect education, occupation, and activities of daily living.

LONG-TERM PROGNOSIS

Long-term prognosis for the seizure disorder in both conditions is good, with <20% suffering from persistent, usually rare, seizures.[10] However, the long-term prognosis for neuropsychological consequences is not nearly as good as was once thought.[17] In general, most patients who suffer from LKS or CSWS have some permanent sequelae that limit their activities. Those with the earliest onset of spike-and-wave discharges and longest persistence over time are most affected.

In 1980 Mantovani and Landau[40] reviewed the long-term prognosis of nine patients with LKS 10 to 28 years after onset. They found that the overall clinical status and language were normal in <50%. Many other studies agree that aphasia persists in the majority.[2,3,14,16,34,53] Only half of patients with a history of LKS are able to live a normal life.[2,34,41,49,53]

Long-term outcome with CSWS has also been reported as poor in most patients.[53] Again, outcome appears to be related to the age of onset and duration of the active phase of spike-and-wave discharges.[68] All four cases reported by Morikawa et al.[45] continue to have neuropsychological sequelae, with IQ ranging from 35 to 60, and require special schools or sheltered workshops.

The Venice colloquium confirmed that permanent neuropsychological sequelae are seen in the majority; in fact, only a few of the 59 children with adequate follow-up intelligence tests achieved a global IQ within the normal range.[44] Disturbances included short attention span, hyperactivity, affective symptoms, and language dysfunction, as well as intellectual impairment. Although there was a global improvement in all intellectual areas after resolution of CSWS, this did not lead to complete restoration of function, particularly in verbal ability, attention, and executive function.[44,53]

SUMMARY AND CONCLUSIONS

LKS and CSWS are two points on a spectrum of age-related functional disorders of childhood characterized by a severe paroxysmal EEG disturbance that can permanently alter critical synaptogenesis by strengthening synaptic contacts that should be pruned. They appear to be linked to other idiopathic localization-related epilepsies by a common pathophysiology. Although prognosis for seizure control is good, cognitive function deteriorates and serious permanent neuropsychological consequences are reported in the majority. At highest risk for permanent sequelae are those with the earliest and longest exposure to the active phase of continuous spike-and-wave discharges during sleep. In LKS the paroxysmal activity permanently affects the posterior temporal area and results in auditory agnosia and language deficits, whereas in CSWS the frontal lobes are more involved and other cognitive disturbances predominate. Aggressive treatment approaches to abolish the paroxysmal disturbance—such as high-dose AEDs, corticosteroids, or, in select LKS patients, surgery—should be seriously considered in the high-risk group.

ACKNOWLEDGMENT

This chapter is dedicated to the life and work of Frank Morrell (1926–1996), our teacher, mentor, colleague, and friend. The ideas and concepts contained in this work were greatly influenced by him.

References

1. Aicardi J, Chevrie JJ. Atypical benign partial epilepsy of childhood. *Dev Med Child Neurol.* 1982;24:281–292.
2. Baynes K, Kegl JA, Brentari D, et al. Chronic auditory agnosia following Landau-Kleffner syndrome: a 23 year outcome study. *Brain Lang.* 1998;63(3):381–425.
3. Beaumanoir A. About continuous or subcontinuous spike-wave activity during wakefulness: electroclinical correlations. In: Beaumanoir A, Bureau M, Deonna T, et al., eds. *Continuous Spikes and Waves During Slow Sleep/Electrical Status Epilepticus During Slow Sleep.* London: John Libbey; 1995:115–118.
4. Beaumanoir A. The Landau-Kleffner syndrome. In: Roger J, Dravet C, Bureau M, et al., eds. *Epileptic Syndromes in Infancy, Childhood and Adolescence.* London: John Libbey; 1985:181–191.
5. Beaumanoir A. The Landau-Kleffner syndrome. In: Roger J, Bureau M, Dravet C, et al., eds. *Epileptic Syndromes in Infancy, Childhood and Adolescence.* 2nd ed. London: John Libbey; 1992:231–243.
6. Beaumanoir A, Bureau M, Deonna T, et al., eds. *Continuous Spikes and Waves During Slow Sleep/Electrical Status Epilepticus During Slow Sleep.* London: John Libbey; 1995.
7. Ben-Zeev B, Kivity S, Pshitizki Y, et al. Congenital hydrocephalus and continuous spike wave in slow-wave sleep—a common association? *J Child Neurol.* 2004;19(2):129–134.
8. Bishop DVM. Age of onset and outcome in "acquired aphasia with convulsive disorder" (Landau-Kleffner syndrome). *Dev Med Child Neurol.* 1985;27:705–712.
9. Bureau M. "Continuous spikes and waves during slow sleep" (CSWS): definition of the syndrome. In: Beaumanoir A, Bureau M, Deonna T, et al., eds. *Continuous Spikes and Waves During Slow Sleep/Electrical Status Epilepticus During Slow Sleep.* London: John Libbey; 1995:17–26.
10. Bureau M. Outstanding cases of CSWS and LKS analysis of the data sheets provided by the participants. In: Beaumanoir A, Bureau M, Deonna T, et al., eds. *Continuous Spikes and Waves During Slow Sleep/Electrical Status Epilepticus During Slow Sleep.* London: John Libbey; 1995:213–216.
11. Caraballa R, Fontana E, Michelizza B, et al. Carbamazepine, assenze atipiche, crisi atoniche e stato di PO continua del sono (POCS). *Boll Lega It Epil.* 1989;66/67:379–381.
12. Cole AJ, Andermann F, Taylor L, et al. The Landau-Kleffner syndrome of acquired epileptic aphasia: unusual clinical outcome, surgical experience, and absence of encephalitis. *Neurology.* 1988;38:31–38.
13. Commission on Classification and Terminology of the International League Against Epilepsy. Proposal for revised classification of epilepsies and epileptic syndromes. *Epilepsia.* 1989;30:389–399.
14. De Negri M. The maturational development of the child: developmental disorders and epilepsy. In: Beaumanoir A, Bureau M, Deonna T, et al., eds. *Continuous Spikes and Waves During Slow Sleep/Electrical Status Epilepticus During Slow Sleep.* London: John Libbey; 1995:3–8.
15. Deonna T. Acquired epileptiform aphasia in children (Landau-Kleffner syndrome). *J Clin Neurophysiol.* 1991;8:288–298.
16. Deonna T, Peter C, Ziegler A-L. Adult follow-up of the acquired aphasia-epilepsy syndrome in childhood. Report of 7 cases. *Neuropediatrics.* 1989;20:132–138.
17. Deonna T, Roulet E. Acquired epileptic aphasia (AEA): definition of the syndrome and current problems. In: Beaumanoir A, Bureau M, Deonna T, et al., eds. *Continuous Spikes and Waves During Slow Sleep/Electrical Status Epilepticus During Slow Sleep.* London: John Libbey; 1995:37–45.
18. Deonna T, Roulet E. Epilepsy and language disorder in children. In: Fukuyama Y, Kamoshita S, Ohtsuka C, et al., eds. *Modern Perspectives of Child Neurology.* Tokyo: The Japanese Society of Child Neurology; 1991:259–266.
19. Deonna T, Ziegler AL, Despland PA. Combined myoclonic-astatic and benign focal epilepsy of childhood (atypical partial epilepsy of childhood)—a separate syndrome? *Neuropediatrics.* 1986;17:144–151.
20. Djabraian AA, Batista MS, deLima MM, et al. Continuous spike-waves during slow waves sleep. A clinical and electroencephalographic study in fifteen children. *Arq Neuro-Psiquiatr.* 1999;57(3A):566–570.
21. Dugas M, Grenet P, Masson M, et al. Aphasie de l'enfant avec épilepsie. Evolution regressive sous traitement antiépileptique. *Rev Neurol (Paris).* 1976;132:489–493.
22. Dugas M, Masson M, Le Heuzey MF, et al. Aphasie "acquise" de l'enfant avec épilepsie (syndrome de Landau et Kleffner). Douze observations personnelles. *Rev Neurol (Paris).* 1982;138:755–780.
23. Dulac O, Billard C, Arthuis M. Aspects électro-cliniques et évolutifs de l'épilepsie dans le syndrome aphasie-épilepsie. *Arch Fr Pediatr.* 1983;40:299–308.
24. Farnarier, G, Kouna P, Genton P. Amplitude EEG mapping in three cases of CSWS. In: Beaumanoir A, Bureau M, Deonna T, et al., eds. *Continuous Spikes and Waves During Slow Sleep/Electrical Status Epilepticus During Slow Sleep.* London: John Libbey; 1995:91–98.
25. Galanopoulou AS, Bojko A, Lado F, et al. The spectrum of neuropsychiatric abnormalities associated with electrical status epilepticus in sleep. *Brain Dev.* 2000;22(5):279–295.
26. Grote CL, VanSlyke P, Hoeppner JA. Language outcome following multiple subpial transaction for Landau-Kleffner syndrome. *Brain.* 1999; 122(Pt 3):561–566.
27. Halasz P, Kelemen A, Clemens B, et al. The perisylvian epileptic network. A unifying concept. (Review) *Ideggyogy Sz.* 2005;58(1–2):21–31.
28. Hirsch E, Maquet P, Metz-Lutz M-N, et al. The eponym "Landau-Kleffner syndrome" should not be restricted to childhood-acquired aphasia with epilepsy. In: Beaumanoir A, Bureau M, Deonna T, et al., eds. *Continuous Spikes and During Slow Sleep/Electrical Status Epilepticus During Slow Sleep.* London: John Libbey; 1995:57–62.
29. Hirsch E, Marescaux C, Maquet P, et al. Landau-Kleffner syndrome: a clinical and EEG study of five cases. *Epilepsia.* 1990;31(6):756–767.
30. Hoeppner TJ, Morrell F, Smith MC, et al. The Landau-Kleffner syndrome: a peri-sylvian epilepsy [Abstract]. *Epilepsia.* 1992;33(Suppl 3):122(abst).
31. Huttenlocher PR, de Courten C. The development of synapses in striate cortex of man. *Hum Neurobiol.* 1987;6:1–9.
32. Huttenlocher PR, de Courten C, Garey LJ, et al. Synaptogenesis in the human visual cortex—evidence for synapse elimination during normal development. *Neurosci Lett.* 1982;33:247–252.
33. Irwin K, Birch V, Lees J, et al. Multiple subpial transaction in Landau-Kleffner syndrome. *Dev Med Child Neurol.* 2001;43(4):248–252.
34. Kaga M. Language disorders in Landau-Kleffner syndrome. *J Child Neurol.* 1999;14(2):118–122.
35. Kanner AM, Byrne R, VanSlyke P, et al. Functional language recovery following a surgical treatment of Landau-Kleffner Syndrome. *Neurology.* 2005;64(Suppl 1):A359.
36. Kolski H, Otsubo H. The Landau-Kleffner syndrome. *Adv Exper Med Biol.* 2002;497:195–208.
37. Landau WM, Kleffner FR. Syndrome of acquired aphasia with convulsive disorder in children. *Neurology.* 1957;7:523–530.

38. Lerman P, Lerman-Sagie T, Kivity S. Effect of early corticosteroid therapy for Landau-Kleffner syndrome. Case reports. *Dev Med Child Neurol.* 1991;33:257–266.
39. Lewine JD, Andrews R, Chez M, et al. Magnetoencephalography patterns of epileptiform activity in children with regressive autism spectrum disorders. *Pediatrics.* 1999;104(3 Pt 1):405–418.
40. Mantovani JF, Landau WM. Acquired aphasia with convulsive disorder: course and prognosis. *Neurology.* 1980;30:524–529.
41. Maquet P, Hirsch E, Metz-Lutz N, et al. Regional cerebral glucose metabolism in children with deterioration of one or more cognitive functions and continuous spike-and-wave discharges during sleep. *Brain.* 1995;118:1497–1520.
42. Marescaux C, Hirsch E, Finck S, et al. Landau-Kleffner syndrome: a pharmacologic study of five cases. *Epilepsia.* 1990;31(6):768–777.
43. McVicar Ka, Shinnar S. Landau-Kleffner syndrome, electrical status epilepticus in slow wave sleep, and language regression in children. *Ment Retard Dev Disabil Res Rev.* 2004;10(2):144–149.
44. Morikawa T, Seino M, Watanabe M. Long-term outcome of CSWS syndrome. In: Beaumanoir A, Bureau M, Deonna T, et al., eds. *Continuous Spikes and Waves During Slow Sleep/Electrical Status Epilepticus During Slow Sleep.* London: John Libbey; 1995:27–36.
45. Morikawa T, Seino T, Yagi K. Long-term outcome of four children with continuous spike-waves during sleep. In: Roger J, Bureau M, Dravet C, et al., eds., *Epileptic Syndromes in Infancy, Childhood and Adolescence.* 2nd ed. London: John Libbey; 1992:257–265.
46. Morrell F. Electrophysiology of CSWS in Landau-Kleffner syndrome. In: Beaumanoir A, Bureau M, Deonna T, et al., eds. *Continuous Spikes and Waves During Slow Sleep/Electrical Status Epilepticus During Slow Sleep.* London: John Libbey; 1995:77–90.
47. Morrell F. Varieties of human secondary epileptogenesis [Review]. *J Clin Neurophysiol.* 1989;6:227–275.
48. Morrell F, Whisler WW, Bleck TP. Multiple subpial transection: a new approach to the surgical treatment of focal epilepsy. *J Neurosurg.* 1989;70:231–239.
49. Morrell F, Whisler WW, Smith MC, et al. Landau-Kleffner syndrome: treatment with subpial intracortical transection. *Brain.* 1995;118:1529–1546.
50. Nass R, Gross A, Wisoff J, et al. Outcome of multiple subpial transactions for autistic epileptiform regression. *Pediatr Neurol.* 1999;21(1):464–470.
51. Paetau R, Granstrom ML, Blomsedt G, et al. Magnetoencephalography in presurgical evaluation of children with the Landau-Kleffner syndrome. *Epilepsia.* 1999;40(3):326–335.
52. Patry G, Lyagoubi S, Tassinari CA. Subclinical "electrical status epilepticus" induced by sleep in children. *Arch Neurol.* 1971;24:242–252.
53. Praline J, Hommet C, Barthez MA, et al. Outcome at adulthood of the continuous spike-waves during slow sleep and Landau-Kleffner syndrome. *Epilepsia.* 2003;44(11):2434–2440.
54. Purves D. *Body and Brain: A Trophic Theory of Neural Connections.* Cambridge: Harvard University Press; 1988.
55. Purves D, Lichtman JW. Elimination of synapses in the developing nervous system. *Science.* 1980;210:153–157.
56. Rapin I, Mattis S, Rowan AJ, et al. Verbal auditory agnosia in children. *Dev Med Child Neurol.* 1977;19:192–207.
57. Robinson RO, Baird G, Robinson G, et al. Landau-Kleffner syndrome: course and correlates with outcome. *Dev Med Child Neurol.* 2001;43(4):243–247.
58. Rossi PG, Parmeggiani A, Posar A, et al. Landau-Kleffner syndrome (LKS): long-term follow-up and links with electrical status epilepticus during sleep (ESES). *Brain Dev.* 1999;21(2):90–98.
59. Sawhney IM, Robinson IJ, Polkey CE, et al. Multiple subpial transaction: a review of 21 cases. *J Neurol Neurosurg Psychiatry.* 1995;58(3):344–349.
60. Sayit E, Dirik E, Durak H, et al. Landau-Kleffner syndrome: relation of clinical, EE and Tc-99m-HMPAO brain SPECT findings and improvement in EEG after treatment. *Annals of Nucl Med.* 1999;13(6):415–418.
61. Sinclair DB, Snyder TJ. Corticosteroids for the treatment of Landau-Kleffner syndrome and continuous spike-wave discharge during sleep. *Pediatr Neurol.* 2005;32(5):300–306.
62. Smith MC, Hoeppner TJ. Epileptic encephalopathy of late childhood: Landau-Kleffner syndrome and the syndrome of continuous spike and waves during slow-wave sleep. *J Clin Neurophysiol.* 2003;20(6):462–472.
63. Smith MC, Pierre-Louis SJC, Kanner AM, et al. Pathological spectrum of acquired epileptic aphasia of childhood. *Epilepsia.* 1992;33(3 Suppl):115.
64. Smith MC, Whisler W, Morrell F. Neurology of epilepsy. *Semin Neurol.* 1989;9:231–248.
65. Sobel DF, Aung M, Otsubo H, et al. Magnetoencephalography in children with Landau-Kleffner syndrome and acquired epileptic aphasia. *Am J Neuroradiol.* 2000;21(2):301–307.
66. Tassinari CA. The problems of "continuous spikes and waves during slow sleep" or "electrical status epilepticus during slow sleep" today. In: Beaumanoir A, Bureau M, Deonna T, et al., eds. *Continuous Spikes and Waves During Slow Sleep/Electrical Status Epilepticus During Slow Sleep.* London: John Libbey; 1995:251–255.
67. Tassinari CA, Bureau M, Dravet C, et al. Epilepsy with continuous spikes and waves during slow sleep. In: Roger J, Dravet C, Bureau M, et al., eds. *Epileptic Syndromes in Infancy, Childhood and Adolescence.* London: John Libbey; 1985:194–204.
68. Tassinari CA, Bureau M, Dravet C, et al. Epilepsie avec pointes-ondes continués pendant le sommeil lent—antérieurement décrite sous le nom d'ESES (épilepsie avec état de mal électroencephalographique pendant le sommeil lent). In: Roger J, Dravet C, Dreifuss FE, et al., eds. *Les Syndromes Épileptiques de l'Enfant et de l'Adolescent.* 2nd ed. Paris: John Libbey Eurotext; 1992:245–256.
69. Tassinari CA, Terzano G, Capocchi G, et al. Epileptic seizures during sleep in children. In: Penry JK, ed. *Epilepsy: The 8th International Symposium.* New York: Raven Press; 1977:345–354.
70. Toso V, Moschini M, Gagnin G, et al. Aphasie acquise de l'enfant avec épilepsie. Trois observations et revue de la littérature. *Rev Neurol (Paris).* 1981;137:425–434.
71. Trevathan E. Seizures and epilepsy among children with language regression and autistic spectrum disorders. *J Child Neurol.* 2004;19(Suppl 1):549–557.
72. Van Lierde A. Therapeutic data. In: Beaumanoir A, Bureau M, Deonna T, et al., eds. *Continuous Spikes and Waves During Slow Sleep/Electrical Status Epilepticus During Slow Sleep.* London.
73. Veggiotti P, Bova S, Granocchio E, et al. Acquired epileptic frontal syndrome as long-term outcome in two children with CSWS. *Neurophsyiol Clin.* 2001;31(6):387–397.
74. World Health Organization. *The ICD-10 Classification of Mental and Behavioural Disorders: Clinical Descriptions and Diagnostic Guidelines.* Geneva: World Health Organization; 1992.

CHAPTER 243 ■ RASMUSSEN'S ENCEPHALITIS (CHRONIC FOCAL ENCEPHALITIS)

FRANÇOIS DUBEAU, FRÉDÉRICK ANDERMANN, HEINZ WIENDL, AND AMIT BAR-OR

INTRODUCTION

Chronic encephalitis is a relentlessly progressive disorder of childhood, associated with hemispheric atrophy, severe intractable focal epilepsy, intellectual decline, and hemiparesis. The etiology of this disorder remains unknown. Neuropathologic features described in the surgical specimens show characteristics of inflammatory changes including perivascular and leptomeningeal lymphocytic infiltration, microglial nodules, astrocytosis, neuronal degeneration, and spongy degeneration. There are variants of this syndrome with regard to age at onset, staging, localization, progression, and outcome. Treatment options are limited: Antiepileptic drugs (AEDs) usually show no significant benefit, and immunotherapy trials, undertaken mostly after the 1990 s, showed modest transient improvement in symptoms and disease progression in some patients. Only surgery, and specifically hemispherectomy, seems to produce persistent relief of seizures and functional improvement.

HISTORICAL PERSPECTIVE

Dr. Theodore Rasmussen (Fig. 1) first described the disorder in 1958, and, together with Jerzy Olszewski and Donald Lloyd-Smith, published the clinical and histopathologic features of three patients with focal seizures due to chronic focal encephalitis.[119] The original proband, F.S., was referred in 1945 to Dr. Wilder Penfield by Dr. Edgar Fincher, chief of neurosurgery at Emory University in Atlanta, GA, because of intractable right-sided focal motor seizures starting at 6 years of age.[120] The child developed a right hemiparesis and underwent, between 1941 and 1956, three surgical interventions (two at the Montreal Neurological Hospital and Institute [MNHI]) at 7, 10, and 21 years in an attempt to control the evolution of the disease. In the first chapter of the monograph on chronic encephalitis published by Dr. Frederick Andermann in 1991, Dr. Rasmussen reported a letter of Dr. Fincher to Dr. Penfield (dated 1956) urging him to consider a more extensive cortical excision and concluded, "I note in your discussion that you list the cause as unknown, but if this youngster doesn't have a chronic low-grade encephalitic process which has likely, by now, burned itself out, I will buy you a new hat." The last intervention was a left hemispherectomy performed by Dr. Rasmussen, and histology showed sparse perivascular inflammation and glial nodules. W. G. remained seizure free until his last follow-up (Fig. 2B). He had a mild intellectual handicap and a fixed right hemiplegia. He developed hydrocephalus as a late complication of the surgical procedure and required a shunt. Dr. Penfield, who was consulted in this case, remained skeptical of the postulate that the syndrome was a primary inflammatory disorder, but raised most of the issues that continue to be debated: If it is an encephalitic process, would it not involve both hemispheres? Is the encephalitic process the result of recurrent seizures due to a small focal lesion in one hemisphere? Why it is that epileptic seizures are destructive in one case and not in another? Dr. Rasmussen himself recognized that Fincher's 1941 diagnosis of chronic encephalitis in FS's case was made 14 years before case two of the original 1958 report (Fig. 2).[119] The story does not say, however, whether Dr. Penfield had to provide his colleague and friend Dr. Fincher with a new hat.[5]

This entity, later recognized as "Rasmussen's encephalitis (RE)," became the subject of extensive discussion in the literature, initially debating the best timing for surgery and best surgical approaches, and, more recently, the etiology and pathogenesis of this unusual and enigmatic disease. A large number of publications can be found in the literature, and two international symposia were held in Montreal, in 1988 and in December 2002, and one in Vienna, in June 2004.[21] The interest in this disease was initially driven by the severity and inescapability of its course, which rapidly led to its description as a prototype of "catastrophic childhood epilepsy."

Physicians and scientists became interested by the unusual pathogenesis and evolution of the syndrome and are now trying to reconcile the apparent focal nature of the disease with the postulated viral and autoimmune etiologies that may or may not be mutually exclusive. This chapter updates a number of issues regarding RE, particularly the putative mechanisms of the disease, the variability of the clinical presentations, and the indications and rationale of new medical therapies, such as immunomodulation and receptor-directed pharmacotherapy.

EPIDEMIOLOGY

There are no data available regarding the incidence of RE in different populations. As the disorder has been increasingly recognized, reports and verbal communications from all parts of the world have emerged. This indicates that RE exists in every area, with the reports depending on the presence of pediatric neurologists and epileptologists. There are, however, no clusters of the disease in any particular region or population.

ETIOLOGY AND PATHOGENESIS OF RASMUSSEN'S ENCEPHALITIS

The etiology and pathogenesis of RE remain unknown. Typical histologic features reported in surgical or autopsy specimens involve perivascular lymphocytic cuffing, microglial proliferation and nodule formation, neuronal loss, and gliosis in the affected

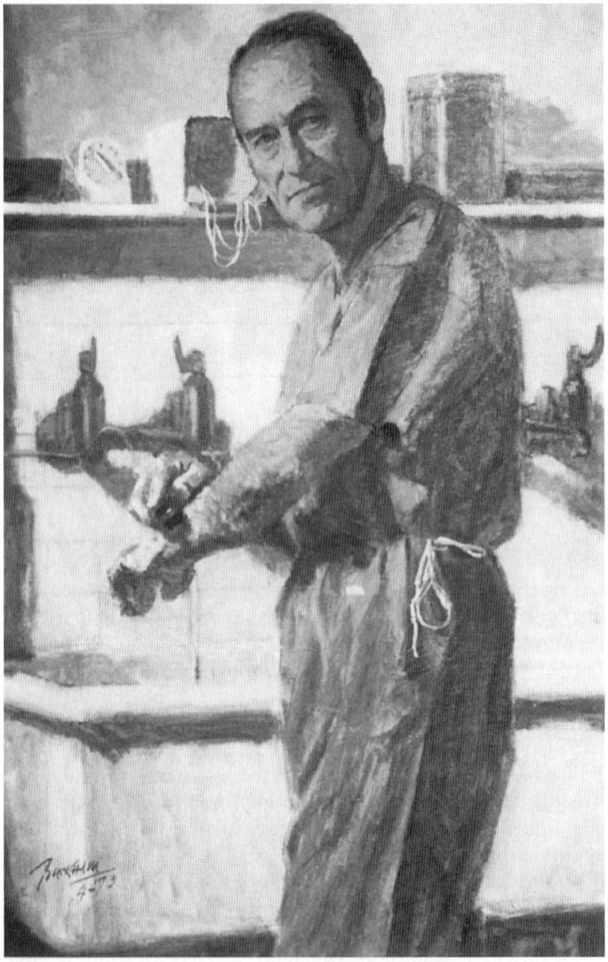

FIGURE 1. Theodore B. Rasmussen, Director Emeritus of the Montreal Neurological Institute.

hemisphere (Fig. 3). The microglial nodules are associated with frequent nonspecific neuronophagia, and occur particularly near perivascular cuffs of lymphocytes and monocytes. There is limited evidence of spongiosis, which is not as widespread as in the true spongiform encephalopathies. Lesions tend to extend in a confluent rather than a multifocal manner. Finally, the main inflammatory changes are found in the cortex, and their intensity is inversely correlated with disease duration with slow progress toward a "burnt-out" stage.[23,122] Three putative immune-mediated (inflammatory) mechanisms, which are not mutually exclusive, have been proposed to explain the initiation and unusual evolution of this rare clinical syndrome: (a) viral infections directly inducing central nervous system (CNS) injury, (b) a viral infection of the CNS that triggers a secondary autoimmune CNS process, and (c) a primary autoimmune CNS process. It remains possible that RE has a noninflammatory origin, and that the observed inflammatory responses merely represent a reaction to another unknown primary injury (Fig. 4).

The observation of inflammatory responses found within the lesions of RE has led to multifaceted approaches to uncover possible infectious or immune-mediated (humoral or cellular) etiologies. In general, epidemiologic studies have not been able to identify clear genetic, geographic, seasonal, or clustering effect, and have failed to demonstrate any association between exposure to various factors, including viruses, and the subsequent development of RE. There appears to be no consistent increase in reports of pre-existent febrile convulsions, nor an association with an infectious illness preceding or associated with the development of RE. Serologic studies to detect antecedent viral infection have been contradictory or inconclusive. [7,8,43,49,77,99,101,115,121,151,154] The search for a pathogenic virus has so far mostly focused on the herpes virus family, and direct brain tissue analysis has also yielded inconsistent results.[7,8,77,99,116] Presently, the role of an infectious agent and the *viral hypothesis* in the causation of RE remains, at best, uncertain. It should be noted, however, that a few patients were reported to improve with antiviral therapy.[35,37,96,100]

Studies of both systemic[62,87,93,118,127,132,133] and cerebrospinal fluid (CSF) compartment immune responses still fail to indicate clear evidence of either ongoing or deficient immune reactivity.[60] A primary role for pathogenic antibodies in the etiology of RE was proposed after Rogers et al.[123] described that rabbits immunized with fusion proteins containing a portion of the GluR3 (glutamate receptor 3 subunit) receptor developed intractable seizures. On histopathologic examination, the brains of these animals exhibited changes characteristic of RE with perivascular lymphocytic infiltrates and microglial nodules. The subsequent finding of autoantibodies to GluR3 in the sera of some affected patients with RE led to the *GluR3 autoantibody hypothesis* of RE and allowed new speculation into disease pathogenesis. GluR3 autoantibodies may cause damage to the brain, and eventually epilepsy, by excitotoxic mechanisms. In the animal model, GluR3 autoantibodies appear to activate the excitatory receptor that leads to massive influx of ions, neuronal cell death, local inflammation, and further disruption of the blood–brain barrier, allowing entry of additional immune mediators.[90,145] Another proposed mechanism suggests that GluR3 autoantibodies can cause damage by activating complement cascades that lead to neuronal cell death and further inflammation.[70,158] These hypotheses prompted a number of open-label therapeutic attempts in order to modulate the immune system of patients, especially by removing or blocking the circulating factors presumably responsible for the disease.[3,6,70,109,123,145,158] Among cases with no detectable anti-GluR3 antibodies, several were also described to respond well to immunosuppressive treatments.[5,66,155] Other reports in several patients showed no response to plasma exchange.[3,82] More recent work, however, has shown that anti-GluR3 antibodies are not specific for RE but can be detected in other neurologic disorders and particularly in non-RE patients with severe epilepsy. Since the sensitivity of detection is low for the RE population and the presence of GluR3 antibodies does not distinguish RE from other forms of epilepsy, the anti-GluR3 antibody test is not useful for RE diagnosis.[12,95,155,159] It remains unclear whether GluR3 or other autoantibodies in various forms of epilepsy are actually responsible for the onset of the seizure disorder, whether their presence contributes to ongoing pathophysiology of an established syndrome, or whether they merely result as an epiphenomenon of an underlying degenerative or inflammatory process.[19,54] Passive transfer of the disease into naïve animals remains unsuccessful so far, and additional animal models of this illness are lacking to finally corroborate the potential pathogenic role of these antibodies.

Various other autoantibodies against neural molecules have been described in RE: Autoantibodies against munc-18,[163] neuronal acetylcholine receptor α-7 subunit,[156] and NMDAAR2 A to 2D—specifically GluR epsilon2[136]—have been reported in a number of patients. Again, however, these autoantibodies were not present in all the RE patients, and they could also be detected in neurologic diseases other than RE. This indicates that none of the described autoantibodies is specifically associated with RE, and that a variety of autoantibodies to neuronal and synaptic structures can be found that may contribute to the inflammatory process, or possibly represent an epiphenomenon of an activated immune system.

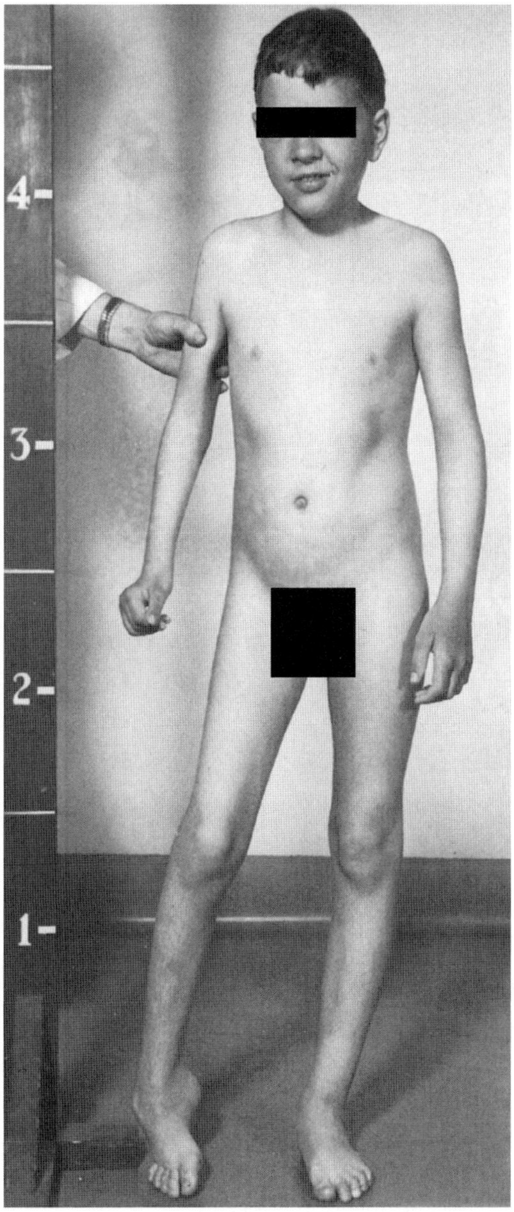

A

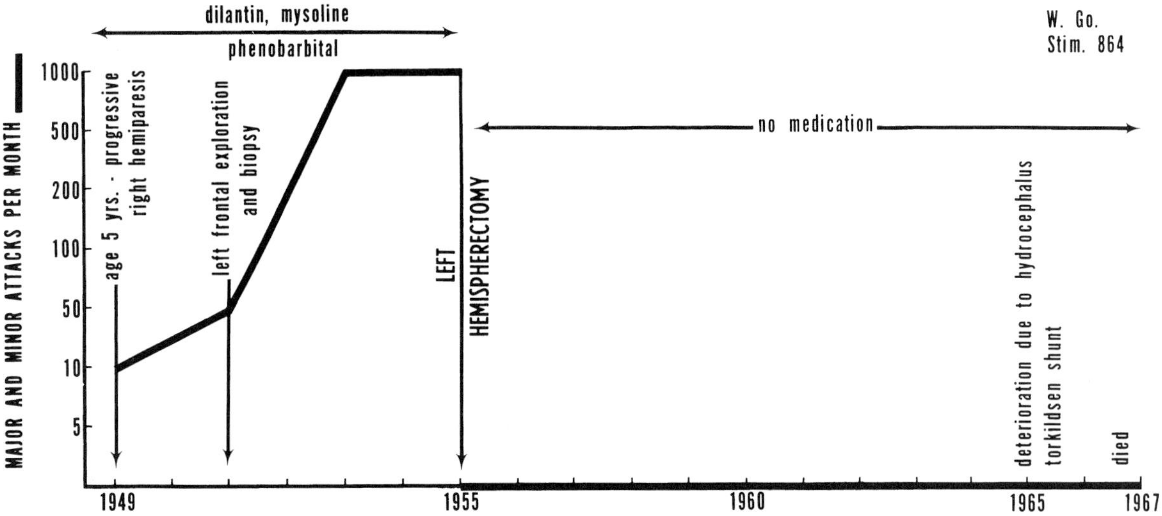

B

FIGURE 2. **A:** W. G., a boy with intractable seizures, right-sided hemiparesis, and hemiatrophy. This is the original patient described by Rasmussen. **B:** The course of W. G.'s illness.

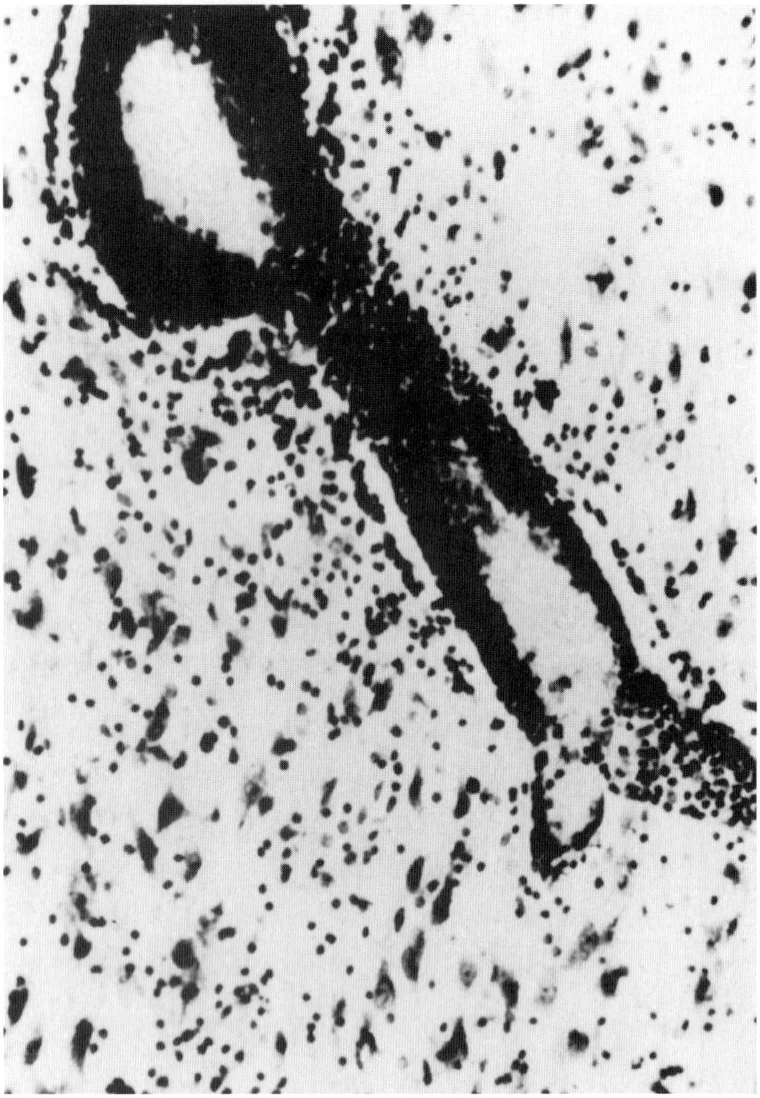

FIGURE 3. Pathologic findings in Rasmussen's syndrome: Perivascular infiltrates, microglial nodules, and neuronophagia.

It is noteworthy that careful analysis of antibody gene rearrangement in lesions of chronic encephalitis patients demonstrated local clonal expansion of antibody producing cells[12]; the exact role of these humoral immune elements in the pathogenetic cascade of RE remains elusive. In the report by Takahashi et al.,[136] anti-GluR epsilon2 antibodies were present only in patients with epilepsia partialis continua (EPC; 15 subjects, including ten with histologically proven or clinical RE, three with acute encephalitis/encephalopathy, and two with nonprogressive EPC), and were directed primarily against cytoplasmic epitopes, suggesting the involvement of T-cell–mediated autoimmunity.

Recent reports have indeed implicated a T-cell–mediated inflammatory response as another potential initiating or perpetuating mechanism in RE. Active inflammatory brain lesions contain large numbers of T lymphocytes,[17] which appear to be recruited early within the lesions, implicating a T-cell–mediated immune response in the early evolution of the disease. Li et al.[91] analyzed T-cell receptor expression in the lesions of patients with RE and found that the local immune response is characterized by restricted T-cell populations that have likely expanded from a small number of precursor T-cell clones, responding themselves to discrete antigenic epitopes. However, the nature of the antigens that trigger such a response is unknown. Recent work provides further credence to the hypothesis that a T-cell–mediated reaction, mainly consisting of cytotoxic $CD8^+$ T-cell responses, may induce damage and apoptotic death of cortical neurons in RE.[13,17,18] The demonstration of such cytotoxic T cells in close apposition to neurons suggests that RE might be a paradigm for a CD8-driven (auto) immune attack against neuronal structures. It is interesting to note that granzyme B, a toxic molecule secreted by $CD8^+$ T cells upon interaction with a target, is capable of generating an antigenic epitope from the glutamate receptor.[53] This observation might indicate a link between cellular and humoral immune components contributing to RE pathogenesis. In an attempt to integrate existing knowledge, several investigators[13,17,19] have proposed a new scheme of pathogenesis. First, a focal CNS event initiates the process (e.g., infection, trauma, immune-mediated brain damage, even focal seizure activity) resulting in an immune reaction, involving antigen presentation in the CNS and entry of cytotoxic T lymphocytes into the CNS across the disrupted blood–brain barrier. Second, activated cytotoxic T lymphocytes attack CNS neurons while the inflammatory process, together with the release of cytokines, causes a spread of the inflammatory reaction and recruitment of more activated cytotoxic T lymphocytes. Third, the generation of potentially antigenic fragments, including GluR3, gives rise to autoantibodies, and may lead to an antibody-mediated "second wave of attack." From an immunologic point of view, the typical adherence of the disease to one hemisphere still remains difficult to explain.

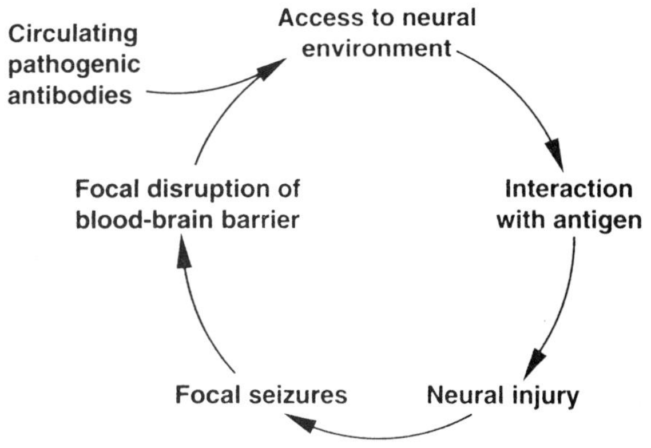

FIGURE 4. The "vicious cycle" hypothesis may explain Rasmussen's encephalitis. Focal blood–brain barrier disruption facilitates entry of antibodies into the brain, with local neural injury and focal seizures. The focal seizures, in turn, cause focal transient blood–brain barrier disruption.

CLINICAL PRESENTATIONS

Typical Course of the Disease

In the early stages of the disease, the major issue is diagnosis. A combination of characteristic clinical, electrophysiologic, and imaging findings aids in the diagnosis. The 48 patients initially studied at the MNHI were collected over a period of 30 years and consisted mostly of cases referred from all over the world. Although now easier to recognize, this entity remains rare. During the last decade, an additional ten patients were studied in our institution, a small number compared to the 100 to 150 patients with intractable focal epilepsy due to other causes studied each year in our center. Typically, the disease starts in healthy children aged 1 to 13 years (mean age, 6.8 years) with 80% developing seizures before the age of 10 years.[106] There is no difference in incidence between the sexes. In approximately half the patients, a history of infectious or inflammatory episode was described 6 months prior to the onset of seizures.

The first sign of the disease is the development of seizures. They are usually partial or secondarily generalized tonic–clonic seizures or status epilepticus (20% of the patients in the MNHI series presented with status epilepticus as the first manifestation). Early seizures could be polymorphic with variable semiology, but motor seizures are almost always reported. Other variable semiology of seizures with somatosensory, autonomic, visual, and limbic features has been described.[58,106] The seizures rapidly become refractory, with little response to AEDs. EPC and other forms of focal motor seizures are particularly unresponsive to AEDs.[39,63,114,142] We reviewed the AED therapy of 25 patients of the MNHI series and found no specific agent or combination therapy that appeared to be more effective or less toxic than other regimens.[39] Our experience with newer AEDs in seven other patients with RE did not support improved effectiveness or tolerability for the new agents (personal data). The new antiepileptic agents levetiracetam and topiramate may theoretically have a role in the treatment of RE, the first because of its efficacy in treating cortical myoclonus[51,56] and the second because of its direct effect on glutamate receptors and release of *N*-methyl-D-glutamine.[103] A variety of seizure types develop over time; the most common are focal motor and EPC (described in 56% of the patients in the MNHI series), with scalp electroencephalogram (EEG) patterns suggesting perirolandic onset. EPC is characterized by recurrent, asynchronous, and persistent (observed during wakefulness and sleep) myoclonias involving different muscle groups of the face, hand, or leg of one hemibody. Secondarily, generalized motor seizures are also described in many patients, but these appear to be easier to control with AEDs. Other less frequent types of motor seizures are a Jacksonian march (12%), posturing (25%), and versive movements of the head and eyes (13%), suggesting involvement of the primary, premotor, and supplementary motor areas. Drop attacks, however, are rare. Focal seizures with somatosensory (22% of patients), visual (16%), or auditory manifestations (2%) are also less frequent and appear later in the course of the disease, suggesting that the epileptogenic process has migrated from frontocentral and temporal regions to more posterior cortical areas, with a characteristic anteroposterior hemispheric march of the disease.[106]

Oguni et al.[106] divided the progression of the disease into three stages: **Stage 1**, from the onset of the seizures and before the development of a fixed hemiparesis (3 months to 10 years, mean duration, 2.8 years); **stage 2**, from the development of a fixed hemiparesis (in 100% of the patients) to the completion of neurologic deterioration, including intellectual decline (in 85%), visual (49%) and sensory (29%) cortical deficits, and speech problems (dysarthria, 23%; dysphasia, 19%) dependent or independent of the burden of seizure activity (2 months to 10 years, mean duration, 3.7 years); and **stage 3**, stabilization of the condition in which further progression no longer occurs, and even the seizures may decrease in severity and frequency or, after some improvement, become again severe, continuous, and debilitating.

A more recent study by Bien et al.[23] presented the clinical natural history of RE in parallel with the time course of brain destruction as measured by serial magnetic resonance imaging (MRI) in a series of 13 patients studied histologically. They separated the progression of the disease into **prodromal, acute,** and **residual stages,** comparable to the three stages of Oguni et al. Bien et al. distinguished two patterns of disease determined by the age at onset of RE: One with an earlier and more severe and rapidly progressive disorder starting during childhood (mean age at first seizure, 4.4 years; range, 1.6 to 6.4 years) and a second with a more protracted and milder course starting during adolescence or adult life (mean age at first seizure, 21.9 years; range, 6.4 to 40.9 years), the second pattern representing a variant of RE repeatedly described, particularly during the last decade.[1,66,82,86,99]

Clinical Variants of Rasmussen's Syndrome

Rasmussen's syndrome has been known for more than 50 years, and over 200 cases have now been reported.[21] After the initial description, it became clear that the disease is clinically heterogeneous despite the pathologic hallmark of nonspecific chronic inflammation in the affected hemisphere. This heterogeneity may be explained by different etiologies (viral, viral- and non–viral-mediated autoimmune disease), by different reactions of the host's immune system to exogenous or endogenous insults (age, genetic background, presence of another lesion, or "double pathology"), and by the modulating effect of a variety of antiviral, immunosuppressant, and immunomodulatory agents, or receptor-directed pharmacotherapy used in variable combinations and durations to treat these patients.

Atypical or unusual clinical features include early onset, usually before 2 years of age, with rapid propagation of the disease; bilateral cerebral involvement; relatively late onset during adolescence or adult life with slow progression; atypical anatomic location of the initial brain MRI findings; focal, protracted, or subcortical variants of RE; and double pathology. Also, two brothers developing bihemispheric disease early in life and with a fatal outcome for one were reported by Silver et al.[128] The brain biopsy of one of the brothers showed changes indistinguishable from the classical form of the disease.

Bilateral Hemispheric Involvement

Usually the disease affects only one hemisphere, and most autopsy studies available confirmed unilateral cerebral involvement.[122] Over time, however, there may be some contralateral ventricular enlargement and cortical atrophy attributed either to the effect of recurrent seizures and secondary epileptogenesis or to wallerian changes.[85] Patients with definite bilateral inflammatory involvement are exceptional, and so far this has been described in no more than a dozen of them.[31,37,67,99,128,135,141] Bilateral disease tends to occur in children with early onset (before 2 years). In these children, the disorder is usually fatal. Bilateral disease was also described in the late-onset adolescent or adult forms and is less severe in these patients. A small number had received high-dose steroids or an intrathecal antiviral agent, which suggested that early aggressive immunologic therapy may have predisposed to contralateral spread of the disease.[37,135]

Late-onset Adolescent and Adult Variants

A number of papers have reported the development of RE in adolescence or adult life as representing approximately 10% of the total number of patients with RE described in the literature over the last 40 years.[1,23,32,50,59,66,71,82,84,86,89,99,104,131,146,147,157,164] In the MNHI series, 9 of 55 patients (16%) collected between 1945 and 2000 started to have seizures after the age of 12 years. The largest series, described by Hart et al.[66] included 13 adults and adolescents collected from five centers. In comparison with the childhood form, late-onset RE has a more variable evolution,[23,66] a generally more insidious onset of focal neurologic defects and cognitive impairment, and an increased incidence of occipital involvement (23% in the series of Hart et al. vs. 7% in children <12 years old in the MNHI series). Hemiparesis and hemispheric atrophy are often late and may not be as severe when compared with the more typical childhood form.[23] Occasionally, however, the outcome in late-onset RE is similar to or worse than in children,[59,99,104,131] but because of the generally more benign and protracted course, hemispherectomy seems less appropriate in this group of patients in whom neurologic deficits are usually less pronounced. Due to lack of brain plasticity in adults, the decision for hemispherectomy is even more complicated due to potential risk of new irreversible postoperative deficits.

Focal and Chronic Protracted Variants

There are rare reports of patients with RE whose seizures were relatively well controlled with AEDs or focal resections, and in whom the neurologic status stabilized spontaneously.[66,71,88,164] Rasmussen had already suggested the existence of a "nonprogressive focal form of encephalitis." With Aguilar, he reviewed 512 surgical specimens from 449 patients and found 32 cases with histologic evidence suggesting the presence of active encephalitis.[1] Twelve patients demonstrated progressive neurologic deterioration compatible with RE, and 20 (4.4%) showed no or mild neurologic deterioration. In his review of patients who underwent temporal resections for intractable focal seizures, Laxer[88] found five patients (3.8% of a series of 160 patients) with what he thought was a benign, focal, nonprogressive form of RE. These patients, children or adults, with no evidence of progression are indistinguishable clinically from those with refractory seizures due to other causes, including mesial temporal sclerosis.[71,88]

Delayed Seizure Onset Variant

Korn-Lubetski et al. recently reported on two children with the typical progressive clinical course and contralateral hemispheric atrophy characteristic for RE, but no clinical and EEG epileptic activity observed for several months.[80] Both children had a brain biopsy (performed before seizure onset) confirming the clinical diagnosis. The focal seizures started in the first child 7 months after initial symptomatology and in the second after 6 months.

Basal Ganglia Involvement

Epilepsia partialis continua and other types of focal motor seizures are a common finding in patients with RE. Chorea, athetosis, and dystonia were infrequently described and may have been overlooked because of the preponderance of the epileptic disorder and of the hemiparesis. In 27 of the 48 patients of the MNHI series who had EPC, nine additionally had writhing or choreiform movements, and a diagnosis of Sydenham chorea was made in three of them early in the disease course.[106] Matthews et al.[97] described a 10-year-old girl with a 1-year history of progressive right-sided hemiparesis, EPC, and secondary generalized seizures. MRI showed diffuse cortical and subcortical changes, maximum in the perisylvian frontotemporoparietal area. At examination, she had choreic movements of the right arm and hand in addition to EPC. Tien et al.[140] were the first to describe in an 8.5-year-old girl with intractable focal motor seizures and atrophy of the caudate and putamen, with abnormal high signals and severe left hemispheric atrophy. They interpreted these findings as the result of gliosis and chronic brain damage. Topçu et al.[142] described a patient who developed hemidystonia as a result of involvement of the contralateral basal ganglia. The movement disorder appeared 3 years after onset of seizures. A rather typical subsequent evolution suggested RE. The movement disorder started during intravenous immunoglobulin (IVIg) and interferon therapy, and did not respond to anticholinergic drugs nor to a frontal resection. Ben-Zeev et al.,[15] Koehn and Zupanc,[79] Frucht,[50] and, finally, Lascelles et al.[87] each reported a case of RE whose clinical presentation was dominated by a hemidyskinesia, with EPC in three of those patients, and progressive hemiparesis. Two cases showed selective frontal cortical and caudate atrophy on MRI, one developed progressive left basal ganglia atrophy and later focal frontotemporoparietal atrophy, and one had only pronounced right caudate, globus pallidus, and putamen atrophy. In the case of Frucht, IVIg dramatically improved both the hyperkinetic movements and the EPC, but the effect was transient, suggesting a common neuroanatomic mechanism or humoral autoimmune process. In a series of 21 patients with RE, Bhatjiwale et al.[16] looked specifically at the involvement of the basal ganglia. Fifteen (71%) showed mild to severe basal ganglia involvement on imaging in three different patterns: Predominantly cortical in six cases, predominantly basal ganglia in six, and with both cortical and basal ganglia involvement in six. In five cases, the changes found in the basal ganglia were static, whereas in the others there was steady progression. The caudate nucleus was generally more prominently involved, usually in association with frontal atrophy. Five cases also showed putaminal involvement, always with temporoinsular atrophy. Interestingly, two of the six patients with prominent basal ganglia involvement had dystonia as a presenting feature. The authors postulated that the disease may proceed from different foci, including cases where RE seems to start in deep gray matter. The Italian Study Group recently described similar findings on Rasmussen's encephalitis,[30] which found basal ganglia atrophy in 9 of 13 patients studied. They suggested that atrophy of the basal ganglia represents secondary changes due to disconnection from the affected overlying frontal and insular cortex.

Brainstem Variant

McDonald et al.[98] reported a 3-year-old boy with RE manifested by chronic brainstem encephalitis. After a prolonged febrile seizure associated with an acute varicella infection, he developed within a few weeks recurrent partial motor seizures, EPC, and left hemiparesis. After a few more weeks, signs of brainstem involvement appeared; repeated MRI showed increased signal in the pons, but a complete infectious and inflammatory evaluation, including brain biopsy, was negative. He died 14 months after the onset of his illness. Neuropathologic findings in the brainstem were typical of those found in RE. Bilateral mesial temporal sclerosis was also present. The authors proposed that this case represents a rare focal form of RE with primary involvement of the brainstem, and hemiparesis and mesial temporal sclerosis resulting from seizure activity. One other patient with brainstem involvement and fatal outcome was included in the MNHI series of 48 patients.[106]

Multifocal Variant

Maeda et al.[94] described a 6-year-old girl with typical RE. One year following the onset of seizures, MRI–fluid-attenuated inversion recovery (FLAIR) sequences showed multiple high-signal-intensity areas in the right hemisphere and a methionine–positron emission tomography (PET) performed at the same time exhibited multifocal methionine uptake areas concordant with the MRI lesions, suggesting multiple independent sites of chronic inflammation. The authors proposed that the inflammatory process in RE may spread from multifocal lesions and not necessarily originate from localized temporal, insular, or frontocentral lesions, as usually described, before spreading across adjacent regions to the entire hemisphere.

Double Pathology

A small number of reports have documented coexisting brain pathologies with RE: A tumor (anaplastic astrocytoma, ganglioglioma, and anaplastic ependymoma) in three patients,[46,65,83] dysgenetic tissue in four,[65,110,122,161] multifocal perivasculitis in seven,[122] and cavernous angiomas with signs of vasculitis in two.[21,51] Double pathology in RE supports the theory of a focal disruption (trauma, infection, or other pathology) of the blood–brain barrier allowing access of antibodies produced by the host to neurons expressing the target receptor and production of focal inflammation.[5,145] So far, however, only one case of double pathology provided reasonable support to this hypothesis.[110] Strongly positive anti-GluR3 antibodies were measured in one case of RE with concomitant cortical dysplasia in a 2.5-year-old girl with catastrophic epilepsy starting at age 2. She underwent a right, partial frontal lobectomy, plasmapheresis, and therapy with IVIg with a transient response, and finally a right functional hemispherectomy with good seizure control. GluR3 antibodies were measured serially throughout the course of her treatment and correlated with her clinical status. They were undetectable 1 year after her last surgery.

There are also reports of coexisting autoimmune diseases such as Parry-Romberg syndrome,[127,133] linear scleroderma,[118,132] and systemic lupus erythematosus[87] with epilepsy and pathologic changes suggestive of RE. The clinical course in these patients, however, was not as severe as that of the classic childhood form. Changes of chronic progressive or smoldering encephalitis have also been described in disorders with impaired immunity such as agammaglobulinemia[93] and multiple endocrinopathies, chronic mucocutaneous candidiasis, and impaired cellular immunity.[62] The occurrence of two conditions presumably due to impaired immunity in the same individual may strengthen the view that immune-mediated mechanisms are responsible for the development of RE.

Lagrange et al.[84] recently reported an interesting case of new-onset seizures and narcolepsy in a previously healthy 40-year-old man. The patient developed within 2 years daytime sleepiness and cataplexy, followed, after a course of few months, by protracted but refractory focal epilepsy and a progressively enlarging lesion in the temporoinsular region. Pathology from a left temporal resection was consistent with RE. An extensive infectious, autoimmune, and paraneoplastic workup was negative, but CSF hypocretin was undetectable and HLA haplotype of the patient was DQB1*0602. The authors proposed a common underlying disease process, possibly autoimmune, to explain in this patient the coincidence of two rare cerebral disorders.

Finally, the rare association of uveitis (three cases) or choroiditis (one case) with typical features of RE have led to the speculation that a viral infection may have been responsible for both.[52,59,69] In all cases, the ocular pathology was ipsilateral to the involved hemisphere that showed chronic encephalitis. In three cases,[59,69] the uveitis or choroiditis was detected 2 to 4 months after epilepsy onset. In one case,[52] ocular diagnosis preceded the onset of chronic encephalitis. In light of these reports, it was hypothesized that a primary ocular infection, in particular a viral infection with herpes simplex virus (HSV), varicella zoster virus (VZV), Epstein-Barr virus (EBV), cytomegalovirus (CMV), measles, or rubella, followed by vascular or neurotropic spread to the brain, was a possible mechanism for development of RE.

DIAGNOSTIC EVALUATION

Electroencephalographic Findings

Few studies specifically reported the EEG changes associated with RE,[10,11,40,58,75,129] and even fewer tried to correlate the clinical and EEG features of the disease over time. So and Gloor[129] reported the scalp and peroperative (electrocorticogram [ECoG]) EEG findings in the MNHI series of patients with RE. They summarized the EEG features as (a) disturbance of background activity in all except one patient with more severe slowing and relative depression of background rhythms in the diseased hemisphere; polymorphic or rhythmic delta activity was found in all (more commonly bilateral with lateralized preponderance); (b) interictal epileptiform activity in 94% of patients, rarely focal (more commonly multifocal and lateralized to one hemisphere or bilateral independent, but strongly lateralized discharges with or without bilateral synchrony); (c) clinical or subclinical seizure onsets were variable and occasionally focal, but more often poorly localized, lateralized, bilateral, or even generalized; and (d) no clear electroclinical correlation apparent in many of the recorded seizures, in particular in EPC. The electrographic lateralization of these abnormalities (focal slowing, progressive deterioration of unilateral background activity, and ictal and multifocal interictal hemispheric activity) was sufficiently concordant with the clinical lateralization to provide essential information about the abnormal hemisphere in 90% of cases. These EEG features, indicative of a widespread destructive and epileptogenic process, in the specific clinical context of catastrophic epilepsy and worsening neurologic deficits involving one hemisphere, suggest the diagnosis of chronic encephalitis.

The evolution of the EEG has been studied longitudinally in a small number of patients.[4,14,26] The studies showed progression of the EEG abnormalities. At the onset of the disease, EEG abnormalities tend to be lateralized and nonspecific, with unilateral impoverishment and slowing of background activity during wakefulness and progressive disappearance of spindles

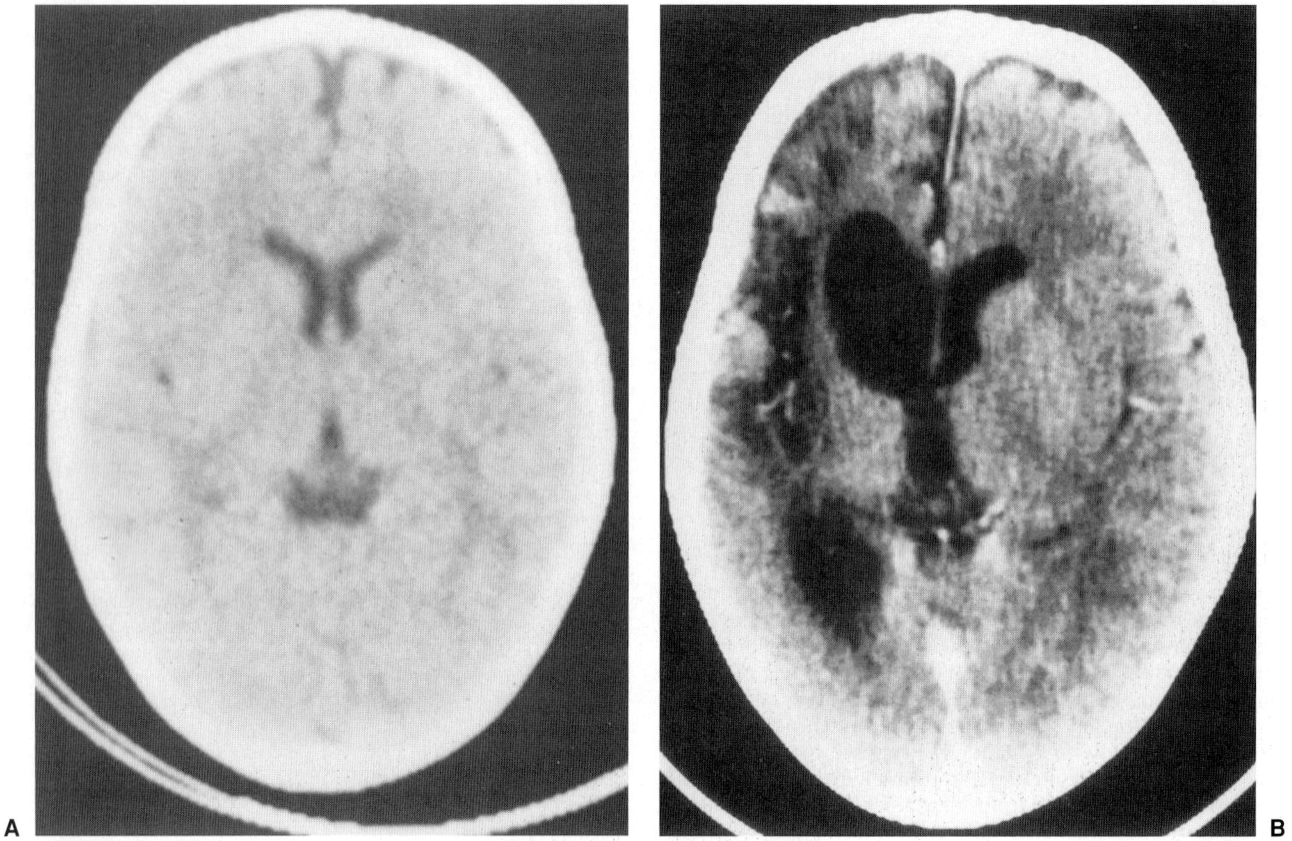

FIGURE 5. Computed tomography scan of a boy with Rasmussen's syndrome. A: Three months after onset of seizures. B: Two years later. Severe parenchymatous atrophy and ventricular enlargement are apparent *on the right*.

during sleep in the diseased hemisphere. As the disorder progressed, the epileptiform and slow-wave abnormalities tend to become bilateral and widespread, multifocal, or synchronous, suggesting a more diffuse hemispheric process, not always confined to one hemisphere. It is not clear if the late bilateralization of the EEG abnormalities represents functional interference, secondary epileptogenesis, or, much less likely, evidence for the inflammatory process directly involving the contralateral hemisphere.

Only one report has been published so far on the usefulness of MEG in the evaluation of patients with RE.[76] MEG may provide insight on cortical function and useful information about cortical reorganization, for instance, before and after hemispherectomy.

Neuroimaging

Anatomic Imaging

Imaging studies, although not specific, are extremely important for the diagnosis of RE. Typically, they show progressive lateralized atrophy coupled with localized or lateralized functional abnormalities.[16,22,23,30,42,45,47,58,76,114,137,140,149] Brain MRI studies early in the course of the illness may be normal, rapidly followed by a combination of characteristic features that parallel the clinical and electrophysiologic deterioration, reflecting the nature of the pathologic process. Recent studies using serial MRIs in a relatively large number of patients with RE provided better insight into the early, progressive, and late gray and white matter changes expected in this disease: Cortical swelling; atrophy of cortical and deep gray matter nuclei, particularly the caudate; a hyperintense signal in gray and white matter; and secondary changes.[16,22,23,30,58] In the early phase of the disease, when the MRI still appears normal, a few studies demonstrated abnormalities of perfusion or metabolism by single photon emission computed tomography (SPECT) or PET, suggesting that these imaging procedures may aid in early identification of the disease and of the abnormal hemisphere.[25,45,47,140] Rapidly on early MRI scans, however, the cortex shows focal hyperintense signals on T2 or FLAIR sequences[30] and may appear swollen. This can be explained by brain edema at the onset of inflammation[22] or, alternatively, it may be due to recurrent focal seizures.[124] Very early signal change in the white matter (within 4 months) is also frequent, usually focal, with or without swelling.[30] Later, progressive atrophy of the affected hemisphere occurs, reflecting the manner in which the disease spreads, and with most of the hemispheric volume loss occurring during the first 2 years[22,30] (Figs. 5 and 6). The cortical atrophy is initially either temporal, frontoinsular, or frontocentral, and more rarely parieto-occipital, later spreading across the hemisphere. Basal ganglia involvement, mostly of the putamen and caudate, is also characteristic and may be due to direct damage by the pathologic process or secondary to changes due to disconnection of the basal ganglia from the affected overlying frontocentral and insular cortices.[16,30] Other secondary changes usually associated with severe hemispheric tissue loss are atrophy of the brainstem, particularly of the cerebral peduncle and pons; thinning of the corpus callosum; and atrophy of the contralateral cerebellar hemisphere.[98] Surprisingly, gadolinium enhancement on MRI is rarely observed.[22,30,45,105,146,161,165]

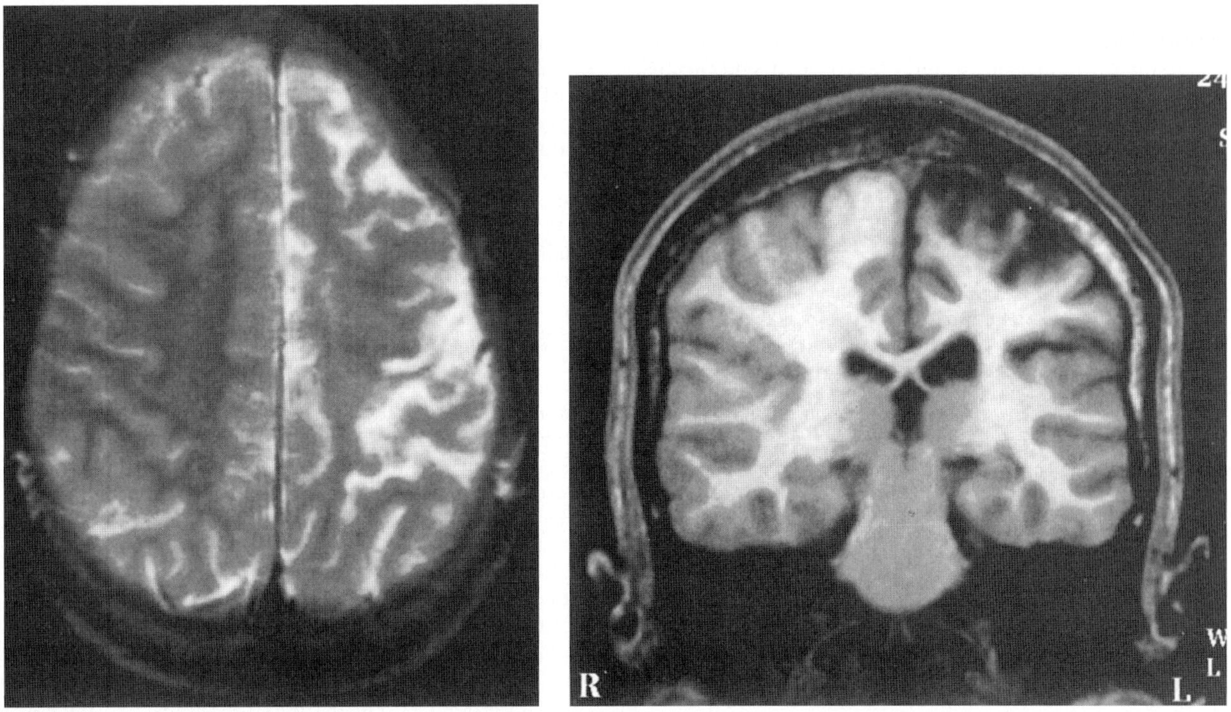

FIGURE 6. Magnetic resonance imaging in a 15-year-old boy with a 7-year history of Rasmussen's syndrome. Axial (A) and coronal (B) images showing hemispheral and focal atrophy *on the left*.

Functional Imaging

Several studies, often case reports, emphasize the utility of functional imaging such as PET, SPECT, and proton magnetic resonance spectroscopy (MRS) in the diagnosis and follow-up. Functional abnormalities may be useful in cases in which MRI is normal, usually at the onset of the disease, or when structural imaging fails to provide satisfactory localizing information. Combined anatomic and functional neuroimaging may serve to focus the diagnostic workup, hasten brain biopsy for definitive diagnosis, or define the appropriate surgical approach. It may be useful to follow the evolution of the disease or the result of treatment. Finally, functional studies may provide insight into the cortical reorganization of speech areas and of motor and somatosensory cortices.

Fiorella et al.[45] reviewed ^{18}F-fluorodeoxyglucose (FDG)-PET and MRI studies of 11 patients with surgically proven RE. All had diffuse, unilateral cerebral hypometabolism on PET images, closely correlated with the distribution of cerebral atrophy on MRI. Even subtle diffuse atrophic changes were accompanied by marked decreases in cerebral glucose utilization that, according to the authors, increased diagnostic confidence and aided in the identification of the abnormal hemisphere. During ictal studies, patients had multiple foci of hypermetabolism, indicative of multifocal seizure activity within the affected hemisphere, and never showed such changes in the contralateral one. Fogarasi et al.[47] also compared MRI and FDG-PET studies in children with RE (five from their own series and eight taken from the literature), emphasizing early metabolic changes and the complementary roles of structural and functional neuroimaging in the early diagnosis of RE. In five cases, the PET changes occurred before any lesions appeared on MRI (the time between seizure onset and functional changes was 1 to 8 months). Similar findings have been reported previously but in smaller series.[30,41,64,74,78,105,140,165] Although MRI alone is generally sufficient to identify the affected hemisphere, FDG-PET unequivocally confirms the findings in each case. Blood flow or perfusion studies using O^{15} PET showed a similar correlation, with regions of perfusion change corresponding with structural MRI changes.[74] Using a specific radioligand ([^{11}C]*(R)*-PK11195) for peripheral benzodiazepine binding sites on cells of mononuclear phagocyte lineage, Banati et al.[9] demonstrated in vivo the widespread activation of microglia in three patients, confirming what is usually found by neuropathologic study.

SPECT was used to study regional blood flow in a number of patients.[2,25,30,41,55,68,74,76,108,114,142,150,162] The findings may be of some help and more sensitive than anatomic neuroimaging early in the disease, but are nonspecific. As with FDG-PET, the regions of functional change usually correlate with anatomic abnormalities. Interictal SPECT scans reveal diminished perfusion in a large zone surrounding the epileptic area shown on EEG. This hypoperfusion may show some variability depending on fluctuation of the epileptic activity. Ictal studies often show zones of hyperperfusion representing likely areas of more intense seizure activity. Sequential scans may be helpful to follow the progression of the disease[42] or the effect of treatment.[150]

MRS has been used in a number of patients with RE.[29,30,97,112,113,125,126,134,144,150] Localized proton MRS was described for the first time in two patients by Matthews et al.[97] They showed reduced *N*-acetylaspartate (NAA) concentrations—a compound exclusively found in neurons and their processes—in diseased areas in both patients, suggesting neuronal loss. In addition, MRS showed increased lactate in a patient with EPC, probably the result of excessive and repetitive seizure activity. Peeling and Sutherland[113] and Cendes et al.[29] confirmed those findings. Peeling and Sutherland also showed that the concentration of NAA in vitro (MRS on tissue obtained from surgical patients) was reduced in proportion to the severity and extent of the encephalitis. Cendes et al. did sequential studies at 1 year in three patients and demonstrated progression of the MRS changes. They noted that those changes were more widespread than the structural changes seen on anatomic MRI. Overall, the studies using NAA indicate that MRS can identify and quantify neuronal damage and loss throughout the affected hemisphere, including areas that appear anatomically normal. In addition to NAA and lactate, other compounds measured included choline, creatine, *myo*-inositol, glutamine, and glutamate. Choline is usually elevated, which probably indicates demyelination and increased membrane turnover.[29,55,126,134] *Myo*-inositol, a glial cell marker, was found to be elevated in a small number of patients,[55,125,144] indicating glial proliferation or prominent gliotic activity. Hypothetically, *myo*-inositol signal should increase with the progression of the disease. Lactate was almost always elevated, and this increase probably results from ongoing or repetitive focal epileptic activity rather than from being a marker of the inflammatory process itself.[95–97,99] The largest peaks in lactate were usually detected in patients with EPC. Glutamine and glutamate levels were also elevated, only in two patients, a finding of interest considering the potential role of excitatory neurotransmitters in the disease.[55]

There are only two reports on diffusion MRI changes observed in three cases of RE.[125,126] These preliminary studies showed that diffusion MRI may provide data on brain tissue integrity and allows easy comparisons between the diseased and normal parenchyma.

DIFFERENTIAL DIAGNOSIS

The clinical changes of RE are nonspecific, particularly at the beginning of the disease, and clearly at this stage the major issue is diagnosis. We have better diagnostic criteria that can lead to early diagnosis (Table 1, and the Vienna consensus statement on RE held at the sixth European Congress on Epileptology, June 2004[21]). The onset in a previously healthy child is of increasing frequency, and severe, simple focal, usually motor seizures often followed by postictal deficit. This, and lack of evidence of anatomic abnormalities on early brain MRI, should raise suspicion regarding the diagnosis of RE. Further course and evaluation with scalp EEG showing unilateral findings with focal or regional slowing, deterioration of background activity, multifocal interictal epileptiform discharges, and seizure onset or EPC, particularly corresponding to the cortical motor area, are major neurophysiologic features in favor of RE. Early MRI characteristics include the association of focal white matter hyperintensity and cortical swelling with hyperintense signal, particularly insular and peri-insular regions. This is later followed by hemispheric atrophy that is usually predominant in the peri-insular and frontal regions and the head of the caudate nucleus contralateral to the clinical manifestations. Functional imaging studies may reveal abnormalities before any visible structural changes. Typically, FDG-PET shows diffuse hemispheric glucose hypometabolism. SPECT shows unilateral interictal hypoperfusion and ictal multifocal areas of hyperperfusion, confirming the lateralized hemispheric nature of the lesion and its extent. MRS may also help in the early detection of brain damage and shows a lateralized decrease in NAA intensity relative to creatine, suggesting neuronal loss or damage in one hemisphere. There is no consistent systemic and CSF response that may contribute to the diagnosis, and, in fact, the most common feature is the lack of cellular or protein response in the CSF of patients with RE. Brain biopsy is often used as a diagnostic tool in many centers for confirming the diagnosis. However, histologic findings in RE are nonspecific chronic inflammatory changes that may be subtle enough to be missed by an inexperienced pathologist. Furthermore, the brain involvement may be patchy, and a normal biopsy does not rule out the diagnosis of RE.[44,111,122] In more experienced centers, brain biopsy is not considered diagnostic of RE, and the key features remain the clinical evolution and the presence of progressive atrophy on repeated MRI scans. The European consensus group proposed a series of diagnostic criteria, and a two-step approach, to help the (early) diagnosis of RE.[21]

The differential diagnosis is from focal cortical dysplasia, hemimegalencephaly and some neurocutaneous disorders (such as tuberous sclerosis, Sturge-Weber syndrome, and

TABLE 1

CRITERIA FOR (EARLY) DIAGNOSIS OF RASMUSSEN'S ENCEPHALITIS

CLINICAL	■ Refractory focal motor seizures rapidly increasing in frequency and severity, and often polymorphic ■ Epilepsia partialis continua ■ Motor, progressive hemiparesis and cognitive deterioration
EEG	■ Focal or regional slow-wave activity contralateral to motor manifestations ■ Multifocal, usually lateralized, interictal and ictal epileptiform discharges ■ Progressive lateralized impoverishment of background activity
IMAGING	■ *MRI*: Focal cortical swelling with hyperintensity and white matter signal hyperintensity, insular cortical atrophy, atrophy of the head of caudate nucleus, and progressive gray and white matter atrophy, unilateral ■ *PET*: Unilateral, hemispheric, but during early stage may be restricted to frontal and temporal regions, glucose hypometabolism ■ *SPECT*: Unilateral interictal hemispheric hypoperfusion and ictal multifocal hyperperfusion ■ *MRS*: Unilateral reduced NAA and increased lactate, choline, *myo*-inositol, and glutamine/glutamate
BLOOD	■ None, except inconsistent finding of anti-GluR3 and other autoantibodies
CSF	■ None, except sometimes presence of oligoclonal bands and inconsistent elevated levels of anti-GluR3 and other autoantibodies
HISTOPATHOLOGY	■ Microglial nodules, perivascular lymphocytic infiltration, neuron degeneration, and spongy degeneration; evidence for local clonal expansion of T cells and antibody-producing cells ■ Combination of active and remote, multifocal, intracortical, and white matter lesions

CSF, cerebrospinal fluid; EEG, electroencephalogram; MRI, magnetic resonance imaging; MRS, magnetic resonance spectroscopy; NAA, *N*-acetylaspartate; PET, positron emission tomography; SPECT, single photon emission computed tomography.

linear sebaceous nevus syndrome), mitochondrial encephalopathy (such as mitochondrial encephalopathy with lactic acidosis and strokelike episodes [MELAS]), brain tumors, cerebral vasculitis, degenerative cortical gray matter diseases (such as Kufs disease and Alpers syndrome), some forms of meningoencephalitis (such as Russian summer meningoencephalitis and subacute sclerosing panencephalitis), some paraneoplastic syndromes, and maybe rare chromosomal epileptogenic disorders (such as the ring-20 chromosome).[21,28] EPC can be found in many of those conditions, but each has its own clinical and laboratory characteristics that usually distinguish it from RE. Although several diagnostic criteria have recently been proposed, especially for an early diagnosis of RE, the correct identification of patients with this disease remains a matter of experience, particularly if specific investigative or therapeutic interventions are considered. When a constellation of clinical and laboratory findings highlights the possibility of RE, close follow-up is necessary to assess progression of the disease and eventually confirm its diagnosis.

TREATMENT AND OUTCOME

The typical evolution of RE is characterized by the development of intractable seizures, progressive neurologic deficits, and intellectual impairment. This has led clinicians to try a variety of empiric treatments, including antiviral agents and immunomodulatory or immunosuppressive therapies. Surgery, and specifically hemispherectomy, appears to be successful in controlling the disease process and arresting the seizures. However, the ensuing neurologic deficits due to surgery usually lead to reluctance to carry out this procedure until significant hemiparesis or other functional deficit has already occurred. Apart from the surgical treatment, there is no established treatment of RE. The natural history suggests that the disease burns itself out with maximal residual deficit and reduction, but not cessation of the seizures. On the other hand, anecdotal evidence suggests that in some patients, long-term recurrent seizures may lead to contralateral epileptogenicity by a mechanism of secondary epileptogenesis as opposed to bilateral disease development.

Antiepileptic Drug Therapy

Guidelines for AED treatment in RE are difficult to define and have always empirical. No AED, or any polytherapy regimen, has been proven to be superior,[114] and the choice of the ideal AED rests on its clinical efficacy and side effect profile. Because of the nature of this disease, the danger of overtreatment is high. AED pharmacokinetics, toxicity, and interactions may be better determinants of AED selection and combination therapy. EPC is particularly difficult to treat, but AEDs can reduce the frequency and severity of other focal and secondarily generalized seizures. Since the original report on AED efficacy in RE,[114] several new agents have been introduced. Drugs such as topiramate that act on excitatory neurotransmitters or those that may affect cortically generated myoclonus, such as levetiracetam in EPC, may have a more specific role in treatment.

Antiviral Therapy

Most treatments directed at aborting the progression of the disease were based on the assumption that RE is an infectious, a viral, or an autoimmune disorder. Examples of antiviral treatments are scarce, and only two reports[37,100] are published: One on the treatment of four patients with ganciclovir, a potent anti-cytomegalovirus drug, and another on the treatment of a single patient with zidovudine. Although definite improvement was documented in four of the five patients, no further reports using antiviral agents in RE have been published.

Immune Therapy

Evidence implicating humoral and cellular immune responses in the pathophysiology of RE has led to various therapeutic initiatives.[19] A number of case reports and small series suggesting potential therapeutic roles of immune-directed interventions have now been published. These included interferon, steroids, IVIg, plasmapheresis, selective IgG immunoadsorption by protein A, and immunosuppression with drugs such as cyclophosphamide or tacrolimus. Rarely, such approaches have been associated with sustained cessation of seizure activity and arrest in the progression of the inflammatory process. In the majority of the cases, only transient or partial improvements due to immunomodulators or immunosuppressors have been noted. Of importance is the observation that, to date, the more aggressive immune therapies have been deferred to later stages of the disease, where the burden of the disease is considered to outweigh the toxicity of these interventions. The challenge is to develop safe therapeutic protocols that can be tested in patients soon after the diagnosis, and at a time when less damage has occurred and the process may have a better chance to respond to therapy. Also, different approaches or protocols may be envisaged depending on the time of onset, progression, severity, and hemispheric localization of the disease.[21,57,67]

Interferon-α

Intraventricular interferon-α has been tried in only two children[35,96] with the rational that interferons have both immunomodulating (enhancement of phagocytic activity of macrophages and augmentation of the cytotoxicity of target-specific lymphocytes) and antiviral activity (inhibition of viral replication in virus-infected cells). In both cases, improvement of the epileptic and neurologic syndrome was observed.

Steroids

Relatively low- and high-dose steroid regimens (dexamethasone, prednisone, methylprednisolone, and adrenocorticotropic hormone [ACTH]) were used either alone or in association with other agents such as IVIg. Initial reports were somewhat disappointing,[93,114] but eventually the use of high-dose IV boluses led to encouraging results. When applied during the first year of the disease, pulse IV steroids appeared effective in suppressing, at least temporarily, the inflammatory process in some patients.[31,67,82,150] The proposed modes of action of steroids include an antiepileptic effect, an improvement of blood–brain barrier function—and hence reduction of entry into the brain of potentially deleterious toxic or immune mediators—and a direct anti-inflammatory effect. Steroids may be helpful when used in pulses to stop status epilepticus.[57] The long-term risk/benefit profile of steroids in RE remains unknown; in the Dulac series of 17 patients treated with steroids, all eventually required treatment by hemispherectomy (O. Dulac, personal communication). Because of a less favorable response and the adverse effects of prolonged high-dose steroids, Hart et al.[67] suggested the use of IVIg as initial treatment followed by high-dose steroids, or both, to control seizures.

Immunoglobulins

Walsh used for the first time IVIg in RE[153] in a 9-year-old child who received repeated infusions of IVIg over a period of several months with initial improvement, but later followed by protracted deterioration and eventual cessation of the treatment. Eight subsequent studies reported on the effect of IVIg, alone or in combination with other treatment modalities.[27,67,82,89,147,150,153,160] These reports have shown similar results with initial benefit, but a much less clear-cut, long-term effect. They indicated variable results, ranging from no benefit to significant improvement, maintained in a single case for a period of close to 4 years.[160] IVIg is usually much better tolerated than steroids. The basis for a potential therapeutic effect of immune globulin in RE is not known, but may reflect the functions of natural antibodies in maintaining immune homeostasis in healthy people. Leach et al.[89] showed a delayed but more persistent response in two adults and suggested that IVIg is more effective in adults than in children. They also proposed that IVIg might have a disease-modifying effect. This phenomenon is probably real, but to date, no one has shown that the early use of immune therapy can modify the long-term outcome of RE. IVIg treatments are usually well tolerated and complications are rare.

Plasmapheresis and Selective IgG Immunoadsorption

Plasma exchange is used with the assumption that circulating factors, likely autoantibodies, are pathogenic in at least some patients.[3,6,82,109,123] The majority of patients treated with apheresis showed repeated, at times dramatic, but transient responses. Because of the lack of long-term efficacy, the complications, and the expense, plasmapheresis should probably be used as adjunctive therapy and may be especially useful in patients with acute deterioration, such as status epilepticus.[3,57]

Immunosuppressive Therapy

One study reported a single patient treated with intermittent cyclophosphamide,[82] suggesting the possibility of steroid-sparing treatment with intermittent pulse IV cyclophosphamide for patients with steroid-responsive RE. The authors proposed that such intermittent cyclophosphamide might well replace steroid therapy because it is associated with less risk of systemic complications. Granata et al.,[57] however, observed no consistent effect in four patients with RE treated with cyclophosphamide for a period of approximately 6 months (range, 2 to 10 months).

Based on the notion that T-cell–mediated processes play a role in the pathogenesis of RE,[13,17,18,53,91] a recent study tested the effects of tacrolimus (FK-506) in RE.[20] Tacrolimus is an immunosuppressant that is successfully used in the prevention of transplantation reactions and preferentially acts on T cells. Seven patients with RE were treated with tacrolimus and followed for a median of 22.4 months. They were compared with 12 historical untreated RE patients (median follow-up, 13.9 months). The tacrolimus-treated patients had a superior outcome regarding neurologic function and progression rate of cerebral hemiatrophy, but no better seizure outcome. None of the treated patients (but 7 of 12 control patients) became eligible for hemispherectomy, suggesting that here again, the immunosuppressive therapy at least modified the natural course of the disease. Tacrolimus appeared to have no major side effects.[20]

Azathioprine (150 mg/day) was used in one of our patients for approximately a year (personal data), 4 years after the beginning of her epilepsy (seizure onset was at 12 years old) and after two limited frontal lobe resections. During the same period, she received IV pulses of steroids and IVIg for periodic acute exacerbations of her epileptic condition. The immunosuppressant drug was finally stopped and replaced by periodic IVIg without significant changes in the course of the disease.

Surgery

The only effective surgical procedure seems to be the resection or disconnection of the abnormal hemisphere.[38,48,81,117,143,148,149] Alternative procedures such as partial corticectomy, subpial transaction, and callosal section have limited results and did not render patients seizure free.[73,102,107,114,130] The recent publications by Kossoff et al.[81] and by Pulsifer et al.[117] clearly demonstrated the benefits of hemispherectomy in children with RE. They showed that 91% of 46 children (mean age at surgery, 9.2 years) with severe RE who underwent hemispherectomy (in the majority hemidecortication) between 1975 and 2002 became seizure free (65%) or had nondisabling seizures (26%) that often did not require medications. Patients were walking independently, and all were talking at the time of their most recent follow-up with relatively minor or moderate residual speech problems. Twenty-one had left-sided pathology (presumably involving the dominant hemisphere) with a mean age at surgery of 8.8 years. A subset of 37 children was further followed to assess cognitive outcome (a mean of 5.5 years after surgery). The majority remained seizure free (73%) at the time of follow-up, and 70% attended school, half only with supportive services.

Hemispherectomy, hemidecortication, functional hemispherectomy, or hemispherotomy have proven efficacy for control of seizures in patients with RE. The decision on how early in the course of the disease surgery should be undertaken depends on the certainty of the diagnosis, the severity and frequency of the seizures, and the impact on the psychosocial development of the patient. The natural evolution of the disease and the severity of the epilepsy often justify early intervention, even prior to maximal neurologic deficit. The decisions about such a radical procedure requires considerable time and thought. The recent use of immunomodulating agents may have been responsible for the considerable reduction in hemiparesis, which increases the difficulty in deciding on hemispherectomy. There is, however, no evidence that these treatments lead to a favorable end-point in the evolution of the disease. Also, the psychological preparation of the patients and their families is essential.[61,149] Finally, involvement of the dominant hemisphere by the disease process provides important observations on brain plasticity, especially on the shift of language.[24,33,34,36,72,92,138,139,152] Recent reports looking at language outcomes after long-term RE, serial Amytal tests, functional MRI studies, and hemispherectomy illustrate the great plasticity of the child's brain and the ability of the nondominant hemisphere to take over some language function even at a relatively late age.

LONG-TERM PROGNOSIS

Progression is characteristic of the disease, although there is some variability in the rate of advance. The advent of immunomodulating therapy has most likely been the reason for lesser tissue loss and atrophy, which leads to maintained motor function. This makes surgical decision difficult. Following hemispherectomy, residual minor seizures, usually involving the face, may persist. Bilateral involvement by the original disease process has been described, mainly in children with early onset. There is, however, no good evidence for eventual contralateral spread over time in most patients. Secondary epileptogenesis without evidence for bilateral disease may occur, and personal observations suggest that this is more likely to happen in children in whom surgical treatment was delayed.

SUMMARY AND CONCLUSIONS

Rasmussen's encephalitis, although a rare disorder, is now much better delineated and understood by both the wider clinical and scientific community. However, recognition of the disease in a naïve patient to make an early diagnosis continues to be a challenge. Although confirmation of the clinical diagnosis of RE rests on pathologic findings, in vivo combinations of diagnostic approaches such as clinical course, scalp EEG findings, and high-resolution repeated MRI suggest the diagnosis with a high degree of accuracy. The syndrome also appears more clinically heterogeneous than initially thought: More localized, protracted, or slowly progressive forms of the disease have now been described, suggesting that distinct pathophysiologic mechanisms may be at play. The different patterns of evolution of the disease observed in children compared to older individuals are probably explained by a higher vulnerability of the developing brain to insults (persistent inflammatory mechanisms and recurrent seizures). Evidence implicating immune responses in the pathophysiology of RE has accumulated involving both B- and T-cell–mediated processes, but the mechanisms by which the immune system is activated remain to be elucidated. The identification of autoantigens provides evidence that RE may be associated with an immune attack on synaptic antigens and impaired synaptic function leading to seizures and cell death. In addition, T-cell–mediated cytotoxicity may lead to neuronal damage and apoptotic death. Identification of the initiating event (possibly the antigen that triggered the autoimmune response) and of the sequence of immune reactivities occurring in the course of the disease will hopefully allow timely and more specific immunotherapy. While pursuit of novel and less toxic immune strategies (such as B-cell depletion with rituximab) remains appealing, at present patients with RE usually present with rapid progression, and questions on the type and timing of surgical intervention are still being raised. It seems clear that most will fare better with earlier surgery, and only hemispherectomy techniques can provide definitive and satisfactory results with good seizure, cognitive, and psychosocial outcome.

References

1. Aguilar MJ, Rasmussen T. Role of encephalitis in pathogenesis of epilepsy. *AMA Arch Neurol.* 1960;2:633–676.
2. Aguilar RF, Rojas BJC, Villanueva PR, et al. SPECT-99mTc-HMPAO en un caso de epilepsia parcial continua y encefalitis focal. *Rev Invest Clin* 1996;48:199–205.
3. Andrews PI, Ditcher MA, Berkovic SF, et al. Plasmapheresis in Rasmussen's encephalitis. *Neurology.* 1996;46:242–246.
4. Andrews PI, McNamara JO, Lewis DV. Clinical and electroencephalographic correlates in Rasmussen's encephalitis. *Epilepsia.* 1997;38:189–194.
5. Antel JP, Rasmussen T. Rasmussen's encephalitis and the new hat. *Neurology.* 1996;46:9–11.
6. Antozzi C, Granata T, Aurisano N, et al. Long-term selective IgG immunoadsorption improves Rasmussen's encephalitis. *Neurology.* 1998;51:302–305.
7. Asher DM, Gadjusek DC. Virologic studies in chronic encephalitis. In: Andermann F, ed. *Encephalitis and Epilepsy: Rasmussen's Syndrome.* Stoneham: Butterworth-Heinneman; 1991:147–158.
8. Atkins MR, Terrell W, Hulette CM. Rasmussen's syndrome: a study of potential viral etiology. *Clin Neuropathol.* 1995;14:7–12.
9. Banati RB, Goerres GW, Myers R, et al. [^{11}C]*(R)*-PK11195 positron emission tomography imaging of activated microglia in vivo in Rasmussen's encephalitis. *Neurology.* 1999;53:2199–2203.
10. Bancaud J, Bonis A, Trottier S, et al. L'épilepsie partielle continue: syndrome et maladie. *Rev Neurol.* 1982;138:803–814.
11. Bancaud J. Kojewnikow's syndrome (epilepsia partialis continua) in children. In: Roger J, Dravet C, Bureau M, et al., eds. *Epileptic Syndromes in Infancy, Childhood and Adolescence.* 2nd ed. London: John Libbey Eurotext; 1992:363–379.
12. Baranzini SE, Laxer K, Saketkhoo R, et al. Analysis of antibody gene rearrangement, usage, and specificity in chronic focal encephalitis. *Neurology.* 2002;58:709–716.
13. Bauer J, Bien CG, Lassmann H. Rasmussen's encephalitis: a role for autoimmune cytotoxic T lymphocytes. *Curr Opin Neurol.* 2002;15:197–200.
14. Beaumanoir A, Grioni D, Kullman G, et al. Anomalies EEG dans la phase prémonitoire du syndrome de Rasmussen. À propos de deux observations. *Neurophysiol Clin.* 1997;27:25–32.
15. Ben-Zeev B, Nass D, Polack S, et al. Progressive unilateral basal ganglia atrophy and hemidystonia: a new form of chronic focal encephalitis. *Neurology.* 1999;S2:A42.
16. Bhatjiwale MG, Polkey C, Cox TCS, et al. Rasmussen's encephalitis: neuroimaging findings in 21 patients with a closer look at the basal ganglia. *Pediatr Neurosurg.* 1998;29:142–148.
17. Bien CG, Bauer J. Neuromolecular medicine, T-cells in human encephalitis. *Neuromolecular Med.* 2005;7(3):243–253.
18. Bien CG, Bauer J, Deckwerth TL, et al. Destruction of neurons by cytotoxic T cells: a new pathogenic mechanism in Rasmussen's encephalitis. *Ann Neurol.* 2002;51:311–318.
19. Bien CG, Elger CE, Wiendl H. Advances in pathogenic concepts and therapeutic agents in Rasmussen's encephalitis. *Expert Opin Investig Drugs.* 2002;11:981–989.
20. Bien CG, Gleissner U, Sassen R, et al. An open study of tacrolimus therapy in Rasmussen's encephalitis. *Neurology.* 2004;62:2106–2109.
21. Bien CG, Granata T, Antozzi C, et al. Pathogenesis, diagnosis and treatment of Rasmussen encephalitis: a European consensus statement. *Brain.* 2005;128:454–471.
22. Bien CG, Urbach H, Deckert M, et al. Diagnosis and staging of Rasmussen's encephalitis by serial MRI and histopathology. *Neurology.* 2003;58:250–257.
23. Bien CG, Widman G, Urbach H, et al. The natural history of Rasmussen's encephalitis. *Brain.* 2002;125:1751–1759.
24. Boatman D, Freeman J, Vining E, et al. Language recovery after left hemispherectomy in children with late-onset seizures. *Ann Neurol.* 1999;46:579–586.
25. Burke GJ, Fifer SA, Yoder J. Early detection of Rasmussen's syndrome by brain SPECT imaging. *Clin Nucl Med.* 1992;17:730–731.
26. Campovilla G, Paladin F, Dalla et al. Rasmussen's syndrome: longitudinal EEG study from the first seizure to epilepsia partialis continua. *Epilepsia.* 1997;38:483–488.
27. Caraballo R, Tenembaum S, Cersosimo R, et al. Sindrome de Rasmussen. *Rev Neurol.* 1998;26:978–983.
28. Carney PR. Rasmussen syndrome: intractable epilepsy and progressive neurological deterioration from a unilateral central nervous system disease. *CNS Spectr.* 2001;6:398–416.
29. Cendes F, Andermann F, Silver K, et al. Imaging of axonal damage in vivo in Rasmussen's syndrome. *Brain.* 1995;118:753–758.
30. Chiapparini L, Granata T, Farina L, et al. Diagnostic imaging in 13 cases of Rasmussen's encephalitis: can early MRI suggest the diagnosis. *Neuroradiology.* 2003;45:171–183.
31. Chinchilla D, Dulac O, Robain O, et al. Reappraisal of Rasmussen's syndrome with special emphasis on treatment with high dose of steroids. *J Neurol Neurosurg Psychiatry.* 1994;57:1325–1333.
32. Coral LC, Haas LJ. Provável síndrome de Rasmussen. Relato de caso. *Arq Neuropsiquiatr.* 1999;54:1032–1035.
33. Curtiss S, de Bode S, Mathern GW. Spoken language outcomes after hemispherectomy: factoring in etiology. *Brain Lang.* 2001;79:379–396.
34. Curtiss S, de Bode S. Age and etiology as predictors of language outcome following hemispherectomy. *Dev Neurosci.* 1999;21:174–181.
35. Dabbagh O, Gascon G, Crowell J, et al. Intraventricular interferon-α stops seizures in Rasmussen's encephalitis: a case report. *Epilepsia.* 1997;38:1045–1049.
36. de Bode S, Firestine A, Mathern GW, et al. Residual motor control and cortical representations of function following hemispherectomy: effects of etiology. *J Child Neurol.* 2005;20:64–75.
37. De Toledo JC, Smith DB. Partially successful treatment of Rasmussen's encephalitis with zidovudine: symptomatic improvement followed by involvement of the contralateral hemisphere. *Epilepsia.* 1994;35:352–355.
38. DeLalande O, Pinard JM, Jalin O, et al. Surgical results of hemispherotomy. *Epilepsia.* 1995;36(Suppl 3):241.
39. Dubeau F, Sherwin A. Pharmacologic principles in the management of chronic focal encephalitis. In: Andermann F, ed. *Encephalitis and Epilepsy: Rasmussen's Syndrome.* Stoneham: Butterworth-Heinneman; 1991:179–192.
40. Dulac O, Dravet C, Plouin P, et al. Aspect nosologique des épilepsies partielles continues chez l'enfant. *Arch F Pediatr.* 1983;40:689–695.
41. Duprez TPJ, Grandin C, Gadisseux JF, et al. MR-Monitored remitting-relapsing pattern of cortical involvement in Rasmussen syndrome: comparative evaluation of serial MR and PET/SPECT features. *J Comput Assist Tomogr.* 1997;21:900–904.
42. English R, Soper N, Shepstone BJ, et al. Five patients with Rasmussen's syndrome investigated by single-photon-emission computed tomography. *Nucl Med Comm.* 1989;10:5–14.

43. Farrell MA, Cheng L, Cornford ME, et al. Cytomegalovirus and Rasmussen's encephalitis. *Lancet.* 1991;337:1551–1552.
44. Farrell MA, Droogan O, Secor DL, et al. Chronic encephalitis associated with epilepsy: immunohistochemical and ultrastructural studies. *Acta Neuropathol Berl.* 1995;89:313–321.
45. Fiorella DJ, Provenzale JM, Coleman RE, et al. ^{18}F-fluorodeoxyglucose positron emission tomography and MR imaging findings in Rasmussen encephalitis. *AJNR Am J Neuroradiol.* 2001;22:1291–1299.
46. Firlik KS, Adelson PD, Hamilton RL. Coexistence of a ganglioglioma and Rasmussen's encephalitis. *Pediatr Neurosurg.* 1999;30:278–282.
47. Fogarasi A, Heguy M, Neuwirth M, et al. Comparative evaluation of concomitant structural and functional neuroimages in Rasmussen's encephalitis. *J Neuroimaging.* 2003;13:339–345.
48. Freeman JM. Rasmussen's syndrome: progressive autoimmune multifocal encephalopathy. *Pediatr Neurol.* 2005;32:295–299.
49. Friedman H, Ch'ien L, Parham D. Virus in brain of child with hemiplegia, hemiconvulsions, and epilepsy. *Lancet.* 1977;ii:666.
50. Frucht S. Dystonia, athetosis, and epilepsia partialis continua in a patient with late-onset Rasmussen's encephalitis. *Mov Disord.* 2002;17:609–612.
51. Frucht SJ, Louis ED, Chuang C, et al. A pilot tolerability and efficacy study of levetiracetam in patients with chronic myoclonus. *Neurology.* 2001;57:1112–1114.
52. Fukuda T, Oguni H, Yanagaki S, et al. Chronic localized encephalitis (Rasmussen's syndrome) preceded by ipsilateral uveitis: a case report. *Epilepsia.* 1994;35:1328–1331.
53. Gahring LC, Carlson NG, Meyer EL, et al. Cutting edge: granzyme B proteolysis of a neuronal glutamate receptor generates an autoantigen and is modulated by glycolysation. *J Immunol.* 2001;166:1433–1438.
54. Ganor Y, Freilinger M, Dulac O, et al. Monozygotic twins discordant for epilepsy differ in the levels of potentially pathogenic autoantibodies and cytokines. *Autoimmunity.* 2005;38:139–150.
55. Geller E, Faerber EN, Legido A, et al. Rasmussen encephalitis: complementary role of multitechnique neuroimaging. *AJNR Am J Neuroradiol.* 1998;19:445–449.
56. Genton P, Gelisse P. Antimyoclonic effect of levetiracetam. *Epileptic Disord.* 2000;2:209–212.
57. Granata T, Fusco L, Gobbi G, et al. Experience with immunomodulatory treatments in Rasmussen's encephalitis. *Neurology.* 2003;61: 1807–1810.
58. Granata T, Gobbi G, Spreafico R, et al. Rasmussen's encephalitis. Early characteristics allow diagnosis. *Neurology.* 2003;60:422–425.
59. Gray F, Serdaru M, Baron H, et al. Chronic localised encephalitis (Rasmussen's) in an adult with epilepsia partialis continua. *J Neurol Neurosurg Psychiatry.* 1987;50:747–751.
60. Grenier Y, Antel JP, Osterland CK. Immunologic studies in chronic encephalitis of Rasmussen. In: Andermann F, ed. *Encephalitis and Epilepsy: Rasmussen's Syndrome.* Stoneham: Butterworth-Heinneman; 1991:125–134.
61. Guimarães CA, Souza EAP, Montenegro MA, et al. Rasmussen's encephalitis. The relevance of neuropsychological assessment in patient's treatment and follow up. *Arq Neuropsiquiatr.* 2002;60:378–381.
62. Gupta PC, Rapin I, Houroupian DS, et al. Smoldering encephalitis in children. *Neuropediatrics.* 1984;15:191–197.
63. Gupta PC, Roy S, Tandon PN. Progressive epilepsy due to chronic persistent encephalitis. Report of 4 cases. *J Neurol Sci.* 1974;22:105–120.
64. Hajek M, Antonini A, Leenders KL, et al. Epilepsia partialis continua studied by PET. *Epilepsy Res.* 1991;9:44–48.
65. Hart Y, Andermann F, Robitaille Y, et al. Double pathology in Rasmussen's syndrome: a window on the etiology? *Neurology.* 1998;50:731–735.
66. Hart YM, Andermann F, Fish DR, et al. Chronic encephalitis and epilepsy in adults and adolescents: a variant of Rasmussen's syndrome? *Neurology.* 1997;48:418–424.
67. Hart YM, Cortez M, Andermann F, et al. Medical treatment of Rasmussen's syndrome (chronic encephalitis and epilepsy): effect of high-dose steroids or immunoglobulins in 19 patients. *Neurology.* 1994;44:1030–1036.
68. Hartley LM, Harkness W, Harding B, et al. Correlation of SPECT with pathology and seizure outcome in children undergoing epilepsy surgery. *Dev Med Child Neurol.* 2002;44:676–680.
69. Harvey AS, Andermann F, Hopkins IJ, et al. Chronic encephalitis (Rasmussen's syndrome) and ipsilateral uveitis. *Ann Neurol.* 1992;32: 826–829.
70. He XP, Patel M, Whitney KD, et al. Glutamate receptor GluR3 antibodies and death of cortical cells. *Neuron.* 1998;20:153–163.
71. Hennessy MJ, Koutroumanidis M, Dean AF, et al. Chronic encephalitis and temporal lobe epilepsy: a variant of Rasmussen's syndrome? *Neurology.* 2001;56:678–681.
72. Hertz-Pannier L, Chiron C, Jambaqué I, et al. Late plasticity for language in a child's non-dominant hemisphere. A pre- and post-surgery fMRI study. *Brain.* 2002;125:361–372.
73. Honavar M, Janota I, Polkey CE. Rasmussen's encephalitis in surgery for epilepsy. *Dev Med Child Neurol.* 1992;34:3–14.
74. Hwang PA, Gilday DL, Spire JP, et al. Chronic focal encephalitis of Rasmussen: functional neuroimaging studies with positron emission tomography and single-photon emission computed tomography scanning. In: Andermann F, ed. *Encephalitis and Epilepsy: Rasmussen's Syndrome.* Stoneham: Butterworth-Heinneman; 1991:61–72.
75. Hwang PA, Piatt J, Cyr L, et al. The EEG of Rasmussen's encephalitis. *Electr Clin Neurophysiol.* 1988;69:51P–52P.
76. Ishibashi H, Simos PG, Wheless JW, et al. Multimodality functional imaging evaluation in a patient with Rasmussen's encephalitis. *Brain Dev.* 2002;24:239–244.
77. Jay V, Becker LE, Otsubo H, et al. Chronic encephalitis and epilepsy (Rasmussen's encephalitis): detection of cytomegalovirus and herpes simplex virus 1 by the polymerase chain reaction and in situ hybridization. *Neurology.* 1995;45:108–117.
78. Kaiboriboon K, Cortese C, Hogan RE. Magnetic resonance and positron emission tomography changes during the clinical progression of Rasmussen encephalitis. *J Neuroimaging.* 2000;10:122–125.
79. Koehn MA, Zupanc ML. Unusual presentation and MRI findings in Rasmussen's syndrome. *Pediatr Neurol.* 1999;21:839–842.
80. Korn-Lubetzski I, Bien CG, Bauer J, et al. Rasmussen encephalitis with active inflammation and delayed seizures onset. *Neurology.* 2004;62:984–986.
81. Kossoff EH, Vining EPG, Pillas DJ, et al. Hemispherectomy for intractable unihemispheric epilepsy. Etiology and outcome. *Neurology.* 2003;61:887–890.
82. Krauss GL, Campbell ML, Roche KW, et al. Chronic steroid-responsive encephalitis without autoantibodies to glutamate receptor GluR3. *Neurology.* 1996;46:247–249.
83. Kumar R, Wani AA, Reddy J, et al. Development of anaplastic ependymoma in Rasmussen's encephalitis: review of the literature and case report. *Childs Ner Syst.* 2006 Apr;22(4):416–419.
84. Lagrange AH, Blaivas M, Gomez-Hassan D, et al. Rasmussen's syndrome and new-onset narcolepsy, cataplexy, and epilepsy in an adult. *Epilepsy Behav.* 2003;4:788–792.
85. Larionov S, König R, Urbach H, et al. MRI brain volumetry in Rasmussen encephalitis: the fate of affected and "unaffected" hemispheres. *Neurology.* 2005;64:885–887.
86. Larner AJ, Smith SJ, Duncan JS, et al. Late-onset Rasmussen's syndrome with first seizure during pregnancy. *Eur Neurol.* 1995;35:172.
87. Lascelles K, Dean AF, Robinson RO. Rasmussen's encephalitis followed by lupus erythematous. *Dev Med Child Neurol.* 2002;44:572–574.
88. Laxer KD. Temporal lobe epilepsy with inflammatory changes. In: Andermann F, ed. *Encephalitis and Epilepsy: Rasmussen's Syndrome.* Stoneham: Butterworth-Heinneman; 1991:135–140.
89. Leach JP, Chadwick DW, Miles JB, et al. Improvement in adult onset Rasmussen's encephalitis with long-term immunomodulatory therapy. *Neurology.* 1999;52:738–742.
90. Levite M, Fleidervish IA, Schwarz A, et al. Autoantibodies to the glutamate receptor kill neurons via activation of the receptor ion channel. *J Autoimmun.* 1999;13:61–72.
91. Li Y, Uccelli A, Laxer KD, et al. Local-clonal expansion of infiltrating T lymphocytes in chronic encephalitis of Rasmussen. *J Immunol.* 1997;158:1428–1437.
92. Loddenkemper T, Wyllie E, Lardizabal D, et al. Late language transfer in patients with Rasmussen encephalitis. *Epilepsia.* 2003;44:870–871.
93. Lyon G, Griscelli C, Fernandez-Alvarez E, et al. Chronic progressive encephalitis in children with X-linked hypogammaglobulinemia. *Neuropaediatrie.* 1980;11:57–71.
94. Maeda Y, Oguni H, Saitou Y, et al. Rasmussen syndrome: multifocal spread of inflammation suggested from MRI and PET findings. *Epilepsia.* 2003;44:1118–1121.
95. Mantegazza R, Bernasconi P, Baggi F, et al. Antibodies against GluR3 peptides are not specific for Rasmussen's encephalitis but are also present in epilepsy patients with severe, early onset disease and intractable seizures. *J Neuroimmnunol.* 2002;131:179–185.
96. Maria BL, Ringdahl DM, Mickle JP, et al. Intraventricular alpha interferon therapy for Rasmussen's syndrome. *Can J Neurol Sci.* 1993;20:333–336.
97. Matthews PM, Andermann F, Arnold DL. A proton magnetic resonance spectroscopy study of focal epilepsy in humans. *Neurology.* 1990;40:985–989.
98. McDonald D, Farrell MA, McMenamin J. Rasmussen's syndrome associated with chronic brain stem encephalitis. *Eur J Paediatr Neurol.* 2001;5:203–206.
99. McLachlan RS, Girvin JP, Blume WT, et al. Rasmussen's chronic encephalitis in adults. *Arch Neurol.* 1993;50:269–274.
100. McLachlan RS, Levin S, Blume WT. Treatment of Rasmussen's syndrome with gancyclovir. *Neurology.* 1996;47:925–928.
101. Mizuno Y, Chou SM, Estes ML, et al. Chronic localized encephalitis (Rasmussen's) with focal cerebral seizures revisited. *J Neuropathol Exp Neurol.* 1985;44:351.
102. Morrell F, Whisler WW, Cremin Smith M. Multiple subpial transection in Rasmussen's encephalitis. In: Andermann F, ed. *Encephalitis and Epilepsy: Rasmussen's Syndrome.* Stoneham: Butterworth-Heinneman; 1991:219–234.
103. Moshé SL. Mechanisms of action of anticonvulsant agents. *Neurology.* 2000;55(Suppl 1):S32–S40.
104. Mourelatos Z, McGarvey M, French JA, et al. 27-year-old female with epilepsy. *Brain Pathol.* 2003;13:233–234.
105. Nakasu S, Isozumi T, Yamamoto A, et al. Serial magnetic resonance imaging findings of Rasmussen's encephalitis. *Neurol Med Chir.* 1997;37: 924–928.

106. Oguni H, Andermann F, Rasmussen T. The natural history of the syndrome of chronic encephalitis and epilepsy: a study of the MNI series of forty-eight cases. In: Andermann F, ed. *Encephalitis and Epilepsy: Rasmussen's Syndrome*. Stoneham: Butterworth-Heinneman; 1991:7–35.
107. Olivier A. Corticectomy for the treatment of seizures due to chronic encephalitis. In: Andermann F, ed. *Encephalitis and Epilepsy: Rasmussen's Syndrome*. Stoneham: Butterworth-Heinneman; 1991:205–212.
108. Paladin F, Capovilla G, Bonazza A, et al. Utility of Tc 99m HMPAO SPECT in the early diagnosis of Rasmussen's syndrome. *Ital J Neurol Sci*. 1998;19:217–220.
109. Palcoux JB, Carla H, Tardieu M, et al. Plasma exchange in Rasmussen's encephalitis. *Ther Apher*. 1997;1:79–82.
110. Palmer CA, Geyer JD, Keating JM, et al. Rasmussen's encephalitis with concomitant cortical dysplasia: the role of GluR3. *Epilepsia*. 1999;40:242–247.
111. Pardo CA, Vining EP, Guo L, et al. The pathology of Rasmussen syndrome: stages of cortical involvement and neuropathological studies in 45 hemispherectomies. *Epilepsia*. 2004;45:516–526.
112. Park YD, Allison JD, Weiss KL, et al. Proton magnetic resonance spectroscopic observations of epilepsia partialis continua in children. *J Child Neurol*. 2000;15:729–733.
113. Peeling J, Sutherland G. 1H magnetic resonance spectroscopy of extracts of human epileptic neocortex and hippocampus. *Neurology*. 1993;43:589–594.
114. Piatt JH Jr, Hwang PA, Armstrong DC, et al. Chronic focal encephalitis (Rasmussen syndrome): six cases. *Epilepsia*. 1988;29:268–279.
115. Power C, Poland SD, Blume WT, et al. Cytomegalovirus and Rasmussen's encephalitis. *Lancet*. 1990;336:1282–1284.
116. Prayson RA, Frater JL. Rasmussen encephalitis. A clinicopathologic and immunohistochemical study of seven patients. *Am J Clin Pathol*. 2002;117:776–782.
117. Pulsifer MB, Brandt J, Salorio CF, et al. The cognitive outcome of hemispherectomy in 71 children. *Epilepsia*. 2004;45:243–254.
118. Pupillo G, Andermann F, Dubeau F. Linear scleroderma and intractable epilepsy: neuropathologic evidence for a chronic inflammatory process. *Ann Neurol*. 1996;39:277–278.
119. Rasmussen T, Olszewski J, Lloyd-Smith D. Focal seizures due to chronic localized encephalitis. *Neurology*. 1958;8:435–445.
120. Rasmussen T. Chronic encephalitis and seizures: historical introduction. In: Andermann F, ed. *Encephalitis and Epilepsy: Rasmussen's Syndrome*. Stoneham: Butterworth-Heinneman; 1991:1–4.
121. Riikonen R. Cytomegalovirus infection and infantile spasms. *Dev Med Child Neurol*. 1978;20:570–579.
122. Robitaille Y. Neuropathological aspects of chronic encephalitis. In: Andermann F, ed. *Encephalitis and Epilepsy: Rasmussen's Syndrome*. Stoneham: Butterworth-Heinneman; 1991:79–110.
123. Rogers SW, Andrews PI, Garhing LC, et al. Autoantibodies to glutamate receptor GluR3 in Rasmussen's encephalitis. *Science*. 1994;265:648–651.
124. Sammaritano M, Andermann F, Melanson D, et al. Prolonged focal cerebral edema associated with partial status epilepticus. *Epilepsia*. 1985;26:334–339.
125. Sener RN. Diffusion and spectroscopy in Rasmussen's encephalitis. *Eur Radiol*. 2003;13:2186–2191.
126. Sener RN. Rasmussen's encephalitis: proton MR spectroscopy and diffusion MR findings. *J Neuroradiol*. 2000;27:179–184.
127. Shah JR, Juhasz C, Kupsky WJ, et al. Rasmussen encephalitis associated with Parry-Romberg syndrome. *Neurology*. 2003;61:395–397.
128. Silver K, Andermann F, Meagher-Villemure K. Familial alternating epilepsia partialis continua with chronic encephalitis: another variant of Rasmussen syndrome? *Arch Neurol*. 1998;55:733–736.
129. So NK, Gloor P. Electroencephalographic and electrocorticographic findings in chronic encephalitis of the Rasmussen type. In: Andermann F, ed. *Encephalitis and Epilepsy: Rasmussen's Syndrome*. Stoneham: Butterworth-Heinneman; 1991:37–45.
130. Spencer SS, Spencer DD. Corpus callosotomy in chronic encephalitis. In: Andermann F, ed. *Encephalitis and Epilepsy: Rasmussen's Syndrome*. Stoneham: Butterworth-Heinneman; 1991:213–218.
131. Stephen LJ, Brodie MJ. An islander with seizures. *Scott Med J*. 1998; 43:183–184.
132. Stone J, Franks AJ, Guthrie JA, et al. Scleroderma 'en coup de sabre': pathological evidence of intracerebral inflammation. *J Neurol Neurosurg Psychiatry*. 2001;70:382–385.
133. Straube A, Padovan CS, Seelos K. Parry-Romberg syndrome and Rasmussen syndrome: only an incidental similarity? *Nervenarzt*. 2001;72:641–646.
134. Sundgren PC, Burtsher IM, Lundgren J, et al. MRI and proton spectroscopy in a child with Rasmussen's encephalitis. Case report. *Neuroradiology*. 1999;41:935–940.
135. Takahashi Y, Kubota H, Fujiwara T, et al. Epilepsia partialis continua of childhood involving bilateral brain hemispheres. *Act Neurol Scand*. 1997;96:345–352.
136. Takahashi Y, Mori H, Mishina M, et al. Autoantibodies to NMDA receptor in patients with chronic forms of epilepsia partialis continua. *Neurology*. 2003;61:891–896.
137. Tampieri D, Melanson D, Ethier R. Imaging of chronic encephalitis. In: Andermann F, ed. *Encephalitis and Epilepsy: Rasmussen's Syndrome*. Stoneham: Butterworth-Heinneman; 1991:47–69.
138. Taylor LB. Neuropsychological assessment of patients with chronic encephalitis. In: Andermann F, ed. *Encephalitis and Epilepsy: Rasmussen's Syndrome*. Stoneham: Butterworth-Heinneman; 1991:111–124.
139. Telfeian AE, Berqvist C, Danielak C, et al. Recovery of language after left hemispherectomy in a sixteen-year-old girl with late-onset seizures. *Pediatr Neurosurg*. 2002;37:19–21.
140. Tien RD, Ashdown BC, Lewis DV Jr, et al. Rasmussen's encephalitis: neuroimaging findings in four patients. *AJR Am J Roentgenol*. 1992;158:1329–1332.
141. Tobias SM, Robitaille Y, Hickey WF, et al. Bilateral Rasmussen encephalitis: postmortem documentation in a five-year-old. *Epilepsia*. 2003;44:127–130.
142. Topçu M, Turanli G, Aynaci FM, et al. Rasmussen encephalitis in childhood. *Childs Nerv Syst*. 1999;15:395–402.
143. Tubbs RS, Nimje SM, Oakes WJ. Long-term follow-up in children with functional hemispherectomy for Rasmussen's encephalitis. *Childs Nerv Syst*. 2005;21:461–465.
144. Tükdogan-Sözüer D, Özek MM, Sav A, et al. Serial MRI and MRS studies with unusual findings in Rasmussen's encephalitis. *Eur Radiol*. 2000;10:962–966.
145. Twyman RE, Gahring LC, Spiess J, et al. Glutamate receptor antibodies activate a subset of receptors and reveal an agonist binding site. *Neuron*. 1995;14:755–762.
146. Valdamudi L, Galton CJ, Jeavons SJ, et al. Rasmussen's syndrome in a 54 year old female: more support for an adult variant. *J Clin Neuroscience*. 2000;7:154–156.
147. Villani F, Spreafico R, Farina L, et al. Immunomodulatory therapy in an adult patient with Rasmussen's encephalitis. *Neurology*. 2001;56:248–250.
148. Villemure JG, Andermann F, Rasmussen TB. Hemispherectomy for the treatment of epilepsy due to chronic encephalitis. In: Andermann F, ed. *Encephalitis and Epilepsy: Rasmussen's Syndrome*. Stoneham: Butterworth-Heinneman; 1991:235–244.
149. Vining EP, Freeman JM, Brandt J, et al. Progressive unilateral encephalopathy of childhood (Rasmussen's syndrome): a reappraisal. *Epilepsia*. 1993;34:639–650.
150. Vinjamuri S, Leach JP, Hart IK. Serial perfusion brain tomographic scans detect reversible focal ischemia in Rasmussen's encephalitis. *Postgrad Med J*. 2000;76:33–40.
151. Vinters HV, Wang R, Wiley CA. Herpesviruses in chronic encephalitis associated with intractable childhood epilepsy. *Hum Pathol*. 1993;24:871–879.
152. Voets NL, Adcock JE, Flitney DE, et al. Distinct right frontal lobe activation in language processing following left hemisphere injury. *Brain*. 2006;129:754–766.
153. Walsh PJ. Treatment of Rasmussen's syndrome with intravenous gammaglobulin. In: Andermann F, ed. *Encephalitis and Epilepsy: Rasmussen's Syndrome*. Stoneham: Butterworth-Heinneman; 1991:201–204.
154. Walter GF, Renella RR. Epstein-Barr virus in brain and Rasmussen's encephalitis. *Lancet*. 1989;i:279–280.
155. Watson R, Jiang Y, Bermudez I, et al. Absence of antibodies to glutamate receptor type 3 (GluR3) in Rasmussen's encephalitis. *Neurology*. 2004;63:43–50.
156. Watson R, Lang B, Bermudez I, et al. Autoantibodies in Rasmussen's encephalitis. *J Neuroimmunol*. 2001;118:148.
157. Wennberg R, Nag S, McAndrews MP, et al. Chronic (Rasmussen') encephalitis in an adult. *Can J Neurol Sci*. 2003;30:263–265.
158. Whitney KD, Andrews JM, McNamara JO. Immunoglobulin G and complement immunoreactivity in the cerebral cortex of patients with Rasmussen's encephalitis. *Neurology*. 1999;53:699–708.
159. Wiendl H, Bien CG, Bernasconi P, et al. GluR3 antibodies: prevalence in focal epilepsy but no specificity for Rasmussen's encephalitis. *Neurology*. 2001;57:1511–1514.
160. Wise MS, Rutledge SL, Kuzniecky RI. Rasmussen syndrome and long-term response to gamma globulin. *Pediatr Neurol*. 1996;14:149–152.
161. Yacubian EMT, Rosemberg S, Marie SKN, et al. Double pathology in Rasmussen's encephalitis: etiological considerations. *Epilepsia*. 1996;37:495–500.
162. Yacubian EMT, Sueli KNM, Valério RMF, et al. Neuroimaging findings in Rasmussen's syndrome. *J Neuroimag*. 1997;7:16–22.
163. Yang R, Puranam RS, Butler LS, et al. Autoimmunity to munc-18 in Rasmussen's encephalitis. *Neuron*. 2000;28:375–383.
164. Yeh PS, Lin CN, Lin HJ, et al. Chronic focal encephalitis (Rasmussen's syndrome) in an adult. *J Formos Med Assoc*. 2000;99:568–571.
165. Zupanc ML, Handler EG, Levine RL, et al. Rasmussen encephalitis: epilepsia partialis continua secondary to chronic encephalitis. *Pediatr Neurol*. 1990;6:397–401.

CHAPTER 244 ■ JUVENILE MYOCLONIC EPILEPSY

ELIANE KOBAYASHI, BENJAMIN G. ZIFKIN, FREDERICK ANDERMANN, AND EVA ANDERMANN

INTRODUCTION

Juvenile myoclonic epilepsy (JME) is a common type of idiopathic generalized epilepsy (IGE). The major landmark of JME is the occurrence of adolescent-onset myoclonic seizures. JME is both genetically and clinically heterogeneous, suggesting that different pathophysiologic mechanisms might be involved.[84]

HISTORICAL PERSPECTIVES

The first description of a patient with JME came from the French literature in 1867 by Herpin,[38] but the myoclonic jerks were only properly characterized in 1899 by Rabot.[63] The intermittent character of these jerks as compared to the myoclonus occurring in progressive myoclonic epilepsy, a neurodegenerative disease, was emphasized by Lundborg[47] in 1903.

The description of JME as a specific IGE syndrome was established almost at the same time by Janz and Christian in Germany[42] and by Castells and Mendilaharsu in Uruguay,[16] almost a century after the first patient was reported in the literature. However, because of varying terminologies employed by previous authors, the syndrome was only recognized as JME in the English-speaking literature in the mid-1980s.[5,22]

DEFINITIONS

JME is the most common form of IGE, and the myoclonic seizures are the hallmark of the syndrome. Isolated myoclonic jerks of the arms, especially shortly after awakening, are characteristic. Generalized tonic–clonic seizures (GTCSs) occur in most patients, and one third of individuals also have absences. Seizure occurrence is more likely with sleep deprivation, fatigue, and alcohol withdrawal. Onset is usually in adolescence but seizures may begin or be diagnosed only in the early 20s. Patients frequently come to medical attention only after a generalized convulsion, and the history of earlier myoclonic jerks is often obtained retrospectively. More recently, myoclonic epilepsy with adult onset (37 to 39 years) has been highlighted by different groups.[20,30,49]

EPIDEMIOLOGY

Prevalence

JME accounts for up to 26% of patients with IGE and up to 10% of all cases of epilepsy,[43] but misdiagnosis and delayed diagnosis remain common.[34]

Based on a 1% population risk for epilepsy by age 20,[36] the Risk of JME in the general population would be 1 per 1,000 to 2,000. It is less frequently seen in children and more frequently in adolescents and adults.[43] In adults with IGE, JME should be strongly considered, and detailed inquiries regarding a history of myoclonus beginning in the teens are essential.

Sex Ratio

Although an equal sex ratio is generally assumed in JME, there is a slight female predominance, with 515 males to 615 females, based on the summation of ten different studies.[43] Only one of the studies showed male preponderance (33 males to 20 females),[22] whereas another study showed marked female preponderance (77 males to 104 females).[24] A recent Irish study also showed significant female predominance for JME.[55] A large family study has also confirmed a very high female-to-male risk ratio.[59]

Age of Onset

The onset of JME is clearly age related. It varies between 8 and 26 years, with the majority between 12 and 18 years.[43] The average age of onset of myoclonic jerks is usually earlier than that of generalized tonic–clonic seizures.[24] The onset age of JME is generally earlier in photosensitive than in nonphotosensitive patients.[70,83]

ETIOLOGY AND BASIC MECHANISMS

The pathophysiology of JME is unknown. Although clinically a well-defined syndrome, detailed investigations of JME suggest that this stereotyped clinical pattern may be the result of different genetic, pathologic, and pathophysiologic processes.[5a,84]

The electroencephalographic (EEG) pattern and other neurophysiologic studies, including those conducted in patients with reflex seizures induced by thinking, writing, or "action programming," suggest a variable focal or regional frontal hyperexcitability in many cases.[84] Even so, although subtle frontal morphologic changes can be found, they are not universal in JME, and neither is sensitivity to various cognitive triggers, which may be absent in a typical case or present in a patient with another IGE syndrome. The association with photosensitivity is also variable.

An association with clinical and EEG findings of a clearly focal epilepsy, namely, idiopathic photosensitive occipital epilepsy (IPOE, described below), also raises questions about the nosologic purity of JME as a generalized epilepsy syndrome.

The classic electrophysiological studies conducted by Gloor[31] led to the corticoreticular theory of generalized epilepsy: This theory postulates an underlying cortical hyperexcitability and abnormal response to thalamocortical input, which would operate in the absence of any lesional substrate. Genetic animal models of generalized epilepsy confirm the role played by thalamocortical circuits in cortical spike-wave generation, and it has been proposed that genetically determined dysfunction of reticular thalamic neurons is responsible for the abnormal excitation. Since then, evidence has also been accumulating suggesting that subtle but probably significant neurochemical and morphologic alterations exist in both cortex and thalamus in IGE. Meencke and Janz[52] and Meencke and Veith[53] described subtle cortical neuropathologic changes in IGE ("microdysgenesis") believed to be migrational disturbances, but this has not been confirmed in other small series.[57]

Furthermore, there is much genetic heterogeneity in JME. A positive family history of epilepsy is common, and there is recent evidence that JME constitutes a single gene syndrome in some families,[19,23] although most families show complex inheritance. Some JME cases are apparently sporadic, others occur in families with other IGE syndromes, and occasional families have a pure autosomal dominant JME phenotype. However, the patients in these various groups are otherwise clinically indistinguishable by usual diagnostic criteria. Different genetic results may relate to different diagnostic criteria, including the importance given to detailed classification of EEG patterns, differing estimates of penetrance, and choice of models for linkage analysis.[9] Linkage to chromosomes 6p and 15q has been described,[25,33,46,79] and mutations in the CACNB4 gene (on chromosome 2q),[26] in the CLCN2 gene (on chromosome 3q),[21,35] in the GABRA1 gene (on chromosome 5q),[19] and in the EFHC1 gene (on chromosome 6p)[71] have been identified in JME patients.

The various mutations suggested for JME are all believed to influence neuronal excitability but involve different mechanisms. Both direct ion channel mechanisms and nonionic mechanisms have been proposed. How these interact with other possible susceptibility genes and with environmental factors is not yet clear. Vijai et al.[77] suggested that a potassium channel gene polymorphism may predispose to JME and that later gene expression of KCNQ3 may account for the striking age dependence that is typical of JME. Another potassium channel gene polymorphism in KCNJ10 has been associated with susceptibility to several common seizure types.[13] Chloride currents, which affect inhibition, are implicated in some studies. Families linked to chromosome 3q and with mutations in the ClCN2 gene, which encodes the ClC-2 voltage-dependent chloride channel, suggest a defect in γ-aminobutyric acid (GABA)-mediated inhibition. Altered GABA-mediated inhibition is also implicated in autosomal dominant JME. The GABRA1 mutation found in autosomal dominant JME encodes a mutant α_1 subunit of the $GABA_A$ receptor, but the functional effect, altered chloride current, and thus altered neuronal inhibition depend on the number of mutant subunits and their position within the pentameric structure of the ligand-gated chloride ion channel.[29]

Mutations in EFHC1 have more complex effects that may be associated with the pathogenesis of JME.[71] In animals, EFHC1 protein is not an ion channel protein but increases calcium currents in R-type voltage-dependent calcium channels and promotes calcium-related apoptosis; these effects are partly reversed by the mutations associated with JME.[71] Such mutations may thus interfere with apoptotic activity and prevent the normal elimination of neurons during postnatal development of the central nervous system in humans. This may result in increased density of neurons and formation of hyperexcitable circuits. Microdysgenesis, reported in JME, may be a visible manifestation of such a process, which may also be associated with age-dependent seizure onset. Mutations may also destabilize calcium homeostasis with resulting effects on sensitivity to sleep deprivation and other clinical triggers of seizures in JME. However, mutations in EFHC1 were found in only 6 of 44 families, and the authors suggested that unidentified mutations may exist in intronic or regulatory regions.[71] Similarly, the BRD2 gene, in which a mutation in JME was reported by Pal et al.,[60] is a putative nuclear transcription regulator and a member of a family of genes that are expressed during development and may thus be relevant to the reported abnormalities in imaging and age-related onset of JME.

CLINICAL PRESENTATION

This is an age-dependent disorder with onset usually in the second decade, but occasionally earlier and not infrequently later. It is important to recognize this group of patients since they are generally fully controlled on valproate in about 80%,[14] but require lifelong treatment.

Myoclonic seizures, mainly involving the arms and occurring preferentially in the postawakening period, are the main feature of JME and are correlated with short bursts of generalized spike-wave or polyspike-wave complexes.[22] The myoclonus is quite variable in intensity, often unreported by patients until a GTCS occurs, and then identified only after specific questioning. It is often not considered to represent a major inconvenience to patients, who frequently prefer not to take medication in order to suppress it. Others, however, prefer not to be frequently reminded of their epilepsy by these minor symptoms. When minor manifestations such as myoclonus or absence coexist with major seizures, treatment with antiepileptic drugs (AEDs) such as valproate or clonazepam is mandatory.

The myoclonus usually responds quite readily to antimyoclonic agents such as valproate, clonazepam, piracetam, or levepiracetam, but it may be difficult to control during certain periods of the patient's life. The reasons for this are not entirely clear, but loss of seizure control may be correlated with emotional factors. The generalized attacks are often precipitated by the concurrence of sleep deprivation and being woken up from sleep, and this sequence should obviously be avoided, if at all possible. Further clinical features are discussed in recent detailed reviews of JME.[75,84]

In an effort to better define syndromes for genetic study, Taylor et al.,[74] working with Berkovic and Scheffer in Australia, showed overlap between the clusters of clinical features used to diagnose JME and IPOE, suggesting a relationship with this focal epilepsy syndrome, especially with respect to visual auras and conscious head version (which are typical of IPOE) in patients with JME. They identified coexistence of myoclonic seizures and occipital EEG spikes in the same individuals in both syndromes. The probands and their families were evaluated in detail by highly skilled observers, and one may suspect that such overlap exists more commonly than is currently realized but that patients are not usually questioned as carefully.

DIAGNOSTIC EVALUATION

Although JME is considered a typical generalized epilepsy, earlier and more recent reports of clinical, EEG, and imaging studies have raised questions regarding the degree to which this classification can be strictly maintained. Clinical and EEG studies of JME and of reflex seizures in generalized epilepsies have suggested localized or regional hyperexcitability in generalized epilepsy syndromes, especially in JME.[5,15,40]

Electroencephalographic Findings

The typical abnormality on EEG is bilateral multiple spike- or polyspike-wave complexes at a rate of four to six per second, with anterior predominance. Photosensitivity occurs in about 30%, especially in women, but the two disorders appear to be inherited separately.

Scalp EEG showed focal interictal epileptiform discharges in 30.3% of JME patients studied in detail by Panayiotopoulos et al.,[61] and focal EEG abnormalities of all kinds in 36.7%.[2] In our experience, frequent unilateral or bilateral temporal EEG abnormalities are seen as patients age.[66] Panayiotopoulos et al.[61] also commented on the precipitation of seizures by mental activation as part of the syndrome, which may represent seizures induced by thinking. Wolf emphasized the typical frontocentral predominance of the ictal EEG activity recorded with the myoclonic jerks of JME.[82] This regional predominance and cognitive activation have been discussed by several authors (for review, see Matsuoka et al.[51]).

Neuroimaging

Although JME is classified under the so-called idiopathic epilepsies, evidence from structural and functional imaging highlights the existence of underlying abnormalities. Studies in patients with JME have shown abnormalities in mesial frontal structures in many[81] and some have more widespread abnormalities of cortical gray matter. Using magnetic resonance spectroscopy (MRS), Savic et al.[68] showed reduction in frontal lobe *N*-acetyl aspartate (NAA) in JME, and later confirmed that frontal NAA was reduced in patients with JME but not in those with generalized epilepsy with tonic–clonic seizures.[69] These investigators also showed reduced thalamic choline and myoinositol concentrations in both IGE syndromes. Mory et al.[54] studied thalamic MRS in JME and reported reduced NAA/phosphocreatine ratios in nine out of ten patients. Similar findings were reported by Bernasconi et al.[11] in 12 out of 20 patients with IGE. Twelve patients had JME, but these cases were not analyzed separately.

Combined EEG and functional magnetic resonance imaging (fMRI) in patients with IGE, including JME, has demonstrated bilateral thalamic activation, with increased blood oxygenation level–dependent (BOLD) signal during bilateral spike-wave activity in most individuals and deactivation in bilateral frontal, parietal, and posterior cingulate regions.[1] Thus, although MRS and fMRI studies support a role for thalamic abnormalities in IGE, they also implicate more localized cortical neuroanatomic mechanisms in JME in particular. MRI and MRS studies thus support the suggestions made on clinical and EEG grounds that the frontal cortex is in some way preferentially involved in JME.

Biochemical Studies

Biochemical studies have also sought evidence of systemic metabolic abnormalities that would, when expressed in the brain, alter cortical function in generalized epilepsy. Platelets have been used as a model of GABAergic neurotransmission. Rainesalo et al.[65] reported reduced platelet GABA uptake in patients with JME and increased activity of the catabolic enzyme GABA-transaminase, which may indicate impaired cerebral GABAergic function. They also reported increased interictal plasma glutamate in JME patients, with no significant change in the postictal period.[64] This study confirms earlier findings in both generalized and focal epilepsies.[41]

Genetic Studies

Genetic studies have also contributed to our understanding of JME. Based on family and twin data, respectively, Andermann,[3] Berkovic et al.,[10] and other investigators concluded that most IGEs, as well as most idiopathic focal epilepsies, are inherited as multifactorial or complex traits, with the additive effects of several or many susceptibility genes and interaction with environmental factors to produce the final phenotype. Even in so-called monogenic epilepsies, the variation in phenotype among family members and between families is attributed to the effects of modifying genes and environmental or developmental factors. Multiple IGE subsyndromes may exist in the same family, even in those with a single gene defect.[4,12] Marini et al.[50] reported that, although childhood and juvenile-onset absence epilepsies share a close genetic relationship, JME appears to be genetically more distinct. A recent study also demonstrated different genetic influences between IGE families with absences and those with myoclonic seizures,[80] and other studies showed different linkage groups for childhood and adolescent absence epilepsy and for JME.[37]

The discovery that some well-defined epilepsy syndromes are channelopathies has also fueled efforts to describe the mechanisms underlying JME. Several genetic models have been proposed for generalized epilepsies and for JME in particular, and mechanisms of epileptogenesis have also been proposed based on these findings. Mulley et al.[56] pointed out that "all but one of the idiopathic epilepsies with a known molecular basis are channelopathies. Where the ion channel defects have been identified, however, they generally account for a minority of families and sporadic cases with the syndrome in question. The data suggest that ion channel mutations of large effect are a common cause of rare monogenic idiopathic epilepsies, but are rare causes of common epilepsies."

When a positive family history of epilepsy can be obtained, most JME occurs in families with a variety of IGE syndromes. Several loci have been mapped for IGE in such families, including 8q, 3p, and 1p (for review, see Gourfinkel-An et al.[32]). Sander et al.,[67] in a large genome-wide scan of families with IGE, reported linkage to chromosome 3q among other loci. The candidate interval on 3q includes the gene ClCN2 coding for the ClC-2 voltage-dependent Cl^- channel, largely expressed in cerebral neurones and inhibited by GABA. Haug et al.[35] reported three different heterozygous mutations in this gene in three unrelated families with IGE. These mutations segregate with the epilepsy phenotype in each family and all cause changes in function associated with neuronal excitability. These authors also detected a novel polymorphism in the ClCN2 gene based on 115 parent–child trios. ClCN2 is the first epilepsy gene with both rare major gene mutations and a common sequence variation (polymorphism) conferring a range of phenotypic effects. Mutations in this gene have also been reported in two other families: In one family the proband had JME and in the other the proband had focal epilepsy, thus confirming ClCN2 as a major gene for more than one type of epilepsy.[21]

Another gene located in the 3q26 region, KCNMB3, codes for regulatory subunits associated with calcium-activated potassium channels (B channels). Four polymorphisms in this gene were detected in a variety of patients with epilepsy including JME. These variants were found to be associated with functional deficits of the BK channel.[39]

A recent genetic study of a large French-Canadian family with autosomal dominant JME (ADJME)[19] showed that affected individuals are heterozygous for a missense mutation (A322D) in the gene coding for the α_1 subunit of the $GABA_A$ receptor (GABRA1) on chromosome 5q34. It is also of interest that this region overlaps the locus for GABRG2, one of the genes responsible for GEFS+ (generalized epilepsy with febrile seizures plus) syndrome as well as for absence epilepsy with febrile seizures.[8,78] As is often the case in genetic studies of epilepsy, autosomal dominant JME accounts for only a small proportion of JME, and studies of other families have yielded different results. Although the same mutation in GABRA1 was not found in a study of Indian JME families,[44] these investigators[77] suggested that polymorphisms in a potassium channel gene, KCNQ3 (EBN2, 8q24), may be important in predisposing to JME in South Indian families. They also suggested that the later expression of the KCNQ3 gene may help to explain the characteristic adolescent onset of JME, as compared with the neonatal onset of seizures in benign familial neonatal convulsions (BFNC) associated with major mutations in KCNQ2. However, major mutations in KCNQ3 have been identified in Mexican-American families with BFNC.[17] Susceptibility to seizures of many kinds has also been proposed in relation to a missense variation in the human potassium ion channel gene KCNJ10.[13]

Other investigators using linkage studies have proposed that susceptibility loci for JME exist at 6p11–12,[6,45,46,62] HLA-6p21.3 region,[33] 15q14,[25] and 5q34.[19] Recent studies conducted in Dutch families narrowed the region on 6p11–12,[62] known as EJM1. Suzuki et al.,[71] reviewing previous studies from Belize, Los Angeles, and Mexico[6,45,46] and extending them, described a novel gene, EFHC1, in this region. Five mutations in EFHC1 segregated with JME in 6 out of 44 families and were not found in healthy control individuals. EFHC1, unlike other epilepsy genes, does not encode ion channels but modulates and interacts with voltage-dependent calcium channels and has apoptotic activity. The authors proposed that EFHC1 is the gene on 6p12 that is associated with JME. Although mutations in both GABRA1 and EFHC1 are rare causes of JME,[48] disease-causing mutations in EFHC1 have been identified by other groups[48,69a] both in JME and in other forms of IGE.

Other families exhibit linkage to the 6p21.3 region associated with HLA rather than to 6p12. Pal et al.[60] suggested that JME at the 6p21 locus may be caused by a mutation in the BRD2 gene. The authors noted that the abnormal MRI in JME[81] would be consistent with involvement of BRD2.

Association studies suggest that the α_{1A} subunit of the voltage-gated calcium channel gene (CACNA1A) may affect susceptibility to IGE.[18] This channel is responsible for seizures and ataxia in tottering and leaner mice[28] and has also been implicated in human episodic ataxia type 2, spinocerebellar ataxia type 6, and a form of familial hemiplegic migraine.[58] Escayg et al.[26] found coding and noncoding variations of the human calcium channel gene CACNB4 in patients with IGE and epithotic etaxia.

In summary, although several major genes have recently been identified for IGE, and for JME in particular, only mutations in the ClCN2 and EFHC1 genes have been replicated by different groups. Furthermore, no consistent genetic pattern has been revealed by association studies for any common idiopathic epilepsy syndrome.[73] A number of association studies of other ion channels in IGE, including JME, have yielded negative results.[7,27,72]

DIFFERENTIAL DIAGNOSIS

Two main differential diagnoses have to be considered here. In the cases where myoclonus is not well characterized, it may be confounded with a partial seizure with motor manifestations and, in this situation, a detailed clinical history is important. The main implication of the misdiagnosis of JME as a partial epilepsy is, of course, the choice of the wrong AED, and further classification of the epilepsy as a refractory one. The second differential diagnosis is for those patients who do not clearly report myoclonus, which may delay the diagnosis of JME. These patients may be diagnosed as having one of the various forms of idiopathic generalized epilepsies with generalized tonic-clonic seizures.[4] Again, a detailed clinical history is the essential tool. Other rare differential diagnoses include the progressive myoclonus epilepsies, especially Lafora disease and Unverricht-Lundborg disease, which also present in adolescence and may resemble JME in the early stages.

TREATMENT AND OUTCOME

Valproate is the drug of choice. The newer AEDs, such as lamotrigine and topiramate, result in variable control of the myoclonus, but good efficacy for the GTCSs in JME. Levetiracetam appears to have significant antimyoclonic effect. Clonazepam is a good add-on drug for myoclonis, and can be used in monotherapy only in patients who have never had GTCs. The lack of responsiveness of JME to AEDs such as carbamazepine or phenytoin with, in some patients, even an increase in myoclonus due to these agents should be emphasized. In the European literature, the activation of minor epileptic manifestations of IGE such as absence or myoclonus by carbamazepine or oxcarbazepine as well as phenytoin, vigabatrin, and gabapentin has been stressed,[76] but this has only recently been accepted in North America.

LONG-TERM PROGNOSIS

The prognosis of myoclonus in this form of epilepsy is not entirely clear. Although AEDs can be withdrawn in only a minority (10% to 20%) of patients,[14,61] it is generally accepted that there may be improvement over time, particularly with respect to myoclonus, and that the process may be less active, but without complete remission in adult life. The great majority of patients responds to treatment with appropriate antimyoclonic and antiepileptic medication, and has an otherwise benign outcome with no other neurologic disturbances. Since most patients continue to be on medication, it is difficult to know how often the myoclonus remits spontaneously over time.

SUMMARY AND CONCLUSIONS

JME is a frequent type of IGE characterized by myoclonic seizures, most often implicating a lifetime use of valproate. Recent work suggests that JME may represent several different disorders with different genetic and pathophysiologic signatures found in patients who are clinically or practically indistinguishable.

References

1. Agakhani Y, Bagshaw AP, Benar CG, et al. fMRI activation during spike and wave discharges in idiopathic generalized epilepsy. *Brain.* 2004;127:1127–1144.
2. Aliberti V, Grunewald RA, Panayiotopoulos CP, et al. Focal electroencephalographic abnormalities in juvenile myoclonic epilepsy. *Epilepsia.* 1994;35:297–301.
3. Andermann E. Multifactorial inheritance of generalized and focal epilepsy. In: Anderson VE, Hauser WA, Penre JK, Sing CS, et al., eds. *Genetic Basis of the Epilepsies.* New York: Raven Press; 1982:355–374.
4. Andermann F, Berkovic S. Idiopathic generalized epilepsy with generalized and other seizures in adolescence. *Epilepsia.* 2001;42:317–320.
5. Asconape J, Penry JK. Some clinical and EEG aspects of benign juvenile myoclonic epilepsy. *Epilepsia.* 1984;25:108–114.

5a. Avoli M, Rogawski MA, Avanzini G. Generalized epileptic disorders: an update. *Epilepsia.* 2001;42:445–457.

6. Bai D, Alonso ME, Medina MT, et al. Juvenile myoclonic epilepsy: linkage to chromosome 6p12 in Mexico families. *Am J Med Genet.* 2002;113:268–274.
7. Bailey MES, Carter SA, Tobias ES, et al. Linkage and candidate gene analysis of idiopathic epilepsies [Abstract]. *Am J Hum Genet.* 2001;69:498(abstr).
8. Baulac S, Huberfeld G, Gourfinkel-An I, et al. First evidence of $GABA_A$ receptor dysfunction in epilepsy: a mutation in the [gamma]2-subunit gene. *Nat Genet.* 2001;28:46–48.
9. Berkovic SF. Genetics of epilepsy syndromes. In: Engel J Jr, Pedley TA, eds. *Epilepsy. A Comprehensive Textbook.* Philadelphia: Lippincott Raven Publishers; 1998:217–224.
10. Berkovic SF, Howell RA, Day DA, et al. Epilepsies in twins: genetics of the major epilepsy syndromes. *Ann Neurol.* 1998;43:435–445.
11. Bernasconi A, Bernasconi N, Natsume J, et al. Magnetic resonance spectroscopy and imaging of the thalamus in idiopathic generalized epilepsy. *Brain.* 2003;126:2447–2454.
12. Bianchi A, Viaggi S, Chiossi E, LICE Episcreen Group. Family study of epilepsy in first degree relatives: data from the Italian Episcreen Study. *Seizure.* 2003;12:203–210.

13. Buono RJ, Lohoff FW, Sander T, et al. Association between variation in the human KCNJ10 potassium ion channel gene and seizure susceptibility. *Epilepsy Res.* 2004;58:175–183.
14. Calleja S, Salas-Puig J, Ribacoba R, et al. Evolution of juvenile myoclonic epilepsy treated from the outset with sodium valproate. *Seizure.* 2001;10(6):424–427.
15. Casaubon L, Pohlmann-Eden B, Khosravani H, et al. Video-EEG evidence of lateralized clinical features in primary generalized epilepsy with tonic-clonic seizures. *Epileptic Disord.* 2003;5:149–156.
16. Castells C, Mendilaharsu C. La epilepsia mioclónica bilateral y consciente. *Acta Neurol Latinoamer.* 1958;4:23–48.
17. Charlier C, Singh NA, Ryan SG, et al. A pore mutation in a novel KQT-like potassium channel gene in an idiopathic epilepsy family. *Nat Genet.* 1998;18:53–55.
18. Chioza B, Wilkie H, Nashef L, et al. Association between the [alpha]$_{1A}$ calcium channel gene CACNA1A and idiopathic generalized epilepsy. *Neurology.* 2001;56:1245–1246.
19. Cossette P, Liu L, Brisebois K, et al. Mutation of GABRA1 in an autosomal dominant form of juvenile myoclonic epilepsy. *Nat Genet.* 2002;31(2):184–189.
20. Cutting S, Lauchheimer A, Barr W, et al. Adult-onset idiopathic generalized epilepsy: clinical and behavioral features. *Epilepsia.* 2001;42(11):1395–1398.
21. D'Agostino D, Bertelli M, Gallo S, et al. Mutations and polymorphisms of the ClCN2 gene in idiopathic epilepsy. *Neurology.* 2004;63:1500–1502.
22. Delgado-Escueta AV, Enrile-Bacsal F. Juvenile myoclonic epilepsy of Janz. *Neurology.* 1984;34:285–294.
23. Delgado-Escueta AV, Suzuki T, Alonso ME, et al. The genetics of juvenile myoclonic epilepsy: where are we going? *Epilepsia.* 2004;45(Suppl 3):28.
24. Durner M. *HLA und Epilepsie mit Impulsiv – petit mal.* Thesis, Freie Universitat, Berlin; 1988.
25. Elmslie FV, Rees M, Williamson MP, et al. Genetic mapping of a major susceptibility locus for juvenile myoclonic epilepsy on chromosome 15q. *Hum Mol Genet.* 1997;6(8):1329–1334.
26. Escayg A, De Waard M, Lee DD, et al. Coding and noncoding variation of the human calcium-channel beta4-subunit gene CACNB4 in patients with idiopathic generalized epilepsy and episodic ataxia. *Am J Hum Genet.* 2000;66(5):1531–1539.
27. Evgrafov OV, Zheng FL, Tabares P, et al. KCNAB1 is not responsible for predisposition to a subgroup of juvenile myoclonic epilepsy [Abstract]. *Am J Hum Genet.* 2002;71:481(abstr).
28. Fletcher CF, Lutz CM, O'Sullivan TN, et al. Absence epilepsy in tottering mutant mice is associated with calcium channel defects. *Cell.* 1996;87:607–617.
29. Gallagher MJ, Song L, Arain F, et al. The juvenile myoclonic epilepsy GABAA receptor [alpha]1 subunit mutation A322D produces asymmetrical, subunit position-dependent reduction of heterozygous receptor currents and [alpha]1 subunit protein expression. *J Neurosci.* 2004;24:5570–5578.
30. Gilliam F, Steinhoff BJ, Bittermann H-J, et al. Adult myoclonic epilepsy: a distinct syndrome of idiopathic generalized epilepsy. *Neurology.* 2000;55:1030–1033.
31. Gloor P. Generalized epilepsy with spike-and-wave discharge: a reinterpretation of its electrographic and clinical manifestations. The 1977 William G. Lennox Lecture, American Epilepsy Society. *Epilepsia.* 1979;20:571–588.
32. Gourfinkel-An I, Baulac S, Nabbout R, et al. Recent insights into the implication of ion channels in familial forms of epilepsies associated or nonassociated to febrile convulsions [in French]. *Rev Neurol (Paris).* 2004;160: S90–S97.
33. Greenberg DA, Delgado-Escueta AV, Widelitz H, et al. Juvenile myoclonic epilepsy (JME) may be linked to the BF and HLA loci on human chromosome 6. *Am J Med Genet.* 1988;31(1):185–192.
34. Grunewald RA, Chroni E, Panayiotopoulos CP. Delayed diagnosis of juvenile myoclonic epilepsy. *J Neurol Neurosurg Psychiatry.* 1992;55:497–499.
35. Haug K, Warnstedt M, Alekov AK, et al. Mutations in CLCN2 encoding a voltage-gated chloride channel are associated with idiopathic generalized epilepsies. *Nat Genet.* 2003;33(4):527–532.
36. Hauser WA, Annegers, JF, Kurland LT. Incidence of epilepsy and provoked seizures in Rochester, Minnesota: 1935–1984. *Epilepsia.* 1993;34: 453–468.
37. Hempelmann A, Taylor KP, Heils A, et al. Exploration of the genetic architecture of idiopathic generalized epilepsies. *Epilepsia.* 2006;47(10):1682–1690.
38. Herpin TH. *Des accès incomplets d'épilepsie.* Paris: Baillière; 1867.
39. Hu S, Labuda MZ, Pandolfo M, et al. Variants of the KCNMB3 regulatory subunit of maxi BK channels affect channel inactivation. *Physiol Genom.* 2003;15:191–198.
40. Inoue Y, Zifkin B. Praxis induction and thinking induction: one or two mechanisms? A controversy. In: Wolf P, Inoue Y, Zifkin B, eds. *Reflex Epilepsies. Current Problems in Epilepsy Series.* Vol. 19. Paris: John Libbey Eurotext; 2004:41–55.
41. Janjua NA, Andermann E, Eeg-Olofsson O, et al. Plasma amino acid and genetic studies in epilepsy. In: Beck-Mannagetta G, Anderson VE, Doose H, Janz D. et al., eds. *Genetics of the Epilepsies.* Berlin: Heidelberg: Springer-Verlag; 1989:162–171.
42. Janz D, Christian W. Impulsiv-Petit mal. *Dtsch Z Nervenheilk.* 1957;176:348–386.
43. Janz D, Durner M. Juvenile myoclonic epilepsy. In: Engel J Jr, Pedley TA, eds. *Epilepsy: A Comprehensive Textbook.* Philadelphia: Lippincott-Raven Publishers; 1998:2389–2400.
44. Kapoor A, Vijai J, Ravishankar HM, et al. Absence of GABRA1 Ala322Asp mutation in juvenile myoclonic epilepsy families from India. *J Genet.* 2003;82:17–21.
45. Liu AW, Delgado-Escueta AV, Serratosa JM, et al. Juvenile myoclonic epilepsy locus in chromosome 6p21.2-p11: linkage to convulsions and electroencephalography trait. *Am J Hum Genet.* 1995;57:368–381.
46. Liu AW, Delgado-Escueta AV, Gee MN, et al. Juvenile myoclonic epilepsy in chromosome 6p12-p11: locus heterogeneity and recombinations. *Am J Med Genet.* 1996;63:438–446.
47. Lundborg M. *Die progressive Myoklonus-Epilepsie (Unverrichts Myoklonie).* Uppsala: Almquist und Wiksell; 1903.
48. Ma S, Blair MA, Abou-Khalil B, et al. Mutations in the GABRA1 and EFHC1 genes are rare in familial juvenile myoclonic epilepsy. *Epilepsy Res.* 2006;71(2–3):129–134.
49. Marini C, King MA, Archer JS, et al. Idiopathic generalised epilepsy of adult onset: clinical syndromes and genetics. *J Neurol Neurosurg Psychiatry.* 2003;74:192–196.
50. Marini C, Scheffer I, Crossland KM, et al. Genetic architecture of idiopathic generalized epilepsy: clinical genetic analysis of 55 multiplex families. *Epilepsia.* 2004;45:467–478.
51. Matsuoka H, Takahashi T, Sasaki M, et al. Neuropsychological EEG activation in patients with epilepsy. *Brain.* 2000;123:318–330.
52. Meencke HJ, Janz D. Neuropathological findings in primary generalized epilepsy. A study of eight cases. *Epilepsia.* 1984;25:8–21.
53. Meencke HJ, Veith G. The relevance of slight migrational disturbances (microdysgenesis) to the etiology of the epilepsies. In: Delgado-Escueta AV, Wilson WA, Olsen RW, et al., eds. *Jasper's Basic Mechanisms of the Epilepsies.* 3rd ed. *Advances in Neurology.* Vol. 79. Philadelphia: Lippincott Williams and Wilkins; 1999:123–131.
54. Mory S, Li LM, Guerreiro CAM, et al. Thalamic dysfunction in juvenile myoclonic epilepsy: a proton MRS study. *Epilepsia.* 2003;44:1402–1405.
55. Mullins GM, O'Sullivan SS. A study of idiopathic generalised epilepsy in an Irish population. *Seizure.* 2007;16(3):204–210.
56. Mulley JC, Scheffer IE, Petrou S, et al. Channelopathies as a genetic cause of epilepsy. *Curr Opin Neurol.* 2003;16:171–176.
57. Opeskin K, Kalnins RM, Halliday G, et al. Idiopathic generalized epilepsy. Lack of significant microdysgenesis. *Neurology.* 2000;55:1101–1106.
58. Ophoff RA, Terwindt GM, Vergouwe MN, et al. Familial hemiplegic migraine and episodic ataxia type 2 are caused by mutations in the Ca^{2+} channel gene CACNL1A4. *Cell.* 1996;87:543–552.
59. Pal DK, Durner M, Klotz I, et al. Complex inheritance and parent-of-origin effect in juvenile myoclonic epilepsy. *Brain Dev.* 2006;28(2):92–98.
60. Pal DK, Evgrafov OV, Tabares P, et al. BRD2 (RING3) is a probable major susceptibility gene for common juvenile myoclonic epilepsy. *Am J Hum Genet.* 2003;73:261–270.
61. Panayiotopoulos CP, Obeid T, Tahan AR. Juvenile myoclonic epilepsy: a 5-year prospective study. *Epilepsia.* 1994;35:285–296.
62. Pinto D, de Haan GJ, Janssen GA, et al. Evidence for linkage between juvenile myoclonic epilepsy-related idiopathic generalized epilepsy and 6p11–12 in Dutch families. *Epilepsia.* 2004;45:211–217.
63. Rabot. *De la myoclonie épileptique.* Paris: Thèse; 1899.
64. Rainesalo S, Keranen T, Palmio J, et al. Plasma and cerebrospinal fluid amino acids in epileptic patients. *Neurochem Res.* 2004;29:319–324.
65. Rainesalo S, Saransaari P, Peltola J, et al. Uptake of GABA and activity of GABA-transaminase in platelets from epileptic patients. *Epilepsy Res.* 2003;53:233–239.
66. Rosati A, Agha Khani Y, Dubeau F, et al. The intractable idiopathic generalized epilepsies [Abstract]. *Epilepsia.* 2002;43(Suppl 7):150.
67. Sander T, Schulz H, Saar K, et al. Genome search for susceptibility loci of common idiopathic generalised epilepsies. *Hum Mol Genet.* 2000;9:1465–1472.
68. Savic I, Lekvall A, Greitz D, et al. MR spectroscopy shows reduced frontal lobe concentrations of N-acetyl aspartate in patients with juvenile myoclonic epilepsy. *Epilepsia.* 2000;41:290–296.
69. Savic I, Österman Y, Helms G. MRS shows syndrome differentiated metabolite changes in human-generalized epilepsies. *NeuroImage.* 2004;21:163–172.
69a. Stogmann E, Lichtner P, Baumgartner C, et al. Idiopathic generalized epilepsy phenotypes associated with different EFHC1 mutations. *Neurology.* 2006;67(11):2029–2031.
70. Sundquist A. Juvenile myoclonic epilepsy: events before diagnosis. *J Epilepsy.* 1990;3:189–192.
71. Suzuki T, Delgado-Escueta AV, Aguan K, et al. Mutations in EFHC1 cause juvenile myoclonic epilepsy. *Nat Genet.* 2004;36:843–849.
72. Tabares PA, Evgrafov OV, Durner M, et al. Mutation in GABA receptor gamma 2 gene is not a frequent cause of idiopathic generalized epilepsies [Abstract]. *Am J Hum Genet.* 2002;71:473(abstr).
73. Tan NCK, Mulley JC, Berkovic SF. Genetic association studies in epilepsy: 'the truth is out there.' *Epilepsia.* 2004;45:1429–1442.
74. Taylor I, Marini C, Johnson MR, et al. Juvenile myoclonic epilepsy and idiopathic photosensitive occipital lobe epilepsy: is there overlap? *Brain.* 2004;127:1878–1886.

75. Thomas P, Genton P, Gelisse P, et al. Epilepsie myoclonique juvenile. In: Roger J, Bureau M, Dravet C, eds. *Les syndromes epileptiques de l'enfant et de l'adolescent*. John Libby & Co.; 2002:335–356.
76. Thomas P, Valton L, Genton P, et al. Absence and myoclonic status epilepticus precipitated by antiepileptic drugs in idiopathic generalized epilepsy. *Brain*. 2006;129(Pt 5):1281–1292.
77. Vijai J, Kapoor A, Ravishankar HM, et al. Genetic association analysis of KCNQ3 and juvenile myoclonic epilepsy in a South Indian population. *Hum Genet*. 2003;113:461–463.
78. Wallace RH, Marini C, Petrou S, et al. Mutant $GABA_A$ receptor [gamma]2-subunit in childhood absence epilepsy and febrile seizures. *Nat Genet*. 2001;28:49–52.
79. Whitehouse WP, Rees M, Curtis D, et al. Linkage analysis of idiopathic generalized epilepsy (IGE) and marker loci on chromosome 6p in families of patients with juvenile myoclonic epilepsy: no evidence for an epilepsy locus in the HLA region. *Am J Hum Genet*. 1993;53(3): 652–662.
80. Winawer MR, Rabinowitz D, Pedley TA, et al. Genetic influences on myoclonic and absence seizures. *Neurology*. 2003;61:1576–1581.
81. Woermann FG, Free SL, Koepp MJ, et al. Abnormal cerebral structure in juvenile myoclonic epilepsy demonstrated with voxel-based analysis of MRI. *Brain*. 1999;122:2101–2107.
82. Wolf P. Regional manifestation of idiopathic epilepsy. Introduction. In: Wolf P, ed. *Epileptic Seizures and Syndromes*. London: John Libbey; 1994:265–267.
83. Wolf P, Goosses R. Relation of photosensitivity to epileptic syndromes. *J Neurol Neurosurg Psychiatry*. 1986;49:1368–1391.
84. Zifkin B, Andermann E, Andermann F. Mechanisms, genetics, and pathogenesis of juvenile myoclonic epilepsy. *Curr Opin Neurol*. 2005;18:147–153.

CHAPTER 245 ■ OVERVIEW: NON–AGE-RELATED AND SPECIAL SYNDROMES

WARREN T. BLUME AND PETER WOLF

INTRODUCTION

Each of the chapters in this section uses a different approach to address one of two challenges in epileptology: (a) the relationship connecting seizure semiology, the structures involved in epileptogenesis, and related lesions and (b) the interplay between predisposing and precipitating factors in igniting seizures. In addition, chapters on familial epilepsies involving the temporal lobe (Chapter 248), frontal lobe (Chapter 249), and variable foci (Chapter 255) reflect the increasingly recognized role of genetics in the etiology of seizure disorders, including those without an apparent familial seizure history.

SEMIOLOGY, EPILEPTOGENESIS, AND RELATED LESIONS

The precise definition of the structures or systems responsible for ictal phenomena has long posed a challenge to the best efforts of distinguished investigators. For Hughlings Jackson, "the study of partial seizures became the starting point for the study of localization of function within the central nervous system."[31] As described by Jasper,[31] Sherrington electrically stimulated the cortex of anthropoid apes to examine functional–structural relationships. The early stimulation studies in humans performed by Foerster[17] preceded the exhaustive studies carried out by Penfield and Jasper in the course of evaluating patients for epilepsy surgery; these culminated in their classic work, *Epilepsy and the Functional Anatomy of the Human Brain.*[31] Interictal electroencephalography (EEG) has provided helpful correlative data to clarify the localizing significance of ictal symptomatology,[11,31] as has intracranial recording.[3] However, Williamson and Engel (see Chapter 246) caution that sophisticated techniques for correlating ictal electrical activity with clinical phenomena have only revealed the complexities of anatomic–symptomatologic relationships.

A second method of identifying structures or systems responsible for ictal phenomena has been to correlate the latter with structural lesions. In Chapter 246, the authors indicate that Hughlings Jackson first recognized the correlation between ictal behavior and the location of structural abnormalities in the brain. Defining "specific lesions" as "discrete focal (or regional) structural pathologies that are associated with chronic partial epilepsy," Chapter 251 examines such relationships. These authors review changes in neurotransmitters in the vicinity of tumors, favoring excitation over inhibition. They cite the finding of Awad et al.[5] that lesionectomy alone more often renders patients seizure free than resection of epileptogenic cortex without regard to lesion, supporting a direct relationship between structure and ictogenesis. Fortunately, improved neuroimaging now more accurately identifies focal or regional epileptogenic lesions (Chapters 247 and 251).

However, several factors complicate such relationships. Penfield[31] demonstrated that the form of the attack is considered to be due to the functional characteristics of the local area of onset within the brain, the strength of initial discharge, and the path of its spread to other brain areas. Rasmussen[32] acknowledged this factor of propagation in elaborating a concept of secondary localizational aspects of epileptic phenomena. His review of seizure-free patients after frontal lobe resection found no correlation between surgery site and seizure characteristics. Variability of propagation patterns is a principal factor in confounding any anatomic classification of seizures.

Williamson[41] indicated that rapid spread of frontal seizures clouds the localizing value of many ictal phenomena. Varying and bilateral motor ictal phenomena may be consequent to multiply targeted intracortical and corticofugal projections within the motor system, including ipsilateral projections to proximal limbs.[8,14,41] Abundant projections from the occipital cortex to anterior temporal areas[24,35] effect the dyscognitive seizures from occipital epileptogenesis. More recently demonstrated temporal-to-occipital projections[4,16,25] are likely among factors producing visual auras from extraoccipital seizure origins.[7] In addition, a seizure disorder beginning while the brain is developing may lead to abnormal patterns of innervation.[19,38] For example, a seizure-related failure of "pruning" through apoptosis may produce a permanently abnormal connectivity.[22]

Moreover, epileptogenic regions may be remote from a lesion that is also epileptogenic (Chapter 251). Temporal epileptogenic regions may coexist with epileptogenic occipital lesions[10,29] or with parietal arteriovenous malformations.[43] For undetermined reasons, lesions may be unevenly epileptogenic around their peripheries. Thus, O'Brien et al. (Chapter 252) cite works indicating that resection of a lesion as well as epileptogenic cortex is necessary for optimal seizure reduction.[6,39,44] A further confounding factor impeding the establishment of structural–semiologic relationships is the possibility that lesions may extend beyond their manifestations on neuroimaging studies. This factor may underlie the relative ineffectiveness of surgery as treatment for epileptogenic neuronal migration disorders (Chapter 251).

Defining seizures or epilepsies according to lobes of the brain is inexact because none is fully functionally distinct from the others. This sharing of functions partially underlies the overlap of symptoms of seizures arising from different regions. Several examples of seizure types that transcend lobar boundaries are described in Chapter 246.

The aforementioned impediments suggest that epileptic seizures should be analyzed according to the systems involved rather than discrete cortical loci. For example, the intimate connections of thalamic nuclei with circumscribed cortical regions suggested to Penfield[31] that the cortex be divided according to thalamic projection areas. Rapid propagation of cortical discharge to related thalamic nuclei[36] and the decrease of cortical discharges by thalamic lesions[15,21,27,28] support this concept. The term "system" is applied here in the same way in which we otherwise speak in neurology about system disorders, actually referring to subsystems of the nervous system.

Probably the best example of an epilepsy involving a system is that of mesial temporal lobe epilepsy with hippocampal sclerosis (MTLE-HS), described in Chapter 247. In contrast to anatomically based descriptions of seizure types, this is a localization-related syndrome with a semiology centered around the limbic system. The characteristic ictal semiology and mesial temporal pathology—hippocampal sclerosis—are the fundamental components of MTLE-HS. This is likely the most common correlate between semiology and structure encountered in practice. However, the persistence of auras after successful temporal lobectomy reflects the complex genesis of symptoms caused by epileptic discharge centered in the mesial temporal regions, which is a further example of a seizure type that transcends lobar boundaries. The system concept is further exemplified by the shared semiology of seizures propagating to the limbic system and those originating in that same system.[9,40] However, ever more precise stereoncephalography can disclose ictal semiologic distinctions within the temporal lobe. Thus, in some studies, laterally originating temporal seizures have been found to be shorter, more likely to have auditory symptoms, and secondarily generalize more than those originating mesially.[26]

The idiopathic localization-related epilepsies afford an additional opportunity to link systems involved in epileptogenesis with seizure symptomatology. Syndromes with focal seizures unrelated to any identifiable or presumed brain pathology but with associated characteristic EEG abnormalities, often in homotopic regions of both hemispheres, and with spontaneous remission have been described principally among children.[2]

Inherited channelopathies are associated with several epilepsy syndromes, usually with onset in childhood.[20] Some become lifelong disorders. "Febrile seizures plus," a genetic disorder involving mutant neuronal sodium channels, begins in childhood as febrile seizures and may continue into adulthood as one or more types of afebrile generalized motor seizures.[33] Similarly, autosomal-dominant nocturnal frontal lobe epilepsy, associated with mutations in genes encoding neuronal nicotinic acetylcholine receptors, begins in childhood but persists into adulthood despite its usually mild nature. Chapters 249 and 256 further describe these entities. The homogeneity of ictal semiology of these conditions and the lack of "contamination" of ictal genesis by associated lesions suggest that such benign conditions may clarify semiologic–structural relationships if newer methods of tracing an ictal pathway—such as functional magnetic resonance imaging—can be applied.

PREDISPOSING AND PRECIPITATING FACTORS IN EPILEPSY

The second group of chapters deals with the complex interplay between predisposition for epileptic seizures and immediate provocative factors. As Dreifuss[13] stated, "The reason a person who is epileptic all the time does not manifest seizures all the time is that the necessary provocation sufficient to trigger the individual seizure is intermittent and is frequently the result of concatenations of circumstances." The proportion of seizures that occur spontaneously is difficult to establish because triggering events may pass unrecognized or unappreciated. Nonetheless, the balance of each pathogenetic component—predisposition and provocation—varies with the epilepsy. These chapters describe various conditions, each with different proportions of predisposing and triggering components.

In posttraumatic seizures (Chapter 253), predisposing components predominate. The authors document forms of trauma that put a patient at a higher risk for the development of late seizures, the common factor being the presence of intracerebral blood. However, stress or lack of sleep may provoke the first late seizure.

Berkovic (see Chapter 252) presents a valuable update on the concepts and data pertinent to the progressive myoclonus epilepsies. These conditions provide convincing evidence of predisposing factors for the development of seizures. Features usually include myoclonic and tonic–clonic seizures, ataxia, and dementia. The distinctive features of each condition producing the syndrome, along with aspects relevant to differential diagnosis, are presented. The increasing importance of obtaining a family history and examining relatives of patients is emphasized. Even in conditions associated with a strong tendency for seizures, provocative factors are involved. Thus, the myoclonus of Unverricht-Lundborg disease may be precipitated by movement, stress, or sensory stimuli. Similar stimuli may evoke the myoclonic seizures of Lafora disease.[1]

Dreifuss' concept[13] of the relationship between predisposing factors and precipitants is again relevant to Chapter 254, in which solitary seizures are defined as events that may occur once in a lifetime or very rarely. Apart from seizures accompanying acute conditions, such as trauma or encephalitis, it may be assumed that a predisposition for an isolated seizure has existed for some time. Indeed, data from Wolf's series disclosed an identifiable predisposing factor in the majority of patients. Moreover, at least one seizure-provoking factor could be identified in 80 of his 104 patients. As in other studies,[18,23] lack of sleep was a common precipitant of isolated seizures.

Chapters 256 and 257 discuss forms of epilepsy in which an identifiable agent, such as fever, flashing lights, lack of sleep, or drug withdrawal, precipitates many or all of the seizures. Most such seizures are of the generalized tonic–clonic type. The relative importance of predisposition and precipitant factors varies among the broad categories described in each chapter, among entities, and among individual patients. In all cases, the sum of these factors intermittently exceeds the seizure threshold. For patients with these epilepsies, avoiding the precipitants helps to control the seizures.

The seizures of simple reflex epilepsies (Chapter 257) are associated with the most apparent and immediate specific provocators. As the authors emphasize, the seizure history must be scrutinized to discern and establish the relationship. Chapter 257 also describes precisely how visual stimulation should be applied during clinical EEG to confirm light- and pattern-sensitive epilepsy and presents clinical data concerning the photoparoxysmal response.

Photosensitive epilepsy is a model for the interplay of factors leading to tonic–clonic seizures. Although a genetic defect specific for photosensitive seizures has not been discovered, data suggest an autosomal-dominant inheritance.[12,30,37] Withdrawal of alcohol and benzodiazepines may be causes of temporary photosensitivity.

Startle epilepsy is a particularly crippling condition; its mechanism and effective management have proved elusive to investigators.

This section concludes with an interesting review of complex reflex epilepsy, in which precipitants also play essential roles in causing seizures. The attacks are triggered by relatively elaborate stimuli whose specific pattern is the determining factor in seizure evocation. Reading, musicogenic, praxis-induction, and thinking epilepsies fall into this group. Because the precipitating stimuli involve higher cortical function, the relationship may be less immediate or obvious and may include anticipation of the stimulus complex. Discovering such epilepsies may be the reward for an ingenious historian or a perceptive patient. As in other precipitant-related epilepsies, these compound stimuli may evoke generalized tonic–clonic seizures. However, they may also elicit more restricted forms, such as myoclonus of the jaw in reading epilepsy and dyscognitive seizures in musicogenic epilepsy. Perhaps even more than the simple reflex epilepsies, the complex variety likely requires participation of several cortical and subcortical regions, further supporting the system concept of epileptogenesis.

It is of special interest, complex precipitating mechanisms like praxis induction of reading and talking seem to be particularly related to the syndrome of juvenile myoclonic epilepsy (JME). Perioral reflex myoclonias provoked by talking and reading are probably related genetic traits that JME shares with primary reading epilepsy, that is, an idiopathic localization-related epilepsy.[34,42] This observation is thought provoking because it seems to open a new view onto ictogenesis in the so-called generalized epilepsies, which are likely also to become redefined according to the concept of system epilepsies.

SUMMARY AND CONCLUSIONS

These chapters examine two relationships in epilepsy of importance to clinicians and basic scientists: (a) epileptogenesis and epileptic lesions on one hand and (b) predisposition and provocation of epileptic seizures on the other.

The intricate interaction between epileptogenic lesion and host, the surrounding brain, exhibits properties common to many patients but often harbors components unique to a particular patient. How this interaction produces the epileptic seizures may be understood by scrutiny of not only the histology and situation of the lesion, but also of the systems so engaged in the epileptogenesis. Several chapters in this section examine these aspects.

Why seizures occur only intermittently in a patient chronically harboring a seizure tendency, that is, predisposition versus provocation of epileptic seizures, is of interest in a second series of chapters. Greater realization of this interaction will improve clinical management and also shed light on several significant pathophysiologic mechanisms.

References

1. Aicardi J, ed. *Epilepsy in Children*. New York: Raven Press; 1986.
2. Aicardi J, ed. *Epilepsy in Children*, 2nd ed. New York: Raven Press; 1994:138.
3. Ajmone Marsan C. Chronic intracranial recording and electrocorticography. In: Daly DD, Pedley TA, eds. *Current Practice of Clinical Electroencephalography*, 2nd ed. New York: Raven Press; 1990:535–560.
4. Albright TD, Stoner GR. Contextual influences on visual processing. *Annu Rev Neurosci.* 2002;25:339–379.
5. Awad IA, Rosenfeld J, Ahl J, et al. Intractable epilepsy and structural lesions of the brain: mapping, resection strategies, and seizure outcome. *Epilepsia.* 1991;32(2):179–186.
6. Berger MS, Kincaid J, Ojemann GA, et al. Brain mapping techniques to maximise resection, safety, and seizure control in children with brain tumors. *Neurosurgery.* 1989;25:786–792.
7. Bien CG, Benninger FO, Urbach H, et al. Localizing value of epileptic visual auras. *Brain.* 2000;123(Pt 2):244–253.
8. Blume WT. Pathogenesis of Lennox-Gastaut syndrome: considerations and hypotheses. *Epileptic Disord.* 2001;3(4):183–196.
9. Blume WT, Girvin JP, Stenerson P. Temporal neocortical role in ictal experiential phenomena. *Ann Neurol.* 1993;33:105–107.
10. Blume WT, Whiting SE, Girvin JP. Epilepsy surgery in the posterior cortex. *Ann Neurol.* 1991;29:638–645.
11. Daly DD. Epilepsy and syncope. In: Daly DD, Pedley TA, eds. *Current Practice of Clinical Electroencephalography*, 2nd ed. New York: Raven Press; 1990:269–334.
12. Doose H, Waltz S. Photosensitivity—genetics and clinical significance. *Neuropediatrics.* 1993;24(5):249–255.
13. Dreifuss FE. The epilepsies: clinical implications of the international classification. *Epilepsia.* 1990; 31(Suppl 3):S3–S10.
14. Erickson TC. Spread of the epileptic discharge; an experimental study of the after-discharge induced by electrical stimulation of the cerebral cortex. *Arch Neurol Psychiatry.* 1940;43:429–452.
15. Feeney DM, Gullotta FP, Pittman JC. Slow-wave sleep and epilepsy: rostral thalamus and forebrain lesion suppress spindles and seizures. *Exp Neurol.* 1977;56:212–226.
16. Felleman DJ, Van Essen DC. Distributed hierarchical processing in the primate cerebral cortex. *Cereb Cortex.* 1991;1(1):1–47.
17. Foerster O. The motor cortex in man in the light of Hughlings Jackson's doctrines. *Brain.* 1936;59:135–159.
18. Friis ML, Lund M. Stress convulsions. *Arch Neurol.* 1974;31:155–159.
19. Gall CM. Seizure-induced changes in neurotrophin expression: implications for epilepsy. *Exp Neurol.* 1993;124(1):150–166.
20. George AL Jr. Inherited channelopathies associated with epilepsy. *Epilepsy Curr.* 2004;4(2):65–70.
21. Gillingham FJ, Watson WF, Donaldson AA, et al. Stereotaxic lesions for the control of intractable epilepsy. *Acta Neurochir (Vienna).* 1976;23(Suppl):263–269.
22. Innocenti GM, Berbel P. Analysis of an experimental cortical network: I). Architectonics of visual areas 17 and 18 after neonatal injections of ibotenic acid; similarities with human microgyria. *J Neural Transplant Plast.* 1991;2(1):1–28.
23. Janz D. Pitfalls in the diagnosis of grand mal on awakening. In: Wolf P, ed. *Epileptic Seizures and Syndromes.* London: John Libbey; 1994: 213–220.
24. Jones EG, Powell TP. An anatomical study of converging sensory pathways within the cerebral cortex of the monkey. *Brain.* 1970;93(4): 793–820.
25. Kastner S, Ungerleider LG. Mechanisms of visual attention in the human cortex. *Annu Rev Neurosci.* 2000;23:315–341.
26. Maillard L, Vignal JP, Gavaret M, et al. Semiologic and electrophysiologic correlations in temporal lobe seizure subtypes. *Epilepsia.* 2004;45(12):1590–1599.
27. Morillo LE, Ebner TJ, Bloedel JR. The early involvement of subcortical structures during the development of a cortical seizure focus. *Epilepsia.* 1982;23:571–585.
28. Mullan S, Vailati G, Karasick J, et al. Thalamic lesions for the control of epilepsy. *Arch Neurol.* 1967;16:277–278.
29. Olivier A, Gloor P, Andermann F, et al. Occipitotemporal epilepsy studied with stereotaxically implanted depth electrodes and successfully treated by temporal resection. *Ann Neurol.* 1982;11:428–432.
30. Parra J, Kalitzin SN, Lopes da Silva FH. Photosensitivity and visually induced seizures. *Curr Opin Neurol.* 2005;18(2):155–159.
31. Penfield W, Jasper H. *Epilepsy and the Functional Anatomy of the Human Brain.* Boston: Little, Brown; 1954.
32. Rasmussen T. Characteristics of a pure culture of frontal lobe epilepsy. *Epilepsia.* 1983;24:482–493.
33. Scheffer IE, Berkovic SF. Generalized epilepsy with febrile seizures plus. A genetic disorder with heterogeneous clinical phenotypes. *Brain.* 1997;120(Pt 3):479–490.
34. Tassinari CA, Wolf P, Inoue Y. Complex reflex epilepsies: reading epilepsy and praxis induction. In: Roger J, Bureau M, Dravet C, et al., eds. *Epileptic Syndromes in Infancy, Childhood and Adolescence*, 4th ed. Montrouge, France: John Libbey; 2005:347–358.
35. Turner BH, Mishkin M, Knapp M. Organization of the amygdalopetal projections from modality-specific cortical association areas in the monkey. *J Comp Neurol.* 1980;191:515–543.
36. Wada JA, Cornelius LR. Functional alteration of deep structures in cats with chronic focal cortical irritative lesions. *Arch Neurol.* 1960;3:425–447.
37. Waltz S, Stephani U. Inheritance of photosensitivity. *Neuropediatrics.* 2000; 31(2):82–85.
38. Wasterlain CG. Effects of neonatal status epilepticus on rat brain development. *Neurology.* 1976;26:975–986.
39. Weber JP, Silbergeld DL, Winn HR. Surgical resection of epileptogenic cortex associated with structural lesions. *Neurosurg Clin North Am.* 1993;4:327–336.
40. Wieser HG, Engel J Jr, Williamson PD, et al. Surgically remediable temporal lobe syndromes. In: Engel J Jr, ed. *Surgical Treatment of the Epilepsies*, 2nd ed. New York: Raven Press; 1993:49–63.
41. Williamson PD. Frontal lobe seizures. Problems of diagnosis and classification. In: Chauvel P, Delgado-Escueta AV, Halgren E, et al., eds. *Advances in Neurology*, Vol. 57. New York: Raven Press; 1992:289–309.
42. Wolf P, Inoue Y, Zifkin B, eds. *Reflex Epilepsies: Progress in Understanding.* Montrouge, France: John Libbey; 2004.
43. Yeh H, Privitera M. Secondary epileptogenesis in humans with cerebral arteriovenous malformations. *Epilepsia.* 1989;30(5):683.
44. Yeh HS, Kashiwagi S, Tew JM, et al. Surgical management of epilepsy associated with cerebral arteriovenous malformations. *J Neurosurg.* 1990;72:216–223.

CHAPTER 246 ■ ANATOMIC CLASSIFICATION OF FOCAL EPILEPSIES

PETER D. WILLIAMSON AND JEROME ENGEL, JR.

INTRODUCTION

The International Classification of Epilepsies, Epileptic Syndromes, and Related Seizure Disorders[2] recognizes five symptomatic localization-related epilepsies, four of which are anatomically defined: Temporal lobe epilepsies, frontal lobe epilepsies, parietal lobe epilepsies, and occipital lobe epilepsies. Only the fifth, chronic progressive epilepsia partialis continua of childhood, is not classified by location. If we accept the definition of an epileptic syndrome as a complex of signs and symptoms, with only one feature being the occurrence of electroclinically characteristic epileptic seizures.[1] then we can make a cogent argument for the existence of a syndrome of mesial temporal lobe epilepsy (MTLE)[47,55,208,218,222] (see Chapter 247). Otherwise, the classification of epilepsies by anatomic lobe appears to refer predominantly to conditions with characteristic seizure types as the only unifying feature. Recent reports of the International League Against Epilepsy (ILAE) argue against the view that these conditions are syndromes rather than seizures.[51] However, as there is as yet no new classification of syndromes, anatomically defined epilepsies with variably specific seizure types will be retained in this chapter. Other than MTLE, there may be a few examples with constellations of findings that do constitute true syndromes. These possible exceptions will be discussed later.

Much effort has gone into creating an anatomic classification of epileptic seizures, based largely on data obtained from epilepsy surgery centers. The anatomic classification has been greatly assisted by the introduction of high-resolution magnetic resonance imaging (MRI) more than 20 years ago, enabling the detection of small, circumscribed, potentially epileptogenic lesions in many patients with symptomatic localization-related epilepsy. Nevertheless, the validity, or for that matter, clinical value of devising an anatomic classification of epileptic disorders remains the topic of considerable debate. This chapter will review the subject, but emphasis, of necessity, will be placed on seizures rather than syndromes.

HISTORICAL PERSPECTIVES

John Hughlings Jackson is credited with being the first neurologist to recognize the correlation between ictal behavior and the location of structural abnormalities in the brain.[190] His work derived largely from observations of ictal signs and symptoms, followed by identification of lesions at postmortem examination, in an era of pioneering investigations of localization of function within the brain.[48] This work led directly to the application of surgical treatment for refractory partial epilepsy,[82] which, in turn, provided opportunities for invasive investigations of the human brain, such as direct stimulation to delineate anatomic substrates of specific ictal manifestations.[151] With the advent of the electroencephalogram (EEG), the location of focal interictal spikes was used as evidence for the site of origin of habitual seizures, and surgical treatment for "temporal lobe epilepsy" was introduced on the basis of EEG evidence alone.[11] Shortly thereafter, the pioneering efforts of Bancaud et al. related intracranial seizure recording to clinical seizure characteristics.[12]

The development of sophisticated electrophysiologic techniques for recording spontaneous seizures with intracranial electrodes and correlating this information precisely with videotaped ictal behavior has made anatomic classification of seizures more, rather than less, controversial. Because of variability of propagation patterns of ictal discharge, the area of brain giving rise to clinical signs and symptoms can be at considerable distance from the actual site of seizure onset. Consequently, virtually no signs or symptoms can be considered pathognomonic of the anatomic localization of the primary epileptogenic region.[4,121,124] Although the timing or sequencing of seizure manifestations may be as important as their presence or absence, this feature fails to localize precisely because of the potential for seizure origin in clinically "silent" brain regions.

Improvements in structural imaging also have not definitively clarified anatomic classification. High-resolution MRI can identify many structural cerebral lesions in patients with localization-related epilepsy,[107] and they are usually indicative of the epileptogenic region.[25] Many patients with partial seizures, however, have normal MRI evaluations; others have lesions that are unrelated to their epilepsy. Furthermore, it has become increasingly apparent from intracranial recordings of patients under evaluation for surgical treatment that a discrete, well-circumscribed epileptogenic region often does not exist in the human brain; instead there are diffuse or multiple areas of functional abnormality capable of generating interictal, and even ictal, discharges, even in patients for whom a specific localized structural lesion has been identified.[46,214,220] For these reasons, anatomically classifying a seizure disorder merely on the basis of the location of an observed structural abnormality is not always justifiable. Nevertheless, a continued effort to categorize epileptic seizures, and even epileptic disorders, according to a presumed anatomic substrate can be considered a reasonable exercise of some value, particularly for devising presurgical diagnostic strategies, as long as the limitations of such a classification are recognized and surgical interventions are not undertaken on the basis of ictal manifestations or MRI lesions alone. Combining clinical seizure characteristics, structural neuroimaging findings, and EEG results, however, has improved our understanding of partial seizures and helped to better define an anatomic classification.

Functional imaging using positron emission tomography (PET) has been employed at a few medical centers for many years and is currently becoming available at many more institutions. While early results in patients with temporal lobe seizures were and still are promising,[28,117] PET utility in patients with seizure origin outside of the temporal lobe has been less consistent.[128] Newer radioligands and improved technologies will almost certainly improve results in extratemporal epilepsy with normal MRI[77,117] (see Chapter 80).

Ictal single positron emission computed tomography (SPECT) is being used widely to help identify regions of seizures origin.[75,92,101,117,130,143,182,201] Early injection is essential, particularly with brief seizures that propagate rapidly.[113,201] The subtraction product of interictal SPECT from ictal SPECT coregistered with MRI improves the resolution of this relatively difficult-to-obtain procedure.[141–143] Ictal SPECT has become an integral part of the presurgical evaluation in some centers. This is particularly relevant when the MRI is normal.

Magnetoencephalography (MEG)[45] superimposed on MRI and EEG-triggered functional MRI[104] have great promise for localizing sources of ictal, as well as interictal, epileptiform activity. In the former, dipole localization is easier than with EEG because differences in conductivity between brain, cerebrospinal fluid (CSF), bone, and skin do not need to be taken into account. In the latter, simultaneous EEG and MRI recording permit MRI acquisition during epileptiform discharges to be subtracted from MRI acquisitions in the absence of epileptiform discharges, so that the difference in blood oxygenation can be used to localize tissue activated during the EEG events of interest. Magnetic resonance spectrometry (MRS) is also being used to identify metabolic changes associated with interictal disturbances, and this has been particularly useful for confirming hippocampal epileptogenic lesions.[109,186]

DEFINITIONS

With the exception of MTLE, the designation of an epileptic condition by anatomic location denotes the occurrence of a specific type of seizure or seizures, rather than a complex of signs and symptoms that would ordinarily constitute a syndrome. In the purest sense, a temporal lobe epilepsy, for example, would be an epileptic condition in which seizures originate somewhere in the temporal lobe, as indicated directly by invasive electrophysiologic monitoring, or inferred indirectly from clinical seizure characteristics, scalp EEG monitoring, perhaps the presence of a discrete lesion on structural neuroimaging, functional disturbances revealed by neurologic examination, neuropsychological testing and functional neuroimaging, and disappearance of habitual events following a temporal lobe resection of some type. There remains some controversy, however, with this terminology. In much of the published literature on temporal lobe epilepsy, some patients are given this diagnosis when extratemporal ictal onsets preferentially project to mesial temporal structures that, in turn, are responsible for mediating the characteristic ictal manifestations. In many cases, such patients are diagnosed as having temporal lobe epilepsy because the extratemporal origin of their seizures is unrecognized, but in others the actual site of the primary epileptogenic region is ignored and classification is based on ictal characteristics.[208] If a temporal lobe seizure is one that is caused by seizures involving temporal lobe structures, then this could result from ictal initiation within the temporal lobe or an extratemporal "silent area" that preferentially projects to the temporal lobe. Thus, if temporal lobe epilepsy is characterized by the existence of temporal lobe seizures, then the broader definition is acceptable. Rather than dwell on the semantic difficulties associated with anatomic classification, this example can be used to argue the folly of attempting to construct an anatomic classification of epileptic disorders at all. On the other hand, if a specific temporal lobe epilepsy syndrome can be defined, then seizures originating elsewhere can, in part, be identified by virtue of not fulfilling all the characteristics of this syndrome.

Attempts to define seizures or epilepsies according to anatomic lobes of the brain are also confounded by the fact that none of the classical four lobes represents functionally homogenous or unique regions. For instance, parts of the frontal lobe, such as the precentral gyrus, are capable of generating specific ictal signs and symptoms, whereas others, such as the orbital frontal cortex, belong, in part, to the limbic system and can give rise to ictal signs and symptoms by virtue of propagation to other frontal regions or mesial temporal structures, or both (see section on frontal lobe seizures). The International Classification of the Epilepsies divides frontal lobe epilepsy into seven anatomic subtypes and temporal lobe epilepsy into two anatomic subtypes, based on the belief that these areas give rise to different characteristic ictal manifestations.[2] However, there are also functional areas of the brain that give rise to relatively stereotyped clinical seizure characteristics, despite the fact that they encompass more than one anatomic lobe. Thus, seizures arising from the perirolandic area can generate indistinguishable signs and symptoms from motor or sensory cortex, and there may be characteristic features associated with ictal discharges in the temporal-parietal-occipital junction, as well as regions of frontal parietal operculum and insula.

Nevertheless, as our understanding of the various specific and anatomically originating seizures improves, there may emerge clearer evidence on how these clinical characteristics can help localize regions of seizure origin, both by virtue of their uniqueness and their masquerading qualities. This may be particularly true of some, but not all, seizures of frontal lobe origin.

EPIDEMIOLOGY

Among the localization-related epilepsies, the relative incidence and prevalence of temporal lobe, frontal lobe, parietal lobe, and occipital lobe epilepsy have not been adequately determined, due largely to the recognized inaccuracies of identifying anatomic substrates without sophisticated diagnostic evaluation. Data from epilepsy surgery centers indicate that temporal lobe epilepsy is by far the most common of the four when only medically refractory patients are considered. In a review of surgical procedures performed worldwide for medically refractory epilepsy, approximately 70% have involved resections of temporal lobe abnormalities, whereas <20% involved resection of extratemporal cortex.[49,162,163,212] Of the latter group, frontal lobe resections are more common than occipital resections, and parietal lobe resections are least commonly performed. It is important to note, however, that these figures reflect the ease of identification of temporal lobe, frontal lobe, occipital lobe, and parietal lobe epileptogenic regions; the degree of intractability and disability of seizures associated with these areas; and the desirability of their surgical resection, as much as they reflect the incidence of epileptogenic abnormalities in these cerebral areas.

Mesial temporal lobe epilepsy may well be the most common epileptic syndrome, partly because of the peculiar epileptogenicity of hippocampal sclerosis (see Chapter 247). Studies of regional differences in epileptogenicity have shown that temporal lobe EEG spike foci are the most likely, and central EEG spike foci the least likely, to be associated with clinical seizures in children,[98] although these data are biased by the inclusion of patients with the benign centrotemporal spike EEG trait.[26] A different pattern of epileptogenicity is revealed by studies of posttraumatic epilepsy, which indicate that injury to the perirolandic region is most likely to give rise to seizures[87] and that frontal and temporal lesions are more epileptogenic than those in parietal and occipital areas.[31,91]

ETIOLOGY AND BASIC MECHANISMS

There are no specific causes or pathophysiologic substrates of the various anatomically defined epileptic disorders, with the exception of hippocampal sclerosis, which underlies most cases of MTLE (discussed in Chapters 13, 41, and 247). Any insult, lesion, or primary genetic abnormality capable of producing a localized epileptogenic region can account for the localization-related epileptic disorders classified by cerebral lobe. There are, for example, variants of the idiopathic benign childhood epilepsy with centrotemporal spikes that appear to originate in other cortical areas.[122]

CLINICAL PRESENTATION

The symptomatic localization-related epilepsies discussed in detail below include only those for which there is reasonable documentation. Much of the information is derived from recently reported series using currently available technologies with localization often confirmed by surgery.

CLINICAL CHARACTERISTICS OF SEIZURES RELATED TO ANATOMIC REGION OF ORIGIN

Temporal Lobe Epilepsy

Wieser[206] extensively evaluated a limited number of carefully studied patients and concluded that there were five different types of "psychomotor" seizures. Four of these were of temporal lobe origin. While this concept failed to achieve wide acceptance, much of what he concluded remains valid, and it did direct attention toward the possibility of different temporal lobe epilepsy syndromes.

Mesial Temporal Lobe Seizures

Currently, temporal lobe epilepsy is divided into two types: Those with seizures originating in the medial temporal structures (MTLE), and those with seizures beginning elsewhere in the temporal lobe (e.g., neocortical temporal lobe epilepsy or lateral temporal lobe epilepsy). MTLE refers to a specific subset of patients with seizures originating in the medial temporal lobe structures (mesial temporal lobe seizures [MTLSs]); MTLE with hippocampal sclerosis (MTLE-HS) comprises the great majority of patients with MTLE. Although MTLE-HS is characterized by many features that are not shared by conditions with MTLS caused by other lesions, the seizures themselves are indistinguishable. For purposes of this chapter on anatomic classification, therefore, MTLE, with and without HS, need not be further discussed here, as the phenomenology is described extensively in Chapter 247. MTLE, however, serves as a prototypical benchmark for localization-related epilepsies. As noted previously, one of the first steps used to identify other anatomic symptomatic focal epilepsies is to examine them in comparison to MTLE to determine how far they stray from the typical syndrome.

Neocortical Temporal Lobe Epilepsy

Since the lateral temporal cortex only comprises a portion of the temporal neocortex, the preferred terms here are neocortical temporal lobe epilepsy (NTLE) and neocortical temporal lobe seizures (NTLSs).

Several reviews of temporal lobe epilepsy do not even attempt to differentiate medial from neocortical temporal lobe seizures.[102,133,208] A review specifically addressing the issue of neocortical temporal lobe epilepsy concludes that currently there is very little information about this type of epilepsy and that distinguishing seizure characteristics do not exist.[203] Patients with neocortical temporal lobe seizure origin are rare, particularly if examples with obvious epileptogenic lesions are excluded. Although exact statistics are not available, a reasonable estimate would be that <10% of patients with temporal lobe epilepsy, who do not have obvious circumscribed lesions, have seizure origin in the temporal neocortex. Patients with seizures due to temporal neocortical lesions are also uncommon. In one study spanning 14 years from a large epilepsy center, only ten examples of neocortical temporal lesional epilepsy were identified.[173]

One study comparing mesial versus neocortical temporal lobe seizures found very little difference in terms of risk factors, demographics, and scalp EEG patterns.[27] The only significant difference was increased lateralized memory impairment during intracarotid Amytal testing in patients with MTLSs. There was a trend toward early risk factors (below age 2 years) in the patients with MTLSs. Clinical seizure characteristics were not examined. An important contribution of this study is that patients with lateral temporal lobe seizure origin (none of whom had detectable lesions) had surgical outcomes as good as those associated with mesial temporal lobe seizure origin. This is in contrast to other studies reporting less favorable postsurgical results in patients with nonlesional lateral temporal lobe epilepsy.[76,184]

Extensive reciprocal connections between lateral temporal neocortex and medial limbic structures might explain why clinical features of seizures could be similar and possibly indistinguishable from both regions.[22,69,207] Even the auras may require participation of both areas.[22,69]

Nevertheless, despite some generally negative results obtained in attempting to define lateral temporal lobe seizures, there are some features that may help identify them. Auditory, vertiginous, and complex visual hallucinations have been equated with lateral temporal origin.[12,212] No one in a large "pure culture" of patients with MTLSs had this type of aura.[55] One study comparing patients with hippocampal sclerosis and temporal lobe tumors, however, did report auditory, visual, and vertiginous auras in both patient groups.[173] Three studies have noted that the motor manifestations observed in MTLSs are less common in lateral temporal seizures.[52,67,173] There are some scalp EEG and neuroimaging findings that might help distinguish the two types of temporal lobe seizures.[43,44,76,202]

During the past 10 years, additional converging evidence has been provided that there are some characteristics that can help differentiate seizures associated with MTLE from those originating in the temporal neocortex.[29,53,68,119,126,148] Patients with NTLSs have no history of febrile convulsions and have experiential auras (auditory and other sensory/experiential illusions and hallucinations, but not fear), early contralateral dystonic posturing in the absence of oral alimentary automatisms, early loss of contact and shorter seizure duration, and greater propensity to generalize compared to patients with MTLSs. Patients with MTLSs often have a history of febrile seizures (usually complicated), younger onset, evidence of hippocampal sclerosis on MRI, auras of visceral sensations, fear or olfactory hallucinations (rare), dreamy state, early oral alimentary automatisms, delayed contralateral dystonic posturing, and less tendency to generalize compared to patients with NTLS. All authors stress the importance of early findings in differentiating the two conditions. Many of the clinical seizure characteristics described in autosomal dominant lateral temporal epilepsy are the same as described here in neocortical temporal lobe seizures.[132]

Frontal Lobe Epilepsy

Patients with seizures originating in the frontal lobes are the second most common to have localized surgical resections.[93,99,161–163,223] Frontal lobe seizures are not rare but, because of lack of familiarity with some of the clinical manifestations, they are often misdiagnosed.[96,205,211,214,217,219,220] Before 1985, scattered reports described different types of frontal lobe seizures,[4,63,65,125,151,193] but during the past 20 years, there has been heightened interest in frontal lobe seizures as reflected in the publications from two symposia specifically concerning this topic.[34,90] A current PubMed search of frontal lobe seizures from 2000 to 2006 yields 907 citations.

Whereas MTLSs are all similar with differences representing variations on a theme, the same is not true for frontal lobe seizures. A number of entirely different seizure types are associated with frontal lobe origin. Initially, because of protean clinical seizure manifestations, frontal lobe seizures seemed to defy classification into subtypes,[213] but recently some order has begun to shape this formerly chaotic situation. Frontal lobe seizures can now be grouped into six broad categories: Focal clonic motor seizures, asymmetric tonic seizures, frontal lobe hyperkinetic (psychomotor, hypermotor, complex partial) seizures, frontal lobe absence seizures, frontal opercular seizures, and frontal lobe seizures that closely resemble typical MTLSs, recognizing that there can be some admixture among the different types.[32,33,92,99,205,211,212]

Focal Clonic Motor Seizures

When focal clonic motor seizures occur in isolation, they are not associated with impaired consciousness and reflect ictal activity in the primary motor area. Focal clonic motor seizures are often part of other frontal and extrafrontal secondary activations of the primary motor cortex. They are discussed in detail in Chapter 44.

Asymmetric Tonic Seizures

Supplementary motor area (SMA) seizures are the classic type of asymmetric tonic seizures. SMA seizures were first described over 50 years ago.[5,150,151] Renewed interest in this relatively uncommon seizure type is reflected in recent publications describing both clinical seizure manifestations and cortical stimulation studies.[13,14,38,56,58,72,92,113,135,159,164,212,214,220] Despite the often dramatic and identifiable clinical seizure manifestations, the frequent absence of EEG abnormalities can still lead to the erroneous diagnosis of nonepileptic psychogenic attacks in patients with SMA seizures.[58,96]

SMA seizures can have subjective symptoms that include bilateral, contralateral, and ipsilateral somatosensory sensations of tightness, pressure, numbness, or tingling. This is fairly common, causing some investigators to prefer the term "supplementary sensorimotor area."[38] A nonspecific general feeling of constriction or tightness can immediately precede visible motor activity. Because the majority of patients do not report specific somatosensory symptoms, the preferred term remains *SMA seizures*.[92] The objective manifestations of SMA seizures usually begin with the sudden, often explosive, assumption of a fixed posture, classically with the arm contralateral to the side of seizure origin abducted at the shoulder, externally rotated, and flexed at the elbow with the head and eyes deviated as if looking at the up-raised hand.[4] The leg on the side contralateral to seizure origin can be held in rigid extension or can be flexed at the hip. Forced vocalization can occur, usually repeated vowel sounds rather than formed words. More often, there is speech arrest. Seizures are brief, lasting seconds, and only rarely last longer than 1 minute. Toward the end of the seizure, there can be clonic motor twitches of the hand or face. These seizures can secondarily generalize into tonic–clonic seizures. Even when generalized convulsive seizures occur, the postictal clinical and EEG suppression is often surprisingly short when compared to other convulsive generalized seizures.[220] If they do not secondarily generalize, they stop as suddenly as they start. They can occur in clusters of many seizures per day. Nocturnal preponderance is common, but there are many exceptions. Patients with SMA seizures are often conscious during seizures. There seems to be no fundamental difference in terms of lateralization or clinical seizure characteristics that determines whether or not consciousness is impaired during SMA seizures. Responsiveness, however, often is not tested during these typically brief seizures. When given test phrases or words during these seizures with intense bilateral motor activity, one is often surprised to discover that patients clearly recall the test phrase during the immediate postictal period.

The classic motor manifestations of SMA seizures are probably the exception rather than the rule. Although to some extent representing variations on a theme, the motor manifestations of SMA seizures among different patients can differ widely, though they are usually stereotyped for a given patient.[14,38,58,92,99,135,145,164,220] Motor manifestations in relatively well-documented examples of SMA seizures can include symmetric tonic or dystonic posturing of both upper and lower extremities; unilateral rigid straight tonic upper extremity posturing; adducted, flexed posturing of the upper extremity with the fist clenched; flailing, thrashing movements of the ipsilateral arm; kicking and stepping activity of the lower extremities; tonic/dystonic posturing involving the contralateral lower extremity; and athetoid dystonic movements of the contralateral hand, arm, leg, or both.[214,217,220] SMA seizures can rarely present with automatisms without tonic motor activity.[92,211]

Startle epilepsy with asymmetric tonic seizures of presumed SMA origin has been the topic of several reports.[36,92,144,177] SMA origin was documented in some, but not all, of the reported patients. Similarly, reflex seizures due to more casual somatosensory stimuli (i.e., movement or rubbing) have been attributed to SMA seizure origin,[95,154] but SMA origin was not documented in any of these patients. In some of these patients seizures probably began in the parietal cortex.[95]

Both positive (tonic) and negative (atonic) motor activity have been attributed to SMA seizure activity.[95,131] Gelastic seizures in the absence of mirth have been described as a part of SMA seizures.[19,33] Finally, many of the features of SMA seizures seen in adults are also seen in children.[13]

Despite a wealth of reports on SMA seizures, some confusion persists, largely because asymmetric tonic seizures can be evoked practically anywhere in the neocortex.[3,83,215,216] In many of the reports of SMA seizures, origin of seizures is not well documented. In a careful study of four patients with asymmetric tonic seizures, various MRI lesions, and good surgical results, seizure origin was documented in the SMA in only one patient.[86] Two of these patients had seizure origin in the lateral frontal regions and the other patient had seizures beginning in the medial parietal cortex. All propagated to the SMA. These authors emphasized that asymmetric "SMA-type" seizures do not equate with SMA origin. These same authors, in a later report, examined clinical progression patterns in ten patients with presumed SMA seizures. SMA origin was based on clinical seizure characteristics and scalp EEG findings. Only three patients had intracranial studies, while two patients had parietal lesions on MRI. In an earlier report, they described two patients with parietal lesions and asymmetric tonic seizures.[83] Another study of SMA seizures with tonic limb posturing found the posturing to have poor localizing and lateralizing results in 14 patients studied with intracranial electrodes. Eleven patients had surgery and only three became free of seizures.[3] The lack of specificity of asymmetric tonic seizures has been well documented in earlier reports.[64,214–216,220] Although it is often assumed that these tonic motor manifestations represent spread to the SMA,[3,83,84] this has seldom been proven[215] and sometimes has been specifically denied.[64]

Considering the sometimes confusing and conflicting data associated with seizures of SMA origin, can they be diagnosed with any degree of accuracy? The scalp EEG in patients with SMA seizures is notoriously inaccurate and may be misleading or completely uninformative.[15,33,54,179,184,200] A recent paper describing ictal and interictal magnetoencephalography in patients with medial/frontal lobe epilepsy reported good results but provided no evidence to verify the findings.[179] Ictal SPECT was used to study eight patients with presumed seizure origin in the SMA.[113] The importance of early (5 seconds or less) isotope injection was emphasized. Excellent results were realized in all eight patients. The ictal SPECT results in part explained the clinical seizure characteristics. Outcome was excellent in the five patients who had surgery. In a recent paper examining frontal lobe seizures in general, seven had seizure origins located in the SMA.[92] While not specifically stated, ictal SPECT was used to direct intracranial electrode placements in many of the patients included in this study. Of the seven patients with SMA seizure onset who had surgery, five are seizure free and one has had brief nocturnal seizures. The one patient with a poor result had a major postoperative complication that resulted in death 2 years later. No seizures occurred after surgery, but the patient was in a persistent vegetative state. Although normal MRI is said to predict less favorable outcomes,[50] the six patients from the Dartmouth series with good outcomes all had normal MRIs.[92] A small series of patients with presumed SMA seizure origin studied with invasive recording all experienced good results following surgery.[14]

SMA seizures, because of associated findings, may be a diagnostic entity. SMA seizures can often be recognized by the company they keep. Patients with brief, asymmetric tonic seizures with a sudden explosive onset and maintenance of consciousness, usually with speech arrest, nocturnal clustering, and normal or nonspecific EEG findings, have what might be considered to be an SMA epilepsy syndrome. This will not define all patients with SMA seizures. One of the seven patients with well-documented SMA seizure origin in the report by Jobst et al.[92] had the bizarre frontal lobe hyperkinetic seizures described in the next section.

A syndrome of autosomal dominant nocturnal frontal lobe epilepsy (ADNFLE) has been well defined recently[37,156] (Chapter 249). This phenotypic expression of ADNFLE is the result of at least three different genetic mutations with the majority of patients having, as yet, no recognized genetic marker. Seizure types associated with ADNFLE include asymmetric tonic seizures and hyperkinetic behavioral seizures described in the next section. Most of these patients respond well to antiepileptic drugs, so documentation of SMA origin has not been possible. Until recently, many of these patients, as well as nonfamilial forms, were thought to be suffering with a sleep disorder labeled nocturnal paroxysmal dystonia.[10,157,175]

Frontal Lobe Hyperkinetic Seizures (Frontal Lobe Seizures with Bizarre Behaviors, Hypermotor Seizures, and Frontal Lobe Complex Partial Seizures)

Certain types of peculiar nonconvulsive frontal lobe seizures occur with prominent motor activity but without tonic posturing. These seizures have been variably labeled frontal lobe complex partial seizures, frontal lobe seizures with bizarre behaviors, hypermotor seizures, and hyperkinetic seizures. The current preferred term is *hyperkinetic seizures*.[23] Isolated reports of these seizures date back to 1972,[193] and hints of their recognition can be found as early as 1954.[151] Several subsequent reports described patients with very unusual seizures of presumed frontal lobe origin.[62,63,65,125] The first detailed report of a series of these patients carefully studied with intracranial electrodes appeared in 1985.[211] Later reports confirmed the existence of this peculiar type of frontal lobe seizure disorder, which has now been extensively well defined.[40,92,103,188,205,213,214,217,220] The peculiar hyperkinetic automatisms are thought to be fairly specific for this type of frontal lobe seizure.[103] A recent report, however, did describe nocturnal hyperkinetic seizures of temporal lobe origin.[140] Although not specifically described, the frontal lobe system responsible for these ictal behaviors can presumably be accessed by other cortical areas as well.

Frontal lobe hyperkinetic seizures (FLHSs) usually occur frequently, often in clusters of many per 24 hours. As with SMA seizures, a nocturnal preponderance is common. The seizures are brief, lasting <1 minute with little or no postictal confusion. Motor automatisms are prominent and complex, beginning suddenly with a frenetic or agitated appearance. In some patients, aggressive sexual activity is a prominent part of the automatic motor activity.[63,185] Vocalization commonly occurs, varying from simple humming to growling and barking to shouted obscenities. Warnings are frequent but usually nonspecific. In approximately half of the patients with FLHSs, there is a history of nonconvulsive status epilepticus, which is often documented during evaluation[92,210] (see also Chapter 59). These attacks have a very bizarre, hysterical appearance, but they are stereotyped for each patient. As with other types of frontal lobe seizures, there can be transition forms between this seizure type and those of SMA origin, with some patients exhibiting components of both. Another important transition form occurs when there is delayed spread to medial temporal structures. In this situation, seizures will begin as FLHSs but then transition into the less dramatic MTLSs.[92] Focal clonic motor activity can also occur, but it is usually not a part of FLHSs. There is no specific region within the frontal lobe in which these seizures originate. They have been described with seizures of orbital frontal origin,[32,92,125,193,211] with seizures of mesial frontal origin (including the SMA),[92,205,211] and with seizures of frontal polar and dorsal convexity origin.[92,160]

Similar to SMA seizures, interictal and even ictal EEGs are often unrevealing in patients with FLHSs. This, coupled with the usually bizarre atypical appearance of these seizures, frequently leads to the erroneous diagnosis of psychogenic, nonepileptic seizures.[211,217] These seizures, however, are recognizable by virtue of their clinical characteristics alone; therefore, awareness of these characteristics is essential. Some specific features may help differentiate frontal lobe seizures in general from psychogenic seizures.[172] Features such as pelvic thrusting, side-to-side head movements, and kicking and a history of psychiatric diseases that have been used to define psychogenic seizures are also seen in FLHSs, whereas nocturnal preponderance, short seizure duration, young age at seizure onset, and prone position during seizures are more characteristic of FLHSs.

Analogous to SMA seizures, FLHSs are associated with a constellation of findings. These include often bizarre but stereotyped seizures, frequent brief seizures that occur in clusters with a nocturnal preponderance, normal or nonspecific interictal and ictal EEG patterns, and often normal MRI. All of these characteristics taken together could also constitute a syndrome. As noted previously, these seizures are also a part of the ADNFLE syndrome (see Chapter 249).

Frontal Lobe Absence Seizures

Rarely, frontal lobe seizures can present with absence seizures.[93,105,112,167] A variety of absence status of the elderly may be of frontal lobe origin.[194,195]

Frontal Opercular Seizures

Seizures beginning in the frontal operculum have been described infrequently.[92,171,180,189] Opercular seizures consist of profuse salivation, oral facial apraxia, and possibly some focal facial clonic activity. To some extent, they resemble the opercular syndrome due to fixed lesions.[35]

Frontal Lobe Seizures Resembling Temporal Lobe Seizures

Seizures confined to the frontal lobes will have features resembling those previously described (i.e., frontal lobe absence, asymmetric tonic seizures, frontal lobe hyperkinetic seizures, and frontal opercular seizures).[93] Some FLHSs, particularly those originating in the orbital frontal region, will spread to the medial temporal structures. As previously discussed clinically, a bizarre FLHS will evolve into a more bland, temporal lobe–type seizure.[214,220] Other examples of orbital frontal seizure origin present with pure temporal lobe seizure manifestations, including scalp EEG findings.[92,178,183] This may be a particular feature of seizure origin in the medial posterior orbital frontal cortex. When this happens in patients without MRI-detected lesions, the potential for diagnostic error is very high.

Occipital Lobe Epilepsy

The prevalence and incidence of occipital lobe epilepsy documented with modern diagnostic technology is not known, but it is generally considered rare. In an older series reported by Gibbs and Gibbs,[66] occipital lobe seizures were thought to occur in 8% of 3,271 cases with focal partial epilepsy. In the large Montreal surgical series between 1928 and 1973, 25 of 1,702 patients without tumors, who underwent surgery for epilepsy, had occipital lobe seizures.[162] Six contemporary series of patients with well-documented occipital lobe seizure origin have been reported: Two examining seizures from the posterior hemispheres[21,39] and four specifically looking at occipital lobe seizures.[24,118,168,216] There have also been several reviews of occipital lobe seizures and epilepsies.[20,169,187,191,219] All contemporary reports on occipital lobe epilepsy are remarkable in the consistency of their findings, recognizing that many of the symptoms have been observed for more than 100 years,[70,71,88] and some of the "newly discovered" observations were reported 50 years ago.[5]

Occipital lobe seizures, as defined by subjective symptoms and objective signs, can be recognized by clinical seizure characteristics in most cases. Some clinical symptoms and signs reflect occipital lobe seizure origin, whereas others are indicative of spread anteriorly from the occipital lobe medially and laterally, above and below the sylvian fissure and contralaterally via the splenium of the corpus callosum with the potential for multiple additional spread patterns.[20,39,168,169,191,216] The manifestations of these multiple and highly variable seizure spread patterns are often the most prominent feature of these seizures, tending to overshadow more subtle findings of occipital lobe origin, leading to diagnostic error.

Elementary visual hallucinations, usually consisting of flashing or steady spots or simple geometric forms, either colored or achromatic, are the most common occipital lobe seizure symptoms. When lateralized, they occur contralateral to the side of seizure origin. They may be stationary or move across the visual field. Ictal amaurosis is the second most common symptom of occipital seizure origin.[24,168,187,216] This symptom, though not universally appreciated, has been consistently described.[7,9,20,149,166,168,198,216] Blindness can be limited to one visual field, but more often is bilateral, consisting of visual blackouts of vision or, rarely, whiteouts.[216] Bilateral (complete) ictal amaurosis implies early spread to the contralateral occipital lobe as previously discussed. An aura of eye movement sensation without detectable eye movement has been reported.[81,216]

Forced blinking or eyelid flutter at the very beginning of seizures can be objective evidence of occipital lobe origin.[24,136,146,216] Both tonic and clonic eye deviation have been noted, with the former much more common than the latter.[18,136,168,216] Concurrent head deviation may or may not be present. Oculoclonic status epilepticus has been reported.[94] Although eye deviation is usually contralateral to the side of seizure origin, ipsilateral eye deviation can occur.[168,216] Other features of occipital lobe epilepsy include ictal vomiting and other autonomic manifestations.[24,73,191] A series of carefully studied surgical patients were examined to determine whether there were differences between medial and lateral occipital seizure origins.[24] The only clear difference was absence of a field cut with lateral onset. There were no clinical seizure features that distinguished the two.

The important fact that seizures originating in the occipital lobe can have the potential for multiple different spread patterns was recognized almost 50 years ago,[5] and has been a consistent finding in recent reports.[20,24,73,118,168,191,216] Symptoms of spread outside of the occipital lobe include somatosensory auras and complex visual and auditory hallucinations. Signs of anterior spread from the occipital lobe include focal clonic activity (lateral, superior), asymmetric tonic seizures (medial superior), and various types of automatisms (inferior). These latter seizures are said to be indistinguishable from those seen in temporal lobe epilepsy.[149,168,169,216] Since most of the clinical seizure characteristics that occur after seizure origin reflect specific spread patterns, occipital lobe seizures can present with a wide variety of clinical patterns that do not reflect occipital lobe seizure origin but that do suggest seizure activity elsewhere. To further confound the issue, some patients exhibit different spread patterns during different seizures, thereby suggesting multifocal disease.[118,216] Static visual field defects, which help identify occipital lobe seizures, are reported in over half the patients in most recent studies.[168,216]

Neuroimaging detects occipital lobe structural abnormalities in up to three quarters of patients with occipital lobe seizures.[118,168,169,216] Focal cortical dysplasia, as a cause of occipital lobe epilepsy, may be undetectable, although newer high-resolution MRI makes this less common. Older literature included birth injury with anoxia in a high proportion of patients with occipital lobe epilepsy.[162] Other causes of occipital lobe seizures include Sturge-Weber variant or celiac disease with occipital lobe calcifications.[9,137,152,197] Occipital lobe seizures can occur in patients with hyperglycemia[78,204] and in women with eclampsia.[155]

Three benign idiopathic childhood epilepsy syndromes with occipital lobe seizures have been described.[59–61,106,110,196] These consist of an early type (Panayiotopoulos syndrome), a late type (Gastaut type), and a juvenile type with photic sensitivity (for a review see Taylor et al.[191]; also see Chapters 236, 237, and 257). The early-onset childhood epilepsy may not always have occipital features.[110] The early type is also noteworthy for the propensity to develop nonconvulsive status with pronounced autonomic features.

The prognosis of occipital lobe epilepsy usually relates to the cause. Permanent cortical blindness can occur following repeated occipital lobe seizures.[7] The prognosis of the benign childhood forms, as the name implies, is usually benign with complete resolution, in most but not all, by 19 years.[61] The clinical characteristics of the late childhood type (Gastaut type) of benign occipital epilepsy are identical to those with chronic symptomatic occipital lobe epilepsy, and the two must be differentiated if surgical intervention is being considered.

Occipital lobe resection can be very effective in controlling medically intractable occipital lobe seizures, particularly when lesions are present.[20,168,169,216] This includes patients with celiac disease and occipital calcifications.[137] Partially or completely intact visual fields contralateral to the side of seizure origin can be converted to complete homonymous hemianopsias. Because most patients adjust to this visual neurologic deficit, homonymous hemianopsia is usually acceptable if medically intractable disabling seizures can be eliminated.[216] However, because postoperative field cuts are often not as severe as would be predicted, there may be reorganization of the visual cortex in some patients.[108] Patients with lateral occipital epileptogenic lesions can often be spared visual field deficits.[24,169] Patients with occipital lobe seizures consistently spreading into the ipsilateral temporal lobe usually do not do well following temporal lobectomy,[149,216] but there are exceptions.[146] Finally, cortical resections in the posterior regions are not associated with cognitive impairments, provided language areas are spared.[123]

Parietal Lobe Epilepsy

Certain clinical characteristics of seizures arising in the parietal lobes have been recognized since antiquity,[192] but patients with these kinds of seizures are uncommon. Parietal lobe seizures constitute no >5% of all partial seizures from surgical series.[162]

There have been several recent reports and reviews examining the clinical seizure characteristics, electroencephalographic findings, and neuroimaging results in patients with well-documented parietal lobe seizure origin.[6,21,30,39,80,100,187,215] Although there were some minor differences among these recent reports on parietal lobe seizures, most findings were consistent.

As with most focal seizures, there are subjective and objective manifestations of parietal lobe seizures. The most common symptoms are paresthesias consisting of numbness and tingling, sometimes described as a "pins and needles" sensation and, less commonly, as a feeling of crawling or itching. Ictal paresthesias, however, occurred in less than half of the patients reported in some series, and were not always correctly lateralizing.[30,80,215] One study, however, found somatosensory auras reliably lateralizing.[89]

Although pain has been recognized as an ictal phenomenon at least since Jackson's time,[88] it is considered rare.[114,199,209,224] Young and Blume[225] examined ictal pain in a series of patients and three types of pain were recognized. The most common was a burning dysesthetic sensation involving part or all of the hemibody opposite to the side of parietal lobe seizure origin. The second type was abdominal pain, sometimes severe, associated with temporal lobe seizure origin. The third type was ictal headache or head pain that had no localizing value. Other reports examining parietal lobe seizures described lateralized abdominal pain.[30,187] Other reports on epileptic pain described lateralized dysesthesias, abdominal pain, and head pain, all in patients with parietal lobe seizure origin.[181,221] Ictal abdominal pain has also been related to an intracranial parietal hemorrhage.[153]

Because pain is not thought to be a cortical sensation, this ictal manifestation might involve activation of corticothalamic circuits. Painful epileptic symptoms, however, have also been equated with seizure activity in the second sensory area,[225] as has widespread numbness.[224] Ictal pain can also be a manifestation of primary sensory cortex involvement.[153]

In a review of parietal lobe seizures, Sveinbjornsdottir and Duncan,[187] in addition to paresthetic, dysesthetic, and painful symptoms, described parietal lobe ictal sensations that included sexual sensations, apraxias, and disturbance of body image. Ictal vertiginous sensations have been attributed to seizure activity in the temporal parietal junction.[97] Gustatory hallucinations have been equated with seizures in the parietal operculum.[79] Some ictal parietal lobe dysfunction would never be detected except in extraordinary circumstances. For example, a patient in the Montreal program[151] had a seizure restricted to the parietal lobe while undergoing electrocorticography under local anesthesia. Two-point discrimination was impaired during the seizure but returned to normal when the seizure terminated. Some parietal lobe seizure symptoms can resemble panic attacks.[8] Parietal lobe seizures can occasionally be induced by complex somatosensory stimulation.[215] There is a case report of hot water–induced seizures related to a focal area of parietal cortical malformation.[116] Other unusual reported findings associated with parietal lobe seizure origin include expressive aprosody and amusica,[16] autoscopy,[127] kinetopsia,[111] and atonic seizures.[170]

Objective manifestations of seizures in the more anterior inferior aspects of the language-dominant parietal lobe would include the expected disorders of speech. If a seizure discharge remained confined to the parietal lobe and produced various apraxias and agnosias, the patient might present in a confused, disoriented state, but this could be true for seizures from almost anywhere. Most objective ictal manifestations of parietal lobe seizures reflect spread of seizure activity anteriorly into the frontal lobe, inferiorly into the temporal lobe, or posteriorly into the occipital lobe.[6] Tonic motor activity, automatisms, or both can occur in patients with documented parietal lobe seizure origin.[64,80,215] In a patient studied with intracranial electrodes, asymmetric tonic posturing occurred with spread to the ipsilateral supplementary motor area,[215] but another study using invasive monitoring did not find that relationship.[64] Subsequently, asymmetric tonic posturing in parietal lobe seizures resembling frontal lobe seizures has been reported repeatedly.[6,100,138] Secondary involvement of the medial temporal structures with associated automatisms has been documented during intracranial recording in patients with parietal lobe seizure origin.[57,64,215] Based on intracranial recording, two patients with unsuspected parietal lobe seizure origin underwent unsuccessful temporal lobectomy in the series reported by Ho et al.,[80] as did two patients from the Yale series.[215] Parietal lobe seizure origin was determined by detecting lesions using previously unavailable MRI and verified by successful surgery in the latter two patients. Ho et al.[80] determined parietal lobe seizure origin in their patients with ictal SPECT, including the two with previous unsuccessful temporal lobectomies.

There is a possible relationship between the location of parietal lobe seizure origin and the clinical seizure manifestations. Anterior parietal lobe lesions or seizure origin can be associated with initial ictal sensorimotor phenomena, whereas posterior seizure origin can be associated with more complex symptomatology.[30,80] Posterior parietal lobe complex partial seizures were described as "psychoparetic,"[80] which implied a psychic aura, such as fear or déjà vu followed by motionlessness and loss of consciousness. Parietal lobe onset seizures are associated with short postictal periods, even if they progress to complex partial seizures or secondarily generalized seizures[80] similar to that reported for frontal lobe seizures.[211,220] Some patients had elementary visual symptoms, presumably due to posterior spread, suggesting occipital lobe onset.[30,215]

Patients from several studies aimed at defining parietal lobe epilepsy all had epileptogenic parietal lobe lesions.[6,30,215] Because most of these patients had no clear lateralizing parietal sensory aura and the clinical seizure manifestations reflected spread outside of the parietal lobe, it can be concluded that a parietal lobe syndrome cannot be well defined. Although it can be argued that patients who present with consistently lateralized paresthesias and dysesthesias and possibly abdominal pain as part of their seizures may be identified as having a high likelihood of having parietal lobe seizure origin, focal tonic seizure activity and seizures with automatisms cannot be considered criteria for or against parietal lobe seizure origin. The salient point regarding parietal lobe seizures is that they can present with all these variable manifestations, and sometimes with more than one seizure type occurring during different seizures in the same patient analogous to that seen in occipital lobe seizures.[100,215,216] Parietal lobe origin should therefore be considered in those patients who do not have clear evidence for seizure origin elsewhere. Ictal SPECT may provide localizing data not otherwise obtainable in these difficult cases[80] (see Chapter 81).

When parietal lobe seizures are refractory to medications, surgery is an option. Because, with the exception of the postrolandic gyrus, much of the parietal lobe is silent with respect to seizure symptoms, initial clinical manifestations will often reflect seizure spread outside of the parietal lobe.[6,139,215] Furthermore, scalp EEG findings may not be helpful and may even be misleading. Therefore, in the absence of a detectable parietal lesion, the presurgical evaluation can proceed in the wrong direction.[80,215] Although ictal SPECT can be helpful, lack of early seizure manifestations could preclude early injections. Nevertheless, when parietal lobe seizure origin could be documented, surgical results were good.[6,21,30,39,100,120,215] There is a report of a remarkable case of atypical Lennox-Gastaut syndrome that was dramatically improved by removing a parietal convexity dysembryoplastic tumor.[158] A patient with painful seizures who developed medically refractory nonconvulsive status epilepticus was cured following a medial parietal resection.[138] New cognitive deficits after parietal surgery have been evaluated and found to be relatively minor.[123]

Insular Lobe Seizures

Insular lobe involvement in temporal lobe seizures is a recognized common spread pattern.[85] In the past, the clinical features of seizures starting in the insula were thought to be indistinguishable from medial temporal lobe seizures, thus accounting for some of the surgical failures following temporal lobectomy.[74,147] Furthermore, surgery was often considered too risky because the insula is located just lateral to the lenticulostriate arteries.[174] Recent reports dispute these assumptions by providing evidence that insular surgery can be done safely, albeit not without risk.[42,86]

Isnard et al.[85,86] described a series of patients with presumed temporal lobe epilepsy who were carefully studied with intracranial electrodes. They found that 10% of these patients had consistent seizure origin in the insula and not the hippocampus. A fairly stereotyped sequence of clinical events was observed, including a sequence of unpleasant, sometimes painful laryngeal constriction followed by dysesthesias, perioral or involving extensive cutaneous areas, then dysarthria, and culminating in focal clonic activity of the face and arm, all with full consciousness. Another case report of insular seizures documented these sensory phenomena and associated them with an unpleasant taste.[165]

Two reports by Duffau et al.[41,42] address the issue of resective surgery in the insular lobe in a series of patients with low-grade gliomas. Postoperative morbidity was high but cleared completely in 3 months in most patients. Three patients, however, were left with a permanent hemiparesis due to compromise of lenticulostriate arteries.

DIAGNOSTIC EVALUATION

Accurate localization of the anatomic substrate of an epileptic disorder, as opposed to identification of a specific pathologic substrate, is only of clinical value when resective surgical treatment is being considered. In this situation, classification merely by lobe is inadequate to plan a resective procedure, and localization by clinical seizure characteristics and interictal scalp EEG is too often misleading to be used alone as an indication for surgical intervention.[120] When a discrete structural lesion is identified on MRI, the ictal clinical characteristics and location of interictal EEG spikes may be sufficient to confirm an anatomic diagnosis, although ictal EEGs are also usually performed prior to surgery to be sure that the intractable habitual seizures are the same as those arising from the presumed epileptogenic lesion. Focal functional deficits, as demonstrated by neurologic examination, neuropsychological testing, and functional neuroimaging such as PET, can offer additional confirmatory evidence when localization is equivocal. Ictal SPECT is becoming increasingly important in presurgical evaluations, particularly when the MRI is normal.[16,75,92,101,182,201]

The importance of very early injection in rapidly propagating neocortical seizures cannot be overemphasized.[115,201] It is important to recognize that structural lesions in patients with localization-related epilepsy occasionally may be fortuitous findings and unrelated to the epileptogenic process, and that interictal EEG spikes can propagate widely to predominate at a distance from the primary epileptogenic region. When localization is uncertain, particularly in patients with focal epilepsy who have normal MRI scans but stereotyped clinical seizure characteristics indicating the likelihood of a single discrete epileptogenic region, chronic recording with intracranial electrodes is generally performed. Depth electrodes are usually preferred when the epileptogenic region is presumed to be in deep limbic structures of the brain, whereas subdural grids or strips are commonly used to delineate neocortical epileptogenic regions. Because all these diagnostic approaches are those used in presurgical evaluation, the reader is referred to the chapters on diagnosis (Chapters 167–175) in the section in this book on surgical treatment for epilepsy. The objective of the presurgical evaluation is to precisely locate and delineate the epileptogenic region, and not merely to make an anatomic diagnosis.[124]

DIFFERENTIAL DIAGNOSIS

No specific issues of differential diagnosis are peculiar to the anatomic classification of focal epilepsies. The distinction between these disorders and those associated with paroxysmal nonepileptic phenomena that can be mistaken for epilepsy is the same as for epilepsy in general. Certain types of focal epilepsies, such as those discussed under frontal lobe epilepsy, are particularly prone to misdiagnosis, and only familiarity with them will prevent mistakes. It is worthwhile to note, however, that seizures can arise from a single anatomic location when MRI reveals a diffuse cerebral structural abnormality that would not permit a discrete anatomic classification. Conversely, patients can have seizures arising from a discrete epileptogenic region that propagate so rapidly that they appear to be generalized from the start, making a correct anatomic classification difficult. An example of the former would be a patient with a large developmental lesion, such as schizencephaly, where only a small part is responsible for generating the habitual ictal events; such patients can often benefit from localized resective surgery,[115] but invasive electrophysiologic recording is usually necessary to characterize the anatomic localization of the epileptogenic region. An example of the latter would be a patient with a localized frontal lobe lesion that gives rise only to generalized seizures that appear to have no electroclinical localizing features. In this situation, evidence of a localized disturbance, either from structural neuroimaging or tests of focal functional deficit, is necessary before invasive electrophysiologic studies can be recommended.

TREATMENT AND OUTCOME

Pharmacotherapy for focal epilepsy is not dependent on anatomic diagnosis, and there is no evidence of differential responses to medication based on anatomic localization of a neocortical epileptogenic region, although mesial temporal lobe epilepsy may be uniquely refractory.[176] In patients with medically refractory seizures, surgical treatment depends largely on precise localization and delineation of the epileptogenic region rather than anatomic diagnosis, and outcome reflects the accuracy of this process and the ability to resect the abnormal tissue completely. Total resection may be limited by involvement of adjacent essential primary neocortex, which cannot be damaged, or by failure to correctly map the epileptogenic substrate, as can often be the case with MRI-negative localization-related epilepsy. When the epileptogenic region involves essential cortex, seizures may be relieved by removal of a structural lesion without cortical margins,[29] or by multiple subpial transection, which is designed to disconnect propagation of epileptic activity along the surface of the brain without disrupting functional columnar cortical organization.[134] Results of the surgical intervention are excellent in a condition where a discrete epileptogenic lesion is identified and a circumscribed adjacent area of epileptogenicity can be delineated; this is considered to be one of the surgically remediable syndromes, with 70% to 80% of patients becoming seizure free,[25] and surgical intervention is recommended as soon as first-line medications fail[50] (Chapters 127 and 168).

LONG-TERM PROGNOSIS

The long-term prognosis of localization-related epilepsy is determined by the pathophysiologic nature of the underlying substrate, and not by its anatomic location. Patients with discrete structural lesions as the cause of medically refractory epilepsy have the greatest chance of becoming seizure free, and remaining seizure free, following surgical resection, as opposed to patients with mesial temporal lobe epilepsy, who have a higher incidence of postoperative simple partial seizures, and patients with cryptogenic localization-related epilepsy, who are much more likely to have postoperative disabling seizures as well.[17,129] However, surgical results in MRI-negative localization-related epilepsy are also improving dramatically in some centers as we gain better understanding of clinical seizure patterns and develop new diagnostic techniques.[92,182]

SUMMARY AND CONCLUSIONS

The International Classification of Epilepsies and Epileptic Syndromes recognizes temporal lobe, frontal lobe, parietal lobe, and occipital lobe epilepsies as subtypes of the focal symptomatic epilepsies. With the exception of mesial temporal lobe epilepsy, these disorders describe seizure types rather than complexes of signs and symptoms that might be considered discrete syndromes. Some conditions with frontal lobe seizures and associated constellations of findings could, however, eventually be recognized as syndromes. A number of different characteristic seizures can be identified as indicative of epileptogenic regions in functionally distinct regions of these broad lobar designations. Furthermore, some seizure types are characteristic of epileptogenic regions that transcend lobar boundaries, particularly those arising in the perirolandic region, the perisylvian operculum and insula, and the temporal-parietal-occipital junction. Anatomic classification is of clinical value when surgical treatment is considered, but much more precise localization of the epileptogenic region is necessary before resection can be performed. In this situation, clinical seizure characteristics, routine EEG, and structural neuroimaging provide important localizing information, but more accurate delineation of a primary epileptogenic region for surgical resection usually requires ictal video-EEG monitoring, functional imaging, other tests of focal functional deficit, and, occasionally, intracranial EEG recording. Treatment and outcome are dependent more upon pathophysiologic substrate than anatomic localization, except in situations where surgical resection is limited by involvement of essential primary cortical areas or an inability to accurately define the boundaries of the epileptogenic region. Patients with medically refractory seizures due to discrete resectable structural lesions have an excellent long-term prognosis; this constitutes a surgically remediable form of epilepsy and is an indication for early surgical intervention. An understanding of the variety of focal seizure manifestations originating in different anatomic locations also helps prevent erroneous diagnoses of nonepileptic seizures by identifying specific unusual epileptic seizure types such as those originating in parts of the frontal lobes.

ACKNOWLEDGMENTS

Original research reported by J. E. was supported in part by Grants NS-02808, NS-15654, NS-33310, and GM-24839, from the National Institutes of Health, and Contract DE-AC03-76-SF00012 from the Department of Energy.

References

1. Commission on Classification and Terminology of the International League Against Epilepsy. Proposal for classification of epilepsies and epileptic syndromes. *Epilepsia*. 1985;26:268–278.
2. Commission on Classification and Terminology of the International League Against Epilepsy. Proposal for revised classification of epilepsies and epileptic syndromes. *Epilepsia*. 1989;30:389–399.
3. Aghakhani Y, Rosati A, Olivier A, et al. The predictive localizing value of tonic limb posturing in supplementary sensorimotor seizures. *Neurology*. 2004;62(12):2256–2261.
4. Ajmone-Marsan C. Clinical-electrographic correlations of partial seizures. In: Wada JA, ed. *Modern Perspectives in Epilepsy, Proceedings of the Inaugural Symposium of the Canadian League Against Epilepsy*. Montreal: Eden Press; 1978:76–98.
5. Ajmone-Marsan C, Ralston BL. *The Epileptic Seizures: Its Functional Morphology and Diagnostic Significance*. Springfield, IL: Charles C Thomas; 1957:211–215.
6. Akimura T, Fuji M, Ideguchi M, et al. Ictal onset and spreading of seizures of parietal lobe origin. *Neurol Med Chir (Tokyo)*. 2003;43:534–540.
7. Aldrich MS, Vanderzant CW, Alessi AG, et al. Ictal cortical blindness with permanent visual loss. *Epilepsia*. 1989;30:1216–1120.
8. Alemayehu S, Bergey GK, Barry E, et al. Panic attacks as ictal manifestations of parietal lobe seizures. *Epilepsia*. 1995;38(8):824–830.
9. Ambrosetto G, Antonini L, Tassinari CA. Occipital lobe seizures related to clinically asymptomatic celiac disease in adulthood. *Epilepsia*. 1992;33(3):476–481.
10. Arroyo S, Santamaria J, Setoain JF, et al. Nocturnal paroxysmal dystonia related to a prerolandic dysplasia. *Epilepsy Res*. 2001;43(1):1–9.
11. Bailey P, Gibbs FA. The surgical treatment of psychomotor epilepsy. *JAMA*. 1951;145:365–370.
12. Bancaud J, Talairach J, Bonis A, et al. *La Stéréo Éectronecephalographie dans l'Épilepsia*. Paris: Masson; 1965.
13. Bass N, Wyllie E, Comair Y, et al. Supplementary sensorimotor area seizures in children and adolescents. *J Pediatr*. 1995;126(4):537–544.
14. Baumgartner C, Flint R, Tuxhorn I, et al. Supplementary motor area seizures: propagation pathways as studied with invasive recordings. *Neurology*. 1996;46:508–514.
15. Bautista RE, Spencer DD, Spencer, SS. EEG findings in frontal lobe epilepsies. *Neurology*. 1998;50(6):1765–1771.
16. Bautista RE, Ciampetti MZ. Expressive aprosody and amusia as a manifestation of right hemisphere seizures. *Epilepsia*. 2003;44(3):466–467.
17. Berkovic SF, McIntosh AM, Kalnins RM, et al. Preoperative MRI predicts outcome of temporal lobectomy: an actuarial analysis. *Neurology*. 1995;45:1358–1363.

18. Beun AM, Beintema DJ, Binnie CD, et al. Epileptic nystagmus. *Epilepsia.* 1984;25(5)609–614.
19. Biraben A, Sartori E, Taussig D, et al. Gelastic seizures: video-EEG and scintigraphic analysis of a case with a frontal focus; review of the literature and pathophysiological hypotheses. *Epileptic Disord.* 1999;4:221–228.
20. Blume WT. Occipital lobe epilepsies. In: Lüders H, ed. *Epilepsy Surgery.* New York: Raven Press; 1991:167–171.
21. Blume WT, Whiting SE, Girvin J P. Epilepsy surgery in the posterior cortex. *Ann Neurol.* 1991;29:638–645.
22. Blume WR, Girvin JP, Stenerson P. temporal neocortical role in ictal experiential phenomena. *Ann Neurol.* 1993;33:105–107.
23. Blume WT, Lüders HO, Mizrahi E, et al. Glossary of descriptive terminology for ictal semiology: report of the ILAE Task Force on Classification and Terminology. *Epilepsia.* 2001;42(9):1212–1218.
24. Blume WT, Wiebe S, Tapsell LM. Occipital epilepsy: lateral versus mesial. *Brain.* 2005;128(Pt 5):1209–1225.
25. Boon PA, Williamson PD, Fried I, et al. Intracranial, intraaxial, space-occupying lesions in patients with intractable partial seizures: an anatomoclinical, neuropsychological, and surgical correlation. *Epilepsia.* 1991;32:467–476.
26. Bray PF, Wiser WC. Evidence for a genetic etiology of temporalcentral abnormalities in focal epilepsy. *N Engl J Med.* 1964;271:926–933.
27. Burgerman RS, Sperling MR, French JA, et al. Comparison of mesial versus neocortical onset temporal lobe seizures: neurodiagnostic findings and surgical outcome. *Epilepsia.* 1995;36(7):662–670.
28. Carne RP, O'Brien TJ, Kilpatrick CJ, et al. MRI-negative PET-positive temporal lobe epilepsy: a distinct surgically remediable syndrome. *Brain.* 2004;127(Pt 10):2276–2285.
29. Cascino GD, Kelly PJ, Hirschorn KA, et al. Stereotactic resection of intra-axial cerebral lesions in partial epilepsy. *Mayo Clinic Proc.* 1990;65:1053–1060.
30. Cascino GD, Hulihan JF, Sharbrough FW, et al. Parietal lobe lesional epilepsy: electroclinical correlation and operative outcome. *Epilepsia.* 1993;34(3):522–527.
31. Caveness WF, Liss HR. Incidence of post-traumatic epilepsy. *Epilepsia.* 1961;2:123–129.
32. Chang C, Ojemann LM, Ojemann GA, et al. Seizures of fronto-orbital origin: a proven case. *Epilepsia.* 1991;32(4):487–491.
33. Chassagnon S, Minotti L, Kremer S, et al. Restricted frontomesial epileptogenic focus generating dyskinetic behavior and laughter. *Epilepsia.* 2003;44(6):859–863.
34. Chauvel P, Delgado-Escueta-Escueta A, Halgren E, et al. *Frontal Lobe Seizures and Epilepsies.* New York: Raven Press; 1992.
35. Christen HJ, Hanefeld F, Kruse E, et al. Foix-Chavany-Marie (anterior operculum syndrome in childhood: a reappraisal of Worster-Drought syndrome. *Dev Med Child Neurol.* 2000;42(2):122–132.
36. Cokar O, Gelisse P, Livet MO, et al. Startle response: epileptic or non-epileptic? The case for "flash" SMA reflex seizures. *Epileptic Disord.* 2001;3(1):7–12.
37. Combi R, Dalpra L, Tenchini ML, et al. Autosomal dominant nocturnal frontal lobe epilepsy—a critical overview. *J Neurol.* 2004;251(8):923–934.
38. Connolly MB, Langill L, Wong PKH, et al. Seizures involving the supplementary sensorimotor area in children: a video-EEG analysis. *Epilepsia.* 1995;36(10):1025–1032.
39. Dalmagro CL, Bianchin MM, Velasco TR, et al. Clinical features of patients with posterior cortex epilepsies and predictors of surgical outcome. *Epilepsia.* 2005;46(9):1142–1449.
40. Delgado-Escueta AV, Swartz B, Maldonado H, et al. Complex partial seizures of frontal lobe origin. In: Wieser HG, Elger CE, eds. *Presurgical Evaluation of Epileptics: Basics, Techniques, Implications.* New York: Springer-Verlag; 1987:268–299.
41. Duffau H, Capelle L, Lopex M, et al. Medically intractable epilepsy from insular low-grade gliomas: improvement after an extended lesionectomy. *Acta Neurochir.* 2002;144:563–573.
42. Duffau H, Taillandier L, Gatignol P, et al. The insular lobe and brain plasticity: lessons from tumor surgery. *Clin Neurol Neurosurg.* 2005;108(6):543–548.
43. Ebersole JS, Wade PB. Spike voltage topography identifies two types of fronto-temporal epileptic foci. *Neurology.* 1991;41:1425–1433.
44. Ebersole JS, Pacia SV. Localization of temporal lobe foci by ictal EEG patterns. *Epilepsia.* 1996;37(4):386–399.
45. Eliashiv DS, Elsas SM, Squires K, et al. Ictal magnetic source imaging as localizing tool in partial epilepsy. *Neurology.* 2002;59(10):1600–1610.
46. Engel J Jr. New concepts of the epileptic focus. In: Wieser HG, Speckmann EG, Engel J Jr, eds. *The Epileptic Focus.* London: John Libbey Eurotext; 1987:83–94.
47. Engel J Jr. Recent advances in surgical treatment of temporal lobe epilepsy. *Acta Neurol Scand.* 1992;86(Suppl 5):71–80.
48. Engel J Jr. Historical perspectives. In: Engel J Jr, ed. *Surgical Treatment of the Epilepsies.* 2nd ed. New York: Raven Press; 1993:695–705.
49. Engel J Jr, Shewmon DA. Overview: who should be considered a surgical candidate? In: Engel J Jr, ed. *Surgical Treatment of the Epilepsies.* 2nd ed. New York: Raven Press; 1993:23–34.
50. Engel J Jr. Current concepts: surgery for seizures. *N Engl J Med.* 1996;334(10):647–652.
51. Engel J Jr. A proposed diagnostic scheme for people with epileptic seizures and with epilepsy: report of the ILAE Task Force on Classification and Terminology. *Epilepsia.* 2001;42:796–803.
52. Foldvary NR, Lee N, Mayes BN. Extrahippocampal temporal lobe epilepsy: clinical manifestations [Abstract]. *Epilepsia.* 1994;35(8):109 (abst).
53. Foldvary N, Lee N, Thwaites G, et al. Clinical and electrographic manifestations of lesional neocortical temporal lobe epilepsy. *Neurology.* 1997;49(3):757–763.
54. Foldvary N, Klem G, Hammel J, et al. The localizing value of ictal EEG in focal epilepsy. *Neurology.* 2001;57(11):2022–2028.
55. French JA, Williamson PD, Thadani VM, et al. Characteristics of medial temporal lobe epilepsy I. Results of history and physical examination. *Ann Neurol.* 1993;34:774–780.
56. Fried I, Katz A, McCarthy G, et al. Functional organization of human supplementary motor cortex studied by electrical stimulation. *J Neurosci.* 1991;11(11):3656–3666.
57. Fujii M, Akimura T, Ozaki S, et al. An angiographically occult arteriovenous malformation in the medial parietal lobe presenting as seizures of medial temporal lobe origin. *Epilepsia.* 1999;40(3):377–381.
58. Fusco L, Iani C, Faedda MT, et al. Mesial frontal lobe epilepsy: a clinical entity not sufficiently described. *J Epilepsy.* 1990;3:123–135.
59. Gastaut H. A new type of epilepsy: benign partial epilepsy of childhood with occipital spike-waves. *Clin Electroencephalogr.* 1982;13:13–22.
60. Gastaut H. Benign epilepsy of childhood with occipital paroxysms. In: Roger J, Dravet C, Bureau M, et al., eds. *Epileptic Syndromes in Infancy, Childhood, and Adolescence.* London: John Libbey Eurotext; 1985:159–170.
61. Gastaut H, Zifkin BG. Benign epilepsy of childhood with occipital spike-and-wave complexes. In: Andermann F, Lugaresi E, eds. *Migraine and Epilepsy.* Boston: Butterworth; 1987:47–82.
62. Geier S, Bancaud J, Talairach J, et al. Clinical note: clinical and tele-stereo-EEG findings in a patient with psychomotor seizures. *Epilepsia.* 1975;16:119–125.
63. Geier S, Bancaud J, Talairach J, et al. Automatisms during frontal lobe epileptic seizures. *Brain.* 1976;99:447–458.
64. Geier S, Bancaud J, Talairach J, et al. Ictal tonic postural changes and automatisms of the upper limb during epileptic parietal lobe discharges. *Epilepsia.* 1977;18:517–524.
65. Geier S, Bancaud J, Talairach J, et al. The seizures of frontal lobe epilepsy: a study of clinical manifestations. *Neurology.* 1977;27:951–958.
66. Gibbs FA, Gibbs EL. *Atlas of Electroencephalography.* Cambridge, MA: Addison-Wesley; 1953:201–225.
67. Gil-Nagel A, Risinger MW. Ictal semiology in hippocampal vs. extrahippocampal temporal lobe epilepsy [Abstract]. *Neurology.* 1993;43: 273(abst).
68. Gil-Nagel A, Risinger MW. Ictal semiology in hippocampal versus extrahippocampal temporal lobe epilepsy. *Brain.* 1997;120(Pt 1):183–192.
69. Gloor P, Olivier A, Quesney LF, et al. The role of the limbic system in experiential phenomena of temporal lobe epilepsy. *Ann Neurol.* 1982;12:129–144.
70. Gowers WR. *Epilepsy and Other Chronic Convulsive Diseases: Their Causes, Symptoms and Treatment.* London: J & A Churchill; 1881:309.
71. Gowers WR. General character of epileptic fits. In: *Epilepsy and Other Chronic Convulsive Diseases: Their Causes, Symptoms, and Treatment.* New York: William Wood; 1885:29–85.
72. Green JR, Angevine JB, White JC, et al. Significance of the supplementary motor area in partial seizures and in cerebral localization. *Neurosurgery.* 1980;6:66–75.
73. Guerrini R, Ferrari AR, Battaglia A, et al. Occipitotemporal seizures with ictus emeticus induced by intermittent photic stimulation. *Neurology.* 1994;44:1253–259.
74. Guillaume J, Mazars G, Mazars, Y. Surgical indications in so-called temporal epilepsy. *Rev Neurol (Paris).* 1953;88(6):461–501.
75. Gupta A, Raja S, Kotagal P, et al. Ictal SPECT in children with partial epilepsy due to focal cortical dysplasia. *Pediatri Neurol.* 2004;31(2):89–95.
76. Hajek M, Antonini A, Leenders KL, et al. Mesiobasal versus lateral temporal epilepsy: metabolic differences in the temporal lobe shown by interictal ^{18}F-FDG positron emission tomography. *Neurology.* 1993;43:790.
77. Hammers A, Koepp MJ, Richardson MP, et al. Grey and white matter flumazenil binding in neocortical epilepsy with normal MRI. A PET study of 44 patients. *Brain.* 2003;126:1300–1318.
78. Harden CL, Rosenbaum DH, Daras M. Hyperglycemia presenting with occipital seizures. *Epilepsia.* 1991;32(2):215–220.
79. Hauser-Hauw C, Bancaud J. Gustatory hallucinations in epileptic seizures: electrophysiological, clinical and anatomical correlates. *Brain.* 1987;110:339–359.
80. Ho SS, Berkovic SF, Newton MR, et al. Parietal lobe epilepsy: clinical features and seizure localization by ictal SPECT. *Neurology.* 1994;44:2277–2284.
81. Holtzman RNN, Goldensohn ES. Sensations of ocular movement in seizures originating in occipital lobe. *Neurology.* 1977;27:554–556.
82. Horsley V. Brain surgery. *BMJ.* 1886;2:670–675.
83. Ikeda A, Matsumoto R, Ohara S, et al. Asymmetric tonic seizures with bilateral parietal lesions resembling frontal lobe epilepsy. *Epileptic Disord.* 2001;3(1):17–22.

84. Ikeda A, Sato T, Ohara S, et al. "Supplementary motor area (SMA) seizure" rather than "SMA epilepsy" in optimal surgical candidates: a document of subdural mapping. *J Neurol Sci*. 2002;202(1–2):43–52.
85. Isnard J, Guenot M, Ostrowsky K, et al. The role of the insular cortex in temporal lobe epilepsy. *Ann Neurol*. 2000;48(4):614–623.
86. Isnard J, Guenot M, Sindou M, et al. Clinical manifestations of insular lobe seizures: a stereo-electroencephalographic study. *Epilepsia*. 2004;45(9):1079–1090.
87. Jabbari B, Vengrow MI, Salazar AM, et al. Clinical and radiological correlates of EEG in the late phase of head injury: a study of 515 Vietnam veterans. *Electroencephalogr Clin Neurophysiol*. 1986;64:285–293.
88. Jackson JH. *Selected Writings of John Hughlings Jackson*. London: Staples Press; 1931.
89. Janszky J, Fogarasi A, Jokeit H, et al. Lateralizing value of unilateral motor and somatosensory manifestations in frontal lobe seizures. *Epilepsy Res*. 2000;43:125–133.
90. Jasper HH, Riggio S, Goldman-Rakic PS. *Epilepsy and the Functional Anatomy of the Frontal Lobe*. New York: Raven Press; 1995.
91. Jennet B. *Epilepsy after Non-Missile Head Injuries*. 2nd ed. Chicago: William Heinemann; 1975.
92. Jobst BC, Siegel AM, Thadani VM, et al. Intractable seizures of frontal lobe origin: clinical characteristics, localizing signs and results of surgery. *Epilepsia*. 2000;41:1139–1152.
93. Jobst BC, Williamson PD. Frontal lobe seizures. In: Riggio S, ed. *Psychiatric Clinics of North America*. Philadelphia: WB Saunders; 2005:635–651.
94. Kanazawa O, Sengoku A, Kawai I. Oculotonic status epilepticus. *Epilepsia*. 1989;30(1):121–123.
95. Kanemoto K, Watanabe Y, Tsuji T, et al. Rub epilepsy: a somatosensory evoked reflex epilepsy induced by prolonged cutaneous stimulation. *J Neurol Neurosurg Psychiatry*. 2001;70(4):541–543.
96. Kanner AM, Morris HH, Lüders H, et al. Supplementary motor seizures mimicking pseudoseizures: some clinic differences. *Neurology*. 1990;40:1404–1407.
97. Karbowski K. Vertigo and epilepsy. *Schweiz Rundsch Med Prax*. 1982;71(41):1600–1604.
98. Kellaway P. The incidence, significance and natural history of spike foci in children. In: Henry C, ed. *Current Clinical Neurophysiology: Update on EEG and Evoked Potentials*. Amsterdam: Elsevier/North Holland; 1980:151–175.
99. Kellinghaus C, Lüders HO. Frontal lobe epilepsy. *Epileptic Disord*. 2004;6(4):223–239.
100. Kim DW, Lee SK, Yun C-H, et al. Parietal lobe epilepsy: the semiology, yield of diagnostic workup, and surgical outcome. *Epilepsia*. 2004;45(6):641–649.
101. Knowlton RC, Lawn ND, Mountz JM, et al. Ictal single-photon emission computed tomography imaging in extra temporal lobe epilepsy using statistical parametric mapping. *J Neuroimaging*. 2004;14(4):324–330.
102. Kotagal P. Seizure symptomatology of temporal lobe origin. In: Lüders H, ed. *Epilepsy Surgery*. New York: Raven Press; 1991:143–155.
103. Kotagal P, Arunkumar G, Hammel J, et al. Complex partial seizures of frontal lobe onset statistical analysis of ictal semiology. *Seizure*. 2003;12(5):268–281.
104. Krakow K, Woermann FG, Symms MR, et al. EEG-triggered functional MRI of interictal epileptiform activity inpatients with partial seizures. *Brain*. 1999;122(Pt 9):1679–1688.
105. Kubota F, Shibata N, Shiihara Y, et al. Frontal lobe epilepsy with secondarily generalized 3 Hz spike-waves: a case report. *Clin Electroencephalogr*. 1997;28(3):166–171.
106. Kuzniecky R, Rosenblatt B. Benign occipital epilepsy: a family study. *Epilepsia*. 1987;28(4):346–350.
107. Kuzniecky RI, Jackson GD. *Magnetic Resonance in Epilepsy*. New York: Raven Press; 1995.
108. Kuzniecky R, Gilliam F, Morawetz R, et al. Occipital lobe developmental malformations and epilepsy: clinical spectrum, treatment, and outcome. *Epilepsia*. 1997;38(2):175–181.
109. Kuzniecky R, Knowlton RC. Neuroimaging of epilepsy. *Semin Neurol*. 2002;22(3):279–288.
110. Lada C, Skiadas K, Theodorou V, et al. A study of 43 patients with Panayiotopoulos syndrome, a common and benign childhood seizure susceptibility. *Epilepsia*. 2003;44(1):81–88.
111. Laff R, Mesad S, Devinsky O. Epileptic kinetopsia: ictal illusory motion perception. *Neurology*. 2003;61(9):1262–1264.
112. Lagae L, Pauwels J, Monte CP, et al. Frontal absences in children. *Eur J Paediatr Neurol*. 2001;5(6):243–251.
113. Laich E, Kuzniecky R, Mountz J, et al. Supplementary sensorimotor area epilepsy. Seizure localization, cortical propagation and subcortical activation pathways using ictal SPECT. *Brain*. 1997;120(Pt 5):855–864.
114. Lancman ME, Asconape JJ, Penry KT, et al. Paroxysmal pain as sole manifestation of seizures. *Pediatr. Neurol*. 1993;9(5):404–406.
115. Landy HJ, Ramsay RE, Ajmone-Marsan C, et al. Temporal lobectomy for seizures associated with unilateral schizencephaly. *Surg Neurol*. 1992;37:477–481.
116. Lee Y-C, Yen D-J, Lirng J-F, et al. Epileptic seizures in a patient by immersing his right hand into hot water. *Seizure*. 2000;9:605–607.
117. Lee JJ, Kang WJ, Lee DS, et al. Diagnostic performance of 18F-FDG PET and ictal ^{99m}Tc-HMPAO SPET in pediatric temporal lobe epilepsy: quantitative analysis by statistical parametric mapping, statistical probabilistic anatomical map, and subtraction ictal SPECT. *Seizure*. 2005;14(3):213–220.
118. Lee S, Lee S, Kim D-W, et al. Occipital lobe epilepsy: clinical characteristics, surgical outcome, and role of diagnostic modalities. *Epilepsia*. 2005;46(5):688–695.
119. Lee SK, Yun CH, Oh JB, et al. Intracranial ictal onset zone in nonlesional lateral temporal lobe epilepsy on scalp ictal EEG. *Neurology*. 2003;61(6):757–764.
120. Lee SK, Lee SY, Kim KK, et al. Surgical outcome and prognostic factors of cryptogenic neocortical epilepsy. *Ann Neurol*. 2005;58(4):525–532.
121. Lee SK, Kim KK, Hong KS, et al. The lateralizing and surgical prognostic value of a single 2-hour EEG in mesial TLE. *Seizure*. 2000;9(5):336–339.
122. Lerman P, Kivity S. The benign partial nonrolandic epilepsies. *J Clin Neurophysiol*. 1991;8:275–287.
123. Luerding R, Boeseback F, Ebner A. Cognitive changes after epilepsy surgery in the posterior cortex. *J Neurol Neurosurg Psychiatry* 2004;75:583–587.
124. Lüders HO, Engel J Jr, Munari C. General principles. In: Engel J Jr, ed. *Surgical Treatment of the Epilepsies*. 2nd ed. New York: Raven Press; 1993:137–153.
125. Ludwig B, Armone-Marsan C, Van Buren J. Cerebral seizures of probable orbitofrontal origin. *Epilepsia*. 1972;16:141–158.
126. Maillard L, Vignal JP, Gavaret M, et al. Semiologic and electrophysiologic correlations in temporal lobe seizure subtypes. *Epilepsia*. 2004;45(12):1590–1599.
127. Maillard L, Vignal JP, Anxionnat R, et al. Semiologic value of ictal autoscopy. *Epilepsia*. 2004;45(4):391–394.
128. Mauguiere F, Ryvlin P. The role of PET in presurgical assessment of partial epilepsies. *Epileptic Disord*. 2004;6(3):193–215.
129. McIntosh AM, Kalnins RM, Mitchell LA, et al. Temporal lobectomy: long-term seizure outcome, late recurrence and risks for seizure recurrence. *Brain*. 2004;127(Pt 9):2018–2030.
130. McNally KA, Paige AL, Varghese G, et al. Localizing value of ictal-interictal SPECT analyzed by SPM (ISAS). *Epilepsia*. 2005;46(9):1450–1464.
131. Meletti S, Tinuper P, Bisulli F, et al. A supplementary sensorimotor area involvement for both negative and positive motor phenomena. Epileptic negative myoclonus and brief asymmetric tonic seizures. *Epileptic Disord*. 2000;3(2):163–168.
132. Michelucci R, Poza JJ, Sofia V, et al. Autosomal dominant lateral temporal epilepsy: clinical spectrum, new epitempin mutations, and genetic heterogeneity in seven European families. *Epilepsia*. 2003;44(10):1289–1297.
133. Mikati MA, Holmes GL. Temporal lobe epilepsy. In: Wyllie, ed. *The Treatment of Epilepsy: Principles and Practice*. Philadelphia: Lea & Febiger; 1993:513–524.
134. Morrell F, Whisler WW, Bleck TP. Multiple subpial transection, a new approach to the surgical treatment of focal epilepsy. *J Neurosurg*. 1989;70:231–239.
135. Morris HH, Dinner DS, Lüders H, et al. Supplementary motor seizures: clinical and electroencephalographic findings. *Neurology*. 1988;38:1075–1082.
136. Munari C, Bonis A, Kochen S, et al. Eye movements and occipital seizures in man. *Acta Neurochir (Wien)*. 1984;33(Suppl):47–52.
137. Nakken KO, Roste GK, Hauglie-Hanssen E. Coeliac disease, unilateral occipital calcifications, and drug-resistant epilepsy: successful lesionectomy. *Acta Neurol Scand*. 2005;111(3):202–204.
138. Ng Y, Kim HL, Wheless JW. Successful neurosurgical treatment of childhood complex partial status epilepticus with focal resection. *Epilepsia*. 2003;44(3):468–471.
139. Niedermeyer E. *Compendium of the Epilepsies*. Springfield, IL: Charles C Thomas; 1974.
140. Nobili L, Cossu M, Mai R, et al. Sleep-related hyperkinetic seizures of temporal lobe origin. *Neurology*. 2004;62(3):482–485.
141. O' Brien TJ, So EL, Mullan BP, et al. Subtraction ictal SPECT co-registered to MRI improves clinical usefulness of SPECT in localizing the surgical seizure focus. *Neurology*. 1998;50(2):445–454.
142. O' Brien TJ, Zupanc ML, Mullan BP, et al. The practical utility of performing peri-ictal SPECT in the evaluation of children with partial epilepsy. *Pediatr Neurol*. 1998;19(1):15–22.
143. O'Brien TJ, So EL, Cascino GD, et al. Subtraction SPECT coregistered to MRI in focal malformations of cortical development: localization of the epileptogenic zone in epilepsy surgery candidates. *Epilepsia*. 2004;45(4):367–376.
144. Oguni H, Hayashi K, Usui N, et al. Startle epilepsy with infantile hemiplegia: report of two cases improved by surgery. *Epilepsia*. 1998;39(1):93–98.
145. Ohara S, Ikeda A, Kunieda T, et al. Propagation of tonic posturing in supplementary motor area (SMA) seizures. *Epilepsy Res*. 2004;62(2–3):179–187.
146. Olivier A, Gloor P, Andermann F, et al. Occipitotemporal epilepsy studied with stereotaxically implanted depth electrodes and successfully treated by temporal resection. *Ann Neurol*. 1982;11:428–432.
147. Ostrowsky K, Isnard J, Ryvlin P, et al. Functional mapping of the insular cortex: clinical implication in temporal lobe epilepsy. *Epilepsia*. 2000;41(6):681–686.
148. Pacia SV, Devinsky O, Perrine K, et al. Clinical features of neocortical temporal lobe epilepsy. *Ann Neurol*. 1996;40(5):724–730.

149. Palmini A, Andermann F, Dubeau F, et al. Occipitotemporal epilepsies: evaluation of selected patients requiring depth electrodes studies and rationale for surgical approaches. *Epilepsia*. 1993;34(1):84–96.
150. Penfield W, Erickson TC. *Epilepsy and Cerebral Localization*. Springfield, IL: Charles C Thomas; 1941:101–103.
151. Penfield W, Jasper H. *Epilepsy and the Functional Anatomy of the Human Brain*. Boston: Little, Brown & Co.; 1954.
152. Pfaender M, D'Souza WJ, Trost N, et al. Visual disturbances representing occipital lobe epilepsy in patients with cerebral calcifications and coeliac disease: a case series. *J Neurol Neurosurg Psychiatry*. 2004;75(11):1623–1625.
153. Phan TG, Cascino GD, Fulgham, J. Ictal abdominal pain heralding parietal lobe haemorrhage. *Seizure*. 2001;10:56–59.
154. Pierelli F, Di Gennaro G, Gherardi M, et al. Movement-induced seizures: a case report. *Epilepsia*. 1997;38(8):941–944.
155. Plazzi G, Tinuper P, Cerullo A, et al. Occipital lobe epilepsy: a chronic condition to transient occipital lobe involvement in eclampsia. *Epilepsia*. 1994;35(3):644–647.
156. Provini F, Plazzi G, Tinuper P, et al Nocturnal frontal lobe epilepsy. A clinical and polygraphic overview of 100 consecutive cases. *Brain*. 1999;122(Pt 6):1017–1031.
157. Provini F, Plazzi G, Lugaresi E. From nocturnal paroxysmal dystonia to nocturnal frontal lobe epilepsy. *Clin Neurophysiol*. 2000;111(Suppl 2):S2–8.
158. Quarato PP, Di Gennaro G, Manfredi M, et al. Atypical Lennox-Gastaut syndrome successfully treated with removal of a parietal dysembryoplastic tumour. *Seizure*. 2002;11:325–329.
159. Quesney LF, Constain M, Fish DR, et al. The clinical differentiation of seizures arising in the parasagittal and anterolaterodorsal frontal convexities. *Arch Neurol*. 1990;47:677–679.
160. Quesney LF, Constain M, Rasmussen T. Seizures from the dorsolateral frontal lobe. In: Chauvel P, Delgado-Escueta AV, Halgren E, et al., eds. *Frontal Lobe Seizures and Epilepsies*. New York: Raven Press; 1992:233–244.
161. Rasmussen T. Surgery for epilepsy arising in regions other than the temporal and frontal lobes. In: Purpura DP, Penry JK, Walter RD, eds. *Neurosurgical Management of the Epilepsies*. New York: Raven Press; 1975:207–226.
162. Rasmussen T. Cortical resection in the treatment of focal epilepsy. In: Purpura DP, Penry RK, Walter RD, eds. *Neurosurgical Management of the Epilepsies*. New York: Raven Press; 1975:139–154.
163. Rasmussen T. Surgery of frontal lobe epilepsy. In: Purpura DP, Penry JK, Walter RD, eds. *Neurosurgical Management of the Epilepsies*. New York: Raven Press; 1975:197–205.
164. Roberts DW, Williamson PD, Thadani VM, et al. Nonlesional supplementary motor area epilepsy: results of evaluation and surgery in four patients [Abstract]. *Epilepsia*. 1995;36(Suppl 4):15 (abst).
165. Rossetti AO, Mortati KA, Black PM, et al. Simple partial seizures with hemisensory phenomena and dysgeusia: an insular pattern. *Epilepsia*. 2005;46(4):590–591.
166. Russell WR, Whitty CWM. Studies in traumatic epilepsy. 3. Visual fits. *J Neurol Neurosurg Psychiatry*. 1955;18:79–96.
167. Sakakibara S, Nakamura F, Demise M, et al. Frontal lobe epilepsy with absence-like and secondarily generalized seizures. *Psychiatry Clin Neurosci*. 2003;57(4):455–456.
168. Salanova V, Andermann F, Olivier A, et al. Occipital lobe epilepsy: electroclinical manifestations, electrocorticography, cortical stimulation, and outcome in 42 patients treated between 1930 and 1991. *Brain*. 1992;115:1655–1680.
169. Salanova V, Andermann F, Rasmussen TB. Occipital lobe epilepsy. In: Wyllie E, ed. *The Treatment of Epilepsy: Principles and Practices*. Philadelphia: Lea & Febiger; 1993:533–540.
170. Satow T, Ikeda A, Yamamoto J, et al. Partial epilepsy manifesting atonic seizure: report of two cases. *Epilepsia*. 2002;43(11):1425–1431.
171. Satow T, Ikeda A, Hayashi N, et al. Surgical treatment of seizures from the peri-Sylvian area by perinatal insult: a case report of ictal hypersalivation. *Acta Neurochir (Wien)*. 2004;146(9):1021–1025; discussion 1026.
172. Saygi S, Katz A, Marks DA, et al. Frontal lobe partial seizures and psychogenic seizures: comparison of clinical and ictal characteristics. *Neurology*. 1992;42:1274–1277.
173. Saygi S, Spencer SS, Scheyer R, et al. Differentiation of temporal lobe ictal behavior associated with hippocampal sclerosis and tumors of temporal lobe. *Epilepsia*. 1994;35:737–742.
174. Schatz CR, Kreth FW, Faist M, et al. Interstitial 125-iodine radiosurgery of low-grade gliomas of the insula of Reil. *Acta Neruochir (Wien)*. 1994;1130(1–4):80–89.
175. Schindler K, Gast H, Bassetti C, et al. Hyperperfusion of anterior cingulate gyrus in a case of paroxysmal nocturnal dystonia. *Neurology*. 2001;57(5):917–920.
176. Semah F, Baulac M, Hasboun D, et al. Is interictal temporal hypometabolism related to mesial temporal sclerosis? A PET/MRI confrontation. *Epilepsia*. 1995;36:447–456.
177. Serles W, Leutmezer F, Pataraia E, et al. A case of startle epilepsy and SSMA seizures documented with subdural recordings. *Epilepsia*. 1999;40(7):1031–1035.
178. Shihabuddin B, Abou-Khalil B, Delbeke D, et al. Orbito-frontal epilepsy masquerading as temporal lobe epilepsy—a case report. *Seizure*. 2001;10(2):134–138.
179. Shiraishi H, Watanabe Y, Watanabe M, et al. Interictal and ictal magnetoencephalographic study in patients with medial frontal lobe epilepsy. *Epilepsia*. 2001;42(7):875–882.
180. Shuper A, Stahl B, Mimouni M. Transient opercular syndrome: a manifestation of uncontrolled epileptic activity. *Acta Neurol Scand*. 2000;101(5):335–338.
181. Siegel AM, Williamson, Roberts DW, et al. Localized pain associated with seizures originating in the parietal lobe. *Epilepsia*. 1999;40(7):845–855.
182. Siegel AM, Jobst BC, Thadani VM, et al. Medically intractable, localization-related epilepsy with normal MRI: presurgical evaluation and surgical outcome in 43 patients. *Epilepsia*. 2001;42(7):883–888.
183. Smith JR, Sillay K, Winkler P, et al. Orbitofrontal epilepsy: electroclinical analysis of surgical cases and literature review. *Stereotact Funct Neurosurg*. 2004;82(1):20–25.
184. So NK. Mesial frontal epilepsy. *Epilepsia*. 1998;39(Suppl 4):S49–61.
185. Spencer SS, Spencer DD, Williamson PD, et al. Sexual automatisms in complex partial seizures. *Neurology*. 1983;33(5):527–533.
186. Stevens TK. Magnetic resonance spectroscopic techniques for localizing epileptogenic zones in refractory partial epilepsy. *Ann Neurol*. 2006;97:285–292.
187. Sveinbjornsdottir S, Duncan JS. Parietal and occipital lobe epilepsy: a review. *Epilepsia*. 1993;34(3):493–521.
188. Swartz B, Delgado-Escueta AV. Complex partial seizures of extratemporal origin: "the evidence for." In: Wieser HG, Speckman EG, Engel J, eds. *The Epileptic Focus*. London: John Libbey; 1987:137–174.
189. Tachikawa E, Oguni H, Shirakawa S, et al. Acquired epileptiform opercular syndrome: a case report and results of single photon emission computed tomography and computer-assisted electroencephalographic analysis. *Brain Dev*. 2001;23(4):246–250.
190. Taylor J, ed. *Selected Writings of John Hughlings Jackson*. Vol. 1. New York: New Basic Books Inc.; 1958.
191. Taylor I, Scheffer IE, Berkovic SF. Occipital epilepsies: identification of specific and newly recognized syndromes. *Brain*. 2003;126(Pt 4):753–769.
192. Temkin O. *The Falling Sickness*. Baltimore: Johns Hopkins Press; 1985.
193. Tharp BR. Orbital frontal seizures: a unique electroencephalographic and clinical syndrome. *Epilepsia*. 1972;13:627–642.
194. Thomas P, Beaumanoir A, Genton P, et al. 'De novo' absence status of late onset: report of 11 cases. *Neurology*. 1992;42(1):104–110.
195. Thomas P, Andermann F, Hirsch E, et al. Late-onset absence status epilepticus is most often situation-related. In: Malafosse A, Genton P, Hirsch E, et al., eds. *Idiopathic Generalized Epilepsies*. London: John Libbey & Company; 1994.
196. Thomas P, Arzimanoglou A, Aicardi J. Benign idiopathic occipital epilepsy: report of a case of the late (Gastaut) type [corrected]. *Epileptic Disord*. 2003;5(1):57–59.
197. Tiacci C, D'Allesandro P, Cantisani TA, et al. Epilepsy with bilateral occipital calcifications: Stürge-Weber variant or a different encephalopathy. *Epilepsia*. 1993;34(3):528–539.
198. Tinuper P, Aguglia U, Pellissier JF, et al. Visual ictal phenomena in a case of Lafora disease proven by skin biopsy. *Epilepsia*. 1983;26(6):577–584.
199. Trevathan E, Cascino GD. Partial epilepsy presenting as focal paroxysmal pain. *Neurology*. 1988;38:329–330.
200. Vadlamudi L, So EL, Worrell GA, et al. Factors underlying scalp-EEG interictal epileptiform discharges in intractable frontal lobe epilepsy. *Epileptic Disord*. 2004;6(2):89–95.
201. van Paesschen, W. Ictal SPECT. *Epilepsia*. 2004;45(Suppl 4):35–40.
202. Walczak R, Bazil C, Lee N, et al. Scalp ictal EEG differs in temporal neocortical and hippocampal seizures [Abstract]. *Epilepsia*. 1994;35:134(abst).
203. Walczak TS. Neocortical temporal lobe epilepsy: characterizing the syndrome. *Epilepsia*. 1995;36(7):633–635.
204. Wang CP, Hsieh PF, Chen CC, et al. Hyperglycemia with occipital seizures: images and visual evoked potentials. *Epilepsia*. 2005;46(7):1140–1144.
205. Waterman K, Purves SJ, Kosaka B, et al. An epileptic syndrome caused by mesial frontal lobe foci. *Neurology*. 1987;37:577–582.
206. Wieser HG. *Electroclinical Features of the Psychomotor Seizure: A Stereo-electroencephalographic Study of Ictal Symptoms and Chronotopographical Seizure Patterns Including Clinical Effects of Intracerebral Stimulation*. London: Butterworths; 1983.
207. Wieser HG. Psychomotor seizures of hippocampal-amygdalar origin. In: Pedley TA, Meldrum BS, eds. *Recent Advances in Epilepsy*. Edinburgh: Churchill Livingston; 1986:57–79.
208. Wieser HG, Engel J Jr, Williamson PD, et al. Surgically remediable temporal lobe syndromes. In: Engel J Jr, ed. *Surgical Treatment of the Epilepsies*. 2nd ed. New York: Raven Press; 1993:49–63.
209. Wilkinson HA. Epileptic pain: an uncommon manifestation with localizing value. *Neurology*. 1973;23:518–520.
210. Williamson PD, Spencer DD, Spencer SS, et al. Complex partial status epilepticus: a depth-electrode study. *Ann Neurol*. 1985;18:647–654.
211. Williamson PD, Spencer DD, Spencer SS, et al. Complex partial seizures of frontal lobe origin. *Ann Neurol*. 1985;18:497–504.

212. Williamson PD, Spencer SS. Clinical and EEG features of complex partial seizures of extratemporal origin. *Epilepsia*. 1986;27(Suppl 2):46–63.
213. Williamson PD. The symptomatic localization-related epilepsies: problems with subclassification. *Yale J Biol*. 1987;60:60–77.
214. Williamson PD. Frontal lobe seizures: problems of diagnosis and classification. In: Chauvel P, Delgado-Escueta AV, Halgren E, et al., eds. *Frontal Lobe Seizures and Epilepsies*. New York: Raven Press; 1992:289–309.
215. Williamson PD, Boon PA, Thadani VM, et al. Parietal lobe epilepsy: diagnostic considerations and results of surgery. *Ann Neurol*. 1992;31:193–201.
216. Williamson PD, Thadani VM, Darcey TM, et al. Occipital lobe epilepsy: clinical characteristics, seizure spread patterns and results of surgery. *Ann Neurol*. 1992;31:3–13.
217. Williamson PD. Psychogenic non-epileptic seizures and frontal seizures: diagnostic considerations. In: Rowan AJ, Gates JR, eds. *Non-epileptic Seizures*. Boston: Butterworth-Heinemann; 1993:55–72.
218. Williamson PD, French JA, Thadani VM, et al. Characteristics of medial temporal lobe epilepsy II. Interictal and ictal scalp electroencephalography, neuropsychological testing, neuroimaging, surgical results and pathology. *Ann Neurol*. 1993;34:781–787.
219. Williamson PD, Van Ness PC, Wieser HG, et al. Surgically remediable extratemporal syndromes. In: Engel J Jr, ed. *Surgical Treatment of the Epilepsies*. New York: Raven Press; 1993:65–76.
220. Williamson PD. Frontal lobe epilepsy: some clinical characteristics. In: Jasper HH, Riggio S, Goldman-Rakic PS, eds. *Epilepsy and the Functional Anatomy of the Frontal Lobe*. New York: Raven Press; 1995:127–152.
221. Williamson PD. Epileptic pain with parietal lobe seizure origin. *Epilepsia*. 1995;36(Suppl 4):158.
222. Williamson PD, Thadani VM, French JA, et al. Medial temporal lobe epilepsy: videotape analysis of objective clinical seizure characteristics. *Epilepsia*. 1998;39:1182–1188.
223. Williamson PD, Wieser HG, Delgado-Escueta AV. Clinical characteristics of partial seizures. In: Engel J Jr, ed. *Surgical Treatment of the Epilepsies*. New York: Raven Press; 1987:101–120.
224. Yamamoto J, Ikeda A, Matsuhashi M, et al. Seizures arising from the interior parietal lobule can show ictal semiology of the second sensory seizure (S11 seizure). *J Neurol Neurosurg Psychiatry*. 2003;74:367–369.
225. Young GB, Blume WT. Painful epileptic seizures. *Brain*. 1983;106:537–554.
226. Young GB, Barr HWK, Blume WT. Painful epileptic seizures involving the second sensory area. *Ann Neurol*. 1986;19(4):412.

CHAPTER 247 ■ MESIAL TEMPORAL LOBE EPILEPSY WITH HIPPOCAMPAL SCLEROSIS

JEROME ENGEL, JR., PETER D. WILLIAMSON, AND HEINZ GREGOR WIESER

INTRODUCTION

The term *temporal lobe epilepsy* (TLE) has been used for many years to denote a variety of conditions associated with complex partial seizures of presumed temporal lobe origin. The 1985 International Classification of Epilepsies and Epileptic Syndromes[21] divided symptomatic localization-related epilepsies according to the cerebral lobe of origin and recognized a syndrome of temporal lobe epilepsy defined purely on an anatomic basis. However, anatomic localization was usually determined purely from electroencephalographic (EEG) evidence, which could be misleading.[39]

It has also been known for many years that the most common pathologic substrate of mesial TLE (MTLE), as loosely defined in the 1985 International Classification, is hippocampal sclerosis (HS).[5] Data have accumulated in recent years strongly suggesting that MTLE with HS (MTLE-HS) represents a discrete syndrome that can usually be recognized in life.[33,47,127,133,138] The International League Against Epilepsy (ILAE) recently convened a workshop of experts to discuss the natural history, pathologic features, pathogenesis, electroclinical, neurophysiologic, neuropsychological, structural, and functional imaging findings of MTLE-HS and to determine whether it should be considered a disease, a single syndrome, or a group of clearly distinct syndromes.[134] Their conclusion was that MTLE-HS should be considered a subtype of a greater syndrome of MTLE due to many causes, and that much more work is needed before MTLE-HS could be specifically characterized. Diagnosis of MTLE, and specifically MTLE-HS, early in the course of the disorder, however, is now considered important because disabling seizures and their consequences can be eliminated by anteromesial temporal lobectomy in 60% to 80% of patients, and early surgical intervention provides the greatest opportunity for complete psychosocial rehabilitation.[34,127,130,133]

HISTORICAL PERSPECTIVES

Bouchet and Cazauvieilh[11] first described the association between epilepsy and a sclerotic hippocampus in 1825, based on gross pathologic examination of brains from patients with "mental alienation seizures." These lesions were believed to be an effect, rather than a cause, of epilepsy, which at that time referred only to generalized convulsions believed to originate in the medulla oblongata. In the latter part of the 19th century, however, Hughlings Jackson[63,64] recognized that partial seizures also represented epileptic phenomena and made an association between limbic-type seizures, which he called "intellectual auras" or "dreamy states," and lesions in mesial temporal structures. During the same period of time, the neuropathologists Sommer[117] and Bratz[12] suggested that HS might be an epileptogenic lesion.

With the advent of EEG, Gibbs et al.[52] reported an ictal discharge pattern that they considered characteristic of psychomotor seizures; however, because they referenced all their electrodes to linked ears, they believed this phenomenon to be generalized. It was Jasper et al.[65,66] who pointed out that interictal and ictal epileptiform EEG abnormalities in psychomotor dreamy states and other phenomena now known to be limbic seizures originated in mesial temporal structures. Bailey and Gibbs[6] were the first to perform anterior temporal lobectomy on the basis of EEG evidence alone, but it was the en bloc resection of Falconer,[43] which included mesial temporal lobe structures, that made it possible to perform systematic pathologic analysis of resected tissue. Not only was HS identified as being present in a high percentage of patients with medically refractory temporal lobe epilepsy, but also surgical outcome in patients in whom this pathologic abnormality was demonstrated was exceptionally good, supporting the argument that this structural lesion was the cause, and not the effect, of recurrent epileptic seizures. Falconer[44,45] also recognized the association between HS and both febrile convulsions and a family history of epilepsy, which suggested the existence of a specific syndrome.

In large part as a result of the success of EEG monitoring in identifying mesial temporal epileptogenic tissue, anterior temporal lobectomy became, and has remained, the most common surgical treatment for medically refractory epilepsy. Crandall et al.[24] subsequently took advantage of the en bloc resection and long-term depth-electrode recording to initiate basic research on temporal lobe epilepsy.[37] HS is now the most studied epileptogenic lesion, and thus the fundamental neuronal mechanisms responsible for MTLE-HS are the best understood of any form of human epilepsy. The elucidation of a unique pathophysiology coupled with characteristic clinical features and an increasing ability to identify hippocampal disturbances noninvasively with functional and structural imaging have all helped to establish MTLE-HS as a discrete epileptic syndrome.[22,134]

DEFINITIONS

Definitions of temporal lobe epilepsy and temporal lobe seizures have varied through the years, and confusion persists concerning their usage.[35] The terms *temporal lobe seizure*, *psychomotor seizure*, and *limbic seizure* are often used interchangeably to denote seizures with signs and symptoms that derive from ictal activation of mesial temporal limbic structures. According to some workers, these terms are reserved only for seizures that originate in mesial temporal structures; other investigators, however, interpret the terms more loosely and use them also to define seizures that might originate in temporal or extratemporal neocortex but rapidly and preferentially propagate to mesial temporal structures.[31]

Whereas the 1970 International Classification of Epileptic Seizures introduced the term *complex partial seizure* in place of *temporal lobe seizure*,[49] the 1981 revision of this classification[20] redefined *simple* and *complex partial seizures* phenomenologically such that the latter term would be used to describe any partial seizure associated with impairment of consciousness. Because partial seizures can be associated with altered consciousness without involvement of mesial temporal limbic structures, not all complex partial seizures are temporal lobe seizures. Furthermore, because ictal discharges limited to one mesial temporal limbic area can produce characteristic symptoms such as epigastric rising, emotional and psychic experiences, and olfactory hallucinations during clear consciousness, temporal lobe seizures can also be simple partial seizures.[54] Consequently, whereas the 1981 International Classification of Epileptic Seizures has had definite clinical utility, the ILAE is now recommending that the concept of simple and complex partial seizures be abandoned. Seizures associated with MTLE are more correctly referred to as limbic seizures, whether or not consciousness is impaired.[36]

The 1985 International Classification of Epilepsies and Epileptic Syndromes divided partial epilepsies according to the cerebral lobe of onset and recognized a number of subcategories of temporal lobe epilepsy based on characteristic patterns of ictal onset and propagation as recorded with depth electrodes.[21,131] Because of controversy regarding the precision of such electrophysiologic localization, the 1989 classification[22] abolished anatomic categorizations but retained a syndrome of temporal lobe epilepsy based on associated clinical features, such as increased incidence of febrile convulsions and family history of epilepsy, as well as characteristic anterior temporal interictal EEG spikes and temporal lobe hypometabolism on positron emission tomography (PET). The term *temporal lobe epilepsy*, however, did not account for various etiologic factors and was used to denote the condition of patients both with and without apparent structural lesions. In some cases, patients with a diagnosis of temporal lobe epilepsy could conceivably have extratemporal epileptogenic regions that preferentially propagated to mesial temporal structures, producing characteristic temporal lobe seizures.

Before the advent of high-resolution magnetic resonance imaging (MRI), the term *cryptogenic temporal lobe epilepsy* had been frequently used to describe the condition of patients with the characteristic features of MTLE but no obvious lesions on structural imaging. Pathologic studies of mesial temporal tissue resected from patients with cryptogenic temporal lobe epilepsy revealed HS in most, so that the adjective *cryptogenic*, as opposed to *lesional*, was used tacitly to denote a subtype of MTLE that has now been more clearly defined as the syndrome of MTLE-HS.

Ammon's horn sclerosis and *mesial temporal sclerosis* are the two most common pathologic terms that have been used more or less synonymously with HS, although strictly speaking they imply different degrees of anatomic involvement.[4] The term *hippocampal sclerosis* refers to a specific type of hippocampal cell loss involving CA1 and hilar neurons most and CA2 neurons least, which distinguishes this entity from nonspecific cell loss with other causes.[5] Other characteristic features, such as mossy fiber sprouting[123] and selective loss of somatostatin and neuropeptide Y–containing hilar neurons,[25] also help to identify this distinct pathologic entity.

EPIDEMIOLOGY

Because the syndrome of MTLE-HS has only recently been clearly defined, and because only the medically refractory forms of this disorder referred to epilepsy surgery centers are usually identified, no epidemiologic information is available. It has been reported that 40% of patients with epilepsy experience complex partial seizures[50]; however, not all these patients necessarily have temporal lobe epilepsy, let alone MTLE-HS. In surgical series, careful pathologic analysis of hippocampal specimens, including cell counts and special staining procedures, reveals that as many as 70% of patients with medically refractory temporal lobe epilepsy may have HS,[5] indicating that the vast majority of patients with medically refractory temporal lobe epilepsy have MTLE-HS. Because of the probable increased incidence of a family history of epilepsy among patients who have MTLE-HS,[133] there may be some relationship between this syndrome and the recently described benign familial form of MTLE, which can also be associated with HS.[10,16] Although it is currently impossible to estimate the number of patients with MTLE-HS whose seizures are adequately controlled by antiepileptic drugs, two studies provide some evidence from nonsurgical series evaluated with high-resolution MRI. Semah et al.[114] reported on patients seen in a Paris epilepsy clinic over a 7-year period, approximately one half of whom had a diagnosis of temporal lobe epilepsy. Of these, half had evidence of hippocampal atrophy on MRI. At least one quarter of their population, therefore, could be given a diagnosis of MTLE-HS, and the percentage was probably higher because not all patients with this condition have sufficient atrophy to be visible on MRI. More importantly, of all the diagnostic categories, the most refractory to antiepileptic drugs was MTLE-HS. Only 11% of patients with this diagnosis, and only 3% with dual pathology (that is, HS and some other MRI lesion), had been seizure free in the previous year. This report suggests that MTLE-HS may be the most common, and most medically refractory, form of epilepsy. Another report from Glasgow by Stephen et al.,[121] however, found a similar proportion of patients with MRI evidence of HS, but only 46% of these were medically refractory (although this group was still the most intractable). The difference may be due to the fact that the Paris clinic included tertiary referral patients. The time at which patients with MTLE were referred may also influence the prevalence of intractability, because this condition typically has a stuttering course with long periods of remission. Berg et al.[8] reported on a large cohort of patients undergoing surgical treatment for medically refractory focal epilepsy, most of whom had MTLE, and found that it took an average of 9 years for the establishment of medical intractability.

ETIOLOGY AND BASIC MECHANISMS

The epileptogenicity of this disorder results from loss of specific neurons in the hippocampus and synaptic reorganization of surviving cellular elements to cause hypersynchronization and hyperexcitability. The characteristic features of cell loss and reorganization, as well as the electrophysiologic aberrations that ultimately give rise to spontaneous seizures, are described in detail in Chapters 13 and 41. Although the pathophysiology of HS in fully developed MTLE-HS has been relatively well defined by studies of patients in epilepsy surgery centers and some very good experimental animal models exist, the events that initiate this process in humans are as yet unknown.

An association between mesial temporal sclerosis and febrile seizures was reported more than 30 years ago,[44] suggesting a causal relationship. Subsequent studies in both animals and humans have challenged this concept; some patients with MTLE-HS do not have a history of febrile convulsions,[47] and prolonged seizures in immature animals do not produce HS.[94] There are methodologic concerns with these studies, however, and more recent series of patients having MTLE-HS report a strong association with early risk factors, with as many as 66% of patients having prolonged febrile convulsions[14,15,47,60,61,115,116,138] and a variety of other early insults, such as trauma and infection.[83] Furthermore, there is evidence that the process, once begun, does not stop after seizures appear but rather continues to progress over time.[47,82]

Also of etiologic importance is the observation that HS is sometimes associated with microdysgenesis[85] and occurs in patients with dysplastic lesions, such as hamartomas and heterotopias, but only rarely in patients with neoplasms.[79] This association, coupled with the increased incidence of a family history of epilepsy and febrile convulsions, suggests a genetic or congenital predisposition to epilepsy. Consequently, familial or congenital disturbances could be a necessary precursor that permits early noxious insult to give rise to the characteristic cell loss and neuronal reorganization necessary for the development of MTLE.

CLINICAL PRESENTATION

The current characteristic clinical features of MTLE-HS are derived almost exclusively from patients with medically intractable seizures who are being evaluated for surgical intervention. Onset of habitual seizures typically begins toward the end of the first decade of life, and seizures often initially respond well to antiepileptic drug treatment. Characteristically, patients do well for several years, but seizures then return in adolescence or even early adulthood and become refractory to medical treatment. Of these patients with medically intractable seizures, the great majority have a history of complicated febrile convulsions or other initial precipitating injury.[47,83]

Evidence for Progression

Debate exists concerning the possibly progressive nature of MTLE-HS despite the fact that some animal models, such as kindling, clearly progress.[124] Based on the known pathophysiology, there is evidence that cell death and neuronal reorganization continue with recurrent seizures.[82] The latent period between occurrence of a precipitating event and onset of habitual seizures, and the period of control between initiation of medical therapy and development of medical intractability, also suggest an ongoing process.[47] The fact that some patients with MTLE-HS have persistent auras following extensive mesial temporal lobe resection that is successful in eliminating disabling complex partial seizures indicates that more than the sclerotic hippocampus is epileptogenic. Evidence that the degree of hippocampal atrophy on MRI[15] and persistence of auras and occasional seizures[38] correlate with duration of MTLE-HS further supports the existence of a progressive process. Progressive worsening of cognitive dysfunction in MTLE-HS, particularly involving memory and learning, has been disputed.[113] However, some degree of cognitive disability can be reversed by successful surgical intervention, indicating that it is related to recurrent seizures.[19,91,98,101,112,120] Although the subject is controversial, much has also been written about the possibility that patients with temporal lobe epilepsy are at greater risk for personality disturbances, depression, and psychosis, and numerous possible neurobiologic mechanisms have been put forth to justify a concept of epilepsy-induced enduring dysfunctions. It is conceivable that progressive changes peculiar to HS could make the appearance and exacerbation of nonepileptic psychologic and psychiatric disturbances reportedly seen in temporal lobe epilepsy a more specific feature of MTLE-HS in particular.

Clinical Seizure Characteristics

Mesial temporal lobe seizures (MTLS) occurring with MTLE-HS are generally thought to be indistinguishable from MTLS resulting from other forms of MTLE and therefore do not characterize the syndrome per se but are an important part of the symptom complex. Recent evidence refutes this concept in part, as there may be some differences between the seizures of MTLE-HS and other varieties of MTLE.[111] For example, ipsilateral limb automatisms, contralateral dystonic posturing, and oral-alimentary automatisms may be characteristic of MTLE-HS but not of MTLE resulting from neoplasms. More work is clearly needed to define this issue better.

The following descriptions of MTLS are based heavily on several reports from a relatively "pure culture" of patients with MTLE-HS,[47,135,138] as well as on recent studies describing various lateralizing or localizing features of these seizures.[1,41,72–74,88,93,99,140,142]

Ictal clinical characteristics can be divided into subjective and objective components. The subjective component in MTLS is the warning or aura. Auras in MTLS are very common, occurring in more than 90% of patients.[47,69] They can occur as the first manifestation of a complex partial seizure, and they often occur in isolation as simple partial seizures.[118,119] Auras in isolation may be a defining feature of MTLE, but not necessarily of MTLE-HS. By far the most common type of aura is a visceral sensation, usually in the epigastrium and often with a rising component.[27,47,81,95,129,132] Fear as an aura is a distant second. Other frequently described auras, such as déjà vu, jamais vu, micropsia, macropsia, olfactory hallucinations, and feelings of depersonalization, do occur, but they are uncommon.[47] Some aura symptoms may not have a counterpart in human experience and cannot be described. Patients who cannot describe their seizures verbally can sometimes do so in writing. Formed visual hallucinations and auditory hallucinations of any kind are not part of these seizures. Some patients have experienced auras in the past but no longer have them. This could be a consequence of seizure-related retrograde amnesia.[30] For example, during intensive monitoring, an occasional patient will consistently press the alarm button at the beginning of a seizure, yet deny any warning afterward.

The objective manifestations of MTLS, described by observers or recorded on videotape, usually occur when consciousness is impaired, so the patient is seldom aware of them. The objective manifestations of MTLS often begin with motor arrest, staring, and pupillary dilation. The seizure may not progress beyond this point (temporal lobe absence), but more often semipurposeful coordinated motor activities (automatisms) are a prominent part of MTLS. Oral-alimentary automatisms, although not seen exclusively in MTLS, are highly characteristic. They consist of lip smacking, chewing, licking, and tooth-grinding movements. Lip smacking can be so pronounced as to be audible on videotaped seizures, as can tooth grinding. Stereotyped automatisms that consist of fumbling, picking, and gesticulating movements are another common feature of MTLS. Automatisms suggesting reactions to environmental objects or situations are also common. Other, less common, automatic activity includes vocalization,[142] spitting,[56,68] and bicycling movements[122]; these, however, are also seen in seizures originating elsewhere. Ictal piloerection has also been reported in patients with MTLS.[26,107]

Emphasis has recently been placed on objective seizure characteristics that may have lateralizing or localizing value. These include lateralized motor manifestations, language signs, and postictal findings.

Head and eye deviation have long been recognized as clinical seizure manifestations,[2,55,97,125] but their lateralizing significance, particularly in MTLS, has been disputed.[92,100,106,140] Many reports suggest that head deviation, eye deviation, or both, occurring in temporal lobe seizures have lateralizing value, but this depends on when during the seizure such deviation takes place.[41,67,73,140] Early, relatively casual head deviation can be ipsilateral to seizure origin, whereas forced head and eye deviation occurring later in the seizure, often as a prelude to a secondarily generalized convulsive seizure, is almost always contralateral.

Unilateral tonic or dystonic posturing occurs in 15% to 70% of patients with MTLS and is reliably contralateral to the side of onset.[41,73,88] Studies using ictal single-photon emission computed tomography (SPECT) have equated this dystonic posturing with increased activity in the basal ganglia ipsilateral to seizure onset.[88] Although unilateral dystonic posturing has been considered a relatively new lateralizing sign, it was actually described 50 years ago.[2,81] Ajmone-Marsan and Ralston[2] provided illustrations of dystonic posturing (and ipsilateral/contralateral head turning) on pages 86 and 95 of their classic monograph, *The Epileptic Seizure*. This posture, termed *larval M2e*, was seen primarily during temporal lobe seizures. Contralateral dystonic posturing can include the leg and even the face and is often associated with ipsilateral automatisms.[73] Ipsilateral automatisms occurring alone are not as consistently lateralizing as dystonic posturing.[73] Conversely, contralateral ictal paresis has recently been reported as a reliable lateralizing sign.[92]

Ictal vomiting in MLTS has been related to right temporal lobe onset.[72,74,87] Unilateral eye blinking reportedly occurs on the same side as seizure origin.[7]

Language disturbance during seizures has been critically examined infrequently. Both ictal aphasia and ictal speech arrest have been equated with seizure onset in the language-dominant temporal lobe.[1,42] Ictal vocalization has been reported to have no lateralizing value,[142] whereas verbalization of coherent speech is associated with seizure onset in the temporal lobe that is not speech dominant.[142] Although uncommon, ictal automatisms with preserved consciousness occur with seizure origin in the nondominant hemisphere.[3,96]

Postictal aphasia as a lateralizing sign in MTLS has been controversial. Two early studies examining clinical features of temporal lobe seizures provided contradictory results: One reported that postictal language disturbances had no localizing value,[128] whereas the other noted highly accurate lateralization of seizure origin to the language-dominant side.[69] The controversy in part must be related to methodology. Postictal language disturbance is often difficult to separate from confusion, and it will be missed completely unless specifically tested for by trained examiners. More recent reports that specifically evaluated postictal language function following temporal lobe seizures confirm that postictal aphasia reliably lateralized seizure origin to the language-dominant side.[42,99] Although seldom evaluated, lateralized postictal motor deficits can occur in patients with MTLS. When detected, they are contralateral to seizure origin and usually follow seizures associated with prominent unilateral dystonic posturing. Patients occasionally wipe their nose at the end of an MTLS, and when they do, they almost always use the hand ipsilateral to ictal onset.[51,78]

Since MTLS with HS usually present with typical seizures, series with this condition in young children do not exist. Two recent reports examined temporal lobe seizures in children, some with documented HS.[103,126] In general, children under the age of 3 have tonic motor and clonic motor activity, while children over 10 years have the same clinical characteristics as adults. In between these years, seizures tend to be relatively simple (hypokinetic seizures) with progressive elaboration of automatisms as they grow older. This pattern was seen in children with HS.[103]

Mesial temporal lobe seizures are typically followed by postictal dysfunction of variable duration, as opposed to some extratemporal seizures with a minimal postictal phase or none.[59,136,137,139] The postictal state is usually obvious at the end of the seizure, often accompanied by visible relaxation; automated semipurposeful motor movements can persist. The postictal state is further characterized by confusion, disorientation, and, as noted above, disturbances of language. Reports have suggested that the duration of the postictal period that follows MTLS beginning in the language-dominant side is much longer than that following seizures originating in the nondominant side.[42,99] This is unquestionably related to gradual clearing of postictal language disturbance.

All these potentially lateralizing signs are helpful during the presurgical evaluation of patients with medically intractable MTLSs. Whether or not these signs also occur in other types of temporal lobe seizures, or in seizures originating outside the temporal lobes, and with what frequency, is not clear, but recent evidence suggests that they occur less often.[46,53,111] Further verification is needed.

DIAGNOSTIC EVALUATION

Results of the neurologic examination are usually normal, with the exception of mild to moderate memory deficit that is generally material specific for the involved hemisphere. Formal neuropsychological testing is useful for demonstrating typical memory and learning disturbances.[139] When surgical treatment is being considered, the neuropsychological evaluation often includes an intracarotid amobarbital procedure to demonstrate that the temporal lobe contralateral to the planned resection is capable of supporting memory.[102] Dysfunction of the ipsilateral mesial temporal structures can be confirmed when injection of amobarbital into the contralateral carotid artery results in a global memory deficit.

Results of routine EEGs in patients with MTLE-HS can be normal or nonspecific, but only rarely will no epileptiform abnormalities be revealed during prolonged monitoring.[138] The characteristic interictal EEG abnormality is anterior temporal sharp waves, spikes, and slow waves. These can be bilaterally independent in up to one third of patients.[33,133,138] The discharges demonstrate a characteristic field with a maximum in basal derivations, such as sphenoidal, true temporal, or earlobe electrodes. Although bilateral synchronous interictal spikes and sharp waves are usually not a part of the MTLE-HS syndrome, occasionally bilateral frontal polar spikes are seen, but they are not considered clinically significant.[108] Ictal EEG onset usually consists of a characteristic unilateral 5- to 7-Hz rhythmic discharge, seen best in one basal electrode derivation and appearing within 30 seconds of the first ictal EEG abnormality.[105] Occasionally the scalp ictal pattern can be seen over the temporal lobe contralateral to obvious HS.[86] In this case, intracranial studies reveal seizure origin in the abnormal hippocampus ("burned-out hippocampus") without spread to the ipsilateral temporal neocortex but with contralateral spread. Specific ictal patterns can help differentiate mesial from lateral temporal lobe epilepsies.[29] Auras are usually not associated with any EEG changes, although frequent interictal spikes may be seen to disappear during the simple partial seizure. Stereotactic depth-electrode studies demonstrate that simple partial seizures usually are associated with hypersynchronous hippocampal discharges, with a transition to a low-voltage fast recruiting rhythm just before contralateral propagation and onset of the clinical complex partial ictal event.[32] Depth-electrode recordings reveal that hypersynchronous hippocampal ictal discharges can also occur without noticeable signs or symptoms.[119]

High-resolution MRI can demonstrate hippocampal atrophy in a high percentage of patients with medically refractory MTLE.[9,75,138] Volumetry is used by some investigators to demonstrate asymmetry,[13] although controversy exists as to the need for this quantitative technique. As technology for structural imaging improves, it may also be possible to diagnose hippocampal sclerosis by loss of the normal architectural pattern. T2-weighted images often show increased signal in the area of hippocampal sclerosis, and this is also a useful finding for confirmation of a diagnosis of MTLE-HS.[9,75]

Positron emission tomography with ^{18}F-fluorodeoxyglucose (FDG-PET) remains the most sensitive interictal imaging technique for identifying the focal functional deficit associated with hippocampal sclerosis.[39,70] The area of hypometabolism can be quite large, involving more than the epileptogenic temporal lobe and including the ipsilateral thalamus, basal ganglia, and other cortical structures.[57] It is not clear at this time, however, whether such patterns might help to distinguish MTLE-HS from MTLE due to other lesions. Other PET tracers demonstrate zones of decreased cerebral perfusion approximating the area of hypometabolism,[141] increased binding of μ-opioid receptors[48] in lateral cortex of the involved temporal lobe, and decreased benzodiazepine receptor binding[117] of the sclerotic hippocampus. Bilateral reduced benzodiazepine binding suggests subtle damage in up to one third of contralateral hippocampi in patients with unilateral HS on MRI.[71] Bilateral limbic system dysfunction was also suggested in patients with unilateral HS by investigating MRI diffusion properties.[23] Interictal SPECT is also capable of showing unilateral temporal hypoperfusion in MTLE-HS, but with a much lower yield than PET. Ictal SPECT, however, demonstrates a characteristic pattern of hyperperfusion of the involved temporal lobe when the tracer is injected during a seizure, and of lateral hypoperfusion with persistent mesial hyperperfusion when it is injected shortly after a seizure, during the early postictal phase.[89,90] Again, it remains to be demonstrated whether this pattern has any specificity for MTLE-HS.

Magnetic resonance spectroscopy has demonstrated that HS is associated with a decrease in *N*-acetylaspartate.[77] Magnetic source imaging (MSI) with magnetoencephalography (MEG) can localize interictal and ictal epileptiform discharges to mesial temporal structures in patients with MTLE.[28]

DIFFERENTIAL DIAGNOSIS

Both MTLE and benign childhood epilepsy with centrotemporal spikes (BCECTS) can first appear in childhood as a single generalized convulsion and interictal temporal EEG epileptiform discharges. The broad centrotemporal spikes of BCECTS with a characteristic transverse dipole are located more posteriorly and superiorly, and morphologically they are easily distinguished from the characteristic, sharper anterior spike and spike-and-wave discharges of MTLE. The partial seizures of the benign childhood syndrome typically begin with sensory or motor phenomena around the mouth or upper extremity, and they are not likely to be confused with the complex partial seizures of mesial temporal origin.

The features of MTLE-HS most likely to distinguish this syndrome from MTLE caused by other lesions in mesial temporal structures include the earlier age of onset, history of complicated febrile convulsions and other early insults, increased incidence of seizures among family members, material-specific memory deficit, characteristic sphenoidal ictal onset pattern, and hippocampal atrophy on MRI. The same features help to distinguish patients with MTLE-HS from patients with complex partial seizures caused by lateral temporal or extratemporal lesions. In addition, the latter may have auras that indicate a site of origin closer to primary sensory or motor cortical areas.

TREATMENT AND OUTCOME

The medical treatment of choice for MTLE-HS includes carbamazepine, oxcarbazepine, lamotrigine, topiramate, and levetiracetam. Seizures usually respond well for several years.[8] However, because a diagnosis of MTLE-HS is rarely made until the condition becomes medically refractory and the patient is referred for surgical treatment, there is no definitive information concerning the percentage of patients who remain adequately controlled with pharmacotherapy.

Once seizures return (usually in adolescence or early adulthood), high-dose monotherapy or combinations of drugs often result in intolerable side effects and fail to control disabling seizures.

Surgical treatment, on the other hand, is now reported to abolish all disabling complex partial seizures in 60% to 80% of patients with MTLE.[40,130] A report that patients with MTLE-HS are more likely to experience late postoperative seizure recurrence than patients with other forms of MTLE has now been refuted.[84] The presurgical evaluation can usually be achieved noninvasively with video-EEG monitoring, MRI, neuropsychological evaluation, and often functional imaging with either PET or SPECT.[34] At most epilepsy centers, surgical resection is now limited to the involved mesial temporal structures, the temporal pole, and only a small amount of lateral neocortex, resulting in no significant additional neurologic deficit. When material-specific memory is already impaired, this does not change postoperatively, but contralateral material-specific memory may improve and IQ may increase.[101] If material-specific memory is intact, however, anteromesial temporal resection will result in a postoperative deficit, particularly when performed on the language-dominant side. This can cause additional disability for highly functional patients who depend on verbal memory.[18,58,76,80,109]

The reason for the 20% to 30% surgical failure rate in MTLE-HS has not been extensively studied. Insular lobe seizure origin has been documented in a few cases,[62] whereas the importance of the temporal polar cortex has been emphasized by others.[17]

LONG-TERM PROGNOSIS

Patients in whom medically refractory MTLE-HS develops have a relatively poor prognosis with medical treatment. Seizures often become worse and interictal behavioral disturbances can ensue. MTLE-HS is, however, the prototype of a surgically remediable syndrome, as presurgical evaluation can now usually be accomplished noninvasively and a high percentage of patients become free of disabling seizures postoperatively.[34,127] Early surgical intervention, as soon as possible following demonstration of failure of two appropriate drugs at maximum tolerable doses, yields the best psychosocial outcome if patients are relieved of disabling seizures before these events interfere with critical social and vocational development during adolescence and early adulthood. If seizures continue through this period, irreversible psychosocial disturbances often result, so that seizures may be abolished by surgical treatment later in life but complete or even partial rehabilitation cannot be achieved, and the patient remains dependent.[104,120]

SUMMARY AND CONCLUSIONS

MTLE-HS is now generally recognized as a distinct syndrome, representing a subtype of MTLE caused by a variety of lesions. The incidence and prevalence of MTLE-HS are unknown, as patients with medically refractory seizures are preferentially identified; however, this is likely to be the most common single form of human epilepsy. Although HS is believed to be the epileptogenic lesion, its etiology is unknown. There is a strong association with an early precipitating insult, particularly complicated febrile convulsions, and a genetic predisposition. The pathophysiology of MTLE-HS is now relatively well understood, and there is evidence that the disturbance can be progressive. The syndrome can be easily recognized in most patients by the characteristic presentation, seizure type, and diagnostic findings, which include increased incidence of febrile convulsions and family history of epilepsy, onset toward the end of the first decade of life, typical simple and complex partial limbic seizures, material-specific memory deficit, anterior temporal interictal EEG spikes and a characteristic ictal EEG onset pattern, temporal hypometabolism on FDG-PET, and hippocampal atrophy on high-resolution MRI. Once seizures become refractory to two appropriate antiepileptic drugs, further pharmacotherapy is not likely to be of benefit; disabling, irreversible psychosocial disturbances can result if aggressive treatment is not instituted. Surgical treatment, however, can abolish disabling seizures in 60% to 80% of patients with MTLE-HS, making this a surgically remediable syndrome. Early surgical intervention, therefore, offers the greatest potential for restoring a patient to a normal life.

ACKNOWLEDGMENTS

Original research reported by Dr. Engel was supported in part by grants NS-02808, NS-15654, NS-33310, and GM-24839 from the National Institutes of Health, and contract DE-AC03-76-SF00012 from the Department of Energy.

References

1. Abou-Khalil B, Welch L, Blumenkopf B, et al. Global aphasia with seizure onset in the dominant basal temporal region. *Epilepsia*. 1994;35:1079–1084.
2. Ajmone-Marsan C, Ralston BL. *The Epileptic Seizure. Its Functional Morphology and Diagnostic Significance*. Springfield, IL: Charles C Thomas; 1957:211–215.
3. Alarcon G, Elwes RD, Polkey CE, et al. Ictal oroalimentary automatisms with preserved consciousness: implications for the pathophysiology of automatisms and relevance to the international classification of seizures. *Epilepsia*. 1998;39:1119–1127.
4. Armstrong DD, Bruton CJ. Postscript: what terminology is appropriate for tissue pathology? How does it predict outcome? In: Engel J Jr, ed. *Surgical Treatment of the Epilepsies*. New York: Raven Press; 1987:541–552.
5. Babb TL, Brown WJ. Pathological findings in epilepsy. In: Engel J Jr, ed. *Surgical Treatment of the Epilepsies*. New York: Raven Press; 1987:511–540.
6. Bailey P, Gibbs FA. The surgical treatment of psychomotor epilepsy. *JAMA*. 1951;145:365–370.
7. Benbadis SR, Kotagal P, Klem GH. Unilateral blinking: a lateralizing sign in partial seizures. *Neurology*. 1996;46:45–48.
8. Berg AT, Langfitt J, Shinnar S, et al. How long does it take for partial epilepsy to become intractable? *Neurology*. 2003;60:186–190.
9. Berkovic SF, Andermann F, Olivier A, et al. Hippocampal sclerosis in temporal lobe epilepsy demonstrated by magnetic resonance imaging. *Ann Neurol*. 1991;29:175–182.
10. Berkovic SF, Howell RA, Hopper JL. Familial temporal lobe epilepsy: a new syndrome with adolescent/adult onset and a benign course. In: Wolf P, ed. *Epileptic Seizures and Syndromes*. London: John Libbey; 1994:257–263.
11. Bouchet C, Cazauvieilh JB. De L'épilepsie considerée dans ses rapports avec l'aliénation mentale. *Arch Gen Med*. 1825;9:510–542.
12. Bratz E. Ammonshornbefunde der epileptischen. *Arch Psychiatr Nervenkr*. 1899;31:820–836.
13. Cascino GD, Jack CR, Parisi JE, et al. Magnetic resonance imaging-based volume studies in temporal lobe epilepsy: pathological correlations. *Ann Neurol*. 1991;30:31–36.
14. Cendes F, Andermann F, Dubeau F, et al. Early childhood prolonged febrile convulsions, atrophy, and sclerosis of mesial structures and temporal lobe epilepsy: an MRI volumetric study. *Neurology*. 1993;43:1083–1087.
15. Cendes F, Andermann F, Gloor P, et al. Atrophy of mesial structures in patients with temporal lobe epilepsy: cause or consequence of repeated seizures? *Ann Neurol*. 1993;34:795–801.
16. Cendes F, Lopes-Cendes I, Andermann E, et al. Familial temporal lobe epilepsy: a clinically heterogeneous syndrome. *Neurology*. 1998;50:554–557.
17. Chabardes S, Kahane P, Minotti L, et al. The temporopolar cortex plays a pivotal role in temporal lobe seizures. *Brain*. 2005;128:1818–1831.
18. Chelune GJ, Naugle RI, Lüders H, et al. Prediction of cognitive change as a function of preoperative ability status among temporal lobectomy patients seen at a 6-month follow-up. *Neurology*. 1991;41:399–404.
19. Chelune GJ, Naugle RI, Lüders H, et al. Individual change after epilepsy surgery: practice effects and base-rate information. *Neuropsychology*. 1993;7:41–52.
20. Commission on Classification and Terminology of the International League Against Epilepsy. Proposal for revised clinical and electroencephalographic classification of epileptic seizures. *Epilepsia*. 1981;22:489–501.
21. Commission on Classification and Terminology of the International League Against Epilepsy. Proposal for classification of epilepsies and epileptic syndromes. *Epilepsia*. 1985;26(Suppl 3):268–278.
22. Commission on Classification and Terminology of the International League Against Epilepsy. Proposal for revised classification of epilepsies and epileptic syndromes. *Epilepsia*. 1989;30:389–399.
23. Concha L, Beaulieu C, Gross DW. Bilateral limbic diffusion abnormalities in unilateral temporal lobe epilepsy. *Ann Neurol*. 2005;57:188–196.
24. Crandall PH, Walter RD, Rand RW. Clinical applications of studies on stereotactically implanted electrodes in temporal lobe epilepsy. *J Neurosurg*. 1963;20:827–840.
25. de Lanerolle NC, Brines ML, Kim JH, et al. Neurochemical remodeling of the hippocampus in human temporal lobe epilepsy. *Epilepsy Res Suppl*. 1992;9:205–220.
26. Dove GH, Buchalter JR, Cascino GD. Acute repetitive pilomotor seizures (goose bumps) in a patient with right mersial temporal sclerosis. *Clin Neurophysiol*. 2005;116:989–990.
27. Duncan JS, Sagar HJ. Seizure characteristics, pathology and outcome after temporal lobectomy. *Neurology*. 1987;37:405–409.
28. Ebersole JS, Eliashiv SD, Smith JR, et al. Applications of magnetic source imaging in evaluation of candidates for epilepsy surgery. *Neuroimaging Clin N Am*. 1995;5:1–22.
29. Ebersole JS, Pacia SV. Localization of temporal lobe foci by ictal EEG patterns. *Epilepsia*. 1996;37:386–399.
30. Engel J Jr. Diagnostic evaluation. In: *Seizures and Epilepsy*. Philadelphia: FA Davis; 1989:303–339.
31. Engel J Jr. *Seizures and Epilepsy*. Philadelphia: FA Davis; 1989.
32. Engel J Jr. Functional explorations of the human epileptic brain and their therapeutic implications. *Electroencephalogr Clin Neurophysiol*. 1990;76:296–316.
33. Engel J Jr. Recent advances in surgical treatment of temporal lobe epilepsy. *Acta Neurol Scand*. 1992;140(Suppl 5):71–80.
34. Engel J Jr. Current concepts: surgery for seizures. *N Engl J Med*. 1996;334:647–652.
35. Engel J Jr. Introduction to temporal lobe epilepsy. *Epilepsy Res*. 1996;26:141–150.
36. Engel J Jr. A proposed diagnostic scheme for people with epileptic seizures and with epilepsy: report of the ILAE Task Force on Classification and Terminology. *Epilepsia*. 2001;42:796–803.
37. Engel J Jr, Babb TL, Crandall PH. Surgical treatment of epilepsy: opportunities for research into basic mechanisms of human brain function. *Acta Neurochir Suppl (Wien)*. 1989;46:3–8.
38. Engel J Jr, Cahan L. Potential relevance of kindling to human partial epilepsy. In: Wada J, ed. *Kindling 3*. New York: Raven Press; 1986:37–51.
39. Engel J Jr, Sutherling WW, Cahan L, et al. The role of positron emission tomography in the surgical therapy of epilepsy. In: Porter RJ, Mattson RH, Ward AA, et al., eds. *Advances in Epileptology: the XVth Epilepsy International Symposium*. New York: Raven Press; 1984:427–432.
40. Engel J Jr, Wiebe S, French J, et al. Practice parameter: temporal lobe and localized neocortical resections for epilepsy. *Neurology*. 2003;60:538–547.
41. Fakhoury T, Abou-Khalil B. Association of ipsilateral head turning and dystonia in temporal lobe seizures. *Epilepsia*. 1995;36:1065–1070.
42. Fakhoury T, Abou-Khalil B, Peguero E. Differentiating clinical features of right and left temporal lobe seizures. *Epilepsia*. 1994;35:1038–1044.
43. Falconer MA. Discussion on the surgery of temporal lobe epilepsy: surgical and pathological aspects. *Proc R Soc Med*. 1953;46:971–974.
44. Falconer MA. Genetic and related etiological factors in temporal lobe epilepsy: a review. *Epilepsia*. 1971;12:13–31.
45. Falconer MA. Mesial temporal (Ammon's horn) sclerosis as a common cause of epilepsy: aetiology, treatment and prevention. *Lancet*. 1974;2:767–770.
46. Foldvary NR, Lee N, Mayes BN. Extrahippocampal temporal lobe epilepsy: clinical manifestations. *Epilepsia*. 1994;35(Suppl 8):109(abst).
47. French JA, Williamson PD, Thadani VM, et al. Characteristics of medial temporal lobe epilepsy I. Results of history and physical examination. *Ann Neurol*. 1993;34:774–780.
48. Frost JJ, Mayberg HS, Fisher RS, et al. Mu-opiate receptors measured by positron emission tomography are increased in temporal lobe epilepsy. *Ann Neurol*. 1988;23:231–237.
49. Gastaut H. Clinical and electroencephalographical classification of epileptic seizures. *Epilepsia*. 1970;11:102–113.
50. Gastaut H, Gastaut JL, Goncalves e Silva GE, et al. Relative frequency of different types of epilepsy: a study employing a classification of the International League Against Epilepsy. *Epilepsia*. 1975;16:457–461.

51. Geyer JD, Payne TA, Faught E, et al. Postictal nose-rubbing in the diagnosis, lateralization, and localization of seizures. *Neurology.* 1999;52:743–745.
52. Gibbs FA, Gibbs EL, Lennox WG. Cerebral dysrhythmias of epilepsy. *Arch Neurol Psychiatry.* 1938;39:298–314.
53. Gil-Nagel A, Risinger MW. Ictal semiology in hippocampal vs. extrahippocampal temporal lobe epilepsy. *Neurology.* 1993;43:273(abst).
54. Gloor P, Olivier A, Quesney LF, et al. The role of the limbic system in experiential phenomena of temporal lobe epilepsy. *Ann Neurol.* 1982;12:129–144.
55. Gowers WR. General character of epileptic fits. In: *Epilepsy and Other Chronic Convulsive Diseases: Their Causes, Symptoms and Treatment.* New York: William Wood; 1885:29–58.
56. Hecker A, Andermann F, Rodin EA. Spitting automatism in temporal lobe seizures. *Epilepsia.* 1972;13:767–772.
57. Henry TR, Mazziotta JC, Engel J Jr. Interictal metabolic anatomy of limbic temporal lobe epilepsy. *Arch Neurol.* 1993;50:582–589.
58. Hermann BP, Seidenberg M, Haltiner A, et al. Relationship of age at onset, chronologic age, and adequacy of preoperative performance to verbal memory change after anterior temporal lobectomy. *Epilepsia.* 1995;36:137–145.
59. Ho SS, Berkovic SF, Newton MR, et al. Parietal lobe epilepsy: clinical features and seizure localization by ictal SPECT. *Neurology.* 1994;44:2277–2284.
60. Hudson LP, Munoz DG, Miller L, et al. Amygdaloid sclerosis in temporal lobe epilepsy. *Ann Neurol.* 1993;33:622–631.
61. Hufnagel A, Elger CE, Pels H, et al. Prognostic significance of ictal and interictal activity in temporal lobe epilepsy. *Epilepsia.* 1994;35:1146–1153.
62. Isnard J, Guenot M, Sindou M, et al. Clinical manifestations of insular lobe seizures: a stereo-electroencephalographic study. *Epilepsia.* 2004;45:1079–1090.
63. Jackson JH. On a particular variety of epilepsy ("intellectual aura"), one case with symptoms of organic brain disease. *Brain.* 1880;11:179–207.
64. Jackson JH. Case of epilepsy with tasting movements and "dreaming state"—very small patch of softening in the left uncinate gyrus. *Brain.* 1898;21:580–590.
65. Jasper H, Kershman J. Electroencephalographic classification of the epilepsies. *Arch Neurol Psychiatry.* 1941;45:903–943.
66. Jasper H, Pertuisset B, Flanigin H. EEG and cortical electrograms in patients with temporal lobe seizures. *Arch Neurol Psychiatry.* 1951;65:272–290.
67. Jayakar P, Duchowny M, Resnick T, et al. Ictal head deviation: lateralizing significance of the pattern of head movement. *Neurology.* 1989;42:1989–1992.
68. Kaplan PW, Kerr DA, Olivi A. Ictus expectoratus: a sign of complex partial seizures usually of non-dominant temporal lobe origin. *Seizure.* 1999;8:480–484.
69. King DW, Ajmone-Marsan C. Clinical features and ictal patterns in epileptic patients with EEG temporal lobe foci. *Ann Neurol.* 1977;2:138–147.
70. Knowlton RC, Laxer KD, Ende G, et al. Presurgical multimodality neuroimaging in electroencephalographic lateralized temporal lobe epilepsy. *Ann Neurol.* 1997;42:829–837.
71. Koepp MJ, Labbe C, Richardson MP, et al. Regional hippocampal [11C] flumazenil PET in temporal lobe epilepsy with unilateral and bilateral hippocampal sclerosis. *Brain.* 1997;120:1865–1876.
72. Kotagal P. Seizure symptomatology of temporal lobe origin. In: Lüders H, ed. *Epilepsy Surgery.* New York: Raven Press; 1991:143–155.
73. Kotagal P, Lüders H, Morris HH, et al. Dystonic posturing in complex partial seizures of temporal lobe onset: a new lateralizing sign. *Neurology.* 1989;39:196–201.
74. Kramer RE, Lüders H, Morris HH, et al. Ictus emeticus: an electroclinical analysis. *Neurology.* 1988;38:1048–1052.
75. Kuzniecky RI, Jackson GD. *Magnetic Resonance in Epilepsy.* New York: Raven Press; 1995.
76. Langfitt JT, Rausch R. Word-finding deficits persist after left anterotemporal lobectomy. *Arch Neurol.* 1996;53:72–76.
77. Laxer KD, Rowley HA, Novotny EJ Jr, et al. Experimental technologies. In: Engel J Jr, ed. *Surgical Treatment of the Epilepsies.* New York: Raven Press; 1993:291–308.
78. Leutmezer F, Series W, Lehrner J, et al. Postictal nose wiping: a lateralizing sign in temporal lobe complex partial seizures. *Neurology.* 1998;51:1175–1177.
79. Levesque MF, Nakasato N, Vinters HV, et al. Surgical treatment of limbic epilepsy associated with extrahippocampal lesions: the problem of dual pathology. *J Neurosurg.* 1991;75:364–370.
80. LoGalbo A, Sawrie S, Roth DL, et al. Verbal memory outcome in patients with normal preoperative verbal memory and left mesial temporal sclerosis *Epilepsy Behav.* 2005;6:337–341.
81. Magnus O, Ponsen L, van Rijn AJ. Temporal lobe epilepsy. *Folia Psychiatr Neurol Neurochir Neerlandica.* 1954;59:264–297.
82. Mathern GW, Babb TL, Vickrey BG, et al. The clinical-pathogenic mechanisms of hippocampal neuron loss and surgical outcomes in temporal lobe epilepsy. *Brain.* 1995;118:105–118.
83. Mathern GW, Pretorius JK, Babb TL. Influence of the type of initial precipitating injury and at what age it occurs on course and outcome in patients with temporal lobe seizures. *J Neurosurg.* 1995;82:220–227.
84. McIntosh AM, Kalnins RM, Mitchell LA, et al. Temporal lobectomy: long-term seizure outcome, late recurrence and risks for seizure recurrence. *Brain.* 2004;127:2018–2030.
85. Meencke H-J, Veith G. Migration Disturbances in Epilepsy. In: Engel J Jr, Wasterlain C, Cavalheiro EA, et al, eds. *Molecular Neurobiology of Epilepsy*, Amsterdam: Elsevier; 1992:31–40.
86. Mintzer S, Cendes F, Soss J, et al. Unilateral hippocampal sclerosis with contralateral temporal scalp ictal onset. *Epilepsia.* 2004;45:792–802.
87. Mitchell WG, Greenwood RS, Messenheimer JA. Cyclic vomiting as the major symptom of simple partial seizures. *Arch Neurol.* 1983;40:251–252.
88. Newton MR, Berkovic SF, Austin MC, et al. Dystonia, clinical lateralization, and regional blood flow changes in temporal lobe seizures. *Neurology.* 1992;42:371–377.
89. Newton MR, Berkovic SF, Austin MC, et al. Postictal switch in blood flow distribution and human temporal lobe seizures. *J Neurol Neurosurg Psychiatry.* 1992;55:891–894.
90. Newton MR, Berkovic SF, Austin MC, et al. SPECT in the localisation of extratemporal and temporal seizure foci. *J Neurol Neurosurg Psychiatry.* 1995;59:26–30.
91. Novelly RA, Augustine EA, Mattson RH, et al. Selective memory improvement and impairment following temporal lobectomy for epilepsy. *Ann Neurol.* 1984;15:64–67.
92. Ochs R, Gloor P, Quesney F, et al. Does head-turning during a seizure have a lateralizing or localizing significance? *Neurology.* 1984;34:884–890.
93. Oestreich LJ, Berg MJ, Bachmann DL, et al. Ictal contralateral paresis in complex partial seizures. *Epilepsia.* 1995;36:671–675.
94. Okada R, Moshe SL, Albala BJ. Infantile status epilepticus and future seizure susceptibility in the rat. *Dev Brain Res.* 1984;15:177–183.
95. Palmini A, Gloor P. The localizing value of auras in partial seizures: a prospective and retrospective study. *Neurology.* 1992;42:801–808.
96. Park SA, Heo K, Koh R, et al. Ictal automatisms with preserved responsiveness in a patient with left mesial temporal lobe epilepsy. *Epilepsia.* 2001;42:1078–1081.
97. Penfield W, Jasper H. *Epilepsy and the Functional Anatomy of the Human Brain.* London: J & A Churchill; 1954.
98. Powell G, Polkey C, McMillian T. The new Maudsley series of temporal lobectomy. I. Short-term cognitive effects. *Br J Clin Psychol.* 1985;24:109–124.
99. Privitera MD, Morris GL, Gilliam F. Postictal language assessment and lateralization of complex partial seizures. *Ann Neurol.* 1991;30:391–396.
100. Quesney LF. Clinical and EEG features of complex partial seizures of temporal lobe origin. *Epilepsia.* 1986;27(Suppl 2):527–545.
101. Rausch R, Crandall PH. Psychological status related to surgical control of temporal lobe seizures. *Epilepsia.* 1982;23:191–202.
102. Rausch R, Silfvenius H, Wieser H-G, et al. Intra-arterial amobarbital procedures. In: Engel J Jr, ed. *Surgical Treatment of the Epilepsies.* New York: Raven Press; 1993:341–357.
103. Ray A, Kotagal P. Temporal lobe epilepsy in children: overview of clinical semiology. *Epileptic Disord.* 2005;7:299–307.
104. Resnick TJ, Duchowny M, Jayakar P. Early surgery for epilepsy: redefining candidacy. *J Child Neurol.* 1994;9(Suppl 2):36–41.
105. Risinger MW, Engel J Jr, Van Ness PC, et al. Ictal localization of temporal lobe seizures with scalp/sphenoidal recordings. *Neurology.* 1989;39:1288–1293.
106. Robillard A, Saint-Hilaire JM, Mercier M, et al. The lateralizing and localizing value of adversion in epileptic seizures. *Neurology.* 1983;33:1241–1242.
107. Sa'adah MA, Shawabkeh A, Sa'adah LM, et al. Pilomotor seizures: symptomatic vs. idiopathic report of two cases and literature review. *Seizure.* 2002;11:455–459.
108. Sadler RM, Blume WR. Significance of bisynchronous spike-waves in patients with temporal lobe spikes. *Epilepsia.* 1989;30:143–146.
109. Sass KJ, Westerveld M, Buchanan CP, et al. Degree of hippocampal neuron loss determines severity of verbal memory decrease after left anteromesiotemporal lobectomy. *Epilepsia.* 1994;35:1179–1186.
110. Savic I, Persson A, Roland P, et al. In vivo demonstration of reduced benzodiazepine receptor binding in human epileptic foci. *Lancet.* 1988;8616:863–866.
111. Saygi S, Spencer SS, Scheyer R, et al. Differentiation of temporal lobe ictal behavior associated with hippocampal sclerosis and tumors of temporal lobe. *Epilepsia.* 1994;35:737–742.
112. Saykin AJ, Robinson LJ, Stafiniak P, et al. Neuropsychological changes after anterior temporal lobectomy: acute effects on memory, language and music. In: Bennett TL, ed. *The Neuropsychology of Epilepsy.* New York: Plenum Press; 1992:263–290.
113. Selwa LM, Berent S, Giordani B, et al. Serial cognitive testing in temporal lobe epilepsy: longitudinal changes with medical and surgical therapies. *Epilepsia.* 1994;35:743–749.
114. Semah F, Picot M-C, Adam C, et al. Is the underlying cause of epilepsy a major prognostic factor for recurrence? *Neurology.* 1998;51:1256–1262.
115. So N, Gloor P, Quesney LF, et al. Depth electrode investigations in patients with bitemporal epileptiform abnormalities. *Ann Neurol.* 1989;25:423–431.
116. So N, Olivier A, Andermann F, et al. Results of surgical treatments in patients with bitemporal epileptiform abnormalities. *Ann Neurol.* 1989;25:432–439.
117. Sommer W. Erkrankung des Ammonschorns als aetiologisches Moment der Epilepsie. *Arch Psychiatr Nervenkr.* 1880;10:631–675.

118. Sperling MR, Lieb JP, Engel J Jr, et al. Prognostic significance of independent auras in temporal lobe seizures. *Epilepsia*. 1989;30:322–331.
119. Sperling MR, O'Connor MJ. Auras and subclinical seizures: characteristics and prognostic significance. *Ann Neurol*. 1990;28:320–328.
120. Sperling MR, O'Connor MJ, Saykin AJ, et al. Temporal lobectomy for refractory epilepsy. *JAMA*. 1996;276:470–475.
121. Stephen LJ, Kwan P, Brodie MJ. Does the cause of localisation-related epilepsy influence the response to antiepileptic drug treatment? *Epilepsia*. 2001;42:357–362.
122. Sussman NM, Jackel RA, Kaplan LR, et al. Bicycling movements as a manifestation of complex partial seizures of temporal lobe origin. *Epilepsia*. 1989;30:527–531.
123. Sutula T, Cascino G, Cavazos J, et al. Mossy fiber synaptic reorganization in the epileptic human temporal lobe. *Ann Neurol*. 1989;26:321–330.
124. Sutula T, He XX, Cavazos J, et al. Synaptic reorganization in the hippocampus induced by abnormal functional activity. *Science*. 1988;239:1147–1150.
125. Temkin O. *The Falling Sickness*. Baltimore: Johns Hopkins Press; 1985.
126. Terra-Bustamante VC, Inuzuca LM, Fernandes RM, et al. Temporal lobe epilepsy surgery in children and adolescents: clinical characteristics and post-surgical outcome. *Seizure*. 2005;14:274–281.
127. Thadani VM, Williamson PD, Berger R, et al. Successful epilepsy surgery without intracranial EEG recording: criteria for patient selection. *Epilepsia*. 1995;36:7–15.
128. Theodore WH, Porter RJ, Penry JK. Complex partial seizures: clinical characteristics and differential diagnosis. *Neurology*. 1983;33:1115–1121.
129. Van Buren JM. The abdominal aura: a study of abdominal sensations occurring in epilepsy and produced by depth stimulation. *Electroencephalogr Clin Neurophysiol*. 1963;15:1–19.
130. Wiebe S, Blume WT, Girvin JP, et al. A randomized, controlled trial of surgery for temporal lobe epilepsy. *N Engl J Med*. 2001;345:311–318.
131. Wieser HG. *Electroclinical Features of the Psychomotor Seizure: A Stereoelectroencephalographic Study of Ictal Symptoms and Chronographic Seizure Patterns Including Clinical Effects of Intracerebral Stimulation*. London: Butterworth; 1983.
132. Wieser HG. Psychomotor seizures of hippocampal-amygdalar origin. In: Pedley TA, Meldrum BS, eds. *Recent Advances in Epilepsy*. Edinburgh: Churchill Livingstone; 1986:57–79.
133. Wieser HG, Engel J Jr, Williamson PD, et al. Surgically remediable temporal lobe syndromes. In: Engel J Jr, ed. *Surgical Treatment of the Epilepsies*. New York: Raven Press; 1993:49–63.
134. Wieser H-G, Özkara Ç, Engel J Jr, et al. Mesial temporal lobe epilepsy with hippocampal sclerosis: report of the ILAE Commission on Neurosurgery of Epilepsy. *Epilepsia*. 2004;45:695–714.
135. Wieser HG, Williamson PD. Ictal semiology. In: Engel J Jr, ed. *Surgical Treatment of the Epilepsies*. New York: Raven Press; 1993:161–172.
136. Williamson PD. Intensive monitoring of complex partial seizures: diagnosis and subclassification. In: Gumnit RJ, ed. *Intensive Neurodiagnostic Monitoring*. New York: Raven Press; 1986:69–84.
137. Williamson PD. Frontal lobe epilepsy: some clinical characteristics. In: Jasper HH, Riggio S, Goldman-Rakic PS, eds. *Epilepsy and the Functional Anatomy of the Frontal Lobe*. New York: Raven Press; 1995:127–152.
138. Williamson PD, French JA, Thadani VM, et al. Characteristics of medial temporal lobe epilepsy II. Interictal and ictal scalp electroencephalography, neuropsychological testing, neuroimaging, surgical results and pathology. *Ann Neurol*. 1993;34:781–787.
139. Williamson PD, Spencer DD, Spencer SS, et al. Complex partial seizures of frontal lobe origin. *Ann Neurol*. 1985;18:497–504.
140. Wyllie E, Lüders H, Morris HH. The lateralizing significance of versive head and eye movements during epileptic seizures. *Neurology*. 1986;36:606–611.
141. Yamamoto YL, Ochs R, Gloor P, et al. Patterns of rCBF and focal energy metabolic changes in relation to electroencephalographic abnormality in the interictal phase of partial epilepsy. In: Baldy-Moulinier M, Ingvar D-H, Meldrum BS, eds. *Cerebral Blood Flow, Metabolism and Epilepsy. Current Problems in Epilepsy.* Vol. 1. London: John Libbey; 1983: 51–62.
142. Yen D, Ming-Shung S, Chun-Hing Y, et al. Ictal speech manifestations in temporal lobe epilepsy: a video-EEG study. *Epilepsia*. 1996;37:45–49.

CHAPTER 248 ■ FAMILIAL TEMPORAL LOBE EPILEPSIES

FERNANDO CENDES, ELIANE KOBAYASHI, ISCIA LOPES-CENDES, FRÉDÉRICK ANDERMANN, AND EVA ANDERMANN

INTRODUCTION

A positive family history of seizures and/or epilepsy is frequently observed among patients with temporal lobe epilepsy (TLE).[67] These families cannot be included in only one group, however, and detailed characterization of affected family members is crucial for defining the familial epilepsy syndrome. Patients with TLE can be identified in the context of familial mesial temporal lobe epilepsy (MTLE),[9,16,19,37,43] familial TLE with auditory features,[34,49,50] familial partial epilepsy with variable foci (FPEVF),[56,69] and generalized epilepsy with febrile seizures plus syndrome (GEFS+).[23,45,55,58,66]

There are two groups of familial TLE, according to the evidence for involvement of mesial or neocortical structures. The majority of affected individuals with *familial MTLE* have a benign clinical course, and in some families all affected members have good seizure control, much like those originally described by Berkovic et al.[9,11] However, as in patients with nonfamilial MTLE, some affected family members may have poor seizure control and require surgical treatment.[19,40] Although hippocampal atrophy (HA) and other signs of hippocampal sclerosis (HS) were more frequent and more severe in those patients with refractory seizures, these changes were also observed in patients with good outcome[41,43] and even in asymptomatic family members (Fig. 1).[42] These are strong indicators that genetic factors play a role in the genesis of hippocampal pathology in patients with *familial MTLE*. The genetic background in familial MTLE, however, does not suggest a more widespread structural abnormality on magnetic resonance imaging (MRI).[25]

Familial TLE with auditory features, also described as *autosomal-dominant partial epilepsy with auditory features* (ADPEAF), and *familial lateral temporal lobe epilepsy* (FLTLE)[38] was first reported by Ottman et al.,[49] and additional families have been described by the same group and by other authors.[34,48,50,52,68] Seizure semiology pointed to an extrahippocampal epileptogenic area in the temporal lobes, and, characteristically, most patients had auditory auras. Patients have good seizure control, and epileptiform discharges may be observed over posterior temporal regions. No clear signs of HA have been described in different series, but abnormalities in the neocortical aspects of the temporal lobes may be present (Figs. 2 and 3).[44] Molecular studies identified linkage to chromosome 10q (ch10q),[49,52,68] and mutations in the *leucine-rich, glioma-inactivated 1* gene (*LGI-1*) have been identified.[34,48,50]

There is no evidence to suggest that partial epilepsy with auditory features, familial partial epilepsy with variable foci, or temporal lobe variants of benign childhood epilepsy with centrotemporal spikes ever evolve into MTLE with HS; this is further evidence for a clear distinction between familial MTLE and these other familial epilepsy syndromes.

HISTORICAL PERSPECTIVE

Genetic factors in epilepsy have long been recognized. Until very recently, however, only generalized epilepsies were thought to be genetic in origin, whereas focal or partial epilepsies were largely attributed to environmental factors, such as birth injuries, infections, postnatal head trauma, and brain lesions such as tumors or vascular insults.

As in the generalized epilepsies, partial epilepsies were found to fit a model of multifactorial inheritance (now termed complex inheritance), in which there is an interaction of one or more genes and environmental factors.[2,3,6]

In the last decade, several autosomal-dominant forms of partial epilepsy were described (reviewed by Berkovic and Steinlein[13] and more recently by Andermann et al[6a]). These include autosomal-dominant nocturnal frontal lobe epilepsy (ADNFLE), familial MTLE, ADPEAF, FPEVF, and autosomal-dominant rolandic epilepsy with speech dyspraxia.

The first description of familial occurrence of TLE was in 1994 by Berkovic et al.; they described it as a benign syndrome with late seizure onset without a history of prolonged febrile seizures (FS) or MRI evidence for mesial temporal sclerosis (MTS). However, in subsequent FTLE series, patients had a less benign clinical course, and a high proportion of individuals with HA were described. Some of these patients required surgical treatment for their epilepsy.[19,40,43] These families showed phenotypic heterogeneity in different family members, as well as between families, with respect to a history of prolonged FS, severity of the epilepsy, and presence of HA. The original series of Berkovic et al.[9,11] was population based, arising from a twin study, whereas the later series were hospital based.

Recently, FTLE was included in the new proposal for classification of epileptic syndromes by the International League Against Epilepsy (ILAE), supporting it as a well-defined syndrome.[22]

With the description of the neocortical form of familial TLE or ADPEAF[49] associated with mutations in the *LGI-1* gene on chromosome 10q,[34,48] the distinction between mesial and lateral forms became more obvious.[7,10,37,38,43,63]

It is important to emphasize that it is impossible to distinguish familial from nonfamilial TLE patients based solely on the clinical presentation, in both mesial and lateral forms. Because the family history is not always accurately documented, many so-called "sporadic" or "isolated" patients may actually have a familial epilepsy syndrome.

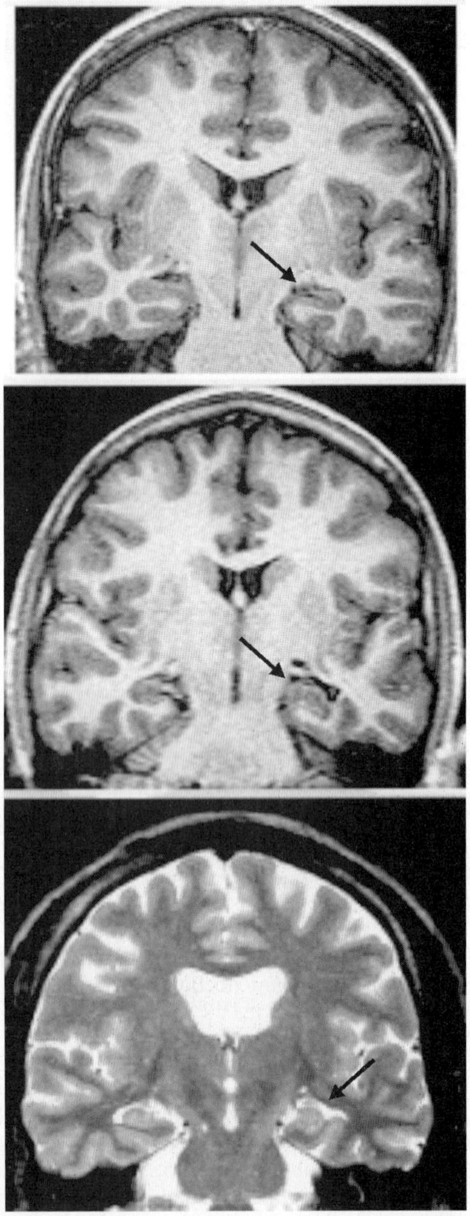

FIGURE 1. Hippocampal abnormalities in three asymptomatic individuals from families with mesial temporal lobe epilepsy. **Top:** Coronal T1-IR image of a 14-year-old boy, showing flattened and atrophic left hippocampus (*arrow*). **Middle:** Coronal T1-IR image from a 15-year-old boy. The left hippocampus is atrophic and bent clockwise and has an abnormal, "irregular" shape (*arrow*). **Bottom:** Coronal T2-FSE image from a 26-year-old man. The left atrophic hippocampus has an abnormal, "rounded" shape (*arrow*). In addition, the fusiform gyrus and collateral sulcus on the left have an abnormal shape. Note also the absence of septum pellucidum. (Reproduced, with permission, from Kobayashi E, Li LM, Lopes-Cendes I, et al. Magnetic resonance imaging evidence of hippocampal sclerosis in asymptomatic first-degree relatives of patients with familial mesial temporal lobe epilepsy. *Arch Neurol.* 2002;59(12):1891–1894. Copyright © 2002, American Medical Association. All rights reserved.)

DEFINITIONS

Familial Mesial Temporal Lobe Epilepsy

The best definition of familial MTLE is based on the familial recurrence of MTLE, according to the ILAE clinical-electroencephalogram (EEG) criteria,[53] in the absence of any suggestion of other partial (including lateral TLE symptoms) or generalized epilepsy syndromes in other affected family members. Thus, the finding of at least two MTLE patients in one family is suggestive of familial MTLE. The observation of an autosomal-dominant inheritance pattern with incomplete penetrance implies the presence of asymptomatic carriers of the genetic abnormalities who can transmit the disease to their offspring. Therefore, we should consider inclusion not only of families with affected first-degree relatives, but also those with affected second- and third-degree relatives. This criterion has not been employed in some reported series, leading to exclusion of many possible familial MTLE kindreds.[51]

Familial Temporal Lobe Epilepsy with Auditory Features

Familial TLE with auditory features is a benign epilepsy syndrome, characterized by auditory auras (buzzing, roaring, radio- or motor-like sounds, distortions in sounds and words). Although other manifestations such as psychic, cephalic, and other sensory and motor phenomena can occur, the auditory auras are a landmark for this syndrome. Sometimes ictal aphasia and visual misperceptions can occur and, in some families, secondarily generalized tonic–clonic seizures (GTCS) are frequent.[16,29,47,52,68] The pattern of inheritance observed is autosomal dominant with incomplete penetrance.

Age of onset is variable, usually in the second or third decade of life, and seizures are easily controlled by antiepileptic drugs (AEDs). EEGs may show posterior temporal epileptiform discharges but are frequently normal. No signs of HA are found on MRI studies, but a lateral temporal malformation pattern has been observed in 45% of affected individuals, including one asymptomatic carrier of the mutation.[44] The left temporal lobes of these individuals seemed enlarged, and sometimes there was protrusion of the brain parenchyma laterally, with an "encephalocele-like" appearance. Anterior temporal lobe volumetry showed a significant global increase in volumes in only two individuals. The epileptogenic significance of these structural abnormalities is unknown.

EPIDEMIOLOGY

The prevalence and incidence of these two forms of familial TLE are unknown. However, familial MTLE is apparently more common than familial TLE with auditory features. There is no predominance in any particular ethnic group. Families with MTLE have been described in Australia, Canada, Brazil, Italy, Belgium, and France. FLTLE has been studied in the United States, Brazil, Japan, Germany, France, Italy, Spain, and Australia. This is probably an underestimate of the real prevalence of both forms of familial TLE worldwide, especially in families with predominantly good outcomes.

Ascertainment of these families requires detailed questioning of patients and family members. This has only been emphasized recently because, in the past, MTLE as well as other partial epilepsies were considered to be symptomatic and due largely to environmental factors. A preliminary hospital-based study found that familial MTLE represented 7% of all MTLE patients.[43]

ETIOLOGY AND BASIC MECHANISMS

The etiology of familial epilepsies is first determined by the genetic pattern that indicates an inherited disease and second

A 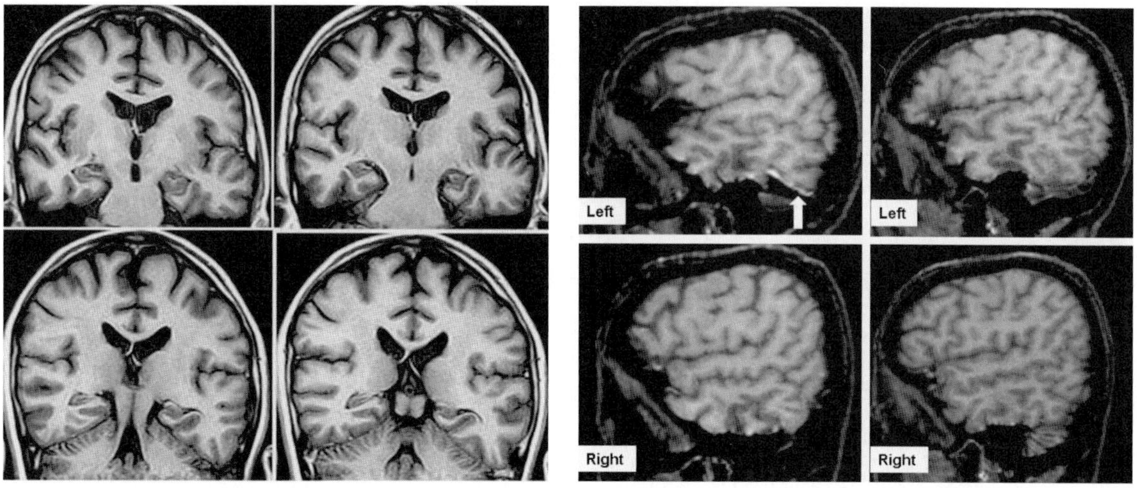 B

FIGURE 2. A: T1-IR coronal images from a patient with *LGI-1* mutation showing left temporal lobe dysgenesis, characterized by enlargement of the lateral temporal lobe, with small gyri (although not characterizing polymicrogyria). B: T1 sagittal images from the same patient showing absence of first and second temporal sulcus on the anterior and middle portions of the left temporal lobe. The posterior basolateral aspect of the left temporal lobe is also abnormal, with a protrusion of parenchyma downward, with an "encephalocele-like" appearance (*arrow*). (Reproduced, with permission, from Kobayashi E, Santos NF, Torres FR, et al. Magnetic resonance imaging abnormalities in familial temporal lobe epilepsy with auditory auras. *Arch Neurol.* 2003;60(11):1546–1551. Copyright © 2002, American Medical Association. All rights reserved.)

by the structural/functional abnormalities that are associated with this genetic background.

Pathogenetic mechanisms underlying familial MTLE remain unknown. Seizures and HS in familial MTLE may result from interactions between genetic and environmental factors. No locus for familial MTLE with HS has been identified.

No single-gene molecular defect has been confirmed, although several loci for familial TLE have been mapped. Digenic inheritance with loci on chromosomes 1q25–q31 and 18qter was described in a large family with febrile seizures and familial TLE without HS,[8] as well as a locus on chromosome 12q22–q23.3 in another large family with autosomal-dominant familial TLE with febrile seizures without HS.[21] Whether these loci represent susceptibility for febrile seizures or for TLE remains to be determined. A more recent locus was described on chromosome 4q in a four-generation kindred with familial MTLE.[31] MRI data, however, did not show signs of HS in this family.[31] Investigation of these loci in other families has not been reported.

No families with familial MTLE were found to have an *LGI-1* mutation, even in those families in which one or more family members had auditory features alone or in association with mesial symptoms.[7,10,54] This further supports the determination that familial MTLE and familial TLE with auditory features constitute distinct genetic syndromes.

Some polymorphisms have been found in association with MTLE,[62] but these could not be replicated in a recent large cohort of patients.[18] Kanemoto et al.[35] found an increased frequency of the T allele at the 511 position of the interleukin 1β gene among TLE patients with HS as compared with TLE patients without HS and with controls. The frequency of this polymorphism was further increased in patients with a history of prolonged FS. Stogmann et al.[59] found an overrepresentation of a functional polymorphism in the prodynorphin gene promoter (possibly related to seizure suppression) in patients with TLE and a positive family history of epilepsy as compared to controls. Gambardella et al.[27] recently demonstrated an overrepresentation of a $GABA_B$ receptor 1 polymorphism (G1465A) in patients with MTLE as compared to the normal population, especially in those with refractory seizures. However, more recent studies failed to replicate these findings.[46,61] The presence of all these polymorphisms would suggest a polygenic or multifactorial mode of inheritance, as first suggested by Andermann.[2–4]

The presence of clear-cut HA in both affected and asymptomatic family members in familial MTLE suggests that the

A 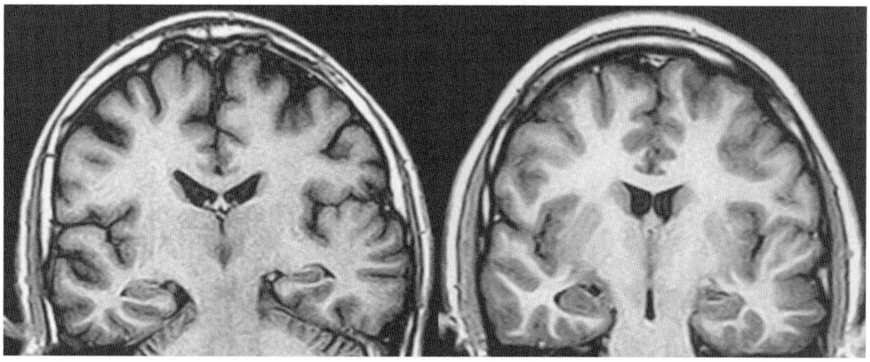 B

FIGURE 3. T1-IR coronal images from two patients with *LGI-1* mutation, showing left temporal lobe malformation, with a dysgenetic aspect of temporal gyri and enlargement of the lateral aspect of the temporal lobe. (Reproduced with permission, from Kobayashi E, Santos NF, Torres FR, et al. Magnetic resonance imaging abnormalities in familial temporal lobe epilepsy with auditory auras. *Arch Neurol.* 2003;60(11):1546–1551. Copyright © 2002, American Medical Association. All rights reserved.)

hippocampal abnormalities themselves could be inherited, and not necessarily lead to epilepsy.[42] The phenotype would then depend on interaction with other modifying factors. Two papers addressed the possibility of inherited hippocampal abnormality. Fernandez et al.[24] studied families of patients with a previous history of FS, including asymptomatic individuals. They observed subtle abnormalities in hippocampal configuration, internal structure, and volume in individuals with and without FS. This suggested the presence of preexisting hippocampal malformations as an associated factor leading to FS and subsequent HS. A study of children with prolonged FS and their monozygotic asymptomatic twins did not confirm these findings.[33] Volumetric studies of the temporal lobes showed similar patterns of atrophy in familial and nonfamilial MTLE patients.[25]

Qualitative pathology from surgical specimens obtained from operated familial MTLE patients showed the typical pattern of MTS: Selective neuronal loss in CA1, CA3, and CA4 with relative preservation of CA2, and variable involvement of the amygdala and parahippocampal region.[40] The observation of MTS in operated familial MTLE patients who became seizure free suggests that MTS represents the epileptogenic substrate, at least in some of these families; analogous to what is observed in nonfamilial or "sporadic" cases.

Most likely, Familial MTLE will be found to have a major gene leading to hippocampal abnormalities, and the phenotype could be influenced by additional genetic and environmental modifying factors.

The mechanism by which LGI-1 causes familial TLE with auditory auras is unknown. LGI-1 is not homologous to any known ion channel, and it is likely to be involved in brain development.[34,50] The *LGI-1* gene was cloned from a glioblastoma cell line and, although previous studies have suggested that *LGI-1* represents a tumor suppressor gene,[20] a more recent study was unable to establish a correlation between the gene and malignant glioma suppression.[28] *LGI-1* codes for a putative membrane-anchored protein of unknown function. The LGI-1 protein is characterized by a central leucine-rich repeat region,[32] which is involved in regulation of cell growth, adhesion, and migration. More recent studies have shown that *LGI-1* mutations in patients with familial TLE with auditory features are associated with loss of function, with the LGI-1 protein either not secreted or unstable.[57] The association of lateral temporal malformation patterns in some families may indicate a probable role of LGI-1 in the development of the temporal lobes.[44]

The *LGI-1* gene is mutated in approximately 50% of families with familial TLE with auditory features.[10,50] Although *LGI-1* mutations appear to be specific for familial TLE with auditory features, the identification of *LGI-1* mutations in only one half of families presenting the typical phenotype[10,50] suggests genetic heterogeneity. No mutations in *LGI-2*, *LGI-3*, and *LGI-4* have been identified in 71 families with various types of TLE, including 4 who had familial TLE with auditory features.[10]

CLINICAL PRESENTATION

Familial Mesial Temporal Lobe Epilepsy

Familial MTLE is a well-characterized syndrome, with different degrees of seizure severity, although the majority of patients have good seizure control.[9,11,19,43] The mode of inheritance is autosomal dominant with incomplete penetrance. Patients with familial MTLE present with simple partial or complex partial seizures (CPS) or both, with characteristics of mesial temporal lobe origin (such as rising epigastric sensation, fear, *déjà vu*, *jamais vu*) that are indistinguishable from the sporadic form of MTLE.[1] Auras of *déjà-vu* and *jamais-vu* are particularly frequent, especially in families with benign outcome, and may be the only feature in some family members.[5] Memory impairment is often associated, even in asymptomatic family members with HA.[1] Secondary GTCSs are uncommon in patients with familial MTLE taking AEDs. Age at onset and the presence of a silent period follow initial febrile seizures are also similar to sporadic MTLE. However, an antecedent of febrile seizures in childhood is less frequent in patients with familial MTLE as compared to sporadic MTLE.[40,41,43]

Familial Temporal Lobe Epilepsy With Auditory Features

Seizure semiology in familial TLE with auditory features is characterized by auditory auras preceding complex partial and secondarily generalized seizures in many, but not all, patients.[50] Visual auras may occur,[52] and ictal aphasia has also been described.[16,29]

The most common initial ictal manifestations are described as buzzing, roaring, radio- or motor-like sounds, and distortions in sounds and words. Sometimes ictal aphasia and visual misperceptions can occur, and, in some families, secondarily generalized seizures are frequent.

The pattern of inheritance is autosomal dominant with incomplete penetrance. Age of onset is variable, usually in the second or third decades of life, and seizures are easily controlled with AEDs.

DIAGNOSTIC EVALUATION

Electroencephalographic Findings

EEGs in patients with familial MTLE show interictal epileptiform discharges over mid- and inferomesial temporal regions with similar characteristics to those of sporadic MTLE. Ictal EEG recordings in familial MTLE patients undergoing presurgical evaluation also show the same pattern observed in sporadic MTLE. A normal EEG, however, does not exclude the diagnosis of familial MTLE.

EEGs in familial TLE with auditory features may show posterior temporal epileptiform discharges but are frequently normal.

Neuroimaging and Other Laboratory Examinations

Familial Mesial Temporal Lobe Epilepsy

MRI evaluation in familial MTLE has shown a high frequency of HA and other signs of HS,[19,41,43] even in individuals with seizure remission and asymptomatic family members (Fig. 1).[42,43] The identification of MRI signs of HS in familial MTLE patients with a benign clinical course confirms that the presence of HA is not always associated with refractory epilepsy.

Data indicate that MRI abnormalities are similar in familial and sporadic MTLE with HS.[25]

Familial Temporal Lobe Epilepsy With Auditory Features

There have been no signs of HS in MRIs of patients from the reported families with *LGI-1* mutation.[10,44,50] Enlargement and abnormal gyration suggesting developmental abnormalities in the lateral cortex of the temporal lobes was described in 53% of affected individuals in one family with *LGI-1* mutation[44] (Figs. 2 and 3), a finding that requires confirmation. However, the MRI findings in that family are clearly distinct from the MRI findings in familial MTLE and are consistent with the distinct seizure semiology in these two forms of familial TLE.[44]

DIFFERENTIAL DIAGNOSIS

A family history of seizures is common among TLE patients. Many of them have one or more relatives who have experienced a single episode compatible with either CPS or GTCS, and a history of FS is also frequently found. Unless there are two individuals in the family with well-defined MTLE, however, a diagnosis of familial MTLE cannot be made.

In addition, there are other familial epilepsy syndromes in which patients with MTLE are found. In FPEVF,[12,17,56,69] most reported families mapped to chromosome 22q, but the gene has not yet been identified. Affected family members may present with various forms of partial epilepsy, including frontal lobe epilepsy and MTLE.[39]

In GEFS+, related to mutations in genes *SCN1A*, *SCN2A*, *SCN1B*, and *GABRG2*,[23,30,45,60,64–66] patients may present heterogeneous epilepsy phenotypes. FS are the most common phenotype, followed by FS plus (FS+), in which individuals have seizures with fever that may persist beyond the age of 6 years and/or may be associated with afebrile GTCS.[55,58] Less frequent phenotypes seen in GEFS+ involve other generalized and partial seizure types, including MTLE.[55,58,65]

A new partial epilepsy syndrome with some individuals presenting seizure semiology consistent with MTLE has been described in one large Brazilian kindred and named partial epilepsy with pericentral spikes.[36] The majority of affected individuals, however, presented hemitonic or hemiclonic seizures, and molecular analysis showed linkage to chromosome 4p15.

It is essential to evaluate the phenotype of all possibly affected individuals before classifying the family as having a specific familial syndrome. In addition, because the severity of the phenotypes in family members may vary, we can never be absolutely sure that an "isolated" or "sporadic" MTLE patient does not have familial MTLE. Molecular studies can be helpful in excluding other familial epilepsies with already identified gene mutations.

The two main differential diagnoses for familial TLE with auditory features are sporadic neocortical TLE and familial MTLE, which can be clarified most of the time with a detailed history and seizure description.

Recently, the presence of patients with neocortical TLE but without a positive family history was highlighted by Bisulli et al.[14] The authors termed this syndrome idiopathic partial epilepsy with auditory features (IPEAF) and performed a clinical and genetic study in 53 sporadic cases. Mutations in *LGI-1* were excluded in all these IPEAF patients, although, except for the absence of family history, these patients had identical clinical manifestations to those seen in familial TLE with auditory features, including the always-good prognosis.[14] After the first description of their large series, the same authors reported a de novo mutation in the *LGI-1* gene in one patient with sporadic neocortical TLE,[15] but another, more recent series of similar patients found no *LGI-1* mutations.[26]

Since the severity of the phenotype in family members with familial TLE with auditory features may vary, and mild cases may not be known to other family members, we can never be absolutely sure that an "isolated" or "sporadic" neocortical TLE patient does not have familial TLE with auditory features. Molecular studies with testing for mutations of the *LGI-1* gene and of other genes associated with related familial epilepsies can be helpful.

In summary, in the differential diagnoses, a familial MTLE and familial LTLE, one may consider familial partial epilepsies with variable foci, temporal lobe variants of benign childhood epilepsy with centrotemporal spikes, and GEFS+.[58]

No family with familial MTLE has been found to have an *LGI-1* mutation, even in those families in which one or more family members had auditory features alone or in association with mesial symptoms.[7,10,54] This further supports the observation that familial TLE with auditory features and familial MTLE constitute separate genetic syndromes.

Patients with TLE are found in other familial epilepsy syndromes. In FPEVF, different family members may present with various forms of partial epilepsy, including TLE,[39] but the focus remains the same in each affected individual. Most reported families mapped to chromosome 22q, but the gene has not been identified.[12,17,56,69]

TREATMENT AND OUTCOME

Treatment should be based on the patient's response to AEDs, and the rationale is similar to that in nonfamilial patients. Familial MTLE patients may have refractory seizures, and surgical treatment should be considered, based on clinical-EEG-MRI data, despite the context of a familial epilepsy syndrome.[19,40]

The majority of patients with familial MTLE have good seizure control, with low doses of AEDs indicated for partial epilepsies.[11,19,43] A large number of patients undergo seizure remission and maintain seizure freedom off medication. However, approximately 24% of our patients with familial MTLE were considered refractory to medical treatment.[19,37,43] Patients with refractory familial MTLE have excellent surgical outcome when unilateral or clearly asymmetric HA is identified on MRI.[40] The investigation of patients with familial MTLE should not differ from that of patients with sporadic MTLE, and the surgical decision should be based on the same clinical-EEG-imaging evidence for seizure lateralization and localization.

Seizures in patients with familial TLE with auditory features are easily controlled with small doses of AEDs indicated for partial epilepsies. Some of the affected family members with *LGI-1* mutation may present only a few seizures during their life time, with clear-cut precipitating factors, such as sleep deprivation or alcohol intake, and a decision to treat these patients with AED should be taken on an individual basis.

LONG-TERM PROGNOSIS

Although the first description of familial MTLE defined it as a benign condition,[9,11] it is now well known that some patients may be refractory to medical treatment. In our series, 81% of familial MTLE patients achieved good seizure control on medication or remitted spontaneously. Refractory seizures were observed in 19%, and surgical treatment was considered in these cases.[40] When unilateral or clearly asymmetric bilateral EEG-MRI abnormalities were observed, familial MTLE patients had an overall likelihood of 85% of becoming seizure free following surgery.[40]

Whether the long-term prognosis for familial MTLE differs from that for sporadic MTLE is still to be determined. For those patients ascertained in epilepsy surgery programs, it appears that the long-term prognosis is similar in the familial and sporadic forms of MTLE. For the majority of patients with familial MTLE who have good seizure control on AEDs or seizure remission, it appears that the long-term prognosis is better than in the sporadic form of MTLE; however, this may represent an ascertainment bias.

Patients with familial MTLE with refractory seizures present a similar degree of memory impairment to patients with sporadic MTLE. In addition, we have shown that individuals with familial MTLE and hippocampal atrophy who have never had seizures also show significant memory-specific impairment on neuropsychological evaluation.[1] It remains to be determined whether this memory impairment in familial MTLE progresses independent of the seizures.

Familial TLE with auditory features has a benign clinical course, with no refractory patients reported.[16,47,49,52,68] Many patients may present only a few episodes and then have spontaneous remission. No neurologic disabilities are known in this syndrome. Long-term prognosis in familial TLE with auditory features is excellent, with most individuals being free of seizures with low doses of AEDs or off medication. There have been no patients with familial TLE with auditory features and *LGI-1* mutation described with refractory seizures requiring surgical treatment.

SUMMARY AND CONCLUSIONS

Two genetically distinct autosomal dominant familial TLE syndromes have been reported: (a) Familial MTLE and (b) Familial TLE with auditory features, ADPEAF, or familial LTLE.

Familial MTLE is a well-characterized syndrome, with different degrees of seizure severity, although the majority of patients have good seizure control. There is a high frequency of MRI signs of HS in affected individuals, including those with seizure remission or who have never developed seizures. The data suggest that the development of hippocampal abnormalities in these families may be related to genetic factors, although there is no gene mutation described so far. Whether familial MTLE without HS is part of the spectrum of the same condition or a distinct syndrome remains to be determined.

Familial TLE with auditory features, ADPEAF, or familial LTLE is characterized by auditory auras preceding complex partial and secondarily generalized seizures. The most common initial ictal manifestations are described as buzzing, roaring, radio- or motor-like sounds and distortions in sounds and words. The clinical course is usually favorable, with most patients being well controlled with AEDs. MRI investigations in this syndrome have not shown signs of HS. Half of the described families have mutations in the *LGI-1* gene, which is probably related to an abnormality in brain development.

It is essential to evaluate the phenotype of all possibly affected individuals before classifying the family as having a specific familial syndrome. To make a diagnosis of familial MTLE or familial TLE with auditory features, at least one family member should have the same clinical syndrome as the probant.

References

1. Alessio A, Kobayashi E, Damasceno BP, et al. Evidence of memory impairment in asymptomatic individuals with hippocampal atrophy. *Epilepsy Behav*. 2004;5(6):981–987.
2. Andermann E. Multifactorial inheritance in the epilepsies. In: Canger R, Angeleri F, Penry JK, eds. *Advances in Epileptology. XII Epilepsy International Symposium*. New York: Raven Press; 1980:297–309.
3. Andermann E. Multifactorial inheritance of generalized and focal epilepsies. In: Anderson VE, Hauser WA, Penry JK, et al., eds. *Genetic Basis of the Epilepsies*. New York: Raven Press; 1982:355–374.
4. Andermann E. Genetic aspects of the epilepsies. In: Sakai T, Tsuboi T, eds. *Genetic Aspects of Human Behavior*. Tokyo: Igaku-Shoin; 1985:129–145.
5. Andermann E, Abou-Khalil B, Berkovic SF, et al. Déja-vu is the characteristic aura in benign familial temporal lobe epilepsy. *Epilepsia*. 1997;38:200.
6. Andermann E, Metrakos JD. EEG studies of relatives of probands with focal epilepsy who have been treated surgically. *Epilepsia*. 1969;10(3):415.

6a. Andermann F, Kobayashi E, Andermann E. Genetic focal epilepsies: state of the art and paths to the future. *Epilepsia*. 2005;46 Suppl 10:61–67.

7. Badhwar A, Racacho LJ, D'Agostino MD, et al. Absence of LGI1 mutations in familial mesial temporal lobe epilepsy with or without auditory features and in sporadic TLE with auditory features. *Neurology*. 2004;62:252.
8. Baulac S, Picard F, Herman A, et al. Evidence for digenic inheritance in a family with both febrile convulsions and temporal lobe epilepsy implicating chromosomes 18qter and 1q25–q31. *Ann Neurol*. 2001;49(6):786–792.
9. Berkovic SF, Howell RA, Hopper JL. Familial temporal lobe epilepsy: a new syndrome with adolescent/adult onset and a benign course. In: Wolf P, ed. *Epileptic Seizures and Syndromes*. London: John Libbey;1994:257–263.
10. Berkovic SF, Izzillo P, McMahon JM, et al. LGI1 mutations in temporal lobe epilepsies. *Neurology*. 2004;62(7):1115–1119.
11. Berkovic SF, McIntosh A, Howell RA, et al. Familial temporal lobe epilepsy: a common disorder identified in twins. *Ann Neurol*. 1996;40(2):227–235.
12. Berkovic SF, Serratosa JM, Phillips HA, et al. Familial partial epilepsy with variable foci: clinical features and linkage to chromosome 22q12. *Epilepsia*. 2004;45(9):1054–1060.
13. Berkovic SF, Steinlein OK. Genetics of partial epilepsies. *Adv Neurol*. 1999;79:375–381.
14. Bisulli F, Tinuper P, Avoni P, et al. Idiopathic partial epilepsy with auditory features (IPEAF): a clinical and genetic study of 53 sporadic cases. *Brain*. 2004;127(Pt 6):1343–1352.
15. Bisulli F, Tinuper P, Scudellaro E, et al. A de novo LGI1 mutation in sporadic partial epilepsy with auditory features. *Ann Neurol*. 2004;56(3):455–456.
16. Brodtkorb E, Gu W, Nakken KO, et al. Familial temporal lobe epilepsy with aphasic seizures and linkage to chromosome 10q22–q24. *Epilepsia*. 2002;43(3):228–235.
17. Callenbach PM, van den Maagdenberg AM, Hottenga JJ, et al. Familial partial epilepsy with variable foci in a Dutch family: clinical characteristics and confirmation of linkage to chromosome 22q. *Epilepsia*. 2003;44(10):1298–1305.
18. Cavalleri GL, Lynch JM, Depondt C, Andermann F. Failure to replicate previously reported genetic associations with sporadic temporal lobe epilepsy: where to from here? *Brain*. 2005;128(Pt 8):1832–1840.
19. Cendes F, Lopes-Cendes I, Andermann E, et al. Familial temporal lobe epilepsy: a clinically heterogeneous syndrome. *Neurology*. 1998;50(2):554–557.
20. Chernova OB, Somerville RP, Cowell JK. A novel gene, *LGI1*, from 10q24 is rearranged and downregulated in malignant brain tumors. *Oncogene*. 1998;17(22):2873–2881.
21. Claes L, Audenaert D, Deprez L, et al. Novel locus on chromosome 12q22–q23.3 responsible for familial temporal lobe epilepsy associated with febrile seizures. *J Med Genet*. 2004;41(9):710–714.
22. Engel J Jr. A proposed diagnostic scheme for people with epileptic seizures and with epilepsy: report of the ILAE Task Force on Classification and Terminology. *Epilepsia*. 2001;42(6):796–803.
23. Escayg A, MacDonald BT, Meisler MH, et al. Mutations of SCN1A, encoding a neuronal sodium channel, in two families with GEFS+2. *Nat Genet*. 2000;24(4):343–345.
24. Fernandez G, Effenberger O, Vinz B, et al. Hippocampal malformation as a cause of familial febrile convulsions and subsequent hippocampal sclerosis. *Neurology*. 1998;50(4):909–917.
25. Ferreira FT, Kobayashi E, Lopes-Cendes I, et al. Structural abnormalities are similar in familial and nonfamilial mesial temporal lobe epilepsy. *Can J Neurol Sci*. 2004;31(3):368–372.
26. Flex E, Pizzuti A, Di Bonaventura C, et al. LGI1 gene mutation screening in sporadic partial epilepsy with auditory features. *J Neurol*. 2005;252(1):62–66.
27. Gambardella A, Manna I, Labate A, et al. GABA(B) receptor 1 polymorphism (G1465A) is associated with temporal lobe epilepsy. *Neurology*. 2003;60(4):560–563.
28. Gu W, Brodtkorb E, Piepoli T, et al. LGI1: a gene involved in epileptogenesis and glioma progression? *Neurogenetics*. 2005;6(2):59–66.
29. Gu W, Brodtkorb E, Steinlein OK. LGI1 is mutated in familial temporal lobe epilepsy characterized by aphasic seizures. *Ann Neurol*. 2002;52(3):364–367.
30. Harkin LA, Bowser DN, Dibbens LM, et al. Truncation of the GABA(A)-receptor gamma2 subunit in a family with generalized epilepsy with febrile seizures plus. *Am J Hum Genet*. 2002;70(2):530–536.
31. Hedera P, Blair MA, Andermann E, et al. Familial mesial temporal lobe epilepsy maps to chromosome 4q13.2–q213. *Neurology*. 2007;68:2107–2112.
32. Hocking AM, Shinomura T, McQuillan DJ. Leucine-rich repeat glycoproteins of the extracellular matrix. *Matrix Biol*. 1998;17(1):1–19.
33. Jackson GD, McIntosh AM, Briellmann RS, et al. Hippocampal sclerosis studied in identical twins. *Neurology*. 1998;51(1):78–84.
34. Kalachikov S, Evgrafov O, Ross B, et al. Mutations in LGI1 cause autosomal-dominant partial epilepsy with auditory features. *Nat Genet*. 2002;30(3):335–341.
35. Kanemoto K, Kawasaki J, Miyamoto T, et al. Interleuklin (IL) 1beta, IL-1alpha, and IL-1 receptor antagonist gene polymorpholisms in patients with temporal lobe epilepsy. *Ann Neurol*. 2000;47:571–574.
36. Kinton L, Johnson MR, Smith SJ, et al. Partial epilepsy with pericentral spikes: a new familial epilepsy syndrome with evidence for linkage to chromosome 4p15. *Ann Neurol*. 2002;51(6):740–749.

37. Kobayashi E, Andermann F, Andermann E. Familial mesial temporal lobe epilepsy. In: Gilman S, ed. *MedLink Neurology*. San Diego, CA: MedLink; 2005.
38. Kobayashi E, Andermann F, Andermann E. Familial lateral temporal lobe epilepsy. In: Gilman S, ed. *MedLink Neurology*. San Diego, CA: MedLink; 2005.
39. Kobayashi E, Andermann F, Andermann E. Familial partial epilepsy with variable foci. In: Gilman S, ed. *MedLink Neurology*. San Diego, CA: MedLink; 2005.
40. Kobayashi E, D'Agostino MD, Lopes-Cendes I, et al. Outcome of surgical treatment in familial mesial temporal lobe epilepsy. *Epilepsia*. 2003;44(8):1080–1084.
41. Kobayashi E, D'Agostino MD, Lopes-Cendes I, et al. Hippocampal atrophy and T2-weighted signal changes in familial mesial temporal lobe epilepsy. *Neurology*. 2003;60(3):405–409.
42. Kobayashi E, Li LM, Lopes-Cendes I, et al. Magnetic resonance imaging evidence of hippocampal sclerosis in asymptomatic first-degree relatives of patients with familial mesial temporal lobe epilepsy. *Arch Neurol*. 2002;59(12):1891–1894.
43. Kobayashi E, Lopes-Cendes I, Guerreiro CA, et al. Seizure outcome and hippocampal atrophy in familial mesial temporal lobe epilepsy. *Neurology*. 2001;56(2):166–172.
44. Kobayashi E, Santos NF, Torres FR, et al. Magnetic resonance imaging abnormalities in familial temporal lobe epilepsy with auditory auras. *Arch Neurol*. 2003;60(11):1546–1551.
45. Lopes-Cendes I, Scheffer IE, Berkovic SF, et al. A new locus for generalized epilepsy with febrile seizures plus maps to chromosome 2. *Am J Hum Genet*. 2000;66(2):698–701.
46. Ma S, Abou-Khalil B, Sutcliffe JS, et al. The GABBR1 locus and the G1465A variant is not associated with temporal lobe epilepsy preceded by febrile seizures. *BMC Med Genet*. 2005;6:13.
47. Michelucci R, Poza JJ, Sofia V, et al. Autosomal dominant lateral temporal epilepsy: clinical spectrum, new epitempin mutations, and genetic heterogeneity in seven European families. *Epilepsia*. 2003;44(10):1289–1297.
48. Morante-Redolat JM, Gorostidi-Pagola A, Piquer-Sirerol S, et al. Mutations in the LGI1/epitempin gene on 10q24 cause autosomal dominant lateral temporal epilepsy. *Hum Mol Genet*. 2002;11(9):1119–1128.
49. Ottman R, Risch N, Hauser WA, et al. Localization of a gene for partial epilepsy to chromosome 10q. *Nat Genet*. 1995;10(1):56–60.
50. Ottman R, Winawer MR, Kalachikov S, et al. LGI1 mutations in autosomal dominant partial epilepsy with auditory features. *Neurology*. 2004;62(7):1120–1126.
51. Picard F, Baulac S, Kahane P, et al. Dominant partial epilepsies. A clinical, electrophysiological and genetic study of 19 European families. *Brain*. 2000;123(Pt 6):1247–1262.
52. Poza JJ, Saenz A, Martinez-Gil A, et al. Autosomal dominant lateral temporal epilepsy: clinical and genetic study of a large Basque pedigree linked to chromosome 10q. *Ann Neurol*. 1999;45(2):182–188.
53. Proposal for revised classification of epilepsies and epileptic syndromes. Commission on Classification and Terminology of the International League Against Epilepsy. *Epilepsia*. 1989;30(4):389–399.
54. Santos NF, Sousa SC, Kobayashi E, et al. Clinical and genetic heterogeneity in familial temporal lobe epilepsy. *Epilepsia*. 2002;43(Suppl 5):136.
55. Scheffer IE, Berkovic SF. Generalized epilepsy with febrile seizures plus. A genetic disorder with heterogeneous clinical phenotypes. *Brain*. 1997;120(Pt 3):479–490.
56. Scheffer IE, Phillips HA, O'Brien CE, et al. Familial partial epilepsy with variable foci: a new partial epilepsy syndrome with suggestion of linkage to chromosome 2. *Ann Neurol*. 1998;44(6):890–899.
57. Senechal KR, Thaller C, Noebels JL. ADPEAF mutations reduce levels of secreted LGI1, a putative tumor suppressor protein linked to epilepsy. *Hum Mol Genet*. 2005;14(12):1613–1620.
58. Singh R, Scheffer IE, Crossland K, et al. Generalized epilepsy with febrile seizures plus: a common childhood-onset genetic epilepsy syndrome. *Ann Neurol*. 1999;45(1):75–81.
59. Stogmann E, Zimprich A, Baumgartner C, et al. A functional polymorphism in the prodynorphin gene promoter is associated with temporal lobe epilepsy. *Ann Neurol*. 2002;51(2):260–263.
60. Sugawara T, Tsurubuchi Y, Agarwala KL, et al. A missense mutation of the Na+ channel alpha II subunit gene Na(v)1.2 in a patient with febrile and afebrile seizures causes channel dysfunction. *Proc Natl Acad Sci U S A*. 2001;98(11):6384–6389.
61. Tan NC, Heron SE, Scheffer IE, et al. Is variation in the GABA(B) receptor 1 gene associated with temporal lobe epilepsy? *Epilepsia*. 2005;46(5):778–780.
62. Tan NC, Mulley JC, Berkovic SF. Genetic association studies in epilepsy: "the truth is out there." *Epilepsia*. 2004;45(11):1429–1442.
63. Vadlamudi L, Scheffer IE, Berkovic SF. Genetics of temporal lobe epilepsy. *J Neurol Neurosurg Psychiatry*. 2003;74(10):1359–1361.
64. Wallace RH, Scheffer IE, Barnett S, et al. Neuronal sodium-channel alpha1-subunit mutations in generalized epilepsy with febrile seizures plus. *Am J Hum Genet*. 2001;68(4):859–865.
65. Wallace RH, Scheffer IE, Parasivam G, et al. Generalized epilepsy with febrile seizures plus: mutation of the sodium channel subunit SCN1B. *Neurology*. 2002;58(9):1426–1429.
66. Wallace RH, Wang DW, Singh R, et al. Febrile seizures and generalized epilepsy associated with a mutation in the Na+-channel beta1 subunit gene SCN1B. *Nat Genet*. 1998;19(4):366–370.
67. Wieser HG. ILAE Commission Report. Mesial temporal lobe epilepsy with hippocampal sclerosis. *Epilepsia*. 2004;45(6):695–714.
68. Winawer MR, Martinelli BF, Barker-Cummings C, et al. Four new families with autosomal dominant partial epilepsy with auditory features: clinical description and linkage to chromosome 10q24. *Epilepsia*. 2002;43(1):60–67.
69. Xiong L, Labuda M, Li DS, et al. Mapping of a gene determining familial partial epilepsy with variable foci to chromosome 22q11–q12. *Am J Hum Genet*. 1999;65(6):1698–1710.

CHAPTER 249 ■ FAMILIAL FRONTAL LOBE EPILEPSIES

FABIENNE PICARD AND EYLERT BRODTKORB

INTRODUCTION

Frontal lobe epilepsies, as with other focal epilepsies, were formerly invariably considered to be the consequence of an overt or obscure brain lesion. However, this view has changed during the last 10 years, as large families comprising several individuals with non–age-related partial seizures without manifest organic cause have been identified. Today, the genetic origin of nonlesional focal epilepsies is well accepted. Several familial focal epilepsy syndromes with an autosomal dominant mode of inheritance have successively been recognized, such as autosomal dominant nocturnal frontal lobe epilepsy (ADNFLE), familial temporal lobe epilepsies, and familial focal epilepsy with variable foci.[46] They are considered idiopathic, like the classical benign localization-related epilepsies of childhood, since affected individuals do not exhibit any other etiology than a presumed genetic cause.

ADNFLE constitutes a reasonably homogeneous clinical syndrome. Mutations have been identified in genes coding for subunits of the cerebral nicotinic acetylcholine receptor (nAChR) in some families, establishing a clear link between ADNFLE and this ion channel. The many cases of sporadic nonlesional nocturnal frontal lobe epilepsy (NFLE) present similar clinical and electroencephalographic features.[66] It is likely that some of them represent unrecognized familial cases or are related to de novo mutations. Yet, others possibly share similar pathophysiologic mechanisms, even if their etiology is not predominantly genetic.

HISTORICAL PERSPECTIVES

In the last 30 years, several reports have described patients with sudden, brief nocturnal episodes of complex motor activity and a family history of similar attacks.[18,27,68] This clinical picture was originally thought to represent a movement disorder, so-called *paroxysmal nocturnal dystonia*,[32,33] but was later recognized as epilepsy.[23,37] In 1993, Vigevano and Fusco used the term *partial idiopathic epilepsy of frontal lobe origin* to describe otherwise healthy children presenting with nocturnal tonic postural seizures with a strong family history of epilepsy.[72] When families with a clear mendelian inheritance later were identified by Scheffer et al. in 1994, this disorder was designated ADNFLE.[59] The first reported families originated in Australia, Canada, and the United Kingdom. In the Australian family, linkage studies revealed mapping to the long arm of chromosome 20.[44] Subsequent sequencing demonstrated a missense mutation in the gene coding for a subunit of the neuronal nAChR.[63] This finding was a surprise, as it was not previously known that this receptor was involved in epileptogenesis. ADNFLE was the first epileptic syndrome with a proven monogenetic origin, a finding that may be considered a milestone in epileptology. Various mutations in genes coding for subunits of nAChRs have later been demonstrated in different families with this condition (Table 1).[4,8,14,21,24,30,34–36,39,42–44,55,56,58,59,62–64]

DEFINITIONS

ADNFLE was first described on the basis of its familial character, but does not differ clinically from the more frequently occurring sporadic cases of nonlesional NFLE. An attempt to define the general characteristics of frontal lobe epilepsy was part of the 1989 Classification of Epilepsies and Epileptic Syndromes by the International League Against Epilepsy (ILAE)[11]:

> "Frontal lobe epilepsies are characterized by simple partial, complex partial, secondarily generalized seizures or combinations of these. Seizures often occur several times a day and frequently occur during sleep. Frontal lobe partial seizures are sometimes mistaken for psychogenic seizures. Status epilepticus is a frequent complication."

A list of features strongly suggestive of the diagnosis was given:

> "(1) generally short seizures, (2) complex partial seizures arising from the frontal lobe, often with minimal or no postictal confusion, (3) rapid secondary generalization (more common in seizures of frontal than of temporal lobe epilepsy), (4) prominent motor manifestations which are tonic or postural, (5) complex gestural automatisms frequent at onset, (6) frequent falling when the discharges are bilateral."

ADNFLE contains several elements from this general outline. However, the unique seizure semiology in this disorder was found to fit poorly with the 1981 ILAE seizure classification.[12,31] Hence, the concept of hypermotor seizures was introduced in the more recent proposal of a semiologic seizure classification[31]:

> "Hypermotor seizures are seizures in which the main manifestations consist of complex movements involving the proximal segments of the limbs and trunk. This results in large movements that appear 'violent' when they occur at high speeds. The 'complex motor manifestations' imitate normal movements, but the movements are inappropriate for the situation and usually serve no purpose. Frequently, the movements are stereotypically repeated in more or less complex sequences (e.g. pedalling). Consciousness may be preserved during these seizures."

Finally, the term hyperkinetic seizure was included in the new glossary of descriptive terminology for ictal semiology by the ILAE Task Force on Classification and Terminology[6]:

> "(1) Involves predominantly proximal limb or axial muscles producing irregular sequential ballistic movements, such as pedalling, pelvic thrusting, thrashing, rocking movements. (2) Increase in rate of ongoing movements or inappropriately rapid performance of a movement"

ADNFLE follows an autosomal dominant inheritance with incomplete penetrance. The first identified families allowed the

TABLE 1

CLINICAL CHARACTERISTICS IN AUTOSOMAL DOMINANT NOCTURNAL FRONTAL LOBE EPILEPSY FAMILIES WITH MUTATIONS IN GENES CODING FOR SUBUNITS OF NICOTINIC ACETYLCHOLINE RECEPTORS

Mutation (references)	Number of patients	Mean age of onset, yr (range)	Pharmacoresistance	Intellectual disability	Psychiatric or behavior disturbance	Siezures while awake	Status epilepticus	Secondary generalization	Abnormal interictal EEG
CHRNA4 mutations									
S248F[44,58,59,63]	27	8.5 (0.2–28)[a]	nr	0/25	nr	nr[b]	nr	nr[b]	nr[b]
S248F[64]	11	8.6 (4–13)	8/11	1/11	1/11	3/11	2/11	8/11	4/11
S248F[56]	11	7.6 (3–12)	4/8	0/11	0/11	0/11	nr	1/9	2/8
S248F[36]	6	12.5 (6–15)	1/6	0/6	In a few	nr	nr	1/6	0/6
776ins3[34,35,39,62]	10	8 (1–11)	1/8	0/10	4/10	2/10	0/10	0/10	1/8
S252L[21,24]	5	(0.3–10)	2/4	2/5	3/5	0/5	0/5	1/5	2/3
S252L[43]	2	1.3 (0.7–2)	1/1	0/2	nr	0/2	nr	0/2	1/1
S252L[55]	3	2.5 (0.5–5)	2/3	0/3	nr	1/3	nr	3/3	0/3
S252L[8]	9	11 (4–14)	6/7	6/6	nr	0/9	nr	1/7	5/9
T265I[30]	2	18 (15–20)	1/2	nr	nr	0/2	0/2	0/2	2/2
CHRNB2 mutations									
V287L[14]	8	9 (8–12)	0/8	nr	nr	0/8	nr	0/8	4/8
V287M[36,42]	10	10 (6–18)	0/10	0/10	In a few	nr	nr	3/10	1/7
I312M[4]	2	7	nr	2/2	2/2	0/2	nr	nr	0/2

EEG, electroencephalogram; nr, not reported.
[a]In the 24 patients in whom age of onset was known.
[b]Data not provided separately for this family.

TABLE 2

MAIN CLINICAL FEATURES OF AUTOSOMAL DOMINANT NOCTURNAL FRONTAL LOBE EPILEPSY

- Onset age is variable, although generally in childhood.
- There are brief hyperkinetic seizures, almost exclusively during sleep.
- Attacks may be numerous every night for long periods.
- Awareness during seizures is often retained.
- The course is nonprogressive and seizures may remit.
- Good response to antiepileptic drugs, especially to carbamazepine, is common.
- Pharmacoresistance occurs in almost one third of patients.
- Clinical neurologic examination and magnetic resonance imaging are normal.
- Cognitive deficits and psychiatric comorbidity may occur.

delineation of the main clinical features,[58] which later have been refined (Table 2). Subsequently, other focal idiopathic epilepsies with an autosomal dominant transmission pattern were described: The familial temporal lobe epilepsies[2] and the autosomal dominant partial epilepsy with variable foci.[60] ADNFLE has together with these syndromes been included within the subgroup of "familial focal epilepsies" in the list of epilepsy syndromes recently proposed by the ILAE Task Force on Classification and Terminology.[15]

EPIDEMIOLOGY

To date, the number of reported ADNFLE families exceeds 100.[4,8,10,14,21,24,25,30,34,35,39–43,45,46,55,58,62] Undoubtedly, they only represent a small fraction of ADNFLE families worldwide and the prevalence of this disorder is obscure. Several known families have probably not been reported when genetic analyses have not been performed or have been inconclusive. In addition, it is likely that there still are families in which the epileptic nature of the paroxysmal nocturnal events has remained unrecognized or misdiagnosed. The reported ADNFLE families all comprise at least two affected first-degree relatives with an inheritance pattern suggestive of autosomal dominant transmission. Twenty-seven affected individuals have been reported in the largest and first described family in Australia.[44] Up until now, mutations have been found in genes encoding subunits of nAChR in 12 families and in one sporadic case (Table 1). Thus, identified mutations currently account for only a minority (10% to 12%) of published ADNFLE families. Sporadic NFLE cases are relatively common,[51] and some may harbor the same mutations that have been identified in ADNFLE.[43]

ETIOLOGY AND BASIC MECHANISMS

ADNFLE was the first idiopathic epilepsy for which a responsible gene was recognized.

Mutations have been identified in the *CHRNA4* gene encoding the nAChR $\alpha4$ subunit and in the *CHRNB2* gene encoding the nAChR $\beta2$ subunit (Table 1). Up until now, four different mutations have been described in *CHRNA4*: (a) S248F, a missense mutation replacing serine with phenylalanine in position 248 in the amino acid sequence, observed in an Australian, a Spanish, a Norwegian, and a Scottish family[36,56,63,64]; (b) 776ins3, an insertion of three nucleotides at nucleotide position 776, leading to the insertion of a leucine in the amino acid sequence, in another Norwegian family[62]; (c) S252L, a missense mutation replacing a serine by a leucine in position 252 in the amino acid sequence in a Japanese, a Polish, and a Korean family, and in a sporadic case of Lebanese origin who subsequently had an affected son[8,21,24,35,43,55]; and (d) T265I, another missense mutation, in a German family.[30] Some authors use an alternative codon numbering, which may cause nomenclature confusion.[10,55,56] Three different mutations (V287L, V287M, and I312M) are described in the *CHRNB2* gene in an Italian, a Scottish, and an English family, respectively.[4,14,42]

The nAChRs are pentameric ligand-gated ion channel receptors consisting of different functional subunit combinations (Fig. 1). When acetylcholine (ACh) binds to the nAChR, the ion channel opens and lets cations enter. The known ADNFLE mutations are located within the second transmembrane domain (M2) of the subunits, which constitutes the walls of the ionic pore, except for the mutation $\beta2$-I312M, which is in the third transmembrane domain. Thus, it appears that mutations with a principally direct effect on the ionic pore may cause ADNFLE. The fact that the major nAChRs in humans are made from an assembly of $\alpha4$ and $\beta2$ subunits explains well that defects in both subunits are associated with the same disorder. The $\alpha4\beta2$ nAChRs are the most abundant form and are found in the entire brain, with a predominance in the thalamus. They may have a presynaptic or a postsynaptic location. The first have a neuromodulatory role (facilitation of neurotransmitter release), whereas the latter induce a depolarization of the postsynaptic neuron. To assess the changes in the electrophysiologic properties of the mutant receptors, a system of

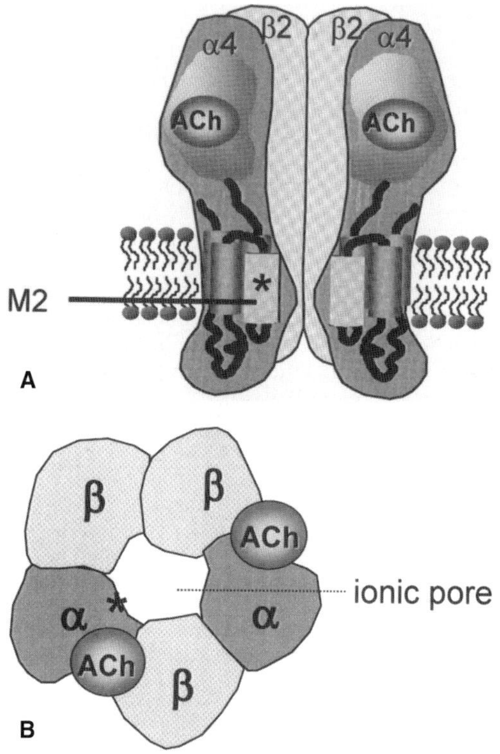

FIGURE 1. Schematic illustration of the neuronal $\alpha4\beta2$ nicotinic acetylcholine receptor (nAChR), a pentameric ion channel. **A:** Coronal section. **B:** Axial section. The $\alpha4\beta2$ nAChR results from the assembly of two α and three β subunits. The wall of the ionic pore is lined by the M2 segment of each subunit (second transmembrane domain). When acetylcholine binds to the nAChR, the ion channel opens and lets cations enter. The *asterisk* indicates the location of the mutations in the $\alpha4$ subunit.

heterologous expression in frog (*Xenopus*) oocytes has been used. These cells were injected with an equivalent amount of the mutant and nonmutant allele, in addition to cDNA coding for the other normal subunit, in order to obtain mutant "heterozygous" receptors mimicking an autosomal dominant disorder. Six different mutations led to a significant increase in sensitivity to ACh of the mutant receptors.[4,5,30,38,42] The seventh mutation, the *CHRNB2* V287L mutation, caused retardation of channel desensitization.[14] Thus, contrary to the first conclusions obtained from the assessment of homozygous mutant receptors, the current studies suggest a gain of function of the mutant nicotinic receptor for the various mutations. In contrast, another study of five mutations proposed a reduction of the Ca^{2+} dependence of the ACh response, which could explain an increase of glutamate release during bouts of synchronous activity, as an alternative common mechanism.[52] However, the precise cellular mechanisms leading to epileptogenesis in ADNFLE remain elusive. In particular, it is not clear how an alteration of an nAChR subtype that is present in the thalamus and in the entire cortex may cause a partial epilepsy.

Currently, it is assumed that the mutant nAChRs alter the activity level of frontal thalamocortical loops, which play a major role during sleep. A positron emission tomography (PET) study using 2-[^{18}F]-F-A-85380, a high-affinity agonist of the heteromeric ($\alpha 4\beta 2$) nAChRs, has recently offered an opportunity to investigate some in vivo consequences of the molecular defect.[48] Eight ADNFLE patients with an identified mutation in nAChRs were studied. Their pattern of nAChR brain distribution was clearly different compared to healthy volunteers. A significant decrease in nAChR density in the right dorsolateral prefrontal region and a significant increase in the epithalamus, ventral mesencephalon, and cerebellum were demonstrated. The regional decrease in the nAChR density in the prefrontal cortex appears congruent with a frontal lobe epilepsy. We propose two explanations for the regional increase in the nAChR number in the mesencephalon: (a) a regional malformation of central nervous system (CNS) circuits, with an increase of synaptic density, since nAChRs may have a role in the migration of neocortical neurons and in synaptogenesis[53]; and (b) a regional nAChR up-regulation, related to the hypersensitivity of the mutant nAChRs to ACh and the richness of local ACh release sites. A consequence of the increased nAChR density in mesencephalon could be an overactivated cholinergic pathway ascending from the brainstem. This pathway acts on postsynaptic nAChRs on thalamocortical cells and participates in "desynchronization" and interruption of the sleep physiologic oscillations at the time of the arousals.[13,28,65] Thus, the findings of the recent PET study[48] support the theory that ADNFLE seizures are due to a defective interruption and a pathologic transformation of synchronized sleep oscillations.

Other in vivo functional studies using transgenic animal models have also enhanced the understanding of ADNFLE pathogenesis. A *CHRNA4* knockout mouse showed increased anxiety compared with the behavioral phenotype of the wild type, but did not exhibit spontaneous seizures.[54] *CHRNB2* knockout mice showed abnormal functional organization in the dorsal lateral geniculate nucleus,[19] reduced sensitivity to nicotine-induced locomotor depression,[70] and reduced fragmentation of non–rapid eye movement (REM) sleep by microarousals.[29] This last phenotypical trait is an interesting finding, as sleep microstructure analysis of NFLE and ADNFLE patients has revealed sleep fragmentation with an increase in arousals and sleep instability in all non-REM sleep stages.[67,74] Knockin mice containing a point mutation in the pore-forming M2 domain of the $\alpha 4$ subunit (Leu9'Ser) showed increased anxiety, increased sensitivity to induced seizures by agonists (such as nicotine, the nicotinic agonist epibatidine, but not the γ-aminobutyric acid $(GABA)_A$ receptor blocker and proconvulsant bicuculline), but no spontaneous epileptic seizures,[16] and also dopaminergic deficits.[26] When tested in oocytes, the $\alpha 4\beta 2$ nAChRs with this specific mutation displayed an increased ACh sensitivity, as observed with the human ADNFLE mutations.[5,26] In addition to these mice models, a new transgenic rat model harboring a true ADNFLE mutation is currently under investigation.[22] This model appears more interesting as it expresses spontaneous seizures resembling those of ADNFLE.

For a long period of time, no other genes than those coding for nAChR subunits were reported to be responsible for this condition. Just recently, mutations have been identified in the promoter of the corticotropin-releasing hormone (CRH) gene.[9] The first mutation, a polymorphism present in 3% of the general population, was detected in three families and in two sporadic cases. The second, not present in 115 healthy subjects, was detected in one ADNFLE proband. However, in vitro the first mutation caused an increase in the protein level, whereas the second resulted in a decrease.[9] Although the nAChRs are known to activate CRH release,[7,57] the pathophysiologic link between CRH and nAChRs in ADNFLE is still obscure.

CLINICAL PRESENTATION

The main clinical features are listed in Table 1. Mean age of onset of ADNFLE varies between 8 and 11.5 years, according to clinical studies. It starts below 20 years in 85% of cases. Onset ages as low as 2 months and as high as 56 years have been reported.[46,58] The penetrance appears to be up to 80%. Males and females are equally affected.[10] Seizures arise from sleep. They are more or less stereotyped in each patient over the years. It is remarkable that sudden arousals are characteristic for ADNFLE[4,39,56,64] in contrast to the reduced consciousness that typically occurs in seizures with medial temporal lobe onset. Some patients describe an aura. They are nonspecific and include a broad variety of phenomena: Somatosensory (shivering/tingling, either diffusely or localized, mostly in the head, sometimes in the limbs; and also epigastric discomfort), special sensory (e.g., sensations of light, auditory hallucinations, vertigo), psychic (fear, malaise, déjà vu, dreaming activity), and autonomic (breathing difficulty).[58,64]

The motor manifestations are characterized by a wide range of clinical features, which in part can be regarded as a release of subcortical activity. Extrapyramidal features are often prominent. Behavior and autonomic elements may reflect limbic overactivity. The mildest form consists only of a sudden awakening with an elevation of head and trunk, often associated with the expression of fear. Abrupt and rapidly changing movements of the limbs and the trunk may occur, leading to a bizarre sequence of various brief dystonic postures, reminiscent of a mechanic puppet. Hyperkinetic activity (frantic movements with bipedal activity, pelvic thrashing) or tonic stiffening are common features. During the seizure, a breathless sensation is reported by many patients.[36,42,43,46,56,58] Seizures usually last less than 1 minute, with a mean duration of 30 seconds,[46,58] but some seizures are prolonged and may take the form of nocturnal wanderings. Postictal symptoms are absent or very brief. Rare secondarily generalized seizures are observed in about half of the patients, but the unusual semiologic pattern may cause classification difficulties. Some patients report that awareness is partly retained even during apparent generalized convulsions, a phenomenon that may wrongly raise the suspicion of psychogenic seizures.

Seizures frequently occur in clusters, predominantly during the first few hours after falling asleep or early in the morning. Some patients have attacks every night, while others report mild and rare symptoms. Periods with high seizure frequency may alternate with seizure-free intervals. In one study, the mean seizure frequency was around eight episodes per night.[58]

Diurnal seizures, apart from during naps, are very rare, but may be observed in the most severe cases, particularly during periods of poor seizure control.[40,46,64] Some patients may also experience status epilepticus. Stress, sleep deprivation, and menstruation may increase seizure frequency. Sensory stimulation during sleep (e.g., shaking the body of the patient or a sudden sound) may sometimes provoke seizures.[24,43,55] On the background of a video-polysomnographic study of a large number of patients, the attacks were classified into four categories according to duration, semiology, and complexity of motor behavior (minimal, minor, major, and prolonged episodes).[40,41] The mildest form is described as paroxysmal arousals, consisting of a sudden awakening with dystonic posturing of upper or lower limbs.[49,50,69] They can recur with a periodic repetition, every 30 seconds to 2 minutes during light sleep. Paroxysmal arousals are probably the most frequent type of seizures, but, due to their short duration, many patients remain unaware of them. The information from relatives about apparently unaffected individuals is thus hampered with a high degree of uncertainty. Structured interviews of all pedigree members and their proxies, particularly their bed partners, are thus necessary to recognize the true penetrance of this disorder. The clinical observation is the major diagnostic tool in NFLE, particularly since even ictal electroencephalograms (EEGs) may be inconclusive. Nocturnal video recordings, preferably with polysomnographic parameters, may be necessary for the clinical diagnosis.

Clinical neurologic examination is normal. A normal intelligence was one of the ADNFLE features originally described.[58] Nevertheless, subsequent descriptions reported neuropsychological deficits in some patients. In four families with typical ADNFLE, most patients also suffered from mild to moderate intellectual disability.[4,8,24,25] Two of these families had an α4-S252L mutation, one the β2-I312M mutation and one no identified mutation. The patient with the de novo α4-S252L mutation was reported to be of low average intellect.[43] Several of the cognitively affected patients had pronounced memory deficits. A neuropsychological study of two other patients from ADNFLE families without identified mutations showed specific frontal lobe neuropsychological disturbances.[46] Currently, it is unknown whether the observed neuropsychological deficits are a consequence of the seizure disorder or a behavioral phenotype primarily associated with the genetic defect. In addition, in some families psychiatric disturbances have been reported in up to half of the patients during the active phase of their epilepsy.[4,24,35,36,46] Behavioral disorders with hyperactivity, irritability, aggressiveness, and impulsive behavior are the most frequent findings, but psychosis have also been reported in some patients.[35] The psychiatric impact may contribute to the diagnostic confusion, which still may occur in this disorder.

No obvious clinical elements seem to differentiate mutation-positive from mutation-negative families.

DIAGNOSTIC EVALUATION

Electroencephalographic Findings

Many patients have a normal interictal EEG. Most studies report waking EEG abnormalities in only 10% to 25% of patients.[8,40,56,58] Other authors who retrospectively looked at all previous EEGs of their patients reported waking EEG abnormalities in up to 60%, mostly recorded during periods of frequent seizures.[46,64] When present, the abnormalities consist of focal intermittent theta or delta slow waves and/or sparse focal sharp waves or spikes. They are usually located over the frontal regions and exceptionally over the temporal areas.[8,46] Interictal sleep EEG sometimes demonstrates abnormalities in patients with a normal waking EEG.[40,46] In a study of 40 patients, 10% had an abnormal waking EEG and 50% an abnormal interictal sleep EEG.[40] When unilateral interictal or ictal EEG abnormalities are identified, they appear to remain lateralized on the same side throughout the evolution of the disorder. Ictal EEG recordings may also fail to show specific discharges. Cortical activity is often concealed by movement artefacts. An ictal pattern appears in 40% to 80% of the patients, according to studies, but rarely consists of clear-cut epileptiform activity in the frontal regions. Most often a diffuse flattening or a rhythmic theta or delta activity with predominance over anterior quadrants is seen. Thus, at least a quarter of the patients have normal interictal as well as ictal scalp EEGs.[40] Video-EEG-polysomnographic recordings show that almost all seizures arise during stage 2 non-REM sleep. Intracerebral EEG recordings performed in a patient with a typical ADNFLE surprisingly demonstrated that seizures originated from the left insular cortex, whereas ictal surface EEG showed diffuse flattening or left frontoprecentral fast activity at the onset of seizures.[46]

Neuroimaging and Other Laboratory Examinations

Brain magnetic resonance imaging (MRI) is normal in all patients with ADNFLE. Functional imaging studies include single photon emission tomography (SPECT) and positron emission tomography (PET) studies. ^{18}F-fluorodeoxyglucose (FDG)-PET was described in eight patients with ADNFLE from three different families.[8,20] The study was considered normal in seven patients and showed a hypometabolism in the frontopolar region in one.[20] A statistical parametric mapping (SPM) analysis was performed in six patients with a normal PET and permitted the detection of glucose hypometabolism in the left superior and middle frontal gyrus in five of them, but also in the left central and parietal regions and the right anterior superior frontal gyrus.[8] Recently, a PET study using a tracer of the nicotinic receptors has been performed in eight ADNFLE patients with an identified mutation[48] (see Etiology and Basic Mechanisms). An interictal SPECT using 123I-IMP (*N*-isopropyl-p-iodoamphetamine) showed no abnormality in a patient from Japan, while an interictal SPECT using 99mTc-ECD (ethyl cysteinate dimer) showed low perfusion in both frontal lobes in another patient from the same family.[24] Another study using ^{99}Tc-HMPAO (technetium-99m hexamethyl-propylamineoxime) showed perfusion changes on interictal and ictal SPECT in the left frontopolar region, congruent with the focal hypometabolism observed in interictal PET in one patient, and right parasagittal, midfrontal hyperperfusion on ictal SPECT with a hypoperfusion in the same area on interictal SPECT in another patient with an identified mutation.[20]

DIFFERENTIAL DIAGNOSIS

Diagnostic difficulties have been recurrent problems in many families with ADNFLE. Nocturnal seizures often occur without eyewitnesses, and if present, the beginning of even dramatic episodes is often not seen. Darkness and covers frequently restrict the detailed observation by bedroom partners. Even ictal EEG recordings may be inconclusive. Previously, many patients with NFLE were considered to suffer from a primary movement disorder termed *paroxysmal nocturnal dystonia*[32,33] (see Historical Perspectives). Misdiagnoses as parasomnias, in the form of night terrors, nightmares, and somnambulism, have been common. Based on the history alone, the differential diagnosis from benign parasomnias may be difficult in children. Attack frequency differs and symptoms usually occur as single or isolated recurrent episodes in the parasomnias in contrast to the frequent clustering of nocturnal frontal lobe seizures. Due to pronounced autonomic and emotional symptoms with arousal and fear, psychiatric disorders such as panic attacks and hysteria may also be suspected. REM behavior disorder is characterized by agitated, sometimes violent movements occurring during REM sleep. The majority is males above age 60 and other neurologic disorders such as Parkinson disease or multisystem atrophy are common.[1,10,24,50,58,69] Other members within the same family can certainly be afflicted with these disorders, but hardly with a distinct autosomal dominant transmission pattern. Besides hypnagogic myoclonias, short nocturnal movements resembling mild seizures can be present in healthy subjects. However, in NFLE the episodes are more stereotypical and include sudden movements with dyskinetic or dystonic components. When characteristic hyperkinetic seizures during sleep are video-recorded, the diagnosis of NFLE is usually readily made.

A careful pedigree analysis confirms the familial occurrence of the disorder and differentiates ADNFLE from the more common sporadic forms of NFLE. Other autosomal dominant focal epilepsies (e.g., from the temporal lobe) may also manifest themselves with nocturnal seizures, but have otherwise different ictal semiologies. However, families with autosomal dominant partial epilepsy with variable foci may contain patients with a seizure pattern similar to NFLE. They can thus wrongly be considered as ADNFLE families before the phenotypic variability is appreciated. In this syndrome, seizures arise from different cortical regions in different family members and a predominance of seizures while awake may be observed in some individuals.[3]

TREATMENT AND OUTCOME

Carbamazepine has been postulated to be the drug of choice in ADNFLE. It has been reported to be more effective than valproate and appears to suppress seizures completely in about two thirds of patients with this syndrome.[46,58] Low doses of carbamazepine (around 600 mg/day in adults) are often sufficient. The detection of an association between nAChR mutations and ADNFLE gave the opportunity to compare the effect of carbamazepine on mutated and wild-type receptors in vitro. Studies in *Xenopus* oocytes demonstrated that carbamazepine most probably acts as an open channel blocker and generally inhibits $\alpha4\beta2$ nAChRs, but that most mutants display a higher sensitivity to this effect.[5,47] Carbamazepine may shut down the mutant receptors, whereas remaining wild-type receptors are less affected.[47,64] Pharmacoresistance to carbamazepine and other antiepileptic drugs has nevertheless been observed in one third of patients. Most reported families have at least had one pharmacoresistant individual, whereas other affected family members have had a good therapeutic response.[10] There is indeed considerable interfamilial and intrafamilial clinical variability concerning epilepsy severity and effect of antiepileptic therapy in this condition.

Acetazolamide was reported to reduce or control seizures in one family without evidence for nAChR mutations.[71] In one single patient with uncontrolled seizures from the original Australian family, transdermal nicotine appeared to be very effective when added to carbamazepine in both an open and a double-blind placebo-controlled fashion.[73] These preliminary data encourage attempts to treat patients who prove to be refractory to standard antiepileptic therapy with these agents.

The effect of surgical treatment has not been reported in ADNFLE in spite of its localization-related clinical manifestations. A priori, resective surgery does not appear to be an appropriate option in disorders caused by mutations affecting receptors with widespread distribution in the brain. Prudence should also be exercised in sporadic NFLE.

LONG-TERM PROGNOSIS

The phenotypic expression of this condition spans from a persistent, severe disability to only a mild intermittent sleep disruption, not recognized as an epileptic manifestation by either the affected individuals or their proxies. Even with frequent seizures, remissions can occur during adolescence and adulthood, without seizure recurrence after discontinuation of drug therapy.[17,34,36,39,42,46,64] However, relapses may occur after many years, and in some families, ADNFLE persists through adult life in many of the affected individuals.[58,62,64,66] Genetic or environmental factors that determine penetrance or remission are not yet identified. The reported efficacy of nicotine administration[73] is interesting in this respect, and to date it is not known to what extent chronic consumption of nicotine could influence the course and prognosis of this disorder. The fact that the attacks are exclusively sleep related in most patients and usually do not change their chronodependency is important when assessing these patients for motor vehicle driving.

SUMMARY AND CONCLUSIONS

ADNFLE was the first idiopathic epilepsy for which a distinct genetic basis was identified. Mutations in two genes (*CHRNA4* and *CHRNB2*) coding for neuronal nicotinic receptor subunits ($\alpha4$ and $\beta2$) have been identified. ADNFLE is characterized by nocturnal attacks that tend to cluster and can recur several times during one night. Seizures have prominent motor features and mainly occur during non-REM sleep, particularly shortly after falling asleep, before waking up in the morning, and during daytime naps. Onset age varies, but is usually within the two first decades of life. Currently, it is hypothesized that the pathogenetic mechanism is linked to overactivity in ascending cholinergic circuits that control arousal, leading to an imbalance of function in the frontal lobes. The ictal symptoms are thought to represent a paroxysmal disinhibition of subcortical activity in the form of automatic motor and limbic activity. The hyperkinetic sleep-related seizure is the clinical hallmark of the disorder. Interictal cognitive and psychiatric symptoms have been described in some families, but it is uncertain whether these features are true phenotypic traits. Most patients respond to antiepileptic therapy, especially carbamazepine, but one third of patients are pharmacoresistant. Some patients report long seizure-free periods. Unknown factors influence penetrance, treatment response, severity, and remission. Further studies, clinical as well as on the molecular level, are needed for a more complete understanding of ADNFLE. Nevertheless, the recent discoveries in ADNFLE have suggested new neurobiologic mechanisms for familial epilepsy and throw new light on the pathogenesis of epilepsy in general.

References

1. Bazil CW. Nocturnal seizures. *Semin Neurol.* 2004;24(3):293–300.
2. Berkovic SF, McIntosh A, Howell RA, et al. Familial temporal lobe epilepsy: a common disorder identified in twins. *Ann Neurol.* 1996;40(2):227–235.
3. Berkovic SF, Serratosa JM, Phillips HA, et al. Familial partial epilepsy with variable foci: clinical features and linkage to chromosome 22q12. *Epilepsia.* 2004;45(9):1054–1060.
4. Bertrand D, Elmslie F, Hughes E, et al. The CHRNB2 mutation I312M is associated with epilepsy and distinct memory deficits. *Neurobiol Dis.* 2005;20(3):799–804.

5. Bertrand D, Picard F, Le Hellard S, et al. How mutations in the nAChRs can cause ADNFLE epilepsy. *Epilepsia*. 2002;43(Suppl 5):112–122.
6. Blume WT, Luders HO, Mizrahi E, et al. Glossary of descriptive terminology for ictal semiology: report of the ILAE task force on classification and terminology. *Epilepsia*. 2001;42(9):1212–1218.
7. Bugajski J, Gadek-Michalska A, Bugajski AJ. Involvement of prostaglandins in the nicotine-induced pituitary-adrenocortical response during social stress. *J Physiol Pharmacol*. 2002;53(4 Pt 2):847–857.
8. Cho YW, Motamedi GK, Laufenberg I, et al. A Korean kindred with autosomal dominant nocturnal frontal lobe epilepsy and mental retardation. *Arch Neurol*. 2003;60(11):1625–1632.
9. Combi R, Dalpra L, Ferini-Strambi L, et al. Frontal lobe epilepsy and mutations of the corticotropin-releasing hormone gene. *Ann Neurol*. 2005;58:899–904.
10. Combi R, Dalpra L, Tenchini ML, et al. Autosomal dominant nocturnal frontal lobe epilepsy–a critical overview. *J Neurol*. 2004;251(8):923–934.
11. Commission on Classification and Terminology of the International League Against Epilepsy. Proposal for revised classification of epilepsies and epileptic syndromes. *Epilepsia*. 1989;30(4):389–399.
12. Commission on Classification and Terminology of the International League Against Epilepsy. Proposal for revised clinical and electroencephalographic classification of epileptic seizures. *Epilepsia*. 1981;22(4):489–501.
13. Curro Dossi R, Pare D, Steriade M. Short-lasting nicotinic and long-lasting muscarinic depolarizing responses of thalamocortical neurons to stimulation of mesopontine cholinergic nuclei. *J Neurophysiol*. 1991;65(3):393–406.
14. De Fusco M, Becchetti A, Patrignani A, et al. The nicotinic receptor beta 2 subunit is mutant in nocturnal frontal lobe epilepsy. *Nat Genet*. 2000;26(3):275–276.
15. Engel J. A proposed diagnostic scheme for people with epileptic seizures and with epilepsy: report of the ILAE Task Force on Classification and Terminology. *Epilepsia*. 2001;42(6):796–803.
16. Fonck C, Nashmi R, Deshpande P, et al. Increased sensitivity to agonist-induced seizures, straub tail, and hippocampal theta rhythm in knock-in mice carrying hypersensitive alpha 4 nicotinic receptors. *J Neurosci*. 2003;23(7):2582–2590.
17. Gambardella A, Annesi G, De Fusco M, et al. A new locus for autosomal dominant nocturnal frontal lobe epilepsy maps to chromosome 1. *Neurology*. 2000;55(10):1467–1471.
18. Godbout R, Montplaisir J, Rouleau I. Hypnogenic paroxysmal dystonia: epilepsy or sleep disorder? A case report. *Clin Electroencephalogr*. 1985;16(3):136–142.
19. Grubb MS, Rossi FM, Changeux JP, et al. Abnormal functional organization in the dorsal lateral geniculate nucleus of mice lacking the beta 2 subunit of the nicotinic acetylcholine receptor. *Neuron*. 2003;40(6):1161–1172.
20. Hayman M, Scheffer IE, Chinvarun Y, et al. Autosomal dominant nocturnal frontal lobe epilepsy: demonstration of focal frontal onset and intrafamilial variation. *Neurology*. 1997;49(4):969–975.
21. Hirose S, Iwata H, Akiyoshi H, et al. A novel mutation of CHRNA4 responsible for autosomal dominant nocturnal frontal lobe epilepsy. *Neurology*. 1999;53(8):1749–1753.
22. Hirose S, Okada M, Zhu G, et al. Transgenic rats harbouring a CHRNA4 mutation exhibit characteristic seizure phenotypes of nocturnal frontal lobe epilepsy [Abstract]. *Epilepsia*. 2005;46(Suppl 6):75(abst).
23. Hirsch E, Sellal F, Maton B, et al. Nocturnal paroxysmal dystonia: a clinical form of focal epilepsy. *Neurophysiol Clin*. 1994;24(3):207–217.
24. Ito M, Kobayashi K, Fujii T, et al. Electroclinical picture of autosomal dominant nocturnal frontal lobe epilepsy in a Japanese family. *Epilepsia*. 2000;41(1):52–58.
25. Khatami R, Neumann M, Schulz H, et al. A family with autosomal dominant nocturnal frontal lobe epilepsy and mental retardation. *J Neurol*. 1998;245(12):809–810.
26. Labarca C, Schwarz J, Deshpande P, et al. Point mutant mice with hypersensitive alpha 4 nicotinic receptors show dopaminergic deficits and increased anxiety. *Proc Natl Acad Sci U S A*. 2001;98(5):2786–2791.
27. Lee BI, Lesser RP, Pippenger CE, et al. Familial paroxysmal hypnogenic dystonia. *Neurology*. 1985;35(9):1357–1360.
28. Lee KH, McCormick DA. Modulation of spindle oscillations by acetylcholine, cholecystokinin and 1S,3R-ACPD in the ferret lateral geniculate and perigeniculate nuclei in vitro. *Neuroscience*. 1997;77(2):335–350.
29. Lena C, Popa D, Grailhe R, et al. Beta2-containing nicotinic receptors contribute to the organization of sleep and regulate putative micro-arousals in mice. *J Neurosci*. 2004;24(25):5711–5718.
30. Leniger T, Kananura C, Hufnagel A, et al. A new Chrna4 mutation with low penetrance in nocturnal frontal lobe epilepsy. *Epilepsia*. 2003;44(7):981–985.
31. Luders H, Acharya J, Baumgartner C, et al. Semiological seizure classification. *Epilepsia*. 1998;39(9):1006–1013.
32. Lugaresi E, Cirignotta F, Montagna P. Nocturnal paroxysmal dystonia. *J Neurol Neurosurg Psychiatry*. 1986;49(4):375–380.
33. Lugaresi E, Cirignotta F. Hypnogenic paroxysmal dystonia: epileptic seizure or a new syndrome? *Sleep*. 1981;4(2):129–138.
34. Magnusson A, Nakken KO, Brubakk E. Autosomal dominant frontal epilepsy. *Lancet*. 1996;347(9009):1191–1192.
35. Magnusson A, Stordal E, Brodtkorb E, et al. Schizophrenia, psychotic illness and other psychiatric symptoms in families with autosomal dominant nocturnal frontal lobe epilepsy caused by different mutations. *Psychiatr Genet*. 2003;13(2):91–95.
36. McLellan A, Phillips HA, Rittey C, et al. Phenotypic comparison of two Scottish families with mutations in different genes causing autosomal dominant nocturnal frontal lobe epilepsy. *Epilepsia*. 2003;44(4):613–617.
37. Meierkord H, Fish DR, Smith SJ, et al. Is nocturnal paroxysmal dystonia a form of frontal lobe epilepsy? *Mov Disord*. 1992;7(1):38–42.
38. Moulard B, Picard F, le Hellard S, et al. Ion channel variation causes epilepsies. *Brain Res Brain Res Rev*. 2001;36(2–3):275–284.
39. Nakken KO, Magnusson A, Steinlein OK. Autosomal dominant nocturnal frontal lobe epilepsy: an electroclinical study of a Norwegian family with ten affected members. *Epilepsia*. 1999;40(1):88–92.
40. Oldani A, Zucconi M, Asselta R, et al. Autosomal dominant nocturnal frontal lobe epilepsy. A video-polysomnographic and genetic appraisal of 40 patients and delineation of the epileptic syndrome. *Brain*. 1998;121(Pt 2):205–223.
41. Oldani A, Zucconi M, Ferini-Strambi L, et al. Autosomal dominant nocturnal frontal lobe epilepsy: electroclinical picture. *Epilepsia*. 1996;37(10):964–976.
42. Phillips HA, Favre I, Kirkpatrick M, et al. CHRNB2 is the second acetylcholine receptor subunit associated with autosomal dominant nocturnal frontal lobe epilepsy. *Am J Hum Genet*. 2001;68(1):225–231.
43. Phillips HA, Marini C, Scheffer IE, et al. A de novo mutation in sporadic nocturnal frontal lobe epilepsy. *Ann Neurol*. 2000;48(2):264–267.
44. Phillips HA, Scheffer IE, Berkovic SF, et al. Localization of a gene for autosomal dominant nocturnal frontal lobe epilepsy to chromosome 20q 13.2. *Nat Genet*. 1995;10:117–118.
45. Phillips HA, Scheffer IE, Crossland KM, et al. Autosomal dominant nocturnal frontal-lobe epilepsy: genetic heterogeneity and evidence for a second locus at 15q24. *Am J Hum Genet*. 1998;63(4):1108–1116.
46. Picard F, Baulac S, Kahane P, et al. Dominant partial epilepsies. A clinical, electrophysiological and genetic study of 19 European families. *Brain*. 2000;123(Pt 6):1247–1262.
47. Picard F, Bertrand S, Steinlein OK, et al. Mutated nicotinic receptors responsible for autosomal dominant nocturnal frontal lobe epilepsy are more sensitive to carbamazepine. *Epilepsia*. 1999;40(9):1198–1209.
48. Picard F, Bruel D, Servent D, et al. Alteration of the in vivo nicotinic receptor density in ADNFLE patients, a PET study. *Brain*. 2006;129:2047–2060.
49. Provini F, Plazzi G, Lugaresi E. From nocturnal paroxysmal dystonia to nocturnal frontal lobe epilepsy. *Clin Neurophysiol*. 2000;111(Suppl 2):S2–8.
50. Provini F, Plazzi G, Montagna P, et al. The wide clinical spectrum of nocturnal frontal lobe epilepsy. *Sleep Med Rev*. 2000;4(4):375–386.
51. Provini F, Plazzi G, Tinuper P, et al. Nocturnal frontal lobe epilepsy. A clinical and polygraphic overview of 100 consecutive cases. *Brain*. 1999;122(Pt 6):1017–1031.
52. Rodrigues-Pinguet N, Jia L, Li M, et al. Five ADNFLE mutations reduce the Ca2+ dependence of the mammalian alpha4beta2 acetylcholine response. *J Physiol*. 2003;550(Pt 1):11–26.
53. Role LW, Berg DK. Nicotinic receptors in the development and modulation of CNS synapses. *Neuron*. 1996;16(6):1077–1085.
54. Ross SA, Wong JY, Clifford JJ, et al. Phenotypic characterization of an alpha 4 neuronal nicotinic acetylcholine receptor subunit knock-out mouse. *J Neurosci*. 2000;20(17):6431–6441.
55. Rozycka A, Skorupska E, Kostyrko A, et al. Evidence for S284L mutation of the CHRNA4 in a white family with autosomal dominant nocturnal frontal lobe epilepsy. *Epilepsia*. 2003;44(8):1113–1117.
56. Saenz A, Galan J, Caloustian C, et al. Autosomal dominant nocturnal frontal lobe epilepsy in a Spanish family with a Ser252Phe mutation in the CHRNA4 gene. *Arch Neurol*. 1999;56(8):1004–1009.
57. Sarnyai Z, Shaham Y, Heinrichs SC. The role of corticotropin-releasing factor in drug addiction. *Pharmacol Rev*. 2001;53(2):209–243.
58. Scheffer IE, Bhatia KP, Lopes-Cendes I, et al. Autosomal dominant nocturnal frontal lobe epilepsy. A distinctive clinical disorder. *Brain*. 1995;118(Pt 1):61–73.
59. Scheffer IE, Bhatia KP, Lopes-Cendes I, et al. Autosomal dominant frontal epilepsy misdiagnosed as sleep disorder. *Lancet*. 1994;343(8896):515–517.
60. Scheffer IE, Phillips HA, O'Brien CE, et al. Familial partial epilepsy with variable foci: a new partial epilepsy syndrome with suggestion of linkage to chromosome 2. *Ann Neurol*. 1998;44(6):890–899.
61. Steinlein OK. Nicotinic acetylcholine receptors and epilepsy. *Curr Drug Targets CNS Neurol Disord*. 2002;1(4):443–448.
62. Steinlein OK, Magnusson A, Stoodt J, et al. An insertion mutation of the CHRNA4 gene in a family with autosomal dominant nocturnal frontal lobe epilepsy. *Hum Mol Genet*. 1997;6(6):943–947.
63. Steinlein OK, Mulley JC, Propping P, et al. A missense mutation in the neuronal nicotinic acetylcholine receptor alpha 4 subunit is associated with autosomal dominant nocturnal frontal lobe epilepsy. *Nat Genet*. 1995;11(2):201–203.
64. Steinlein OK, Stoodt J, Mulley J, et al. Independent occurrence of the CHRNA4 Ser248Phe mutation in a Norwegian family with nocturnal frontal lobe epilepsy. *Epilepsia*. 2000;41(5):529–535.

65. Steriade M, Datta S, Pare D, et al. Neuronal activities in brain-stem cholinergic nuclei related to tonic activation processes in thalamocortical systems. *J Neurosci*. 1990;10(8):2541–2559.
66. Tenchini ML, Duga S, Bonati MT, et al. SER252PHE and 776INS3 mutations in the CHRNA4 gene are rare in the Italian ADNFLE population. *Sleep*. 1999;22(5):637–639.
67. Terzano MG, Monge-Strauss MF, Mikol F, et al. Cyclic alternating pattern as a provocative factor in nocturnal paroxysmal dystonia. *Epilepsia*. 1997;38(9):1015–1025.
68. Tinuper P, Cerullo A, Cirignotta F, et al. Nocturnal paroxysmal dystonia with short-lasting attacks: three cases with evidence for an epileptic frontal lobe origin of seizures. *Epilepsia*. 1990;31(5):549–556.
69. Tinuper P, Provini F, Bisulli F, et al. Hyperkinetic manifestations in nocturnal frontal lobe epilepsy. Semeiological features and physiopathological hypothesis. *Neurol Sci*. 2005;26(Suppl 3):210–214.
70. Tritto T, McCallum SE, Waddle SA, et al. Null mutant analysis of responses to nicotine: deletion of beta2 nicotinic acetylcholine receptor subunit but not alpha7 subunit reduces sensitivity to nicotine-induced locomotor depression and hypothermia. *Nicotine Tob Res*. 2004;6(1):145–158.
71. Varadkar S, Duncan JS, Cross JH. Acetazolamide and autosomal dominant nocturnal frontal lobe epilepsy. *Epilepsia*. 2003;44(7):986–987.
72. Vigevano F, Fusco L. Hypnic tonic postural seizures in healthy children provide evidence for a partial epileptic syndrome of frontal lobe origin. *Epilepsia*. 1993;34(1):110–119.
73. Willoughby JO, Pope KJ, Eaton V. Nicotine as an antiepileptic agent in ADNFLE: an N-of-one study. *Epilepsia*. 2003;44(9):1238–1240.
74. Zucconi M, Oldani A, Smirne S, et al. The macrostructure and microstructure of sleep in patients with autosomal dominant nocturnal frontal lobe epilepsy. *J Clin Neurophysiol*. 2000;17(1):77–86.

CHAPTER 250 ■ HYPOTHALAMIC HAMARTOMA WITH GELASTIC SEIZURES

A. SIMON HARVEY, ORVAR EEG-OLOFSSON, AND JEREMY L. FREEMAN

INTRODUCTION

The syndrome of hypothalamic hamartoma (HH) with gelastic (laughing) seizures (GSs) is a rare but important epileptic syndrome (HHGS), being one of the most refractory, disabling, and poorly understood seizure disorders affecting children and adults. Over the last decade, much has been learned about the nature of HH and its often progressive neurologic and behavioral manifestations, and effective surgical treatments have also been developed.

HISTORICAL PERSPECTIVES

Le Marquand and Russell[44] first used the term hamartoma in 1934 to describe a tumor-like lesion of the hypothalamus found at postmortem in a boy with precocious puberty. Chronic epilepsy associated with a hypothalamic lesion, designated an astrocytoma but likely an HH, was first reported 2 years earlier[86] in a boy with precocious puberty and mental retardation who died from status epilepticus. The first report of GS in a patient with HH was in 1938,[18] the patient also having precocious puberty and pervasive developmental delay. Isolated reports of probable or proven HH with gelastic seizures followed.[27,45,50,59,60,66,78] In 1988, the association was better characterized by Berkovic et al. as a recognizable and possibly progressive epileptic syndrome, their series incorporating neuroimaging diagnosis.[4] The first report of a patient surviving surgical resection of an HH was in 1967,[59] but it was not until the mid-1990s that GSs were shown conclusively to arise in the HH[39,41,54] and surgical treatment for refractory seizures flourished. Over the last 10 years, there has been great interest in the nature of HH and its association with GSs, and great efforts in developing minimally invasive surgical techniques for treatment of the refractory seizure disorder. For further details concerning GSs, see Chapter 53.

DEFINITIONS

A hamartoma is a focal malformation that resembles a neoplasm, composed of an abnormal mixture or proportion of tissue elements normally present in that site, which develop and grow at virtually the same rate as normal tissue.[71] HHs are usually spherical in shape with a diameter between 0.5 and 4 cm, in most cases <1.5 cm. HHs arise from the tuber cinereum or from one or both mammillary bodies, and if large, may bulge into the third ventricle and compress (but not disrupt) the hypothalamic nuclei and fiber tracts.[45] Asymmetric location and attachment are seen in about two thirds of patients.[21]

Several anatomic classifications of HH based on magnetic resonance imaging (MRI) features have been proposed, distinguishing different sizes and patterns of hamartoma attachment to the hypothalamus.[1,8,15,85] The most important separation from clinical, pathophysiologic, and surgical perspectives seems to be the distinction between HHs sitting within the third ventricle that are attached to the mammillary bodies and/or the hypothalamic walls (sessile, intraventricular, intrahypothalamic) from those HHs beneath the third ventricle with attachment to the tuber cinereum (pedunculated, extraventricular, parahypothalamic). HHs associated with epilepsy are almost always intraventricular, at least in part, with a significant mammillary body attachment.

Histologically, HHs resemble normal gray matter,[57] though some neurons may show variation in size and shape[8,14,37,59,62,75] and may appear in discrete nests or nodules of cells.[8,29,59] Fibrillary gliosis is also found,[8] and cystic changes have been observed in large lesions.[70] Dysplastic neurons and balloon cells are not seen in HHs.

EPIDEMIOLOGY

HHGS is an uncommon epileptic syndrome, with a prevalence in childhood of about 0.5 in 100,000.[9] Most early reports of HHs were in patients with central precocious puberty,[91] but most recent reports concern HHs and GSs. The current literature is biased toward surgical patients with severe seizure and other neurologic manifestations, making it hard to determine the proportion of patients with different clinical features. Also, it is likely that there are patients with HHs who are asymptomatic or have only mild or undiagnosed seizure manifestations,[81] leading to underreporting of HH. A greater number of males with HHs and epilepsy is reported.[82]

ETIOLOGY AND BASIC MECHANISMS

HHs are a nonfamilial, congenital malformation usually occurring in isolation. They are rarely associated with other intracranial malformations such as callosal dysgenesis, heterotopias, arachnoid cysts, and microgyria.[8,21,30] Rarely, HHs may occur as part of a multiple congenital malformation syndrome, most notably the autosomal dominant Pallister-Hall syndrome, which includes HH, polydactyly, hypopituitarism, imperforate anus, and dysplastic nails.[7] Seizures occur in about 15% of patients with Pallister-Hall syndrome and are often mild, despite HHs often being very large. Patients with Pallister-Hall syndrome have mutations of the zinc-finger transcription factor gene *GLI3* on chromosome 7p13,[35,40] but the role of *GLI3* mutation in patients with sporadic HHs[24] is unconfirmed and so the etiology of sporadic HHs remains uncertain.

The genesis of seizures associated with HH is also incompletely understood. Mechanical irritation or distortion of the adjacent hypothalamus or midbrain by the HH was initially believed to be the cause of seizures.[45] The severity and generalized nature of seizures and associated neurologic and behavioral problems in many patients with HHs, and the early poor results of HH surgery,[10,49,69,75] led to speculation that patients with HHs had widespread occult cerebral dysgenesis.[4,79] GSs were eventually shown to arise from the HH by stereotactic depth electroencephalographic (EEG) recording of seizures from the HH, by reproduction of symptoms with electrical stimulation of the HH, and by demonstration of HH hyperperfusion with ictal single photon emission computed tomography (SPECT).[34,36–39,41,54] This led to a change in view from the HH simply being an epiphenomenon to the HH being intrinsically epileptogenic.[6] Such intrinsic hyperexcitability has been documented with single cell studies of small neurons within cell clusters in resected HHs exhibiting pacemaker-like spontaneous repetitive firing,[90] similar to that seen in focal cortical dysplasia.[48,63]

The reasons for marked variability of the neurologic manifestations of HHs, and the relationship between the size and attachment of the HH, and the neurologic manifestations remain uncertain. Some reports suggest that seizures are more frequent or severe in patients with larger HHs.[47,81] A connection of the HH with the mammillary bodies seems to be integral to epileptogenesis.[1,21,85] Tonic seizures that develop in a proportion of children do not seem to arise from the HH,[37] but rather occur as a related but independent neocortical phenomenon. The whole electroclinical picture of symptomatic generalized epilepsy, with slow spike-wave on EEG and generalized tonic seizures, may develop in patients with HHGS as a consequence of secondary epileptogenesis in the neocortex.[22]

CLINICAL PRESENTATION

GSs are the characteristic epileptic manifestation of HH, occurring in nearly all patients (see Chapter 53). Early onset of GSs is characteristic[9,82] and onset from the day of life is well known.[4,16,17,41,62,78] The sound produced during GSs associated with HH is described variously as laughter, chuckling, or giggling, often qualified by words such as unnatural, mechanical, mirthless, and inappropriate. Dacrystic (crying) seizures are noted in many patients,[10,28,37,45,65,78,80,87,89] invariably accompanied by GSs. Very frequent, brief GSs occurring during wakefulness and sleep are common in infancy. A mild form of GSs is described in adults with small HHs, the patients sometimes describing only a "pressure to laugh"[81] or an "urge to giggle."[52] Consciousness is said to be preserved during brief gelastic seizures.[4,12,78] Often accompanying laughter in gelastic seizures are autonomic features such as facial flushing and pupillary dilation, hypermotor automatisms, oro-alimentary automatisms, head and eye deviation, and tonic or clonic facial contraction.[4,78]

West syndrome is reported in association with HH,[3,9,22,53] such that HH should be included in the differential diagnosis of infants presenting with epileptic spasms.

An epileptic progression with development of focal seizures, tonic/atonic seizures, and tonic–clonic seizures occurs in more than half of patients.[82] Many patients develop Lennox-Gastaut syndrome with disabling drop attacks. There is a paucity of detailed clinical and EEG descriptions of these associated seizures occurring in patients with HHs, in contrast to GSs. The interrelationship of these different seizure types is uncertain, but focal seizures associated with HHs often have frontal and temporal lobe features, tonic seizures and spasms associated with HHs often have focal motor features, and laughter may precede or follow all of these.

Cognitive and behavioral impairments are common in patients with HHGS who have seizures beginning in childhood, especially refractory seizures that begin in infancy and evolve to focal and generalized seizures with marked EEG disturbances. These vary in severity from mild impairments of memory, attention, and learning[4,20,52,81] to severe intellectual disability.[15,33,62] Aggressive behavior, rage attacks, and other psychiatric comorbidities are widely reported in patients with HHGS.[4,88] The relationship of behavior disturbance to GSs and intrinsic hypothalamic dysfunction is uncertain.

Central precocious puberty is common in patients with HHGS (see below), occurring in 30% to 40% of patients with epilepsy,[21,82] usually following the onset of seizures and associated with larger HH size and involvement of the tuber cinereum.[21] Treatment of central precocious puberty with gonadotropin-releasing hormone (GnRH) agonists is usually effective, and patients rarely undergo surgery for this indication alone.

DIAGNOSTIC EVALUATION

The diagnosis of HHGS is usually based on the recognition of pathologic laughter attacks and the finding of an HH on MRI; EEG is rarely informative early in the course of the epilepsy. The diagnostic evaluation for patients undergoing epilepsy surgery is similar to that for patients with refractory epilepsy of cortical origin except for the need for perioperative endocrine assessment, the need for precise anatomic imaging of midline brain structures, and less attention paid to scalp EEG localization of seizures and interictal discharges.[32]

EEG Findings

Scalp EEG in patients with HHs is variable, reflecting the age of the patient and the evolution of the seizure disorder. In young children with only GSs, and in adults with mild symptoms, the interictal EEG is usually normal,[60] potentially leading to missed diagnosis. Interictal EEG abnormalities may not appear until later childhood,[46] coinciding with the appearance of additional seizure types.[82] Initially, the interictal record may only be abnormal during sleep.[12] Spike-wave activity is prominent over the frontal and temporal regions initially and may be bilaterally synchronous or predominantly unilateral.[11,82] Unilateral abnormalities tend to occur on the side of predominant HH attachment. In patients with tonic and other generalized seizures, background slowing is common and multifocal or generalized spike-wave activity, paroxysmal fast activity, and electrodecremental patterns are recorded, often with electrical status in sleep.[22] The interictal EEG abnormalities in patients with HH must be secondary neocortical phenomena, as a small mass of nonlayered gray matter deep in the middle of the cranium cannot generate electrical potentials of significant amplitude to be recorded on the scalp surface. In fact, intracranial EEG recordings show that interictal discharges arise independently in the HH and the neocortex.[22,37] Furthermore, interictal discharges persist over the neocortex immediately following resection of the HH,[22] though they may subside in the weeks and months that follow successful surgery.

Ictal scalp EEG may show no change during brief GSs,[60] or just a desynchronization of the background activity.[9] Later, as tonic seizures and interictal slow spike-waves develop, GSs are marked by suppression of the interictal discharges and attenuation of background rhythms, with or without widespread low-voltage fast activity.[4] In patients with partial seizures, ictal EEG recordings may show focal rhythms or spike-wave activity, either unilaterally or bilaterally. Misleading focal ictal onsets in the frontal or anterior temporal lobes of patients studied with intracranial EEG recordings, but without electrodes in the HH, once led to unsuccessful focal cortical resections.[11] Depth EEG recordings from the HH[37–39,41,54] show that GSs are associated with an ictal discharge within the HH that, in most

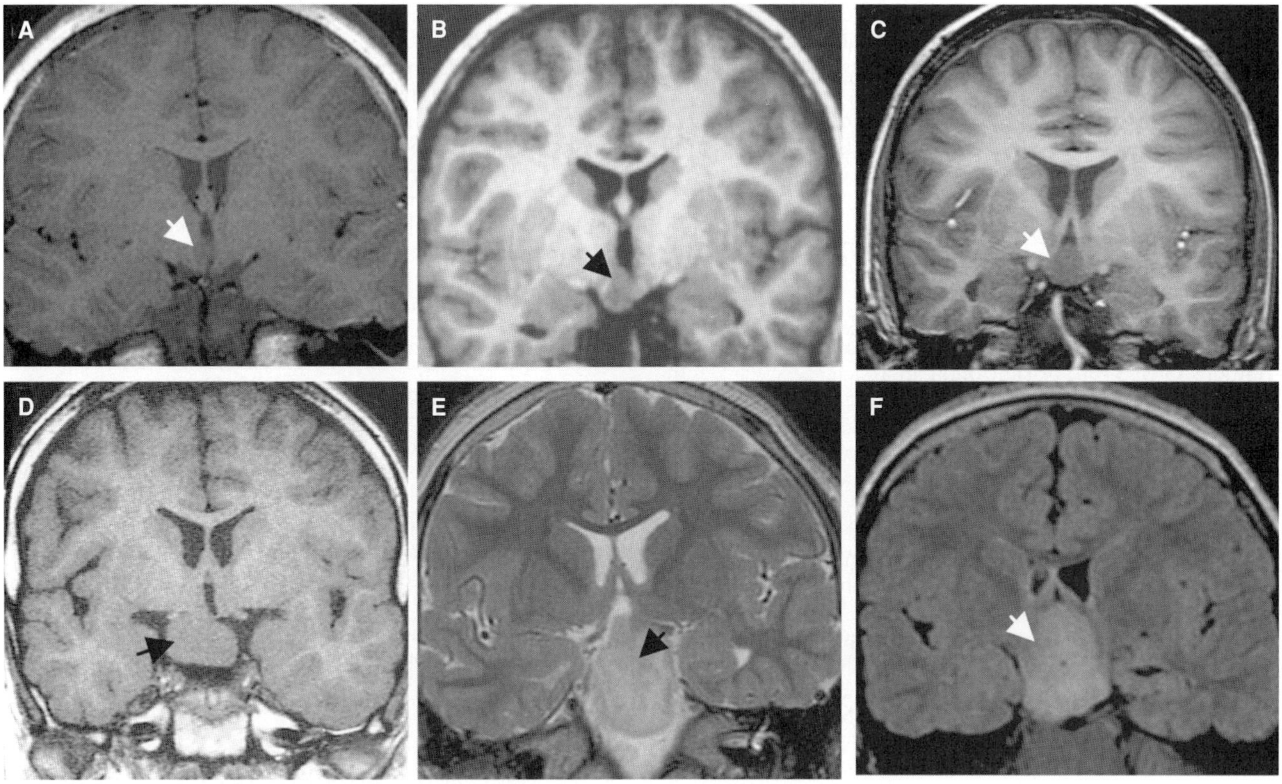

FIGURE 1. Coronal magnetic resonance images of six patients with gelastic seizures and hypothalamic hamartoma (HH) of different sizes and attachments. **A, B:** Small, unilateral, intraventricular HHs. **C:** A moderate size, bilateral, intraventricular HH. **D, E:** Large, unilateral HHs attached broadly to the ventricular wall and tuber cinereum. **F:** A large, bilateral, intraventricular HH, which distorts the hypothalamus and extends into the interpeduncular cistern.

cases, remains confined to the HH. Electrical stimulation of the HH via the depth electrodes in these cases may provoke the characteristic ictal laughter. In contrast, depth EEG recording of tonic seizures reveals discharges remote from the HH involving various cortical areas.[37]

MRI

MRI (Fig. 1) is far superior to computed tomography (CT) of the brain in revealing and characterizing HHs.[4] Small HHs may be difficult to detect unless the hypothalamic region is specifically examined. HHs usually have increased signal compared to gray matter on T2-weighted and fluid-attenuated inversion recovery (FLAIR) sequences, and low signal on T1, but do not enhance with contrast and remain in proportion with the rest of the brain over time.[21] T2-weighted sequences in the three orthogonal planes are well suited to displaying the high-signal HHs in relation to the low-signal, heavily myelinated hypothalamic nuclei and tracts. Proton magnetic resonance spectroscopy suggests neuronal attenuation and relative gliosis compared with normal gray matter.[21]

PET and SPECT Imaging

Positron emission tomography (PET) studies are few and show either scattered areas of focal cortical or regional hypometabolism, with lateralization usually being concordant with the side of HH attachment.[62,74] Ictal SPECT studies during GSs demonstrate focal hyperperfusion in the region of the HH[17,34,41,43]; HH hypermetabolism is reported in a patient studied with ^{18}F-fluorodeoxyglucose (FDG)-PET during status epilepticus.[64] Asymmetric cerebral perfusion during seizures is common in HHGS,[9] with hyperperfusion ipsilateral to the side of predominant HH attachment, suggesting preferential cortical spread of seizure activity from the HH.[23]

DIFFERENTIAL DIAGNOSIS

Pathologic laughter is reported as an epileptic and nonepileptic manifestation of various lesions and processes affecting the temporal lobe, frontal lobe, and brainstem (see Chapter 53). Craniopharyngiomas and tumors of the hypothalamus and third ventricle are imaging differentials of HHs but are generally distinguishable on MRI and rarely present with chronic epilepsy. A search for associated cerebral malformations on MRI and a clinical examination for midline malformations and polydactyly should be undertaken in a patient with seemingly isolated HHs to look for syndromic features.

SURGERY AND OUTCOME

Antiepileptic medications are generally ineffective in the management of epilepsy associated with HHs.[4,9] While they may have some impact on the severity or frequency of partial and generalized seizures, antiepileptic drugs generally have little impact on GSs. Vagal nerve stimulation may provide partial benefit in some patients.[9,55]

Early attempts at HH removal were not particularly successful,[10,69,75,78] but with refinements in technique and advances in technology, epilepsy surgery has since become the accepted treatment of choice for refractory epilepsy associated with HHs.[5,6,31,68] Several operative approaches are currently reported, including open craniotomy (pterional, frontotemporal, paramedian) for either microsurgical or endoscopic resection or disconnection of the HH, and minimally invasive stereotactic approaches with endoscopic, radiofrequency, or radiosurgical ablation.

Open Craniotomy

Pterional and large frontotemporal craniotomies provide access to the inferior part of the HH via a transsylvian, transfrontal, subtemporal, or subfrontal approach.[15,46,51,58,62,85] In some cases the temporal pole or orbital cortex is resected. Such surgical approaches to HHs have proven ineffective in many cases, as only the subventricular component of the HH can be removed, leaving the intraventricular component attached to the mammillary bodies.[5,6,62] Furthermore, there is significant risk of endocrine complications, stroke, and oculomotor paresis with these approaches.[15,62] Delalande proposed disconnection as a safer alternative to resection during frontotemporal approaches.[15]

An interhemispheric, transcallosal approach to intraventricular resection of HHs was developed by Rosenfeld et al.,[73] with superior results and fewer neurovascular complications reported. This approach passes between the columns of the fornices to access the HH within the third ventricle, allowing direct vision of the intraventricular component of the HH under the operating microscope, and complete or near-complete resection or disconnection of the intraventricular HH with the ultrasonic aspirator (Fig. 2). In a series of 29 consecutive young patients undergoing transcallosal surgery for HHs, complete or near-complete resection was achieved in 22. Seizure freedom was achieved in 15 patients and >90% seizure reduction in seven.[33] Most striking in this series was the improvement in patients with symptomatic generalized epilepsy, in whom tonic seizures were frequently abolished and generalized, multifocal spike-wave on scalp EEG was improved, and improved language and behavior were observed.[22,33] "Running down" of generalized seizures was observed in several patients.[22,33] These results dispel the notion that these HHGS have diffuse and irreversible cerebral dysfunction or dysplasia. Morbidity consisted of short-term memory impairment, weight gain, hypothyroidism, and transient hypernatremia.[25,33] Similar results are reported from another center.[56]

Stereotactic Radiofrequency Ablation

Stereotactic radiofrequency thermocoagulation was employed early in the development of surgical treatments for HHs with intractable epilepsy.[26,41,65] Multiple lesions are produced in the HH, often after seizures are recorded from the implanted electrode and symptoms are reproduced with electrical stimulation. The need for repeat procedures is not uncommon and low seizure-free rates are reported, most likely reflecting the limited impact of the small lesions induced. Stereotactic radiofrequency thermocoagulation may only be suitable for small HHs.[42]

Neuroendoscopy

Neuroendoscopy is being increasingly utilized to resect or disconnect HHs,[13,15,42,62] with access to the third ventricle being obtained via a transcortical approach through the frontal horn of the lateral ventricle and the foramen of Monro.

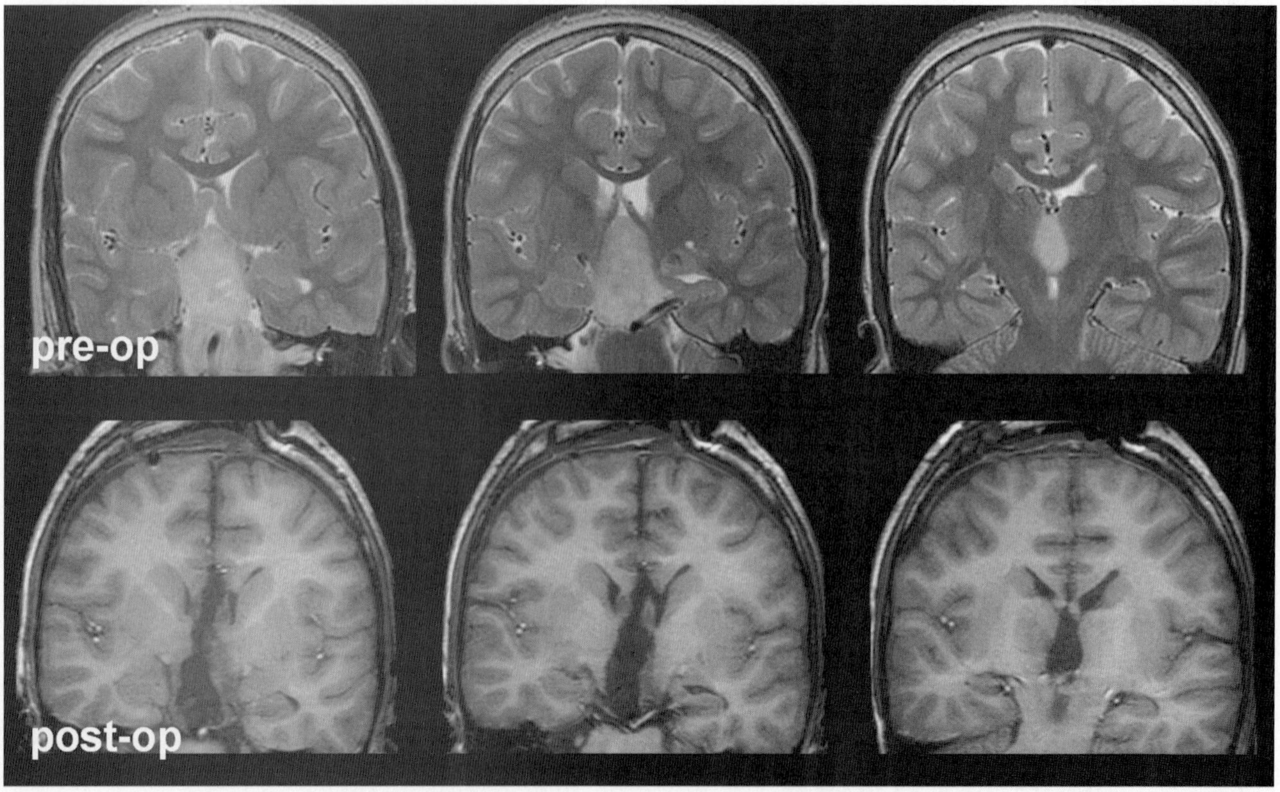

FIGURE 2. Coronal magnetic resonance images of a child with a large bilateral hypothalamic hamartoma and intractable gelastic seizures, before (**top row**) and after (**bottom row**) transcallosal resection.

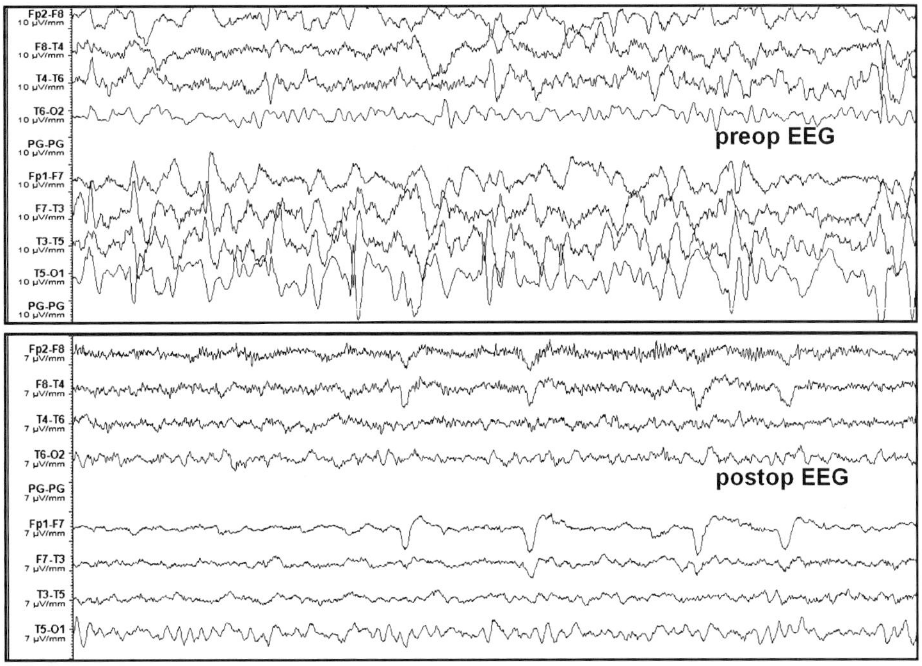

FIGURE 3. Interictal scalp electroencephalographic (EEG) recordings in a child with gelastic seizures and hypothalamic hamartoma who underwent transcallosal resection of the hamartoma. The preoperative awake EEG 8 days before surgery (**top**) showed multifocal epileptiform discharges predominantly on the left, which were abolished on the postoperative awake EEG 21 days following surgery (**bottom**).

Radiofrequency thermocoagulation can be combined with endoscopic access to disconnect or lesion HHs. Postoperative hospital stay is reduced with such minimally invasive procedures, but whether efficacy and safety are comparable with open craniotomy and resection is yet to be demonstrated in large series.

Stereotactic Radiosurgery

Stereotactic radiosurgery, such as with the Gamma Knife, delivers high-dose, ionizing radiation to a stereotactically defined intracranial target, with a steep radiation fall-off outside of the treated volume. Gamma Knife radiosurgery has been extensively applied to the treatment of HHs.[2,19,72,83,84] Like stereotactic radiofrequency ablation, Gamma Knife surgery is probably best suited for small HHs or for the hypothalamic attachment of larger HHs. Minimal morbidity and short hospital stays are clear advantages, whereas delayed seizure reduction is a disadvantage. Seizure-free rates are difficult to determine as large series are lacking. Stereotactic implantation of ^{125}I seeds into the HH is an alternative radiosurgical approach.[76,77]

Surgery Outcomes

If seizure outcomes are compared in patients undergoing only one surgical technique, and analysis is confined to series with adequate reporting and minimum 1-year follow-up, Engel class I or II outcome (seizure freedom, auras only, rare seizures only) is reported in 66% of patients undergoing transcallosal resection, 60% of patients undergoing endoscopic procedures, 38% of patients undergoing Gamma Knife surgery, 36% of patients undergoing pterional or frontotemporal approaches to resection or disconnection, and 27% of patients undergoing stereotactic radiofrequency ablation.[31] Neurovascular complications are significantly greater for operative compared with stereotactic approaches, especially for pterional and frontotemporal approaches. Endocrine and memory disturbances appear to be more common with the transcallosal approach. Seizure outcome does not seem to be related to patient age, the presence of generalized seizures, or HH size[33] such that all patients with HHs and refractory epilepsy should be considered for surgery. More data with longer patient follow-up are required to properly evaluate radiosurgery. Callosotomy and neocortical resection are failed operative approaches that are no longer advocated in patients with HHs.[11,61]

Improvements in behavior, school performance, and aspects of development are reported in many patients undergoing HH surgery, regardless of approach and seizure outcome. Amelioration of autistic features has also been noted in one case with postoperative seizure freedom.[67] Reduction of interictal spike-wave following HH surgery is reported[22] (Fig. 3) and is associated with improvements in alertness, language, and behavior. However, reversal of intellectual impairment is not reported.

LONG-TERM PROGNOSIS

In patients with HHs in whom seizures begin early in childhood, the prognosis for seizure control and neurologic development and behavior seem poor, especially if seizures begin in infancy and there is early evidence of seizure evolution. Favorable treatment outcomes seem only to occur in patients who undergo successful surgery early in childhood, before the development of severe neurologic sequelae.

SUMMARY AND CONCLUSIONS

A rare, severe, and once untreatable epileptic syndrome, HHGS is now better understood and being effectively treated with surgery. Early diagnosis is important and requires recognition of pathologic laughter and adequate MRI imaging and interpretation. While controlled trials of surgical treatments are unlikely, greater experience with transcallosal, endoscopic, and radiosurgical approaches should lead to a better understanding of the most effective and safe treatment for this condition.

References

1. Arita K, Ikawa F, Kurisu K, et al. The relationship between magnetic resonance imaging findings and clinical manifestations of hypothalamic hamartoma. *J Neurosurg*. 1999;91:212–220.

2. Arita K, Kurisu K, Iida K, et al. Subsidence of seizure induced by stereotactic radiation in a patient with hypothalamic hamartoma. Case report. *J Neurosurg*. 1998;89:645–648.
3. Asanuma H, Wakai S, Tanaka T, et al. Brain tumors associated with infantile spasms. *Pediatr Neurol*. 1995;12:361–364.
4. Berkovic SF, Andermann F, Melanson D, et al. Hypothalamic hamartomas and ictal laughter: evolution of a characteristic epileptic syndrome and diagnostic value of magnetic resonance imaging. *Ann Neurol*. 1988;23:429–439.
5. Berkovic SF, Arzimanoglou A, Kuzniecky R, et al. Hypothalamic hamartoma and seizures: a treatable epileptic encephalopathy. *Epilepsia*. 2003;44:969–973.
6. Berkovic SF, Kuzniecky RI, Andermann F. Human epileptogenesis and hypothalamic hamartomas: new lessons from an experiment of nature. *Epilepsia*. 1997;38:1–3.
7. Biesecker LG, Graham JM Jr. Pallister-Hall syndrome. *J Med Genet*. 1996;33:585–589.
8. Boyko OB, Curnes JT, Oakes WJ, et al. Hamartomas of the tuber cinereum: CT, MR, and pathologic findings. *AJNR Am J Neuroradiol*. 1991;12:309–314.
9. Brandberg G, Raininko R, Eeg-Olofsson O. Hypothalamic hamartoma with gelastic seizures in Swedish children and adolescents. *Eur J Paediatr Neurol*. 2004;8:35–44.
10. Breningstall GN. Gelastic seizures, precocious puberty, and hypothalamic hamartoma. *Neurology*. 1985;35:1180–1183.
11. Cascino GD, Andermann F, Berkovic SF, et al. Gelastic seizures and hypothalamic hamartomas: evaluation of patients undergoing chronic intracranial EEG monitoring and outcome of surgical treatment. *Neurology*. 1993;43:747–750.
12. Cerullo A, Tinuper P, Provini F, et al. Autonomic and hormonal ictal changes in gelastic seizures from hypothalamic hamartomas. *Electroencephalogr Clin Neurophysiol*. 1998;107:317–322.
13. Choi JU, Yang KH, Kim TG, et al. Endoscopic disconnection for hypothalamic hamartoma with intractable seizure. Report of four cases. *J Neurosurg*. 2004;100:506–511.
14. Culler FL, James HE, Simon ML, et al. Identification of gonadotropin-releasing hormone in neurons of a hypothalamic hamartoma in a boy with precocious puberty. *Neurosurgery*. 1985;17:408–412.
15. Delalande O, Fohlen M. Disconnecting surgical treatment of hypothalamic hamartoma in children and adults with refractory epilepsy and proposal of a new classification. *Neurol Med Chir (Tokyo)*. 2003;43:61–68.
16. Diebler C, Ponsot G. Hamartomas of the tuber cinereum. *Neuroradiology*. 1983;25:93–101.
17. DiFazio MP, Davis RG. Utility of early single photon emission computed tomography (SPECT) in neonatal gelastic epilepsy associated with hypothalamic hamartoma. *J Child Neurol*. 2000;15:414–417.
18. Dott NM. Surgical aspects of the hypothalamus. In: Le Gros Clark WE, Beattie J, Riddoch G, et al., eds. *The Hypothalamus: Morphological, Functional, Clinical, and Surgical Aspects*. Edinburgh: Oliver and Boyd; 1938:131–185.
19. Dunoyer C, Ragheb J, Resnick T, et al. The use of stereotactic radiosurgery to treat intractable childhood partial epilepsy. *Epilepsia*. 2002;43:292–300.
20. Frattali CM, Liow K, Craig GH, et al. Cognitive deficits in children with gelastic seizures and hypothalamic hamartoma. *Neurology*. 2001;57:43–46.
21. Freeman JL, Coleman LT, Wellard RM, et al. MR imaging and spectroscopic study of epileptogenic hypothalamic hamartomas: analysis of 72 cases. *AJNR Am J Neuroradiol*. 2004;25:450–462.
22. Freeman JL, Harvey AS, Rosenfeld JV, et al. Generalized epilepsy in hypothalamic hamartoma: evolution and postoperative resolution. *Neurology*. 2003;60:762–767.
23. Freeman JL, Reutens DC, Bailey CA, et al. Seizure origin and propagation in hypothalamic hamartoma: evidence from subtraction ictal SPECT. *Epilepsia*. 2004;45(Suppl 7):S271.
24. Freeman JL, Wallace RH, Izzillo PA, et al. Hypothalamic hamartoma due to a somatic mutation in transcription factor gene *GLI3*. *Epilepsia*. 2003;44(Suppl 9):S68–S69.
25. Freeman JL, Zacharin M, Rosenfeld JV, et al. The endocrinology of hypothalamic hamartoma surgery for intractable epilepsy. *Epileptic Disord*. 2003;5:239–247.
26. Fukuda M, Kameyama S, Wachi M, et al. Stereotaxy for hypothalamic hamartoma with intractable gelastic seizures: technical case report. *Neurosurgery*. 1999;44:1347–1350.
27. Gascon GG, Lombroso CT. Epileptic (gelastic) laughter. *Epilepsia*. 1971;12:63–76.
28. Gomibuchi K, Ochiai Y, Kanraku S, et al. [Infantile spasms and gelastic seizure due to hypothalamic hamartoma]. *No To Hattatsu*. 1990;22:392–394.
29. Guibaud L, Rode V, Saint-Pierre G, et al. Giant hypothalamic hamartoma: an unusual neonatal tumor. *Pediatr Radiol*. 1995;25:17–18.
30. Gulati S, Gera S, Menon PS, et al. Hypothalamic hamartoma, gelastic epilepsy, precocious puberty—a diffuse cerebral dysgenesis. *Brain Dev*. 2002;24:784–786.
31. Harvey AS, Freeman JL. Newer operative and stereotactic techniques and their application to hypothalamic hamartoma. In: Wyllie E, ed. *The Treatment of Epilepsy: Principles and Practice*. Philadelphia: Lippincott Williams & Wilkins; 2005.
32. Harvey AS, Freeman JL, Berkovic SF. Presurgical evaluation in patients with hypothalamic hamartomas. In: Rosenow F, Lüders HO, eds. *Presurgical Assessment of the Epilepsies with Clinical Neurophysiology and Functional Imaging*. Amsterdam: Elsevier; 2004:441–450.
33. Harvey AS, Freeman JL, Berkovic SF, et al. Transcallosal resection of hypothalamic hamartomas in patients with intractable epilepsy. *Epileptic Disord*. 2003;5:257–265.
34. Harvey AS, Rosenfeld JV, Wrennall J. Hypothalamic hamartoma and intractable epilepsy: ictal SPECT localization and surgical resection of hamartoma in four children. *Epilepsia*. 1998;39(Suppl 6):S65.
35. Johnston JJ, Olivos-Glander I, Killoran C, et al. Molecular and clinical analyses of Greig cephalopolysyndactyly and Pallister-Hall syndromes: robust phenotype prediction from the type and position of GLI3 mutations. *Am J Hum Genet*. 2005;76:609–622.
36. Kahane P, Di Leo M, Hoffmann D, et al. Ictal bradycardia in a patient with a hypothalamic hamartoma: a stereo-EEG study. *Epilepsia*. 1999;40:522–527.
37. Kahane P, Munari C, Minotti L, et al. The role of the hypothalamic hamartoma in the genesis of gelastic and dacrystic seizures. In: Tuxhorn I, Hothausen H, Boenigk H, eds. *Paediatric Epilepsy Syndromes and Their Surgical Treatment*. London: John Libbey; 1997:447–461.
38. Kahane P, Ryvlin P, Hoffmann D, et al. From hypothalamic hamartoma to cortex: what can be learnt from depth recordings and stimulation? *Epileptic Disord*. 2003;5:205–217.
39. Kahane P, Tassi L, Hoffmann D, et al. Crises dacrystiques et hamartome hypothalamique. A propos d'une observation vidéo-stéréo-EEG. *Epilepsies*. 1994;6:259–279.
40. Kang S, Graham JM Jr, Olney AH, et al. GLI3 frameshift mutations cause autosomal dominant Pallister-Hall syndrome. *Nat Genet*. 1997;15:266–268.
41. Kuzniecky R, Guthrie B, Mountz J, et al. Intrinsic epileptogenesis of hypothalamic hamartomas in gelastic epilepsy. *Ann Neurol*. 1997;42:60–67.
42. Kuzniecky RI, Guthrie BL. Stereotactic surgical approach to hypothalamic hamartomas. *Epileptic Disord*. 2003;5:275–280.
43. Kuzniecky RI, Knowlton R, Lawn N, et al. Ictal single-photon emission computed tomography (SPECT) findings in hypothalamic hamartomas and intractable seizures. *Epilepsia*. 2001;42(Suppl 7):S101.
44. Le Marquand HS, Russell DS. A case of pubertas praecox (macrogenitosomia praecox) in a boy associated with a tumour in the floor of the third ventricle. *Roy Berks Hosp Rep*. 1934;3:31–61.
45. List CF, Dowman CE, Bagchi BK, et al. Posterior hypothalamic hamartomas and gangliogliomas causing precocious puberty. *Neurology*. 1958;8:164–174.
46. Machado HR, Hoffman HJ, Hwang PA. Gelastic seizures treated by resection of a hypothalamic hamartoma. *Childs Nerv Syst*. 1991;7:462–465.
47. Mahachoklertwattana P, Kaplan SL, Grumbach MM. The luteinizing hormone-releasing hormone-secreting hypothalamic hamartoma is a congenital malformation: natural history. *J Clin Endocrinol Metab*. 1993;77:118–124.
48. Mattia D, Olivier A, Avoli M. Seizure-like discharges recorded in human dysplastic neocortex maintained in vitro. *Neurology*. 1995;45:1391–1395.
49. Matustik MC, Eisenberg HM, Meyer WJ III. Gelastic (laughing) seizures and precocious puberty. *Am J Dis Child*. 1981;135:837–838.
50. Money J, Hosta G. Laughing seizures with sexual precocity: report of two cases. *Johns Hopkins Med J*. 1967;3:326–336.
51. Mottolese C, Stan H, Bret P, et al. Hypothalamic hamartoma: the role of surgery in a series of eight patients. *Childs Nerv Syst*. 2001;17:229–236.
52. Mullatti N. Hypothalamic hamartoma in adults. *Epileptic Disord*. 2003;5:201–204.
53. Mullatti N, Selway R, Nashef L, et al. The clinical spectrum of epilepsy in children and adults with hypothalamic hamartoma. *Epilepsia*. 2003;44:1310–1319.
54. Munari C, Kahane P, Francione S, et al. Role of the hypothalamic hamartoma in the genesis of gelastic fits (a video-stereo-EEG study). *Electroencephalogr Clin Neurophysiol*. 1995;95:154–160.
55. Murphy JV, Wheless JW, Schmoll CM. Left vagal nerve stimulation in six patients with hypothalamic hamartomas. *Pediatr Neurol*. 2000;23:167–168.
56. Ng Y-T, Rekate HL, Prenger EC, et al. Transcallosal Resection of Hypothalamic Hamartoma for Intractable Epilepsy. *Epilepsia*. 2006;47:1192–1202.
57. Nishio S, Fujiwara S, Aiko Y, et al. Hypothalamic hamartoma. Report of two cases. *J Neurosurg*. 1989;70:640–645.
58. Nishio S, Morioka T, Fukui M, et al. Surgical treatment of intractable seizures due to hypothalamic hamartoma. *Epilepsia*. 1994;35:514–519.
59. Northfield DW, Russell DS. Pubertas praecox due to hypothalamic hamartoma: report of two cases surviving surgical removal of the tumour. *J Neurol Neurosurg Psychiatry*. 1967;30:166–173.
60. Paillas JE, Roger J, Toga M, et al. Hamartome de l'hypothalmus: étude clinique, radiologique, histologique: résultats de l'exérèse. *Rev Neurol (Paris)*. 1969;120:177–194.
61. Pallini R, Bozzini V, Colicchio G, et al. Callosotomy for generalized seizures associated with hypothalamic hamartoma. *Neurol Res*. 1993;15:139–141.
62. Palmini A, Chandler C, Andermann F, et al. Resection of the lesion in patients with hypothalamic hamartomas and catastrophic epilepsy. *Neurology*. 2002;58:1338–1347.
63. Palmini A, Gambardella A, Andermann F, et al. Intrinsic epileptogenicity of human dysplastic cortex as suggested by corticography and surgical results. *Ann Neurol*. 1995;37:476–487.
64. Palmini A, Van Paesschen W, Dupont P, et al. Status gelasticus after temporal lobectomy: ictal FDG-PET findings and the question of dual

pathology involving hypothalamic hamartomas. *Epilepsia.* 2005;46:1313–1316.
65. Parrent AG. Stereotactic radiofrequency ablation for the treatment of gelastic seizures associated with hypothalamic hamartoma. Case report. *J Neurosurg.* 1999;91:881–884.
66. Pendl G. Gelastic epilepsy in tumours of the hypothalamic region. *Adv Neurosurg.* 1975;3:442–449.
67. Pérez-Jiménez A, Villarejo FJ, Fournier del Castillo MC, et al. Continuous giggling and autistic disorder associated with hypothalamic hamartoma. *Epileptic Disord.* 2003;5:31–37.
68. Polkey CE. Resective surgery for hypothalamic hamartoma. *Epileptic Disord.* 2003;5:281–286.
69. Ponsot G, Diebler C, Plouin P, et al. Hamartomes hypothalamiques et crises de rire. A propos de 7 observations. *Arch Fr Pediatr.* 1983;40:757–761.
70. Prasad S, Shah J, Patkar D, et al. Giant hypothalamic hamartoma with cystic change: report of two cases and review of the literature. *Neuroradiology.* 2000;42:648–650.
71. Pugh MB, Stedman TL. *Stedman's Medical Dictionary.* 27th ed. Philadelphia: Lippincott Williams & Wilkins; 2001.
72. Régis J, Bartolomei F, de Toffol B, et al. Gamma knife surgery for epilepsy related to hypothalamic hamartomas. *Neurosurgery.* 2000;47:1343–1351.
73. Rosenfeld JV, Harvey AS, Wrennall J, et al. Transcallosal resection of hypothalamic hamartomas, with control of seizures, in children with gelastic epilepsy. *Neurosurgery.* 2001;48:108–118.
74. Ryvlin P, Ravier C, Bouvard S, et al. Positron emission tomography in epileptogenic hypothalamic hamartomas. *Epileptic Disord.* 2003;5:219–227.
75. Sato M, Ushio Y, Arita N, et al. Hypothalamic hamartoma: report of two cases. *Neurosurgery.* 1985;16:198–206.
76. Schulze-Bonhage A, Homberg V, Trippel M, et al. Interstitial radiosurgery in the treatment of gelastic epilepsy due to hypothalamic hamartomas. *Neurology.* 2004;62:644–647.
77. Schulze-Bonhage A, Quiske A, Homberg V, et al. Effect of interstitial stereotactic radiosurgery on behavior and subjective handicap of epilepsy in patients with gelastic epilepsy. *Epilepsy Behav.* 2004;5:94–101.
78. Sher PK, Brown SB. Gelastic epilepsy. Onset in neonatal period. *Am J Dis Child.* 1976;130:1126–1131.
79. Sisodiya SM, Free SL, Stevens JM, et al. Widespread cerebral structural changes in two patients with gelastic seizures and hypothalamic hamartomata. *Epilepsia.* 1997;38:1008–1010.
80. Striano S, Meo R, Bilo L, et al. Gelastic epilepsy: symptomatic and cryptogenic cases. *Epilepsia.* 1999;40:294–302.
81. Sturm JW, Andermann F, Berkovic SF. "Pressure to laugh": an unusual epileptic symptom associated with small hypothalamic hamartomas. *Neurology.* 2000;54:971–973.
82. Tassinari CA, Riguzzi P, Rizzi R, et al. Gelastic seizures. In: Tuxhorn I, Hothausen H, Boenigk H, eds. *Paediatric Epilepsy Syndromes and Their Surgical Treatment.* London: John Libbey; 1997:429–446.
83. Unger F, Schrottner O, Feichtinger M, et al. Stereotactic radiosurgery for hypothalamic hamartomas. *Acta Neurochir Suppl.* 2002;84:57–63.
84. Unger F, Schrottner O, Haselsberger K, et al. Gamma knife radiosurgery for hypothalamic hamartomas in patients with medically intractable epilepsy and precocious puberty. Report of two cases. *J Neurosurg.* 2000;92:726–731.
85. Valdueza JM, Cristante L, Dammann O, et al. Hypothalamic hamartomas: with special reference to gelastic epilepsy and surgery. *Neurosurgery.* 1994;34:949–958.
86. Vickers W, Tidswell F. A tumour of the hypothalamus. *Med J Aust.* 1932;2:116–117.
87. Wakai S, Nikaido K, Nihira H, et al. Gelastic seizure with hypothalamic hamartoma: proton magnetic resonance spectrometry and ictal electroencephalographic findings in a 4-year-old girl. *J Child Neurol.* 2002;17:44–46.
88. Weissenberger AA, Dell ML, Liow K, et al. Aggression and psychiatric comorbidity in children with hypothalamic hamartomas and their unaffected siblings. *J Am Acad Child Adolesc Psychiatry.* 2001;40:696–703.
89. Williams M, Schutt W, Savage D. Epileptic laughter with precocious puberty. *Arch Dis Child.* 1978;53:965–966.
90. Wu J, Xu L, Kim DY, et al. Electrophysiological properties of human hypothalamic hamartomas. *Ann Neurol.* 2005;58:371–382.
91. Zñiga OF, Tanner SM, Wild WO, et al. Hamartoma of CNS associated with precocious puberty. *Am J Dis Child.* 1983;137:127–133.

CHAPTER 251 ■ LOCALIZATION-RELATED EPILEPSIES DUE TO SPECIFIC LESIONS

NOOJAN J. KAZEMI, TERENCE J. O'BRIEN, AND GREGORY D. CASCINO

INTRODUCTION

The localization-related epilepsies are epileptic syndromes in which seizures arise in a geographically restricted area within a part of one or alternate hemisphere(s) (partial or focal seizures).[30] Lesional localization-related epilepsies are the most common group of medically intractable epilepsies seen in adults and are also an important cause of intractable seizures in children.[58,162] Magnetic resonance imaging (MRI) is the most sensitive and specific modality for imaging lesions in patients with focal epilepsies and has greatly improved our understanding of the nature and frequency of these lesions.[19,31,72,85]

Approximately 30% of patients who undergo surgical treatment for intractable epilepsy have a foreign tissue lesion detected on pathologic examination.[6] There is a strong correlation between the site of the lesion and the site of the epileptogenic zone.[5,14,25,119] The identification of an epileptogenic lesion on MRI has been cited as being as predictive of a poor response to antiepileptic drugs.[43] Furthermore, such patients are more likely to become seizure free postoperatively than those in whom no structural abnormality is found.[94,127,144] In a randomized, controlled trial for surgery versus medical treatment for medically refractory mesiotemporal lobe epilepsy, 58% of those treated surgically in addition to drugs were seizure free at 12 months compared with 8% in the only conservatively treated group.[159]

HISTORICAL PERSPECTIVES

Focal structural lesions, particularly brain tumors, have been recognized as a cause of seizures since ancient times.[148] Hughlings Jackson[73] wrote extensively of the relationship between partial seizures and underlying focal brain pathology. He stressed that seizures could be the first and only manifestation of the tumor, that ictal behavior may predict the cerebral localization of the lesion, and that the severity and type of seizures were not predictive of the nature of the underlying pathology. Horsley in 1886[66] reported three patients who had been cured of seizures by surgical excision of an underlying focal structural lesion. In the earlier part of this century, it was particularly the work of Penfield and colleagues[87,121] at the Montreal Neurological Institute (MNI) and of Falconer and Serafetinides[48] in London that advanced our understanding of localized cerebral lesions and epilepsy and of the surgical treatment of these conditions. It has been only since the advent of modern neuroimaging, however, that the true importance of local structural lesions as a common, surgically treatable cause of both temporal and extratemporal focal epilepsy has been appreciated.[6]

DEFINITIONS

For the purposes of this chapter, "specific lesions" are defined as discrete local (or regional) structural pathologies that are associated with chronic focal epilepsy. These local lesions most commonly occur in an otherwise structurally normal brain. More diffuse cerebral pathologies that may be associated with partial seizures but do not typically present as discrete mass lesions (e.g., diffuse neuronal migration disorders, Rasmussen encephalitis) are discussed elsewhere (Chapters 259 and 243). Mesial temporal sclerosis is discussed fully in Chapter 247.

EPIDEMIOLOGY

A large surgical series of patients with focal structural lesions comes from the MNI; Table 1 summarizes the results of this series and other selected epilepsy surgery series along with reported pathology. Surgical series, however, are subject to significant biases because patients with a known mass lesion are more likely to be referred to an epilepsy center and then proceed to surgery.[101] There is also a bias regarding the sites of the lesions reported in these series, with patients having temporal lobe seizures more likely to undergo epilepsy surgery. Furthermore, most of the patients in these series were collected before the advent of modern neuroimaging, when only large masses could be detected preoperatively. It is important to note that a number of pathologies associated with focal epilepsy, notably focal cortical dysplasias (FCDs) and dysembryoplastic neuroepithelial tumors (DNETs), were not recognized until the advent of high-quality magnetic resonance imaging.

Studies using high-resolution MRI have the potential to reduce some of the biases of these surgical series, and they may give a more accurate representation of the incidence and sites of occurrence of neocortical lesions in focal epilepsy. Because these series also come from large epilepsy referral centers, however, they are subject to some of the same referral biases. Table 2 summarizes four large, high-resolution MRI series. In comparison with the pathologic series, it is noteworthy that the proportion of extratemporal lesions is higher, as is the incidence of certain types of lesions, particularly FCDs and DNETs.

Epidemiologic population-based studies of epilepsy have the potential to reduce the biases seen in both the surgical and MRI series.[57,71] Hauser and Kurland,[58] in one of the largest such studies (Rochester, Minnesota, from 1935 through 1967), found a focal mass lesion in only 27 (5.2%) of 516 cases given a diagnosis of epilepsy during this period. Of these patients, 21 had brain tumors (18 primary and 3 metastatic), 4 had vascular malformations, and 1 patient had tuberous sclerosis. This study was also performed before the advent of modern neuroimaging, however, and therefore it is likely to have underestimated the true incidence of lesions because most are indolent and produce

TABLE 1

SELECTED SERIES OF LESIONS DETECTED ON PATHOLOGIC EXAMINATION FOLLOWING SURGERY FOR INTRACTABLE PARTIAL SEIZURES

	Le Blanc and Rasmussen 1974	Spencer et al. 1984	Wolf et al. 1993[a]	Fried et al. 1994[b]	Britton et al. 1994[a]	Xiao et al. 2004
Reference	87	140	163	52	15	166
Number of cases (% Total Cases)[c]	265 (20%)	27 (15%)	125 (58.1%)	65	51	1,650
Institution	MNI	Yale	Bonn	Yale	Mayo Clinic	Xiangya
Time Period	1928–1966	1972–1982	1987–1993	1978–1991	1984–1990	1991–2000
Site						
Temporal	NS	12 (41.3%)	125 (100%)[a]	41 (63%)	39 (76%)	904 (55%)
Extratemporal	NS	15 (58.7%)	—	24 (37%)	12 (24%)	746 (45%)
Frontal	NS	7	—	7	10	—
Frontoparietal	NS	3	—	—	—	—
Parietal	NS	1	6	2	—	—
Occipital	NS	2	—	11	—	—
Other	NS	2	—	—	—	—
Pathology						
Primary brain tumors	171 (79.5%)	19 (70.3%)	75 (60%)	65 (100%)[c]	51 (100%)	247 (15%)
Low-grade astrocytoma	127	8	23	40	18	117
Oligodendroglioma	NS	3	9	5	15	76
Ganglioglioma	NS	1	34	4	4	24
Miscellaneous low-grade gliomes	44	1	2	5	10	—
Glioblastoma	24	3	1	11	—	—
DNET	NS	NS	6	—	4	—
Meningiomas	20	2	—	—	—	30
Other	—	1	—	—	—	—
Vascular malformations	NS	3 (11.1%)	13 (10.4%)	—	—	292 (17.7%)
Arteriovenous malformations	14 (5%)	3	2	—	—	70
Cavernous hemangiomas	NS	—	11	—	—	222
Disorders of cortical development	—	—	1 (3.2%)	29 (23.2%)	—	122 (7.4%)
Cystic lesions	—	3 (11.1%)	4 (3.2%)	—	—	63 (3.8%)
Metastatic tumor	6 (2%)	—	—	—	—	—
Miscellaneous lesions	20 (8%)	1 (3.7%)	4 (3.2%)	—	—	926 (56.1%)[d]

DNET, dysembryoplastic neuroepithelial tumors; MNI, Montreal Neurological Institute; NS, not stated.
[a]This series reported temporal lobe specimens only.
[b]This series was restricted to glial tumors.
[c]Number of cases of lesional epilepsy and percentage of total surgical specimens examined.
[d]Miscellaneous lesions included scar, hippocampal sclerosis, gliosis, infection, calcification and encephalomalacia lesions.

no focal clinical impairment or electroencephalographic (EEG) slowing.[150]

The incidence of cerebral tumors in children undergoing epilepsy surgery may be higher than in adults, with estimates as high as 46%.[13,101] Studies using MRI also suggest that before the age of 12 years, lesional epilepsy, particularly gangliomas and disorders of cortical development (DCDs), may be more common and mesial temporal sclerosis (MTS) less common.[85,119,122]

ETIOLOGY AND BASIC MECHANISMS

The pathophysiologic mechanisms by which intracranial mass lesions cause chronic seizure activity is poorly understood, but a number of theories have been advocated. One proposed mechanism is "denervation hypersensitivity," which results from the partial isolation of a part of the neocortex through tumor growth or brain scarring, thus creating enhanced excitatory status and epileptogenic potential.[41] The degree of mass effect of the lesion, however, is unrelated to the incidence of epilepsy.[8,95] There is some evidence that there may be a familial predisposition to epilepsy developing with mass lesions, but much of the data on this are conflicting.[14,109]

Low-grade tumors, which predominate in series of chronic lesional epilepsy, are rarely associated with pathologic evidence of hemorrhage, necrosis, inflammation, or ischemia, nor are they usually associated with significant mass effect.[101] Cerebral tumors may induce changes in the surrounding neocortex that affect the balance of neurotransmitter levels, synaptic receptors (especially for *N*-methyl-D-aspartate [NMDA] or γ-aminobutyric acid [GABA]), or ion channels (e.g., increased leakage of axonal calcium or chloride channels).[21] In support of this theory, Bateman et al.[8] demonstrated an increased concentration of glutamine (the precursor to the excitatory neurotransmitter glutamate) in the gliomas of patients with epilepsy compared with gliomas from patients without seizures. Glutamine has been shown to be released and taken up by glioma cells.[106,156] Decreases in concentrations of the inhibitory

TABLE 2

SELECTED SERIES OF HIGH-RESOLUTION MAGNETIC RESONANCE IMAGING IN PATIENTS WITH PARTIAL EPILEPSY

	Jackson 1994	Li et al. 1995	O'Brien et al. 1996	Velasco et al. 2006
Reference	72	91	109	153
Total number of cases	340	341	468	512
Number of Lesional cases	117 (34.4%)	117 (34.3%)	213 (45.6%)	179 (35%)
Site				
Temporal	58 (58%)[a]	28 (23.9%)	36 (62.1%)[b]	NS
Extratemporal	42 (42%)[a]	89 (76.1%)	22 (37.9%)[b]	NS
Frontal lobe	NS	41	15	—
Central lobe	NS	—	4	—
Parietal lobe	NS	19	1	—
Occipital lobe	NS	5	2	—
Multilobar	NS	24	—	—
Lesion Type				
Low-grade tumor	46 (39.3%)	40 (34.1%)	58 (27.2%)	51 (28.5%)
Disorders of cortical development	35 (29.9%)	43 (36.8%)	82 (38.5%)	62 (34.6%)
Focal cortical dysplasia	NS	NS	71	NS
Nodular heterotopia	NS	NS	11	NS
Vascular malformations	14 (12.0%)	28 (23.9%)	39 (18.3%)	2 (1.1%)
Cavernous hemangiomas	12	NS	NS	NS
Arteriovenous malformations	—	2	NS	NS
Cystic lesions	5 (4.3%)	—	10 (4.7%)	33 (18.4%)[d]
Focal encephalomalacia	—	20 (17.1%)	20 (9.4%)	31 (17.3%)
Miscellaneous	17 (14.5%)	—	4 (1.9%)	—

NS, not stated.
[a]Sites are not given for patients with miscellaneous lesions.
[b]Figures for the sites in this study are for 58 lesional patients with complex partial seizures proved by video telemetry.
[c]Figures available for "brain tumors" only.
[d]Includes porencephaly and neurocysticercosis cases.
[e]Defined as gliosis.

neurotransmitter GABA have also been demonstrated in gliomas of patients with seizures[8] and in the surrounding non–tumor-infiltrated neocortex.[10] Expanding tumors may also interfere with vascularization of the surrounding cerebral cortex, creating a region of relative cerebral ischemia having an increased epileptogenic potential.[126]

In vascular malformations, pathologic studies have shown the presence of neuronal loss, gliosis, demyelination, and hemosiderin deposition in the surrounding cerebral cortex, which may act as a focus for epileptogenesis.[97,145] It has been suggested that the increased epileptogenic potential associated with these lesions is caused at least in part by the effects of repeated subclinical hemorrhage and resultant hemosiderin deposition.[21,145,169] Dodick et al.,[38] however, showed that hemosiderin deposition could not be the sole mechanism of epileptogenesis in patients with vascular malformations. Alternatively, ischemia in the brain surrounding an arteriovenous malformation (AVM) caused by arteriovenous shunting of blood may result in an area of epileptogenic encephalomalacia.[167]

CLINICAL PRESENTATION

It has been appreciated for more than a century that the clinical history and ictal behavior may give a clue to the site of the underlying epileptogenic lesion.[73] Since the advent of MRI, however, it has become clear that a large overlap exists in the ictal symptomatology produced by lesions at different cortical locations. Lesions at any site may result in simple partial, complex partial, or secondarily generalized seizures. Complex partial seizures are often thought to indicate temporal lobe seizures, but in a study of high-resolution MRI in 129 consecutive patients with video-EEG-proven complex partial seizures, discrete neocortical lesions were detected in 58 (45%), of which 22 (37.9%) were extratemporal (15 frontal, 4 frontoparietal, 1 parietal, and 2 occipital).[108] Boon et al.,[14] in 51 patients with lesions, found that although all patients with temporal lesions had complex partial seizures, 74% of patients with extratemporal lesions also had complex partial seizures. This study also found that although visual auras may give a clue to the presence of an occipital lesion, the nature of the aura was not otherwise useful in predicting the location of the lesion.

The clinical features, including seizure type, age of patient at onset, and duration of epilepsy, response to antiepileptic drugs, and findings of neurologic examination, are not useful in predicting the nature of the underlying lesion.[126] Patients tend to have a long history of seizures before surgery, and even patients with tumors do not commonly have an increasing frequency of seizures.[87,101,140] Careful neurologic examination in patients with low-grade tumors may occasionally detect focal signs, such as visual field loss, unilateral facial weakness, or progressive sensory loss or hemiparesis, but findings are normal in the vast majority of patients.[21,101]

DIAGNOSTIC EVALUATION

The identification of a lesion in a patient with intractable epilepsy is not sufficient grounds to proceed directly to surgical excision, because the zone of seizure onset may occasionally be at a site remote from the lesion.[5,14,20,85]

Furthermore, patients with potentially epileptogenic lesions have been found after evaluation to have idiopathic generalized epilepsy or nonepileptic seizures. It is therefore important that all patients with intractable epilepsy have a comprehensive presurgical evaluation to ensure that the identified lesion is the source of the seizures. A great deal of caution, however, should be exercised before determining that the MRI lesion is *not* the source of the seizures; both extracranial and intracranial EEG can be misleading in lesional epilepsy,[5,23] and if the apparent epileptogenic zone is excised without the lesion, the results are likely to be poor in these patients.[50] Of course the reverse also holds true. The second important aspect of the presurgical evaluation is precise definition of the location and extent of the lesion, so that an operative strategy can be planned allowing maximal potential for a seizure-free outcome while minimizing the chance of a disabling postsurgical neurologic deficit.

Clinical Evaluation

As with all epilepsy patients, it is very important that a thorough history be taken. Questions should specifically be asked about factors that may suggest another source of seizures than the identified lesion—for example, a history of febrile convulsions, significant head trauma, intracranial infections, other neurologic disorders, or a family history of epilepsy. A careful neurologic examination should be performed in which focal deficits that may help to localize or lateralize the lesion are sought with particular care. It is now generally accepted practice that all patients also undergo visual perimetry, neuropsychological, and psychiatric evaluation before undergoing epilepsy surgery.

Neuroimaging

High-resolution MRI seizure protocols have virtually a 100% detection rate for tumors and vascular malformations, and improvements in technique have allowed the vast majority of focal DCDs also to be detected.[31,71] It may be difficult from the MRI appearance to predict the precise histologic tumor type, and FCD can sometimes be difficult to distinguish from low-grade cortical tumors.[71] The presence of a lesion on MRI concordant with the site of seizure onset has proved to be the best prognostic factor for a good postsurgical outcome if the lesion is included within the planned resection.[5,12,14,23,60,139]

The MRI data should be acquired using a seizure protocol that includes thin (1.5 or 1.6 mm), T_1-weighted volumetric slices of the *whole brain*.[71] This maximizes structural resolution and allows for reformatting, which is essential for the accurate detection of small cortical dysplasias, in which the only abnormality may be a subtle thickening of the cortex that is difficult to distinguish from volume averaging of normal cortical gyration.[31,71] T_2-weighted spin-echo and spin-density sequences may reveal areas of high signal in small cortical tumors, cortical dysplasias, and cortical sclerosis in some patients that are not obvious on the T_1 images.[71] Certain pulse sequences, especially fast fluid inversion recovery imaging (FLAIR), may increase the sensitivity for small cortical abnormalities.[132]

Even after the detection of one lesion, the whole-brain MRI needs to be carefully examined for the presence of coexistent hippocampal atrophy or a second neocortical lesion because a number of patients with lesional epilepsy may have dual pathology.[6,21,26,51] Cendes et al.[26] found that 15% of 167 patients with lesional epilepsy also had hippocampal atrophy. The incidence was particularly high in patients having DCDs (25%), porencephalic cysts (31%), and reactive gliosis (23.5%) compared with those having tumors (2%) or vascular malformations (9%), which suggests a common etiology during embryogenesis or early development. The identification of coexistent hippocampal atrophy in a patient with lesional epilepsy can alter the surgical strategy because these patients may have a worse outcome following lesionectomy alone.[24,51]

A carefully analyzed high-resolution MRI is essential for presurgical planning and accurate definition of the site and extent of the lesion.[31] This is especially important if a stereotactic lesionectomy is planned rather than epilepsy surgery with excision of the surrounding epileptogenic cortex.[25] Functional MRI can be used to localize eloquent cortex when the planned excision may impinge on these areas.[86]

Functional Neuroimaging

^{18}F-Fluorodeoxyglucose Positron Emission Tomography

There is evidence from studies of patients with MTS that the focal region of hypometabolism seen on ^{18}F-fluorodeoxyglucose positron emission tomography (FDG-PET) in many patients with focal epilepsy represents a functional rather than a structural change.[60,110] Therefore, FDG-PET may potentially have a role in defining the extent of the surrounding epileptogenic zone in lesional epilepsy. Traditionally, studies had found a poor correlation between the extent of the hypometabolic area and the extent of electrically abnormal cortex.[42] Due to major technical improvements in PET imaging, however, recent studies have demonstrated correct localization of the seizure focus, as correlated with MRI or EEG, in 62% to 100% of patients.[76,103,146,164] O'Brien et al.[107] demonstrated that FDG-PET had a significant effect on changing management in 45% of patients with intractable epilepsy, with a further 13% benefiting through increased confidence in localization and ultimately epilepsy surgery, despite the availability of other localizing information. The evidence is suggestive that localization of epileptogenic lesions by PET is greater for temporal lobe lesions than for extratemporal lobe lesions, especially when PET is assessed visually.[100,107]

Single Photon Emission Computed Tomography

Weis et al.[158] found that in temporal lobe epilepsy (TLE), the sensitivity of ictal single photon emission computed tomography (SPECT), in which the radiotracer (^{99m}Tc-D,L-hexamethylpropylene amine oxime [HMPAO]) is injected during a seizure, was lower in patients with structural lesions of the temporal lobe (56%) than in those with MTS (92%) or a normal MRI (88%). Coregistration of the ictal SPECT and MRI (SISCOM) constructs a difference image between the ictal and interictal SPECT and then coregisters it to the patient's MRI for anatomic localization. SISCOM aids in accurately identifying the regions of activation with ictal SPECT and also provides an objective way to quantitatively compare images from different patients or groups of patients.[111–115] SISCOM can play a role in lesional epilepsy when other data about the relationship of the structural lesion to the epileptogenic zone are conflicting and might aid in identifying the epileptogenic lesion in the case of dual pathology, but this requires further study.

Interictal Electroencephalography

Focal polymorphic delta activity, which is said to be the EEG hallmark of cerebral mass lesions, is relatively uncommon in patients with chronic lesional epilepsy.[14,67,140] Boon et al.[14]

found that interictal focal sharp waves were more common than focal slow waves, but that 34% of patients had neither. O'Brien et al.,[109] comparing TLE patients having temporal neocortical lesions with those having MTS, found that the lesional patients have a higher incidence of interictal epileptiform activity (60% vs. 37%) and focal slowing (66% vs. 41%). However, no interictal EEG abnormality was found in 27% of lesional patients.

Boon et al.[14] found that unilateral temporal spikes predicted the side of the lesion correctly in 29 of 30 patients; however, the correlation of location of the spikes with site of the lesion was poor, being correct in only 30% of patients. A similar proportion of patients with temporal and extratemporal lesions had ipsilateral temporal spikes (44% vs. 39%), with bilateral independent spikes occurring in 22%. Other studies have also demonstrated that bilateral independent temporal spikes are not uncommon with unilateral lesions but that this does not correlate with a poor surgical outcome.[21,125,127]

Video-electroencephalography

Closed-circuit video-EEG is an important part of the routine presurgical evaluation of a patient with lesional epilepsy. At least one typical seizure should be recorded. In most cases, careful analysis of the seizure semiology and the ictal EEG will allow a confident determination that the site of seizure onset is concordant with the site of the lesion.[21,162] It is important to note, however, that extratemporal neocortical lesions can spread rapidly to the mesial temporal structures, producing semiology and ictal EEG findings that are indistinguishable from those of temporal seizures.[50,160,161]

The scalp ictal EEG is often poorly localizing in patients with lesional epilepsy.[21] O'Brien et al.,[109] analyzing 46 seizures in 15 patients with temporal neocortical lesions, found a clearly localized ictal EEG onset in only 14 (30.4%), with another 15 (32.6%) having an onset that began diffusely in the temporal lobes. The ictal EEG was more accurate in lateralization, with the onset being correctly lateralized in 31 (78%), nonlateralized in 8 (20%), and incorrectly lateralized in only 1 (3%). However, Boon et al.[14] found an unequivocally lateralized scalp ictal EEG in only 58% of their patients, and one of these cases was falsely lateralized. Morris and Estes[101] reported that in their series of patients with brain tumor, the combination of ictal and interictal EEG agreed with the lobe of the lesion in 72% of cases and was correctly lateralized in another 17%.

Intracranial Electroencephalography

Intracranial EEG monitoring is not routinely required for all patients with lesional epilepsy.[21] If the results of the noninvasive evaluation are concordant with the site of the lesion, then surgery can be recommended without invasive studies being required. Intracranial studies are principally reserved for two situations: (a) Results of the noninvasive evaluation give conflicting information or suggest that the lesion is remote from the source of the seizures, and (b) preoperative mapping of the eloquent cortex using subdural strips is required when the planned resection may involve these areas.

Unfortunately, even intracranial EEG is often nonlocalizing or misleading in patients with lesional epilepsy.[41] Williamson et al.[160] studied 9 patients having parietal mass lesions with depth electrodes, parietal grids, or both, and consistently found a localized seizure onset in the parietal lobe in only 3. In 4 patients, the onset was diffuse and poorly localized, and in 2 the seizures were apparently of mesial temporal onset (1 bilateral independent).

Intraoperative Neurophysiologic Techniques

Intraoperative electrical cortical stimulation can accurately define the speech area and the motor strip and allows the cortical resection to be performed to within 1 cm of these areas.[101] Intraoperative mapping requires a very cooperative patient, however, because it is performed under local anesthetic, and the complexity of the language tasks that can be tested is limited. Intraoperative somatosensory-evoked potentials can also be helpful in defining the motor strip.[102] Functional mapping can also be performed using an implanted subdural electrode array.[14,94] This technique has the dual advantage of enabling the recording of interictal and ictal intracranial EEG and allowing the patient to be evaluated in a more comfortable setting with more complex and extensive tests.[21]

DIFFERENTIAL DIAGNOSIS

Tumors

Epilepsy caused by brain tumors represents 3.5% to 5% of all cases of epilepsy and 16% of cases seen in adults, and tumors are the most common cause for new-onset epilepsy in persons between the ages of 35 and 55 years.[46] Low-grade or slow-growing or indolent tumors are the most highly epileptogenic.[157] In their review of the MNI series, Le Blanc and Rasmussen[87] determined that the incidence of epilepsy in patients with supratentorial tumors was approximately 50%. The site of tumors in the hemispheres is related to their epileptogenicity; individuals with tumors of the centrotemporoparietal region have the highest incidence of epilepsy (approximately 75%). Lund[95] found in 615 cases that the depth of the tumor also was related to the incidence of epilepsy, with epilepsy occurring in association with 63% of "superficial and cortical" tumors and only 29% of "deep and noncortical" tumors.

Gliomas

Gliomas account for 72% to 88% of tumors in patients with chronic epilepsy, of which 50% to 70% are low-grade astrocytomas; oligodendrogliomas, gangliomas, and mixed gliomas account for the remainder.[80,127] Le Blanc and Rasmussen[87] found that oligodendrogliomas had the highest epileptogenic potential (92%), followed by astrocytomas (70%) and glioblastomas (35%). High-grade glial neoplasms and metastatic tumors are rare in series of patients with chronic epilepsy.

Astrocytomas most often appear in the third and fourth decades, and seizures are the most common clinical manifestation.[101] Oligodendrogliomas tend to appear in the fourth to fifth decades, although they can occur in children.[28,93] Some calcification is present in up to 90% of patients, and therefore many are seen on CT. Gangliomas represent only 0.7% to 6% of brain tumors overall, but they are overrepresented in series of patients with chronic focal epilepsy, with estimates of their incidence ranging from 10% to 50%.[4,81,101,163] These tumors seem to occur preferentially in the temporal and frontal lobes.[70]

Meningiomas

Meningiomas are the most common benign intracranial tumor, especially in middle age, representing about 15% of all primary brain tumors.[46] Seizures are estimated to occur in 60% to 75% of all patients with these tumors.[79,87]

Dysembryoplastic Neuroepithelial Tumors

Dysembryoplastic neuroepithelial tumors are an important cause of focal epilepsy that has only relatively recently been recognized.[35] A number of the patients that were classified as having low-grade gliomas or hamartomas in older series probably had DNETs. A recent series of 216 temporal lobectomies found that DNETs comprised 8% of lesional cases.[163] They have a predilection for the temporal lobes, but they also often occur extratemporally, especially in the frontal lobes.[35] These lesions usually develop within dysplastic cortex, and it is thought by some authors that they would be better classified as a neuronal migration disorder rather than as a tumor.[71]

Disorders of Cortical Development

Taylor et al.[147] first recognized cortical dysplasia in their pathologic study of postsurgical specimens of patients with intractable epilepsy. The importance of DCDs as a cause of focal epilepsy, however, has been widely appreciated only since the development of high-resolution MRI. The derangement of cortical structure associated with these lesions can be relatively subtle and is not well detected by CT or earlier MRI methods.[31,71,85,119] Even with high-resolution MRI, these lesions are easily overlooked because they are often difficult to detect on standard planar images acquired with thick slices (see Chapter 79 for further discussion).

The DCDs have been classified according to MRI findings as generalized, unilateral hemispheric, and focal.[20] In this chapter, the focal DCDs are emphasized; these include FCDs, focal subependymal heterotopias, polymicrogyria, and schizencephaly (see Chapter 259 for a more complete discussion).[20,85,119] In a series of 49 patients with DCD and chronic focal epilepsy reported by Andermann and Palmini,[3] 30 had unilateral localized areas of abnormalities (either FCD or tuberous sclerosis in forme fruste), 10 had bilateral abnormalities, and 9 had a generalized DCD.

Focal cortical dysplasias, schizencephaly, and microdysgenesis usually have no apparent inheritance pattern and are likely caused by cerebral insults occurring during perinatal development.[71] The initial seizures in patients with focal DCD usually occur in the first decade of life.[119,147]

Focal cortical dysplasia is the most common type of focal DCD. Definitions of the term *cortical dysplasia* have varied from a subtle degree of disorganized cortical architecture with or without neuronal cytomegaly to profound abnormalities, such as lissencephaly and polymicrogyria.[154] Tuberous sclerosis in forme fruste is usually classified as a DCD because clinical and imaging studies cannot reliably differentiate it from FCD, and pathologically it is also often very difficult to make the distinction.[80]

Neuronal heterotopias may include several patterns, but nodular and laminar heterotopias are most frequently associated with epilepsy.[80] Nodular heterotopias consist of discrete, isolated regions of gray matter that occur in the periventricular region. They may also be associated with other abnormalities, such as polymicrogyria or pachygyria. Laminar heterotopias are elongated islands of neurons that occur as bands in the white matter separated from the cortex or ventricular wall. Heterotopias are believed to result form an arrest during neuronal migration.

Focal schizencephaly is characterized by a communication between the ventricle and the surface of the brain, which is often lined by polymicrogyrous cortex.[3] Focal unilateral schizencephaly is commonly associated with epilepsy, and surgical excision of the most epileptogenic areas can lead to a reduction in seizure frequency.[89]

Cerebral Vascular Malformations

The estimated seizure risk in patients with vascular malformations is 1.5%/person-yr.[34] The types of vascular malformations are, in decreasing order of frequency, arteriovenous malformations (AVMs), cavernous hemangiomas, venous angiomas, and capillary telangiectasias.[142] Venous angiomas and capillary telangiectasias are only rarely associated with seizures.[6]

Arteriovenous Malformations

Arteriovenous malformations are congenital vascular abnormalities consisting of communicating arteries and veins without intervening capillary beds. Seizures represent the second-most-common presenting feature of AVMs after cerebral hemorrhage (17%–40% of cases).[63,88,168] In an international multicenter trial, Hofmeister et al.[63] demonstrated that 30% of all patients with AVMs experienced generalized seizures, with 10% experiencing focal seizures. Hoh et al.[64] reported that male gender, age <65 years, AVM size <3 cm, and temporal lobe AVM location were significantly associated with an increased incidence of seizures. Posterior fossa and deep locations were not statistically associated with seizures.

Others have also confirmed that patients with larger AVMs (>3 cm) are more likely to have seizures.[88,123] Seizures are more frequent with AVMs situated in the posterofrontal and temporal lobes.[123]

Cavernous Angiomas

This benign vascular anomaly consists of a tangled mass of tightly arranged abnormal vessels made of common hypocellular walls,[80] and it represents about 5% to 20% of all vascular malformations of the central nervous system.[49] Seizures, estimated to occur in 40% to 70% of patients, are often the most common and only clinical manifestation of cavernous angiomas,[29,151] typically commencing in the 30- to 40-year age group.[49] On MRI, these lesions have a characteristically high T_2 signal core surrounded by a low signal halo (caused by hemosiderin deposition in macrophages), which results in a "targetlike" appearance.[141] It is theorized that the excess iron deposition may act as an electron donor providing free radicals and lipid peroxides, which can lead to neuronal excitability and hence seizures.[82,155] In some patients the coexistence of hippocampal sclerosis may be present (dual pathology), complicating potential surgical management.[24]

Cysts

Several studies have found a higher-than-expected frequency of seizures in patients with porencephalic cysts.[1,149] Porencephalic cysts have also been found in surgical specimens from patients undergoing resective surgery for intractable partial seizures.[1] One study of 10 patients with arachnoid cysts and intractable seizures found no other explanation for the seizures in 8.[129] Accurate localization of the epileptogenic foci has been difficult traditionally, and hence either surgical resection has been discouraged or functional hemispherectomy has been performed, especially on patients with significant deficits.[62,68]

Infectious Lesions

Neurocysticercosis

In countries where it is endemic, neurocysticercosis may affect from 2% to 4% of the population.[36] It is estimated that 50% to 70% of patients with neurocysticercosis have epilepsy, and it is the most common cause of adult-onset epilepsy in developing countries.[37,99] It is now being increasingly recognized as a cause of epilepsy in Western countries as a result of increased migration from endemic areas and of improved neuroimaging, which can detect the typical multiple cystic lesions.[126] In most patients with neurocysticercosis, epilepsy is the only clinical manifestation, with only a minority of patients having focal neurologic symptoms or signs.[37]

Cerebral Tuberculoma

Cerebral tuberculomas are now very rare in Western countries, but they still represent up to 20% to 40% of intracranial tumors in developing countries.[126] They can appear even after the apparently successful treatment of systemic or central nervous system tuberculosis, and seizures are not uncommonly the first manifestation.[56]

TREATMENT AND OUTCOME

Antiepileptic Drugs

The medical treatment of lesional epilepsy does not essentially differ from that of other localization-related epilepsies. Monotherapy with carbamazepine or phenytoin is generally accepted as the first line of treatment in many countries, and the drugs are probably of equal efficacy.[96] Valproic acid, alone or in combination with one of the aforementioned drugs, is also effective in some patients. Phenobarbital and primidone may control seizures, but they frequently result in unacceptable behavior and cognitive disturbances and therefore are no longer recommended as first-line therapy. Many patients with lesional epilepsy continue to have poorly controlled seizures despite treatment with antiepileptic drugs (AEDs),[43] and these patients need not be subjected to prolonged, unsuccessful trials of multiple different drugs, or polypharmacy, before surgical therapy is considered.

Surgical Treatment

It is well documented that surgery is a successful treatment for medically intractable localization-related seizures associated with structural lesions.[21,39,55,159] As mentioned previously, in a randomized, controlled trial comparing surgical resection with medical treatment for intractable temporal lobe epilepsy, 58% of those undergoing surgery in addition to continued AED treatment were seizure free compared with 8% in the purely medical group at 12 months.[159] The greatest controversy in the surgical treatment of lesional epilepsy is the relative importance of excision of the structural lesion as opposed to the epileptogenic zone. The nature of the relationship between the two is relatively poorly understood, and hence the surgical strategy lacks an irrefutable physiologic basis.[51]

Resection of the Epileptogenic Region

A number of series have found that up to 90% of patients with intractable seizures secondary to tumors become seizure free when both the structural lesion and the epileptogenic cortex are resected ("seizure surgery").[10,13–15,18,165] There is some evidence that epileptogenic cortex may develop independently secondary to a noncontiguous structural lesion and that the epileptogenic zone may not be restricted to the lesion site.[5,39,54] Some authors have also found that complete excision of both structural lesion and epileptogenic cortex is necessary for worthwhile seizure reduction.[11,135,167]

However, resection of the epileptogenic zone in addition to the structural lesion involves a larger area of brain excision. The rate of operative morbidity increases dramatically when eloquent cortex is removed in an attempt to resect the epileptogenic zone,[117] and this approach does not necessarily improve postoperative seizure control.[128,138] Resection of the epileptogenic cortex alone, without the structural lesion, is likely to result in an unfavorable outcome. Siegel et al.[135] found that seizure freedom occurred in their patients only when a second operation was performed to resect an epileptogenic zone surrounding a previously resected cavernous angioma. Fish et al.[50] found that of 19 patients with small posterior structural lesions who had had resections limited to the epileptogenic zone in the anterior temporal lobe, only 2 became seizure free. The epileptogenic zone is likely to be a direct consequence of the structural lesion,[157] and therefore epilepsy surgery should include excision of the structural lesion whenever possible.

Lesionectomy

Patients often become seizure free, or have a decrease in seizure frequency, after simple lesionectomy.[22,61] Furthermore, the structural impact of the lesion appears to be reversible in some patients following lesionectomy, so that the previously epileptogenic cortex is free of electrical activity.[157] In addition, Falconer et al.[47] showed that even when the EEG abnormalities remain after the structural lesion is removed, clinical seizures often do not persist.

The studies of both Casazza et al.[17] and Zevgaridis et al.[171] did not find that the additional excision of hemosiderin-stained tissue around a cavernous angioma improved seizure freedom compared with resection of the lesion alone. Goldring et al.,[55] in a study evaluating the surgical outcome of 20 patients undergoing temporal lobe lesionectomy mainly for low-grade tumors, found that only one patient continued to have long-term postoperative seizures. Awad et al.[5] found that 79% of patients became seizure free when the epileptogenic cortex was completely resected without regard to the structural lesion, compared with 90% following lesionectomy alone regardless of complete excision of epileptogenic brain tissue. An alternative to standard neurosurgical lesionectomy is stereotactic lesionectomy. This is particularly useful in reducing morbidity in patients with deep-seated intra-axial lesions and lesions encroaching on functional cortex.[2,25,78] Cascino et al.[25] found that 74% of 23 patients who underwent stereotactic lesionectomy had a marked reduction in seizure activity, with 5 patients able to discontinue antiepileptic drugs.

Unfortunately, few studies have directly compared lesionectomy with more extensive epilepsy surgery. Awad et al.[5] found no significant difference in seizure-free outcome between patients who underwent simple lesion removal and those who underwent surgery directed at removal of the epileptogenic zone (Tables 3 and 4). Weber et al.[157] used meta-analysis to compare studies reporting outcomes of simple lesionectomy with those reporting more extensive epilepsy surgery, and found that more patients were seizure free 2 years after "seizure surgery" than after lesionectomy. Tables 3 and 4 compare selected studies reporting postsurgical outcome in patients undergoing lesionectomy alone and those undergoing surgery involving resection of the epileptogenic cortex.

TABLE 3

RESULTS OF SURGICAL SERIES OF PATIENTS UNDERGOING LESIONECTOMY ONLY

Study (ref.)	Structural lesion	Number of cases	Follow-up	Seizure free (%)
al-Rodhan et al. 1992[2]	Mixed lesions	30	24–66 mo	50
Awad et al. 1991[5]	Mixed lesions	18	20–114 mo	94
Baumann et al. 2006[9]	Cavernous angiomas	14	12–36 mo	77
Cascino 1990[8]	Mixed lesions	30	3–46 mo	53
Fried et al. 1994[52,a]	Glial tumors	54[a]	>12 mo (median, 46 mo)	85
Giulioni et al. 2006[53]	Gangliogliomas	21	1.25–10 yr	67
Goldring et al. 1986[55]	Mixed lesions	35	12–120 mo	82
Kalyan-Raman and Olivero 1987[77]	Ganglioglioma	8	30–84 mo	50
Murphy 1985[104]	AVM	20	2–36 yr	55
Silver et al. 1991[136]	Ganglioglioma	14	1–19 yr	50

AVM, arteriovenous malformation.
[a]Only patients with complete lesion excision were included.

Treatment and Outcome for Different Lesions

Tumors

Older AEDs, including phenytoin, carbamazepine, and phenobarbital, have been reported to produce more idiosyncratic effects in patients with brain tumors than in the general epilepsy population.[130] These anticonvulsants induce cytochrome P450 enzymes, and it has therefore been proposed that they interfere with other commonly used drugs and increase chemotherapeutic agent clearance.[152] Most cerebral tumors are considered for surgical resection. In 51 patients who were operated on at the Mayo Clinic for intractable epilepsy caused by low-grade neoplasms, 66% were rendered seizure free and 88% experienced a significant reduction in seizure frequency.[15] Le Blanc and Rasmussen[87] reported that of 171 patients with astrocytomas and other low-grade cerebral neoplasms treated with tumor resection and excision of the epileptogenic cortex, 41% were rendered seizure free and 70% had at least a marked reduction in seizure frequency. Most patients in this study also had postoperative radiotherapy; this is of unproven benefit, however, in patients with low-grade gliomas in whom a complete tumor resection has been achieved and is generally reserved for cases of tumor recurrence.[101] In patients with unresectable gliomas, radiotherapy alone, after biopsy conformation of the pathologic diagnosis, may result in a significant reduction in seizure frequency, with some patients being rendered seizure free.[55,131]

Complete resection of meningiomas is usually curative.[46] Surgical excision of meningiomas can achieve seizure freedom in up to 63% of patients.[92] Patients with gangliomas generally have a good postsurgical prognosis with regard to seizures, and Otsubo et al.[118] found that 22 of 25 surgically treated children were either seizure free or had >50% reduction in seizures. In a series of 29 adult and pediatric patients experiencing intractable seizures associated with gangliogliomas, Im et al.[69] reported that 76% were rendered seizure free and 59% had completely ceased anticonvulsant medications after surgical resection.

Radiotherapy is usually reserved for patients with postsurgical tumor recurrence, or the rare patient with an anaplastic ganglioma.[74] Complete surgical excision is usually curative for DNETs, and an excellent outcome with respect to seizures can be expected in about 90% of patients.[35] Chan et al.[27] demonstrated that temporal lobectomy for DNETs was significantly better associated with seizure freedom than was lesionectomy (83% Engel class 1). In contrast, however, only 10% of patients with glioblastomas and other aggressive malignant lesions become seizure free postoperatively.[128]

TABLE 4

RESULTS OF SURGICAL SERIES INVOLVING PATIENTS UNDERGOING RESECTION OF THE EPILEPTOGENIC CORTEX

Study (ref.)	Structural lesion	Number of cases	Follow-up (mo)	Seizure free (%)
Awad et al. 1991[5]	Mixed lesions	6	20–114	83
Baumann et al. 2006[9]	Cavernous angiomas	17	12–36	65
Daumas-Duport et al. 1988[35]	DNET	37	12–216	81
Estes et al. 1988[45]	Mixed lesions	11	6–72	82
Jooma et al. 1995[75]	Mixed lesions	14	12–84	93
Nakasato et al. 1992[105]	Glioma	11	12–348	64
Rasmussen 1975[128]	Mixed lesions	261	NS	47
Wyllie et al. 1987[165]	Mixed lesions	6	12–42	83
Yeh et al. 1990[167]	AVM	27	24–72	78

AVM, arterivenous malfromation; DNET; dysembryoplastic neuropeithelial tumors.

Disorders of Cortical Development

There is some evidence that focal DCD have a worse outcome following epilepsy surgery than other lesional types, with only 2 of 26 patients reported by Andermann and Palmini[3,119] becoming seizure free and 9 having >90% reduction in seizure frequency. They found a good correlation between outcome and amount of the lesion removed. Sisodiya et al.[137] demonstrated that in 15 of 18 patients with FCD, the abnormalities in distribution of gray and subcortical white matter volumes extended beyond the margins of the lesions as visualized on MRI. Therefore, the apparently worse outcome in patients with focal DCD may be a result of the lesion often being more extensive than the region of surgical excision. More recently, other authors report better postsurgical results, with Kral et al.[83] finding that 38 of 53 patients with focal cortical dysplasia who had cortical resections became seizure free postoperatively; a similarly good outcome was found by Hong et al.[65]

Vascular Malformations

Arteriovenous malformations are associated with a significant lifelong risk of hemorrhage and a significant risk of morbidity and mortality; prevention of this complication is the most common indication for surgical excision in these patients.[16] The efficacy of surgery in treating seizures associated with AVMs is more controversial. A number of earlier authors report disappointing results, with some even finding an increase in seizure frequency postoperatively.[33,104,120] Most recent surgical series, however, have found that many patients with AVMs have a good postoperative outcome with respect to seizures.[38,64,123,150,167,169] Dodick et al.[38] found that three fourths of patients with epilepsy secondary to a vascular malformation were seizure free after lesion resection, and most of the remaining patients had a significant reduction in seizure frequency. Yeh et al.[169] found that several factors correlated with outcome, including age at seizure onset, duration of seizures, location of lesions, and cortical excision of the epileptogenic zone. Radiosurgery is an accepted treatment measure for AVMs not suitable for surgical resection and is largely reserved for lesions <3 cm in size.

In cases of intractable seizures caused by cavernous hemangiomas, Cohen et al.[29] advocated lesionectomy alone for patients having fewer preoperative seizures and shorter seizure histories (<1 year) but an increased margin of resection for patients with longer seizure histories or more frequent seizures. In cases of dual pathology, however, lesionectomy has not resulted in seizure control, and subsequent resection of the mesial temporal structures is necessary to achieve a satisfactory outcome.[17,24,90]

Neurocysticercosis

Patients with inactive calcified neurocysticercosis can usually be adequately controlled on standard monotherapy for most localization-related epilepsy, for example, with carbamazepine or phenytoin. However, Del Brutto et al.[37] found that seizure control was significantly improved in patients with active neurocysticercosis by simultaneous treatment with anticysticercal drugs (praziquantel or albendazole), with 83% of such treated patients remaining seizure free compared with only 26% of those treated with antiepileptic drugs alone. In patients with multiple cysts, increased seizures and neurologic signs may develop soon after commencement of anticysticercal drugs as a result of an intense inflammatory reaction to the dying cysticerci in the surrounding brain. Coadministration of corticosteroids may minimize this complication.[36] Occasionally, large cysts causing significant mass effect may require surgical removal (see also Chapter 265).

LONG-TERM PROGNOSIS

When seizures are adequately controlled with antiepileptic drugs, patients must usually continue to take them indefinitely. Recurrence of seizures will occur in most patients on withdrawal of antiepileptic drugs because they merely suppress seizures, whereas the underlying epileptogenic lesion remains unchanged.

Following epilepsy surgery, patients who have discrete structural lesions (including mesial temporal sclerosis) have a better long-term outcome with respect to seizures than those who do not.[44] An earlier study by Berkovic et al.[12] using actuarial analysis to assess the outcome at 60 months in 135 surgically treated patients with TLE found that 69% of patients with a foreign tissue lesion on the preoperative MRI had no postoperative seizures, compared with 50% of those with hippocampal sclerosis and 21% of those with normal findings on MRI. In a more recent publication by the same group assessing long-term outcome, 328 patients underwent anterior temporal lobectomy over a 20-year period.[98] This study reported that 59.6% of lesional patients achieved seizure freedom at 10 years, with 47% of patients with hippocampal sclerosis achieving the same in this time period. The group with no discernible lesions on preoperative studies did most poorly, with 18.2% achieving seizure freedom at 10-year follow-up. These results are confirmed by other studies.[40,170]

Tumors

As previously discussed, tumors resulting in chronic epilepsy are usually of low grade and slowly growing. In patients with gliomas in whom seizures are the sole clinical manifestation, the clinical course tends to be more protracted and indolent than in other patients with gliomas, and survival for 10 to 20 years is not uncommon.[124,134] Depending on the grade, patients with oligodendrogliomas have been reported as demonstrating 5-year survival of 73% and 10-year survival of 49%,[59] with median survival time of 11.6 years.[116] Overall, patients with gangliogliomas have a better prognosis for long-term survival than those with histologically similar astrocytomas or mixed glial tumors, but gangliogliomas arising in the midline may be more aggressive and are associated with a poorer prognosis.[74]

Serial MRI is mandatory to follow patients with low-grade tumors in whom surgery has not been performed, and the appearance of such lesions can remain remarkably constant on repeated examinations over time.[55,140] An increase in size, mass effect, or degree of contrast enhancement of the lesion or the development of surrounding cerebral edema, however, suggests transformation to a higher-grade tumor. Serial MRI is also mandatory in following patients who have had surgery because recurrence of the tumor may be an indication for further treatment such as radiotherapy. Tumor recurrence may also be suggested by return of seizures in a patient who was initially rendered seizure free following surgery.[101]

Disorders of Cortical Development

Most patients with DCD reported in the literature have had medically intractable seizures, but this is likely to reflect at least in part a selection bias because almost all these series are from large epilepsy referral centers.[3] More recent studies report that among patients with focal cortical dysplasia, up to 72% may be rendered seizure free with epilepsy surgery.[84] Routinely, studies examining outcome from medical treatment alone report lower rates of seizure freedom, ranging from 24% to 54%.[7,133,143]

Vascular Malformations

Crawford et al.,[32] in a long-term follow-up study of 217 patients with unoperated AVMs, found that those without a history of hemorrhage in whom epilepsy was the primary clinical manifestation have a somewhat lower long-term risk for hemorrhage than other patients with AVMs (30% vs. 42% at 20 years). If there was a history of hemorrhage, however, the risk for a further hemorrhage increased to 51% at 20 years. Of the patients in this study who had a hemorrhage during the follow-up period, 25% died as result of that hemorrhage. The risk for cerebral hemorrhage with cavernous hemangiomas is lower than that for AVMs but is reported to occur in 10% to 30% of patients.[49]

Hoh et al.[64] demonstrated that in AVMs treated via a multidisciplinary approach, short seizure history, seizures linked to intracranial hemorrhage, generalized tonic–clonic seizures, deep and posterior fossa AVMs, and surgical resection and complete AVM obliteration were associated with Engel class 1 seizure frequency outcome. Thorpe et al.[150] found that multiple seizures and poor neurologic outcome postoperatively were independent factors predictive of the incidence of postoperative seizures.

Neurocysticercosis

Despite the fact that excellent control of seizures is usually obtained with antiepileptic and anticysticercal drugs, achievement of a long-term seizure-free state without drug therapy is difficult. Del Brutto et al.[37] found that 16 of 21 patients with epilepsy and neurocysticercosis who had been seizure free for 2 years while taking antiepileptic drugs relapsed when the drugs were withdrawn.

SUMMARY AND CONCLUSIONS

Of all patients who undergo surgery for chronic intractable epilepsy, 30% have a discrete structural lesion. There is a strong correlation between the site of epileptogenesis and the epileptogenic zone. Common structural lesions include low-grade neoplasms, vascular malformations, and disorders of cortical development. Cysticercosis and tuberculomas are increasingly being seen in developed countries and they are still a prevalent cause of epilepsy in endemic regions.

The pathophysiology of lesional epilepsy is uncertain, but a number of explanations have been proposed, and the mechanisms may vary for different lesional types.

Magnetic resonance imaging is the most sensitive and specific investigation in the detection of structural lesions. Evaluation for surgery involves careful clinical assessment, structural neuroimaging, and video-EEG in all patients. Intracranial monitoring, functional neuroimaging, and intraoperative neurophysiologic techniques may be useful in some cases.

Epilepsy surgery is the treatment of choice for intractable partial seizures caused by focal structural lesions. In most reported series, more than 50% of patients are rendered seizure free. It is controversial whether resection of the epileptogenic cortex in addition to the structural lesion is required for optimal seizure control. Stereotactic lesionectomy is a useful technique for minimizing morbidity with deep-seated lesions and those involving eloquent cortex.

References

1. Adams C, Hwang PA, Gilday DL, et al. Comparison of SPECT, EEG, MRI, and pathology in partial epilepsy. *Paediatric Neurology*. 1992;8:97–103.
2. al-Rodhan NR, Kelly PJ, Cascino GD, et al. Surgical outcome in computer assisted stereotactic resection of intra-axial cerebral lesions for partial epilepsy. *Stereotact Funct Neurosurg*. 1992;58:172–177.
3. Andermann F, Palmini AL. Neuronal migration disorders, tuberous sclerosis, and Sturge-Weber syndrome. In: Lüders H, ed. *Epilepsy Surgery*. New York: Raven Press; 1991:203–211.
4. Armstrong DD. The neuropathology of temporal lobe epilepsy. *J Neuropathol Exp Neurol*. 1993;52:433–443.
5. Awad IA, Rosenfield J, Ahl H, et al. Intractable epilepsy and structural lesions of the brain: mapping, resection strategies and seizure outcome. *Epilepsia*. 1991(32):179–186.
6. Babb TL, Brown WJ. Pathological findings in epilepsy. In: Engel J Jr, ed. *Surgical Treatment of the Epilepsies*. New York: Raven Press; 1987:511–540.
7. Bast T, Ramantani G, Seitz A, et al. Focal cortical dysplasia: prevalence, clinical presentation and epilepsy in children and adults. *Acta Neurol Scand*. 2006;113(2):72–81.
8. Bateman DE, Hardy JA, McDermott JR, et al. Amino acid neurotransmitter levels in gliomas and their relationship to the incidence of epilepsy. *Neurol Res*. 1988;10:112–114.
9. Baumann CR, Schuknecht B, Lo Russo G, et al. Seizure outcome after resection of cavernous malformations is better when surrounding hemosiderin-stained brain also is removed. *Epilepsia*. 2006;47(3):563–566.
10. Berger MS, Ghatan S, Geyer JR, et al. Seizure outcome in children with hemispheric tumors and associated intractable epilepsy: the role of tumor removal combined with seizure foci resection. *Paediatr Neurosurg*. 1991;17:185–191.
11. Berger MS, Kincaid J, Ojemann GA, et al. Brain mapping techniques to maximise resection, safety, and seizure control in children with brain tumors. *Neurosurgery*. 1989;25:786–792.
12. Berkovic SF, McIntosh AM, Kalnins RM, et al. Preoperative MRI predicts outcome of temporal lobectomy: an actuarial analysis. *Neurology*. 1995;45:1358–1363.
13. Blume WT, Girvin JP, Kaufmann JCE. Childhood brain tumors presenting as chronic, uncontrolled seizure disorders. *Ann Neurol*. 1982;12:538–541.
14. Boon PA, Williamson PD, Fried I, et al. Intracranial, intraaxial, space occupying lesions in patients with intractable partial seizures: an anatomoclincial, neuropsychological and surgical correlation. *Epilepsia*. 1991;32:467–476.
15. Britton JW, Cascino GD, Sharbrough FW, et al. Low-grade glial neoplasms and intractable partial epilepsy: efficacy of surgical treatment. *Epilepsia*. 1994;35:1130–1135.
16. Brown RD Jr, Wieberg DO, Forbes G. The natural history of ruptured intracranial arteriovenous malformations. *J Neurosurg*. 1988;68:352–357.
17. Casazza M, Broggi G, Franzini A, et al. Supratentorial cavernous angiomas and epileptic seizures: preoperative course and postoperative outcome. *Neurosurgery*. 1996;39(1):26–32; discussion, 32–34.
18. Cascino GD. Epilepsy and brain tumors: implications for treatment. *Epilepsia*. 1990;31(Suppl 3):S37–S44.
19. Cascino GD. Commentary: how has neuroimaging improved patient care? *Epilepsia*. 1994;35:S103–S107.
20. Cascino GD. Structural neuroimaging in partial epilepsy. *Neurosurg Clin North Am*. 1995;6:455–464.
21. Cascino GD, Boon PAJM, Fish DR. Surgically remediable lesional syndromes. In: Engel J Jr, ed. *Surgical Treatment of the Epilepsies*, 2nd ed. New York: Raven Press; 1993:77–86.
22. Cascino GD, Hirschorn KA, Jack CR, et al. Gadolinium-DTPA enhanced MRI in intractable partial epilepsy. *Neurology*. 1989;39:1115–1118.
23. Cascino GD, Jack CR, Parisi JE, et al. MRI in the presurgical evaluation of patients with frontal lobe epilepsy and children with temporal lobe epilepsy: pathological correlation and prognostic importance. *Epilepsy Res*. 1992;11:51–59.
24. Cascino GD, Jack CR, Parisi JE, et al. Operative strategy in patients with MRI-identified dual pathology and temporal lobe epilepsy. *Epilepsy Res*. 1993(14):175–182.
25. Cascino GD, Kelly PJ, Sharbrough FW, et al. Long-term follow-up of stereotactic lesionectomy in partial epilepsy: predictive factors and electroencephalographic results. *Epilepsia*. 1992;33(4):639–644.
26. Cendes F, Cook MJ, Watson C, et al. Frequency and characteristics of dual pathology in patients with lesional epilepsy. *Neurology*. 1995;45:2058–2064.
27. Chan CH, Bittar RG, Davis GA, et al. Long-term seizure outcome following surgery for dysembryoplastic neuroepithelial tumor. *J Neurosurg*. 2006;104(1):62–69.
28. Chin HW, Hazel JJ, Kim TH, et al. Oligodendrogliomas: I, a clinical study of cerebral oligodendrogliomas. *Cancer*. 1980;45:1458–1466.
29. Cohen DS, Zubay GP, Goodman RR. Seizure outcome after lesionectomy for cavernous malformations. *J Neurosurg*. 1995;83(2):237–242.
30. Commission on Classification and Terminology of the International League Against Epilepsy. Proposal for revised classification of epilepsies and epileptic syndromes. *Epilepsia*. 1989;30:389–399.

31. Cook M, Stevens JM. Imaging in epilepsy. In: Hopkins A, Shorvon S, Cascino G, eds. *Epilepsy,* 2nd ed. London: Chapman & Hall; 1995:143–169.
32. Crawford PM, West CR, Chadwick DW, et al. Arteriovenous malformations of the brain: natural history in unoperated patients. *J Neurol Neurosurg Psychiatry.* 1986;49(1):1–10.
33. Crawford PM, West CR, Shaw MDM, et al. Cerebral arteriovenous malformations and epilepsy: factors in the development of epilepsy. *Epilepsia.* 1986;27:270–275.
34. Curling OD Jr, Kelly DL Jr, Elster AD, et al. An analysis of the natural history of cavernous angioma. *J Neurosurg.* 1991;75:702–708.
35. Daumas-Duport C, Scheithauer BW, Chodkiewicz JP, et al. Dysembryoplastic neuroepithelial tumor: a surgically curable tumor of young patients with intractable partial seizures. *Neurosurgery.* 1988;23:545–556.
36. Davis LE, Kornfeld M. Neurocysticercosis: neurologic, pathologic, diagnostic and therapeutic aspects. *Eur Neurol.* 1991;31:229–240.
37. Del Brutto OH, Santibanez R, Noboa CA, et al. Epilepsy due to neurocysticercosis: analysis of 203 patients. *Neurology.* 1992;42:389–392.
38. Dodick DW, Cascino GD, Meyer FB. Vascular malformations and intractable epilepsy: Outcome after surgical treatment. *Mayo Clin Proc.* 1994;69:741–745.
39. Drake J, Hoffman HJ, Kobayashi J, et al. Surgical management of children with temporal lobe epilepsy and mass lesions. *Neurosurgery.* 1987;21:792–797.
40. Eliashiv SD, Dewar S, Wainwright I, et al. Long-term follow-up after temporal lobe resection for lesions associated with chronic seizures. *Neurology.* 1997;48(5):1383–1388; Erratum, *Neurology.* 1997;49(3):904.
41. Engel J Jr. Basic mechanisms of epilepsy. In: Engel J Jr, ed. *Seizures and Epilepsy.* Philadelphia: FA Davis; 1989:71–111.
42. Engel J Jr, Kuhl D, Phelps M. Interictal cerebral glucose metabolism in partial epilepsy and its relationship to EEG changes. *Ann Neurol.* 1982;12:510–517.
43. Engel J Jr, Shewmon DA. Overview: who should be considered a surgical candidate? *Surgical Pathology of the Nervous System and Its Coverings.* New York: Churchill Livingstone; 1991:23–26.
44. Engel J Jr, Van Ness P, Rasmussen T, et al. Outcome with respect to epileptic seizures. In: Engel J, ed. *Surgical Treatment of the Epilepsies.* New York: Raven Press; 1993:609–621.
45. Estes ML, Morris HH 3rd, Luders H, et al. Surgery for intractable epilepsy. Clinicopathologic correlates in 60 cases. *Cleve Clin J Med.* 1988;55(5):441–447.
46. Ettinger AB. Structural causes of epilepsy: Tumors, cysts, stroke, and vascular malformation. *Neurol Clin.* 1994;12:41–56.
47. Falconer MA, Driver MV, Serafetinides EA. Temporal lobe epilepsy due to distant lesions. *Brain.* 1962;85:521–534.
48. Falconer MA, Serafetinides EA. A follow-up study of surgery in temporal lobe epilepsy. *J Neurol Neurosurg Psychiatry.* 1963;26:154–165.
49. Farmer JP, Cosgrove JR, Villemure JG, et al. Intracerebral cavernous angiomas. *Neurology.* 1988;38:1699–1704.
50. Fish MD, Andermann F, Olivier A. Complex partial seizures and small posterior temporal or extratemporal structural lesions: surgical management. *Neurology.* 1991;41:1781–1784.
51. Fried I, Kim JH, Spencer DD. Hippocampal pathology in patients with MRI-identified dual pathology and temporal lobe epilepsy. *J Neurosurg.* 1992(76):735–740.
52. Fried I, Kim JH, Spencer DD. Limbic and neocortical gliomas associated with intractable seizures: a distinct clinicopathological group. *Neurosurgery.* 1994;34(5):815–823; discussion, 23–24.
53. Giulioni M, Gardella E, Rubboli G, et al. Lesionectomy in epileptogenic gangliogliomas: seizure outcome and surgical results. *J Clin Neurosci.* 2006;13(5):529–535.
54. Goldring S, Gregorie E. Surgical management of epilepsy using epidural recordings to localise the seizure focus. *J Neurosurg.* 1984;60:457–466.
55. Goldring S, Rich RM, Picker S. Experience with gliomas in patients presenting with a chronic seizure disorder. *Clin Neurosurg.* 1986;33:15–42.
56. Gulati P, Jena A, Tripathi RP, et al. Magnetic resonance imaging in childhood epilepsy. *Indian Pediatr.* 1991;28:761–765.
57. Hauser WA. Seizure disorders: the changes with age. *Epilepsia.* 1992; 33(Suppl 4):S6–S14.
58. Hauser WA, Kurland LT. The epidemiology of epilepsy in Rochester, Minnesota, 1935 through 1967. *Epilepsia.* 1975;16:1–16.
59. Henderson KH, Shaw EG. Randomized trials of radiation therapy in adult low-grade gliomas. *Semin Radiat Oncol.* 2001;11(2):145–151.
60. Henry TR, Babb TL, Engel J Jr, et al. Hippocampal neuronal loss and regional hypometabolism in temporal lobe epilepsy. *Ann Neurol.* 1994;36:925–927.
61. Hirsch JF, Sainte Rose C, Pierre-Kahn A, et al. Benign astrocytic and oligodendrocytic tumors of the cerebral hemispheres in children. *J Neurosurg.* 1989;70:568–572.
62. Ho SS, Kuzniecky RI, Gilliam F, et al. Congenital porencephaly and hippocampal sclerosis. Clinical features and epileptic spectrum. *Neurology.* 1997;49(5):1382–1388.
63. Hofmeister C, Stapf C, Hartmann A, et al. Demographic, morphological, and clinical characteristics of 1289 patients with brain arteriovenous malformations. *Stroke.* 2000;31:1307–1310.
64. Hoh BL, Chapman PH, Loeffler JS, et al. Results of multimodality treatment for 141 patients with brain arteriovenous malformations and seizures: factors associated with seizure incidence and seizure outcomes. *Neurosurgery.* 2002;51(2):303–309.
65. Hong SC, Kang KS, Seo DW, et al. Surgical treatment of intractable epilepsy accompanying cortical dysplasia. *J Neurosurg.* 2000;93(5):766–773.
66. Horsley V. Brain surgery. *Br Med J.* 1886;2:670–675.
67. Hughes JR, Zak SM. EEG and clinical changes in patients with chronic seizures associated with slowly growing brain tumors. *Arch Neurol.* 1987;44:540–543.
68. Iida K, Otsubo H, Arita K, et al. Cortical resection with electrocorticography for intractable porencephaly-related partial epilepsy. *Epilepsia.* 2005;46(1):76–83.
69. Im SH, Chung CK, Cho BK, et al. Supratentorial ganglioglioma and epilepsy: postoperative seizure outcome. *J Neuro-Oncol.* 2002;57(1):59–66.
70. Isla A, Alvarez F, Gutierrez M, et al. Gangliogliomas: clinical study and evolution. *J Neurosurg Sci.* 1991;35:193–197.
71. Jack CR. Magnetic resonance imaging: neuroimaging and anatomy. *Neuroimaging Clin North Am.* 1995;5:597–622.
72. Jackson GD. New techniques in magnetic resonance and epilepsy. *Epilepsia.* 1994;35:S2–S13.
73. Jackson JH. Localized convulsions from tumor of the brain. *Brain.* 1882;5:364–374.
74. Johannsson JH, Rekate HL, Roessmann U. Ganglioglioma: pathological and clinical correlation. *J Neurosurg.* 1981;54:58–63.
75. Jooma R, Yeh HS, Privitera MD, et al. Lesionectomy versus electrophysiologically guided resection for temporal lobe tumors manifesting with complex partial seizures. *J Neurosurg.* 1995;83(2):231–236.
76. Juhasz C, Chugani DC, Muzik O, et al. Alpha-methyl-L-tryptophan PET detects epileptogenic cortex in children with intractable epilepsy. *Neurology.* 2003;60(6):960–968.
77. Kalyan-Raman UP, Olivero WC. Ganglioglioma: a correlative clinicopathological and radiological study of ten surgically treated cases with follow-up. *Neurosurgery.* 1987;20:428–433.
78. Kelly PJ. Volumetric stereotactic surgical resection of intra-axial brain mass lesions. *Mayo Clinic Proc.* 1988;63:1186–1198.
79. Ketz E. Brain tumors and epilepsy. In: Vinken PJ, Bruyn GW, eds. *Handbook of Clinical Neurology.* Amsterdam: North-Holland; 1974:254–269.
80. Kim JH. Pathology of seizure disorders. *Neuroimag Clin North Am.* 1995;5:527–545.
81. Kirkpatrick PJ, Honavar M, Janota I, et al. Control of temporal lobe epilepsy following en bloc resection of low grade tumors. *J Neurosurg.* 1993(78):19–25.
82. Kraemer DL, Awad IA. Vascular malformations and epilepsy: clinical considerations and basic mechanisms. *Epilepsia.* 1994;35(Suppl 6):S30–S43.
83. Kral T, Clusmann H, Blumcke I, et al. Outcome of epilepsy surgery in focal cortical dysplasia. *J Neurol Neurosurg Psychiatry.* 2003;74(2):183–188.
84. Kral T, Clusmann H, Blumcke I, et al. Outcome of epilepsy surgery in focal cortical dysplasia. *J Neurol Neurosurg Psychiatry.* 2003;74(2):183–188.
85. Kuzniecky RI, Cascino GD, Palmini A, et al. Structural neuro-imaging. In: Engel J Jr, ed. *Surgical Treatment of the Epilepsies,* 2nd ed. New York: Raven Press; 1993.
86. Latchaw RE, Hu X. Functional MR imaging in the evaluation of the patient with partial epilepsy: functional localization. *Neuroimaging.* 1995;5:683–693.
87. Le Blanc FE, Rasmussen T. Cerebral seizures and brain tumors. In: Vinken PJ, Bruyn GW, eds. *Handbook of Clinical Neurology.* Amsterdam: North-Holland; 1974:295–301.
88. Le Blanc R, Feindel W, Ethier R. Epilepsy from cerebral arteriovenous malformations. *Can J Neurol Sci.* 1983;10:91–95.
89. Le Blanc R, Tampieri D, Robitaille Y, et al. Surgical treatment of intractable epilepsy associated with schizencephaly. *Neurosurgery.* 1991;29:421–429.
90. Li LM, Cendes F, Andermann F, et al. Surgical outcome in patients with epilepsy and dual pathology. *Brain.* 1999;122(Pt 5):799–805.
91. Li LM, Fish DR, Sisodioya SM, et al. High resolution resonance imaging in adults with partial or secondarily generalised epilepsy attending a tertiary referral unit. *J Neurol Neurosurg Psychiatry.* 1995;59:384–387.
92. Lieu AS, Howng SL. Intracranial meningiomas and epilepsy: incidence, prognosis and influencing factors. *Epilepsy Res.* 2000;38(1):45–52.
93. Lindegaard KF, Mork SJ, Eide GE, et al. Statistical analysis of clinicopathological features, radiotherapy, and survival in 170 cases of oligodendroglioma. *J Neurosurg.* 1987;67:224–230.
94. Luders H, Lesser RP, Dinner DS, et al. Commentary: chronic intracranial recording and stimulation with subdural electrodes. In: Engel J Jr, ed. *Surgical Treatment of the Epilepsies.* New York: Raven Press; 1987:297–321.
95. Lund M. Epilepsy in association with intracranial tumor. *Acta Neurol Scand.* 1952;81(Suppl):87–106.
96. Mattson RH, Cramer JA, Collins JF, et al. Comparison of carbemazepine, phenobarbital, phenytoin, and primidone in partial and secondarily generalised tonic–clonic seizures. *N Engl J Med.* 1985;313:145–151.
97. McCormick WF. The pathology of vascular ('arteriovenous') malformations. *J Neurosurg.* 1966;24:807–816.
98. McIntosh AM, Kalnins RM, Mitchell LA, et al. Temporal lobectomy: long-term seizure outcome, late recurrence and risks for seizure recurrence. *Brain.* 2004;127:2018–2030.

99. Medina MT, Rosas E, Rubino-Donnadieu F, et al. Neurocysticercosis as the main cause of epilepsy in Mexico. *Arch Int Med.* 1990;150:325–327.
100. Meyer PT, Cortes-Blanco A, Pourdehnad M, et al. Inter-modality comparisons of seizure focus lateralization in complex partial seizures. *Eur J Nucl Med.* 2001;28(10):1529–1540.
101. Morris HH III, Estes ML. Brain tumors and chronic epilepsy. In: Wyllie E, ed. *The Treatment of Epilepsy: Principles and Practice.* Philadelphia: Lea & Febiger; 1993:659–665.
102. Morris HH III, Luders H, Hahn JF, et al. Neuropsysiological techniques as an aid to surgical treatment of primary brain tumors. *Ann Neurol.* 1986;19:559–567.
103. Murphy MA, O'Brien TJ, Morris K, et al. Multimodality image-guided surgery for the treatment of medically refractory epilepsy. *J Neurosurg.* 2004;100(3):452–462.
104. Murphy MJ. Long-term follow-up of seizures associated with cerebral arteriovenous malformations. Results of therapy. *Arch Neurol.* 1985;42:477–479.
105. Nakasato N, Levesque MF, Babb TL. Seizure outcome following standard temporal lobectomy: correlation with hippocampal neuron loss and extrahippocampal pathology. *J Neurosurg.* 1992;77(2):194–200.
106. Nicklasi WJ, Browning ET. Amino acid metabolism in glial cells: homeostatic regulation of intra- and extracellular milieu by C-6 glioma cells. *J Neurochem.* 1978;30:955–963.
107. O'Brien TJ, Hicks RJ, Ware R, et al. The utility of a 3-dimensional, large-field-of-view, sodium iodide crystal–based PET scanner in the presurgical evaluation of partial epilepsy. *J Nucl Med.* 2001;42(8):1158–1165.
108. O'Brien TJ, Kazemi NJ, Cascino GD. Localization-related epilepsies due to specific lesions. In: Engel J Jr,Pedley TA, eds. *Epilepsy: A Comprehensive Textbook.* Philadelphia: Lippincott-Raven; 1997:2433–2446.
109. O'Brien TJ, Kilpatrick C, Murrie V, et al. Temporal lobe epilepsy caused by mesial temporal sclerosis and temporal neocortical lesions. *Brain.* 1996;119:2133–2141.
110. O'Brien TJ, Newton MR, Cook MJ, et al. Hippocampal atrophy is not a major determinant of regional hypometabolism in temporal lobe epilepsy. *Epilepsia.* 1997;38:74–80.
111. O'Brien TJ, O'Connor MK, Mullan BP, et al. Subtraction ictal SPECT co-registered to MRI in partial epilepsy: description and technical validation of the method with phantom and patient studies. *Nucl Med Commun.* 1998;19(1):31–45.
112. O'Brien TJ, So EL, Cascino GD, et al. Subtraction SPECT coregistered to MRI in malformations of cortical development: localization of the epileptogenic zone in epilepsy surgery candidates. *Epilepsia.* 2004;45:367–376.
113. O'Brien TJ, So EL, Mullan BP, et al. Subtraction ictal SPECT co-registered to MRI improves clinical usefulness of SPECT in localizing the surgical seizure focus. *Neurology.* 1998;50(2):445–454.
114. O'Brien TJ, So EL, Mullan BP, et al. Subtraction SPECT co-registered to MRI improves postictal SPECT localization of seizure foci. *Neurology.* 1999;52(1):137–146.
115. O'Brien TJ, So EL, Mullan BP, et al. Subtraction peri-ictal SPECT is predictive of extratemporal epilepsy surgery outcome. *Neurology.* 2000;55(11):1668–1677.
116. Ohgaki H, Kleihues P. Population-based studies on incidence, survival rates, and genetic alterations in astrocytic and oligodendroglial gliomas. *J Neuropathol Exp Neurol.* 2005;64(6):479–489.
117. Ojemann LM, Ojemann GA, Bauggh-Brookman C. What is the optimal extent of the medical resection in interior temporal lobe epilepsy? *Epilepsia.* 1986;27:636.
118. Otsubo H, Hoffman HJ, Humphreys RP, et al. Detection and management of gangliogliomas in children. *Surg Neurol.* 1992;38(5):371–378.
119. Palmini A, Andermann F, Oliver A, et al. Focal neuronal migration disorders and intractable partial epilepsy: a study of 30 patients. *Ann Neurol.* 1991;30:741–749.
120. Parkinson D, Bachers G. Arteriovenous malformations. Summary of 100 consecutive supratentorial cases. *J Neurosurg.* 1980;53:285–299.
121. Penfield WS, Jasper H. *Epilepsy and the Functional Anatomy of the Human Brain.* Boston: Little, Brown; 1954.
122. Peretti P, Raybaud C, Dravet C, et al. MRI in partial epilepsy of childhood. *J Neuroradiol.* 1989;16:308–316.
123. Piepgras DG, Sundt TM, Ragoowansi AT, et al. Seizure outcome in patients with surgically treated cerebral arteriovenous malformations. *J Neurosurg.* 1993;78:5–11.
124. Piepmeier JM. Observations on the current treatment of low-grade astrocytic tumors of the cerebral hemispheres. *J Neurosurg.* 1987;67(2):177–181.
125. Quesney L. Extratemporal epilepsy: clinical presentation, pre-operative EEG localization and surgical outcome. *Acta Neurol Scand Suppl.* 1992;140:81–94.
126. Radhakrishnan K, Cascino GD. Surgery of neoplastic, vascular and infective mass lesions. In: Shorvon S, Dreifuss F, Fish D, et al., eds. *The Treatment of Epilepsy.* Oxford: Blackwell Science; 1996:649–668.
127. Rasmussen T. Cortical excision for medically refractory cortical epilepsy. In: Harris P, Maudsley C, eds. *Epilepsy.* Edinburgh: Churchill Livingstone; 1974:227–239.
128. Rasmussen T. Surgery of epilepsy associated with brain tumours. In: Purpura DP, Penry JK, Walter RD, eds. *Advances in Neurology: Neurosurgical Management of the Epilepsies.* New York: Raven Press; 1975:227–239.
129. Rengachary SS. Intracranial arachnoid and ependymal cysts. In: Wilkins RH, Rengachary SS, eds. *Neurosurgery.* New York: McGraw-Hill; 1985:2160–2172.
130. Riva M. Brain tumoral epilepsy: a review. *Neurol Sci.* 2005;26(Suppl 1):S40–S42.
131. Rossi GF, Scerrati M, Roselli R. Epileptogenic cerebral low-grade tumours: effect of interstitial stereotactic irradiation on seizures. *Appl Neurophysiol.* 1985;48:127–132.
132. Ruggieri P, Comair Y, Ross J, et al. The utility of fast flair imaging in epilepsy. *Epilepsia.* 1995;36(Suppl 4):S25.
133. Semah F, Picot MC, Adam C, et al. Is the underlying cause of epilepsy a major prognostic factor for recurrence? *Neurology.* 1998;51(5):1256–1262.
134. Shaw EG, Scheithauer BW, Gilbertson DT, et al. Post operative radiotherapy of supratentorial low grade gliomas. *Int J Radiat Oncol Biol Phys.* 1989;16:663–668.
135. Siegel AM, Roberts DW, Harbaugh RE, et al. Pure lesionectomy versus tailored epilepsy surgery in treatment of cavernous malformations presenting with epilepsy. *Neurosurg Rev.* 2000;23(2):80–83.
136. Silver JM, Rawlings CE 3rd, Rossitch E Jr, et al. Ganglioglioma: a clinical study with long-term follow-up. *Surg Neurol.* 1991;35(4):261–266.
137. Sisodiya SM, Free SL, Stevens JM, et al. Widespread cerebral structural changes in patients with cortical dysgenesis and epilepsy. *Brain.* 1995;118:1039–1050.
138. So N, Olivier A, Andermann F, et al. Results of surgical treatment in patients with bitemporal epileptiform abnormalities. *Ann Neurol.* 1989;25:432–439.
139. Spencer DD. Strategies for focal resection in medically intractable epilepsy. *Epilepsy Res Suppl.* 1992;5:157–168.
140. Spencer DD, Spencer SS, Mattson RH, et al. Intracerebral masses in patients with partial epilepsy. *Neurology.* 1984;34:432–436.
141. Stefan H, Hammen T. Cavernous haemangiomas, epilepsy and treatment strategies. *Acta Neurol Scand.* 2004;110(6):393–397.
142. Stein BM, Mohr JP. Vascular malformations of the brain [Editorial]. *N Engl J Med.* 1988;319:368–369.
143. Stephen LJ, Kwan P, Brodie MJ. Does the cause of localisation-related epilepsy influence the response to antiepileptic drug treatment? *Epilepsia.* 2001;42(3):357–362.
144. Sutherling WW, Risinger MW, Crandall PH, et al. Focal functional anatomy of dorsolateral frontocentral seizures. *Neurology.* 1990;40(1):87–98.
145. Takashima S, Becker LE. Neuropathology of cerebral arteriovenious malformations in children. *J Neurol Neurosurg Psychiatry.* 1980;43:380–385.
146. Tatlidil R, Luther S, West A, et al. Comparison of fluorine-18 deoxyglucose and O-15 water PET in temporal lobe epilepsy. *Acta Neurol Belg.* 2000;100(4):214–220.
147. Taylor DC, Falconer MA, Brutin CJ, et al. Focal cortical dysplasia of the cerebral cortex in epilepsy. *J Neurol Neurosurg Psychiatry.* 1971;34:369–387.
148. Temkin O. *The Falling Sickness.* Baltimore: Johns Hopkins Press; 1945:380.
149. Theodore WH, Holmes MD, Dorwart RH. Complex partial seizures. Cerebral structure and cerebral function. *Epilepsia.* 1986;27:576–582.
150. Thorpe ML, Cordato DJ, Morgan MK, et al. Postoperative seizure outcome in a series of 114 patients with supratentorial arteriovenous malformations. *J Clin Neurosci.* 2000;7(2):107–111.
151. Vaquero J, Salazar J, Martinez R, et al. Cavernomas of the central nervous system: clinical syndromes, CT scan diagnosis, and prognosis after surgical treatment in 25 cases. *Acta Neurochir (Vienna).* 1987;85(1–2):29–33.
152. Vecht CJ, Wagner GL, Wilms EB. Interactions between antiepileptic and chemotherapeutic drugs. *Lancet Neurol.* 2003;2(7):404–409.
153. Velasco TR, Zanello PA, Dalmagro CL, et al. Calcified cysticercotic lesions and intractable epilepsy: a cross sectional study of 512 patients. *J Neurol Neurosurg Psychiatry.* 2006;77(4):485–488.
154. Vinters HV, Armstrong DL, Babb TL, et al. The neuropathology of human symptomatic epilepsy. In: Engel J Jr, ed. *Surgical Treatment of the Epilepsies.* New York: Raven Press; 1993:593–608.
155. Volterra A, Trotti D, Tromba C, et al. Glutamate uptake inhibition by oxygen free radicals in rat cortical astrocytes. *J Neurosci.* 1994;14(5 Pt 1):2924–2932.
156. Walum F. Counter transport of glutamine and choline in cultures of human glioma cells. *Biochem Biophys Res Commun.* 1979;88:1271–1274.
157. Weber JP, Silbergeld DL, Winn HR. Surgical resection of epileptogenic cortex associated with structural lesions. *Neurosurg Clin North Am.* 1993;4:327–336.
158. Weis M, Feistel H, Stefan H. Utility of ictal SPECT: peri-ictal, post-ictal. *Acta Neurol Scand.* 1994(Suppl)152:145–147.
159. Wiebe S, Blume WT, Girvin JP, et al. A randomized, controlled trial of surgery for temporal-lobe epilepsy. *N Engl J Med.* 2001;345(5):311–318.
160. Williamson PD, Boon PA, Thadani VM, et al. Parietal lobe epilepsy: diagnostic considerations and results of surgery. *Ann Neurol.* 1992;31:193–201.
161. Williamson PD, French JA, Thadani VM, et al. Occipital lobe epilepsy: clinical characteristics, seizure spread patterns, and the results of surgery. *Ann Neurol.* 1992;31:1–13.

162. Williamson PD, Wieser HG, Delgado-Escueta AV. Clinical characteristics of partial seizures. In: Engel J Jr, ed. *Surgical Treatment of the Epilepsies*. New York: Raven Press; 1987:101–120.
163. Wolf HK, Zentner J, Hufnage A, et al. Surgical pathology of temporal lobe epilepsy. Experience with 216 cases. *J Neuropathol Exp Neurol*. 1993;52:499–506.
164. Won HJ, Chang KH, Cheon JE, et al. Comparison of MR imaging with PET and ictal SPECT in 118 patients with intractable epilepsy. *AJNR Am J Neuroradiol*. 1999;20(4):593–599.
165. Wyllie E, Luders H, Morris HH, et al. Clinical outcome after complete or partial resection for intractable epilepsy. *Neurology*. 1987;37:1634–1641.
166. Xiao B, Huang ZL, Zhang H, et al. Aetiology of epilepsy in surgically treated patients in China. *Seizure*. 2004;13(5):322–327.
167. Yeh HS, Kashiwagi S, Tew JM, et al. Surgical management of epilepsy associated with cerebral arteriovenous malformations. *J Neurosurg*. 1990;72:216–223.
168. Yeh HS, Tew JM. Management of arteriovenous malformations of the brain. *Contemp Neurosurg*. 1988;9:1–8.
169. Yeh HS, Tew JM, Gartner M. Seizure control after surgery on cerebral arteriovenous malformations. *J Neurosurg*. 1993;78:12–18.
170. Yoon HH, Kwon HL, Mattson RH, et al. Long-term seizure outcome in patients initially seizure-free after resective epilepsy surgery. *Neurology*. 2003;61(4):445–450.
171. Zevgaridis D, van Velthoven V, Ebeling U, et al. Seizure control following surgery in supratentorial cavernous malformations: a retrospective study in 77 patients. *Acta Neurochir (Vienna)*. 1996;138(6):672–677.

CHAPTER 252 ■ PROGRESSIVE MYOCLONUS EPILEPSIES

SAMUEL F. BERKOVIC

INTRODUCTION

Progressive myoclonus epilepsy (PME) is an uncommon epilepsy syndrome caused by a large number of rare specific disorders. In its fully developed form with florid, unremitting myoclonic seizures and progressive neurologic deterioration, the syndrome can hardly be missed. Diagnosis of the PME syndrome can be more difficult in the early stages, and confusion with more benign epilepsies is common. Diagnosis of the specific type of PME is challenging, as most individual clinicians' experience with these rare disorders is limited. Molecular genetics has had an enormous impact on the clinical approach to these disorders, and PME is the clinical syndrome par excellence showing the value of careful clinicomolecular correlations leading to advances in practical clinical diagnosis and fundamental biologic understanding. This chapter will focus on diagnosis of the PME syndrome and of the more common specific causes.

HISTORICAL PERSPECTIVES

The rarity and complexity of the disorders causing PME have resulted in a confusing literature since the first description by Unverricht in 1891 (Fig. 1).[130] Eponymous names were used in conflicting ways, and there were often erroneous putative clinicopathologic correlations. In particular, the term *Ramsay Hunt syndrome* generated enormous confusion (for review see references 11, 18, 84, and 95).

Pathologic studies since the 1930s established that there were at least three separate pathologic substrates of the PME syndrome: Lafora bodies, lipid storage, and "degenerative" changes.[36,54,56] However, in clinical practice, PME was often the final clinical diagnosis, as there was no way to diagnose specific forms during life.

Over the last three decades a number of clinical, pathologic, genetic, biochemical, and molecular advances have led to considerable clarification of this subject, allowing a sophisticated and rational approach to diagnosis in life of the patient with PME.[7,14,46,84,116] First, in many of the specific causes of PME, characteristic clinical patterns have been recognized. Second, ethnic and geographic clusters of certain disorders have been identified, accounting for the different perspective of PME by authors in various countries. Third, the broad pathologic group of "lipidoses" causing PME has been classified by clinical, biochemical, and pathologic studies into neuronal ceroid lipofuscinoses, sialidoses, and Gaucher disease. Fourth, the mitochondrial disorder MERRF (myoclonus epilepsy and ragged red fiber syndrome) was discovered and found to be a major cause of PME. Fifth, the "degenerative" type of PME was found to be heterogeneous, comprising at least three distinct conditions: Unverricht-Lundborg disease, MERRF, and dentatorubral-pallidoluysian atrophy. Sixth, minimally invasive methods for diagnosis during life were developed. Finally, important molecular genetic findings have further refined understanding of these disorders and are playing an increasing role in routine diagnosis.

DEFINITIONS

The syndrome of PME consists of myoclonic seizures, tonic–clonic seizures, and progressive neurologic dysfunction, particularly ataxia and dementia. Onset can be at any age, but is usually in late childhood or adolescence. There are a large number of causes of the PME syndrome; most are due to specific genetic disorders, which can now be accurately diagnosed in life.[7,46]

Myoclonus in PME is typically fragmentary and multifocal, and often precipitated by posture, action, or external stimuli such as light, sound, or touch. It is particularly apparent in facial and distal limb musculature. Bilateral massive myoclonic jerks, which tend to involve proximal limb muscles, may also occur.

The origin of and generators for myoclonus in PME is a confusing and controversial area. Neurophysiologic studies show that some but not all myoclonic jerks are accompanied by obvious electroencephalographic (EEG) spikes, polyspikes, or spike-and-wave complexes. Where EEG accompaniments of jerks are not obvious, back-averaging techniques may reveal preceding EEG changes. These data, coupled with the frequent finding of giant somatosensory-evoked potentials (SSEPs) and of evidence suggesting abnormal cortical hyperexcitability using transcranial magnetic stimulation, suggest that the myoclonic jerks are often of cortical origin—*cortical reflex myoclonus*. Electrophysiologic studies of bilateral jerks suggest that some are generated in the cortex unilaterally and spread rapidly contralaterally via the corpus callosum, whereas others may be generated in the brainstem—*reticular reflex myoclonus*.[50,109,118,119] The lack of demonstrable EEG change with some jerks might lead to the conclusion that these are examples of "nonepileptic" myoclonus, akin to that seen in certain movement disorders. Unfortunately, no absolute clinical or indeed experimental technique exists to determine the epileptic nature or otherwise of particular jerks. Moreover, the coexistence of "epileptic" and "nonepileptic" myoclonus in one patient is counterintuitive. From a pragmatic clinical viewpoint, therefore, "epileptic" myoclonus can be diagnosed in cases where tonic–clonic or other seizures coexist or where obvious epileptiform discharges accompany some, but not necessarily all, myoclonic jerks.

EPIDEMIOLOGY

PMEs account for <1% of people with epilepsy seen at specialist centers.[46] Series from different countries reveal considerable

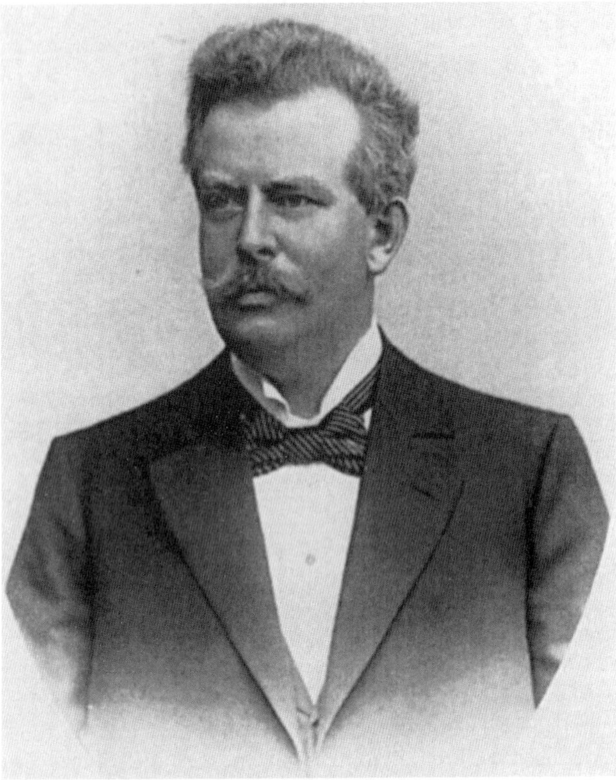

FIGURE 1. Heinrich Unverricht of Magdeberg (1853–1912). First clinical description of progressive myoclonus epilepsy in 1891. (Reproduced from Berkovic SF, Andermann F. The progressive myoclonus epilepsies. In: Pedley TA, Meldrum BS, eds. Recent advances in Epilepsy. Edinburgh: Churchill Livingstone; 1986:157–187.)

geographic and ethnic variability in the occurrence of specific types of PMEs.[1,36,40,46] Details of known geographic clusters of specific PMEs are given below. Knowledge of the patient's ethnic background can provide an essential clue to the likely differential diagnosis of the type of PME.

The incidence and prevalence of specific PMEs are largely unknown. In Finland, Unverricht-Lundborg disease has an incidence of at least 1 per 20,000,[95] but outside the Baltic region the incidence is probably at least an order of magnitude less, although a recent study in The Netherlands using molecular methods suggested that Unverricht-Lundborg disease is underdiagnosed.[35]

SPECIFIC DISORDERS

Unverricht-Lundborg Disease

Etiology and Basic Mechanisms

Unverricht-Lundborg disease is the prototypic cause of PME.[65,77,130] No storage material is present but there is neuronal loss and gliosis particularly affecting the cerebellum, medial thalamus, and spinal cord.[51]

It is an autosomal recessive condition[95] initially recognized as a geographic cluster in Finland and eastern Sweden (*Baltic myoclonus*). An erroneous, but frequently held, view is that this disorder is confined to the Baltic region. Clusters of a phenotypically identical disorder occur in Southern Europe and North Africa, so-called "Mediterranean myoclonus."[47] It is also found sporadically worldwide in Caucasians, Blacks, and Japanese.[40,84] Indeed, it appears that Unverricht's original family was of Baltic German extraction, and not Estonian as widely believed.

The disorder was linked to the long arm of chromosome 21 in Finnish cases in 1991[71] and cystatin B was identified as the responsible gene in 1996.[104] The clinical prediction that similar cases seen outside the Baltic region have the same condition was confirmed by showing the identification of mutations in cystatin B (*CSTB*) in families from around the world. The most common mutation, responsible for about 90% of abnormal alleles, is an unstable expansion of a dodecamer repeat in the 5′ untranslated promoter region. The remaining mutations are missense mutations.[69,70,72] CSTB is a cysteine protease inhibitor. The *CSTB* mutations lead to marked reduced expression of *CSTB* mRNA. Development of a mouse model with targeted disruption of the mouse *Cstb* gene has shown increased apoptosis affecting particularly cerebellar granule cells. It has been suggested that deficiency of CSTB protein results in increased activity of cathepsins with increased apoptosis in specific neuronal cell types.[72,103,117]

A variant has been described where *CTSB* has been excluded as the causative gene. This form maps to chromosome 12 but the gene is presently unknown.[15]

Clinical Presentation

Clinical onset is with myoclonus or tonic–clonic seizures between the ages of 8 and 13 (mean 10, range 6 to 16 years). The myoclonus is usually quite severe and may be precipitated by movement, stress, and sensory stimuli. Repetitive morning myoclonus is also typical, frequently building up and culminating in a major tonic–clonic seizure.[63,64] Seizures may be difficult to control, but progression in terms of ataxia and dementia is mild and late. The clinical course is variable and there may be considerable intrafamily variation in the severity of the seizures. Some patients are relatively mildly affected and survive to old age.[78] A more fulminant course with death within a few years of onset has been observed; this outcome is rarely if ever seen now and may have been due to unrecognized deleterious effects of phenytoin.[40,58]

The EEG background may show some diffuse theta that increases over years, as well as some frontal beta activity. Epileptic activity comprises 3- to 5-Hz spike-wave or multiple spike-wave activity with the maximum field being anterior. Sporadic focal spikes, particularly in the occipital region, may be seen but are usually not prominent (Fig. 2). Photosensitivity is typically marked. During non–rapid eye movement (REM) sleep the spike-wave activity is diminished.[18,64]

Diagnostic Evaluation

Unverricht-Lundborg disease is recognized clinically by its characteristic age of onset and clinical pattern, with an absence of other clinical or pathologic features. Diagnosis is confirmed by molecular analysis of the cystatin B gene.

Myoclonus Epilepsy and Ragged Red Fibers

Etiology and Basic Mechanisms

The MERRF syndrome has emerged as one of the most common causes of PME. It may be familial or sporadic. Most familial cases of MERRF are transmitted through the maternal line and are examples of mitochondrial inheritance.[111] The peculiarities of mitochondrial inheritance provide an explanation for the wide phenotypic variability in patients with MERRF and for the extraordinary intrafamily variation.

A single base substitution at nucleotide pair 8344 of mitochondrial DNA, causing an A-to-G substitution in the

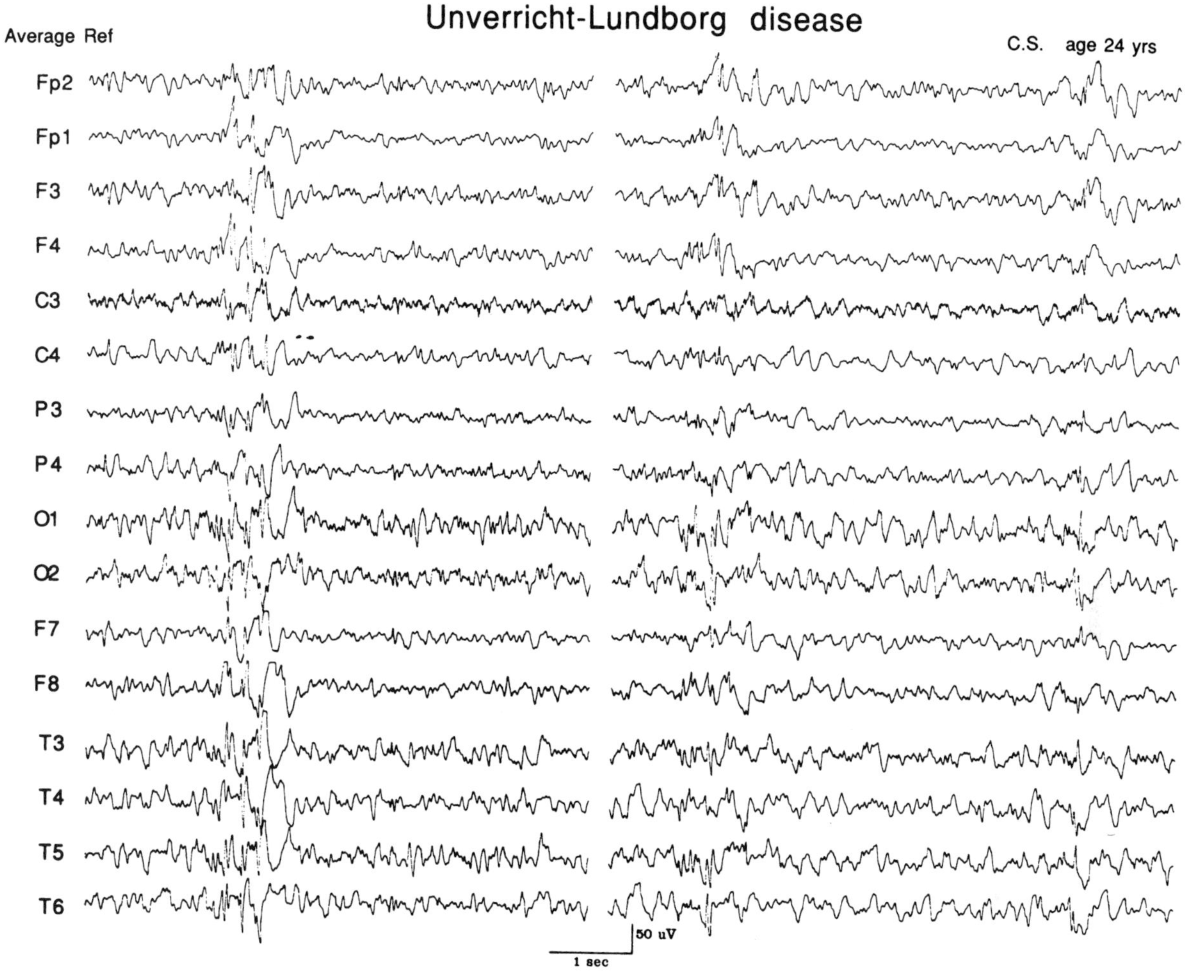

FIGURE 2. Unverricht-Lundborg disease. Waking electroencephalogram in a 24-year-old woman showing generalized polyspike-and-wave discharges on a slow background (**left panel**) with occasional focal occipital discharges (**right panel**).

tRNA^{Lys} gene, occurs in many familial cases of MERRF.[120] The fact that this mutation affects tRNA, rather than a gene for a respiratory enzyme, probably explains the heterogeneous results for respiratory enzyme assays reported in MERRF. This tRNA^{Lys} mutation appears to underlie most, but not all, familial cases and some sporadic examples of MERRF.[17,52,53,138] Other rare identified molecular causes of MERRF also affect the tRNA^{Lys} gene.[121] Recently, autosomal recessive mutations in the nuclear encoded mitochondrial gene polymerase-γ (POLG) have been identified in some MERRF cases.[129]

Pathologically the brain shows "degenerative" changes, particularly affecting the dentate nucleus and inferior olive. In more severely affected cases, lesions typical of Leigh disease are also found. Positron emission tomography shows decreased metabolism for glucose and oxygen with relatively preserved cerebral blood flow, findings compatible with a respiratory chain defect.[13] Phosphorus magnetic resonance spectroscopy of the brain is normal but studies of resting muscle show an increase of inorganic phosphate and a decrease of the phosphocreatine-to-inorganic phosphate concentration ratio.[86]

Clinical Presentation

MERRF was first described in cases with a florid clinical myopathy and myoclonus epilepsy.[43,128] It is now clear that the clinical spectrum of MERRF is extremely broad. It should be suspected in a wide variety of situations, even when clinical and pathologic evidence of myopathy is absent.[8,13] Symptoms can begin at any age and there may be marked intrafamily variation in the age of onset and clinical severity.[13,111] The clinical features include myoclonus, tonic–clonic seizures, dementia, ataxia, and less common findings of myopathy, neuropathy, deafness, and optic atrophy. Some cases show striking axial lipomas. Occasional patients or families have focal neurologic events and there is an overlap with the syndrome of mitochondrial encephalomyopathy, lactic acidosis, and strokelike episodes (MELAS), where strokelike episodes frequently preceded by migrainous headaches with vomiting are characteristic.[8,102]

It has been previously suggested that a wide variety of cases of PME known by eponyms, clinical signs, or particular patterns of system degeneration were examples of mitochondrial disease.[4,7,13] This has now been confirmed for PME with lipomas,[13,39] and for at least some cases of PME and deafness[87,131] and of so-called Ramsay Hunt syndrome.[4,10,84] PME with Friedreich ataxia[122] and PME with deafness, focal cerebral deficits, alopecia, and a transient response to biotin[21] may also be due to mitochondrial disease.

The EEG shows slowly progressive background slowing paralleling degree of clinical deterioration. There are generalized spike-and-wave discharges at 2 to 5 Hz or multiple spike-and-wave discharges. Sporadic occipital spikes and sharp waves may be seen. Prominent photosensitivity may occur. Non-REM sleep is disorganized and spike-and-wave discharges are diminished.[18,123]

Diagnostic Evaluation

The unifying feature of these cases is dysfunction in the mitochondrial respiratory chain. This is most simply demonstrated by ragged red fibers in skeletal muscle, although these can be absent. Biochemical assays of the mitochondrial respiratory enzymes may show abnormalities, but these too may be normal.[13,134]

Diagnosis can usually be suspected clinically and may be difficult to confirm with laboratory markers. The clinical clues to the diagnosis include deafness, optic atrophy, myopathy, lipomas, intrafamily variation in age of onset and severity, and a pattern of inheritance compatible with maternal transmission.[13] Serum lactate, ragged red fibers, and respiratory enzyme activities in muscle can all be normal in patients known to be affected (e.g., family members of proven cases). Magnetic resonance spectroscopy of muscle may show elevated levels of inorganic phosphate and a decrease of the phosphocreatine-to-inorganic phosphate concentration ratio.[86] Molecular defects in mitochondrial DNA or POLG can be detected, when present, in peripheral blood or muscle.[53,138] Screening for the mitochondrial DNA 8344 mutation should be done first; if negative, then more extensive DNA testing of mitochondrial DNA or POLG may be indicated.

Lafora Disease

Etiology and Basic Mechanisms

Lafora disease is characterized by the presence of Lafora bodies, which are polyglucosan inclusions found in neurons and in a variety of other sites including heart, skeletal muscle, liver, and sweat gland duct cells[25,68] (Fig. 3).

It is an autosomal recessive condition. The largest series have been reported from Southern Europe,[125] but it is found worldwide, apparently without a marked racial or ethnic predilection. Approximately 90% of cases have mutations in the gene *EPM2A*, which encodes a dual phosphatase known as laforin,[89,114] or in *EPM2B* (also called *NHLRC1*), which codes for an E3 ubiquitin ligase known as malin.[28,48] There is evidence for a third as yet unknown locus.[27]

Clinical Presentation

Onset is between the ages of 10 and 18 years with a mean age of onset of 14. Clinical features are myoclonus, tonic–clonic seizures, and relentless cognitive decline. Focal seizures, particularly arising from the occipital regions, occur in about half the patients. Recognition of Lafora disease in its fully developed form is not difficult. At the onset, however, the disorder can resemble a typical benign adolescent generalized epilepsy with no evidence of cognitive decline. It may also present as a dementing illness with relatively infrequent seizures, or it may mimic a nonspecific secondary generalized epilepsy because myoclonus is not obvious.[11,107,110] The prognosis of Lafora disease is dismal, with death occurring 2 to 10 years after onset and the mean age of death being 20 years.

The clinical picture, including the relatively narrow age range of onset and relentlessly progressive course to death within 2 to 10 years of onset, is constant in all reports with the exception of a few cases. These cases, sometimes erroneously labelled as "type Lundborg," had symptoms beginning in late adolescence or early adult life with a milder protracted course.[36,60,66] Certain mutations in *EPM2B* may cause a milder course.[6] Conversely, an early-onset form with marked cognitive decline has been reported with mutations in exon 1 of *EPM2A*.[44]

At onset the EEG background is well organized and there are multiple spike-and-wave discharges that are increased by intermittent photic stimulation. Erratic myoclonus is seen without EEG correlation. Spike-and-wave discharges are not accentuated during sleep. Over the next few months to years, the background deteriorates, the physiologic elements of sleep become disrupted, and only REM sleep can be identified. Multifocal, particularly posterior, epileptiform abnormalities appear in addition to the generalized bursts, and in the terminal phase of the illness the EEG is quite disorganized.[125]

Diagnostic Evaluation

The age of onset, eventual inexorable dementia, and frequent occurrence of focal occipital seizures are clinical clues to the diagnosis.[110,127] Lafora bodies can be demonstrated in many tissues, but diagnosis is most simply made by examination of eccrine sweat gland ducts by a simple skin biopsy[25] and can

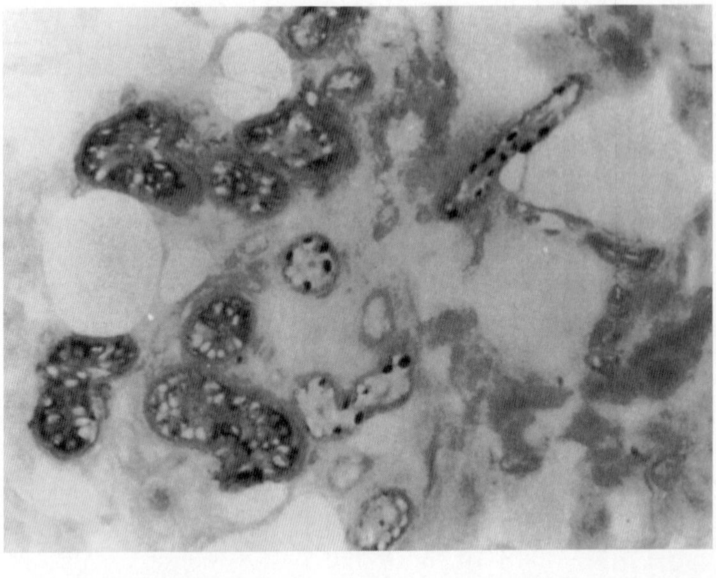

FIGURE 3. Lafora disease, skin biopsy. Cryostat section of skin stained with periodic acid-Schiff showing oval densely staining inclusions in eccrine duct cells. The secretory ascini (on the **left**) show normal glycogen staining (×225). (Reproduced from Berkovic SF, Andermann F. The progressive myoclonus epilepsies. In: Pedley TA, Meldrum BS, eds. Recent advances in Epilepsy. Edinburgh: Churchill Livingstone; 1986:157–187.)

now be confirmed in most cases by molecular study of *EPM2A* and *EPM2B*.[57]

Neuronal Ceroid Lipofuscinoses

Etiology and Basic Mechanisms

The neuronal ceroid lipofuscinoses (NCLs) are characterized by the accumulation of abnormal amounts of lipopigment in lysosomes. There are four classical clinical forms: Infantile, late-infantile (Jansky-Bielschowsky), juvenile (Spielmeyer-Vogt-Sjögren), and adult NCL (Kufs), of which all but the infantile form may present as a PME syndrome. The infantile form presents differently with regression, hypotonia, and impaired vision and is not considered here. The childhood forms are sometimes collectively referred to as Batten disease.

The various forms are genetically distinct and occur worldwide, but with peculiar patterns of geographic clustering. In Finland there are large numbers of infantile and juvenile cases, whereas in Newfoundland late-infantile and juvenile cases are seen with increased frequency.[3,108] All forms have autosomal recessive inheritance. Kufs disease, however, also occurs in families with dominant inheritance.[20]

The storage material proved extremely difficult to characterize, and for many years was thought to be lipid. Subunit c of mitochondrial adenosine triphosphate (ATP) synthase, a very hydrophobic protein, was subsequently identified as the major storage protein in an ovine model[99] and in human late-infantile, juvenile, and adult cases.[49,98] Clinicomolecular studies have now designated eight variants (*CLN1 to 8*) for which the gene has been isolated in six.[90]

Clinical Presentation

The classic late-infantile form (*CLN2*) has an onset between $2\frac{1}{2}$ and 4 years. Seizures are usually the first manifestation with myoclonic seizures, tonic–clonic seizures, atonic seizures, and atypical absences. Within a few months of onset, ataxia and psychomotor regression are seen with visual failure generally developing late. Examination of the optic fundi reveals attenuated retinal vessels and macular degeneration. The seizures are usually intractable, dementia is relentless, and there is progressive spasticity with death about 5 years after onset.[11,107] The EEG shows background slowing and disorganization with generalized epileptiform discharges. Photosensitivity is marked and single flashes may provoke giant posterior-evoked responses. Visual-evoked potentials (VEPs) are abnormally broad and of high amplitude, and SSEPs are enlarged. The electroretinogram (ERG) becomes progressively attenuated.[101,107,136] *CLN2* encodes a lysosomal enzyme tripetidyl peptidase (TPP1).[90]

The late-infantile variant form, described in Finland (*CLN5*), differs in the following ways. Onset is later, between 5 and 7 years; psychomotor regression and visual failure occur earlier, with myoclonic and tonic–clonic seizures generally appearing at around age 8 years; and progression is somewhat slower.[113] Electrophysiologic findings are similar to those of the late-infantile form except that the marked response to photic stimulation develops around age 7 to 8 years and disappears by ages 10 to 11 years, and the visual-evoked response (VER), which is initially large, progressively attenuates.[113] *CLN5* encodes a glycosylated lysosomal protein.[90]

CLN6 encodes a membrane protein found in the endoplasmic reticulum and is associated with a late-infantile variant form, which presents between 5 and 7 years with seizures and motor impairment, while visual failure occurs later. This disorder has been described in many countries.[90] Late-infantile cases are frequent in Turkey; some have mutations in *CLN8*, which encodes a membrane protein found in the endoplasmic reticulum, and others have been designated as *CLN7*, but the gene has not been identified.[90]

Juvenile NCL (*CLN3*) begins between the ages of 4 and 10 years. The majority of patients present with visual failure, and have the gradual development of dementia and extrapyramidal features, with seizures being a relative minor manifestation. Funduscopy reveals optic atrophy, macular degeneration, and attenuated vessels. Inheritance is autosomal recessive. The course is variable, with death about 8 years after onset.[107] The EEG shows background slowing and generalized epileptiform discharges that are often of the slow spike-and-wave type. Sleep activates the epileptic abnormality but photic stimulation does not. VEPs are of low amplitude and sometimes cannot be elicited. The ERG is flat.[101,107,136] The gene encodes a glycosylated membrane protein probably localized to lysosomes.[90]

The adult form (*CLN4*) is considerably rarer. It can present as a PME syndrome around the age of 30, although other cases present with a picture of dementia and extrapyramidal or cerebellar disturbance. Visual auras may occur before some seizures. Blindness is notably absent and the optic fundi are normal. The clinical course from onset to death is approximately 12 years.[12] The EEG shows generalized fast spike-and-wave discharges with marked photosensitivity. Single flashes may evoke paroxysmal discharges. The background activity may be normal in the early stages, and ERGs are normal.[9,12] The genes have not been identified.

Diagnostic Evaluation

Diagnosis can often be suspected clinically, particularly if there are visual changes. The electrophysiologic findings described above can be helpful. Vacuolated lymphocytes may be noted in the juvenile form. Neuroradiologic studies show cerebral and particularly cerebellar atrophy. Diagnosis can be made by the demonstration of characteristic inclusions by electron microscopy. These can be found in a variety of cell types including eccrine secretory cells. The inclusions take various forms, with curvilinear profiles being characteristic of a late-infantile NCL, fingerprint profiles being usual in the juvenile and adult forms, and granular osmiophilic deposits occurring in the infantile form (Fig. 4). A number of variations occur, however, such as rare cases of the adult and juvenile cases showing granular osmiophilic deposits. Considerable expertise may be required in the pathologic interpretation of the electron micrographs.[24,26] In the case of suspected *CLN2*, enzymatic assays for TPP1 are available and molecular testing can be performed for *CLN2*, *CLN3*, *CLN5*, *CLN6*, and *CLN8*.[90]

Sialidoses

Etiology and Basic Mechanisms

The sialidoses are the least common of the major forms of PME. They are autosomal recessive disorders associated with deficiencies of α-*N*-acetyl-neuraminidase. Sialidosis type I is due to a primary deficiency in a neuraminidase. Many of the published cases were of Italian origin.[75] Sialidosis type I is due to mutations in the α-*N*-acetyl-neuraminidase gene *(NEU1)* on chromosome 6.[115]

Sialidosis type II comprises a complex group of phenotypes. The juvenile form presents as a PME and occurs predominantly in Japan. In addition to the neuraminidase deficiency, a partial deficiency of β-galactosidase is also found in most if not all cases.[75,85] The combination of neuraminidase and β-galactosidase deficiency (galactosialidosis) is due to a lack of a 32-kilodalton protein that is required to protect

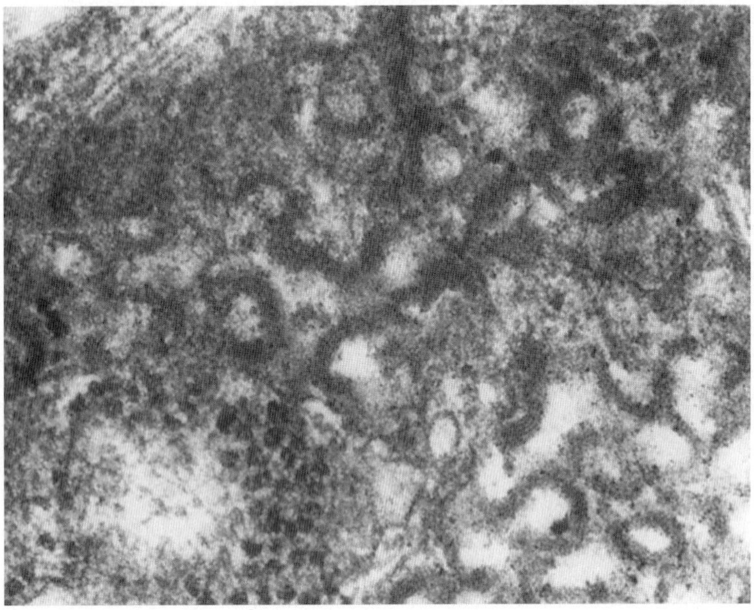

FIGURE 4. Late-infantile neuronal ceroid lipofuscinosis, skin biopsy. Electron micrograph of a skin biopsy showing curvilinear profiles from an eccrine secretory cell (×120,000). (Reproduced from Berkovic SF, Andermann F. The progressive myoclonus epilepsies. In: Pedley TA, meldrum BS, eds. Recent advances in Epilepsy. Edinburgh: Churchill Living Stone; 1986:157–187.)

galactosidase from degradation and is essential for the catalytic action of neuraminidase.[34,100] Missense mutations in the gene lysosomal protective protein/cathepsin A (PPCA) on chromosome 20 cause the juvenile form with PME.[91,139]

Clinical Presentation

In sialidosis type I (*cherry red spot-myoclonus syndrome*), there is onset in adolescence with myoclonus, gradual visual failure, tonic–clonic seizures, ataxia, and a characteristic cherry-red spot in the fundus. The myoclonus is usually very severe. Lens opacities and a mild peripheral neuropathy with burning feet may occur. Dementia is absent.[42,75,106,107,124]

Juvenile sialidosis type II presents as a PME with features like sialidosis type I except that onset is sometimes a little later. There may be additional features of coarse facies, corneal clouding, dysostosis multiplex, hearing loss, and low intellect, which can be present from early life.[75,85]

The EEG background comprises low-voltage fast activity, but some slowing can be seen in demented patients. Generalized spike-and-wave bursts are absent or infrequent; rather massive myoclonus is associated with trains of 10- to 20-Hz small vertex positive spikes preceding the EMG artefact. Non-REM sleep is disorganized, and although myoclonus diminishes, the vertex spikes persist and become very frequent in deep sleep.[41,107]

Diagnostic Evaluation

Sialidoses should be identified clinically because of the characteristic optic fundus. Periodic acid-Schiff–positive inclusions may be seen in lymphocytes, bone marrow cells, neurons, and Kupffer cells. Diagnosis is confirmed by grossly elevated urinary sialyloligosaccharides and by a deficiency of cryolabile α-*N*-acetylneuraminidase in leucocytes or cultured fibroblasts.[75]

RARE CAUSES OF PROGRESSIVE MYOCLONUS EPILEPSY

Dentatorubral-pallidoluysian atrophy (DRPLA) is an autosomal dominant condition that has been extensively studied in Japan. It is caused by a triplet repeat expansion in a gene on chromosome 12p; the function of the gene is as yet unknown.[62,93] DRPLA has a distinct pathology with neuronal loss and gliosis in the dentatorubral and pallidoluysian systems. A variety of clinical phenotypes occur, which may all be seen in one family. PME is one mode of presentation and tends to occur in cases with onset in childhood or adolescence. Other patients, usually with onset in adulthood, present with ataxic-choreoathetoid or chorea-dementia (mimicking Huntington disease) phenotypes.[59,94] Diagnosis is by detection of the abnormal triplet repeat expansion. DRPLA was previously thought to be extraordinarily rare outside Japan. Molecular diagnosis has recently revealed a number of non-Japanese families, although the PME phenotype appears to be uncommon.[23,105,135]

Noninfantile neuronopathic Gaucher disease presents as a PME, with supranuclear gaze palsy and splenomegaly without dementia. Neurologic manifestations may appear in childhood or as late as 38 years.[61,137] Pancytopenia, elevated serum acid phosphatase, and low leukocyte β-glucocerebrosidase activity are found. Inheritance is autosomal recessive. The glucocerebrosidase gene is on chromosome 1. A large variety of mutations causing disease have been identified.[19]

Atypical inclusion body disease has inclusions that are limited to the brain and are histochemically and ultrastructurally different from Lafora bodies.[30,37] Clinical onset is between 7 and 31 years, and dementia is prominent. Diagnosis requires brain biopsy. The initially reported cases were sporadic, but it has been suggested that at least some of these cases may be related to familial encephalopathy with neuroserpin inclusion bodies.[32,33]

A remarkable autosomal recessive disorder has been described in French Canadians with tremor and a PME syndrome beginning at around the age of 19, followed shortly by renal failure with proteinuria. Dementia is absent. An unusual pattern of pigment deposition is seen in astrocytes. EEGs show typical features of a PME with marked photosensitivity.[2] This condition has recently been recognized outside French Canada in a number of countries.[5,132]

Neuroaxonal dystrophy rarely presents in late childhood or adolescence as a PME. Additional clinical features include dementia, ataxia, chorea, and lower motor neuron involvement.[38,126] Diagnosis is made by demonstrating the presence of axon spheroids, which may be seen in peripheral nerves, in brain and by electron microscopy around eccrine secretory coils.

Celiac disease can be associated with generalized myoclonus, seizures, and ataxia,[76] although palatal myoclonus, rather than a PME syndrome, is more common in the malabsorptive disorders of celiac and Whipple diseases. Other very rare causes of PME are atypical late-infantile or juvenile forms of GM_2 gangliosidosis,[22] an unusual form of β-galactosidase deficiency with normal neuraminidase activity,[92] familial encephalopathy with neuroserpin inclusion bodies,[33] and possibly pantothenate kinase-associated neurodegeneration.[112] Alzheimer disease beginning in the third or fourth decade can present as a typical PME.[16]

DIFFERENTIAL DIAGNOSIS

Distinguishing Progressive Myoclonus Epilepsy from Other Epilepsies and Myoclonic Syndromes

It is usually not difficult to diagnose the syndrome of PME some years after onset with the distinctive diagnostic triad of myoclonic seizures, tonic–clonic seizures, and progressive neurologic decline. At the beginning of the illness, however, the clinical and EEG features may be similar to that of benign idiopathic generalized epilepsies, particularly mimicking juvenile myoclonic epilepsy. Response to therapy may be relatively favorable initially. With the passage of time, however, seizures may become more frequent, and progressive neurologic decline occurs. Failure to respond to therapy and progressive neurologic signs should lead to consideration of the presence of a PME. Conversely, the clinical picture of patients with idiopathic generalized epilepsies may mimic those of PME if they are inappropriately treated and intoxicated with antiepileptic drugs leading to ataxia, impaired cognitive function, and poorly controlled seizures.

Myoclonus in PMEs is usually quite severe, but in some patients, it may be relatively inobvious with convulsive seizures and intellectual decline dominating the clinical picture, leading to a misdiagnosis of a nonspecific symptomatic (secondary) generalized epilepsy or Lennox-Gastaut syndrome. In such cases, a careful search for myoclonus should lead to consideration of the PME syndrome.

Neurophysiologic assessment may also provide clues to the presence of a PME. The EEG background rhythm may be relatively well preserved in the early phases, but as the condition progresses generalized slow activity appears. This is particularly so in those forms of PME associated with relentless dementia, such as Lafora disease and NCL. Generalized epileptiform abnormalities are seen during the resting record, usually in the form of fast spike-and-wave, multiple spike-and-wave, or multiple spike discharges. Photosensitivity is common and may be marked. Focal, particularly posterior, epileptiform abnormalities are common in Lafora disease but also may occur in other forms.[18] SSEPs frequently show giant responses.[118,119]

PMEs should be distinguished from degenerative disorders where seizures and/or myoclonus can occur but do not form part of the clinical core or usual initial presentation of the disorder. The causes of such progressive encephalopathies with seizures are numerous and include GM_2 gangliosidosis, nonketotic hyperglycinemia, Niemann-Pick type C, juvenile Huntington disease, and Alzheimer disease. The distinction between this diverse group of disorders and the PMEs, while not absolute, is clinically useful and provides a practical framework on which to begin specific differential diagnosis.[11] For example, typical Alzheimer disease may have myoclonus as a relatively late feature, and would not be confused with a PME. Rare early-onset cases may, however, present as a PME in early adult life. Myoclonus is also prominent in certain static encephalopathies, of which postanoxic myoclonus (Lance-Adam syndrome) is the best known. The absence of progression and the usual clear history of the causative encephalopathy enable clear distinction from PME.

The PME syndrome should also be distinguished from the progressive myoclonic ataxias. This term was introduced to denote a group of patients, usually adults, with progressive ataxia and myoclonus but with few if any tonic–clonic seizures and little or no evidence of dementia.[84] Previously, some authors used the term *Ramsay Hunt syndrome* for these patients, although others used this term for quite different clinical groups, leading to considerable confusion in the literature.[4,83] The causes of progressive myoclonic ataxia partially overlap with the causes of PME but also include spinocerebellar degenerations, celiac disease, and Whipple disease. While it is now possible to specifically diagnose most patients with the PME syndrome in life (see below), a larger proportion of carefully studied cases with progressive myoclonic ataxia remain without a specific cause being established.[82,84]

Japanese authors have highlighted a condition of benign myoclonic epilepsy of adulthood. In this autosomal dominant disorder, onset is usually between 20 and 40 years, with myoclonus and rare tonic–clonic seizures.[88] Generalized epileptiform EEG abnormalities and giant SSEPs are present, but there is little or no evidence of progression. A number of other families have been described, under various names, that share adult onset, distal action tremor and myoclonus, epileptic seizures, autosomal dominant inheritance, benign course, effectiveness of antiepileptic drugs, and possibly cognitive decline, and the term *familial cortical myoclonic tremor with epilepsy* has been suggested.[133] This condition may be the same or similar to that previously described in the German literature as myoclonus epilepsy of Hartung type.[36]

Finally, the condition of benign familial myoclonus needs to be distinguished. In this autosomal dominant disorder, nonepileptic myoclonus begins in the first three decades of life, but is not associated with major seizures, epileptiform EEG abnormalities, or neurologic deterioration.[31,80]

Diagnosing the Specific Type of Progressive Myoclonus Epilepsy

Once the clinician is convinced that a patient has the PME syndrome, the critical question is to determine which specific disorder is present. This is essential for proper clinical and genetic counseling of the family (see below).

It is now possible to provide a specific diagnosis in life for the vast majority of patients with PME using clinical methods and minimally invasive investigations. An approach to this problem has been described previously.[7,14] The clinician should first consider the five major disorders causing PME, with the addition of DRPLA in patients of Japanese origin. Once these conditions are excluded, the rarer disorders should be considered.

Clinical Features

Although patients with the PME syndrome may appear superficially to have similar clinical features, knowledge of the specific clinical patterns of the common causes of PME often allows the differential diagnosis to be narrowed. Age at onset of symptoms provides some guidance in making the diagnosis, although MERRF may begin at any age. Certain seizure patterns are helpful; very prominent myoclonus suggests Unverricht-Lundborg disease, MERRF, or sialidosis. Partial seizures, particularly of occipital origin, can occur in a variety of the disorders but are often noted in Lafora disease. Characteristic fundal changes are almost invariable in sialidosis and are frequent in the neuronal ceroid lipofuscinosis. Dementia is a constant feature of Lafora disease, the neuronal ceroid lipofuscinoses, and neuroaxonal dystrophy, whereas it is characteristically absent or mild in Unverricht-Lundborg disease, sialidosis type I, noninfantile Gaucher disease, and the action myoclonus-renal failure syndrome. The presence of deafness, lipomas, optic atrophy, myopathy, or neuropathy is a clinical pointer to MERRF. Neuropathy may also occur in sialidosis and neuroaxonal dystrophy. Dysmorphic features are usual in sialidosis type II and may occur in MERRF. Chorea can occur in dentatorubral-pallidoluysian atrophy, neuroaxonal dystrophy, and MERRF. Splenomegaly and supranuclear gaze palsy suggest Gaucher disease. Transient alopecia was seen in biotin-responsive encephalopathy.

Family History

A detailed family history, including examination of relatives, is essential. Recessive inheritance is usual, and the finding of parental consanguinity or early clinical signs in asymptomatic siblings would support this pattern. Maternal transmission is characteristic of MERRF. In MERRF and in the autosomal dominant disorders, older relatives may be found to have mild, incomplete forms of the condition.[14]

Neurophysiology

Findings that may be useful in specific diagnosis include the finding of vertex spikes as the main epileptiform abnormality in sialidosis, activation of epileptiform abnormalities in non-REM sleep in the sialidoses and the late-infantile and juvenile forms of NCL, photosensitivity to single flashes in late-infantile and adult NCL, and absent ERG in late-infantile and juvenile NCL.[18]

Laboratory Findings

Hematologic examination may reveal lymphocyte vacuolation in sialidosis and in certain cases of neuronal ceroid lipofuscinosis. Pancytopenia is common in Gaucher disease.

Routine biochemical tests are not helpful, with the exception of findings of elevated lactate levels in blood and cerebrospinal fluid in some cases of MERRF, elevated serum tartrate-resistant isozymes of acid phosphatase in Gaucher disease, and proteinuria with impaired renal function in the action myoclonus-renal failure syndrome. More sophisticated testing includes assays for TPP1 in leukocytes or fibroblast culture to diagnose late-infantile NCL, urinary thin-layer chromatographic oligosaccharide screen to detect sialidosis, urinary organic acid estimation for biotin-responsive encephalopathy, and β-hexosaminidase A and B screens of serum and leukocytes for GM_2 gangliosidosis. Specific enzyme assays for the sialidoses (α-*N*-acetylneuraminidase and β-galactosidase) and Gaucher disease β-glucocerebrosidase) and definitive assays for the various forms of β-hexosaminidase deficiency in GM_2 gangliosidosis using fibroblast cultures and special substrates are performed only when the relevant diagnosis is strongly suspected.

Pathologic Studies

A tissue diagnosis is essential for a number of these disorders. Skin biopsy with or without skeletal-muscle biopsy is the initial procedure. Lafora disease can be reliably diagnosed by examining eccrine sweat gland duct cells with stains for polysaccharides.[25] The diagnosis of neuronal ceroid lipofuscinosis may be suggested by an acid phosphatase stain, but electron microscopy of the skin biopsy specimen is essential for the definitive identification of inclusions. These inclusions are detectable in many cell types in the late-infantile form of the disease, but in the juvenile and adult varieties, diagnostic lesions may be limited to eccrine secretory cells.[24] False-negative skin biopsies in Lafora disease and in late-infantile and juvenile NCL are, in our experience, due to failure to examine the appropriate cell type properly. In suspected Lafora disease it is essential to ensure that sweat gland ducts are included in the biopsy and properly examined. Where doubt remains, skin biopsy should be repeated because of the serious prognostic implications of the diagnosis of Lafora disease. The reliability of diagnosis of Kufs disease from skin biopsy is not yet clear.

Axon spheroids may be seen in autonomic terminals around eccrine secretory coils in cases of neuroaxonal dystrophy, but the sensitivity of this finding has not been established. Study of muscle biopsy specimens with modified Gomori trichome and oxidative enzyme reactions may demonstrate ragged red fibers in MERRF. Abnormal mitochondria may be identified in muscle or skin using electron microscopy. Normal light and electron microscopic studies of muscle do not rule out the diagnosis of MERRF and, in clinically suspicious cases, a second biopsy may be indicated.

Molecular Genetic Studies

Molecular genetic studies are playing an increasing role in the diagnosis of the PMEs. Simple DNA tests for the dodecamer repeat in Unverricht-Lundborg disease and mitochondrial DNA mutations in MERRF and for the triplet repeat expansion in DRPLA are readily available. Testing for mutations associated with Lafora disease, neuronal ceroid lipofuscinoses, and sialidoses is available from more specialized or research-orientated laboratories (see http://www.genetests.org).

TREATMENT AND OUTCOME

Treatment of these disorders may be distressingly difficult. Accurate diagnosis is the first step as informed genetic counseling must be given. It is very important to distinguish MERRF, which may show maternal inheritance, from autosomal recessive disorders such as Unverricht-Lundborg disease, Lafora disease, sialidoses, and the neuronal ceroid lipofuscinoses, and from dominant disorders such as DRPLA, familial encephalopathy with neuroserpin inclusion bodies, and rare dominant families with Kufs disease. Genetic counseling may now be extended to prenatal diagnosis in some cases. Specific diagnosis also allows an accurate prognosis to be given, including a realistic appraisal of the educational and vocational goals of the patient.

For symptomatic control of myoclonus, valproate and/or clonazepam should be used. Phenytoin has a clear deleterious effect in Unverricht-Lundborg disease.[40,58] Phenytoin should not be used in the other PMEs either. Small doses of barbiturates may be helpful, but sedation should be avoided. Piracetam may be useful in certain cases.[96] Care must be taken not to render the patient intoxicated with drugs, although there is some evidence that carefully monitored polytherapy may be more effective in some patients as opposed to the usual practice of aiming for monotherapy.[97] Combinations of L-tryptophan or 5-hydroxytryptophan with carbidopa have been used[73,74] but are not generally of long-term benefit. Zonisamide[55,67] and levetiracetam[29,79,81] may be quite effective. Drugs that may exacerbate myoclonus, including carbamazepine, vigabatrin, and gabapentin, should be avoided.

Programs of physical therapy may be of benefit, and attempts should be made to search for strategies allowing movement without precipitating myoclonus in individual patients. Alcohol may provide symptomatic benefit in some patients, but must be used judiciously.[45]

Strategies for replacing enzymes in the storage disorders and for augmenting mitochondrial function in the mitochondrial disorders are being developed, but presently they remain in the experimental phase and results to date have been disappointing.

LONG-TERM PROGNOSIS

The prognosis of all the PMEs is poor, and is discussed under the specific diseases. In general, the worst prognosis is seen in the storage disorders (NCL and Lafora), where there is an associated relentless dementia. The prognosis is somewhat better in Unverricht-Lundborg disease, where some patients can remain ambulant and active for many years or even decades after diagnosis. The prognosis of MERRF is highly variable; cases with an earlier onset generally have a more rapid course.

SUMMARY AND CONCLUSIONS

The PMEs are a group of rare genetic disorders previously shrouded in nosologic confusion. Recent advances have clarified the features of these disorders and provided a rational approach to diagnosis. The major causes of PME are now known to be Unverricht-Lundborg disease, MERRF, Lafora disease, neuronal ceroid lipofuscinoses, and sialidoses. In the last 15 years a series of molecular genetic findings have further refined the understanding of the PMEs. The genes responsible for most forms of PME have been identified. Precise diagnosis in life is now possible in virtually all cases using clinical methods, biochemical tests, skin and muscle biopsies, and molecular genetic techniques. Accurate diagnosis allows determination of prognosis, rational genetic counseling, possible prenatal diagnosis, and consideration of emerging therapeutic strategies. Although the PMEs are among the rarest of the inherited epilepsies, because of molecular genetic discoveries, they are best understood at a molecular level. It is hoped that the great strides that have recently been made in the biochemical and molecular genetics of these disorders will soon transfer into rational and effective therapeutics.

References

1. Acharya JN, Satishchandra P, Shankar SK. Familial progressive myoclonus epilepsy: clinical and electrophysiologic observations. *Epilepsia.* 1995;36:429–434.
2. Andermann E, Andermann F, Carpenter S. Action myoclonus-renal failure syndrome. In: Fahn S, Marsden CD,Van Woert MH, eds. *Myoclonus.* New York: Raven Press; 1986:87–103.
3. Andermann E, Jacob JC, Andermann F, et al. The Newfoundland aggregate of neuronal ceroid-lipofuscinosis. *Am J Med Genet Suppl.* 1988;5:111–116.
4. Andermann F, Berkovic S, Carpenter S, et al. The Ramsay Hunt syndrome is no longer a useful diagnostic category. *Mov Disord.* 1989;4:13–17.
5. Badhwar A, Berkovic SF, Dowling JP, et al. Action myoclonus-renal failure syndrome: characterization of a unique cerebro-renal disorder. *Brain.* 2004;127:2173–2182.
6. Baykan B, Striano P, Gianotti S, et al. Late-onset and slow-progressing Lafora disease in four siblings with EPM2B mutation. *Epilepsia.* 2005;46:1695–1697.
7. Berkovic SF, Andermann F, Carpenter S, et al. Progressive myoclonus epilepsies: specific causes and diagnosis. *N Engl J Med.* 1986;315:296–305.
8. Berkovic SF, Andermann F, Karpati G, et al. Mitochondrial encephalomyopathies: recognition of the associated epileptic syndromes. In: Manelis J, ed. *Advances in Epileptology.* New York: Raven Press; 1989:257–260.
9. Berkovic SF, Andermann F, Shoubridge EA, et al. Mitochondrial dysfunction in multiple symmetrical lipomatosis. *Ann Neurol.* 1991;29:566–569.
10. Berkovic SF, Andermann F. Ramsay Hunt syndrome: to bury or to praise. *J Neurol Neurosurg Psychiatry.* 1990;53:89–90.
11. Berkovic SF, Andermann F. The progressive myoclonus epilepsies. In: Pedley TA, Meldrum BS, eds. *Recent Advances in Epilepsy.* Edinburgh: Churchill Livingstone; 1986:157–187.
12. Berkovic SF, Carpenter S, Andermann F, et al. Kufs' disease: a critical reappraisal. *Brain.* 1988;111(Pt 1):27–62.
13. Berkovic SF, Carpenter S, Evans A, et al. Myoclonus epilepsy and ragged-red fibres (MERRF). 1. A clinical, pathological, biochemical, magnetic resonance spectrographic and positron emission tomographic study. *Brain.* 1989;112:1231–1260.
14. Berkovic SF, Cochius J, Andermann E, et al. Progressive myoclonus epilepsies: clinical and genetic aspects. *Epilepsia.* 1993;34:S19–30.
15. Berkovic SF, Mazarib A, Walid S, et al. A new clinical and molecular form of Unverricht-Lundborg disease localized by homozygosity mapping. *Brain.* 2005;128:652–658.
16. Berkovic SF, Melanson M, Andermann F. Dementia and myoclonus: differential diagnosis of early-onset Alzheimer's disease. *Ann Neurol.* 1995;37:412.
17. Berkovic SF, Shoubridge EA, Andermann F, et al. Clinical spectrum of mitochondrial DNA mutation at base pair 8344. *Lancet.* 1991;338:457.
18. Berkovic SF, So NK, Andermann F. Progressive myoclonus epilepsies: clinical and neurophysiological diagnosis. *J Clin Neurophysiol.* 1991;8:261–274.
19. Beutler E. Gaucher disease: new molecular approaches to diagnosis and treatment. *Science.* 1992;256:794–799.
20. Boehme DH, Cottrell JC, Leonberg SC, et al. A dominant form of neuronal ceroid-lipofuscinosis. *Brain.* 1971;94:745–760.
21. Bressman S, Fahn S, Eisenberg M, et al. Biotin-responsive encephalopathy with myoclonus, ataxia, and seizures. In: Fahn S, Marsden CD,Van Woert MH, eds. *Advances in Neurology.* New York: Raven Press; 1986:119–125.
22. Brett EM, Ellis RB, Haas L, et al. Late onset GM2-gangliosidosis. Clinical, pathological, and biochemical studies on 8 patients. *Arch Dis Child.* 1973;48:775–785.
23. Burke JR, Wingfield MS, Lewis KE, et al. The Haw River syndrome: dentatorubropallidoluysian atrophy (DRPLA) in an African-American family. *Nat Genet.* 1994;7:521–524.
24. Carpenter S, Karpati G, Andermann F, et al. The ultrastructural characteristics of the abnormal cytosomes in Batten-Kufs' disease. *Brain.* 1977;100(Pt 1):137–156.
25. Carpenter S, Karpati G. Sweat gland duct cells in Lafora disease: diagnosis by skin biopsy. *Neurology.* 1981;31:1564–1568.
26. Carpenter S. Morphological diagnosis and misdiagnosis in Batten-Kufs disease. *Am J Med Genet Suppl.* 1988;5:85–91.
27. Chan EM, Omer S, Ahmed M, et al. Progressive myoclonus epilepsy with polyglucosans (Lafora disease): evidence for a third locus. *Neurology.* 2004;63:565–567.
28. Chan EM, Young EJ, Ianzano L, et al. Mutations in NHLRC1 cause progressive myoclonus epilepsy. *Nat Genet.* 2003;35:125–127.
29. Crest C, Dupont S, Leguern E, et al. Levetiracetam in progressive myoclonic epilepsy: an exploratory study in 9 patients. *Neurology.* 2004;62:640–643.
30. Dastur DK, Singhal BS, Gootz M, et al. Atypical inclusion bodies with myoclonic epilepsy. *Acta Neuropathol (Berl).* 1966;7:16–25.
31. Daube JR, Peters HA. Hereditary essential myoclonus. *Arch Neurol.* 1966;15:587–594.
32. Davis RL, Holohan PD, Shrimpton AE, et al. Familial encephalopathy with neuroserpin inclusion bodies. *Am J Pathol.* 1999;155:1901–1913.
33. Davis RL, Shrimpton AE, Carrell RW, et al. Association between conformational mutations in neuroserpin and onset and severity of dementia. *Lancet.* 2002;359:2242–2247.
34. D'Azzo A, Hoogeveen A, Reuser AJ, et al. Molecular defect in combined beta-galactosidase and neuraminidase deficiency in man. *Proc Natl Acad Sci U S A.* 1982;79:4535–4539.
35. de Haan GJ, Halley DJ, Doelman JC, et al. Univerricht-Lundborg disease: underdiagnosed in the Netherlands. *Epilepsia.* 2004;45:1061–1063.
36. Diebold K. Four genetic and clinical types of progressive myoclonus epilepsies. *Arch Psychiatr Nervenkr.* 1972;215:362–375.
37. Dolman CL. Atypical myoclonus body epilepsy (adult variant). *Acta Neuropathol (Berl).* 1975;31:201–206.
38. Dorfman LJ, Pedley TA, Tharp BR, et al. Juvenile neuroaxonal dystrophy: clinical, electrophysiological, and neuropathological features. *Ann Neurol.* 1978;3:419–428.
39. Ekbom K. Hereditary ataxia, photomyoclonus, skeletal deformities and lipoma. *Acta Neurol Scand.* 1975;51:393–404.
40. Eldridge R, Iivanainen M, Stern R, et al. "Baltic" myoclonus epilepsy: hereditary disorder of childhood made worse by phenytoin. *Lancet.* 1983;2:838–842.
41. Engel J Jr, Rapin I, Giblin DR. Electrophysiological studies in two patients with cherry red spot–myoclonus syndrome. *Epilepsia.* 1977;18:73–87.
42. Franceschetti S, Uziel G, Di Donato S, et al. Cherry-red spot myoclonus syndrome, and alpha-neuraminidase deficiency: neurophysiological, pharmacological, and biochemical study in an adult. *J Neurol Neurosurg Psychiatry.* 1980;43:934–940.
43. Fukuhara N, Tokiguchi S, Shirakawa K, et al. Myoclonus epilepsy associated with ragged-red fibres (mitochondrial abnormalities): disease entity or a syndrome? Light-and electron- microscopic studies of two cases and review of literature. *J Neurol Sci.* 1980;47:117–133.
44. Ganesh S, Delgado-Escueta AV, Suzuki T, et al. Genotype-phenotype correlations for EPM2A mutations in Lafora's progressive myoclonus epilepsy: exon 1 mutations associate with an early-onset cognitive deficit subphenotype. *Hum Mol Genet.* 2002;11:1263–1271.
45. Genton P, Guerrini R. Antimyoclonic effects of alcohol in progressive myoclonus epilepsy. *Neurology.* 1990;40:1412–1416.
46. Genton P, Malafosse A, Moulard B, et al. Progressive myoclonic epilepsies. In: Roger J, Bureau M, Dravet C, et al., eds. *Epileptic Syndromes in*

Infancy, Childhood and Adolescence. 4th ed. London: John Libbey; 2005: 25.
47. Genton P, Michelucci R, Tassinari CA, et al. The Ramsay Hunt syndrome revisited: Mediterranean myoclonus versus mitochondrial encephalomyopathy with ragged-red fibers and Baltic myoclonus. *Acta Neurol Scand*. 1990;81:8–15.
48. Gentry MS, Worby CA, Dixon JE. Insights into Lafora disease: malin is an E3 ubiquitin ligase that ubiquitinates and promotes the degradation of laforin. *Proc Natl Acad Sci U S A*. 2005;102:8501–8506.
49. Hall NA, Lake BD, Dewji NN, et al. Lysosomal storage of subunit c of mitochondrial ATP synthase in Batten's disease (ceroid-lipofuscinosis). *Biochem J*. 1991;275(Pt 1):269–272.
50. Hallett M. Myoclonus: relation to epilepsy. *Epilepsia*. 1985;26(Suppl 1): S67–77.
51. Haltia M, Kristensson K, Sourander P. Neuropathological studies in three Scandinavian cases of progressive myoclonus epilepsy. *Acta Neurol Scand*. 1969;45:63–77.
52. Hammans SR, Sweeney MG, Brockington M, et al. The mitochondrial DNA transfer RNA(Lys)A–>G(8344) mutation and the syndrome of myoclonic epilepsy with ragged red fibres (MERRF). Relationship of clinical phenotype to proportion of mutant mitochondrial DNA. *Brain*. 1993;116(Pt 3): 617–632.
53. Hammans SR, Sweeney MG, Brockington M, et al. Mitochondrial encephalopathies: molecular genetic diagnosis from blood samples. *Lancet*. 1991;337:1311–1313.
54. Harriman DG, Millar JH, Stevenson AC. Progressive familial myoclonic epilepsy in three families: its clinical features and pathological basis. *Brain*. 1955;78:325–349.
55. Henry TR, Leppik IE, Gumnit RJ, et al. Progressive myoclonus epilepsy treated with zonisamide. *Neurology*. 1988;38:928–931.
56. Hodskins M, Yakovlev P. Anatomico-clinical observations on myoclonus in epileptics and on related symptom complexes. *Am J Psychiatry*. 1930;86:827–848.
57. Ianzano L, Zhang J, Chan EM, et al. Lafora progressive myoclonus epilepsy mutation database-EPM2A and NHLRC1 (EPM2B) genes. *Hum Mutat*. 2005;26:397.
58. Iivanainen M, Himberg JJ. Valproate and clonazepam in the treatment of severe progressive myoclonus epilepsy. *Arch Neurol*. 1982;39:236–238.
59. Iizuka R, Hirayama K, Maehara KA. Dentato-rubro-pallido-luysian atrophy: a clinico-pathological study. *J Neurol Neurosurg Psychiatry*. 1984;47:1288–1298.
60. Kaufman MA, Dwork AJ, Willson NJ, et al. Late-onset Lafora's disease with typical intraneuronal inclusions. *Neurology*. 1993;43:1246–1248.
61. King JO. Progressive myoclonic epilepsy due to Gaucher's disease in an adult. *J Neurol Neurosurg Psychiatry*. 1975;38:849–854.
62. Koide R, Ikeuchi T, Onodera O, et al. Unstable expansion of CAG repeat in hereditary dentatorubral-pallidoluysian atrophy (DRPLA). *Nat Genet*. 1994;6:9–13.
63. Koskiniemi M, Donner M, Majuri H, et al. Progressive myoclonus epilepsy. A clinical and histopathological study. *Acta Neurol Scand*. 1974;50:307–332.
64. Koskiniemi M, Toivakka E, Donner M. Progressive myoclonus epilepsy. Electroencephalographical findings. *Acta Neurol Scand*. 1974;50:333–359.
65. Koskiniemi M. Myoclonus. In: Fahn S, Marsden CD,Van Woert MH, eds. *Advances in Neurology*. New York: Raven Press; 1986:57–64.
66. Kraus-Ruppert R, Ostertag B, Hafner H. A study of the late form (type Lundborg) of progressive myoclonic epilepsy. *J Neurol Sci*. 1970;11:1–15.
67. Kyllerman M, Ben-Menachem E. Zonisamide for progressive myoclonus epilepsy: long-term observations in seven patients. *Epilepsy Res*. 1998;29:109–114.
68. Lafora G, Glueck B. Beitrag zur Histopathologie der myoklonischen Epilepsie. *Z Gesamte Neurol Psychiatr*. 1911;6:1–14.
69. Lafreniere RG, Rochefort DL, Chretien N, et al. Unstable insertion in the 5′ flanking region of the cystatin B gene is the most common mutation in progressive myoclonus epilepsy type 1, EPM1. *Nat Genet*. 1997;15:298–302.
70. Lalioti MD, Scott HS, Antonarakis SE. What is expanded in progressive myoclonus epilepsy? *Nat Genet*. 1997;17:17.
71. Lehesjoki A-E, Koskiniemi M, Sistonen P, et al. Localization of a gene for progressive myoclonus epilepsy to chromosome 21q22. *Proc Natl Acad Sci U S A*. 1991;88:3696–3699.
72. Lehesjoki AE. Molecular background of progressive myoclonus epilepsy. *EMBO J*. 2003;22:3473–3478.
73. Leino E, MacDonald E, Airaksinen MM, et al. L-tryptophan-carbidopa trial in patients with long-standing progressive myoclonus epilepsy. *Acta Neurol Scand*. 1981;64:132–141.
74. Leino E. Open trial with levodopa-carbidopa combination to patients with long-standing progressive myoclonus epilepsy. *Acta Neurol Scand*. 1981;63:389–394.
75. Lowden JA, O'Brien JS. Sialidosis: a review of human neuraminidase deficiency. *Am J Hum Genet*. 1979;31:1–18.
76. Lu CS, Thompson PD, Quinn NP, et al. Ramsay Hunt syndrome and coeliac disease: a new association? *Mov Disord*. 1986;1:209–219.
77. Lundborg H. *Die progressive Myoclonus-Epilepsie (Unverrict's Myoclonie)*. Uppsala: Almqvist and Wiksell; 1903.
78. Magaudda A, Ferlazzo E, Nguyen VH, et al. Unverricht-Lundborg disease, a condition with self-limited progression: long-term follow-up of 20 patients. *Epilepsia*. 2006;47:860–866.
79. Magaudda A, Gelisse P, Genton P. Antimyoclonic effect of levetiracetam in 13 patients with Unverricht-Lundborg disease: clinical observations. *Epilepsia*. 2004;45:678–681.
80. Mahloudji M, Pikielny RT. Hereditary essential myoclonus. *Brain*. 1967;90:669–674.
81. Mancuso M, Galli R, Pizzanelli C, et al. Antimyoclonic effect of levetiracetam in MERRF syndrome. *J Neurol Sci*. 2006;243:97–99.
82. Marsden CD, Harding AE, Obeso JA, et al. Progressive myoclonic ataxia (the Ramsay Hunt syndrome). *Arch Neurol*. 1990;47:1121–1125.
83. Marsden CD, Obeso JA. The Ramsay Hunt syndrome is a useful clinical entity. *Mov Disord*. 1989;4:6–12.
84. Marseille Consensus Group. Classification of progressive myoclonus epilepsies and related disorders. *Ann Neurol*. 1990;28:113–116.
85. Matsuo T, Egawa I, Okada S, et al. Sialidosis type 2 in Japan. Clinical study in two siblings' cases and review of literature. *J Neurol Sci*. 1983;58:45–55.
86. Matthews PM, Berkovic SF, Shoubridge EA, et al. In vivo magnetic resonance spectroscopy of brain and muscle in a type of mitochondrial encephalomyopathy (MERRF). *Ann Neurol*. 1991;29:435–438.
87. May DL, White HH. Familial myoclonus, cerebellar ataxia, and deafness. Specific genetically-determined disease. *Arch Neurol*. 1968;19:331–338.
88. Mikami M, Yasuda T, Terao A, et al. Localization of a gene for benign adult familial myoclonic epilepsy to chromosome 8q23.3-q24.1. *Am J Hum Genet*. 1999;65:745–751.
89. Minassian BA, Lee JR, Herbrick JA, et al. Mutations in a gene encoding a novel protein tyrosine phosphatase cause progressive myoclonus epilepsy. *Nat Genet*. 1998;20:171–174.
90. Mole SE, Williams RE, Goebel HH. Correlations between genotype, ultrastructural morphology and clinical phenotype in the neuronal ceroid lipofuscinoses. *Neurogenetics*. 2005;6:107–126.
91. Mueller OT, Henry WM, Haley LL, et al. Sialidosis and galactosialidosis: chromosomal assignment of two genes associated with neuraminidase-deficiency disorders. *Proc Natl Acad Sci U S A*. 1986;83:1817–1821.
92. Mutoh T, Sobue I, Naoi M, et al. A family with beta-galactosidase deficiency: three adults with atypical clinical patterns. *Neurology*. 1986;36:54–59.
93. Nagafuchi S, Yanagisawa H, Sato K, et al. Dentatorubral and pallidoluysian atrophy expansion of an unstable CAG trinucleotide on chromosome 12p. *Nat Genet*. 1994;6:14–18.
94. Naito H, Oyanagi S. Familial myoclonus epilepsy and choreoathetosis: hereditary dentatorubral-pallidoluysian atrophy. *Neurology*. 1982; 32:798–807.
95. Norio R, Koskiniemi M. Progressive myoclonus epilepsy: genetic and nosological aspects with special reference to 107 Finnish patients. *Clin Genet*. 1979;15:382–398.
96. Obeso JA, Artieda J, Luquin MR, et al. Antimyoclonic action of piracetam. *Clin Neuropharmacol*. 1986;9:58–64.
97. Obeso JA, Artieda J, Rothwell JC, et al. The treatment of severe action myoclonus. *Brain*. 1989;112(Pt 3):765–777.
98. Palmer DN, Fearnley IM, Medd SM, et al. Lysosomal storage of the DCCD reactive proteolipid subunit of mitochondrial ATP synthase in human and ovine ceroid lipofuscinoses. *Adv Exp Med Biol*. 1989;266:211–222; discussion 223.
99. Palmer DN, Martinus RD, Cooper SM, et al. Ovine ceroid lipofuscinosis. The major lipopigment protein and the lipid-binding subunit of mitochondrial ATP synthase have the same NH2-terminal sequence. *J Biol Chem*. 1989;264:5736–5740.
100. Palmeri S, Hoogeveen AT, Verheijen FW, et al. Galactosialidosis: molecular heterogeneity among distinct clinical phenotypes. *Am J Hum Genet*. 1986;38:137–148.
101. Pampiglione G, Harden A. So-called neuronal ceroid lipofuscinosis. Neurophysiological studies in 60 children. *J Neurol Neurosurg Psychiatry*. 1977;40:323–330.
102. Pavlakis SG, Phillips PC, DiMauro S, et al. Mitochondrial myopathy, encephalopathy, lactic acidosis, and strokelike episodes: a distinctive clinical syndrome. *Ann Neurol*. 1984;16:481–488.
103. Pennacchio LA, Bouley DM, Higgins KM, et al. Progressive ataxia, myoclonic epilepsy and cerebellar apoptosis in cystatin B-deficient mice. *Nat Genet*. 1998;20:251–258.
104. Pennacchio LA, Lehesjoki A-E, Stone NE, et al. Mutations in the gene encoding cystatin B in progressive myoclonus epilepsy (*EPM1*). *Science*. 1996;271:1731–1734.
105. Potter NT, Meyer MA, Zimmerman AW, et al. Molecular and clinical findings in a family with dentatorubral-pallidoluysian atrophy. *Ann Neurol*. 1995;37:273–277.
106. Rapin I, Goldfischer S, Katzman R, et al. The cherry-red spot–myoclonus syndrome. *Ann Neurol*. 1978;3:234–242.
107. Rapin I. Myoclonus in neuronal storage and Lafora diseases. In: Fahn S, Marsden CD,Van Woert MH, eds. *Myoclonus*. New York: Raven Press; 1986:65–85.
108. Rapola J, Santavuori P, Savilahti E. Suction biopsy of rectal mucosa in the diagnosis of infantile and juvenile types of neuronal ceroid lipofuscinoses. *Hum Pathol*. 1984;15:352–360.

109. Reutens DC, Puce A, Berkovic SF. Cortical hyperexcitability in progressive myoclonus epilepsy: a study with transcranial magnetic stimulation. *Neurology*. 1993;43:186–192.
110. Roger J, Pellissier JF, Bureau M, et al. [Early diagnosis of Lafora disease. Significance of paroxysmal visual manifestations and contribution of skin biopsy]. *Rev Neurol (Paris)*. 1983;139:115–124.
111. Rosing HS, Hopkins LC, Wallace DC, et al. Maternally inherited mitochondrial myopathy and myoclonic epilepsy. *Ann Neurol*. 1985;17:228–237.
112. Rozdilsky B, Cumings JN, Huston AF. Hallervorden-Spatz disease. Late infantile and adult types, report of two cases. *Acta Neuropathol (Berl)*. 1968;10:1–16.
113. Santavuori P, Rapola J, Sainio K, et al. A variant of Jansky-Bielschowsky disease. *Neuropediatrics*. 1982;13:135–141.
114. Serratosa J, Gomez-Garre P, Gallardo M, et al. A novel protein tyrosine phosphatase gene is mutated in progressive myoclonus epilepsy of the Lafora type (EPM2). *Hum Mol Genet*. 1999;8:345–352.
115. Seyrantepe V, Poupetova H, Froissart R, et al. Molecular pathology of NEU1 gene in sialidosis. *Hum Mutat*. 2003;22:343–352.
116. Shahwan A, Farrell M, Delanty N. Progressive myoclonic epilepsies: a review of genetic and therapeutic aspects. *Lancet Neurol*. 2005;4:239–248.
117. Shannon P, Pennacchio LA, Houseweart MK, et al. Neuropathological changes in a mouse model of progressive myoclonus epilepsy: cystatin B deficiency and Unverricht-Lundborg disease. *J Neuropathol Exp Neurol*. 2002;61:1085–1091.
118. Shibasaki H, Yamashita Y, Neshige R, et al. Pathogenesis of giant somatosensory evoked potentials in progressive myoclonic epilepsy. *Brain*. 1985;108(Pt 1):225–240.
119. Shibasaki H, Yamashita Y, Tobimatsu S, et al. Electroencephalo-graphic correlates of myoclonus. In: Fahn S, Marsden CD,Van Woert MH, eds. *Myoclonus*. New York: Raven Press; 1986:357–372.
120. Shoffner JM, Lott MT, Lezza AMS, et al. Myoclonic epilepsy and ragged-red fiber disease (MERRF) is associated with a mitochondrial DNA $tRNA^{Lys}$ mutation. *Cell*. 1990;61:931–937.
121. Silvestri G, Moraes CT, Shanske S, et al. A new mtDNA mutation in the tRNA(Lys) gene associated with myoclonic epilepsy and ragged-red fibers (MERRF). *Am J Hum Genet*. 1992;51:1213–1217.
122. Smith NJ, Espir ML, Matthews WB. Familial myoclonic epilepsy with ataxia and neuropathy with additional features of Friedreich's ataxia and peroneal muscular atrophy. *Brain*. 1978;101:461–472.
123. So N, Berkovic S, Andermann F, et al. Myoclonus epilepsy and ragged-red fibres (MERRF). 2. Electrophysiological studies and comparison with other progressive myoclonus epilepsies. *Brain*. 1989;112:1261–1276.
124. Steinman L, Tharp BR, Dorfman LJ, et al. Peripheral neuropathy in the cherry-red spot-myoclonus syndrome (sialidosis type I). *Ann Neurol*. 1980;7:450–456.
125. Tassinari CA, Bureau-Paillas M, Dalla Bernardina B, et al. (Lafora disease [author's transl]). *Rev Electroencephalogr Neurophysiol Clin*. 1978;8:107–122.
126. Thibault J. Neuroaxonal dystrophy. A case of non pigmented type and protracted course. *Acta Neuropathol (Berl)*. 1972;21:232–238.
127. Tinuper P, Aguglia U, Pellissier JF, et al. Visual ictal phenomena in a case of Lafora disease proven by skin biopsy. *Epilepsia*. 1983;24:214–218.
128. Tsairis P, Engel WK, Kark P. Familial myoclonic epilepsy syndrome associated with skeletal-muscle mitochondrial abnormalities. *Neurology*. 1973;23:408.
129. Tzoulis C, Engelsen BA, Telstad W, et al. The spectrum of clinical disease caused by the A467T and W748S POLG mutations: a study of 26 cases. *Brain*. 2006;129:1685–1692.
130. Unverricht H. *Die Myoclonie*. Leipzig: Franz Deuticke; 1891.
131. Vaamonde J, Muruzabal J, Tunon T, et al. Abnormal muscle and skin mitochondria in family with myoclonus, ataxia, and deafness (May and White syndrome). *J Neurol Neurosurg Psychiatry*. 1992;55:128–132.
132. Vadlamudi L, Vears DF, Hughes A, et al. Action myoclonus-renal failure syndrome: a cause for worsening tremor in young adults. *Neurology*. 2006;67:1310–1311.
133. van Rootselaar AF, van Schaik IN, van den Maagdenberg AM, et al. Familial cortical myoclonic tremor with epilepsy: a single syndromic classification for a group of pedigrees bearing common features. *Mov Disord*. 2005;20:665–673.
134. Wallace DC, Zheng XX, Lott MT, et al. Familial mitochondrial encephalomyopathy (MERRF): genetic, pathophysiological, and biochemical characterization of a mitochondrial DNA disease. *Cell*. 1988;55:601–610.
135. Warner TT, Williams L, Harding AE. DRPLA in Europe. *Nat Genet*. 1994;6:225.
136. Westmoreland BF, Groover RV, Sharbrough FW. Electrographic findings in three types of cerebromacular degeneration. *Mayo Clin Proc*. 1979;54:12–21.
137. Winkelman MD, Banker BQ, Victor M, et al. Non-infantile neuronopathic Gaucher's disease: a clinicopathologic study. *Neurology*. 1983;33:994–1008.
138. Zeviani M, Amati P, Bresolin N, et al. Rapid detection of the A—G(8344) mutation of mtDNA in Italian families with myoclonus epilepsy and ragged-red fibers (MERRF). *Am J Hum Genet*. 1991;48:203–211.
139. Zhou XY, van der Spoel A, Rottier R, et al. Molecular and biochemical analysis of protective protein/cathepsin A mutations: correlation with clinical severity in galactosialidosis. *Hum Mol Genet*. 1996;5:1977–1987.

CHAPTER 253 ■ POSTTRAUMATIC SEIZURES

FREDERICK G. LANGENDORF, TIMOTHY A. PEDLEY, AND NANCY R. TEMKIN

INTRODUCTION

The risk for epilepsy is increased at least threefold in patients with head injury compared with the general population.[4] Head injury is a major risk factor, comparable with bacterial meningitis, heroin abuse, or a family history of seizures.[32,33] Each year in the United States, about 1.5 million people sustain a traumatic brain injury.[64] Although trauma accounts for only about 5% of all epilepsy cases, this is still a problem of considerable magnitude. More importantly, it is a potentially preventable cause of epilepsy.

The link between head trauma and epilepsy raises a number of important issues. A rational approach to treatment and prevention requires knowledge of the incidence of posttraumatic seizures and the specific aspects of injury that are associated with the development of epilepsy. How should posttraumatic seizures be treated, and is there a role for prophylactic antiepileptic drug therapy? Finally, because seizures develop after a known injury to the brain, posttraumatic seizures offer the opportunity to investigate mechanisms of epileptogenesis.

HISTORICAL PERSPECTIVES

That head injuries could be associated with acute seizures was known to Hippocrates. Duretus (1527–1586) attributed epilepsy in an 18-year-old man to a skull fracture that had occurred 6 years earlier. Head injury appears in 19th-century tabulations of causes of epilepsy, although it ranked well behind fright and masturbation in importance.[61] Modern concepts of head injury and epilepsy derive from studies of British and American veterans of four major 20th-century wars.[11,55]

DEFINITIONS

Implicit in the designation *posttraumatic seizures* is the notion that the injury not only preceded, but also caused the seizures. Posttraumatic seizures are classified as *early* (occurring within 1 week of injury) or *late* (occurring more than 1 week after injury); in some studies "early" encompasses a longer interval, or means the phase of recovery from the acute effects of injury. Early seizures include a subgroup of immediate or impact seizures, which occur at the time of, or immediately after, the injury. Early seizures are acute symptomatic seizures. Late seizures are remote symptomatic seizures; they may be single or multiple. Conventionally, only recurrent late seizures represent *posttraumatic epilepsy*. In practice, posttraumatic seizures and posttraumatic epilepsy are sometimes used interchangeably.

Head injuries have traditionally been divided into two categories: *Penetrating* injuries from "missile" damage (mostly gunshot wounds) and *closed* injuries from "blunt" trauma (mostly caused by falls, motor vehicle accidents, and assaults not involving firearms). There has not been uniform agreement about what constitutes mild, moderate, and severe head injury. *Mild* injury generally excludes evidence of intracranial structural pathology and neurologic abnormalities other than brief loss of consciousness or amnesia. *Severe* injury implies significant structural damage to the brain (either focal or diffuse), or coma, encephalopathy, or amnesia lasting more than 24 hours. Victims of head injury can be stratified more objectively based on the neurologic examination using the Glasgow Coma Scale.[36]

EPIDEMIOLOGY

Head Injury

In the United States, the annual incidence of hospitalization or death from traumatic brain injury is about 100 per 100,000 population.[64,65] Men are more often affected than women. The age-related incidence peaks are in young adults 15 to 24 years of age and in the elderly. Next most affected are young children. The incidence of fatal head injury is about 20 per 100,000. Among survivors of moderate to severe head injury, only about half recover to baseline in such functional domains as home management, financial independence, and social integration.[18] It is estimated that 5.3 million Americans (2% of the population) are living with disability as a result of a traumatic brain injury.[64]

Seizure Studies

It is difficult to establish the incidence of posttraumatic seizures accurately because of a number of methodologic pitfalls. Case ascertainment varies from study to study. For example, head injuries may be noticed only because of a seizure. In some patients, other risk factors for seizures may be present, including pre-existing epilepsy, previous head injury, or alcoholism. Ascribing acute seizures to the effects of brain injury may be confounded by alcohol withdrawal, medication toxicity, or metabolic encephalopathy. In determining the incidence of late posttraumatic seizures, acute symptomatic seizures should be excluded, and the expected incidence of unprovoked seizures occurring in the general population must be taken into account. Many patients are lost to follow-up, and these may not be representative of the study population. As a result of all of these pitfalls, estimates of posttraumatic epilepsy tend to be inflated.

Early Seizures

Early seizures occur in 2% to 5% of all patients with head injuries,[3,15,37] and they are more common in children than adults. After severe head injury, the frequency of early seizures is 10% to 15% for adults and 30% to 35% for children.[3,28,58] Most early seizures occur within 24 hours of injury.

Late Seizures

In the Vietnam Head Injury Study,[55] 53% of veterans who suffered a missile injury eventually experienced at least one seizure, with multiple seizures occurring in the great majority. The relative risk in the first year was 580. In about half the patients, the first seizure occurred within 12 months of injury, but in more than 15% of patients, seizures did not develop until 5 or more years later and the relative risk remained elevated at 10 years. In earlier studies of veterans with military head injuries, late seizures occurred in 35% to 45%.[11]

In Jennett's large series of patients in Oxford and Glasgow who were hospitalized because of nonpenetrating head injury, late seizures occurred in 5%.[34] However, of those patients with severe trauma, late seizures occurred in up to 35%.

In a seminal work, Annegers et al. studied civilian head injury (mostly, but not exclusively, nonpenetrating injury) in Olmsted County, Minnesota, and determined the incidence of late seizures, taking into account the incidence of unprovoked seizures in the general population.[3,4] Children under 15 constituted 38% of the study population. The 5-year cumulative probability of seizures for mild, moderate, and severe injury was 0.7%, 1.2%, and 10%, respectively (Fig. 1). Late seizures occurred in 7.4% of children and 13.3% of adults with severe trauma, with the elderly at still greater risk. The relative risk of late seizures (single or multiple) for mild, moderate, and severe injury was 1.5, 2.9, and 17.0, respectively. After severe injury, about half of the first seizures occurred in the first year, but the risk of a first late seizure remained elevated even 10 years later. After mild injury, this risk had largely subsided at 4 years.

The demonstration (for the first time) of a link between mild head injury and seizures is tempered by the very low relative risk. It follows from a relative risk of 1.5 that an unprovoked seizure following a mild head injury is twice as likely to be unrelated to the injury as it is to be related.

Seizure Recurrence

Early seizures are followed by late seizures in 25% to 35% of adults; early seizures are less predictive of late seizures in children.[3,16,37] The relative risk is in the range of 3 to 5,[4,5,19] but risk factors for early and late seizures are similar, and early seizures did not appear to confer a large independent risk of late seizures in a multivariate analysis.[4]

A first late seizure will have a high risk of recurrence.[3,12,55] In one study of moderately to severely injured patients (penetrating and nonpenetrating) with a first late seizure, recurrence occurred in 47% at 1 month and 86% at 2 years, with at least four additional late seizures in half of these patients.[30]

Immediate seizures have been studied phenomenologically and epidemiologically in Australian rugby players. When not associated with other evidence of significant injury, they appear not to significantly increase the risk for later seizures. They may be no more than a transient symptom of concussion.[45,46]

Risk Factors

For penetrating injury, retained metal fragments, intracranial hematoma, persistent neurologic deficits, and degree of brain volume loss as estimated from computed tomography (CT) images were all associated with increased seizure risk.[55] For nonpenetrating injury, depressed skull fracture and intracranial hematoma (both subdural and intracerebral) are risk factors for both early and late seizures.[4,15,34] Multiple cerebral contusions may place a patient at particularly high risk.[20] The presence of parenchymal blood, whether caused by trauma or stroke,[39] appears to be an important element in the development of seizures. Coma duration and Glasgow Coma Scale score correlate with occurrence of both early and late seizures.[20] There is some controversy as to whether intracerebral hemorrhage[14,16] or severity of diffuse encephalopathy[42] best predicts seizures. Seizures are seen in a higher proportion of abusive injuries than accidental injuries in children; the abusive injuries were more serious by other measures as well.[8]

Genetic influences have long been suspected as a factor in the development of posttraumatic seizures. Although some investigators have reported that a family history of epilepsy is more common in subjects in whom epilepsy does develop following head injury than in those in whom it does not,[12,21] the most careful studies to date were unable to demonstrate any increase in the frequency of seizures among relatives of probands with head injury.[50,56] Similarly, the Vietnam Head Injury Study failed to show any increase in family history of seizures among those in whom posttraumatic epilepsy developed.[55] Despite a lack of evidence, it is possible that genetic susceptibility increases the risk for epilepsy in people with milder injuries, individuals who constitute a small proportion of the posttraumatic seizure population.

The use of seat belts and helmets substantially decreases the severity of brain injuries resulting from bicycle, motorcycle,

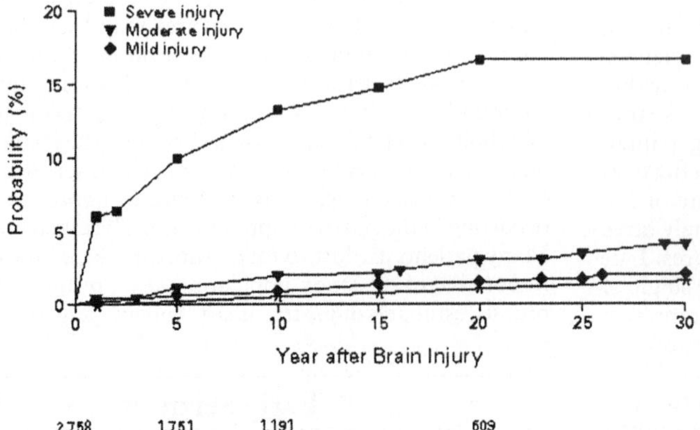

NO. OF PATENTS

Mild injury	2,758	1,751	1,191	609
Moderate injury	1,455	934	660	351
Severe injury	328	181	136	74
Total	4,541	2,866	1,987	1,034

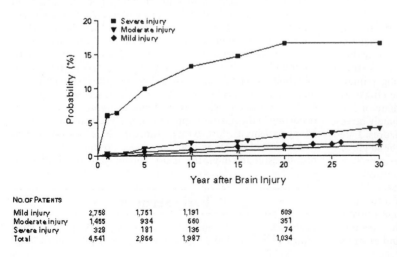

FIGURE 1. Cumulative probability of unprovoked seizures in 4,541 patients with traumatic brain injuries, according to the severity of the injury and the incidence of seizures in the general population. The cumulative incidence in the population was derived from incidence rates with the use of the density method to convert the rates to risk estimates. The *asterisks* indicate the incidence in the general population at specified points in time. (From Annegers JF, Hauser WA, Coan SP, et al. A population-based study of seizures after traumatic brain injuries. *N Engl J Med.* 1998;338:20–24, with permission.)

and automobile accidents.[1,49,63] Although it has not yet been shown directly that these measures also reduce the occurrence of late posttraumatic seizures, a mitigating effect can be assumed. The current proliferation of firearms ominously forecasts an increase in the most severe category of head injury, with a consequent increase in posttraumatic epilepsy. Firearm deaths related to head injury are clearly increasing in the United States.[64]

ETIOLOGY AND BASIC MECHANISMS

Trauma produces many structural, physiologic, and biochemical changes in the brain. Acceleration and rotational forces shear nerve fiber tracts, rupture blood vessels, and produce diffuse axonal injury characterized histologically by gliosis, microglial scar formation, axonal retraction balls, and wallerian degeneration.[25] Both contusions (focal injuries characterized by a mixture of blood, edema, and necrosis) and frank hemorrhage may occur. Damage to the hippocampus, especially the CA1 region, occurs in a high proportion of fatal head injuries[40] and may be important in the development of epilepsy in survivors. Interestingly, Lowenstein et al.[43] demonstrated that even a brief, relatively minor percussive blow to the dura of rats could result in selective hilar cell loss and hyperexcitability of granule cells that may be a necessary substrate for some kinds of partial seizures. In another rat model of head injury, selective hippocampal cell loss (hilus and area CA3), granule cell hyperexcitability, and mossy fiber sprouting could be seen, and these rats demonstrated enhanced susceptibility to seizures.[23] The findings in the hippocampus are similar to those of mesial temporal lobe epilepsy.

Parenchymal blood with subsequent hemosiderin deposition is a major risk factor for epilepsy, and experimental studies have demonstrated that neocortical injection of ferrous or ferric chloride produces focal electroencephalographic (EEG) epileptiform discharges and seizures.[70] The epileptogenic effect of iron is related to the formation of free radicals, and development of seizures can be blocked by antiperoxidant compounds.[27,71,72] The exact mechanisms of this process are unknown. Low levels of hemoglobin-binding protein have been described in families with epilepsy (although not posttraumatic epilepsy).[52] Because individuals with low levels of hemoglobin-binding protein may clear intracerebral blood less efficiently, this could prolong iron exposure and increase the risk for posttraumatic seizures.

In rats, seizures occurring immediately or shortly after traumatic injury are accompanied by increased glutamate and aspartate levels,[48] a finding documented with seizure onset in humans as well.[54] Excitatory amino acids are highly epileptogenic as well as cytotoxic to neurons; these effects can be blocked by *N*-methyl-D-aspartate (NMDA) antagonists.[13] Release of excitatory amino acids may also be responsible for the large, calcium-dependent increase in extracellular potassium seen after experimental brain injury.[38] Increased extracellular potassium further increases neuronal excitability and may contribute to interictal–ictal transitions. It is unlikely, however, that a unitary mechanism for posttraumatic seizures will be found.

That there is generally a latent or "silent" period between the actual brain injury and first seizure has been known since Gowers. It is most likely that trauma initiates a dynamic epileptogenic process that progressively alters neuronal excitability, establishes or obliterates critical interconnections, and perhaps results in critical structural remodeling so that an epileptogenic network of sufficient size is established, resulting in clinical seizures. It is also possible, however, that head injury resets the seizure threshold downward relatively rapidly. In this case, the delay between injury and the first posttraumatic seizure would not necessarily reflect a progressive, evolving process but rather the outer fringe of a probabilistic spread of first seizure latencies.

With head injury (unlike brain tumor), the moment of onset of a potentially epileptogenic process is known with precision. This would allow for the early initiation of neuroprotective agents. There appears to be a critical period for intervention in rats.[24] However, the successful use of antioxidants and NMDA receptor blockers as neuroprotective agents in rats, as mentioned above, has not so far translated into human head injury trials.

CLINICAL PRESENTATION

Seizures caused by head injury have similar semiologies to those occurring in other contexts. Thus, the full spectrum of simple and complex partial seizures as well as generalized tonic–clonic seizures can be seen following head injury. Both cortical ("epileptic") myoclonus[29] and epilepsia partialis continua[62] have been described. Generalized absence seizures probably do not occur as a consequence of head injury.

Because individual patients may have both partial and generalized seizures, it is difficult to estimate the relative frequency of different seizure types with accuracy. Recognized early seizures are predominantly generalized tonic–clonic in type,[15,41,44] particularly seizures on the very first day.[6] A study of continuous EEG monitoring for an average of 1 week after moderate to severe injury revealed electrical seizures without clinical accompaniment in 11 of 94 patients.[66] These subclinical, typically unrecognized seizures could not, however, be temporally correlated with increased intracranial pressure or decreased cerebral perfusion pressure, nor did they predict poorer outcome. The majority of patients with late posttraumatic seizures have at least one generalized tonic–clonic convulsion.[34,55] Perhaps a quarter will have complex partial seizures,[6] though this particular seizure type is probably underrecognized in the head-injured population.

DIAGNOSTIC EVALUATION

Electroencephalographic Findings

Electroencephalography plays only a limited role in the evaluation of early posttraumatic seizures. It is usually most useful in clarifying the basis of intermittent behavioral changes in obtunded or semicomatose patients. It is not of value in predicting the development of posttraumatic epilepsy.[35] The EEG is also less helpful in predicting recurrence after a first late posttraumatic seizure than it is in predicting recurrence after a first idiopathic seizure.[9]

Neuroimaging and Other Laboratory Examinations

The initial diagnostic approach to head trauma is based on the characteristics of the injury and the assessment of the patient's neurologic and general medical status. Patients with moderate or severe head injury require urgent CT imaging. Because intracerebral hemorrhage, subdural hematoma, and hydrocephalus may be delayed, repeated imaging is mandatory in patients who do not improve as expected or deteriorate in the face of appropriate treatment. Development of seizures after the initial CT scan is also an indication for repeated imaging. The role of brain imaging after mild head injury is more controversial, but it is certainly indicated if a seizure occurs or if there is any other unexpected turn in a patient's course. In a large study of adults with mild head injuries,[41] 47% of those with early seizures had intracranial abnormalities; 7% of these required surgical intervention. In a meta-analysis, seizures predicted intracranial pathology in relatively mild injuries.[19] The need for magnetic resonance imaging (MRI) in the acute phase depends on factors other than the presence of seizures.

The first late seizure should be evaluated as any new, unprovoked seizure, including consideration of other etiologies.

DIFFERENTIAL DIAGNOSIS

Fluctuations in level of consciousness and intermittent changes in behavior may pose diagnostic problems, especially in the first 1 to 2 weeks after injury, when patients with severe head injuries are likely to be encephalopathic or otherwise neurologically abnormal. Momentary lapses without other symptoms or signs, emotional outbursts without alteration of consciousness, and attacks of directed violence should not be attributed to seizures. Persistent emotional, cognitive, or behavioral changes are likewise unlikely to be caused by seizure activity. On the other hand, the behavior of an individual with frontal lobe partial seizures may be bizarre, and such seizures are frequently misdiagnosed as nonepileptic events. Even the more typical complex partial seizures may be hard to recognize if they occur in a setting clouded by underlying encephalopathy. Determining which changes may be caused by seizure activity is important for management. Video-EEG monitoring may be necessary for definitive diagnosis in some cases.

Nonepileptic seizures (NESs; also psychogenic seizures, pseudoseizures) can occur in head-injured adults[7,69] and children.[51] Indeed, head injury seems to be a risk factor for NES, though the precipitating head injury is usually minor. Most head-injured NES patients have pre-existing or concomitant psychiatric disorders. Some may be malingering or involved in litigation.

TREATMENT AND OUTCOME

Patients with moderate and severe head injuries are often medically unstable and especially vulnerable to such physiologic consequences of seizures as metabolic acidosis, sudden increases in cerebral blood flow and intracranial pressure, and compromised respiratory function, including pulmonary edema. Convulsive movements may further injure a patient with multiple trauma. Postictal depression complicates neurologic assessment. For these reasons, antiepileptic medication is appealing, at least in the early phase.

Several prospective, randomized, controlled trials[47,53,58,59,73,74] examined the efficacy of antiepileptic drugs in preventing early or late seizures, with mixed results owing to methodologic problems, particularly underpowering. The topic of antiepileptic drug prophylaxis was, for some time, controversial. The most comprehensive studies are those of Temkin et al. In a study of phenytoin in head injury patients at high risk for seizures,[58] phenytoin levels were maintained in the high therapeutic range; side effects were modest.[31] Phenytoin was very effective in suppressing early seizures, with a relative risk of 0.25 at 1 week. However, phenytoin was ineffective in reducing the incidence of late seizures, with no difference between treated and untreated groups at 2 years (Fig. 2). In a second study, valproate was not statistically different from phenytoin in preventing early seizures (though with a trend to less efficacy), but was ineffective late, after 6 months of treatment.[59] For unclear reasons, the valproate group had a trend toward higher mortality. An earlier study found that carbamazepine was also ineffective in preventing development of late seizures.[22] These data imply that although phenytoin, valproate, and carbamazepine are useful *antiseizure* drugs, they do not affect mechanisms involved in the development of posttraumatic epilepsy—they are not *antiepileptogenic* drugs. The situation is similar in patients with other disease processes that promote epileptogenesis, such as brain tumors: long term antiepileptic drug prophylaxis does not prevent the development of a first seizure.

The use of glucocorticoids was examined in the data set of the phenytoin study described above. The early exposure to glucocorticoids did not appear to affect the rate at which late seizures developed.[68] A study of magnesium sulfate has recently been completed. It showed no positive effects on late seizures or neurobehavioral outcome. Almost all participants received phenytoin for the first week, so the early seizure rate was too low to evaluate any effect of magnesium on early seizures.[60]

Recommendations

Patients with severe head injuries should be treated with phenytoin for the first week after injury to minimize complications from seizures occurring during acute management. Phenytoin (or fosphenytoin) should be given intravenously in a dose equivalent to 20 mg/kg; subsequent doses should be adjusted to an unbound ("free") blood level of 2.0 to 2.5 μg/mL. It is not appropriate to continue phenytoin beyond 1 week or the acute phase of injury, if no seizures have occurred, given its neurobehavioral effects.[17] Phenytoin is the drug of choice for preventing and treating early seizures because of its demonstrated efficacy and the availability of an effective formulation for intravenous administration. The hepatic metabolism of phenytoin may be increased and its plasma protein binding decreased in patients with severe head injury.[10,26,75] It is therefore advisable to monitor unbound ("free") phenytoin levels in these patients. While the cause of increased mortality in valproate-treated patients is unclear, it makes valproate a much less attractive alternative to phenytoin. The clearance of valproate in head-injured patients is increased.[2]

In patients who have a single posttraumatic seizure, treatment decisions should be based on the anticipated risk for further seizures. Late seizures follow early posttraumatic seizures no more often than they do a first unprovoked seizure in the general population.[3,9,16,22,37] Thus, long-term antiepileptic drug treatment after early seizures is usually not indicated. In contrast, a first late posttraumatic seizure is usually followed by recurrent seizures, and long-term treatment is usually indicated. There is no settled doctrine on duration of treatment. Antiepileptic drug treatment of early seizures can usually be stopped after a period of weeks or months. Treatment of late seizures, particularly recurrent late seizures, would generally continue for a minimum of 2 years.

Standard antiepileptic medications should all be effective for late seizures; a choice is made as in other contexts, with particular attention to the sedating and behavioral effects of the medications.

Status epilepticus related to head injury is treated in the same manner as in other contexts.

LONG-TERM PROGNOSIS

The same problems that plague incidence studies of late seizures make it difficult to assess prognosis. About half of head-injured patients with late seizures have prolonged remissions,

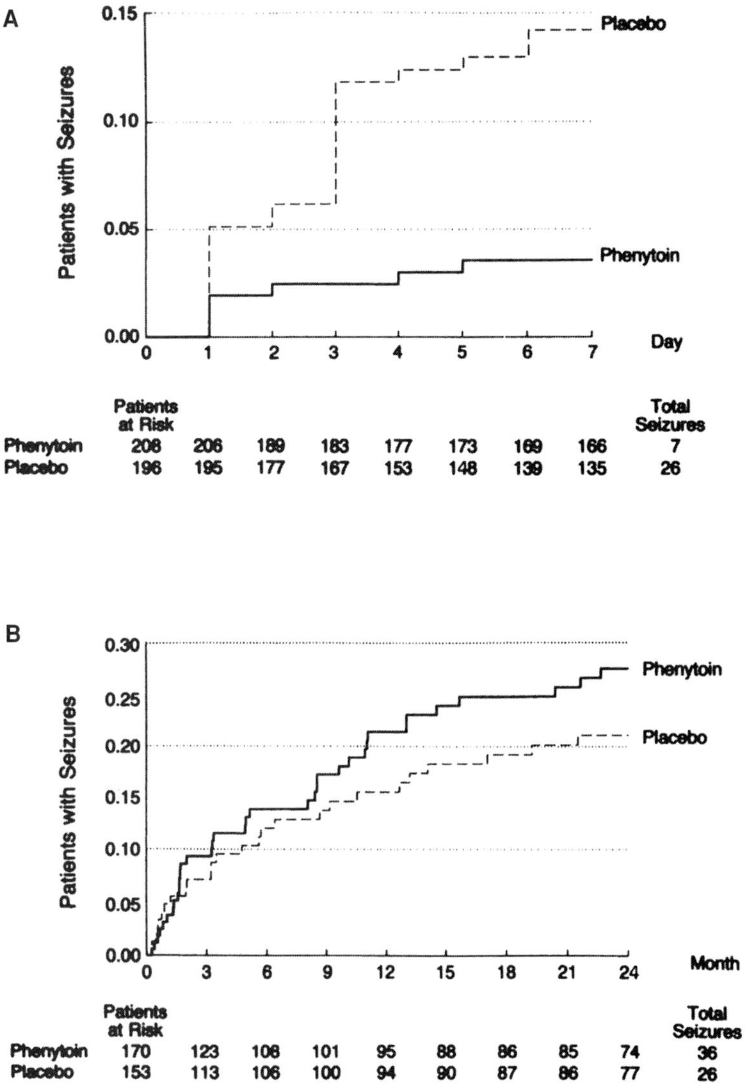

FIGURE 2. Treatment of patients with severe head injury with phenytoin or placebo. Cumulative fraction of patients with early (**A**) or late (**B**) seizures in the two groups. (From Temkin NR, Dikmen SS, Wilensky AJ, et al. A randomized, double-blind study of phenytoin for the prevention of post-traumatic seizures. *N Engl J Med.* 1990;323:497–502, with permission.)

although it is not always clear if patients with early seizures or single seizures were excluded.[12,55,67] Remission rates for epilepsy are somewhat higher (70% or so) in the general population.[32] In the Vietnam Head Injury Study, the average duration of active seizures was 93 months.[55] Intracranial hematoma, partial seizures, and frequent seizures during the first year substantially decrease the chance for extended remission.

SUMMARY AND CONCLUSIONS

Seizures complicate about 50% of penetrating head injuries and about 5% of closed head injuries. Early seizures are related to the acute effects of trauma and are more common in children than adults. The risk for both early and late seizures is increased by depressed skull fracture, intracranial hematoma, and severe encephalopathy. Early seizures increase the likelihood of late seizures, and late seizures have a high recurrence rate. Iron deposition related to hemosiderin, cytotoxic effects of excitatory amino acids, and free radical formation may all play a role in the pathogenesis of posttraumatic seizures. Phenytoin is effective in reducing the chance of early seizures but does not prevent development of posttraumatic epilepsy.

References

1. Agran PF, Dunkle DE, Winn DG. Effects of legislation on motor vehicle injuries to children. *Am J Dis Child.* 1987;141:959–964.
2. Anderson GD, Awan AB, Adams CA, et al. Increases in metabolism of valproate and excretion of 6β-hydroxycortisol in patients with traumatic brain injury. *Br J Clin Pharmacol.* 1998;45:101–105.
3. Annegers JF, Grabow JD, Groover RV, et al. Seizures after head trauma: a population study. *Neurology.* 1980;30:683–689.
4. Annegers JF, Hauser WA, Coan SP, et al. A population-based study of seizures after traumatic brain injuries. *N Engl J Med.* 1998;338:20–24.
5. Asikainen I, Kaste M, Sarna S. Early and late posttraumatic seizures in traumatic brain injury rehabilitation patients: brain injury factors causing late seizures and influence of seizures on long-term outcome. *Epilepsia.* 1999;40:584–589.
6. Barry E, Bergey GK, Krumholz A, et al. Posttraumatic seizure types vary with the interval after head injury. *Epilepsia.* 1997;38(Suppl 8):49–50.
7. Barry E, Krumholz A, Bergey GK, et al. Nonepileptic posttraumatic seizures. *Epilepsia.* 1998;39:427–431.
8. Bechtel K, Stoessel K, Leventhal JM, et al. Characteristics that distinguish accidental from abusive injury in hospitalized young children with head trauma. *Pediatrics.* 2004;114:165–168.
9. Berg AT, Shinnar S. The risk of seizure recurrence following a first unprovoked seizure: a quantitative review. *Neurology.* 1991;41:965–972.
10. Boucher BA, Kuhl DA, Fabian TC, et al. Pharmacokinetics and drug disposition: effect of neurotrauma on hepatic clearance. *Clin Pharmacol Ther.* 1991;50:487–497.
11. Caveness WF, Walker AE, Ascroft PB. Incidence of post-traumatic epilepsy in Korean veterans as compared with those from World War I and World War II. *J Neurosurg.* 1962;19:122–129.

12. Caveness WF. Onset and cessation of fits following craniocerebral trauma. *J Neurosurg*. 1963;10:570–582.
13. Chapman AG, Meldrum BS. Excitatory amino acid antagonists and epilepsy. *Biochem Soc Trans*. 1993;21:106–110.
14. D'Alessandro R, Ferrara R, Benassi G, et al. Computed tomographic scans in post-traumatic epilepsy. *Arch Neurol*. 1988;45:42–43.
15. Desai BT, Whitman S, Coonley-Hoganson R, et al. Seizures and civilian head injuries. *Epilepsia*. 1983;24:289–296.
16. De Santis A, Sganzerla E, Spagnoli D, et al. Risk factors for late post-traumatic epilepsy. *Acta Neurochir*. 1992;55(Suppl):64–67.
17. Dikmen SS, Temkin NR, Miller B, et al. Neurobehavioral effects of phenytoin prophylaxis of posttraumatic seizures. *JAMA*. 1991;265:1271–1277.
18. Dikmen SS, Machamer JE, Powell JM, et al. Outcome 3 to 5 years after moderate to severe traumatic brain injury. *Arch Phys Med Rehabil*. 2003;84:1449–1457.
19. Dunning J, Batchelor J, Stratford-Smith P, et al. A meta-analysis of variables that predict significant intracranial injury in minor head trauma. *Arch Dis Child*. 2004;89:653–659.
20. Englander J, Bushnik T, Duong TT, et al. Analyzing risk factors for late posttraumatic seizures: a prospective, multicenter investigation. *Arch Phys Med Rehabil*. 2003;84:365–373.
21. Evans JH. Post-traumatic epilepsy. *Neurology*. 1962;12:665–674.
22. Glötzner FL, Haubitz I, Miltner F, et al. Epilepsy prophylaxis with carbamazepine in severe brain injuries. *Neurochirurgia*. 1983;26:66–79.
23. Golaria G, Greenwood AC, Feeney DM, et al. Physiologic and structural evidence for hippocampal involvement in persistent seizure susceptibility after traumatic brain injury. *J Neurosci*. 2001;21:8523–8537.
24. Graber KD, Prince DA. A critical period for prevention of posttraumatic neocortical hyperexcitability in rats. *Ann Neurol*. 2004;55:860–870.
25. Graham DI, Adams JH, Gennarelli TA. Pathology of brain damage in head injury. In: Cooper PR, ed. *Head Injury*. 2nd ed. Baltimore: Williams & Wilkins; 1987:72–88.
26. Griebel ML, Kearns GL, Fiser DH, et al. Phenytoin protein binding in pediatric patients with acute traumatic injury. *Crit Care Med*. 1990;18:385–391.
27. Gupta YK, Chaudhary G, Sinha K, et al. Protective effect of resveratrol against intracortical FeCl3-induced model of posttraumatic seizures in rats. *Methods Find Exp Clin Pharmacol*. 2001;23:241–244.
28. Hahn YS, Fuchs S, Flannery AM, et al. Factors influencing post-traumatic seizures in children. *Neurosurgery*. 1988;22:864–867.
29. Hallett M, Chadwick D, Marsden CD. Cortical reflex myoclonus. *Neurology*. 1979;29:1107–1125.
30. Haltiner AM, Temkin NR, Dikmen SS. Risk of seizure recurrence after the first late posttraumatic seizure. *Arch Phys Med Rehabil*. 1997;78:835–840.
31. Haltiner AM, Newell DW, Temkin NR, et al. Side effects and mortality associated with use of phenytoin for early posttraumatic seizure prophylaxis. *J Neurosurg*. 1999;91:588–592.
32. Hauser WA, Hesdorffer DC. *Epilepsy: Frequency, Causes and Consequences*. New York: Demos; 1990.
33. Hauser WA, Annegers JF. Risk factors for epilepsy. In: Anderson VE, Hauser WA, Leppik IE, et al., eds. *Genetic Strategies in Epilepsy Research*. Amsterdam: Elsevier; 1991:45–52.
34. Jennett B. *Epilepsy After Non-Missile Head Injuries*. 2nd ed. Chicago: William Heinemann; 1975.
35. Jennett B, van de Sande J. EEG prediction of post-traumatic epilepsy. *Epilepsia*. 1975;16:251–256.
36. Jennett B, Teasdale G. *Management of Head Injuries*. Philadelphia: FA Davis; 1981.
37. Jennett WB, Lewin W. Traumatic epilepsy after closed head injuries. *J Neurol Neurosurg Psychiatry*. 1960;23:295–301.
38. Katayama Y, Becker DP, Tamura T, et al. Massive increases in extracellular potassium and the indiscriminate release of glutamate following concussive brain injury. *J Neurosurg*. 1990;73:889–900.
39. Kilpatrick CJ, Davis SM, Tress BM, et al. Epileptic seizures in acute stroke. *Arch Neurol*. 1990;47:157–160.
40. Kotapka MJ, Graham DI, Adams JH, et al. Hippocampal damage in fatal paediatric head injury. *Neuropathol Appl Neurobiol*. 1993;19:128–133.
41. Lee S-T, Lui T-N. Early seizures after mild closed head injury. *J Neurosurg*. 1992;76:435–439.
42. Lewis RJ, Yee L, Inkelis SH, et al. Clinical predictors of post-traumatic seizures in children with head trauma. *Ann Emerg Med*. 1993;22:1114–1118.
43. Lowenstein DH, Thomas MJ, Smith DH, et al. Selective vulnerability of dentate hilar neurons following traumatic brain injury: a potential mechanistic link between head trauma and disorders of the hippocampus. *J Neurosci*. 1992;12:4846–4853.
44. Martins da Silva A, Nunes B, Vaz AR, et al. Posttraumatic epilepsy in civilians: clinical and electroencephalographic studies. *Acta Neurochir*. 1992;55(Suppl):56–63.
45. McCrory PR, Bladin PF, Berkovic SF. Retrospective study of concussive convulsions in elite Australian rules and rugby league footballers: phenomenology, aetiology, and outcome. *BMJ*. 1997;314:171–174.
46. McCrory PR, Berkovic SF. Video analysis of acute motor and convulsive manifestations in sport-related concussion. *Neurology*. 2000;54:1488–1491.
47. McQueen JK, Blackwood DHR, Harris P, et al. Low risk of late post-traumatic seizures following severe head injury: implications for clinical trials of prophylaxis. *J Neurol Neurosurg Psychiatry*. 1983;46:899–904.
48. Nilsson P, Ronne-Engstrom E, Flink R, et al. Epileptic seizure activity in the acute phase following cortical impact trauma in rat. *Brain Res*. 1994;637:227–232.
49. Nurchi GC, Golino P, Flaris F, et al. Effect of the law on compulsory helmets in the incidence of head injuries among motorcyclists. *J Neurosurg Sci*. 1987;31:141–143.
50. Ottman R, Lee JH, Risch N, et al. Clinical indicators of genetic susceptibility to epilepsy. *Epilepsia*. 1996;37:353–361.
51. Pakalnis A, Paolicchi J. Psychogenic seizures after head injury in children. *J Child Neurol*. 2000;15:78–80.
52. Panter SS, Sadrzadeh MH, Halloway PE, et al. Hypohaptoglobinemia associated with familial epilepsy. *J Exp Med*. 1985;161:748–754.
53. Pechadre JC, Lauxerois M, Colnet G, et al. Prévention de l'épilepsie post-traumatique tardive par phénytoine dans les traumatismes craniens graves. *Presse Med*. 1991;20:841–845.
54. Ronne-Engstrom E, Hillered L, Flink R, et al. Intracerebral microdialysis of extracellular amino acids in the human epileptic focus. *J Cereb Blood Flow Metab*. 1992;12:873–876.
55. Salazar AM, Jabbari B, Vance SC, et al. Epilepsy after penetrating head injury. I. Clinical correlates: a report of the Vietnam Head Injury Study. *Neurology*. 1985;35:1406–1414.
56. Schaumann BA, Annegers JF, Johnson SB, et al. Family history of seizures in post-traumatic and alcohol-associated seizure disorders. *Epilepsia*. 1994;35:48–52.
57. Smith KR, Goulding PM, Wilderman D, et al. Neurobehavioral effects of phenytoin and carbamazepine in patients recovering from brain trauma: a comparative study. *Arch Neurol*. 1994;51:653–660.
58. Temkin NR, Dikmen SS, Wilensky AJ, et al. A randomized, double-blind study of phenytoin for the prevention of post-traumatic seizures. *N Engl J Med*. 1990;323:497–502.
59. Temkin NR, Dikmen SS, Anderson GD, et al. Valproate therapy for prevention of posttraumatic seizures: a randomized trial. *J Neurosurg*. 1999;91:593–600.
60. Temkin NR, Anderson GD, Winn HR, et al. Magnesium sulfate for neuroprotection after traumatic brain injury: a randomized trial. *Lancet Neurol*. 2007;6:29–38.
61. Temkin O. *The Falling Sickness*. Baltimore: The Johns Hopkins University Press; 1945.
62. Thomas JE, Reagan TJ, Klass DW. Epilepsia partialis continua. A review of 32 cases. *Arch Neurol*. 1977;34:266–275.
63. Thompson RS, Rivara FP, Thompson DC. A case-control study of the effectiveness of bicycle safety helmets. *N Engl J Med*. 1989;320:1361–1367.
64. Thurman DJ, Alverson C, Dunn KA, et al. Traumatic brain injury in the United States: a public health perspective. *J Head Trauma Rehabil*. 1999;14:602–615.
65. Thurman D, Guerrero J. Trends in hospitalization associated with traumatic brain injury. *JAMA*. 1999;282:954–957.
66. Vespa PM, Nuwer MR, Nenov V, et al. Increased incidence and impact of nonconvulsive and convulsive seizures after traumatic brain injury as detected by continuous electroencephalographic monitoring. *J Neurosurg*. 1999;91:750–760.
67. Walker AE, Erculei F. Post-traumatic epilepsy 15 years later. *Epilepsia*. 1970;11:17–26.
68. Watson NF, Barber JK, Doherty MJ, et al. Does glucocorticoid administration prevent late seizures after head injury? *Epilepsia*. 2004;45:690–694.
69. Westbrook LE, Devinsky O, Geocadin R. Nonepileptic seizures after head injury. *Epilepsia*. 1998;39:978–982.
70. Willmore LJ, Sypert GW, Munson JB. Recurrent seizures induced by cortical iron injection: a model of posttraumatic epilepsy. *Ann Neurol*. 1978;4:329–336.
71. Willmore LJ, Rubin JJ. Antiperoxidant pretreatment and iron-induced epileptiform discharges in the rat: EEG and histopathologic studies. *Neurology*. 1981;31:63–69.
72. Willmore LJ. Post-traumatic epilepsy: cellular mechanisms and implications for treatment. *Epilepsia*. 1990;31(Suppl 3):S67–73.
73. Young B, Rapp RP, Norton JA, et al. Failure of prophylactically administered phenytoin to prevent early post-traumatic seizures. *J Neurosurg*. 1983;58:231–235.
74. Young B, Rapp RP, Norton JA, et al. Failure of prophylactically administered phenytoin to prevent late post-traumatic seizures. *J Neurosurg*. 1983;58:236–241.
75. Zielmann S, Mielck F, Kahl R, et al. A rational basis for the measurement of free phenytoin concentration in critically ill trauma patients. *Ther Drug Monit*. 1994;16:139–144.

CHAPTER 254 ■ ISOLATED SEIZURES

PETER WOLF

INTRODUCTION

All epilepsies begin with a first seizure. However, a first seizure does not necessarily mean that epilepsy will develop (Chapters 7 and 122). It may turn out to be an isolated event, symptomatic of some other pathologic condition (Chapter 8), or indicative of an inherent increased risk for development of epilepsy and the need to prevent such development.

This chapter does not deal with the first of these possibilities—the epileptic seizure as an acute symptomatic event—but rather with the second, which is often discussed under the heading of "first unprovoked seizures." The discussion of these has mostly addressed two questions: How probable is it that a first "unprovoked" seizure signifies epilepsy, and should treatment begin after a first seizure? In this literature, treatment is always conceived of as pharmacotherapy, and a thorough definition of seizure provocation is rarely given. Important as these aspects may be, the theoretically more interesting question of nosology—the relation of isolated seizures to the established epileptic syndromes—is asked rarely, if at all, although apart from dealing with the occasional patient in such a situation, physicians hear about isolated seizures perhaps most frequently when taking the family histories of patients with epilepsy.

HISTORICAL PERSPECTIVES

The statement of Gowers[10] that "we have no means of ascertaining, on any considerable scale, the frequency with which a single epileptic fit occurs without successors" clearly shows that he and his contemporaries were quite aware of the possibility of isolated seizures. However, this was not a major concern with the classic epileptologic writers. Apart from the specific subgroup of febrile seizures in infants, isolated seizures mostly were mentioned in epidemiologic and genetic investigations. These were briefly reviewed by Janz[16] in a section on *Gelegenheits-Epilepsien*. His remarkable conclusion was that this is "at the same time the most frequent and mildest form of epilepsy, and the one with the highest rate of heredity."

It was mainly for epidemiologic, prognostic, and similar statistical purposes and quantitative studies of therapy that epilepsy was defined as a minimum of two unprovoked seizures. This definition left isolated seizure events as a separate group that logically—and provided that the diagnosis of an epileptic seizure was reliable—had to be included in the classification of epilepsies and epileptic syndromes.[4] The new International League Against Epilepsy (ILAE) and International Bureau for Epilepsy (IBE) definition of epilepsy as a disorder "characterized by an enduring predisposition to generate epileptic seizures" and requiring "the occurrence of at least one epileptic seizure"[9] gives the possibility in certain instances of coming to a diagnosis of epilepsy even after one seizure, but these cases will probably be the exception rather than the rule.

DEFINITIONS AND NOSOLOGIC PLACE

Isolated seizures can be defined as solitary seizure events that may occur once in a lifetime or very rarely, at lengthy intervals. A seizure event according to this definition would be one single seizure or a short series of two or more seizures in the course of 24 hours, or an isolated episode of status epilepticus.[14]

The best-known type of isolated seizure, febrile convulsions of early childhood, is considered to be a separate entity and is not discussed here.

The relationship of isolated seizures to other epilepsy syndromes has rarely been given much attention, let alone systematically considered. However, it appears that the rare recurrences of seizures in later life among patients with idiopathic localization-related childhood epilepsies are usually isolated generalized tonic–clonic seizures.[19] The same seems to be true for another benign idiopathic epilepsy syndrome, benign familial neonatal convulsions,[22] and isolated seizures may be found in the pedigree of patients with this syndrome.[3]

EPIDEMIOLOGY

Stress convulsions, defined as epileptic attacks in adults exposed to various "stressing" exogenous influences who have not previously had unprovoked epileptic attacks, were diagnosed in 37 of 1,250 patients with convulsive disorders studied during a 13-year period by Laue Friis and Lund.[18] These patients can be considered a subset of the patients discussed here.

Hauser et al.[12] reported 244 patients with a first idiopathic or remote symptomatic seizure. These were drawn from a total of 1,047 patients with newly diagnosed seizures who had been enrolled during a 4 1/2-year period. They compared them with 334 patients who had acute symptomatic seizures and 435 who had had two or more seizures at first diagnosis; 34 patients were excluded from study. After 36 months of follow-up, seizures had recurred in 27% of the persons with only one seizure—that is, in 73%, the seizure had been an isolated event.

In the National General Practice Study of Epilepsy,[23] which was a prospective, population-based cohort study of 1,195 patients with newly diagnosed or suspected epileptic seizures, 220 patients had febrile seizures, and definite epileptic seizures were diagnosed in 564. Of these, 252 were registered at the time of their first seizure, 89 of whom were followed for 3 or more years. Of the latter group, 56% had had a seizure recurrence at 3 years of follow-up—that is, in 44%, the seizure had remained isolated.[11]

The focus of these and similar studies, however, differs slightly but significantly from the subject of this chapter. They were aimed at establishing the risk for recurrence after a first seizure and did not ask whether a second seizure signifies epilepsy or is only the recurrence of an isolated event, or *Gelegenheitsanfall*.

When seizure types are considered, it turns out that in all studies of this matter, generalized tonic–clonic seizures are by far the most frequent type. Percentages ranged between 61% (27% with simple and 10% with complex partial seizures; the remainder were unclassified, although these figures apply only to the cryptogenic group, the semiology of remote symptomatic seizures not being recorded)[12] and 97.5%.[15] This important difference from the usual distribution of seizure types in clinical cohorts is probably attributable to the fact that with minor and less frightening seizures, a physician is frequently not seen after a first seizure, but is seen only later. These cases are frequently lost for studies of first seizures.

However, as Loiseau et al. pointed out, partial seizures also may occur as isolated events, and these have been reported in several studies.[20]

ETIOLOGY AND BASIC MECHANISMS

Apart from the bias toward generalized tonic–clonic seizures, it would appear that these patients are not nosologically homogeneous. Rather, they comprise both a group with an innate risk for development of some type of idiopathic generalized epilepsy and a mixed bag of patients at risk for development of symptomatic localization-related epilepsies of various etiologies.

Of the 564 patients with first seizures in the series of Sander et al.,[23] the seizures of 346 were classified as idiopathic/cryptogenic, those of 119 as remote symptomatic, those of 83 as acute symptomatic, and those of 16 as associated with neurologic deficit.

In the extended follow-up study of Hauser et al.[13] of 208 patients with first seizures, the seizures of 149 were diagnosed as idiopathic and those of 59 as remote symptomatic. There were no acute symptomatic cases in this study.

The prospective cohort of adolescents and adults with first seizures of Wolf[26] comprised 104 patients as of January 31, 2002. Of these, 26 (25%) had a positive family history of epilepsy or febrile convulsions. Febrile convulsions were a previous manifestation of seizure susceptibility in 5 (4.8%), and 1 patient had had benign rolandic epilepsy in childhood. Twenty-five (24%) were photosensitive and thus revealed a trait most frequently seen in association with idiopathic generalized epilepsy syndromes.[24] In an additional 20 (19.2%), the electroencephalogram (EEG) showed some other type of generalized epileptiform discharge. On the other hand, indications of a remote symptomatic etiology were present in 15 (14.4%), and 41 (39.4%) displayed some focal trait (clinical, EEG, or both). In 16 patients (15.4%), no definite indicators of either a focal or a bihemispheric onset were found.

CLINICAL PRESENTATION

There is good reason to assume that the manifestation of epilepsy of any type is often preceded by a stage of increased risk for development of seizures. This risk may be discovered on EEG if for some reason it happens to be performed. More often, risk becomes apparent through a first seizure. In a continuum stretching from no risk through low risk and high risk to active epilepsy, an isolated seizure would identify a person as belonging to a high-risk group for development of any type of epilepsy.

Risk for Relapse

The usual approach to this issue is to define the risk for relapse after a first seizure, which is the inverse expression of the chance of its remaining isolated. The discussion of this risk is highly controversial. The percentages in various recent studies vary from a low of 16% in the first year of follow-up and 27% in 3 years[12] to a maximum of 67% after 1 and 78% after 3 years.[11]

The reasons for these variances are not entirely clear. They could not be explained by differences in therapy. In the study of Annegers et al.,[1] 60.6% of 424 patients received drugs. In cryptogenic ("idiopathic" in the authors' terminology) cases, the relapse rates in patients taking drugs were considerably higher after 3 years (44% vs. 36%) and 5 years (60% vs. 41%), whereas in remote symptomatic cases there was no difference (70% for each group at 3 years and 80% vs. 76% at 5 years). In the Royal College of Physicians Study,[15] 41 of 306 patients (13.4%) had had drugs prescribed by their family doctor or neurologist, and this had no influence on the relapse rate.

It has been suggested that the figures for recurrence in the optimistic studies were unrealistically low because the patients who had already had a second seizure were excluded from them at the onset of a prospective follow-up—thus excluding the group with the highest risk for relapse.[8] This is certainly true, but when Hauser et al.[13] in a second study included such patients who had been excluded from their previous one, only a minor increase in the relapse rate resulted. According to Berg and Shinnar,[2] with retrospective ascertainment, the success of follow-up may depend on the outcome because the patients who have recurrence are easier to find and follow. In addition, they pointed out that in such studies, "the investigator may have little control over the quality of the initial assessment."

A serious methodologic weakness of the British studies showing a high relapse rate is indeed that most[15] or even all[11] patients were not given their diagnoses by the investigators; rather, the diagnoses of other physicians were relied on, and no special precautions were taken to exclude the possibility that a patient with a first major seizure leading to a diagnosis had previously been subject to minor seizures. Some of these, such as absences, myoclonic seizures in juvenile myoclonic epilepsy, or isolated auras, can easily escape the attention of an inexperienced observer. In the study of Sander et al.,[23] which relied on information collected by general practitioners, only 3% of 564 patients with "definite epileptic seizures" were given diagnoses of "true absences or myoclonic jerks with or without generalized tonic–clonic seizures." Obviously, these diagnoses were frequently missed, as can also be seen in another article from the same investigation.[21] In this study of 1,195 primarily registered patients, only 9% were excluded because it was determined that they had already had seizures. In contrast, in the investigation of Hauser et al.,[13] who are the only authors who discussed this problem and provided for it, 74% of patients "with newly identified unprovoked seizures had experienced multiple seizure episodes prior to their first medical contact"; these authors even excluded 13 patients referred by neurologists after a "first seizure" because a history of complex partial seizures had been overlooked—a diagnosis that would be thought hard to miss. It cannot be ruled out and seems even probable that the studies reporting high relapse rates comprise an unknown and potentially large number of patients with established but undiagnosed epilepsy.

Several studies have tried to identify subgroups with higher and lower risks for relapse. Hauser et al.[12] reported that risk was significantly higher in patients with remote symptomatic than with cryptogenic seizures. In the latter group, it was increased if the patients had generalized slow-wave activity in the EEG ($n = 13$) but not focal EEG abnormalities ($n = 61$). (These results may very well be a question of numbers.) Risk was increased if patients had a sibling with seizures ($n = 17$) but not a parent with seizures ($n = 6$).

Annegers et al.[1] found that the risk increased for patients whose seizures had a presumed etiology, and among their "idiopathic" (cryptogenic) cases, EEG abnormalities, neurologic findings, and initial partial seizures were significant independent predictors of higher recurrence risks.

In the study of Hopkins et al.,[15] the only clinical variable associated with recurrence was seizure occurrence between midnight and 9:00 AM.

According to Hauser et al.,[13] the risk for recurrence was increased by the history of an identified insult to the central nervous system. Further factors in cryptogenic cases were generalized slow-wave activity in the EEG, a history of acute symptomatic seizures, and a sibling with epilepsy; in remote symptomatic cases, they were a history of acute symptomatic seizures, a history of status epilepticus or multiple seizures, and Todd's paresis.

In the National General Practice Study,[11] the risk was increased when the age at first seizure was <16 or >59 years, when a neurologic deficit was presumed present at birth, or when the first seizure was simple or complex partial. (Seizures of partial onset evolving to generalized tonic–clonic seizures seem in this study for unexplained reasons to have been lumped together with primarily generalized tonic–clonic seizures.) The risk was decreased in this study when the seizure was precipitated acutely by an insult to the brain (occurring within 3 months) or by alcohol. In this same study, relative risks are given for many subgroups (etiology, seizure type, age, index seizure first, or subsequent seizure).

Donselaar et al.[5] found that against an overall 2-year risk for relapse of 40% in 151 patients, 15 of 16 patients with epileptiform discharge in the standard EEG and 12 of 19 additional patients with discharge in the EEG after sleep deprivation had a relapse. They concluded that "the decision to initiate or delay treatment should be based on EEG findings." In this investigation, however, no particular efforts were made to exclude a history of minor seizures, and no steps were taken to ensure that the epileptiform EEG activity was only subclinical. Especially in the case of generalized spike-and-wave discharges, absences may be difficult to rule out. Sometimes this requires a video-EEG investigation with tests of reaction and awareness, which were not part of this study.

In the study of Wolf,[26] in which all measures, including those mentioned in the preceding paragraph, were taken to exclude preexisting epilepsy with difficult-to-diagnose seizures, the relapse rate was not influenced by EEG, antecedents, or focal versus generalized seizure onset.

Of course, the ultimate question behind these studies is not how often a second seizure occurs, and the concept of "isolated seizures" is not identical to the concept of one single seizure in a whole lifetime. The substantial question is how often epilepsy develops. However, most studies stop at the second seizure, probably because two unprovoked seizures, in studies of epidemiology and therapy, are often considered sufficient for a diagnosis of epilepsy, and "unprovoked" is frequently understood to mean no indication of an acute symptomatic background.

Elwes et al.,[7] however, looked at retrospective sequences of up to five initial generalized tonic–clonic seizures in 183 patients. They found that the intervals between seizures of 82 patients with more than two seizures decreased in 48 individuals, did not change in 16, and increased in 18. They concluded that "in many patients ... an accelerating disease process may occur at least in the early stages." However, they also believed that this was not an invariable phenomenon, and "as well as processes of acceleration of epilepsy the brain may generate processes of remission."

Donselaar et al.[5] investigated the outcome of 58 of 151 patients with an idiopathic first seizure and no drug treatment who had had a relapse during the 2 following years. Of these, 6 had no further seizures although they remained untreated, 25 were started on drug treatment immediately after their second seizure, and 26 were started on drugs following additional seizures. One patient refused drugs despite several recurrences and was excluded. Forty patients (70%) became seizure free (including the aforementioned untreated 6), and 17 (30%) continued to have seizures—only sporadically in 8 cases.

An analysis of factors influencing the risk for relapse after a first seizure would thus suggest that a variety of candidate factors exist, some of which have reached statistical significance in some studies and some in others. None of them is surprising, and none would sort out isolated seizures in any specific way. Rather, they seem to corroborate the conclusion of the previous nosologic considerations that across epileptic syndromes, isolated seizures characterize a group of patients with an increased relative risk for the development of seizures and, eventually, some specific syndrome.

The question arises whether this risk can be enhanced by any specific or nonspecific precipitating factors. The more important the influence of nonspecific precipitating factors, the closer we come to the concept of isolated seizures, and the more important the influence of specific precipitating factors, the closer we come to the concept of reflex epilepsies.

Provocation of Isolated Seizures

Provocation of the first seizure is an aspect not uniformly dealt with in the literature. Some studies exclude all provoked seizures, others some, and still others none. More important, there is no uniform definition of seizure provocation. Seizures occurring "in the context of uncertain precipitants such as sleep deprivation or 'stress' were considered unprovoked" by Hauser et al.[13]

Sander et al.[23] stated that "the circumstances of the ... first seizure [in 252 cases] were explored but did not suggest any striking precipitating factors"—a surprising statement from an investigation that did not include any expert interviews and had therefore no means to look into this question seriously.

Others[16,17,25] consider lack of sleep as a potent and common seizure precipitant. Even if many of the provoking factors have not yet been discovered, some epileptologists could imagine that provocation of seizures is the rule.[6]

In addition to such nonspecific provocative or facilitating factors of seizures, the role of specific sensory precipitants has received little attention in the literature, although early identification of such risk factors for the development of reflex epilepsy is, of course, important.

In the most recent update of the follow-up study of Wolf,[26] on January 31, 2002, at least one facilitating or precipitating factor could be identified in 80 of 104 patients (Table 1), and this knowledge was used therapeutically (see later discussion). In only 10 patients (9.6%) was the seizure unprovoked beyond suspicion.

Epilepsy Evolving From a First Seizure

Berg and Shinnar[2] tried to distinguish methodologically between "first-seizure" studies and "new-onset epilepsy" studies, but this distinction is not always as clear as these authors would have us believe. All epilepsy starts with a first seizure, and it is a mere convention when physicians start to call a condition *epilepsy*. It is surprising to see what little attention the question

TABLE 1

FACILITATING OR PRECIPITATING FACTORS OF FIRST SEIZURE IN LIFE IN 104 ADOLESCENTS AND ADULTS

Nonspecific (facilitating)		
Disturbances of the sleep–wake cycle	69	(66.3%)
Extraordinary physical or emotional stress	23	(22.0%)
Acute excessive intake of alcohol	11	(10.6%)
Fever, infectious disease	3	(2.9%)
Hunger, hypoglycemia	3	(2.9%)
Miscellaneous (migraine, hyperhydration)	3	(2.9%)
Specific (precipitating or reflex epileptic)		
Intermittent lights (environmental) and television	14	(13.5%)
Video games, praxis induction	4	(4.8%)
Other specific movement, complex visual)	2	(2.0%)
Questionable	14	(13.5%)
No probable or suspected factors	10	(9.6%)

of how epilepsy evolves from a first seizure has received from modern writers.

Not much progress seems to have been made since Gowers,[10] who, in his chapter on the course of epilepsy, differentiated three modes of onset. The first is:

> by minor seizures which occur alone for months and years before there are severe attacks.... The second mode of commencement is by severe fits recurring at short intervals, without any preceding *petit mal*.... The third mode of onset is with a single severe fit, and no other fit or sign of epilepsy for months and even years, when another attack occurs, after which they usually become frequent. Between the last two forms there is every gradation of varying interval between the first and second fit.

The situation addressed in this chapter clearly is closest to the third mode of onset.

Elwes et al.[7] pointed out the possible interaction of factors of "acceleration" and remission in the development of epilepsy, and according to Janz,[17] the development of epilepsy with grand mal on awaking is characterized by a shift from initial seizures with clearly exogenous precipitating factors to a much more spontaneous mode of seizure recurrence. Would it, then, be possible to prevent the development of at least this particular type of epilepsy by "isolating" the first one or few seizures by preventing further recurrences? This question is discussed later.

DIAGNOSTIC EVALUATION

The first and immediate question to be answered after a first epileptic seizure is whether it was the symptom of an acute or undiscovered progressive illness. Alcoholic and other toxic/metabolic causes have to be ruled out. The diagnostic program, beyond history and physical investigation, normally comprises the usual tests for exclusion of an acute inflammatory disorder; the EEG, mainly in view of possible signs of acute conditions such as encephalitis or metabolic-toxic disorders, or indicators of existing epilepsy or such specific traits as photosensitivity; and magnetic resonance imaging (MRI), now the most reliable method for detecting any morphologic changes. Only if MRI is unavailable or in case of emergency would computerized tomography (CT) be performed.

DIFFERENTIAL DIAGNOSIS

Frequently, when a first seizure takes everybody by surprise, there is little reliable information about what really has happened. Often there is no witness at all, or only a fraction of the seizure has been seen, perhaps by a poor observer. Patients may give the most important clues when they remember a typical—epileptic or vasomotor—aura. Indirect indicators of an epileptic seizure are a sudden fall without an aura, lateral tongue biting and enuresis (infrequent!), a slow recovery with Todd's paresis, feelings of physical exhaustion or muscular aches, and periocular petechiae. It is better to leave the diagnosis unresolved when the obtainable information is poor than to jump to rapid conclusions and take incorrect therapeutic measures. When a seizure is unmistakably a generalized tonic–clonic seizure, it is extremely important to remember that a first convulsive seizure may be just the tip of an iceberg and that minor seizures may long have been present. Intense, pointed, knowledgeable, and sometimes repeated questioning is often required. Isolated epileptic auras and absences are the types that most frequently go unnoticed by patients and relatives, and the jerks of juvenile myoclonic epilepsy are the type that physicians most often forget to ask about. They are practically never volunteered by patients, who usually are unaware that they are a pathologic phenomenon.

The EEG may be an important indicator of established epilepsy. Seemingly subclinical groups of bilateral spikes-and-waves require intensive monitoring, including video registrations and cognitive tests (tapping, counting, response to an acoustic stimulus), to be sure that they do not represent actual seizures. It is quite amazing how many patients with a presumed first seizure actually have epilepsy!

TREATMENT AND OUTCOME

After a first seizure, "secondary prevention" rather than "therapy" seems the appropriate term for the recommended interventions because no disease has yet developed. The controversial question of whether antiepileptic pharmacotherapy should be recommended after a first seizure is discussed in Chapter 122.

In the longitudinal investigation of Wolf,[26] the only systematic interventions were the detailed and close instructions given to patients regarding avoidance of precipitating factors that had been identified individually. These were given verbally to patients and, if at all possible, to relatives or friends. In addition, patients received a printed memorandum (Table 2) explaining the significance of a single epileptic seizure, the risk for development of epilepsy, and the necessity and principles of preventing recurrences.[25] The question of drugs was not treated dogmatically. Possible benefits and risks of available antiepileptic drugs were explained, as well as the necessity, if drugs were to be given, of regular intake for a period of at least 2 years. The patients were invited to make their own choice regarding drug treatment. However, if no precipitating factor for the seizure could be defined, drug treatment was recommended. Of the 104 patients in this study, 29 (27.9%) were already taking some antiepileptic drug at enrollment, and these all chose to continue taking drugs for variable periods of time.

As of January 31, 2002, 87 patients of this cohort had been followed for a minimum of 12 months and a maximum of 10 years. Because 35 of these patients had already had more than one seizure when they were enrolled, the expected number of recurrences in the first year of follow-up was 35.7 (41%),

TABLE 2

ITEMS TO BE DISCUSSED WITH PATIENT AND HANDED OUT IN PRINT

Single seizures (*Gelegenheitsanfälle*) do not yet mean the diagnosis is epilepsy.
They indicate a high risk that epilepsy will develop unless preventive measures are taken.
Every additional seizure is one step in the development of epilepsy.
A special danger with seizures is the risk for accidents; even a single seizure means temporary unfitness for driving.
Drug treatment is not always necessary but may be advisable, depending on the individual circumstances.
Several antiepileptic drugs are available; they are usually well tolerated, but no effective drug is without possible untoward effects.
Even in the best case, drug treatment has to be pursued for several years, and regular intake every day is necessary; missed doses mean a risk for withdrawal seizures.
In most instances, first seizures do not occur "out of the blue sky" but are precipitated by factors such as disturbances of the sleep–wake cycle; recurrences can often be prevented by control of precipitating factors.
Rules to be followed concerning the use of alcohol.
Rules to be followed concerning sleep–wake habits on workdays and holidays. Night shifts must be discontinued, if applicable.
Rules to be followed concerning specific precipitating mechanisms (e.g., photosensitivity).

calculated from the respective risk rates reported by Hart et al.[11] for patients with one and with more than one seizure (Table 3). A slightly higher rate would have been expected from Hauser et al.,[13] who estimated the recurrence rate after more than one seizure to be greater than 65%. In contrast, the observed rate was 15, or 17%. Sixty-three of these patients had been followed for at least 2 years, and 6 cases of recurrence were observed in the second year. Forty-six patients were followed for at least 3 years, and another 5 recurrences were observed in the third year. The majority of recurrences were provoked by factors similar to those associated with the previous seizure, and this was true for all of the few recurrences after >3 years. Spontaneously recurrent seizures requiring treatment, that is, epilepsy, developed in 13 patients (15% of those followed for at least 1 year), 2 with a diagnosis of idiopathic generalized epilepsy, 1 with an idiopathic focal epilepsy (a remanifestation at age 33 years after a history of probable childhood rolandic epilepsy), 2 with generalized tonic–clonic seizures without clear focal or generalized signs, 1 with both generalized and focal signs, and 7 with symptomatic or cryptogenic focal epilepsy. Considering that 42 of these patients at onset presented with generalized signs and symptoms, 27 with focal ones, and 18 could not be assigned to either category, a relapse in the presence of focal features is more likely to indicate the establishment of epilepsy, whereas in the presence of generalized features it is more likely to represent another isolated seizure or *Gelegenheitsanfall.*

TABLE 3

CALCULATED AND OBSERVED RECURRENCES IN FIRST YEAR OF FOLLOW-UP IN PATIENTS WHOSE TREATMENT CONSISTED OF AVOIDING PRECIPITATING FACTORS

Fifty-Two patients with 1 seizure expected rate of 37%	19.2
Thirty-five patients with >1 seizure expected rate of 47%	16.5
Total recurrences expected	35.7 (41%)
Total recurrences observed	15 (17%)

Eighty-seven patients were followed for ≥1 year; the expected rates of recurrence are according to Hart et al.[11]

It can therefore be concluded that appropriate preventive measures taken after first seizures, including the avoidance of specific and nonspecific precipitating factors and, probably, administration of antiepileptic drugs in selected cases, can be highly successful in keeping seizures isolated and preventing the transition to epilepsy, especially in the patients who are at risk of developing an idiopathic generalized type of epilepsy.

LONG-TERM PROGNOSIS

In the majority of cases, the question of whether a first seizure will remain isolated or mark the onset of epilepsy is resolved within 1 to 2 years. If by then epilepsy has not developed, a good prognosis can be expected. The data from existing studies do not indicate that epilepsy is likely to develop once this period of time has elapsed after one or a few isolated seizures. On the other hand, there are sufficient observations of late recurrences of isolated seizures to indicate that the increased risk for seizures is lifelong (see also Chapter 7).

SUMMARY AND CONCLUSIONS

A first seizure may signify the onset of epilepsy, but it may also remain an isolated event. Isolated seizures can be defined as solitary seizure events that may occur once in a lifetime or very rarely, at lengthy intervals. In the literature, the most common approach is to define the risk for recurrence after a first seizure, which is the inverse expression of the chance of its remaining isolated. However, most studies of first seizures analyze recurrence risk but not the development of epilepsy with ongoing seizures. Therefore, the epidemiology of isolated seizures cannot be definitely determined at present. Their relation to other epileptic syndromes has never been systematically investigated. Isolated seizures, apart from the febrile seizures of early childhood, may not be a separate syndrome, but rather they may represent, across syndromes, the group of patients having the most benign course and the lowest risk for seizures.

In studies of first seizures, by far the most common seizure type is generalized tonic–clonic. The most important and often rather difficult diagnostic task, besides exclusion of an acute symptomatic or progressive etiology, is to make sure that the patient does not already have epilepsy, hitherto manifested only as unrecognized minor seizures. Once this possibility is safely ruled out, the therapeutic aim is the secondary prevention of epilepsy in those patients who, by having had a first seizure, can be identified as individuals with a clearly increased risk for epilepsy.

The indication for antiepileptic drug treatment after an isolated seizure is controversial. An often neglected aspect is the precipitation of isolated seizures by specific or nonspecific factors. Control of these seems to be the most important therapeutic intervention, and it drastically reduces the risk for recurrence, especially in patients with a risk of idiopathic generalized epilepsy.

References

1. Annegers JF, Shirts SB, Hauser WA, et al. Risk of recurrence after an initial unprovoked seizure. *Epilepsia.* 1986;27:43–50.
2. Berg AT, Shinnar S. The risk of recurrence following a first unprovoked seizure: a quantitative review. *Neurology.* 1991;41:965–972.
3. Berkovic SF, Reutens DC, Andermann E, et al. The epilepsies: specific syndromes or a neurobiological continuum. In: Wolf P, ed. *Epileptic Seizures and Syndromes.* London: John Libbey; 1994:25–37.
4. Commission on Classification and Terminology of the International League Against Epilepsy. A revised proposal for the classification of epilepsies and epileptic syndromes. *Epilepsia.* 1989;30:268–278.
5. Donselaar CA van, Geerts AT, Schimsheimer RJ. Idiopathic first seizure in adult life: who should be treated? *Br Med J.* 1991;302:620–623.
6. Dreifuss FE. Current problems of the international seizure classification being addressed by the ILAE Commission on Classification and Terminology. In: Wolf P, ed. *Epileptic Seizures and Syndromes.* London: John Libbey; 1994:21–23.
7. Elwes RDC, Johnson AL, Reynolds EH. The course of untreated epilepsy. *Br Med J.* 1988;297:948–950.
8. Elwes RDC, Reynolds EH. Should people be treated after a first seizure? *Arch Neurol.* 1988;45:490–491.
9. Fisher RS, van Emde Boas W, Blume W, et al. Epileptic seizures and epilepsy: definitions proposed by the International League Against Epilepsy (ILAE) and the International Bureau for Epilepsy (IBE). *Epilepsia.* 2005;46:470–472.
10. Gowers WR. *Epilepsy, and Other Chronic Convulsive Diseases.* London: Churchill; 1881.
11. Hart YM, Sander JWAS, Johnson AL, et al. National General Practice Study of Epilepsy. *Lancet.* 1990;336:1271–1274.
12. Hauser WA, Anderson VE, Loewenson RB, et al. Seizure recurrence after a first unprovoked seizure. *N Engl J Med.* 1982;307:522–528.
13. Hauser WA, Rich SS, Annegers JF, et al. Seizure recurrence after a first unprovoked seizure: an extended follow-up. *Neurology.* 1990;40:1163–1170.
14. Heintel H. *Status Epilepticus. Etiology, Clinical Aspects, and Lethality. A Clinical-Statistical Analysis.* Stuttgart: Gustav Fischer; 1972.
15. Hopkins A, Garman A, Clarke C. The first seizure in adult life. *Lancet.* 1988;1:721–726.
16. Janz D. *Die Epilepsien. Spezielle Pathologie und Therapie.* Stuttgart: Thieme; 1969.
17. Janz D. Pitfalls in the diagnosis of grand mal on awakening. In: Wolf P, ed. *Epileptic Seizures and Syndromes.* London: John Libbey; 1994:213–220.
18. Laue Friis M, Lund M. Stress convulsions. *Arch Neurol.* 1974;31:155–159.
19. Loiseau P,Duché B, Cohadon S. The prognosis of benign localized epilepsy in early childhood. In: Degen R,Dreifuss FE, eds. *Localized and Generalized Epilepsies of Early Childhood.* Amsterdam: Elsevier; 1992:75–82.
20. Loiseau P, Jallon P, Wolf P. Isolated partial seizures of adolescence. In: Roger J, Bureau M, Dravet C, et al., eds. *Epileptic Syndromes in Infancy, Childhood and Adolescence,* 4th ed. Montrouge, France: John Libbey; 2005:359–362.
21. Manford M, Hart YM, Sander JWAS, et al. National General Practice Study of Epilepsy: the syndromic classification of the International League Against Epilepsy applied to epilepsy in a general population. *Arch Neurol.* 1992;49:801–808.
22. Plouin P. Benign idiopathic neonatal convulsions (familial and nonfamilial). In: Roger J, Bureau M, Dravet C, et al., eds. *Epileptic Syndromes in Infancy, Childhood and Adolescence,* 2nd ed. London: John Libbey; 1992:3–11.
23. Sander JWAS, Hart YM, Johnson AL, et al. National General Practice Study of Epilepsy: newly diagnosed epileptic seizures in a general population. *Lancet.* 1990;336:1267–1271.
24. Wolf P, Goosses R. Relation of photosensitivity to epileptic syndromes. *J Neurol Neurosurg Psychiatry.* 1986;49:1386–1391.
25. Wolf P. Der erste epileptische Anfall bei Jugendlichen und Erwachsenen. *Epilepsie-Blätter.* 1993;3:59–64.
26. Wolf P. Nonmedical treatment of first epileptic seizures in adolescence and adulthood. *Seizure.* 1995;4:87–94.

CHAPTER 255 ■ FAMILIAL PARTIAL (FOCAL) EPILEPSY WITH VARIABLE FOCI

ELIANE KOBAYASHI, FRÉDÉRICK ANDERMANN, AND EVA ANDERMANN

INTRODUCTION

Familial partial (focal) epilepsy with variable foci (FPEVF) is a distinct syndrome among the familial partial epilepsies, in that different clinical and electroencephalographic (EEG) features can be observed in different family members, suggesting that different epileptic foci may be determined by the same genetic mutation. On the other hand, the epileptic focus in any one individual remains the same.

Recently, FPEVF was included in the new diagnostic scheme for epileptic syndromes proposed by the International League Against Epilepsy (ILAE). Although it is displayed as a syndrome in development, this inclusion supports its uniqueness.[8]

HISTORICAL PERSPECTIVES

FPEVF is a unique syndrome first reported in 1998 in an Australian kindred by Scheffer et al,[28] and in the following year in two French–Canadian kindreds by Xiong et al.[36] Other more homogeneous familial partial epilepsy syndromes, including autosomal-dominant nocturnal frontal lobe epilepsy (ADNFLE),[27] familial temporal lobe epilepsy (FTLE),[1a,2] and autosomal-dominant partial epilepsy with auditory features (ADPEAF)[21] had been described (reviewed in Andermann et al.[1]). To date, only 10 pedigrees of FPEVF have been identified and reported in the literature.[3,4,25,28,35,36]

DEFINITIONS

Due to its uniqueness, FPEVF can only be defined on the basis of family rather than individual phenotypes. The occurrence of at least two different partial epilepsy syndromes in first- and second-degree relatives with no identifiable structural brain abnormality and segregating in a sufficient number of individuals in more than one generation is suggestive of FPEVF. Nevertheless, it has to be highlighted that, since the first report by Scheffer and colleagues,[28] many small families have been ascertained that could indeed have represented FPEVF, but both the diagnosis and the inheritance pattern could not be definitely confirmed.

EPIDEMIOLOGY

FPEVF kindreds have been identified in Australia, Canada, Spain, Holland and other European countries. Three of the 10 families are French-Canadian, originating from the region around Quebec City and sharing the same haplotype on chromosome (chr) 22q, suggesting a founder effect (Figs. 1 and 2).[3,35] Figure 2 demonstrates that a Spanish family has a completely different haplotyes than the French-Canadian families. Several small families have also been identified in the Eastern Townships region of Quebec, where linkage to the same region on chr22 is suggested, but these families have a different haplotype (P. Cossette, personal communication). Another Spanish family, which links to chr22, has also been described.[19] This family originates from a different region of Spain and has a different haplotype from the first Spanish family (J. Serratosa, personal communication).

Due to the variable seizure pattern among affected family members and the usually benign clinical outcome, FPEVF might often be underdiagnosed, as is the case for other familial partial epilepsy syndromes. It seems to be less frequent than other familial partial epilepsies, but, in the absence of genetic confirmation, it is impossible to estimate its frequency at present.

ETIOLOGY AND BASIC MECHANISMS

In terms of etiology, it should again be emphasized that only 10 pedigrees have been reported in the literature.[3,4,25,28,35,36] All are compatible with an autosomal-dominant inheritance pattern with approximately 70% penetrance. Two different loci have been associated with FPEVF, the first with suggestive linkage on chr 2q,[28] and the second on chr 22q.[36] However, the gene(s) have not been cloned. Only one reported kindred had suggestive linkage to chr 2q,[28] but the family was not large enough to confirm linkage. Although linkage to chr 22q has now been confirmed in six families,[3,4,19,35,36] the gene has not been identified. Sequencing with mutation analysis has excluded the coding regions of >60 genes in the region on chr22q (A. Kerstin Lindblad-Toh, personal communication).

The mechanisms by which these molecular abnormalities can present as different types of idiopathic partial epilepsy within the same family are intriguing. Modifying genes and environmental factors should be further investigated.

CLINICAL PRESENTATION

In FPEVF, affected family members may present with different types of partial epilepsy, which are, however, invariable within each subject. Frontal lobe seizures are the most frequent manifestation, but they have a different pattern in FPEVF as compared to that observed in ADNFLE (Table 1): The seizures are less frequent, clusters and auras are rare, and daytime seizures as well as secondarily generalized seizures are more frequent.[3] Age at seizure onset is variable; onset usually occurs in the first three decades, with two peaks at approximately 5 and 25 years of age.[35,36] Although temporal lobe seizures are also commonly found, centroparietal and occipital seizures are less frequent. There is also marked intrafamilial heterogeneity in seizure severity and outcome.

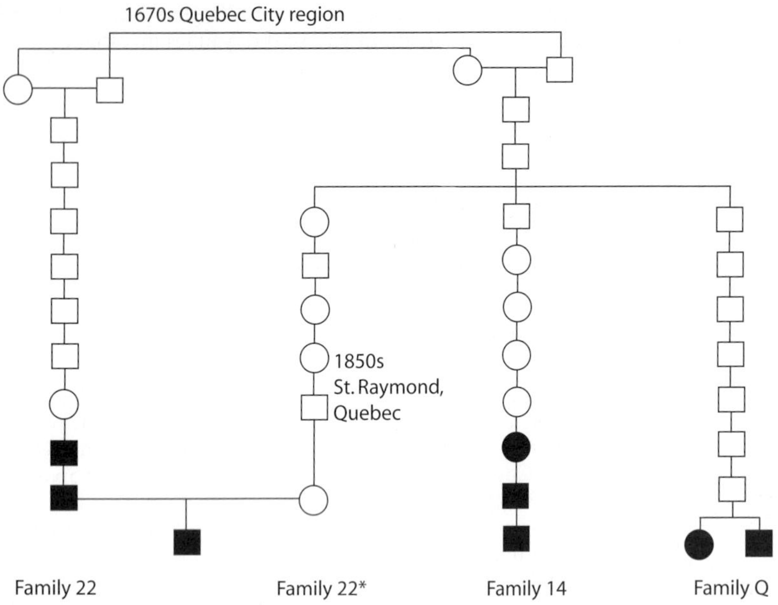

FIGURE 1. Genealogic representation of three French-Canadian families (F22, F22*, F14) demonstrating a founder effect.

DIAGNOSTIC EVALUATION

A detailed clinical evaluation with clear description of the seizures by the patient and close relatives is the first important requirement for diagnosis of FPEVF.

Electroencephalographic Findings

Electroencephalograms (EEGs) in patients with FPEVF may disclose temporal, frontal, and, less frequently, occipital and centroparietal foci. Although the variable foci are a landmark of this familial syndrome, the focus remains stable throughout life in each affected patient.

Neuroimaging and Other Laboratory Examinations

No structural magnetic resonance imaging abnormalities have been described in kindreds with FPEVF. In large families, studies to search for linkage to the chr 2 or chr 22 loci can be performed. In French-Canadian families with two or more individuals having different forms of focal epilepsy, origin from the same geographic region and/or the finding of the same haplotype as described in the original three families[36] is strongly suggestive of the diagnosis.

DIFFERENTIAL DIAGNOSIS

Sporadic benign partial epilepsies constitute the main differential diagnosis, but it is impossible at present to know whether these individuals may have mutations in the same gene or genes as patients with FPEVF. It should be noted that some sporadic patients could in fact be part of an FPEVF kindred in which the other family members are only mildly affected and sometimes unrecognized. In the case of sporadic French-Canadian patients, however, origin from the same region of Quebec and/or identification of the same haplotype on chr 22q as in the previously reported French-Canadian families[3,35,36] constitutes a high probability for a positive diagnosis of FPEVF. Even in smaller families, linkage to the two loci for FPEVF can be excluded but not confirmed.

For differential diagnosis of the two commonest clinical presentations FPEVF patients might have, genetic testing to exclude mutations in the known genes for ADNFLE and FTLE could also be helpful.

3.8 cM/ 5,222Mb (S1163–S1175)

centr → tel	S420	GCT10	S421	S1154	S1167	S1144	**S1163**	**S689**	**S275**	**S1150**	**S1176**	**S273**	**S1175**	S280	S1172	S1162	S685	S1147	S1152	S683	S422	S1158	S277	S283	S272	S244
F22	6	5	6	4	7	2	6	2	2	7	7	6	3	4	5	2	3	4	5	10	9	3	5	11	4	3
F22*	1	3	4	4	7	2	6	2	2	7	7	6	3	2	5	7	6	11	5	12	9	8	6	13	1	3
F14	3	2	6	4	7	2	6	2	2	7	7	6	3	2	5	7	6	11	5	12	9	8	6	13	1	3
Family Q	3	-	4	-	7	2	6	2	2	7	7	-	-	2	-	7	6	-	-	-	-	-	-	13	1	3
Family S	-	-	-	-	-	5	6	7	6	9	8	-	-	6	-	6	5	1	-	-	-	10	8	7	-	4

FIGURE 2. Disease haplotypes in familial partial epilepsy with variable foci (FPEVF) families. The order of markers is based on the DNA sequence of chromosome 22. F22, F22*, F14, and family Q all represent haplotypes of French-Canadian families from the Quebec City region (same families as shown in Fig. 1). Shared haplotype portions are shaded. Note that the Spanish family (S) has a totally different haplotype. Markers within the candidate interval defined by recombination analysis are in bold. The 3.8-cM candidate region is marked by an arrow. Dashes indicate that the marker was not typed. (From Berkovic SF, Serratosa JM, Phillips HA, et al. Familial partial epilepsy with variable foci: clinical features and linkage to chromosome 22q12. *Epilepsia.* 2004;45(9):1054–1060, with permission.)

Among the genetically determined partial epilepsies, the most important differential diagnosis is ADNFLE because frontal lobe seizures are the most frequent type found in affected family members with FPEVF. However, frontal lobe seizures have a different pattern in FPEVF as compared to that observed in ADNFLE: The seizures are less frequent, clusters and auras are rare, and daytime seizures as well as secondarily generalized seizures are more frequent (Table 1).[3,36]

For ADNFLE, three loci and two genes have been identified: ENFL1 (chr 20q13.2), with four different mutations in the *CHRNA4* gene, coding for the alpha 4 subunit of the neuronal nicotinic acetylcholine receptor (nAchR)[12,17,23,30]; ENFL2 (chr 15q24, gene unknown)[24]; and the *CHRNB2* gene on the ENFL3 locus (chr 1q), coding for the beta 2 subunit of the AchR.[7,10,22] However, most families with ADNFLE do not map to any of these loci and do not have mutations in either the *CHRNA4* or the *CHRNB2* gene. Thus, in the absence of genetic confirmation, the differential diagnosis between FPEVF and ADNFLE should be based on the clinical and EEG characteristics of the frontal lobe seizures, as well as family members with seizure patterns that indicate foci outside the frontal regions in the former.

The familial temporal lobe epilepsies, both familial mesial temporal lobe epilepsy (FMTLE)[1a,2,5,6,14,16] and familial lateral temporal lobe epilepsy (FLTLE) or ADPEAF,[5,15,21] also should be considered in the differential diagnosis if one or more affected individuals in the family presents clinical and EEG features of temporal lobe epilepsy.[5] A confirmed extratemporal focus in a family member would exclude the diagnosis of FMTLE or FLTLE and suggest FPEVF. Genetic testing is only possible for FLTLE, in which mutations in the *LGI1* gene on chr 10q[13,20] have been found in about half of the families investigated.

In generalized epilepsy with febrile seizure plus (GEFS+), related to mutations in genes *SCN1A*,[9,18,32] *SCN2A*,[31] *SCN1B*,[33,34] and *GABRG2*,[11] different family members also present heterogeneous epilepsy phenotypes, as in FPEVF. Febrile seizures (FS) are the most common phenotype, followed by FS+, in which individuals have seizures with fever that may persist beyond the age of 6 years and/or may be associated with afebrile generalized tonic–clonic seizures.[26,29] Less frequent phenotypes seen in GEFS+ involve other generalized and partial seizure types, including MTLE.[5,16,26,29,33]

TREATMENT AND OUTCOME

Treatment should be based on the patient's response to antiepileptic drugs (AEDs), and the rationale is similar to that in nonfamilial patients with partial epilepsies. Usually, patients with FPEVF are well controlled with small doses of the same AEDs indicated in other partial epilepsies, and the seizures may remit spontaneously.

LONG-TERM PROGNOSIS

FPEVF has an overall benign clinical course, although some patients with refractory seizures have been reported. One of our refractory French-Canadian patients was homozygous for

TABLE 1

COMPARISON OF CLINICAL AND GENETIC FEATURES IN TWO FORMS OF FAMILIAL PARTIAL EPILEPSY WITH VARIABLE FOCI (FPEVF) AND AUTOSOMAL-DOMINANT NOCTURAL FRONTAL LOBE EPILEPSY (ADNFLE)

	ADNFLE	FPEVF	
Genetics			
Inheritance	AD	AD	AD
Penetrance	~70%	~70%	~60%
Linkage (gene if known)	20q (*CHRNA4*) 1q (*CHRNB2*)	22q	?2q
Age at onset			
Mean	12yr	12 yr	13 yr
Median	8 yr	10 yr	10 yr
Range	2 mo–35 yr	1 mo–52 yr	9 mo–43 yr
Seizure features			
Frontal origin	Always	Often	Often
Temporal origin	No	Often	Often
Centroparietal origin	No	Rare	Rare
Occipital origin	No	Occasional	Rare
Nocturnal clusters	Almost always	Occasional	No
Seizures when awake	Very rare	Present in some	Common
Secondarily generalized	Rare	Common	Common
Interictal discharges			
Frequency	Rare	Occasional	Common
Localization	Frontal	Variable foci or poorly localized	Variable foci
Structural imaging	Normal	Normal	Normal
Intrafamily variation			
Seizure localization	No	Yes	Yes
Epilepsy severity	Yes	Yes	Yes

AD, autosomal dominant.
(From Berkovic SF, Serratosa JM, Phillips HA, et al. Familial partial epilepsy with variable foci: clinical features and linkage to chromosome 22q12. *Epilepsia*. 2004;45(9):1054–1060, with permission.)

the haplotype, having received it from both parents,[35,36] although only one of the parents had epilepsy (1 and 2). Only one individual from another French-Canadian family underwent a temporal lobectomy, but this was not effective in controlling his seizures.[3,35] No neurologic disabilities are known in this syndrome.

SUMMARY AND CONCLUSIONS

FPEVF is a characteristic epilepsy syndrome with different types and localization of focal epilepsy within families, in the absence of any structural lesion.[28,36] Seizures and epileptic EEG abnormalities are consistent over time in each affected family member and may be frontal, temporal, or occipital, but they vary among family members, which may lead to the misdiagnosis of other familial partial epilepsy syndromes. Two different loci have been associated with FPEVF, an unconfirmed locus on chr 2q,[28] and a confirmed locus on chr 22q.[36] The gene(s) have not yet been identified.

References

1. Andermann F, Kobayashi E, Andermann E. Genetic focal epilepsies: state of the art and paths to the future. *Epilepsia.* 2005;46 Suppl 10:61–67.

1a. Berkovic SF, Howell RA, Hopper JL. Familial temporal lobe epilepsy: a new syndrome with adolescent/adult onset and a benign course. In: Wolf P, ed. *Epileptic Seizures and Syndromes.* London: John Libbey; 1994;257–263.

2. Berkovic SF, McIntosh A, Howell RA, et al. Familial temporal lobe epilepsy: a common disorder identified in twins. *Ann Neurol.* 1996;40(2):227–235.
3. Berkovic SF, Serratosa JM, Phillips HA, et al. Familial partial epilepsy with variable foci: clinical features and linkage to chromosome 22q12. *Epilepsia.* 2004;45(9):1054–1060.
4. Callenbach PM, van den Maagdenberg AM, Hottenga JJ, et al. Familial partial epilepsy with variable foci in a Dutch family: clinical characteristics and confirmation of linkage to chromosome 22q. *Epilepsia.* 2003;44(10):1298–1305.
5. Cendes F, Kobayashi E, Lopes-Cendes I, et al. Familial temporal lobe epilepsies. In: Engel J, Pedley TA, eds. *Epilepsy: A Comprehensive Textbook,* 2nd ed. Philadelphia: Lippincott 2008;2487–2494.
6. Cendes F, Lopes-Cendes I, Andermann E, et al. Familial temporal lobe epilepsy: a clinically heterogeneous syndrome. *Neurology.* 1998;50(2):554–557.
7. De Fusco M, Becchetti A, Patrignani A, et al. The nicotinic receptor beta 2 subunit is mutant in nocturnal frontal lobe epilepsy. *Nat Genet.* 2000;26(3):275–276.
8. Engel J Jr. A proposed diagnostic scheme for people with epileptic seizures and with epilepsy: report of the ILAE Task Force on Classification and Terminology. *Epilepsia.* 2001;42(6):796–803.
9. Escayg A, MacDonald BT, Meisler MH, et al. Mutations of *SCN1A,* encoding a neuronal sodium channel, in two families with GEFS+2. *Nat Genet.* 2000;24(4):343–345.
10. Gambardella A, Annesi G, De Fusco M, et al. A new locus for autosomal dominant nocturnal frontal lobe epilepsy maps to chromosome 1. *Neurology.* 2000;55(10):1467–1471.
11. Harkin LA, Bowser DN, Dibbens LM, et al. Truncation of the GABA(A)-receptor gamma2 subunit in a family with generalized epilepsy with febrile seizures plus. *Am J Hum Genet.* 2002;70(2):530–536.
12. Hirose S, Iwata H, Akiyoshi H, et al. A novel mutation of CHRNA4 responsible for autosomal dominant nocturnal frontal lobe epilepsy. *Neurology.* 1999;53(8):1749–1753.
13. Kalachikov S, Evgrafov O, Ross B, et al. Mutations in LGI1 cause autosomal-dominant partial epilepsy with auditory features. *Nat Genet.* 2002;30(3):335–341.
14. Kobayashi E, Andermann F, Andermann E. Familial mesial temporal lobe epilepsy. In: Gilman S, ed. *MedLink Neurology.* San Diego, CA: MedLink; 2007.
15. Kobayashi E, Andermann F, Andermann E. Familial lateral temporal lobe epilepsy. In: Gilman S, ed. *MedLink Neurology.* San Diego, CA: MedLink; 2007.
16. Kobayashi E, Lopes-Cendes I, Guerreiro CA, et al. Seizure outcome and hippocampal atrophy in familial mesial temporal lobe epilepsy. *Neurology.* 2001;56(2):166–172.
17. Leniger T, Kananura C, Hufnagel A, et al. A new *Chrna4* mutation with low penetrance in nocturnal frontal lobe epilepsy. *Epilepsia.* 2003;44(7):981–985.
18. Lopes-Cendes I, Scheffer IE, Berkovic SF, et al. A new locus for generalized epilepsy with febrile seizures plus maps to chromosome 2. *Am J Hum Genet.* 2000;66(2):698–701.
19. Morales-Corraliza J, Gomez-Garre P, Gutierrez-Delicado E, et al. Familial partial epilepsy with variable foci in a Spanish family with linkage to chromosome 22q12. *Epilepsia.* 2003;44(Suppl 8):166–167.
20. Morante-Redolat JM, Gorostidi-Pagola A, Piquer-Sirerol S, et al. Mutations in the LGI1/epitempin gene on 10q24 cause autosomal dominant lateral temporal epilepsy. *Hum Mol Genet.* 2002;11(9):1119–1128.
21. Ottman R, Risch N, Hauser WA, et al. Localization of a gene for partial epilepsy to chromosome 10q. *Nat Genet.* 1995;10(1):56–60.
22. Phillips HA, Favre I, Kirkpatrick M, et al. CHRNB2 is the second acetylcholine receptor subunit associated with autosomal dominant nocturnal frontal lobe epilepsy. *Am J Hum Genet.* 2001;68(1):225–231.
23. Phillips HA, Scheffer IE, Berkovic SF, et al. Localization of a gene for autosomal dominant nocturnal frontal lobe epilepsy to chromosome 20q 13.2. *Nat Genet.* 1995;10(1):117–118.
24. Phillips HA, Scheffer IE, Crossland KM, et al. Autosomal dominant nocturnal frontal-lobe epilepsy: genetic heterogeneity and evidence for a second locus at 15q24. *Am J Hum Genet.* 1998;63(4):1108–1116.
25. Picard F, Baulac S, Kahane P, et al. Dominant partial epilepsies. A clinical, electrophysiological and genetic study of 19 European families. *Brain.* 2000;123(Pt 6):1247–1262.
26. Scheffer IE, Berkovic SF. Generalized epilepsy with febrile seizures plus. A genetic disorder with heterogeneous clinical phenotypes. *Brain.* 1997; 120(Pt 3):479–490.
27. Scheffer IE, Bhatia KP, Lopes-Cendes I, et al. Autosomal dominant frontal epilepsy misdiagnosed as sleep disorder. *Lancet.* 1994;343(8896): 515–517.
28. Scheffer IE, Phillips HA, O'Brien CE, et al. Familial partial epilepsy with variable foci: a new partial epilepsy syndrome with suggestion of linkage to chromosome 2. *Ann Neurol.* 1998;44(6):890–899.
29. Singh R, Scheffer IE, Crossland K, et al. Generalized epilepsy with febrile seizures plus: a common childhood-onset genetic epilepsy syndrome. *Ann Neurol.* 1999;45(1):75–81.
30. Steinlein OK, Mulley JC, Propping P, et al. A missense mutation in the neuronal nicotinic acetylcholine receptor alpha 4 subunit is associated with autosomal dominant nocturnal frontal lobe epilepsy. *Nat Genet.* 1995;11(2):201–203.
31. Sugawara T, Tsurubuchi Y, Agarwala KL, et al. A missense mutation of the Na+ channel alpha II subunit gene *Na(v)1.2* in a patient with febrile and afebrile seizures causes channel dysfunction. *Proc Natl Acad Sci USA.* 2001;98(11):6384–6389.
32. Wallace RH, Scheffer IE, Barnett S, et al. Neuronal sodium-channel alpha1-subunit mutations in generalized epilepsy with febrile seizures plus. *Am J Hum Genet.* 2001;68(4):859–865.
33. Wallace RH, Scheffer IE, Parasivam G, et al. Generalized epilepsy with febrile seizures plus: mutation of the sodium channel subunit SCN1B. *Neurology.* 2002;58(9):1426–1429.
34. Wallace RH, Wang DW, Singh R, et al. Febrile seizures and generalized epilepsy associated with a mutation in the Na+-channel beta1 subunit gene *SCN1B. Nat Genet.* 1998;19(4):366–370.
35. Xiong L. *Identification, clinical characterization, and molecular genetic studies of familial partial epilepsy with variable foci.* Ph.D. dissertation, McGill University, Montreal; 2002.
36. Xiong L, Labuda M, Li DS, et al. Mapping of a gene determining familial partial epilepsy with variable foci to chromosome 22q11–q12. *Am J Hum Genet.* 1999;65(6):1698–1710.

CHAPTER 256 ■ GENERALIZED (GENETIC) EPILEPSY WITH FEBRILE SEIZURES PLUS

INGRID E. SCHEFFER AND SAMUEL F. BERKOVIC

INTRODUCTION

Generalized epilepsy with febrile seizures plus (GEFS$^+$) is a familial epilepsy syndrome characterized by heterogeneous epilepsy subsyndromes or phenotypes within families.[50] GEFS$^+$ has been key in advancing understanding of the genetic interrelationship between epilepsy and febrile seizures. The clinical concept of GEFS$^+$ led directly to the discovery of the role of sodium channels in epilepsy and has also highlighted the importance of γ-aminobutyric acid (GABA)$_A$ receptor subunits in causing seizure disorders.

The majority of families with GEFS$^+$ have generalized seizure types and generalized spike-wave activity on the electroencephalogram (EEG) in addition to febrile seizures.[7,9,37,45,50,54,55] Studies of families around the world have highlighted that focal seizures may also occur, leading some authors to question the nomenclature of "generalized" in generalized epilepsy with febrile seizures plus.[3,7,9,30,51,58] We suggest that the nomenclature be altered to "*genetic* epilepsy with febrile seizures plus" to reflect this observation. It must be emphasized that generalized epilepsies are considerably more frequent in GEFS$^+$ families.

HISTORICAL PERSPECTIVES

GEFS$^+$ was originally described in 1997 in a large Australian family comprising many affected individuals who showed a spectrum of phenotypic severity.[50] The phenotypes ranged from febrile seizures to mild generalized epilepsies to the severe end of the GEFS$^+$ spectrum, which included myoclonic-astatic epilepsy (MAE, or Doose syndrome; see Chapter 232). This work built on the extensive clinical genetic studies of Doose, where he concluded that MAE was a polygenic disorder.[17] Doose showed that family members of MAE probands most commonly had febrile and afebrile convulsions in early childhood. Evidence to support Doose's hypothesis that MAE has a genetic basis has been gained from the conclusive findings of mutations found in some GEFS$^+$ families, including family members with MAE.

Subsequently, the clinical spectrum of GEFS$^+$ was further elucidated in a study of nine families, the majority of whom were identified through probands with MAE.[54] The clinical genetics of GEFS$^+$ were extrapolated further with the study of probands of families with severe myoclonic epilepsy of infancy (SMEI, or Dravet syndrome; see Chapter 230) where family members with seizure disorders had GEFS$^+$ phenotypes.[53,60]

In 1998, the first gene for GEFS$^+$ was discovered in another large Australian family. This was a mutation of the sodium channel $\beta 1$ subunit gene, *SCN1B*,[64] and was the first time that sodium channel genes were implicated in epilepsy. In 2000, Escayg et al. reported mutations in *SCN1A*, the gene encoding the $\alpha 1$ subunit of the sodium channel, in GEFS$^+$ families,[21] a finding later confirmed by other groups.[3,20,30,63] The recognition that patients with SMEI, also known as Dravet syndrome, began with febrile seizures led Claes et al. to find that all seven of their patients with Dravet syndrome had *SCN1A* mutations.[13] This work led many others to replicate the findings, highlighting the importance of *SCN1A* in the severe epileptic encephalopathies[47] as well as in milder GEFS$^+$ phenotypes.

The GABA$_A$ receptor $\gamma 2$ subunit gene, *GABRG2*, has also been implicated in GEFS$^+$ in several kindreds.[7,27,62] More recently, mutations in possible "susceptibility genes" have been reported in the GABA$_A$ receptor δ subunit gene *GABRD* and the calcium channel subunit gene *CACNA1H*; these observations require confirmation.[16,29]

DEFINITIONS

GEFS$^+$ is defined as a "familial epilepsy syndrome." This syndrome is diagnosed on the basis of more than one individual within a family with a history of seizures that fits into a specific subsyndrome or phenotype of the GEFS$^+$ spectrum (Fig. 1). It remains to be seen whether the phenotype of febrile seizures plus (see below) can be diagnosed in isolation and whether the same genes will be implicated. GEFS$^+$ is best conceptualized as a spectrum of phenotypes seen within a family ranging in severity from mild to severe seizure disorders.

Febrile seizures (FSs) are defined as convulsive seizures with fever above 38°C that occur between 3 months and 6 years of age at their broadest limits.[2]

The phenotype of febrile seizures plus (FS$^+$) refers to a number of different presentations. The most straightforward example is where febrile seizures continue past the defined upper limit of FS of 6 years. Rarely, seizures with fever may start before 3 months of age and would also be called FS$^+$. Additionally, afebrile convulsions may occur in the setting of a child who has febrile seizures. These afebrile seizures may occur during the typical age range of FS (i.e., from 3 months to 6 years), or alternatively, they may follow on from the febrile seizures after 6 years. The afebrile convulsions may also occur after a break of several years after the last febrile seizure.

FS or FS$^+$ may occur with afebrile generalized or partial seizures. For example, individuals may have FS/FS$^+$ and absence, myoclonic, or atonic seizures or a constellation of generalized seizure types.[50]

Partial seizures emanating from the temporal or frontal lobes may also occur with FS or FS$^+$.[3,7,30,52] Although temporal lobe epilepsy (TLE) may occur in the context of hippocampal sclerosis (HS), presumably secondary to FS/FS$^+$, TLE may also occur with normal neuroimaging and pathology and in the absence of preceding FS.[51]

At the severe end of the GEFS$^+$ spectrum are MAE and the epileptic encephalopathy Dravet syndrome.[18,26] It is unusual for a family to have multiple severely affected individuals with

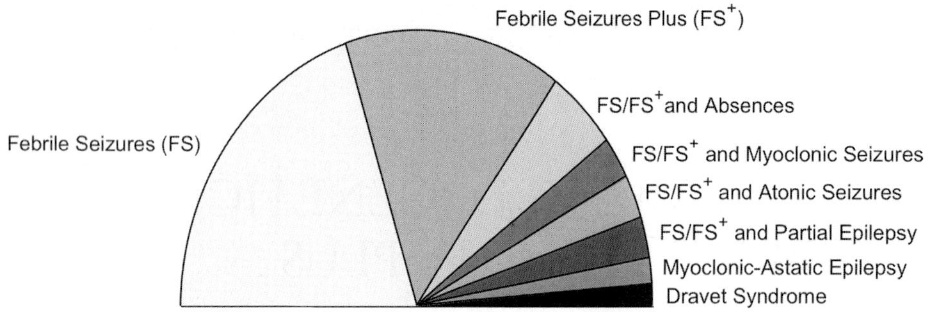

FIGURE 1. Generalized epilepsy with febrile seizures plus (GEFS+) spectrum: The spectrum illustrates the phenotypic heterogeneity seen in GEFS+ families ranging from benign phenotypes such as febrile seizures to severe epileptic encephalopathies such as Dravet syndrome.

these syndromes, as most family members have more benign phenotypes.

EPIDEMIOLOGY

The idiopathic generalized epilepsies (IGEs) account for about 15% to 20% of all epilepsies.[28,32] The IGEs can be divided into two major subgroups: The classic IGE and GEFS+. Families in which a number of individuals have IGE typically show phenotypic heterogeneity. However, GEFS+ families show different phenotypic patterns compared with the classic IGE where childhood absence epilepsy, juvenile absence epilepsy, juvenile myoclonic epilepsy, and "generalized tonic–clonic seizures alone" segregate within families.[1,42] Although overlap between the classic IGE and GEFS+ phenotypes does occur within families,[41,54] this is not frequent, suggesting that these major subgroups arise due to distinct, but at times overlapping, groups of genes. No formal epidemiologic studies of GEFS+ have been performed.

ETIOLOGY AND BASIC MECHANISMS

GEFS+ is a genetic disorder that has been recognized through study of large multiplex families where there is clinical genetic evidence of a gene of major effect. It sometimes is erroneously stated that GEFS+ is an autosomal dominant syndrome based on the initial genetic discoveries. Whilst autosomal dominant families do occur, the majority of GEFS+ families have clinical genetic evidence of complex inheritance. The rare dominant families led to the appreciation of the phenotypic variation seen in GEFS+ families and the genetic relationship between these phenotypes. However, even in these large kindreds, there is evidence for "complex monogenic" inheritance, which would explain why one family member has a benign phenotype such as FS while another has MAE or Dravet syndrome. In these latter cases, presumably other genes, with or without environmental factors, contribute to produce a severe phenotype.

Mutations of a number of ion channel genes have been identified in GEFS+ kindreds. These include sodium channel subunit and $GABA_A$ receptor subunit genes. The most frequently reported is *SCN1A,* which encodes the pore-forming α subunit of the sodium channel and comprises four transmembrane domains. Missense mutations spread throughout the gene have been associated with the full spectrum of GEFS+ phenotypes including MAE, Dravet syndrome, partial seizures, FS, and FS+ with other generalized seizure types.[3,20,21,30,63]

In contrast, *SCN1A* mutations usually arise de novo in Dravet syndrome and are truncation mutations in at least 50% of cases. Only about 5% of *SCN1A* mutations occur in patients with Dravet syndrome who have familial missense mutations where other family members have milder GEFS+ phenotypes.[22,47,48] Recent reports of low levels of parental somatic and germline mosaicism explain cases of apparently de novo mutations in affected siblings; the parent may be unaffected or have a mild phenotype such as FS.[15,23]

Studies of the functional effects of *SCN1A* mutations yield variable results, with some mutations leading to loss of channel function while others suggest gain of function.[38,39,57] Indeed, different functional effects have been demonstrated using the same mutation in different expression systems.[4,39] In general, missense mutations may lead to gain of channel function, whereas truncation mutations in Dravet syndrome cause loss of function; however, this is by no means universal.[44] Computer simulation of the effects of several GEFS+ mutations suggests a unifying functional endpoint, with each showing an increased propensity to fire repetitive action potentials and thus hyperexcitability.[56]

The first gene implicated in GEFS+ was *SCN1B,* which encodes the $\beta 1$ subunit of the sodium channel, the auxiliary subunit with a role in channel-gating kinetics and localization of the ion channel.[43] There are now four different mutations of *SCN1B* reported, three missense and one deletion mutation.[6,51,61,64] An analysis of six families with *SCN1B* mutations highlighted that the most common of the known mutations, C121W, is associated with TLE, including patients with and without HS.[51] Functional studies suggest that these mutations cause loss of function.[6,64] The C121W mutant causes subtle effects on channel function and subcellular distribution; initial studies suggested that the major effect was due to slowing of the sodium current inactivation time course.[64] More recent studies showed increased sodium channel availability at hyperpolarized membrane potentials and reduced sodium channel rundown during high-frequency channel activity, as well as altered protein–protein interactions critical for sodium channel localization.[43]

One small family with a GEFS+-like phenotype has been reported with a missense mutation in the sodium channel gene *SCN2A,*[59] and there is one report of a more severe childhood encephalopathy in a child with a nonsense *SCN2A* mutation.[34] Missense mutations in *SCN2A* have been clearly associated with the benign familial neonatal-infantile seizure syndrome, which is unrelated to GEFS+, and in our experience, SCN2A mutations have not been found in GEFS+ families.[8]

The second group of genes associated with GEFS+ encodes subunits of the $GABA_A$ receptor, the ligand-gated chloride channel, which mediates fast synaptic inhibition. The $\gamma 2$ subunit gene, *GABRG2,* has been confirmed to play a role in GEFS+ families, in some cases in association with classic childhood absence epilepsy.[7,27,41,62] The latter is an intriguing finding given the key role of $GABA_A$ receptors in corticothalamic pathways that mediate generalized spike-wave activity. Functional studies of *GABRG2* mutations suggest loss of function or abnormal trafficking, whereby the receptors do not reach the cell surface.[7,10,27,35,36,40]

Although GEFS+ has been recognized through large dominant families, in most cases GEFS+ follows complex inheritance where a number of genes are presumed to be involved with or without an environmental contribution. Initial insights into susceptibility genes that contribute to complex inheritance are just developing through discovery of alleles in small kindreds where there is evidence of a functional effect of gene variants. It is not known how many such susceptibility genes are needed to produce a $GEFS^+$ phenotype, either for a mild picture such as FS or a severe one such as MAE.

Interestingly, different changes in the *GABRD* gene encoding the δ subunit of the $GABA_A$ receptor were found in small families with $GEFS^+$ and IGE.[16] These changes showed reduction of GABA current, suggesting increased excitability given the central role of GABA in inhibition. The δ subunit confers different characteristics to the heteropentameric $GABA_A$ receptor compared with the $\gamma 2$ subunit. The δ-containing receptor has a perisynaptic or extrasynaptic localization and has a role in tonic inhibition, whereas the $\gamma 2$-containing receptor is subsynaptic and mediates phasic inhibition.[16] The finding of *GABRD* changes in $GEFS^+$ and the classic IGE reinforces the concept that $GABA_A$ receptor subunits are involved in both major subgroups of IGE, whereas sodium channel subunits appear to be primarily involved with $GEFS^+$ phenotypes.

The genes currently known for $GEFS^+$ account for <20% of large families studied[44,63]; thus, there remain many genes of major effect to be discovered. Moreover, the number of genes contributing to complex inheritance is not known, nor is the effect size of each gene. Does a $GEFS^+$ phenotype require five or ten genes? Do the molecular permutations and combinations explain phenotypic differences? How do we distill the environmental effects that may underlie aspects of phenotypic heterogeneity? Current molecular and mechanistic insights into $GEFS^+$ highlight how much we are yet to understand regarding the neurobiology of this complex familial syndrome.

CLINICAL PRESENTATION

Clinical evaluation in $GEFS^+$ involves a detailed history and examination with careful attention to the presence of a documented fever, rather than the presumption of a fever, when attacks occur. This may require sourcing the ambulance and emergency department notes to determine if a fever was present as families often equate fever with the observation that a child feels hot, yet the child may be afebrile when his or her temperature is formally taken.

The nature of the attacks needs to be determined ideally through an eyewitness account. Many attacks may mimic febrile seizures such as febrile delirium, febrile syncope, rigors, and breath-holding attacks. It is important to accurately determine that a convulsion occurred. Clues to unwitnessed convulsions should also be sought such as a bitten tongue or rare enuresis in a child not prone to enuresis.

Specific questioning regarding other seizure types is necessary as myoclonic seizures, atonic seizures, or staring spells may not be mentioned spontaneously; indeed, a child may just be considered to be a day-dreamer, "nervous," or jumpy. Absence seizures may be less frequent than in typical childhood absence epilepsy, with rare but definite attacks lasting <30 seconds and occurring several times per year, rather than several times per day. Symptoms of focal seizures should also be sought with emphasis on temporal lobe auras and complex partial seizures.

When considering phenotypes at the severe end of the $GEFS^+$ spectrum, the electroclinical presentation of syndromes such as myoclonic-astatic epilepsy of Doose and Dravet syndromes is quite specific (see Chapters 232 and 230).

Family History

The key to a diagnosis of $GEFS^+$ is the family history as this is a *familial* epilepsy syndrome and requires at least two affected individuals in a family to have $GEFS^+$ phenotypes.

The family history should explore the presence of seizures in family members and consanguinity. One should always ask specifically about febrile seizures or febrile convulsions in addition to epilepsy, as families often do not think the former is of relevance. Frequently the matriarchs of the family hold the key to this knowledge and the family should be encouraged to speak with older family members and report back to the clinician at subsequent visits. Where there is controversy about attacks, the clinician may need to directly contact family members, with the permission of the proband's family, to understand the nature of the attacks in other branches of the family. This aids in diagnosing whether a specific individual's phenotype is likely to be part of the $GEFS^+$ spectrum. As epilepsy is common, it is not unusual for an individual with epilepsy in a $GEFS^+$ family to have an unrelated seizure disorder such as symptomatic epilepsy; this must be carefully considered when performing and interpreting genetic studies.[64]

DIAGNOSTIC EVALUATION

Electroencephalographic Findings

Although no systematic EEG studies in $GEFS^+$ have been performed, the EEG is often normal in the milder phenotypes in $GEFS^+$. Irregular generalized spike wave can occur in FS^+ individuals and is likely to be an age-dependent abnormality. Similar changes were reported in a cohort of children with seizures with fever; it is possible this cohort included cases that we would now regard as FS^+.[5] With the more severe phenotypes, the EEG findings are as anticipated by their seizure types. For example, epileptiform discharges emanating from the region in which the seizures originate may occur in focal seizures. Similarly, fast generalized spike wave would be seen in MAE, and generalized spike wave and focal discharges in Dravet syndrome.[19,25]

Neuroimaging and Other Laboratory Examinations

Magnetic resonance imaging (MRI) of the brain is almost always normal in $GEFS^+$ phenotypes. Where ongoing focal seizures occur, MRI is indicated as HS has been found in certain cases, including some with known sodium channel mutations, and has typically followed a history of FS or FS^+.[31,51] Some patients with TLE and *SCN1B* mutations have been rendered seizure free following anterior temporal lobectomy,[51] but they still require comprehensive presurgical characterization as with other patients undergoing epilepsy surgery.

Mutational analysis of *SCN1A* is indicated in Dravet and related syndromes such as the borderline variant of Dravet syndrome. Mutations are found in about 70% to 80% of children with classic Dravet syndrome, and around 95% arise de novo. Very recently, exonic deletion of *SCN1A* has been shown to be a novel mechanism underlying Dravet syndrome, responsible for some patients negative by conventional mutational analysis.[46] In these children, the discovery of a mutation obviates the need for other potentially invasive investigations such as lumbar puncture and muscle and liver biopsy. It also supports more aggressive strategies to achieve seizure control to potentially improve developmental outcome.

Mutational analysis in GEFS+ is more controversial. While mutations have been found in GEFS+ in sodium channel and $GABA_A$ receptor subunits, these are uncommon and do not modify treatment approaches. Further research is needed, as with current knowledge the presence of a familial mutation does not inform the clinician regarding phenotype or outcome. Indeed, the finding of a mutation in a family does not explain the phenotypic heterogeneity that is the hallmark of GEFS+. Deeper understanding of the complex genetics of GEFS+ is necessary to explain why one family member has a benign versus a severe phenotype.

DIFFERENTIAL DIAGNOSIS

The differential diagnosis of GEFS+ includes an understanding of the phenotypic variation that occurs in GEFS+ families and those phenotypes that are not regarded as part of the spectrum. For example, malformations are not seen in GEFS+ and are unlikely to be due to the same genetic mutations.

Diagnosis of FS requires an understanding of attacks that can be misdiagnosed as FS such as febrile delirium and febrile syncope. It cannot be emphasized sufficiently that a clear description of the event is necessary, ideally from an eyewitness. Moreover, distinction of different phenotypes within GEFS+ may require additional effort, such as establishing whether a fever was actually present at the time of the attack.

There are many childhood epilepsy syndromes that are not characteristically seen in GEFS+ families. These include benign childhood epilepsy with centrotemporal spikes and the benign occipital epilepsies of childhood. As they are relatively common disorders, they may occur in a GEFS+ family just by chance; a mutation common to both disorders would need to be demonstrated to prove a molecular relationship.

TREATMENT AND OUTCOME

Children with FS and FS+ usually do not require medication. Recognition of FS+ allows the clinician to defer antiepileptic therapy where infrequent brief convulsions with fever persist after 6 years in a developmentally normal child. If, on the other hand, frequent or afebrile seizures occur at any age, the clinician should consider antiepileptic therapy. There are no trials of the efficacy of treatment; however, our experience suggests that valproate is effective in FS+ or where the child has FS/FS+ with other generalized seizure types. If seizures are refractory to valproate monotherapy, lamotrigine should be considered. The usual principle of treating the child until he or she has been seizure free for 2 years should guide therapy. If convulsions are prolonged, benzodiazepines may be considered acutely. If convulsions occur frequently, interval use of benzodiazepines may be used when fever occurs prophylactically.[49]

For the phenotypes at the more severe end of the GEFS+ spectrum, choice of antiepileptic drug should be based on the seizure types and syndromes. For example, seizures in Dravet syndrome may be exacerbated by lamotrigine,[24] whereas, seizure control is often better with clobazam and topiramate.[14] The experimental drug stiripentol was effective in one double-blinded study of Dravet syndrome suggestive of a syndrome-specific effect.[12]

LONG-TERM PROGNOSIS

The outcome is usually good, with most GEFS+ phenotypes being benign. Seizures settle by adolescence in FS+, although rare adult convulsions may occur under conditions of stress or sleep deprivation. Where other generalized or focal seizures occur in addition to febrile convulsions, the outcome is often, but not universally, good. For example, TLE may cease by mid-childhood or, alternatively, prove refractory, warranting surgical consideration.[51]

MAE is known for its variable cognitive outcome from normal to severe intellectual disability, and this is clearly evident where MAE occurs in GEFS+ families.[54] Seizure frequency improves with age although may not cease altogether. The majority of patients with Dravet syndrome have poor cognitive outcome, although rare individuals have normal intellect. Seizures typically continue into adult life and comprise nocturnal tonic–clonic seizures, although partial, absence, and myoclonic seizures may also occur.[33] These patients often have pyramidal signs and ataxia, and rarely manage to live independently as adults.

GENETIC COUNSELING

Genetic counseling is an important aspect of management of patients and families with GEFS+. The diagnosis of a GEFS+ phenotype acknowledges the relationship with other familial seizure disorders but does not allow the clinician to predict prognosis. A finding of a mutation, if present, cannot be used alone to offer prognostic counseling because of the wide phenotypic and outcome variability; thus, prognostic counseling should be based on the clinical phenotype. Familial mutations are usually associated with a penetrance of 60% to 80%, so it is difficult to predict the outcome in carrier offspring.[37,54]

Genetic counseling is critical in Dravet syndrome, where *SCN1A* mutations are found in 70% to 80% of children with Dravet syndrome and 95% arise de novo. It is rare for families to have two children with severe phenotypes such as Dravet syndrome and the borderline variant of Dravet syndrome. This rare occurrence has recently been explained by the finding of parental germline and somatic mosaicism.[15,23]

A recent pertinent issue is the risk to offspring of adults with Dravet syndrome who have an essentially normal cognitive outcome. Such questions have only arisen since recognition that this may occur.[11,33] For example, in the case of a familial GEFS+ mutation where the patient has Dravet syndrome, the outcome for offspring may be relatively good as the severe phenotype is likely to have a polygenic basis. On the other hand, where the adult has a de novo *SCN1A* mutation, it is more likely that offspring may have a similarly severe phenotype. Whether this is indeed the correct interpretation will depend on careful observation of such patient groups.

SUMMARY AND CONCLUSIONS

GEFS+ is an important form of idiopathic epilepsy recognized throughout the world and forms one of the major subgroups of the IGEs. GEFS+ is a clinical diagnosis that depends on recognition of the clinical syndrome in the familial context. The concept of a familial epilepsy syndrome aids in understanding the interrelationships of seizure disorders such as epilepsy and febrile seizures. Recognition of the phenotypes that fit into the GEFS+ spectrum helps in diagnosis and may inform investigations, treatment selection, and prognostic and genetic counseling.

GEFS+ led directly to the discovery of mutations of sodium channels and GABA receptors in epilepsy, further reinforcing the key role of ion channels in the pathophysiology of the epilepsies. The finding of *SCN1A* mutations in Dravet syndrome is of significant clinical importance and is the key investigation in these individuals. Nevertheless, the diagnosis of Dravet syndrome is based on electroclinical features and is not dependent on molecular testing. Equally, the finding of an *SCN1A* mutation does not necessarily mean that a child has Dravet syndrome; this diagnosis depends on the clinical setting. New genetic counseling issues are arising with recent discoveries. GEFS$^+$ has opened many doors to understanding the genetics of the epilepsies but has also highlighted the large task ahead in solving this complex area.

ACKNOWLEDGMENTS

The authors are grateful to the many patients and families who have participated in their research studies. Funding has been received from the National Health and Medical Research Council of Australia and Bionomics Ltd.

References

1. Concordance of clinical forms of epilepsy in families with several affected members. Italian League Against Epilepsy Genetic Collaborative Group. *Epilepsia.* 1993;34(5):819–826.
2. Practice parameter: the neurodiagnostic evaluation of the child with a first simple febrile seizure (American Academy of Pediatrics Provisional Committee on Quality Improvement, Subcommittee on Febrile Seizures). *Pediatrics.* 1996;97(5):769–772; discussion (technical report summary), 773–775.
3. Abou-Khalil B, Ge Q, Desai R, et al. Partial and generalized epilepsy with febrile seizures plus and a novel SCN1A mutation. *Neurology.* 2001;57(12):2265–2272.
4. Alekov AK, Rahman MM, Mitrovic N, et al. Enhanced inactivation and acceleration of activation of the sodium channel associated with epilepsy in man. *Eur J Neurosci.* 2001;13(11):2171–2176.
5. Alvarez N, Lombroso CT, Medina C, et al. Paroxysmal spike and wave activity in drowsiness in young children: its relationship to febrile convulsions. *Electroencephalogr Clin Neurophysiol.* 1983;56(5):406–413.
6. Audenaert D, Claes L, Ceulemans B, et al. A deletion in SCN1B is associated with febrile seizures and early-onset absence epilepsy. *Neurology.* 2003;61(6):854–856.
7. Baulac S, Huberfeld G, Gourfinkel-An I, et al. First genetic evidence of GABA(A) receptor dysfunction in epilepsy: a mutation in the gamma2-subunit gene. *Nat Genet.* 2001;28(1):46–48.
8. Berkovic SF, Heron SE, Giordano L, et al. Benign familial neonatal-infantile seizures: characterization of a new sodium channelopathy. *Ann Neurol.* 2004;55(4):550–557.
9. Bonanni P, Malcarne M, Moro F, et al. Generalized epilepsy with febrile seizures plus (GEFS+): clinical spectrum in seven Italian families unrelated to SCN1A, SCN1B, and GABRG2 gene mutations. *Epilepsia.* 2004;45(2):149–158.
10. Bowser DN, Wagner DA, Czajkowski C, et al. Altered kinetics and benzodiazepine sensitivity of a GABAA receptor subunit mutation [gamma 2(R43Q)] found in human epilepsy. *Proc Natl Acad Sci U S A.* 2002;99(23):15170–15175.
11. Buoni S, Orrico A, Galli L, et al. SCN1A (2528delG) novel truncating mutation with benign outcome of severe myoclonic epilepsy of infancy. *Neurology.* 2006;66(4):606–607.
12. Chiron C, Marchand MC, Tran A, et al. Stiripentol in severe myoclonic epilepsy in infancy: a randomised placebo-controlled syndrome-dedicated trial. STICLO study group. *Lancet.* 2000;356(9242):1638–1642.
13. Claes L, Del-Favero J, Ceulemans B, et al. De novo mutations in the sodium-channel gene SCN1A cause severe myoclonic epilepsy of infancy. *Am J Hum Genet.* 2001;68(6):1327–1332.
14. Coppola G, Capovilla G, Montagnini A, et al. Topiramate as add-on drug in severe myoclonic epilepsy in infancy: an Italian multicenter open trial. *Epilepsy Res.* 2002;49(1):45–48.
15. Depienne C, Arzimanoglou A, Trouillard O, et al. Parental mosaicism can cause recurrent transmission of SCN1A mutations associated with severe myoclonic epilepsy of infancy. *Hum Mutat.* 2006;27(4):389.
16. Dibbens LM, Feng HJ, Richards MC, et al. GABRD encoding a protein for extra- or peri-synaptic GABAA receptors is a susceptibility locus for generalized epilepsies. *Hum Mol Genet.* 2004;13(13):1315–1319.
17. Doose H. Myoclonic astatic epilepsy of early childhood. In: Roger J, Bureau M, Dravet C, et al., eds. *Epileptic Syndromes in Infancy, Childhood and Adolescence.* 2nd ed. London: John Libbey & Company Ltd; 1992:103–114.
18. Dravet C, Bureau M, Oguni H, et al. Severe myoclonic epilepsy in infancy (Dravet syndrome). In: Roger J, Bureau M, Dravet C, et al., eds. *Epileptic Syndromes in Infancy, Childhood and Adolescence.* 3rd ed. Eastleigh: John Libbey & Co Ltd; 2002:81–103.
19. Dravet C, Bureau M, Oguni H, et al. Severe myoclonic epilepsy in infancy (Dravet syndrome). In: Roger J, Bureau M, Dravet C, et al., eds. *Epileptic Syndromes in Infancy, Childhood and Adolescence.* 4th ed. Mountrouge: John Libbey Eurotext Ltd; 2005:89–113.
20. Escayg A, Heils A, MacDonald BT, et al. A novel *SCN1A* mutation associated with generalized epilepsy with febrile seizures plus–and prevalence of variants in patients with epilepsy. *Am J Hum Genet.* 2001;68(4):866–873.
21. Escayg A, MacDonald BT, Meisler MH, et al. Mutations of SCN1A, encoding a neuronal sodium channel, in two families with GEFS+2. *Nat Genet.* 2000;24(4):343–345.
22. Fujiwara T, Sugawara T, Mazaki-Miyazaki E, et al. Mutations of sodium channel alpha subunit type 1 (SCN1A) in intractable childhood epilepsies with frequent generalized tonic-clonic seizures. *Brain.* 2003;126(Pt 3):531–546.
23. Gennaro E, Santorelli FM, Bertini E, et al. Somatic and germline mosaicisms in severe myoclonic epilepsy of infancy. *Biochem Biophys Res Commun.* 2006;341(2):489–493.
24. Guerrini R, Dravet C, Genton P, et al. Lamotrigine and seizure aggravation in severe myoclonic epilepsy. *Epilepsia.* 1998;39s:508–512.
25. Guerrini R, Parmeggiani L, Bonanni P, et al. Myoclonic astatic epilepsy. In: Roger J, Bureau M, Dravet C, et al., eds. *Epilepsy Syndromes in Infancy, Childhood and Adolescence.* 4th ed. Montrouge: John Libbey Eurotext Ltd; 2005:115–124.
26. Guerrini R, Parmeggiani L, Kaminska A, et al. Myoclonic astatic epilepsy. In: Roger J, Bureau M, Dravet C, et al., eds. *Epileptic Syndromes in Infancy, Childhood and Adolescence.* 3rd ed. Eastleigh: John Libbey & Co Ltd; 2002:105–112.
27. Harkin LA, Bowser DN, Dibbens LM, et al. Truncation of the GABA(A)-receptor gamma2 subunit in a family with generalized epilepsy with febrile seizures plus. *Am J Hum Genet.* 2002;70(2):530–536.
28. Hauser WA, Annegers JF, Kurland LT. Incidence of epilepsy and unprovoked seizures in Rochester, Minnesota: 1935–1984. *Epilepsia.* 1993;34(3):453–468.
29. Heron SE, Phillips HA, Mulley JC, et al. Genetic variation of CACNA1H in idiopathic generalized epilepsy. *Ann Neurol.* 2004;55(4):595–596.
30. Ito M, Nagafuji H, Okazawa H, et al. Autosomal dominant epilepsy with febrile seizures plus with missense mutations of the (Na+)-channel alpha 1 subunit gene, SCN1A. *Epilepsy Res.* 2002;48(1–2):15–23.
31. Jackson GD, McIntosh AM, Briellmann RS, et al. Hippocampal sclerosis studied in identical twins. *Neurology.* 1998;51(1):78–84.
32. Jallon P, Latour P. Epidemiology of idiopathic generalized epilepsies. *Epilepsia.* 2005;46(Suppl 9):10–14.
33. Jansen FE, Sadleir LG, Harkin LA, et al. Severe myoclonic epilepsy of infancy (Dravet syndrome): recognition and diagnosis in adults. *Neurology.* 2006;67:2224–2226.
34. Kamiya K, Kaneda M, Sugawara T, et al. A nonsense mutation of the sodium channel gene SCN2A in a patient with intractable epilepsy and mental decline. *J Neurosci.* 2004;24(11):2690–2698.
35. Kang JQ, Macdonald RL. The GABAA receptor gamma2 subunit R43Q mutation linked to childhood absence epilepsy and febrile seizures causes retention of alpha1beta2gamma2S receptors in the endoplasmic reticulum. *J Neurosci.* 2004;24(40):8672–8677.
36. Kang JQ, Shen W, Macdonald RL. Why does fever trigger febrile seizures? GABAA receptor gamma2 subunit mutations associated with idiopathic generalized epilepsies have temperature-dependent trafficking deficiencies. *J Neurosci.* 2006;26(9):2590–2597.
37. Lerche H, Weber Y, Baier H, et al. Generalized epilepsy with febrile seizures plus (GEFS+): evidence for clinical and genetic heterogeneity in a large family. *Epilepsia.* 2001;42(Suppl 2):70.
38. Lossin C, Rhodes TH, Desai RR, et al. Epilepsy-associated dysfunction in the voltage-gated neuronal sodium channel SCN1A. *J Neurosci.* 2003;23(36):11289–11295.
39. Lossin C, Wang DW, Rhodes TH, et al. Molecular basis of an inherited epilepsy. *Neuron.* 2002;34(6):877–884.
40. Macdonald RL, Gallagher MJ, Feng HJ, et al. GABA(A) receptor epilepsy mutations. *Biochem Pharmacol.* 2004;68(8):1497–1506.
41. Marini C, Harkin LA, Wallace RH, et al. Childhood absence epilepsy and febrile seizures: a family with a GABA(A) receptor mutation. *Brain.* 2003;126(Pt 1):230–240.
42. Marini C, Scheffer IE, Crossland KM, et al. Genetic architecture of idiopathic generalized epilepsy: clinical genetic analysis of 55 multiplex families. *Epilepsia.* 2004;45(5):467–478.
43. Meadows LS, Malhotra J, Loukas A, et al. Functional and biochemical analysis of a sodium channel beta1 subunit mutation responsible for generalized epilepsy with febrile seizures plus type 1. *J Neurosci.* 2002;22(24):10699–10709.
44. Meisler MH, Kearney JA. Sodium channel mutations in epilepsy and other neurological disorders. *J Clin Invest.* 2005;115(8):2010–2017.
45. Moulard B, Guipponi M, Chaigne D, et al. Identification of a new locus for generalized epilepsy with febrile seizures plus (GEFS$^+$) on chromosome 2q24-q33. *Am J Hum Genet.* 1999;65:1396–1400.
46. Mulley JC, Nelson P, Guerrero S, et al. A new molecular mechanism for severe myoclonic epilepsy of infancy: exonic deletions in SCN1A. *Neurology.* 2006;67(6):1094–1095.
47. Mulley JC, Scheffer IE, Petrou S, et al. SCN1A mutations and epilepsy. *Hum Mutat.* 2005;25(6):535–542.
48. Nabbout R, Gennaro E, Dalla Bernardina B, et al. Spectrum of SCN1A mutations in severe myoclonic epilepsy of infancy. *Neurology.* 2003;60(12):1961–1967.
49. Sadleir LG, Scheffer IE. Febrile seizures. *BMJ.* 2007;334:307–311.

50. Scheffer IE, Berkovic SF. Generalized epilepsy with febrile seizures plus. A genetic disorder with heterogeneous clinical phenotypes. *Brain*. 1997;120:479–490.
51. Scheffer IE, Harkin LA, Grinton BE, et al. Temporal lobe epilepsy and GEFS+ phenotypes associated with SCN1B mutations. *Brain*. 2007;130:100–109.
52. Scheffer IE, Wallace R, Wellard MR, et al. Temporal lobe epilepsy and febrile seizures associated with a sodium channel beta 1 subunit (SCN1B) mutation. *Epilepsia*. 2000;41(Suppl 7):71.
53. Singh R, Andermann E, Whitehouse WPA, et al. Severe myoclonic epilepsy of infancy: Extended spectrum of GEFS+? *Epilepsia*. 2001;42(7):837–844.
54. Singh R, Scheffer IE, Crossland K, et al. Generalized epilepsy with febrile seizures plus: a common, childhood onset, genetic epilepsy syndrome. *Ann Neurol*. 1999;45(1):75–81.
55. Singh R, Scheffer IE, Whitehouse W, et al. Severe myoclonic epilepsy of infancy is part of the spectrum of generalized epilepsy with febrile seizures plus (GEFS^{+}). *Epilepsia*. 1999;40:175.
56. Spampanato J, Aradi I, Soltesz I, et al. Increased neuronal firing in computer simulations of sodium channel mutations that cause generalized epilepsy with febrile seizures plus. *J Neurophysiol*. 2004;91(5):2040–2050.
57. Spampanato J, Escayg A, Meisler MH, et al. Generalized epilepsy with febrile seizures plus type 2 mutation W1204R alters voltage-dependent gating of Na(v)1.1 sodium channels. *Neuroscience*. 2003;116(1):37–48.
58. Sugawara T, Mazaki-Miyazaki E, Ito M, et al. *Na(v)1.1* mutations cause febrile seizures associated with afebrile partial seizures. *Neurology*. 2001;57(4):703–705.
59. Sugawara T, Tsurubuchi Y, Agarwala KL, et al. A missense mutation of the Na+ channel alpha II subunit gene Na(v)1.2 in a patient with febrile and afebrile seizures causes channel dysfunction. *Proc Natl Acad Sci U S A*. 2001;98(11):6384–6389.
60. Veggiotti P, Cardinali S, Montalenti E, et al. Generalized epilepsy with febrile seizures plus and severe myoclonic epilepsy in infancy: a case report of two Italian families. *Epileptic Disord*. 2001;3(1):29–32.
61. Wallace R, Scheffer IE, Parasivam G, et al. Generalised epilepsy with febrile seizures plus: mutation of the sodium channel subunit *SCN1B*. *Neurology*. 2002;58(9):1426–1429.
62. Wallace RH, Marini C, Petrou S, et al. Mutant GABA(A) receptor gamma2-subunit in childhood absence epilepsy and febrile seizures. *Nat Genet*. 2001;28(1):49–52.
63. Wallace RH, Scheffer IE, Barnett S, et al. Neuronal sodium-channel alpha1-subunit mutations in generalized epilepsy with febrile seizures plus. *Am J Hum Genet*. 2001;68(4):859–865.
64. Wallace RH, Wang DW, Singh R, et al. Febrile seizures and generalized epilepsy associated with a mutation in the Na+ channel beta1 subunit gene SCN1B. *Nat Genet*. 1998;19(4):366–370.

CHAPTER 257 ■ REFLEX SEIZURES

BENJAMIN G. ZIFKIN, RENZO GUERRINI, AND PERRINE PLOUIN

INTRODUCTION

Reflex seizures are reliably triggered by some identifiable factor.[200] Reviews include Beaumanoir et al., Zifkin et al., and Wolf et al.[11,210,213] The identification of a patient with reflex epilepsy depends on the physician's awareness and on the observations of the patient and witnesses. The epileptogenic trigger must occur often enough in everyday life so that its relation to the resulting seizures can be suspected. If the trigger is ubiquitous, however, the seizures appear to occur by chance or with no obvious antecedent.

The study of reflex seizures has also furthered understanding of cortical organization in man and has implications for our understanding of how and why some apparently generalized seizures may begin.

DEFINITION AND HISTORY

Seizures induced by light stimulation were known from classical antiquity, and in the 20th century before the electroencephalographic (EEG) era.[166,189] The use of the term *reflex* has been controversial. Hall[85] first applied it to epilepsy in 1850. Arguing that no reflex arc is involved in reflex epilepsy, others proposed terms such as *sensory precipitation*[65,156] or *stimulus-sensitive epilepsies*.[42] Wieser noted that sensory precipitation epilepsy is a misnomer because some reflex seizures, for example, those triggered by cognition, are not precipitated by sensory stimuli.[197] In the 19th century, Brown-Séquard[27] noted that "certain parts of the central nervous system possess an elevated excitability so that any minimal stimulation may cause a crisis." Both Gowers[77] and Hughlings Jackson[95] described reflex seizures triggered by various causes including sudden noise, bright sunlight, movement, and tapping the head, which are still accepted reflex seizure types. In the 20th century, Adrian and Matthews[1] first documented the effect of light on the normal EEG. The stroboscope became available after World War II and rapidly led to further progress as flicker stimulation and its clinical and EEG effects could be easily studied. Important studies by Walter and Walter,[195] and later by groups led by Gastaut in France and by Bickford in America, yielded basic information about those EEG responses to stroboscopic flicker (intermittent photic stimulation [IPS]), which were reliably linked to seizures. Television screens and sunlight are the most common environmental triggers of visual-sensitive seizures; triggering by television broadcasts and video games has become notorious in recent years, leading to increased interest in reflex seizures.

CLASSIFICATION

Some earlier classifications and the publications on which they were based described "simple" and "complex" reflex epilepsies. Binnie[19] noted: "A distinction should be made between seizures evoked by simple, unstructured sensory stimuli and those precipitated by complex cognitive activities, often with an emotional component. The former are interpretable in terms of known physiological events (not strictly reflex processes) following a stimulus, whereas the latter may offer insights into the complex mechanisms underlying cognition." Wolf and Inoue[209] described reading epilepsy and praxis induction as complex reflex epilepsies.

Complex reflex epilepsies are characterized by seizures triggered by relatively elaborate stimuli whose specific pattern is the determining factor in seizure evocation. The attacks are precipitated by stimuli involving integration of higher cortical function, rather than by relatively simple sensory stimuli, and may be evoked by anticipation of the stimulus. Latency from stimulus onset to the clinical seizure or evoked abnormal paroxysmal EEG activity is typically longer than in simple reflex epilepsies, such as photosensitive epilepsy, in which the response to flicker is usually almost immediate. These properties, enunciated in the 1985 proposal for classification of epilepsies,[42] had been systematically described in the pioneering work of Forster.[61] To avoid confusion, it should also be emphasized that the term *complex*, as applied to reflex epilepsy, does not refer to a classification of the induced seizures. Although many varieties are not accepted as epileptic syndromes in the current international classification, partly because of the occurrence of spontaneous seizures in the same patients, they are described as "epilepsies characterized by specific modes of seizure precipitation."[43] Despite this, the induction of attacks in these patients is prominent and often quite stereotyped, and the Commission's 1989 definition of a syndrome—"a cluster of signs and symptoms customarily occurring together"—may be met. In others, for example, with "language-induced seizures," the clinical pattern may overlap other more clearly defined entities.

The current classification proposal[55] defines reflex epilepsy syndromes as those "... in which all epileptic seizures are precipitated by sensory stimuli. Reflex seizures that occur in focal and generalized epilepsy syndromes that are also associated with spontaneous seizures are listed as seizure types." Thus, this proposal also recognizes few reflex epilepsy syndromes:

- Idiopathic photosensitive occipital lobe epilepsy
- Other visual-sensitive epilepsies
- Startle epilepsy
- Primary reading epilepsy
- Musicogenic epilepsy

Reflex seizures are often classified according to the stimuli that trigger them rather than by the type of seizure that is triggered. The classification proposal also includes, under seizure types, a list of precipitating stimuli for reflex seizures. These stimuli are:

- Visual stimuli
- Flickering light—color to be specified when possible
- Patterns
- Other stimuli
- Thinking

- Praxis
- Reading
- Somatosensory
- Proprioceptive
- Eating
- Music
- Hot water
- Startle

It is important to note that reflex seizures are not distinguishable from spontaneous seizures except for the fact that they are triggered in some identifiable way; that is, a reflex generalized tonic–clonic seizure is clinically the same as one that occurs spontaneously.

BASIC MECHANISMS OF REFLEX EPILEPSY

Animal Models

There are two types of animal model of reflex epilepsy. In the first, diffuse or regional cortical hyperexcitability is induced chemically or by the creation of a lesion. The second model involves naturally occurring reflex epilepsies or seizures induced by specific sensory stimulation in genetically predisposed animals.

The first approach has been used since 1929, when Clementi[38] induced convulsions with intermittent photic stimulation after applying strychnine to the canine visual cortex. Strychninization of auditory,[39] gustatory,[40] and olfactory cortex[140] also produced focal irritative lesions that could produce seizures with the appropriate afferent stimulus. EEG studies showed that the clinical seizures (chewing movements), which were induced by photic stimulation in rabbits with strychnine lesions of the visual cortex, resulted from rapid transmission of the epileptic discharge from the visual cortex to masticatory areas.[190] Paroxysmal discharge from visual cortex may also spread to frontorolandic areas during seizures.[63,66] The ictal EEG spread was thought to represent corticocortical conduction,[38,63] although later work with pentylenetetrazol also implicated thalamic relays[66] and demonstrated spread of the visual-evoked potential to the brainstem reticular formation.[64] Hunter and Ingvar[96] identified a subcortical pathway involving the thalamus and reticular system and an independent corticocortical system for radiation of visual-evoked responses to the frontal lobe. In cats and monkeys, the frontorolandic region was also shown to receive spreading-evoked paroxysmal activity from auditory and other stimuli.[18,28]

The second approach, the study of naturally occurring or induced reflex seizures in genetically susceptible animals, has been pursued in chickens with photosensitivity,[45,105] rodents susceptible to sound-induced convulsions,[35] the E1 mouse sensitive to vestibular stimulation,[179] and the Mongolian gerbil sensitive to a variety of stimuli.[126,127] Most of these are of limited relevance to human epilepsy but are of interest to the drug industry as rodent models are useful as relatively cheap and standardized methods for testing possible antiepileptic drugs.

The only species in which naturally occurring reflex seizures and EEG findings are similar to those in humans is the baboon Papio papio,[113] but the light-induced epileptic discharges in baboons occur in the frontorolandic area, rather than in the occipital lobe as they do in human photosensitive epilepsy.[112] EEG, visual-evoked potentials, intracerebral recording, and lesion and pharmacologic studies show that visual afferents are necessary to trigger frontorolandic light-induced epileptic discharges in these animals. Unlike human photosensitivity in which the occipital cortex is hyperexcitable, in the baboon the occipital lobe does not generate this abnormal activity, but sends corticocortical visual afferents to hyperexcitable frontal cortex, which is responsible for the epileptiform activity.[137] The interhemispheric synchronization of the light-induced paroxysmal EEG activity and seizures depends mainly on the corpus callosum and not on the brainstem. Brainstem reticular activation depends initially on frontal cortical mechanisms until a seizure is about to begin, at which point the cortex can no longer control reticular activation. The genetically determined hyperexcitability may be related to cortical biochemical abnormalities, involving regulation of extracellular calcium concentration,[51,161] or an imbalance between excitatory and inhibitory neurotransmitter amino acids[124] similar to those described in feline generalized penicillin epilepsy and in human epilepsy.[74]

VISUAL-SENSITIVE EPILEPSIES AND SEIZURES

Reflex seizures and epilepsies sensitive to visual stimulation, especially flashing light, are the commonest and longest known, and will be described first. Visual sensitivity has been defined as "having seizures evoked by the physical characteristics of a visual stimulus in daily life or by IPS."[111] Recognition of seizures induced by flashing light predates the EEG. Before clinical EEG, seizures were reported with environmental flicker or with sudden changes in light intensity. Gastaut et al. reported an early series of patients investigated with stroboscopic IPS during EEG recording.[68] Historically, photosensitivity has meant an abnormal response to light and since the development of the stroboscope, an abnormal response to flicker stimulation during EEG recording is generally called photosensitivity. This flicker sensitivity is common to different types of seizures induced by visual stimuli, but subtypes in which patients are reproducibly sensitive to more complex visual stimuli can be distinguished among patients, who are almost always sensitive to intermittent photic stimulation at some time. Pure photosensitive epilepsy, in which seizures occur only with environmental light stimulation, is the most common reflex epilepsy. The induction of focal occipital lobe seizures by the same types of visual stimuli is more common than previously thought. Television and sunlight are the most common environmental triggers of visual-sensitive seizures; triggering by television broadcasts and video games has become notorious in recent years. Visual-sensitive epilepsy is included as a reflex epilepsy syndrome in the most recent proposed classification of epilepsy syndromes.[55]

Several types of EEG response to flicker have been described. An epileptiform EEG response to IPS is a photoparoxysmal response (PPR). These may be restricted to the occipital area or be apparently generalized. Different responses may occur in the same patient depending on the stimulator used, the stimulation protocol, age, and medication effects. In untreated subjects, only generalized paroxysmal epileptiform discharges in response to IPS (spikes, polyspikes, and spike-and-wave complexes) are clearly linked to epilepsy: Apart from those with idiopathic photosensitive occipital epilepsy (IPOE), less is known about patients with clinically evident visually triggered seizures but who have only focal occipital PPRs. These responses are most common with stimulation from 10 to 30 flashes per second.

Epidemiology of Visual Sensitivity

Most studies are retrospective and target specific patient groups. Following seizures triggered by the video game Mario World in 1992, Quirk et al.[163] prospectively studied the incidence of visually-induced seizures and PPRs in newly diagnosed epilepsy patients in the United Kingdom. For all ages, a conservative estimate was that the incidence of epilepsy with PPRs was 1.1 per 100,000, about 2% of all new cases of epilepsy. Incidence rose to 5.7 per 100,000, or 10% of all new cases, in patients from 7 to 19 years old.

PPRs and clinical photosensitivity show marked age dependency. They are very rare before age 2 years. In Dravet syndrome (severe myoclonic epilepsy of infancy), responses may be abnormal before age 2 but without evident seizures, and Oguni et al.[148] reported a subgroup in whom myoclonic seizures and atypical absences could be triggered by constant illumination, rather than by IPS, depending on the brightness of the light. This sensitivity tended to disappear before age 5 years. Only one case has been reported of an infant aged 15 months who experienced about 20 seizures in 3 weeks when brought into a bathroom with bright white walls and shiny bright chromed plumbing; he showed the following symptoms: Motion arrest, deviation of the head and eyes to the left, jerks of the eyelids, looking afraid, and right occipital seizure on the EEG. He had no further seizures until he was 11, when occipital seizures recurred.[172]

Both PPRs and visually induced seizures show a clear female preponderance of about 60% of cases, and photosensitivity appears to peak at around puberty. Whether photosensitivity declines with age in patients is debated; several report that it declines in the third decade, while others found no decline with age.[111] PPRs occur in normal subjects, especially in children up to 16 years old, in whom a prevalence of 1.3% has been reported, and this photosensitivity declines with age. Studies in young adult male aircrew candidates in several countries yielded PPR rates of 0.5% to 0.7%.

Genetics of Photoparoxysmal Responses

Genetic studies of photosensitivity have been hampered by differences in stimulation methods and in classification of the EEG responses. The reduction of sensitivity with age, especially in asymptomatic children, also makes transgenerational studies impossible or difficult to interpret. Monozygotic twins have shown almost 100% concordance for PPRs. Waltz and Stephani reported that photosensitivity is significantly more common in 5- to 10-year-old siblings of proband offspring of a photosensitive parent (50%) than in siblings of photosensitive children without parental photosensitivity (14%). The highest risk of seizure (33%) was in photosensitive siblings of a proband with parental photosensitivity, and the lowest (4%) in nonphotosensitive siblings of probands without parental photosensitivity.[196]

A single gene for photosensitivity has not yet been identified. Three different loci have been found, one on each of chromosomes 2 (in a single family), 7q32, and 16p13, and the last two in families with prominent myoclonic epilepsy.[158] Photosensitivity occurring in some patients with identifiable epileptic syndromes (e.g., juvenile myoclonic epilepsy [JME]) is inherited separately from the other epileptic disorder.

Clinical Aspects of Visual Sensitivity

The proposed classification recognizes idiopathic photosensitive occipital lobe epilepsy and "other" visual-sensitive epilepsies as reflex epilepsy syndromes, requiring that all seizures be triggered. Other cases are classified as seizure types, which are more common, and it is not specified whether these represent generalized or focal epilepsy.

Pure Photosensitive Epilepsy

Pure photosensitive epilepsy is characterized by seizures exclusively provoked by flicker. These patients do not have spontaneous seizures. Forty percent of patients with seizures and photosensitivity studied by Jeavons and Harding, Binnie et al., and Kasteleijn-Nolst Trenité et al. are reported to fall into this group. In one study, 84% of patients had seizures reported as generalized tonic–clonic, whereas absences occurred in only 6%, partial motor seizures (possibly asymmetric myoclonus in some cases or unrecognized idiopathic photosensitive occipital epilepsy) in 2.5%, and myoclonic seizures in 1.5% of patients.[104] However, these proportions are subject to bias; patients will come to medical attention after a convulsion in front of the television but may have already had many subtle unobserved reflex seizures with brief myoclonic or absence-like events. Patient self-reporting of these triggered seizures can be extremely inaccurate: Over half of known photosensitive epilepsy patients questioned immediately after stimulation denied having had brief but clear-cut seizures induced by IPS and documented by video-EEG monitoring.[110] In laboratory studies with video monitoring, most events are myoclonic jerks[110] and patients commonly report eye pain and feelings of eyestrain. The developmental and neurologic examinations are normal.

Idiopathic Photosensitive Occipital Epilepsy

IPOE[84] is recognized as a reflex epilepsy syndrome in the proposed diagnostic scheme. IPOE is a relatively benign, age-related syndrome without spontaneous seizures. Seizures evoked by visual stimuli were formerly thought to be almost exclusively generalized despite the clear occipital localization of visual function, though asymmetric myoclonus could occur. Induction of partial seizures by visual stimulation, including typical complex partial seizures, is now well recognized.[92] Intermittent photic stimulation can induce clear-cut partial seizures originating in the occipital lobe.[81,92] As in more typical photosensitive subjects, environmental triggers include television and video games. The symptoms may remain localized to the occipital area for several minutes even after the stimulus has ceased: Visual blurring, blindness, or elementary visual hallucinations may occur.[81,169,188] The clinical seizure pattern depends on the pattern of spread. The initial reflex visual symptoms may be followed by versive movements and motor seizures. Myoclonus is not typical, but migraine-like symptoms of throbbing headache, nausea, and, sometimes, vomiting are common and can lead to delayed or incorrect diagnosis.

Photosensitive Epilepsy with Spontaneous Seizures

The remaining 60% of patients with epilepsy and photosensitivity also have spontaneous seizures, and photosensitivity gives rise to attacks precipitated by environmental visual stimulation in 33% of the total. A further 7% have demonstrable seizures during IPS but report no visually precipitated attacks in everyday life. Thus, 80% of photosensitive people with epilepsy have some form of visually precipitated seizures. These are often associated with idiopathic generalized epilepsies and especially with juvenile myoclonic epilepsy, in which 30% to 48% are photosensitive, and childhood absence epilepsy, in which 18% were reportedly photosensitive.[125,208] Typical absence seizures may be triggered by IPS: These are rare and may be resistant to treatment.[10]

Photosensitivity in Other Epileptic Disorders

Photosensitivity may be found in several epileptic disorders. It is rare in symptomatic occipital epilepsies but has been described with triggered focal occipital seizures in patients with occipital calcifications and celiac disease.[4] It also may occur with symptomatic generalized epilepsies such as severe myoclonic epilepsy of infancy (SMEI, Dravet syndrome); with the progressive myoclonus epilepsies such as Lafora disease, Unverricht-Lundborg disease, Kufs disease; or with the neuronal ceroid lipofuscinoses, in which photosensitivity at low flash frequencies such as 1/s is typical. These syndromes are associated with photic cortical reflex myoclonus, and the patients also have clear-cut action myoclonus.

Pattern-sensitive Seizures

Pattern-sensitive epilepsy consists of seizures triggered by viewing patterns, typically stripes. The seizures are generalized convulsions, absences, or brief myoclonic attacks provoked by viewing patterns such as patterned video screen content, escalator steps, striped wallpaper, or patterned clothing.[22] Television is now the most common precipitant, reported in 41% of 73 patients.[165]

Initially described in a single child by Bickford, it was considered an interesting rarity. Bickford et al.[17] reported a low rate of EEG sensitivity to stationary pattern of 0.25% in 40,000 patients. Chatrian showed that the nature of the pattern affected its epileptogenicity, and the classic studies of Wilkins et al.[22] further described the characteristics of epileptogenic patterns. With stimuli designed for maximum effect, pattern sensitivity is more common than previously reported, found in 17% to 54% of photosensitive subjects with static patterns.[21,109,144,160] Patterns oscillating orthogonal to their line orientation are more provocative and elicit sensitivity in 60% to 70%.[21] Clinical pattern sensitivity is much less common, found in about 2% of photosensitive subjects by Jeavons and Harding[104] and in 6% by Kasteleijn-Nolst Trenité.[109] Some subjects sensitive to pattern are not sensitive to flicker.[90] Radhakrishnan et al.[165] noted this in 11% of 73 subjects, but their first EEGs were performed in 1950 and this may be partly related to different methods of IPS and age-related changes in photosensitivity.

Interictal epileptiform EEG activity has been reported in 84%. Two thirds had generalized epileptiform activity with pattern stimulation, and in one third, this was confined to posterior head regions.[165] These authors also found that 14 of 73 (19%) had JME, three had progressive myoclonus epilepsy, and one had SMEI.

Other

Some photosensitive patients are sensitive to eye closure alone. Reflex absences or brief myoclonic attacks, and visual disturbances ("scotosensitive seizures") can occur with eye closure or in darkness in patients not sensitive to intermittent photic stimulation and are thought to be precipitated in some by the abolition of central vision and fixation.[151,152] Others may not require total darkness or abolition of fixation. However, most subjects with the florid posterior epileptiform EEG activity abolished by fixation, and typical of the Panayiotopoulos and Gastaut types of idiopathic childhood occipital epilepsy, do not have reflex seizures.

Eyelid myoclonia with absences, described by Jeavons[103] and reviewed by Gobbi,[75] is characterized by eyelid jerks with eye closure in a photosensitive patient, with bilateral fast spike-and-wave EEG activity. The seizures can occur even in darkness. Some have no spontaneous seizures. Often, only the EEG change can be seen. Not all patients have absences and not all are photosensitive. It is not yet clear whether this forms a discrete clinical entity: The trigger mechanisms are complex and not well defined, and many may have another epileptic disorder such as JME. Harding and Jeavons[90] suggested that most such cases were examples of self-induction, but a detailed definition of a syndrome of eyelid myoclonia with absences has been suggested by Panayiotopoulos.[153]

Seizures reportedly triggered by eye movement[183,191] are a heterogeneous group. Some may represent scotosensitivity, and others may be cases of self-induction. Others triggered by conjugate eye movement may depend on proprioceptive input, and anterior, occipital, and parietal EEG discharges have been reported with these.

Self-induction of Visual-sensitive Seizures

Patients with all types of visually induced seizures may induce attacks with visual stimulation and may be compulsively drawn to sources of flicker or pattern stimulation such as television screens. Patients sensitive to eye closure may use a compulsively repeated eye rolling and eyelid flicker movement to self-stimulate.[47] Monitoring has shown that the stimulatory behaviors indeed trigger the seizures rather than being manifestations of the seizures. Intensely pleasurable sensations have been reported with these, and some patients induce seizures to relieve stress or to gain attention.[188] Monitoring indicates that 24% to 30%[21] engage in self-induction when placed in a well-lit environment, particularly if stressed. Diagnostic features are:[19]

1. The eye movement precedes the epileptiform EEG discharge.
2. The oculographic artifact is larger and slower than that accompanying normal spontaneous eye closure and often shows a superimposed ocular tremor at about 6 Hz.
3. The maneuver is carried out less frequently in darkness, where it fails to produce epileptiform discharge.
4. The behavior is increased by stress.
5. Patients display guilt when the phenomenon is discussed.
6. Patients admit to carrying out the maneuver, variously describing it as voluntary or compulsive.
7. A pleasant sensation is often reported; this may have a sexual component leading to orgasm in some subjects.
8. There may be a history of seizures induced by hand waving in the past, or patients may use hand waving in combination with slow eye closure to enhance or prolong the discharge, as documented on film by Ames.[5]

These can be distinguished by EEG monitoring from nonepileptic paroxysmal eyelid movements that may occur in children and adults with generalized photosensitive epilepsy. These may be mistaken for absence seizures. There is often a family history of eyelid movements.[29]

Seizures Triggered by Television and Video Displays

Reflex seizures triggered by television, computer screens, and video games have become notorious. The Pocket Monsters cartoon episode that triggered a nationwide outbreak of photosensitive seizures in Japan is a well-known example,[87,102] but broadcasting of dangerous screen content had already led to outbreaks of photosensitive seizures, and guidelines to prevent the broadcasting of screen content likely to trigger seizures were already in place in the United Kingdom. These have become more widespread since the Pocket Monsters episode. Many of these events represent pure photosensitive epilepsy with or without pattern sensitivity. Some have occurred in subjects not previously known to have epilepsy, and others have occurred in known photosensitive patients. Some were likely focal occipital visual reflex seizures with autonomic manifestations (see IPOE above). Ferrie et al.[59] found that 29% of a group of subjects with video game–induced seizures had photosensitive partial seizures. In patients with seizures recurring after an initial Pocket Monster seizure, juvenile myoclonic epilepsy was the most common diagnosis in those not known to have epilepsy before the triggered event, while those with a history of epilepsy and recurrent seizures often had frontal lobe epilepsy.[149]

Guidelines in Japan and the United Kingdom now prohibit such program material.[91] These have been shown to successfully control potentially harmful TV screen content.[186] Special electronic filter devices are also effective in reducing PPRs induced by television.[185] Seizures associated with video screens may also have occurred by chance or in nonphotosensitive individuals in relation to other reflex seizure triggers, such as thinking, with or without manipulation of objects (action programming or praxis, see below) during computer use or game play.

Mechanisms of Visual-sensitive Seizures

Several approaches have been taken to studying human photosensitivity and seizures induced by visual stimuli. Visual stimulation resembling reported environmental stimuli such as video games can be modified and responses studied. Properties of elementary and subthreshold visual stimuli can be manipulated to enable inferences to be drawn about physiologic trigger mechanisms in both EEG and evoked potential studies and more recently in magnetic resonance and magnetoencephalography studies.

Television-induced seizures and others triggered by video displays can be understood in relation to the properties of video screens and to the images on the screen. Visual reflex seizures and the characteristics of the effective triggers have been recently reviewed.[214] Flicker rate, pattern, luminous intensity, size, location, and duration of the stimulus need to be considered. A television screen produces flicker at the alternating current (AC) frequency, effectively generating IPS at 60 Hz in North America and 50 Hz in Europe. Photosensitivity is more common at the lower frequency, with nearly 50% of patients sensitive to 50-Hz intermittent photic stimulation,[104] and television sensitivity has indeed been a greater problem in Europe than in North America. Television-induced seizures, however, are not only related to AC frequency flicker. Wilkins et al. studied patients who were not sensitive to this flicker but who responded to the vibrating pattern of interleaved lines at half the AC frequency (25 Hz in Europe and 30 Hz in North America) to which about 75% of photosensitive subjects are sensitive and which can be discerned only close to the screen.[205] Special 100-Hz television screens, marketed in Europe, reduce the risk of television-induced seizures.[169] Color is important even without luminance changes; photoparoxysmal EEG responses can be elicited in sensitive subjects by non–color-opponent stimuli even if they are isoluminant.[88] Sensitivity is greater with red stimulation at wavelengths greater than 700 nm, and red stimulation was important in the Japanese cartoon incident.[87] Red-cyan flicker, even when isoluminant, is reportedly even more provocative of epileptic discharge.[180] Thus, seizures can be triggered even at greater distances and by 100-Hz TV sets and modern noninterlaced screens without intrinsic flicker. Flashing or patterned screen content has been implicated in these. Although the 50-Hz television screen is an important determinant of screen sensitivity and 100-Hz screens reduce the ability of the screen to trigger seizures, it is important to note that all systems are equally dangerous if dangerous screen content is broadcast.

Most patients sensitive to IPS can be shown to be sensitive to pattern, and studies on pattern-sensitive patients have enabled several inferences to be drawn, based also on animal studies of single unit responses. These have recently been reviewed by Wilkins et al.[203] and can be summarized as follows:

The seizure trigger involves cortical cells. A paroxysmal EEG response occurs in the majority of patients with a history of photosensitive seizures when they are exposed to IPS. In about 30% of patients, bright, large, continuously illuminated patterns of high-contrast stripes evoke a similar, though usually less pronounced, response. The response is probabilistic and depends on the spatial and temporal properties of the visual stimuli that evoke it. Studies of length of line contour of effective patterns, pattern orientation, and the effect of binocularity indicate a cortical trigger. Further evidence comes from studies of effects of spatial frequency and of pattern motion: These suggest that the trigger involves neurons whose spatial tuning is independent of position in the visual field, and the first point at which this independence occurs is at the level of the complex cell in the visual cortex. EEG studies using patterns presented in only part of the visual field, such as hemifield stimulation, are also consistent with an occipital cortical event, and also indicate that seizure onset involves one cerebral hemisphere or both hemispheres independently. Often the response is generalized, involving many brain areas other than the visual cortex, but even in these circumstances the trigger may be cortical and unilateral because when the response is suppressed with sodium valproate, focal occipital activity can remain.[48] All these are consistent with an epileptic discharge triggered in the visual cortex, which sometimes remains within the visual cortex and sometimes spreads to involve other areas.

The triggering mechanism requires the physiologic activation of a critical area of cortical tissue. Any region of the visual cortex can evoke an epileptiform discharge, provided a sufficiently large area is stimulated. Wilkins[201] noted that the probability of a response to patterns differs in each patient, but in such a way as to indicate that each patient's threshold can be expressed in terms of the area of cortex necessary to trigger a discharge.

Synchronization of the physiologic activation is necessary for epileptogenesis. Patterns that vibrate back and forth, orthogonal to their line orientation, become more epileptogenic, but a pattern that drifts steadily in the same direction ceases to be epileptogenic. This difference suggests an important role for the synchronization of large neuronal aggregates in the induction of a discharge. When the pattern alternately changes direction, the neurons sensitive to one direction of motion should fire, followed by a period during which cells sensitive to the opposite direction of motion should fire. The very marked difference in the epileptogenic properties of drifting and vibrating patterns suggests that the synchronization that occurs with a vibrating or phase-reversing pattern is critical at the initiation of the epileptic discharge.

The trigger involves the magnocellular pathways, but the resulting discharge may be more diffuse and involve both magnocellular and parvocellular divisions. Several characteristics of epileptogenic patterns suggest this involvement. The stripes differ in brightness rather than color, and are more epileptogenic if they move in certain ways and fuse in binocular vision. They have a rather low spatial frequency. Magnocellular neurons do not generally code for color, are directionally coded, and are tuned for binocular disparity. They have a lower spatial resolution and a higher temporal resolution than parvocellular neurons. The magnocellular system is thought to be part of the "dorsal stream," and in pattern-sensitive patients, the isolated spikes in response to a pattern tend to be most marked over parietal electrodes. The cortical hyperexcitability need not be confined to this system but the discharge may start there. Harding and Fylan[88] also provide evidence for the participation of the parvocellular system.

The visual system in visual-sensitive epilepsies is normal with respect to acuity, stereopsis, and color vision. However, evidence of visual cortical abnormality is found in pattern reversal visual-evoked potentials; these show a lack of luminance contrast gain control at low spatial frequencies in subjects with IPOE.[159] This is seen only at temporal frequencies lower than those that are typically epileptogenic. Functional magnetic resonance imaging (fMRI)[94] and magnetoencephalography

(MEG)[154,168] also suggest regional occipital cortical hyperexcitability, regional activations, and abnormal neuronal synchronization in photosensitive subjects. MEG in photosensitive subjects showed enhanced phase synchrony in the gamma band (30 to 120 Hz) preceding those photic stimulation trials that evolve into PPR compared with trials not followed by PPR and compared with phase synchrony in nonphotosensitive controls, possibly reflecting a pathologic synchronization of gamma oscillation that mediates the transition to PPR.[154]

An important feature of most visual-sensitive seizures and of pattern sensitivity in particular is that a stimulus that activates a well-defined cortical area subserving a specific function will produce seizures usually thought of as generalized and often occurring within a typical generalized epilepsy syndrome such as JME. This paradigm will be encountered with complex reflex seizures, discussed below, and appears to operate in seizures induced by thinking and praxis and in many cases of reading epilepsy. Studies of reflex seizures suggest that cognitive triggering occurs mostly with idiopathic generalized epilepsy (IGE). These and other observations in both reflex and spontaneous epileptogenesis[20,58] suggest that the postulated cortical hyperexcitability in IGE is not necessarily uniform: Specific activities can activate specific cortical systems and produce focal discharges or partial seizures, which may generalize. This does not invalidate a diagnosis of underlying generalized epilepsy but shows that the biologic substrate of generalized epilepsy can be complicated.

Treatment of Visual-Sensitive Seizures

All reflex seizures may be treated by avoiding the triggering stimulus. This is not always practical or possible, but modification of the stimulus may reduce or eliminate its epileptogenicity. Increasing the distance from the television set, watching a small screen in a well-lighted room, using a remote control so that the set need not be approached, and monocular viewing or the use of polarized eyeglasses to block one eye should provide protection.[204] Colored eyeglasses may be useful in selected cases.[32,202] Prevention of seizures induced by video screens is effective but requires adherence to guidelines that reduce the likelihood of a visually triggered seizure or the use of special electronic filter devices, which is less practical as these would be required on all screens. A recent draft consensus developed by the Epilepsy Foundation of America[91] noted:

> "A pattern with the potential for provoking seizures contains clearly discernible stripes, numbering more than five light–dark pairs of stripes in any orientation. When the light–dark stripes of any pattern collectively subtend at the eye from the minimal-expected viewing distance a solid angle of >0.006 steradians, the luminance of the lightest stripe is >50 cd/m2, and the pattern is presented for ≥ 0.5 s, then the pattern should display no more than five light–dark pairs of stripes, if the stripes change direction, oscillate, flash, or reverse in contrast; if the pattern is unchanging or smoothly drifting in one direction, no more than eight stripes."

Drug treatment is needed if preventive measures are impractical or unsuccessful, if photosensitivity is severe, or if spontaneous attacks occur. The drug of choice is valproate, which in one study[89] abolished photosensitivity in 54% of patients and markedly reduced it in a further 24%. Lamotrigine, topiramate, ethosuximide, benzodiazepines such as clobazam,[34] and levetiracetam[111] also may be useful. Quesney et al.[162] proposed a dopaminergic mechanism in human epileptic photosensitivity based on the transient abolition of photosensitivity with apomorphine, and bromocriptine and parenteral L-dopa have been reported to alleviate photosensitivity.[37,139] Appropriate treatment for photosensitivity is generally successful and noncompliance or self-induction should be considered if it is not.

STARTLE EPILEPSY

Startle epilepsy is characterized by seizures triggered by unexpected sensory stimuli, usually auditory. Startle epilepsy was described in the 1989 International Classification of Epilepsies and Epileptic Syndromes as a symptomatic epilepsy in which seizures occur with a specific mode of precipitation. The most recent proposed classification[55] includes startle epilepsy as a reflex epilepsy syndrome. The effective stimulus is usually a sudden sound.[3] Most patients are sensitive to a single sensory modality but the suddenness of the stimulation, which must be unexpected, is crucial. The seizures usually last <30 seconds and consist of a startle response followed by a brief tonic posture, which is usually asymmetric. Many subjects fall, and clonic jerks may occur. Injury is common when the seizures occur in patients who are standing or able to fall while seated, or while they are in bathtubs or similar risky locations. The seizures may be frequent but habituation is typical: If the stimulus is repeatedly presented over several minutes, it becomes temporarily ineffective. Patients with startle epilepsy usually have static cerebral lesions arising prenatally or within the first 2 years of life and intellectual handicap. Many are hemiparetic; in these, the weak side is preferentially involved in the seizure. Spontaneous seizures occur, reportedly in all cases, but may be infrequent. Startle epilepsy is typically intractable.

Brain imaging may show localized lesions (mesial hypodensity) or diffuse lesions.[2,82] The lateralized lesions usually involve sensorimotor and premotor cortex and white matter, but normal scans have been reported without neurologic deficit.[128] Such patients have precentral or perisylvian dysplastic lesions on MRI. Schizencephaly has also been found. Startle epilepsy often occurs with Down syndrome.

Scalp EEG ictal recording shows an initial vertex discharge followed by diffuse relative flattening or low-voltage rhythm at about 10 Hz. Ictal depth electrode recordings have shown an initial high-amplitude evoked response over motor areas corresponding to the vertex scalp activity, followed by ictal EEG discharge, which begins in lesioned motor or premotor cortex and spreads to mesial frontal, parietal, and contralateral frontal regions.[12,13,192] Subdural recordings in a patient with a small lesion next to the right supplementary sensorimotor area showed seizure onset in the right dorsolateral premotor cortex and the right supplementary sensorimotor area.[178]

The seizures resemble supplementary motor seizures. Localized lesions and seizure onset often involve that area or its surroundings: The epileptogenic lesion may be in the dorsolateral frontal lobe or in the perirolandic area (for a recent example with video illustration see Nolan et al.[146]).

Differential diagnosis includes startle disease (hyperekplexia).[6] Touch-evoked or tap seizures in children[50,212] may have a startle component, but are not startle epilepsy as currently defined. Startle stimuli can cause nonepileptic falls in Coffin-Lowry syndrome. Startle myoclonus, though not clearly startle epilepsy, has been reported in association with GM2 gangliosidosis[143] and startle epilepsy has been reported with aspartylglucosaminuria.[119] Seizures induced by sudden dousing with hot water may also have a startle component at some time in their course but are not to be confused with startle epilepsy.[15,174] Other reflex seizures, produced by cutaneous or proprioceptive stimulation, should also be distinguished from startle epilepsy.[107,192]

Startle epilepsy can be treated with drugs appropriate for focal seizures. Reports discuss carbamazepine, lamotrigine, clobazam, and clonazepam.[2,41,56,119,171] Psychological intervention has also been proposed.[136] Startle epilepsy is usually intractable, however, and surgery has been reported to control startle epilepsy associated with infantile hemiplegia.[33,131,147]

READING EPILEPSY

Primary reading epilepsy (RE) consists of seizures triggered exclusively by reading, without spontaneous seizures.[17] The current proposed diagnostic scheme defines it as a reflex epilepsy syndrome without specifying a generalized or focal subtype.[55] Seizures usually begin in adolescence. Patients report jaw jerking or clicking and other sensations or movements in orofacial muscles, usually after reading for some time, representing partial seizures or localized myoclonus. They may thus appear to stutter.[138] If reading then continues, even for a very short time in some patients, a generalized convulsion may occur. Seizures are not induced by mental activity without reading. The developmental history, neurologic examination, interictal EEG, and computed tomography (CT) scan are normal. A family history of epilepsy is common, and familial reading epilepsy may occur.[134,209] The syndrome is relatively benign and often goes undiagnosed, mistaken for harmless tics or stuttering.

Both unilateral and bilateral orofacial myoclonus may be triggered by reading and either may be seen with unilateral or bilateral EEG discharges.[209] In an important review of 111 patients by Wolf and Inoue,[209] 77% had triggered epileptiform discharges consisting of short bursts of sharp waves, spikes, or spike-and-wave complexes that are bilateral and symmetric in 32%, bilateral but asymmetric in 38%, and unilateral or focal in 30%. Lateralization is more frequent to the language-dominant hemisphere (78%), preferentially over the temporoparietal region (80%).

Radhakrishnan et al.[164] found generalized and symmetric ictal discharges in 15 of 20 patients (75%) with RE and asymmetric or unilateral discharges in five (25%) with lateralization to the dominant hemisphere. They suggested that RE be classified among the idiopathic generalized epilepsies. Mayer and Wolf[135] found that the triggered perioral reflex myoclonus thought to be exclusive to RE was also found with bilateral spike-and-wave EEG activity in juvenile myoclonic epilepsy, and was also recorded, triggered by talking more than by reading, in patients with a variety of epileptic disorders.[211] Koutroumanidis et al.[117] monitored 17 patients with RE. During the triggered myoclonic jerks, eight had bilateral synchronous epileptic discharges. Two patients had alexia or possibly speech arrest as the only ictal manifestation, associated on the EEG with focal abnormalities over the left posterior temporal area.

Koepp et al.[115] performed [11C]-diprenorphine positron emission tomography (PET) in a patient with RE and found decreased peri-ictal opioid binding in both temporal lobes and the left frontal lobe, regions that had shown PET activation during normal reading. Archer et al.[7] performed spike-triggered fMRI in a patient with reading epilepsy. During activation tasks, spike-related activity was found in the left precentral gyrus and bilaterally in the central sulcus and globus pallidus. Comparison of fMRI activation seen during spiking with that during reading showed overlap in the posterior dorsolateral prefrontal cortex. This area was shown to be activated during specific cognitive tasks with a working memory component, and evidence for the involvement of this region in RE also comes from a patient who developed RE after removal of a left premotor arteriovenous malformation.[170] Archer postulated that the ictal activity of RE spread from working memory into nearby motor cortex. The facial myoclonus typical of RE may also be triggered by language tasks in symptomatic epilepsies.[30]

Thus, it appears that reading can activate generalized epilepsies, similar to activation by pattern sensitivity with its occipital trigger. RE is not, however, exclusively a generalized epileptic phenomenon but involves a functional system over both hemispheres. Reading requires bihemispheric cooperation, with dominant hemisphere predominance for phonologic processing and nondominant hemisphere predominance for semantic representation. Pegna et al.[155] reported a case of RE and suggested lexical and nonlexical forms of RE, and RE seems less common in Japanese, which uses a logographic writing system.

Language-induced epilepsy involves seizure precipitation by speaking, reading, and writing.[71] The seizures are similar to those of primary reading epilepsy, and patients may report one or several seizure triggers related to language (e.g., recitation or writing only).[8,93] The nosologic position of language-induced epilepsy is not clear: Reported cases most closely resemble reading epilepsy but are more heterogeneous than those of primary reading epilepsy, whose definition should probably be expanded to include them.

RE may be treated by partial avoidance of the stimulus, especially if the patient does not develop generalized seizures or has a useful delay before one occurs. Interruption or limitation of reading can then be effective. Maneuvers that briefly disrupt comprehension or increase arousal may be helpful, but social and educational handicap may arise from all of these. Audiotaped texts may be useful. Text masking may help those in whom pattern or eye movement contribute to seizure occurrence.[206] Wolf and Inoue[209] reported that valproate is the drug of choice and that clonazepam can be a useful adjunct.

MUSICOGENIC SEIZURES

Induction of seizures in humans by unstructured sound apart from startle stimuli is very unusual. Musicogenic epilepsy is characterized by seizures induced by hearing certain sounds, typically music.[9,46] Patients with musicogenic seizures alone may have a reflex epilepsy syndrome, but most also have spontaneous seizures. The reflex seizures then often begin over a year after the onset of the spontaneous attacks.[198] Seizures have also been reported while the subject is exposed to the musical trigger during sleep or while thinking about it. The effective stimulus can be stereotyped for each patient. It can be restricted to a single musical work, but there is no clear common pattern among patients. An affective component of the stimulus must be present in some, yet nonmusical sounds, such as whirring machinery, can be effective triggers in others. The seizures are of simple or complex partial type, with interictal and ictal epileptiform activity recorded from either temporal region,[176] usually the right. Often, the seizure does not begin immediately and the patient must be exposed to the trigger for several seconds or minutes. Musicogenic seizures have been reported in infancy.[122] Some patients with autosomal dominant lateral temporal lobe epilepsy have reported triggering by sound or by hearing speech.[26]

A right temporal predominance for musicogenic seizures has been reported by several authors.[69,70,198] They also documented right anterior and mesial hyperperfusion during ictal single photon emission computed tomography (SPECT) of musicogenic seizures.

The mechanism of musicogenic seizures is not clear. Although cortical processing of music has been studied extensively, subjects have been normal controls or patients with lesions or intractable spontaneous seizures. Chronic temporal lobe depth electrode studies in epileptic subjects without musicogenic epilepsy suggest different lateralizations for different components of a musical stimulus.[199] Creutzfeldt and Ojemann showed that musical stimuli may have widespread effects on neuronal activity in human temporal lobes extending well beyond the primary auditory area,[44,121] that different components of music have different effects possibly with specialized lateralization and localization, and that the effects of music are different from those of speech. Studies of the cerebral representation and processing of music have been extended, and are reviewed in Peretz and Zatorre.[157] PET studies in patients and others[106] show predominant involvement of right hemisphere structures in networks involved in processing musical information, extending well beyond the classical auditory cortex of the Heschl gyrus. Studies in subjects with musical hallucinations show that the primary auditory cortex is not "a sufficient substrate for higher-order pattern perception."[79]

The primate auditory cortex consists of a central core of primary cortex that receives thalamic projections, linked to several "belt" areas. Primary cortex has multiple tonotopically organized areas and is especially sensitive to pure tones. Belt regions are more sensitive to complex stimuli and are less tonotopically organized.[106] Zifkin and Zatorre also noted that more complex musical processing tasks activate more cortical and subcortical territory bilaterally but with right hemisphere predominance.[215] Thus, hyperexcitable cortical areas could be stimulated to different degrees and extents by different musical stimuli in patients sensitive to musical triggers. Gloor suggested that responses to limbic stimulation in epileptic subjects depend on widespread neuronal matrices linked through connections that have become strengthened through repeated use, of interest in considering the delay from seizure onset to the development of sensitivity to music.[73]

Musicogenic seizures can be treated by stimulus avoidance or modification in many cases, especially if there is a useful latency from stimulus onset to seizure onset or if the stimulus is very specific. If this is not possible or effective, or if spontaneous seizures occur, drugs for focal seizures are indicated and intractable cases should be assessed for surgical treatment.

REFLEX SEIZURE TYPES USUALLY ASSOCIATED WITH GENERALIZED EPILEPSIES

Touch-evoked ("Tap") Seizures

Otherwise normal infants and toddlers may develop seizures induced by tapping, often by a single touch on the head ("tap epilepsy") or by a sudden sound.[50,212] Age of onset is usually from 6 months to 3 years. These are typically manifestations of an idiopathic generalized epilepsy and consist of an initial blink followed by bilateral myoclonic jerks mostly involving the arms, with flexion of the head and upward deviation of the eyes. If intense, they can cause a fall. They can occur isolated or in clusters. The interictal EEG is usually normal and there is no photosensitivity. The ictal EEG shows bilateral spike-and-wave EEG discharges usually predominant anteriorly. Differential diagnosis includes hyperekplexia, symptomatic disorders such as startle epilepsy and focal reflex seizures induced by cutaneous stimulation, and benign myoclonic epilepsy of infancy, which is not triggered and has somewhat later onset and longer duration of the disorder with other seizure types.[54] Imaging is normal. These seizures appear to represent an early-onset idiopathic generalized epilepsy, and many such cases remit without drug treatment. Valproate may be used when drug treatment is needed. These attacks are not remarkably different from the benign early infantile reflex absence seizures illustrated with video recording by Voskuil.[194]

Seizures Induced by Thinking and Praxis

Seizures induced by thinking[207] occur in response to higher cortical function and have been reported with a variety of stimuli, including arithmetic, drawing, playing cards or chess, decision making, solving Rubik's cube, and using the soroban (a Japanese abacus). Goossens et al.,[76] in an extensive review, have proposed this as a separate epileptic syndrome. These patients are not sensitive to reading. Although a patient may report only a single trigger, detailed testing shows that about 80% have more than one effective stimulus. Unlike those with primary reading epilepsy, most have spontaneous seizures, and the reflex and spontaneous attacks include bilateral myoclonus, absences, and generalized tonic–clonic seizures. Partial seizures have been reported but are the exception. Seizures related to "praxis," clinically and electroencephalographically similar to these,[98] have been reported, strongly associated with juvenile myoclonic epilepsy (Herpin-Janz syndrome) and at times with other generalized epilepsies. Patients with seizures induced by thinking almost always have an idiopathic generalized epilepsy syndrome but without any specific variety associated.

Seizures induced by thinking are typically associated with both spontaneous and evoked generalized bilaterally synchronous spike or multiple spike-and-wave complexes. These may reappear only after reduction of medications in some patients. Though patients often report mental arithmetic as a trigger, other effective stimuli have included parts of standard neuropsychological test batteries such as Block Design. While occasional patients have temporoparietal or frontal spontaneous nonspecific EEG abnormalities, typically over the right side, these are at times mixed with generalized epileptiform activity. Clearly localized induced epileptiform activity is very unusual.[76]

The essential component in the seizure trigger appears to be nonverbal thought, the processing of numeric or spatial information, and possibly sequential decision making. Recent studies provide more detail on the cerebral representation of calculation and spatial thought and document a bilateral functional network activated by such tasks.[181]

The term *praxis induction* was introduced by Japanese authors who described seizures triggered when subjects "are obliged to contemplate complicated spatial tasks in a sequential fashion, to make decisions, and to practically respond using a part of their body."[99] Writing is reported to be a frequent precipitating factor[98] although reading is not. Hand or finger movements without "action-programming activity" (defined as "higher mental activity requiring hand movement" and apparently synonymous with praxis) are not effective triggers. Matsuoka et al.[132,133] noted, "The dependence of hand movements in the seizure-inducing tasks differentiates the action-programming activity from the thinking activity." Reflex upper limb myoclonus occurs and may spread. This pattern occurs very predominantly in juvenile myoclonic epilepsy. It does not seem prominent in patients with thinking-induced seizures who do not also have prominent myoclonic reflex attacks. In its milder or most restricted forms, such as the morning myoclonic jerk of the arm manipulating a utensil, this phenomenon resembles cortical reflex myoclonus as part of a "continuum of epileptic activity centered on the sensorimotor cortex,"[192] and back-averaging of chess-induced spikes with unilateral myoclonia in a patient with JME has shown localization to bilateral frontocentral regions.[129] The motor component, either imagined or performed, is crucial in praxis induction, whereas seizures induced by thinking are activated by tasks such as purely mental calculation of orally presented arithmetic tasks with no motor component in either the stimulus or the response.

Seizures induced by thinking and praxis, many cases of reading epilepsy, and photosensitive epilepsy are all examples of specific brain activities involving definable cortical areas triggering generalized seizures or epileptiform EEG activity, often in the context of known idiopathic generalized epilepsy. Inoue and Kubota[97] postulated on the basis of MEG and sensory-evoked potential studies that increased, but spatially different cortical hyperexcitability operates in photosensitivity and praxis sensitivity. Binnie[20] has discussed the implications of such studies of reflex seizures for the understanding of generalized epilepsy.

Treatment of Seizures Induced by Thinking and Praxis

Avoidance of triggering stimuli is usually impractical. These seizures are almost always found as part of an idiopathic generalized epilepsy, particularly juvenile myoclonic epilepsy, and drugs appropriate for these syndromes are the treatment of choice.

REFLEX SEIZURE TYPES USUALLY ASSOCIATED WITH FOCAL EPILEPSIES

Seizures Induced by Eating

Eating epilepsy is characterized by seizures closely related to one or several parts of eating. Although described as eating epilepsy, seizures triggered by eating often occur in patients who also have spontaneous seizures and are not now classified as a separate epileptic syndrome but as a seizure type in the most recent proposal.[55] Some cases may be described as epilepsies characterized by specific modes of seizure precipitation.[43] A prevalence of approximately 1 per 1,000 to 2,000 epileptic patients has been reported.[142,193] The unusually high figures reported for Sri Lanka[177] may be related to ascertainment methods. Seizures induced by eating have been reported in childhood, youth, and adult life. The clinical triggers of a seizure are usually stereotyped for each patient but may have a few points in common. Thus, some patients have seizures at the very sight or smell of food, while others may have them immediately after a heavy meal. Most typically, the seizure occurs shortly after beginning to eat and does not recur during the same meal. In some, the seizures may be related to emotional or autonomic components of eating, and in others to gastric distension or to stimulation of the mouth or pharynx and with possible participation of autonomic, somatosensory, or proprioceptive afferents.

Seizures with eating are typically of complex or simple partial type, almost always related to a symptomatic localization-related epilepsy. Rémillard et al.[167] suggest that patients with temporolimbic seizures activated by eating have fewer spontaneous attacks and are more likely to have such attacks from the onset of their epilepsy than are those with extralimbic, usually suprasylvian, seizure onset who have less constant activation by eating, more obvious extratemporal structural lesions, and possible activation by specific thalamocortical afferents. The latter may also have seizures with other forms of buccal stimulation such as tooth brushing or kissing and may represent particular examples of sensitivity to somatosensory or proprioceptive stimulation. Koutroumanidis et al. reported a case of adult-onset sensitivity to tooth brushing only, with normal imaging and interictal left frontal epileptiform activity, and suggested that this was a cryptogenic reflex epilepsy.[118] The role of malformations of cortical development in reflex seizures has been recently discussed by Palmini et al.,[150] who found eating-related seizures in patients with perisylvian lesions and noted functional anatomic correlation with the reflex seizure types.

Eating epilepsy is usually associated with localized or regional epileptiform activity either from temporolimbic structures or from suprasylvian regions in association with larger lesions. Patients considered to have idiopathic generalized epilepsies are exceptional, and cases in which seizures have been shown to be generalized from the start are less frequent.[60,116]

The seizures of eating epilepsy can be affected by modifying the trigger. It is our impression that patients with eating epilepsy and extralimbic seizure onset are more sensitive to either somatosensory or proprioceptive stimuli during eating and are more likely to report that seizure induction can be prevented by altering the sensory characteristics of their food. Some will drink through a straw rather than from a cup or will avoid biting into a whole fruit by cutting it into small pieces. Such stimulus modification can reduce seizure frequency in what may otherwise be an intractable or socially disabling condition. Some patients also take advantage of a refractory period after a reflex seizure and will induce an attack in private to avoid having a seizure later in a more embarrassing setting. Some patients have prolonged periods of heightened susceptibility to reflex attacks and may then refuse to eat adequately. Drugs effective for partial seizures are usually necessary, but medically intractable patients should be recognized early and assessed for surgical treatment.

Seizures induced by eating in infancy are unusual, may present as acute life-threatening events (ALTEs), and appear to have a poor prognosis. Navelet et al.[145] reported four infants with onset before 6 months, attacks provoked by meals, cyanosis, hypo- or hypertonia, and apnea followed by clonic movements of the limbs. Gastroesophageal reflux (GER) was present in the four cases but attacks remained frequent despite anti-GER treatment and all infants developed a severe epilepsy. The first interictal EEG was normal but repeated polygraphic EEG recordings documented the seizures. The trigger in these patients is unknown and the relationship between GER, ALTEs, and epilepsy remains unclear. One of us (P.P.) studied three children with epileptic spasms beginning in the first year who developed seizures with the approach or ingestion of food at 3 to 4 years old. The triggered seizures were spasms in two cases and tonic seizures in one. The last child had cryptogenic epilepsy, the others had symptomatic epilepsy with early large opercular lesions, and all had lateralized or regionally predominant ictal and interictal EEG abnormalities. They continued to have reflex and spontaneous seizures. It is possible that a network responsible for the reflex attacks may not have matured until several years of age.

Seizures Induced by Proprioceptive Stimuli (Movement Induced)

Reflex seizures apparently induced by movement were reported before the EEG era.[78] Early reports emphasized induction by movement,[123] but later experiments showed the determinant role of proprioceptive afferents.[36,72] Thus, seizures originally described as movement induced or gait induced are usually more accurately described as "proprioceptive induced." These reflex seizures are rare[192] and may be most commonly seen as a transient occurrence with nonketotic hyperglycemia.[23]

Proprioceptive-induced seizures involve the sensorimotor area of the hemisphere contralateral to the clinical seizure onset. This has been confirmed by imaging and intensive monitoring. The supplementary motor area may also be involved. Maximum EEG electronegativity appears to be at the central vertex electrode in a published EEG of seizures induced by walking.[101] Cerebral lesions are often evident and may have occurred long before the onset of attacks. Acute cerebral lesions or acute diffuse encephalopathies may also be accompanied by self-limited proprioceptive-induced seizures. In nonketotic hyperglycemia or other metabolic encephalopathies, neurologic deficit related to a remote lesion may be transiently unmasked during the period of seizures.[23] New-onset proprioceptive-induced seizures thus require rapid medical and neurologic evaluation.

Reflex drop attacks elicited by walking[53] are seen rarely in patients with reflex interictal spikes evoked by percussion of the foot.[49,187] These may be a variety of seizures induced by proprioceptive stimulation. However, individuals with these evoked spikes, generally considered a benign finding, do not usually have epilepsy or reflex seizures.[120] This disorder likely represents a form of idiopathic focal epilepsy of childhood, distinct because of the parietal lobe involvement. Participation of a more elaborate network involved in motor programming cannot be excluded in some cases, especially if the effective stimulus seems restricted to activities such as walking, although "gait epilepsy"[101] is not now a recognized seizure type or epilepsy syndrome.

Seizures Induced by Somatosensory Stimuli

Seizures induced by somatosensory stimulation are typically triggered by repeatedly tapping, rubbing, or pricking part of the body. There is often a localized or regional cutaneous trigger zone. The seizures begin with a sensory aura; a sensory jacksonian seizure occurs often followed by tonic motor manifestations suggesting a supplementary motor area seizure. Generalization may occur. Consciousness is preserved at least at the onset. Ictal pain and autonomic disturbances have also been reported.[175] Compulsive somatosensory self-stimulation with self-induced epileptic spasms has also been demonstrated in children with severe developmental delay.[83] Somatosensory-induced seizures typically occur in patients with postrolandic cortical lesions that may be subtle.[192] Malformations of cortical development have also been implicated.[150] Normal MR imaging has been reported in patients with "rub" epilepsy, but detailed imaging was not described[107] and current imaging methods are more refined.

These focal-onset seizures must be distinguished from the typically more benign generalized reflex seizures induced by tapping in infants and young children (see above) that are not associated with lesions. Patients with somatosensory reflex seizures must be investigated for brain lesions and treatment is as for other symptomatic or cryptogenic focal epilepsies.

Hot Water Epilepsy

Seizures induced by immersion in or contact with hot water have until recently been reported predominantly in older children and adolescents from south India, where ritual bathing involves repeatedly pouring hot water over the head from a jug.[173,174] Indian patients are typically boys, with adolescence-onset complex partial or generalized tonic–clonic seizures during ritual bathing. Hot water epilepsy (HWE) has been thought to be a relatively benign age- and situation-related disorder akin to febrile seizures. This is often so when seizures start in infancy or early childhood. Ictal recordings are rare and interictal EEG abnormalities have been recorded over temporal areas in half of the patients. Imaging has been unremarkable in most, but focal cortical malformations have been reported.[80] Differential diagnosis includes nonepileptic events such as startle and vasovagal syncope, and startle epilepsy. Some older patients report pleasurable feelings with these events, and self-induction has been reported. Prophylactic clobazam is reportedly helpful.[52] Studies in non-Indian subjects[15,100] report onset from infancy to adult life and spontaneous seizures in 62% of patients in whom onset was after infancy. These series include younger children than in India, with complex partial seizures occurring as soon as the child is immersed in hot water rather than when hot water is poured over the head; sensitivity often diminishes with time.[100]

HWE beginning in infancy appears to have a better prognosis. Seizures begin in the first year and are always triggered by immersion in hot bath water with a temperature around 37.5°C. Parents describe some nonspecific malaise and when recorded these are complex partial seizures; general pediatricians may be unfamiliar with these seizures in such young children.

In infantile HWE, the neurologic and developmental examinations are always normal. There is no personal or family history of epilepsy. Interictal EEG is normal, including during sleep. CT scan and MRI are reported as normal, and no interictal or ictal SPECT has been reported in these infants. Treatment is by lowering the temperature of the bath. No antiepileptic drugs are needed and in more than 3 years of follow-up, no further seizures have developed in five cases we have evaluated (P.P.), some of whom were also reported by Ioos et al.[100] Differential diagnosis of HWE in infants includes gastroesophageal reflux, which, however, would be rare in the bath; syncope; startle events; and aquagenic urticaria. Sensitivity to visual stimuli such as the light reflections in the bathroom or the color of the bathtub would not be expected in otherwise normal children at this age.

A mechanism involving defective thermoregulation has been proposed.

MISCELLANEOUS REFLEX SEIZURES

Psychogenic seizures are triggered by specific thoughts, either self-induced attacks (e.g., by thinking sad thoughts) or those unintentionally triggered by specific mental activity.[57] This use of the term *psychogenic* does not refer to nonepileptic seizures. A report of temporal lobe seizures induced by thinking of the family home documented such seizures during monitoring and a subtle malformation of cortical development in the resected temporal structures.[130]

Seizures with extremely specific visual stimuli have been reported. Recurring self-induced brief tonic seizures triggered by looking at round objects occurred in an 18-month-old boy. Later he developed sensitivity to other patterns and secondary generalized seizures, which were difficult to control. He was not photosensitive.[25] A child with generalized seizures self-induced by looking at his own hand was reported. By 4 years of age, medications were withdrawn, and no further seizures, reflex or otherwise, occurred in 26 years of follow-up.[114] The EEG was said to be normal. A similar case has been reported.[62]

Vestibular stimuli, caloric or rotatory, have been reported to produce EEG discharges, generally nonspecific but at times in the contralateral temporal region,[14,24,31,141] but seizures induced by these stimuli, as distinguished from startle effects or syncopal events, appear to be very rare.[16,108]

Olfactory stimuli have elicited seizures in experimental animals.[140] Stevens[182] reported that strong odors increased interictal epileptiform EEG activity in 26% of patients with temporal lobe epilepsy, but triggering of seizures is much rarer.[184]

Presumed enteroceptive seizures are very unusual. Occasionally, seizures induced by eating may be shown to depend on gastric distension,[67] but this is not typical. Defecation has been reported to induce seizures, confirmed by EEG, but not immediately after emptying the rectum,[86] and was the most common trigger reported by Schubert and Cracco[175] in a case of induction by tactile stimuli.

SUMMARY AND CONCLUSIONS

Reflex seizures have been considered interesting rarities, but are probably more frequent than we realize, especially in some relatively common syndromes that are now believed to be generalized epilepsies. Study of reflex seizures has been important in understanding some basic brain mechanisms of seizure occurrence. Neurologists, pediatricians, and family or general practitioners can expect to encounter patients with these seizures. A detailed history is the first step to proper diagnosis of seizure type and epilepsy syndrome, so that effective treatment may be prescribed.

ACKNOWLEDGEMENT

We are grateful to Ms Faye Rourke-Frew for her help in preparing this manuscript.

References

1. Adrian ED, Matthews BHC. The Berger rhythm: potential changes from the occipital lobes in man. *Brain.* 1934;57:355–384.
2. Aguglia U, Tinuper P, Gastaut H. Startle-induced epileptic seizures. *Epilepsia.* 1984;25:712–720.
3. Alajouanine T, Gastaut H. La syncinésie-sursaut et l'épilepsie-sursaut à déclenchement sensoriel ou sensitif inopiné. *Rev Neurol.* 1955;93:29–41.
4. Ambrosetto G, Antonini L, Tassinari CA. Occipital lobe seizures related to clinically asymptomatic celiac disease in adulthood. *Epilepsia.* 1992;33:476–481.
5. Ames FR. Cinefilm and EEG recording during "handwaving" attacks of an epileptic, photosensitive child. *Electroencephalogr Clin Neurophysiol.* 1974;37:301–304.
6. Andermann F, Andermann E. Excessive startle syndromes: startle disease, jumping, and startle epilepsy. *Adv Neurol.* 1986;43:321–338.
7. Archer JS, Briellmann RS, Syngeniotis A, et al. Spike-triggered fMRI in reading epilepsy: involvement of left frontal cortex working memory area. *Neurology.* 2003;60:415–421.
8. Asbury A, Prensky A. Graphogenic epilepsy. *Trans Am Neurol Assoc.* 1963;88:193–194.
9. Avanzini G. Musicogenic seizures. *Ann N Y Acad Sci.* 2003;999:95–102.
10. Baykan B, Matur Z, Gurses C, et al. Typical absence seizures triggered by photosensitivity. *Epilepsia.* 2005;46:159–163.
11. Beaumanoir A, Gastaut H, Naquet R. *Reflex Seizures and Reflex Epilepsies.* Genéve: Éditions Médecine et Hygiène; 1989.
12. Bancaud J, Talairach J, Bonis A. Physiopathogénie des épilepsies-sursaut (à propos d'une épilepsie de l'aire motrice supplémentaire). *Rev Neurol.* 1967;117:441–453.
13. Bancaud J, Talairach J, Lamarche M, et al. Hypothèses neurophysiopathologiques sur l'épilepsie-sursaut chez l'homme. *Rev Neurol.* 1975;131:559–571.
14. Barac B. The clinical value of vestibular activation of EEG. *Electroencephalogr Clin Neurophysiol.* 1977;43:514.
15. Bebek N, Gurses C, Gokyigit A, et al. Hot water epilepsy: clinical and electrophysiologic findings based on 21 cases. *Epilepsia.* 2001;42:1180–1184.
16. Behrman S, Wyke BD. Vestibulogenic seizures: a consideration of vertiginous seizures, with particular reference to convulsions produced by stimulation of labyrinthine receptors. *Brain.* 1958;81:529–541.
17. Bickford RG, Whelan JL, Klass DW, et al. Reading epilepsy: clinical and electro-encephalographic studies of a new syndrome. *Trans Am Neurol Assoc.* 1956;81:100–102.
18. Bignall KE, Imbert M. Polysensory and corticocortical projections to the frontal lobe of squirrel and rhesus monkey. *Electroencephalogr Clin Neurophysiol.* 1969;26:206–215.
19. Binnie CD. Simple reflex seizures. In: Engel J Jr, Pedley TA, eds. *Epilepsy: A Comprehensive Textbook.* Philadelphia: Lippincott-Raven Publishers; 1997:2489–2505.
20. Binnie CD. Evidence of reflex epilepsy on functional systems in the brain and "generalized" epilepsy. In: Wolf P, Inoue Y, Zifkin B, eds. *Reflex Epilepsy: Progress in Understanding.* Montrouge: John Libbey; 2004:7–14.
21. Binnie CD, Darby CE, Kasteleijn-Nolst Trenité DGA, et al. Photosensitive epilepsy: clinical features. In: Beaumanoir A, Gastaut H, Naquet R, eds. *Reflex Seizures and Reflex Epilepsies.* Geneva: Éditions Médecine et Hygiène; 1989:163–170.
22. Binnie CD, Wilkins AJ. Visually induced seizures not caused by flicker (intermittent light stimulation). In: Zifkin BG, Andermann F, Beaumanoir A, et al., eds. *Reflex Epilepsies and Reflex Seizures. Advances in Neurology.* Vol. 75. Philadelphia: Lippincott-Raven Publishers; 1998:123–138.
23. Brick JF, Gutrecht JA, Ringel RA. Reflex epilepsy and nonketotic hyperglycemia in the elderly: a specific neuroendocrine syndrome. *Neurology.* 1989;39:394–399.
24. Brinar V, Barac B. Correlation of influences of intermittent light stimulation (ILS) and vestibular caloric stimulation in focal EEG abnormalities. *Electroencephalogr Clin Neurophysiol.* 1977;43:515.
25. Brockmann K, Huppke P, Karenfort M, et al. Visually self-induced seizures sensitive to round objects. *Epilepsia.* 2005;46:786–789.
26. Brodtkorb E, Michler RP, Gu W, et al. Speech-induced aphasic seizures in epilepsy caused by LGI1 mutation. *Epilepsia.* 2005;46:963–966.
27. Brown-Séquard E. *Researches on Epilepsy.* Boston: David Clapp; 1857.
28. Buser P, Ascher P, Bruner J, et al. Aspects of sensory motor reverberations to acoustic and visual stimuli: the role of primary specific cortical areas. In: Moruzzi G, Fessard A, Jasper HH, eds. *Brain Mechanisms. Progress in Brain Research.* Amsterdam: Elsevier; 1963:294–322.
29. Camfield CS, Camfield PR, Sadler M, et al. Paroxysmal eyelid movements: a confusing feature of generalized photosensitive epilepsy. *Neurology.* 2004;63:40–42.
30. Canevini MP, Vignoli A, Sgro V, et al. Symptomatic epilepsy with facial myoclonus triggered by language. *Epileptic Disord.* 2001;3:143–146.
31. Cantor FK. Vestibular-temporal lobe connections demonstrated by induced seizures. *Neurology.* 1971;21:507–516.
32. Capovilla G, Beccaria F, Romeo A, et al. Effectiveness of a particular blue lens on photoparoxysmal response in photosensitive epileptic patients. *Ital J Neurol Sci.* 1999;20:161–166.
33. Caraballo R, Semprino M, Cersosimo R, et al. Hemiparetic cerebral palsy and startle epilepsy (in Spanish). *Rev Neurol.* 2004;38:123–127.
34. Chapman AG, Horton RW, Meldrum BS. Anticonvulsant action of a 1,5 benzodiazepine, clobazam, in reflex epilepsy. *Epilepsia.* 1978;19:293–299.
35. Chapman AG, Meldrum BS. Epilepsy-prone mice: genetically determined sound-induced seizures. In: Jobe PC, Laird HE II, eds. *Neurotransmitters and Epilepsy.* Clifton, NJ: Humana Press; 1987.
36. Chauvel P, Lamarche M. Analyse d'une 'épilepsie du mouvement' chez un singe porteur d'un foyer rolandique. *Neurochirurgie.* 1975;21:121–137.
37. Clemens B. Dopamine agonist treatment of self-induced pattern-sensitive epilepsy: a case report. *Epilepsy Res.* 1988;2:340–343.
38. Clementi A. Stricninizzazione della sfera corticale visiva ed epilessia sperimentale da stimoli acustici. *Arch Fisiol.* 1929;27:388–414.
39. Clementi A. Stricninizzazione della sfera corticale visiva ed epilessia sperimentale da stimoli luminosi. *Arch Fisiol.* 1929;27:356–387.
40. Clementi A. Sfera gustativa della corteccia cerebrale del cane ed epilessia sperimentale riflessa a tipo sensoriale gustativo. *Boll Soc Ital Biol.* 1935;10:902–904.
41. Cokar O, Gelisse P, Livet MO, et al. Startle response: epileptic or non-epileptic? The case for "flash" SMA reflex seizures. *Epileptic Disord.* 2001;3:7–12.
42. Commission on Classification and Terminology of the International League Against Epilepsy. Proposal for classification of epilepsies and epileptic syndromes. *Epilepsia.* 1985;26:268–278.
43. Commission on Classification and Terminology of the ILAE. Proposal for revised classification of epilepsies and epileptic syndromes. *Epilepsia.* 1989;30:389–399.
44. Creutzfeldt O, Ojemann G. Neuronal activity in the human lateral temporal lobe. III. Activity changes during music. *Exp Brain Res.* 1989;77: 490–498.
45. Crichlow EC, Crawford RD. Epileptiform seizures in domestic fowl, II: intermittent light stimulation and the electroencephalogram. *Can J Physiol Pharmacol.* 1974;52:424–429.
46. Critchley M. Musicogenic epilepsy. I. The beginnings. In: Critchley M, Henson RA, eds. *Music and the Brain.* London: William Heinemann; 1977:344–353.
47. Darby CE, De Korte RA, Binnie CD, et al. The self-induction of epileptic seizures by eye closure. *Epilepsia.* 1980;21:31–42.
48. Darby CE, Park DM, Wilkins AJ. EEG characteristics of epileptic pattern sensitivity and their relation to the nature of pattern stimulation and the effects of sodium valproate. *Electroencephalogr Clin Neurophysiol.* 1986;63:517–525.
49. de Marco P, Tassinari CA. Extreme somatosensory evoked potential (ESEP): an EEG sign forecasting a possible occurrence of seizures in children. *Epilepsia.* 1981;22:569–575.
50. Deonna T. Reflex seizures with somatosensory precipitation. Clinical and electroencephalographic patterns and differential diagnosis, with emphasis on reflex myoclonic epilepsy of infancy. In: Zifkin BG, Andermann F, Beaumanoir A, et al., eds. *Reflex Epilepsies and Reflex Seizures. Advances in Neurology.* Vol 75. Philadelphia: Lippincott-Raven Publishers; 1998:193–206.
51. DeSarro GB, Nistico G, Meldrum BS. Anticonvulsant properties of flunarizine on reflex and generalized models of epilepsy. *Neuropharmacology.* 1986;25:695–701.
52. Dhanaraj M, Jayavelu A. Prophylactic use of clobazam in hot water epilepsy. *J Assoc Physicians India.* 2003;51:43–44.
53. Di Capua M, Vigevano F, Tassinari CA. Drop seizures reflex to walking. In: Beaumanoir A, Gastaut H, Naquet R, eds. *Reflex Seizures and Reflex Epilepsies.* Geneva: Éditions Médecine et Hygiène; 1989:83–88.
54. Dravet C, Bureau M, Roger J. Benign myoclonic epilepsy in infants. In: Roger J, Bureau M, Dravet C, et al., eds. *Epileptic Syndromes in Infancy,*

Childhood and Adolescence. 2nd ed. London, Paris: John Libbey Eurotext Ltd; 1992:67–74.
55. Engel J Jr. A proposed diagnostic scheme for people with epileptic seizures and epilepsy: report of the ILAE Task Force on Classification and Terminology. *Epilepsia*. 2001;42:796–803.
56. Faught E. Lamotrigine for startle-induced seizures. *Seizure*. 1999;8:361–363.
57. Fenwick P. Self-generation of seizures by an action of mind. In: Zifkin BG, Andermann F, Beaumanoir A, et al., eds. *Reflex Epilepsies and Reflex Seizures. Advances in Neurology*. Vol. 75. Philadelphia: Lippincott-Raven Publishers; 1998:87–92.
58. Ferlazzo E, Zifkin BG, Andermann E, et al. Cortical triggers in generalized reflex seizures and epilepsies. *Brain*. 2005;128:700–710.
59. Ferrie CD, De Marco P, Grunewald RA, et al. Video game-induced seizures. *J Neurol Neurosurg Psychiatry*. 1994;57:925–931.
60. Fiol ME, Leppik IE, Pretzel K. Eating epilepsy: EEG and clinical study. *Epilepsia*. 1986;27:441–445.
61. Forster FM. The classification and conditioning treatment of the reflex epilepsies. *Int J Neurol*. 1972;9:73–86.
62. Forster FM. *Reflex Epilepsy, Behavioral Therapy and Conditional Reflexes*. Springfield, IL: Charles C Thomas; 1977:318.
63. Fulchignoni S. Contributo alla conoscenza dell'epilessia sperimentale riflessa per stimoli luminosi. *Riv Pat Nerv Ment*. 1938;51:154.
64. Gastaut H. L'épilepsie photogénique. *Rev Prat*. 1951;1:105–109.
65. Gastaut H. Reflex mechanisms in the genesis of epilepsy. *Epilepsia*. 1962;3:457–460.
66. Gastaut H, Hunter J. An experimental study of the mechanism of photic activation in idiopathic epilepsy. *Electroencephalogr Clin Neurophysiol*. 1950;2:263–287.
67. Gastaut H, Poirier F. Experimental, or "reflex," induction of seizures: report of a case of abdominal (enteric) epilepsy. *Epilepsia*. 1964;5:256–270.
68. Gastaut H, Roger J, Gastaut Y. Les formes expérimentales de l'épilepsie humaine. 1. L'épilepsie induite par la stimulation lumineuse intermittente rhythmée ou épilepsie photogénique. *Rev Neurol*. 1948;80:162–183.
69. Gelisse P, Thomas P, Padovani R, et al. Ictal SPECT in a case of pure musicogenic epilepsy. *Epileptic Disord*. 2003;5:133–137.
70. Genc BO, Genc E, Tastekin G, et al. Musicogenic epilepsy with ictal single photon emission computed tomography (SPECT): could these cases contribute to our knowledge of music processing? *Eur J Neurol*. 2001;8:191–194.
71. Geschwind N, Sherwin I. Language-induced epilepsy. *Arch Neurol*. 1967;16:25–31.
72. Giovanni Y, Everett J, Lamarche M. The transcortical reflex triggered by cutaneous or muscle stimulation in the cat with a penicillin epileptic focus: relative importance of regions 3a and 4. *Exp Brain Res*. 1983;51:57–64.
73. Gloor P. Experiential phenomena of temporal lobe epilepsy. Facts and hypotheses. *Brain*. 1990;113:1673–1694.
74. Gloor P, Metrakos J, Metrakos K, et al. Neurophysiological, genetic and biochemical nature of the epileptic diathesis. In: Broughton RJ, ed. *Henri Gastaut and the Marseilles School's Contribution to the Neurosciences*. Amsterdam: Elsevier; 1982:45–56.
75. Gobbi G, Bruno L, Mainetti A, et al. Seizures induced by eye closure. In: Beaumanoir A, Gastaut H, Naquet R, eds. *Reflex Seizures and Reflex Epilepsies*. Geneva: Éditions Médecine et Hygiène; 1989:181–192.
76. Goossens LA, Andermann F, Andermann E, et al. Reflex seizures induced by calculation, card or board games, and spatial tasks: a review of 25 patients and delineation of the epileptic syndrome. *Neurology*. 1990;40:1171–1176.
77. Gowers WR. *Epilepsy and Other Chronic Convulsive Diseases: Their Causes, Symptoms and Treatment*. New York: Wood and Co; 1885.
78. Gowers WR. *Epilepsy and Other Chronic Convulsive Diseases: Their Causes, Symptoms and Treatment*. London: Churchill; 1901.
79. Griffiths TD. Musical hallucinosis in acquired deafness. Phenomenology and brain substrate. *Brain*. 2000;123:2065–2076.
80. Grosso S, Farnetani MA, Francione S, et al. Hot water epilepsy and focal malformation of the parietal cortex development. *Brain Dev*. 2004;26:490–493.
81. Guerrini R, Bonanni P, Parmeggiani L, et al. Induction of partial seizures by visual stimulation. In: Zifkin BG, Andermann F, Beaumanoir A, et al., eds. *Reflex Epilepsies and Reflex Seizures. Advances in Neurology*. Vol. 75. Philadelphia: Lippincott-Raven Publishers; 1998:159–178.
82. Guerrini R, Genton P, Bureau M, et al. Reflex seizures are frequent in patients with Down syndrome and epilepsy. *Epilepsia*. 1990;31:406–417.
83. Guerrini R, Genton P, Dravet C, et al. Compulsive somatosensory self-stimulation inducing epileptic seizures. *Epilepsia*. 1992;33:509–516.
84. Guerrini R, Dravet C, Genton P, et al. Idiopathic photosensitive occipital lobe epilepsy. *Epilepsia*. 1995;36:883–891.
85. Hall M. *Synopsis of the Diastaltic Nervous System*. London: Joseph Mallet; 1850:112.
86. Harbord MG, Mitchell C. Reflex seizures induced by defecation, with an ictal EEG focus in the left frontotemporal region. *Epilepsia*. 2002;43:946–947.
87. Harding GFA. TV can be bad for your health. *Nat Med*. 1998;4:265–267.
88. Harding GFA, Fylan F. Two visual mechanisms of photosensitivity. *Epilepsia*. 1999;40:1446–1451.
89. Harding GFA, Herrick CE, Jeavons PM. A controlled study of the effect of sodium valproate on photosensitive epilepsy and its prognosis. *Epilepsia*. 1979;19:555–565.
90. Harding GFA, Jeavons PM. *Photosensitive Epilepsy*. 2nd ed. London: MacKeith Press; 1994.
91. Harding GFA, Wilkins AJ, Erba G, et al. Epilepsy Foundation of America Working Group. Photic- and pattern-induced seizures: expert consensus of the Epilepsy Foundation of America Working Group. *Epilepsia*. 2005;46:1423–1425.
92. Hennessy M, Binnie CD. Photogenic partial seizures. *Epilepsia*. 2000;41:59–64.
93. Herskowitz J, Rosman NP, Geschwind N. Seizures induced by singing and recitation. A unique form of reflex epilepsy in childhood. *Arch Neurol*. 1984;41:1102–1103.
94. Hill RA, Chiappa KH, Huang-Hellinger F, et al. Hemodynamic and metabolic aspects of photosensitive epilepsy revealed by functional magnetic resonance imaging and magnetic resonance spectroscopy. *Epilepsia*. 1999;40:912–920.
95. Hughlings Jackson J. Fits following touching the head. *Lancet*. 1895;1:274.
96. Hunter J, Ingvar D. Pathways mediating Metrazol-induced irradiation of visual impulses. *Electroencephalogr Clin Neurophysiol*. 1955;7:39–60.
97. Inoue Y, Kubota H. Juvenile myoclonic epilepsy with praxis-induced seizures. In: Schmitz B, Sander T, eds. *Juvenile Myoclonic Epilepsy. The Janz Syndrome*. Petersfield U.K.: Wrightson Biomedical; 2000:73–81.
98. Inoue Y, Seino M, Kubota H, et al. Epilepsy with praxis-induced seizures. In: Wolf P, ed. *Epileptic Seizures and Syndromes*. London: John Libbey; 1994:81–91.
99. Inoue Y, Zifkin B. Praxis induction and thinking induction: one or two mechanisms? A controversy. In: Wolf P, Inoue Y, Zifkin B, eds. *Reflex Epilepsies. Current Problems in Epilepsy*. Vol. 19. Paris: John Libbey Eurotext; 2004:41–55.
100. Ioos C, Fohlen M, Villeneuve N, et al. Hot water epilepsy: a benign and unrecognized form. *J Child Neurol*. 2000;15:125–128.
101. Iriarte J, Sanchez-Carpintero R, Schlumberger E, et al. Gait epilepsy. A case report of gait-induced seizures. *Epilepsia*. 2001;42:1087–1090.
102. Ishida S, Yamashita Y, Matsuishi T, et al. Photosensitive seizures provoked while viewing "pocket monsters," a made-for-television animation program in Japan. *Epilepsia*. 1998;39:1340–1344.
103. Jeavons PM. Nosological problems of myoclonic epilepsies of childhood and adolescence. *Dev Med Child Neurol*. 1977;19:3–8.
104. Jeavons PM, Harding GFA. *Photosensitive Epilepsy*. London: Heinemann; 1975.
105. Johnson DD, Davis HL. Drug responses and brain biochemistry of the Epi mutant chicken. In: Ookawa T, ed. *The Brain and Behavior of the Fowl*. Tokyo: Japan Scientific Society Press; 1983:281–296.
106. Johnsrude IS, Giraud AL, Frackowiak RS. Functional imaging of the auditory system: the use of positron emission tomography. *Audiol Neurootol*. 2002;7:251–276.
107. Kanemoto K, Watanabe Y, Tsuji T, et al. Rub epilepsy: a somatosensory evoked reflex epilepsy induced by prolonged cutaneous stimulation. *J Neurol Neurosurg Psychiatry*. 2001;70:541–543.
108. Karbowski K. Pathophysiologie des Vestibularis-Schwindels. In: Karbowski K, ed. *Der Schwindel aus Interdisziplinärer Sicht*. Heidelberg: Springer; 1981:1–19.
109. Kasteleijn-Nolst Trenité DGA. Photosensitivity in epilepsy: electrophysiological and clinical correlates. *Acta Neurol Scand (Suppl)*. 1989;125.
110. Kasteleijn-Nolst Trenité DGA, Binnie CD, Meinardi H. Photosensitive patients: symptoms and signs during intermittent photic stimulation and their relation to seizures in daily life. *J Neurol Neurosurg Psychiatry*. 1987;50:1546–1549.
111. Kasteleijn-Nolst Trenité DGA, Pinto D, Hirsch E, et al. Photosensitivity, visual induced seizures and epileptic syndromes. In: Roger J, Bureau M, Dravet C, et al., eds. *Epileptic Syndromes in Infancy, Childhood and Adolescence*. 4th ed. Montrouge: John Libbey Eurotext; 2005:395–422.
112. Killam KF, Killam EK, Naquet R. An animal model of light sensitive epilepsy. *Electroencephalogr Clin Neurophysiol*. 1967;22(Suppl):497–513.
113. Killam KF, Killam EK, Naquet R. Mise en évidence chez certains singes d'un syndrome myoclonique. *C R Acad Sci (Paris)*. 1966;262:1010–1012.
114. Klass DW. Self-induced seizures: long-term follow-up of two unusual cases. In: Beaumanoir A, Gastaut H, Naquet R, eds. *Reflex Seizures and Reflex Epilepsies*. Geneva: Éditions Médecine et Hygiène; 1989:369–378.
115. Koepp MJ, Hansen ML, Pressler RM, et al. Comparison of EEG, MRI and PET in reading epilepsy: a case report. *Epilepsy Res*. 1998;29:251–257.
116. Koul R, Koul S, Razdan S. Eating epilepsy. *Acta Neurol Scand*. 1989;80:78–80.
117. Koutroumanidis M, Koepp MJ, Richardson MP, et al. The variants of reading epilepsy. A clinical and video-EEG study of 17 patients with reading-induced seizures. *Brain*. 1998;121:1409–1427.
118. Koutroumanidis M, Pearce R, Sadoh DR, et al. Tooth brushing-induced seizures: a case report. *Epilepsia*. 2001;42:686–688.
119. Labate A, Barone R, Gambardella A, et al. Startle epilepsy complicating aspartylglucosaminuria. *Brain Dev*. 2004;26:130–133.
120. Langill L, Wong PK. Tactile-evoked rolandic discharges: a benign finding? *Epilepsia*. 2003;44:221–227.

121. Liegeois-Chauvel C, Musolino A, Chauvel P. Localization of the primary auditory area in man. *Brain*. 1991;114:139–151.
122. Lin KL, Wang HS, Kao PF. A young infant with musicogenic epilepsy. *Pediatr Neurol*. 2003;28:379–381.
123. Lishman WA, Symonds CP, Whitty CW, et al. Seizures induced by movement. *Brain*. 1962;85:93–108.
124. Lloyd KG, Scatton B, Voltz C, et al. Cerebrospinal fluid amino acid and monoamine metabolite levels of Papio papio: correlation with photosensitivity. *Brain Res*. 1986;363:390–394.
125. Loiseau P, Duché B. Childhood absence epilepsy. In: Duncan JS, Panayiotopoulos CP, eds. *Typical Absences and Related Epileptic Syndromes*. London: Churchill Livingstone; 1995:152–160.
126. Löscher W, Schmidt D. Which animal models should be used in the search for new antiepileptic drugs: a proposal based on experimental and clinical considerations. *Epilepsy Res*. 1988;2:145–181.
127. Loskota WJ, Lomax P, Rich ST. The gerbil as a model for the study of the epilepsies: seizure patterns and ontogenesis. *Epilepsia*. 1974;15:109–119.
128. Manford MR, Fish DR, Shorvon SD. Startle-provoked epileptic seizures: features in 19 patients. *J Neurol Neurosurg Psychiatry*. 1996;61:151–156.
129. Mann MW, Gueguen B, Guillou S, et al. Chess-playing epilepsy: a case report with video-EEG and back averaging. *Epileptic Disord*. 2004;6:293–296.
130. Martinez O, Reisin R, Andermann F, et al. Evidence for reflex activation of experiential complex partial seizures. *Neurology*. 2001;56:121–123.
131. Martinez-Manas R, Daniel RT, Debatisse D, et al. Intractable reflex audiogenic epilepsy successfully treated by peri-insular hemispherotomy. *Seizure*. 2004;13:486–490.
132. Matsuoka H, Takahashi T, Sasaki M, et al. Neuropsychological EEG activation in patients with epilepsy. *Brain*. 2000;123:318–330.
133. Matsuoka H, Nakamura M, Ohno T, et al. The role of cognitive-motor function in precipitation and inhibition of epileptic seizures. *Epilepsia*. 2005;46(Suppl 1):17–20.
134. Matthews WB, Wright FK. Hereditary primary reading epilepsy. *Neurology*. 1967;17:919–921.
135. Mayer T, Wolf P. Reading epilepsy: related to juvenile myoclonic epilepsy? *Epilepsia*. 1997;38(Suppl 3):18–19.
136. McCusker CG, Hicks EM. Psychological management of intractable seizures in an adolescent with learning disability. *Seizure*. 1999;8: 358–360.
137. Menini C, Silva-Barrat C. The photosensitive epilepsy of the baboon. A model of generalized reflex epilepsy. In: Zifkin BG, Andermann F, Beaumanoir A, et al., eds. *Reflex Epilepsies and Reflex Seizures. Advances in Neurology*. Vol. 75. Philadelphia: Lippincott-Raven Publishers; 1998:29–47.
138. Michel V, Burbaud P, Taillard J, et al. Stuttering or reflex seizure? A case report. *Epileptic Disord*. 2004;6:181–185.
139. Morimoto T, Hayakawa T, Sugie H, et al. Epileptic seizures precipitated by constant light, movement in daily life, and hot water immersion. *Epilepsia*. 1985;26:237–242.
140. Moruzzi G. *L'Epilessia sperimentale*. Bologna, Italy: Nicolo Zanichelli; 1946:128.
141. Münter M, Götze W, Krokowski G. Telemetrische EEG: Untersuchungen während rotatorische Vestibularisreizung. *Dtsch Z Nervenheilkd*. 1964;186:137–148.
142. Nagaraja D, Chand RP. Eating epilepsy. *Clin Neurol Neurosurg*. 1984;86:95–99.
143. Nalini A, Christopher R. Cerebral glycolipidoses: clinical characteristics of 41 pediatric patients. *J Child Neurol*. 2004;19:447–452.
144. Naquet R, Bancaud J, Bostem F, et al. Activation and provocation methods in clinical neurophysiology. In: Rémond A, ed. *Handbook of Electroencephalography and Clinical Neurophysiology*. Vol. 3. Amsterdam: Elsevier; 1976:89–104.
145. Navelet Y, Wood C, Robieux I, et al. Seizures presenting as apnoea. *Arch Dis Child*. 1989;64:357–359.
146. Nolan MA, Otsubo H, Iida K, et al. Startle-induced seizures associated with infantile hemiplegia: implication of the supplementary motor area. *Epileptic Disord*. 2005;7:49–52.
147. Oguni H, Hayashi K, Usui N, et al. Startle epilepsy with infantile hemiplegia: report of two cases improved by surgery. *Epilepsia*. 1998;39: 93–98.
148. Oguni H, Hayashi K, Awaya Y, et al. Severe myoclonic epilepsy in infants—a review based on the Tokyo Women's Medical University series of 84 cases. *Brain Dev*. 2001;23:736–748.
149. Okumura A, Watanabe K, Negoro T, et al. Epilepsies after Pocket Monster seizures. *Epilepsia*. 2005;46:980–982.
150. Palmini A, Halasz P, Scheffer IE, et al. Reflex seizures in patients with malformations of cortical development and refractory epilepsy. *Epilepsia*. 2005;46:1224–1234.
151. Panayiotopoulos CP. Fixation-off, scotosensitive, and other visual-related epilepsies. In: Zifkin BG, Andermann F, Beaumanoir A, et al., eds. *Reflex Epilepsies and Reflex Seizures. Advances in Neurology*. Vol. 75. Philadelphia: Lippincott-Raven Publishers; 1998:139–157.
152. Panayiotopoulos CP. *A Clinical Guide to Epileptic Syndromes and Their Treatment*. Chipping Norton, U.K.: Bladon Medical Publishing; 2002.
153. Panayiotopoulos CP. Idiopathic generalized epilepsies. In: Panayiotopoulos CP, ed. *The Epilepsies: Seizures, Syndromes, and Management*. Oxford: Bladon Medical Publishing; 2005:271–348.
154. Parra J, Kalitzin SN, Iriarte J, et al. Gamma-band phase clustering and photosensitivity: is there an underlying mechanism common to photosensitive epilepsy and visual perception? *Brain*. 2003;126:1164–1172.
155. Pegna AJ, Picard F, Martory MD, et al. Semantically-triggered reading epilepsy: an experimental case study. *Cortex*. 1999;35:355–356.
156. Penfield W, Erickson T. *Epilepsy and Cerebral Localization*. Springfield, IL: Charles C Thomas; 1941:28.
157. Peretz I, Zatorre R, eds. *The Cognitive Neuroscience of Music*. Oxford: Oxford University Press; 2003.
158. Pinto D, Westland B, de Haan GJ, et al. Genome-wide linkage scan of epilepsy-related photoparoxysmal electroencephalographic response: evidence for linkage on chromosomes 7q32 and 16p13. *Hum Mol Genet*. 2005;14:171–178.
159. Porciatti V, Bonanni P, Fiorentini A, et al. Lack of cortical contrast gain control in human photosensitivity epilepsy. *Nat Neurosci*. 2000;3:259–263.
160. Porter AC. Pattern sensitivity testing in routine EEG. *J Electrophysiol Technol*. 1985;11:153–155.
161. Pumain R, Menini C, Heinemann U, et al. Chemical synaptic transmission is not necessary for epileptic seizures to persist in the baboon Papio papio. *Exp Neurol*. 1985;89:250–258.
162. Quesney LF, Andermann F, Gloor P. Dopaminergic mechanism in generalized photosensitive epilepsy. *Neurology*. 1981;31:1542–1544.
163. Quirk JA, Fish DR, Smith SJM, et al. First seizures associated with playing electronic screen games: a community-based study in Great Britain. *Ann Neurol*. 1995;37:733–737.
164. Radhakrishnan K, Silbert PL, Klass DW. Reading epilepsy. An appraisal of 20 patients diagnosed at the Mayo Clinic, Rochester, Minnesota, between 1949 and 1989, and delineation of the epileptic syndrome. *Brain*. 1995;118:75–89.
165. Radhakrishnan K, St Louis EK, Johnson JA, et al. Pattern-sensitive epilepsy: electroclinical characteristics, natural history, and delineation of the epileptic syndrome. *Epilepsia*. 2005;46:48–58.
166. Radovici A, Misirliou V, Gluckman M. Épilepsie réflexe provoquée par excitations optiques des rayons solaires. *Rev Neurol*. 1932;1:1305–1308.
167. Rémillard GM, Andermann F, Zifkin BG, et al. Eating epilepsy. A study of ten surgically treated patients suggests the presence of two separate syndromes. In: Beaumanoir A, Gastaut H, Naquet R, eds. *Reflex Seizures and Reflex Epilepsies*. Genève: Éditions Médecine et Hygiène; 1989:289–300.
168. Ricci GB, Chapman RM, Erne SN, et al. Neuromagnetic topography of photoconvulsive response in man. *Electroencephalogr Clin Neurophysiol*. 1990;75:1–12.
169. Ricci S, Vigevano F, Manfredi M, et al. Epilepsy provoked by television and video games: safety of 100-Hz screens. *Neurology*. 1998;50:790–793.
170. Ritaccio AL, Hickling EJ, Ramani V. The role of dominant premotor cortex and grapheme to phoneme transformation in reading epilepsy. A neuroanatomic, neurophysiologic, and neuropsychological study. *Arch Neurol*. 1992;49:933–939.
171. Saenz-Lope E, Herranz-Tanarro FJ, Masdeu JC, et al. Hyperekplexia: a syndrome of pathological startle responses. *Ann Neurol*. 1984;15: 36–41.
172. Santanelli P. Idiopathic partial epilepsy with reflex visual seizures and both multifocal and generalized EEG changes. In: Beaumanoir A, Gastaut H, Naquet R, eds. *Reflex Seizures and Reflex Epilepsies*. Genève: Éditions Médecine et Hygiène; 1989:229–232.
173. Satishchandra P. Hot-water epilepsy. *Epilepsia*. 2003;44(Suppl 1):29–32.
174. Satishchandra P, Ullal GR, Shankar SK. Hot water epilepsy. In: Zifkin BG, Andermann F, Beaumanoir A, et al., eds. *Reflex Epilepsies and Reflex Seizures. Advances in Neurology*. Vol. 75. Philadelphia: Lippincott-Raven Publishers; 1998:283–293.
175. Schubert R, Cracco JB. Familial rectal pain: a type of reflex epilepsy? *Ann Neurol*. 1992;32:824–826.
176. Scott DF. Musicogenic epilepsy. (2) The later story: its relation to auditory hallucinatory phenomena. In: Critchley M, Henson RA, eds. *Music and the Brain*. London: William Heinemann; 1977:354–364.
177. Senanayake N. Eating epilepsy—a reappraisal. *Epilepsy Res*. 1990;5:74–79.
178. Serles W, Leutmezer F, Pataraia E, et al. A case of startle epilepsy and SSMA seizures documented with subdural recordings. *Epilepsia*. 1999;40:1031–1035.
179. Seyfried TN, Glaser GH. A review of mouse mutants as genetic models of epilepsy. *Epilepsia*. 1985;26:143–150.
180. Shirakawa S, Funatsuka M, Osawa M, et al. A study of the effect of color photostimulation from a cathode-ray tube (CRT) display on photosensitive patients: the effect of alternating red-cyan flicker stimulation. *Epilepsia*. 2001;42:922–929.
181. Stanescu-Cosson R, Pinel P, van de Moortele PF, et al. Understanding dissociations in dyscalculia. A brain imaging study of the impact of number size on the cerebral networks for exact and approximate calculation. *Brain*. 2000;123:2240–2255.

182. Stevens JR. Central and peripheral factors in epileptic discharge. *Arch Neurol.* 1962;7:330–338.
183. Takahashi T. EEG activation by movement of the eyelids and eyes. *Clin EEG.* 1976;18:334–344.
184. Takahashi T. Seizures induced by odorous stimuli. *Clin EEG (Osaka).* 1975;17:769.
185. Takahashi T, Kamijo K, Takaki Y, et al. Suppressive efficacies by adaptive temporal filtering system on photoparoxysmal response elicited by flickering pattern stimulation. *Epilepsia.* 2002;43:530–534.
186. Takahashi Y, Fujiwara T. Effectiveness of broadcasting guidelines for photosensitive seizure prevention. *Neurology.* 2004;62:990–993.
187. Tassinari CA, DeMarco P, Plasmati R, et al. Extreme somatosensory evoked potentials (ESEPs) elicited by tapping of hands or feet in children: a somatosensory cerebral evoked potentials study. *Neurophysiol Clin.* 1988;18:123–128.
188. Tassinari CA, Rubboli G, Rizzi R, et al. Self-induction of visually induced seizures. In: Zifkin BG, Andermann F, Beaumanoir A, et al., eds. *Reflex Epilepsies and Reflex Seizures. Advances in Neurology.* Vol. 75. Philadelphia: Lippincott-Raven Publishers; 1998:179–192.
189. Temkin O. The Falling Sickness. *A History of Epilepsy from the Greeks to the Beginnings of Modern Neurology.* Baltimore: Johns Hopkins University Press; 1971.
190. Terzian H, Terzuolo C. Richerche electrofisiologiche sull'epilessia fotica di Clementi. *Arch Fisiol.* 1951;5:301–320.
191. Vignaendra V, Lim CL. Epileptic discharges triggered by eye convergence. *Neurology.* 1978;28:589–591.
192. Vignal JP, Biraben A, Chauvel PY, et al. Reflex partial seizures of sensorimotor cortex (including cortical reflex myoclonus and startle epilepsy). In: Zifkin BG, Andermann F, Beaumanoir A, et al., eds. *Reflex Epilepsies and Reflex Seizures. Advances in Neurology.* Vol. 75. Philadelphia: Lippincott-Raven Publishers; 1998:207–226.
193. Vizioli R. The problem of human reflex epilepsy and the possible role of masked epileptic factors. *Epilepsia.* 1962;3:293–302.
194. Voskuil PH. Benign early infantile reflex absence seizures. *Epileptic Disord.* 2002;4:29–33.
195. Walter WG, Walter VJ, Gastaut H, et al. Une forme électroencéphalographique nouvelle de l'épilepsie, l'épilepsie photogénique. *Rev Neurol.* 1948;80:613–614.
196. Waltz S, Stephani U. Inheritance of photosensitivity. *Neuropediatrics.* 2000;31:82–85.
197. Wieser HG. Seizure-inducing and preventing mechanisms. In: Beaumanoir A, Gastaut H, Naquet R, eds. *Reflex Seizures and Reflex Epilepsies.* Geneva: Éditions Médecine et Hygiène; 1989:49–60.
198. Wieser HG, Hungerbühler H, Siegel AM, et al. Musicogenic epilepsy: review of the literature and case report with ictal single photon emission computed tomography. *Epilepsia.* 1997;38:200–207.
199. Wieser HG, Mazzola G. Musical consonances and dissonances: are they distinguished independently by the right and left hippocampi? *Neuropsychologia.* 1986;24:805–812.
200. Wilkins AJ. Available at: http://privatewww.essex.ac.uk/~arnold/epilepsy.html.
201. Wilkins AJ. Towards an understanding of reflex epilepsy and the absence. In: Duncan JS, Panayiotopoulos CP, eds. *Typical Absences and Related Epileptic Syndromes.* London: Churchill Livingstone; 1995:196–205.
202. Wilkins AJ, Baker A, Amin D, et al. Treatment of photosensitive epilepsy using coloured glasses. *Seizure.* 1999;8:444–449.
203. Wilkins AJ, Bonanni P, Porciatti V, et al. Physiology of human photosensitivity. *Epilepsia.* 2004;45(Suppl 1):7–13.
204. Wilkins AJ, Darby CE, Binnie CD. Optical treatment of photosensitive epilepsy. *Electroencephalogr Clin Neurophysiol.* 1977;43:577.
205. Wilkins AJ, Darby CE, Binnie CD. Neurophysiological aspects of pattern-sensitive epilepsy. *Brain.* 1979;102:1–25.
206. Wilkins AJ, Lindsay J. Common forms of reflex epilepsy: physiological mechanisms and techniques for treatment. In: Pedley TA, Meldrum BS, eds. *Recent Advances in Epilepsy II.* Edinburgh: Churchill Livingstone; 1985:239–271.
207. Wilkins AJ, Zifkin B, Andermann F, et al. Seizures induced by thinking. *Ann Neurol.* 1982;11:608–612.
208. Wolf P, Goosses R. Relation of photosensitivity to epileptic syndromes. *J Neurol Neurosurg Psychiatry.* 1986;49:1386–1391.
209. Wolf P, Inoue Y. Complex reflex epilepsies: reading epilepsy and praxis induction. In: Roger J, Bureau M, Dravet C, et al., eds. *Epileptic Syndromes in Infancy, Childhood and Adolescence.* 4th ed. Montrouge: John Libbey Eurotext; 2005:347–358.
210. Wolf P, Inoue Y, Zifkin BG, eds. *Reflex Epilepsies. Current Problems in Epilepsy.* Vol. 19. Paris: John Libbey Eurotext; 2004.
211. Wolf P, Mayer T. Juvenile myoclonic epilepsy: a syndrome challenging syndromic concepts? In: Schmitz B, Sander T, eds. *Juvenile Myoclonic Epilepsy. The Janz Syndrome.* Petersfield, U.K.: Wrightson Biomedical; 2000: 33–39.
212. Zafeiriou D, Vargiami E, Kontopoulos E. Reflex myoclonic epilepsy in infancy: a benign age-dependent idiopathic startle epilepsy. *Epileptic Disord.* 2003;5:121–122.
213. Zifkin BG, Andermann F, Beaumanoir A, et al., eds. *Reflex Epilepsies and Reflex Seizures. Advances in Neurology.* Vol. 75. Philadelphia: Lippincott-Raven Publishers; 1998.
214. Zifkin B, Inoue Y. Visual reflex seizures induced by complex stimuli. *Epilepsia.* 2004;45(Supp 1):27–29.
215. Zifkin BG, Zatorre R. Musicogenic epilepsy. In: Zifkin BG, Andermann F, Beaumanoir A, et al., eds. *Reflex Epilepsies and Reflex Seizures. Advances in Neurology.* Vol. 75. Philadelphia: Lippincott-Raven Publishers; 1998:273–281.

CHAPTER 258 ■ OVERVIEW: DISEASES ASSOCIATED WITH EPILEPSY

TIMOTHY A. PEDLEY

INTRODUCTION

Seizures and epilepsy are common manifestations of disturbed cerebral function; thus, they may be symptoms of other diseases that involve the brain and not of epilepsy *sui generis*. This association has long been recognized in the case of brain tumors and tuberous sclerosis, for example, but the modern era of brain imaging and molecular diagnosis has greatly expanded our recognition of specific disease entities in which epilepsy is a major feature. This section reviews major categories of disease that present with seizures or in which epilepsy constitutes a significant aspect of the illness. Certain presentations or evolution should always raise the question of a specific underlying disorder.

CLUES FROM EPILEPSY SYNDROMES

The diagnosis of infantile spasms (West syndrome; Chapter 229) or Lennox-Gastaut syndrome (Chapter 241) should always lead to a search for a specific cause. Both syndromes can occur as either idiopathic or symptomatic conditions, and therein lies one of the disadvantages of the current classification. Both are electroclinical syndromes and therefore etiologically heterogeneous. Neither is a singular pathologic entity, and cerebral malformations, perinatal asphyxia, anoxic encephalopathy from cardiopulmonary arrest, central nervous infection, postimmunization encephalopathy, and progressive degenerative or metabolic syndromes have all been implicated in individual children. Tuberous sclerosis is the most common disease entity causing infantile spasms,[7] but untreated phenylketonuria, nonketotic hyperglycinemia, and other metabolic and structural disorders are also encountered occasionally.[4] A small subgroup of children with spasms but no identifiable causes have normal developmental outcome and may represent an idiopathic condition.[3] Similar disorders are found in children with Lennox-Gastaut syndrome (Chapter 241),[1,8] and of course infantile spasms and Lennox-Gastaut syndrome are not fully independent entities: The 6-year-old child designated as having Lennox-Gastaut syndrome may well have carried a diagnosis of West syndrome as an infant. Indeed, with computed tomographic (CT) and magnetic resonance (MR) brain imaging and the availability of sophisticated and highly specific biochemical and genetic tests, the percentage of cryptogenic cases has steadily declined.

INTRACTABLE EPILEPSY

Persistent seizures despite appropriate therapy are often an indication to consider medical illnesses or treatments that can contribute to or cause recurrent seizures, such as systemic lupus erythematosus, hypoglycemia, drug abuse, and theophylline toxicity (Chapters 127, 191, and 192). The use of molecular techniques to establish linkage or a gene defect has clearly demonstrated that variability in phenotype is common and that syndromic fidelity, defined traditionally by seizure semiology and electroencephalographic (EEG) features, is not invariable. Thus, older children and even adults with seemingly stable (or only very slowly progressive) neurologic abnormalities are now found to have progressive metabolic or degenerative encephalopathies due to adrenoleukodystrophy, ceroid lipofuscinosis, storage diseases such as Tay-Sachs or sialidosis, various aminoacidurias and urea cycle disorders, or one of the progressive myoclonus epilepsies. Other genetic disorders (also referred to as chromosomal abnormalities), including trisomy 13 and 21, fragile X syndrome, and Aicardi syndrome, as well as cortical malformations such as lissencephaly (e.g., Miller-Dieker syndrome) and Angelman ("happy puppet") syndrome, may present with seizures that prove to be drug resistant (Chapter 261). Associated physical abnormalities often provide clues to the diagnosis in most of these conditions.

Seizures are a common manifestation of the mitochondrial encephalopathies, although the frequency is highly variable among the different mitochondrial syndromes. Specific gene defects in many of these disorders have been identified, and they include both mitochondrial and nuclear mutations. In some cases, the type of mutation is quite different in patients that commonly present with seizures than in those in which epilepsy is rare. Thus, seizures are the rule in MELAS (mitochondrial encephalopathy, lactic acidosis, and stroke-like episodes) and MERRF (myoclonus epilepsy with ragged red fibers), which are almost always associated with point mutations in the $tRNA^{Lys}$ gene.[10] However, seizures are rare in Kearns-Sayres syndrome, which is related to large deletions or duplications of mtDNA. Hirano and colleagues (Chapter 262) believe that the spatial distribution within the brain of the mitochondrial mutation underlies the association of particular mutations with epilepsy.

Seizures occur in the majority of children with Rett syndrome,[6] and these can sometimes be intractable. Some of these patients also have syncopal episodes that are occasionally misdiagnosed as epilepsy, and the characteristic stereotypic movements (e.g., hand-wringing) also may be erroneously considered to reflect seizure activity.

IMPORTANCE OF BRAIN DEVELOPMENTAL ABNORMALITIES

Except for major malformations such as anencephaly, holoprosencephaly, and schizencephaly, abnormalities of cortical development were largely unrecognized as a common cause of epilepsy until high-resolution MR brain imaging became widely available and part of the routine diagnostic evaluation of patients with seizures. Cortical developmental malformations are now known to be common, especially as a cause of intractable epilepsy. They are found in up to 20% of adults[2] and >50% of children referred to epilepsy centers because of drug-resistant seizures or as possible surgical candidates.[5] Of equal interest is the growing recognition that cortical dysgenesis can be found in a wide spectrum of patients, including some without seizures, in patients with only one or a few seizures, and as associated pathology in patients with temporal lobe epilepsy due to mesial temporal sclerosis. The movement of cortical developmental abnormalities from the domain of the neuropathologist to that of the neurologist has been one of the most significant changes in modern epileptology (Chapter 259). Some critical questions are beginning to be addressed:

1. To what extent is cortical dyplasia in a given patient coincidental, an associated marker of epileptogenic mechanisms, or the direct cause of seizures?
2. Why do seizures often seem to arise from a single epileptogenic region even when the developmental abnormalities are multifocal or bilateral?
3. How do developmental malformations cause epilepsy?

MISCELLANEOUS CONSIDERATIONS

Seizures are the presenting symptom in the majority of patients with astrocytomas and oligodendrogliomas, but they are also common at some point in the course of more malignant brain tumors (Chapter 264). With slowly growing neoplasms, seizures typically occur early, when there may be no other clinical symptoms or signs to suggest a tumor. CT may be normal at the time of a first seizure caused by well-differentiated, relatively benign tumors, so MRI is essential. Seizures are also common in many infectious and inflammatory diseases (Chapter 265). Parasitic, bacterial, and viral agents all cause various syndromes in which seizures or chronic epilepsy are common, including as the presenting manifestation. Both mental retardation and cerebral palsy (Chapter 263) are major risk factors for epilepsy, probably because they are markers of brain damage, and the risk for epilepsy is additive when both conditions are present. Alcohol and drug abuse are common causes of symptomatic seizures, but alcohol use itself is also a dose-dependent risk for chronic epilepsy (Chapter 268). Heroin and cocaine, but usually not marijuana, also raise the risk of unprovoked seizures, although symptomatic seizures related to acute toxic effects on the brain are far more common.

SUMMARY AND CONCLUSIONS

Certain epileptic syndromes, associated neurologic abnormalities, age at first seizure, drug resistance, and associated morphologic or systemic abnormalities should warrant a search for a specific diagnosis. High-resolution brain MR imaging will generally establish structural causes of epilepsy, including cortical developmental malformations and brain tumors, although serial scans and special imaging sequences may be necessary fully to define the abnormality. In those circumstances in which epilepsy is due to or associated with an underlying disease, proper treatment, genetic and prognostic counseling, and clinical investigation depend on accurate diagnosis.

References

1. Aicardi J, Levy Gomes A. The Lennox-Gastaut syndrome: clinical and electroencephalographic features. In: Niedermeyer E, Degen R, eds. *The Lennox-Gastaut Syndrome. Neurology and Neurobiology,* Vol. 45. New York: Alan R Liss; 1988:25–46.
2. Barkovich AJ, Kuzniecky RI, Jackson G, et al. A developmental and genetic classification for malformations of cortical development. *Neurology.* 225;65:1873–1887.
3. Dulac O, Plouin P, Jambaque I. Predicting favorable outcome in idiopathic West syndrome. *Epilepsia.* 1993;34:747.
4. Jeavons PM, Livet MO. West syndrome: infantile spasms. In: Roger J, Bureau M, Dravet C, et al, eds. *Epileptic Syndromes in Infancy, Childhood, and Adolescence,* 2nd ed. London: John Libbey; 1992:53–65.
5. Kuzniecky RI, Murro A, King D, et al. Magnetic resonance imaging in childhood intractable partial epilepsies: pathologic correlations. *Neurology.* 1993;43:681–687.
6. Moser SJ, Weber P, Lütschg J. Rett syndrome: clinical and electrophysiologic aspects. *Pediatr Neurol.* 2007;36:95–100.
7. Riikonen R, Simell O. Tuberous sclerosis and infantile spasms. *Dev Med Child Neurol.* 1990;32:203–209.
8. Roger J, Gambarelli-Dubois D. Neuropathological studies of the Lennox-Gastaut syndrome. In: Niedermeyer E, Degen R, eds. *The Lennox-Gastaut Syndrome. Neurology and Neurobiology,* Vol. 45. New York: Alan R Liss; 1988:73–93.
9. Rett Syndrome Diagnostic Criteria Work Group. Diagnostic criteria for Rett syndrome. *Ann Neurol.* 1988;23:425–428.
10. Silvestri G, Moraes CT, Shanske S, et al. A new mtDNA mutation in the $tRNA^{Lys}$ gene associated with myoclonic epilepsy and ragged-red fibers (MERRF). *Am J Hum Genet.* 1992;51:1213–1217.

CHAPTER 259 ■ MALFORMATIONS OF CORTICAL DEVELOPMENT

RUBEN I. KUZNIECKY AND GRAEME D. JACKSON

INTRODUCTION

The development of the human brain is a long and complex process that begins with the induction of the neural plate from the undifferentiated surface ectoderm and continues after birth.[115] Any disruption of the normal mechanisms responsible for the formation of the cerebral structures can result in malformations due to abnormal cortical development.[81,85] A wide variety of genetic and environmental factors can cause disturbances in these developmental processes and can therefore lead to an abnormality in the mature brain.

Until the advent of high-resolution magnetic resonance (MR), malformative disorders of the nervous system were almost exclusively the domain of the pathologist. With magnetic resonance imaging (MRI), abnormalities of cortical development can be identified in life, and understanding these conditions, their clinical consequences, and outcome has become essential for appropriate management. The physician's goal is to diagnose these disorders accurately, using information that is available in the clinical setting. This chapter presents an approach that we believe is helpful to clinicians dealing with these disorders, especially in the setting of epilepsy.

The clinical circumstances in which these disorders are encountered are many but primarily involve developmental delay, epilepsy, skin lesions in specific neurocutaneous disorders, and associated organ malformations. From the perspective of epilepsy, there are two common presentations. First, a patient with epilepsy has an abnormal MR brain scan suggesting a malformation of cortical development (MCD). In this case, the issue is largely one of diagnosis, appropriate classification, knowledge of the relevant condition, and genetic testing, if available. This is important for prognosis, treatment, and genetic counseling. Second, a patient with epilepsy has a "normal" brain MR scan, but the clinician suspects, perhaps on the basis of family history, seizure intractability, or other findings on clinical examination, that there may be an underlying abnormality of cortical development. In this case, one is usually dealing with a subtle, localized cortical malformation, and the challenge is to identify the abnormal brain region(s). This is not an uncommon problem for epilepsy centers that deal with surgical treatment.

CLINICAL PRESENTATION

Disorders of cortical development encompass many types of malformations with a comparably wide range of etiologies that produce different effects depending on the stage of brain development that is affected. Not surprisingly, then, clinical presentations are quite heterogeneous and can manifest at almost any age. As a result, the practical problem is that because there are actually many disorders of cortical development, there are no specific clinical features associated with MCDs when considered as a group.

While MCDs are a common cause of epilepsy, there are many cases in which seizures are not a feature of these disorders. Why almost identical brain abnormalities can have such variable clinical phenotypes is not known. Yet while there are no clinical features that are specific for MCDs taken as a whole, there are within this group some specific syndromes recognized on the basis of characteristic patterns of genetic, clinical, and imaging findings.

Seizure type usually reflects the topology of the malformations. That is, focal seizures occur with focal or multifocal MCD, and secondarily generalized seizures with diffuse or bilateral MCDs.

Almost any epilepsy presentation, at almost any age, can be due to an MCD. However, in focal epilepsy, some features create a strong suspicion of an underlying MCD and encourage thorough investigation to exclude this possibility if no other cause has been identified. These features include developmental delay, static focal neurologic deficits, a family history of developmental delay or epilepsy, frequent seizures from onset, and focal status epilepticus. While the presence of such elements may raise the suspicion of an MCD, it must be emphasized that none of them is specific. In surgical series of patients, such characteristics will likely lead to detailed high-resolution MRI with special techniques in an effort to define an abnormality of cortical development.

The severity of seizures in patients with MCDs also varies greatly. There are many individuals with extensive cortical malformations who have no seizures. On the other hand, some individuals with apparently small developmental malformations have severe and intractable epilepsy. The mechanisms of epileptogenesis associated with these abnormalities are complex and generally poorly understood.

EPIDEMIOLOGY

Few studies have addressed the epidemiology of MCDs in detail, and little information can be obtained from studies using the modalities, including MRI, that are currently available. One series based on pathology findings revealed that 46.5% of patients had developmental malformations at autopsy.[95] A case ascertainment study of lissencephaly showed a prevalence of 11.7 per million births.[40] No data are available for heterotopia, focal cortical dysplasia, or other malformations of cortical development.

Recent clinical and neuroimaging studies in special populations have suggested that cortical malformations are much more common than was previously appreciated. In children referred to epilepsy centers for intractable seizures, more than half have some type of developmental abnormality, with focal cortical dysplasia discovered in approximately 25% of those with intractable focal seizures.[79] The prevalence of these disorders in the adult population with intractable focal epilepsy is 15% to 20%.[6,10]

TERMS AND DEFINITIONS

A number of terms are commonly used in referring to patients with developmental malformations.[10] For example, *dysplasia* in this context is an encompassing term that usually means abnormalities of the cortex that have a particular histopathology and are developmental in origin. *Neuronal migration disorder* is generally used in a similar context, but this is clearly incorrect as a general term, as it describes only one embryologic stage in cortical development. We consider all of these disorders to be *malformations of cortical development* and prefer this as the general term for referring to this category of conditions. All of these disorders seem to result from disturbed organogenesis (and, hence, are malformations), and all involve cells that under normal circumstances would participate in formation of the cerebral cortex. The most common malformative disorders involve abnormal stem cell formation in the germinative zone or abnormal cortical organization. Some result from faulty neuronal migration, whereas still others are postmigratory in origin.

We believe that establishing a single nomenclature and classification system for these disorders is essential to their understanding and management. The classification proposed in the following discussion provides a means by which similar disorders can be logically grouped together.[10]

CLASSIFICATION PRINCIPLES

MCDs can be classified according to a number of different criteria emphasizing clinical phenotype, imaging findings, pathology, and genetic defects. The overall classification scheme that we favor (Table 1) is based on the three fundamental events of cortical formation: (a) proliferation of neurons and glia in the ventricular zone and subventricular zones; (b) multidirectional migration of immature but postmitotic neurons to the developing cerebral cortex; and (c) cortical organization, which consists of vertical and horizontal organization of neurons within the cortex and elaboration of axonal and dendritic ramifications. For those malformations with abnormalities involving more than one of these processes, classification is based on the first identified abnormal step. Diffuse and focal malformations that were classified separately in the past are no longer separated since genetic studies have shown that the same gene defects can cause focal or generalized MCDs.

Thus, with advances in molecular genetics, we have moved from a purely phenotypic approach to a combined phenotypic/genetic classification. The basis of this change has been the recognition that malformations of varying severity can result from the same underlying processes, specifically from mutations of the same causative genes. This was shown first for classical lissencephaly[38,93,94,111–114,123] and more recently in the brain malformations associated with congenital muscular dystrophies.[15–17,88,89,108,132–134] For example, patients with large deletions and truncations of the *LIS1* and *DCX* mutations have diffuse or severe lissencephaly, while those with less severe *LIS1* mutations may only have posterior pachygyria or posterior-predominant subcortical band heterotopia. Those with less severe *DCX* mutations have anterior pachygyria or frontal subcortical band heterotopia of variable thickness,[27,49–51,87,92,111,114,123] or they may even have normal brain MRI scans.[57] Further support for this approach has been the recent discovery of mutations of multiple genes each causing very similar clinical syndromes, and the finding that mutations of different genes can cause the phenotype of Walker-Warburg syndrome or muscle-eye-brain disease.[123]

TABLE 1

CLASSIFICATION SCHEME OF MALFORMATIONS OF CORTICAL DEVELOPMENT

- I. Malformations due to abnormal neuronal and glial proliferation or apoptosis
  - A. Decreased proliferation/increased apoptosis or increased proliferation/decreased apoptosis—abnormalities of brain size
    - 1. Microcephaly with normal to thin cortex
    - 2. Microlissencephaly (extreme microcephaly with thick cortex)
    - 3. Microcephaly with extensive polymicrogyria
    - 4. Macrocephalies
  - B. Abnormal proliferation (abnormal cell types)
    - 1. Nonneoplastic
      - a. Cortical hamartomas of tuberous sclerosis
      - b. Cortical dysplasia with balloon cells
      - c. Hemimegalencephaly
    - 2. Neoplastic (associated with disordered cortex)
      - a. Dysembryoplastic neuroepithelial tumor
      - b. Ganglioglioma
      - c. Gangliocytoma
- II. Malformations due to abnormal neuronal migration
  - A. Lissencephaly/subcortical band heterotopia spectrum
  - B. Cobblestone complex/congenital muscular dystrophy syndromes
  - C. Heterotopia
    - 1. Subependymal (periventricular)
    - 2. Subcortical (other than band heterotopia)
    - 3. Marginal glioneuronal
- III. Malformations due to abnormal cortical organization (including late neuronal migration)
  - A. Polymicrogyria and schizencephaly
    - 1. Bilateral polymicrogyria syndromes
    - 2. Schizencephaly (polymicrogyria with clefts)
    - 3. Polymicrogyria or schizencephaly as part of multiple congenital anomaly/mental retardation syndromes
  - B. Cortical dysplasia without balloon cells
  - C. Microdysgenesis
- IV. Malformations of cortical development, not otherwise classified
  - A. Malformations secondary to inborn errors of metabolism
    - 1. Mitochondrial and pyruvate metabolic disorders
    - 2. Peroxisomal disorders
  - B. Other unclassified malformations
    - 1. Sublobar dysplasia
    - 2. Others

DEVELOPMENTAL MALFORMATIONS ASSOCIATED WITH EPILEPSY: SPECIFIC DISORDERS

We have restricted the following discussion to an overview of the most common and relatively distinct entities that affect patients with epilepsy.

Focal Cortical Dysplasia

Focal cortical dysplasia (FCD) is probably the most common form of focal developmental disorder diagnosed in patients with intractable focal epilepsy.[24,67,83,86,100] The lesions consist of disruption of cortical lamination with poorly differentiated glial cell elements. Since its original description, FCD has been recognized to encompass a spectrum of changes.[130] These range from mild cortical disruption without apparent giant neurons to the most severe forms in which cortical dyslamination, large bizarre cells, and astrocytosis are present.[75,79,130] It is the presence of balloon cells that differentiates FCD type I (without balloon cells) from FCD type II (with balloon cells) and that lead to the distinction in our classification scheme (see Table 1).

The clinical manifestations of patients with cortical FCD are variable. Seizures usually begin between the ages of 2 and 10 years. Sometimes, however, seizures may be the presenting clinical problem in the second decade or even later. Focal and secondarily generalized attacks are common. Interestingly, seizures often occur in clusters, but generalized status epilepticus is rare except in patients with FCD involving the central region.[76] In our experience, the majority of patients have extratemporal cortical dysplasias that affect the pre- and postcentral regions most often. Interictal scalp electroencephalography (EEG) may demonstrate focal subclinical ictal discharges over the dysplastic lesions, underscoring the high epileptogenicity of these lesions.[103] FCD involving the frontal lobe has also been reported, and lesions can occur in both mesial and lateral neocortical structures as well.[77]

The MRI findings consist of abnormal gyral thickening with underlying T2-weighted white matter changes. These abnormalities are often circumscribed in nature, and they can sometimes be extensive, involving more than one gyrus or lobe. High-resolution MRIs with thin slices and multiplanar reconstruction are often necessary to identify these[24,25,55] (Fig. 1). Location can be quite unpredictable, as in the example of a very small lesion that was restricted to the bottom of a sulcus. Correlating clinical manifestations with the spectrum of changes seen in FCD has been limited, because histopathology is usually required before subtypes of FCD (e.g., FCD without balloon cells and microdysgenesis) can be firmly established.[10]

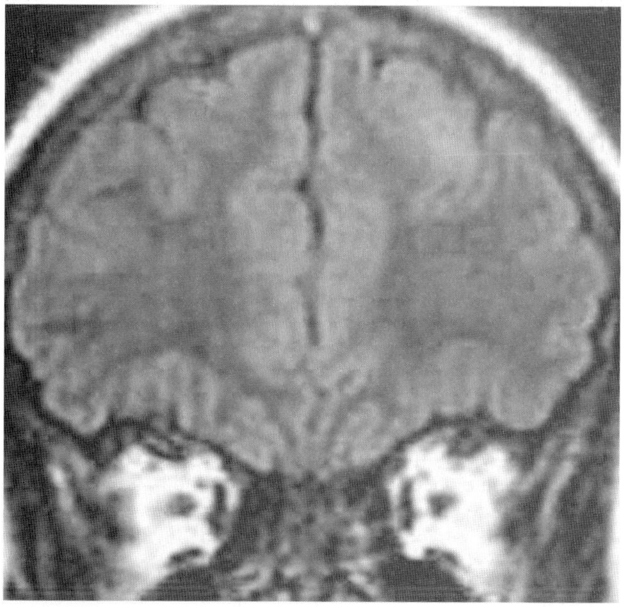

FIGURE 1. Focal cortical dysplasia (FCD). Left frontal lobe shows in this coronal fluid-attenuated inversion recovery magnetic resonance image a subtle signal abnormality and thickened cortex representing FCD. Pathology showed balloon cells.

Hemimegalencephaly

Hemimegalencephaly is a rare malformation characterized by predominantly unilateral cerebral pathology typically associated with an enlarged hemisphere. It can be seen in isolation or in association with epidermal nevus syndrome[105] or hypomelanosis of Ito.[91,104,128] Pathologic findings are diverse and include cortical dysplasia, white matter abnormalities with abnormal cell types, or polymicrogyria usually restricted to one hemisphere. Most children with hemimegalencephaly associated with cortical malformations have not had other associated congenital anomalies.

Seizures and hemiparesis are common presenting symptoms.[101,107,118] Developmental delay is also common. Seizures usually appear within the first 6 months of life. They are often unilateral but can secondarily generalize, and they are frequently intractable to medical therapy. Continuing seizure activity is associated with the appearance or worsening of unilateral neurologic findings, such as hemiparesis and hemianopias. Occasionally there is only minimal neurologic dysfunction.

Diagnosis is based on the predominantly focal epileptic syndrome, the unilateral hemispheric EEG discharges, and the presence of unilateral neurologic abnormalities. MRI findings provide definitive diagnosis. Mild to severe enlargement of at least one lobe is present in all patients (Fig. 2). In more than half of the patients, the entire hemisphere is enlarged with thick gray

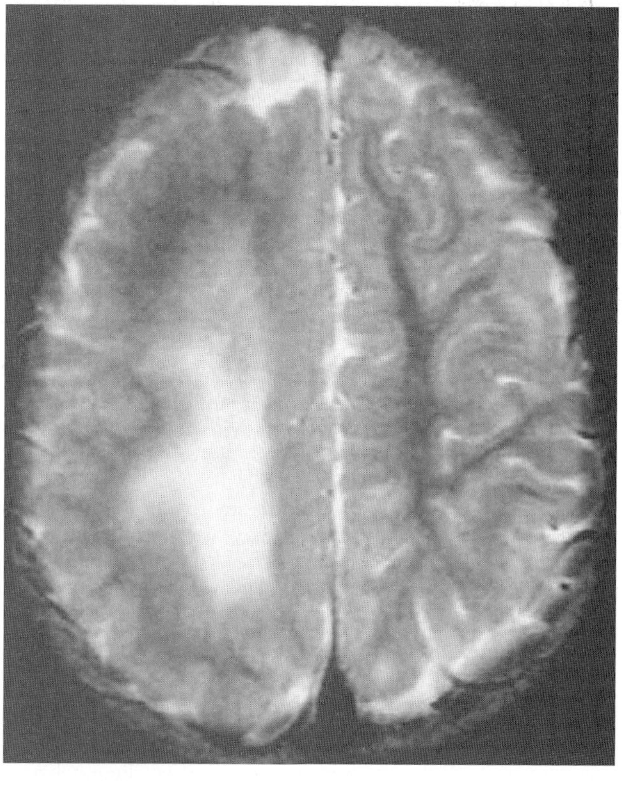

FIGURE 2. Hemimegalencephaly. Axial T2-weighted magnetic resonance image shows abnormal left hemisphere with smooth cortex and white matter changes.

matter and broad, flat gyri.[23,83,136] The underlying hemispheric white matter usually demonstrates abnormal MRI signal intensity. Heterotopia and other malformations are sometimes detected throughout the abnormal hemisphere, and there may be ipsilateral ventricular enlargement.

Focal Transmantle Dysplasia

Transmantle dysplasia is a developmental malformation characterized by abnormal brain tissue that extends through the entire mantle of the cerebrum, from the pia to the ventricular surface.[12] On MRI brain scans, areas of signal abnormality extend radially inward from the cortical surface toward the lateral ventricle. When the imaging plane is parallel to the tract, the T2 imaging signal abnormality involves the deep cortex and subcortical white matter.

Patients with this malformation present with focal seizures at different ages. Ictal semiology and neurologic deficits resemble those that accompany FCD. EEG abnormalities are usually lateralized to the areas of cortical malformations. Mild motor signs may be present if the lesions are in close proximity to the central cortical area. This malformation likely represents a subtype of FCD as pathology obtained during resections for epilepsy show a lack of normal cortical lamination, neuronomegaly, and hypomyelination with atypical reactive astrocytosis in the white matter.

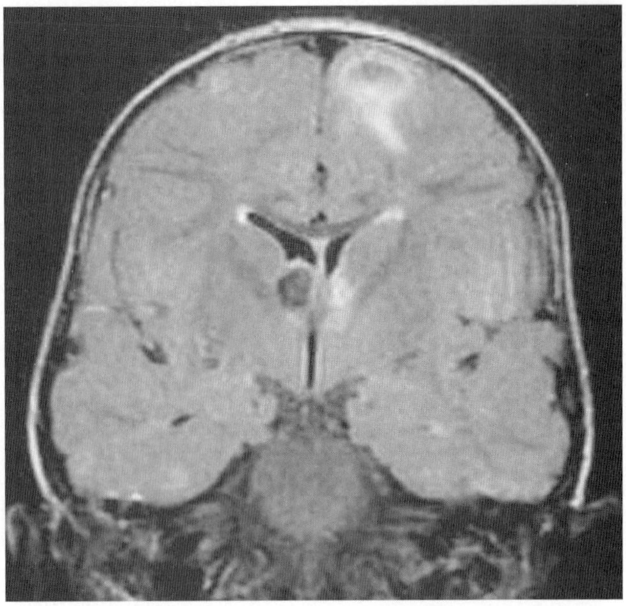

FIGURE 3. Tuberous sclerosis complex. Coronal fluid-attenuated inversion recovery magnetic resonance image shows multiple hamartomas and a large subependymal nodule.

Tuberous Sclerosis

Tuberous sclerosis (TS) is an autosomal dominant, genetically determined multisystem disorder with high penetrance and variable expression.[35–37,71] Genetic heterogeneity is observed with gene defects reported in both chromosome 9q34 and chromosome 16p13 with genetic classification into TSC1 and TSC2.

Pathologically, TS is a disorder of cellular migration, proliferation, and differentiation, resulting in hamartomata formation that involves a large number of neural crest derivatives. Histologically, two major abnormalities are seen. Cortical tubers are characterized by cortical dyslamination, large cells (neurons and glial cells or neuroastrocytes), and abnormal neuropil with hypomyelination. Subcortically, subependymal nodules projecting into the ventricles are typical. Microscopically, densely aggregated larger cells are present, often resembling neoplasms. Electron microscopic (EM) studies of cortical tubers have demonstrated that glial cells predominate near the pial surface, whereas small neurons are more prevalent inferiorly. Underneath the tubers, a rudimentary cortical plate is seen. The presence of the most undifferentiated cell types in the subependymal zone (giant cells) and more differentiated cells in the cortical tubers with intermediate lesions between them suggest a spectrum of abnormalities in neural and glial differentiation and migration.

Seizures are the most common neurologic symptom in TS: More than 90% of patients have seizures during their lifetimes.[71,120,142] Infantile spasms and partial seizures are highly prevalent, and secondary generalization occurs more often after age 2 years. Myoclonic seizures and mental retardation are very frequent. Over time, clinical deterioration is common, with seizures becoming more frequent and difficult to treat.

MRI scans often demonstrate subependymal nodules with varying degrees of contrast enhancement. Calcifications are frequent and are best demonstrated using gradient-echo sequences. Cortical tubers, ranging in size from 1 to 2 cm, are located at the gray–white matter interface. The parietal and frontal lobes are affected most often (Fig. 3). Tubers are isointense on T1 images but hyperintense using T2 sequences. Gyral core tubers may resemble an empty gyrus due to hypointensity of the white matter.[3,48,129]

The location of certain size tubers appears to correlate with EEG epileptogenic foci and prognosis. Patients with posteriorly located lesions have early onset of seizures as opposed to those with frontal lesions.[31] The presence of multiple and large cortical tubers, early onset of multiple seizure types, and multifocal EEG abnormalities correlate with unfavorable prognosis.

Lissencephalies

Lissencephaly refers to brains without normal sulcation (i.e., smooth brains).[43,72] The lissencephalies are a group of different disorders with distinct pathologic substrates and multiple causes. The major distinction is between classical lissencephaly and cobblestone lissencephaly, terms that reflect the appearance of the brain and that, in turn, derive from different genes. The various types of lissencephaly are classified according to the gene defect and associated malformations. For example, instead of classifying *LIS1* mutations and *DCX* mutations as subcategories of the isolated lissencephaly sequence, the classification includes Miller-Dieker syndrome, isolated lissencephaly syndrome, and subcortical band heterotopia as subcategories under *LIS1* mutations.[10] Instead of listing *POMT1* mutations and *FKRP* mutations under Walker-Warburg syndrome, the classification lists muscle-eye-brain disease and Walker-Warburg syndrome under *FKRP* mutations. As a result of this reclassification, many syndromes are listed more than once. For example, isolated lissencephaly sequence and band heterotopia are listed under both *LIS1* and *DCX* mutations and Walker-Warburg syndrome is listed under *POMT, FKRP,* and *FCMD* mutations.

Classical Lissencephaly

Classical lissencephaly or generalized agyria-pachygyria is a severe brain malformation manifested by a smooth cerebral surface, abnormally thick cortex with four abnormal layers, diffuse neuronal heterotopia, enlarged ventricles, and often hypoplasia of the corpus callosum. Mutations in the *LIS1* gene result in Miller-Dieker syndrome (MDS), isolated lissencephaly sequence (ILS), and subcortical band heterotopia (SBH). Similar phenotypes also occur with *DCX* mutations, although in patients with *DCX* mutations, the frontal lobes are most affected; whereas in patients with *LIS1* mutations, the posterior areas are more involved. Mutations of the *ARX* gene cause X–linked lissencephaly with ambiguous genitalia and anomalies of the corpus callosum.[65,69,70,127]

Children with classical lissencephaly present with feeding difficulties or hypotonia. By 6 months of life, most of these children will have seizures, and the evolution of the epilepsy is similar in all patients. Infantile spasms with hypsarrhythmia and typical paroxysmal fast activity on the EEG appear in the first year of life. Response to treatment with adrenocorticotropic hormone (ACTH) or other anticonvulsants is variable, but most children will continue to have frequent seizures accompanied by severe developmental delay. Typical seizure types also include myoclonic, tonic, and tonic–clonic seizures. Profound mental retardation and spastic quadriplegia are present.

Diagnosis of classic lissencephaly is based on the typical clinical, EEG, and MRI features. MRI demonstrates a thickened cortex, loss of white matter, and vertical sylvian fissures, which result in the typical 8-shaped appearance of the brain (Fig. 4). Cortical thickness is in the range of 11 to 20 mm compared to 3.5 mm in normal controls.[11] In some patients there are regions of pachygyric cortex. Barkovich et al.[11] have also reported the presence of incomplete inversion of the hippocampi, a marker of arrest of neuronal migration.

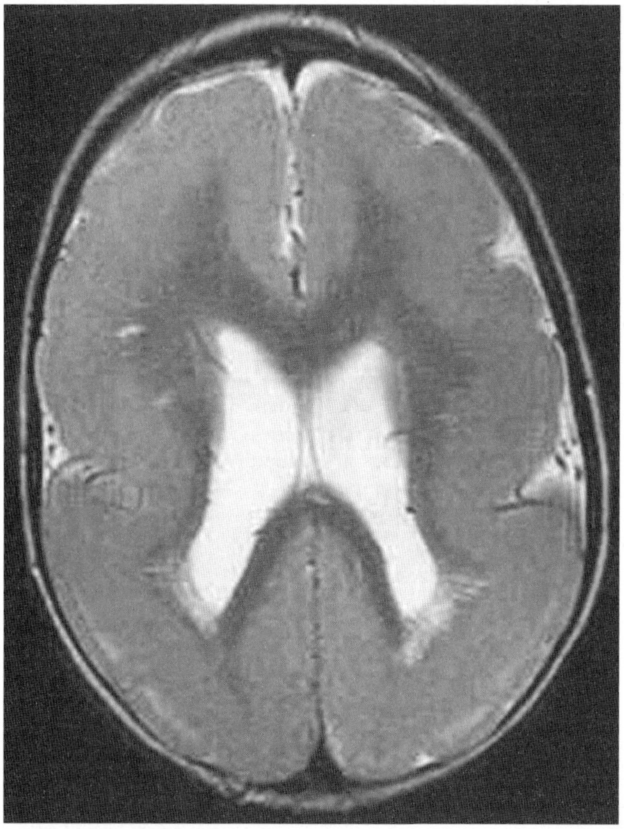

FIGURE 4. Lissencephaly. Miller-Dieker syndrome. *LIS1* mutation. Axial T2-weighted image shows smooth cortex.

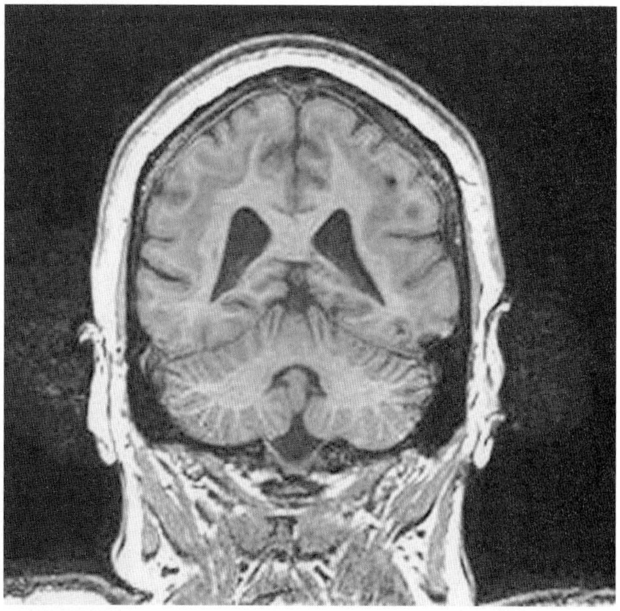

FIGURE 5. Subcortical band heterotopia (SBH). Coronal T1-weighted image shows typical subcortical band of gray matter with relative normal cortical infolding; *DCX* mutation.

Band Heterotopia (Double Cortex)

Subcortical band heterotopia or "double cortex syndrome" (Fig. 5) consists of symmetric and circumferential bands of gray matter located just beneath the cortex and separated from it by a thin band of white matter. The inner margin of the band is usually smooth, while the outer margin may be smooth or follow the interdigitations of the true cortex and white matter. Pathologic specimens have demonstrated normal lamination in cortical layers one through four; layers five and six usually cannot be seen; and layer six is merged with the U-fibers of the white matter.[90] Underneath, clusters of ganglion cells are present. Cortical thickness overlying the heterotopia is mildly increased or normal, and the temporal lobes, in particular the hippocampal structures, are normal as opposed to lissencephaly.

Band heterotopia is an X-linked recessive trait, and thus it is usually found only in females, although a few affected males have survived.[112] The risk for carrier females is high: 50% of their sons will have lissencephaly, and 50% of their daughters will have band heterotopia. Patients have mild to moderate developmental delay, upper motor neuron signs, and, in some, dysarthria. Full-scale IQs ranging from severely low to normal have been reported.[5] EEG investigations usually demonstrate frequent bilateral focal and multifocal spikes, although generalized discharges are also seen, including slow spike-wave patterns.

MRI findings are fairly stereotyped and demonstrate a circumferential band of subcortical gray matter heterotopia underlying the cortical mantle and separated from it by a thin rim of white matter. This is usually more obvious over the frontocentral parietal region. Barkovich et al. have suggested that the thickness of the heterotopic gray matter correlates with severity of the clinical syndrome.[5,66,90]

Cobblestone Lissencephaly Complex

Cobblestone lissencephaly, so called because of the pebbled appearance of the cortical surface due to leptomeningeal neuronal and glial heterotopia, is less common than classical

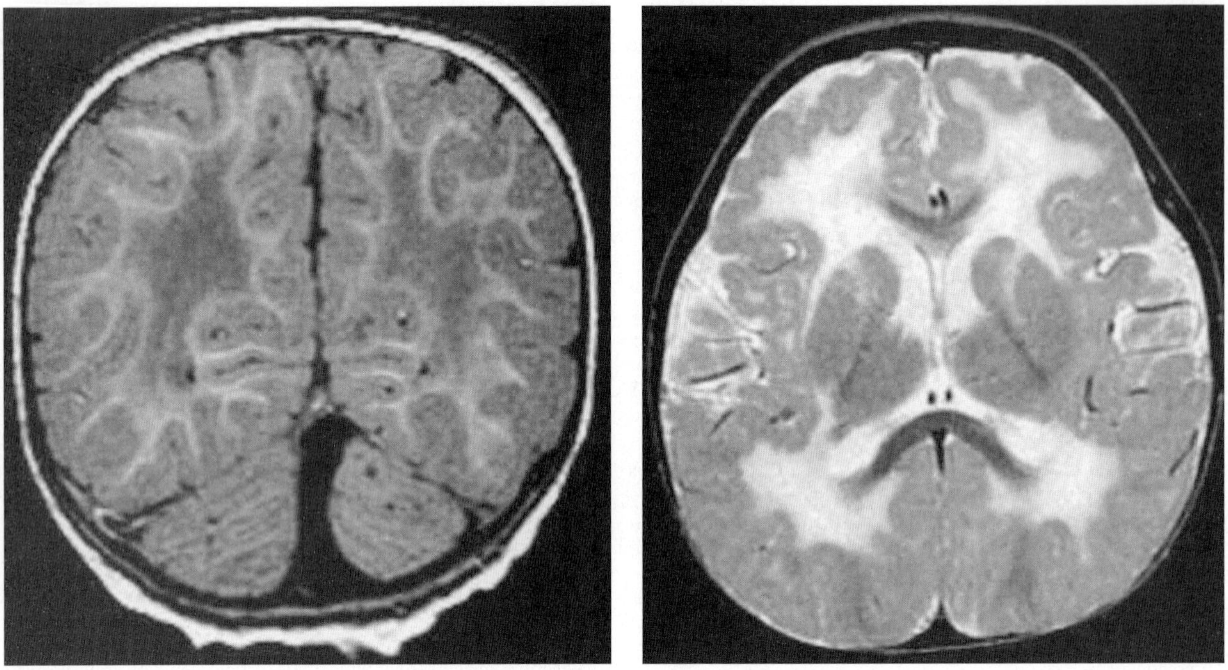

FIGURE 6. Cobblestone lissencephaly in Fukuyama congenital muscular dystrophy with *FKTN* mutation. Note white matter changes, smooth cortex, and cerebellar cyst.

lissencephaly. It is a complex brain malformation that consists of cobblestone cortex, polymicrogyria, pachymicrogyria, abnormal white matter, enlarged ventricles, small brainstem, and cerebellar vermian atrophy with cerebellar polymicrogyria.[43] It is often associated with eye malformations and congenital muscular dystrophy.

Syndromes associated with cobblestone lissencephaly include Fukuyama congenital muscular dystrophy (FCMD) (Fig. 6), muscle-eye-brain disease (MEB), and Walker- Warburg syndrome (WWS). The classification of cobblestone lissencephalies changed significantly when it was discovered that congenital muscular dystrophies result from abnormalities of protein glycosylation.[2,22,143] Mutations in any of the genes involved can cause several different clinical syndromes. For example, Fukutin-related protein *(FKRP)* mutations can cause the clinical phenotypes of limb-girdle muscular dystrophy, muscle-eye-brain disease, and Walker-Warburg syndrome.[15] Fukuyama *(FCMD)* mutations can cause Walker-Warburg syndrome in addition to FCMD and MEB (Fukuyama CMD plus retinal abnormality) phenotypes.[14,124] Thus, the clinical phenotype may be related more to the severity of the mutation than to the precise gene.

Most children with cobblestone lissencephaly have severe mental retardation and hypotonia, mild distal spasticity, and often poor vision. Most patients do not survive beyond the first decade. Seizures have not been well studied.

Heterotopia

Heterotopia is, by definition, the presence of normal cells in improper locations.[8,47] In cases of epilepsy associated with MCDs, this definition usually refers to neurons within the periventricular or subcortical white matter. At the present time, there are two major groups of heterotopia that are recognized as syndromes: Periventricular nodular heterotopia (PNH) and focal subcortical heterotopia.

Periventricular Nodular Heterotopia

Periventricular nodular heterotopia, or subependymal nodular heterotopia, is the most common form of developmental disorder seen in patients with epilepsy.[8,21,44,58,68] The condition is caused by the failure of a group of neurons to either initiate or complete the migration process toward the cortical mantle. PNH can range from a few nodular clusters of neurons to diffuse lining of the ependymal regions. Bilateral periventricular nodular heterotopias (BPNHs) are usually contiguous and symmetric but occasionally are isolated and asymmetric. Ninety percent of reported patients with PNH had diffuse, narrow involvement of all subventricular regions.[44,63,84]

Patients with PNH usually have normal neurologic development. A few have had symptoms that were probably overlooked, such as headaches or psychiatric complaints, while other persons discovered during family evaluations have been asymptomatic. The majority of patients have normal intellectual and motor function or mild mental retardation. Seizures are common, and epilepsy occurs in almost 80% of cases. Interestingly, seizures usually begin in adolescence. In patients with seizures, temporal and parieto-occipital symptomatology is common. EEG findings are generally nonspecific, and interictal discharges are infrequent.[57]

Typical MRI features consist of multiple smooth ovoid nodules of cortical gray matter lining the lateral ventricles but sparing the third and fourth ventricles (Fig. 7). Approximately 75% of patients have bilateral lesions, and 30% have additional focal subcortical heterotopia. Callosal and cerebellar malformations are present in 25% of cases. Signal intensity from the nodules is isointense with gray matter in all MRI sequences, and the nodules do not enhance with contrast, distinguishing features from subependymal hamartomas seen in tuberous sclerosis. In 20% of patients, other cortical malformations may be detected.

Classic PNH can be associated with FILA (Filamin) mutation on chromosome Xq28.[46] Because it is an X-linked mutation, men are only rarely affected.[45,57,59,97] Most pregnancies carrying male fetuses terminate in spontaneous abortions.

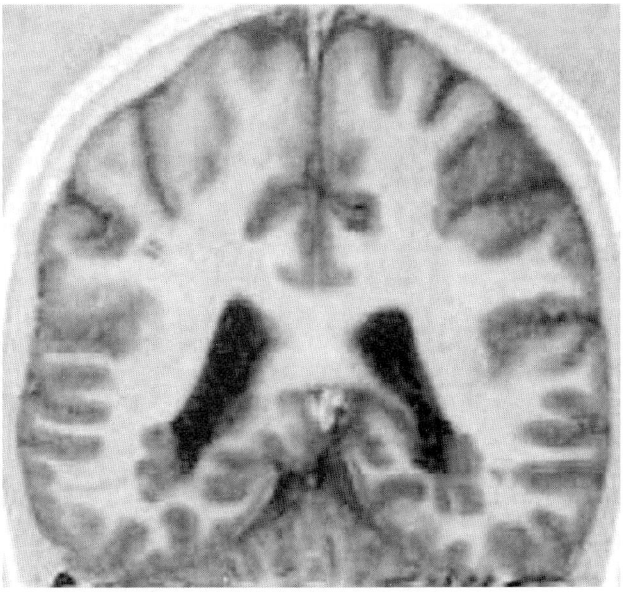

FIGURE 7. Periventricular nodular heterotopia due to Filamin 1 mutation. Note periventricular gray matter nodules.

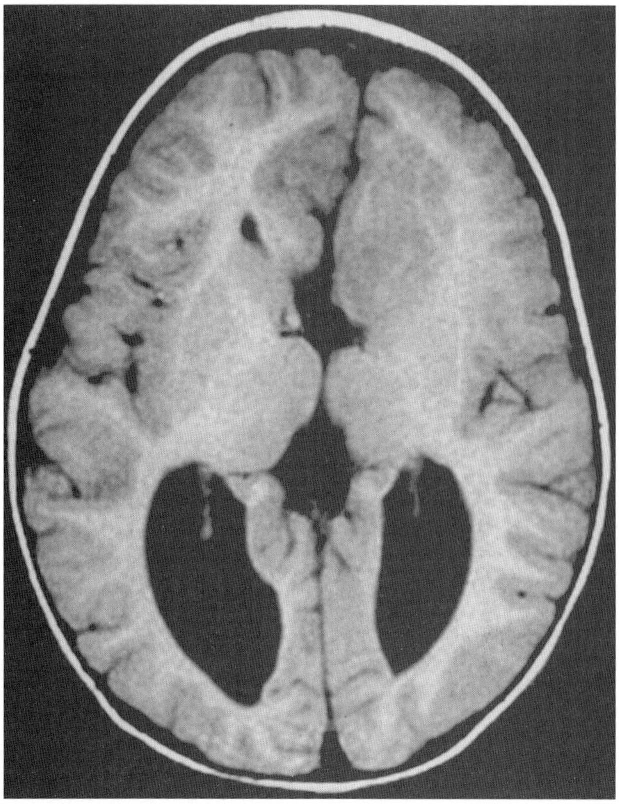

FIGURE 8. Subcortical nodular heterotopia. Axial T1-weighted magnetic resonance image shows large subcortical mass of gray matter in the mesial frontal lobe associated with partial agenesis of corpus callosum and ventricular changes.

Focal Subcortical Heterotopia

Although the majority of patients with subependymal heterotopia have diffuse nodular lesions, occasionally patients may present with few focal lesions involving one hemisphere. According to reviews,[13,45,83] the frequency of focal subcortical heterotopia is <20%. In a patient without neurologic symptoms, such lesions may be just coincidental findings, but the true incidence of seizures in these patients is unknown. Most patients have been sporadic occurrences, and subcortical heterotopias are probably secondary to mosaic mutations or to true environmental injuries.

Clinically, patients may present with normal development, but at times, depending on the size of the lesions, contralateral pyramidal signs may be present. Approximately 50% of patients with focal subcortical heterotopia are developmentally and cognitively delayed. Developmental delay is more common among patients who have concomitant callosal agenesis. Speech appears to be normal in some patients, but when lesions are extensive and involve the dominant hemisphere, speech delay is observed. Seizures in these patients are a mixture of focal motor and secondary generalized convulsions. Infantile spasms have also been described. The ultimate neurologic and seizure outcome not only depends on the type, location, and size of lesions, but also on the type of developmental disorder.

Imaging features in these patients are quite characteristic. Heterotopia appears as clusters of nodules of gray matter with irregular margins (Fig. 8). The surrounding white matter is usually normal and has normal-intensity signal. At times, the heterotopia may appear as masses with ventricular compression. On some occasions, cerebrospinal fluid (CSF) signal may be seen within these malformations. Corpus callosum abnormalities have also been reported.

Polymicrogyria

Polymicrogyria (PMG) refers to an abnormal macroscopic appearance of brain gyration that is characterized by excessive numbers of small gyri. In some cases, the gyri are shallow and very small, separated by slight sulci, whereas in other cases the gyri are wider.[1,86,108]

The histologic changes in polymicrogyria are midcortical laminar necrosis in layer five resembling ischemic change. Superficial to this cortical band, the cortex consists of normal layers four, three, and two. Because late-migrating neurons reach their normal positions before laminar necrosis takes place, this type of malformation most likely originates in some cases after the 20th fetal week and is thus postmigratory in origin.

Histologic classification divides polymicrogyria into four-layered and unlayered types. Although most of the experimental data and pathologic findings in human fetuses suggest that polymicrogyria is the result of a postmigratory ischemic mechanism, this has been disputed and some investigators[1,99] have postulated that at least some forms of PMG are premigratory in origin. In fact, the best known cause in humans is intrauterine cytomegalovirus (CMV) infection, which is also usually associated with diffuse or patchy white matter changes and often diffuse or multifocal calcifications.

Several new unilateral and bilateral polymicrogyria syndromes have recently been described, and several others have had the causative genes mapped or identified. Reports of *bilateral perisylvian polymicrogyria* had commented on a significant male preponderance.[96] This was subsequently confirmed in a large series that localized a gene to Xq28.[135] Unilateral and bilateral perisylvian polymicrogyria has been observed in several chromosomal aneuploidy syndromes, most prominently with deletion of the chromosome 22q11.2 DiGeorge syndrome critical region,[18,19] and in families with presumed X-linked inheritance.[20] Additional bilateral polymicrogyria syndromes include bilateral *frontal polymicrogyria,*[60] *bilateral parasagittal parieto-occipital polymicrogyria,*[61] *bilateral lateral parietal*

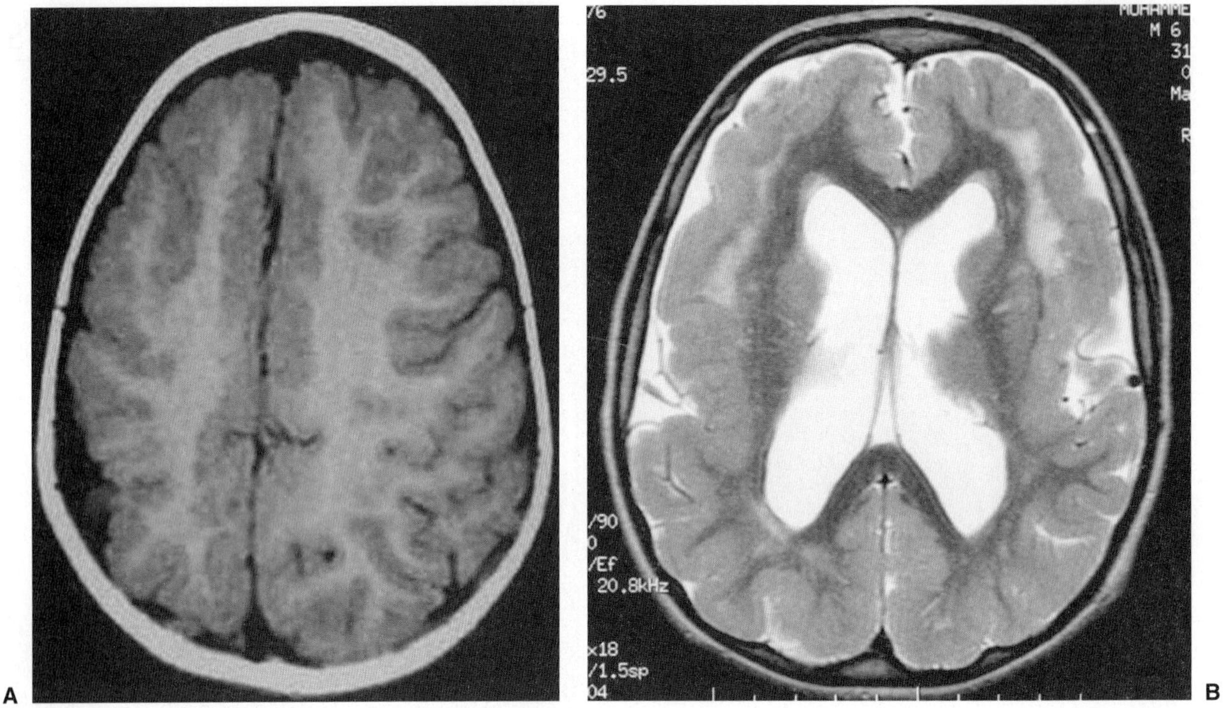

FIGURE 9. **A:** Unilateral polymicrogyria (PMG). Note extensive atrophy and PMG cortex in the left hemisphere. **B:** Bifrontal PMG syndrome with *GPR56* mutation. Note PMG and abnormal white matter changes.

polymicrogyria,[7] *bilaterally generalized polymicrogyria,*[30] and two distinct malformations with periventricular nodular heterotopia and overlying polymicrogyria, one with frontal-perisylvian predominance and another with posterior-temporal predominance. A recent report described a malformation designated *bilateral frontoparietal polymicrogyria* associated with abnormalities of myelination and dysplasia of the cerebellum and brainstem.[29] This has been mapped to chromosome 16q12.2-21 and subsequently associated with mutations of the *GPR56* gene.[109]

The clinical presentation depends on the location and extent of polymicrogyria, and whether the contralateral hemisphere is involved. It is thus highly variable. Diffuse polymicrogyria may present with severe developmental delay, microcephaly, and hypotonia. Polymicrogyria can be limited to one hemisphere (*unilateral hemispheric polymicrogyria*) (Fig 9); it can also be one of the pathologic changes associated with hemimegalencephaly.

MRI findings demonstrate a seemingly thick cortex that can be interpreted as pachygyria. However, cortical thickness in polymicrogyria is less than that observed in pachygyria. The sulci are shallow, and the underlying white matter may show abnormal T2 signal. (Figs. 9 and 10).

As indicated by the foregoing descriptions, PMG syndromes have been classified by the anatomic distribution of the abnormal gyri. Some syndromes can also now be identified on the basis of clinical and imaging features. The most common of these is *bilateral perisylvian polymicrogyria,* also known as *congenital bilateral perisylvian syndrome* (CBPS).[52,56,73,74,98] Clinical features include congenital pseudobulbar paresis, intellectual delay, and characteristic bilateral lesions on computed tomography (CT) or MRI. Almost 90% of patients present with seizures, and half of them have intractable epilepsy. A unique seizure pattern consists of perioral and bilateral facial involvement. Other seizure types include atypical absences attacks, tonic/atonic seizures, and generalized tonic–clonic seizures. EEG findings include generalized spike-wave or multifocal abnormalities, but 20% have had localized epileptogenic discharges. The diagnosis can be made on the basis of the clinical features; brain MRI provides confirmation.[74] The imaging findings are distinctive with involvement of the sylvian,

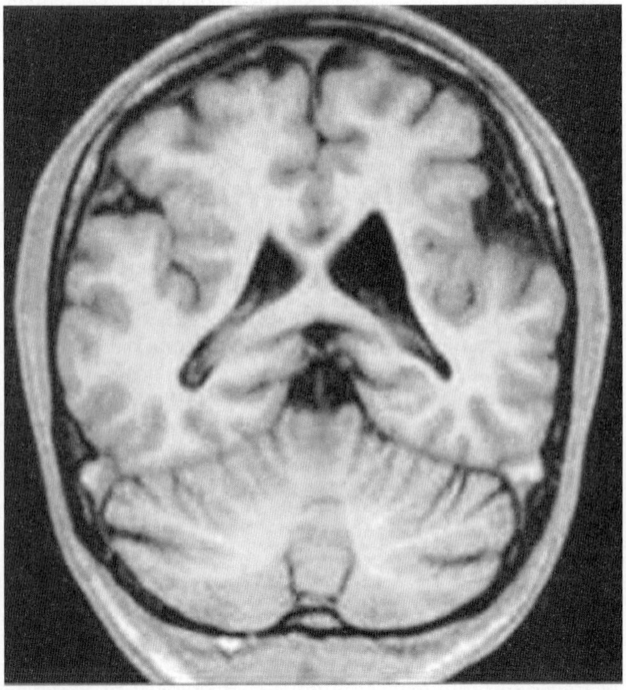

FIGURE 10. Polymicrogyria (PMG), bilateral perisylvian syndrome. Coronal T1- weighted magnetic resonance image shows bilateral perisylvian PMG.

opercular, and perisylvian regions (Fig. 10). Except for unilateral hemispheric polymicrogyria, the other bilateral polymicrogyria syndromes do not have characteristic clinical or EEG features.

Schizencephaly

Although schizencephaly has been considered a condition different from polymicrogyria, most authorities today classify them as *polymicrogyria/schizencephaly complex*. The term *schizencephaly* is used to describe clefts in the cerebral hemispheres that are lined with gray matter and extend from the pia to the ependymal lining.[42,54,64] The clefts may be in apposition to each other (closed lip or type I schizencephaly) or separated (open lip or type II schizencephaly).[126] The cortex surrounding the clefts can be normal or have underlying polymicrogyria. The gray matter lining the cleft itself is usually composed of polymicrogyric cortex. Subependymal heterotopias are common. The pathogenesis of schizencephaly is probably similar to that of polymicrogyria and porencephaly. It is, rather, the extent of cortical injury that determines if a lesion becomes polymicrogyria or schizencephaly. Injuries that extend more deeply into the cortex and destroy the superficial portions of the glial fibers produce cortical infoldings lined by polymicrogyria. When the injury involves the entire thickness of the developing hemisphere, schizencephaly results. The septum pellucidum is absent in 70% to 90% of patients.[9,117]

Schizencephaly has many features resembling those of polymicrogyria. As with polymicrogyria, schizencephaly can be bilateral or unilateral. Furthermore, bilateral lesions can be either symmetric or asymmetric. In our experience, approximately 30% to 40% of patients with schizencephaly have bilateral lesions. They are often asymmetric, however, with type I schizencephalic lesions in one hemisphere and type II lesions in the opposite hemisphere (Fig 11).

Patients with bilateral schizencephaly often have a moderate to severe spastic quadriparesis. Severe mental retardation and language disorders are also common. Infantile spasms may be the presenting seizure type in these patients, and focal motor seizures with and without secondary generalization are common. A minority of patients with bilateral lesions are controlled on drugs.

Unilateral schizencephalies are evenly distributed between the two hemispheres. The frequency of type I versus type II lesions is similar. Developmental delay, intellectual impairment, and hemiparesis contralateral to the cleft are common findings. We have not observed any significant differences in language dysfunction between left and right dominance in persons with schizencephaly, probably because these patients most likely transfer language to the more normal hemisphere. Seizures are usually focal motor, but sensory and complex partial seizures also occur. EEG investigations may reveal focal temporal discharges when the lesions are localized to the temporal-parietal convexity. However, EEG spikes may occur beyond the area of malformation, including the opposite hemisphere (see below). The location of lesions by MRI appears to be evenly distributed, with the majority located in pre- and postcentral regions.

An interesting issue concerning patients with unilateral polymicrogyria or schizencephaly is the presence of subtle cortical developmental malformations of the opposite hemisphere. The contralateral lesions are usually present in the mirror regions of the opposite hemisphere. This may explain why some patients with unilateral lesions may present with severe developmental delay. These findings underscore the possible pathogenic mechanism for cortical dysplasia, polymicrogyria, and schizencephaly.

MANAGEMENT OF PATIENTS WITH MALFORMATIONS OF CORTICAL DEVELOPMENT

The first step is to make a correct diagnosis of the specific MCD. This is important for several reasons. First, accurate identification of the underlying MCD permits proper genetic counseling. Second, a syndromic classification assists in making rational decisions about the medical and surgical treatment for seizures. The best example of such a case is the congenital bilateral perisylvian syndrome. Third, proper diagnosis may permit assessment of ultimate prognosis. In the following section we will discuss management issues pertaining to specific problems and conditions.

Infantile Spasms and Malformations of Cortical Development

MCD is recognized with increasing frequency in children with infantile spasms (ISs) because high-resolution imaging has permitted improvement in the detection of MCDs. In fact, MCDs are the most frequent cause of ISs. However, the ultimate prognosis for these children is variable and more likely to be associated with the extent and type of underlying MCD (see Chapter 229, West Syndrome).

A number of observations have modified the treatment options in patients with ISs and MCDs.[36] It is likely that corticosteroids may be the treatment of choice in patients with focal developmental lesions and ISs associated with hypsarrhythmia. In contrast, open studies have shown that vigabatrin (VGB) is effective in patients with diffuse malformations such as TS. VGB in combination with carbamazepine or benzodiazepines is effective in TS. The response to drug treatment in patients with ISs and diffuse malformations such as lissencephaly is poor.

Surgical treatment of patients with ISs and MCDs is dependent on the underlying condition. The presence of a tumor or porencephalic cyst is usually associated with good results.[4,138] Large multifocal resections have provided improvement in a number of children with ISs and focal features.[32,33] Modified hemispherectomy is also effective in patients with ISs and hemimegalencephaly.[39,106] Callosal sections performed in some children with diffuse MCDs and ISs have given disappointing results.[140]

Other Seizure Types

Apart from the clear difference in response of TS patients with ISs to VGB treatment, there have been no randomized drug trials to prove that any particular drug regimen is superior in treating patients with MCDs.

The response to antiepileptic drugs (AEDs) is generally dismal in diffuse malformations such as Aicardi syndrome; it is more variable among patients with lissencephaly. Among patients with bilateral lesions or focal malformations, about 35% respond to AEDs.[125] It is estimated that the response rate to AEDs is approximately 35%. Valproic acid and other broad-spectrum drugs are generally chosen in patients with diffuse malformations.

Surgical Strategies

In some cases of MCDs, depending on the specific clinical and investigative findings, surgical procedures may be appropriate

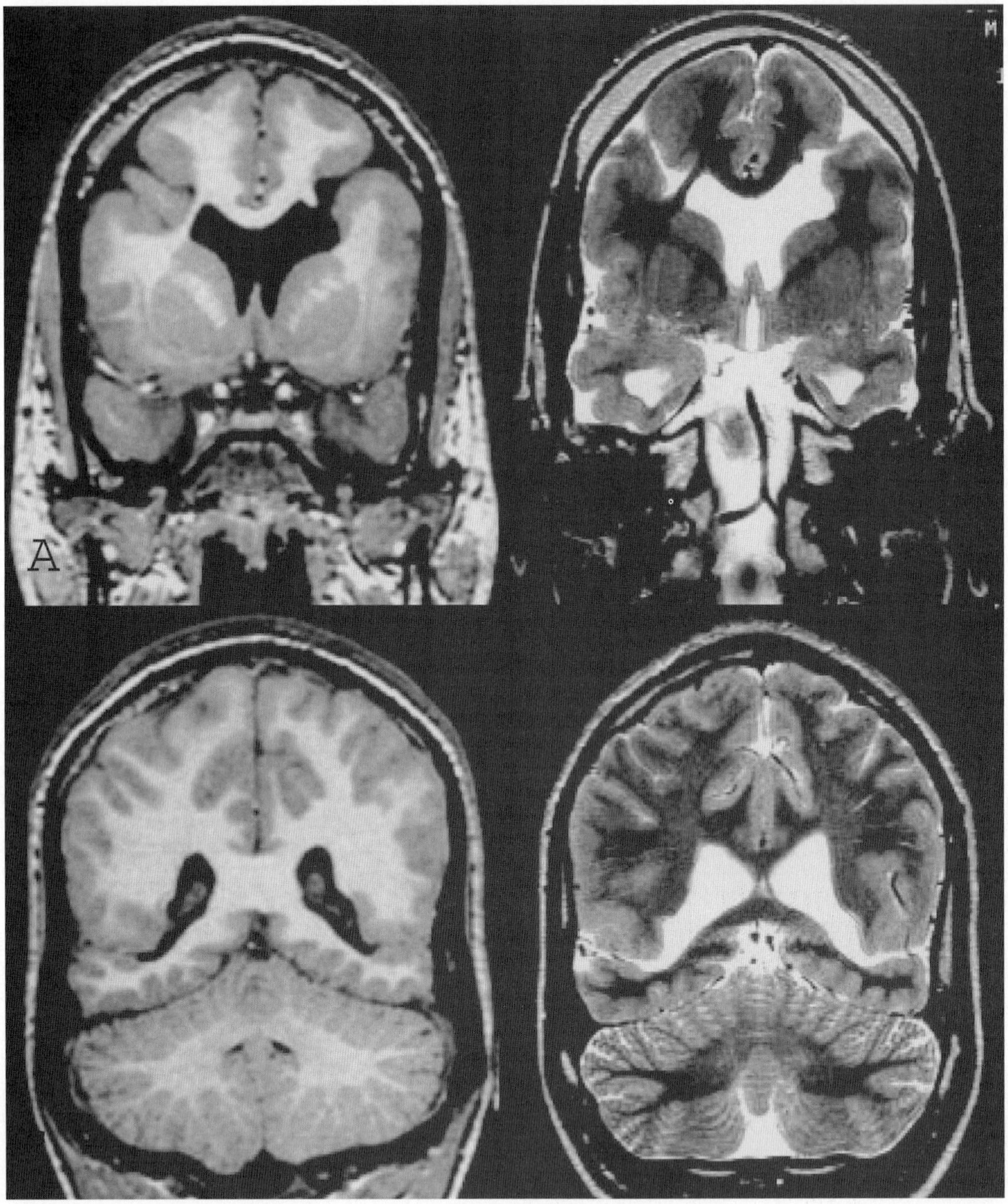

FIGURE 11. Schizencephaly/polymicrogyria syndrome, bilateral symmetric clefts involving frontal and parietal regions.

for treatment (see Chapters 178 and 179). In general, any defined abnormality (usually on MRI) is only a small part of the disturbance of the brain due to abnormal development. Therefore, resections need to extend beyond just the clearly defined abnormality; outcome is generally not as good as that following resections of focal lesions such as benign tumors or cavernomas.

Focal resections in patients with MCDs have been performed with variable results. Several groups[78,80,102,137,139,141] reported good outcome if the visualized lesions were completely resected. In our experience, the best outcome is seen among patients with small developmental abnormalities in the temporal lobe. Unfortunately, focal MCDs are commonly localized in the perisylvian region, and thus, motor or language vital cortical areas limit resections. In such cases, outcome is more variable. Recent data have indicated that 52% of patients with temporal lobe dysplasias were seizure free compared with 29% of those with frontal lobe dysplasias.[102] reported excellent outcome when ictal-like EEG activity was eliminated by surgery. Therefore, it would appear that the outcome following surgical resection of focal MCDs depends on the extent of lesion removal and elimination of highly epileptogenic discharges on EEG.

In cases of hemimegalencephaly, high seizure-free rates have been reported with early hemispherectomy.[119] Although there has been controversy regarding the optimal timing of surgery, an increasing number of investigators advocate early surgical intervention with the aim of protecting the normal hemisphere from the damaging effects of seizures and subsequent abnormal development. Another point of contention has related to the type of surgery. Some have argued that complete hemispherectomy is the procedure of choice,[34,119] whereas others recommend functional hemispherectomy.[28,34,131] Unfortunately, there have been no randomized trials to assess this issue. The complications of complete hemispherectomy, which include hydrocephalus and hemosiderosis, appear to be higher than with functional hemispherectomy.

Callosotomy has been used in patients with severe diffuse MCDs, but the results have been disappointing. However, benefit has been observed in some patients with specific types of malformations. For example, we previously reported good outcome in cases of congenital bilateral perisylvian syndrome,[73] although results have not been predictable. Recent experience with individual patients suggests that multiple subpial transactions may be a potential treatment for selected patients with bilateral lesions. In such cases, the surgical approach should be viewed as a palliative procedure that offers the possibility of a good outcome. Finally, vagus nerve stimulation (VNS) has been carried out in patients with various types of MCDs. Although some reports have described improved seizure control, there are no prospective studies. Our own experience indicates that outcome with VNS is unpredictable.

Genetic Counseling

MCDs often affect children, and thus, genetic counseling becomes extremely important for their families. Much has been learned about the genetics of MCDs, but diagnostic testing is available for only a few (Table 2). Among malformations of neuronal and glial proliferation/apoptosis, routine tests are only available for the two causal genes for tuberous sclerosis (*TSC1* and *TSC2*).

All forms of lissencephaly/subcortical band heterotopia are genetic, and tests are available that are applicable to at least 80% of patients, although this varies with the specific phenotype. When lissencephaly is suspected, chromosome analysis and fluorescent in situ hybridization (FISH) using a probe that contains the *LIS1* gene should be done followed by sequencing of *LIS1* and then *DCX* if *LIS1* is negative. When band

TABLE 2

GENETIC BASIS OF MALFORMATIONS OF CORTICAL DEVELOPMENT

Syndrome	Locus	Gene (Testing)	Protein
ARMCP^{MCPH1}	8p23	**MCPH1** *(R)*	Microcephalin
ARMCP^{ASPM}	1q31	**ASPM** *(R)*	Abnormal spindle—like microcephaly
ARMCP^{CDK5RAP2}	9q34	**CDK5RAP2** *(R)*	Cyclin-dependent kinase 5 regulatory associated protein 2
ARMCP^{CENPJ}	13q12.2	**CENPJ** *(R)*	Centromere associated protein J
ARPHM	20q13.13	**ARFGEF2** *(R)*	ARFGEF2
MCPHA	17q25.3	SLC25A19 (R)	Nuclear mitochondrial deoxynucleotide carrier
SCKL1	3q22-q24	**ATR** *(R)*	FRAP-related protein 1
ILS^{DCX}	Xq22.3-q23	*DCX=XLIS* (C)	DCX or doublecortin
SBH^{DCX}	Xq22.3-q23	*DCX=XLIS* (C)	DCX or doublecortin
MDS	17p13.3	Several contiguous	PAFAH1B1, 14–3–3ϵ, and others
ILS^{LIS1}	17p13.3	*LIS1* (C)	PAFAH1B1
SBH^{LIS1}	17p13.3	*LIS1* (C)	PAFAH1B1
LCH^{RELN}	7q22	*RELN* (R)	Reelin
XLAG^{ARX}	Xp22.13	*ARX* (C)	Aristaless-related homeobox protein
FCMD^{FCMD}	9q31	*FCMD* (R)	FCMD or Fukutin
MEB^{POMGnT1}	1p33-34	**POMGnT1** *(C)*	Unknown
MEB^{FKRP}	19q13.3	**FKRP** *(R)*	Fukutin-related protein
MDC1C^{FKRP}	19q13.3	**FKRP** *(R)*	Fukutin-related protein
MDC1D^{LARGE}	22q12.3-q13.1	**LARGE** *(R)*	
WWS^{POMT}	9q34.1	**POMT1** *(R)*	O-mannosyl-transferase 1
WWS^{FKRP}	19q13.3	**FKRP** *(R)*	Fukutin-related protein
WWS^{FCMD}	9q31	**FCMD** *(R)*	FCMD
BPNH^{FLNA}	Xq28	*FLNA* (R)	Filamin-A
BPNH with microcephaly	20q13.3	**ARFGEF2** *(R)*	BIG2
BPNH^{5p}	5p15	Unknown	Unknown
TSC1	9q32	*TSC1* (C)	Hamartin
TSC2	16p13.3	*TSC2* (C)	Tuberin
BFPP	16q13	*GPR56* (R)	Unknown
WARBM1	2q21.3	RAB3GAP (R)	
BPSP	Xq28	Unknown	Unknown

ARMCP, autosomal recessive microcephaly; ARPHM, autosomal recessive periventricular heterotopia and microcephaly; BFPP, bilateral frontoparietal polymicrogyria; BPNH, bilateral periventricular nodular heterotopia; BPSP, bilateral perisylvian polymicrogyria; C, clinical testing available for gene; FCMD, Fukuyama congenital muscular dystrophy; ILS, isolated lissencephaly sequence; LCH, lissencephaly with cerebellar hypoplasia; MCPHA, Amish lethal microcephaly; MDC, congenital muscular dystrophy; MDS, Miller-Dieker syndrome; MEB, muscle-eye-brain disease; R, research testing available for gene; SBH, subcortical band heterotopia; SCKL1, Seckel syndrome 1; WWS, Walker Warburg syndrome.

heterotopia is suspected, the order of testing should be changed to sequencing of *DCX*, followed by FISH with a probe containing *LIS1*, and finally sequencing of *LIS1*. In a child with lissencephaly whose brain imaging also reveals callosal agenesis, or whose physical examination demonstrates abnormal genitalia, *ARX* testing should be done first. When mutations of any of the aforementioned genes are found, parents should generally be tested to determine their carrier status, as this is important for genetic counseling. Parental testing is especially important for the two X-linked genes, *ARX* and *DCX*, as mothers are often carriers. The frequency of postzygotic mosaicism is high in mothers, probably at least 5%, which must be taken into account for genetic counseling. When genetic tests for lissencephaly or band heterotopia are negative, later siblings have nonetheless been affected in several instances.[41,50,82,116] Counseling should include acknowledging a 10% to 15% risk in such situations. Without testing, counseling is more difficult.

Two genes associated with PNH, *FLNA* and *ARFGEF2*, have been discovered, but no labs currently offer clinical testing. Classic PNH with cerebellar hypoplasia and no dysmorphic features occurs much more frequently in females than in males, and mutations of the X-linked *FLNA* gene account for >80% of familial PNH, ~20% of sporadic PVNH in females, and ~10% in sporadic males.[121] The large size of the gene, which would make clinical testing very expensive, probably accounts for the lack of testing by clinical labs. Among women carriers, ~50% have de novo mutations of *FLNA*, whereas the remaining 50% have inherited mutations. Although maternal transmission is much more likely, father-to-daughter transmission is possible, implying that either parent can transmit the mutation to a female proband.[62] An affected man with PNH caused by an *FLNA* mutation would be expected to transmit the mutation to all of his daughters unless somatic mosaicism is present. To date, all individuals harboring *FLNA* mutations have been found to have PNH, although they can be asymptomatic. Because germline mosaicism of *FLNA* has never been reported in PNH, the recurrence risk is probably low when a mutation is found in the proband but neither parent is a carrier. Microcephaly with PNH is a rare malformation associated with mutations of *ARFGEF2* in a few patients.[122]

So far, five genes have been identified that are associated with the cobblestone cortical malformation found in Fukuyama congenital muscular dystrophy, muscle-eye-brain disease, and Walker-Warburg syndrome (*FCMD*, *FKRP*, *LARGE*, *POMGnT1*, and *POMNT1*). Testing is not yet available clinically. However, enzyme analysis has been developed for POMGnT1 in muscle,[144] and it should be possible to use the same assay in fibroblasts. Similar assays for other enzymes in this group could be developed as well.

There are few laboratory tests to identify genes associated with malformations of late migration and cortical organization. A few patients with perisylvian polymicrogyria have had small chromosomal deletions or duplications, the most common being deletion of chromosome 22q11.2. We therefore recommend chromosome analysis, FISH using a probe from 22q11.2, and FISH using a subtelomeric probe set. The yield with the 22q11.2 probe appears to be high if the polymicrogyria is asymmetric. The causal gene for bilateral frontoparietal polymicrogyria has been identified (*GPR56*),[110] but it cannot yet be tested for clinically. Several years ago, mutations of the *EMX2* gene were reported in a few patients with schizencephaly,[26,53] but these results have not been confirmed. There is now doubt that *EMX2* is a causal gene for schizencephaly.

SUMMARY AND CONCLUSIONS

Malformations of cortical development are an important cause of drug-resistant epilepsy. High-resolution MRI now permits detection and classification of MCDs, and advances in molecular genetics are identifying causal gene mutations. It is important today to view MCDs within a coherent framework that integrates the clinical phenotype, imaging findings, and genetic cause (if known). Antiepileptic drug treatment provides benefit in some cases, and surgical intervention is useful in others. However, treatment is often frustrating and the results of various therapeutic interventions unpredictable.

References

1. Andermann F. Cortical dysplasias and epilepsy: a review of the architectonic, clinical, and seizure patterns. *Adv Neurol.* 2000;84:479–496.
2. Aravind L, Koonin EV. The fukutin protein family–predicted enzymes modifying cell-surface molecules. *Curr Biol.* 1999;9(22):R836–837.
3. Asano E, et al. Multimodality imaging for improved detection of epileptogenic foci in tuberous sclerosis complex. *Neurology.* 2000;54(10):1976–1984.
4. Asano E, et al. Surgical treatment of West syndrome. *Brain Dev.* 2001;23(7):668–676.
5. Barkovich AJ, et al. Band heterotopia: correlation of outcome with magnetic resonance imaging parameters. *Ann Neurol.* 1994;36(4):609–617.
6. Barkovich AJ, et al. Focal transmantle dysplasia: a specific malformation of cortical development. *Neurology.* 1997;49(4):1148–1152.
7. Barkovich AJ, Hevner R, Guerrini R. Syndromes of bilateral symmetrical polymicrogyria. *AJNR Am J Neuroradiol.* 1999;20:1814–1821.
8. Barkovich AJ, Kjos BO. Gray matter heterotopias: MR characteristics and correlation with developmental and neurologic manifestations. *Radiology.* 1992;182:493–499.
9. Barkovich AJ, Kjos BO. Schizencephaly: correlation of clinical findings with MR characteristics. *AJNR Am J Neuroradiol.* 1992;13(1):85–94.
10. Barkovich AJ, Kuzniecky R, Jackson G, et al. A developmental and genetic classification for malformations of cortical development. *Neurology.* 2005;65:1873–1887.
11. Barkovich AJ, Kuzniecky RI, Dobyns WB. Radiologic classification of malformations of cortical development. *Curr Opin Neurol.* 2001;14(2):145–149.
12. Barkovich AJ, Kuzniecky R, Bollen AW, et al. Focal transmantle dysplasia: a specific malformation of cortical development. *Neurology.* 1997;49:1148–1151.
13. Barkovich AJ. Subcortical heterotopia: a distinct clinicoradiologic entity. *AJNR Am J Neuroradiol.* 1996;17(7):1315–1322.
14. Beltran-Valero de Bernabe D, et al. A homozygous nonsense mutation in the fukutin gene causes a Walker-Warburg syndrome phenotype. *J Med Genet.* 2003;40(11):845–848.
15. Beltran-Valero de Bernabe D, et al. Mutations in the FKRP gene can cause muscle-eye-brain disease and Walker-Warburg syndrome. *J Med Genet.* 2004;41:e61.
16. Beltran-Valero de Bernabe D, et al. Mutations in the O-mannosyltransferase gene POMT1 give rise to the severe neuronal migration disorder Walker-Warburg syndrome. *Am J Hum Genet.* 2002;71:1033–1043.
17. Beltran-Valero de Bernabe D, Voit T, Longman C, et al. Mutations in the FKRP gene can cause muscle-eye-brain disease and Walker-Warburg syndrome. *J Med Genet.* 2004;41:e61.
18. Bingham PM, et al. Polymicrogyria in chromosome 22 deletion syndrome. *Neurology.* 1998;51:1500–1502.
19. Bird LM, Scambler P. Cortical dysgenesis in 2 patients with chromosome 22q11 deletion. *Clin Genet.* 2000;58:64–68.
20. Borgatti R, et al. Bilateral perisylvian polymicrogyria in three generations. *Neurology.* 1999;52:1910–1913.
21. Borgatti R, et al. Unilateral periventricular nodular heterotopia associated with diffuse areas of cerebral functional abnormalities. *J Child Neurol.* 2000;15(9):622–626.
22. Brockington M, et al. Mutations in the fukutin-related protein gene (FKRP) cause a form of congenital muscular dystrophy with secondary laminin alpha2 deficiency and abnormal glycosylation of alpha-dystroglycan. *Am J Hum Genet.* 2001;69(6):1198–1209.
23. Brodtkorb E, et al. Epilepsy and anomalies of neuronal migration: MRI and clinical aspects. *Acta Neurol Scand.* 1992;86(1):24–32.
24. Bronen RA, et al. Focal cortical dysplasia of Taylor, balloon cell subtype: MR differentiation from low-grade tumors. *AJNR Am J Neuroradiol.* 1997;18(6):1141–1151.
25. Bronen RA, Spencer DD, Fulbright RK. Cerebrospinal fluid cleft with cortical dimple: MR imaging marker for focal cortical dysgenesis. *Radiology.* 2000;214(3):657–663.
26. Brunelli S, et al. Germline mutations in the homeobox gene EMX2 in patients with severe schizencephaly. *Nat Genet.* 1996;12:94–96.
27. Cardoso C, et al. The location and type of mutation predict malformation severity in isolated lissencephaly caused by abnormalities within the LIS1 gene. *Hum Mol Genet.* 2000;9:3019–3028.
28. Carreno M, et al. Seizure outcome after functional hemispherectomy for malformations of cortical development. *Neurology.* 2001;57(2):331–333.

29. Chang B, et al. Bilateral frontoparietal polymicrogyria: clinical and radiological features in 10 families with linkage to chromosome 16. *Ann Neurol.* 2003;53:596–606.
30. Chang BS, et al. Bilateral generalized polymicrogyria (BGP): a distinct syndrome of cortical malformation. *Neurology.* 2004;62(10):1722–1728.
31. Chugani HT, Conti JR. Etiologic classification of infantile spasms in 140 cases: role of positron emission tomography. *J Child Neurol.* 1996;11(1):44–48.
32. Chugani HT, et al. Surgery for intractable infantile spasms: neuroimaging perspectives. *Epilepsia.* 1993;34(4):764–771.
33. Chugani HT, et al. Surgical treatment of intractable neonatal-onset seizures: the role of positron emission tomography. *Neurology.* 1988;38(8):1178–1188.
34. Cook SW, et al. Cerebral hemispherectomy in pediatric patients with epilepsy: comparison of three techniques by pathological substrate in 115 patients. *J Neurosurg.* 2004;100(2 Suppl Pediatrics):125–141.
35. Crino PB, Henske EP. New developments in the neurobiology of the tuberous sclerosis complex. *Neurology.* 1999;53(7):1384–1390.
36. Curatolo P. Neurological manifestations of tuberous sclerosis complex. *Childs Nerv Syst.* 1996;12(9):515–521.
37. Cusmai R, et al. Bourneville syndrome in children: relationships between EEG and MRI. *Boll Lega Ital Epilessia.* 1988;63(115).
38. D'Agostino M, et al. Subcortical band heterotopia (SBH) in males: clinical, imaging and genetic findings in comparison with females. *Brain.* 2002;125:2507–2522.
39. D'Agostino MD, et al. Posterior quadrantic dysplasia or hemi-hemimegalencephaly: a characteristic brain malformation. *Neurology.* 2004;62(12):2214–2220.
40. de Rijk-van Andel J, et al. Epidemiology of lissencephaly type I. *Neuroepidemiology.* 1991;10:200–204.
41. Deconinck N, et al. Familial bilateral medial parietooccipital band heterotopia not related to DCX or LIS1 gene defects. *Neuropediatrics.* 2003;34:146–148.
42. Denis D, et al. Schizencephaly: clinical and imaging features in 30 infantile cases. *Brain Dev.* 2000;22(8):475–483.
43. Dobbyns W. Smooth, rough and upside-down neocortical development. *Curr Opin Genet Dev.* 2002;12(3):320–327.
44. Dobyns WB, et al. X-linked malformations of neuronal migration. *Neurology.* 1996;47(2):331–339.
45. Dubeau F, et al. Periventricular and subcortical nodular heterotopia. A study of 33 patients. *Brain.* 1995;118(Pt 5):1273–1287.
46. Eksioglu Y, et al. Periventricular heterotopia: an x-linked dominant epilepsy locus causing aberrant cerebral cortical development. *Neuron.* 1996;16:77–87.
47. Eksioglu YZ, et al. Periventricular heterotopias: an X-linked dominant epilepsy locus causing aberrant cortical development. *Neuron.* 1996;16:77–87.
48. Evans JC, Curtis J. The radiological appearances of tuberous sclerosis. *Br J Radiol.* 2000;73(865):91–98.
49. Gleeson JG, et al. Genetic and neuroradiological heterogeneity of double cortex syndrome. *Ann Neurol.* 2000;47(2):265–269.
50. Gleeson JG, et al. Genetic and neuroradiological heterogeneity of double cortex syndrome. *Ann Neurol.* 2000;47:265–269.
51. Gleeson JG, et al. Somatic and germline mosaic mutations in the doublecortin gene are associated with variable phenotypes. *Am J Hum Genet.* 2000;67:574–581.
52. Gordon N. Worster-drought and congenital bilateral perisylvian syndromes. *Dev Med Child Neurol.* 2002;44(3):201–204.
53. Granata T, et al. Familial schizencephaly associated with EMX2 mutation. *Neurology.* 1997;48:1403–1406.
54. Granata T, et al. Schizencephaly: neuroradiologic and epileptologic findings. *Epilepsia.* 1996;37(12):1185–1193.
55. Grant PE, et al. High-resolution surface-coil MR of cortical lesions in medically refractory epilepsy: a prospective study. *AJNR Am J Neuroradiol.* 1997;18(2):291–301.
56. Gropman AL, et al. Pediatric congenital bilateral perisylvian syndrome: clinical and MRI features in 12 patients. *Neuropediatrics.* 1997;28(4):198–203.
57. Guerrini R, Carrozzo R. Epileptogenic brain malformations: clinical presentation, malformative patterns and indications for genetic testing. *Seizure.* 2001;10(7):532–543; quiz 544–547.
58. Guerrini R, Carrozzo R. Epileptogenic brain malformations: clinical presentation, malformative patterns and indications for genetic testing. *Seizure.* 2002;11(Suppl A):532–543; quiz 544–547.
59. Guerrini R, Dobyns WB. Bilateral periventricular nodular heterotopia with mental retardation and frontonasal malformation. *Neurology.* 1998;51(2):499–503.
60. Guerrini R, et al. Bilateral frontal polymicrogyria. *Neurology.* 2000;54:909–913.
61. Guerrini R, et al. Bilateral parasagittal parietooccipital polymicrogyria and epilepsy. *Ann Neurol.* 1997;41:65–73.
62. Guerrini R, et al. Germline and mosaic mutations of FLN1 in men with periventricular heterotopia. *Neurology.* 2004;63(1):51–56.
63. Guerrini R, Sicca F, Parmeggiani L. Epilepsy and malformations of the cerebral cortex. *Epileptic Disord.* 2003;5(Suppl 2):S9–26.
64. Gulati P, et al. Schizencephaly–imaging by MRI. *Indian Pediatr.* 1992;29(12):1570–1572.
65. Hartmann H, UG, Gross C, et al. X-linked lissencephaly with abnormal genitalia associated with renal phosphate wasting. *Neuropediatrics.* 2004;35(3):202–205.
66. Hashimoto R, et al. The 'double cortex' syndrome on MRI. *Brain Dev.* 1993;15(1):57–59; discussion 83–84.
67. Ho SS, et al. Temporal lobe developmental malformations and epilepsy: dual pathology and bilateral hippocampal abnormalities. *Neurology.* 1998;50(3):748–754.
68. Huttenlocher PR, Taravath S, Mojtahedi S. Periventricular heterotopia and epilepsy. *Neurology.* 1994;44(1):51–55.
69. Kato M, et al. Mutations of ARX are associated with striking pleiotropy and consistent genotype-phenotype correlation. *Hum Mutat.* 2004;23(2):147–159.
70. Kitamura K., et al. Mutation of ARX causes abnormal development of forebrain and testes in mice and X-linked lissencephaly with abnormal genitalia in humans. *Nat Genet.* 2002;32:359–369.
71. Kotagal P, Luders HO. Recent advances in childhood epilepsy. *Brain Dev.* 1994;16(1):1–15.
72. Kurlemann G, et al. Lissencephaly syndromes: clinical aspects. *Childs Nerv Syst.* 1993;9(7):380–386.
73. Kuzniecky R, Andermann F, Guerrini R. Congenital bilateral perisylvian syndrome: study of 31 patients. *Lancet.* 1993;341:608–612.
74. Kuzniecky R, Andermann F. Congenital bilateral perisylvian syndrome: imaging findings in a multicenter study. *AJNR Am J Neuroradiol.* 1994;15:139–144.
75. Kuzniecky R, et al. Cortical dysplasia in TLE: MRI correlations. *Ann Neurol.* 1991;29:293–298.
76. Kuzniecky R, et al. Focal cortical myoclonus and rolandic cortical dysplasia: clarification by magnetic resonance imaging. *Ann Neurol.* 1988;23(4):317–325.
77. Kuzniecky R, et al. Frontal and central lobe focal dysplasia: clinical, EEG and imaging features. *Dev Med Child Neurol.* 1995;37(2):159–166.
78. Kuzniecky R, et al. Intrinsic epileptogenesis of hypothalamic hamartomas in gelastic epilepsy. *Ann Neurol.* 1997;42:60–67.
79. Kuzniecky R, et al. Magnetic resonance imaging in childhood intractable partial epilepsies: pathologic correlations. *Neurology.* 1993;43:681–687.
80. Kuzniecky R, et al. Occipital lobe developmental malformations and epilepsy: clinical spectrum, treatment and outcome. *Epilepsia.* 1997;38(2):175–181.
81. Kuzniecky RI, Barkovich AJ. Malformations of cortical development and epilepsy. *Brain Dev.* 2001;23(1):2–11.
82. Kuzniecky RI. Familial diffuse cortical dysplasia. *Arch Neurol.* 1994;51:307–310.
83. Kuzniecky RI. Magnetic resonance imaging in developmental disorders of the cerebral cortex. *Epilepsia.* 1994;35(Suppl 6):S44–56.
84. Kuzniecky RI. Malformations of cortical development and epilepsy, part 1: diagnosis and classification scheme. *Rev Neurol Dis.* 2006;3(4):151–162.
85. Kuzniecky RI. MRI in cerebral developmental malformations and epilepsy. *Magn Reson Imaging.* 1995;13(8):1137–1145.
86. Leventer RJ, et al. Clinical and imaging features of cortical malformations in childhood. *Neurology.* 1999;53(4):715–722.
87. Leventer RJ, et al. LIS1 missense mutations cause milder lissencephaly phenotypes including a child with normal IQ. *Neurology.* 2001;57:416–422.
88. Longman C, et al. Mutations in the human LARGE gene cause MDC1D, a novel form of congenital muscular dystrophy with severe mental retardation and abnormal glycosylation of alpha-dystroglycan. *Hum Mol Genet.* 2003;12(21):2853–2861.
89. Louhichi N, et al. New FKRP mutations causing congenital muscular dystrophy associated with mental retardation and central nervous system abnormalities. Identification of a founder mutation in Tunisian families. *Neurogenetics.* 2004;5:27–34.
90. Mai R, et al. A neuropathological, stereo-EEG, and MRI study of subcortical band heterotopia. *Neurology.* 2003;60(11):1834–1838.
91. Malherbe V, et al. Central nervous system lesions in hypomelanosis of Ito: an MRI and pathological study. *J Neurol.* 1993;240(5):302–304.
92. Matsumoto N, et al. Mutation analysis of the DCX gene and genotype/phenotype correlation in subcortical band heterotopia. *Eur J Hum Genet.* 2001;9:5–12.
93. Matsumoto N, et al. Mutation analysis of the DCX (XLIS) gene and X chromosome inactivation in females with subcortical band heterotopia. *Eur J Hum Genet.* 2001;9:5–12.
94. Matsumuro K, et al. A case of cerebrotendinous xanthomatosis with convulsive seizures. *Clin Neurol.* 1990;30(2):207–209.
95. Meencke HJ. Neuron density in the molecular layer of the frontal cortex in primary generalized epilepsy. *Epilepsia.* 1985;26(5):450–454.
96. Montenegro MA, et al. Interrelationship of genetics and prenatal injury in the genesis of malformations of cortical development. *Arch Neurol.* 2002;59(7):1147–1153.
97. Moro F, et al. Familial periventricular heterotopia: missense and distal truncating mutations of the FLN1 gene. *Neurology.* 2002;58(6):916–921.
98. Nevo Y, et al. Worster-Drought and congenital perisylvian syndromes-a continuum? *Pediatr Neurol.* 2001;24(2):153–155.
99. Olive M, et al. [Polymicrogyria and ulegyria. Diagnosis by magnetic resonance.] *Neurologia.* 1992;7(5):117–119.
100. Palmini A, et al. Focal neuronal migration disorders and intractable partial epilepsy: a study of 30 patients. *Ann Neurol.* 1991;30(6):741–749.

101. Palmini A, et al. Operative strategies for patients with cortical dysplastic lesions and intractable epilepsy. *Epilepsia*. 1994;35(Suppl 6):S57–S71.
102. Palmini A, et al. Operative strategies for patients with cortical dysplastic lesions and intractable epilepsy. *Epilepsia*. 1994;35(6):S57–S71.
103. Palmini A, Gambardella A, Andermann F. Intrinsic epileptogenicity of human dysplastic cortex as suggested by corticography and surgical results. *Ann Neurol*. 1995;37:476–487.
104. Pascual-Castroviejo I, et al. Hypomelanosis of ITO. A study of 76 infantile cases. *Brain Dev*. 1998;20(1):36–43.
105. Pavone L, et al. Epidermal nevus syndrome: a neurologic variant with hemimegalencephaly, gyral malformation, mental retardation, seizures, and facial hemihypertrophy. *Neurology*. 1991;41(2 Pt 1):266–271.
106. Pedespan JM, et al. Surgical treatment of an early epileptic encephalopathy with suppression-bursts and focal cortical dysplasia. *Epilepsia*. 1995;36(1):37–40.
107. Pelayo R, et al. Progressively intractable seizures, focal alopecia, and hemimegalencephaly. *Neurology*. 1994;44(5):969–971.
108. Piao X, CB, Bodell A, et al. Genotype-phenotype analysis of human frontoparietal polymicrogyria syndromes. *Ann Neurol*. 2005;58(5):680–687.
109. Piao X, et al. An autosomal recessive form of bilateral frontoparietal polymicrogyria maps to chromosome 16q12.2–21. *Am J Hum Genet*. 2002;70:1028–1033.
110. Piao X, et al. G protein-coupled receptor-dependent development of human frontal cortex. *Science*. 2004;303:2033–2036.
111. Pilz D, et al. Subcortical band heterotopia in rare affected males can be caused by missense mutations in DCX (XLIS) or LIS1. *Hum Mol Genet*. 1999;8:1757–1760.
112. Pilz D, et al. Subcortical band heterotopia in rare affected males can be caused by missense mutations in DCX or LIS1. *Hum Mol Genet*. 1999;8:2029–2037.
113. Pilz D, Stoodley N, Golden JA. Neuronal migration, cerebral cortical development, and cerebral cortical anomalies. *J Neuropathol Exp Neurol*. 2002;61(1):1–11.
114. Pilz DT, et al. LIS1 and XLIS (DCX) mutations cause most classical lissencephaly, but different patterns of malformation. *Hum Mol Genet*. 1998;7(13):2029–2037.
115. Rakic P. Principles of neural cell migration. *Experientia*. 1990;46:822–891.
116. Ramirez D, et al. Autosomal recessive frontotemporal pachygyria. *Am J Med Genet*. 2004;124A:231–238.
117. Raybaud C, et al. Schizencephaly: correlation between the lobar topography of the cleft(s) and absence of the septum pellucidum. *Childs Nerv Syst*. 2001;17(4–5):217–222.
118. Sasaki M. [Hemimegalencephaly.] *Ryoikibetsu Shokogun Shirizu*. 2002;(37 Pt 6):141–144.
119. Schramm J. Hemispherectomy techniques. *Neurosurg Clin N Am*. 2002; 13(1):113–134,ix.
120. Seri S, et al. Frontal lobe epilepsy associated with tuberous sclerosis: electroencephalographic-magnetic resonance image fusioning. *J Child Neurol*. 1998;13(1):33–38.
121. Sheen V, et al. Mutations in the X-linked filamin 1 gene cause periventricular nodular heterotopia in males as well as in females. *Hum Mol Genet*. 2001;10:1775–1783.
122. Sheen VL, et al. Mutations in ARFGEF2 implicate vesicle trafficking in neural progenitor proliferation and migration in the human cerebral cortex. *Nat Genet*. 2004;36(1):69–76.
123. Sicca F, et al. Mosaic mutations of the LIS1 gene cause subcortical band heterotopia. *Neurology*. 2003;61:1042–1046.
124. Silan F, et al. A new mutation of the fukutin gene in a non-Japanese patient. *Ann Neurol*. 2003;53(3):392–396.
125. Sisodiya SM, et al. Drug resistance in epilepsy: human epilepsy. *Novartis Found Symp*. 2002;243:167–174; discussion 174–179,180–185.
126. Srikanth SG, Jayakumar PN, Vasudev MK. Open and minimally open lips schizencephaly. *Neurol India*. 2000;48(2):155–157.
127. Suri M. The phenotypic spectrum of ARX mutations. *Dev Med Child Neurol*. 2005;47(2):133–137.
128. Tagawa T, et al. [Hypomelanosis of Ito associated with hemimegalencephaly.] *No To Hattatsu*. 1994;26(6):518–521.
129. Tamaki K, et al. Magnetic resonance imaging in relation to EEG epileptic foci in tuberous sclerosis. *Brain Dev*. 1990;12(3):316–320.
130. Taylor DC, et al. Focal dysplasia of the cerebral cortex in epilepsy. *J Neurol Neurosurg Psychiatry*. 1971;34:369–387.
131. Tinuper P, et al. Functional hemispherectomy for treatment of epilepsy associated with hemiplegia: rationale, indications, results, and comparison with callosotomy. *Ann Neurol*. 1988;24:27–34.
132. Topaloglu H, et al. FKRP gene mutations cause congenital muscular dystrophy, mental retardation, and cerebellar cysts. *Neurology*. 2003;60:988–992.
133. van Reeuwijk J, Janssen M, van den Elzen C, et al. POMT2 mutations cause alpha-dystroglycan hypoglycosylation and Walker-Warburg syndrome. *J Med Genet*. 2005;42(12):907–912.
134. Vervoort VS, et al. POMGnT1 gene alterations in a family with neurological abnormalities. *Ann Neurol*. 2004;56:143–148.
135. Villard L, et al. A locus for bilateral perisylvian polymicrogyria maps to Xq28. *Am J Hum Genet*. 2002;70:1003–1008.
136. Wilms G, et al. [Computed tomography and magnetic resonance imaging in anomalies of neuronal migration.] *J Radiol*. 1989;70(1):1–6.
137. Wygold T, Kurlemann G, Schuierer G. [Kohlschutter syndrome–an example of a rare progressive neuroectodermal disease. Case report and review of the literature.] *Klin Padiatr*. 1996;208(5):271–275.
138. Wyllie E, et al. Epilepsy surgery in infants. *Epilepsia*. 1996;37(7):625–637.
139. Wyllie E, et al. Epilepsy surgery in the setting of periventricular leukomalacia and focal cortical dysplasia. *Neurology*. 1996;46(3):839–841.
140. Wyllie E. Surgery for catastrophic localization-related epilepsy in infants. *Epilepsia*. 1996;37(Suppl 1):S22–25.
141. Wyllie E. Surgical treatment of epilepsy in pediatric patients. *Can J Neurol Sci*. 2000;27(2):106–110.
142. Yeung RS. Tuberous sclerosis as an underlying basis for infantile spasm. *Int Rev Neurobiol*. 2002;49:315–332.
143. Yoshida A, et al. Muscular dystrophy and neuronal migration disorder caused by mutations in a glycosyltransferase, POMGnT1. *Dev Cell*. 2001;1(5):717–724.
144. Zhang W, et al. Enzymatic diagnostic test for muscle-eye-brain type congenital muscular dystrophy using commercially available reagents. *Clin Biochem*. 2003;36:339–344.

CHAPTER 260 ■ CHROMOSOMAL ABNORMALITIES

RENZO GUERRINI, AGATINO BATTAGLIA, ROMEO CARROZZO, GIUSEPPE GOBBI, ELENA PARRINI, TIZIANO PRAMPARO, AND ORSATTA ZUFFARDI

INTRODUCTION

About 30 years ago, chromosomal abnormalities, as detectable by classic cytogenetics, were estimated to cause approximately 6% of central nervous system (CNS) malformations.[31] Today, the use of current techniques such as high-resolution chromosome banding, fluorescent in situ hybridization (FISH), and molecular genetics would certainly increase this percentage; it was estimated recently that genome-wide molecular cytogenetics techniques (array-CGH) can detect cryptic deletions/duplications in no less than 20% of individuals with mental retardation and dysmorphic features but apparently normal karyotype (Fig. 1).[139] It is likely that array-CGH at higher resolution will increase this percentage even further.

Most syndromes associated with chromosomal abnormalities are caused by duplications (with duplication of a segment of chromosome), deletions (absence of a segment), or breakpoint disruptions (only one or a few genes are disrupted). Virtually all known chromosomal abnormalities lead to anatomic and functional impairment of the CNS and, especially those involving autosomes, are accompanied by mental retardation. Tharapel and Summit[155] found 6.2% of cases of mental retardation to be associated with chromosomal abnormalities, as contrasted with the 0.7% rate found in controls.

The risk of epilepsy is greater in individuals with chromosomopathy than in the general population.[74] However, chromosomal abnormalities do not represent a frequent cause of epilepsy.[78]

Epilepsy as a complication of a chromosomal abnormality syndrome should be considered in a twofold perspective. First, symptomatic epilepsies have a high probability of causing intractable seizures, leading to further disability in these patients. Severe epilepsy may significantly reduce a low-IQ patient's potential for autonomy in everyday life.[64] Second, when seizures are the main manifestation of a chromosomal disorder or present with peculiar electroclinical patterns, it is important to establish whether these associations result from structural CNS abnormalities caused by the chromosomal changes or from the effect of loci that specifically affect seizure susceptibility. Careful attention to chromosomal abnormalities associated with seizures, together with detailed analysis of electroclinical patterns, may help to detect specific genes affecting seizure susceptibility.[2,142] It seems likely that the association between cryptic deletions/duplications and epilepsy will improve our ability to clone new critical genes.

Only those chromosomal abnormalities of special importance for their high frequency or association with epilepsy are considered in this chapter.

STANDARD CYTOGENETIC AND MOLECULAR TECHNIQUES FOR DIAGNOSTICS

Standard Karyotype and High-Resolution Chromosome Analysis

The karyotype of an individual can be ascertained from readily accessible somatic cells, such as peripheral blood lymphocytes or skin fibroblasts. Each chromosome can be identified by special staining techniques, using fluorescent dyes or Giemsa staining after treatment with a proteolytic enzyme (trypsin). A typical standard karyotype from metaphase cells contains 400 to 550 bands per haploid genome. "High-resolution" chromosome analysis makes it possible to visualize up to 2,000 bands, although a high-resolution chromosome analysis of standard quality allows the detection of about 850 bands. Given the greatly increased amount of work, the difficulty of the analysis, and the cost, high-resolution chromosome analysis should not be considered as a routine cytogenetic assay.

Molecular Karyotyping with Array-CGH

Several techniques defined as molecular cytogenetics have, over the course of the last 10 years, improved the resolution capability of the chromosome banding. The latest technology is the array-CGH, which represents a powerful modification of classical comparative genomic hybridization (CGH) based on metaphases. Using CGH, the DNA of a patient (to be tested) and the DNA of a control are labeled with green and red fluorochromes, respectively, and hybridized on metaphase spreads. The images of both fluorescence signals are captured, and the ratio of DNA intensities quantified using a dedicated software along each chromosome. The chromosome regions represented in the same amount in both DNAs (patient and control) appear yellow, the deleted regions appear red, and the duplicated regions appear green. The difficulty of obtaining sufficiently long metaphases limits the resolution power of this technique to a maximum of 3 Mb. Array-CGH technology replaces the use of chromosome spreads with clones or oligomers (targets) that cover the entire genome, and its resolution power depends only on the amount of targets and their distribution. Recently, microarrays using bacterial artificial chromosome (BAC) clones separated by 100 Kb have been used. Other platforms, using oligomers as targets, have a higher resolution that theoretically can reach up to a few hundreds of base pairs. The use of these arrays might allow the detection of deletions and duplications below the size of 1 Mb and precisely define their

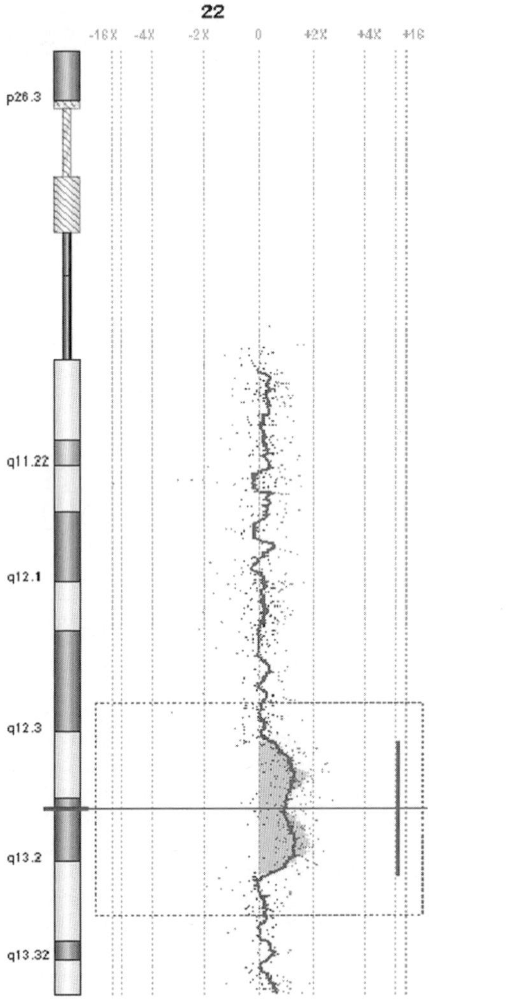

FIGURE 1. Eight-year-old girl with early-onset focal epilepsy and dysmorphic features. 6.9 Mb duplication at 22q13.1q13.2 detected through oligo-array-CGH at 75 kb resolution; log2 ratio of signals intensity is increased in the duplication region where red signals are located more proximal to the +2x line than are the remaining ones. This interstitial duplication had not been detected at conventional karyotyping nor, obviously, after FISH with subtelomeric probes. (See color insert.)

breakpoints (Fig. 1). This technology has also revealed that the human genome may harbor deletions and duplications, having an average size of 2 Mb and being devoid of phenotypic effects, which may play a role in multifactorial diseases. It seems obvious that microarray-CGH will have a crucial role in pre- and postnatal cytogenetics as well as in oncology; its potential in the etiologic diagnosis of epilepsy associated with mental disability and dysmorphic features is extremely high.

Fluorescent in Situ Hybridization

The hybridization of a labeled DNA probe for spreading metaphase chromosomes allows the detection of small deletions, duplications, or cryptic translocations involving the chromosomal segment complementary to a probe labeled with a fluorochrome. The probe signal can be visualized by fluorescence microscopy. Double or multiple hybridizations can be carried out at the same time using different fluorochromes. Although this is a sensitive technique, it allows the investigation of only a few loci in one experiment, thus it can be requested when the clinician already has a specific clinical suspicion known to be associated with the deletion/duplication of that gene/region (i.e., Angelman syndrome and 15q11–q13 deletion).

Southern Blot Analysis

Differences in the DNA sequences at the same locus in different individuals can be detected by restriction enzyme digestion and Southern blot analysis. The diversity in DNA sequences among different individuals will result in either the introduction or loss of specific restriction sites, thereby causing DNA fragments of different sizes. The DNA is subsequently electrophoresed on an agarose gel, denatured with alkali, transferred to a nylon filter, and hybridized with a radiolabeled probe. The resulting X-ray film permits a comparison among the segments of DNA from different individuals.

Polymerase Chain Reaction

Polymerase chain reaction (PCR) allows the amplification of DNA fragments of 100 to 2,000 bp in length. The reaction is carried out in the presence of oligonucleotides flanking the region of interest, free deossinucleotides, template DNA, thermostable DNA polymerase from *Thermophilus aquaticus* (TAQ), and an appropriate saline buffer. The reaction requires 25 to 35 cycles of denaturing, annealing, and synthesizing DNA strands complementary to the template, thus allowing an exponential increase in the amount of target DNA for each cycle. The PCR product can be visualized on an agarose gel stained with ethidium bromide or labeled with a radioisotope, run on a polyacrylamide gel, and detected after exposure of the gel to an X-ray film.

MAIN CHROMOSOMAL ABNORMALITIES ASSOCIATED WITH EPILEPSY

Trisomy 21 (Down Syndrome)

General Clinical Findings

Down syndrome (DS) has an approximate incidence of 1 in 650 births.[144] In 95% of cases, the cause is a nondisjunction of chromosomes 21 during meiosis; in about 4% of cases, there is an unbalanced translocation. Approximately 1% of patients are mosaics and show a less severe phenotype. The region that, if triplicated, results in the typical phenotype maps to 21q22.3.[41] The risk of carrying a child with DS increases with increasing maternal age and with very young maternal age.[79]

The main clinical features of this condition include growth retardation, mental retardation of variable degree, hypotonia, flat facies, brachycephaly with flat occiput, upward-slanting eyes, epicanthal folds, small ears, speckling of the iris (Brushfields spots), simian crease, and hypogonadism. About 40% of patients have congenital heart disease. There is a marked risk of leukemia. All individuals above the age of 35 years show features of Alzheimer disease.

Epilepsy

Epilepsy in DS has been extensively investigated.[45,60,66,83,135,147] The incidence of epilepsy in children with DS was estimated to be 1.4%.[153] However, the overall prevalence of epilepsy increases with age, reaching 12.2% in patients over 35 years

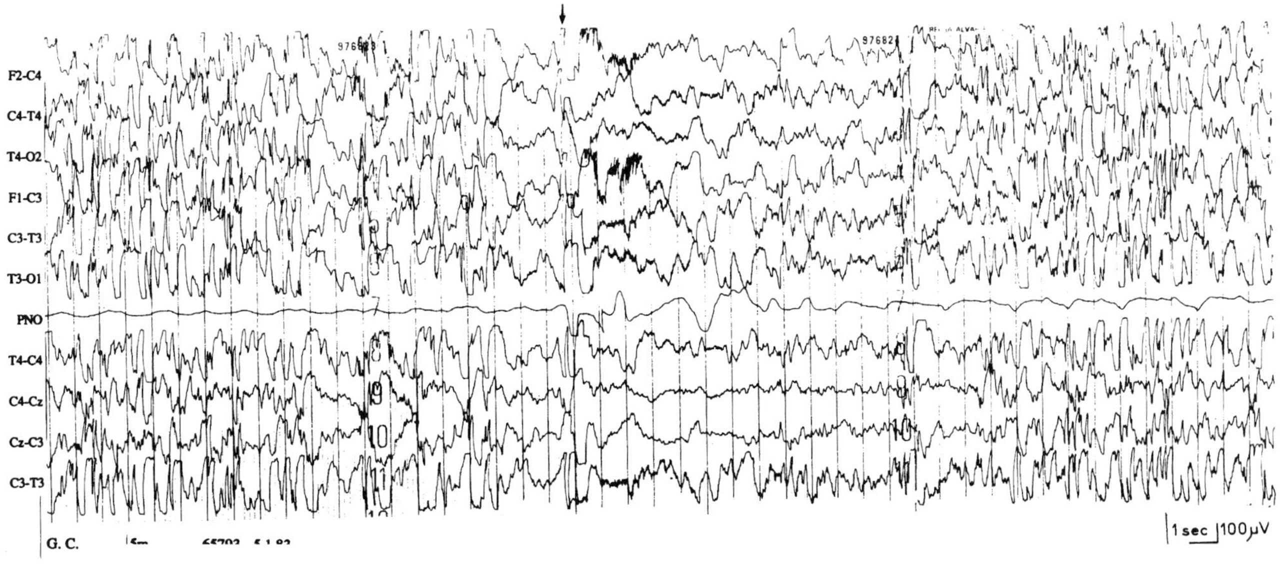

FIGURE 2. Five-month-old girl with Down syndrome and infantile spasms. Typical and symmetrical hypsarrhythmia that is interrupted after a spasm (*arrow*) initiating a cluster of spasms (not shown). Note rapid rebuilding of hypsarrhythmia after the spasm.

of age.[159] About 40% of patients have seizures since the first year of life, and another 40% experience their first seizure during the third decade.[116] This trend seems to be related to the early medical complications of DS, such as hypoxic ischemic encephalopathy and congenital heart disease,[129] and the development of neuropathologic changes typical of Alzheimer disease[36] have a specific etiology, most often related to common medical complications of DS such as hypoxic–ischemic perinatal suffering, hypoxia from congenital heart disease, or infection. Febrile seizures have a low frequency (0.9%) in comparison with the general population.[60,93,129,153] When only cases without known causes were considered, 2.5% of patients presented with seizures, a frequency still greater than that in the general population. Although many patients in both groups had their first seizure in the first year of life, seizures occurred significantly later in infants without a known etiology. Generalized tonic–clonic (GTC) seizures predominated in both the known and unknown etiology groups. Myoclonic seizures and infantile spasms with hypsarrhythmia were also common, the latter predominating in the unknown etiology group. Partial seizures usually occurred in patients with an identifiable etiology. Prognosis for recurrent seizures varied with the etiology. Patients with seizures related to cardiovascular disease were usually well controlled by anticonvulsants. Neonates with hypoxic–ischemic injury had poor outcomes. None of the patients who developed seizures as a result of CNS infection had persistent attacks. Patients with idiopathic seizures had generally good outcomes. The authors concluded that children with DS have an increased susceptibility to seizures early in life, and superimposed systemic illness increased the risk.

In a review of studies in which population estimates were possible, infantile spasms occurred in 0.6% to 13% of children with DS, representing 4.5% to 47% of all seizures (reviewed by Stafstrom and Konkol[146]). Infantile spasms probably represent the most common seizure type in DS and, in most children, they appear without any evidence of additional brain damage.[60,113,141,146] Prognosis is usually good with regard to seizure control. Remission was obtained on conventional antiepileptic drugs (AEDs), adrenocorticotropic hormone (ACTH), or steroids, without relapse of seizures[60,113,146] or with later onset of pharmacologically controllable, age-related generalized seizure disorders[141] (Fig. 2). Conversely, spasms proved to be resistant, progressing to other forms of intractable epilepsy in most of the patients who suffered hypoxic insults.[60,146]

The occurrence of reflex seizures in the context of startle epilepsy is particularly frequent (Fig. 3).[54,66,115,130] Age at seizure onset is variable, and there is usually no evidence for etiologic factors other than DS. Most of the patients described presented "pure" forms of reflex epilepsies, with almost all seizures being precipitated by acoustic or tactile stimuli. However, the epileptic syndrome varied in type and severity, with a predominance of Lennox-Gastaut–type patterns.[66] The mechanism leading a high incidence of reflex phenomena in DS patients is unclear. A central deficit of inhibition of afferent stimuli has been proposed.[29]

Lennox-Gastaut syndrome (LGS) has been well documented in DS, but is not frequent. Quite characteristic is its de novo appearance at a mean age of 10 years, not preceded by other forms of epilepsy.[60,66]

Only a few studies have analyzed adult or late-onset epilepsy in DS, despite its high frequency.[90,159,164] Although in most late-onset epilepsies seizures appeared infrequently but were intractable,[60] no precise indications on seizure severity are available. Late-onset generalized epileptic myoclonus has also been reported.[53]

Neuropathology and Neurogenetic Basis of Seizures

Brain weight is in the lower normal range, and the gyral pattern is simplified.[39] A narrow superior temporal gyrus is observed in about 50% of patients. The insula is exposed because of hypoplasia of the inferior frontal gyrus.[86] Changes typical of Alzheimer disease appear above the age of 30 years.[51,64] Several cytoarchitectonic abnormalities have been found from birth, including a 20% to 50% decrease in the number of small granule cells, mainly inhibitory γ-aminobutyric acid (GABA)ergic interneurons, with lower neuronal density, abnormal neuronal distribution, and dysgenesis of dendritic spines.[18,81,98,127,166] The relation among these structural abnormalities and increased susceptibility to certain seizure types, particularly infantile spasms and reflex seizures, is poorly understood.

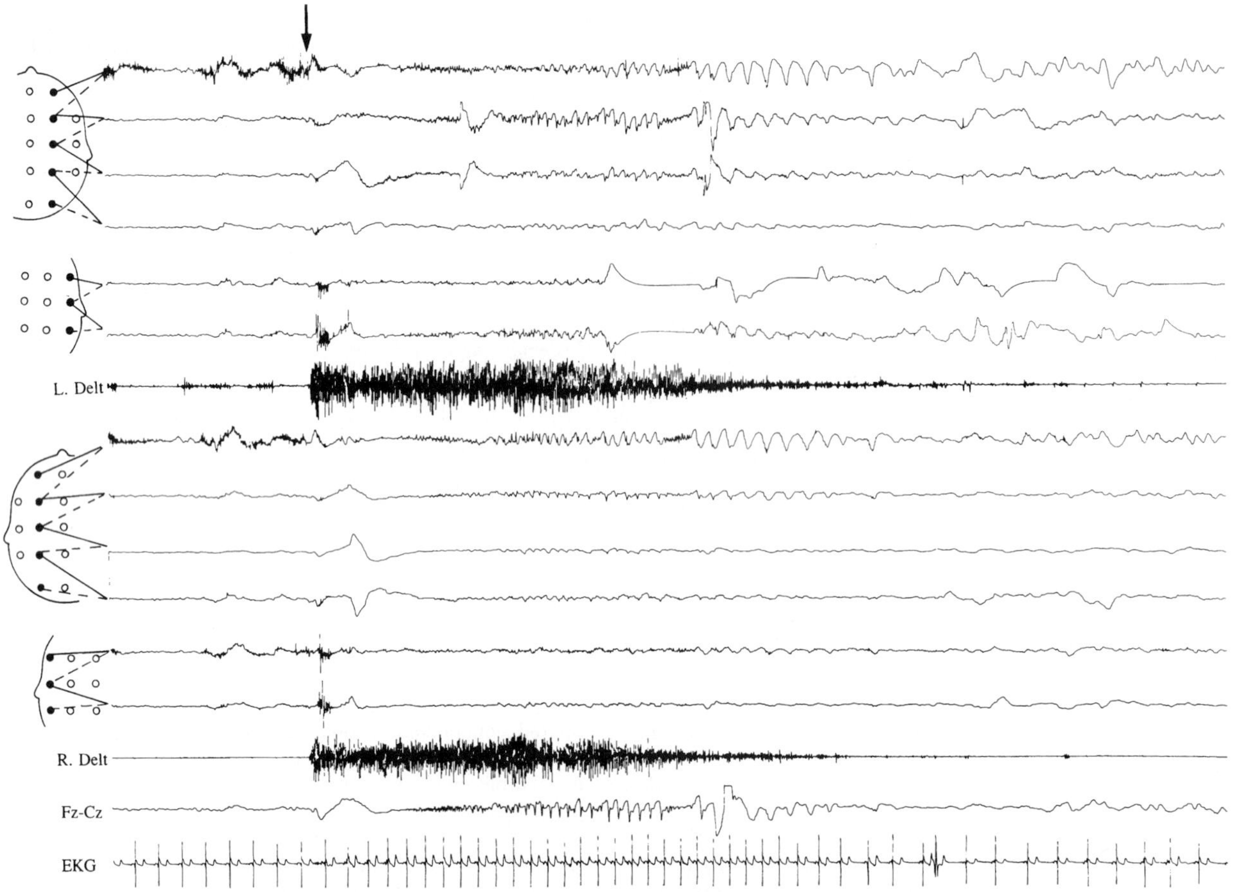

FIGURE 3. Twenty-year-old male Down syndrome patient with startle epilepsy. A sudden, unexpected noise induces a tonic seizure lasting 15 seconds, accompanied by tachycardia; the patient, who is sitting on the bed, is projected violently backward. Tonic contraction, visible on the deltoid muscles (R and L Delt), is accompanied on the EEG by a decremental event, followed by low-voltage fast activity, with increasing amplitude and decreasing frequency, well recognizable over the vertex and frontocentral electrodes, more on the right.

Diagnostic Evaluation

Most patients have a free trisomy 21, detectable on standard chromosome analysis. In such circumstances, chromosome study in the parents is not indicated. Parents should be given a 1% recurrence risk, based on the calculation of the recurrence of DS in a sibship. This slightly higher recurrence risk, when compared to the expectation based on the maternal age is likely due to a germinal mosaicism present in a few parents or to a general failure in the chromosomal disjunction mechanisms normally occurring at meiosis.[110]

If DS results from a translocation, this usually occurs between acrocentric chromosomes, termed a *robertsonian translocation*. In such circumstances, one of the parents might be a balanced carrier of the translocation, and a chromosomal study is strongly indicated for both parents. The most common robertsonian translocation found in healthy carriers involves chromosomes 14 and 21. Virtually all the (21;21) translocations are de novo. The involvement of chromosome 21 in translocations with nonacrocentric chromosomes[101] is very rare. The calculation of the recurrence risk for DS in the carriers of robertsonian translocation is based on the gender of the transmitting parent and the chromosome involved.

Fragile-X Syndrome

General Clinical Findings

Fragile-X syndrome has an approximate incidence of 1 in 1,500 males[163] and is the most common chromosomal abnormality associated with heritable mental retardation. Both genders may be affected, but the phenotype is notably more severe in males. It is estimated that 1 in 1,000 females are carriers.[23] The X-chromosome of patients affected with the syndrome shows a "fragile" site at Xq27.3 when cells are grown in a folic-deprived medium. The condition results from a dynamic mutation in heritable unstable DNA,[124] because of variation in the copy number of a trinucleotide repeat p(CCG)n within the *FMR1* gene. This fragile site is termed *FRAXA*. The disorder has an unusual mode of inheritance. About 20% of males who carry the mutation are clinically and cytogenetically normal (normal transmitting males). About 30% of female carriers have mental impairment. Transmission is consistent with an X-linked semidominant condition. The main clinical features include moderate mental retardation, poor language, hypotonia, growth retardation, macrocephaly, prominent forehead, long, narrow facies, large ears, macroorchidism, pectus excavatum, a floppy mitral valve, and hyperactive or autistic behavior.[50,165]

Epilepsy

The prevalence of epileptic seizures is approximately 25%.[167] Seizures usually appear before the age of 15 and tend to disappear during the second decade of life.[65,167] In most patients, seizures are fairly rare or are controllable with simple drug regimens.[59,65,105,167] The most frequently mentioned seizure types are generalized tonic–clonic seizures.[50,165] However, no specific epilepsy syndrome is observed.[65] Background electroencephalographic (EEG) activity is slow.[105,167] An EEG pattern of midtemporal spikes, possibly age related, similar to the waveform of benign rolandic epilepsy, has been described in some affected males, with or without seizures.[104] This EEG pattern has been confirmed by other investigators, but only in a minority of cases.[60,167] The fragile-X locus has been excluded as the candidate gene for benign rolandic epilepsy.[118]

Neuropathology and Neurogenetic Basis of Seizures

The variety in seizure types in the fragile-X syndrome may reflect extreme clinical polymorphism as a consequence of the variability of amplification of the trinucleotide repeat among patients.[52] A somatic variation in DNA amplification during development is also possible.[168] Little is known of the neuropathology. Anomalous synapses and abnormal development of dendritic spines have been observed using Golgi impregnation.[129,167] Neuroimaging studies have shown hypoplasia of the cerebellar vermis[121] and periventricular heterotopia in rare patients.[103]

Diagnostic Evaluation

The fragile site at Xq27.3 is not expressed in cell culture media employed for standard karyotypes. The induction of the fragile site in stimulated lymphocytes can be achieved using culture media free of folic acid and thymidine. The fragile site is detected only in a proportion of metaphase cells, with most fragile-X males expressing their fragile site in only 5% to 50% of their lymphocytes. Normal transmitting males usually do not express the fragile site. Fragile-X females with mental impairment express their fragile site, but in a lower proportion of cells than do fragile-X males. The majority of female carriers do not express the fragile site, but some of them might show an expression in 5% or less of their cells. The fragile-X syndrome is due to the expansion of a p(CGG)n repeat within the 5′ untranslated region of the *FMR1* gene. Normal chromosomes are polymorphic, containing 6 to 52 copies of this repeat, whereas males with more than 200 copies have the disease (full mutation). Normal transmitting males have 50 to 200 copies (premutation). Females bearing the premutation are phenotypically normal and do not express the fragile site. Females with more than 200 copies may be normal or mentally retarded and can show facial features of fragile-X syndrome. Premutations tend to expand when transmitted to offspring through female carriers, and the risk of expansion to a full mutation correlates with the size of the premutation.[52,73] In association with the full mutation, the promoter region of the *FMR1* gene is hypermethylated, and the transcription of the gene is repressed.[112,160] DNA studies have improved the accuracy of testing for fragile-X syndrome. By looking at the size of the trinucleotide repeat segment, as well as the methylation status of the *FMR1* gene, the genotype can be determined for both affected individuals and suspected carriers. Two main approaches are used: Polymerase chain reaction (PCR) and Southern blot analysis. PCR analysis utilizes flanking primers to amplify a fragment of DNA spanning the repeat region. Thus, the sizes of the PCR products are indicative of the approximate number of repeats present in each allele of the individual being tested. The efficiency of the PCR reaction is inversely related to the number of CGG repeats, so that large mutations are more difficult to analyze and may fail to yield a detectable product in the PCR assay. An additional limitation to the PCR approach is due to the fact that it provides no information about *FMR1* methylation. On the other hand, PCR analysis permits accurate sizing of alleles in the normal and premutation size ranges. *FMR1* analysis by Southern blotting allows both size of the repeat segment and methylation status to be assayed simultaneously. A methylation-sensitive restriction enzyme that fails to cleave methylated sites is used to distinguish between methylated and unmethylated alleles. Southern blot analysis is more labor intensive than PCR and requires larger quantities of genomic DNA. Southern blot accurately detects alleles in all size ranges, but precise sizing is not possible. Many laboratories can use both methods, and choose the type of analysis that is most appropriate to the circumstances. A few patients with fragile-X harboring deletions in the *FMR1* have been described.[117,152]

Two additional fragile sites reside in the distal Xq, termed *FRAXE* and *FRAXF*. Although *FRAXF* is not clearly associated with a specific phenotype, those with *FRAXE* show mental impairment, usually milder than that observed in patients with *FRAXA* mutations. Because no clinical overlap occurs between patients with mutations at the *FRAXA* and the *FRAXE* loci, other than mental retardation, the details about the diagnostic procedures for identifying *FRAXE* will not be discussed here.

Del 4p (Wolf-Hirschhorn) Syndrome

General Clinical Findings and Genetic Background

Wolf-Hirschhorn syndrome (WHS) is a multiple congenital anomalies/mental retardation syndrome[34] with a frequency of 1 in 50,000 births and a female:male predilection of 2:1.[57,96] It is caused by partial loss of material from the distal portion of the short arm of chromosome 4. The minimal deleted segment causing the phenotype is 4p16.3.[96] Although about 75% of patients have a de novo deletion[96] of preferential paternal origin,[38,157] about 12% have an unusual chromosome abnormality (such as ring 4), and about 13% have a deletion of 4p16 resulting from an inherited unbalanced chromosome rearrangement from a parent with a balanced rearrangement. The main features of monosomy 4p are the typical "Greek warrior helmet appearance of the nose," microcephaly, pre- and postnatal growth delay, congenital hypotonia, severe mental retardation, and seizures.[13] In at least one-third of cases, death occurs during the first year of life because of severe systemic malformations, cardiac failure, or pulmonary infection.

Epilepsy

Seizures constitute a major medical concern during the first years of life, and occur in 50% to 100% of patients.[10,13,32,40,68,149] Seizure onset usually occurs within the first 2 years of life, with a peak incidence around 9 to 10 months of age. These seizures may be clonic or tonic, unilateral with or without secondary generalization, or generalized tonic–clonic from the onset.[5,8–13,47,108,119] They are frequently triggered by fever, may be prolonged, and often occur in clusters.[5,11,12,136,171] More than 50% of the patients experience early unilateral or generalized clonic or tonic–clonic status epilepticus (SE), despite adequate treatment.[13] Two-thirds of the subjects develop, between 1 and 5 years of age,

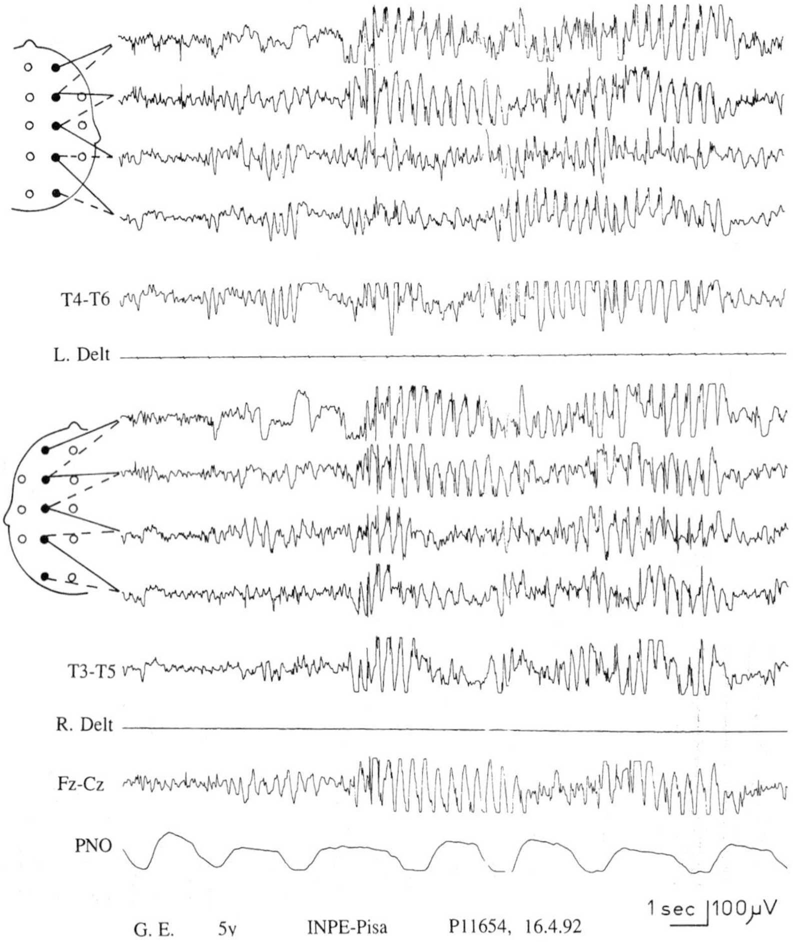

FIGURE 4. Five-year-old girl with 4p- syndrome. An atypical absence seizure is accompanied by diffuse atypical slow spike-and-wave complexes. Interictal EEG preceding the episode shows multifocal spikes and spikes and spike-and-wave complexes.

atypical absences, often accompanied by a mild myoclonic component, mainly involving the eyelids and axorizomelic muscles.[5,11–14,136] Such episodes are accompanied by generalized slow spike-and-wave complexes. The interictal EEG shows high-amplitude, fast spikes, polyspikes, and wave complexes over the posterior third of the head on eye closure. Other seizure types have been described in a minority of patients (Fig. 4).[80,171]

In our experience, the seizures observed in WHS can be effectively controlled by valproate alone or associated with ethosuximide and, in patients who continue to have seizures, add-on benzodiazepines are usually effective. Carbamazepine may cause seizure worsening. Despite early severity, the long-term outcome of epilepsy is relatively good, because seizures tend to disappear with age.[7,10]

Neuropathology and Neurogenetic Basis of Seizures

Corpus callosum hypoplasia is the most frequent brain abnormality (rarely associated with decreased white matter volume) and hypoplasia or agenesis of the posterior lobe of the cerebellum also is seen. Hypoplastic brain with narrow gyri, heterotopia, and dysplasia of nuclear structures has been described in some cases.[58,92]

The $GABA_A$ receptor gene maps proximal to the critical deletion region (WHSCR), specifically, 4p12–p13[27] and is probably not involved in epileptogenesis in this condition. *LETM1*, a gene possibly involved in calcium (Ca^{2+}) signaling or homeostasis, seems to be a good candidate for seizures and neuromuscular problems in WHS.[46,158] Initially, *LETM1* was suggested to flank the WHSCR,[13,46] but a recent report implies that it falls within the newly proposed critical region of WHS nearer the telomere.[173]

Diagnostic Evaluation

Standard cytogenetics detects about 60% to 70% of deletions, whereas FISH (using the WHSCR probe) detects more than 95%. Subtelomeric FISH analysis can be useful to determine if a deletion is the result of an unbalanced translocation.[14]

Partial Monosomy 15q (Angelman Syndrome)

General Clinical Findings

Angelman syndrome (AS) has a prevalence of about one in 12,000 to 20,000 of the population,[148] accounting for up to 6% of all cases with severe mental retardation and epilepsy.[87] The main clinical features of AS may not be apparent early in life. All patients have developmental delay, which becomes apparent by 6 to 12 months of age, microcephaly, severely impaired expressive language, ataxic gait, tremulousness of limbs, and a typical behavioral profile including a happy demeanor, hypermotoric behavior, and low attention span. About 90% have epilepsy.[3,161,174]

Seventy percent of patients show a deletion involving the maternally inherited chromosome 15q11–q13, encompassing a cluster of GABA receptor subunit genes; 5% show chromosome 15 paternal uniparental disomy (UPD); 5% harbor a mutation in the imprinting center (IC), a transcriptional regulatory element; and 10% harbor intragenic mutations of the *UB3A* gene. A few patients have no detectable genetic abnormality. The rare cases of familial recurrence of AS show either IC or *UBE3A* mutations.[62]

Epilepsy

It is estimated that about 90% of patients have epilepsy.[174] Viani et al.[161] reviewed 155 published patients, of whom 130 (84%) had experienced seizures. Viani's review[161] and subsequent reports suggest that the first seizures occur between the ages of 3 months and 20 years,[63,100,150,161,174] although onset is in infancy or early childhood in most. The first seizures are often precipitated by fever.[100,150] Infantile spasms are exceptional. Complex partial seizures with eye deviation and vomiting, possibly indicating occipital lobe origin, were estimated to occur frequently.[161] Atypical absences, myoclonic seizures, GTC, and unilateral seizures are among the main seizure types.[63,100,150,161] Over half of the patients suffer from episodes of decreased alertness and hypotonia lasting days or weeks, described as nonconvulsive SE.[100,150] Often there is concomitant mild jerking, rhythmic or not,[37,63] typical of myoclonic status. Polygraphic recordings reveal diffuse, slow, irregular spike-and-wave complexes at about 2 Hz, accompanied in some patients by myoclonic potentials that are time locked to the EEG spikes (Fig. 5). This clinical and EEG pattern has also been described by Dalla Bernardina et al.[37] as *myoclonic status* in nonprogressive encephalopathies. In other patients, myoclonus may remain erratic, showing no apparent relation with EEG discharges. Myoclonic jerks typically cease during sleep.[63,161] Myoclonic status is rare after the age of 6 years. In addition to myoclonic seizures or status, AS patients exhibit quasicontinuous rhythmic cortical myoclonus at about 11 Hz, mainly involving hands and face, and producing a mild jerking or twitching, easily mistaken for tremor (see Fig. 5).[63]

Individuals with chromosome 15q11–q13 deletions have more severe impairment and are more prone to develop severe epilepsy. Uniparental disomy, IC, and *UB3A* mutations are associated with a milder phenotype.[62,102]

Although seizures are generally difficult to treat in infancy and early childhood, they are usually less severe in later childhood,[174] although complete seizure remission is rare.[89] The exact percentage of patients continuing to suffer seizures as adults is unknown.

Episodes of myoclonic status and of nonconvulsive status are usually stopped with intravenous benzodiazepines,[63,161] although they frequently relapse.[100] Chronic treatment using benzodiazepines achieve fairly effective control of myoclonus. Particularly effective is the association clobazam-valproate for the long-term treatment of epilepsy.[63,161] Valproate and ethosuximide in association are also effective in patients presenting recurrent myoclonic status.[37] Worsening of myoclonus and absence seizures may be produced by carbamazepine or vigabatrin.[85,161] If cortical myoclonus is particularly disabling, generous doses of piracetam are often effective in reducing it.[63]

Neuropathology and Neurogenetic Basis of Seizures

Neuroimaging does not disclose conspicuous CNS abnormalities.[63,174] Available neuropathologic data derive from the study of the brains in two patients in whom the AS had not

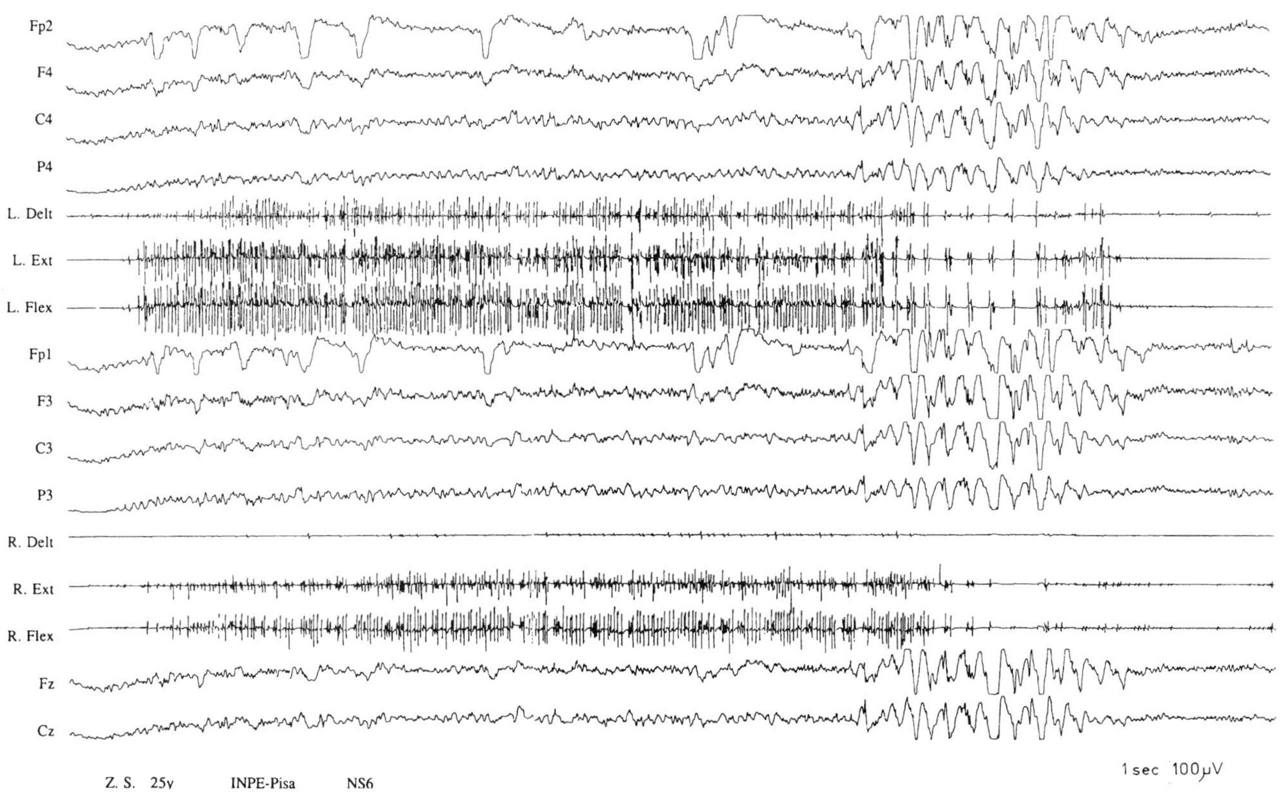

FIGURE 5. Twenty-five-year-old female patient with Angelman syndrome and 15q11–13 deletion. Polygraphic recording. Rhythmic 12- to 15-Hz myoclonus (fast-bursting cortical myoclonus) involving all muscles recorded, is accompanied by 5- to 7-Hz rhythmic activity recorded from all EEG electrodes. A discharge of generalized, irregular polyspike-and-wave complexes lasting 3 seconds is accompanied by rhythmic bursts of two or three myoclonic potentials; each burst is time-locked with the spike component of the discharge. Clinically, the fast-bursting cortical myoclonus resembles tremor. The generalized spike-and-wave discharge is accompanied by a short myoclonic absence.

been confirmed by genetic analysis. Jay et al.[77] found cerebellar atrophy with loss of Purkinje and granule cells and extensive Bergman gliosis. Neurochemical study of the cerebellar cortex demonstrated markedly reduced GABA content, possibly related to failure to develop or a loss of Purkinje cells and inhibitory GABAergic interneurons. Kyriakides et al.[88] reported small temporal and frontal lobes with disorganized and irregular gyri, irregular distribution of neurons in layer 3, and minor cell heterotopia in both the cerebrum and cerebellum. There is some evidence that the motor cortex in AS is hyperexcitable. Because the deletion involving the maternal 15q11–13 chromosome eliminates a cluster of $GABA_A$ receptor genes ($\beta 3$, $\alpha 5$, $\gamma 3$), it has been suggested that cortical hyperexcitability might result from reduced GABAergic inhibition.[63] A 60% to 80% reduction in benzodiazepine binding has been shown in most brain regions of a mutant mouse exhibiting a deletion involving a chromosomal region that is syntenic to the AS region.[106] The antiabsence and antimyoclonic action of benzodiazepines, which is based on their GABAergic properties, is confirmed in AS.[62]

Diagnostic Evaluation

About 80% of cases are detected through the CpG methylation at 15q11.q13 genes through "bisulfite" tests, which allows the detection of deletions, UPD, and IC mutations. The test is based on the different parentally derived methylation patterns at specific loci. If the methylation test is abnormal, a FISH assay should be run in the search of a 15q11–q13 deletion. If the FISH assay is normal, a UPD study should be performed to distinguish UPD from an IC mutation. If an IC mutation is suspected, the case should be referred to a research laboratory for the identification of the IC mutation. Mutation analysis of the *UBE3A* gene should be performed in those cases matching the clinical criteria for AS in the presence of a normal methylation test. This analysis is not 100% sensitive, because mutations involving the promoter or intronic regions might remain undetected.

The results of genetic testing have important implications for genetic counseling, because de novo deletions and UPD can be assigned a very low recurrence risk, whereas IC mutations and *UB3A* mutations can be inherited in a dominant fashion and may be causative disease mutations according to the gender of the transmitting parent. It is important to point out that about 5% of patients do not show any molecular or cytogenetic abnormality. Most such cases are sporadic but, due to the few reported familial cases, recurrence risk in siblings may be as high as 50%.

Ring Chromosome 20 Syndrome

General Clinical Findings and Genetic Background

Ring chromosome 20 (r20) is a rare chromosomal disorder, of which epilepsy is a striking feature. Although some patients may have microcephaly, mild to moderate mental retardation, and behavioral abnormalities,[114] the lack of specific phenotypic features in most individuals makes diagnosis difficult. Dysmorphic signs are exceptional. Psychomotor development tends to be initially normal. The description of about 50 cases has drawn attention to the uniqueness of the electroclinical presentation,[142] which should always prompt a request for karyotype. The chromosomal abnormality can occur in mosaic. Most cases are sporadic, but a few are familial.[30] The severity of cognitive impairment seems to correlate with the percentage of mosaicism, whereas that of epilepsy does not.[76]

Epilepsy

Seizures occur in almost all subjects, with onset between infancy and age 17 years, and these seizures are usually refractory to treatment.[142,175] The typical presentation is with repetitive episodes of confusional state, lasting from several minutes to 30 minutes, also described as "complex partial" or "nonconvulsive" status, during which patients appear to be confused and unresponsive to a variable degree. Motionlessness and staring or, conversely, complex automatisms or wandering have been described.[76,142] Perioral jerking and eyelid myoclonus are often observed.[30,76,91,111,142] Such episodes often occur daily and are accompanied on the EEG by long bursts or trains of rhythmic θ-waves and high-amplitude, 2- to 3-Hz rhythmic, notched slow waves with frontal predominance.[30,76,111] Typical spike-and-wave discharges are rarely seen. Hyperventilation, specific mental activities, or adverse psychological situations can act as triggers in some children.[128] Frontal lobe ictal-onset was shown by means of subdural electrodes during typical confusional episodes.[76] On the basis of ictal single positron emission computed tomography (SPECT) studies, a possible role of subcortical structures has been hypothesized in the genesis of such a characteristic ictal pattern. Mainly in young children, the prolonged seizures are misinterpreted as behavioral nonepileptic manifestations, unless video-EEG recording is available.[76] Partial motor and generalized tonic–clonic seizures have also been reported. Interictal EEG, normal in some individuals, can show spikes over both frontotemporal areas in others.

Diagnostic Evaluation

A standard karyotype should be performed examining at least 100 mitoses, considering that the percentage of lymphocytes carrying the chromosome rearrangement may be low.[128] In most cases, the locus of fusion between the deleted short and long arms in the ring chromosome was p13q13, p13q13.3, or p13q13.33.[76,142] The loss of telomeric material on both arms of chromosome 20 is usually identified by FISH.[26] Cases with a mosaicism for r20 have also been observed.

Del 1p36 Syndrome

General Clinical Findings and Genetic Background

The incidence of del 1p36 syndrome is estimated to be 1 in 5,000 to 1 in 10,000, with a female predilection of 1.5:1.[17,71,137] About 100 cases have been reported.[71,97] It appears that 1p36 deletions account for as much as 0.5% to 0.7% of "idiopathic" mental retardation.[56] Intrauterine growth retardation and/or postnatal growth deficiency,[19,21,55,69,82,97,120,125,138,143,170] as well as obesity and hyperphagia[48,82,132,138] have been observed.

The craniofacial features represent a hallmark of the disorder, and are characterized by microbrachycephaly, large and late-closing anterior fontanel, prominent forehead, straight eyebrows, deep-set eyes, short palpebral fissures, broad/flat nasal bridge, midface hypoplasia, pointed chin, abnormal ears, and short hands and feet.[17,71,120,138] Moderate to profound mental retardation and very poor language skills are observed in most individuals.[17,71,137,138]

Epilepsy

Seizures occur in over 50% of patients.[17,71] Different seizure types, such as infantile spasms, simple and complex partial seizures, generalized tonic–clonic, myoclonic, and absence seizures, have been reported.[21,55,82,84,120,125,138,143] Infantile spasms associated with a hypsarrhythmic EEG are observed in about 50% of cases and are usually responsive to ACTH.[4] In about 30% of patients, complex partial seizures or tonic seizures may occur, often having a favorable outcome.[17,48,143] Seizure onset is usually within the third year of life. Background EEG shows poverty of the usual rhythmic activities. Interictal EEG abnormalities are variable, including hypsarrhythmia, focal and multifocal spikes, generalized slow spike-and-wave complexes.[15]

Neuropathology and Neurogenetic Basis of Seizures

Cerebral atrophy, ventricular dilatation, hydrocephalus, delay in myelination, focal cortical dysplasia, and a leukodystrophic picture have been documented on brain neuroimaging.[6,17,49,69,72,82,125,138,143,170] A severe seizure phenotype has been associated with hemizygosity for the voltage-gated potassium (K^+) channel β-subunit gene, *KCNAB2*.[72]

Diagnostic Evaluation

Monosomy 1p36 may be the result of pure terminal deletions, interstitial deletions,[169] derivative chromosome 1, and more complex rearrangements.[6,17,71] Conventional cytogenetics may not detect these different rearrangements, particularly those that are derivative chromosomes. FISH analysis with subtelomeric region-specific probes is necessary in most cases. CGH microarray can be used as an alternative. Determination of the parental origin has provided discordant results.[17,71] Overall, deletions of paternal origin seem to be larger than deletions derived from the maternally inherited chromosome.[17,71]

OTHER CHROMOSOMAL DISORDERS ASSOCIATED WITH SEIZURES

Inv Dup(15) or Idic(15) Syndrome

The chromosome region 15q11–q13 is known for its instability,[43] and many rearrangements may occur in this imprinted segment, such as deletions, translocations, inversions, and supernumerary marker chromosomes formed by the inverted duplication of proximal 15. Interstitial duplications and triplications are much less frequent. The inv dup(15) accounts for about 60% of supernumerary marker chromosomes.[35] Of the two identified cytogenetic types, one is a metacentric chromosome, smaller or similar to a G group chromosome, not containing the PWS/AS critical region (PWS/ASCR); it is found in children without dysmorphic features who are usually studied because of mild mental retardation or behavioral abnormalities.[75] However, a normal phenotype is also possible. The second type of inv dup(15) is as large as or larger than a G group chromosome, contains the PWS/ASCR,[22,126] and is associated with an abnormal phenotype.[16] Its cytogenetic description is dic(15)(q12 or q13). Most dic(15)(q12 or q13) derive from the two homologous maternal chromosomes at meiosis and are associated with increased maternal age at conception. The presence of large inv dup(15) results in tetrasomy 15p and partial tetrasomy 15q. Incidence at birth is estimated to be 1 to 30,000, with an equal sex ratio.[133]

Patients with large inv dup(15), extending to q15, usually have severe epilepsy, mental retardation, autistic-like behavior, and minor dysmorphic features.[16,25,28,151] A clinical presentation of infantile spasms in children with minor dysmorphic features has been reported in some patients, whereas LGS with very poor outcome has been observed by several authors.[16,28,151,156] Focal epilepsy has also been reported.[25] Milder presentations with mild mental retardation, generalized epilepsy with onset in adolescence of absence seizures, and an interictal pattern of generalized spike-and-wave discharges have been reported even in patients with large duplications.[33]

Various genetic mechanisms have been hypothesized to explain clinical heterogeneity (beyond the size of chromosomal duplication), including dosage effect of genes located within the duplication.[33,156] Considering that a mild epilepsy phenotype is possible, it has been suggested that inv dup(15) be ruled out as a possible, although rare, cause of "cryptogenic" or seemingly idiopathic generalized epilepsy.[33]

To distinguish between inv dup(15)s and the other supernumerary marker chromosomes, the simple distamycin A/4′-6′-diamidino-2-pheylindole hydrochloride (DA-DAPI) staining technique is sufficient, but FISH or array-CGH may be useful, although more expensive. The majority of inv dup(15)s are dicentric, with one centromere inactivated; these are also referred to as *pseudodicentric chromosome 15* or *SMC(15)*. By conventional cytogenetics, they can be classified into two main groups: (a) small SMC(15)s, which are metacentric chromosomes without euchromatic material; and (b) large SMC(15)s, which are acrocentric chromosomes containing two copies of the 15q11–q13 region. Small SMC(15)s can be familial or de novo. In contrast, large SMC(15)s are almost always de novo in origin, maternally derived, and associated with an abnormal phenotype that includes severe mental retardation, developmental delay, behavioral problems, and epilepsy. For this reason, it is important to discriminate between small and large inv dup(15), especially in prenatal diagnosis. To this aim, FISH performed on a gene within the critical Prader Willi/Angelman syndrome region allows the precise discrimination of whether the supernumerary chromosome is harmful or without any effect. However, the molecular confirmation that inv dup(15) belongs to the "small" category is not sufficient to exclude that the fetus will be affected by Prader Willi or Angelman syndrome, because cases have been reported with small inv dup(15) associated with uniparental disomy for chromosome 15 or with 15q11–q13 deletions.[94]

Ring Chromosome 14

Ring chromosome 14 (r14) is a rare chromosomal abnormality consistently associated with epilepsy. Reviews of reported cases suggest that early onset epilepsy, which is often intractable, is a constant feature of the syndrome, but does not have typical clinical or EEG features.[142] Generalized tonic–clonic seizures, myoclonic, and complex partial seizures have been reported.[95,134] General clinical features include moderate to severe mental retardation, microcephaly and facial dysmorphism with narrow elongated face and retrognathia.[122] Ocular abnormalities involving cataract and retinal pigmentation have been observed in about 50% of cases.[172] Most patients show a mosaic chromosomal abnormality. Familial occurrence is possible.[99] There is no indication of the brain histopathology that underlies such severe neurologic presentation, and neuroimaging seems to be of little help.[109]

Trisomy 12p and Tetrasomy 12 (Pallister-Killian Syndrome)

Trisomy of the short arm of chromosome 12 can be caused either by a malsegregation of a balanced parental chromosomal rearrangement or can occur de novo.[1]

Trisomy 12p is characterized by severe mental retardation, early hypotonia, turricephaly, flat occiput, short neck, round facies with prominent cheeks, prominent forehead, hypertelorism, epicanthal folds, and other dysmorphic facial features. Lateralized microgyria, internal hydrocephalus, cortical dysplasia, and ectopic glial tissue in the leptomeninges have been reported.[107]

Particularly striking was the finding of generalized 3-Hz spike-and-wave discharges in four patients, three of whom had childhood onset myoclonic absences or myoclonic seizures that appeared well controlled by AEDs.[44,61] It is of interest that three voltage-gated K^+ channel genes are clustered together, probably in the 12p13 band.

Pallister-Killian syndrome (PKS) is a rare, sporadic disorder caused by a mosaic supernumerary isochromosome 12p (i[12p]). The i(12p) is infrequently present in peripheral lymphocytes, but it is found in cultured fibroblasts and other tissues such as bone marrow and lungs. Children present with peculiar dysmorphic features including coarse and flat facies, prominent forehead, scarcity of scalp hair over frontal and temporal regions, hypertelorism, broad nasal bridge, small nose with anteverted nostrils, highly arched palate, microretrognathia, cupid bow-shaped upper lip, and low-set ears.[20,70,123] A combination of these features, with severe to profound cognitive impairment and epilepsy, characterizes the syndrome.[20,70,123,145,162] Seizures have been reported in 40% of 67 cases,[20] but their frequency is probably underestimated because most patients had a short follow-up.[20,123,145,162] For the same reason, no information is available on the seizure semiology and electrophysiologic correlates of epilepsy in these patients. Epileptic spasms have been reported in some patients.[131]

Klinefelter Syndrome (XXY Syndrome)

The prevalence of seizures in Klinefelter syndrome ranges from 2% to 10% in major series.[67] Some patients have been reported with generalized epilepsy with absence seizures or generalized tonic–clonic seizures, and a 3-Hz spike-and-wave EEG pattern.[24] However, the most common profile of patients with Klinefelter syndrome and seizures includes mental retardation, behavioral problems, epileptiform EEGs, and generalized tonic–clonic seizures. In one series, the seizures of six of 11 patients with epilepsy were well controlled with AEDs; the electroclinical spectrum was heterogenous, and outcome with AED treatment was often favorable.[154]

Partial Monosomy 17p (Miller-Dieker Syndrome)

The main clinical and genetic findings of Miller-Dieker lissencephaly are discussed in Chapter 228. We present here some guidelines for diagnostic evaluation of patients with both Miller-Dieker syndrome (MDS) and lissencephaly related to chromosome 17p (more severe in the posterior part of the brain). More than 90% of the MDS patients show a cytogenetically visible or a submicroscopic deletion involving the 17p13.3 band. About 40% with the LIS1-type lissencephaly show a submicroscopic deletion at the same chromosomal locus. Because these deletions are not observed under standard chromosome banding analysis, they are referred to as "submicroscopic." *LIS1*, a gene mapping to 17p13.3 and encoding for the noncatalytic 45-Kd subunit of the platelet-activating factor (PAF) acetylhydrolase, is the lissencephaly causative gene, based on the finding of subtle mutations involving this gene in some patients with LIS1-type lissencephaly.

FISH using commercial probes containing the *LIS1* gene is required in all patients in whom a chromosome 17 lissencephaly is suspected on the basis of the appearance of magnetic resonance imaging (MRI).[42] In particular, it is recommended that a FISH study be performed using the *LIS1*-specific probe PAC 95H6. The search for point mutations consists of the direct sequencing of the *LIS1* gene, following PCR amplification of the entire coding region. About 25% of patients with classic lissencephaly show an intragenic mutation of *LIS1*. Gene sequencing is not 100% sensitive because the promoter and transcription regulatory regions of the gene are not routinely investigated, and a mutation in these regions could be missed. Southern blot analysis reveals gross rearrangements of the *LIS1* gene, which can be detected in about 4% of patients. The recent demonstration of mosaic mutations of the *LIS1* gene in individuals with posterior band heterotopia-pachygyria[140] suggests that a highly sensitive technique, such as denaturing high pressure liquid chromatography (DHPLC), can be useful in identifying low-level mosaicism that may escape recognition by direct sequencing or other standard techniques.

SUMMARY AND CONCLUSIONS

Chromosomal abnormalities are relatively common, genetically determined conditions that increase the risk of epilepsy. However, the likelihood of developing seizures varies greatly among the different chromosomal disorders. Chromosomal abnormalities almost constantly result in rearrangements or deletions/duplications that affect the function of more than one gene. As a consequence, even when very high-resolution techniques, such as microarray-CGH, are used, patients with chromosomal abnormalities always have a combination of clinical features and only exceptionally have isolated epilepsy. The ring chromosome 20 syndrome represents the most striking example in which a highly specific epilepsy phenotype can be the only expression of the chromosomal disorder. Most often, mental retardation and dysmorphic features, even subtle, coexist with epilepsy. Although some conditions are associated with a risk for epilepsy only slightly greater than that of the general population, others carry a risk of close to 100%, and the epilepsy is part of the phenotype. Some chromosomal abnormalities result in intractable seizures, whereas others have a more favorable epilepsy prognosis. Susceptibility to developing epilepsy does not necessarily correlate with the severity of structural abnormalities in the brain or with the extent of the chromosomal derangement. Depending on the specific genes involved, seizure susceptibility is more likely to be related to factors that alter cortical excitability, such as gene dosage effect in genes involved in ion channel and neurotransmitter function or neural development. Awareness of the associations between syndromes due to chromosomal abnormalities and epilepsy, together with knowledge of their response to treatment and the expected outcome, should be of help in planning rational treatment and counseling families.

References

1. Allen TL, Brothman AR, Carey JC, et al. Cytogenetic and molecular analysis in trysomy 12p. *Am J Med Genet.* 1996;63:250–256.
2. Anderson EV, Hauser WA. Genetics. In: Dam M, Gram M, eds. *Comprehensive Epileptology*. New York: Raven Press; 1990: 57–74.
3. Angelman H. "Puppet" children: A report on three cases. *Dev Med Child Neurol.* 1965;7:681–683.
4. Bahi-Buisson N, Ville D, Eisermann M, et al. Epilepsy in chromosome aberrations. *Arch Pediatr.* 2005;12:449–458.
5. Battaglia A. Sindrome di Wolf-Hirschhorn (4p-): Una causa di ritardo mentale grave di difficile diagnosi. *Riv Ital Pediatr (IP).* 1997;23:254–259.
6. Battaglia A. Del 1p36 syndrome: A newly emerging clinical entity. *Brain Dev.* 2005;27:358–361.
7. Battaglia A. Wolf-Hirschhorn (4p-) Syndrome. In: Cassidy SB, Allanson JE. *Management of Genetic Syndromes.* Hoboken: John Wiley & Sons; 2005: 667–676.
8. Battaglia A, Carey JC. Health supervision and anticipatory guidance of individuals with Wolf-Hirschhorn syndrome. *Am J Med Genet. (Semin Med Genet).* 1999;89:111–115.
9. Battaglia A, Carey JC. Update on the clinical features and natural history of Wolf-Hirschhorn syndrome (WHS): Experience with 48 cases. *Am J Hum Genet.* 2000;6:127.

10. Battaglia A, Carey JC. Seizure and EEG patterns in Wolf-Hirschhorn (4p-) syndrome. *Brain Dev.* 2005;27:362–364.
11. Battaglia A, Carey JC, Cederholm P, et al. Storia naturale della sindrome di Wolf-Hirschhorn: Esperienza con 15 casi. *Pediatrics (edizione Italiana-Milano).* 1999;11:236–242.
12. Battaglia A, Carey JC, Cederholm P, et al. Natural history of Wolf-Hirschhorn syndrome: Experience with 15 cases. *Pediatrics.* 1999;103:830–836.
13. Battaglia A, Carey JC, Wright TJ. Wolf-Hirschhorn (4p-) syndrome. *Adv Pediatr.* 2001;48:75–113.
14. Battaglia A, Carey JC, Wright TJ. Wolf-Hirschhorn syndrome. In: *GeneReviews: Genetic Disease Online Reviews at GeneTests – GeneClinics (database online).* University of Washington, Seattle; 2002–2004. Available at: http.//www.geneclinics.org.
15. Battaglia A, Guerrini R. Chromosomal disorders associated with epilepsy. *Epileptic Disord.* 2005;7:181–192.
16. Battaglia A, Gurrieri F, Bertini E, et al. The inv dup(15) syndrome: A clinically recognizable syndrome with altered behaviour, mental retardation and epilepsy. *Neurology.* 1997;48:1081–1086.
17. Battaglia A, Viskochil DH, Lewin SO, et al. 1p deletion syndrome: Further clinical characterisation of a common, important and often missed cause of developmental delay/mental retardation. *Proceed Greenwood Genet Ctr.* 2004;23:140–141.
18. Becker LE, Armstrong DL, Chan F. Dendritic atrophy in children with Down's syndrome. *Ann Neurol.* 1986;20:520–526.
19. Biegel JA, White PS, Marshall HN. Constitutional 1p36 deletion in a child with neuroblastoma. *Am J Hum Genet.* 1993;52:176–182.
20. Bielanska MM, Khalifa MM, Duncan AMV. Pallister–Killian syndrome: A mild case diagnosed by fluorescence in situ hybridization. Review of the literature and expansion of the phenotype. *Am J Med Genet.* 1996;65:104–108.
21. Blennow E, Bui TH, Wallin A, et al. Monosomy 1p36.31–33pter due to a paternal reciprocal translocation: Prognostic significance of FISH analysis. *Am J Med Genet.* 1996;65:60–67.
22. Blennow E, Nielsen KB, Telenius H, Carter NP, Kristoffersson U, Holmberg E, et al. Fifty probands with extra structurally abnormal chromosomes characterized by fluorescence in situ hybridization. *Am J Med Genet.* 1995;55:85–94.
23. Blomquist HK, Gustavson KH, Holmgren G, et al. Fragile X syndrome in mildly retarded children in a northern Swedish county. *Clin Genet.* 1983;24:393–398.
24. Boltshauser E, Meyer M, Deonna T. Klinefelter's syndrome and neurological disease. *J Neurol.* 1978;219:253–259.
25. Borgatti R, Piccinelli P, Passoni D, et al. Relationship between clinical and genetic features in "inverted duplicated chromosome 15" patients. *Pediatr Neurol.* 2001;24:111–116.
26. Brandt CA, Kierkegaard O, Hindkjaer J, et al. Ring chromosome 20 with loss of telomeric sequences detected by multicolour PRINS. *Clin Genet.* 1993;44:26–31.
27. Buckle VJ, Fujita N, Ryder-Cook AS, et al. Chromosomal localization of GABA(A) receptor beta-a-3–subunit gene. *Neuron.* 1989;3:647–654.
28. Cabrera JC, Marti M, Toledo L, et al. West's syndrome associated with inversion duplication of chromosome 15. *Rev Neurol (Spain).* 1998;26:77–79.
29. Calner DA, Dustman RE, Madsen JA, et al. Life span changes in the averaged evoked responses of Down syndrome and nonretarded patients. *Am J Ment Def.* 1978;4:398–405.
30. Canevini MP, Sgro V, Zuffardi O, et al. Chromosome 20 ring: A chromosomal disorder associated with a particular electroclinical pattern. *Epilepsia.* 1998;39:942–951.
31. Carter CO. Genetics of common single malformations. *Br Med Bull.* 1977;32:21–28.
32. Centerwall WR, Thompson WP, Allen IE, et al. Translocation 4p- syndrome. *Am J Dis Child.* 1975;129:366–370.
33. Chifari R, Guerrini R, Pierluigi M, et al. Mild generalized epilepsy and developmental disorder associated with large inv dup(15). *Epilepsia.* 2002;43:1096–1100.
34. Cooper H, Hirschhorn K. Apparent deletion of short arms of one chromosome (4 or 5) in a child with defects of midline fusion. *Mammalian Chrom Newsl.* 1961;4:14.
35. Crolla JA, Youings SA, Ennis S, et al. Supernumerary marker chromosomes in man: Parental origin, mosaicism and maternal age revisited. *Eur J Hum Genet.* 2005;13:154–160.
36. Cutler NR, Heston LL, Davies P, et al. Alzheimer's disease and Down syndrome: New insights. *Ann Intern Med.* 1985;103:566–578.
37. Dalla Bernardina B, Zullini E, Fontana E, et al. Sindrome di Angelman: Studio EEG-poligrafico di 8 casi. *Boll Lega It Epil.* 1992;79/80:257–259.
38. Dallapiccola B, Mandich P, Bellone E, et al. Parental origin of chromosome 4p deletion in Wolf-Hirschhorn syndrome. *Am J Med Genet.* 1993;47:921–924.
39. Davidoff LM. The brain in mongolian idiocy: A report of ten cases. *Arch Neurol Psychiatry.* 1928;20:1229–1257.
40. De Grouchy J, Turleau C. *Clinical Atlas of Human Chromosomes,* 2nd ed. New York: John Wiley, 1984.
41. Delabar JM, Theophile D, Rahmani Z, et al. Molecular mapping of twenty-four features of Down syndrome on chromosome 21. *Europ J Hum Genet.* 1993;1:114–124.
42. Dobyns WB, Truwit CL, Ross ME, et al. Differences in the gyral pattern distinguish chromosome 17–linked and X-linked lissencephaly. *Neurology.* 1999;53:270–277.
43. Donlon TA, Lalande M, Wyman A, Bruns G, Latt SA. Isolation of molecular probes associated with the chromosome 15 instability in the Prader-Willi syndrome. *Proc Natl Acad Sci USA.* 1986;83:4408–4412.
44. Elia M, Musumeci SA, Ferri R, et al. Trisomy 12p and epilepsy with myoclonic absences: A new case. *Epilepsia.* 1995;36(Suppl 3):52.
45. Ellingson RJ, Eisen JD, Ottersberg G. Clinical and electroencephalographic observations of institutionalized mongoloids confirmed by karyotype. *Electroencephalogr Clin Neurophysiol.* 1973;34:193–196.
46. Endele S, Fuhry M, Pak SJ, et al. LETM1, a novel gene encoding a putative EF-Hand Ca-binding protein, flanks the Wolf-Hirschhorn syndrome (WHS) critical region and is deleted in most WHS patients. *Genomics.* 1999;60:218–225.
47. Estabrooks LL, Lamb AN, Aylsworth AS, et al. Molecular characterization of chromosome 4p deletions resulting in Wolf-Hirschhorn syndrome. *J Med Genet.* 1994;31:103–107.
48. Eugster EA, Berry SA, Hirsch B. Mosaicism for deletion 1p36.33 in a patient with obesity and hyperphagia. *Am J Med Genet.* 1997;70:409–412.
49. Faivre L, Morichon-Delvallez N, Vior G, et al. Prenatal detection of a 1p36 deletion in a fetus with multiple malformations and a review of the literature. *Pren Diagn.* 1999;19:49–53.
50. Finelli PF, Pueschel SM, Padre-Mendoza T, et al. Neurological findings in patients with fragile-X syndrome. *J Neurol Neurosurg Psychiatry.* 1985;48:150–153.
51. Friede RL. *Developmental Neuropathology,* 2nd ed. Heidelberg: Springer-Verlag, 1989.
52. Fu YH, Kuhl DPA, Pizzuti A, et al. Variation of the CGG repeat at the fragile X site results in genetic instability: Resolution of the Sherman paradox. *Cell.* 1991;67:1047–1059.
53. Genton P, Paglia G. Epilepsie myoclonique sénile? Myoclonies épileptiques d'apparition tardive dans le syndrome de Down. *Epilepsies.* 1994;1:5–11.
54. Gimenez-Roldàn S, Martin M. Startle epilepsy complicating Down syndrome during adulthood. *Ann Neurol.* 1980;7:78–80.
55. Giraudeau F, Aubert D, Young I, et al. Molecular cytogenetic detection of a deletion of 1p36.3. *J Med Genet.* 1997;34:314–317.
56. Giraudeau F, Taine L, Biancalana V, et al. Use of a set of highly polymorphic minisatellite probes for the identification of cryptic 1p36.3 deletions in a large collection of patients with idiopathic mental retardation. *J Med Genet.* 2001;38:121–125.
57. Gorlin RJ, Cohen MM, Levin LS. *Syndromes of the Head and Neck.* New York: Oxford University Press; 1990: 46–48.
58. Gottfried M, Lavine L, Roessmann U. Neuropathological findings in Wolf-Hirschhorn (4p-) syndrome. *Acta Neuropathol (Berl).* 1981;55:163–165.
59. Guerrini R, Battaglia A, Mattei MG, et al. Epilessia e crisi epilettiche nella sindrome del cromosoma X fragile. *Boll Lega It Epil.* 1992;79–80:73–74.
60. Guerrini R, Battaglia A, Stagi P, et al. Caratteristiche elettrocliniche dell'epilessia nella Sindrome di Down. *Boll Lega It Epil.* 1989;66–67:317–319.
61. Guerrini R, Bureau M, Mattei MG, et al. Trisomy 12p syndrome: A chromosomal disorder associated with generalized 3–Hz spike and wave discharges. *Epilepsia.* 1990;31:557–566.
62. Guerrini R, Carrozzo R, Rinaldi R, et al. Angelman syndrome: Etiology, clinical features, diagnosis, and management of symptoms. *Paediatr Drugs.* 2003;5:647–661.
63. Guerrini R, De Lorey TM, Bonanni P, et al. Cortical myoclonus in Angelman syndrome. *Ann Neurol.* 1996;40:39–48.
64. Guerrini R, Dravet C, Bureau M, et al. Diffuse and Localized Dysplasias of Cerebral Cortex: Clinical Presentation, Outcome, and Proposal for a Morphologic MRI Classification Based on a Study of 90 Patients. In: Guerrini R, Andermann F, Canapicchi R, Roger J, Zifkin B, Pfanner P, eds. *Dysplasias of Cerebral Cortex and Epilepsy.* Philadelphia: Lippincott-Raven; 1996: 255–269.
65. Guerrini R, Dravet C, Ferrari AR, et al. Evoluzione dell'epilessia nelle più frequenti forme genetiche con ritardo mentale (sindrome di Down e sindrome dell'X fragile). *Ped Med Chir.* 1993;15:19–22.
66. Guerrini R, Genton P, Bureau M, et al. Reflex seizures are frequent in patients with Down syndrome and epilepsy. *Epilepsia.* 1990;31:406–417.
67. Guerrini R, Gobbi G, Genton P, et al. Chromosomal Abnormalities In: Engel J, Pedley TA. *Epilepsy,* Vol.3. Philadelphia: Lippincott-Raven; 1997: 2533.
68. Guthrie RD, Aase IM, Asper AC, et al. The 4p- syndrome: A clinically recognizable chromosomal deletion syndrome. *Am J Dis Child.* 1971;122:421–425.
69. Hain D, Leversha M, Campbell N. The ascertainment and implications of an unbalanced translocation in the neonate: Familial 1:15 translocation. *Austr Paediatr J.* 1980;16:196–200.
70. Hall BD. Syndrome identification case report 103. Trescher-Nicola/Killian syndrome: A sporadic case in an 11–year-old male. *J Clin Dysmorphol.* 1983;1:14–17.

71. Heilstedt HA, Ballif BC, Howard LA, et al. Physical map of 1p36, placement of breakpoints in monosomy 1p36, and clinical characterisation of the syndrome. *Am J Hum Genet.* 2003;72:1200–1212.
72. Heilstedt HA, Burgess DL, Anderson AE, et al. Loss of the potassium channel beta-subunit gene, KCNAB2, is associated with epilepsy in patients with 1p36 deletion syndrome. *Epilepsia.* 2001;42:1103–1111.
73. Heitz D, Devys D, Imbert G. Inheritance of the fragile X premutation is a major determinant of transition to full mutation. *J Med Genet.* 1992;29:794–801.
74. Holmes GL. Genetics of Epilepsy. In: Holmes GL, eds. *Diagnosis and Management of Seizures in Children.* Philadelphia: WB Saunders; 1987: 56–71.
75. Hou JW, Wang TR. Unusual features in children with inv dup(15) supernumerary marker: A study of genotype-phenotype correlation in Taiwan. *Eur J Pediatr.* 1998;157:122–127.
76. Inoue Y, Fujiwara T, Matsuda KS, et al. Ring chromosome 20 and non convulsive status epilepticus. A new epileptic syndrome. *Brain.* 1997;120:939–953.
77. Jay V, Becker LE, Chan F-W, et al. Puppet-like syndrome of Angelman: A pathologic and neurochemical study. *Neurology.* 1991;41:416–422.
78. Jennings MT, Bird TD. Genetic influences in the epilepsies. *Am J Dis Child.* 1981;135:450–457.
79. Jones KL. *Smith's Recognizable Patterns of Human Malformations,* 4th ed. Philadelphia: WB Saunders; 1988.
80. Kanazawa O, Irie N, Kawai I. Epileptic seizures in the 4p- syndrome: Report of two cases. *Jpn J Psychiatry Neurol.* 1991;45:653–659.
81. Kemper TL. Neuropathology of Down's Syndrome. In: Nadel L, eds. *The Psychobiology of Down's Syndrome.* Cambridge: MIT Press; 1988: 145–164.
82. Keppler-Noreuil KM, Carroll AJ, Finley WH, et al. Chromosome1p terminal deletion: Report of new findings and confirmation of two characteristic phenotypes. *J Med Genet.* 1995;32:619–622.
83. Kirkam BH. Epilepsy in mongolism. *Arch Dis Child.* 1951;26:501–503.
84. Knight-Jones E, Knight S, Heussler H, et al. Neurodevelopmental profile of a new dysmorphic syndrome associated with submicroscopic partial deletion of 1p36.3. *Dev Med Child Neurol.* 2000;42:201–206.
85. Kuenzle Ch, Steinlin M, Wohlrab G, et al. Adverse effects of vigabatrin in Angelman syndrome. *Epilepsia.* 1998;39:1213–1215.
86. Kumar AJ, Naidich TP, Stetten G, et al. Chromosomal disorders: Background and neuroradiology. *AJNR.* 1992;13:577–593.
87. Kyllerman M. On the prevalence of Angelman syndrome. *Am J Med Genet.* 1995;59:405.
88. Kyriakides T, Hallam LA, Hockey A, et al. Angelman's syndrome: A neuropathological study. *Acta Neuropathol (Berl).* 1992;83:675–678.
89. Laan LAEM, Renier WO, Arts WFM, et al. Evolution of epilepsy and EEG findings in Angelman syndrome. *Epilepsia.* 1997;38:195–199.
90. Lai F, Williams RS. Prospective study of Alzheimer disease in Down syndrome. *Arch Neurol.* 1989;46:849–853.
91. Lancman ME, Penry JK, Asconape JJ, et al. Number 20 ring chromosome: A case with complete seizure control. *J Child Neurol.* 1993;8:186–187.
92. Lazjuk GI, Lurie IW, Ostrowskaja TI, et al. The Wolf-Hirschhorn syndrome. II. Pathologic anatomy. *Clin Genet.* 1980;18:6–12.
93. Le Berre C, Jorunel H, Lucas J, et al. L'épilepsie chez le trisomique 21. *Ann Pediatr (Paris).* 1986;33:579–585.
94. Liehr T, Brude E, Gillessen-Kaesbach G, et al. Prader-Willi syndrome with a karyotype 47,XY,+min(15)(pter->q11.1:) and maternal UPD 15—case report plus review of similar cases. *Eur J Med Genet.* 2005;48:175–181.
95. Lippe BM, Sparkes RS. Ring 14 chromosome: Association with seizures. *Am J Med Genet.* 1981;9:301–305.
96. Lurie IW, Lazjuk GI, Ussova YI, et al. The Wolf-Hirschhorn syndrome. *Clin Genet.* 1980;17:375–385.
97. Magenis RE, Brown MG, Lacy DA, et al. Is Angelman syndrome an alternate result of del (15) (q11–q13)? *Am J Med Genet.* 1987;28:829–838.
98. Marin-Padilla M. Pyramidal cell abnormalities in the motor cortex in a child with Down's syndrome: A Golgi study. *J Compar Neurol.* 1976;167:63–81.
99. Matalon R, Supple P, Wyandt H, et al. Transmission of ring 14 chromosome from mother to two sons. *Am J Med Genet.* 1990;36:381–385.
100. Matsumoto A, Kumagai T, Miura K, et al. Epilepsy in Angelman syndrome associated with chromosome 15q deletion. *Epilepsia.* 1992;33:1083–1090.
101. Mikkelsen M. Down's syndrome. Current stage of cytogenetic research. *Hum Genet.* 1971;12:1–28.
102. Minassian B, DeLorey T, Olsen RW, et al. The epilepsy of Angelman syndrome due to deletion, disomy, imprinting center and UB3A mutations. *Ann Neurol.* 1998;43:485–493.
103. Moro F, Pisano T, Dalla Bernardina B, et al. Periventricular heterotopia in fragile X syndrome. *Neurology.* 2006;67(4):713–715.
104. Musumeci SA, Colognola RM, Ferri R, et al. Fragile-X syndrome: A particular epileptogenic EEG pattern. *Epilepsia.* 1988;29:41–47.
105. Musumeci SA, Ferri R, Elia M, et al. Epilepsy and fragile X syndrome: A follow-up study. *Am J Med Genet.* 1991;38:511–513.
106. Nakatsu Y, Tyndale RF, DeLorey TM, et al. A cluster of three $GABA_A$ receptor subunit genes is deleted in a neurological mutant of the mouse p locus. *Nature.* 1993;364:448–450.
107. Nielsen J, Venter M, Holm V, et al. A newborn child with caryotype 47,XX,+der(12) (12pter >12q12::8q24 >8qter),t(8;12) (q24;q12)pat. *Hum Genet.* 1977;35:357–362.
108. Ogle R, Sillence DO, Merrick A, et al. The Wolf-Hirschhorn syndrome in adulthood: Evaluation of a 24-year-old man with a rec(4) chromosome. *Am J Med Genet.* 1996;65:124–127.
109. Ono J, Nishiike K, Imai K, et al. Ring chromosome 14 complicated with complex partial seizures and hypoplastic corpus callosum. *Pediatr Neurol.* 1999;20:70–72.
110. Pangalos CG, Talbot CC, Lewis JG, et al. DNA polymorphism analysis in families with recurrence of free trisomy 21. *Am J Hum Genet.* 1992;51:1015–1027.
111. Petit J, Roubertie A, Inoue Y, et al. Non-convulsive status in the ring chromosome 20 syndrome: A video illustration of 3 cases. *Epileptic Disord.* 1999;1:237–241.
112. Pieretti M, Zhang FP, Fu YH, et al. Absence of expression of the FMR-1 gene in fragile X syndrome. *Cell.* 1991;66:817–822.
113. Pollack MA, Golden GS, Schmidt R, et al. Infantile spasms in Down syndrome: A report of 5 cases and review of the literature. *Ann Neurol.* 1978;3:406–408.
114. Porfirio B, Valorani MG, Giannotti A, et al. Ring 20 chromosome phenotype. *J Med Genet.* 1987;24:375–377.
115. Pueschel SM, Louis S. Reflex seizures in Down syndrome. *Childs Nerv Syst.* 1993;9:23–24.
116. Pueschel SM, Louis S, McKnight P. Seizure disorders in Down syndrome. *Arch Neurol.* 1991;84:318–320.
117. Quan F, Zonana J, Gunter K, et al. An atypical case of fragile X syndrome caused by a deletion that includes the *FMR1* gene. *Am J Hum Genet.* 1995;56:1042–1051.
118. Rees M, Diebold U, Parker K, et al. Benign childhood epilepsy with centrotemporal spikes and the focal sharp wave trait is not linked to the fragile X region. *Neuropediatrics.* 1993;24:211–213.
119. Reid I, Morrison N, Barron L, et al. Familial Wolf-Hirschhorn syndrome resulting from a cryptic translocation: A clinical and molecular study. *J Med Genet.* 1996;33:197–202.
120. Reish O, Berry SA, Hirsch B. Partial monosomy of chromosome 1p36.3: Characterisation of the critical region and delineation of a syndrome. *Am J Med Genet.* 1995;59:467–475.
121. Reiss AL, Aylward E, Freund LS, et al. Neuroanatomy of fragile X syndrome: The posterior fossa. *Ann Neurol.* 1991;29:26–32.
122. Rethore MO, Caille B, Huet de Barochez Y, et al. Ring chromosome 14. II. A case report of r(14) mosaicism. The r(14) phenotype. *Ann Genet.* 1984;27:91–95.
123. Reynolds JF, Daniel A, Kelly TE, et al. Isochromosome 12p mosaicism (Pallister aneuploidy or Pallister–Killian syndrome): Report of 11 cases. *Am J Med Genet.* 1987;27:257–274.
124. Richards RI, Sutherland GR. Dynamic mutations: A new class of mutations causing human disease. *Cell.* 1992;70:709–712.
125. Riegel M, Castellan C, Balmer D, et al. Terminal deletion, del(1)(p36.3), detected through screening for terminal deletions in patients with unclassified malformation syndromes. *Am J Med Genet.* 1999;82:249–253.
126. Robinson WP, Binkert F, Gine R, et al. Clinical and molecular analysis of five inv dup (15) patients. *Eur J Hum Genet.* 1993;1:37–50.
127. Ross MH, Galaburda AM, Kemper TL. Down's syndrome: Is there a decreased population of neurons? *Neurology.* 1984;34:909–916.
128. Roubertie A, Petit J, Genton P. Chromosome 20 en anneau: Un syndrome épileptique identifiable. *Rev Neurol.* 2000;156:149–153.
129. Rudelli RD, Brown WT, Wisniewski K, et al. Adult fragile X syndrome: Clinico-neuropathologic findings. *Acta Neuropathol (Berl).* 1985;67:289–295.
130. Sàenz-Lope E, Herranz FJ, Marsden JC. Startle epilepsy: A clinical study. *Ann Neurol.* 1984;16:78–81.
131. Sanchez-Carpintero R, McLellan A, Parmeggiani L, et al. Pallister-Killian syndrome: An unusual cause of epileptic spasms. *Dev Med Child Neurol.* 2005;47:776–779.
132. Sandlin CJ, Dodd BS, Dumars KW, et al. Phenotypes associated with terminal deletion of the short arm of chromosome1. *Am J Hum Genet.* 1995;57:A125.
133. Schinzel A, Niedrist D. Chromosome imbalances associated with epilepsy. *Am J Med Genet (Semin Med Genet).* 2001;106:119–124.
134. Schmidt R, Eviatar L, Nitowski HM, et al. Ring chromosome 14: A distinct clinical entity. *J Med Genet.* 1981;18:304–307.
135. Seppalainen AM, Kivalo E. EEG findings in Down's syndrome. *J Ment Def Res.* 1967;11:116–125.
136. Sgrò V, Riva E, Canevini MP, et al. 4p- Syndrome: A chromosomal disorder associated with a particular EEG pattern. *Epilepsia.* 1995;36:1206–1214.
137. Shaffer LG, Heilstedt HA. Terminal deletion of 1p36. *Lancet.* 2001;358:S9.
138. Shapira SK, McCaskill C, Northrup H, et al. Chromosome 1p36 deletions: The clinical phenotype and molecular characterisation of a common newly delineated syndrome. *Am J Hum Genet.* 1997;61:642–650.
139. Shaw-Smith C, Redon R, Rickman L, et al. Microarray based comparative genomic hybridisation (array-CGH) detects submicroscopic chromosomal deletions and duplications in patients with learning disability/mental retardation and dysmorphic features. *J Med Genet.* 2004;41:241–248.
140. Sicca F, Kelemen A, Genton P, et al. Mosaic mutations of the LIS1 gene cause subcortical band heterotopia. *Neurology.* 2003;61:1042–1046.
141. Silva ML, Cieuta C, Guerrini R, et al. Early clinical and EEG features of infantile spasms in Down syndrome. *Epilepsia.* 1996;37:977–982.

142. Singh R, Gardner RJ, Crossland KM, et al. Chromosomal abnormalities and epilepsy: A review for clinicians and gene hunters. *Epilepsia*. 2002;43:127–140.
143. Slavotinek A, Shaffer LG, Shapira SK. Monosomy 1p36. *J Med Genet*. 1999;36:657–663.
144. Smith GF, Berg JM. *Down's Anomaly,* 2nd ed. Edinburgh: Churchill Livingstone, 1976.
145. Speleman F, Leroy JG, Van Roy N, et al. Pallister–Killian syndrome: Characterization of the isochromosome 12p by fluorescent in situ hybridization. *Am J Med Genet*. 1991;41:381–387.
146. Stafstrom CE, Konkol RJ. Infantile spasms in children with Down syndrome. *Dev Med Chil Neurol*. 1994;36:576–585.
147. Stafstrom CE, Patxot CE, Gilmore HE, et al. Seizures in children with Down syndrome: Etiology, characteristics and outcome. *Dev Med Child Neurol*. 1991;33:191–200.
148. Steffenburg S, Gillberg CL, Steffenburg U, et al. Autism in Angelman syndrome: A population-based study. *Pediatr Neurol*. 1996;14:131–136.
149. Stengel-Rutkowski S, Warkotsch A, Schimanek P, et al. Familial Wolf's syndrome with a hidden 4p deletion by translocation of an 8p segment. Unbalanced inheritance from a maternal translocation (>4; 8) (p15.3;p22). Case report, review and risk estimates. *Clin Genet*. 1984;25:500–521.
150. Sugimoto T, Araki A, Yasuhara A, et al. Angelman syndrome in three siblings: Genetic model of epilepsy associated with chromosomal DNA deletion of the $GABA_A$ receptor. *Jpn J Psychiatry Neurol*. 1994;42:271–273.
151. Takeda Y, Baba A, Nakamura F, et al. Symptomatic generalized epilepsy associated with an inverted duplication of chromosome 15. *Seizure*. 2000;9:145–150.
152. Tarleton J, Richie R, Schwartz C, et al. An extensive de novo deletion removing *FMR1* in a patient with mental retardation and the fragile X syndrome phenotype. *Hum Molec Genet*. 1993;2:1973–1974.
153. Tatsuno M, Hayashi M, Iwamoto H, et al. Epilepsy in childhood Down syndrome. *Brain Dev*. 1984;6:37–44.
154. Tatum WO 4th, Passaro EA, Elia M, et al. Seizures in Klinefelter's syndrome. *Pediatr Neurol*. 1998;19:275–278.
155. Tharapel AT, Summit RL. A cytogenetic study of 200 unclassifiable mentally retarded children with congenital anomalies and 200 normal human subjects. *Hum Genet*. 1977;37:329–332.
156. Torrisi L, Sangiorgi E, Russo L, et al. Rearrangements of chromosome 15 in epilepsy. *Am J Med Genet (Semin Med Genet)*. 2001;106:125–128.
157. Tupler R, Bortotto L, Buhler EM, et al. Paternal origin of the de novo deleted chromosome 4 in Wolf-Hirschhorn syndrome. *J Med Genet*. 1992;29:53–55.
158. Van Buggenhout G, Melotte C, Dutta B, et al. Mild Wolf-Hirschhorn syndrome: Micro-array CGH analysis of atypical 4p16.3 deletions enables refinement of the genotype-phenotype map. *J Med Genet*. 2004;41:691–698.
159. Veall RM. The prevalence of epilepsy among mongols related to age. *J Ment Def Res*. 1974;18:99–106.
160. Verheij C, Bakker CE, de-Graaf E, et al. Characterization and localization of the FMR-1 gene product associated with fragile X syndrome. *Nature*. 1993;363:722–724.
161. Viani F, Romeo A, Viri M, et al. Seizure and EEG patterns in Angelman's syndrome. *J Child Neurol*. 1995;10:467–471.
162. Warburton D, Anyane-Yeboa K, Francke U. Mosaic tetrasomy 12p: Four new cases and confirmation of the chromosomal origin of the supernumerary chromosome in one of the original Pallister mosaic syndrome cases. *Am J Med Genet*. 1987;27:275–283.
163. Webb TP, Bundey SE, Thacke AI, et al. Population incidence and segregation ratios in the Martin-Bell syndrome. *Am J Med Genet*. 1986;23:573–580.
164. Wisniewski KE, Dalton AJ, McLachlan DRC, et al. Alzheimer's disease in Down syndrome: Clinicopathologic studies. *Neurology*. 1985;35:957–961.
165. Wisniewski KE, French JH, Fernando S, et al. Fragile X syndrome: Associated neurological abnormalities and developmental disabilities. *Ann Neurol*. 1985;18:665–669.
166. Wisniewski KE, Schmidt-Sidor B. Myelination in Down's syndrome brains (pre- and post-natal maturation and some clinical-pathologic correlation). *Ann Neurol*. 1986;20:429–430.
167. Wisniewski KE, Segan SM, Miezejesji EA, et al. The Fra (X) syndrome: Neurological, electrophysiological, and neuropathological abnormalities. *Am J Med Genet*. 1991;38:476–480.
168. Wöhrle D, Kotzot D, Hirst MC, et al. A microdeletion of less than 250 kb, including the proximal part of the FMR-1 gene and the fragile-X site, in a male with the clinical phenotype of fragile-X syndrome. *Am J Hum Genet*. 1992;51:299–306.
169. Wu YQ, Heilstedt HA, Bedell JA, et al. Molecular refinement of the 1p36 deletion syndrome reveals size diversity and a preponderance of maternally derived deletions. *Hum Mol Genet*. 1999;8:313–321.
170. Yunis E, Quintero L, Lebovici M. Monosomy 1pter. *Hum Genet*. 1981;56:279–282.
171. Zankl A, Addor MC, Maeder-Ingvar M, et al. A characteristic EEG pattern in 4p- syndrome: Case report and review of the literature. *Eur J Pediatr*. 2001;160:123–127.
172. Zelante L, Torricelli F, Calvano S, et al. Ring chromosome 14 syndrome: Report of two cases, including extended evaluation of a previously reported patient and review. *Ann Genet*. 1991;34:93–97.
173. Zollino M, Lecce R, Fischetto R, A et al. Mapping the Wolf-Hirschhorn syndrome phenotype outside the currently accepted WHS critical region and defining a new critical region, WHSCR-2. *Am J Hum Genet*. 2003;72:590–597.
174. Zori RT, Hendrickson J, Woolven S, et al. Angelman syndrome: Clinical profile. *J Child Neurol*. 1992;7:270–280.
175. Zuberi SM, Biraben AJ. Presentation, clinical evaluation and outcome in ring chromosome 20 syndrome. *Brain Dev*. 2004;26:554–555.

CHAPTER 261 ■ INHERITED METABOLIC DISORDERS

DOUGLAS R. NORDLI JR. AND DARRYL C. DE VIVO

INTRODUCTION

There are a wide variety of disorders of metabolism, approximately 50 of which are associated with seizures or epilepsy. From the epileptologist's perspective, many present similarly, with indistinguishable seizure semiology and electroencephalographic (EEG) findings. The clinical presentation may be influenced more by the age of the child than the specific etiology. In some children with inborn errors of metabolism and recurrent seizures, the epilepsy can be categorized into one of the recognized epileptogenic encephalopathies, such as early myoclonic epilepsy or West syndrome. In other cases, precise syndromes are lacking and terms like "generalized symptomatic epilepsy, not otherwise specified" and "epilepsies with focal and generalized features" are used. Clearly, more work needs to be done to accurately identify children with inborn errors, and we suspect that there are novel epilepsy syndromes yet to be described in this interesting group of patients. In the meantime, useful clues sometimes present that might alert one to the correct diagnosis. In some cases, this might be a relatively unique clinical feature, in others a characteristic of the epilepsy, and, finally, in some, a particular detail of the interictal EEG (Table 1). We have tried wherever possible to include these details, but we recognize that these definitive features seldom present themselves. For this reason, it is usually necessary to consider a relatively broad differential diagnosis. To organize the thought process, it is useful to think in terms of the age of the child and broad characteristics of the presentation. These have been organized into a table for ready reference (Table 2). The differential can be refined with the use of judiciously chosen screening tests. The results of these tests further guide the selection of definitive enzyme studies or genetic testing.

The acquisition of genetic information is proceeding at an exciting pace. Although this is stimulating to the neurologist, it presents a challenge for the traditional textbook format to contain up-to-date information. For this reason, we include a reference number from the Online Mendelian Inheritance of Man (OMIM) Web site so that the interested reader can quickly obtain the most current data (this source also links to Medline references). Wherever applicable, the OMIM number is given in parentheses in each heading. Another useful site is http://www.genetests.org, which provides a comprehensive listing of gene tests and the associated laboratories.

METABOLIC DISORDERS OF THE NEONATAL PERIOD

The neonatal period comprises the first month of postnatal life, and a number of metabolic disorders that appear at this time include seizures as a major clinical feature.

Nonketotic Hyperglycinemia (#605899)

In this condition, glycine accumulates in the central nervous system and elsewhere in the body because of a primary biochemical defect involving the glycine cleavage system. There are four enzymes that cleave glycine: (a) P protein, a pyridoxal phosphate–dependent glycine decarboxylase (GLDC), (b) T protein, a tetrahydrofolate-requiring enzyme (GCST), (c) H protein, a lipoic acid–containing protein (GCSH), and (d) L protein, a lipoamide dehydrogenase. Disease can be caused by defects in any of these enzymes, although mutations involving GLDC and GCST are most common. Mutations that involve the pore region of the T protein appear to particularly impair function.[7] The mode of transmission is autosomal recessive, with an estimated prevalence of 1/250,000. Neonatal nonketotic hyperglycinemia (NKH) is characterized by an initial variable symptom-free interval of 1 to 42 days. Clinical symptoms are at first lethargy, poor feeding, apneic spells, altered muscular tone, and intermittent ophthalmoparesis that occasionally progresses to bilateral external ophthalmoplegia. Erratic myoclonus is another major symptom that may appear early; hiccups and coma follow. The electroencephalogram (EEG) demonstrates a suppression-burst pattern that correlates with brainstem-evoked potential abnormalities and intrinsic brainstem pathology seen on postmortem examination (Fig. 1).[54] Similar EEG abnormalities are characteristic of phenylketonuria, maple syrup urine disease, and molybdenum cofactor deficiency (Table 2). Clinical seizure patterns include infantile spasms and generalized tonic seizures. Progressive brain atrophy, delayed myelination, incomplete development of the corpus callosum, gyral malformations, cerebellar hypoplasia, and culpocephaly are common. Elevated glycine concentrations in the cerebrospinal fluid (CSF) during the first hours of life and a partial suppression-burst EEG pattern detected as early as 30 minutes after delivery in an asymptomatic patient indicate that the abnormal glycine metabolism has been present prenatally. A CSF-to-plasma glycine ratio >0.08 is diagnostic of nonketotic hyperglycinemia. The disease usually has a severe outcome, but milder cases have been reported. Some of these are due to abnormal splicing with slightly preserved enzyme function.[72] Transient nonketotic hyperglycinemia is associated with similar clinical and biochemical findings initially, but glycine concentrations normalize between 2 and 8 weeks of life, and the prognosis is generally more favorable.[10]

Treatment of NKH has focused on three compounds: (a) glycine, (b) benzoate, and (c) carnitine. Glycine is known to stimulate the *N*-methyl-D-aspartic acid (NMDA) receptor, and dextromethorphan is a noncompetitive agonist of this same receptor, which has been used with some clinical success. High doses of benzoate can lower the CSF concentration of glycine, and there are anecdotal reports of responses. Carnitine deficiency has been documented in patients treated with benzoate,

TABLE 1

METABOLIC DISORDERS IN LATE INFANCY

Disorder	Seizure frequency	Seizure type	EEG	Dysmorphism	Neuroimaging	Laboratory findings	Treatment
Metachromatic leukodystrophy	++/+++	P	Diffuse slowing; asymmetric, slow-wave activity	Absent	White-matter lesions	High CSF protein; arylsulfatase deficiency	Not available (bone marrow transplant)
Schindler disease	+++	GTC, M	Multifocal spike-and-wave complexes	Absent	Severe atrophy of cerebellum, brainstem, and cervical spinal cord	Abnormal oligosaccharide pattern; α-*N*-acetylgalactos-aminidase deficiency	Not available
Mucopoly-saccharidoses	++	G	No specific pattern	Present	Cortical atrophy; ventricular dilation	Abnormal oligosaccharide pattern; several enzyme defects	Bone marrow transplant
CDG syndrome	+++	IS (CDG type III), P	Focal slow activity; hypsarrhythmia	Absent	Cerebellar atrophy; pons atrophy; demyelination (type III)	Low thyroxine-binding protein; abnormal serum and CSF disialotransferrin; phosphomannomutase deficiency	Not available

+, 0%–25% seizure activity; CDG, carbohydrate-deficient glycoprotein; CSF, cerebrospinal fluid; EEG, electroencephalogram; G, generalized; GTC, generalized tonic–clonic; IS, infantile spasms; M, myoclonic; P, partial.

TABLE 2

METABOLIC DISORDERS IN THE NEONATAL PERIOD

Disorder	Seizure frequency	Seizure type	EEG	Dysmorphism	Neuroimaging	Laboratory findings	Treatment
Urea cycle	++	P	Theta/delta waves; suppression-burst	Absent	Cerebral edema	High ammonia; low plasma urea	Dietary and pharmacologic
Nonketotic hyperglycinemia	++++	M, G, IS	Suppression-burst	Absent	CNS malformations	High CSF/plasma glycine ratio	Symptomatic
Maple syrup urine disease	++	M, P	Suppression-burst; comblike rhythm activity	Absent	Cerebral edema	Elevated Leu, Ile, Val; abnormal OA pattern	Dietary
Pyroxidine dependency	++++	P, G, M, IS	Multifocal spikes	Absent	Normal	Low CSF GABA	Pyridoxine
Organic acidurias	++	P, G	Trace alternans pattern; delta-wave paroxysms	Absent	Cerebral edema, white-matter hypodensity	Metabolic acidosis/ketosis; abnormal OA pattern	Dietary and pharmacologic
Pyruvate dehydrogenase deficiency	++	P, G, M	Bursts of slow spikes-and-waves	Present	CNS malformations; high CSF and plasma lactate	Metabolic acidosis	Symptomatic
Molybdenum cofactor deficiency	++++	P, G, M	Suppression-burst; multifocal paroxysms	Present	Progressive atrophy	Abnormal plasma and urinary amino acid profile: *S*-sulfocysteine and taurine	Not available
Peroxisomal disorders	++++	P, G, M	Multifocal paroxysms	Present	Cerebral dysplasia	High VLCFA	Not available
Fructose-1, 6-diphosphatase deficiency	+++	P, G	Diffuse slowing; intermittent burst; fast activity	Absent	Normal	Hypoglycemia; lactic acidosis; ketosis	Dietary
Biotin disorders	+/++	P, M	Suppression-burst; multifocal paroxysms	Absent	Cerebral edema	Ketoacidosis; hyperammonemia; organic aciduria	Biotin

+, 0%–25% seizure activity; CNS, central nervous system; CSF, cerebrospinal fluid; EEG, electroencephalogram; G, generalized; GABA, γ-aminobutyric acid; IS, infantile spasms; M, myoclonic; OA, organic acids; P, partial; VLCFA, very-long-chain fatty acids.

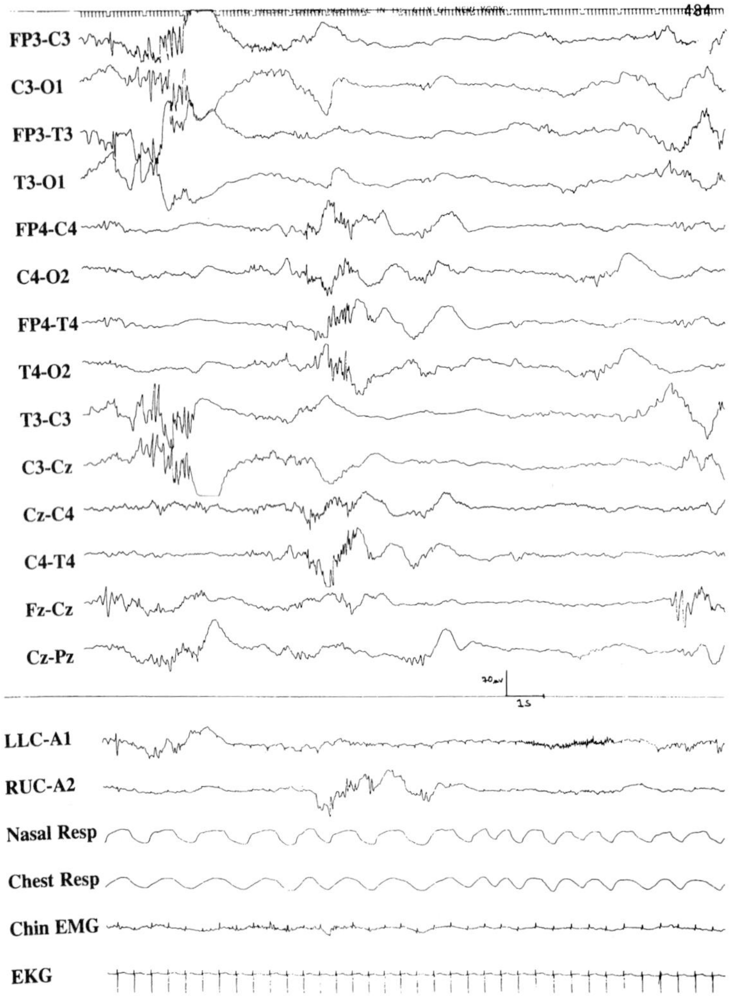

FIGURE 1. Suppression-burst electroencephalogram with interhemispheric asynchrony in a newborn. The suppression-burst pattern is characteristic of a variety of disorders, including nonketotic hyperglycinemia, phenylketonuria, maple syrup urine disease, and molybdenum cofactor deficiency. EKG, electrocardiogram; EMG, electromyogram; Resp, respiration.

and therefore supplementation with L-carnitine has been advocated in patients receiving benzoate. Despite prompt administration of these treatments, some children may still suffer lasting neurologic sequelae.[8]

Pyridoxine-dependent Epilepsy (#266100)

This disorder, transmitted as an autosomal-recessive trait, was previously believed to be due to a defect involving glutamic acid decarboxylase, but linkage studies have excluded this enzyme and implicated other pathways that do not appear to be primarily involved with this reaction.[5] Instead, mutations in an enzyme, antiquitin, in the lysine degradation pathway are responsible for the condition. An accumulated substrate inactivates pyridoxal 5-phosphate by forming a Knoevenagel condensation. The diagnosis can be suspected by finding elevated pipecolic acid in the blood, urine, or CSF.[41]

Typically, recurrent and long-lasting seizures occur in the neonatal period that are refractory to treatment with conventional antiepileptic drugs. The seizure types vary, and include persistent partial seizures with variable preservation of consciousness, recurrent status epilepticus, generalized myoclonic and atonic seizures, and infantile spasms. Progressive irritability, restlessness, and vomiting often precede seizures. The EEG may be diagnostic, showing an unusual paroxysmal pattern consisting of bursts of diffuse but asynchronous high-voltage delta activity intermixed with spikes or sharp waves. Other EEG findings include focal and multifocal spikes, bursts of generalized delta waves, and paroxysmal complexes of sharp and slow waves.[40] Intravenous administration of pyridoxine usually produces rapid control of seizures, but some cases may require several days of oral administration to show clinical effect. Patients remain dependent on pyridoxine supplementation to maintain seizure control and normal neurologic development.

Atypical cases of pyridoxine dependency have been described. Onset may be delayed into early infancy. As a rule, all infants of this age who have idiopathic seizures should be given a test dose of pyridoxine (75–100 mg) to determine responsiveness. Occasionally, a patient with vitamin B6–dependent conditions will become apneic after the test dose is administered, and so it is important to anticipate the need for transient respiratory support. Decreased concentration of γ-aminobutyric acid (GABA) in the CSF is the defining biochemical abnormality. This finding, coupled with elevated CSF concentration of glutamate and response to administration of pyridoxine, is diagnostic.

Some patients with neonatal encephalopathies do not respond to B6 but do respond to pyridoxal phosphate.[9,67] Pyridoxal phosphate is the biologically active form of the B6 vitamins, but the defect in these patients is not precisely known. Some advocate giving neonates or infants with intractable seizures and encephalopathy a test dose of pyridoxal phosphate (either 50 mg for a neonate or 30–50 mg/kg/d for infants) for 2 weeks because of these rare cases of pyridoxine resistance and the observation that pyridoxal phosphate appears to be superior to B6 in idiopathic epilepsies.[4,68]

Dihydropyrimidine Dehydrogenase Deficiency (#274270)

Dihydropyrimidine dehydrogenase (DPD) is used in the first step of the pyrimidine degradation pathway, converting uracil and thymine to β-alanine and the R-enantiomer of β-aminoisobutyric acid. This conversion primarily takes place in the liver, and DPD is the rate-limiting enzyme of the catabolism. This enzyme is absent in the brain, but it is believed that alanine may be converted from carnosine owing to the presence of tissue carnosinase in brain. There is a wide range of clinical presentation, but nearly all children present with neurologic abnormalities, including hypertonia, hyperreflexia, tremor, seizures, and developmental delay. Severely affected children present as newborns with hypertonia, stiffness, and feeding difficulties.[2] Details of the EEG features and characteristics of the seizures have yet to be described. In our own patient, erratic myoclonias were present. The EEG showed bursts of semirhythmic delta and attenuation of the expected background complexity over either hemisphere with shifting laterality. Multifocal interictal epileptiform discharges were present (Fig. 2). No treatment has been shown to be effective.

Molybdenum Cofactor Deficiency (#252150)

This condition is exceedingly rare. Molybdenum is a trace element that serves as an essential cofactor for the reactions of three different enzymes: (a) sulfite oxidase, (b) xanthine dehydrogenase, and (c) aldehyde oxidase. Deficiency of molybdenum cofactor can result from mutations in four separate genes: *MOCS1*, *MOCS2* (which codes for molybdopterin synthase), *MOSC3*, and *GEPH* (which codes for gephyrin).[36] Absence of hepatic molybdenum cofactor results in a combined enzyme deficiency. A progressive encephalopathy develops in affected infants, with recurrent and refractory seizures appearing shortly after birth. Focal seizures, diffuse tonic seizures, and erratic myoclonic jerks are common. Jitteriness, abnormal cry, and intermittent irritability are other neurologic findings. Dysmorphic features, ectopia lentis, and hepatomegaly are associated somatic manifestations. The EEG is characterized by multifocal paroxysms and a suppression-burst pattern. Brain magnetic resonance imaging (MRI) demonstrates initial signal changes consistent with white matter edema, then curvilinear signal changes in the gray–white junction suggestive of hemorrhage and laminar necrosis, and ultimately multiple subcortical cystic areas scattered throughout the brain.[16]

Isolated sulfite oxidase deficiency is clinically and pathologically indistinguishable from molybdenum cofactor deficiency, suggesting that decreased sulfite oxidase activity is central to the clinical syndrome.[59] In both conditions, the serum concentration of uric acid is abnormally low, and sulfur-containing

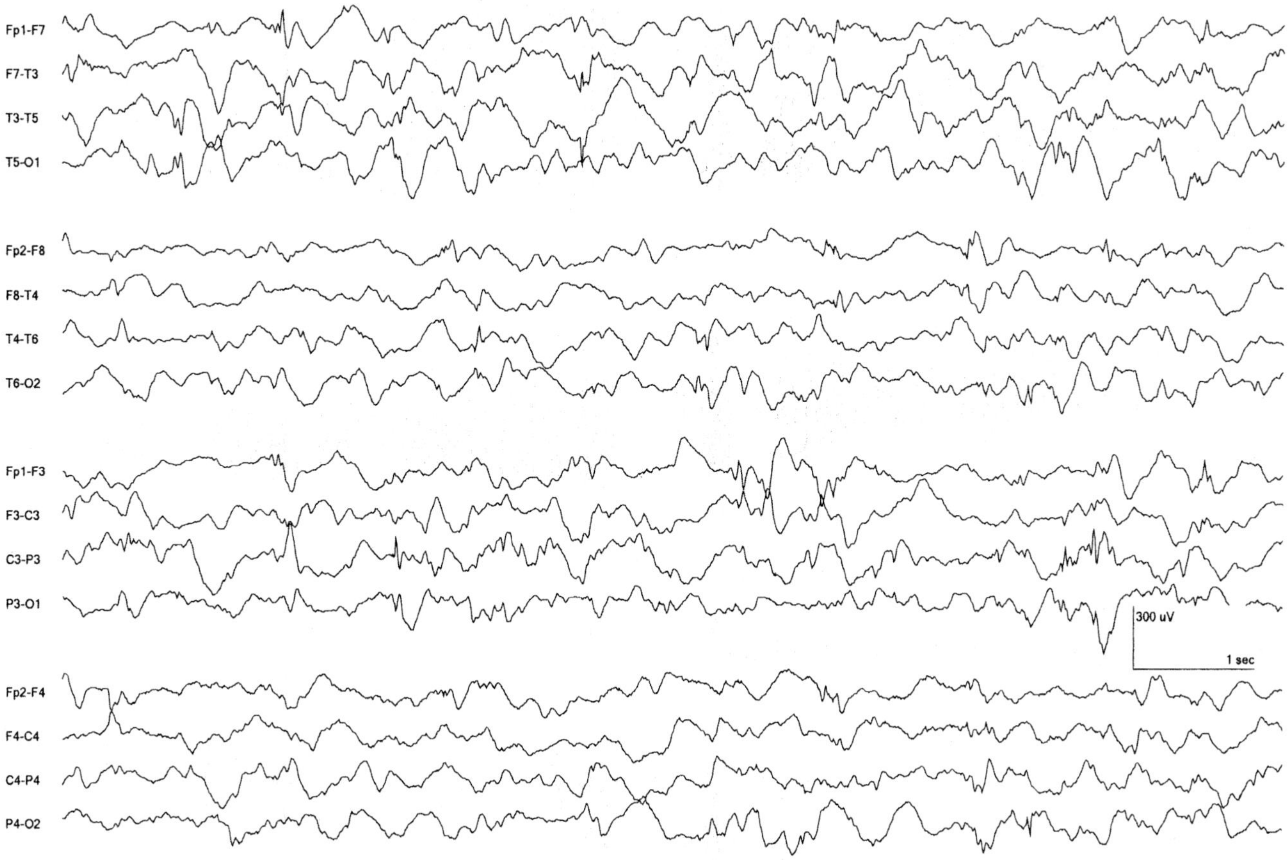

FIGURE 2. Electroencephalogram (EEG) in a patient with dihydropyrimidine dehydrogenase deficiency. The infant is 6 months old. Note the background slowing, the asymmetry with reduced complexity on the right, and the presence of multifocal spikes. A prior EEG had shown reduced complexity on the left, indicating that this feature presents with shifting laterality. (Courtesy of Dr. Kent R. Kelley.)

products are evident in the urine. Serum urate may be the more sensitive screening test.[3] There is no effective treatment for this condition. Recent work suggests that sulfites might have a direct impact on glutamate dehydrogenase function, thereby reducing the adenosine triphosphate (ATP)-producing capacity of cells.[75] In theory, a severe impairment of energy production could account for the MRI appearance and the burst-suppression pattern apparent on EEG tracings.

Peroxisomal Diseases

These disorders are invariably associated with seizures in the neonatal period. Zellweger (cerebrohepatorenal) syndrome (ZS) is the prototype of this group of conditions. Neonatal adrenoleukodystrophy and infantile Refsum disease are progressively milder presentations. Most cases of ZS are caused by mutations in the *PEX1* gene, and the severity of the mutation correlates with the clinical severity, although to an imperfect degree.[66] Severe encephalopathy with failure to thrive, hypotonia, hyporeflexia or areflexia, and seizures are the major features. Seizures develop in the neonatal period in 80% of patients. Seizure types include focal, myoclonic, and atypical flexor spasms. The EEG shows multifocal spikes or, less frequently, hypsarrhythmia. Dysmorphic features are distinctive and often permit diagnosis by inspection. These include a high, prominent forehead; shallow orbital ridges; high palatal arch; deformities of the external ear; micrognathia; presence of epicanthal folds; low, broad nasal bridge; and redundant skin folds of the neck. Cataracts, glaucoma, pigmentary retinopathy, optic nerve dysplasia, and amaurosis are usually present, as are hepatomegaly, polycystic kidneys, and calcific stippling of the patellae. Laboratory abnormalities include absence of peroxisomes on liver biopsy and high levels of very-long-chain fatty acids in the serum.

Disorders of the Urea Cycle

These conditions involve 1/30,000 live births.[24] Except for ornithine transcarbamoylase deficiency, which is transmitted as an X-linked dominant trait, the other five urea cycle disorders are autosomal-recessive diseases. Hyperammonemia, respiratory alkalosis, absence of ketoacidosis, and decreased blood urea nitrogen concentrations are laboratory findings that strongly suggest a urea cycle disorder. The concentrations of citrulline and argininosuccinic acid in the plasma and of orotic acid in the urine help to differentiate among six different enzyme defects of the urea cycle.

Approximately 60% of infants with urea cycle defects become symptomatic within 24 to 72 hours of birth. Symptoms include progressive lethargy, vomiting, hypothermia, and hyperventilation. Seizures are not usually seen initially but are manifested later, as cerebral edema develops. The EEG is characterized by low-voltage, asymmetric delta and theta activity. A suppression-burst pattern may develop, and the duration of intervals between bursts may correlate with the degree of hyperammonemia. Brain imaging reveals cerebral edema with small ventricles, and intracranial hemorrhage has been reported. Primary treatment is dietary, with various drugs administered to lower the blood and tissue concentrations of ammonia.

Maple Syrup Urine Disease (#248600)

There are five subtypes of maple syrup urine disease (MSUD), but the classic severe neonatal form presents with poor sucking, lethargy, and coma, beginning sometime between the fourth and seventh days of life. Intermittent hypertonus and opisthotonus, gross tremor, myoclonic jerks, and repetitive flexion–extension movements of the limbs are common. It is the result of a defect of the branched-chain α-ketoacid dehydrogenase complex, and mutations in at least four different genes can cause the clinical syndrome. This mutation is expressed as an autosomal-recessive trait, with an estimated prevalence of 1/200,000 live births. The branched-chain amino acids (leucine, isoleucine, and valine) accumulate together with the α-ketoacid derivatives. Clear focal seizures, seizures with diffuse clinical expression, and uncontrolled cerebral edema are common in untreated subjects. A mu-like rhythm characterized by bursts of 7- to 9-Hz spindle-like sharp waves of moderate amplitude is distinctive.[18] Fast rolandic rhythms have also been described.

Organic Acidurias

The disorders of organic acid metabolism comprise a large number of inborn errors, including isovaleric aciduria and several ketotic hyperglycinemic syndromes (propionic acidemia, methylmalonic acidemia, and β-ketothiolase deficiency).

Symptoms develop during the neonatal period in approximately 50% of children who have isovaleric aciduria (#243500), with poor feeding, vomiting, dehydration, and a progressive encephalopathy manifested by lethargy, tremors, seizures, and coma. Cerebral edema is present, and seizures are most often focal motor or diffuse tonic posturing. The EEG shows dysmature features during sleep. Distinctive biochemical findings include metabolic acidosis, ketosis, lactic acidosis, hyperammonemia, and transient bone marrow suppression. Isovalerylglycinuria is diagnostic. The disorder is due to a defect in isovaleryl CoA dehydrogenase. It is of note that recent newborn screening has led to the identification of asymptomatic individuals with identical genetic mutations. This is important information for genetic counseling.[44]

The symptoms of propionic acidemia (#606054) also appear during the neonatal period, and 20% of affected newborns have seizures as the first symptom. The defect is in propionyl-CoA carboxylase. Again, both focal seizures and manifestations that appear more diffuse have been reported. The EEG shows diffuse delta wave activity, with generalized or focal temporal spikes during the encephalopathic phase. Intractable epilepsy may develop. In 40% of affected children, generalized convulsions and myoclonic seizures develop in later infancy, and older children may have atypical absence seizures. A recent workshop showed that modern mortality rates are about one in three, but the degree of dietary protein restriction used as treatment varies considerably among centers worldwide.[65] Biochemical findings include metabolic acidosis, ketosis, and elevation of branched-chain amino acids and propionic acid.

Methylmalonic acidemia is the metabolic signature of several biochemically distinct entities, all of which show decreased activity of methylmalonyl-CoA mutase.[48] Stomatitis, glossitis, developmental delay, failure to thrive, and seizures are the major features. Diffuse tonic postures and focal seizures with apparent secondary generalization are the most frequently described seizure types. Methylmalonic acidemia also occurs in association with homocystinuria. Seizures involve repetitive clonic eyelid blinking and simultaneous upward deviation of the eyes. Lesions of the globus pallidus on computed tomography (CT) or MRI are classic.[57]

Defects of carnitine palmitoyltransferase types I and II may be manifested in the newborn period by diffuse neurologic signs and seizures.[39] Hypsarrhythmia has been described in one case. Deficiency of carnitine acylcarnitine translocase also may produce seizures, apnea, and bradycardia in the neonatal period, and seizures may occur in other defects of fatty acid oxidation.[28]

Pyruvate Dehydrogenase Deficiency (#312170) and Pyruvate Carboxylase Deficiency (#266150)

The clinical manifestations of pyruvate dehydrogenase (PDH) deficiency are extremely heterogeneous. The spectrum ranges from neonatal lactic acidosis with severe neurologic dysfunction to a slowly progressive, chronic neurodegenerative disorder.[6] Structural abnormalities, such as agenesis of the corpus callosum, are frequently revealed by brain imaging. Mutations most often affect the E_1 α subunit gene located on the short arm of chromosome X.[11] The pyruvate dehydrogenase complex catalyzes the irreversible conversion of pyruvate into acetyl-CoA. The PDH complex is composed of multiple copies of three enzymes: E1 (PDHA1), dihydrolipoyl transacetylase (DLAT or E2), and dihydrolipoyl dehydrogenase (DLD or E3). The E1 enzyme is made up of two α and two β subunits. The E1 α subunit contains the active site and plays a key role in the function of the PDH complex. Complex malformations of the nervous system are common in girls with neonatal onset, and seizures are a frequent feature, including infantile spasms and myoclonic seizures. Electroencephalographic abnormalities are usually severe and include multifocal slow spike-and-wave discharges. Patients with defects in E2 have been recently reported. The clinical expression is quite different, and affected individuals may present with episodic dystonia and few or none of the classical features of PDH deficiency.[26] Patients are treated with the ketogenic diet because use of ketone bodies for oxidative metabolism bypasses the primary defect. A zebrafish model was developed that demonstrates the effectiveness of this approach.[60]

Pyruvate carboxylase deficiency also may be devastating in the neonatal period, being associated with severe lactic acidosis, hypotonia, failure to thrive, and seizures.[11] The combination of lactic acidosis and ketosis is a distinctive metabolic disturbance, and when hyperammonemia, citrullinemia, and hyperlysinemia are also present, it is diagnostic of the disorder. Seizures are related to the associated hypoglycemia and failure of the Krebs cycle. Treatment with adrenocorticotropic hormone (ACTH) can worsen infantile spasms associated with this disorder, and treatment with the ketogenic diet can be lethal.[52]

Other disturbances of mitochondrial function have been linked to Leigh syndrome (LS) and Alpers syndrome. Symptoms of these two syndromes, which appear in infancy, include convulsions. Leigh syndrome is better understood and may be related to various biomolecular defects.[14] Maternally inherited Leigh syndrome (MILS) is frequently associated with convulsions and pigmentary retinopathy. The common mutation associated with MILS is a thymine–guanine transition at nucleotide position 8993 in complex V of the mitochondrial genome. Other mitochondrial DNA mutations may produce the MILS phenotype. Leigh syndrome associated with deficiency of pyruvate dehydrogenase is characterized by convulsions about 50% of the time. In contrast, convulsions occur infrequently (7% of cases) in LS associated with cytochrome *c* oxidase.

The pathophysiology of Alpers syndrome is more obscure. This condition is transmitted as an autosomal-recessive trait and is invariably associated with convulsions. Liver failure with cirrhosis follows in the Huttenlocher variant.[27] Whether Alpers syndrome is mitochondrial in origin had been a subject of debate.[24] Mutations in the POLG gene have been reported.[45]

Disorders of Carbohydrate Metabolism

Hypoglycemia in the neonatal period is often caused by an inborn error of gluconeogenesis, such as deficiency of fructose-1,6-bisphosphatase. Fifty percent of affected children show symptoms during the first week of life, including periodic hyperventilation, hepatomegaly, irritability, apnea, somnolence, and coma. Other patients become symptomatic during the early infantile period. Seizures are common, and the initial EEG reveals diffuse slowing and low-amplitude background activity with intermittent bursts of fast activity. Less frequently, there are multifocal sharp waves and spikes. Profound hypoglycemia, lactic acidosis, ketosis, elevated plasma concentrations of alanine, and presence of abnormal urinary organic acids with glycerol and glycerol-3-phosphate are characteristic biochemical findings. The diagnosis can be made using cultured lymphocytes, thereby eliminating the need for a liver biopsy.[31] Neurologic symptoms and permanent brain damage can be avoided by preventing hypoglycemia.

Other disorders are caused by abnormalities of fructose and galactose metabolism. Galactosemia can be caused by defects in the products of three genes. The most commonly involved enzyme is galactose-1-phosphate uridyltransferase (#230400). Deficiency occurs in 1/62,000 births. The precise cause of the neurologic disability is not known. Despite prompt recognition and appropriate dietary management, long-term disability may still result.[55] Hyperchloremic metabolic acidosis, hyperaminoaciduria, albuminuria, abnormal liver function, and elevated blood concentrations of galactose are diagnostic of this condition. Neonatal screening can be performed.

Disorders of Biotin Metabolism

These conditions may produce seizures in the neonatal period (Table 2).[7] Holocarboxylase synthetase binds biotin covalently to four apocarboxylases (propionyl-CoA carboxylase, pyruvate carboxylase, β-methylcrotonyl-CoA carboxylase, and acetyl-CoA carboxylase) (#253270). The gene map locus is 21q22.1. Biotinidase, in turn, cleaves biotin from biocytin, a short biotinylated peptide that is formed during the proteolytic degradation of the holocarboxylases. Holocarboxylase synthetase deficiency is also known as early-onset multiple carboxylase deficiency, and biotinidase deficiency is also termed late-onset multiple carboxylase deficiency. Symptoms of holocarboxylase synthetase deficiency appear in the neonatal period; diffuse tonic seizures, brief focal motor seizures, and multifocal myoclonic jerks develop in 25% to 50% of cases. In addition, Thoene et al.[61] reported lactic acidosis, alopecia, keratoconjunctivitis, and perioaral erosions. Seizures are usually refractory to treatment with antiepileptic drugs but may improve with large doses of biotin. The EEG shows a suppression-burst pattern and multifocal spikes (Fig. 1).

METABOLIC DISORDERS OF EARLY INFANCY

Several inborn metabolic errors of which seizures are a manifestation become symptomatic after the first month of life. All patients with GM_2 gangliosidosis, disorders of folate metabolism, glucose transporter protein deficiency, fumarase deficiency, and Menkes disease have seizures as part of the clinical picture. In the other metabolic disorders of early infancy, seizures occur in 25% to 75% of cases (Table 3).

Lysosomal Disorders

GM_2 gangliosidosis is a lysosomal disorder that invariably includes seizures as a prominent feature. The infantile form of GM_2 gangliosidosis includes Tay-Sachs disease (#272800), caused by deficiency of hexosaminidase A, and Sandhoff disease, caused by deficiency of hexosaminidase A and B. Classic

TABLE 3

METABOLIC DISORDERS IN EARLY INFANCY

Seizure disorder	Seizure frequency	type	EEG	Dysmorphism	Neuroimaging	Laboratory findings	Treatment
GM_2 gangliosidosis	++++	SM, P, M	Multifocal paroxysms	Absent	Progressive ventriculomegaly	Abnormal urinary oligosaccharide pattern; hexosaminodase A deficiency	Not available
Krabbe disease	+++	M, SM, IS	Asynchronous spike-polyspike paroxysms	Absent	White-matter demyelination	Increased CSF protein; galactosylceramidase deficiency	Not available
Biotinidase deficiency	+++	G, M, IS	Suppression-burst; spike-and-slow-wave paroxysms	Absent	Nonspecific	Abnormal urinary OA pattern	Biotin
Folate disorders	+++/ ++++	IS, M, P	Multifocal paroxysms; hypsarrhythmia	Absent	Cortical atrophy; leukoencephalopathy; calcifications	Abnormal amino acid pattern: homocystinuria, low methionine, normal or low CSF folate	Folate, betaine
Glucose transporter protein deficiency	++++	M, A	Normal	Absent	Normal	Low CSF glucose and lactate; normal serum glucose	Ketogenic diet
Branched-chain organic acidurias	+++	P, G, M, IS	Generalized or focal delta slowing	Present (3-OH-isobutyric aciduria)	Cerebral edema; hypodensity BG; heterotopias; cerebral dysplasia	Ketonuria or hypoketosis; hypoglycemia; abnormal urinary OA	Dietary, carnitine
Fumarase deficiency	++++	P, IS, M	Multifocal spikes; spike-and-wave complexes; hypsarrhythmia	Absent	CNS malformations	Lactic acidosis; fumaric aciduria	Symptomatic
Hyperpheny-alninemias	+++	G, P, M, IS	Generalized or focal paroxysms; hypsarrhythmia	Absent	White-matter lesions; cerebral atrophy	High phenylalanine; abnormal CSF biopterin ratio	Dietary, biopterin
Fructose-1, 6-biphosphatase deficiency	+++	P, G	Diffuse slowing; intermittent burst; fast activity	Absent	Normal	Hypoglycemia; lactic acidosis; ketosis	Dietary
HHH syndrome	+++	G, P, M, IS	Spike-and-wave complexes; diffuse slowing	Absent	Normal	Increased orotic acid, glutamate, alanine; homocitrullinuria; hyperammonemia	Dietary
Urea cycle	++	P, G	Generalized theta-wave paroxysms	Absent	Cerebral edema; white-matter lesions	Hypera-mmonemia; abnormal amino acid pattern	Dietary, phenyl-butyrate
Menkes disease	++++	M	Multifocal paroxysms	Absent	Cerebral, cerebellar atrophy; focal areas of necrosis	Low serum copper and ceruloplasmin	Symptomatic
Histidinemia	+++	M, IS, SM	Atypical hypsarrhythmia	Absent	Normal	High histidine	Symptomatic, histidine restriction
Hyper-prolinemia	++	P, IS	Slow delta-wave activity	Absent	Normal; leukodystrophy (1 case)	High proline	Symptomatic

+, 0%–25% seizure activity; BG, basal ganglia; CNS, central nervous system; CSF, cerebrospinal fluid; EEG, electroencephalogram; G, generalized; IS, infantile spasms; M, myoclonic; OA, organic acids; P, partial; SM, startle myoclonic.

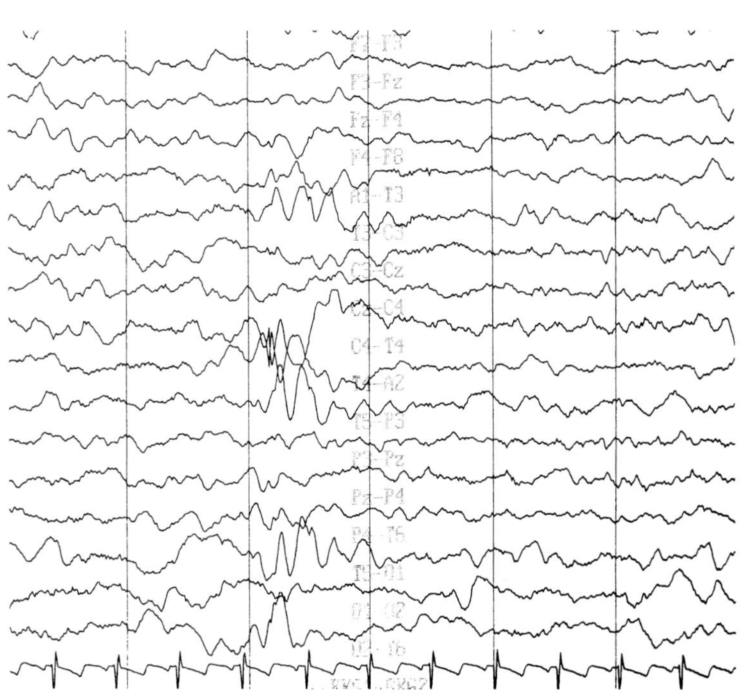

FIGURE 3. Electroencephalographic tracing showing very fast central spikes in an infant with Tay-Sachs disease.

Tay-Sachs disease is characterized by developmental regression, paralysis, blindness, seizures, and death in the second or third year of life.[46] An exaggerated startle response, often associated with myoclonic jerks, is one of the earliest neurologic signs, and is a distinctive feature of this disorder. Focal and atypical absence seizures have been described and respond poorly to antiepileptic drugs. The EEG shows central spikes with a very sharp morphology (Fig. 3). The classic cherry red spot is present in the ocular fundi of nearly all patients. One report in the literature based on autopsy findings suggested an exaggerated sensitivity to phenytoin neurotoxicity.[42] Nonetheless, phenytoin should be avoided in patients with Tay-Sachs disease because of the high incidence of myoclonus and the availability of other agents effective against multiple seizure types.

Other lysosomal disorders occurring at this age include globoid-cell leukodystrophy (Krabbe disease; #245200), caused by a deficiency of galactocerebrosidase. Presentation in early infancy is characterized by developmental regression, increasing irritability, progressive spasticity, and opisthotonic posturing.[20] Myoclonic jerks, startle myoclonus, and extensor spasms are common, and infantile spasms with hypsarrhythmia have been reported in several cases. The EEG is usually characterized by increasingly severe bilateral, symmetric delta activity and asynchronous spike-polyspike discharges. Increased CSF protein and peripheral neuropathy are distinctive features of this disease of white matter. In contrast to what is observed in most classic white-matter diseases, seizures occur early in the course of 50% to 75% of infants with Krabbe disease. Bone marrow transplantation has been used and is most promising in the presymptomatic newborns.[17,70]

Disorders of Vitamin Metabolism

Disorders of vitamin metabolism with symptoms that appear in early infancy include biotinidase deficiency (#253260) and disorders of folic acid. As described in a previous section, biotinidase deficiency produces multiple carboxylase deficiency. Thirteen different mutations have been described in the gene.[73] Seizures occur in 50% to 75% of patients and are the presenting clinical symptoms in one third of cases. Apparently generalized clonic seizures, infantile spasms, and myoclonic seizures are seen. Electroencephalographic findings may include a suppression-burst pattern, absence of physiologic sleep patterns, poorly organized and slow waking background activity, and frequent spike and spike-and-slow-wave discharges. A deficiency of biotinidase is diagnostic, and patients respond dramatically to supplementation with high-dose biotin. Newborn screening is used to make the diagnosis, but not all individuals identified will develop clinical symptoms.[74]

Methelyne tetrahydrofolate reductase deficiency (#236250) is the most common inborn error of folate metabolism, with a clinical spectrum from early neurologic deterioration and death to asymptomatic adults, even within the same family.[25] In affected individuals, a progressive neurologic syndrome develops with regression in infancy. Clinical features include acquired microcephaly and seizures. Intractable infantile spasms, generalized atonic and myoclonic seizures, and partial motor seizures are seen. Electroencephalographic findings vary from diffuse slowing of background activity to continuous spike-and-wave complexes or multifocal spikes. The early-onset form differs from the late-onset form. The latter presents with progressive motor deterioration, schizophrenia-like psychiatric symptoms, and recurrent strokes; seizures are uncommon. Homocystinuria and elevated serum concentrations of homocystine and methionine are the main biochemical features. Treatment with folate can reverse white matter lesions, but this response may be variable, even within families of affected members.[58]

Defects in methionine biosynthesis are also associated with seizures. Convulsions are frequent and are predominantly generalized, although myoclonic seizures with a hypsarrhythmia on the EEG have been reported. Diagnostic laboratory findings are megaloblastic anemia, homocystinuria, decreased methionine, and normal folate and cobalamin concentrations in the absence of methylmalonic aciduria.

Seizures are common in congenital folate malabsorption, a rare condition that is believed to be caused by a defect in the folate transporter system. Folate is concentrated in the nervous system, and the CSF concentrations of folate are higher than serum concentrations. Sometimes, calcifications form in the occipital lobes and basal ganglia. Without folate supplementation, a slowly progressive encephalopathy develops with refractory seizures. Other clinical features include megaloblastic anemia, diarrhea, mouth ulcers, and failure to thrive. High-dose folate or folinic acid may improve seizure control.

Inherited defects of vitamin B12 metabolism also may produce severe megaloblastic anemia in early infancy. Generalized tonic convulsions occur almost invariably and are refractory to conventional treatment. Methylmalonic aciduria without homocystinuria suggests this diagnosis.

Glucose Transporter Type 1 Deficiency Syndrome

The glucose transporter type 1 deficiency syndrome is a prototypic example of a defect in energy supply.[12,64] Affected infants become encephalopathic, with seizures and delayed motor and mental development. Seizures typically begin after the second month of life and are of diverse types but are probably multifocal in origin. Later, generalized nonconvulsive seizures, myoclonic jerks, and atypical absence seizures are common. Developmental clumsiness, impaired early language and behavioral development, and deceleration of head growth with acquired microcephaly are additional findings. Low CSF glucose and lactate concentrations in the presence of a normal blood sugar concentration are diagnostic. The EEG is often normal early in the course or may show scattered multifocal interictal epileptiform discharges (Fig. 4B). As the child matures, bursts of generalized spike-and-wave discharges are seen in about one third of patients (Fig. 4A).[35] Another useful EEG clue to the diagnosis is the marked enhancement of the interictal epileptiform abnormalities in the fasting state and, in turn, the marked improvement of the EEG after a meal.[29] The disease can be diagnosed by assaying glucose transport in isolated intact erythrocytes. Seizures generally respond well to a ketogenic diet, but they tend to be refractory to conventional antiepileptic drugs. Phenobarbital should be avoided because of its potential to interfere with transport of glucose into the nervous system.[34]

Early infantile seizures can be seen in other disorders of carbohydrate metabolism, including hereditary fructose intolerance, d-glyceric aciduria, and galactokinase deficiency.

Congenital Disorders of Glycosylation

Congenital disorders of glycosylation (CDGs) are caused by deficiencies in glycoprotein biosynthesis and usually result in severe cognitive dysfunction. CDG type I (CDG-I) disorders are an increasingly expanding group of conditions caused by disturbances in the synthesis of the lipid linked glycan precursor or in the attachment of glycans to proteins. CDG-II disorders are caused by impairments of either the trimming of the protein-bound oligosaccharide or the addition of sugars. Seizures can be seen in infants with CDG-IE and CDG-IL. Patients with CDG-IE have had onset of seizures within the first year of life. Additional features are development delay, hypotonia, and acquired microcephaly. Laboratory evaluations showed hypoglycosylation on serum transferring and cerebral spinal fluid β-trace protein. The disorder is due to dolichol phosphate mannose synthase (DPM1) mutations.[32] Detailed descriptions of the seizures and EEG features are not available. CDG-IL is caused by deficiency of the ALG9 α1,2-mannosyltransferase enzyme and results in delay, seizures, hypotonia, diffuse brain atrophy with delayed myelination, failure to thrive, pericardial effusion, cystic renal disease, hepatosplenomegaly, esotropia, and inverted nipples. Detailed descriptions of the seizures are lacking. One report stated that the initial EEG shortly after onset of seizures was normal.[71] Febrile seizures are a common feature of CDG-IA, but afebrile seizures are only variably seen in this disorder.[33]

Organic Acidurias

Seizures in early infancy may be the presenting symptom of branched-chain organic acidurias. These include isovaleric aciduria, 3-methylcrotonyl-CoA carboxylase deficiency, 3-methylglutaconic aciduria with normal 3-methylglutaconyl-CoA hydratase, and 3-hydroxy-3-methylglutaryl CoA lyase deficiency (#246450).[76] In the latter condition, the urine has been observed to smell like a cat. The common mutation associated with this condition may alter the three-dimensional structure of the enzyme.[50] Seizures, including convulsions and infantile spasms, tend to be prominent in 3-methylcrotonyl-CoA carboxylase deficiency. The typical abnormal organic acid includes 3-hydroxyisovaleric acid and 3-methylcrotonyl glycine. Serum concentrations of free carnitine are very low.

Severe developmental delay, progressive encephalopathy, and seizures are the most common features of 3-methylglutaconic aciduria, but the biochemical features can also be identified in asymptomatic individuals.[1,19] Seizures occur in one third of cases, and infantile spasms have been reported early on. The typical organic acid abnormality includes marked elevations of 3-methylglutaconic acid and 3-methylglutaric acid in the urine.

Seizures are the presenting symptom in 10% of patients with 3-hydroxy-3-methylglutaric aciduria, a metabolic disorder caused by a deficiency of the lyase enzyme that mediates the final step of leucine degradation and plays a pivotal role in hepatic ketone body production.

Infantile spasms have been reported in patients with 3-hydroxybutyric aciduria. Facial dysmorphism and brain dysgenesis are prominent manifestations. The enzyme deficiency causing this condition is unknown. Urinary excretion of 3-hydroxyisobutyric acid in the absence of ketosis is diagnostic.

Glutaric acidemia type I is a more common autosomal recessive disorder of lysine metabolism that is caused by a deficiency of glutaryl-CoA dehydrogenase. Seizures often are the first clinical signs of metabolic decompensation following a febrile illness. Valproate and carnitine with a low-protein diet and riboflavin supplementation are recommended.

Aminoacidurias

Phenylketonuria (PKU; #261600) is typical of several disorders of amino acid metabolism whose symptoms appear in early infancy.[2] Phenylketonuria is caused by phenylalanine hydroxylase deficiency and is associated with mental retardation, microcephaly, psychotic behavior, and seizures.[47] Generalized seizures occur in 25% of patients. The majority of children with classic PKU who are treated early will have normal EEGs.[51] Focal and generalized slowing and epileptiform discharges have been reported in patients with abnormal EEGs. Increased delta activity may occur with oral phenylalanine loading. PKU may be successfully treated by dietary restriction of phenylalanine.

A hyperphenylalaninemic state may be the consequence of disorders of phenylalanine metabolism or tetrahydrobiopterin (BH_4) homeostasis. A disorder of BH_4 recycling produces severe neurologic regression and epilepsy that is refractory to antiepileptic drugs. Recurrent episodes of status epilepticus have been reported during the first year of life. The EEG may show hypsarrhythmia in early infancy. The typical biochemical profile is hyperphenylalaninemia, associated with decreased urinary and CSF biogenic amines.

A disorder of BH_4 synthesis secondary to deficiency of guanosine triphosphate cyclohydrolase (#233910) produces

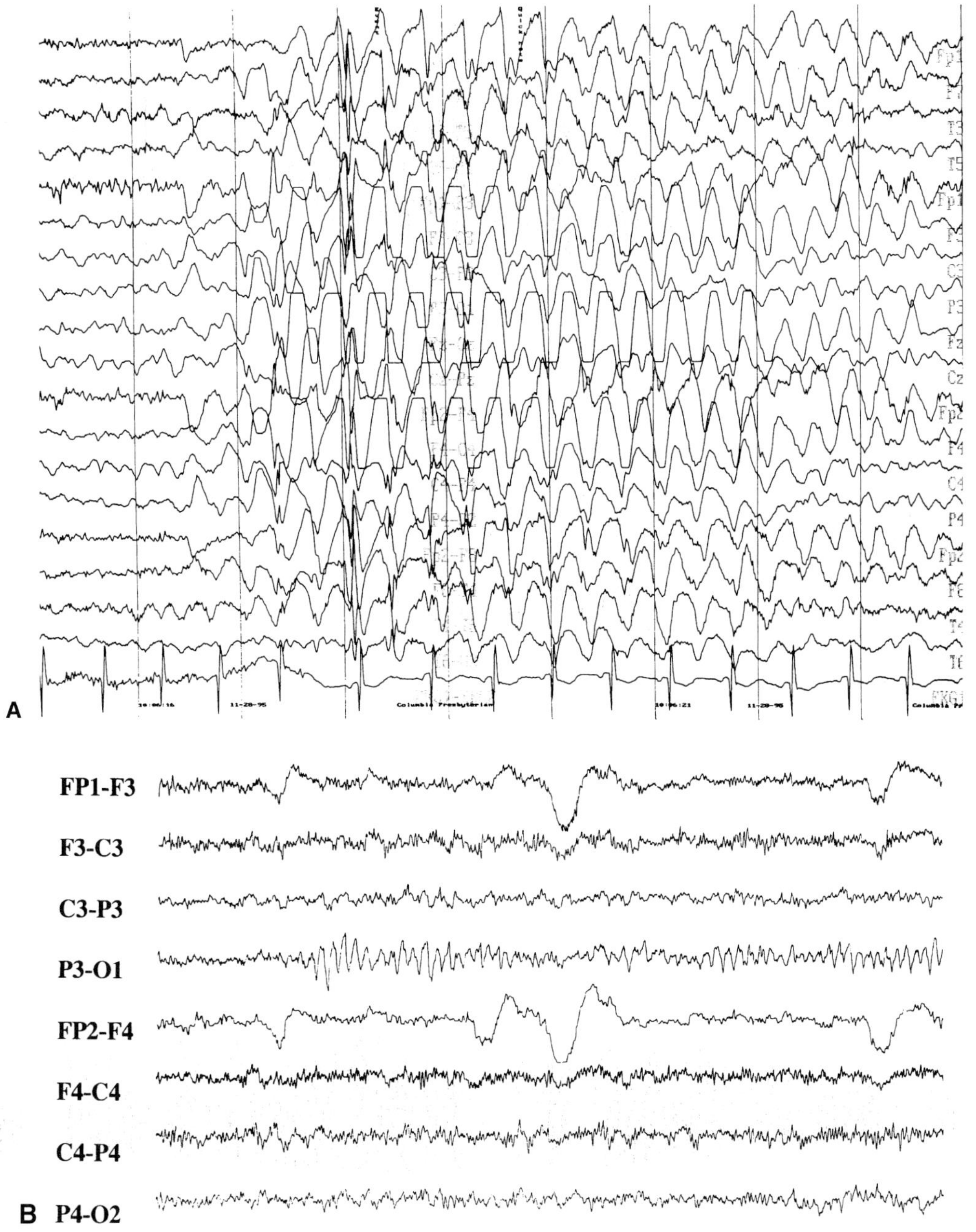

FIGURE 4. Typical electroencephalogram from a patient with glucose transporter type 1 deficiency syndrome. **A:** Bursts of generalized irregular spike-and-wave discharges and runs of rhythmic delta activity are associated with altered responsiveness. Similar discharges have been encountered in approximately one third of patients with glucose transporter protein deficiency. In other patients (not shown), multifocal spikes with very sharp morphology, rapid repetition, and a proclivity for the posterior head regions have been seen. **B:** Electroencephalogram showing a depression of the alpha rhythm on the right, consistent with a focal disturbance of cerebral function in the right posterior head region.

early developmental regression and infantile spasms. Control of seizures and improvement in the clinical condition can follow BH_4 replacement. Central replenishment of dopamine and serotonin can also lead to further improvement. The EEG of a patient followed at our institution revealed diffuse background slowing and multifocal spikes (Fig. 5). Deficiency of 6-pyruvoyal tetrahydrobiopterin synthase is characterized by progressive encephalopathy, pyramidal and extrapyramidal signs, and myoclonic seizures. Treatment with BH_4 and central neurotransmitter precursors controls seizures and normalizes the EEG.

Inborn errors of tyrosine metabolism cause seizures in patients of this age group. Tyrosinemia type III (4-hydroxyphenylpyruvate dioxygenase deficiency) was reported in a newborn with recurrent seizures and in children in whom infantile spasms developed. Electroencephalographic findings included generalized voltage attenuation with single-spike and polyspike discharges in the parietal-occipital areas.

Mental retardation and seizures occur with histidinemia or histidase deficiency. Infantile spasms and myoclonic seizures are frequent. Delayed development and an exaggerated startle response are additional features. Seizures are refractory to the

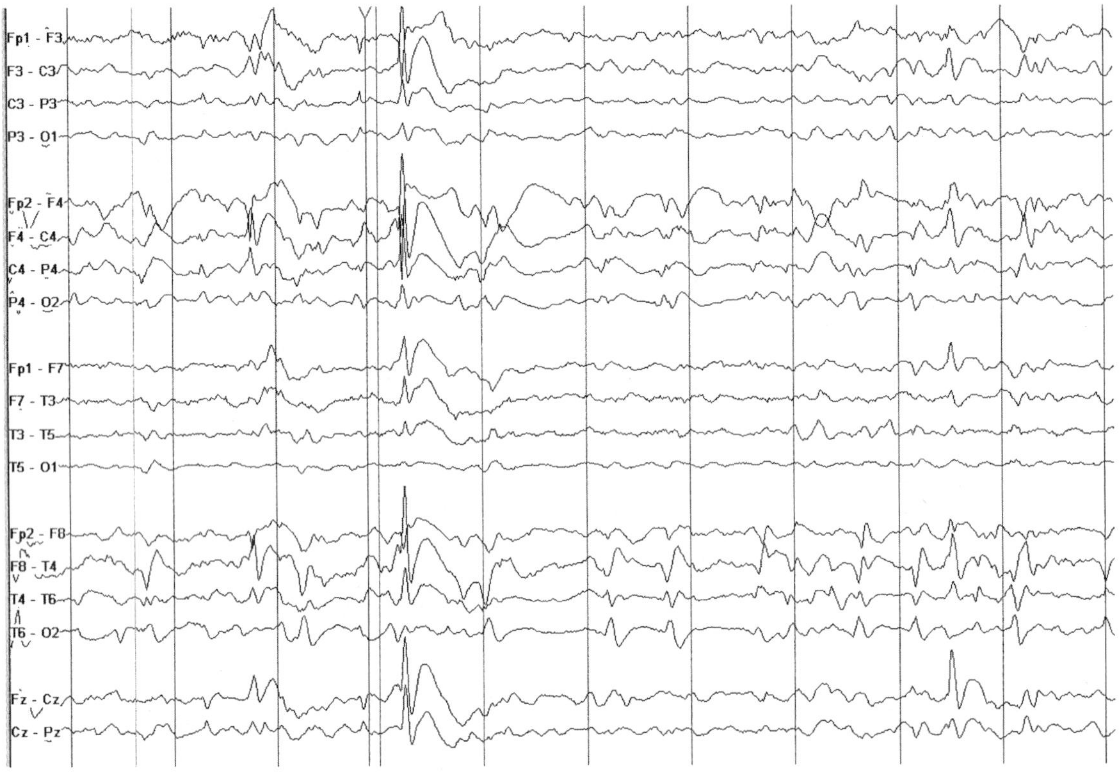

FIGURE 5. A 9-year-old child with guanosine triphosphate cyclohydrolase deficiency. Note severe background slowing with admixed multifocal spikes.

usual drugs, and only one patient has responded to a diet low in histidine. A few patients with hyperprolinemia type I (proline oxidase deficiency) have mental retardation, seizures, and severe encephalopathy. Hyperornithinemia-hyperammonemia-homocitrullinuria (HHH) syndrome is manifested by ataxia, myoclonus, chorea, spasticity of gait, mental retardation, and seizures.[15] Infantile spasms have been reported in association with this defect of intramitochondrial ornithine transport. Restriction of protein and supplementation with ornithine, arginine, and citrulline are recommended as treatment.

Defects of the Urea Cycle

Presenting symptoms of disorders of the urea cycle and disorders of branched-chain amino acid and keto acid metabolism can appear either in the neonatal period, as discussed previously, or during infancy.

Disorders of γ-Aminobutyric Acid Metabolism

4-Hydroxybutyric aciduria is an example of an inborn error of GABA metabolism that results from a defect in succinic semialdehyde dehydrogenase function (#271980).[30] Psychomotor retardation, language delay, hypotonia, and ataxia develop in affected children between the ages of 6 months and 11 years. Seizures may be the presenting symptom in about 50% of patients. Accumulation of 4-hydroxybutyric acid in urine, plasma, and CSF and variable elevations of glycine are characteristic. Valproic acid is effective in controlling the seizures. Although it should theoretically work, our personal experience with vigabatrin treatment in one case was very disappointing. Others have also found lack of a good effect.[20,22]

Menkes Disease

This is an X-linked inherited disorder that results from a defect in the Cu^{2+}-transporting ATPase α polypeptide.[39] As a result, copper-dependent enzymes, including cytochrome *c* oxidase, are catalytically less active. The disturbance in cerebral oxidative metabolism is reflected in elevated CSF concentrations of lactic acid. Affected infants have a progressive encephalopathy with characteristic facial features, abnormalities of the hair, and various skin manifestations, including cutis laxa, seborrheic dermatitis, recurrent rash, and hypopigmentation. Myoclonic seizures are common during the first 2 months of life and are generally refractory to treatment. The EEG shows multifocal epileptiform discharges. Details regarding the EEG findings are not often reported, but evolution to infantile spasms has been observed.[56] Copper histidinate, the only available treatment, may be effective if begun in the presymptomatic phase.

METABOLIC DISORDERS OF LATE INFANCY

In general, metabolic diseases that cause seizures in late infancy are disorders affecting the structural components of the nervous system. These conditions are inexorably progressive, and the most important ones are lysosomal (Table 1).

Metachromatic Leukodystrophy

Metachromatic leukodystrophy is the result of a deficiency of arylsulfatase A. There are at least five allelic forms, including the characteristic late-infantile variant. Gait disorder and ataxia are the most common presenting symptoms, which are followed by a progressive decline in mental and motor skills.[21]

Partial seizures develop late in the clinical course in 25% of patients with the late-infantile form of metachromatic leukodystrophy and in 50% to 60% of patients with the juvenile-onset form. Electroencephalographic findings include diffuse high-voltage slowing and occasional bursts of spikes. Slow-frequency activity may be asymmetric. Focal interictal epileptiform discharges predominate in the late-infantile form.[69]

Schindler disease (#609241) results from a deficiency of α-*N*-acetylgalactosaminidase and is an extraordinarily rare condition.[62] Affected patients appear normal at birth, but progressive neurologic decline becomes evident after 1 year of age. Manifestations include spasticity, cerebellar signs, and extrapyramidal dysfunction. Generalized tonic–clonic seizures and myoclonic jerks are common. Electroencephalographic abnormalities include multifocal spikes and spike-and-wave complexes.

Mucopolysaccharidoses

The mucopolysaccharidoses are a family of lysosomal storage disorders caused by the deficiency of several enzymes involved in the degradation of glycosaminoglycans. The various mucopolysaccharidoses share many clinical features, including a chronic and progressive course, multisystem involvement, organ enlargement, dysostosis multiplex, and abnormal facial features. The most frequently occurring mucopolysaccharidosis is Sanfilippo syndrome; four different subtypes have been described, each associated with a different enzymatic defect. Generalized seizures develop in about 40% of patients with Sanfilippo syndrome, but these are often easily controlled by antiepileptic drugs. Progressive dementia and severe behavioral disorders are other features. Bone marrow transplantation has been successful in several cases.

Neuronal Ceroid Lipofuscinoses

The neuronal ceroid lipofuscinoses (NCL) are a group of diseases with the common feature of storage of lipopigments in the brain and other tissues. At least seven clinical subtypes as well as additional rare atypical forms have been reported, and virtually all these are transmitted as autosomal-recessive traits.[53] Infantile NCL (#256730), also referred to as Santavuori-Haltia-Hagberg disease, is particularly common in Finland, with an incidence of 1/13,000 live births. The disease is caused by a defect in palmitoyl-protein thioesterase (PPT). Infants are normal in the neonatal period, but at about 1 year of age, rapid neurologic deterioration with ataxia occurs. Initially, patients may be given a misdiagnosis of Rett syndrome because of the deceleration of head growth and stereotypic abnormal hand movements. However, myoclonic jerks become increasingly evident, and the appearance of macular and retinal degeneration with optic atrophy allows cases of infantile NCL to be distinguished clinically from cases of Rett syndrome. The electroretinographic findings are abnormal, and the EEG shows progressive slowing and loss of amplitude. Some cases of Lennox-Gastaut syndrome have been caused by NCL. Symptoms of the late-infantile form of NCL, known as Jansky-Bielschowsky disease (#204500), appear in late infancy or early childhood, and epilepsy is the dominant clinical manifestation. This is due to a mutation in the CLN2 gene. Other features are ataxia and dementia. The EEG shows multifocal spikes and slow background rhythm and a highly characteristic response to photic stimulation. Stroboscopic light flashed at rates of <4/s produce high-voltage spike discharges over the posterior scalp regions. Visual-evoked potentials and somatosensory-evoked potentials are also of very high voltage. A pseudoperiodic pattern with absence of sleep spindles may be highly suggestive of the disorder in the early stages of presentation.[63] Seizures are difficult to control, and the diagnosis may be hard to establish. Skin or conjunctival biopsy specimens demonstrate abnormal cytosomes containing curvilinear bodies.

METABOLIC DISORDERS OF CHILDHOOD AND ADOLESCENCE

Numerous metabolic disorders make their presence known in later childhood or adolescence. These conditions largely represent variants of disorders discussed in the preceding sections. Seizures may occur, but not invariably, as shown in Table 4.

Homocystinuria

Disorders of transulfuration include cystathionine β-synthase deficiency, the most frequent cause of homocystinuria (#603174). Some patients respond to pyridoxine administration. Mental retardation, behavioral disturbances, and seizures are manifestations of nervous system involvement; ectopia lentis, osteoporosis, and scoliosis are other common clinical findings. Generalized seizures occur in about 20% of patients with pyridoxine-nonresponsive homocystinuria and in 16% of patients with the pyridoxine-responsive form. Electroencephalographic abnormalities are more common than seizures and may consist of either mild diffuse background slowing or focal interictal epileptiform discharges. These abnormalities may not respond to B6 administration.[13] Thromboembolism, malar flush, and livedo reticularis reflect vascular system involvement. Biochemical abnormalities include homocystinemia, methioninemia, decreased cystine concentration, and homocystinuria.

Diabetes Mellitus

Diabetes mellitus is the most common metabolic disorder. Seizures are generally not a feature except during metabolic crisis with ketoacidosis and cerebral edema. Nonketotic hyperosmolar diabetic coma has a high mortality, and generalized or partial seizures are common in this setting. Epilepsia partialis continua has been reported with nonketotic hyperglycinemia. Generalized tonic–clonic seizures have also been reported in a patient with diabetes mellitus who had an intracerebral hemorrhage during ketoacidosis.

Adrenoleukodystrophy

There are seven different clinical presentations of adrenoleukodystrophy (#300100).[43] It is caused by mutation in the *ABCD1* gene, which encodes an ATPase-binding-cassette protein. Symptoms of the X-linked form of adrenoleukodystrophy classically appear in early childhood. Partial motor seizures, often with secondary generalization, and generalized tonic–clonic seizures are common in this peroxisomal disorder. Status epilepticus has been the initial presenting symptom, and epilepsia partialis continua has also been reported. The EEG is characteristic, with high-voltage polymorphic delta activity and loss of faster frequencies over the posterior regions.[38]

Lysosomal Disorders

An example of this group of diseases is neuraminidase deficiency (#256550), characterized by progressive loss of vision, presence of a macular cherry red spot, and progressive and

TABLE 4

METABOLIC DISORDERS IN CHILDHOOD AND ADOLESCENCE

Disorder	Seizure frequency	Seizure type	EEG	Dysmorphism	Neuroimaging	Laboratory findings	Treatment
Tyrosinemia type I	+/++	G	Slow-wave acitvity in acute phase	Absent	Cerebral edema (rare)	Hyponatremia; aminoaciduria; high tyrosine; abnormal coagulation profile	Dietary, liver transplant
Homocystinuria	+/++	GTC	No specific abnormalities	Marfan-like; ectopia lentis	Normal	High methionine and homocysteine; low cystine; homocystinuria	Pyroxidine
Diabetes mellitus	++	P, EPC (nonketotic hyperglycemia), GTC	Diffuse or focal slow activity; focal paroxysms (sharp/slow wave)	Absent	Cerebral edema	Hyperglycemia; hyponatremia; hyperosmolarity	Mannitol therapy; fluid restriction
Pyrimidine disorders	+++	GTC, A	Generalized paroxysms; photic response	Absent	Hypoplasia CC; BG calcifications	High thymine and uracil	Symptomatic
X-linked adrenoleukodystrophy	+++	P, GTC, SE, EPC	Slow theta-delta waves of large amplitude	Absent	White-matter lesions	High VLCFA	Symptomatic; immunosuppression; bone marrow transplant
Sialidosis	+++ (type 1)	M	Abnormal background	Present (type II)	Cerebral, cerebellar atrophy	Abnormal urinary oligosaccharide pattern	Symptomatic
Niemann-Pick type C	++	GTC, P, akinetic	Diffuse theta slowing; bursts of spike-and-wave complexes; multifocal spikes	Absent	Cerebellar atrophy; large fourth ventricle; white-matter lesions	Accumulation of unesterified cholesterol; normal or elevated sphingomyelinase activity	Drug therapy
Gaucher disease	+++	P, GTC	Slow background; spike-and-wave paroxysms	Absent	Normal	Glucocerebrosidase deficiency	Enzyme replacement; bone marrow transplant
Krabbe disease	++	M, atonic, RSE	No specific pattern	Absent	White-matter lesions; enhancement of the splenium CC; low-density gray matter	Galactosylceramidase deficiency	Not available
Galactosialidosis	+++	M, GTC	Multiple spike-and-slow-wave paroxysms	Present	Normal	Abnormal oligosaccharides; combined β-galactosidase and neuraminidase deficiency	Not available
GM_2 gangliosidosis	++	P, GTC, M, gelastic	Spike-and-wave complexes; slow waves (anterior region)	Absent	Cerebellar atrophy	Abnormal oligosaccharides; hexosaminidase A deficiency	Not available

+, 0%–25% seizure activity; BG, basal ganglia; CC, corpus callosum; EEG, electroencephalogram; EPC, epilepsia partialis continua; G, generalized; GTC, generalized tonic-clonic; M, myoclonic; P, partial; RSE, recurrent status epilepticus; SE, status epilepticus; VLCFA, very-long-chain fatty acids.

disabling myoclonus but relative preservation of cognition. The condition is also known as the cherry red spot-myoclonus syndrome. Generalized seizures are common, and the EEG is characterized by low-voltage, fast background activity and positive spikes that correlate with massive myoclonic jerks. This form of neuraminidase deficiency is referred to as sialidosis type I. Sialidosis type II is subdivided into two groups, an infantile form with early onset and a juvenile form with early normal development.[37] The infantile form is characterized by progressive encephalopathy, visceromegaly, course facial features, dysostosis multiplex, and presence of macular cherry red spots. Seizures are uncommon. Symptoms of the juvenile form appear in childhood, and include progressive mental regression, myoclonus, short stature, dysostosis multiplex, course facial features, and cherry red spots. The EEG is abnormal in 50% of patients, with an irregular slow background activity and spike-and-wave complexes.

Niemann-Pick disease type C is an autosomal recessive lipidosis caused by a defect in cholesterol esterification (#257220), specifically a mutation in either the *NPC1* or *NPC2* gene.[49] The sphingomyelinase activity is normal or elevated. Neurologic manifestations are striking and include a progressive ataxia, supranuclear vertical gaze palsy, progressive extrapyramidal symptoms, and seizures.[27] Complex partial seizures, partial seizures with secondary generalization, and primary generalized tonic–clonic convulsions occur frequently. Akinetic seizures, often precipitated by sudden laughter, are less frequent but suggestive of the disorder. Conventional antiepileptic drugs are rarely effective.

Gaucher disease is another lysosomal disorder; it results from a deficiency of acid β-glucosidase. There are three clinical types. Type I (#230800) is characterized by hepatosplenomegaly, hypersplenism, and bone lesions. Type II (#230900) involves the nervous system, with early onset of progressive encephalopathy and visceromegaly. Type III (#23100) represents an intermediate form, characterized by early normal development, ocular apraxia, and slowly progressive mental and motor deterioration with ataxia. Complex partial seizures and generalized tonic–clonic seizures occur almost invariably. Some patients have early progressive myoclonus. Current treatment is enzyme protein replacement and bone marrow transplantation.

Finally, GM_2 gangliosidosis may appear in early to late childhood as a progressive ataxic syndrome associated with mental and motor deterioration and seizures. Partial complex seizures and generalized tonic or tonic–clonic seizures are particularly common. Generalized atonic seizures and gelastic seizures also have been described. Seizures are generally refractory to treatment.

DIAGNOSTIC INVESTIGATION

The diagnosis of genetically determined metabolic diseases is straightforward in many instances but complicated in others. For example, the classic aminoacidopathies and organic acidurias, once suspected, can be easily diagnosed by appropriate blood or urine measurements. Conversely, the diagnosis of an obscure condition, such as the carbohydrate-deficient glycoprotein syndrome, may require specific isoelectric focusing of the serum sialotransferrin isoform pattern in a specialized research laboratory.[23] Before obtaining appropriate metabolic, biochemical, or tissue specimens, the physician must have a reasonable differential diagnosis. Age of onset, clinical findings, family history, and neurologic examination continue to be the cornerstones of diagnosis. Experienced neurologists can often diagnose many of the disorders discussed in this chapter at the first clinical encounter. In such situations, laboratory studies serve only to confirm the clinical diagnosis. The presence of macular cherry red spots, abnormal appearance of the hair, or a peculiar distribution of fat over the posterior flanks or thighs immediately suggests the diagnosis of Tay-Sachs disease, Menkes disease, or the carbohydrate-deficient glycoprotein syndrome. Deceleration of head growth during infancy with consequent acquired microcephaly implies a defect of energy metabolism, the infantile form of NCL, or Rett syndrome, among other possibilities. Dislocated lenses and a seizure followed by a stroke are virtually diagnostic of homocystinuria. Genetically determined metabolic diseases often have a saltatory historical pattern, in contrast to neurodegenerative diseases, which are inexorably progressive.

A complete blood cell count with differential and platelet count should be obtained in every case. Bone marrow depression occurs in the ketotic hyperglycinemic syndromes. A review of the peripheral smear may reveal important clues, such as a macrocytic anemia or vacuolated lymphocytes. A complete serum chemistry profile will uncover carbohydrate and electrolyte disturbances or specific organ dysfunction. Calcium and magnesium concentrations should be determined in every case. Low uric acid concentration raises the possibility of molybdenum cofactor deficiency, and low blood urea nitrogen suggests a defect involving the urea cycle. Quantitative measurement of plasma and urinary amino acids is necessary to identify the various aminoacidopathies. A urinary organic acid profile should be obtained based on the first morning urine specimen.

A lumbar puncture is required to measure various CSF metabolites. Elevated CSF protein concentration is characteristic of metachromatic leukodystrophy and globoid-cell encephalopathy. Low CSF glucose concentration is consistent with hypoglycemia caused by a defect of gluconeogenesis or a defect in the transport of glucose across the blood–brain barrier (glucose transporter type 1 deficiency syndrome). Low CSF folate concentration suggests a defect involving folate metabolism. The presence in CSF of amino acids, specifically glycine, glutamate, and GABA, may be diagnostic of nonketotic hyperglycinemia or pyridoxine-dependent epilepsy. Lactate and pyruvate values are elevated in CSF in disorders of cerebral energy metabolism, including pyruvate dehydrogenase deficiency, pyruvate carboxylase deficiency, numerous disturbances of the respiratory chain, and Menkes disease. A low CSF lactate value may be seen in the glucose transporter protein deficiency syndrome. Abnormal findings on measurement of CSF biogenic amine and measurement of biopterin metabolism suggest several disorders associated with the hyperphenylalaninemic state.

Tissue biopsy specimens also provide important information in establishing a diagnosis. Specimens of skin, conjunctiva, rectum, peripheral nerve, and skeletal muscle may provide useful clues. Only rarely would a brain biopsy be necessary.

Electroencephalographic abnormalities are frequently helpful in establishing a diagnosis. A suppression-burst pattern is characteristic of nonketotic hyperglycinemia, phenylketonuria, maple syrup urine disease, and molybdenum cofactor deficiency. Distinctive EEG features include the comblike rhythm with 7- to 9-Hz central activity in maple syrup urine disease, vertex positive spikes in sialidosis type I, bioccipital polymorphic delta activity in X-linked adrenoleukodystrophy, and 14- to 22-Hz invariant activity with infantile neuroaxonal dystrophy.

Structural brain imaging provides important information, although findings are frequently nonspecific. Progressive atrophy is characteristic of NCL. White-matter signal abnormalities are characteristic of metachromatic leukodystrophy, globoid-cell encephalopathy, phenylketonuria, some mitochondrial diseases, Canavan disease, and some organic acidurias. Calcification of the cerebral cortex and basal ganglia is seen with many inherited metabolic diseases. Magnetic resonance spectroscopy may demonstrate elevated concentrations of lactate in brain tissue in various mitochondrial diseases or elevated concentrations of *N*-acetylaspartic acid in Canavan disease.

TREATMENT

The treatment of seizures associated with inherited metabolic diseases should focus primarily on the metabolic disturbance whenever possible. For example, seizures associated with a hypoglycemia are correctly treated with administration of glucose to maintain a normal blood glucose concentration. Similarly, seizures associated with hyponatremia, hypocalcemia, or hypomagnesemia respond best to correction of these electrolyte disturbances. Dietary treatment is appropriate for many inherited metabolic diseases, including defects of the urea cycle, defects of fatty acid oxidation, gluconeogenic defects, aminoacidopathies, organic acidurias, and the glucose transporter deficiency syndrome. The ketogenic diet is effective in controlling seizures in patients with the glucose transporter protein deficiency syndrome, and it provides some benefit in the management of patients with pyruvate dehydrogenase deficiency. Phenylketonuria can be well treated with a diet low in phenylalanine. Protein restriction is recommended for defects of the urea cycle, and fat restriction is advised for defects involving fatty acid oxidation. Pyridoxine-dependent epilepsy and other vitamin-responsive syndromes can be cured by early diagnosis and prompt administration of the specific vitamin or cofactor. Enzyme protein replacement has proved to be effective in Gaucher disease. Bone marrow transplantation has been used effectively to treat patients with mucopolysaccharidoses and adrenoleukodystrophy. Conventional antiepileptic drugs are useful adjuncts to these more direct therapeutic interventions but are often ineffective by themselves. Patients with certain inherited metabolic diseases (e.g., defects of fatty acid oxidation) may be less tolerant of some antiepileptic drugs, notably valproic acid, particularly because it interferes with fatty acid oxidation and depletes tissue stores of carnitine.

SUMMARY AND CONCLUSIONS

Seizures often are part of the clinical picture of inherited metabolic disorders, particularly when these conditions first appear in the neonatal period or during infancy. Why seizures commonly accompany some metabolic diseases and are infrequent in others is incompletely understood, but certain correlations are intuitively obvious. Defects of energy metabolism commonly are associated with seizures—witness the hypoglycemic syndromes and defects involving pyruvate metabolism, the Krebs cycle, and the respiratory chain. In addition, seizures frequently accompany inherited metabolic disorders that affect neurotransmission, such as nonketotic hyperglycinemia and pyridoxine-dependent epilepsy. A more fundamental common mechanism may be operative in many of these conditions. For example, an alteration in the ratio of glutamic acid to GABA may exist in conditions associated with cerebral energy failure and in conditions affecting the GABA shunt. Any inherited metabolic condition in which the extracellular glutamate concentration is elevated and the extracellular GABA concentration is lowered would lower the seizure threshold. Recent studies have confirmed this speculation in cases of symptomatic hypoglycemia, nonketotic hyperglycinemia, and pyridoxine-dependent epilepsy.

In contrast, defects of fatty acid oxidation are less likely to be associated with epilepsy. Fatty acids do not serve as oxidizable fuels for brain metabolism. Brain function is compromised principally when the patient is subjected to fasting and hypoketotic hypoglycemia develops. Under these conditions, the brain is deprived of its two primary fuels—glucose and ketone bodies. Disturbed consciousness and seizures may occur under these circumstances.

All infants and young children seen with unexplained seizures should be evaluated for an inherited metabolic disorder. A positive family history may provide an important clue, and careful studies of blood, urine, and CSF may uncover important diagnostic clues. Primary correction of the metabolic disturbance is the optimal treatment of the associated seizure disorder, even though conventional antiepileptic drugs may blunt the expression of the seizure disorder. In certain situations, antiepileptic drugs are ineffective, as is the case with the glucose transporter protein deficiency syndrome. Providing an alternative fuel source for brain metabolism by placing the patient on a ketogenic diet is effective in controlling seizures in this syndrome, whereas conventional antiepileptic drugs are ineffective.

It can reasonably be assumed that seizures in the neonatal period or infancy have a metabolic basis until it is proved otherwise. Careful study of this patient population will continue to identify novel inherited metabolic disorders and lead to more direct and effective treatments of these conditions.

References

1. al Aqeel A, Rashed M, Ozand PT, et al. 3-Methylglutaconic aciduria: ten new cases with a possible new phenotype. *Brain Dev*. 1994;16(Suppl):23–32.
2. Al Sanna'a NA, Van Kuilenburg AB, Atrak TM, et al. Dihydropyrimidine dehydrogenase deficiency presenting at birth. *J Inherit Metab Dis*. 2005;28(5):793–796.
3. Aukett A, Bennett MJ, Hosking GP. Molybdenum co-factor deficiency: an easily missed inborn error of metabolism. *Dev Med Child Neurol*. 1988;30(4):531–535.
4. Baxter P. Pyridoxine or pyridoxal phosphate for intractable seizures? *Arch Dis Child*. 2005;90(5):441–442.
5. Bennett CL, Huynh HM, Chance PF, et al. Genetic heterogeneity for autosomal recessive pyridoxine-dependent seizures. *Neurogenetics*. 2005;6(3):143–149.
6. Brown GK, Otero LJ, LeGris M, et al. Pyruvate dehydrogenase deficiency. *J Med Genet*. 1994;31(11):875–879.
7. Bruns J Jr, Hauser WA. The epidemiology of traumatic brain injury: a review. *Epilepsia*. 2003;44(Suppl 10):2–10.
8. Chien YH, Hsu CC, Huang A, et al. Poor outcome for neonatal-type nonketotic hyperglycinemia treated with high-dose sodium benzoate and dextromethorphan. *J Child Neurol*. 2004;19(1):39–42.
9. Clayton PT, Surtees RA, DeVile C, et al. Neonatal epileptic encephalopathy. *Lancet*. 2003;361(9369):1614.
10. Correa Leite ML, Nicolosi A, Cristina S, et al. Dietary and nutritional patterns in an elderly rural population in Northern and Southern Italy: (II). Nutritional profiles associated with food behaviours. *Eur J Clin Nutr*. 2003;57(12):1522–1529.
11. De Vivo DC, Hirano M, DiMauro S. Mitochondrial disorders. In: Moser HW, ed. *Handbook of Clinical Neurology*. Amsterdam: Elsevier; 1997:389–446.
12. De Vivo DC, Trifiletti RR, Jacobson RI, et al. Defective glucose transport across the blood–brain barrier as a cause of persistent hypoglycorrhachia, seizures, and developmental delay. *N Engl J Med*. 1991;325(10):703–709.
13. Del Giudice E, Striano S, Andria G. Electroencephalographic abnormalities in homocystinuria due to cystathionine synthase deficiency. *Clin Neurol Neurosurg*. 1983;85(3):165–168.
14. DiMauro S, Andreu AL, De Vivo DC. Mitochondrial disorders. *J Child Neurol*. 2002;17(Suppl 3):3S35–3S45.
15. Dionisi VC, Bachmann C, Gambarara M, et al. Hyperornithinemia-hyperammonemia-homocitrullinuria syndrome: low creatine excretion and effect of citrulline, arginine, or ornithine supplement. *Pediatr Res*. 1987;22(3):364–367.
16. Dublin AB, Hald JK, Wootton-Gorges SL. Isolated sulfite oxidase deficiency: MR imaging features. *AJNR Am J Neuroradiol*. 2002;23(3):484–485.
17. Escolar ML, Poe MD, Provenzale JM, et al. Transplantation of umbilical-cord blood in babies with infantile Krabbe's disease. *N Engl J Med*. 2005;352(20):2069–2081.
18. Friedman JR, Thiele EA, Wang D, et al. Atypical GLUT1 deficiency with prominent movement disorder responsive to ketogenic diet. *Mov Disord*. 2006;21(2):241–245.
19. Gibson KM, Sherwood WG, Hoffman GF, et al. Phenotypic heterogeneity in the syndromes of 3-methylglutaconic aciduria. *J Pediatr*. 1991;118(6):885–890.

20. Gordon N. Succinic semialdehyde dehydrogenase deficiency (SSADH) (4-hydroxybutyric aciduria, gamma-hydroxybutyric aciduria). *Eur J Paediatr Neurol.* 2004;8(5):261–265.
21. Greenfield JG. Form of progressive cerebral sclerosis in infants associated with primary degeneration of interfascicular glia. *Proc R Soc Med.* 1933;26:690–697.
22. Gropman A. Vigabatrin and newer interventions in succinic semialdehyde dehydrogenase deficiency. *Ann Neurol.* 2003;54(Suppl 6):S66–S72.
23. Hagberg BA, Blennow G, Kristiansson B, et al. Carbohydrate-deficient glycoprotein syndromes: peculiar group of new disorders. *Pediatr Neurol.* 1993;9(4):255–262.
24. Harding BN. Progressive neuronal degeneration of childhood with liver disease (Alpers-Huttenlocher syndrome): a personal review. *J Child Neurol.* 1990;5(4):273–287.
25. Haworth JC, Dilling LA, Surtees RA, et al. Symptomatic and asymptomatic methylenetetrahydrofolate reductase deficiency in two adult brothers. *Am J Med Genet.* 1993;45(5):572–576.
26. Head RA, Brown RM, Zolkipli Z, et al. Clinical and genetic spectrum of pyruvate dehydrogenase deficiency: dihydrolipoamide acetyltransferase (E2) deficiency. *Ann Neurol.* 2005;58(2):234–241.
27. Huttenlocher PR, Solitare GB, Adams G. Infantile diffuse cerebral degeneration with hepatic cirrhosis. *Arch Neurol.* 1976;33(3):186–192.
28. Iafolla AK, Thompson RJ Jr, Roe CR. Medium-chain acyl-coenzyme A dehydrogenase deficiency: clinical course in 120 affected children. *J Pediatr.* 1994;124(3):409–415.
29. Ito Y, Gertsen E, Oguni H, et al. Clinical presentation, EEG studies, and novel mutations in two cases of GLUT1 deficiency syndrome in Japan. *Brain Dev.* 2005;27(4):311–317.
30. Jakobs C, Bojasch M, Monch E, et al. Urinary excretion of gamma-hydroxybutyric acid in a patient with neurological abnormalities. The probability of a new inborn error of metabolism. *Clin Chim Acta.* 1981;111(2–3):169–178.
31. Kikawa Y, Shin YS, Inuzuka M, et al. Diagnosis of fructose-1,6-bisphosphatase deficiency using cultured lymphocyte fraction: a secure and noninvasive alternative to liver biopsy. *J Inherit Metab Dis.* 2002;25(1):41–46.
32. Kim S, Westphal V, Srikrishna G, et al. Dolichol phosphate mannose synthase (DPM1) mutations define congenital disorder of glycosylation Ie (CDG-Ie). *J Clin Invest.* 2000;105(2):191–198.
33. Kjaergaard S, Schwartz M, Skovby F. Congenital disorder of glycosylation type Ia (CDG-Ia): phenotypic spectrum of the R141H/F119L genotype. *Arch Dis Child.* 2001;85(3):236–239.
34. Klepper J, Fischbarg J, Vera JC, et al. GLUT1-deficiency: barbiturates potentiate haploinsufficiency in vitro. *Pediatr Res.* 1999;46(6):677–683.
35. Leary LD, Wang D, Nordli DR Jr, et al. Seizure characterization and electroencephalographic features in Glut-1 deficiency syndrome. *Epilepsia.* 2003;44(5):701–707.
36. Leimkuhler S, Charcosset M, Latour P, et al. Ten novel mutations in the molybdenum cofactor genes *MOCS1* and *MOCS2* and in vitro characterization of a *MOCS2* mutation that abolishes the binding ability of molybdopterin synthase. *Hum Genet.* 2005;117(6):565–570.
37. Lowden JA, O'Brien JS. Sialidosis: a review of human neuraminidase deficiency. *Am J Hum Genet.* 1979;31(1):1–18.
38. Mamoli B, Graf M, Toifl K. EEG, pattern-evoked potentials and nerve conduction velocity in a family with adrenoleucodystrophy. *Electroencephalogr Clin Neurophysiol.* 1979;47(4):411–419.
39. Menkes JH, Alter M, Steigleder GK, et al. A sex-linked recessive disorder with retardation of growth, peculiar hair, and focal cerebral and cerebellar degeneration. *Pediatrics.* 1962;29:764–779.
40. Mikati MA, Trevathan E, Krishnamoorthy KS, et al. Pyridoxine-dependent epilepsy: EEG investigations and long-term follow-up. *Electroencephalogr Clin Neurophysiol.* 1991;78(3):215–221.
41. Mills PB, Struys E, Jakobs C, et al. Mutations in antiquitin in individuals with pyridoxine-dependent seizures. *Nat Med.* 2006;12(3):307–309.
42. Moriwaki S, Takashima S, Yoshida H, et al. Histological observation of the brain of Tay-Sachs disease with seizure and chronic DPH intoxication—report of an autopsy case. *Acta Pathol Jpn.* 1977;27(3):387–407.
43. Moser HW, Loes DJ, Melhem ER, et al. X-Linked adrenoleukodystrophy: overview and prognosis as a function of age and brain magnetic resonance imaging abnormality. A study involving 372 patients. *Neuropediatrics.* 2000;31(5):227–239.
44. Naini A, Kaufmann P, Shanske S, et al. Hypocitrullinemia in patients with MELAS: an insight into the "MELAS paradox." *J Neurol Sci.* 2005;229–230:187–193.
45. Nguyen KV, Ostergaard E, Ravn SH, et al. POLG mutations in Alpers syndrome. *Neurology.* 2005;65(9):1493–1495.
46. Okada S, O'Brien JS. Tay-Sachs disease: generalized absence of a beta-D-N-acetylhexosaminidase component. *Science.* 1969;165(894):698–700.
47. Paine RS. The variability in manifestations of untreated patients with phenylketonuria (phenylpyruvic aciduria). *Pediatrics.* 1957;20(2):290–302.
48. Pascual JM, Lecumberri B, Wang D, et al. Type 1 glucose transporter (Glut1) deficiency: manifestations of a hereditary neurological syndrome [in Spanish]. *Rev Neurol.* 2004;38(9):860–864.
49. Patterson MC. A riddle wrapped in a mystery: understanding Niemann-Pick disease, type C. *Neurologist.* 2003;9(6):301–310.
50. Puisac B, Lopez-Vinas E, Moreno S, et al. Skipping of exon 2 and exons 2 plus 3 of HMG-CoA lyase (HL) gene produces the loss of beta sheets 1 and 2 in the recently proposed (beta-alpha)8 TIM barrel model of HL. *Biophys Chem.* 2005;115(2–3):241–245.
51. Rolle-Daya H, Pueschel SM, Lombroso CT. Electroencephalographic findings in children with phenylketonuria. *Am J Dis Child.* 1975;129(8):896–900.
52. Rutledge SL, Snead OC III, Kelly DR, et al. Pyruvate carboxylase deficiency: acute exacerbation after ACTH treatment of infantile spasms. *Pediatr Neurol.* 1989;5(4):249–252.
53. Santavuori P, Vanhanen SL, Autti T. Clinical and neuroradiological diagnostic aspects of neuronal ceroid lipofuscinoses disorders. *Eur J Paediatr Neurol.* 2001;5(Suppl A):157–161.
54. Scher MS, Bergman I, Ahdab-Barmada M, et al. Neurophysiological and anatomical correlations in neonatal nonketotic hyperglycinemia. *Neuropediatrics.* 1986;17(3):137–143.
55. Schweitzer-Krantz S. Early diagnosis of inherited metabolic disorders towards improving outcome: the controversial issue of galactosaemia. *Eur J Pediatr.* 2003;162(Suppl 1):S50–S53.
56. Sfaello I, Castelnau P, Blanc N, et al. Infantile spasms and Menkes disease. *Epileptic Disord.* 2000;2(4):227–230.
57. Shanske S, Pancrudo J, Kaufmann P, et al. Varying loads of the mitochondrial DNA A3243G mutation in different tissues: implications for diagnosis. *Am J Med Genet A.* 2004;130(2):134–137.
58. Tallur KK, Johnson DA, Kirk JM, et al. Folate-induced reversal of leukoencephalopathy and intellectual decline in methylene-tetrahydrofolate reductase deficiency: variable response in siblings. *Dev Med Child Neurol.* 2005;47(1):53–56.
59. Tan WH, Eichler FS, Hoda S, et al. Isolated sulfite oxidase deficiency: a case report with a novel mutation and review of the literature. *Pediatrics.* 2005;116(3):757–766.
60. Taylor MR, Hurley JB, Van Epps HA, et al. A zebrafish model for pyruvate dehydrogenase deficiency: rescue of neurological dysfunction and embryonic lethality using a ketogenic diet. *Proc Natl Acad Sci USA.* 2004;101(13):4584–4589.
61. Thoene J, Sweetman L, Yoshino M. Biotin-responsive multiple carboxylase deficiency [Abstract]. *Am J Hum Genet.* 1979;31:64A.
62. van Diggelen OP, Schindler D, Willemsen R, et al. alpha-*N*-Acetylgalactosaminidase deficiency, a new lysosomal storage disorder. *J Inherit Metab Dis.* 1988;11(4):349–357.
63. Veneselli E, Biancheri R, Buoni S, et al. Clinical and EEG findings in 18 cases of late infantile neuronal ceroid lipofuscinosis. *Brain Dev.* 2001;23(5):306–311.
64. Wang D, Pascual JM, Yang H, et al. Glut-1 deficiency syndrome: clinical, genetic, and therapeutic aspects. *Ann Neurol.* 2005;57(1):111–118.
65. Wang D, Pascual JM, Yang H, et al. Glut-1 deficiency syndrome: clinical, genetic, and therapeutic aspects. *Ann Neurol.* 2005;57(1):111–118.
66. Wang D, Sun RP, Wang X, et al. Progress in studies on the glucose transporter deficiency syndrome [in Chinese]. *Zhonghua Er Ke Za Zhi.* 2004;42(10):756–758.
67. Wang H, Kuo M. Pyridoxine sometimes fails to be activated to pyridoxal phosphate. *Brain Res Bull.* 2002;58(6):541.
68. Wang HS, Kuo MF, Chou ML, et al. Pyridoxal phosphate is better than pyridoxine for controlling idiopathic intractable epilepsy. *Arch Dis Child.* 2005;90(5):512–515.
69. Wang PJ, Hwu WL, Shen YZ. Epileptic seizures and electroencephalographic evolution in genetic leukodystrophies. *J Clin Neurophysiol.* 2001;18(1):25–32.
70. Weinberg KI. Early use of drastic therapy. *N Engl J Med.* 2005;352(20):2124–2126.
71. Weinstein M, Schollen E, Matthijs G, et al. CDG-IL: an infant with a novel mutation in the ALG9 gene and additional phenotypic features. *Am J Med Genet A.* 2005;136(2):194–197.
72. Winawer MR, Rabinowitz D, Pedley TA, et al. Genetic influences on myoclonic and absence seizures. *Neurology.* 2003;61(11):1576–1581.
73. Wolf B, Jensen KP, Barshop B, et al. Biotinidase deficiency: novel mutations and their biochemical and clinical correlates. *Hum Mutat.* 2005;25(4):413.
74. Wolf B, Norrgard K, Pomponio RJ, et al. Profound biotinidase deficiency in two asymptomatic adults. *Am J Med Genet.* 1997;73(1):5–9.
75. Zhang X, Vincent AS, Halliwell B, et al. A mechanism of sulfite neurotoxicity: direct inhibition of glutamate dehydrogenase. *J Biol Chem.* 2004;279(41):43035–43045.
76. Zoghbi HY, Spence JE, Beaudet AL, et al. Atypical presentation and neuropathological studies in 3-hydroxy-3-methylglutaryl-CoA lyase deficiency. *Ann Neurol.* 1986;20(3):367–369.

CHAPTER 262 ■ MITOCHONDRIAL DISEASES

MICHIO HIRANO, WOLFRAM S. KUNZ, AND SALVATORE DIMAURO

INTRODUCTION

Since the initial discovery of mitochondrial DNA mutations in 1988, our understanding of the mitochondrial encephalomyopathies has advanced at an astoundingly rapid pace. Numerous scientific and clinical reports have documented the discoveries, while review articles[19,23] and even several books[20,104] have summarized much of this progress. The purpose of this chapter is not to describe the mitochondrial encephalomyopathies comprehensively, but rather, to illustrate some of the fundamental clinical and scientific themes in these diverse disorders that often manifest epilepsy.

Mitochondria are vital organelles, because they (a) produce energy in the form of adenosine triphosphate (ATP) through oxidative-phosphorylation of carbohydrates, fats, and amino acids,[57,70,128] (b) are essential for intracellular calcium homeostasis,[28] (c) contribute to the synthesis of important metabolic precursors [e.g., uridine,[54] amino acids, and iron-sulfur (Fe-S) clusters[34]], and (d) finally, participate in cell death pathways.[39] Much has been learned about the functions of these organelles, and defects of specific processes provide an elegant and rational biochemical classification system of the mitochondrial diseases (Table 1). A prime example of a specific biochemical defect of mitochondria is carnitine palmityl transferase (CPT) II deficiency.[21] Transport of fatty acids through the mitochondrial membranes is impaired by specific mutations in CPT II. By contrast, mitochondrial respiratory chain disorders often do not conform to single-enzyme defects because multiple enzymes can be affected; therefore, this biochemical classification scheme has limitations.

Molecular genetics provides an alternative perspective of mitochondrial diseases. One can gain a better understanding of mitochondrial disorders by considering the several unique genetic characteristics of mitochondria. Mitochondria are unique mammalian organelles because they possess their own genetic material, mitochondrial DNA (mtDNA), which is a small (16.5 kilobases) circular molecule encoding 13 polypeptides, 22 transfer RNAs (tRNA), and two ribosomal RNAs (rRNA).[4] The mtDNA-encoded polypeptides are vital subunits of the respiratory chain. In addition, more than 1,000 mitochondrial proteins are encoded in the nuclear DNA (nDNA). Because mitochondria are the products of two genomes, defects in either genome can cause mitochondrial dysfunction. To date, most of the respiratory chain defects that have been characterized at the molecular genetic level are due to mtDNA mutations.[19,20,23]

An important principle of mtDNA genetics is *heteroplasmy.* Each mitochondrion contains two to ten copies of mtDNA and, in turn, each cell contains multiple mitochondria; therefore, there are hundreds to thousands of mtDNA molecules in each cell. Alterations of mtDNA may be present in some of the mtDNAs (heteroplasmy) or in all of the molecules (*homoplasmy*). As a consequence of heteroplasmy, the proportion of a deleterious mtDNA mutation can vary widely. An individual who harbors a large proportion of mutant mtDNA will be more severely afflicted by the mitochondrial dysfunction than a person with a low percentage of the same mutation. As a consequence, a given mtDNA mutation can produce a diverse spectrum of clinical severity among patients.

A second factor that can influence the expression of a mtDNA mutation in a person is the *tissue distribution* of that mutation. The best example of tissue distribution variation is offered by large-scale mtDNA deletions. Infants with a high proportion of deleted mtDNA in their blood can develop Pearson syndrome, a sideroblastic anemia often accompanied by exocrine pancreatic dysfunction.[68,92] Presumably, these infants have a high proportion of deleted mtDNA in the bone marrow stem cells. Some children survive the anemia with blood transfusions and subsequently recover, because the stem cells with a high proportion of deleted mtDNA are eliminated through a negative selection bias. Later in life, however, those children may develop the multisystem mitochondrial disorder Kearns-Sayre syndrome (KSS), characterized by ophthalmoplegia, pigmentary retinopathy, and cardiac conduction block.[53,93] Thus, variable tissue distribution broadens the clinical spectrum of pathogenic mtDNA mutations.

The third factor that determines clinical expression of a mtDNA mutation is tissue *threshold effect.* Cells with high metabolic activities are more severely affected by relatively lower levels of mtDNA mutations; therefore, these disorders tend to affect disproportionately the brain and muscles (encephalomyopathies).

A fourth unusual characteristic of mtDNA is *maternal inheritance.* During the formation of the zygote, the mtDNA is derived exclusively from the oocyte. Thus, mtDNA is transmitted vertically in a nonmendelian fashion from the mother to both male and female progeny. A single exception to this rule has been described; a man with exercise intolerance and two base-pair deletions in the mitochondrial-encoded gene for subunit 2 of complex I (nicotinamide adenine dinucleotide [NAD] dehydrogenase 2 [ND2]) showed paternal inheritance of mtDNA in skeletal muscle.[56,108] Because paternal inheritance of mtDNA appears to be exceedingly rare,[29,109,122] maternal inheritance is important to recognize in determining whether a family is likely to harbor a mtDNA mutation. A caveat to this principle is the fact that maternal relatives who have lower percentages of a mtDNA mutation may have fewer symptoms (oligosymptomatic) than the proband, or they may even be asymptomatic. Therefore, in taking the family history, it is important to ask about the presence of subtle symptoms or signs in maternally related family members who might be oligosymptomatic.

These peculiar features of "mitochondrial genetics" contribute to the clinical complexity of human mitochondrial

TABLE 1

BIOCHEMICAL CLASSIFICATION OF MITOCHONDRIAL ENCEPHALOMYOPATHIES

1. **Defects of transport**
   (a) CPT deficiency
   (b) Carnitine deficiency
   (c) Defects of FAD uptake (?)
2. **Defects of substrate utilization**
   (a) Pyruvate carboxylase deficiency
   (b) Pyruvate dehydrogenase complex deficiency
   (c) Defects of β-oxidation
3. **Defects of the Krebs cycle**
   (a) Fumarase deficiency
   (b) α-Ketoglutarate dehydrogenase (dihydrolipoyl dehydrogenase) deficiency
4. **Defects of oxidation-phosphorylation coupling**
   (a) Luft syndrome (loose coupling of muscle mitochondria)
5. **Defects of the respiratory chain**
   (a) Complex I deficiency
   (b) Complex II deficiency
   (c) Complex III deficiency
   (d) Complex IV deficiency
   (e) Complex V deficiency
   (f) Combined defects of respiratory chain components

From DiMauro S, et al. Mitochondrial encephalomyopathies. *Neurol Clin.* 1990;8:483–506, with permission.

disorders. Variable heteroplasmy of mtDNA mutations produces an extensive range of disease severity, whereas tissue distribution and tissue threshold of mtDNA mutations explain the frequent but variable involvement of multiple organ systems.

In addition to mtDNA mutations, nuclear DNA (nDNA) defects can also cause mitochondrial dysfunction. In fact, nDNA encodes most of the components of the respiratory chain and, since 1995, many nDNA mutations associated with defects in oxidative-phosphorylation have been identified.[19,20] In this chapter, we review the major mitochondrial encephalomyopathy syndromes associated with seizures. We will not quote or summarize the vast literature on mitochondrial encephalomyopathies; rather, we will try to convey some of the principles of evaluation, diagnosis, and treatment of these disorders with emphasis on epilepsy.

CLINICAL DESCRIPTION

The mitochondrial encephalomyopathies comprise a heterogenous group of multisystem disorders that typically affect infants, children, or young adults. Among these diverse conditions, specific clinical syndromes were recognized. Because clinicians are confronted with patients, the clinical classification of the mitochondrial disorders is of pragmatic significance in guiding the diagnostic evaluation, determining prognosis, and in directing therapy. The discovery of distinct mtDNA and nDNA mutations has demonstrated that, in general, clinical phenotypes have specific genotypes; however, some patients do not fit into any clinical syndrome, or they have an atypical presentation for a particular mutation.

Common to all mitochondrial disorders with prominent epilepsy is involvement of the central nervous system (CNS), particularly the cortex. Imaging techniques have confirmed that gray matter involvement is an early feature of myoclonus epilepsy with ragged-red fibers (MERRF) and of mitochondrial encephalomyopathy, lactic acidosis, and stroke-like episodes (MELAS); white matter abnormalities are also seen at later stages, but usually not in isolation.[15] Maternal inheritance is pathognomonic of mtDNA point mutations, whereas patients with single large-scale rearrangements tend to be sporadic. In addition, phenotypic variability in families is the general rule rather than the exception with pathogenic mtDNA point mutations.

Mitochondrial Encephalomyopathies Associated with mtDNA Mutations

Kearns-Sayre Syndrome

Rowland and colleagues defined Kearns-Sayre syndrome (KSS) by the obligate triad of ophthalmoplegia, pigmentary retinopathy, and onset before age 20, with at least one of the following additional features: Cardiac conduction block, ataxia, and cerebrospinal fluid (CSF) levels of greater than 100 mg/dL.[93] The existence of KSS as a clinical entity is supported by the fact that more than 150 patients with these characteristics have been reported.[43] About 90% of the KSS patients have single large-scale rearrangements of the mtDNA, either deletions, duplications, or both.[72,85] Typically, KSS patients are sporadic, because the mtDNA rearrangements seem to originate in oogenesis or early zygote formation. Despite the clear evidence of encephalopathy (dementia, basal ganglia calcifications, and spongy changes of the brain white matter), seizures are uncommon in KSS (5/156 patients) (Table 2).[43]

Myoclonus Epilepsy with Ragged-Red Fibers Syndrome

In contrast to KSS, MERRF includes epilepsy as a defining clinical feature. In addition, these patients have myoclonus, ataxia, and ragged-red fibers in the muscle biopsy.[32] Other common clinical manifestations associated with MERRF are hearing loss, dementia, peripheral neuropathy, short stature, exercise intolerance, lipomas, and lactic acidosis.[118] The majority of MERRF patients have a history of affected maternally related family members, although not all have the full syndrome.

In 1990, Shoffner et al. identified a mtDNA A-to-G transition mutation at nucleotide (nt) 8344 of the *tRNA*^{Lys} gene[113]; that mutation has been found in about 90% of MERRF patients tested.[118] This mutation was the first molecular genetic defect to be associated with a hereditary epilepsy syndrome. A second mutation in the same gene at nt-8356 was identified in a pedigree with typical MERRF[117] and in another family with overlap features of MERRF and MELAS.[134] In addition, a mutation at nt-611 in the *tRNA*^{Phe} gene has

TABLE 2

SEIZURE INCIDENCE IN SPECIFIC MITOCHONDRIAL ENCEPHALOMYOPATHY SYNDROMES

Syndrome	Incidence	Percent	References
MERRF	62/62	100	44
MELAS	97/102	96	43
KSS	5/156	3	44

MERRF, myoclonus epilepsy with ragged-red fibers; MELAS, mitochondrial encephalomyopathy, lactic acidosis and stroke-like episodes; KSS, Kearns-Sayre syndrome.

been also associated with MERRF.[63] Within families with a MERRF proband, oligosymptomatic and asymptomatic members harbor the same mtDNA mutation, but the phenotype is presumably attenuated by heteroplasmy and tissue distribution of the mtDNA mutation.[118]

Mitochondrial Encephalomyopathy, Lactic Acidosis, and Stroke-like Episodes Syndrome

MELAS is another maternally inherited disorder whose defining clinical features include (a) stroke-like episodes at a young age (typically before age 40); (b) encephalopathy manifest as seizures, dementia, or both; and (c) mitochondrial dysfunction with lactic acidosis, ragged-red fibers, or both.[44,82] Other commonly encountered manifestations include normal early development, migraine headaches, myopathic weakness, exercise intolerance, myoclonus, ataxia, short stature, and hearing loss.[44,82] It is uncommon for more than one family member to have the full MELAS syndrome; in most pedigrees, there is only one MELAS patient with oligosymptomatic or asymptomatic relatives in the maternal lineage.

Other Mitochondrial Encephalomyopathies with Epilepsy Caused by mtDNA Point Mutations

In addition to the three aforementioned common and well-defined phenotypes of mitochondrial diseases, several other epilepsy syndromes have been associated with point mutations of mtDNA (Table 3). These mutations reside predominantly in mitochondrial tRNA genes.[50,64,78,86,99,106,114,115,125] Although less common, mutations in polypeptide-coding mitochondrial genes have also been reported in patients with epilepsy.[11,13,17,65,75,124,130] Some of these mutations are associated with multisystem disorders such as maternally inherited Leigh syndrome (MILS),[17,115] neuropathy ataxia retinitis pigmentosa (NARP),[13] or Leber hereditary optic neuropathy

TABLE 3

MTDNA MUTATIONS ASSOCIATED WITH EPILEPSY

Phenotype	Gene	Nucleotide	Mutation	References
MELAS	$tRNA^{Leu(UUR)}$	3243	A-to-G	35
	$tRNA^{Leu(UUR)}$	3271	T-to-C	36
	$tRNA^{Leu(UUR)}$	3252	A-to-G	73
	$tRNA^{Leu(UUR)}$	3256	C-to-T	102
	$tRNA^{Leu(UUR)}$	3260	A-to-G	79
	$tRNA^{Leu(UUR)}$	3291	T-to-C	38
	$tRNA^{Phe}$	583	G-to-A	40
	$tRNA^{Val}$	1642	G-to-A	121
	$tRNA^{Gln}$	4332	G-to-A	5
	$tRNA^{Cys}$	5814	A-to-G	65
	$tRNA^{Lys}$	8296	A-to-G	95
	$tRNA^{Lys}$	8316	T-to-C	12
	$tRNA^{Lys}$	8356	T-to-C	134
	COX III	9957	T-to-C	64
	ND5	13513	G-to-A	100
	ND6	14453	G-to-A	88
	Cyt b	14787–90	4-bp del	16
MERRF	$tRNA^{Lys}$	8344	A-to-G	113
	$tRNA^{Lys}$	8356	T-to-C	117, 134
	$tRNA^{Phe}$	611	G-to-A	63
Atypical MERRF	$tRNA^{Leu(UUR)}$	3255	G-to-A	78
	$tRNA^{Ser(UCN)}$	7472	Ins C	86
	$tRNA^{Asp}$	7543	A-to -G	114
	$tRNA^{Lys}$	8342	G-to-A	126
	$tRNA^{His}$	12147	G-to-A	124
	ND3	10191	T-to-C	122
	ND5	13042	G-to-A	75
Seizures, PEO, diabetes, and deafness	$tRNA^{Leu(UUR)}$	3256	A-to-G	72
Cardiomyopathy, deafness, and seizures	$tRNA^{Ile}$	4269	A-to-G	120
	$tRNA^{Ile}$	4320	C-to-T	99
ME with recurrent episodes of epilepsia partialis continua	$tRNA^{Ser}$	7512	T-to-C	50, 106
	COX I	6489	C-to-A	130
Leigh syndrome	*ATP 6*	8993	T-to-G	13
		8993	T-to-C	17
	$tRNA^{Lys}$	8363	G-to-A	115
LHON	*ND1*	3460	G-to-A	11
	ND2	4640	C-to-A	11

(LHON).[11] In addition to epilepsy, other common manifestations include dementia, cardiomyopathy (typically hypertrophic) skeletal myopathy, and hearing loss.[99,120]

Mitochondrial Encephalomyopathies Associated with Nuclear Mutations

Leigh Syndrome

Subacute necrotizing encephalomyelopathy was originally described in 1951 by Dr. Denis Leigh, who reported a 6.5-month-old infant presenting with developmental regression that progressed quickly and led to death 6 weeks later.[61] At autopsy, Dr. Leigh observed multiple symmetric foci of spongy degeneration with microvascular proliferation in the brainstem tegmentum, thalami, cerebellum, posterior columns of the spinal cord, and optic nerves. He astutely noted that the neuropathologic alterations resembled those of Wernicke syndrome but spared the mamillary bodies, a consistent feature that distinguishes the two disorders.

The clinical presentations of Leigh syndrome (LS) are heterogeneous, due to variations in age-at-onset, rates of progression, frequency of epilepsy, and presence or absence of pigmentary retinopathy. The onset is often acute and may coincide with a febrile illness or may follow a seizure. Most LS patients present in infancy with psychomotor regression, whereas some present in childhood or adolescence. Adult-onset LS is uncommon. In infants with LS, in addition to developmental regression, generalized hypotonia, feeding problems, progressive vision loss due to optic neuropathy or pigmentary retinopathy, progressive external ophthalmoplegia, hearing loss, nystagmus, ataxia, and seizures are typical manifestations. In addition, failure to thrive, dysarthria, vomiting, and diarrhea are common manifestations. Respiratory dysfunction is often prominent and frequently causes death. Most infantile-onset LS patients die before age 2 years. In older infants or young children, LS may begin with ataxia, dystonia, or intellectual decline.

The clinical diagnosis of LS is usually made by brain magnetic resonance imaging (MRI) scans, which reveal increased signals in the basal ganglia and brainstem on T2-weighted or FLAIR images. The lesions are typically symmetric and commonly affect the putamen, globus pallidus, caudate, thalami, substantia nigra, inferior olivary nuclei, periaqueductal gray matter, and brainstem tegmentum. Magnetic resonance spectroscopy (MRS) scans reveal decreased N-acetylaspartate and increased lactate in the affected brain regions.

The causes of LS are biochemically heterogeneous and, to an even greater extent, genetically diverse (Table 4). LS has been associated with defects of pyruvate carboxylase, pyruvate dehydrogenase complex (PDHC), and mitochondrial respiratory chain complexes I, II, IV, and V.[10,98,126,129,135] The inheritance pattern depends on the specific mutated gene, but may

TABLE 4

MITOCHONDRIAL ENCEPHALOMYOPATHIES WITH EPILEPSY DUE TO NUCLEAR DNA MUTATIONS

Biochemical defect	Clinical phenotype	Defective gene or gene product
1. *Mutations in genes encoding structural subunits of respiratory chain enzymes*		
Complex I deficiency	Encephalomyopathy or Leigh syndrome	*NDUFS1, NDUFS2, NDUFS3, NDUFS4, NDUFS6, NDUFS7, NDUFS8, NDUFV1, NDUFV2*
Complex II deficiency	Leigh syndrome	Flavoprotein subunit of SDH
2. *Mutations in genes encoding assembly factors for respiratory chain enzymes*		
Complex I deficiency	Encephalopathy	*B17.2*
Complex III deficiency	Encephalopathy, tubulopathy, and hepatopathy	*BCS1L*
Complex IV deficiency	Leigh syndrome	*SURF1*
	Infantile cardioencephalopathy	*SCO2*
	Infantile encephalopathy	*SCO1, COX10*
3. *Defects of intergenomic communication*		
Autosomal recessive PEO with multiple Δ-mtDNA	MNGIE	Thymidine phosphorylase
	arPEO	*POLG1*
	ARCO	Unknown
Autosomal dominant PEO with multiple Δ-mtDNA	adPEO	*ANT1*, Twinkle, *POLG1*
MtDNA depletion	Infantile encephalopathy and hepatopathy	dGK
	Alpers disease	*POLG1*
	Infantile encephalomyopathy	ADP-forming succinyl-CoA synthase
4. *Defects of the mitochondrial membrane*		
Coenzyme Q10 deficiency	Myoglobinuria, encephalopathy, ragged-red fibers	Unknown
	Cerebellar ataxia	Unknown
	Infantile encephalomyopathy nephropathy	CoQ2

be autosomal recessive, X-linked recessive, or, as previously mentioned, maternally inherited.

Alpers Syndrome

Alpers or Alpers-Huttenlocher syndrome was reported in 1931 by Bernard Alpers, who described a previously healthy 3-month-old girl, who developed intractable seizures, blindness, and became stuporous before dying at age 4 months.[3] Neuropathology revealed widespread degeneration of the cortex and basal ganglia. Huttenlocher et al. described the pathologic findings in liver, which included microvesicular steatosis, proliferation of bile ducts, and cirrhosis.[48] Clinically, Alpers syndrome is characterized by autosomal recessive inheritance, normal early development, episodic neurodegeneration with psychomotor regression, seizures that become intractable, and hepatopathy. The occipital lobe is frequently affected, leading to cortical blindness. Onset is usually in infancy or childhood, but can be as late as 25 years. In patients with Alpers disease, valproic acid should be avoided because this drug can precipitate fulminant hepatopathy.

Ultrastructurally abnormal mitochondria in cerebral neurons suggested that the disease might be a mitochondrial encephalomyopathy[97]; this notion was confirmed by the identification of mtDNA depletion in association with pathogenic mutations in the gene encoding the catalytic subunit of mitochondrial DNA polymerase-γ (*POLG1*).[77]

Coenzyme Q_{10} Deficiency

Coenzyme Q_{10} (CoQ_{10}) is a small lipophilic molecule located in the inner mitochondrial membrane and composed of a quinone group and a poly-isoprenoid tail.[127] CoQ_{10} transfers reducing equivalents from complexes I and II to complex III. Deficiency of CoQ_{10} in skeletal muscle has been associated with four major phenotypes. A predominantly myopathic form is characterized by the triad of recurrent myoglobinuria, ragged-red fibers, and encephalopathy with seizures, ataxia, or mild mental retardation.[81] A more common ataxic form presents with cerebellar ataxia and atrophy with variable involvement of the peripheral nerves, muscle, and other CNS functions.[59,74] The third variant is a rare infantile encephalomyopathy with nephropathy.[92,96] Finally, a pure myopathic variant without epilepsy exists.[58] Presumably, all the CoQ_{10} deficiencies are due to defects of biosynthesis. The first mutation directly affecting CoQ_{10} biosynthesis was identified in a pair of siblings with the infantile form; the homozygous missense mutation resides in the *COQ2* gene, which encodes *para*-hydroxybenzoate-polyprenyl transferase.[87] It is important for clinicians to recognize patients with CoQ_{10} deficiency because the syndrome responds dramatically to CoQ_{10} supplementation (150–3,000 mg daily in adult patients).

EPILEPTIC SEIZURES

Seizures are a common manifestation of mitochondrial encephalomyopathies (Table 2). As with other clinical features, the frequency and severity of seizures varies with the syndrome and even among affected individuals within a family with a single mtDNA point mutation.

Kearns-Sayre Syndrome

Seizures have been rarely described in KSS. Of 156 reported patients, only five (3%) were noted to have seizures and, in four of these, epilepsy was attributed to electrolyte imbalance secondary to hypoparathyroidism.[43] The infrequency of epileptic seizures in KSS illustrates an important clinical point; although seizures are a common feature of MELAS and a defining symptom of MERRF, their relative absence in KSS reinforces the concept that distinct clinical syndromes do exist although overlap features sometimes occur. It is very likely that the spatial distribution of the mitochondrial defect in the CNS is the responsible factor that determines the association of certain mtDNA mutations with epilepsy.[56,123] This seems to be in line with the fact that KSS is a white matter disorder affecting preferentially brainstem tegmentum, white matter of cerebellum and cerebrum, cervical spinal cord, basal ganglia, and diencephalon,[56] which are brain areas with low epileptogenicity.

Myoclonus Epilepsy with Ragged-Red Fibers

Myoclonus epilepsy with ataxia comprises a classical neurologic triad originally described by Ramsey Hunt as *dyssynergia cerebellaris myoclonica*.[47] We now label idiopathic cases of that triad as Ramsey Hunt syndrome, which is one form of progressive myoclonus epilepsy (PME).[6] PME syndromes include a well-characterized set of disorders that are described earlier in this volume. Since 1980, when Fukuhara et al.[32] first defined MERRF, this syndrome has been increasingly recognized as a major form of PME.

Symptoms and signs in isolated MERRF patients may be clinically indistinguishable from other PME disorders such as Unverricht-Lundborg disease and Lafora body disease. The myoclonus typically affects limbs, and can be severe enough to interfere with normal voluntary functions such as writing, speaking, or walking.[7,32,91] The myoclonus can be virtually constant,[91] but is usually spontaneous and intermittent, and it may be photosensitive.[60] In one unusual patient, the myoclonus correlated with EEG spikes: Both manifestations were seen with eyes closed and disappeared when the patient opened her eyes.[33]

Patients with MERRF typically have generalized tonic–clonic seizures, which are responsive to conventional antiepileptic therapy. Focal clonic and akinetic seizures have been reported.[7,60] Visual or somatosensory auras may precede the generalized seizures.[7] Both myoclonus and seizures may be precipitated by photic stimulation, such as watching television.[33,91]

Mitochondrial Encephalomyopathy, Lactic Acidosis, and Stroke-Like Episodes

Patients with MELAS frequently manifest seizures, myoclonus, and ataxia; therefore, they may closely resemble individuals with MERRF. In a review of 110 reported MELAS patients, myoclonus was noted in 38% (23/72), seizures in 96% (97/102), and ataxia in 33% (23/70)[44]; however, stroke is the distinguishing clinical feature of MELAS.

Seizures are extremely common in MELAS patients and are not infrequently the initial clinical manifestation (28% in one series).[44] The seizures are sometimes associated with stroke-like episodes. It is possible that the increased metabolic demands imposed by the seizures provoke some MELAS strokes, and it is likely that the cerebral lesions cause the seizures, thus establishing a vicious cycle. Sometimes, febrile episodes accompany the seizures, raising the hypothetical possibility that the added metabolic stress of the febrile illness can precipitate seizures.

Information about seizures was available in 42 of the 110 reported MELAS patients we identified.[44] Of those patients, 26 had both generalized and partial seizures, and 10 had generalized epilepsy (including one patient with absence seizures).[22,31,46,49,66,67,80,103] Partial seizures were predominantly motor, (21 patients), and, less commonly, visual (six patients), temporal (three patients), auditory (one patient), or sensory (one patient).[22,31,46] At least six individuals developed status epilepticus.[22] Myoclonus is generally less common and less severe in MELAS patients than in MERRF patients.[44]

Other Mitochondrial Encephalomyopathies with Epilepsy Due to mtDNA Point Mutations

In addition to the common clinically delineated mitochondrial conditions, atypical or overlap encephalomyopathy syndromes with epilepsy—atypical MELAS, atypical MERRF, MELAS/MERRF, or MERRF/KSS—have been reported in association with mutations in genes encoding $tRNA^{Ser}$,[86] $tRNA^{Leu}$,[78] $tRNA^{Lys}$,[125] $tRNA^{Asp}$,[115] $tRNA^{His}$,[123] and the polypeptides ND3[124] and ND5.[75] Epileptic seizures have been also described in patients harboring mtDNA mutations that typically cause clinical syndromes without epilepsy, such as LHON.[11] Although more frequently caused by nDNA mutations, LS can be a manifestation of mtDNA point mutations[13,17,115] and is often associated with epilepsy. Furthermore, mitochondrial encephalomyopathies with recurrent episodes of epilepsia partialis continua have been linked to mutations in $tRNA^{Ser}$ genes[50,106] and subunit 1 of cytochrome C oxidase (COX) (CO1).[130]

Mitochondrial Encephalomyopathies Associated with Nuclear Mutations

Leigh Syndrome

Seizures are common in LS, but are particularly frequent in patients with MILS due to the T8993G or T8993C NARP mutations or with PDHC deficiency.[98] In contrast, seizures are less prominent in LS due to COX deficiency.

Alpers Syndrome

In Alpers syndrome, seizures are a clinical hallmark and include simple and complex partial, generalized tonic–clonic, epilepsia partialis continua, and status epilepticus. The seizures typically become intractable. EEGs often reveal very slow activity (≤ 1 Hz) of high-amplitude (0.2–1 mV) with polyspikes of lower amplitude.[41] In patients with this condition, valproic acid should be avoided because this drug can precipitate fulminant hepatopathy.

Coenzyme Q_{10} Deficiency

Seizures have been observed in three of the four clinical phenotypes associated CoQ_{10} deficiency: The predominantly myopathic form, the ataxic form, and the infantile encephalomyopathy with nephropathy.[59,74,81,92,96] Although detailed descriptions of the epileptic syndromes in CoQ_{10} deficiency are lacking, complex partial and generalized seizures have improved with oral CoQ10 supplementation.[18,74,96]

DIAGNOSTIC INVESTIGATION

Clinical Issues

As with any patient with a neurologic disorder, one must begin with the clinical evaluation. These disorders are typically multisystemic and clinically variable. The wide clinical diversity provides diagnostic challenges even for experienced neurologists. In obtaining the medical history of patients suspected to have a mitochondrial encephalomyopathy, clinicians should inquire about the following clinical features: Normal infancy and early development, premature exercise-induced fatigue, migraine headaches, diabetes mellitus, short stature, and hearing loss. Multiple lipomas are not uncommon in MERRF syndrome and hypoparathyroidism in KSS. Family history is important, but may be very subtle when dealing with a mtDNA point mutation. For example, in families with MELAS syndrome, relatives in the maternal lineage may have migraine-like headaches or diabetes mellitus as the only manifestation of the genetic defect.

A careful physical examination may reveal subtle clues to the correct diagnosis. Patients are often short and thin. Multiple lipomatosis can be disfiguring in patients with MERRF or in their maternal relatives.[7] Dementia can be a prominent finding in KSS, MELAS, and MERRF.[43] Cranial nerve functions may be impaired and affect particularly extraocular muscles, with ptosis and progressive external ophthalmoplegia (PEO), which are necessary to diagnose KSS, but are sometimes seen in MELAS patients. Funduscopy may reveal pigmentary retinopathy in KSS and, less commonly, in MELAS and MERRF. Optic atrophy is sometimes detected in MERRF patients. Peripheral neuropathy is frequent in MERRF and MELAS. Sensorineural hearing loss is common in many mitochondrial encephalomyopathies.

Clinical Laboratory Tests

The laboratory evaluation should begin with routine blood tests, including complete blood count, serum electrolytes (including calcium and phosphate), liver function tests, blood urea nitrogen, creatinine, lactate, and pyruvate. These tests may reveal parathyroid, kidney, or liver dysfunction. Lactate and pyruvate at rest are commonly elevated in patients with mitochondrial encephalomyopathies, and these values may increase dramatically after moderate exercise.

Electrocardiograms may reveal preexcitation in MELAS or MERRF, and heart block in KSS or MELAS. Lumbar puncture may show elevated CSF protein, especially in KSS patients, in whom it is often greater than 100 mg/dL. CSF may also reveal elevated lactate and pyruvate levels. Electromyography and nerve conduction studies are typically consistent with a myogenic process, although neurogenic changes may be detected in MERRF or MELAS. Brain imaging with CT or MRI scans may reveal basal ganglia calcifications and atrophy in all three major syndromes. In MELAS patients, neuroimaging often reveals lesions compatible with strokes that typically affect the posterior cerebrum and generally do not conform to the distribution of major arteries.[1,2,67]

Electroencephalogram findings are usually not specific. Of 27 MELAS patients with seizures, EEG demonstrated diffuse slowing in 20 individuals and focal slowing in seven; epileptic activity was diffuse in 12 patients and focal in 15.[22] One MELAS patient had clinical and radiologic evidence of a left occipital stroke and a normal EEG.[67]

In 62 reported MERRF patients, we were able to identify descriptions of 32 EEGs; all were considered abnormal.[7,9,25,27,30,32,33,44,60,62,76,84,89–91,110,118,119,132] Although details of the EEGs were not available in all cases, 13 showed slowing (12 generalized, one focal and generalized) and 14 revealed epileptiform activity (12 generalized, one focal, one bitemporal). Photic stimulation was elicited in seven of nine MERRF patients, whereas hyperventilation produced epileptiform activity in one of three patients. The relationship of myoclonus and EEG discharges was unclear in several cases.[119] As in other forms of progressive myoclonus epilepsy, somatosensory evoked responses typically reveal giant cortical evoked responses.[119]

Special Laboratory Tests

Clinical research has contributed greatly to our understanding of mitochondrial disorders and to our diagnostic capabilities. Specialized evaluation for oxidative-phosphorylation defects has evolved from laboratory research and includes histology (particularly skeletal muscle), measurement of oxidative-phosphorylation enzyme activities, and molecular genetic analyses.

Histology

Histology has focused on skeletal muscle, but mitochondrial changes have been noted in other tissues. In the mid-1960s, Shy, Gonatas, and Perez described the typical ultrastructural alterations seen in mitochondrial myopathies.[116] These changes include (a) an overabundance of ultrastructurally normal mitochondria ("pleoconial myopathy"), (b) enlarged mitochondria with disoriented cristae ("megaconial myopathy"), and (c) "paracrystalline" and "osmiophilic" inclusions within mitochondria.[116] Engel and Cunningham developed a modified Gomori trichrome stain,[24] which has been commonly used to identify fibers with subsarcolemmal accumulations of mitochondria, which are commonly referred to as "ragged-red fibers."

Histochemical stains for mitochondrial enzymes are also used to identify excessive mitochondrial proliferation and to demonstrate specific enzyme defects. These stains include succinate dehydrogenase (SDH), nicotinamide dehydrogenase-tetrazolium reductase (NADH-TR), and cytochrome *c* oxidase (COX). Immunohistochemical techniques are used to identify defects in specific mitochondrial polypeptides.

In KSS, MELAS, and MERRF, RRF with ultrastructurally abnormal mitochondria are almost always identified in skeletal muscle by the Gomori trichrome stain. SDH histochemistry reveals mitochondrial proliferation as hyperintense staining in subsarcolemmal regions of muscle fibers. In MELAS patients, excessive SDH staining often occurs within blood vessel walls, so-called strongly SDH-reactive vessels or SSVs.[42,94] Another characteristic of skeletal muscle from MELAS patients is the relative preservation of COX staining in RRF, in contrast to muscle from KSS and MERRF, which generally shows an abundance of COX-negative RRF on serial or double-stained (SDH and COX) sections. Nevertheless, histologic abnormalities in skeletal muscle biopsies are absent in some patients with MERRF[113] or other mitochondrial disorders.[45,46]

Unfortunately for clinicians, the histologic abnormalities described are neither specific nor sensitive enough to define all mitochondrial diseases. Morphologically abnormal muscle mitochondria have been detected in many conditions that are not primary oxidative-phosphorylation defects, for example, inflammatory myopathies[14] and myotonic dystrophy.[26] Conversely, some conditions with defects of respiratory chain enzymes do not have morphologically abnormal mitochondria, including LHON, LS, and Alpers syndrome.

Biochemistry (Enzyme Assays)

Activities of mitochondrial respiratory chain enzymes can be measured in vitro using crude extracts or isolated mitochondria. In KSS, MELAS, and MERRF, one can detect various combinations of respiratory chain enzyme deficiencies; however, the pattern is often not consistent, and normal enzyme activities have been reported. Factors influencing the activities of mitochondrial respiratory chain enzymes are the degree of heteroplasmy[37] and the distribution pattern of the mutation within the skeletal muscle biopsy sample.[38]

Molecular Genetics

Since the initial discoveries of the first mtDNA point mutation and large-scale deletions in 1988,[45,131,133] there has been an outburst of information relating molecular genetic defects to human disorders. Numerous mtDNA mutations have been identified including duplications, depletion, single and multiple deletions, and more than 100 pathogenic point mutations.[19,20,23]

Holt et al. first identified large-scale mtDNA deletions in mitochondrial myopathy patients[45] and, soon thereafter, Zeviani et al. pointed out the specific association with KSS.[133] Approximately 90% of KSS patients have large-scale mtDNA deletions, duplications, or both.[72,85] The mtDNA deletions generally range from about 2.0 to 10.4 kb in length,[45,72] and are mainly confined to an 11-kb region that does not include the origins of mtDNA replication or mtDNA promoter regions. About one-third of the mtDNA deletions involve an identical 4,977 base pair (bp) segment, which is often referred to as the "common deletion."[72] The majority of the mtDNA deletions are flanked by direct DNA sequence repeats, which suggests that they may originate from homologous recombination events.[45,51,69,105,112] The large-scale mtDNA deletions are often undetectable in leukocytes, so that molecular diagnosis requires muscle biopsy.

MERRF was the first multisystemic disorder to be associated with a mtDNA point mutation, specifically, A8344G in the transfer RNA lysine ($tRNA^{Lys}$) gene.[113] A second $tRNA^{Lys}$ mutation at nt-8356 was associated with both MERRF and MERRF-MELAS phenotypes,[117,134] and a $tRNA^{Phe}$ mutation at nt-611 has been associated with MERRF.[86] These point mutations can be easily identified in blood leukocytes from patients.

MELAS was also associated with a specific mtDNA point mutation, an adenine-to-guanine transition in the $tRNA^{Leu(UUR)}$ gene at nt3243 (A3243G). About 80% to 90% of MELAS patients have been found to harbor this mutation. Fifteen other mtDNA mutations have been identified in patients with MELAS, and a large number of other mtDNA point mutations have been associated with epilepsy (Table 3). As in MERRF, blood leukocytes can be screened for epilepsy-associated mtDNA point mutations.

Although the identification of mtDNA mutations has simplified diagnosis in most cases of mitochondrial encephalomyopathies, it has created new dilemmas. Genetic counseling of patients and their maternal relatives is difficult because heteroplasmy and variability of mutation loads in different tissues make clinical outcome predictions tenuous. Similarly, prenatal diagnosis is also perilous. The molecular genetic information should be handled carefully, because it can adversely affect medical insurability, employment opportunities, and the emotional status of patients.

TREATMENT

The medical management of mitochondrial myopathy has lagged behind research and diagnostic knowledge. Treatment can be divided into two types: Symptom management and metabolic therapy.

Symptom Management

Seizures in MERRF and MELAS typically respond to conventional antiepilepsy drugs[119]; however, they may be difficult to control in the setting of metabolic disarray. There have been reports that valproate therapy can cause adverse effects in certain patients with mitochondrial encephalomyopathies and particularly in individuals with Alpers syndrome.[8,107] The electrolyte disturbances related to hypoparathyroidism and diabetes mellitus should be corrected. Thyroid hormone replacement will alleviate the hypothyroidism. Cardiac pacemaker placement can prolong life in KSS patients with cardiac conduction defects.

Metabolic Therapy

Treatments aimed at the primary biochemical defects in mitochondrial encephalomyopathies have been tried; however, the evidence of efficacy has been anecdotal. We generally recommend CoQ_{10}, 50 to 200 mg t.i.d. and L-carnitine, 1,000 mg t.i.d. Idebenone, a related quinone, has also been administered to patients and has the theoretical advantage of better crossing the blood–brain barrier.

Dichloroacetate, a lactate-lowering agent, was shown to cause or exacerbate peripheral neuropathy, which overshadowed potential benefit in a randomized double-blind placebo-controlled trial in MELAS patients.[52] Vitamins that may donate electrons directly to COX include phylloquinone (vitamin K_1), menadione (vitamin K_3), and ascorbic acid (vitamin C).[111] Vitamin C has also been used as an antioxidant because the impaired oxidative-phosphorylation pathway may generate increased amounts of free radicals. Nicotinamide and riboflavin have been used to improve electron chain functions.[83]

In cultured human cells, ketone body treatment reduced the amount of deleted mtDNA.[101] This finding, coupled with the fact that ketogenic treatment has been effective in children with intractable epilepsy,[55] suggests that a ketogenic diet may be an effective treatment for patients with heteroplasmic mtDNA mutations and seizure disorders, but clinical trials have not yet been conducted to demonstrate safety and clinical efficacy.

SUMMARY AND CONCLUSIONS

Since the seminal publications of the first pathogenic human mtDNA mutations in 1988, the field of mitochondrial encephalomyopathies has expanded at a rapid rate. Molecular genetic research has led the way through the identification of numerous mutations including more than 100 different mtDNA point mutations, numerous single mtDNA large-scale deletions and duplications, multiple mtDNA deletions, mtDNA depletion, and a growing number of nuclear DNA mutations. Seizures are common manifestations, and the first epilepsy syndrome to be defined at the molecular genetic level was MERRF.[113] Modern histology with histochemistry, immunohistochemistry, and ultrastructural analysis has provided further insight into the pathogenesis of these disorders. Correlations of genotypes and phenotypes revealed general relationships between specific mutations and clinical syndromes; however, we learned that there can be wide variability of the clinical manifestations of a given mtDNA mutation. Due to this clinical complexity, neurologists must carefully evaluate patients with suspected mitochondrial encephalomyopathies to reach the correct diagnosis. Genetic counseling is important, but is imprecise in families with heteroplasmic mtDNA point mutations. Treatment is primarily symptomatic, and seizures are generally amenable to conventional antiepileptic agents. Clearly, there is a large gap in our understanding of how the mtDNA defects lead to human disease; however, as our knowledge expands, more rational and specific therapies may develop.

References

1. Abe K, Inui T, Hirono N, et al. Fluctuating MR images with mitochondrial encephalopathy, lactic acidosis, stroke-like syndrome (MELAS). *Neuroradiology*. 1990;32:77.
2. Allard J, Tilak S, Carter A. CT and MR of MELAS syndrome. *Am J Neurorad*. 1988;9:1234–1238.
3. Alpers BJ. Diffuse progressive degeneration of the grey matter of the cerebrum. *Arch Neurol Psychiatry*. 1931;25:469–505.
4. Anderson S, Bankier AT, Barrel BG, et al. Sequence and organization of the human mitochondrial genome. *Nature*. 1981;290:457–465.
5. Bataillard M, Chatzoglou E, Rumbach L, et al. Atypical MELAS syndrome associated with a new mitochondrial tRNA glutamine point mutation. *Neurology*. 2001;56:405–407.
6. Berkovic S, Andermann F, Carpenter S, et al. Progressive myoclonus epilepsies: Specific causes and diagnosis. *N Engl J Med*. 1986;315:296–305.
7. Berkovic SF, Carpenter S, Evans A, et al. Myoclonus epilepsy and ragged-red fibres (MERRF): A clinical, pathological, biochemical, magnetic resonance spectrographic and positron emission tomographic study. *Brain*. 1989;112:1231–1260.
8. Bicknese AR, May W, Hickey WF, et al. Early childhood hepatocerebral degeneration misdiagnosed as valproate hepatotoxicity. *Ann Neurol*. 1992;32:767–775.
9. Bindoff L, Desnuelle C, Birch-Machin M, et al. Multiple defects of the mitochondrial respiratory chain in a mitochondrial encephalopathy (MERRF): A clinical, biochemical and molecular study. *J Neurol Sci*. 1991;102:17–24.
10. Bourgeron T, Rustin P, Chretien D, et al. Mutation of a nuclear succinate dehydrogenase gene results in mitochondrial respiratory chain deficiency. *Nature Genet*. 1995;11:144–149.
11. Brown MD, Zhadanov S, Allen JC, et al. Novel mtDNA mutations and oxidative phosphorylation dysfunction in Russian LHON families. *Hum Genet*. 2001;109:33–39.
12. Campos Y, Lorenzo G, Martin MA, et al. A mitochondrial tRNA(Lys) gene mutation (T8316C) in a patient with mitochondrial myopathy, lactic acidosis, and stroke-like episodes. *Neuromuscul Disord*. 2000;10:493–496.
13. Canafoglia L, Franceschetti S, Antozzi C, et al. Epileptic phenotypes associated with mitochondrial disorders. *Neurology*. 2001;56:1340–1346.
14. Carpenter S, Karpati G, Eisen AA. A morphologic study of muscle in polymyositis: Clues to pathogenesis of different types. In: Amsterdam: Excerpta Medica, 1975;374–379.
15. Cock H, Schapira AH. Mitochondrial DNA mutations and mitochondrial dysfunction in epilepsy. *Epilepsia*. 1999;40 Suppl 3:33–40.
16. De Coo IF, Renier WO, Ruitenbeek W, et al. A 4–base pair deletion in the mitochondrial cytochrome b gene associated with parkinsonism/MELAS overlap syndrome. *Ann Neurol*. 1999;45:130–133.
17. de Vries DD, van Engelen BG, Gabreels FJ, et al. A second missense mutation in the mitochondrial ATPase 6 gene in Leigh's syndrome. *Ann Neurol*. 1993;34:410–412.
18. Di Giovanni S, Mirabella M, Spinazzola A, et al. Coenzyme Q10 reverses pathological phenotype and reduces apoptosis in familial CoQ10 deficiency. *Neurology*. 2001;57:515–518.
19. DiMauro S, Hirano M. Mitochondrial encephalomyopathies: An update. *Neuromuscul Disord*. 2005;15:276–286.
20. DiMauro S, Hirano M, Schon EA. *Mitochondrial Medicine*. London: Taylor & Francis, 2006.
21. DiMauro S, Melis-DiMauro PM. Muscle carnitine palmitoyl-transferase deficiency and myoglobinuria. *Science*. 1973;182:929–931.
22. DiMauro S, Ricci E, Hirano M, et al. Epilepsy in mitochondrial encephalomyopathies. *Elsevier Science Publishers B*. In: Anderson VE, Hauser WA, Leppik IE, et al. Genetic Strategies in Epilepsy. Amsterdam. 1991:173–180.
23. DiMauro S, Schon EA. Mitochondrial respiratory-chain diseases. *N Engl J Med*. 2003;348:2656–2668.
24. Engel WK, Cunningham CG. Rapid examination of muscle tissue: An improved trichrome stain method for fresh-frozen biopsy sections. *Neurology*. 1963;13:919–923.
25. Estournet B, Duyckaerts C, Marsac C, et al. Encephalopathie mitochondriale familiale. Etude clinicopathologique. *Rev Neurol*. 1991;147:491–496.
26. Fardeau M. Ultrastructural lesions in progressive muscular dystrophies: A critical study of their specificity. In: Canal N, Scarlato G, Walton JN. Muscle Diseases. Amsterdam: Excerpta Medica, 1970;98–108.
27. Federico A, Cornelio F, DiDonato S, et al. Mitochondrial encephalo-neuromyopathy with myoclonus epilepsy, basal nuclei calcifications and hyperlactacidemia. *Ital J Neurol Sci*. 1988;9:65–71.
28. Filippin L, Magalhaes PJ, Di Benedetto G, et al. Stable interactions between mitochondria and endoplasmic reticulum allow rapid accumulation of calcium in a subpopulation of mitochondria. *J Biol Chem*. 2003;278:39224–39234.
29. Filosto M, Mancuso M, Vives-Bauza C, et al. Lack of paternal inheritance of muscle mitochondrial DNA in sporadic mitochondrial myopathies. *Ann Neurol*. 2003;54:524–526.

30. Fitzsimons RB, Clifton-Bligh P, Wolfenden WH. Mitochondrial myopathy and lactic acidemia with myoclonic epilepsy, ataxia and hypothalamic infertility: A variant of Ramsay-Hunt syndrome? *J Neurol Neurosurg Psychiatry*. 1981;44:79–82.
31. Förster C, Hubner G, Muller-Hocker J, et al. Mitochondrial angiopathy in a family with MELAS. *Neuropediatrics* 1992;23:165–168.
32. Fukuhara N, Tokigushi S, Shirakawa K, et al. Myoclonus epilepsy associated with ragged-red fibers (mitochondrial abnormalities): Disease entity or syndrome? Light and electron microscopic studies of two cases and review of the literature. *J Neurol Sci*. 1980;47:117–133.
33. Garcia Silva MT, Aicardi J, Goutiéres F, et al. The syndrome of myoclonic epilepsy with ragged-red fibers. Report of a case and review of the literature. *Neuropediatr*. 1987;18:200–204.
34. Gerber J, Lill R. Biogenesis of iron-sulfur proteins in eukaryotes: Components, mechanism and pathology. *Mitochondrion*. 2002;2:71–86.
35. Goto Y-I, Nonaka I, Horai S. A mutation in the tRNA(Leu)(UUR) gene associated with the MELAS subgroup of mitochondrial encephalomyopathies. *Nature*. 1990;348:651–653.
36. Goto Y-I, Nonaka I, Horai S. A new mtDNA mutation associated with mitochondrial myopathy, encephalopathy, lactic acidosis and stroke-like episodes (MELAS). *Biochim Biophys Acta*. 1991;1097:238–240.
37. Goto Y-I, Tojo M, Tohyama J, et al. A novel point mutation in the mitochondrial $tRNA^{Leu(UUR)}$ gene in a family with mitochondrial myopathy. *Ann Neurol*. 1992;31:672–675.
38. Goto Y-I, Tsugane K, Tanabe Y, et al. A new point mutation at nucleotide pair 3291 of the mitochondrial $tRNA^{Leu(UUR)}$ gene in a patient with mitochondrial myopathy, encephalopathy, lactic acidosis, and stroke-like episodes (MELAS). *Biochem Biophys Res Comm*. 1994;202:1624–1630.
39. Green DR. Apoptotic pathways: Ten minutes to dead. *Cell*. 2005;121:671–674.
40. Hanna MG, Nelson IP, Morgan-Hughes JA, et al. MELAS: A new disease associated mitochondrial DNA mutation and evidence for further genetic heterogeneity. *J Neurol Neurosurg Psychiatry*. 1998;65:512–517.
41. Harding BN. Progressive neuronal degeneration of childhood with liver disease (Alpers-Huttenlocher syndrome): A personal review. *J Child Neurol*. 1990;5:273–287.
42. Hasegawa H, Matsuoka T, Goto I, et al. Strongly succinate dehydrogenase-reactive blood vessels in muscles from patients with mitochondrial myopathy, encephalopathy, lactic acidosis, and stroke-like episodes. *Ann Neurol*. 1991;29:601–605.
43. Hirano M, DiMauro S. Clinical Features of Mitochondrial Myopathies and Encephalomyopathies. In: Lane R, ed. *Handbook of Muscle Disease*. New York: Marcel Dekker; 1996:479–504.
44. Hirano M, Pavlakis S. Mitochondrial myopathy, encephalopathy, lactic acidosis, and strokelike episodes (MELAS): Current concepts. *J Child Neurol*. 1994;9:4–13.
45. Holt IJ, Cooper JM, Morgan Hughes JA, et al. Deletions of muscle mitochondrial DNA [letter]. *Lancet*. 1988;1:1462.
46. Horiguchi Y, Fujii T, Imamura S. Purpuric cutaneous manifestations in mitochondrial encephalomyopathy. *J Dermatol*. 1991;18:295–301.
47. Hunt J. Dyssynergia cerebellaris myoclonia-primary atrophy of the dentate system: A contribution to the pathology and symptomatology of the cerebellum. *Brain*. 1921;44:490–538.
48. Huttenlocher PR, Solitare GB, Adams G. Infantile diffuse cerebral degeneration with hepatic cirrhosis. *Arch Neurol*. 1976;33:186–192.
49. Inui K, Fukushima H, Tsukamoto H, et al. Mitochondrial encephalomyopathies with the mutation of the mitochondrial tRNALeu(UUR) gene. *J Pediatr*. 1992;120:62–66.
50. Jaksch M, Klopstock T, Kurlemann G, et al. Progressive myoclonus epilepsy and mitochondrial myopathy associated with mutations in the tRNA(Ser(UCN)) gene. *Ann Neurol*. 1998;44:635–640.
51. Johns DR, Rutledge SL, Stine OC, et al. Directly repeated sequences associated with pathogenic mitochondrial DNA deletions. *Proc Natl Acad Sci USA*. 1989;86:8059–8062.
52. Kaufmann P, Engelstad K, Wei Y, et al. Dichloroacetate causes toxic neuropathy in MELAS: A randomized, controlled clinical trial. *Neurology*. 2006;66(3):324–330.
53. Kearns TP, Sayre GP. Retinitis pigmentosa, external ophthalmoplegia, and complete heart block. *Arch Ophthalm*. 1958;60:280–289.
54. King MP, Attardi G. Human cells lacking mtDNA: Repopulation with exogenous mitochondria by complementation. *Science*. 1989;246:500–503.
55. Kossoff EH, McGrogan JR. Worldwide use of the ketogenic diet. *Epilepsia*. 2005;46:280–289.
56. Kraytsberg Y, Schwartz M, Brown TA, et al. Recombination of human mitochondrial DNA. *Science* 2004;304:981.
57. Krebs HA, Kornberg HL. Energy transformations in living matter. *Erge Physiol*. 1957;49:212.
58. Lalani SR, Vladutiu GD, Plunkett K, et al. Isolated mitochondrial myopathy associated with muscle coenzyme Q10 deficiency. *Arch Neurol*. 2005;62:317–320.
59. Lamperti C, Naini A, Hirano M, et al. Cerebellar ataxia and coenzyme Q10 deficiency. *Neurology*. 2003;60:1206–1208.
60. Larsson N-G, Tulinius M, Holme E, et al. Segregation and manifestations of the mtDNA $tRNA^{Lys}$ A->$G^{(8344)}$ mutation of myoclonus epilepsy and ragged-red fibers (MERRF) syndrome. *Am J Hum Genet*. 1992;51:1201–1212.
61. Leigh D. Subacute necrotizing encephalomyelopathy in an infant. *J Neurol Neurosurg Psychiatry*. 1951;14:216–221.
62. Lombes A, Mendell JR, Nakase H, et al. Myoclonic epilepsy and ragged-red fibers with cytochrome *c* oxidase deficiency: Neuropathology, biochemistry, and molecular genetics. *Ann Neurol*. 1989;26:20–33.
63. Mancuso M, Filosto M, Mootha VK, et al. A novel mitochondrial tRNAPhe mutation causes MERRF syndrome. *Neurology*. 2004;62:2119–2121.
64. Manfredi G, Schon EA, Bonilla E, et al. Identification of a mutation in the mitochondrial $tRNA^{Cys}$ gene associated with mitochondrial encephalopathy. *Hum Mutat*. 1996;7:158–163.
65. Manfredi G, Schon EA, Moraes CT, et al. A new mutation associated with MELAS is located in a mitochondrial DNA polypeptide-coding gene. *Neuromusc Disord* 1995;5:391–398.
66. Martinuzzi A, Bartolomei L, Carrozzo R, et al. Correlation between clinical and molecular features in two MELAS families. *J Neurol Sci*. 1991;113:222–229.
67. Matthews PM, Tampieri D, Berkovic SF, et al. Magnetic resonance imaging shows specific abnormalities in the MELAS syndrome. *Neurology*. 1991;41:1043–1046.
68. McShane MA, Hammans SR, Sweeney M, et al. Pearson syndrome and mitochondrial encephalomyopathy in a patient with a deletion of mtDNA. *Am J Hum Genet*. 1991;48:39–42.
69. Mita S, Rizzuto R, Moraes CT, et al. Recombination via flanking direct repeats is a major cause of large-scale deletions of human mitochondrial DNA. *Nucl Acids Res*. 1990;18:561–567.
70. Mitchell P. Coupling of phosphorylation to electron and hydrogen transfer by a chemiosmotic type of mechanism. *Nature*. 1961;191:144–148.
71. Moraes CT, Ciacci F, Bonilla E, et al. Two novel pathogenic mtDNA mutations affecting organelle number and protein synthesis: Is the tRNA-Leu(UUR) gene an etiologic hot spot? *J Clin Invest*. 1993;92:2906–2915.
72. Moraes CT, DiMauro S, Zeviani M, et al. Mitochondrial DNA deletions in progressive external ophthalmoplegia and Kearns-Sayre syndrome. [See comments.] *N Engl J Med*. 1989;320:1293–1299.
73. Morten KJ, Cooper JM, Brown GK, et al. A new point mutation associated with mitochondrial encephalomyopathy. *Hum Mol Genet*. 1993;2:2081–2087.
74. Musumeci O, Naini A, Slonim AE, et al. Familial cerebellar ataxia with muscle coenzyme Q10 deficiency. *Neurology*. 2001;56:849–855.
75. Naini AB, Lu J, Kaufmann P, et al. Novel mitochondrial DNA ND5 mutation in a patient with clinical features of MELAS and MERRF. *Arch Neurol*. 2005;62:473–476.
76. Nakano T, Sakai H, Amano N, et al. An autopsy case of degenerative type myoclonus epilepsy associated with Friedreich's ataxia and mitochondrial myopathy. *Brain Nerve*. 1982;34:321–332.
77. Naviaux RK, Nguyen KV. POLG mutations associated with Alpers' syndrome and mitochondrial DNA depletion. *Ann Neurol*. 2004;55:706–712.
78. Nishigaki Y, Tadesse S, Bonilla E, et al. A novel mitochondrial tRNA(Leu(UUR)) mutation in a patient with features of MERRF and Kearns-Sayre syndrome. *Neuromuscul Disord*. 2003;13:334–340.
79. Nishino I, Komatsu M, Kodama S, et al. The 3260 mutation in mitochondrial DNA can cause mitochondrial myopathy, encephalopathy, lactic acidosis, and strokelike episodes (MELAS). *Muscle Nerve*. 1996;19:1603–1604.
80. Obermaier-Kusser B, Paetzke-Brunner I, Enter C, et al. Respiratory chain activity in tissues from patients (MELAS) with a point mutation of the mitochondrial genome [$tRNA^{Leu(UUR)}$]. *FEBS*. 1991;286:67–70.
81. Ogasahara S, Engel AG, Frens D, et al. Muscle coenzyme Q deficiency in familial mitochondrial encephalomyopathy. *Proc Nat Acad Sci USA*. 1989;86:2379–2382.
82. Pavlakis SG, Phillips PC, DiMauro S, et al. Mitochondrial myopathy, encephalopathy, lactic acidosis, and strokelike episodes: A distinctive clinical syndrome. *Ann Neurol*. 1984;16:481–488.
83. Penn AMW, Lee JWK, Thuillier P, et al. MELAS syndrome with mitochondrial tRNALeu(UUR) mutation: Correlation of clinical state, nerve conduction, and muscle 31P magnetic resonance spectroscopy during treatment with nicotinamide and riboflavin. *Neurology*. 1992;42:2147–2152.
84. Petty RKH, Harding AE, Morgan-Hughes JA. The clinical features of mitochondrial myopathy. *Brain*. 1986;109:915–938.
85. Poulton J, Deadman ME, Gardiner RM. Duplications of mitochondrial DNA in mitochondrial myopathy. *Lancet*. 1989;1:236–240.
86. Pulkes T, Liolitsa D, Eunson LH, et al. New phenotypic diversity associated with the mitochondrial tRNA(SerUCN) gene mutation. *Neuromuscul Disord*. 2005;15:364–371.
87. Quinzii CM, Naini A, Salviati L, et al. A mutation in *Para*-hydroxybenozoate-polyprenyl transferase (*COQ2*) causes primary coenzyme Q_{10} deficiency. *Am J Hum Genet*. 2006;78:345–349.
88. Ravn K, Wibrand F, Hansen FJ, et al. An mtDNA mutation, 14453G->A, in the NADH dehydrogenase subunit 6 associated with severe MELAS syndrome. *Eur J Hum Genet*. 2001;9:805–809.
89. Riggs JE, Schochet S Jr, Fakadej AV, et al. Mitochondrial encephalomyopathy with decreased succinate- cytochrome c reductase activity. *Neurology*. 1984;34:48–53.
90. Roger J, Pellissier JF, Dravet C, et al. Dégénérescence spino-cérébelluese—atrophie optique épilepsie-myoclonies-myopathie mitochondriale. *Rev Neurol*. 1982;138:187–200.

91. Rosing HS, Hopkins LC, Wallace DC, et al. Maternally inherited mitochondrial myopathy and myoclonic epilepsy. *Ann Neurol.* 1985;17:228–237.
92. Rotig A, Appelkvist EL, Geromel V, et al. Quinone-responsive multiple respiratory-chain dysfunction due to widespread coenzyme Q10 deficiency. *Lancet.* 2000;356:391–395.
93. Rowland LP, Hays AP, DiMauro S, et al. Diverse Clinical Disorders Associated with Morphological Abnormalities of Mitochondria. In: Cerri C, Scarlato G, eds. *Mitochondrial Pathology in Muscle Diseases.* Padua: Piccin Editore; 1983:141–158.
94. Sakuta R, Honzawa S, Murakami N, et al. Atypical MELAS associated with mitochondrial tRNA(Lys) gene A8296G mutation. *Pediatr Neurol.* 2002;27:397–400.
95. Sakuta R, Nonaka I. Vascular involvement in mitochondrial myopathy. *Ann Neurol.* 1989;25:594–601.
96. Salviati L, Sacconi S, Murer L, et al. Infantile encephalomyopathy and nephropathy with CoQ10 deficiency: A CoQ10–responsive condition. *Neurology.* 2005;65:606–608.
97. Sandbank U, Lerman P. Progressive cerebral poliodystrophy—Alpers' disease. Disorganized giant neuronal mitochondria on electron microscopy. *J Neurol Neurosurg Psychiatry.* 1972;35:749–755.
98. Santorelli FM, Mak SC, Vazquez-Acevedo M, et al. A novel mitochondrial DNA point mutation associated with mitochondrial encephalocardiomyopathy. *Biochem Biophys Res Commun.* 1995;216:835–840.
99. Santorelli FM, Shanske S, Macaya A, et al. The mutation at nt 8993 of mitochondrial DNA is a common cause of Leigh syndrome. *Ann Neurol.* 1993;34:827–834.
100. Santorelli FM, Tanji K, Kulikova R, et al. Identification of a novel mutation in the mtDNA ND5 gene associated with MELAS. *Biochem Biophys Res Commun.* 1997;238:326–328.
101. Santra S, Gilkerson RW, Davidson M, et al. Ketogenic treatment reduces deleted mitochondrial DNAs in cultured human cells. *Ann Neurol.* 2004;56:662–669.
102. Sato W, Hayasaka K, Shoji Y, et al. A mitochondrial tRNA(Leu)(UUR) mutation at 3,256 associated with mitochondrial myopathy, encephalopathy, lactic acidosis, and stroke-like episodes (MELAS). *Biochem Mol Biol Int.* 1994;33:1055–1061.
103. Satoh M, Ishikawa N, Yoshizawa T, et al. N-isopropyl-p-[^{123}I]Iodoamphetamine SPECT in MELAS syndrome: Comparison with CT and MR imaging. *J Comput Assist Tomogra.* 1991;15:77–82.
104. Schapira AHV, DiMauro S. *Mitochondrial Disorders in Neurology.* Oxford: Butterworth-Heinemann Ltd., 1994.
105. Schon EA, Rizzuto R, Moraes CT, et al. A direct repeat is a hotspot for large-scale deletions of human mitochondrial DNA. *Science.* 1989;244:346–349.
106. Schuelke M, Bakker M, Stoltenburg G, et al. Epilepsia partialis continua associated with a homoplasmic mitochondrial tRNA(Ser(UCN)) mutation. *Ann Neurol.* 1998;44:700–704.
107. Schwabe MJ, Dobyns WB, Burke B, et al. Valproate-induced liver failure in one of two siblings with Alpers disease. *Pediatr Neurol.* 1997;16:337–343.
108. Schwartz M, Vissing J. Paternal inheritance of mitochondrial DNA. *N Engl J Med.* 2002;347:576–580.
109. Schwartz M, Vissing J. No evidence for paternal inheritance of mtDNA in patients with sporadic mtDNA mutations. *J Neurol Sci.* 2004;218:99–101.
110. Seibel P, Degoul F, Bonne G, et al. Genetic, biochemical and pathophysiological characterization of a familial mitochondrial encephalomyopathy (MERRF). *J Neurol Sci.* 1991;105:217–224.
111. Shoffner J, Wallace D. Oxidative Phosphorylation Diseases. In: Schriver C, Beaudet A, Sly W, Valle D, eds. *The Metabolic and Molecular Bases of Inherited Diseases,* 7th ed. New York: McGraw-Hill Inc.; 1995:1535–1609.
112. Shoffner JM, Lott MT, Lezza A, et al. Myoclonic epilepsy and ragged-red fiber disease (MERRF) is associated with a mitochondrial DNA tRNALys mutation. *Cell.* 1990;61:931–937.
113. Shoffner JM, Lott MT, Voljavec AS, et al. Spontaneous Kearns-Sayre/chronic external ophthalmoplegia plus syndrome associated with a mitochondrial DNA deletion: A slip-replication model and metabolic therapy. *Proc Natl Acad Sci USA.* 1989;86:7952–7956.
114. Shtilbans A, El-Schahawi M, Malkin E, et al. A novel mutation in the mitochondrial DNA transfer ribonucleic acidAsp gene in a child with myoclonic epilepsy and psychomotor regression. *J Child Neurol.* 1999;14:610–613.
115. Shtilbans A, Shanske S, Goodman S, et al. G8363A mutation in the mitochondrial DNA transfer ribonucleic acidLys gene: Another cause of Leigh syndrome. *J Child Neurol.* 2000;15:759–761.
116. Shy GM, Gonatas NK, Perez M. Childhood myopathies with abnormal mitochondria. I. Megaconial myopathy- pleoconial myopathy. *Brain.* 1966;89:133–158.
117. Silvestri G, Ciafaloni E, Santorelli F, et al. Clinical features associated with the A>G transition at nucleotide 8344 of mtDNA ("MERRF" mutation). *Neurology.* 1993;43:1200–1206.
118. Silvestri G, Moraes CT, Shanske S, et al. A new mtDNA mutation in the tRNALys gene associated with myoclonic epilepsy and ragged-red fibers (MERRF). *Am J Hum Genet.* 1992;51:1213–1217.
119. So N, Berkovic S, Andermann F, et al. Myoclonus epilepsy and ragged-red fibres (MERRF). *Brain.* 1989;112:1261–1276.
120. Taniike M, Fukushima H, Yanagihara I, et al. Mitochondrial $tRNA^{Ile}$ mutation in fatal cardiomyopathy. *Biochem Biophys Res Comm.* 1992;186:47–53.
121. Taylor RW, Chinnery PF, Haldane F, et al. MELAS associated with a mutation in the valine transfer RNA gene of mitochondrial DNA. *Ann Neurol.* 1996;40:459–462.
122. Taylor RW, McDonnell MT, Blakely EL, et al. Genotypes from patients indicate no paternal mitochondrial DNA contribution. *Ann Neurol.* 2003;54:521–524.
123. Taylor RW, Schaefer AM, McDonnell MT, et al. Catastrophic presentation of mitochondrial disease due to a mutation in the tRNA(His) gene. *Neurology.* 2004;62:1420–1423.
124. Taylor RW, Singh-Kler R, Hayes CM, et al. Progressive mitochondrial disease resulting from a novel missense mutation in the mitochondrial DNA ND3 gene. *Ann Neurol.* 2001;50:104–107.
125. Tiranti V, Carrara F, Confalonieri P, et al. A novel mutation (8342G–>A) in the mitochondrial tRNA(Lys) gene associated with progressive external ophthalmoplegia and myoclonus. *Neuromuscul Disord.* 1999;9:66–71.
126. Tiranti V, Hoertnagel K, Carrozzo R, et al. Mutations of SURF-1 in Leigh disease associated with cytochrome *c* oxidase deficiency. *Am J Hum Genet.* 1998;63:1609–1621.
127. Turunen M, Olsson J, Dallner G. Metabolism and function of coenzyme Q. *Biochim Biophys Acta.* 2004;1660:171–199.
128. Tzagoloff A. *Mitochondria.* New York: Plenum Press, 1982.
129. Ugalde C, Janssen RJ, van den Heuvel LP, et al. Differences in assembly or stability of complex I and other mitochondrial OXPHOS complexes in inherited complex I deficiency. *Hum Mol Genet.* 2004;13:659–667.
130. Varlamov DA, Kudin AP, Vielhaber S, et al. Metabolic consequences of a novel missense mutation of the mtDNA CO I gene. *Hum Mol Genet.* 2002;11:1797–1805.
131. Wallace DC, Singh G, Lott MT, et al. Mitochondrial DNA mutation associated with Leber's hereditary optic neuropathy. *Science.* 1988;242:1427–1430.
132. Zeviani M, Amati P, Bresolin N, et al. Rapid detection of the A->G(8344) mutation of mtDNA in Italian families with myoclonus epilepsy and ragged-red fibers (MERRF). *Am J Hum Genet.* 1991;48:203–211.
133. Zeviani M, Moraes CT, DiMauro S. Deletions of mitochondrial DNA in Kearns-Sayre syndrome. *Neurology.* 1988;38:1339–1346.
134. Zeviani M, Muntoni F, Savarese N, et al. A MERRF/MELAS overlap syndrome with a new point mutation in the mitochondrial DNA tRNALys gene. *Eur J Hum Genet.* 1993;1:80–87.
135. Zhu S, Yao J, Johns T, et al. *SURF1,* encoding a factor involved in the biogenesis of cytochrome *c* oxidase, is mutated in Leigh syndrome. *Nat Genet.* 1998;20:337–343.

CHAPTER 263 ■ CEREBRAL PALSY

JOHN B. P. STEPHENSON

INTRODUCTION

Understanding epilepsy is a necessary part of the management of individuals with cerebral palsy.[45] Epilepsy is common in all types of cerebral palsy and, in some varieties, it is the rule.

DEFINITIONS

The definitions of *epileptic seizures, symptomatic epileptic seizures*, and *epilepsy* are the same as those used in other chapters throughout this book. The definition of *cerebral palsy* (CP) is a little more difficult, insofar as some variation occurs in the way in which the term is used between different authors and different studies. The most frequent definition of *cerebral palsy* is "a disorder of posture and movement due to a static lesion of the developing brain." Most authors include cerebral malformations as examples of static lesions of the brain but, in at least one study, cerebral malformations were excluded.[20] Many authors include the aftereffects of acute cerebral insults and injuries in infancy and even in early childhood, whereas others would exclude from the CP definition any condition presumed not to have been present before the age of 4 weeks.[20] There is considerable force in the argument for limiting the definition of cerebral palsy in this way, insofar as the prognosis with respect to epilepsy differs between those whose brain lesion is of perinatal or prenatal origin and those children with unequivocally postnatal cerebral insults.

A new definition of cerebral palsy was proposed in 2005[5]: "Cerebral palsy (CP) describes a group of disorders of the development of movement and posture, causing activity limitation, that are attributed to nonprogressive disturbances that occurred in the developing fetal or infant brain. The motor disorders of cerebral palsy are often accompanied by disturbances of sensation, cognition, communication, perception, and/or behavior, and/or by a seizure disorder." From the point of view of this chapter, it is disappointing to see the term "seizure disorder" employed. This sloppy and ambiguous term deserves to be deleted from scientific discourse.[38]

Authors have exhibited some variability on the definition of the various subtypes of CP but, on the whole, these differences in classification do not materially affect the understanding of epilepsy in the context of CP. The main divisions in the Edinburgh classification were[23]: (a) hemiplegia, (b) bilateral hemiplegia, (c) diplegia (which might vary from virtually paraplegic to tetraplegic), (d) ataxic CP (including ataxic diplegia and ataxia), (e) dyskinesia (including dystonia and athetosis), and (f) any other form of CP, including mixed forms. Many authors now include ataxic diplegia within the diplegia categories. Certainly, for the purposes of discussion of epilepsy, dystonic CP should be strongly distinguished from athetoid CP, insofar as the liability to epilepsy may be high in the former and low in the latter type. The group described by the Edinburgh School as bilateral hemiplegia will have severe mental retardation, as discussed in the section Risk Factors for Epilepsy.[13]

Recent studies[31,37] of the etiology of CP (with or without epilepsy) have shown a much higher diagnostic yield than was thought likely in the past. This should make one wary of the CP label without firm foundation.

PROBLEMS IN DIAGNOSIS OF CEREBRAL PALSY

Many conditions can masquerade as cerebral palsy but turn out to be something else.[21,40] Most such conditions are individually rare, but parents do not commonly judge the rarity of a condition as a justification for pediatricians or neurologists to make an incorrect diagnosis. Fortunately for the present issue, cerebral palsy imitators complicated by epilepsy or epileptiform attacks are few. Pelizaeus-Merzbacher disease is one such confusing condition.[6] One might argue that this is actually an example of cerebral palsy but, of course, the important point is that it is an X-linked disorder and may recur in a future male child.

Another condition with an unequivocally progressive cerebral pathology is the Aicardi-Goutières syndrome.[39] Affected children may behave much like patients with cerebral palsy without regression.[39] Confirmation of the diagnosis of Aicardi-Goutières syndrome depends on finding elevated cerebrospinal fluid (CSF) and serum α-interferon in the absence of any congenital viral infection.

Another confusing condition is hyperekplexia[47] in which affected neonates may be very stiff and troubled by severe nonepileptic convulsions. When a family history of dominantly inherited startle disease is present, the diagnosis presents no difficulty, but in sporadic cases it can be difficult.

Rare, potentially treatable inborn errors of metabolism leading to cerebral palsy and epilepsy have been described. These include defective serine biosynthesis[24] deficiency,[4] and GAMT deficiency.[28a]

New conditions will continue to be recognized, and it behooves the child neurologist to question the diagnosis in every patient with "cerebral palsy." This is particularly so in so-called *ataxic cerebral palsy*, which some have suggested should not be called cerebral palsy at all,[26] insofar as genetic etiologies abound.

PROBLEMS IN EPILEPSY DIAGNOSIS

Having cerebral palsy is no insurance against exhibiting or suffering from the various nonepileptic attacks that may affect the general population.[38] We suspect that children with cerebral palsy are more at risk of having epilepsy misdiagnosed in this way because epilepsy is common in cerebral palsy and so expected to be seen. For example, a young child with spastic diplegia may have what we term *reflex anoxic seizures*[38] after falling over and bumping his head just like anyone else who is similarly genetically predisposed. In addition, patients with cerebral palsy may have a predilection for various movements having a superficial resemblance to epileptic seizures. In all these situations, keen clinical judgment must be used. The interictal electroencephalogram (EEG) cannot be relied on to assist in the differential diagnosis. Although it has been attested that spikes or epileptiform discharges are more common in children with cerebral palsy who have epileptic seizures, cerebral palsy individuals who have never had epileptic seizures may not uncommonly show spike discharges also.[35] When an individual with cerebral palsy has had one or more previous epileptic seizures, it is even less rational to expect that an EEG examination will help to diagnose a new unexplained paroxysmal event.[38] On the other side of the coin, those with startle epilepsy[36] may not show spikes at all in the ictal EEG; however, such individuals always have other epileptic seizures without the startle provocation.[28]

Nonepileptic Paroxysmal Disorders in Sleep

It is particularly important not to mistake nonepileptic paroxysmal phenomena associated with sleep for epileptic seizures. Repetitive sleep starts are serial, sleep-related nonepileptic jerks or spasms that may occur in young neurologically impaired children.[16] As these children may *also* have epilepsy,[16] the recognition of these nonepileptic sleep starts is necessary to avoid needless increases in antiepileptic therapy.

Second, because of their cerebral palsy, affected individuals may have obstructive sleep apnea with tonic nonepileptic seizures, easily misdiagnosed as the expected nocturnal epileptic seizures.[3]

In both these clinical situations polygraphy during sleep may be necessary, recording EEG, electrocardiogram (ECG), respiration, and electromyogram (EMG).[3,16]

Anoxic-Epileptic Seizures: Epileptic Seizures Induced by Syncope

Epileptic seizures induced by syncopes—what we call anoxic-epileptic seizures—may not be rare in children.[22] When this occurs in cerebral palsy, diagnosis may be exceptionally difficult. A recent report describes a boy with Cornelia de Lange syndrome diagnosed as having symptomatic epilepsy until it was realized that his clonic and hemi-clonic epileptic seizures—including status epilepticus—were always triggered by obstructive apnea[29] and ceased without the need for antiepileptic medication once recurrent upper airways obstruction was prevented.[29]

PROBLEMS IN COMBINED CEREBRAL PALSY AND EPILEPSY DIAGNOSIS

The Special Case of Glucose Transporter Deficiency

It has become apparent that one of the most important etiologies of "cerebral palsy" and epilepsy or "epilepsy" is the genetic disorder of glucose transport now known as GLUT-1 deficiency syndrome or GLUT1DS.[46] The importance lies not in the frequency of this disorder but in its potential treatment by ketogenic diet, albeit such treatment is not universally successful.[25] Affected individuals mostly—but not always[34]—have epilepsy, and many have a motor disorder that could be described as cerebral palsy. Presumed nonepileptic movement disorders and other paroxysmal events are also seen.[46] Insofar as the ketogenic diet is potentially useful for the treatment of these various phenomena, clinicians should consider this disorder early and make careful simultaneous measurements of fasting blood and CSF glucose when in doubt.[46]

RISK FACTORS FOR EPILEPSY

The early studies of Ellenberg and Nelson[14] indicated that knowledge of the etiology of epilepsy not associated with cerebral palsy was very limited. A number of later studies have addressed such a question in various ways.

Goulden et al.[20] studied a cohort of mentally retarded individuals born in Aberdeen, Scotland, between 1951 and 1955. By 22 years, 15% of these had epilepsy. With their definition of *cerebral palsy* as "having a presumed prenatal or perinatal onset," the cumulative risk for epilepsy was 28%, 31%, and 38% at 5, 10, and 22 years of age, respectively. This compared with a much lower risk for individuals with mental retardation and no associated disabilities, and a much higher risk of epilepsy in those with postnatal brain injury (defined as a significant brain insult after 28 days of life which might reasonably account for the child's later functioning). This particular study included a separate group with cerebral malformations but, in fact, the only malformation determined was described as an occipital meningocele.

A careful Italian study[9] focused on the risk factors for the co-occurrence of partial epilepsy, cerebral palsy, and mental retardation. In a studied population of 64 children with these three conditions, neuroimaging identified 32 with cerebral malformations and 32 without but with encephalomalacia, periventricular leukomalacia, or diffuse atrophy. These two groups were compared with a much larger population of normal children. The definitions in this study were as follows:

Partial epilepsy met the International League Against Epilepsy (ILAE) criteria. Such seizures had to have begun in the first 3 years of life. Apparently generalized seizures at onset did not exclude a child if persistent partial motor or complex partial seizures appeared within the first 3 years, but partial seizures in West syndrome or Lennox-Gastaut syndrome excluded a child from this study. *Cerebral palsy* was defined as "a disorder characterized by abnormal control of movement or posture starting early in life and without any recognized underlying progressive disease." *Mental retardation* was defined as an IQ of less than 70.

Significant relative risks were found for both familial factors and for maternal and neonatal factors. Any kind of epilepsy occurred in 0.5% of first-degree relatives of controls, whereas in both the groups with cerebral malformation and without cerebral malformation, the epilepsy risk in first-degree relatives was over 7% (95% confidence interval did not include one). Similarly significant maternal and neonatal factors for both groups (with and without cerebral malformation) were: Maternal diseases in the 2 years before pregnancy (such as diabetes, heart disease, hyperthyroidism, and gynecologic disorders), placental pathology, prematurity with delivery later than 31 weeks' gestation in those who were small for their gestational age, and neonatal convulsions. An enormously increased risk was found for those born at or before 31 weeks' gestation, all of these from the group without cerebral malformation. The need for cardiopulmonary resuscitation in the neonatal period, used as a measure of presumed asphyxia, was a high risk factor in the group without cerebral malformation, but not a risk factor in those with cerebral malformation. The findings of this study indicate that a number of genetic and prenatal risk factors interact in the genesis of early partial epilepsy with cerebral palsy and mental retardation.

Ottman et al.[32,33] looked at the etiology of epilepsy from a different perspective. In this study of about 2,000 individuals, all had epilepsy but none had severe mental retardation. Of these, 80% had either idiopathic or cryptogenic epilepsy; 18% had postnatal symptomatic epilepsy, defined as having had a cerebral insult 7 or more days before the first unprovoked seizure. Of interest in the present context was the smallest group with neuro deficits (1%). This group consisted of 28 individuals with cerebral palsy and one with mild intellectual impairment. Although the 95% confidence intervals did not include one because of small numbers, the standard morbidity ratios for epilepsy or for idiopathic or cryptogenic epilepsy was 3 or over in the group with neuro deficits from birth. This was no different from the standard morbidity ratios in the case of those with idiopathic or cryptogenic epilepsy, but different from the situation in postnatal symptomatic epilepsy, where the standardized morbidity ratio was 1.

These studies are consistent with other results such as those of Aicardi[1] in demonstrating that, whereas postnatal brain damage is frequently the cause of subsequent epilepsy, similar genetic and prenatal factors underlie both cerebral palsy not of postnatal origin and epilepsy when it coexists.

The relationship of mental retardation is complex. Those with mental retardation are more likely to have epilepsy if they also have cerebral palsy, and those with cerebral palsy are more likely to have epilepsy if they are mentally retarded. To a certain extent, these relationships reflect a common etiology, but by no means is enough known. A simple method of demonstrating the relationship of neurologic deficit severity to IQ has been proposed for individuals with childhood hemiplegia.[19]

The risk of epilepsy in different subtypes of cerebral palsy also varies. It is highest[13] in those with what some call *double hemiplegia* and some *quadriplegia*, perhaps not surprisingly. Those with dystonic cerebral palsy who may not be easily distinguishable from those in the former group will also have a high incidence. In those with spastic hemiplegia, the relative incidence is intermediate,[42] with the lowest frequency in those with preterm related diplegia or athetoid cerebral palsy.

CLINICAL FEATURES OF THE EPILEPSY

Considerable difficulties arise in classifying the epilepsies in individuals with cerebral palsy, according to the previous international classification. It might be argued that the epilepsies in cerebral palsy ought to be either partial or localization-related, or secondarily generalized. However, there is no *a priori* reason why genetic epilepsy, such as the primary generalized epilepsies, or even benign partial epilepsy, such as benign rolandic epilepsy,[27] should not occur in those with cerebral palsy, with or without mental retardation. For instance, typical absences with 3 per second spike-and-wave can be seen in children with cerebral palsy,[1] and one cannot on clinical and EEG grounds say whether that individual has secondary generalized absences or whether there is coincident primary generalized absence epilepsy. This applies to many of the epilepsies in the context of cerebral palsy. Perhaps the argument is specious insofar as, as indicated earlier in the sections Problems in Combined Cerebral Palsy and Epilepsy and Risk Factors for Epilepsy, a common genetic etiology may exist for the cerebral palsy and the epilepsy.

Certain seizure types, such as infantile or juvenile spasms (otherwise called *periodic spasms*[17]), or atonic or startle seizures,[36] may be more likely to occur in those with cerebral palsy, but almost any type of epileptic seizure is possible.[1,2] It is important to recognize that although normal intellect may be preserved when cerebral palsy and epilepsy are combined (see Case 2) even with startle epilepsy,[30] intellectual stagnation or decline may occur (see Case 4).

A study from London[44] showed that in children with hemiplegic cerebral palsy and overall intelligence within normal limits, the presence of epileptic seizures in the first 5 years of life was associated with defects of cognition, language, and memory. In this study, when hemiplegia was unaccompanied by early seizures, nonverbal functions were almost exclusively impaired. The authors inferred that language displaced spatial abilities. By contrast, when hemiplegia was accompanied by early seizures, nearly all measures of psychologic function were affected, nonverbal and verbal alike. The presence of seizures seemed to be more important than the presence of EEG discharges. Furthermore, the presence of early seizures was more important than the size of the lateralized lesion on imaging: Children with severe neuroradiologic deficits and no seizures did better on verbal IQ, memory quotient, and third-trial paired associate learning than did those with mild neuroradiologic deficit and early seizures. Case 4 provides a more extreme example with documented regression and loss of skills.

THERAPY OF THE EPILEPSY AND OF THE CEREBRAL PALSY

The principles of medical therapy of the epilepsies complicating cerebral palsy are generally similar to those that pertain in other clinical contexts. Little has been written about the use of corticosteroid, but this is alluded to in a case example below (Case 4). The use of rectal diazepam or buccal midazolam has become widespread in the management of children with cerebral palsy and epilepsy, perhaps in part because of the frequency of long hemiclonic seizures.

The place of epilepsy surgery in cerebral palsy has remained rather small, despite impressive reports on the value of hemispherectomy in refractory epilepsy with complicating hemiplegia (see Chapter 178). Section of the corpus callosum and subpial transection are discussed elsewhere (see Chapters 180 and 182). An impressive recent report from Utrecht has shown that epilepsy surgery in children and adolescents with or without prior spasticity does not harm motor performance.[43]

Baclofen by intrathecal route has increased in popularity as a treatment for spastic and other forms of cerebral palsy. There has been concern that this use of baclofen—insofar as it is a GABA-B antagonist—might be epileptogenic. However, a recent controlled study concluded that in children with spasticity of cerebral origin intrathecal baclofen does not seem to aggravate or induce epilepsy.[7]

PROGNOSIS

The prognosis of the neurodevelopmental features, in particular cognitive function and the development of mental retardation, has been discussed earlier in "Risk Factors for Epilepsy." This section focuses on the prognosis for the epilepsy, with brief mention of mortality.

Prognosis of the Epilepsy

Clinical impression of the intractability and unremitting continuation of epileptic seizures in many children with cerebral palsy is undoubtedly biased by patient referral and differential follow-up of those with good and bad outcomes. In a report[11] from Dallas, around 25% (531 of 2,086 children with cerebral palsy actively followed) had epilepsy at the time of writing or previously had epilepsy. Since 1985, only 69 or 13% of these children with cerebral palsy and epilepsy had been seizure free for 2 years or more. These children were studied prospectively on antiepileptic drug withdrawal. Electroencephalography was done before the antiepileptic drug discontinuation. In all children, therapy was tapered off by 15% to 20% every 2 weeks. Four were lost to follow-up, but the remaining 65 were followed after antiepileptic drug discontinuation until seizure relapse or until at least 2 years without seizures. In the event, the seizure relapse rate was about 41% (i.e., the remission rate was about 60%). Many factors appeared to have no significant effect on whether remission would or would not take place, although, as the authors point out, nonsignificance means only that we are yet unable to state with a high degree of confidence that the factor does have prognostic value. Paradoxically, there is a higher frequency of relapse in those with normal mental development than in those with mental retardation, but this was likely due to the higher incidence of epilepsy relapse in those with hemiplegic cerebral palsy. In this study spastic hemiparesis was the only factor identified that significantly increased the risk of epilepsy relapse after discontinuation of antiepileptic drug therapy. These hemiplegic individuals were more likely to have normal intelligence than were those having other forms of cerebral palsy.

Thus, the vast majority of children with cerebral palsy do not become seizure free, but of those who do, the majority will be able to discontinue antiepileptic drugs. Children with hemiplegic cerebral palsy seem to be an exception to this rule.

Mortality

Epilepsy significantly increases the mortality rate in those with mental retardation,[15] and it has been shown[8] that independent predictors of this increased mortality are: The type of cerebral palsy (spastic quadriplegia and double hemiplegia having the worst prognosis); the presence of epilepsy (of any type); and the presence of severe or profound mental retardation. In remote symptomatic epilepsy as a whole mortality is increased,[10] seizure severity seemingly a factor.[41] By contrast, the prognosis for survival in those with hemiplegic cerebral palsy and epilepsy but without mental retardation is excellent (96% at 30 years).[8]

CASE EXAMPLES

For those who appreciate the value of detailed clinical observations on individual children, four case studies are provided in this section. One child represents a condition that successfully masquerades as cerebral palsy but has different implications. The other three case studies are of three children with congenital left spastic hemiplegia, with different trajectories and outcomes. These clinical studies may suggest to others further ways of refining the excellent type of epidemiologic studies referred to earlier.

Case 1: Progressive "Cerebral Palsy"

A girl was born at term in 1991 to unrelated parents who had two previous normal children. She presented at age 10 weeks because she was not holding up her head and did not smile. Her left limbs jerked repetitively as she fell asleep. Her development was very slow, but her parents and medical attendants did not observe loss of skills. She smiled once at 3 months and then more so at 9 months, smiling very readily at age 3 years. Initial hypotonia changed to spastic tetraplegia from her second year of life. Seizures consisting of extension of her limbs with quivering for about a minute occurred daily in infancy, at which time the EEG was normal, but diminished to once a week at age 3 years, EEG then showing a considerable quantity of slow spike-and-wave activity. Chilblains (pernio) were prominent, particularly on her toes. The only clinical evidence of a progressive disorder was failure of head growth. Initially, head circumference was on the mean, albeit 2 cm below that expected from her parental and sibling head circumferences, but after age 4 months, growth further declined; by 4 years of age, head circumference was 4 standard deviations below the mean.

Computed tomography head scans demonstrated progressive encephalopathy with periventricular calcifications, later also in basal ganglia and dentate locations, associated with white matter hypointensity. Cerebrospinal fluid contained 40 lymphocytes/mM^3. There was no evidence of viral infection, and the huge level of cerebrospinal fluid α-interferon confirmed the diagnosis of autosomal recessive Aicardi-Goutières syndrome.[35a, 39]

Comment

Epilepsy, yes; cerebral palsy, no!

Case 2: Hemiplegic Cerebral Palsy, West Syndrome, and Good Outcome

A first-born male did not show signs of asphyxia after a long labor but was very jumpy at noise at the age of 2 hours and from age 2 days had a tendency to tenseness of his left limbs, with his fontanel bulging when he was upset. Thereafter, his behavior and development seemed normal except that there was a tendency for his left hand to be fisted.

When he presented at the age of 7.5 months, his parents said that about a month previously he had lost his happy disposition and had become lethargic, docile, and unsmiling. At about the same time, he had begun to have runs of spasms five or so times a day, with ten or more spasms in each run about 10 seconds apart. On admission to the hospital, runs of spasms were observed, sometimes with a degree of asymmetry. His head circumference was on the second percentile, and his skull transilluminated excessively on the right. He had a left hemianopia and absent optokinetic nystagmus when the drum or tape was moved to his right. His left hand did not have full voluntary control, only briefly retaining an object. Brain imaging was not done at that time, but years later showed infarction in the right middle cerebral territory. Electroencephalography showed hypsarrhythmia without convincing asymmetry.

He was treated with adrenocorticotropic hormone (ACTH) gel, 40 units daily for 2 weeks, and nitrazepam 1 mg twice daily. He had no further infantile spasms after the first dose of ACTH, and 3 days later he was smiling and taking an interest in his toys again. Repeat EEG after 2 weeks showed no discharges but reduced rhythmic activity over the right.

He received nitrazepam in the same dose until the age of 2 years. He developed intellectually, having a verbal comprehension at the age of 1.5 years of more than 2 standard deviations above the mean. He had left spastic hemiparesis and required lengthening of his Achilles tendon at the age of 3 years. An additional medical complication was an atrial septal defect, which was closed without use of blood at the age of 9 years.

From the age of 4 years, he had occasional episodes of altered consciousness, sometimes with some motor disturbance on the left. These tended to be preceded by a "funny feeling in his tummy"; instances of "sick tummy" were more frequent. Antiepileptic therapy for these simple and complex partial seizures was not required until the age of 11 years, when carbamazepine was introduced. At the age of 12 years, he replied to a letter sent to his parents inquiring about him: "Thank you for the letter of interest. My Mum and Dad thought that it would be appropriate for me to write because I am the person you are so considerate of..." At about age 15 years, he began to have startle-induced alterations in the tone of his left limbs, lasting 15 to 30 seconds, the startle stimulus being solely an accidental scuffing of the toe of his left foot on the ground. He was improved by an increase of carbamazepine dose in the sustained release form. At the age of 17 years, he had two episodes of left limb stiffness without startle, but since the addition of vigabatrin, 500 mg daily, he has remained seizure free.

When he was aged 17 years, he discovered that he would have difficulty obtaining a driving license because of his left hemianopia. However, the combination of a life-long habit of frequently shifting his gaze to the left and training in blind sight in his left visual field has enabled him to drive commercially and to achieve complete independence.

When in his 20s, he suffered several attacks of loss of consciousness, preceded by a funny feeling in his abdomen. These were misdiagnosed as a return of his epilepsy, and an EEG was inappropriately requested. In fact, his mother had a long history of vasovagal syncopes with an identical abdominal aura.[38]

Comment

Aside from illustrating determined human qualities, this case illustrates that neither symptomatic West syndrome nor epilepsy complicating hemiplegic cerebral palsy are bars to intellectual achievement and success in life.[18]

It is also a powerful reminder that individuals who have had epilepsy may have syncopes as well.

Case 3: Congenital Hemiplegia with Secondary Generalized Myoclonic Epilepsy

This boy's mother sustained a motor vehicle accident in pregnancy at 22 weeks' gestation, after which she was unconscious for 2 hours and required an infusion to maintain her blood pressure. He was born normally at term, but a left hemiparesis became apparent later in the first year of life. His development appeared to be otherwise normal.

At age 3.5 years, he first had simultaneous head nods with right arm jerk. Soon after, he had one clonic epileptic seizure from sleep. At age 4 years, jerks became very frequent daily. They appeared to involve head nodding and abrupt dropping of the right upper limb, suggesting negative myoclonus (although surface EMG polygraphy was not undertaken). Interictal EEG showed very frequent runs of high-voltage 2/sec spike-and-wave; this slow spike-and-wave was generalized but of even higher voltage on the right. Computed tomography brain scan showed a smaller right cerebral hemisphere with abnormal gyration and a deep cleft consistent with polymicrogyria. His attentiveness varied with the frequency of his seizures but intellectual assessment showed normal intelligence.

Carbamazepine was associated with worsening of his seizures, and sodium valproate with or without lamotrigine had no consistent beneficial effect. A 2-week course of betamethasone led to marked reduction in seizures and an increase in attentiveness; he went into normal school and has continued on lamotrigine monotherapy with only occasional jerks.

Comment

An example of prenatal origin hemiplegic cerebral palsy with intelligence in the normal range despite severe secondary generalized epilepsy, probably negative myoclonic.[7a] Selective learning difficulties were expected to become more apparent in school years.

Case 4: Congenital Hemiplegia with Epileptic Encephalopathy

After an uneventful pregnancy, this girl was born at term by emergency cesarean section because of a maternal straight sacrum. There was said to be fetal distress with meconium staining and type 2 dips in labor. The APGAR score was 3 at 1 minute, and she was intubated at 3 minutes for 2 minutes. However, she was well as a neonate except that when about 1 week old, it was noted that whenever she fought out of her shawl or cot covers, it was always with the right hand. Thereafter, although she developed evidence of a left spastic hemiparesis (shown later to be due to a large right middle cerebral infarct), her general development was distinctly advanced, and she spoke many meaningful words, including "what's that?" before the age of 1 year.

Just after the age of 2.5 years, she had an episode of staring with left hand twitching. At the age of 3.5 years, she had a bilateral clonic seizure of at least 25 minutes' duration. At the age of 4 years, she began to have blanks, which increased in frequency and began to be described as periods of confusion. EEG from before the age of 4 years showed runs of generalized spike-and-wave discharges, which were nearer to 2 per second but were often at 2.5 to 3 per second with blinking and probable absence. By the age of 5 years, there was also bifrontal slow activity. She received sodium valproate in a dose of 400 mg daily from 4 years 4 months, and 800 mg daily from 4 years 8 months, changing to ethosuximide 500 mg daily, 2 months later.

Cognitive and behavioral decline was noticed by her mother from about the age of 4 years 4 months. Although there was some fluctuation, the girl would no longer sit down and draw people and faces if requested but would run about most of the time. Professional evaluation confirmed the decline. At the age of 4 years 2 months, her expressive language was well above average, and her verbal comprehension not less than 4 years 9 months (the ceiling had not been reached in the tests). By 4 years 11 months, both expressive language and verbal comprehension had dropped to 2 years 6 months. She had also become disorientated and declined in nonverbal skills, and had various behavioral abnormalities.

Short courses of betamethasone initially reduced spike-and-wave activity on EEG and were associated with improved cognition and behavior such that, for example, her Stanford-Binet intelligence was raised from 2 years 11 months at 5 years 2 months up to 3 years 11 months at 5 years 5 months, but such improvements became less and of shorter duration after each successive betamethasone course. In due course, although the atypical absences were eliminated by the betamethasone, her cognition and behavior did not much improve. Over the next 5 years, these atypical absences fluctuated and were often not observed. Very occasional night seizures, possibly tonic–clonic, were reported, but there have been no further seizures of any type observed since the age of 10 years on ethosuximide monotherapy. At the age of 15 years, she has just begun to read but has no road sense, is too friendly with strangers, and has other behavioral difficulties.

Comment

In this previously very intelligent girl with hemiplegic cerebral palsy, severe cognitive and behavioral decline was associated with rather subtle epileptic manifestations. Although corticosteroid administration at first led to improvement, this was temporary, and she is now not likely to be able to live independently, despite remission of her epilepsy. Whether more modern medical or surgical antiepileptic approaches might have prevented this dismal prognosis remains speculative. A good discussion of cognitive and behavioral disturbances as epileptic manifestations is to be found elsewhere.[12]

SUMMARY AND CONCLUSIONS

It is essential to make sure that the diagnosis of cerebral palsy is correct and that the diagnosis of the epilepsy is correct. In the case of cerebral palsy diagnosis, both genetic disorders with high recurrence risk and rare treatable cerebral disorders should be excluded. In the case of the epilepsy diagnosis, special attention should be paid to nonepileptic events in patients with cerebral palsy that masquerade as epileptic seizures. Even epileptic seizures do not always imply epilepsy, as the section on anoxic-epileptic seizures has illustrated. Obviously, antiepileptic therapy should be avoided when it is not appropriate.

It appears that cerebral palsy and epilepsy are linked both by etiology and prognosis. The outlook is not universally bad, but we have little evidence on which to make improvements. Especially terrible are regressions in mental capacity linked in some way to the epileptic component of the cerebral palsy.

References

1. Aicardi J. Epilepsy in brain-injured children. *Dev Med Child Neurol.* 1990;32:191–202.
2. Aksu F. Nature and prognosis of seizures in patients with cerebral palsy. *Dev Med Child Neurol.* 1990;32:661–668.
3. Arzimanoglou A, Guerrini R, Aicardi J. *Aicardi's Epilepsy in Children,* 3rd ed. Philadelphia: Lippincott Williams & Wilkins; 2004: 329.
4. Bass N. Cerebral palsy and neurodegenerative disease. *Curr Opin Pedatr.* 1999;11:504–507.
5. Bax M, Goldstein M, Rosenbaum P, et al. , and the Executive Committee for the Definition of Cerebral Palsy. Proposed definition and classification of cerebral palsy, April 2005. *Dev Med Child Neurol.* 2005;47:571–576.
6. Boulloche J, Aicardi J. Pelizaeus-Merzbacher disease: Clinical and nosological study. *J Child Neurol.* 1986;1:233–239.
7. Buonaguro V, Scelsa B, Curci D, et al. Epilepsy and intrathecal baclofen therapy in children with cerebral palsy. *Pediatr Neurol.* 2005;33:110–113.

7a. Caraballo R, Cersosimo R, Fejerman N. A particular type of epilepsy in children with congenital hemiparesis associated with unilateral polymicrogria. *Epilepsia.* 1999;40:865–871.

8. Crighton JU, Mackinnon M, White CP. The life-expectancy of persons with cerebral palsy. *Dev Med Child Neurol.* 1995;37:567–576.
9. Curatolo P, Arpino C, Stazi MA, et al. Risk factors for the co-occurrence of partial epilepsy, cerebral palsy and mental retardation. *Dev Med Child Neurol.* 1995;37:776–782.
10. Day SM, Wu YW, Strauss DJ, et al. Causes of death in remote symptomatic epilepsy. *Neurology.* 2005;65:216–222.
11. Delgado MR, Riela AR, Mills J, et al. Discontinuation of antiepileptic drug treatment after two seizure-free years in children with cerebral palsy. *Pediatrics.* 1996;97:192–197.
12. Deonna T, Roulet-Perez E. *Cognitive and Behavioural Disorder of Epileptic Origin in Children.* MacKeith Press: London; 2005 Cognitive and behavioural disturbances as epileptic manifestations in children: An overview. *Semin Pediatr Neurol.* 1995;2:254–260.
13. Edebol-Tysk K. Epidemiology of spastic tetraplegic cerebral palsy in Sweden. I. Impairment and disabilities. *Neuropediatrics.* 1989;20:41–45.
14. Ellenberg JH, Nelson KB. Birth weight and gestational age in children with cerebral palsy or seizure disorders. *Am J Dis Child.* 1979;133:1044–1048.
15. Forsgren L, Edvinsson S-O, Nystrom L, et al. Influence of epilepsy on mental retardation: An epidemiologic study. *Epilepsia.* 1996;37:956–963.
16. Fusco L, Pachatz C, Cusmai R, et al. Repetitive sleep starts in neurologically impaired children: An unusual non-epileptic manifestation in otherwise epileptic subjects. *Epileptic Disord.* 1999;1:63–67.
17. Gobbi G, Bruna L, Pina A, et al. Periodic spasms: An unclassified type of epileptic seizure in childhood. *Dev Med Child Neurol.* 1987;29:766–775.
18. Golomb MR, Carvalho KS, Garg BP. A 9-year-old boy with a history of large perinatal stroke, infantile spasms, and high academic achievement. *J Child Neurol.* 2005;20:444–446.
19. Goodman R, Yule C. IQ and its predictors in childhood hemiplegia. *Dev Med Child Neurol.* 1996;38:881–890.
20. Goulden KJ, Shinnar S, Koller H, et al. Epilepsy in children with mental retardation: A cohort study. *Epilepsia.* 1991;32:690–697.
21. Gupta R, Appleton RE. Cerebral palsy: Not always what it seems. *Arch Dis Child.* 2001;85:356–360.
22. Horrocks IA, Nechay A, Stephenson JBP, et al. Anoxic-epileptic seizures: Observational study of epileptic seizures induced by syncopes. *Arch Dis Child.* 2005;90:1283–1287.
23. Ingram TTS. The neurology of cerebral palsy. *Arch Dis Child.* 1966;41: 337–357.
24. Jaeken J, Detheux M, Van Maldergem L, et al. 3-Phosphoglycerate dehydrogenase deficiency: An inborn error of serine biosynthesis. *Arch Dis Child.* 1996;74:542–545.
25. Klepper J, Scheffer H, Leindecker B, et al. Seizure control and acceptance of the ketogenic diet in GLUT1 deficiency syndrome: A 2- to 5-year follow-up of 15 children enrolled prospectively. *Neuropediatrics.* 2005;36:302–308.
26. Krageloh-Mann I. Magnetic Resonance Imaging in Cerebral Palsy. In: Neville B, Albright AL. *The Management of Spasticity Associated with the Cerebral Palsies in Children and Adolescents.* New Jersey: Churchill Communications; 2000: 60.
27. Lerman P, Kivity S. The Benign Focal Epilepsies of Childhood. In: Pedley TA, Meldrum BS, eds. *Recent Advances in Epilepsy*, Vol. 3. Edinburgh: Churchill Livingstone; 1986: 137–156.
28. Manford MRA, Fish DR, Shorvon SD. Startle provoked epileptic seizures: Features in 19 patients. *J Neurol Neurosurg Psychiatry.* 1996;61:151–156.

28a. Mercimek-Mahmutoglu S, Stoeckler-Ipsiroglu S, Adami A, et al. GAMT deficiency: features, treatment, and outcome in an inborne error of creatine synthesis. *Neurology* 2006;67:480–484. Epub 2006 Jul 19.

29. Nechay A, Smulska N, Chepiga L. Anoxic-epileptic seizures in Cornelia de Lange syndrome: Case report of epileptic seizures induced by obstructive apnea. *Eur J Paediatr Neurol.* 10:142–144. Epub 2006 May 19.
30. Nolan MA, Otsubo H, Iida K, et al. Startle-induced seizures associated with infantile hemiplegia: Implication of the supplementary motor area. *Epileptic Disord.* 2005;7:49–52.
31. Oskoui M, Shevell MI. Profile of pediatric hemiparesis. *J Child Neurol.* 2005;20:471–476.
32. Ottman R, Annegers JF, Risch N, et al. Relations of genetic and environmental factors in the etiology of epilepsy. *Ann Neurol.* 1996;39:442–449.
33. Ottman R, Lee JH, Risch N, et al. Clinical indicators of genetic susceptibility to epilepsy. *Epilepsia.* 1996;37:353–361.
34. Overweg-Plandsoen WC, Groener JE, Wang D, et al. GLUT-1 deficiency without epilepsy—an exceptional case. *J Inherit Metab Dis.* 2003;26:559–563.
35. Perlstein MA, Gibbs EL, Gibbs FA. The electroencephalogram in infantile cerebral palsy. *Am J Phys Med.* 1953;34:477–496.

35a. Rice G, Patrick T, Parmer R, et al. Clinical and Molecular phenotype of Aicardi-Goutières syndrome. *Am J Hum Genet.* 2007 (in press).

36. Saenz-Lope E, Herranz FJ, Masdeu JC. Startle epilepsy: A clinical study. *Ann Neurol.* 1984;16:78–81.
37. Shevell MI, Majnemer A, Morin I. Etiologic yield of cerebral palsy: A contemporary case series. *Pediatr Neurol.* 2003;28:352–359.
38. Stephenson JBP. *Fits and Faints.* London: MacKeith Press, 1990.
39. Stephenson JBP. Aicardi-Goutières syndrome: Observations of the Glasgow school. *Eur J Paediatr Neurol.* 2002;6(Suppl A):A67–70.
40. Stephenson JBP, King MD. *Handbook of Neurological Investigations in Children.* London: Butterworth-Heinemann; 1991.
41. Strauss DJ, Day SM, Shavelle RM, et al. Remote symptomatic epilepsy: Does seizure severity increase mortality? *Neurology.* 2003;60:395–399.
42. Uvebrant P. Hemiplegic cerebral palsy. Aetiology and outcome. *Acta Paediatr Scand.* 1988;345(Suppl):1–82.
43. van Empelen R, Jennekens-Schinkel A, Gorter JW, et al, and the Dutch Collaborative Epilepsy Surgery Programme. Epilepsy surgery does not harm motor performance of children and adolescents. *Brain.* 2005;128:1536–1545.
44. Vargha-Khadem F, Isaacs E, Van der Werf S, et al. Development of intelligence and memory in children with hemiplegic cerebral palsy. *Brain.* 1992;115:315–329.
45. Wallace SJ. Epilepsy in cerebral palsy. *Dev Med Child Neurol.* 2001;43:713–717.
46. Wang D, Pascual JM, Yang H, et al. Glut-1 deficiency syndrome: Clinical, genetic, and therapeutic aspects. *Ann Neurol.* 2005;57:111–118.
47. Zhou L, Chillag KL, Nigro MA. Hyperekplexia: A treatable neurogenetic disease. *Brain Dev.* 2002;24:669–674.

CHAPTER 264 ■ NEOPLASTIC DISEASES

LAWRENCE D. RECHT AND MICHAEL GLANTZ

INTRODUCTION

Seizures are frequently the first symptom in patients with brain tumors, and they represent an important cause of potentially preventable morbidity. They thus present a clinical problem requiring specific treatments that do not necessarily affect the course of the brain tumor but that generally improve quality of life.

HISTORICAL PERSPECTIVES

The first reports of a relationship between brain tumor and epilepsy were published before the 18th century, and a number of clinicians, including J. Russell Reynolds, drew attention to this problem in the early 19th century. Hughlings Jackson, however, was the first to point out a direct association between partial epilepsy and tumors.[40] Jackson also recognized the relationship between epileptogenicity and tumor involvement of the cortical gray matter.[40,41]

Since then, the evolution of neurosurgical techniques and the development of new imaging techniques have greatly facilitated the management of tumor-associated epilepsy. Nevertheless, controversy over optimal pharmacologic and surgical therapies persists, and seizures still represent one of the more commonly encountered problems in neuro-oncology.

EPIDEMIOLOGY

Although neoplasms of the brain account for only 1% of cases of epilepsy, seizures occur in approximately 50% of children with supratentorial tumors,[4,39,50] and seizures develop in approximately 35% to 40% of adults with brain tumors.[48] The rate is much lower for tumors of the infratentorial or pituitary region, and consequently even higher for supratentorial lesions. Furthermore, because physicians who are not neurologists are apt to miss seizures with other than motor manifestations, these figures are probably underestimates.

In the majority of patients with supratentorial low-grade gliomas, seizure is the initial manifestation.[47,66] Seizures occur especially commonly in association with oligodendrogliomas. A recent retrospective study found seizures to be the first symptom in three quarters of patients with oligodendrogliomas.[91] Seizures are also commonly encountered in patients with meningiomas. Although earlier workers reported that seizures were less frequently encountered in cases of more malignant glial neoplasms,[27] recent studies demonstrate that up to 60% of patients with malignant gliomas experience seizures at some time during their clinical course.[57] In contrast, the incidence of seizures in patients with cerebral metastasis is much lower; most reports suggest an incidence of 20% at time of presentation.[18,28,63,96]

CLINICAL PRESENTATION

Clinical Correlates of Tumor-Associated Epilepsy

Despite the variable frequency of seizures as a function of histologic subtype, the most important factor associated with the development of seizure is probably tumor location.[44,52] Seizures occur much more frequently in supratentorial (22%–68%) than infratentorial (6%) lesions.[31,64,78] Moreover, the incidence of seizures increases as the site of tumor approaches the rolandic fissure.[90] As the distance from the central sensorimotor region increases, early-onset seizures are less likely to occur.[65] Similarly, superficial and cortical tumors are associated with a much higher incidence of epilepsy than are noncortical deep lesions (63% vs. 29%), and lesions entirely within the white matter infrequently produce seizures.

Other factors aside from location are also probably important determinants. Both the chronicity of tumor growth and patient age affect the incidence of epilepsy in intra-axial supratentorial neoplasms.[23,24,25,30,31,34,54,64,69,70] Slowly growing tumors, such as gangliogliomas and dysembryoplastic neuroepithelial tumors, are overrepresented in patients with brain tumors who have seizures, whereas more rapidly growing tumors are less often epileptogenic. Thus, a seizure incidence of 70% is reported for astrocytoma, but only 37% for glioblastoma multiforme.[4,70,90] Young age also is correlated with the presence of epilepsy.[91]

Seizure Types in Tumor-Associated Epilepsies

Since Jackson first noted, at the end of the last century, the relationship between uncinate seizures and tumors of the frontotemporo-orbital regions, many reports have documented the important relationship between the type of seizure and the presence of tumor. Despite occasional disagreement,[48,86] a correlation between a specific seizure type and either a particular neoplasm or specific tumor location has been commented on repeatedly. In an analysis of psychomotor attacks in 80 untreated patients with and without tumor, for example, olfactory and gustatory hallucinations were very suggestive of tumor.[43,52] Muller (cited in Jackson[40]) noted olfactory hallucinations, increasing frequency of attacks, and random variations in the type of attack (especially of motor seizures) to be particularly characteristic of tumor. For children, the probability of diagnosing an underlying tumor is higher in those with complex partial seizures (10%–46%) than in those with other seizure types.[7,82,90]

In a recent series of patients with oligodendroglial tumors, seizures were approximately equally divided between generalized, partial, and mixed types.[91] In contrast, localization-related motor seizures, characterized by a clonic jerking of the face or one extremity, are often characteristic of patients with intracranial metastases or malignant gliomas,[44,48] and these seizures are almost always seen in association with focal neurologic abnormalities.[57] Multifocal or bilateral neoplasms more often produce seizures than solitary neoplasms do,[57] and seizures tend to occur more frequently with lesions of the central nervous system (CNS) caused by metastatic melanoma, because these lesions involve gray matter and tend to be multiple.[11] Furthermore, partial seizures in patients with brain tumors are clinically significant, because they are rarely falsely localizing and thus provide a clue to tumor location.[1] Following partial or secondarily generalized seizures, many patients with underlying brain tumors exhibit a significant Todd's paralysis; although usually transient, this may be permanent.[56]

DIAGNOSTIC EVALUATION

Because seizures are a presenting complaint in approximately 20% of patients with newly diagnosed brain metastases,[68] neuroimaging, preferably magnetic resonance imaging (MRI), is required in every patient with cancer in whom seizures develop. Since seizures also occur in up to 40% of neutropenic patients with infectious meningitis,[51] are a common manifestation of leptomeningeal carcinomatosis, and have been reported as an early manifestation of limbic encephalitis, a spinal fluid analysis with careful assessment of the patient's prior clinical course for possible epileptogenic drugs and metabolic aberrations is always indicated.

Before the advent of modern neuroimaging, the significance of a seizure as a first manifestation of brain tumor was insufficiently recognized, and the average delay between first seizure and tumor diagnosis was about 3 years.[16,44,89] In recent years, however, scanning with computed tomography (CT) and MRI has made it possible to document that many low-grade gliomas have relatively benign pathologic features and, although they produce chronic epilepsy, tend to be associated with long survival.[26,71] Furthermore, low-grade gliomas are serendipitously noted in up to 20% of resected surgical specimens from the brains of patients with chronic temporal lobe epilepsy.[10,58,79,84] Therefore, it is the authors' recommendation that all patients with a first seizure have a CNS imaging study, preferably an MRI scan, at the time of presentation.

Electroencephalography (EEG) is also useful in assessing these patients. Findings correlate with tumor location, and in approximately 40% of patients, the EEG abnormalities are lateralized to the side of the tumor.[17] On the other hand, in the authors' experience,[32] EEG does not predict in which patients with supratentorial lesions late seizures will develop. Nevertheless, because EEG is relatively inexpensive and helps to localize the epileptogenic foci by a method different from neuroimaging, it remains a useful test for attempting to localize the physiologic seizure focus.

DIFFERENTIAL DIAGNOSIS

In patients with established cancer, the differential diagnosis of either isolated or multiple seizures includes more than just mass lesions, and the appropriate work-up must be designed accordingly. Although the differential diagnoses of a seizure in cancer patients are similar to those in patients without cancer, certain etiologies are specific to or more frequent in a patient with preexisting cancer. For example, hyponatremia, hypomagnesemia, and hypocalcemia all occur more frequently in patients with cancer owing to a number of factors, including dehydration and chemotherapy. These metabolic aberrations in turn predispose to seizures. Similarly, the immunosuppression associated with cancer and its treatment predisposes patients to meningitis, often with less common etiologic agents, such as *Listeria* and *Cryptococcus*. A partial list of potential causes of seizures in patients with cancer is given in Table 1.

TREATMENT AND OUTCOME

Pharmacotherapeutic Aspects of Tumor-Associated Epilepsy

Seizures can be especially detrimental to patients with tumors because they can lead to breakdown of the blood—brain barrier[61] and subsequent formation of brain edema. This process is probably related to seizure-induced arterial hypertension. Because the increase in blood flow and blood volume may worsen elevated intracranial pressure, leading to focal ischemia and sometimes infarction, the Todd's paralysis that frequently follows these seizures tends to be more protracted (even permanent on occasion) than that occurring in patients with partial seizures and no tumor. This potential complication alone justifies instituting aggressive antiepileptic measures for these patients once a seizure has occurred.

As in the treatment of idiopathic seizures and secondary seizures not related to tumor, however, the efficacy of anticonvulsant therapy for tumor-associated epilepsy falls well short of complete control. Tumor-associated epilepsy tends to be relatively refractory to antiepileptic drugs (AEDs), and significant remission of seizures is rare.[34,57,78] Primary tumors tend to be more difficult to control than metastatic lesions (M. Glantz, *unpublished observations*), but seizures with onset late in a patient's clinical course tend to be easier to control than those that are an initial manifestation of tumor.[57]

A number of unique problems also complicate the use of AEDs in cancer patients. For example, a rash develops in approximately 25% of patients taking either phenytoin or carbamazepine, a figure twice the reported incidence in the population without tumors.[57] Even more serious, both of these agents have been reported to cause Stevens-Johnson syndrome, particularly in patients who receive radiation therapy while taking a decreasing dose of steroids.[19]

Moreover, it is difficult to maintain therapeutic levels of conventional AEDs (e.g., phenytoin, carbamazepine, phenobarbital) in cancer patients. A number of chemotherapeutic agents, including bischloroethylnitrosourea (BCNU), cisplatin, carboplatin, and Taxol, cause antiepileptic drug levels to decrease, either because of induction of microsomal enzymes or decreased absorption.[9,22,29,36,60] Complex mutual interactions of these agents with the commonly coadministered dexamethasone also exist; as a result, corticosteroid requirements are increased[15,38] and phenytoin levels are decreased, necessitating close monitoring of antiepileptic drug levels.[93] To compensate for lower AED levels, dosages may have to be increased, only to have the level overshoot into the toxic range. Toxicity, in turn, may mimic the symptoms of brain tumor progression, including seizure.[12,81] Lethargy and cognitive dysfunction do not occur only as manifestations of drug toxicity; they can also occur when drug levels are in the therapeutic range. Finally, in approximately 20% of patients with brain tumor who are taking phenobarbital, pain and dysfunction develop in the shoulder and sometimes the entire upper extremity (shoulder-hand syndrome) on the tumor-affected side.[83]

Furthermore, AEDs address only a minority of the possible pathophysiologic mechanisms purported to be important in generating tumor-associated epilepsy. Specifically, these agents tend to act on excitatory mechanisms by blocking and inactivating Na^+ or Ca^{++} channels or on inhibitory ones through

TABLE 1

CAUSES OF SEIZURES OTHER THAN TUMOR MASSES IN CANCER PATIENTS

Etiology	Setting	Comment
Metabolic	Hypomagnesemia	Occurs 2–7 days after cisplatin chemotherapy.
	Hyponatremia	Often occurs after craniotomy. Usually caused by hydration with hypotonic fluids. Sometimes occurs with vincristine chemotherapy.
	Hypocalcemia	Occurs after cisplatin chemotherapy.
Drug-induced	Methotrexate	Especially with concurrent RT and in patients with abnormal CSF flow.
	Cisplatin	May be caused by electrolyte disturbance.
	Ifosfamide	Especially common in setting of renal failure.
	BCNU (high-dose), IL-2, VP-16 (high-dose)	Uncommon.
	Anticonvulsants	Associated with abrupt decreases or increases; frequently caused by interactions with other drugs.
Intracranial hemorrhage	Coagulopathy	Also occurs with chemotherapy-induced thrombocytopenia.
Radiation	Radiation necrosis	May mimic recurrent tumor.
Infectious	Meningitis	Especially *Listeria*; occurs frequently in patients with ventricular reservoirs.
Neoplastic	Leptomeningeal carcinomatosis	
Paraneoplastic	Limbic encephalitis	Most common with small-cell cancer of lung; very rare.

RT, radiation therapy; CSF, cerebrospinal fluid; BCNU, bischloroethylnitrosourea (carmustine); IL-2, interleukin-2; VP-16, etoposide.

increasing γ-aminobutyric acid (GABA)ergic activity.[21] They do not address other possible causative factors such as morphological changes, altered receptor and connexin patterns and changes in cytokine expression.[73]

To complicate matters even further, no published studies address whether AEDs prevent further seizures in patients with brain metastases or whether any one epileptic agent is superior. In earlier work, Posner[68] recommended phenytoin as an initial agent, followed by carbamazepine, phenobarbital, and valproate. However, because brain tumor patients with epilepsy suffer from a number of neuropsychological and psychological problems that are aggravated not only by the severity of epilepsy, but also by the intensity of treatment,[46] use of some of the newer agents such as levetiracetam, which has less allergenicity and fewer medical interactions, seems an attractive alternative that is more frequently being recommended.[85] However, no agent has been proven clearly superior, and the failure of one agent does not predict failure of another.

Should Patients with Brain Tumors Receive Prophylactic Antiepileptic Drugs?

Although the risk for perioperative seizures after neurosurgical procedures is 10% to 15% in the first week,[20,55] this does not necessarily justify the long-term use of prophylactic antiepileptic drugs in patients with brain tumors. Only one study suggests that prophylactic administration of antiepileptic drugs can prevent seizures in patients with glioma.[8] Other retrospective studies have failed to demonstrate decreased seizure frequency in patients with brain metastases or gliomas treated with antiepileptic drugs.[18,53,57] Recently, two prospective studies also failed to indicate a difference in the frequency of first seizures in patients having either primary or metastatic tumors treated with either phenytoin or valproic acid.[32,88] A similar recommendation was made for patients with malignant gliomas by Moots et al.,[57] who recommend that these agents be withheld except for patients at high risk (multiple or hemorrhagic lesions). This has led to a general consensus that was published as an American Academy of Neurology practice parameter that prophylactic drugs not be prescribed in this situation,[33] a recommendation further supported by a subsequent controlled study on the topic.[24]

The practice of the authors therefore has been not to prescribe antiepileptic drugs until a seizure occurs. On the other hand, prophylactic antiepileptic drugs have proved effective in at least one specific instance: Prevention of contrast-induced seizures at the time of CT. Five to ten milligrams of diazepam given orally 30 minutes before contrast administration decreases the likelihood of seizures.[62]

Surgical Treatment of Tumor-Associated Epilepsies

Tumor-associated epilepsies can also be ameliorated by resection. Even a lesion in or near the sensorimotor or language cortex is not an absolute contraindication to surgery.[34] Intractable seizures can often be controlled by gross total removal.[13,34,79] Of patients with low-grade gliomas, for example, 40%

become seizure-free and another 30% have a marked reduction in seizure frequency after surgery.[48] Tumor removal or lesionectomy alone provides effective relief in many patients. In numerous series, from 30% to 60% of patients with brain tumors are rendered seizure free after surgery,[3,13,14,25,34,35,39,74] even though up to 35% of these patients retain their auras after surgery.[80] When surgery failed to control seizures, incomplete resection of the lesion was usually found.

The most favorable seizure-free outcomes following lesionectomy have been reported for patients with indolent glial neoplasms. Complete seizure remission can be obtained in 65% to 80% of these patients, and doses of antiepileptic drugs can be tapered in half of them.[13,14,39] When surgery involves subtotal lobectomy and removal of the medial temporal or frontal structures, at least a 95% reduction in seizure frequency is seen in virtually every patient.[79] Best results are seen in patients undergoing extensive resections soon after the development of epilepsy.[2,94,95] Results are poorer, however, for patients with meningiomas and malignant gliomas.[48] Seizures in patients with brain tumors can also be reduced using either radiation therapy[34,72] or chemotherapy.

Lesionectomy Versus More Extensive Surgery

Although lesionectomies are generally effective, many investigators feel that more extensive surgery produces better results. This contention is supported by the frequent finding on intraoperative electrocorticography in patients with low-grade gliomas of epileptogenic foci remote from the tumor nidus that are devoid of tumor infiltration.[6] Furthermore, a statistically significant decrease in both GABA and somatostatin neurons has been noted in epileptogenic tissue not infiltrated by tumor, compared with nonepileptic cortex not infiltrated by tumor.[37] These findings suggest that cortex surrounding a slowly growing tumor may become isolated, lose inhibitory neurotransmitters, and develop into an independent, tumor-free epileptogenic cortical focus. The not infrequent persistence of seizures following complete tumor resection further suggests that the epileptogenic zone responsible for the initiation and propagation of seizures is sometimes separate from the area of tumor-involved brain removed during lesionectomy.

Whether resection of separate seizure foci, using intraoperative electrocorticography, in addition to radical resection of tumor optimizes seizure outcome remains controversial. Penfield et al.[64] demonstrated a seizure-free outcome in only 21% of patients undergoing lesionectomy and therefore subsequently recommended electrocorticography and more extensive surgery.[65] Many other workers have since reported optimal results when both tumor and epileptogenic foci are identified and removed. If the region of epileptogenicity involves the amygdala-hippocampal complex, results can be improved even further.[5,42,45,67] Furthermore, others[3,34,39,91,92] have reported that routine tumor resection performed without electrocorticography is inferior to more monitored procedures in terms of attaining postoperative seizure control, but this issue remains unsettled.

Part of the difficulty in attaining remission of epilepsy associated with brain tumor can be attributed to progressive, reactive changes taking place in the brain surrounding the lesion, in contrast to the regressive neuronal changes commonly found in seizure foci in idiopathic epilepsies. Thus, failure to control seizures is usually related to persistent disease. In some patients, an initially satisfactory result is followed by a relapse; second surgeries tend to be ineffective.[91] In this situation, if electrocorticography is used, large contiguous and noncontiguous areas of brain surrounding the lesion are found to be dysrhythmic. Paradoxically, however, in patients whose focal neurologic deficits become worse, seizure disorders frequently become easier to control, presumably because of progressive neuronal loss in previously epileptogenic brain.[91]

PROGNOSIS

Although the Brain Tumor Cooperative Group (BTCG) trials for patients with malignant gliomas did not demonstrate a correlation between the occurrence of seizures at diagnosis and improved survival,[77,87] a number of other observations suggest that at least for patients with primary brain tumors, presentation with a seizure is a favorable prognostic sign. In the era before CT, for example, reports of cases of long-standing seizures in patients with benign tumors of the temporal lobe abound. List[49] and Penfield et al.[64] both felt that the prognosis of patients with brain tumors who had seizures was better, because less aggressive neoplasms are commonly seen in these patients. This observation has been substantiated in recent years. Convulsions tend to occur more frequently and earlier in patients with lower-grade gliomas, whereas more malignant tumors tend to produce other signs first. Tumor calcification, which occurs more frequently in lower-grade neoplasms, also correlates with seizure frequency.[76] In fact, a number of recent studies have identified presentation with a seizure as a favorable prognostic sign.[59,75,78] Possible explanations for this observation include relative surgical accessibility (because tumors tend to have a cortical location), earlier detection and diagnosis, and overrepresentation of lower-grade tumors. Interestingly, although most glial neoplasms producing intractable epilepsy are not clinically aggressive, almost 20% have anaplastic histologic features.[26]

SUMMARY AND CONCLUSIONS

Seizures are frequently the first symptom in patients with brain tumors, or seizures develop later in the clinical course. Thus, they represent an important cause of potentially preventable morbidity in these patients. Determining the cause of the seizure using neuroimaging and other diagnostic tests is critical, because multiple potential etiologies exist in patients with cancer. Unfortunately, pharmacologic therapies are often ineffective in the absence of surgery or other antitumor therapy, and no one antiepileptic drug is clearly superior in terms of efficacy. Furthermore, antiepileptic drugs probably do not prevent seizures from occurring in those patients with brain tumors who have not yet had a seizure. Therefore, for most patients, prophylactic antiepileptic drugs are not recommended. In contrast, surgery, either lesionectomy or more extensive epilepsy-type surgery, frequently produces long-lasting remission of epilepsy, especially in patients with lower-grade primary tumors of the brain.

References

1. Arseni C, Maretsis M. Focal epileptic seizures ipsilateral to the tumour. *Acta Neurochir*. 1979;49:47–60.
2. Aronica E, Leenstra S, van Veelen CW, et al. Glioneuronal tumors and medically intractable epilepsy: A clinical study with long-term follow-up of seizure outcome after surgery. *Epilepsy Res*. 2001;43:179–191.
3. Awad IA, Rosenfeld J, Ahl J, et al. Intractable epilepsy and structural lesion of the brain: Mapping, resection strategies, and seizure outcome. *Epilepsia*. 1991;32:179–186.
4. Backus RE, Millichap JG. The seizure as a manifestation of intracranial tumor in childhood. *Pediatrics*. 1962;29:978.
5. Berger MS, Ghatan S, Geyer JR, et al. Seizure outcome in children with hemispheric tumors and associated intractable epilepsy: The role of tumor removal combined with seizure foci resection. *Pediatr Neurosurg*. 1991/2;17:185–191.

6. Berger MS, Ghatan S, Haglund MM, et al. Low-grade gliomas associated with intractable epilepsy: Seizure outcome utilizing electrocorticography during tumor resection. *J Neurosurg*. 1993;79:62–69.
7. Blume WT, Girvin JP, Kaufmann JC. Childhood brain tumors presenting as chronic uncontrolled seizure disorders. *Ann Neurol*. 1982;12: 538–541.
8. Boarini DJ, Beck DW, Van Gilder JC. Postoperative prophylactic anticonvulsant therapy in cerebral gliomas. *Neurosurgery*. 1985;16:290–292.
9. Bollini P, Riva R, Albani F, et al. Decreased phenytoin level during antineoplastic therapy: A case report. *Epilepsia*. 1983;24:75–76.
10. Boon PA, Williamson PD, Fried I, et al. Intracranial, intra-axial, space-occupying lesions in patients with intractable partial seizures: An anatomoclinical, neuropsychological, and surgical correlation. *Epilepsia*. 1991;32:467–476.
11. Byrne TN, Cascino TL, Posner JB. Brain metastases from melanoma. *J Neuro-oncol*. 1983;1:313–317.
12. Callahan DJ, Noetzel MJ. Prolonged absence status epilepticus associated with carbamazepine therapy, increased intracranial pressure, and transient MRI abnormalities. *Neurology*. 1992;42:2198–2201.
13. Cascino G. Epilepsy and brain tumours: Implications for treatment. *Epilepsia*. 1990;31(Suppl 3):S37–S44.
14. Cascino GD, Kelly PJ, Hirschorn KA, et al. Stereotactic resection of intra-axial cerebral lesions in partial epilepsy. *Mayo Clin Proc*. 1990;65:1053–1060.
15. Chalk JB, Ridgeway K, Brophy T, et al. Phenytoin impairs the bioavailability of dexamethasone in neurological and neurosurgical patients. *J Neurol Neurosurg Psychiatry*. 1984;47:1087–1090.
16. Chin HW, Haxel JJ, Kim TH, et al. Oligodendrogliomas. 1. A clinical study of cerebral oligodendrogliomas. *Cancer*. 1980;45:1458–1466.
17. Chiofalo N, Armenjol V, Fuentes A, et al. Electroencephalographical-anatomical correlation of brain tumors in infancy and childhood. *Child's Brain*. 1981;8:417–422.
18. Cohen N, Strauss G, Lew R, et al. Should prophylactic anticonvulsants be administered to patients with newly diagnosed cerebral metastases. A retrospective analysis. *J Clin Oncol*. 1988;6:1621–1624.
19. Delattre J-Y, Safai B, Posner JB. Erythema multiforme and Stevens-Johnson syndrome in patients receiving cranial irradiation and phenytoin. *Neurology*. 1988;38:194–198.
20. Deutschman CS, Haines SJ. Anticonvulsant prophylaxis in neurological surgery. *Neurosurgery*. 1985;17:510–517.
21. Dichter MA. Mechanisms of action of new antiepileptic drugs. *Adv Neurol*. 1998;76:1–9.
22. Dofferhoff AS, Berendsen HH, Naalt VD, et al. Decreased phenytoin level after carboplatin treatment. *Am J Med*. 1990;89:247–248.
23. Falconer MA, Serafetinides EA, Corsellis JA. Etiology and pathogenesis of temporal lobe epilepsy. *Arch Neurol*. 1964;10:233–248.
24. Forsyth PA, Weaver S, Fulton D, et al. Prophylactic anticonvulsants in patients with brain tumour. *Can J Neurol Sci*. 2003;30:106–112.
25. Franceschetti S, Binelli S, Casazza M, et al. Influence of surgery and antiepileptic drugs on seizures symptomatic of cerebral tumours. *Acta Neurochir*. 1990;103:47–51.
26. Fried I, Kim JH, Spencer DD. Limbic and neocortical gliomas associated with intractable seizures: A distinct clinicopathological group. *Neurosurgery*. 1994;34:815–824.
27. Gaertner J. Statistische Untersuchungen an 654 intrakraniellen raumfordernden Prozessen. *Zentralbl Neurochir*. 1955;15:33.
28. Gamache FW, Posner JB, Paterson RH. Involvement of the Central Nervous System by Metastatic Tumor. In: Youmans JR, ed. *Neurological Surgery*, 2nd ed. Philadelphia: WB Saunders, 1979.
29. Ghosh C, Lazarus HM, Hewlett JS, et al. Fluctuation of serum phenytoin concentrations during autologous bone marrow transplant for primary central nervous system tumors. *J Neuro-oncol*. 1992;12:25–32.
30. Gibbs FA. Symptoms of brain tumors. *Arch Neurol (Chicago)*. 1932;28:969–989.
31. Gilles FH, Sobell E, Leviton A, et al. Epidemiology of seizures in children with brain tumors. *J Neuro-oncol*. 1992;12:53–68.
32. Glantz MJ, Cole BF, Friedberg MH, et al. A randomized, blinded, placebo-controlled trial of divalproex sodium prophylaxis in adults with newly diagnosed brain tumors. *Neurology*. 1996;46:985–991.
33. Glantz MJ, Cole BF, Forsyth PA, et al. Practice parameter: Anticonvulsant prophylaxis in patients with newly diagnosed brain tumors. *Neurology*. 2000;54:1886–1893.
34. Goldring S, Rich KM, Picker S. Experience with Gliomas in Patients Presenting with a Chronic Seizure Disorder. In: Little JR, ed. *Clinical Neurosurgery*. Baltimore: Williams & Wilkins; 1986: 15–42 (Vol. 33).
35. Gonzalez D, Elvidge AR. On the occurrence of epilepsy caused by astrocytoma of the cerebral hemispheres. *J Neurosurg*. 1962;19:470–482.
36. Grossman SA, Sheidler VR, Gilbert MR. Decreased phenytoin levels in patients receiving chemotherapy. *Am J Med*. 1989;87:505–510.
37. Hagland MM, Berger MS, Kunkel DD, et al. Changes in gamma-aminobutyric acid and somatostatin in epileptic cortex associated with low-grade gliomas. *J Neurosurg*. 1992;77:209–216.
38. Haque N, Thrasher K, Werk E, et al. Studies on dexamethasone metabolism in man. Effect of diphenylhydantoin. *J Clin Endocrinol Metab*. 1972;34:44–50.
39. Hirsch JF, Saint Rose C, Pierre-Kahn A, et al. Benign astrocytic and oligodendrocytic tumors of the cerebral hemispheres in children. *J Neurosurg*. 1989;70:568–572.
40. Jackson JH. Localised convulsions from tumor of the brain. *Brain*. 1882;5:364–384.
41. Jackson H. On Convulsive Seizures. In: Taylor J, ed. *Selected Writings of John Hughlings Jackson*. New York: Basic Books, 1958(Vol. 1).
42. Jooma R, Yeh H-S, Privitera MD, Gartner M. Lesionectomy versus electrophysiologically guided resection for temporal lobe tumors manifesting with complex partial seizures. *J Neurosurg*. 1995;83:231–236.
43. Ketz E. *Zum klinischen Aspekt der psychomotoischen Epilepsie*. Heidelberg: Dr. Alfred Huthig; 1968.
44. Ketz E. Brain Tumors and Epilepsy. In: Vinken PJ, Bruyn GW, eds. *Handbook of Clinical Neurology*. New York: Elsevier; 1974: 254–269 (Vol. 16).
45. Kirkpatrick PJ, Honavar M, Janota I, et al. Control of temporal lobe epilepsy following *en bloc* resection of low-grade tumors. *J Neurosurg*. 1993;78:19–25.
46. Klein M, Engelberts N, van der Ploeg H, et al. Epilepsy in low-grade gliomas: The impact on cognitive function and quality of life. *Ann Neurol*. 2003;54:514–520.
47. Laws ER, Taylor WF, Clifton MB, et al. Neurosurgical management of low-grade astrocytoma of the cerebral hemispheres. *J Neurosurg*. 1984;61:665–673.
48. LeBlanc FE, Rasmussen T. Cerebral Seizures and Brain Tumors. In: Vinken PJ, Bruyn GW, eds. *Handbook of Clinical Neurology*. New York: Elsevier; 1974: 295–301 (Vol. 15).
49. List CF. Epileptiform attacks in cases of glioma of the cerebral hemispheres. *Arch Neurol Psychiatry (Chicago)*. 1936;35:323.
50. Low NL, Correll JW, Hammill JF. Tumors of the cerebral hemispheres in children. *Arch Neurol*. 1965;13:547–554.
51. Lukes SA, Posner JB, Nielsen S, et al. Bacterial infections of the CNS in neutropenic patients. *Neurology*. 1984;34:269–275.
52. Lund M. Epilepsy in association with intracranial tumour. *Acta Psychiatr (Kbh) Suppl*. 1952;81.
53. Mahaley MS, Dudka L. The role of anticonvulsant medications in the management of patients with anaplastic gliomas. *Surg Neurol*. 1981;16:399–401.
54. Mathieson G. Pathologic aspects of epilepsy with special reference to the surgical pathology of focal cerebral seizures. *Adv Neurol*. 1975;8:107–138.
55. Matthew E, Sherwin AL, Weiner SA, et al. Seizures following intracranial surgery: Incidence in the first post-operative week. *Can J Neurol Sci*. 1980;7:285–290.
56. Meyer JS, Portnoy HD. Post-epileptic paralysis. A clinical and experimental study. *Brain*. 1959;82(Pt 2):162–185.
57. Moots PL, Maciunas RJ, Eisert DR, et al. The course of seizure disorders in patients with malignant gliomas. *Arch Neurol*. 1995;52:717–724.
58. Morris HH, Estes ML, Gilmore R, et al. Chronic intractable epilepsy as the only symptom of primary brain tumor. *Epilepsia*. 1993;34:1038–1043.
59. MRC Brain Tumour Working Party. Prognostic factors for high-grade malignant glioma: Development of a prognostic index. *J Neuro-oncol*. 1990;9:47–55.
60. Neef C, der Straaten I. An interaction between cytostatic and anticonvulsant drugs. *Clin Pharmacol Ther*. 1988;43:372–375.
61. Nitsch C, Klatzo J. Regional patterns of blood-brain barrier breakdown during epileptiform seizures induced by various convulsive agents. *J Neurol Sci*. 1983;59:305–322.
62. Pagani JJ, Hayman LA, Bigelow RH, et al. Diazepam prophylaxis of contrast media-induced seizures during computed tomography of patients with brain metastases. *Am J Neuroradiol*. 1983;140:787–792.
63. Paillas JE, Pellet W. Brain Metastasis. In: Vinken PJ, Bruyn GW, eds. *Handbook of Clinical Neurology*. New York: Elsevier; 1976,Vol. 18.
64. Penfield W, Erickson TC, Tarlov I. Relation of intracranial tumors and symptomatic epilepsy. *Arch Neurol Psychiatry (Chicago)*. 1940;44:300–315.
65. Penfield W, Jasper H. *Epilepsy and the Functional Anatomy of the Human Brain*. Boston: Little, Brown, 1954.
66. Piepmeier JM. Observations on the current treatment of low-grade astrocytic tumors of the cerebral hemispheres. *J Neurosurg*. 1987;67:177–181.
67. Pilcher WH, Silbergeld DC, Berger MS, et al. Intraoperative electrocorticography during tumor resection: Impact on seizure outcome in patients with ganglioglioma. *J Neurosurg*. 1993;78:891–902.
68. Posner JB. *Neurologic Complications of Cancer*. Philadelphia: FA Davis, 1995.
69. Rasmussen T. Cortical resection in the treatment of focal epilepsy. *Adv Neurol*. 1975;8:139–154.
70. Rasmussen T. Surgery of epilepsy associated with brain tumors. *Adv Neurol*. 1975;8:227–239.
71. Recht LD, Smith TW, Lew RA. Suspected low-grade glioma: How safe is deferring treatment? *Ann Neurol*. 1992;31:431–436.
72. Rogers LR, Morris HH, Lupica K. Effect of cranial irradiation on seizure frequency in adults with low-grade astrocytoma and medically intractable epilepsy. *Neurology*. 1993;43:1599–1601.
73. Schaller B, Ruegg SJ. Brain tumor and seizures: Pathophysiology and its implications for treatment revisited. *Epilepsia*. 2003;44:1223–1232.
74. Schisano G, Tori D, Nordenstamm H. Spongioblastoma polare of the cerebral hemisphere. *J Neurosurg*. 1963;20:241–251.

75. Scott GM, Gibberd FB. Epilepsy and other factors in the prognosis of gliomas. *Acta Neurol Scand.* 1980;61:227–239.
76. Shady JA, Black P, Kupsky WJ, et al. Seizures in children with supratentorial astroglial neoplasms. *Pediatr Neurosurg.* 1994;21:23–30.
77. Shapiro WR, Green SB, Burger PC, et al. Randomized clinical trial of three chemotherapy regimens and two radiotherapy regimens in postoperative treatment of malignant glioma. *J Neurosurg.* 1989;71:1–9.
78. Smith DF, Hutton JL, Sandermann D, et al. The prognosis of primary intracerebral tumours presenting with epilepsy: The outcome of medical and surgical management. *J Neurol Neurosurg Psychiatry.* 1991;54:915–920.
79. Spencer DD, Spencer SS, Mattson RH, et al. Intracerebral masses in patients with intractable partial epilepsy. *Neurology.* 1984;34:432–436.
80. Sperling MR, Cahan LD, Brown WJ. Relief of seizures from a predominantly posterior temporal tumor with anterior temporal lobectomy. *Epilepsia.* 1989;30:559–563.
81. Stilman N, Masdeu JC. Incidence of seizures with phenytoin toxicity. *Neurology.* 1985;35:1769–1772.
82. Suarez JC, Sfaello, Viano JC. Epilepsy and brain tumors in infancy and adolescence. *Child's Nerv Syst.* 1986;2:169–174.
83. Taylor LP, Posner JB. Phenobarbital rheumatism in patients with brain tumor. *Ann Neurol.* 1989;25:92–94.
84. Theodore WH, Katz D, Kufta C, et al. Pathology of temporal lobe foci: Correlation with CT, MRI, and PET. *Neurology.* 1990;40:797–803.
85. Vecht CJ, Wagner GL, Wilms EB. Interactions between antiepileptic and chemotherapeutic drugs. *Lancet Neurol.* 2003;2:404–409.
86. Vignaendra V, Ng KK, Lim CL, et al. Clinical and electroencephalographic data indicative of brain tumours in a seizure population. *Postgrad Med J.* 1978;54:1–5.
87. Walker MD, Alexander E, Hunt WE, et al. Evaluation of BCNU and/or radiotherapy in the treatment of anaplastic gliomas. *J Neurosurg.* 1978;49:333–343.
88. Weaver S, Forsyth P, Fulton D, et al. A prospective randomized study of prophylactic anticonvulsants (AC) in patients with primary brain tumors (PBT) or metastatic brain tumors (MBT) and without prior seizures (Sz): A preliminary analysis of 67 patients. *Neurology.* 1995;45(Suppl 4):A263.
89. Weir B, Elvidge AR. Oligodendrogliomas: An analysis of 63 cases. *J Neurosurg.* 1968;29:500–505.
90. White JC, Liu CT, Mixter WJ. Focal epilepsy: A statistical study of its causes and the results of surgical treatment. I. Epilepsy secondary to intracranial tumors. *N Engl J Med.* 1948;438:891–899.
91. Whittle IR, Beaumont A. Seizures in patients with supratentorial oligodendroglial tumours. Clinicopathological features and management considerations. *Acta Neurochir.* 1995;135:19–24.
92. Whittle IR, Clarke M, Cull RE. Intraoperative electrocorticographic findings during brain tumour resection. *Br J Neurosurg.* 1994;8:263–264.
93. Wong DD, Longenecker RG, Liepman M, et al. Phenytoin-dexamethasone: A potential drug interaction (Letter). *JAMA.* 1985;254:2062–2063.
94. Zaatreh MM, Firlik KS, Spencer DD, et al. Temporal lobe tumoral epilepsy. Characteristics and predictors of surgical outcome. *Neurology.* 2003;61:636–641.
95. Zentner J, Hufnagel A, Wolf HK, et al. Surgical treatment of neoplasms associated with medically intractable epilepsy. *Neurosurgery.* 1997;41:378–387.
96. Zimm S, Wampler G, Stablein D, et al. Intracerebral metastases in solid-tumor patients. Natural history and results of treatment. *Cancer.* 1981;48:384–394.

CHAPTER 265 ■ INFECTION AND INFLAMMATORY DISEASES

OSCAR H. DEL BRUTTO

INTRODUCTION

Infectious and inflammatory diseases of the central nervous system (CNS) cause a wide range of clinical manifestations, including decreased level of consciousness, behavioral changes, increased intracranial pressure, focal neurologic deficits, and seizures. The latter may occur as the primary manifestation of the disease or as part of a diffuse encephalopathy. Pathogenesis of the seizure disorder varies widely from one disease to another. In some of these conditions, seizures appear in close temporal association with the acute disease process, although in others, seizures may occur from several weeks to months later, and tend to recur over the following years. Recognition of infectious- or inflammatory-related acute or remote symptomatic seizures has important therapeutic and prognostic implications. Here, we review the most common CNS infectious and inflammatory disorders associated with seizures.

PARASITIC INFECTIONS

Neurocysticercosis

Neurocysticercosis (NCC) is defined as the infection of the CNS by the larval stage of *Taenia solium*. The disease occurs when humans become intermediate hosts in the life cycle of this cestode after ingesting its eggs in contaminated food or by the fecal–oral route in individuals harboring the adult parasite in the intestine. Although the former was previously considered the most common form of transmission, recent studies showing clustering of NCC patients around taeniasic individuals have changed previous concepts crediting food and the environment as the main sources of human contamination with *T. solium* eggs.[21] *Taenia* carriers are contagious sources of cysticercosis, endangering everyone coming into contact with them. Human cysticercosis must be considered a disease resulting from contagion from an infected human; therefore, the patient's close environment should be investigated to eradicate the source of contagion.

NCC constitutes a threat to millions of people in Latin America, sub-Saharan Africa, and Asia. Massive immigration of people from endemic areas has also caused a recent increase in the prevalence of this parasitic disease in the United States and some European countries.[68] NCC is a leading cause of late-onset epilepsy and a major cause of seizures in developing countries, where the prevalence of active epilepsy is twice that seen in industrialized nations. Indeed, population-based studies have shown that NCC accounts for up to 30% of this excess fraction of epilepsy in the developing world.[14,39,41] It is estimated that 50,000 deaths due to NCC occur every year, and many times that number of patients survive but are left with irreversible brain damage. Despite the magnitude of these numbers, they are but the "tip of the iceberg" because the actual prevalence of NCC is not known.

Pathophysiology

Cysticerci may be located in brain parenchyma, subarachnoid space, ventricular system, and spinal cord. After entering the CNS, cysticerci elicit few inflammatory changes in the surrounding tissues. In many patients, cysticerci remain in this vesicular stage for years. In others, parasites enter, as the result of the host's immune attack, in a process of degeneration. Stages of involution through which cysticerci pass during this process are called colloidal, granular, and calcified. Inflammatory reaction around cysticerci induce pathological changes in the CNS serving as a substratum for the further development of seizures. Within the brain parenchyma, such a reaction is usually associated with edema and reactive gliosis. At the subarachnoid space level there is thickening of the leptomeninges with entrapment of cranial nerves and blood vessels located at the base of the skull. Luschka and Magendie's foramina may be occluded with the subsequent development of hydrocephalus. Ventricular cysticerci elicit a local inflammatory reaction if they are attached to the ventricular wall. In such cases, ependymal cells proliferate and may block cerebrospinal fluid (CSF) transit at the level of the cerebral aqueduct or Monro's foramina; this process of granular ependymitis causes obstructive hydrocephalus.[49]

Epilepsy is more frequently observed in patients with cysticerci located in the brain parenchyma or in the depth of cortical sulci. Cysticerci in all stages of involution may induce seizures, although the mechanisms of epileptogenesis are different. Vesicular cysts cause seizures due to compression of the surrounding brain parenchyma and colloidal cysts cause seizures due to acute inflammatory changes. In contrast, granular and calcified cysticerci cause seizures due to the intense astrocytic gliosis that usually surrounds these lesions.[44]

The concept that cysticerci play a role in epileptogenesis comes from epidemiological studies showing a correlation between populations with increased prevalence of both cysticercosis and epilepsy, and from neuroimaging studies showing NCC in patients with epilepsy in the absence of other etiologies. Also, the episodic appearance of edema surrounding cysticerci after a seizure episode unquestionably links cysticerci with seizures (Fig. 1). This phenomenon occurs not only in patients with living cysts but also in those with calcifications, suggesting that calcified cysticerci should not be seen as inert lesions causing no symptoms.

The pathogenesis of edema around calcified cysticerci is not fully understood.[44] One hypothesis is that periodic remodeling of calcifications exposes the host's immune system to residual antigens still present in these lesions. Direct calcium toxicity is another possibility as it has been suggested that brain lesions that calcify are associated with increased seizure activity compared to those that fail to calcify. It is also possible that brain gliosis left during the death of the parasite explain recurrent

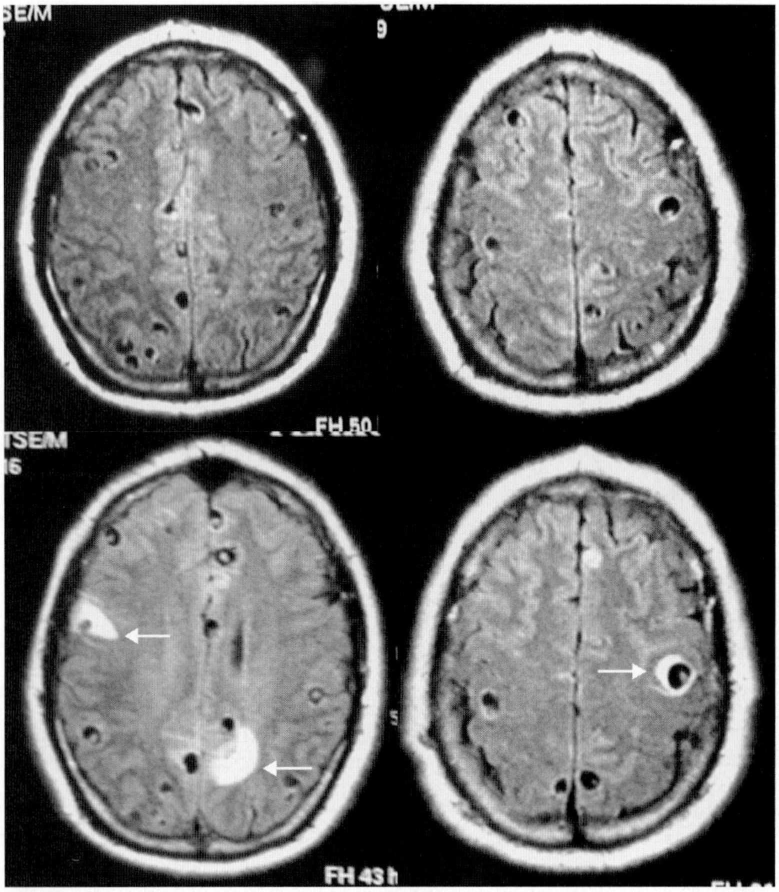

FIGURE 1. Fluid attenuated inversion recovery MRI of patient with parenchymal NCC before (*upper panel*) and 6 hours after (*lower panel*) a seizure episode, showing new hyperintense areas in brain parenchyma, some of which are surrounding cystic lesions (*arrows*).

seizure activity. Another hypothesis is that edema is not the cause but the result of the seizure, as has been documented in a few patients after a cryptogenic partial status epilepticus. However, this is improbable because the magnetic resonance imaging (MRI) pattern of perilesional edema in cysticercosis is most consistent with vasogenic edema resulting from breakdown of the blood–brain barrier, and does not have the imaging appearance of cytotoxic edema resulting from cell swelling associated with prolonged seizures.

Clinical Manifestations

NCC is highly pleomorphic owing to individual differences in the number and location of the lesions. Seizures, focal deficits, cognitive decline, and increased intracranial pressure are common manifestations of NCC. Seizures occur in more than 70% of NCC patients.[15] Most of these patients have a normal neurologic examination, and differ from patients with epilepsy due to other cerebral lesions, who usually present with focal signs.

Seizures due to NCC are most commonly simple partial or generalized tonic-clonic, although some patients may present with complex partial or myoclonic seizures. The seizure type has been considered to be related to the number and location of the parasites, whereby patients with a single lesion present with partial seizures, although patients with multiple lesions have generalized seizures.[15] However, other studies have shown no difference in the frequency of partial seizures in patients with single cysts as compared with those with multiple cysts.[40] It is possible that most NCC patients with generalized seizures actually have partial seizures with rapid secondary generalization, an assumption based on the fact that focal brain lesions rarely course with genuine generalized seizures. Not all NCC patients with seizures develop epilepsy. Indeed, there are some patients with a single colloidal cyst who after a bout of two or three seizures remain free of seizures even without antiepileptic drug (AED) therapy.[53] Nevertheless, if we consider the population of patients with NCC-related seizures at large, the vast majority actually have epilepsy because the epileptogenic focus is already developed when the patient is first seen.

Diagnosis

NCC is often diagnosed on the basis of information provided by neuroimaging studies and serology. Both computed tomography (CT) and MRI give objective information on the number and location of lesions as well as on the stage of evolution of cysticerci.[19] Although MRI has better accuracy than CT, it may miss some small calcifications and has the shortcoming of being less available in endemic areas for NCC. From the many immune diagnostic tests, current evidence favors the use of serum immunoblot using purified glycoprotein antigens.[21] A major problem using the immunoblot is that almost 50% of patients with a single intracranial cyst may test negative, and that some patients with taeniasis (but not NCC) may test positive. A set of diagnostic criteria has been proposed to homogenize the diagnosis of NCC.[13] Proper interpretation of these criteria permit two degrees of diagnostic certainty, definitive or probable (Table 1).

Treatment

Characterization of NCC according to the viability and location of lesions is important for a rational therapy, which usually includes a combination of symptomatic and cysticidal drugs, surgical resection of lesions, or placement of ventricular shunts.[20] Albendazole and praziquantel have changed the prognosis of most patients with parenchymal brain and

TABLE 1

DIAGNOSTIC CRITERIA FOR NEUROCYSTICERCOSIS

DIAGNOSTIC CRITERIA

Absolute Criteria:
- Histologic demonstration of the parasite from biopsy of a brain or spinal cord lesion.
- Cystic lesions showing the scolex on CT or MRI.
- Direct visualization of subretinal parasites by funduscopic examination.

Major Criteria:
- Lesions highly suggestive of neurocysticercosis on neuroimaging studies.
- Positive serum immunoblot for the detection of anticysticercal antibodies.
- Resolution of cystic lesions after therapy with albendazole or praziquantel.
- Spontaneous resolution of small single enhancing lesions.

Minor Criteria:
- Lesions compatible with neurocysticercosis on neuroimaging studies.
- Clinical manifestations suggestive of neurocysticercosis.
- Positive CSF enzyme-linked immunosorbent assay (ELISA) for detection of anticysticercal antibodies or cysticercal antigens.
- Cysticercosis outside the central nervous system.

Epidemiologic Criteria:
- Evidence of household contact with *T. solium* infection.
- Individuals coming from or living in an area where cysticercosis is endemic.
- History of frequent travel to disease-endemic areas.

DEGREES OF DIAGNOSTIC CERTAINTY

Definitive Diagnosis:
- Presence of one absolute criterion.
- Presence of two major plus one minor and one epidemiologic criteria.

Probable Diagnosis:
- Presence of one major plus two minor criteria.
- Presence of one major plus one minor and one epidemiologic criteria.
- Presence of three minor plus one epidemiologic criteria.

subarachnoid cysts presenting with seizures. However, because pioneer studies of NCC therapy focused on the number of cysts before and after the trial, some authors affirmed that cyst disappearance did not necessarily mean improved clinical outcome. Thereafter, two studies showed a strong association between cysticidal treatment and fewer seizures in NCC patients, a finding that was also questioned due to the non-randomized design of these studies.[15,66] During the past few years, placebo-controlled trials have shown that the use of cysticidal drugs not only results in better resolution of lesions but in a lesser risk of seizure recurrence in patients with NCC, providing Class I evidence favoring therapy in these cases.[2,22]

The control of epilepsy in NCC patients not only depends on the use of cysticidal drugs, but on the chronicity of the disorder and the presence of brain calcifications. These patients must be treated with an AED regardless of the use of cysticidal drugs. The optimal length of AED therapy has not been settled. A prospective study showed that up to 50% of NCC patients had relapses after AED withdrawal.[11] Such patients had been free of seizures during two years, and their brain cysts had been successfully destroyed with albendazole. Prognostic factors associated with seizure recurrence included the development of calcifications, and the presence of both recurrent seizures and multiple brain cysts before cysticidal drug therapy.[11,52] Calcified cysticerci are potentially active epileptogenic foci that may cause recurrent seizures after AED withdrawal. Although epilepsy due to NCC may be easily controlled with AEDs, a seizure-free state without medications cannot always be achieved.

Cerebral Malaria

Of the four species of malaria parasites, only *Plasmodium falciparum* invades the CNS and causes cerebral malaria. Because all species may cause fever associated with delirium or seizures, definition of cerebral malaria requires all of the following conditions to be present: unarousable coma, evidence of acute infection with *P. falciparum*, and no other identifiable cause of coma.[69] Humans acquire the infection when parasites are inoculated through the skin during a blood meal by a female *Anopheles* mosquito. Malaria is a public health problem around the world. Up to 500 million people are infected by *Plasmodium spp*. every year, with 3 million fatal cases, most of which occur in African children. Due to increased travel, many cases of cerebral malaria have also been recently recognized in developed countries.[63]

Pathophysiology

The brain of patients dying from cerebral malaria shows diffuse swelling and small ring hemorrhages in the subcortical white matter. These are related to extravasation of erythrocytes resulting from endothelial damage which, in turn, is caused by the liberation of cytokines and vasoactive substances. Another common neuropathologic finding in cerebral malaria is the plugging of capillaries by parasitized erythrocytes due to an increased adherence of these cells to the endothelium. This causes brain damage as a result of obstruction of the cerebral microvasculature, increased concentrations of lactic acid, and ischemic hypoxia.[53]

Clinical Manifestations

Cerebral malaria is an acute encephalopathy characterized by headache, seizures, somnolence or agitation that rapidly progresses to stupor and coma, and extensor posturing. Seizures occur in up to 70% of cases, and are most often tonic-clonic generalized, although some patients present with partial seizures.[54] Pulmonary edema, renal failure, hypoglycemia, and disseminated intravascular coagulation are common during the acute phase of the disease. Most patients who do not die during the first few days recover without sequelae. Some others are left with hemiplegia, blindness, psychiatric symptoms, speech disturbances, recurrent seizures, and extrapyramidal manifestations.[69]

Diagnosis

P. falciparum may be seen by examining blood smears with Giemsa stain; repeated examinations may be needed, because parasitemia is cyclic. Dipstick antigen-capture assay may be of diagnostic value in patients with low levels of parasitemia.[67] Although the cytochemical analysis of CSF is normal in these patients, a spinal tap is mandatory to exclude other causes of encephalopathy. Neuroimaging studies may show brain swelling, hypodense areas in the thalamus or cerebellum, small hemorrhages, or dural sinus thrombosis.[36]

Treatment

Because of chloroquine-resistant strains of *P. falciparum*, quinine is the drug of choice for cerebral malaria.[6] The association of quinine plus pentoxifylline may be better than quinine alone for therapy of cerebral malaria in adults. Mefloquine is effective against *P. falciparum* but has not been evaluated in patients with cerebral malaria. Recent evidence favors the use of artemether as a first-line therapeutic agent for cerebral malaria.[43] Symptomatic therapy includes fluid replacement, sedatives, and osmotic diuretics. Corticosteroids are harmful to comatose patients with cerebral malaria and should be avoided. Although phenobarbital is often used to treat malaria-related seizures in endemic areas, the common loading dose of 20 mg/kg may be deleterious for children with cerebral malaria. A recent study suggested that an initial dose of 15 mg/kg followed by two doses of 2.5 mg/kg after 24 and 48 hours is safe and effective in these patients.[30] Despite therapy, up to 25% of patients with cerebral malaria die. Factors adversely affecting the prognosis include coma, retinal hemorrhages, recurrent seizures, renal failure, disseminated intravascular coagulation, respiratory distress, arterial hypotension, severe anemia, hypoglycemia, altered liver function tests, presence of malaria pigment in peripheral white blood cells, high levels of parasitemia, and co-infection with HIV.[8,69]

Other Parasitic Diseases of the Central Nervous System

Almost any parasite invading the CNS may cause seizures. These may occur as the result of the pressure effects of a parasite growing within the brain parenchyma (as in the case of cerebral hydatid disease or coenurosis), due to the irritative effects of a larva migrating through the brain (as in gnathostomiasis or sparganosis), or as part of a diffuse encephalopathy (as in patients with cerebral amebiasis or African trypanosomiasis). In any case, seizures may occur during the acute phase of the disease or as a chronic sequelae of the infection.[12,58] AED therapy should be promptly started in these cases to stop seizures and to avoid recurrences, irrespective of the specific therapy used for each of these conditions. Duration of AED therapy and the risk of seizure recurrence after AED withdrawal will vary depending on the severity of the initial infection and the occurrence of residual structural brain damage.

BACTERIAL INFECTIONS

Pyogenic Meningitis

Causal agents of pyogenic meningitis vary according to the age and the immune status of the patient, and the route by which the infection gains access to the CNS. *Haemophilus influenzae*, *Neisseria meningitidis*, and *Streptococcus pneumoniae* are the most common pathogens causing this condition. Bacteria may reach the subarachnoid space by the hematogenous route from a remote infection, or by contiguity from an infection of paranasal sinuses or ears.[56]

Pathophysiology

Pyogenic bacteria induce the formation of a purulent exudate within the subarachnoid space related to migration of neutrophils and other immune cells.[53] Such exudate, together with direct effects of bacterial toxins, may cause seizures by a number of pathogenetic mechanisms, including: (a) occlusion of small pial arteries with the subsequent development of cortical infarctions, (b) venous thrombosis, (c) diffuse brain swelling, (d) toxic effects of bacteria accumulation within the subpial space, and (e) acute metabolic changes.

Clinical Manifestations

Pyogenic meningitis is an acute disease mainly characterized by fever, headache, cloudiness of consciousness, and seizures. Neurologic examination usually shows neck stiffness or other signs of meningeal irritation. Less common signs include cranial nerve palsies, papilledema or focal deficits. Acute symptomatic seizures occur in up to 40% of patients and are more often of the tonic-clonic generalized type, although some patients present with partial seizures. Only a few patients develop chronic epilepsy after the acute infection. In two large series of children with pyogenic meningitis, epilepsy occurred in 2% and 7% of cases, and was most often associated with the occurrence of permanent neurologic deficits.[50,64]

Diagnosis

A spinal tap usually shows a turbid CSF under increased opening pressure. CSF examination reveals increased polymorphonuclear cells (>1,000 mm^3), decreased glucose levels (<20 mg/dL), and high protein contents (from 100–500 mg/dL). Gram stains and cultures are helpful for identifying the offending microorganism but may be negative in some patients, especially in those receiving antibiotics prior to admission. Polymerase chain reaction (PCR) amplification techniques are useful for detecting bacterial antigens in patients with partially treated infections.[17] CT or MRI should be performed to rule out a cerebral abscess.

Treatment

Patients must be treated with antibiotics according to the causal agent. When the etiology is not know, antibiotics should be chosen according to the age of the patient and the suspected portal of entry of bacteria.[56] Current knowledge does not favor the routine use of corticosteroids in most cases. Acute seizures should be treated with intravenous phenytoin of fosphenytoin; most of these patients will not need long-term AED therapy. However, patients with late seizures should be managed according to the guidelines of treatment of symptomatic epilepsies. Some patients, particularly those developing mesial temporal sclerosis as a late sequela may course with intractable epilepsy, and may require surgery for seizure control.[33]

Brain Abscess

Abscesses are localized infections occurring as the result of invasion of the brain parenchyma by pyogenic bacteria. Most common causal agents include *Bacteroides spp.*, *Staphylococcus aureus*, *Streptococcus spp.*, *Proteus spp.*, and *Enterobacter spp.* These lesions are most often related to the direct spread of bacteria from an adjacent focus of infection (paranasal sinuses, ears, orbits, or teeth), but may also be the result of hematogenous spread of microorganisms from distant foci of infection, usually located in the heart and lungs.[7]

Pathophysiology

Most abscesses are located in the cerebral hemispheres at the cortico-subcortical junction. These lesions evolve into four stages: Early cerebritis (days 1–3), late cerebritis (days 4–9), early capsule formation (days 10–13), and late capsule formation (after 14 days). Once fully developed, an abscess consists of a necrotic center and a capsule composed of fibroblasts, macrophages, and collagen fibers. The surrounding brain parenchyma shows severe swelling and gliosis, providing a substrate for the occurrence of seizures.[31]

Clinical Manifestations

A brain abscess may cause fever, signs and symptoms of increased intracranial pressure, and focal deficits that vary according to the location of the lesion.[7] Fever may be lacking, especially in the elderly or immunosuppressed patients. Seizures occur in more than 50% of patients during the acute phase of the disease, and almost 40% of survivors are left with residual epilepsy. A retrospective series showed that brain abscesses located in the temporal lobe were associated with the highest risk of developing late epilepsy.[31]

Diagnosis

Abscesses appear on CT and MRI as ring enhancing lesions surrounded by edema. The rim of enhancement is usually thicker at the cortical than at the ventricular side of the abscess. Lesions may be multilobulated, due to the formation of the so-called "daughter abscesses" (Fig. 2). New MRI techniques such as MR spectroscopy, diffusion-weighted imaging, and apparent diffusion coefficient (ADC) maps have been shown to be of value in the differentiation of abscesses from other space-occupying brain lesions such as brain tumors and tuberculomas.[24] The purulent center of a brain abscess has a reduced ADC as opposed to necrotic or cystic brain tumors presenting with elevated ADC values (Fig. 3).

Treatment

Patients usually require a combination of medical and surgical management. Antibiotics must be started without knowing the causal agent and their spectrum of action should cover both aerobic and anaerobic bacteria.[4] Increased intracranial pressure should be treated with mannitol or corticosteroids; the latter may reduce the concentration of antibiotics in the necrotic center of the lesion. Seizure prophylaxis is indicated as soon as a brain abscess is diagnosed, and most patients will require prolonged AED therapy.

Empyemas

Empyemas are collections of purulent material at the subdural and epidural spaces. They occur as the result of direct

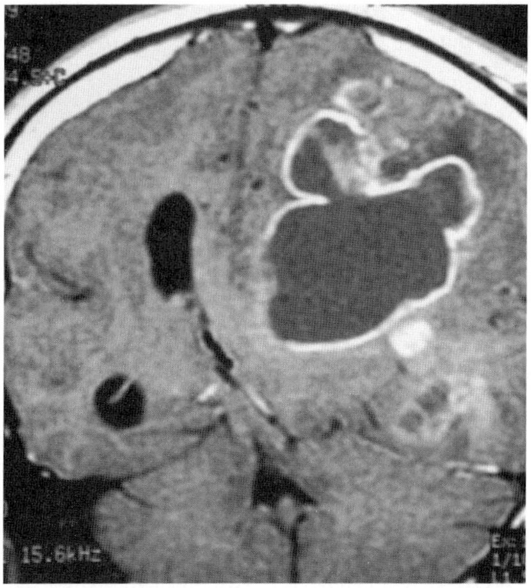

FIGURE 2. Gadolinium-enhanced, T1-weighted MRI of patient with brain abscess showing multilobulated ring-enhancing lesion displacing midline structures.

spread from an adjacent focus of infection and, in cases of brain abscesses, empyemas are most often caused by anaerobic bacteria.[28]

Pathophysiology

Empyemas distend the dura and cause septic thrombosis of intracranial dural sinuses. Cortical veins may also be occluded with the subsequent development of cortical infarctions. Seizures may occur as the result of these infarctions or due to direct irritation of the cerebral cortex by the infectious process, as occurred in patients with meningitis.

Clinical Manifestations

Intracranial hypertension and seizures are common manifestations of empyemas.[16] Focal neurologic deficits occur in patients with cortical venous infarctions. Careful examination usually reveals an infectious process of paranasal sinuses, orbits, or ears.

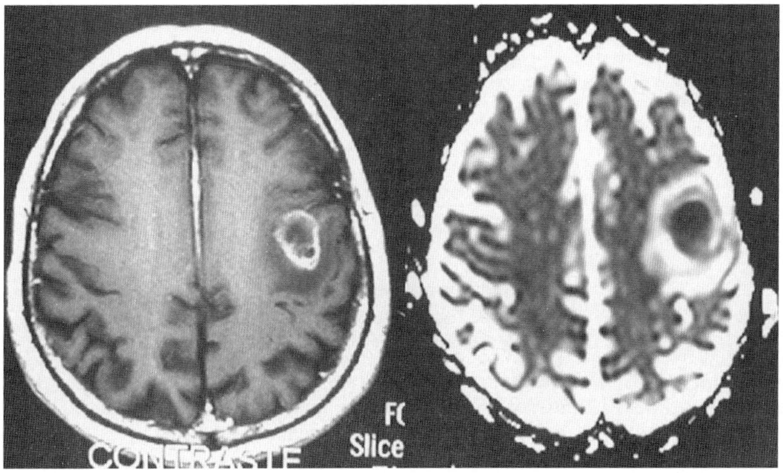

FIGURE 3. Gadolinium-enhanced, T1-weighted MRI (*left*) and apparent diffusion coefficient (ADC) map (*right*) of patient with brain abscess. Reduced ADC helps to differentiate abscesses from brain tumors (courtesy of Dr. Julio Lama, Guayaquil, Ecuador).

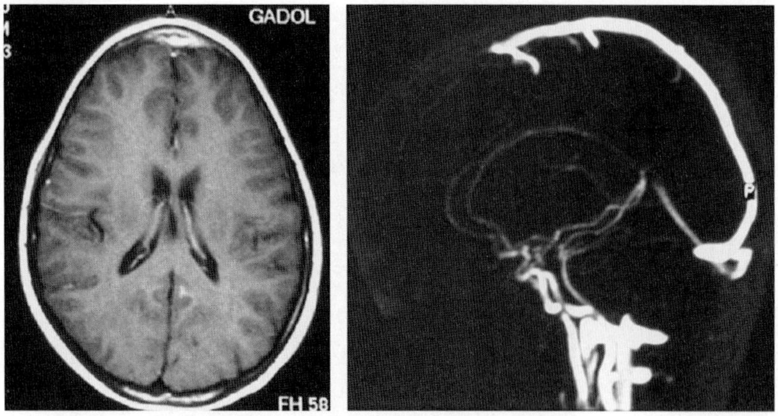

FIGURE 4. Gadolinium-enhanced, T1-weighted MRI (*left*) and MR angiography (*right*) showing epidural empyema and occlusion of anterior half of superior sagittal sinus in patient presenting with tonic–clonic generalized status epilepticus.

Diagnosis

Neuroimaging studies usually allow the visualization of the empyema and the extent of compromise of intracranial dural sinuses (Fig. 4). A spinal tap is contraindicated in these patients due to the high risk of cerebral herniation.

Treatment

Most patients require surgical drainage of the purulent collection.[4,60] Broad-spectrum antibiotics should be given for several weeks, especially if osteomyelitis is present. AEDs should be started in all cases due to the high risk of seizures during the acute disease. The need of long-term AED therapy will be guided by the development of cortical infarctions.

Tuberculosis of the Central Nervous System

Tuberculosis is most often caused by *Mycobacterium tuberculosis*, an acid-fast bacillus that enters the body through the respiratory tract, settles in the lungs, and then reaches the CNS by the hematogenous route. The first step of brain invasion is the formation of small parenchymal brain tubercles called Rich foci. Then, tubercles may rupture into the subarachnoid space to cause meningoencephalitis or may grow in the brain parenchyma to form tuberculomas.[23]

Pathophysiology

Tuberculous meningitis is characterized by the formation of a thick exudate that encroaches cranial nerves and subarachnoid blood vessels causing arterial narrowing and cerebral infarctions. Luschka and Magendie's foramina may be occluded with the subsequent development of hydrocephalus. Also, damage of the cerebral cortex adjacent to areas of subarachnoid exudate may occur. These pathological changes are responsible for the occurrence of seizures as well as other manifestations of the disease.[47] Intracranial tuberculomas are space-occupying lesions composed of a core of caseation necrosis and a capsule of collagen tissue and inflammatory cells. The surrounding brain parenchyma shows edema and astrocytic proliferation, providing a substrate for the occurrence of seizures.[10]

Clinical Manifestations

Tuberculous meningitis is a subacute disease characterized by fever, malaise, behavioral changes, headache, seizures, focal neurologic signs, and stupor or coma. The disease has been classified into three stages according to its severity (Table 2). Seizures occur in approximately 20% of cases, are more common in children than in adults, and may represent a predictor of poor outcome.[26,65] Intracranial tuberculomas present as mass lesions, with increased intracranial pressure, focal signs, and seizures.[23]

Diagnosis

Data provided by CSF analysis and neuroimaging studies usually allows a correct diagnosis of tuberculous meningitis.[23] The CSF shows lymphocytic pleocytosis, low glucose levels, and increased protein contents. Acid-fast bacilli may be seen in less than 50% of cases, but cultures are positive in 80%. PCR detection of mycobacterial antigens is of diagnostic value in doubtful cases. CT and MRI show hydrocephalus, abnormal leptomeningeal enhancement, and small cerebral infarctions.[45] In contrast, diagnosis of intracranial tuberculomas is more complex because they resemble other space-occupying lesions on neuroimaging studies, and CSF examination is most often unrevealing. On MRI, some tuberculomas are visualized with a hypointense center surrounded by concentric rims of different intensities (Fig. 5).

Treatment

Prompt therapy with antituberculous drugs is associated with decreased morbidity and mortality in patients with meningitis. Corticosteroids ameliorate the inflammatory reaction and reduce the risk of angiitis. Tuberculomas should also be treated medically because of the risk of disseminated disease after surgery. AED therapy is indicated in patients with seizures.

TABLE 2

BRITISH MEDICAL RESEARCH COUNCIL CLASSIFICATION OF SEVERITY OF TUBERCULOUS MENINGITIS

STAGE I
- Fully conscious and rational patient, who does not have any neurologic sign.

STAGE II
- Confused but not comatose patient, who may present with some focal neurologic signs such as hemiparesis or a single cranial nerve palsy.

STAGE III
- Stuporous or comatose patient, who has hemiplegia, paraplegia, or multiple cranial nerve palsies.

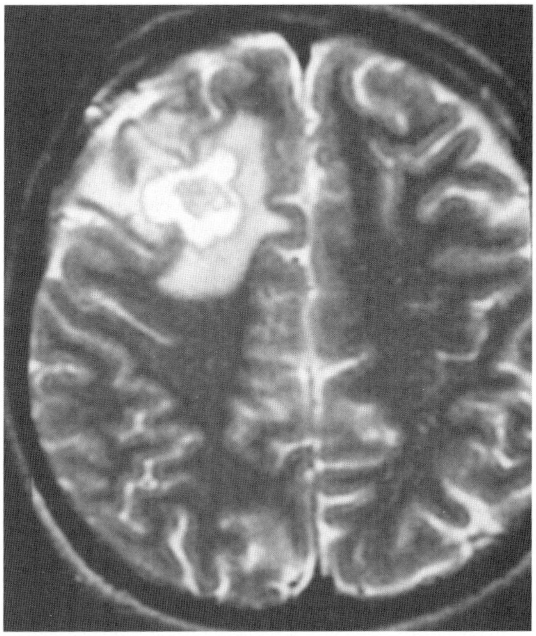

FIGURE 5. T2-weighted MRI of patient with intracranial tuberculoma showing characteristic "target" appearance of lesion.

VIRAL INFECTIONS

Viral Encephalitis

A number of viruses may cause encephalitis, defined as a diffuse inflammation of the brain parenchyma.[57] Some of these conditions are mosquito-borne, whereas others are transmitted by rodents, ticks, non-human primates, or by direct human-to-human contagion. Some encephalitides result from direct viral invasion of the CNS, whereas others are related to the occurrence of postinfectious immune disorders. In some other cases, reactivation of a latent viral infection may cause encephalitis. Viral encephalitis may occur sporadically or in epidemic bouts, and some are cosmopolitan whereas others are restricted to certain areas. Herpes simplex virus type 1 (HSV-1) is the most common cause of sporadic viral encephalitis worldwide. Of the geographically restricted viral encephalitis, the most important are Japanese B encephalitis, Venezuelan equine encephalitis, Eastern equine encephalitis, and West Nile virus encephalitis, a formerly restricted disease that is currently spreading from Africa to Europe and America.[38]

Pathophysiology

Once in the CNS, viruses spread to involve the cerebral cortex, basal ganglia, cerebellum, and brainstem. Severity of brain damage is influenced by both the virulence of the offending agent and the immune status of the host. Pathological abnormalities in the brain parenchyma of patients with viral encephalitis include diffuse swelling, vascular congestion, demyelination, inflammatory infiltrates of mononuclear cells, microglial proliferation, formation of glial nodules, and diffuse necrosis of the cerebral cortex and basal ganglia. These changes explain clinical manifestations of viral encephalitis, including seizures.

Clinical Manifestations

Viral encephalitides usually have an acute or subacute onset followed by a rapidly progressive course that may kill the patient in a few days. Occasionally, encephalitis evolves over months, causing a slowly progressive brain damage. Clinical manifestations include fever, seizures, behavioral changes, cloudiness of consciousness, rigidity, and focal neurologic deficits related to the development of cerebral infarctions.[1,29] Some patients present myalgias, sore throat, conjunctivitis, skin rash, bleeding diathesis, and respiratory dysfunction.[9,29] Seizures may be generalized or partial, are most often recurrent, and may persist after the acute disease, especially in patients left with permanent brain damage.

Diagnosis

Viral encephalitis is diagnosed on the basis of virus isolation or detection of specific antibodies in serum, in the proper epidemiological context.[62] CSF examination is abnormal in about 90% of patients, and usually shows a lymphocytic pleocytosis associated with mildly increased protein contents and normal glucose levels.[57] Neuroimaging studies most often show diffuse brain swelling or multiple small cerebral infarctions. In some conditions, MRI findings may suggest the diagnosis by showing hyperintense lesions in the temporal lobe, as in the case of HSV-1 encephalitis (Fig. 6), or bilateral necrosis of the thalamus and striatum, as in patients with Japanese B and other flaviviruses encephalitis.[18,51]

Treatment

Antiviral agents are of value in some conditions such as in HSV-1 encephalitis (acyclovir or foscarnet), cytomegalovirus

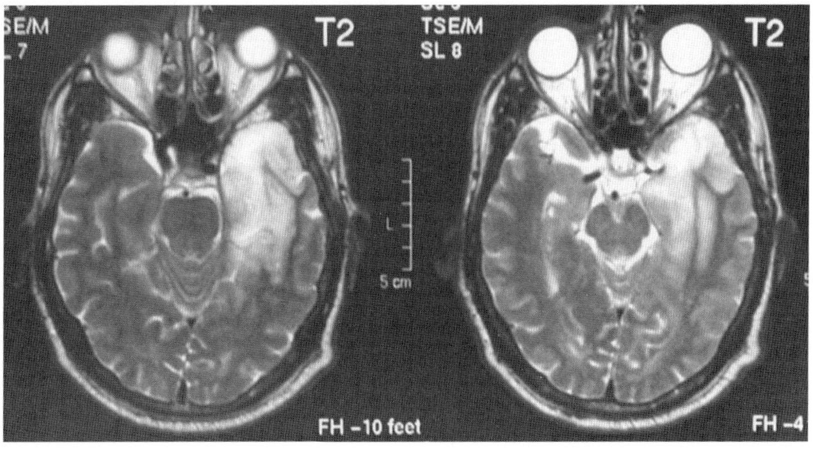

FIGURE 6. T2-weighted MRI of patient with herpes simplex virus type 1 encephalitis showing hyperintense lesion in left temporal lobe.

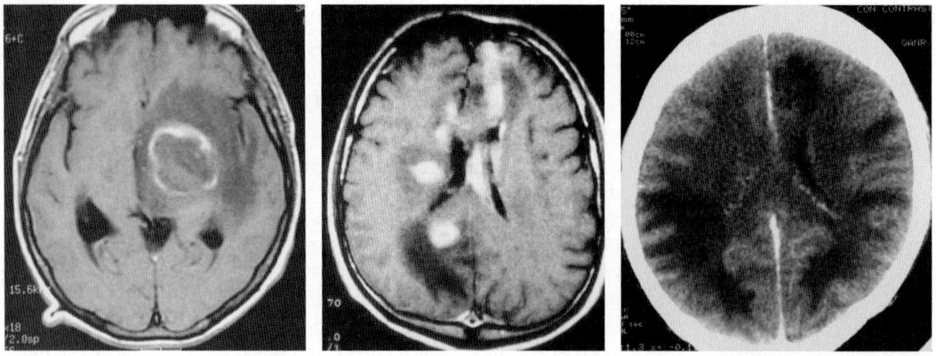

FIGURE 7. Neuroimaging findings in AIDS patients with seizures. Gadolinium-enhanced, T1-weighted MRI showing toxoplasma brain abscess (*left*) and intracranial lymphoma (*center*), and contrast-enhanced CT showing progressive multifocal leukoencephalopathy (*right*).

encephalitis (ganciclovir and foscarnet), and Lassa fever (ribavirin). Other viral encephalitides as well as those in which the etiology cannot be established may be treated initially with acyclovir and then with foscarnet if the patient deteriorates despite therapy.[29] Seizures must be aggressively treated with intravenous AEDs.

Acquired Immunodeficiency Syndrome

Acquired immunodeficiency syndrome (AIDS) affects millions of people worldwide. It represents the late stage of infection with the human immunodeficiency virus (HIV), a nononcogenic retrovirus that is acquired by sexual contact, blood transfusions, needle sharing, or vertically from the mother to the fetus. Neurologic complications of AIDS are protean, and may be caused by the HIV itself or by a number of opportunistic microorganisms or neoplasias.[37] Seizures may occur as the result of different pathogenetic mechanisms, including direct neuronal damage induced by HIV, the presence of space-occupying infectious or tumoral lesions within the brain, metabolic abnormalities, or even as a collateral effect of antiretroviral therapy.[55] Seizures may be the presenting symptoms of CNS involvement or may occur late in the course of the disease. It has been estimated that seizures occur 10 times more frequently in HIV-positive patients than in the general population.[25] In most cases, neuroimaging studies show toxoplasma brain abscesses, lymphomas, or progressive multifocal leukoencephalopathy (Fig. 7). Some patients presenting with seizures and no discernible mass lesion develop HIV-related encephalopathy in the short-term.[25,70]

HIV-positive patients with seizures must be treated with AEDs because of the high risk of recurrences. However, traditional AEDs should not be used. Phenytoin is associated with an increased prevalence of cutaneous reactions, valproic acid may favor HIV replication, and carbamazepine or phenobarbital interact with protease inhibitors.[25,27,42] Newer AEDs, such as topiramate or gabapentin, are the preferred drugs in these patients.[55]

NONINFECTIOUS INFLAMMATORY DISORDERS

Rasmussen Encephalitis

Rasmussen encephalitis (RE) is a sporadic focal encephalopathy of unknown cause. A viral etiology has been postulated but never proved, and it has been suggested that the disease may be related to autoimmune mechanisms or to depletion of cellular immunity.[5] These hypotheses are supported by the fact that most patients had an infectious disease before the start of symptoms.

Pathophysiology

The brain of patients with RE shows astrocytic gliosis, microglial nodules, spongy degeneration, and perivascular inflammation. Pathological changes are always localized to the cerebral cortex of one hemisphere.[46] There is no sound pathogenetic mechanism explaining these findings, although it has been suggested that antibodies against subunit 3 of the inotropic glutamate receptor (GluR3) cause brain damage.[5] Those antibodies would be produced after an infectious process, and would enter the brain through a focal breach in the blood–brain barrier, thus explaining the unilateral nature of RE.

Clinical Manifestations

The disease most often affects children and has an acute onset characterized by partial seizures, followed by progressive hemiparesis and cognitive decline. Epilepsia partialis continua is common, with many patients dying with severe intellectual deterioration a few years after the onset of symptoms.[59]

Diagnosis

RE should be considered in children with a typical clinical picture in whom neuroimaging studies show unilateral cerebral atrophy. Electroencephalograms (EEGs) may show delta waves or multifocal spikes in the affected cerebral hemisphere. CSF examination reveals a mild mononuclear pleocytosis associated with increased protein contents.

Treatment

Antiviral agents, interferon-α, immunoglobulins, plasmapheresis, and corticosteroids have been empirically used in some cases. Many patients develop intractable seizures despite aggressive AED therapy, and will require cerebral hemispherectomy.[48]

Neurosarcoidosis

Sarcoidosis is a systemic granulomatous disease that more often affects African-American, middle-aged women. Although the etiology is unknown, it is accepted that exposure to certain infectious agents or environmental toxins triggers, in a susceptible host, a severe inflammatory response leading to noncaseating granuloma formation.[71] Sarcoidosis usually affects the lungs, the liver, and the eyes. CNS involvement occurs in 5% of cases, and does not necessarily occur in patients with systemic manifestations of the disease. Neurosarcoidoses usually present with cranial nerve palsies, peripheral neuropathy, or diabetes insipidus. Seizures may occur in patients who develop parenchymal brain or subdural granulomas.[34,61] Children are more prone to develop seizures than adults

(15% vs. 40% of cases, respectively).[3,32] Diagnosis is difficult in patients who do not have systemic disease, and is often disclosed after a brain biopsy.[34] Therapy includes corticosteroids and AEDs. The risk of developing recurrent seizures is related to the occurrence of fibrotic scars in the brain parenchyma after granuloma resolution.

SUMMARY AND CONCLUSIONS

Almost any infectious agent invading the CNS, and a number of inflammatory conditions affecting the brain parenchyma, may cause seizures. In this setting, seizures may be related to the pressure effects of a focal infection growing within the brain, to the irritative effects of a given infectious agent, or as part of a diffuse encephalopathy. In any case, seizures may occur during the acute phase of the disease or as a chronic sequelae of the infection. Initial therapy should be directed to stop seizures and to treat the specific infection. In many cases, AEDs must be given for years to avoid seizure recurrences irrespective of the successful management of the infectious process. Duration of AED therapy and the risk of seizure recurrence after AED withdrawal vary according to the severity of the infection and the occurrence of structural brain damage.

References

1. Arciniegas DB, Anderson CA. Viral encephalitis: Neuropsychiatric and neurobehavioral aspects. *Curr Psychiatry Rep.* 2004;6:372–379.
2. Baranwal AK, Singhi PD, Khandelwal N, Singhi SC. Albendazole therapy in children with focal seizures and single small enhancing computerized tomographic lesions: A randomized, placebo-controlled, double-blind trial. *Pediatr Infect Dis J.* 1998;17:696–700.
3. Baumann RJ, Robertson WC Jr. Neurosarcoid presents differently in children than in adults. *Pediatrics.* 2003;112:e480–486.
4. Bernardini GL. Diagnosis and management of brain abscess and subdural empyema. *Curr Neurol Neurosci Rep.* 2004;4:448–456.
5. Bien CG, Granata T, Antozzi C, et al. Pathogenesis, diagnosis and treatment of Rasmussen encephalitis. A European consensus statement. *Brain.* 2005;128:454–471.
6. Birbeck GL. Cerebral malaria. *Curr Treat Options Neurol.* 2004;6:125–137.
7. Calfee DP, Wispelwey B. Brain abscess. *Semin Neurol.* 2000;20:353–360.
8. Chirenda J, Siziya S, Tshimanga M. Association of HIV infection with the development of severe and complicated malaria cases at a rural hospital in Zimbabwe. *Cent Afr J Med.* 2000;46:5–9.
9. Cummins D. Arenaviral haemorragic fevers. *Blood Rev.* 1991;5:129–137.
10. Dastur DK. Neurosurgically relevant aspects of pathology and pathogenesis of intracranial and intraspinal tuberculomas. *Neurosurg Rev.* 1983;6:103–110.
11. Del Brutto OH. Prognostic factors for seizure recurrence after withdrawal of antiepileptic drugs in patients with neurocysticercosis. *Neurology.* 1994;44:1706–1709.
12. Del Brutto OH. Helminthic Infections. In Roos KL, ed. *Principles of Neurologic Infectious Diseases.* New York: McGraw-Hill; 2005: 241–261.
13. Del Brutto OH, Rajshekhar V, White AC Jr, et al. Proposed diagnostic criteria for neurocysticercosis. *Neurology.* 2001;57:177–183.
14. Del Brutto OH, Santibañez R, Idrovo L, et al. Epilepsy and neurocysticercosis in Atahualpa: A door-to-door survey in rural coastal Ecuador. *Epilepsia.* 2005;46:583–587.
15. Del Brutto OH, Santibañez R, Noboa CA, et al. Epilepsy due to neurocysticercosis. Analysis of 203 patients. *Neurology.* 1992;42:389–392.
16. Dill SR, Cobbs CG, McDonald CK. Subdural empyemas: Analysis of 32 cases and review. *Clin Infect Dis.* 1995;20:372–386.
17. du Plessis M, Smith AM, Klugman KP. Rapid detection of penicillin-resistant *Streptococcus pneumoniae* in cerebrospinal fluid by a seminested-PCR strategy. *J Clin Microbiol.* 1998;36:453–457.
18. Einsiedel L, Kat E, Ravindran J, et al. MR findings in Murray Valley encephalitis. *Am J Neuroradiol.* 2003;24:1379–1382.
19. Garcia HH, Del Brutto OH. Imaging findings in neurocysticercosis. *Acta Trop.* 2004;87:71–78.
20. García HH, Del Brutto OH, Nash TE, et al. New concepts in the diagnosis and management of neurocysticercosis (*Taenia solium*). *Am J Trop Med Hyg.* 2005;72:3–9.
21. García HH, Gonzalez AE, Evans CAW, et al., for the Cysticercosis Working Group in Peru. *Taenia solium* cysticercosis. *Lancet.* 2003;361:547–556.
22. García HH, Pretell EJ, Gilman RH, et al. A Trial of Antiparasitic Treatment to Reduce the Rate of Seizures Due to Cerebral Cysticercosis. *N Engl J Med.* 2004;350:249–258.
23. García-Monco JC. CNS Tuberculosis and Mycobacteriosis. In Roos KL, ed. *Principles of Neurologic Infectious Diseases.* New York: McGraw-Hill; 2005: 195–213.
24. Gupta RK, Hasan KM, Mishra AM, et al. High fractional anisotropy in brain abscesses versus other cystic intracranial lesions. *Am J Neuroradiol.* 2005;26:1107–1114.
25. Holtzman DM, Kaku DA, So YT. New-onset seizures associated with human immunodeficiency virus infection: Causation and clinical features in 100 cases. *Am J Med.* 1989;87:173–177.
26. Hosoglu S, Geyik MF, Balik I, et al. Predictors of outcome in patients with tuberculous meningitis. *Int J Tuberc Lung Dis.* 2002;6:64–70.
27. Hugen PW, Burger DM, Brinkman K, et al. Carbamazepine-indinavir interaction causes antiretroviral therapy failure. *Ann Pharmacother.* 2000;34:465–470.
28. Kaufman DM, Litman N, Miller MH. Sinusitis-induced subdural empyema. *Neurology.* 1983;33:123–132.
29. Kennedy PGE. Viral encephalitis: Causes, differential diagnosis, and management. *J Neurol Neurosurg Psychiatry.* 2004;75(Suppl 1):I10–I15.
30. Kokwaro GO, Ogutu BR, Muchohi SN, et al. Pharmacokinetics and clinical effect of phenobarbital in children with severe falciparum malaria and convulsions. *Br J Clin Pharmacol.* 2003;56:453–457.
31. Koszewski W. Epilepsy following brain abscess. The evaluation of possible risk factors with emphasis on new concepts of epileptic focus formation. *Acta Neurochir.* 1991;113:110–117.
32. Krumholz A, Stern BJ, Stern EG. Clinical implications of seizures in neurosarcoidosis. *Arch Neurol.* 1991;48:842–844.
33. Lancman ME, Morris HH III. Epilepsy and central nervous system infection: Clinical characteristics and outcome after epilepsy surgery. *Epilepsy Res.* 1996;25:285–290.
34. Larner AJ, Ball JA, Howard RS. Sarcoid tumour: Continuing diagnostic problems in the MRI era. *J Neurol Neurosurg Psychiatry.* 1999;66:510–512.
35. Leib SL, Tauber MC. Pathogenesis of bacterial meningitis. *Infect Dis Clin North Am.* 1999;13:527–547.
36. Looareesuwan S, Wilairatana P, Krishna S, et al. Magnetic resonance imaging of the brain in patients with cerebral malaria. *Clin Infect Dis.* 1995;21:300–309.
37. McArthur JC. Neurologic manifestations of AIDS. *Medicine (Balt).* 1987;66:407–437.
38. McCarthy M. Newer viral encephalitis. *Neurologist.* 2003;9:189–199.
39. Medina MT, Durón RM, Martínez L, et al. Prevalence, incidence, and etiology of epilepsies in rural Honduras: The Salamá study. *Epilepsia.* 2005;46:124–131.
40. Medina MT, Rosas E, Rubio-Donnadieu F, et al. Neurocysticercosis as the main cause of late-onset epilepsy in Mexico. *Arch Intern Med.* 1990;150:325–327.
41. Montano SM, Villaran MV, Ylquimiche L, et al. Neurocysticercosis. Association between seizures, serology, and brain CT in rural Peru. *Neurology.* 2005;65:229–234.
42. Moog C, Kuntz-Simon G, Caussin-Schwemling C, et al. Sodium valproate, an anticonvulsant drug, stimulates human immunodeficiency virus type 1 replication independently of glutathione levels. *J Gen Virol.* 1996;77:1993–1999.
43. Mturi N, Musumba CO, Wamola BM, et al. Cerebral malaria: Optimising management. *CNS Drugs.* 2003;17:153–165.
44. Nash TE, Del Brutto OH, Butman JA, et al. Calcific neurocysticercosis and epileptogenesis. *Neurology.* 2004;62:1934–1938.
45. Ozates M, Kemaloglu S, Gurkan F, et al. CT of the brain in tuberculous meningitis. A review of 289 patients. *Acta Radiol.* 2000;41:13–17.
46. Pardo CA, Vining EP, Guo L, et al. The pathology of Rasmussen syndrome: Stages of cortical involvement and neuropathological studies in 45 hemispherectomies. *Epilepsia.* 2004;45:516–526.
47. Patwari AK, Aneja S, Ravi RN, et al. Convulsions in tuberculous meningitis. *J Trop Pediatr.* 1996;42:91–97.
48. Piatt JH Jr, Hwang PA, Armstrong DC, et al. Chronic focal encephalitis (Rasmussen syndrome): Six cases. *Epilepsia.* 1988;29:268–279.
49. Pitella JEH. Neurocysticercosis. *Brain Pathol.* 1997;7:681–693.
50. Pomeroy SL, Holmes SJ, Dodge PR, et al. Seizures and other neurologic sequelae of bacterial meningitis in children. *N Engl J Med.* 1990;323:1651–1657.
51. Prakash M, Kumar S, Gupta RK. Diffusion-weighted MR imaging in Japanese encephalitis. *J Comput Assist Tomogr.* 2004;28:756–761.
52. Rajshekhar V, Jeyasselan L. Seizure outcome in patients with a solitary cerebral cysticercus granuloma. *Neurology.* 2004;62:2236–2240.
53. Román GC. Cerebral malaria: The unsolved riddle. *J Neurol Sci.* 1991;101:1–6.
54. Roman GC, Senanayake N. Neurologic manifestations of malaria. *Arq Neuropsiquiatr.* 1992;50:3–9.
55. Romanelli F, Ryan M. Seizures in HIV-seropositive individuals. Epidemiology and treatment. *CNS Drugs.* 2002;16:91–98.
56. Roos KL. Acute bacterial meningitis. *Semin Neurol.* 2000;20:293–306.
57. Roos KL. Encephalitis. In Roos KL, ed. *Principles of Neurologic Infectious Diseases.* New York: McGraw-Hill; 2005: 65–76.
58. Schmutzhard E. Protozoal Infections. In Roos KL, ed. *Principles of Neurologic Infectious Diseases.* New York: McGraw-Hill; 2005: 263–306.

59. Snook R. Rasmussen's Encephalitis. In Roos KL, ed. *Principles of Neurologic Infectious Diseases*. New York: McGraw-Hill; 2005: 517–522.
60. Southwick FS, Richardson EP Jr, Swartz NM. Septic thrombosis of the dural venous sinuses. *Medicine (Balt)*. 1986;65:82–106.
61. Sponsler JL, Werz MA, Maciunas R, Cohen M. Neurosarcoidosis presenting with partial seizures and solitary enhancing mass: Case reports and review of the literature. *Epilepsy Behav*. 2005;6:623–630.
62. Steiner I, Budka H, Chaudhuri A, et al. Viral encephalitis: A review of diagnostic methods and guidelines for management. *Eur J Neurol*. 2005;12:331–343.
63. Stoppacher R, Adams SP. Malaria deaths in the United States: Case report and review of deaths, 1979–1998. *J Forensic Sci*. 2003;48:404–408.
64. Taylor HG, Mills EL, Clampi A, et al. The sequelae of *Haemophilus influenzae* meningitis in school-age children. *N Engl J Med*. 1990;323:1657–1663.
65. Tung YR, Lai MC, Lui CC, et al. Tuberculous meningitis in infancy. *Pediatr Neurol*. 2002;27:262–266.
66. Vazquez V, Sotelo J. The course of seizures after treatment for cerebral cysticercosis. *N Engl J Med*. 1992;327:696–701.
67. Verle P, Binh LN, Lieu TT, et al. ParaSight-F test to diagnose malaria in hypo-endemic and epidemic prone regions of Vietnam. *Trop Med Int Health*. 1996;1:794–796.
68. Wallin TW, Kurtzke JF. Neurocysticercosis in the United States. Review of an important emerging infection. *Neurology*. 2004;63:1559–1564.
69. Warrell DA. Cerebral Malaria. In Shakir RA, Newman PK, Poser CM, eds. *Tropical Neurology*. London: W.B. Saunders; 1996: 213–245.
70. Wong MC, Suite ND, Labar DR. Seizures in human immunodeficiency virus infection. *Arch Neurol*. 1990;47:640–642.
71. Wu JJ, Schiff KR. Sarcoidosis. *Am Fam Physician*. 2004;70:312–322.

CHAPTER 266 ■ CONNECTIVE TISSUE DISEASES

BARBARA S. KOPPEL

INTRODUCTION

Seizures occur in several connective tissue diseases, most frequently systemic lupus erythematosus (SLE), and in forms of vasculitis that involve the brain. Often, however, seizures are not due to the primary disease process itself, but rather to secondary conditions. For example, seizures may occur in the setting of hypoxic or metabolic encephalopathy. Chronic hypertension and accelerated atherosclerosis, even in the absence of antiphospholipid syndrome or cerebral vasculitis, increase the risk of stroke and hemorrhage, which in turn predispose to seizures. Both the underlying disease and its treatment with immunosuppressive drugs increase the risk of brain or meningeal infection, which can cause seizures. Finally, some therapeutic agents used in the management of collagen-vascular disease or vasculitis, such as tacrolimus and cyclosporine, cause an encephalopathy of which seizures are a manifestation.[29]

This chapter reviews the incidence of seizures in connective tissue and vasculitic diseases; when in the course of these illnesses, and under what circumstances, seizures can be expected; and pathophysiology, diagnostic testing, and treatment guidelines. The role of antiepileptic drugs in causing chemical and clinical signs of lupus is also discussed briefly.

GENERAL PRINCIPLES OF AUTOIMMUNITY IN EPILEPSY

Seizures occur in autoimmune disorders of the brain such as Hashimoto encephalopathy, Rasmussen encephalitis, paraneoplastic limbic encephalitis, and probably Landau-Kleffner syndrome.[87] In addition, in the absence of structural pathology, antibodies against membranes or ion channels have been proposed as causes for some cases of epilepsy. Some antibodies that are found may be just disease markers, but if there is a clinical response to treatments that lower antibody levels, or if animals immunized with the target antigen develop signs similar to those of the human disease, pathogenesis due to an immune reaction to a targeted antibody is confirmed.[105] In a study of 139 epilepsy patients, 26 had known autoimmune diseases (most often SLE and antiphospholipid syndrome) with antibodies to nuclear antigens. Although these antibodies did not correlate closely with seizure frequency, patients with antibodies against voltage-gated potassium channels and glutamic acid decarboxylase (GAD) generally had more seizures. This suggests a role for these antibodies in causing seizures, especially given that antibodies to voltage-gated calcium channels, gangliosides, glutamic receptor 3, and cardiolipins were not found.[70]

SYSTEMIC LUPUS ERYTHEMATOSUS

Clinical Manifestations

Collagen-vascular disorders, including SLE, rarely present with seizures. Seizures almost always appear later in the course of active disease, especially during flares of systemic and central nervous system (CNS) lupus.[79] SLE is one of the most common autoimmune diseases, with an annual incidence of 1.8 to 7.6/100,000 and a prevalence of 39 to 51/100,000.[79] Onset is most common in early adult life, women account for 80% of patients, and non-whites (Asians and African-Americans) are disproportionately affected.[62,81] In addition to the nervous system, SLE affects, in order of frequency, joints, mucous membranes and skin (discoid lupus, malar rash, photosensitivity, alopecia), kidneys, pleura, heart, and bone marrow. Neurologic or neuropsychiatric complications have been reported in all series since Kaposi[53] first described them in 14% to 75% of patients >100 years ago.[2,13,46,71] Psychiatric symptoms include depression and psychosis. Neurologic syndromes include dementia, aseptic meningitis, seizures, stroke, movement disorders (especially chorea), myelopathy, and peripheral neuropathy.[2,14,37] Headache can be prominent due to benign intracranial hypertension, aseptic meningitis, and venous thrombosis.[46,61] Even in the absence of dementia or depression, neuropsychological testing reveals high frequencies of cognitive dysfunction.[46,47,71,72] Neurologic complications are a common cause of hospitalization in patients with SLE[89] and the second leading cause of death.[14,107] Early neurologic involvement, especially stroke, has a worse prognosis, but seizures also contribute to poor outcome when they occur in children with arthritis.[90] Seizures double the rate of mortality when found with nephritis in adults.[107]

Both partial and generalized seizures occur in SLE. Generalized seizures can be the sole evidence of brain involvement in diffuse CNS lupus [the term "cerebritis" is no longer used by the American College of Rheumatology (ACR) due its lack of specific pathologic findings], or they may occur as part of hypertensive or metabolic encephalopathy. Status epilepticus also occurs, especially in critically ill patients, in whom it may be a preterminal event.[109] Partial seizures can be a manifestation of cerebrovascular complications (hemorrhage, ischemic stroke, venous thrombosis), abscess, or meningitis.[110] Reflex epilepsy induced by acoustic and patterned visual stimuli has been reported,[16] as has photosensitive myoclonic epilepsy,[74] both in children with SLE. Psychiatric symptoms, especially psychosis and delirium, commonly coexist with seizures[14] and are reported to occur at some time in up to 50% of patients. Partial complex (nonconvulsive) status epilepticus presents with confusion, delirium, or hallucinations; electroencephalographic monitoring is often necessary to confirm the diagnosis,[14,86] which suggests that it may have been missed in the past.

Because of the multiple causes of neuropsychiatric symptoms, it is difficult to obtain meaningful incidence figures for seizures occurring in SLE. However, the fact that seizures are listed first on the SLE activity index devised by the ACR,[12] even after this was updated to separate persistent from acute symptoms,[40] indicates their importance in this condition. In one series of 91patients with SLE, 22% experienced generalized seizures and an additional 5% had partial seizures.[37] Multiple factors, including renal failure, coagulopathy, and hypertension, contributed to seizure occurrence, whereas 3 patients had seizures completely unrelated to SLE. Of interest, 2 patients had seizures only during flares of their SLE, and 8 of the 14 patients who had had strokes experienced seizures during the course of their illness. Most series do not provide sufficient detail to conclude whether the reported seizures are due to SLE or to other conditions.

Diagnostic Tests

In patients with seizures, brain imaging should be done promptly to look for evidence of intracranial hemorrhage (parenchymal or subarachnoid), cerebral infarction, or other structural pathology. Hemorrhage is associated with vasculitis, which occurs in only a minority of patients with SLE.[78] Cortical atrophy is a frequent finding[46,49] and may relate to either long-term steroid use or disease duration.[41] Abnormalities detected by brain magnetic resonance imaging (MRI) scans have been reported in up to 75% of patients with active disease, but the findings are frequently nonspecific subcortical and periventricular punctuate areas of increased T2 signal that most likely reflect small-vessel disease or, possibly, demyelination with gliosis.[41,92] In patients with chronic SLE, abnormal MRI scans were found in 57% of cases; many of the findings were clinically silent.[41] SLE patients with neuropsychiatric symptoms have increased cerebral atrophy and more T1- and T2-weighted lesions compared to both controls and SLE patients without such symptoms.[3] However, only 4 of 43 patients had seizures in this study. Similar lesions have been reported in neurologically asymptomatic patients.[13] Acute inflammatory lesions are enhanced with gadolinium, and in symptomatic patients, serial MRI scans can document loss of enhancement or complete resolution as clinical improvement occurs.[71,110] MR venography and computed tomography (CT) angiography are useful in detecting thrombosis, especially given the dangers of invasive angiography in patients with anticardiolipin antibodies. Transcranial Doppler can be used to follow ischemic changes over time.[57]

Functional brain imaging modalities that have been used in patients with SLE include single photon emission computed tomography (SPECT), positron emission tomography (PET), and MR spectroscopy.[27,92,108] SPECT is abnormal in patients with ischemic stroke, showing focally reduced perfusion in areas that correlate well with both CT and clinical findings. At times, SPECT may be an even more sensitive indicator of cerebral ischemia than MRI, with hypoperfusion preceding clinical symptoms in patients undergoing serial scans.[50,111] Loss of the vascular response to acetazolamide detects marginally perfused areas that are at risk for infarction.[43] In patients with psychosis, SPECT has revealed decreased perfusion in the frontal lobes.[56] PET scans using fluorodeoxyglucose (FDG) demonstrate hypometabolic areas in regions of ischemia or infarction.[22,92]

Serologic markers have been studied in both generalized and CNS lupus. Positive antinuclear antibody (ANA) is found in 95% of patients with SLE, and anti–double-stranded DNA is found in 30% to 75%.[76] Although anti-Sm (smith) antibody is found in <30% of patients, it is specific for SLE. Other laboratory abnormalities that are useful in following active disease are elevated CSF complement 3 and 4,[52] and anti–single- or anti–double-stranded RNA.[33] Serum markers of autoantibodies, especially antiphospholipids (aPL), are increased in SLE patients with neuropsychiatric symptoms compared to those without them.[110] The tests most often used to distinguish among the different connective tissue disorders and types of vasculitis are summarized in Table 1. Anticardiolipin antibody levels, especially immunoglobulin G (IgG), correlate with the occurrence of seizures,[48] whereas antiribosomal P seems to be a marker of psychosis without other neurologic symptoms or signs.[14,33,113] The presence of antibodies to native DNA rather than to the histone complex favors idiopathic rather than drug-induced lupus.[16,21,36,79] Although antineuronal antibodies reflect diffuse pathology and have been reported in 60% of patients with neuropsychiatric SLE, they are also found in patients without neurologic symptoms, raising doubt as to their role in "cerebritis."[27,71,99]

In patients with cerebral ischemia or infarction, the following findings on blood tests can be helpful: The presence of anticardiolipin antibodies, of which IgG is more significant for stroke[79,116] protein S or C deficiency (this is sometimes caused by the nephrotic syndrome[61] when kidney damage is prominent); thrombocytopenia; and lupus anticoagulant using kaolin clotting time or lupus anticoagulant (LAC)-prolonged activated partial thromboplastin time (aPTT). Echocardiography can assist in determining whether there is a cardiac source for cerebral emboli, although marantic (Libman-Sacks) endocarditis is only rarely responsible for stroke in SLE.[46]

Lumbar puncture is required whenever infection is suspected, although significant thrombocytopenia or other clotting abnormalities need to be corrected before it can be performed to avoid producing a lumbar epidural hematoma. Up to one third of patients undergoing a lupus flare with CNS involvement have nonspecific findings in the cerebrospinal fluid (CSF) including increased numbers of white cells (usually lymphocytic) and elevated protein levels.[46] CSF antiribosomal-P and anticardiolipin antibodies correlate with disease activity,[112] but they can also be related to vascular damage that produces breakdown of the blood–brain barrier. Similarly, CSF interleukin-6 (IL-6), a regulator of autoantibody production, can be elevated in patients with infection and is thus best viewed as a nonspecific inflammatory marker.[46,103,112] CSF antineuronal antibody, oligoclonal bands (seen in 25% of one series, produced locally in half),[72] and IgG levels decline with treatment,[110] suggesting that they play a role in the pathogenesis of neuropsychiatric symptoms.

Electroencephalographic abnormalities have been reported in up to 65% of patients with SLE,[69] including those without symptomatic cerebral involvement.[110] The most common finding is generalized slowing, which correlates better with cognitive dysfunction than with the occurrence of seizures.[14,46] For example, in one series of 42 patients, 11 of whom had seizures, EEG recordings did not reveal epileptiform activity in any, although focal slowing was present in 29%, and diffuse slowing was seen in 26%.[49] In contrast, however, a study of 120 patients with SLE found that epileptiform activity occurred in one third, but none of these patients had seizures.[69] Monitoring critically ill SLE patients using continuous EEG is useful in discovering reversible causes of altered mental state or coma, including seizures and metabolic encephalopathy.[86]

Pathophysiology

There are diverse causes of seizures in patients with SLE. Cerebral involvement by lupus itself results in seizures through immune, vascular, and inflammatory mechanisms. Generalized seizures, often accompanied by neuropsychiatric symptoms

TABLE 1

FEATURES OF SYNDROMES WITH PRIMARY OR SECONDARY VASCULITIS

Disease	Patients (%) CNS	Patients (%) Seizures	When	Vessel size	Laboratory	Radiology
PACNS	95	30	Anytime	Small, medium, large; granulomata, stenosis, beads	CSF: > 10 WBC, Pro > 100; culture, Ag, Ab, + oligoclonal bands	MR: subcortical $\uparrow$signal T2, meningeal enhancement, mass lesion +/-MRA, SPECT changes
SLE	11–75	12–50	Early or with flares	Small artery vein, capillary Rare stenoses in large arteries (vasculitis rare)	Pancytopenia, +ANA, +/- anticardiolipin, + n-dsDNA (homogeneous), + Sm or RNP (speckled) + RNA (nucleolar), antiribosomal P, $\downarrow$complement during flare; CSF: $\uparrow$protein, few lymphs, $\uparrow$IgG, oligoclonal bands	Hemorrhage with vasculitis; CT, MRI: nonspecific $\uparrow$signals; wm, resembles hypertensive; rare abnormal angiogram; MRA; atrophy (diffuse involvement) PET $\downarrow$ metabolism
APA			With CVA	Rare vasculitis, medium, large, thrombosis	+ Antiocardiolipin Ab (IgG, IgM), +LA or $\uparrow$pTT, $\downarrow$plt	Multiple cortical and subcortical strokes, SPECT diffuse and focal $\downarrow$ uptake
WG	3		Late	Arteriole, venule, rare medium large	Anti-cANCA>>pANCA; kidney, lung, sinus involvement	Sinusitis
RA	Rare	<1	Anytime	Any size, near involved meninges	+RF	Enhanced meninges, granuloma, or pachymeningeal plaque, hemorrhage
SS	Rare	<1	Anytime	Small outside CNS	Anemia, $\uparrow$ESR, +RF, +ANA, anti-Ro(SSA), La(SSB), hyperyglobulinemia	MS-like lesions
Behçet	5–20	<1	With flare	Capillories, veins, often brainstem	Mucous membrane lesions, uveitis, CSF: few L or N, sl $\uparrow$ Pro, oligoclonal bands	Meningeal thickening; small irregular lesions brainstem; spinal cord, deep wm
Cogan	3–5	<1	Rare	Aorta, any	Eye findings, CSF lymphs	Rare cavernous sinus thrombosis
PAN	3–28	1.5	Rare	Small, medium, branch-point aneurysms	$\uparrow$ESR, $\uparrow$WBC, anemia + HepB, HepC, HIV, pANCA	Single or multiple strokes, often normal, irregular vessels with aneurysms on angiogram
MPA	8	<1	Rare	Small artery, capillary, venule	+pANCA, no Hep B	CXR pulmonary hemorrhage, normal CNS studies usually
TA	1.5	<1	Anytime	Medium, large carotid (external) rare intracranial	$\uparrow$ESR, $\uparrow$CRP	Rare infarct, angiogram beading

Ab, antibody; ANA, antinuclear antibody; APA, antiphospholipid antibody; cANCA, cytoplasmic-staining antineutrophil cytoplasmic autoantibody; CNS, central nervous system; CRP, C-reactive protein; CSF, cerebrospinal fluid; CT, computed tomography; CVA, cerebrovascular accident; CXR, chest x-ray; ESR, erythrocyte sedimentation rate; GA, granulomatous angiitis; HepB, hepatitis B; HepC, hepatitis C; IgG, immunoglobulin G; IgM, immunoglobulin M; L, lymphocyte; LA, lupus anticoagulant; La(SSB); MPA, microscopic polyangiitis; MR, magnetic resonance; MRA, magnetic resonance angiography; MRI, magnetic resonance imaging; MS, multiple sclerosis; N, neutrophil; n-dsDNA, non double stranded DNA; PACNS, primary angiitis central nervous system; PAN, polyarteritis nodosa; pANCA, perinuclear staining antineutrophil cytoplasmic autoantibody; PET, positron emission tomography; plt, platelet; Pro, protein; PT, prothrombin time; pTT, partial thromboplastin time; RA, rheumatoid arthritis; RF, rheumatoid factor; RNP, ribonuclear protein; Ro(SSA); sl, slight; SLE, systemic lupus erythematosus; Sm, Smith antibody; SS, Sjogren syndrome; SPECT, single photon emission computed tomography; TA, temporal arteritis; WBC, white blood cells; WG, Wegener granulomatosis; wm, white matter and headache, are associated with increased titers of antineuronal antibodies, elevated levels of CSF IgG, and oligoclonal bands,[72] as well as cytokine production.[46] Whether these are simply markers of cerebral lupus or are actually pathogenic is not known,[110] although loss of self-tolerance leading to increased cytokine and T- and B-cell production undoubtedly plays some role. Antibodies against brain reactive antibodies,[99] synaptosomes,[46] and gangliosides[67,88] are also increased, especially in patients with seizures or psychosis.[99] Anticardiolipin antibodies from patients with SLE reduce γ-aminobutyric acid (GABA)-mediated chloride currents in snail neurons, a finding that may be relevant to development of seizures.[64]

After brain involvement by lupus itself, the next-most-common cause of partial and secondarily generalized seizures is cerebral infarction. Infection may also occasionally be a cause. Infarcts can occur from vasculitis caused by immune-complex deposition, emboli from Libman-Sacks endocarditis, enhanced platelet aggregation—due either to endothelial damage or antiphospholipid antibodies—and hypercoagulable states.[14,37,61,109] Cerebral hemorrhage is associated with hypertension, renal failure, and vasculitis. Ironically, accelerated atherosclerosis in patients receiving long-term corticosteroid therapy also contributes to increased risk of cerebrovascular disease, although the role of inflammation promoters (cytokines, proteases, adhesion molecules) is probably paramount.[66] Cerebral ischemia of any cause can be associated with seizures, either at the time the infarct occurs (acute symptomatic seizures) or much later (remote symptomatic seizures). Microinfarcts due to vasculopathy contribute to generalized seizures and depression of mental status.

Seizures can occur as symptoms of a metabolic encephalopathy that is most often related to uremia[109] or as a consequence of lupus-related cardiac disease causing heart block with secondary cerebral ischemia.[75] Because multiple potential causative factors can contribute to seizures even in individual patients, it is frequently difficult to identify SLE as the primary cause. For example, in a review of 91 SLE patients with neurologic dysfunction, more than one third of those with seizures had had a stroke, 2 patients had probable idiopathic epilepsy, and 1 had posttraumatic seizures.[37] Two patients had seizures only during lupus flares.

Treatment

Antiepileptic drug (AED) therapy is not always needed, especially in circumstances in which underlying causes, such as metabolic abnormalities, hypertension, or infection, can be quickly and successfully treated.[93] Seizures occurring with systemic lupus exacerbations often respond to intravenous pulsed methylprednisolone alone. When seizures are frequent, short-term treatment with AEDs is necessary until the lupus flare is suppressed. Seizures occurring in the context of neuropsychiatric symptoms without other factors indicate cerebral parenchymal involvement by lupus and require immunosuppression.[79] Children with SLE who have depression or behavior problems almost always respond to corticosteroids, which suggests that immune-mediated neuronal dysfunction, not a reactive psychiatric condition, is responsible.[62] The incidence of steroid-induced psychosis is often exaggerated. Most patients who develop hallucinations and other psychotic symptoms require increased doses of steroids, not a decrease.[25,55] In addition to oral and intravenous steroids, other immunosuppressive drugs in common use include cyclophosphamide, azathioprine, and cyclosporine.[102] Cyclosporine must be used with caution in patients with seizures both because it can provoke seizures and because it interacts with antiepileptic drugs that are hepatic enzyme inducers. Intravenous immunoglobulin has also been effective.[101] Stroke prevention includes anticoagulation, with or without antiplatelet aggregants.[79,81] Patients with remote-symptomatic seizures generally require long-term antiepileptic drug therapy.

Drug-Induced Lupus

SLE has been attributed to almost all anticonvulsant drugs, as well as to other medications such as procainamide, chlorpromazine, isoniazid, and hydralazine.[7,21,32,39] Clinical manifestations are mild, appear only when the suspected medication is being used, and subside quickly after it is discontinued. Symptoms and signs are usually limited to the skin and joints with accompanying fever and malaise. Visceral, kidney, and CNS involvement is extremely rare. The immune mechanisms underlying drug-induced lupus have been reviewed recently.[117] Although antibodies to the histone complex of DNA are present in 90% of drug-induced cases, they are also found in up to one third of idiopathic SLE patients. Other laboratory abnormalities that drug-induced cases share with idiopathic SLE include cytopenia, positive ANA, prolonged PTT, and rheumatoid factor.[32] Antibodies to single-stranded DNA are common in drug-induced lupus, but antibodies to native double-stranded DNA do not occur. Complement levels are normal.[36] Symptoms resolve soon after the offending drug has been withdrawn, although antibody production may persist for months. In patients with SLE and seizures, AEDs should be prescribed as clinically indicated without undue concern about exacerbating the underlying condition, because only isolated cases of drug-induced lupus attributed to AEDs have been reported.[15,36,110]

CEREBRAL VASCULITIS: CLINICAL SYNDROMES

Vasculitis with CNS involvement occurs alone or in combination with several diseases, all of which produce symptoms by inflammatory mechanisms that create structural damage to blood vessels that may lead to ischemia or hemorrhage. In addition to primary autoimmune processes, vasculitis is seen with several collagen-vascular diseases, infections, tumors, or paraneoplastic syndromes, as a consequence of amphetamine, cocaine, or other stimulant use, and with other drugs. The annual incidence of vasculitis is about 4/100,000.[78] Ischemia results from several pathologic processes, including deposition of antigen–antibody complexes in vessel walls, infiltration of blood vessel walls by inflammatory cells, and formation of antibodies to platelets and other cell-mediated immune mechanisms.[17,63,78,115,116] Different conditions affect blood vessels of a particular size and at various sites.[111] Some types of vasculitis affect the brain primarily; others are systemic and involve multiple organs, including the brain. In addition to ischemic strokes, hemorrhage can occur, especially in the presence of aneurysm.[78,80] When many small blood vessels become occluded, diffuse encephalopathy and even coma results. Other symptoms include fluctuating level of consciousness and systemic signs such as fever, diffuse muscle or joint pains, weight loss, anemia, and headache.[17,78] An international consensus group recently updated the classification of the various forms of vasculitis.[98] Several types (polyarteritis nodosa, Churg-Strauss syndrome, temporal arteritis) mainly involve the skin, peripheral nerves, and muscle.[59] Seizures occur as complications of cerebral infarction, metabolic encephalopathy related to hepatic or renal failure, or steroid encephalopathy.[59] Seizures occur in about 4% of patients with polyarteritis nodosa.[28] Although brain involvement is common in Behçet disease, seizures are rare.[23,80] Electroencephalography may be necessary to exclude subclinical seizures in patients with confusion, behavioral changes, and depressed levels of consciousness.[4,86] Some authors have suggested that a vasculitis may be the cause of Landau-Kleffner syndrome,[87] although the evidence for this is weak (see Chapter 242). In general, children who have cerebral vasculitis are less likely to have seizures than are adults.[8]

Connective tissue diseases are among the causes of secondary CNS vasculitis that can lead to seizures. Arteritis is also a complication of some infections (most notably cytomegalovirus, tuberculosis, herpes simplex, herpes zoster, and aspergillosis), vasoactive drugs (phenylpropanolamine, ergotamine, amphetamines, and cocaine), malignancies (lymphoma), and drug hypersensitivity reactions.[17,45,98,114] In these conditions, patients usually have a subacute or chronic course characterized by headache, behavioral or psychiatric symptoms, confusion and altered mentation, as well as generalized seizures. Large-vessel ischemia produces prominent focal neurologic signs and partial seizures. The presence of systemic signs such as fever, nausea, weight loss, and fatigue is variable.

GRANULOMATOUS ANGIITIS (PRIMARY CENTRAL NERVOUS SYSTEM ANGIITIS)

Seizures are most often a feature of primary (isolated) granulomatous angiitis of the brain: They occur in 20% to 44% of patients.[1,17,19] Seizures are less often encountered in a recently described "benign" form of granulomatous angiitis that often lacks angiographic evidence of vasculitis and is associated with a better outcome.[20] The incidence of seizures is much higher than can be accounted for by stroke alone, which occurs in no more than 15% of cases, usually those with medium- and large-vessel involvement. Onset of the disorder is subacute, and the course is consistent with a progressive encephalopathy. Focal signs are common but can be transient. Children with primary angiitis have seizures, cumulative neurologic deficits, and headache due to granulomatous invasion of small cerebral vessels.[60] Laboratory findings include CSF pleocytosis and high protein content with normal glucose.[17,114] Meningeal or brain biopsy is required for definitive diagnosis because similar clinical and arteriographic findings can occur in other inflammatory and neoplastic diseases.[17,114]

Diagnostic Tests

When cerebral vasculitis is suspected as a cause of seizures, laboratory testing should be directed to obtaining evidence of an autoimmune disorder and to determining whether there is systemic as well as brain involvement. Blood tests should include erythrocyte sedimentation rate (ESR), C-reactive protein,[66] autoantibody titers (antinuclear, antineutrophil, anticardiolipin), complement levels, creatinine, liver enzymes, and creatine phosphokinase.[98] In granulomatous angiitis, the ESR is normal in 30% of patients.[45,78] Cerebrospinal fluid should be obtained for evidence of inflammation and to exclude infection and neoplasia. In up to 80% of patients with granulomatous angiitis, the CSF shows a lymphocytic pleocytosis, elevated protein, and normal glucose.[45] Brain MRI may show findings consistent with small-vessel disease and stroke,[111] gyral or parameningeal enhancement and edema, and mass lesions in 10% of cases that may mimic abscess or sarcoid.[79,111] Cerebral angiography, although insensitive for changes affecting smaller vessels, can sometimes be helpful and generally should be performed.[45,54,106] Brain and meningeal biopsies are necessary for definitive diagnosis,[31] although these have a false-negative rate of about 25%.[17,114]

Treatment

Treatment of cerebral vasculitis is based on immunosuppression using corticosteroids or cytotoxic agents such as cyclophosphamide.[1,18,44,45,77,98] There is little evidence, however, that these drugs are effective in primary granulomatous angiitis of the brain. When vasculitis is secondary to an infection or neoplasia, the underlying disease must be treated. Plasmapheresis has helped in some cases of steroid failure.[26] Seizures can generally be controlled by carbamazepine or phenytoin; there is less experience with newer AEDs. Because encephalopathy is usually present, benzodiazepines and barbiturates, which can further depress mental status, should be avoided.

WEGENER DISEASE

Wegener granulomatosis results from immune-mediated necrotizing granuloma formation in the mouth, nose, ears, upper and lower respiratory tract, and sinuses, sometimes accompanied by vasculitis and glomerulonephritis.[84] Neurologic complications occur in one third of patients. Cranial or peripheral neuropathies are most common, but stroke and seizures are not rare.[84] Multifocal myoclonus has been described in one child.[44] Wegener granulomatosis is associated with seizures in up to 10% of patients.[84] Vasculitis involving small and medium blood vessels is the presumed etiology of both strokes and seizures, although renal hypertension is associated with cerebral hemorrhage. Direct intracranial extension of the granulomatous pathology can occur from involved sinuses. Seizures are also seen as a preterminal event in patients with severe pulmonary or renal disease, sepsis, and disseminated intravascular coagulation.[104]

Diagnosis of Wegener granulomatosis is based on demonstration of oral ulcers or purulent, bloody nasal discharge, pulmonary involvement with a characteristic X-ray picture, microhematuria, and biopsy demonstrating perivascular granulomatous inflammation. The condition is classically associated with antineutrophil cytoplasmic antibodies (ANCA) in many but not all patients.[42] Cytoplasmic antibodies (cANCA) are more frequent than perinuclear antibodies (pANCA).[51] ANCA titers decline following immunosuppressive treatment but do not correlate reliably with disease activity. CT or MRI of the brain may show meningeal disease or parenchymal destruction consistent with stroke.[100] The most common MRI finding is diffuse white matter hyperintense signals on T2-weighted images[44] that are maximal posteriorly.[85] Treatment includes corticosteroids and cyclophosphamide, with immune globulin reported as having helped one child.[97]

BEHÇET SYNDROME

Behçet syndrome is a form of vasculitis that affects small, medium, and large vessels; both arteries and veins can be involved. This disease occurs mainly in young adults, men more often than women, and classically manifests with the triad of mouth ulcers, genital ulcers, and inflammatory iritis, uveitis, or keratoconjunctivitis. The brain, especially the brainstem, is involved in about 5% of cases.[23] The picture is one of meningoencephalitis. Cranial nerve palsies, focal cerebral signs (aphasia, hemiparesis), encephalopathy, and seizures have been reported. Neurologic dysfunction appears late in the course, although rarely it is the presenting problem.[73] In one study, seizures occurred in 4.5% of 223 patients with CNS involvement.[9] Half of these patients had other risk factors for seizures, such as insertion of ventriculoperitoneal shunts, brain biopsy, or unrelated surgical interventions. Patients with seizures had a high mortality rate, attributable to the underlying meningoencephalitis.

RHEUMATOID ARTHRITIS

Rheumatoid arthritis is an inflammatory disease that produces erosive arthritis of many joints; the viscera are occasionally involved. Neurologic manifestations, although uncommon, sometimes occur in patients with long-standing disease. Cases of polyneuropathy, myopathy, atlantoaxial dislocation with spinal cord compression, myelopathy caused by rheumatoid nodules in the spinal dura, meningitis, and, rarely, rheumatoid nodules in the brain parenchyma[15] have been described in addition to secondary complications of vasculitis.[24,83] Seizures are extremely rare, and when they occur, they are most often a consequence of stroke caused by immunoglobulin, complement, or amyloid deposition in arterioles. Seizures have also been attributed to parenchymal rheumatoid nodules.[15] Rheumatoid cerebral involvement is treated by immunosuppressive therapy such as cyclophosphamide.[79] When seizures are present, AEDs are usually required.

SARCOIDOSIS

The nervous system is involved in approximately 5% of patients with sarcoidosis.[91,96] Neurologic symptoms usually appear within the first 2 years following diagnosis, although in Sponsler et al.'s review of the literature, they occurred late in the course in almost one third of patients.[95] Seizures occur in about 20% of patients with CNS sarcoidosis. Partial seizures suggest a mass lesion.[58,95] Most, however, are secondarily generalized.[96] Generalized seizures accompanying meningitis or hydrocephalus are associated with a poor prognosis and increased mortality,[30,58] a correlation that presumably reflects more severe parenchymal involvement. Focal seizures that are related to isolated mass lesions have a better prognosis.[95] Seizures occur at higher frequency in children <13 years of age (38% of one series) than in adults[10] without deleterious effect on prognosis. Seizures may also be symptomatic of hyponatremia due to hypothalamic dysfunction or inappropriate antidiuretic hormone (ADH) secretion due to lung disease.[96] Patients with sarcoid are at risk for opportunistic infections and malignancies that may also cause seizures.

Angiotensin-converting-enzyme (ACE) levels are usually elevated in the serum and may be increased in the CSF as well.[94] Brain MRI demonstrates inflammatory changes and granulomata in the majority of patients with neurologic symptoms or signs.[94] Oligoclonal bands are found in the CSF in about one half of these patients.[72]

Patients with sarcoidosis who have seizures require treatment with AEDs, but seizures are often refractory until the underlying disease remits.[30,65]

SCLERODERMA

Neurologic manifestations of scleroderma (also known as *progressive systemic sclerosis*) are uncommon and usually limited to myopathy and neuropathy. Seizures or other manifestations of brain involvement are rare,[11,49] probably because the antigenic targets in scleroderma are components of collagen, which in the brain occurs only in the basement membrane of some blood vessels and in the leptomeninges.[49]

In the few published case reports, seizure etiology has been unclear but may have been stroke related, due to carotid or intracranial arteritis, or due to hypoperfusion secondary to cardiac involvement.[82]

SJÖGREN SYNDROME

Sjögren syndrome is common and often complicates other connective tissue diseases.[118] Diagnostic criteria include dry mouth (xerostomia), lack of tearing (keratoconjunctivitis sicca) causing dry eyes (xerophthalmia), and characteristic pathologic findings in a salivary gland biopsy. It has been estimated that Sjögren syndrome affects 3% of adults, mostly women.[5] The most common neurologic complications are peripheral neuropathy and polymyositis. CNS manifestations are rare,[34,49] although meningitis and cerebral involvement with cognitive impairment and mental symptoms were seen in 15% of patients with Sjögren syndrome at one tertiary referral center.[5]

Seizures have been estimated to occur in up to 1.5% of patients and are most often partial or secondarily generalized. They are usually attributed to vascular involvement,[6] although autopsy findings in one patient with partial seizures were limited to leptomeningeal lymphocytic infiltrates and laminar cortical necrosis and gliosis without evidence of vasculitis.[38]

MRI scans are abnormal in up to 80% of patients with Sjögren syndrome who have CNS symptoms.[68] Findings include multiple, small, T2-weighted signal abnormalities in the subcortical white matter and periventricular areas (similar to findings in multiple sclerosis), as well as cerebral infarcts and cortical atrophy. The white matter lesions do not resolve with treatment. Cerebral angiography demonstrates changes consistent with arteritis in about 20% of CNS cases.[5] EEG abnormalities are common, and both epileptiform and nonspecific changes have been described.[5,49] Patients with CNS involvement frequently have anti-Ro antibodies in serum.

The pathophysiology of the neurologic manifestations of Sjögren syndrome is unknown, although immune-mediated damage to blood vessels is hypothesized.[5] Vasculitis is commonly presumed to be present, although neither immune-complex deposition nor vasospasm has been excluded as possible mechanisms. Anti-Ro (SSA) antibodies have been implicated; antineuronal antibodies have not been found. Treatment includes corticosteroids, plasmapheresis, and monthly injections of cyclophosphamide.[34]

SNEDDON SYNDROME

Sneddon syndrome was identified in 1965 in patients who had livedo reticularis (a fishnet-like mottling of the skin) and vasculitis involving medium-sized cerebral blood vessels.[35] About one half the patients have antiphospholipid (aPL) antibodies, which are associated with strokes in patients <45 years of age, headache, and chorea. Seizures have been reported to occur more often in aPL-positive patients (14%–37%) than in aPL-negative patients (0%–11%). They have not been associated with clinical or MRI ischemic events, which suggests an immune etiology. Some patients with Sneddon syndrome have features of SLE. Treatment with steroids can worsen vascular complications; antiplatelet agents have been as effective as anticoagulation with warfarin in aPL-positive patients.[35]

SUMMARY AND CONCLUSIONS

Seizures can occur in many connective tissue diseases and vasculitis syndromes, although the incidence varies considerably across the different disorders. Seizures are seen most often as a feature of SLE and primary granulomatous angiitis of the brain. Generalized seizures are usually associated with signs of encephalopathy reflecting diffuse brain involvement by the vasculitis or metabolic or infectious complications. Partial seizures usually indicate ischemic complications or, less often, inflammatory lesions. An infectious cause must always be considered before starting or intensifying immunosuppressive regimens. AED therapy must be individualized, based on usual clinical practice. Drug-induced lupus is rarely serious or permanent.

References

1. Abu-Shakra M, Khraishi M, Grosman H, et al. Primary angiitis of the CNS diagnosed by angiography. *Q J Med.* 1994;87:351–358.
2. Afeltra A, Garzia P, Mitterhofer AP, et al. Neuropsychiatric lupus syndromes. Relationship with antiphospholipid antibodies. *Neurology.* 2003;61:108–110.
3. Ainiala H, Dastidar P, Loukkola J, et al. Cerebral MRI abnormalities and their association with neuropsychiatric manifestations in SLE: a population-based study. *Scand J Rheumatol.* 2005;34(5):376–382.
4. Akman-Demir G, Baykan-Kurt B, Serdaroglu P, et al. Seven-year follow-up of neurologic involvement in Behçet syndrome. *Arch Neurol.* 1996;53:691–694.
5. Alexander EL. Neurologic disease in Sjögren's syndrome: mononuclear inflammatory vasculopathy affecting central/peripheral nervous system and muscle. *Rheum Dis Clin North Am.* 1993;19(4):869–908.
6. Alexander EL, Provost TT, Stevens MB, et al. Neurologic complications of primary Sjögren's syndrome. *Medicine.* 1982;61:247–257.
7. Asconape JJ, Manning KR, Lancman ME. Systemic lupus erythematosus associated with use of valproate. *Epilepsia.* 1994;35:162–163.
8. Athreya BH. Vasculitis in children. *Pediatr Clin North Am.* 1995;42:1239–1261.
9. Aykutlu E, Baykan B, Serdaroğlu P, et al. Epileptic seizures in Behçet disease. *Epilepsia.* 2002;43(8):832–835.
10. Baumann RJ, Robertson WC Jr. Neurosarcoid presents differently in children than in adults. *Pediatrics.* 2003;112:480–486.
11. Bhardwaj A, Badesha PS. Seizures in a patient with diffuse scleroderma. *Postgrad Med J.* 1995;71:687–689.
12. Bombardier C, Gladman DD, Urowitz MB, et al. , and the Committee on Prognosis Studies in SLE. Derivation of the SLEDAI. A disease activity index for lupus patients. *Arthritis Rheum.* 1992;35(9):630–640.
13. Boumpas DT, Austin III HA, Fessler BJ, et al. Systemic lupus erythematosus: emerging concepts. *Ann Int Med.* 1995;122(12):940–950.
14. Bourke BE. Central nervous system involvement in systemic lupus erythematosus. Are we any further forward? [Editorial]. *Br J Rheumatol.* 1993;32:267–268.
15. Brick JE, Brick JF. Neurologic manifestations of rheumatologic disease. *Neurol Clin North Am.* 1989;7:629–639.
16. Brinciotti M, Ferrucci G, Trasatti G, et al. Reflex seizures as initial manifestations of systemic lupus erythematosus in childhood. *Lupus.* 1993;2:281–283.
17. Calabrese LH. Vasculitis of the central nervous system. *Rheum Dis Clin North Am.* 1995;21:1059–1076.
18. Calabrese LH. Therapy of systemic vasculitis. *Neurol Clinic North Am.* 1997;15:973–992.
19. Calabrese LH. Clinical management issues in vasculitis. Angiographically defined angiitis of the central nervous system: diagnostic and therapeutic dilemmas. *Clin Exp Rheumatol.* 2003;21(Supp 32):S127–S130.
20. Calabrese LH, Gragg LA, Furlan AJ. Benign angiopathy: a distinct subset of angiographically defined primary angiitis of the central nervous system. *J Rheumatol.* 1993;20:2046–2050.
21. Caramaschi P, Biasi D, Carletto A, et al. Clobazam-induced systemic lupus erythematosus. *Clin Rheumatol.* 1995;14(1):116.
22. Carbotte RM, Denburg SD, Denburg JA, et al. Fluctuating cognitive abnormalities and cerebral glucose metabolism in neuropsychiatric systemic lupus erythematosus. *J Neurol Neurosurg Psychiatry.* 1992;55(11):1054–1059.
23. Chajek T, Fainaru M. Behçet's disease. Report of 41 cases and a review of the literature. *Medicine.* 1975;54(3):179–196.
24. Chang DJ, Paget SA. Neurologic complications of rheumatoid arthritis. *Rheum Dis Clin North Am.* 1993;19(4):955–973.
25. Chau SY, Mok CC. Factors predictive of corticosteroid psychosis in patients with systemic lupus erythematosus. *Neurology.* 2003;61:104–107.
26. Chen CL, Chiou YH, Wu CY, et al. Cerebral vasculitis in Henoch-Schonlein purpura: a case report with sequential magnetic resonance imaging changes and treated with plasmapheresis alone. *Pediatr Nephrol.* 2000;15(3–4):276–278.
27. Colamussi P, Giganti M, Cittanti C, et al. Brain single-photon emission tomography with 99mTc-HMPAO in neuropsychiatric systemic lupus erythematosus: relations with EEG and MRI findings and clinical manifestations. *Eur J Nucl Med.* 1995;22:17–24.
28. Cupps TR, Fauci AS. The vasculitic syndromes. *Adv Int Med.* 1982;27:315–344.
29. De Groen PC, Aksamit AJ, Rakela J, et al. Central nervous system toxicity after liver transplantation. *N Engl J Med.* 1987;317:861–866.
30. Delaney P. Neurologic manifestations in sarcoidosis: review of the literature, with a report of 23 cases. *Ann Int Med.* 1977;87:336–345.
31. Duna GF, Calabrese LH. Limitations of invasive modalities in the diagnosis of primary angiitis of the central nervous system. *J Rheumatol.* 1995;22(4):662–667.
32. Echaniz-Laguna A, Thiriaux A, Ruolt-Olivesi I, et al. Lupus anticoagulant induced by the combination of valproate and lamotrigine. *Epilepsia.* 1999;40(11):1661–1663.
33. Elkon KB, Bonfa E, Weissbach H, et al. Antiribosomal antibodies in SLE, infection and following deliberate immunization. *Adv Exp Med Biol (Immunobiol Proteins Peptides VII).* 1994;347:81–92.
34. Escudero D, Latorre P, Codina M, et al. Central nervous system disease in Sjögren's syndrome. *Ann Med Interne* 1995;146(4):239–242.
35. Francès C, Piette JC. The mystery of Sneddon syndrome: relationship with antiphospholipid syndrome and systemic lupus erythematosus. *J Autoimmunity.* 2000;15:139–143.
36. Fritzler MJ. Drugs recently associated with lupus syndromes. *Lupus.* 1994;3:455–459.
37. Futrell N, Schultz LR, Millikan C. Central nervous system disease in patients with systemic lupus erythematosus. *Neurology.* 1992;42:1649–1657.
38. Gerraty RP, McKelvie PA, Byrne E. Aseptic meningoencephalitis in primary Sjögren's syndrome. *Acta Neurol Scand.* 1993;88:309–311.
39. Gigli GL, Scalise A, Pauri F, et al. Valproate-induced systemic lupus erythematosus in a patient with partial trisomy of chromosome 9 and epilepsy. *Epilepsia.* 1996;37(6):587–588.
40. Gladman DD, Ibañez D, Urowitz MB. Systemic lupus erythematosus disease activity index 2000. *J Rheumatol.* 2002;29:288–291.
41. Gonzalez-Crespo MR, Blanco FJ, Ramos A, et al. Magnetic resonance imaging of the brain in systemic lupus erythematosus. *Br J Rheumatol.* 1995;34:1055–1060.
42. Gross WL, ed. *ANCA-Associated Vasculitides. Immunological and Clinical Aspects.* New York: Plenum Press; 1993.
43. Grünwald F, Schomburg A, Badali A, et al. 18FDG SPET and acetazolamide-enhanced 99mTc-HMPAO SPECT in systemic lupus erythematosus. *Eur J Nucl Med.* 1995;22:1073–1077.
44. Haas JP, Metzler M, Ruder H, et al. An unusual manifestation of Wegener's granulomatosis in a 4-year-old girl. *Pediatr Neurol.* 2002;27(1):71–74.
45. Hajj-Ali RA, Ghamande S, Calabrese LH, et al. Central nervous system vasculitis in the intensive care unit. *Crit Care Clin.* 2002;18:897–914.
46. Hanly JG. Evaluation of patients with CNS involvement in SLE. *Ballière's Clin Rheumatol.* 1998;12(3):415–431.
47. Hanly JG, Liang MH. Cognitive disorders in systemic lupus erythematosus: epidemiologic and clinical issues. *Ann N Y Acad Sci.* 1997;823:60–68.
48. Herranz MT, Rivier G, Khamashta MA, et al. Association between antiphospholipid antibodies and epilepsy in patients with systemic lupus erythematosus. *Arthritis Rheum.* 1994;37:568–571.
49. Hietaharju A, Jäntti V, Korpela M, et al. Nervous system involvement in systemic lupus erythematosus, Sjögren syndrome and scleroderma. *Acta Neurol Scand.* 1993;88:299–308.
50. Huang JL, Yeh KW, You DL, et al. Serial single photon emission computed tomography imaging in patients with cerebral lupus during acute exacerbation and after treatment. *Pediatr Neurol.* 1997;17(1):44–48.
51. Jaffe IA. Wegener's granulomatosis and ANCA syndromes. *Neurol Clin North Am.* 1997;15(4):887–892.
52. Jongen PJH, Doesburg WH, Ibrahim-Stappers JLM, et al. Cerebrospinal fluid C3 and C4 indexes in immunological disorders of the central nervous system. *Acta Neurol Scand.* 2000;101:116–121.
53. Kaposi MK. Neue Beiträge zur Kenntniss des Lupus erythematosus. *Arch Derm Syph.* 1872;36–78.
54. Kissel JT. Neurologic manifestations of vasculitis. *Neurol Clin North Am.* 1989;7:655–673.
55. Kohen M, Asherson RA, Gharavi AE, et al. Lupus psychosis: differentiation from the steroid-induced state. *Clin Exp Rheumatol.* 1993;11:323–326.
56. Kovacs JAJ, Urowitz MB, Gladman DD, et al. The use of single photon emission computerized tomography in neuropsychiatric SLE: a pilot study. *J Rheumatol.* 1995;22:1247–1253.
57. Kron J, Hamper UM, Petri M. Prevalence of cerebral microemboli in systemic lupus erythematosus: transcranial Doppler. *J Rheumatol.* 2001;28(10):2222–2225.
58. Krumholz A, Stern BJ, Stern EG. Clinical implications of seizures in neurosarcoidosis. *Arch Neurol.* 1991;48:842–844.
59. Lanham JG, Elkon KB, Pusey CD, et al. Systemic vasculitis with asthma and eosinophilia: a clinical approach to the Churg-Strauss syndrome. *Medicine.* 1984;63:65–79.
60. Lanthier S, Lortie A, Michaud J, et al. Isolated angiitis of the CNS in children. *Neurology.* 2001;56:837–842.
61. Laversuch CJ, Brown MM, Clifton A, et al. Cerebral venous thrombosis and acquired protein S deficiency: an uncommon cause of headache in systemic lupus erythematosus. *J Rheumatol.* 1995;34:572–575.
62. Lehman TJA. A practical guide to systemic lupus erythematosus. *Pediatr Clin North Am.* 1995;42:1223–1237.
63. Lie JT. Classification and histopathologic spectrum of central nervous system vasculitis. *Neurol Clin North Am.* 1997;15(4):805–820.

64. Liou HH, Wang CR, Chou HC, et al. Anticardiolipin antisera from lupus patients with seizures reduce a GABA receptor–mediated chloride current in snail neurons. *Life Sci*. 1994;54:1119–1125.
65. Maeda J, Moriwaki Y, Tamura S, et al. A case of central nervous system sarcoidosis, presenting with psychomotor seizure. *Nippon Kyobu Shikkan Gakkai Zasshi*. 1992;30:2002–2006.
66. Maksimowicz-McKinnon K, Bhatt DL, Calabrese LH. Recent advances in vascular inflammation: C-reactive protein and other inflammatory biomarkers. *Curr Opin Rheumatol*. 2004;16(1):18–24.
67. Martinez X, Tintore M, Montalban J, et al. Antibodies against gangliosides in patients with SLE and neurological manifestations. *Lupus*. 1992;1:299–302.
68. Mataro M, Escudero D, Ariza M, et al. Magnetic resonance abnormalities associated with cognitive dysfunction in primary Sjogren syndrome. *J Neurol*. 2003;250(9):1070–1076.
69. Matsukawa Y, Nishinarita S, Hayama T, et al. Clinical significance of electroencephalography in patients with systemic lupus erythematosus. *Ryumachi*. 1993;33:20–28.
70. McKnight K, Jiang Y, Hart Y, et al. Serum antibodies in epilepsy and seizure-associated disorders. *Neurology*. 2005;65:1730–1736.
71. McLean BN. Neurological involvement in systemic lupus erythematosus. *Curr Opin Neurol*. 1998;11(3):247–251.
72. McLean BN, Miller D, Thompson EJ. Oligoclonal banding of IgG in CSF, blood–brain barrier function, and MRI findings in patients with sarcoidosis, systemic lupus erythematosus, and Behçet's disease involving the nervous system. *J Neurol Neurosurg Psychiatry*. 1995;58:548–554.
73. Mead S, Kidd D, Good C, et al. Behçet's syndrome may present with partial seizures. *J Neuro Neurosurg Psychiatry*. 2000;68:388–399.
74. Mecarelli O, deFeo MR, Accornero N, et al. Systemic lupus erythematosus and myoclonic epileptic manifestations. *Ital J Neurol Sci*. 1999;20:129–132.
75. Mevorach D, Raz E, Shalev O, et al. Complete heart block and seizures in an adult with systemic lupus erythematosus. *Arthritis Rheum*. 1993;36:259–262.
76. Moder KG. Use and interpretation of rheumatologic tests: a guide for clinicians. *Mayo Clin Proc*. 1996;71:391–396.
77. Moore PM. Diagnosis and management of isolated angiitis of the central nervous system. *Neurology*. 1989;39:167–173.
78. Nadeau SE. Neurologic manifestations of systemic vasculitis. *Neurol Clin North Am*. 2002;20(1):123–150.
79. Nadeau SE. Neurologic manifestations of connective tissue disease. *Neurol Clin North Am*. 2002;20(1):151–178.
80. Nakasu S, Kaneko M, Matsuda M. Cerebral aneurysms associated with Behçet's disease: a case report. *J Neurol Neurosurg Psychiatry*. 2001;70:682–684.
81. Navarette MG, Brey RL. Neuropsychiatric systemic lupus erythematosus. *Curr Treat Options Neurol*. 2000;2:473–485.
82. Navon P, Halevi A, Brand A, et al. Progressive systemic sclerosis "sine" scleroderma in a child presenting as nocturnal seizures and Raynaud's phenomenon. *Acta Paediatr*. 1993;82:122–123.
83. Neamtu L, Belmont M, Miller DC, et al. Rheumatoid disease of the CNS with meningeal vasculitis presenting with a seizure. *Neurology*. 2001;56(6):814–815.
84. Nishino H, Rubino FA, DeRemee RA, et al. Neurological involvement in Wegener's granulomatosis: an analysis of 324 consecutive patients at the Mayo Clinic. *Ann Neurol*. 1993;33:4–9.
85. Ohta T, Sakano T, Shiotsu M, et al. Reversible posterior leukoencephalopathy in a patient with Wegener granulomatosis. *Pediatr Nephrol*. 2004;19:442–444.
86. Pang T, Hirsch LJ. Treatment of convulsive and nonconvulsive status epilepticus. *Curr Treat Options Neurol*. 2005;7(4):247–259.
87. Pascual-Castroviejo I, Lopez Martin V, Martinez Bermejo A, et al. Is cerebral arteritis the cause of the Landau-Kleffner syndrome? Four cases in childhood with angiographic study. *Can J Neurol Sci*. 1992;19:46–52.
88. Pereira RM, Yoshinari NH, DeOliveira RM, et al. Antiganglioside antibodies in patients with neuropsychiatric systemic lupus erythematosus. *Lupus*. 1992;1:175–179.
89. Petri M, Genovese M. Incidence of and risk factors for hospitalizations in systemic lupus erythematosus: a prospective study of the Hopkins Lupus Cohort. *J Rheumatol*. 1992;19(10):1559–1565.
90. Rood MJ, ten Cate R, van Suijlekom-Smit LWA, et al. Childhood—onset systemic lupus erythmatosus. *Scand J Rheumatol*. 1999;28:222–226.
91. Sakuta M. Neurosarcoidosis. *Nippon Rinsho*. 1994;52:1590–1594.
92. Sibbitt WL Jr, Sibbitt RR. Magnetic resonance spectroscopy and positron emission tomography scanning in neuropsychiatric systemic lupus erythematosus. *Rheum Dis Clin North Am*. 1993;19:851–868.
93. Sibley JT, Olszynski WP, Decoteau WE, et al. The incidence and prognosis of central nervous system disease in systemic lupus erythematosus. *J Rheumatol*. 1992;19:47–52.
94. Spencer TS, Campellone JV, Maldonado I, et al. Clinical and magnetic resonance imaging manifestations of neurosarcoidosis. *Semin Arthritis Rheum*. 2004;34:649–661.
95. Sponsler JL, Werz MA, Maciunas R, et al. Neurosarcoidosis presenting with simple partial seizures and solitary enhancing mass: case reports and review of the literature. *Epilepsy Behav*. 2005;6:623–630.
96. Stern BJ, Krumholz A, Johns C, et al. Sarcoidosis and its neurological manifestations. *Arch Neurol*. 1985;42:909–917.
97. Taylor CT, Buring SM, Taylor KH. Treatment of Wegener's granulomatosis with immune globulin: CNS involvement in an adolescent female. *Ann Pharmacother*. 1999;33:1055–1059.
98. Tervaert JWC, Kallenberg C. Neurologic manifestations of systemic vasculitides. *Rheum Dis Clin North Am*. 1993;19:913–940.
99. Tin SK, Xu Q, Thumboo J, et al. Novel brain reactive autoantibodies: prevalence in systemic lupus erythematosus and association with psychoses and seizures. *J Neuroimmunol*. 2005;169:153–160.
100. Tishler S, Williamson T, Mirra SS, et al. Wegener granulomatosis with meningeal involvement. *Am J Neuroradiol*. 1993;14:1248–1252.
101. Tomer Y, Schoenfeld Y. Successful treatment of psychosis secondary to SLE with high dose intravenous immunoglobulin. *Clin Exp Rheumatol*. 1992;10:391–393.
102. Trevisani VFM, Castro AA, Neves Neto JF, et al. Cyclophosphamide versus methylprednisolone for treating neuropsychiatric involvement in systemic lupus erythematosus. *Cochrane Database Syst Rev*. 2000;(3):CD002265.
103. Tsai CY, Wu TH, Tsai ST, et al. Cerebrospinal fluid interleukin-6, prostaglandin E2 and autoantibodies in patients with neuropsychiatric systemic lupus erythematosus and central nervous system infections. *Scand J Rheumatol*. 1994;23:57–63.
104. Ulsinki T, Martin H, MacGregor B, et al. Fatal neurologic involvement in pediatric Wegener's granulomatosis. *Pediatr Neurol*. 2005;32(4):278–281.
105. Vernino S. Neurologic autoantibodies. Cautious enthusiasm. *Neurology*. 2005;65:1688–1689.
106. Vollmer TL, Guarnaccia J, Harrington W, et al. Idiopathic granulomatous angiitis of the central nervous system. Diagnostic challenges. *Arch Neurol*. 1993;50:925–930.
107. Ward MM, Pyun E, Studenski S. Causes of death in systemic lupus erythematosus. *Arthritis Rheum*. 1995;38:1492–1499.
108. Weiner SM, Otte A, Schumacher M, et al. Diagnosis and monitoring of central nervous system involvement in systemic lupus erythematosus: value of F-18 flurodeoxyglucose PET. *Ann Rheum Dis*. 2000;59:377–385.
109. West SG. Neuropsychiatric lupus. *Rheum Dis Clin North Am*. 1994;20:129–158.
110. West SG, Emlen W, Wener MH, et al. Neuropsychiatric lupus erythematosus: a 10-year prospective study on the value of diagnostic tests. *Am J Med*. 1995;99:153–163.
111. Wynne PJ, Younger DS, Khandji A, et al. Radiographic features of central nervous system vasculitis. *Neurol Clin North Am*. 1997;15(4):779–804.
112. Yeh TS, Wang CR, Jeng GW, et al. The study of anticardiolipin antibodies and interleukin–6 in cerebrospinal fluid and blood of Chinese patients with systemic lupus erythematosus and central nervous system involvement. *Autoimmunity*. 1994;18:169–175.
113. Yoshio T, Masuyama J, Ikeda M, et al. Quantification of antiribosomal PO protein antibodies by ELISA with recombinant PO fusion protein and their association with central nervous system disease in systemic lupus erythematosus. *J Rheumatol*. 1995;22:1681–1687.
114. Younger DS, Calabrese LH, Hayes AP. Granulomatous angiitis of the nervous system. *Neurol Clin North Am*. 1997;15(4):821–834.
115. Younger DS, Kass RM. Vasculitis and the nervous system: historical perspective and overview. *Neurol Clin North Am*. 1997;15(4):737–758.
116. Younger DS, Sacco RL, Khandji AG, et al. Major cerebral vessel occlusion in SLE due to circulating anticardiolipin antibodies. *Stroke*. 1994;25:912–914.
117. Yung RL, Quddus J, Chrisp CE, et al. Mechanism of drug-induced lupus. I. Cloned Th2 cells modified with DNA methylation inhibitors in vitro cause autoimmunity in vivo. *J Immunol*. 1995;154:3025–3035.
118. Zufferey P, Meyer OC, Bourgeois P, et al. Primary systemic Sjögren syndrome (SS) preceding systemic lupus erythematosus: a retrospective study of 4 cases in a cohort of 55 SS patients. *Lupus*. 1995;4:23–27.

CHAPTER 267 ■ ELECTROLYTE, SPORADIC METABOLIC, AND ENDOCRINE DISORDERS

GIUSEPPE GOBBI, SALVATORE GROSSO, GIANNA BERTANI, AND ANTONELLA PINI

INTRODUCTION

Acute and chronic metabolic, electrolyte, and endocrine disorders may cause dysfunction or impairment of the central nervous system, including epileptic seizures.

Occasional seizures resulting from metabolic and electrolyte imbalances are typical and well-recognized events in neonates. However, seizures may develop in later childhood and adulthood as the presenting symptom of an endocrine or metabolic disturbance, and these have been reported with increasing frequency, sometimes in newly recognized clinical conditions such as primary magnesium deficiency. Metabolic disorders in which seizures are one of the main symptoms also occur with liver and kidney transplantation.[4]

Epilepsy as an initial and prominent symptom of unrecognized gastrointestinal disease has been described in cases of gluten intolerance.[11,31,88202] Finally, there have been anecdotal reports of patients affected by concomitant endocrine, metabolic, and gastrointestinal disorders in whom seizures were the presenting manifestation.

In this chapter, the main metabolic, endocrine, and gastrointestinal disorders in which seizures or epilepsy may occur are reviewed based on the literature. The following conditions are considered:

- Electrolyte disorders of sodium (hyponatremia) and magnesium (hypomagnesemia).
- Renal failure (uremic encephalopathy, aluminum encephalopathy, dialysis disequilibrium syndrome, dialysis encephalopathy syndrome).
- Endocrine disorders, including pituitary disorders, hypothalamic hamartoma, thyroid disorders (primary hyperthyroidism, primary hypothyroidism, Hashimoto encephalopathy), parathyroid disorders (hypoparathyroidism, hyperparathyroidism), pancreatic disorders (diabetes mellitus or nonketotic hyperglycemia, diabetic and nondiabetic hypoglycemia), and reproductive disorders.
- Gastrointestinal diseases (celiac disease, orthotopic liver transplantation).

ELECTROLYTE DISORDERS

Electrolyte disorders can be associated with seizures especially in neonates, but also in children and adults. Seizures may be the presenting symptom of an isolated disorder or of a disorder associated with renal or endocrine disease. Seizures may be present in cases of sodium, magnesium, and calcium imbalance. Seizures associated with sodium and magnesium imbalance are described in this section on electrolyte disorders; disturbances of calcium balance are discussed in the section on endocrine disorders.

Sodium Electrolyte Disorders: Hyponatremia

General Findings

Hypotonic hyponatremia is an electrolyte disturbance characterized by low plasma osmolality (<280 mosm/kg).[29] Hyponatremia may be mild (serum sodium concentration <130 mEq/L) or severe (serum sodium concentration <120 mEq/L). Mild hyponatremia commonly occurs in about 3% to 5% of hospitalized patients[14] and in 1.5% of hospitalized children.[37] Usually, it is asymptomatic and requires no specific therapy. Severe hyponatremia is rare (occurring in only 0.2%),[37] but it must be corrected immediately because of the risk for severe neurologic sequelae.[14] Hypotonic hyponatremia may be hypovolemic, euvolemic, or hypervolemic (Table 1).

The clinical consequences of hyponatremia uncommonly manifest primarily as neurological symptoms but may occur in cases of *acute (symptomatic) hypotonic hyponatremia.* In this condition serum sodium concentration falls rapidly (in <24 hours) to levels <120 mEq/L, without the brain having time to adapt to the electrolyte disturbance. When an osmotic gradient occurs in the brain within a few hours, equilibrium is restored by movement of water molecules into both extracellular fluid and cells. Cerebral edema consequently develops, inducing convulsions followed by tentorial herniation, respiratory arrest, and death. The rate of change is a key element in the appearance of convulsions, and is more important than the degree of hyponatremia. The same mechanism causes seizures during rapid rehydration in cases of hypernatremia.[17] Some authors[18] have suggested that the ability of the brain to adapt to hyponatremia is gender related and that androgens may augment such adaptation. In children, in whom hormonal concentrations are minimal or absent, no gender difference has been found.[19] Of course, the pathogenesis is complicated, and there may be other contributing factors, such as concomitant hypomagnesemia,[180] a combination of hypokalemia and elevated levels of antidiuretic hormone (ADH) (diuretic-induced hyponatremia), a combination of excessive water intake and impaired renal excretion of free water caused by inappropriate secretion of ADH syndrome (SIADH),[19] increased tubular sensitivity to ADH (e.g., in psychotic patients taking neuroleptics),[52] and a combination of extensive extrarenal loss of electrolyte-containing fluids and intravenous replacement with hypotonic fluids in the presence of ADH activity (as in postsurgical patients).

Epileptic seizures have been reported in cases of *diuretic-induced acute hyponatremia*, *SIADH acute hyponatremia*, and *acute water intoxication.*

TABLE 1

CLASSIFICATION OF HYPOTONIC HYPONATREMIA

Hypovolemic hypotonic hyponatremia	Extrarenal losses	Vomiting, diarrhea, sweating, pancreatitis, peritonitis, ascites, burns, muscle trauma	Low urinary sodium concentration (<20 mEq/L)	Loss of sodium exceeds loss of water
	Renal losses	Primary renal disease, drug- and hormone-induced renal dysfunction	High urinary sodium concentration (>20 mEq/L)	Loss of sodium exceeds loss of water
Euvolemic hypotonic hyponatremia		Excess of ADH (SIADH), reset osmostat, water intoxication, endocrine disturbances	High urinary sodium concentration (>20 mEq/L)	Near-normal total body sodium and slightly increased extracellular fluid volume
Hypervolemic hypotonic hyponatremia		Acute renal failure, chronic renal failure	High urinary sodium concentration (>40 mEq/L)	Water retention markedly exceeds sodium retention
		Congestive heart failure, cirrhosis of the liver, nephrotic syndromes	Low urinary sodium concentration (<20 mEq/L)	Water retention exceeds sodium retention

ADH, antidiuretic hormone; SIADH, syndrome of inappropriate secretion of ADH.

Diuretic-induced acute hyponatremia may be caused by a thiazide or a combination of hydrochlorothiazide and amiloride.[141]

The syndrome of inappropriate secretion of ADH (SIADH) is a form of chronic hyponatremia sustained by constant or intermittent secretion of ADH that is inappropriate in relation to both osmotic and volume stimuli.[37] SIADH is characterized by hyponatremia without extracellular dehydration and edema and by plasma hypo-osmolality without urinary hypo-osmolality. Renal, thyroid, or adrenal insufficiency is absent. Causes of SIADH may be any of the following: Central nervous system disorders (infections, trauma, tumor, sarcoid psychosis), tumors (leukemia; lymphosarcoma; and carcinoma of prostate, ureter, pancreas, or duodenum), drugs (vincristine, vinblastine, carbamazepine, oxcarbazepine, barbiturates, amitriptyline), or pulmonary diseases (infection, tumors, asthma, pneumothorax).[37] In particular, acute hyponatremia and generalized tonic–clonic seizures have been observed in infants with respiratory syncytial virus bronchiolitis. Therefore, fluid therapy in these vulnerable infants should be tailored to reduce the risk of hyponatremia.[93] The syndrome has also been observed in postoperative patients with water retention caused by heart, liver, or kidney failure and in cases of excess salt depletion, as occurs in adrenal insufficiency, malnutrition, or diuretic therapy. Seizures have been reported only in cases of SIADH acute hyponatremia associated with *Salmonella* infection,[47] ingestion of 3,4-methylenedioxymethylamphetamine (MDMA, "ecstasy"), or febrile convulsions.[178]

Acute water intoxication is a rare condition occurring in a variety of clinical settings, all of which involve excessive and rapid intake of free water resulting in a sudden fall of serum sodium levels to <120 mEq/L. Acute oral water intoxication is increasing in frequency, especially in infants <6 months of age, in whom it follows inappropriate administration of low-solute formula or excessive administration of water to infants who are denied formula or breast-feeding.[140] In some cases, water had been given because of mistaken ideas about the correct management of diarrhea in infants or because of infant irritability (perhaps caused by neglect).[140] The risk for this problem may be increased among infants of parents living in poverty. Oral water intoxication is rarer in children (0.4%) and adults (1%–4%); it has been reported in cases of children being forced to drink water or swallowing swimming pool water[114] and of psychogenic polydipsia.[95] Acute non-oral water intoxication has been reported following tap water enemas or excessive parenteral administration of water in hospitalized patients receiving intravenous fluid.[114] It is also seen in postoperative patients with extrarenal loss of electrolyte-containing fluids undergoing parenteral replacement with hypotonic fluid, which normally leads to an increased plasma ADH concentration and a decrease in urinary output.[74] In postoperative patients, excessive ADH secretion may be caused by pain or emotional stress. Most of these patients have a superimposed condition that impairs excretion of free water.[37] Acute hyponatremia followed by seizures may also occur after desmopressin treatment. Desmopressin is an ADH analogue used to improve hemostasis in patients with bleeding disorders and in patients suffering from nocturnal enuresis. Therefore, fluid restriction, avoidance of hypo-osmolar fluid, and close monitoring of fluid and electrolytes are recommended in patients who undergo desmopressin therapy.[59,143] The risk of imipramine administration also has to be taken into account in patients who are given desmopressin.[92]

In *chronic hyponatremia*, the osmotic gradient occurs gradually, so that diffusion of sodium chloride is sufficient and the respective volumes are kept constant. As a result cerebral edema and convulsions do not occur. On the other hand, during these adaptive changes, sodium and potassium are lost from the brain, rendering it susceptible to dehydration during correction of hypersalinity if this occurs more rapidly than the brain can recover solute.[195] The suddenly higher plasma osmolality may cause dehydration and injury of the brain, leading to *osmotic demyelination syndrome* with central pontine myelinolysis and extrapontine demyelination.[195]

In addition, acute or chronic hyponatremia may occur as a side effect of antiepileptic drugs. Oxcarbazepine and carbamazepine are able to lower serum levels of sodium in 29.9% and 13.5% of patients, respectively.[65] Symptomatic hyponatremia may also be induced by levetiracetam.[149]

Clinical Description

Typical neurologic manifestations of acute symptomatic hyponatremia consist of generalized tonic–clonic seizures, hypothermia, and respiratory failure. Nausea, vomiting, muscular twitching, and, in later phases, coma may also occur.

In diuretic-induced acute hyponatremia, hyponatremic seizures are usually generalized tonic–clonic, with frequent progression to status epilepticus.[110] In SIADH acute hyponatremia, neurologic manifestations are headache, incoordination, disturbances of consciousness, and especially generalized tonic–clonic seizures.[47,178] Persistent simple partial motor seizures and multifocal seizures have been reported in a patient with SIADH, acute intermittent porphyria, hyponatremia, and hypomagnesemia; seizures were controlled by magnesium therapy.[180]

Infants affected by acute oral water intoxication exhibit persistent, severe generalized tonic–clonic seizures, usually with progression to status epilepticus. The seizures are intermixed with periods of reduced responsiveness, which have been considered to represent a postictal state or persistent, clinically unapparent seizures.[114] Seizures may be preceded by twitching of the eyes. Brief seizures lasting <10 minutes are rare (9% in the series of Farrar et al.[74]). Clinical features may also include opisthotonic posturing, restlessness, weakness, nausea, vomiting, diarrhea, polyuria or olyguria, and muscle fasciculations. Seizures are rare in older children and adults. However, in 84 of 121 cases in the literature with psychogenic self-induced acute water intoxication, generalized tonic–clonic seizures were the presenting symptom.[52] Partial jacksonian seizures were reported in only one case.[108] In contrast to oral water intoxication, acute nonoral water intoxication is not characterized by seizures as the presenting symptom, and generalized tonic–clonic seizures lasting several minutes have been reported only anecdotally as the presenting symptom.[39] Seizures are similar to those of oral acute intoxication.

A relationship has been demonstrated between lower serum sodium levels and an increased risk of developing recurrent seizures within the same febrile illness. In fact, sodium levels were significantly lower in children with recurrent "simple" febrile seizures as compared with single febrile seizures.[117] Because this finding has not been confirmed by other authors, the American Academy of Pediatrics Practice Parameter does not recommend routinely obtaining electrolytes in patients with febrile convulsions.[200]

The outcome is usually favorable, and in series of both infants and adults, almost all patients recovered completely after prompt correction of the electrolyte imbalance; severe brain damage is usually prevented.[52] Coma and death resulting from respiratory failure, brainstem herniation, and permanent brain damage occurred only in patients who underwent treatment after respiratory failure and coma had already occurred. Permanent brain damage may take the form of diabetes mellitus, central diabetes insipidus, mental retardation, or vegetative status.[18,19] Mortality has been reported in 50% of adult patients, especially women,[18] and 8.4% of children.[19] Vulnerability to water intoxication seems to be greater in postoperative patients, especially children[19] and adult women,[18] in whom the incidence of death or permanent brain damage is higher. These figures appear to be an overestimate, however, because a more recent review found a much lower mortality rate and only few cases of permanent neurologic sequelae.[74]

Chronic hyponatremia is less symptomatic, brain edema is not severe, and neurologically these patients may experience only minor symptoms. Nonetheless, osmotic demyelination syndrome may occur during the correction phase, producing convulsions, fluctuating levels of consciousness, and behavioral disturbances that progress to pseudobulbar palsy.[195] Thus, patients with chronic hyponatremia may be more likely to become permanently impaired than those with acute hyponatremia.

Diagnostic Evaluation

Because acute hyponatremia was the cause of seizures in 56% of infants <2 years of age who experienced seizures without any obvious cause,[74] a diagnosis of hyponatremia should be strongly considered in infants with long-lasting seizures or status epilepticus that is poorly responsive to antiepileptic drugs in whom evidence of another cause is lacking. Similarly, generalized seizures in psychogenic patients should be suggestive of acute hyponatremia. An accurate history is useful in investigating the vast number of possible causes of acute hyponatremia but not in emergent cases, for which only laboratory evaluations are of diagnostic value. Clinically, hypothermia associated with drug-resistant seizures or status epilepticus (in contrast to the more common situation of a rising temperature in such cases) may be a predictor of hyponatremia.[74]

Moreover, because hyponatremic seizures are usually occasional seizures that occur only once either as an isolated attack or in the form of repeated convulsions, a correct diagnostic evaluation first must consider all the main causes of occasional seizures, such as bacterial and viral infections, intoxication, trauma, cerebrovascular diseases and accidents, burn encephalopathy, and metabolic disturbances, including electrolyte imbalance. Laboratory determinations of serum electrolytes, urea nitrogen, creatinine, glucose, and osmolality and of urinary electrolytes, urea, creatinine, and osmolality are more important and may provide sufficient data for a correct diagnosis. In general, a condition characterized by hypovolemia and low plasma osmolality (<280 mosm/kg) together with excessive levels of total body water and sodium and an abnormally high urinary sodium concentration (>20 mEq/L) is suggestive of a primary renal disorder or of drug- or hormone-induced renal dysfunction, which is associated with renal salt wasting. Low serum sodium associated with low urinary sodium concentration (<20 mEq/L) is caused by extrarenal losses, such as vomiting, diarrhea, sweat, pancreatitis, peritonitis, ascites, burns, and muscle trauma. Water intoxication is confirmed by euvolemia associated with low plasma osmolality (<280 mosm/kg), dilute urine, and low serum sodium levels despite normal or near-normal total body sodium, whereas low serum sodium levels with high urinary sodium concentration (>20 mEq/L) suggest SIADH. A full clinical and laboratory examination is needed to investigate all the possible causes of SIADH, and the diagnosis is confirmed by normal adrenal, pituitary, thyroid, and renal excretory function. Finally, excessive levels of total body water and sodium with low plasma osmolality and low urinary sodium concentration (<20 mEq/L) may suggest nephrotic syndromes, congestive heart failure, or cirrhosis.

Electroencephalographic (EEG) examinations have not been commonly performed in acute water intoxication. Nevertheless, lack of alpha activity and presence of high-voltage slow waves requiring long periods to disappear[155] and diffuse and bilateral periodic lateralizing epileptiform discharges (PLEDs) occurring in relation to hemispheric ischemic disturbance have been reported.[108]

Treatment

Acute hyponatremia must be promptly corrected, even when the cause is unknown, because rapid correction of sodium levels is usually well tolerated before brain adaptation against osmotic swelling is complete.[199] The empiric use of hypertonic saline solution (2–6 mL of 3% sodium solution per kilogram of body weight),[52] producing a rapid increase of 3 to 5 mmol/L in the serum sodium concentration, corrects hyponatremia within 4 hours, may prevent death and brain damage,[183] and should be strongly considered. Further correction toward a normal serum sodium concentration should be continued during the next 20 to 48 hours. Similar successful correction of acute hyponatremia has been demonstrated in psychogenic water drinkers, either by saline infusion alone or by a combination of saline infusion and fluid restriction,[52] although cases of presumed pontine myelinolysis following fast correction of self-induced water intoxication have been reported in alcoholic, malnourished psychogenic water drinkers.[199] Patients who are potentially more vulnerable to osmotic demyelination are similar to patients with polydipsia-hyponatremia syndrome, which is a chronic hyponatremic condition. Even though they experience episodes of acute water intoxication, these patients may be at risk for osmotic demyelination syndrome if an aggressive therapeutic approach with hypertonic saline solution is administered.[195] Therefore, a more conservative approach, with slow correction of hyponatremia, must be taken. In addition to hypertonic correction, treatment may include intubation and assisted mechanical ventilation in cases of respiratory failure.[19] Finally, special care must be taken if carbamazepine or barbiturates have been administered as treatment of recurrent seizures before hyponatremia was diagnosed. These drugs may cause SIADH, which induces water retention and complicates the clinical outcome. On the other hand, phenytoin has been reported to be the therapy of choice for SIADH, reducing seizures in neonates with SIADH developing refractory hyponatremic seizures.[154]

Magnesium Electrolyte Disorders: Hypomagnesemia

General Findings

The location of magnesium in the body is chiefly intracellular, and about half of the body content is located in bone, with high concentrations also in liver, muscle, and brain. Magnesium is the second-most-abundant intracellular cation in the body and plays an important role in neuromuscular excitability. Magnesium produces a curare-like action on neuromuscular function and has a depressant effect on the central nervous system. A direct correlation between low plasma magnesium concentrations, seizure frequency, and status epilepticus has been demonstrated in generalized idiopathic epilepsies.[33] However, the reason that hypomagnesemia causes seizures is unknown. It has been suggested that hypomagnesemia may remove an inhibitory influence from the *N*-methyl-D-aspartate (NMDA) glutamate receptors. Then, this process may trigger neuronal depolarization. Magnesium specifically inhibits sodium flux through NMDA-type glutamate receptors.[64] Chronic hypomagnesemia, as an isolated abnormality, may be caused by a reduced intestinal absorption due to transport defect or a reduced tubular filtration rate. It may be asymptomatic or symptomatic, depending on the patient's age.[77] Normal serum concentration is between 1.6 and 2.1 mEq/L. In cerebrospinal fluid the normal concentration is 2.4 mEq/L because of active transport of the ion. Symptomatic magnesium deficiency is an electrolyte disturbance defined as a serum magnesium concentration of $<$1.4 mEq/L (usually between 0.7 and 1.4 mEq/L). A secondary hypocalcemia caused by the inhibitory effects of magnesium deficiency on the parathyroid gland[12] is frequently present, and it is associated with inappropriately low parathyroid hormone levels for the degree of hypocalcemia, as has been found in both primary and secondary hypomagnesemia.[26,175]

Primary hypomagnesemia (*congenital hypomagnesemia, familial hypomagnesemia or primary hypomagnesemia with secondary hypocalcemia, isolated intestinal magnesium malabsorption*) is a rare condition in infants. Phenotypic characterization of clinically affected patients and experimental studies of appropriate animal models have contributed to a growing knowledge of renal magnesium transport mechanisms. In that context, both autosomal-dominant and recessive models of inheritance have been reported. The autosomal-dominant variant has been found to be associated with hypocalciuria and linked to the gene *FXYD2* on chromosome 11q23, which codes for a subunit of the basolateral Na-K-ATPase on the distal collecting tubule.[120] In the recessive variant, defects and mechanisms for hypomagnesemia are unknown.

Hypomagnesemia may also be associated with other abnormalities in the context of specific syndromes. For example, hypomagnesemia in association with hypokalemia is suggestive of Gitelman syndrome, which also manifests with metabolic alkalosis and high renin and aldosterone levels. Gitelman syndrome is caused by an inactivating mutation in the electroneutral cation-chloride–coupled cotransporter gene *SLC12A3*, which is located on human chromosome 16q13 and functions as a sodium/chloride thiazide-sensitive cotransporter.[138]

Familial hypomagnesemia with secondary hypocalcemia is an autosomal-recessive inherited disorder related to mutations in the *TRPM6* gene located on chromosome 9q21, which encodes for a transient receptor potential ion channel and leads to defects in both intestinal and renal handling of magnesium.

Finally, hypomagnesemia, hypercalciuria, and nephrocalcinosis also comprise a rare autosomal-recessive disorder in which polyuria and hyperuricemia may occur. Mutations in the paracellin-1 or *CLDN16* gene located on chromosome 3q, which encodes for paracellular transport pathways, have been found.[64]

Secondary hypomagnesemia has been reported after removal of parathyroid neoplasm and in cases of diabetic acidosis, malabsorption syndromes caused by intestinal injury, bowel resection (for carcinoma, enteritis, mesenteric thrombosis), prolonged loss of gastrointestinal fluids, hyperaldosteronism,[10] excessive use of diuretics, prolonged treatment with platinum compounds,[26] and closed heart surgery.[184] Frequently, it is associated with concurrent metabolic disorders, such as electrolyte deficiencies, hypo-osmolality, and septicemia, which may make it difficult to recognize hypomagnesemia. In neonates, transient hypomagnesemia is known to occur in children of toxemic and diabetic mothers, intrauterine growth retardation (IUGR) infants, or infants with transient hypoparathyroidism or maternal hypomagnesemia due to celiac disease.

Generalized or partial seizures have also been described in patients with hypomagnesemia induced by the ketogenic diet for intractable epilepsy,[9] cyclosporin A therapy,[9] and ibuprofen overdose.[7]

Clinical Description

In general, magnesium depletion is characterized by an epileptic syndrome consisting of generalized seizures or partial seizures with single or multiple foci. There is a complicated symptomatology associated with neuromuscular irritability resulting in action-intention tremor, myoclonic jerks, startle response, generalized tendon hyperreflexia, Chvostek's sign without concomitant Trousseau's sign or carpopedal spasm (which may be found in primary hypomagnesemia with secondary hypocalcemia; see later discussion), tachycardia, and rarely athetoid and choreiform movements.

Infant patients are classically seen with partial seizures that have one or multiple foci. They are conscious and hyperactive. Diarrhea and secondary hypocalcemia are present.[3] Seizures occur repeatedly and are resistant to antiepileptic drugs. Stiffness of all four extremities and hypertonia also have been reported.[50] In children and adults, generalized tonic–clonic seizures associated with nonepileptic massive myoclonic jerks and carpopedal spasm, without diarrhea, were the presenting symptoms.[175] Sudden-onset aphasia and no clear initial motor seizure activity have also been reported.[64]

Convulsions and diarrhea are intractable, and children may die if the magnesium disorder is not recognized and corrected early.[3] Otherwise, the prognosis is relatively good with normal psychomotor development as long as magnesium supplements are maintained.

Diagnostic Evaluation

Hypomagnesemia should be strongly suspected in infants with generalized or partial seizures with one or multiple foci of unknown cause that are resistant to treatment and are associated with diarrhea and tetany that do not respond to calcium replacement. Given that older patients are less symptomatic, isolated magnesium malabsorption has to be investigated at any age. Finally, complete investigation of magnesium metabolism should also be considered in cases of idiopathic epilepsy because of reports[91,193] concerning a direct correlation between low levels of serum magnesium and the frequency of seizures and status epilepticus in patients with idiopathic generalized epilepsies.

Intestinal malabsorption of magnesium is confirmed by markedly elevated fecal magnesium levels and low serum magnesium levels, even if serum magnesium concentrations do not reflect total body magnesium stores. A 24-hour urine collection and intravenous magnesium loading test for total body magnesium determination are very sensitive. When facilities for serum magnesium determinations are not available, a trial of parenteral magnesium sulfate may serve as a therapeutic test if renal function is not impaired. Comprehensive intestinal and renal investigations to detect intestinal malabsorption and renal failure or tubulopathy, hormone and electrolyte determinations to detect hypoparathyroidism, hyperaldosteronism, and conditions associated with hypokalemia or hypocalcemia, and X-ray of the carpal bones to detect other metabolic diseases are also required.

In addition, because of the associated movement disorders, specific investigations to detect disease of the basal ganglia (computed tomography, magnetic resonance imaging, neurophysiologic evaluations, and laboratory tests for liver disease, metabolic disorders, and immunologic disease) should be considered.

Treatment

Elective therapy in isolated magnesium malabsorption consists of high-dose oral or parenteral magnesium supplements. Typically, magnesium administration alone controls convulsions and low serum levels of magnesium and calcium in primary hypomagnesemia; administration of calcium and vitamin D is not effective. The major complication of magnesium supplementation appears to be diarrhea caused by the magnesium itself.

RENAL FAILURE

Renal failure leads to disturbances in the function of every organ system in the body. Complications of renal failure become increasingly prevalent as the glomerular filtration rate decreases below 5 mL/min/1.73 m^2 , the level of function that defines end-stage renal disease. Neurologic disorders remain an important source of morbidity and mortality in this vulnerable patient population. With the introduction of dialysis and renal transplantation, the spectrum of neurologic complication has changed. On one hand, the incidence and severity of uremic encephalopathy, neuropathy, and myopathy have declined.[40] On the other hand, dialytic regimen or renal transplantation may determine neurologic disorders such as dialysis dementia, dialysis dysequilibrium syndrome, cerebrovascular accident, and hypertensive encephalopathy, which are thought to be the consequence of ultrafiltration-related arterial hypotension directly related to dialysis. Moreover, hemorrhagic stroke, subdural hematoma, osmotic myelinolysis, opportunistic infections, intracranial hypertension, Wernicke encephalopathy and peripheral neuropathy can also occur. In patients who undergo renal transplantation, immunosuppressive drugs may cause encephalopathy, movement disorders, opportunistic infections, neoplasms, myopathy, and atherosclerosis. The neurologic manifestations of renal failure are summarized in Table 2.

TABLE 2

NEUROLOGIC MANIFESTATIONS OF RENAL FAILURE

Neurologic manifestations of uremia
Uremic encephalopathy
Hypertensive encephalopathy
Aluminum encephalopathy in infancy and childhood
Uremic polyneuropathy
Cranial nerve dysfunctions
Autonomic dysfunctions
Neurologic complications of uremia treatment
Dialysis disequilibrium syndrome
Dialysis encephalopathy syndrome
Neurologic complications of transplantation
Rejection encephalopathy

This section discusses epileptic seizures in *uremic encephalopathy*, *aluminum encephalopathy in infancy and childhood*, *dialysis disequilibrium syndrome*, and *dialysis encephalopathy syndrome*.

Neurologic Manifestations of Uremia

Uremic Encephalopathy

General Findings. Uremia can be defined as "systemic intoxication caused by severe glomerular deficiency associated with disturbances in tubular and endocrine functions of the kidney. It is characterized by retention of toxic metabolites derived mainly from proteins associated with changes in volume and electrolyte composition of the body fluids and excess or deficiency of various hormones."[35] The pathophysiology of uremic encephalopathy is complex and poorly understood. Renal failure results in a gradual accumulation of several substances, but no single metabolite has been identified as the sole cause of uremic encephalopathy.[204] Accumulation of urea, uric and hippuric acids, phenols and conjugates of phenols, phenolic and indolic acids, glucuronic acid, various amino acids, polyamines, polypeptides, carnitine, sulfates, phosphates, and "middle molecules" has been observed.[61] It may also depend on guanidino compounds; acidosis; hyperhydration and dehydration; electrolyte disorders (hyponatremia, hypomagnesemia, hypocalcemia, hyperkalemia); hormonal disturbances (parathyroid hormone, thyrotropin, prolactin, luteinizing hormone, growth hormone, insulin, and glucagon); disturbances of cerebral amino acid metabolism; decreased concentration of γ-aminobutyric acid (GABA); increased concentrations of dopamine and serotonin; diminished cerebral uptake of glutamine, valine, and isoleucine; and increased extraction of glycine and cystine.[38] Seizures may be related to hypertension, electrolyte imbalance, aluminum toxicity, drug toxicity, and infections. Inhibition of cerebral sodium-potassium adenosine triphosphatase (ATPase) has been demonstrated in experimental animals, which might be correlated with elevation of intracellular sodium and seizure activity.[142] A main role is thought to be played by guanidino compounds such as methylguanidine and guanidinosuccinic acid, which were found to be highly increased in cerebrospinal fluid (CSF) and brain of uremic patients.[61] They may also induce a disorder similar to the "twitch-convulsive" syndrome, including epilepsy.[144] Activation of the excitatory NMDA receptors and concomitant inhibition of inhibitory $GABA_A$-ergic neurotransmission have been pointed out as underlying mechanisms.[61] Intrahippocampal guanidinosuccinic acid injection in unanesthetized rats triggered partial clonic seizures leading to generalized tonic–clonic seizures and eventually status epilepticus.[158] Moreover, inhibition of cerebral sodium-potassium-ATPase was shown in experimental uremic animals.[42] This might correlate with the elevation of intracellular sodium and might therefore be associated with the epileptogenicity affecting this population.[40] In this context, the pathophysiologic role of parathyroid hormone should also be considered. Although the mechanisms are unknown, parathyroid hormone is able to facilitate the entry of calcium in brain tissue.[42] Because calcium is an essential mediator of neurotransmitter release and plays a major role in intracellular metabolic and enzymatic processes, alterations in brain calcium may possibly take part in determining cerebral dysfunction and seizures. Focal or multifocal and stimulus-sensitive myoclonus is supposed to originate in the brainstem reticular formation.[49] Uremic encephalopathy is reversible on correction of renal insufficiency, consistent with the failure of histopathologic studies to find a specific anatomic lesion.[156]

Clinical Description. Uremic encephalopathy almost invariably complicates both chronic and acute uremia, its severity depending on the rate of renal failure. Neurologic manifestations of acute and chronic renal failure do not differ qualitatively, but clinical symptomatology is usually more severe and progresses more rapidly in patients with an acute deterioration of renal function.[42] The clinical course is characterized by variability from day to day. Presenting symptoms may be subtle and represented by apathy, irritability, inattentiveness, clumsiness, and fatigue. Tests show that attention span is impaired at this stage.[42] "Frontal lobe" dysfunction manifests with deficient abstract thinking, behavioral disorders, paratonia, and palmomental reflex.[42] Recent memory deficits indicate a more advanced stage of disease. Later, remote memory fails, and confusion, lethargy, stupor, and ultimately coma develop. Typical features of delirium (toxic psychosis), such as hallucinations, agitation, confusion, and disorientation, are especially frequent in acute renal failure. Mental impairment is greater in children who experience onset of chronic renal failure during the first year of life, especially within the first 2 months.[166] Psychomotor and mental development are delayed, and a small head circumference and progressive decrease in IQ may be encountered, even in the absence of neurologic signs.[4] Even in patients who have been treated with renal replacement therapy, memory deficits and sleep disturbances are not uncommon. Neuropsychological investigations showed significant deviation from normal controls in areas of attention/response speed, learning and memory, and perceptual coding.[42] Movement disorders and epilepsy constitute a very characteristic clinical feature of uremic encephalopathy and define the so-called "*uremic twitch-convulsive*" syndrome,[2] which consists of intense asterixis and multifocal myoclonic jerks that are accompanied by fasciculations, muscle twitches, and seizures.[60] Early manifestations include muscle cramps, tremors, and asterixis. Muscle fasciculations and myoclonus appear in advanced encephalopathy. Asterixis or "flapping tremor" is probably caused by sudden loss of tonus, originating from cortical dysfunction and clinically consists of multifocal action-induced jerks that can even mimic drop attacks in severe cases. In uremia, both spontaneous action myoclonus and stimulus-sensitive myoclonus with good response to benzodiazepines can occur. Uremic myoclonus may be caused by a dysfunction in the lower brainstem reticular formation due to water-electrolyte imbalance leading to microcirculatory and degenerative changes.[40] Thiamine deficiency is thought to determine chorea by interfering with basal ganglia function.[106] "Alternating hemiparesis" can occur in up to 45% of patients.[42]

Epileptic seizures have been reported in about one third of patients with uremic encephalopathy. In cases of chronic renal failure, they are most often a late manifestation and sometimes a preterminal event.[169] In acute renal failure, seizures occur within the first 15 days of disease.[60] Late-onset seizures have been rarely observed in association with hemiparesis and transient blindness as a result of a posterior reversible encephalopathy syndrome.[34] Usually, seizures are generalized tonic–clonic or myoclonic, but focal motor seizures and even epilepsia partialis continua have also been reported.[60] Nonconvulsive status epilepticus characterized by acute confusion or stupor without motor seizures has also been observed in patients with end-stage renal failure.[53]

Neurophysiologic Investigations. The EEG is abnormal in the setting of acute encephalopathy due to renal failure. EEG background activity becomes progressively disorganized. Decreased alpha activity is associated with the appearance of intermittent paroxysmal bursts of bilaterally synchronous slow waves, with largest amplitudes over the frontal regions (projected rhythm). In chronic renal failure, changes are less dramatic. As the uremic state progresses, the EEG becomes slower, with a recognizable correlation between the percentage of frequencies <7 Hz and the increase in creatinine. Bilateral spike and wave complexes, in the absence of evident clinical seizure activity, have been reported in up to 14% of patients with chronic renal failure.[42] A paradoxical response to eye opening and an abnormal arousal response to afferent stimuli consisting of bursts of slow waves may occur. Photic driving, photomyogenic response, and photosensitivity manifested by paroxysmal epileptiform discharges are more characteristic of uremic encephalopathy. They may be elicited just before the onset of convulsions. Electroencephalographic features correlate with alteration in consciousness to a greater degree than with the degree of uremia, electrolyte imbalance, and acidosis.[185] Asterixis is electromyographically characterized by typical silence, which follows a biphasic wave in the backaveraged EEG activity.

The N75 and P100 components of one visual-evoked potential (VEP) are significantly prolonged in chronic renal failure.[57] Peak V and I–V and III–V interpeak latencies of brainstem auditory-evoked responses (BAERs) were significantly prolonged in one third of chronic renal failure patients.[176] Unfortunately, no significant correlations have been documented between the degree of prolongation of various VEP or BAER component latencies and the severity of chronic renal failure or its associated metabolic complications.

Visually-evoked event-related potentials (ERPs) in neurologically asymptomatic patients affected by chronic renal failure clearly showed an increased P3 latency and decreased P3 amplitude. After hemodialysis, P3 latency showed a significant decrease, and P3 latency habituation during the ERP measurement was also significantly decreased. These data suggested that impaired cognitive processing can be disclosed by ERP even in neurologically asymptomatic chronic renal disease. Removal of uremic toxins by hemodialysis leads to an improvement in cognitive function.[73]

Somatosensory-evoked potentials (SEPs) after median nerve stimulation are enhanced bilaterally. Both the biphasic wave and the giant SEP are believed to have a common origin in the sensorimotor cortex in brain-mapping recordings.[22]

Diagnostic Evaluation. A combination of clinical signs of depression and signs of cerebral excitation, such as multifocal myoclonus and epilepsy, is strongly suggestive of uremia.

When seizures are present, a series of investigations, including determination of bone and plasma aluminum concentrations and plasma and urinary electrolyte concentrations, osmolality, volume, and levels of ADH, has to be performed to exclude other, superimposed causes of seizures, such as hypertensive encephalopathy, electrolyte imbalance (water intoxication, hypocalcemia, hyponatremia, hypomagnesemia), or aluminum encephalopathy. Computed tomography followed by lumbar puncture (unless intracranial pressure is increased), which may show elevated protein concentrations or pleocytosis, can aid in the diagnosis of infection of the central nervous system. Papilledema, focal neurologic signs, and elevated opening pressure at lumbar puncture may suggest hypertensive encephalopathy or intracranial hemorrhage. If no causes are demonstrated, an idiopathic seizure disorder must be differentiated. When a patient with acute or chronic renal failure experiences an unexpected onset of seizures, asterixis, myoclonus, and behavioral disturbances such as agitation and confusion (toxic psychosis), a drug-induced encephalopathy should be suspected. In the case of renal failure, the availability of certain drugs, such as vigabatrin, acyclovir, chlorpromazine, cyproheptadine, salicylates, phenytoin, barbiturates, and benzodiazepines or their metabolites, is increased by the diminished urinary elimination of active metabolites or diminished protein binding, which increases their plasma concentrations. Immunosuppressive-associated encephalopathy has been described with cyclopsorin,[51] tacrolimus,[161] and muromonab-CD3.[159] The clinical picture involves tremor, cerebellar and and/or extrapyramidal signs, and headache. Sometimes a reversible posterior leukoencephalopathy syndrome may complicate the clinical course,[161] with white matter changes. Subcortical and cortical involvement has also been described.[31] Recognition of immunosuppressant-associated encephalopathy is crucial because modulation in immunosuppressive drugs administration may result in resolution of clinical symptoms and neuroimaging abnormalities.

Finally, possible thyroid disorders have to be investigated (see section on endocrine disorders). Video-polymyographic-EEG recordings and electromyographic (EMG) examinations must be performed to differentiate epileptic events from other, nonepileptic movement disorders such as asterixis, tremor, and myoclonus.

Treatment. Clinical symptoms of uremic encephalopathy may improve following dialysis and renal transplantation. The development of uremic encephalopathy is an indication for prompt initiation of dialysis and consideration of renal transplantation.

Seizures may be treated with standard antiepileptic drugs, taking into account the changes in renal excretion and reductions in plasma protein binding that may occur in renal insufficiency. Therefore, monitoring of blood levels of drugs is advisable; levels of unbound antiepileptic drugs, which increase during renal disease, are most informative. In general, oral doses of all the antiepileptic drugs should be reduced and the intervals of administration modified. Sodium and magnesium valproate and phenytoin free plasma fractions increase, whereas lamotrigine clearance is not significantly modified in renal disease. Carbamazepine (which may exert a significant antidiuretic effect, causing increased danger of fluid retention), vigabatrin, and felbamate (which are excreted almost entirely by the kidneys) should not be given.[129] Benzodiazepines, and especially clonazepam, are effective against myoclonus,[4] whereas piracetam and l-5-hydroxytryptophan cannot be used in renal failure. Sedative hypnotics and antipsychotic tranquilizers, which may cause toxic psychosis,[122] and antibiotics, which may induce myoclonus, asterixis, seizure, and coma, must be administered with extreme care.[172] With respect to the newer antiepileptic drugs, zonisamide and oxcarbazepine are cleared by both the renal and hepatic routes. The clearance of both drugs has been shown to decrease with decreasing creatinine clearance. No specific guidelines for dose adjustment have been provided for zonisamide. Oxcarbazepine should be initiated at one half of the usual starting dose and increased to achieve clinical response.[41,128] More than two thirds of levetiracetam and topiramate is excreted in the urine. A reduction in the dosing rate for both drugs is recommended for patients with moderate or severe renal impairment.[41]

Aluminum Encephalopathy Syndrome in Infancy and Childhood

General Findings. Aluminum encephalopathy syndrome is a progressive encephalopathy that tends to occur in infants and children with chronic renal failure following prolonged exposure to aluminum-containing solutions and compounds, such as aluminum-containing phosphate binders.[165] It has also been described in adults.[177] Although the mechanisms for the entry of aluminum into the central nervous system (CNS) are poorly understood,[174] the aluminum content of brain gray matter of these patients has been found to be markedly elevated in comparison with controls.[6] It has mainly been found in the nerve cells of the cerebral cortex.[6] Neuropathologically, the brain shows cortical atrophy and stromal spongiosis.[190] The mechanisms associated with the pathogenesis of the neurotoxicity of aluminum are unknown.[174] The increased bioavailability of aluminum in chronic renal failure seems to be related to decreased urinary excretion and enhanced gastrointestinal aluminum uptake induced, in turn, by secondary hyperparathyroidism, which is common in infants and children with chronic renal failure. Aluminum in individuals with chronic renal failure is stored in bone tissue, from which it may be mobilized during intercurrent stress, thereby causing acute aluminum intoxication.

Clinical Description. Usually, aluminum encephalopathy syndrome develops in children with chronic renal failure who have been exposed to aluminum for several years. Clinically, aluminum encephalopathy syndrome is closely similar to both uremic encephalopathy and dialysis dementia syndrome. Features are a progressive encephalopathy with arrest or regression of psychomotor development, disturbances of motor function (such as dysmetria, tremor, hypotonia, focal or generalized myoclonus), seizures, speech disturbances, and ultimately vegetative status. Seizures are usually generalized, but simple and complex partial seizures with secondary generalization have also been reported.[177] Subacute aluminum encephalopathy with loss of consciousness, myoclonic jerks, and status epilepticus leading to the exitus was related to the direct exposure of CNS to aluminum.[170] Computed tomography shows cortical atrophy. Electroencephalographic features, which evolve simultaneously with clinical features, consist of diffuse slowing of background activity with superimposed bursts of high-amplitude slow waves and multiple paroxysms of triphasic contoured waves, sharp waves, and complexes of spikes and slow waves.[103]

Diagnostic Evaluation. The presence of typical clinical features in children with chronic renal failure who have been taking aluminum-containing phosphate binding gels or formulas suggests aluminum encephalopathy syndrome. Computed tomography showing cortical atrophy, presence of specific EEG features, and demonstration of high bone and plasma aluminum concentrations confirm the diagnosis. Aluminum encephalopathy syndrome has to be differentiated from uremic encephalopathy, which also causes mental retardation, myoclonus, and seizures. This differential diagnosis is very important because uremic encephalopathy promptly improves with dialysis, whereas aluminum encephalopathy syndrome does not in all cases. Electrolyte determinations may differentiate aluminum encephalopathy syndrome from acute hypercalcemia, severe phosphate depletion, and other electrolyte imbalances that may complicate chronic renal failure. Finally, aluminum encephalopathy syndrome must be differentiated from the rare cases of aluminum intoxication in nonuremic patients.[102,174] Video-polymyographic-EEG recordings and EMG examinations are mandatory in the differential diagnosis of movement disorders, such as asterixis, tremor, and myoclonus, and other epileptic events.

Treatment. Prompt discontinuation of the use of aluminum gels is indicated. Dramatic improvement in advanced stages has been achieved by aluminum chelation (deferoxamine). The combined use of deferoxamine and appropriately timed hemodialysis has been proposed in the rare patients presenting with severe acute aluminum intoxication.[147] Common antiepileptic drugs and especially benzodiazepines are effective in the treatment of myoclonus and seizures, but the same risks are encountered as in the treatment of uremic encephalopathy (see earlier discussion). Because the main cause of aluminum encephalopathy syndrome is gastrointestinal absorption of aluminum, infant diets should consist of low-phosphate formulas with the addition of calcium carbonate. Calcium citrate– and aluminum-containing antacids should be avoided.

Neurologic Complications of Uremia Treatment

Dialysis Dysequilibrium Syndrome

General Findings. Dialysis dysequilibrium syndrome is an acute reversible neurologic syndrome caused by exacerbation of the neurologic manifestations of renal failure during a patient's first few dialysis maintenance treatments. Dialysis disequilibrium syndrome has been attributed to the "reverse urea effect" during rapid hemodialysis. Urea is believed to be cleared less rapidly from the brain than from the blood, producing an osmotic gradient and shift of extracellular water into the brain to cause cerebral edema.[115] Experimental data showed a reduced expression of urea transporter (UT-B) and increased expression of aquaporins in brain cells. Urea exit from astrocytes is therefore delayed during rapid removal of extracellular urea through fast dialysis. An osmotic driving force that promotes water entry into the cells is also favored by abundant expression of aquaporins.[203] Moreover, it has been demonstrated that cerebral edema may result from the generation of idiogenic osmoles in association with a decrease in intracellular pH of the cerebral cortex.

Clinical Description. The symptoms of dialysis dysequilibrium syndrome are irritability, restlessness, headache, nausea, emesis, hypertension, blurred vision, epileptic seizures, muscular twitchings, fasciculations, asterixis, and confusion. Seizures usually are generalized tonic–clonic, and status epilepticus may also occur.[189] When delirium appears, it tends to persist for several days. Death from brainstem herniation has been reported in the past, while in more recent years only milder symptoms have been reported. After a general trend toward normalization, marked EEG changes may develop during dialysis, consisting of increased slow-wave activity, bursts of bilateral symmetric rhythmic slow waves, and increased photosensitivity.[185] Patterns of VEPs are exaggerated, with abnormal prolongation of P100;[57] BAER latencies are abnormal.[176] Computed tomography demonstrates cerebral edema. Brain magnetic resonance imaging (MRI) may show white matter changes in the posterior area mimicking a reversible posterior leukoencephalopathy syndrome (RPLS).[189] Central pontine and extrapontine myelinolysis has also been reported in children.[25]

Diagnostic Evaluation. Diagnostic evaluation must exclude all other causes of irritability, headache, nausea, hypertension, muscular twitchings, fasciculations, asterixis, confusion, and seizures that can occur in patients on maintenance dialysis. Seizures are a key symptom. When seizures occur with various degrees of impairment of consciousness, headache, nausea and vomiting, hypertensive encephalopathy, intracranial hemorrhage, and subdural hematoma[127] should be investigated. Papilledema, focal neurologic signs, typical findings on computed tomography, and elevated opening pressure at lumbar puncture confirm the diagnosis of these conditions. When seizures are generalized or partial and are associated with irritability, headache, restlessness, or twitchings, special consideration must be given to disorders of electrolyte imbalance, including hyponatremia and hypernatremia (which in renal insufficiency may induce seizures more frequently than hyponatremia), hypocalcemia and hypercalcemia, hypophosphatemia, abrupt increase in blood pH (which can lower the serum concentration of ionized calcium), and nonketotic hyperosmolal coma in nondiabetic patients, which is caused by increasing levels of glucose after repeated peritoneal dialysis. Determination of plasma and urinary electrolyte concentration, glucose concentration, osmolality, volume, ADH levels, and presence of acidemia may aid in the differential diagnosis. Full neurophysiologic monitoring is useful to differentiate epileptic myoclonus and seizures from other, nonepileptic movement disorders and detect any sudden changes of central nervous system electrical activity during dialysis.

Treatment. If a patient experiences seizures during dialysis, treatment must be discontinued immediately until vital signs have stabilized. Standard therapy of movement disorders and epileptic seizures may improve the patient's course but must be monitored carefully in renal failure (see earlier discussion of treatment of uremic encephalopathy). Hypocalcemic seizures may be controlled with calcium gluconate administration.

Dialysis Encephalopathy Syndrome

General Findings. Dialysis encephalopathy syndrome has been described in patients receiving maintenance hemodialysis. The syndrome usually occurs in patients dialyzed for periods >3 years. It is considered to be the most dramatic manifestation of aluminum toxicity, and is caused by an increase in brain levels of aluminum secondary to a high content of this metal in the dialysis bath.[6] Its incidence has sharply decreased with the use of aluminum-free water.[4]

Clinical Description. Presenting symptoms consist of dysarthria, apraxia, and slurred speech with stuttering and hesitation. The speech disorder is intensified during and immediately after dialysis and at first may be seen only during these periods. Cognitive disturbance usually occurs, and the EEG shows bursts of high-amplitude slow waves in the frontal regions. Within months, myoclonus, asterixis, movement dyspraxia, seizures, memory loss, personality changes, and psychosis develop.[78] In most cases, the disease progresses to apneic spells, tonic–clonic seizures, focal neurologic deficits, and death within months from sepsis or suicide.[6]

After a short and transient improvement, usually following dialysis, the EEG shows progressive abnormalities that become indistinguishable from those seen in aluminum encephalopathy syndrome (see earlier discussion).[185]

Diagnostic Evaluation. Dysarthria, myoclonus, delirium, and seizures are possible symptoms of clinical conditions that may exist concomitantly with hemodialysis, such as acute hypercalcemia[173] and severe hypophosphatemia,[164] and these must be differentiated from dialysis encephalopathy syndrome. Video-polymyographic-EEG recordings and EMG examinations must be performed to differentiate epileptic myoclonus from other, nonepileptic movement disorders.[105] Water-soluble vitamin deficiency, especially pyridoxine deficiency (removed from blood during hemodialysis), should always be considered in cases of drug-resistant seizures. Clinical and EEG features similar to those of dialysis encephalopathy syndrome have been described in patients not on dialysis who are receiving large quantities of aluminum salts.[187] The CSF is unremarkable. No distinct abnormalities have been found in brain at autopsy. In all these cases, only the history and laboratory investigations may aid in the differential diagnosis.

Treatment. The presence of clinical and EEG evidence of dialysis encephalopathy syndrome is a clear indication for discontinuation of aluminum-containing phosphate binders (especially in infants with chronic renal failure) and initiation of chelation therapy. Dramatic improvement in advanced stages has been achieved by aluminum chelation (deferoxamine). Associated myoclonus responds well to clonazepam and diazepam, which are also able to improve speech disorders. Common antiepileptic drugs may be effective in the treatment of seizures, but as with other conditions of renal failure, special care must be taken. Phenytoin usually is used for tonic–clonic seizures. Because a relatively little amount is removed by hemodialysis, it can be given intravenously in loading doses to maintain a desired plasma concentration. Pyridoxine supplementation must be administered in cases of pyridoxine deficiency. Before initiating dialysis, avoidance of aluminum-containing formulas should be recommended. It is also mandatory to test for secondary hypoparathyroidism (frequent in children with chronic renal failure) and iron-deficiency anemia to minimize gastrointestinal absorption of aluminum and restrict dietary phosphate to prevent hyperphosphatemia. Finally, in patients undergoing maintenance dialysis, the aluminum concentration of the dialysate should be monitored periodically.

ENDOCRINE DISORDERS

Epileptic seizures may occur in patients affected by many endocrine disorders and sometimes constitute the presenting symptom. Epileptic seizures may be caused directly by hormones (as in thyrotoxicosis) or indirectly by metabolic disequilibrium associated with hypoglycemia, hyperglycemia, or electrolyte imbalance (hyponatremia, hypomagnesemia, hypocalcemia), which causes an increase in neuronal excitability. Alternatively, as in the case of hypothalamic-pituitary tumors, epilepsy can result from a temporal lobe extension of the tumor or from the tumor itself (i.e., hypothalamic hamartoma). Finally, epilepsy and an endocrine disorder may both result from one genetic immunologic disease. In general, seizure control is obtained with correction of the endocrine disorder or the related metabolic disturbances. If not, administration of antiepileptic drugs may become necessary, with the associated risk for adverse effects on the endocrine system.

Endocrine disorders associated with epileptic seizures or epilepsy are summarized in Table 3.

TABLE 3

ENDOCRINE DISORDERS ASSOCIATED WITH EPILEPTIC SEIZURES OR EPILEPSY

Hypothalamic-pituitary
Pituitary neoplasms/hypoplasia
Hypothalamic hamartoma/precocious puberty
Inappropriate secretion of antidiuretic hormone (ADH) syndrome
Thyroid
Primary hyperthyroidism/thyrotoxicosis
Primary hypothyroidism/myxedema
Hashimoto encephalopathy
Parathyroid
Hypoparathyroidism
Hyperparathyroidism
Pancreas
Diabetes mellitus
Reproductive system
Polycystic ovaries/hypogonadotropic hypogonadism

Hypothalamic-Pituitary Disorders

Pituitary Disorders

Pituitary disorders can occasionally be associated with epileptic seizures, as in conditions of the posterior pituitary affecting water metabolism, such as SIADH, or in panhypopituitarism with hypoglycemia. Generalized epileptic seizures have been anecdotally reported as the presenting or unique symptom in a case of incidental pituitary macroadenomas or incidentalomas,[48] in a case of normotensive primary aldosteronism with hypopituitarism,[122] and in an infant with panhypopituitarism secondary to hypoplasia of the anterior pituitary.[55] Temporal lobe epilepsy resulting from pituitary adenoma with temporal extension has also been described. Temporal extension of an adenoma might disturb the uncinate gyrus and the medial surface of the temporal lobe, resulting in complex partial seizures.[27]

Hypothalamic Hamartoma

General Findings

Hypothalamic hamartomas (HHs) are nonneoplastic, heterotopic nodules resembling the normal gray matter of the hypothalamus. They mainly consist of mature neurons and rare large dysplastic neurons, intermingled with glial cells. Myelinated and unmyelinated fibers have been identified, and some of these connect to hypothalamic nuclei.[20] Mature and differentiated ectopic neurosecretory cells secreting luteinizing hormone–releasing hormone (LH-RH) have also been observed. Etiology of HHs is unknown. No genetic anomaly has been found, except for patients with Pallister-Hall syndrome (PHS).

The two main manifestations of HHs are central precocious puberty (CPP) and seizures, and the latter may be the predominant clinical symptom (see Chapter 250). Among 277 sporadic patients with HHs, 63% had CPP, 61% presented with seizures (of any type), and 25% had both CPP and seizures.[151] Typical seizures consist of brief stereotyped attacks of laughter, also known as gelastic seizures (GS) (see Chapter 53). Although a neocortical origin has been found in some cases, GS are pathognomonic of HHs.[36,151] The pathogenesis of the epileptic syndrome occurring in HHs is unknown. It has been suggested that it may result from a general dysgenetic process that includes cortical abnormalities. The size of the lesion and the secondary mechanical compression on hypothalamus and the mammillary bodies seem to play roles in generating seizures.[20] However, several pieces of evidence suggest that the source of GS is HHs per se. In fact, when associated with GS, HH tissues contain predominantly small GABAergic inhibitory neurons that exhibit intrinsic "pacemaker-like" behavior.[213] Moreover, the HH can have a pedunculated stalk or a sessile one. The latter is associated with epilepsy, whereas the former is associated only with precocious puberty. It appears that the epileptiform activity generated inside the hamartoma leads to clinical manifestations only when a sessile attachment to the hypothalamus allows its propagation to the diencephalon.

Clinical Description. The characteristic epileptic syndrome occurring with HHs begins in infancy, even in the first days of life. Brief episodes of pleasant laughter or giggling last a few seconds, and at the beginning occur without loss of consciousness, recurring many times a day, with both diurnal and nocturnal attacks.[36] In the clinical course, GS are more frequently associated with alteration of consciousness and associated with autonomic phenomena, automatisms, epigastric auras, déjà vu, déjà vecu, and motor symptoms. Some patients may also show a pattern of symptomatic generalized epilepsy. Absence, tonic, atonic, and tonic–clonic seizures occur mimicking Lennox-Gastaut syndrome with intractable seizures, progressive cognitive impairment, and severe behavioral disturbances.[196] HHs may determine a less severe epileptic disorder. Indeed, only some cases progress to an epileptic encephalopathic picture, and cognitive disturbances may be mild or absent. Therefore, the severity of the epilepsy syndrome related to HHs may range from mild, drug-resistant epilepsy with a simple "pressure to laugh" in otherwise normal patients up to a catastrophic epileptic encephalopathy.[13,196] Pathogenetically, such an evolution has been related to the anatomic and physiologic connections of the hypothalamus to the thalamus and cortex.[182] Interictal EEG shows generalized and focal frontal or temporal spikes.[36] Neurophysiologic and clinical studies have demonstrated that when the hamartoma connects to the mamillary bodies, a secondary involvement of the temporal lobe is present, suggesting that the projection of the paroxysmal activity to the cortex is due to a specific pathway connecting the hypothalamus with the temporal lobe. By contrast, when the hamartoma connects to the medial hypothalamus, a frontal lobe epileptic activity is recorded. The existence of direct projections of several neuronal groups in the middle and posterior supramamillary hypothalamus to the frontal lobes (bilaterally) has been described, which could provide such a selective propagation of spike activity.[182]

Initially there are no significant EEG abnormalities detected during a gelastic seizure. Subsequently, generalized onset with low-voltage rhythmic fast activity, generalized suppression of background rhythms, or both, sometimes preceded by single or multiple generalized spike-and-wave complexes, are recorded.[36]

Diagnostic Evaluation. Diagnosis of HH can be evoked in patients affected by gelastic epilepsy and/or PP. The presence on MRI of a nonprogressive, noncalcified, nonenhancing hypothalamic mass that appears isointense to gray matter on T1-weighted images, isointense to mildly hyperintense on proton density-weighted images, and often hyperintense on T2-weighted images confirms the diagnosis.[151] As the seizures become more complex with clinical features of secondary generalized epilepsy, background activity can show variable diffuse slowing, and interictal findings can include unilateral or bilateral temporal/frontal independent epileptiform discharges and/or irregular generalized slow spike-and-wave discharges. Ictally, diffuse nonlocalizing electrographic changes such as generalized low-voltage rhythmic fast activity (LVFA) and/or generalized suppression of background activity have been described. Intracranial studies can be misleading if the hypothalamic lesion is not sampled itself. Depth electrodes advanced into the lesion have revealed LVFA discharges well localized in the hamartoma during GS and more widely extended LVFA in atonic seizures.[151]

Treatment. The therapeutic approach must consider the risk for death after attempted operative removal and the very slow-growing or nonprogressive nature of the hamartoma. The precocious sexual development can be controlled by treatment with LH-RH agonists, but epileptic seizures are usually resistant to antiepileptic drugs and deaths from status epilepticus have been reported.[36] However, focal seizures and tonic and atonic attacks are at best moderately controlled by antiepileptic drugs. Treatment with clonazepam and, more recently, lamotrigine has resulted in significant abatement of seizures. Epilepsy surgery may be considered when drop attacks occur.[36]

Long-lasting control of seizures can be achieved by complete removal, destruction, or disconnection of the hamartoma. The debate has therefore shifted to the best means of treatment with a variety of surgical approaches and the possibility of destruction of the lesion with radiofrequency probes or gamma-knife surgery. A transcallosal approach reaching the lesion from above through the third ventricle has been performed with low morbidity. At 1 year, 90% of cases are free or essentially free of all seizures. Marked behavioral improvement has been reported, and cognitive decline appears to stop. Dissection of the hamartoma from the wall of the third ventricle and infundibulum or mammillary bodies may be achieved in selected patients under direct vision. All forms of surgery can be associated with transient diabetes insipidus, but no other major endocrinologic or hypothalamic complications have emerged as hazards of these procedures. Destruction of the lesion by focused ionizing radiation (gamma knife) is an approach that does not require conventional surgery. Although the follow-up periods are short, early results suggest an excellent seizure response. Gamma knife has the lowest morbidity rate of all treatments with comparable seizure-free rates. Concerns exist about the long-term effects of radiation in the hypothalamic region. Overall, authors agree that the surgical approach must be tailored to the specific surgical anatomy of the hamartoma.[13]

Thyroid Disorders

Primary Hyperthyroidism

General Findings. Studies of experimental animals and humans have provided evidence that thyroid hormones can lower seizure thresholds.[198] Epileptic EEG discharges have been found in many patients with *thyrotoxicosis*. Epileptic seizures associated with thyrotoxicosis have been considered an infrequent event: 9% of all admitted patients with thyrotoxicosis.[109] Nevertheless, epilepsy associated with thyrotoxicosis remains a possible infrequent event,[167,181] and thyrotoxicosis must be considered among the causes of adult-onset epileptic disorders.[121]

Thyrotoxicosis (or thyrotoxic crisis) is an uncommon but severe complication of hyperthyroidism that occurs in *Graves disease* (an autoimmune disorder associated with the HLA-DQA1*0501 allele and characterized by thyrotoxicosis and ophthalmopathy in the presence of autoantibodies to thyroglobulin, microsome, or thyroid peroxidase[30]) and *toxic multinodular goiter*, which is almost always precipitated by an intercurrent illness.[181] *Iatrogenic thyrotoxicosis* may occur after treatment of hypothyroidism.[109] The association between juvenile myoclonic epilepsy and Graves disease may be not fortuitous but rather an indication of a shared genetic immunologic etiology.[198]

Clinical Description. Both generalized tonic–clonic and partial motor epileptic seizures (including visual-adversive and partial motor seizures with secondary generalization and prolonged postictal coma) associated with or followed by signs of hyperthyroidism (irritability, tachycardia, tremor, anxiety, confusional state) have been reported as presenting symptoms of thyrotoxicosis.[109,167] Juvenile myoclonic epilepsy has recently been reported in two unrelated patients with untreated Graves disease.[198] Typically, in these cases epilepsy begins during adolescence with characteristic clinical, laboratory, and ictal EEG findings; the latter consist of 3- to 3.5-Hz diffuse polyspikes-and-waves and spike-and-wave bursts. Often epilepsy in hyperthyroidism may be secondary to neurologic disorders such as stroke, Moyamoya disease, and superior sagittal sinus thrombosis induced by thyrotoxicosis rather than to hyperthyroidism per se.[116,168] Recurrent generalized seizures, preceded by an encephalopathy state, coinciding with relapses of the thyrotoxicosis have been reported in a patient. EEG showed bilateral slowing of activity. Characteristically, antithyroid drug treatment was able to control symptoms. Convulsive[126]and nonconvulsive status epilepticus[132] may also represent the first manifestation of thyrotoxicosis. In this context, status epilepticus is often resistant to conventional antiepileptic drugs.[181] The situation is obviously life threatening, requiring vigorous and comprehensive management.

Interictal EEG findings of thyrotoxicosis consist of diffuse slowing, sharp discharges, and occasional bilateral triphasic waves.[167]

Diagnostic Evaluation. Although seizures are not especially frequent in thyrotoxicosis, thyroid hormone levels should be evaluated during diagnostic investigation at the onset of an epileptic disease.

Differential diagnosis must exclude other metabolic (nonketotic hyperosmolal state) or endocrine (hypoparathyroidism) disorders that may significantly increase focal cerebral excitation.

Treatment. Treatment of thyrotoxic crisis should begin as soon as the diagnosis is suspected. The aim is to correct both severe thyrotoxicosis and any precipitating intercurrent illness and to provide general supportive therapy. Effective therapy of the endocrine disorder and epileptic seizures comprises administration of antithyroid drugs (propylthiouracil, methimazole, or both), dialysis, plasmapheresis, hemoperfusion (to lower circulating levels of thyroid hormones), administration of glucocorticoids and adrenergic antagonists, supportive therapy (intravenous administration of glucose, saline, vitamin B complex, and sedatives), and correction of hyperpyrexia and heart failure.[181] Common antiepileptic drugs may be useful in controlling seizures, but careful evaluation of other organ systems is required to estimate the risk for adverse effects of antiepileptic therapy.

Primary Hypothyroidism

General Findings. *Primary hypothyroidism* is characterized by the combination of low levels of thyroid hormone and high levels of thyroid-stimulating hormone (TSH). Possible causes are Hashimoto thyroiditis (see later discussion), treatment with radioiodine, thyroidectomy, drugs, and thyroid lymphoma; primary hypothyroidism may also be congenital. Decreased TSH resulting from tumor or infiltrative disease of the pituitary causes secondary hypothyroidism.[125] Decreased thyrotropin-releasing hormone (TRH) resulting from hypothalamic tumor causes tertiary hypothyroidism.[125] The most important consequence of *primary congenital hypothyroidism* is impaired brain development, which, if not treated, leads to severe mental retardation. Psychotic manifestations and terminal myxedematous coma are the most common central nervous system manifestations in *primary acquired hypothyroidism*; epileptic seizures only rarely occur. In these cases, convulsions may be the presenting symptom or may occur in untreated cases of myxedema of long duration.[43]

A paroxysmal triad consisting of high fever, seizures, and coma with a flulike prodrome can rarely occur in patients with scleromyxedema and is termed "dermato-neuro" syndrome. It has been found that the incidence of febrile convulsions among patients with congenital hypothyroidism under therapy with L-thyroxine since the age of 1 month was significantly lower than that of normal control children. It seems therefore that patients with congenital hypothyroidism on regular L-thyroxine replacement are less prone to experience febrile convulsions.[23]

Although epileptic seizures do not usually occur in *primary hypothyroidism*, experimental data demonstrated that the number of stimuli necessary to produce lidocaine-kindling seizures (i.e., tonic attacks followed by tonic–clonic movements) in congenital hypothyroid rats was significantly lower than in the control group for both ages.[157] Moreover, it is well known that early-onset hypothyroidism produces audiogenic seizure susceptibility in rodents, in which TR $\alpha 1$ and TR β thyroid hormone receptors seem to play a role.[150]

Clinical Description. In primary acquired hypothyroidism, generalized tonic–clonic seizures and EEG findings of low-voltage slow waves and dysrhythmic background suggest a nonspecific encephalopathy. Seizures may be characterized by an unexplained prolonged postictal recovery.[43]

Diagnostic Evaluation. Although hypothyroidism is an uncommon cause of epilepsy, thyroid assessment must be considered in the etiologic diagnosis of cryptogenic generalized seizures, especially when followed by a prolonged postictal recovery. Differential diagnosis should exclude other metabolic or endocrine disorders. However, coarse facies, bradycardia, dry skin, and hair loss (when present) are clearly suggestive of hypothyroidism.

Treatment. Treatment with L-thyroxine leads to normalization of the endocrine disorder and abatement of epilepsy. Therefore, antiepileptic drug treatment seems to be unnecessary. However, it should be remembered that rapid correction of a hypothyroid state during administration of thyroxine might constitute a risk for thyrotoxicosis, with epileptic seizures as a consequence. In fact, a causal relationship has been presumed between high-dosage thyroxine therapy and a nonconvulsive status epilepticus characterized by absence seizures with eyelid and distal myoclonic twitchings, triggered by spontaneous or passive eye closure and generalized convulsive seizures.[109] These seizures appeared to respond to valproate. Thyroxine-induced epilepsy with hypermotor seizures was also controlled by reducing thyroxine doses.[24]

Hashimoto Encephalopathy

General Findings. Hashimoto encephalopathy (HE) is a steroid-responsive neurologic disorder associated with antithyroid antibodies. Frequently, epileptic seizures are a presenting symptom.[28,83,98] The term "Hashimoto encephalopathy" is not considered appropriate by some authors because the thyroid condition has not been proved to have a direct relationship with the neurologic process, and the role of thyroid antibodies in the pathogenesis of encephalopathy has not been defined. The term "autoimmune encephalopathy associated with Hashimoto thyroiditis" is considered a more accurate definition. "Nonvasculitic autoimmune encephalopathy" and "corticosteroid-responsive encephalopathy associated with Hashimoto thyroiditis" are also used. In fact, although in some patients thyroiditis is diagnosed before Hashimoto encephalopathy, the disease may affect euthyroid patients with normal levels of thyroid hormones and TSH. At present, HE is suspected whenever symptoms of acute or subacute encephalopathy or myelopathy are associated with high serum levels of antithyroid antibodies.[28]

Several theories have been proposed to explain the pathogenesis of HE. They include autoimmune vasculitis, autoimmune reaction to common antigens between the thyroid gland and the CNS, cerebral hypoperfusion, and toxic effects of thyrotropin-releasing hormone. The presence of antithyroid antibodies in CSF of patients with encephalopathy and myelopathy associated with Hashimoto disease was reported, and indirect evidence was provided to suggest intrathecal synthesis of antithyroid antibodies. Therefore, it has been proposed that the diagnosis of Hashimoto encephalopathy should be based on this CSF finding.[76,83] Specific high reactivity against human α-enolase has been found to be in patients with Hashimoto encephalopathy. Some authors suggest that the detection of an anti–α-enolase antibody is useful for defining encephalopathy-related pathology.[153]

Postmortem examination in a patient with Hashimoto encephalopathy complicated by fatal status epilepticus demonstrated mild perivascular lymphocytic infiltration throughout the brain and leptomeninges with diffuse gliosis of gray matter in the cortex, basal ganglia, thalamus, and hippocampus.[66]

Clinical Description. The clinical picture of Hashimoto encephalopathy with epilepsy includes generalized and partial seizures as distinguishing features. Myoclonus, tremor, choreic movements, central nystagmus, gait disturbance and ataxia, and hallucinations may be present, as well as transient aphasia or somnolence, headache, fatigue, confusion, and unilateral sensory loss. Strokelike episodes, palatal tremor, musical hallucination, and cerebellar dysfunction have also been reported in some cases. The symptoms may improve spontaneously or after corticosteroid therapy. Two distinct clinical forms of HE have been suggested: (a) a *vasculitic type* characterized by multiple strokelike episodes and (b) a *diffuse progressive* type characterized by dementia and psychiatric symptoms. Both forms may be associated with tremor, seizures, stupor, and myoclonus. The myoclonic syndrome may be so prominent that Hashimoto encephalopathy has also been defined as *Hashimoto myoclonic encephalopathy*.[28,83]

Recurrent generalized convulsive status epilepticus and recurrent generalized absence status with blinking and/or twitching resistant to antiepileptic medications but successfully treated with corticosteroids have been reported.[139]

The interictal EEG findings are also variable. Most commonly the EEG shows generalized abnormalities including generalized slow wave activity, slow posterior background, and frontal intermittent rhythmic delta activity (FIRDA). Triphasic waves and focal slow waves have been described in some patients. The EEG findings seem to subside with the improvement of the encephalopathy, although the EEG tends to lag behind the clinical improvement.

Ictal recordings showed bitemporal discharges and focal mesial-basal temporal seizure discharges. In the latter patient, the ictal seizure semiology, with gradual onset and slow secondary generalization, was consistent with a temporal onset.[16,83,98,205] Ghika-Schmid et al. considered the clonazepam-induced synchronous paroxysmal monomorphic rhythmic delta activity associated with transient myoclonus recorded in a patient as a peculiar finding and suggested caution in the administration of antiepileptic drugs.[83]

Magnetic resonance imaging findings vary. A review of MRI findings on 82 patients found abnormalities in 49%. Findings are nonspecific and include subcortical white matter abnormality and T2 cortical signal abnormalities and are reversible with recovery or after corticosteroid therapy.

Cerebral angiography has been reported to be normal; in contrast, cerebral blood flow single-photon emission computed tomography (SPECT) scans have shown areas of reduced perfusion in cortical areas and basal ganglia.

Brain biopsy findings were normal in one patient. Patchy myelin pallor, scant perivascular chronic inflammation, mild gliosis, and lymphocytic infiltration of the venous brain system have been reported.[75,152]

Diagnostic Evaluation. An adult-onset encephalopathy of unknown origin with focal neurologic signs, myoclonus, drug-resistant epileptic seizures, and mental impairment is strongly suggestive of Hashimoto thyroiditis. Therefore, screening for antithyroid antibodies should be performed. Viral and bacterial infections must be excluded. The CSF protein concentrations are high in 78% of patients. Mild lymphocytic pleocytosis may be present occasionally. Differential diagnosis between movement disorders (tremor and myoclonus) and epilepsy requires video-polygraphic-EEG recordings and EMG examination. EEG anomalies are found in 98% of patients. The progressive chronic evolution associated with seizures, myoclonus, and strokelike episodes[98] may cause problems in the differential diagnosis of mitochondrial encephalopathy. Finally, possible kidney disorders must be investigated (see section on renal failure).

Treatment. Although some patients have been found to be corticosteroid nonresponsive, both high doses of oral prednisone and shorter courses of intravenous methylprednisolone were reported to be very effective in controlling HE symptoms.[83,98] Azathioprine, methotrexate, cyclophosphamide and hydroxychloroquine sulfate, plasmapheresis, and intravenous immunoglobulin have been used with clinical benefit. Spontaneous improvement without corticosteroid therapy occurred in some cases.[75] Because of this rapid seizure control, antiepileptic drugs are not usually given.

Parathyroid Disorders

Hyperparathyroidism

Hyperparathyroidism, characterized by hypercalcemia and elevated levels of parathyroid hormone (PTH), is not usually associated with epileptic seizures. However, a *grand mal* epileptic seizure associated with psychiatric symptoms has been reported anecdotally in patients with hypercalcemia secondary to neoplastic hyperparathyroidism and basal ganglia calcifications.[70]

Hypoparathyroidism

General Findings. Hypoparathyroidism is a clinical disorder characterized by hypocalcemia and hyperphosphatemia. It manifests when PTH secreted from the parathyroid glands is insufficient to maintain normal extracellular fluid calcium concentrations or, less commonly, when PTH is unable to function optimally in target tissues, despite adequate circulating levels. Deficiency of PTH may occur following thyroidectomy or other surgical procedures involving the neck. Infections, glandular infiltrations by granulomatous processes, heavy metals, or more commonly autoimmune disorders may cause deficiency of PTH. Congenital parathyroid hypoplasia or agenesis causes congenital hypoparathyroidism. Autosomal-dominant and autosomal-recessive familial idiopathic hypothyroidism have also been identified. Hypocalcemia is the characteristic biologic consequence of hypoparathyroidism. Because low calcium levels result in hyperexcitability of neural membranes, the prominent clinical neurologic manifestations of hypoparathyroidism are those related to hypocalcemia with neuromuscular irritability, perioral paresthesias, tingling of the fingers and toes, and tetany. Generalized tonic–clonic seizures and laryngeal spasm also occur. In a chronic setting, hypocalcemia can be asymptomatic. Alternatively, mild neuromuscular irritability, calcification of the basal ganglia, extrapyramidal disorders, cataracts, alopecia, abnormal dentition, mental retardation, or behavior disorders may be present. From a biochemical point of view, hypoparathyroidism is mainly characterized by hypocalcemia and hyperphosphatemia with normal renal function. Serum levels of PTH are low, except in the setting of PTH resistance, in which case levels are high-normal or elevated. Serum levels of 1,25-dihydroxyvitamin D are usually low or low-normal. The 24-hour urinary excretion of calcium is decreased. Nephrogenous cAMP excretion is low, whereas renal tubular reabsorption of phosphorus is elevated.

DiGeorge syndrome, 10p deletion syndrome, Hallermann-Streiff syndrome, and familial nephrosis with nerve deafness constitute different genetic syndromes with congenital hypoparathyroidism. In particular, hypoparathyroidism with short stature, mental retardation, and seizures (or Sanjad-Sakati syndrome) is characterized by congenital hypoparathyroidism, growth and mental retardation, and seizures as a prominent finding. Recent studies demonstrated that both Sanjad-Sakati syndrome and the autosomal recessive Kenny-Caffey syndrome are allelic variants caused by mutations in the *TBCE* gene.[160]

Anecdotal reports describe the association between idiopathic hypoparathyroidism and systemic lupus erythematosus[82] or subacute sclerosing panencephalitis,[54] in which the authors suggest a common pathogenetic mechanism. In these reports, epileptic seizures occurred in the period of idiopathic hypoparathyroidism.

Here we present data regarding epileptic seizures in hypoparathyroidism occurring after the neonatal period.

Clinical Description. Typically, clinical signs of hypoparathyroidism include tetany, epileptic seizures, and, when basal ganglia calcifications are present, hemichorea, choreoathetosis, and parkinsonism.[146] Epileptic seizures may occur at any age and are usually generalized tonic–clonic with loss of consciousness.[54,81,82] Nonconvulsive status epilepticus has also been described in this group of patients.[118]

Seizures may be the presenting symptom, preceding other signs of hypocalcemia such as chorea and tetany. Normally, tetany develops after calcium levels decline further. Generalized convulsive epileptic seizures may also be the presenting symptom in elderly patients with hypoparathyroidism, in association with confusion and then with signs of tetany. In fact, iatrogenic hypoparathyroidism needs to be considered in the differential diagnosis of adult-onset, generalized tonic–clonic seizures even if the thyroidectomy was performed years earlier.[145] Several types of partial motor seizures, including jacksonian seizures, may also be observed. If not treated, the outcome of these conditions may be very severe. Among the members of a familial idiopathic hypoparathyroidism, some untreated members died in infancy because of convulsions. Paroxysmal kinesigenic choreoathetosis and convulsions occurring in clusters at age 2.5 months have been observed in a child with idiopathic hypothyroidism. The clinical picture was indistinguishable from that of infantile convulsions and choreoathetosis syndrome.[96] Reported EEG findings show irregular high-voltage delta activity that is increased on hyperventilation. Paroxysmal abnormalities may also occur during wakefulness and sleep.[111]

Diagnostic Evaluation. Hypoparathyroidism with hypocalcemia as a cause of epileptic seizures should be considered and investigated in patients of any age. The condition can be treated successfully, whereas if it is untreated, it may be fatal in infants. Tetany, generalized epileptic seizures, and movement disorders may occur at the same time in hypocalcemic states, posing problems of differential diagnosis. Differential diagnosis of partial epileptic seizures and hemitetanic carpopedal spasm may be difficult, as may be the differential diagnosis of reflex epilepsy and paroxysmal kinesigenic choreoathetosis associated with hypoparathyroidism.[29] Finally, the differential diagnosis of primary hypomagnesemia with secondary hypocalcemia must be considered (see section on electrolyte disorders). In all these cases, correct diagnosis requires direct observation of the motor phenomena and ictal EEG investigation during hyperventilation maneuvers. Computed tomography and magnetic resonance imaging of the brain are mandatory to investigate basal ganglia lesions.

Treatment. The aim of therapy in all hypoparathyroid states is to restore serum calcium to levels sufficient to alleviate symptoms of acute hypocalcemia and prevent the complications of chronic hypocalcemia and hypercalcemia. The main pharmacologic agents available are calcium and vitamin D preparations. Neurologic findings disappear on normalization of calcium levels with calcium supplementation and vitamin D therapy in all cases, including those with extrapyramidal signs and basal ganglia calcifications. Magnesium replacement should also be considered routinely in patients with hypocalcemia because hypomagnesemia induces functional hypoparathyroidism. When antiepileptic drugs are required, it must be emphasized that they may lower circulating calcium concentrations. Regular monitoring of plasma calcium levels is recommended.

Disorders of the Pancreas

Diabetes Mellitus

The most important disease of the pancreas associated with epileptic seizures is diabetes mellitus. Seizures may be induced in diabetes mellitus during nonketotic hyperglycemia or during hypoglycemia resulting from iatrogenic hyperinsulinism; in ketotic hyperglycemia, epileptic seizures are rare.

Nonketotic Hyperglycemia

General Findings. Seizures associated with nonketotic hyperglycemia were first reported in 1965.[133] Many other subsequent reports confirmed the occurrence of seizures in nonketotic hyperglycemia. Cases in non–insulin-dependent diabetes mellitus may exhibit a spectrum from asymptomatic hyperglycemia without ketosis (which may be clinically asymptomatic for months or years[90]) to hyperosmolal nonketotic diabetic coma (representing the extreme end of a biochemical continuum). Hyperosmolar nonketotic diabetic coma is associated with a high mortality in adults (range, 20%–70%) and children, but it is more common in the elderly and rarer in children.[208] Diabetes is often detected before severe hyperosmolality develops. Neurologic manifestations such as seizures, focal neurologic signs (usually postictal), myoclonic twitches, nystagmus, and meningeal signs often provide the first clinical clues to the presence of nonketotic hyperglycemia.[133] Age at onset of nonketotic hyperglycemia ranges between 48 and 72 years. Epileptic seizures have been rarely reported in juvenile nonketotic hyperglycemia.[179] As a rule, seizures occur when hyperglycemia is not severe and osmolality is normal or only slightly increased, with normal to moderately decreased sodium levels.[191] In this phase, patients are usually alert. If diabetes mellitus is not treated, however, hyperosmolality with progressive impairment of consciousness develops while seizures stop. The pathogenetic mechanism of the association between hyperglycemia and seizures is still debated. Most authors attribute the partial seizures to a preexisting structural lesion activated by hyperosmolality and hyperglycemia.[56,133] An entirely metabolic cause of epilepsy, such as hypertonicity or hyperglycemia, appears unlikely because in diabetic ketoacidosis partial seizures are rare. However, experimental studies demonstrated that susceptibility to clonic and tonic–clonic flurothyl-induced seizures positively correlates with blood glucose concentrations and that the increased glucose concentration is associated with proconvulsant effects.

Similarly, in the in vitro experiments, epileptiform activity was promoted by increased and suppressed by decreased glucose concentrations. Therefore, extracellular glucose itself has proconvulsant activity even without a previous focal lesion.[186] Hyperglycemia may precipitate seizures by lowering γ-aminobutyric acid levels, resulting in a lower seizure threshold. Moreover, the parietal lobe seems to play a role in epilepsia partialis continua, which is often associated with nonketotic hyperglycemia. Ictal SPECT studies in humans[104] and experimental studies, which found that diabetic hyperglycemic animals have more severe neuronal necrosis in the parietal cortex than do normoglycemic animals,[130] corroborate that hypothesis. The apparently protective effect of ketoacidosis may be attributed to an increase in GABA bioavailability secondary to acidosis, which is known to increase glutamic acid decarboxylase activity.[56,94]

Clinical Description. Seizures occur in about 25% of patients and are the chief initial manifestation in 6%.[94] Seizures are most often partial motor seizures, occurring in 75% to 86% of cases.[94] The seizures are frequent and repetitive and are often followed by transient postictal paralysis.[90] Occipital visual and adversive seizures have been described[92] and have been considered to be a relatively common early manifestation of nonketotic hyperglycemia. Typical jacksonian seizures have also been reported.[97] Epilepsia partialis continua has been described in some cases as the initial symptom of nonketotic hyperglycemia.[56,99,179] Contrary to data in the literature, in some of these cases epilepsia partialis continua could not be attributed to any structural cerebral lesion but seemed to be caused solely by metabolic dysfunction; results of neuroimaging were normal.[56] Nonconvulsive status epilepticus of frontal origin has also been observed.[113,201] Generalized tonic–clonic seizures have been described less frequently.[94] Some patients have reflex or posture-induced epileptic seizures.[99,207] Such seizures are relatively rare and have been defined as kinesigenic seizures[99] or fencing-posture seizures.[207] Characteristically, the seizures are partial, simple, or complex in type, last <5 minutes, and appear within seconds after onset of the triggering maneuver. This maneuver may consist of passive or active elevation of an arm or leg or walking. Seizures are followed by a refractory period during which no further seizures can be elicited.[207] Gaze-evoked sensory visual occipital seizures have been described in an anecdotal case.[67] Ictal stereotypic visual experiences consist of flashing lights followed by formed objects or unfamiliar human faces and may be consistently elicited by having the patient look to one side. Usually, the EEG is normal in uncomplicated diabetes. Focal EEG abnormalities have been found only in nonketotic hyperglycemia, related to an underlying focal cortical lesion, likely vascular in nature, as a consequence of hyperglycemia and hyperosmolarity.[112,133]

Diagnostic Evaluation. Patients with partial seizures, fencing-posture seizures, and even epilepsia partialis continua without any detectable cause and with normal findings on neuroimaging examinations should be investigated for diabetes mellitus. Consequently, it is very important to check glucose levels in all patients with seizures, especially if they are elderly, to detect the early manifestations of nonketotic hyperglycemia associated with mild or minimal hyperosmolality. In cases of occipital seizures, celiac disease must be excluded (see section on gastrointestinal diseases). Of course, neuroimaging investigations must be performed in patients with partial seizures and epilepsia partialis continua to detect more frequent causes, such as cerebral tumor, infarction, encephalitis, brain malformations, and abscess. CT scans in cases of nonketotic hyperglycemia–related seizures often fail to reveal relevant focal cerebral disease. Hyperintensities in T_2 and fluid attenuated inversion recovery (FLAIR) related to seizure activity have frequently been seen in the cortices. Transient $T_2$and FLAIR subcortical hypointensity with or without abnormalities in the overlying cortex in the setting of partial status epilepticus associated with NKH was reported in three patients. The mechanisms of T_2 and FLAIR hypointensities are unclear. These changes may be due to an accumulation of free radicals and iron deposition, as has been described in early cortical ischemia. The decreased N-acetyl-aspartate in the same region observed in some patients suggests reduced vital neuronal tissue.[56,188]

Treatment. As long as biochemical disturbances remain uncorrected, the seizures are refractory to antiepileptic drug therapy. Patients become seizure free after administration of insulin and rehydration, and they remain seizure free while the diabetes mellitus is controlled. Moreover, patients who receive prompt treatment, before nonketotic hyperglycemic coma develops, have a better prognosis. If antiepileptic drugs are used for seizures, it should be noted that plasma free fractions of valproate are increased in diabetes mellitus, and phenytoin should be avoided because it inhibits insulin secretion and may aggravate hyperglycemia and nonketotic hyperglycemia, precipitating diabetic ketoacidosis.[94]

Diabetic Hypoglycemia

General Findings. Diabetic hypoglycemia is a common problem in adults and children with diabetes who are treated with insulin and other oral hypoglycemic agents.[123]

Nondiabetic hypoglycemia may have many causes, such as alcoholism, sepsis, fasting, terminal neoplasms, and insulin-secreting neoplasms. There are also anecdotal reports of patients affected by gastroenteritis with diarrhea and dehydration, hypoparathyroidism, and adrenocortical insufficiency.[81,123]

Clinical Description. Initial clinical symptoms of hypoglycemia are caused by excessive adrenergic activity; patients may be dizzy, tremulous, anxious, and profusely sweating. Hypotonia, motor restlessness, and generalized seizures appear later. Confusion, bizarre behavior, obtundation, stupor, or coma occur in more severe degrees of hypoglycemia. At times, for unknown reasons, the neurologic deficits are of a focal nature, producing partial motor epileptic seizures, focal sensory deficit, and hemiplegia with or without dysphasia.[79,123] Some authors[123,210] have suggested that several mechanisms, including selective sensitivity of neurotransmitters, selective neuronal vulnerability, and loss of autoregulation of cerebral blood flow leading to vasospasm are involved in hypoglycemia associated with focal neurologic deficits.

Hypoglycemic seizures occur in 10% to 20% of adults and more frequently in children.[107] Usually, seizures are generalized, tonic, and tonic–clonic in type. Partial seizures typically occur in adults.[79] There are only two reports of nocturnal partial seizures in children,[123,210] one of them with transient postictal hemiparesis (Todd paralysis).[123] It is well known that unrecognized nocturnal hypoglycemic events are frequent in diabetics, with blood glucose levels returning to normal by morning (Somogyi effect). Therefore, unrecognized nocturnal hypoglycemic seizures may occur in patients with no previous history of fits and hypoglycemic symptoms during waking hours.[123] It appears that severe hypoglycemic events mainly affect the youngest patients and boys (the latter of all ages) rather than adolescents girls, who mainly suffer from ketoacidosis.[171] In this context, Strudwick et al.[197] investigated whether severe hypoglycemic episodes in young children with early-onset type 1 diabetes (T1DM) were associated with subsequent abnormalities in cognitive status. They found that there was no clear evidence that episodes of seizure or coma, even those occurring in very early childhood, resulted in broad cognitive dysfunction, nor was there evidence of specific memory difficulties at the time of testing in children and adolescents with early-onset T1DM.

From a pathogenetic point of view, elegant experimental studies demonstrated that insulin doses of 8 IU/kg were able to induce seizures in 100% of animals and that insulin-induced hypoglycemic convulsions could be mediated by serotoninergic, dopaminergic, and excitatory amino acid pathways.[15]

Interictal EEG findings show different degrees of generalized slowing of background activity, exaggerated response to hyperventilation, increasing of preexisting epileptiform abnormalities, and/or appearance of paroxysmal patterns, such as 3-Hz spike-and-wave discharges or focal abnormalities.[185,192] Blood sugar levels of 50 to 80 mg/dL are associated with slowing of background activity and appearance of diffuse theta activity. At lower glucose levels, EEG shows intermittent bursts of bisynchronous slow waves.[185] Electroencephalographic abnormalities are more frequent in hypoglycemic children, especially younger ones, and in the case of repeated severe hypoglycemic episodes.[192] Usually, these abnormalities disappear rapidly when blood sugar levels return to normal levels, but they may persist after more severe and prolonged hypoglycemic events.[123] The pathogenesis of these EEG abnormalities is unknown. Repeated hypoglycemic episodes alone do not seem to be the major factor in causing EEG abnormalities, and it has been hypothesized that a diabetic encephalopathy caused by microvascular lesions may be involved.[69]

Diagnostic Evaluation. Nocturnal generalized or partial seizures in diabetic patients should be strongly considered as evidence of possible unrecognized insulin-induced hypoglycemia. It has been postulated that these seizures are more common than generally thought and that they may be a presenting symptom of diabetes mellitus.[123] Because such seizures are not symptomatic of a brain lesion and because results of computed tomography were normal in all patients,[79,123] seizures could mistakenly be diagnosed as idiopathic epilepsy, leading to unnecessary treatment with antiepileptic drugs, which must be administered with special care to diabetic patients (see section on nonketotic hyperglycemia). Because of its characteristic pattern, the EEG may aid significantly in the diagnosis. Otherwise, laboratory and clinical investigations are strongly recommended to rule out all other causes of hypoglycemia, especially neoplasms secreting insulin.

Treatment. Reducing the daily dose of insulin and other oral hypoglycemic agents is strongly advised because this is sufficient to prevent hypoglycemia. Antiepileptic drugs should not be considered as elective therapy and must be monitored closely, and it should be remembered that various drugs interact with insulin and other hypoglycemic agents, such as phenothiazine, aspirin, phenylbutazone, sulfa drugs, haloperidol, propranolol, and lithium.

Reproductive Endocrine Disorders

Epileptic seizures as a symptom of reproductive endocrine disorders are problematic. Although there is evidence that reproductive endocrine disorders (especially hypogonadotropic hypogonadism with infertility, hyperprolactinemia, and polycystic ovarian syndrome) and epilepsy (especially temporal lobe epilepsy) frequently occur together, the pathogenesis is controversial.[101,214] Experimental evidence that the temporal lobe modulates sexual, reproductive, and neuroendocrine functions has been obtained in animals, and anatomic-functional pathways connecting the amygdala and hypothalamus have also been defined.[100] Thus, in temporal lobe epilepsy associated with reproductive endocrine disorders, altered impulses arising as epileptiform discharges from the amygdala have been postulated to disrupt normal secretion of gonadotropins and prolactin. In this context, endocrine disorders can be considered as secondary to temporal lobe epilepsy, and so they are beyond the scope of this chapter. However, because experimental animal and human clinical evidence suggests that estrogen and testosterone may precipitate epileptic seizures, and because there are many patients who have temporal lobe epilepsy and reproductive endocrine disorders without taking antiepileptic drugs, it is possible that the presence of a reproductive endocrine disorder may favor the development of temporal lobe epilepsy.[101]

Finally, because of the frequent familial occurrence, a possible contribution of genetic factors to the development of both temporal lobe epilepsy and reproductive endocrine disorders has been hypothesized.[101] A relationship between the type of endocrine disorder and the laterality of temporal epileptiform EEG discharges in women with temporal lobe epilepsy occurs, suggesting the existence of a lateralized asymmetry in cerebral influences on reproductive endocrine function.[100]

GASTROINTESTINAL DISEASES

The relationship between epilepsy and gastrointestinal diseases is a very intriguing problem. Apart from vomiting, which may be a common symptom of either gastrointestinal illness or neurologic disturbances such as migraine, epilepsy, increased intracranial pressure, and metabolic disorders, epilepsy and epileptic seizures may be the presenting symptom in some gastrointestinal diseases. Some authors have reported seizures associated with gastroesophageal reflux and suggested that it could be a part of the autonomic dysfunction that accompanies temporal lobe seizures. Afebrile partial or generalized seizures as a presenting symptom have been reported in children with mild gastroenteritis.[119] Generalized tonic–clonic seizures are nearly the most common extraintestinal manifestation of shigellosis.[46] The reported incidence ranges from 12% to 45%.[87]

Epilepsy and epileptic seizures may be a relevant symptom in celiac disease and orthotopic liver transplantation.

Celiac Disease

General Findings

Celiac disease (CD) is characterized by permanent gluten intolerance. Clinically, the "classical or typical" form appears in the first 2 years of life with diarrhea, weight loss, dystrophic appearance, and anorexia. Irritability and vomiting occur in one third of patients. On the other hand, CD may be silent, latent, or potential. These "atypical" forms are more frequent in children older than 2 years and may present with extraintestinal features such as dermatitis herpetiformis and dental enamel defects. Neurologic disorders have been extensively observed in patients with CD. Among them, epilepsy is the most frequent, and its prevalence in CD patients has been estimated to be between 1.2% and 5%. In 7% of newly diagnosed CD patients, neurologic disorders may be the presenting symptoms of the disease, especially in the case of silent and latent CD.[58,67,88,136] Epilepsy as a presenting symptom of celiac disease has also been reported.[88]

In the case of epilepsy and CD, three groups of patients have been identified: (a) patients with celiac disease, epilepsy, and cerebral calcifications (CEC), or "typical form"; (b) patients with celiac disease and epilepsy without cerebral calcifications; and (c) patients with celiac disease and cerebral calcifications without epilepsy. The latter two groups are considered "atypical forms." There is a fourth group of patients with epilepsy and cerebral calcifications without celiac disease, who are believed to be affected by a latent or silent form of celiac disease.[87]

The *CEC syndrome* was first hypothesized in 1988 and then defined in 1992.[86,88] The majority of patients reported in the literature came from Italy, Spain, and Argentina.[87] Fewer patients have been reported in Australia, Canada, Israel, and Sweden. On the other hand, patients from outside Italy do not have an Italian origin. These data demonstrate that this syndrome, although most widespread in Italy, is generally found all over the world. The Italian diet is rich in gluten, but there may be other reasons for the reported high incidence of CEC in the Italian population, such as the particular interest in this condition in Italy. Whether the association between CD and epilepsy and cerebral calcifications is merely a coincidence or a genetic condition, or whether epilepsy and/or cerebral calcifications are a consequence of an untreated CD, still has to be demonstrated. On one hand, clinical and histopathologic findings, which seem to be the expression of vascular calcified malformation instead of the inflammatory lesion, of CEC syndrome are similar to those found in Sturge-Weber syndrome.[202] On the other hand, the high number of cases reported in the literature and the much higher-than-expected frequency of CD (77.5% of cases in the series of the Italian Working Group on Celiac Disease and Epilepsy[88]) in patients with cerebral calcifications and epilepsy, the progressive growth of cerebral calcifications or their late occurrence during evolution before the adoption of a gluten-free diet,[5,44] and the increasing prevalence with age of epilepsy and cerebral calcifications in patients with undiagnosed CD (from 0.79% at mean age of 5.9 years to 3.5% at mean age of 10 years[206]) lead us to consider that the two conditions are related. Epilepsy and cerebral calcifications might be the consequence of an autoimmune disorder affecting the central nervous system triggered by gliadin in predisposed subjects (HLA phenotype) and originating from the jejunal mucosa. In fact, it has been suggested that an altered expression of jejunal mucosa–activated circulating T cells, secreted cytokines, and tissue transglutaminase may initiate an immune response in the CNS tissue and might play a pathogenetic key role in seizures and cerebral calcifications in these patients.[85]

Concerning the genetic predisposition, CD is strongly associated with HLA class II genes. HLA-DQ2 was found in 90% of CD patients and HLA-DQ8 in 10% of cases. Another association with CD is the DR53 heterodimer, which seems to have affinity with gliadin-A peptides. In a minor percentage of patients, DQ2 is not present and CD is associated with DQ8 heterodimer. Those rare CD patients lacking these HLA markers may exhibit the DR4 allele.[85] It has been suggested that different aspects of the syndrome (with or without CD, with or without epilepsy, and with or without cerebral calcifications) might depend on involved genes and their combination.[80]

Epileptogenesis in CD patients does not appear to be directly dependent on the local deposit of calcium. In fact, seizures may occur early in CD patients before the development of cerebral calcifications.[21] Cerebral calcifications might depend also on deposit of calcium due to chronic immune complex–related endothelial inflammation. Chronic folic acid deficiency has also been hypothesized, similar to what occurs in non-CD conditions such as congenital disease, methotrexate therapy, and radiotherapy. Chronic folic acid deficiency could also depend on the effect of antiepileptic drugs, but that seems less probable because antiepileptic drug–induced folate deficiency is rare.[85] Preferential occipital involvement is an unexplained issue, but it could be related to a selective vulnerability of the occipital lobe.[97] According to Martinez-Bermejo et al.,[137] considering that most CEC patients are from the Mediterranean area (Italy and Spain) and Argentina, it could be hypothesized that CEC may represent a genetic, noninherited, ethnically and geographically restricted syndrome associated with environmental factors.

Atypical forms include patients with celiac disease, epilepsy without cerebral calcifications, and patients with CD and cerebral calcifications without epilepsy. Sixty-nine patients of the latter group were reported up to 1996,[87] and one third of them had partial occipital epilepsy. Labate et al.[122a] found that in a cohort of 72 newly diagnosed patients with idiopathic partial epilepsy, 9% of those with occipital epilepsy were affected by silent CD. Of course, it is possible that cerebral calcifications were lacking because of the early age at diagnosis of celiac disease. In fact, it is well known that some CEC patients with an initial normal CT scan may develop bilateral parieto–occipital calcifications later during the evolution.[44,85–87,124,135]

Finally, 9 cases in the Italian Working Group (IWG) series and 24 literature patients[87] had *epilepsy and cerebral calcifications without celiac disease*. Some of these patients had strong similarities with the CEC patients. In fact, imaging characteristics of cerebral calcifications overlapped those of CEC patients, appearing to be progressive in one case, and epilepsy was localization related in 24 cases (7 from the IWG and 17 from the literature). Of these, 18 showed partial occipital epilepsy, with evolution toward epileptic encephalopathy in 2. The fact that 7 of 9 cases of the Italian Working Group series had the HLA DQW2 and DR3 phenotype, as in CEC patients, suggested that some of these patients might be affected by a CEC syndrome in which CD is in a latent state, perhaps with mucosal patchiness.[85,87]

Recently, Pengiran Tengah et al.[162] ascertained the prevalence of active epilepsy in a cohort of 801 CD patients by patient interviews and retrospective case note review. All the CD patients had diagnostic confirmation by small bowel biopsy. Twenty-one patients had a history of epileptic seizures, but only 9 (1.1%) had active epilepsy. No specific epileptic syndrome was identified, suggesting that a causal relation between gluten sensitivity and active epilepsy is unlikely.

Clinical Description

In CEC syndrome, epilepsy may start at any age, with a peak between 5 and 6 years. In a more recent Argentinean series, mean age at onset of epilepsy was 6.13 years (range 1–16 years).[21] On the basis of clinical and EEG findings and evolution, the epilepsy was classified as localization related in 109 cases. Among them, 78 patients had occipital epilepsy. The semiology of the seizures may consist of versive and/or visual seizures (simple hallucinations, amaurosis, blurred vision, loss of focus, vision of colored dots, complex visual hallucinations such as seeing unfamiliar faces or scenes).[163] Visual seizures followed by complex seizures or secondary generalization may also occur. Two anecdotal cases had reflex epilepsy, with reading reflex seizures in one[87] and eating-induced seizures in the other.[134] The remaining 31 cases showed other varieties of partial epilepsy, with complex seizures in 15, motor seizures in 9, and partial seizures with secondary generalization in 7.[85] Although clinically heterogeneous, epilepsy in these patients is usually pharmacoresistant, frequently characterized by an early and apparently benign initial phase followed by an epileptic encephalopathy after a seizure-free interval.[89] Nevertheless, in many cases the evolution is benign (20 cases in a review of the literature).[87] In 9 benign cases, the outcome of occipital epilepsy was similar to that of early- and late-onset benign childhood epilepsy with occipital paroxysms. Progressive myoclonic ataxia syndrome with a cortical myoclonus has been reported in 7 cases.[32] Progressive mental impairment has been found in patients having epilepsy with a severe evolution. Typical generalized epilepsies have also been reported.

In patients with CD and epilepsy without cerebral calcifications, one third had partial occipital epilepsy and one half had a benign evolution of the seizures. Some of these patients were believed to have a form of benign occipital epilepsy. In two patients, occipital epilepsy was progressive toward epileptic encephalopathy.

Electroencephalographic recordings mainly showed focal occipital spike-and-wave abnormalities; rarely, focal abnormalities were outside the occipital regions. Bilateral slow spike-and-wave activity occurred in the cases of occipital epilepsy with progression toward epileptic encephalopathy. The EEG normalized in patients in whom the seizures disappeared.[88]

Typical CT features of CEC syndrome consist of bilaterally subcortical, roughly symmetric or asymmetric, occipital calcifications, absence of contrast enhancement, and absence of brain atrophy. Calcifications may also be observed in the frontal region, and scattered cases of unilateral occipital calcifications have been reported.[21,85,88,134] Calcifications are extremely variable in size, and no correlation between the extension of calcifications and the severity of disease has been demonstrated.[88]

Diagnostic Evaluation

Considering the apparently specific involvement of the occipital lobe in patients with untreated celiac disease, careful investigation of CD in all patients with occipital epilepsy of unknown cause, even if cerebral calcifications are absent, should be performed.[11] Testing for celiac disease is strongly advised also because, as stated earlier, CD is a gluten-dependent syndrome that may be silent, latent, or potential, and clinical signs of malabsorption may be lacking. Pediatric neurologists may be the only specialists who can detect CD early in these patients.[88]

Complete evaluation to identify CD includes xylose load test, determination of serum folic acid, antigliadin immunoglobulin G (IgG) and IgA antibodies, and antiendomysium antibodies (EmA). Transglutaminase antigen (tTG) has recently been identified as the main autoantigen recognized by antiendomysial antibodies in celiac disease. Low CSF folate levels with alteration in the CSF/serum folate ratio associated with increased CSF and serum levels of cystathionine have been described.[45] Peroral biopsy (with a Crosby capsule) of the jejunal mucosa at the ligament of Treitz (crypt hyperplasia and unequivocal flat mucosa were accepted as markers of celiac disease according to the criteria of Dunnill and Whitehead[68]) should be performed before luten-free diet and 1 year later. Determination of HLA phenotype also should be included in the diagnostic evaluation process.

Moreover, all other known causes of cerebral calcifications must be excluded, including encephalitis, purulent meningitis, ossifying meningoencephalitis, leukemia, chemotherapy, neonatal hemorrhage, congenital infections, TORCH group (toxoplasmosis, rubella, cytomegalovirus, herpes simplex) diseases, and disturbances of calcium and phosphate metabolism. The following examinations should be performed: hematology; urinalysis; blood chemistry; serum electrolytes (sodium, potassium, calcium, and phosphate); serum parathyroid hormone; calcitonin; urinary oligosaccharides and mucopolysaccharides; lysosomal enzyme activities; blood antibodies to herpes simplex virus, cytomegalovirus, mumps virus (parotitis), rubella virus, measles virus, Epstein-Barr virus, and *Toxoplasma*; and vitamin B12.

Finally, enhanced CT scan and MRI must be performed to differentiate these cases from the other phacomatoses, such as tuberous sclerosis complex and Sturge-Weber syndrome, especially when port wine facial nevus is absent. In particular, in patients with celiac disease there is no enlargement of the choroid plexus or local or diffuse brain atrophy, which are common imaging findings in Sturge-Weber syndrome.[88]

Treatment

The epilepsy is usually drug resistant, sometimes evolving into epileptic encephalopathy; it is only rarely benign. Reduced efficacy of common antiepileptic drugs because of malabsorption has been supposed but not demonstrated.

The role and the effectiveness of a gluten-free diet as therapy for epilepsy have yet to be established, although there is no doubt that a correct diet may prevent long-term health risks in unrecognized celiac disease.[103] Nevertheless, it has been demonstrated that the chances of seizure control after gluten-free diet (GFD) seem to be significantly inversely related to the duration of epilepsy before GFD, the age at onset of epilepsy, and the age at the beginning of GFD.[88] When GFD is started late during the evolution, epilepsy may be more severe and epileptic encephalopathy may develop.[63,134]

Lesionectomy might be considered in those patients with drug-resistant epilepsy related to unilateral occipital calcifications.[148]

Hepatic Disorders: Orthotopic Liver Transplantation

General Findings

Seizures are not reported in hepatic encephalopathy, which is usually characterized by varying degrees of confusion, tremor, dysarthria, ataxia, and asterixis. In contrast, seizures are a frequent complication of liver transplantation, even though this procedure usually produces a striking improvement in brain function in patients who have preoperatively hepatic encephalopathy. Nevertheless, neurologic complications are frequent and important causes of morbidity and mortality following orthotopic liver transplantation (OLT). The frequency of neurologic complications after a second OLT is significantly greater than after a first or a third transplant.[131] Seizures represent a main complication of OLT. Although seizures may often be related to focal brain injury, metabolic abnormalities may represent a predisposing factor in these patients. Commonly, underlying factors causing seizures in OLT patients include metabolic derangements, drugs such as cyclosporine and muromonab-CD3 (OKT3), hypoxic–ischemic injury, cerebral structural lesions, and infection. The more frequent electrolyte disturbances in these patients are represented by hypomagnesemia, hypocalcemia, and hyponatremia. Hypomagnesemia may also be secondary to cyclosporin A, which can cause magnesium wasting. The latter drug as well as other immunosuppressant medications (OKT3 and tacrolimus [FK 506]) may trigger seizures per se. Dose reduction or discontinuation of the drug usually leads to complete recovery. It has also been hypothesized that the high dose of steroids used in the therapy of graft rejection may play a role in causing seizures. Cerebral structural lesions that may occur in OLT patients, such as cerebral infarction, pontine or extrapontine myelinolysis, hemorrhagic or ischemic infarct, intracerebral hemorrhage, subarachnoid hemorrhage, and brain abscess and viral and mycosis infections of the central nervous system may also contribute to seizures.[1,71,72,131,194,212] In addition, several reports in the transplantation literature link seizures and other neurologic signs such as confusion, blindness or other visual abnormalities, tremor and paresthesias to immunosuppressive therapy, especially with cyclosporine.[1,101a,131,136a,209] Because of MRI findings (see further on), this has been referred to as a "reversible posterior leukoencephalopathy syndrome." Children seem to be more susceptible than adults to cyclosporine-related seizures[1,206] especially in the presence of synergistic factors such as electrolyte disturbances, structural damage, high-dose steroid treatment for rejection,[8] or low serum cholesterol levels.[62]

Clinical Description

Epileptic seizures are a frequent neurologic complication of liver transplantation, affecting 10% to 29% of cases.[131,209] Single or recurrent generalized tonic–clonic seizures are the most common ictal manifestation. Myoclonic seizures, partial motor seizures, partial seizures with secondary generalization, and status epilepticus have been reported.[1,72,131,209] Unlike hepatic encephalopathy, an increased frequency of seizures may occur within the first week after transplantation, especially after the second orthotopic liver transplantation, but not after subsequent transplant procedures.[131] The cause is undetermined. Conversely, alteration in mental status may increase with each successive orthotopic liver transplantation, progressing to coma. Only a few reports describe the postoperative EEG after orthotopic liver transplantation. Usually, the EEG shows nonspecific generalized slowing of cerebral activity consistent with the development of a metabolic encephalopathy. Interictal generalized or focal spikes and sharp waves have been reported.[1,72,209,211] These epileptiform abnormalities have not been found in all patients. They are associated with serious, often irreversible brain damage, and their incidence has been estimated as fivefold higher in patients who died than in those who survived.[211] EEG was performed after seizure onset in the majority of patients, and partial and generalized electroclinical seizures have also been recorded.[211]

Diagnostic Evaluation

Development of seizures after orthotopic liver transplantation should alert the clinician to investigate for one of the cerebral complications listed earlier. Case history and laboratory tests may aid in the differential diagnosis with other associated metabolic disorders. Usually, computed tomographic findings are described as normal in orthotopic liver transplantation patients.[209] In some patients receiving immunosuppressive drugs (e.g. cyclosporine, tacrolimus), MRI scans show extensive bilateral white matter abnormalities consistent with edema involving mainly the parietal-occipital regions that resolve within 2-3 weeks if immunosuppressive therapy can be reduced, changed or withdrawn. This has been termed a *reversible posterior leukoencephalopathy*.[1,62,101a,136a] MRI is difficult to obtain in these critically ill patients, particularly when they are intubated or unable to remain still.[212] Electroencephalographic monitoring is indicated for its prognostic value.[211]

Treatment

Treatment of the underlying cause of the seizures should always be undertaken together with the administration of anticonvulsant medication. Special attention should be given to the correction of electrolyte imbalances, treatment of infection, and intracranial hemorrhage. Neurosurgical management may be necessary in selected cases such as those with cerebral abscess or subdural hematoma.[212]

Usually, seizures can be controlled by antiepileptic drugs such as phenytoin, phenobarbital, carbamazepine, or benzodiazepines.[1,72] However, phenobarbital, diazepam, phenytoin, and lamotrigine, which are highly bound to albumin, and carbamazepine and ethosuximide, which are primarily eliminated by hepatic oxidation, must be administered carefully because their metabolism is impaired in liver insufficiency, and doses need to be reduced. The most useful anticonvulsant in OLT patients remains phenytoin. Higher doses (18–20 mg/kg) than usual may be necessary to achieve high therapeutic levels. Both total and free phenytoin levels should be measured because hypoalbuminemia and decreased protein binding of phenytoin may result in a toxic free phenytoin level even when the total level is in the subtherapeutic range. Phenobarbital can also be considered. However, because of the excessive sedation, hypotension, and respiratory suppression that may occur during intravenous administration, phenytoin remains the drug of choice. The intravenous loading dose of phenobarbital is not well established, but it is generally in the range of 8 to 20 mg/kg. Carbamazepine can be used in patients with a history of epilepsy and on carbamazepine preoperatively. Carbamazepine, phenobarbital, phenytoin, and primidone may decrease cyclosporine blood levels by induction of P450IIIA (cyclosporine oxidase).[212] Sodium and magnesium valproate and felbamate should be avoided because of their hepatotoxic effects. Gabapentin and vigabatrin, which are not metabolized in the liver, are not bound to albumin, and are exclusively excreted by the kidneys, may also be preferable for these patients.[129]

Anecdotal reports showed that levetiracetam might be an attractive treatment because of its efficacy, lack of hepatic enzyme induction, and rapid attainment of serum levels. It is significant that levetiracetam-treated patients require significantly lower doses of immunosuppressant medications to achieve an equivalent antirejection effect.[84]

SUMMARY AND CONCLUSIONS

Occasional seizures due to metabolic electrolyte and endocrine disorders may occur more frequently in neonates but are also seen in children and adults. Based on the review of the literature presented in this chapter, three different situations must be considered. First, seizures may be an occasional and transient event concomitant with the toxic effect of a metabolic or endocrine disorder; in this case, they usually disappear following correction of the disorder, as in uremic encephalopathy,[156] electrolyte disturbances,[74,195] hypoparathyroidism, hyperthyroidism, and hypothyroidism,[43,167,181] and hypoglycemia and nonketotic hyperglycemia. Second, seizures may be the symptom of a brain lesion produced either by the toxic effect of a metabolic or endocrine disorder on cerebral tissue, as in hyperglycemia and hyperosmolarity,[133] aluminum encephalopathy,[165] and dialysis disequilibrium syndrome,[127] or by an immune-mediated mechanism, as in Hashimoto thyroiditis and probably celiac disease.[88] Third, brain tumors that cause an endocrine or metabolic disorder, as in pituitary incidentalomas and hypothalamic hamartomas, may produce seizures by a mechanical effect on the cortex.

All of these disorders indicate that epilepsy may be a symptom not only of a disease that primarily affects the brain, but also of systemic disorders or diseases that primarily affect other organ systems. Frequently, epileptic seizures may be the presenting symptom in these systemic disorders and also the predominant or sole clinical manifestation.

Consequently, in the presence of new-onset epileptic seizures, clinicians should carefully investigate not only for brain disease, but also for metabolic, endocrine, or gastrointestinal diseases that may be clinically silent. Such investigations may improve the etiologic diagnosis and thereby indicate a more correct therapeutic approach.

References

1. Adams DH, Posford S, Gunson B, et al. Neurological complications following liver transplantation. *Lancet*. 1987;1:949–951.
2. Adams RD, Victor M. *Principles of Neurology*, 3rd ed. New York: McGraw-Hill; 1985.
3. Adulrazzaq YM, Smigura FC, Wettrell G. Primary infantile hypomagnesemia: report of two cases and review of the literature. *Eur J Pediatr*. 1989;148:459–461.
4. Aicardi J. *Diseases of the Nervous System in Childhood*. London: MacKeith Press; 1992:1241–1278.
5. Aldao del Rosario M. Oligosymptomatic coeliac disease and progressive cerebral calcifications with seizures. *Pediatr Neurol*. 1992;8:392.
6. Alfrey AC, Le Gendre GR, Kaehney WD. The dialysis encephalopathy syndrome: possible aluminum intoxication. *N Engl J Med*. 1976;294:184–188.
7. al-Harbi NN, Domrongkitchaiporn S, Lirenman DS. Hypocalcemia and hypomagnesemia after ibuprofen overdose. *Ann Pharmacother*. 1997;31:432–434.
8. Allen RD, Hunnisett AG, Morris PJ. Cyclosporin and magnesium. *Lancet*. 1985;1:1283.
9. Al-Rasheed AK, Blaser SI, Minassian BA, et al. Cyclosporine A neurotoxicity in a patient with idiopathic renal magnesium wasting. *Pediatr Neurol*. 2000;23:353–356.
10. Amarenco P, Roullet E, Nordlinger B, et al. Tremblement d'attitude et encéphalopathie révélateurs d'un syndrome de Conn. *Presse Med*. 1989;18:131.
11. Ambrosetto G, Antonini L, Tassinari CA. Occipital lobe seizures related to clinically asymptomatic celiac disease in adulthood. *Epilepsia*. 1992;33:476–481.

12. Anast CS, Mohs JM, Kaplan SL, et al. Evidence for parathyroid failure in magnesium deficiency. *Science*. 1972;177:606–608.
13. Andermann F, Arzimanoglou A, Berkovic SF. Hypothalamic hamartoma and epilepsy: the pathway of discovery. *Epileptic Disord*. 2003;5:173–175.
14. Anderson RJ, Chung HM, Kluge R, et al. Hyponatremia: a prospective analysis of its epidemiology and the pathogenetic role of vasopressin. *Ann Intern Med*. 1985;102:164–168.
15. Anuradha K, Hota D, Pandhi P. Investigation of central mechanism of insulin induced hypoglycemic convulsions in mice. *Indian J Exp Biol*. 2004;42:368–372.
16. Arain A, Abou-Khalil B, Moses H. Hashimoto's encephalopathy: documentation of mesial temporal seizure origin by ictal EEG. *Seizure*. 2001;10:438–441.
17. Arieff AI. Effects of water, acid–base and electrolyte disorders on the central nervous system. In: Arieff AI, De Fronzo RA, eds. *Fluid, Electrolyte and Acid–Base Disorders*. New York: Churchill Livingstone; 1985:969–1040.
18. Arieff AI. Hyponatremia, convulsions, respiratory arrest, and permanent brain damage after elective surgery in healthy women. *N Engl J Med*. 1986;314:1529–1535.
19. Arieff AI, Ayus JC, Fraser CL. Hyponatraemia and death or permanent brain damage in healthy children. *Br Med J*. 1992;304:1218–1222.
20. Arita K, Kurisu K, Kiura Y, et al. Hypothalamic hamartoma. *Neurol Med Chir* (Tokyo). 2005;45:221–231.
21. Arroyo H, De Rosa S, Ruggieri V, et al. Epilepsy, occipital calcifications, and oligosymptomatic celiac disease in childhood. *J Child Neurol*. 2002;17:800–806.
22. Artieda J, Muruzabal J, Larumbe R, et al. Cortical mechanisms mediating asterixis. *Mov Disord*. 1992;3:209–216.
23. Asami T, Sasagawa F, Kyo S, et al. Incidence of febrile convulsions in children with congenital hypothyroidism. *Acta Paediatr*. 1998;87:623–626.
24. Aydin A, Cemeroglu AP, Baklan B. Thyroxine-induced hypermotor seizure. *Seizure*. 2004;13:61–65.
25. Aydin OF, Uner C, Senbil N, et al. Central pontine and extrapontine myelinolysis owing to disequilibrium syndrome. *J Child Neurol*. 2003;18:292–296.
26. Bachmeyer C, Decroix Y, Medioni J, et al. Coma, crise convulsive et troubles de l'oculomotricité hypomagnésémiques et hypocalcémiques après chimiothérapie par sels de platine. *Rev Med Intern*. 1996;17:467–469.
27. Bairamian D, Di Chiro G, Blume H, et al. Pituitary adenoma with seizures: PET demonstration of reduced glucose utilization in the medial temporal lobe. *J Comput Assist Tomogr*. 1986;10:529–532.
28. Balestri P, Grosso S, Garibaldi G. Alternating hemiplegia of childhood or Hashimoto's encephalopathy? *J Neurol Neurosurg Psychiatry*. 1999;66:548–549.
29. Barabas G, Tucker SM. Idiopathic hypoparathyroidism and paroxysmal dystonic choreoathetosis [Letter]. *Ann Neurol*. 1988;24:585.
30. Barlow ABT, Wheatcroft N, Watson P, et al. Association of HLA-DQA1*0501 with Grave's disease in English Caucasian men and women. *Clin Endocrinol*. 1996;44:73–77.
31. Bartynski WS, Zeigler Z, Spearman MP, et al. Etiology of cortical and white matter lesions in cyclosporin-A and FK-506 neurotoxicity. *AJNR Am J Neuroradiol*. 2001;22:1901–1914.
32. Bathia KP, Brown P, Gregory R, et al. Progressive myoclonic ataxia associated with coeliac disease. *Brain*. 1995;118:1087–1093.
33. Benga I, Baltescu V, Tilinca R, et al. Plasma and cerebrospinal fluid concentrations of magnesium in epileptic patients. *J Neurol Sci*. 1985;67:29–34.
34. Bennett B, Booth T, Quan A. Late onset seizures, hemiparesis and blindness in hemolytic uremic syndrome. *Clin Nephrol*. 2003;59:196–200.
35. Bergstrom J. Uremia is an intoxication. *Kidney Int*. 1985;28(Suppl 17):S2–S4.
36. Berkovic SF, Andermann F, Melanson D, et al. Hypothalamic hamartomas and ictal laughter: evolution of a characteristic epileptic syndrome and diagnostic value of magnetic resonance imaging. *Ann Neurol*. 1988;23:429–439.
37. Berry PL, Belsha CW. Hyponatremia. *Pediatr Clin North Am*. 1990;37:351–363.
38. Biasoli S, D'Andrea G, Feriani M, et al. Uremic encephalopathy: an updating. *Clin Nephrol*. 1986;25:57–63.
39. Blanchard P, Brossien JP. Convulsions due to severe hyponatremia following desmopressin as treatment for enuresis. *Arch Fr Pediatr*. 1991;48:589.
40. Brouns R, De Deyn PP. Neurological complications in renal failure: a review. *Clin Neurol Neurosurg*. 2004;107:1–16.
41. Bruno A, Adams HP Jr. Neurologic problems in renal transplant patients. *Neuro Clin*. 1988;6:305–325.
42. Burn DJ, Bates D. Neurology and the kidney. *J Neurol Neurosurg Psychiatry*. 1998;65:810–821.
43. Bryce GM, Poyner F. Myxedema presenting with seizures. *Postgrad Med J*. 1992;68:35–36.
44. Bye AME, Andermann F, Robitaille I, et al. Cortical vascular abnormalities in the syndrome of celiac disease, epilepsy, bilateral occipital calcification, and folate deficiency. *Ann Neurol*. 1993;34:399–403.
45. Calvani M, Parisi P, Guaitolini C, et al. Latent coeliac disease in a child with epilepsy, cerebral calcifications, drug-induced systemic lupus erythematosus and intestinal folic acid malabsorption associated with impairment of folic acid transport across the blood–brain barrier. *Eur J Pediatr*. 2001;160:288–292.
46. Carson FR, Susman JL. Convulsions associated with shigellosis in children. *Am Fam Physician*. 1989;39:217–218.
47. Castanet J, Taillan B, Garnier G, et al. Crise d'épilepsie révélatrice d'un syndrome de sécrétion inappropriée d'hormone anti-diurétique au cours d'un lupus érythémateux aigu disséminé. *Rev Med Intern*. 1993;14:194–195.
48. Chacko AG, Chandy MJ. Incidental pituitary macroadenomas. *Br J Neurosurg*. 1992;6:233–236.
49. Chadwick D, French AJ. Uraemic myoclonus: an example of reticular reflex myoclonus? *J Neurol Neurosurg Psychiatry*. 1979;42:52–55.
50. Challa A, Papaefstathiou I, Lapatsanis D, et al. Primary idiopathic hypomagnesium in two female siblings. *Acta Paediatr*. 1994;84:1075–1078.
51. Chang SH, Lim CS, Low TS, et al. Cyclosporine-associated encephalopathy: a case report and literature review. *Transplant Proc*. 2001;33:3700–3701.
52. Cheng JC, Zikos D, Skopicki HA, et al. Long-term neurologic outcome in psychogenic water drinkers with severe symptomatic hyponatremia: the effect of rapid correction. *Am J Med*. 1990;88:561–566.
53. Chow KM, Wang AY, Hui AC, et al. Nonconvulsive status epilepticus in peritoneal dialysis patients. *Am J Kidney Dis*. 2001;38:400–405.
54. Cianchetti C, De Virgiliis S, Marrosu MG, et al. Subacute sclerosing panencephalitis and hypoparathyroidism. *Eur Neurol*. 1985;24:149–152.
55. Cianfarani S, Vitale S, Stanhope R, et al. Imperforate anus, bilateral hydronephrosis, bilateral undescended testes and pituitary hypoplasia: a variant of Hall-Pallister syndrome or a new syndrome? *Acta Paediatr*. 1995;84:1322–1344.
56. Cochin JP, Hannequin D, Delangre T, et al. Épilepsie partielle continuée révélatrice d'un diabète sucré. *Rev Neurol* (Paris). 1994;150:239–241.
57. Cohen SN, Syndulko K, Rever B, et al. Visual evoked potentials and long-latency event-related potentials in chronic renal failure. *Neurology*. 1983;33:1219–1222.
58. Cooke WT, Holmes GKT. Neurological and psychiatric complications. In: Cooke WT, Holmes GKT, eds. *Coeliac Disease*. Edinburgh: Churchill Livingstone; 1984:202–220.
59. Das P, Carcao M, Hitzler J. DDAVP-induced hyponatremia in young children. *J Pediatr Hematol Oncol*. 2005;27:330–332.
60. De Deyn PP, D'Hooge R, Van Bogaert PP, et al. Endogenous guanidino compounds as uremic neurotoxins. *Kidney Int Suppl*. 2001;78:77–83.
61. De Deyn PP, Saxena VK, Abts H, et al. Clinical and pathophysiological aspects of neurological complications in renal failure. *Acta Neurol Belg*. 1992;92:191–206.
62. De Groen PC, Aksamit AJ, Rakela J, et al. Central nervous system toxicity after liver transplantation. The role of cyclosporine and cholesterol. *N Engl J Med*. 1987;317:861–866.
63. Del Giudice E. Gluten free diet and evolution of the seizures in coeliac disease and epilepsy. In: Gobbi G, Andermann F, Naccarato S, et al., eds. *Epilepsy and Other Neurological Disorders in Coeliac Disease*. London: Libbey; 1997:89–92.
64. Dharnidharka VR, Carney PR. Isolated idiopathic hypomagnesemia presenting as aphasia and seizures. *Pediatric Neurol*. 2005;33:61–65.
65. Dong X, Leppik IE, White J, et al. Hyponatremia from oxcarbazepine and carbamazepine. *Neurology*. 2005(27);65:1976–1978.
66. Duffey P, Yee S, Reid IN, et al. Hashimoto's encephalopathy: postmortem findings after fatal status epilepticus. *Neurology*. 2003;61:1124–1126.
67. Duncan MB, Jabbari B, Rosenberg ML. Gaze-evoked visual seizures in nonketotic hyperglycemia. *Epilepsia*. 1991;32:221–224.
68. Dunnill MS, Whitehead R. A method for the quantification of small intestinal biopsy specimen. *J Clin Pathol*. 1972;25:243–245.
69. Eeg-Olofson O, Petersen I. Childhood diabetic neuropathy. A clinical and neurophysiological study. *Acta Paediatr Scand*. 1966;55:163–176.
70. El Maghraoui A, Birouk N, Zaim A, et al. Syndrome de Fahr et dysparathyroidie. *Presse Méd*. 1995;24:1301–1304.
71. Estol CJ, Faris AA, Martinez AJ, et al. Central pontine myelinolysis after liver transplantation. *Neurology*. 1989;39:493–498.
72. Estol CJ, Lopez O, Brenner RP, et al. Seizures after transplantation: a clinicopathologic study. *Neurology*. 1989;39:1297–1301.
73. Evers S, Tepel M, Obladen M, et al. Influence of end-stage renal failure and hemodialysis on event-related potentials. *J Clin Neurophysiol*. 1998;15:58–63.
74. Farrar CH, Chande VT, Fitzpatrick DF, et al. Hyponatremia as the cause of seizures in infants: a retrospective analysis of incidence, severity, and clinical predictors. *Ann Emerg Med*. 1995;26:42–48.
75. Fatourechi V. Hashimoto's encephalopathy: myth or reality? An endocrinologist's perspective. *Best Pract Res Clin Endocrinol Metab*. 2005;19:53–66.
76. Ferracci F, Bertiato G, Moretto G. Hashimoto's encephalopathy: epidemiologic data and pathogenetic considerations. *J Neurol Sci*. 2004;217:165–168.
77. Flink EB. Magnesium deficiency. Etiology and clinical spectrum. *Acta Med Scand*. 1981;647(Suppl):125–137.
78. Foley CM, Polinsky MS, Gruskin AB, et al. Encephalopathy in infants and children with chronic renal disease. *Arch Neurol*. 1981;38:656–658.

79. Foster JW, Hart RG. Hypoglycemic hemiplegia: two cases and clinical review. *Stroke*. 1987;18:944–946.
80. Fromager G, Viader F. Epilepsy, bi-occipital calcifications and celiac disease. *Rev Neurol*. 2001;157:116–118.
81. Gazarian M, Cowell CT, Bonney M, et al. The 4A syndrome: adrenocortical insufficiency associated with achalasia, alacrima, autonomic and other neurological abnormalities. *Eur J Pediatr*. 1995;154:18–23.
82. Gazarian M, Laxer RM, Kooh SW, et al. Hypoparathyroidism associated with systemic lupus erythematosus. *J Rheumatol*. 1995;22:2156–2158.
83. Ghika-Schmid F, Ghika J, Regli F, et al. Hashimoto's myoclonic encephalopathy: an underdiagnosed treatable condition? *Mov Disord*. 1996;11:555–562.
84. Glass GA, Stankiewicz J, Mithoefer A, et al. Levetiracetam for seizures after liver transplantation. *Neurology*. 2005;64:1084–1085.
85. Gobbi G. Coeliac disease, epilepsy and cerebral calcifications. *Brain Dev*. 2005;27:189–200.
86. Gobbi G, Ambrosetto P, Zaniboni MG, et al. Celiac disease, posterior cerebral calcifications and epilepsy. *Brain Dev*. 1992;14:23–29.
87. Gobbi G, Bertani G. Coeliac disease and epilepsy. In: Gobbi G, Andermann F, Naccarato S, et al., eds. *Epilepsy and Other Neurological Disorders in Coeliac Disease*. London: Libbey; 1997:65–80.
88. Gobbi G, Bouquet F, Greco L, et al. Coeliac disease, epilepsy and cerebral calcifications. *Lancet*. 1992;340:439–443.
89. Gobbi G, Sorrenti G, Santucci M, et al. Epilepsy with bilateral occipital calcifications: a benign onset with progressive severity. *Neurology*. 1988;38:913–920.
90. Grant C, Warlow C. Focal epilepsy in diabetic nonketotic hyperglycaemia. *Br Med J*. 1985;290:1204–1205.
91. Gupta SK, Manhas AS, Gupta VK, et al. Serum magnesium levels in idiopathic epilepsy. *J Assoc Physicians India*. 1994;42:456–457.
92. Hamed M, Mitchell H. Hyponatremic convulsion associated with desmopressin and imipramine treatment. *Br Med J*. 1993;306:1169.
93. Hanna S, Tibby SM, Durward A, et al. Incidence of hyponatraemia and hyponatraemic seizures in severe respiratory syncytial virus bronchiolitis. *Acta Paediatr*. 2003;92:430–434.
94. Harden CL, Rosenbaum DH, Daras M. Hyperglycemia presenting with occipital seizures. *Epilepsia*. 1991;32:215–220.
95. Hariprasad MK, Eisinger RP, Nadler IM, et al. Hyponatremia in psychogenic polydipsia. *Arch Intern Med*. 1980;140:1639–1642.
96. Hattori H, Yorifuji T. Infantile convulsions and paroxysmal kinesigenic choreoathetosis in a patient with idiopathic hypoparathyroidism. *Brain Dev*. 2000;22:449–450.
97. Hauser RA, Lacey M, Knight MR. Hypertensive encephalopathy: magnetic resonance imaging demonstration of reversible cortical and white matter lesions. *Arch Neurol*. 1988;45:1078–1083.
98. Henchey R, Cibula J, Helveston W, et al. Electroencephalographic findings in Hashimoto's encephalopathy. *Neurology* 1995;45:977–981.
99. Hennis A, Corbin D, Fraser H. Focal seizures and non-ketotic hyperglycaemia. *J Neurol Neurosurg Psychiatry*. 1992;55:195.
100. Herzog AG. A relationship between particular reproductive endocrine disorders and the laterality of epileptiform discharges in women with epilepsy. *Neurology* 1993;43:1907–1910.
101. Herzog AG, Seibel MM, Schomer DL, et al. Reproductive endocrine disorders in men with partial seizures of temporal lobe origin. *Arch Neurol*. 1986;43:347–350.
101a. Hinchey J, Chaves C, Appignani B, et al. A reversible posterior leukoencephalopathy syndrome. *N Engl J Med*. 1996;334:494–500.
102. Hoang-Xuan K, Perrotte P, Dubas F, et al. Myoclonic encephalopathy after aluminum exposure. *Lancet*. 1996;347:910–911.
103. Holmes GKT, Prior P, Lane MR, et al. Malignancy in coeliac disease—effect of a gluten free diet. *Gut*. 1989;30:333–338.
104. Huang CW, Hsieh YJ, Pai MC, et al. Nonketotic hyperglycemia-related epilepsia partialis continua with ictal unilateral parietal hyperperfusion. *Epilepsia*. 2005;46:1843–1844.
105. Hughes JR, Schreeder MT. EEG in dialysis encephalopathy. *Neurology*. 1980;30:1148–1154.
106. Hung SC, Hung SH, Tarng DC, et al. Thiamine deficiency and unexplained encephalopathy in hemodialysis and peritoneal dialysis patients. *Am J Kidney Dis*. 2001;38:941–947.
107. Hypoglycaemia and the nervous system. *Lancet*. 1985;2:759–760.
108. Itoh M, Matsui N, Matsui S. Periodic lateralized epileptiform discharges in EEG during recovery from hyponatremia: a case report. *Clin Electroencephalogr*. 1994;25:164–169.
109. Jabbary B, Huott AD. Seizures in thyrotoxicosis. *Epilepsia*. 1980;21:91–96.
110. Johnston C, Webb L, Daley J, et al. Hyponatraemia and Moduretic *grand mal* seizures: a review. *J R Soc Med*. 1989;82:479–483.
111. Jorens PG, Appel BJ, Hilte FA, et al. Basal ganglia calcifications in postoperative hypoparathyroidism: a case with unusual characteristics. *Acta Neurol Scand*. 1991;83:137–140.
112. Kang HC, Chung da E, Kim DW, et al. Early- and late-onset complications of the ketogenic diet for intractable epilepsy. *Epilepsia*. 2004;45(9):1116–1123.
113. Karmochkine M, Woimant F, Chaine P, et al. État de mal partiel au cours de l'hyperglycémie sans cétose. *Presse Méd*. 1990;19:869.
114. Keating JP, Schears GJ, Dodge PR. Oral water intoxication in infants. *Am J Dis Child*. 1991;145:985–990.
115. Kerr DNS. Clinical and pathophysiologic changes in patients on chronic dialysis: the central nervous system. *Adv Nephrol*. 1980;9:109–132.
116. Kim JY, Kim BS, Kang JH. Dilated cardiomyopathy in thyrotoxicosis and Moyamoya disease. *Int J Cardiol*. 2001;80:101–103.
117. Kiviranta T, Airaksinen EM. Low sodium levels in serum are associated with subsequent febrile seizures. *Acta Paediatrica*. 1995;84:1372–1374.
118. Kline CA, Esekogwu VI, Henderson SO, et al. Non-convulsive status epilepticus in a patient with hypocalcemia. *J Emerg Med*. 1998;16:715–718.
119. Komori H, Wada M, Eto M, et al. Benign convulsions with mild gastroenteritis: a report of 10 recent cases detailing clinical varieties. *Brain Dev*. 1995;17:334–337.
120. Konrad M, Weber S. Recent advances in molecular genetics of hereditary magnesium-losing disorders. *J Am Soc Nephrol*. 2003;14:249–260.
121. Korczyn AD, Bechar M. Convulsive fits in thyrotoxicosis. *Epilepsia*. 1976;17:33–34.
122. Kuroda T, Okamura K, Yoshinari M, et al. A case of normotensive primary aldosteronism with hypopituitarism, epilepsy, and medullary sponge kidney. *Acta Endocrinol*. 1989;121:797–801.
122a. Labate A, Gambardella A, Messina D, et al. Silent celiac disease in patients with childhood localization-related epilepsis. *Epilepsia* 2001;42:1153–1155.
123. Lahat E, Barr J, Bistritzer T. Focal epileptic episodes associated with hypoglycemia in children with diabetes. *Clin Neurol Neurosurg*. 1995;97:314–316.
124. Lambertini A, Zaniboni MG, Mayer M, et al. Epilepsy and cerebral calcifications with normal jejunal mucosa: latent coeliac disease? In: Gobbi G, Banchini G, Naccarato S, et al., eds. *Epilepsy and Other Neurological Disorders in Coeliac Disease*. London: John Libbey; 1997:83–88.
125. Lazarus JH. Investigation and treatment of hypothyroidism. *Clin Endocrinol*. 1996;44:129–131.
126. Lee TG, Ha CK, Lim BH. Thyroid storm presenting as status epilepticus and stroke. *Postgrad Med J*. 1997;73:61.
127. Leonard A, Shapiro FL. Subdural hematoma in regularly hemodialyzed patients. *Ann Intern Med*. 1975;82:650–658.
128. Leppik IE. Zonisamide. *Epilepsia*. 1999;40(Suppl 5):S23–S29.
129. Levy RH, Mattson RH, Meldrum BS, eds. *Antiepileptic Drugs*, 4th ed. New York: Raven Press; 1995.
130. Li C, Li PA, He QP, et al. Effects of streptozotocin-induced hyperglycemia on brain damage following transient ischemia. *Neurobiol Dis*. 1998;5:117–128.
131. Lopez OL, Estol C, Colina I, et al. Neurological complications after liver transplantation. *Hepatology*. 1992;16:162–166.
132. Lopez-Medrano F, Garcia Gil ME, Ruiz Valdepenas P, et al. Non convulsive status epilepticus: exceptional first manifestation of hyperthyroidism. *Med Clin* (Barcelona). 2002;118:118–119.
133. Maccario M, Messis CP, Vastola EF. Focal seizures as a manifestation of hyperglycemia without ketosis. *Neurology*. 1965;15:195–206.
134. Magaudda A, Dalla Bernardina B, Magazzu' G, et al. Frequency of occipital bilateral calcifications and epilepsy in coeliac patients. In: Gobbi G, Andermann F, Naccarato S, et al., eds. *Epilepsy and Other Neurological Disorders in Coeliac Disease*. London: John Libbey; 1997:121–130.
135. Maki M, Holm K, Kosmies S, et al. Normal small bowel biopsy followed by coeliac disease. *Arch Dis Child*. 1990;65:1137–1141.
136. Mantovani V, Zaniboni MG, Collina E, et al. HLA in coeliac disease and epilepsy. In: Gobbi G, Andermann F, Naccarato S, et al., eds. *Epilepsy and Other Neurological Disorders in Coeliac Disease*. London: John Libbey; 1997:143–146.
136a. Marchiori PE, Mies S, Scaff M. Cyclosporine A-induced ocular opsoclonus and reversible leukoencephalopathy after orthotopic liver transplantation: brief report. *Clin Neuropharmacol* 2004;27:195–197.
137. Martinez-Bermejo A, Polanco I, Royo A, et al. A study of Gobbi's syndrome in Spanish population. *Rev Neurol*. 1999;29:105–110.
138. Mastroianni N, De Fusco M, Zollo M, et al. Molecular cloning, expression pattern, and chromosomal localization of the human Na–Cl thiazide-sensitive cotransporter (SLC12A3). *Genomics*. 1996;35:486–493.
139. McKeon A, McNamara B, Sweeney B. Hashimoto's encephalopathy presenting with psychosis and generalized absence status. *J Neurol*. 2004;251:1025–1027.
140. Medani CR. Seizures and hyponatremia due to dietary water intoxication in infants. *South Med J*. 1987;80:421–425.
141. Millson D, Borland C, Murphy P, et al. Hyponatraemia and Moduretic. *Br Med J*. 1984;289:1308–1309.
142. Minkoff L, Gaerther G, Darab M, et al. Inhibition of brain sodium-potassium-ATPase in uremic rats. *J Lab Clin Med*. 1972;80:71–78.
143. Molnar Z, Farkas V, Nemes L, et al. Hyponatraemic seizures resulting from inadequate post-operative fluid intake following a single dose of desmopressin. *Nephrol Dial Transplant*. 2005;20:2265–2267.
144. Mori A. Biochemistry and neurotoxicology of guanidino compounds. History and recent advances. *Pavlov J Biol Sci*. 1987;22:85–94.

145. Mrowka M, Knake S, Klinge H, et al. Hypocalcemic generalised seizures as a manifestation of iatrogenic hypoparathyroidism months to years after thyroid surgery. *Epileptic Disord*. 2004;6:85–87.
146. Muenter MD, Whisnant JP. Basal ganglia calcification, hypoparathyroidism, and extrapyramidal motor manifestation. *Neurology*. 1968;18:1075–1083.
147. Nakamura H, Rose PG, Blumer JL, et al. Acute encephalopathy due to aluminum toxicity successfully treated by combined intravenous deferoxamine and hemodialysis. *J Clin Pharmacol*. 2000;40:296–300.
148. Nakken KO, Roste GK, Hauglie-Hanssen E. Celiac disease, unilateral occipital calcifications, and drug-resistant epilepsy: successful lesionectomy. *Acta Neurol Scand*. 2005;111:202–204.
149. Nasrallah K, Silver B. Hyponatremia associated with repeated use of levetiracetam. *Epilepsia*. 2005;46:972–973.
150. Ng L, Pedraza PE, Faris JS, et al. Audiogenic seizure susceptibility in thyroid hormone receptor beta-deficient mice. *Neuroreport*. 2001;12:2359–2362.
151. Nguyen D, Singh S, Zaatreh M, et al. Hypothalamic hamartomas: seven cases and review of the literature. *Epilepsy Behav*. 2003;4:246–258.
152. Nolte KW, Unbehaun A, Sieker H, et al. Hashimoto encephalopathy: a brainstem vasculitis? *Neurology*. 2000;54:769–770.
153. Ochi H, Horiuchi I, Araki N, et al. Proteomic analysis of human brain identifies alpha-enolase as a novel autoantigen in Hashimoto's encephalopathy. *FEBS Lett*. 2002;528:197–202.
154. Okamoto M, Nako Y, Tachibana A, et al. Efficacy of phenytoin against hyponatremic seizures due to SIADH after administration of anticancer drugs in a neonate. *J Perinatol*. 2002;22:247–248.
155. Okura M, Okada H, Nagoumi I, et al. Electroencephalographic changes in acute water intoxication. *Jpn J Psychiatr Neurol*. 1990;44:729–734.
156. Olsen S. The brain in uremia. *Acta Psychiatr Neurol Scand*. 1961;36:1–122.
157. Pacheco-Rosado J, Hernandez-Garcia A, Ortiz-Butron R. Perinatal hypothyroidism increases the susceptibility to lidocaine-kindling in adult rats. *Neurosci Lett*. 2004;367:186–188.
158. Pan JC, Pei YQ, An L, et al. Epileptiform activity and hippocampal damage produced by intrahippocampal injection of guanidinosuccinic acid in rat. *Neurosci Lett*. 1996;209:121–124.
159. Parizel PM, Snoeck HW, van den Hauwe L, et al. Cerebral complications of murine monoclonal CD3 antibody (OKT3): CT and MR findings. *AJNR Am J Neuroradiol*. 1997;18:1935–1938.
160. Parvari R, Hershkovitz E, Grossman N, et al. Mutation of TBCE causes hypoparathyroidism-retardation-dysmorphism and autosomal recessive Kenny-Caffey syndrome. *Nature Genet*. 2002;32:448–452.
161. Parvex P, Pinsk M, Bell LE, et al. Reversible encephalopathy associated with tacrolimus in pediatric renal transplants. *Pediatr Nephrol*. 2001;16:537–542.
162. Pengiran Tengah DS, Holmes GK, Wills AJ. The prevalence of epilepsy in patients with celiac disease. *Epilepsia*. 2004;45:1291–1293.
163. Pfaender M, D'Souza WJ, Trost N, et al. Visual disturbances representing occipital lobe epilepsy in patients with cerebral calcifications and celiac disease: a case series. *J Neurol Neurosurg Psychiatry*. 2004;75:1623–1625.
164. Pierides AM, Ward MK, Kerr DNS. Haemodialysis encephalopathy: possible role of phosphate depletion. *Lancet*. 1976;1:1234–1235.
165. Pillion G, Loirat C, Blum C, et al. Aluminum encephalopathy: a potential risk of aluminum gels in children with chronic renal failure. *Int J Pediatr Nephrol*. 1981;2:29–32.
166. Polinsky MS, Kaiser BA, Stover JR, et al. Neurologic development of children with severe chronic renal failure from infancy. *Pediatr Nephrol*. 1987;1:157–165.
167. Primavera A, Brusa G, Novello P. Thyrotoxic encephalopathy and recurrent seizures. *Eur Neurol*. 1990;30:186–188.
168. Ra CS, Lui CC, Liang CL, et al. Superior sagittal sinus thrombosis induced by thyrotoxicosis. Case report. *J Neurosurg*. 2001;94:130–132.
169. Raskin NA, Fishman RA. Neurologic disorders in renal failure (part I). *N Engl J Med*. 1976;294:143–148.
170. Reusche E, Pilz P, Oberascher G, et al. Subacute fatal aluminum encephalopathy after reconstructive otoneurosurgery: a case report. *Hum Pathol*. 2001;32:1136–1140.
171. Rewers A, Chase HP, Mackenzie T, et al. Predictors of acute complications in children with type 1 diabetes. *JAMA*. 2002;287:2511–2518.
172. Richet G, Lopez de Noveles E, Verroust P. Drug intoxication and neurologic episodes in chronic renal failure. *Br Med J*. 1979;1:394–395.
173. Rivera-Vasquez AB, Noriega-Sanchez A, Ramirez-Gonzales R, et al. Acute hypercalcemia in hemodialysis patients: distinction from dialysis dementia. *Nephron*. 1980;25:243–246.
174. Rob PM, Niederstadt C, Reusche E. Dementia in patients undergoing long-term dialysis: aetiology, differential diagnoses, epidemiology and management. *CNS Drugs*. 2001;15:691–699.
175. Romero R, Meacham LR, Winn KT. Isolated magnesium malabsorption in a 10-year-old boy. *Am J Gastroenterol*. 1996;91:611–613.
176. Rossini PM, Di Stefano E, Febro A, et al. Brain stem auditory evoked responses (BAERs) in patients with chronic renal failure. *Electroencephalogr Clin Neurophysiol*. 1984;57:507–514.
177. Russo LS, Beale G, Sandroni S, et al. Aluminum intoxication in undialysed adults with chronic renal failure. *J Neurol Neurosurg Psychiatry*. 1992;55:697–700.
178. Rutter N, O'Callaghan MJ. Hyponatraemia in children with febrile convulsions. *Arch Dis Child*. 1978;53:85–87.
179. Sabharwal RK, Gupta M, Sharma D, et al. Juvenile diabetes manifesting as epilepsia partialis continua. *J Assoc Physicians India*. 1989;37:603–604.
180. Sadeh M, Blatt I, Martonovits A, et al. Treatment of porphyric convulsions with magnesium sulfate. *Epilepsia*. 1991;32:712–715.
181. Safe AF, Griffiths KD, Maxwell RT. Thyrotoxic crisis presenting as status epilepticus. *Postgrad Med J*. 1990;66:150–152.
182. Saper CB. Hypothalamic connections with the cerebral cortex. *Prog Brain Res*. 2000;126:39–48.
183. Sarnaik AP, Meert K, Hackbarth R, et al. Management of hyponatremic seizures in children with hypertonic saline: a safe and effective strategy. *Crit Care Med*. 1991;19:758–762.
184. Satur CMR, Jenning A, Walker DR. Hypomagnesaemia and fits complicating paediatric cardiac surgery. *Ann Clin Biochem*. 1993;30:315–317.
185. Saunders MG, Westmoreland BF. The EEG in evaluation of disorders affecting the brain diffusely. In: Klass DW, Daly DD, eds. *Current Practice of Clinical Electroencephalography*. New York: Raven Press; 1979:343–379.
186. Schwechter EM, Veliskova J, Velisek L. Correlation between extracellular glucose and seizure susceptibility in adult rats. *Ann Neurol*. 2003;53:91–101.
187. Sedman AB, Wilkening GM, Warady BM, et al. Encephalopathy in childhood secondary to aluminum toxicity. *J Pediatr*. 1984;105:836–838.
188. Seo DW, Na DG, Na DL, et al. Subcortical hypointensity in partial status epilepticus associated with nonketotic hyperglycemia. *J Neuroimaging*. 2003;13:259–263.
189. Sheth KN, Wu GF, Messe SR, et al. Dialysis disequilibrium: another reversible posterior leukoencephalopathy syndrome? *Clin Neurol Neurosurg*. 2003;105:249–252.
190. Shirabe T, Irie K, Uchida M. Autopsy case of aluminum encephalopathy. *Neuropathology*. 2002;22:206–210.
191. Singh BM, Strobos RJ. Epilepsia partialis continua associated with nonketotic hyperglycemia: clinical and biochemical profile of 21 patients. *Ann Neurol*. 1980;8:155–160.
192. Soltész G, Acsadi G. Association between diabetes, severe hypoglycaemia, and electroencephalographic abnormalities. *Arch Dis Child*. 1989;64:992–996.
193. Sood AK, Handa R, Malhotra RC, et al. Serum, CSF, RBC, and urinary levels of magnesium and calcium in idiopathic generalized tonic–clonic seizures. *Indian J Med Res*. 1993;98:152–154.
194. Stein DP, Lederman RJ, Vogt DP, et al. Neurological complications following liver transplantation. *Ann Neurol*. 1992;31:644–649.
195. Sterns RH, Riggs JE, Schochet SS Jr. Osmotic demyelination syndrome following correction of hyponatremia. *N Engl J Med*. 1986;314:1535–1542.
196. Striano S, Striano P, Sarappa C, et al. The clinical spectrum and natural history of gelastic epilepsy-hypothalamic hamartoma syndrome. *Seizure*. 2005;14:232–239.
197. Strudwick SK, Carne C, Gardiner J, et al. Cognitive functioning in children with early onset type 1 diabetes and severe hypoglycemia. *J Pediatr*. 2005;147:680–685.
198. Su YH, Izumi T, Kitsu M, et al. Seizures threshold in juvenile myoclonic epilepsy with Graves' disease. *Epilepsia*. 1993;34:488–492.
199. Tanneau RS, Henry A, Rouhart F, et al. High incidence of neurologic complications following rapid correction of severe hyponatremia in polydipsic patients. *J Clin Psychiatry*. 1994;8:349–354.
200. Thoman JE, Duffner PK, Shucard JL. Do serum sodium levels predict febrile seizure recurrence within 24 hours? *Pediatr Neurol*. 2004;31:342–344.
201. Thomas P, Zifkin B, Migneco O, et al. Nonconvulsive status epilepticus of frontal origin. *Neurology*. 1999;52:1174–1183.
202. Tiacci C, D'Alessandro P, Cantisani TA, et al. Epilepsy with bilateral occipital calcifications: Sturge-Weber variant or a different encephalopathy? *Epilepsia*. 1993;34:528–539.
203. Trinh-Trang-Tan MM, Cartron JP, Bankir L. Molecular basis for the dialysis disequilibrium syndrome: altered aquaporin and urea transporter expression in the brain. *Nephrol Dial Transplant*. 2005;20(9):1984–1988.
204. Vanholder R, Glorieux G, De Smet R, et al.; European Uremic Toxin Work Group. New insights in uremic toxins. *Kidney Int Suppl*. 2003;84:6–10.
205. Vasconcellos E, Pina-Garza JE, Fakhoury T, et al. Pediatric manifestations of Hashimoto's encephalopathy. *Pediatr Neurol* 1999;20:394–398.
206. Vascotto M, Fois A. Frequency of epilepsy in coeliac disease and frequency of coeliac disease in epilepsy. In: Gobbi G, Banchini G, Naccarato S, et al., eds. *Epilepsy and Other Neurological Disorders in Coeliac Disease*. London: John Libbey; 1997:105–110.
207. Venna N, Sabin TD. Tonic focal seizures in nonketotic hyperglycemia of diabetes mellitus. *Arch Neurol*. 1981;38:512–514.
208. Vernon DD, Postellon DC. Nonketotic hyperosmolal diabetic coma in a child: management with low-dose insulin infusion and intracranial pressure monitoring. *Pediatrics*. 1986;77:770–772.
209. Vogt DP, Lederman RJ, Carey WD, et al. Neurologic complications of liver transplantation. *Transplantation*. 1988;45:1057–1061.

210. Waine EA, Dean HJ, Booth F, et al. Focal neurologic deficits associated with hypoglycemia in children with diabetes. *J Pediatr*. 1990;117:575–577.
211. Wszolek ZK, Aksamit AJ, Ellingson RJ, et al. Epileptiform electroencephalographic abnormalities in liver transplant recipients. *Ann Neurol* 1991;30:37–41.
212. Wszolek ZK, Stegt, R. E. Seizures after orthotopic liver transplantation. *Seizure*. 1997;6:31–39.
213. Wu J, Xu L, Kim do Y, et al. Electrophysiological properties of human hypothalamic hamartomas. *Ann Neurol*. 2005;58:371–382.
214. Ziegelbaum MM. Hypogonadotropic hypogonadism and temporal lobe epilepsy. *Urology*. 1991;3:235–236.

CHAPTER 268 ■ ALCOHOL AND DRUG ABUSE

JOHN C. M. BRUST

INTRODUCTION

Worldwide, a variety of drugs are used recreationally, and they differ in their ability to produce either psychic dependence (compulsive drug-seeking behavior, "craving," "addiction") or physical dependence (an adaptive state in which cessation of drug use or administration of an antagonist produces physical withdrawal signs).[5] Many of these agents, by either indirect or direct mechanisms, increase the risk of seizures. This chapter addresses those drugs most often used recreationally in North America and Europe, exclusive of tobacco and caffeine (Table 1). Although agents are discussed individually, it is important to recognize that polydrug use (including ethanol) is common and, in fact, a person may be simultaneously overdosed on one drug while withdrawing from another.

INDIRECT MECHANISMS

Drug users are frequent victims of cerebral trauma: in alcoholics usually associated with intoxication and in illicit drug users with lawlessness and violence. Post-traumatic seizures can be early or late in onset, and, depending on the agent, intoxication or withdrawal can further reduce seizure threshold.

Parenteral drug abusers are subject to systemic and central nervous system (CNS) infection. Endocarditis causes meningitis, brain abscess, and infected ("mycotic") aneurysm. Seizures in patients with AIDS may reflect opportunistic CNS infection or neoplasm, or direct infection of the brain by human immunodeficiency virus (HIV). Illicit drug users and alcoholics are often immunocompromised in the absence of HIV infection.

Independent of endocarditis, illicit drug users are at risk for ischemic and hemorrhagic stroke; mechanisms include embolization of foreign material, vasculitis, coagulopathy, and, with psychostimulants (especially cocaine), hypertensive crisis and direct cerebral vasoconstriction. Although mild-to-moderate doses of ethanol are protective against ischemic stroke, high doses increase risk, and any dose of ethanol is a risk factor for hemorrhagic stroke.[51]

Metabolic derangements are frequently encountered in drug users, including hyponatremia, hypocalcemia, and renal failure. In particular, hypoglycemic seizures, which in alcoholics tend to occur during binges, are often mistakenly attributed to ethanol withdrawal.

Direct Mechanisms: Toxicity, Withdrawal, and Individual Agents

Opioids

Opioid drugs include a large number of agonists, antagonists, and mixed agonists/antagonists (Table 2). Heroin, the most commonly abused opioid, can be injected, snorted, or smoked. Commercial street heroin contains a variety of pharmacologically active and inactive adulterants.

Heroin overdose, with coma, pinpoint pupils, and respiratory depression, is sometimes associated with seizures, but their occurrence in that setting is so unusual that other possible causes such as concomitant cocaine use, ethanol withdrawal, or CNS infection should be sought. In a case-control study, heroin use, either past or current, was a risk factor for new-onset seizures independent of head trauma, infection, stroke, ethanol, or other drugs.[45] For provoked seizures (i.e., caused by an underlying precipitant such as infection or trauma) the odds ratio (OR) was 3.65; for unprovoked seizures it was 2.57. The risk was greatest if heroin had been used on the same day as the seizure, but in no patient was there clinical evidence of overdose, and the risk persisted after a year of abstinence.

The pharmacologic basis of this risk is unclear. In animals, opioids are variably proconvulsant or anticonvulsant depending on species, seizure model, rate of administration, and particular agent (e.g., μ-, δ-, or κ-agonist). In some models, effects are blocked by the antagonist naloxone; in others they are not.[4,55]

Seizures or myoclonus are a well-recognized feature of meperidine toxicity, attributable to its active metabolite normeperidine.[29] Seizures are also anecdotally described as a toxic effect of fentanyl, pentazocine, and propoxyphene.

Except in neonates seizures are not a feature of opioid withdrawal, which produces flu-like symptoms and intense craving. In newborns of opioid-dependent mothers, withdrawal causes tremor, screaming, fever, tachypnea, tachycardia, vomiting, explosive diarrhea, and sometimes death.[21] Seizures and myoclonus are described, but can be difficult to distinguish from jitteriness. The diagnosis requires exclusion of hypoglycemia, hypocalcemia, intracranial hemorrhage, CNS infection, and withdrawal from other drugs or ethanol.

Psychostimulants

Psychostimulant drugs include amphetamine-like agents, whose principal action is to release monoamines at synaptic nerve endings, and cocaine, which blocks monoamine synaptic reuptake (Table 3). Cocaine is the only recreationally used psychostimulant with local anesthetic properties, which probably contributes to its epileptogenicity. Amphetamine-like drugs are taken parenterally or orally, and methamphetamine is often smoked. Cocaine hydrochloride is taken parenterally or intranasally; alkaloidal cocaine ("crack") is smoked.[5]

Amphetamine-like drugs tend to cause seizures in the setting of obvious overdose (fever, hypertension, cardiac arrhythmia, delirium, or coma).[3] With cocaine, seizures more often occur in the absence of other signs of toxicity; they can appear immediately or several hours after use, perhaps attributable to pharmacologically active metabolites.[25,34,43] A focal signature to seizures suggests a structural lesion such as cocaine-related

TABLE 1

CATEGORIES OF RECREATIONAL DRUGS

Opioids
Psychostimulants
Sedatives/hypnotics
Cannabis
Hallucinogens
Inhalants
Phencyclidine
Anticholinergics
Ethanol
Tobacco

intracerebral hemorrhage. Status epilepticus (SE) following cocaine use is often refractory to conventional anticonvulsant therapy.

In different reports, the prevalence of seizures among cocaine-intoxicated patients ranged from 1% to 9.3%.[8,34,48,52] Seizures are more likely to occur after smoking crack than after snorting cocaine hydrochloride, probably a dosage effect. A seizure can be new onset with no other contributing factor than cocaine, or it can be triggered by cocaine in a known epileptic.[48] In animals (and probably humans), repeated administration of cocaine progressively lowers seizure threshold until seizures occur at doses that were originally subthreshold ("kindling," "reverse tolerance").[13,41]

Methylenedioxymethamphetamine ("ecstasy") has pharmacological properties of both amphetamine-like psychostimulants and hallucinogenic agents such as mescaline. Popular on college campuses, it is usually taken orally in groups, including "rave" parties (dancing to loud fast music for hours at a time). Overdose can cause seizures, delirium, coma, and death.[30,59]

Phenylpropanolamine, available over-the-counter as a decongestant or appetite suppressant, and sold by mail order as a "legal stimulant," was banned by the U. S. Food and Drug Administration (FDA) after it was shown to increase the risk of stroke. Seizures are described at recommended doses.[42]

"Dietary supplements" containing ephedra alkaloids ("ma huang") became popular in North America and Europe during the 1990s, and both seizures and stroke were described in users. In 2003, the FDA banned these products.[24]

TABLE 2

MAJOR OPIOIDS

Agonist
Camphorated tincture of opium (paregoric)
Morphine
Heroin
Methadone
Fentanyl
Meperidine
Oxymorphone
Hydromorphone
Codeine
Oxycodone
Hydrocodone
Levorphanol
Antagonist
Naloxone
Naltrexone
Mixed agonist-antagonist
Pentazocine
Butorphanol
Buprenorphine

TABLE 3

MAJOR PSYCHOSTIMULANTS

Dextroamphetamine
Methamphetamine
Methylphenidate
Pemoline
Ephedrine
Pseudoephedrine
Phenmetrazine
Diethylpropion
Benzphetamine
Phenylpropanolamine
Methylenedioxymethamphetamine (ecstasy)
Cocaine

Sedatives and Hypnotics

Sedative/hypnotic agents include barbiturates, benzodiazepines, and nonbarbiturate/nonbenzodiazepine agents. Recreational barbiturate use is either parenteral or oral; short-acting agents are most popular. Although available as street drugs, benzodiazepines have much less abuse potential. Other sedative drugs vary in their addiction liability. Glutethimide, for example, is a well-recognized street drug, often combined with codeine ("hits," "loads"). Buspirone, by contrast, does not appear to be abused.[5]

Barbiturates and benzodiazepines potentiate γ-aminobutyric acid (GABA) neurotransmission through stereospecific receptors on the GABA receptor–chloride channel complex. GABA receptor downregulation is probably a major mechanism of seizures during barbiturate or benzodiazepine withdrawal.

Short-acting barbiturates are most likely to produce seizures on the second or third day of abstinence; full-blown delirium tremens sometimes follows. In a study of human volunteers, abrupt withdrawal from secobarbital or pentobarbital after several months of a daily dose of 400 mg produced paroxysmal EEG changes without symptoms in one-third of the subjects. Withdrawal from 600 mg daily produced minor symptoms in half the subjects and a seizure in 10%. Withdrawal from 900 mg daily produced seizures in three-fourths and delirium tremens in two-thirds.[20]

Following withdrawal from benzodiazepines, anxiety and tremor are common but can be difficult to distinguish from the symptoms for which the drug was being taken in the first place. Seizures and delirium tremens do occur, however, usually within 24 hours of stopping a short-acting agent and within several days of stopping a long-acting agent.[18] As with barbiturates, seizures are dose-related and unlikely in patients taking recommended therapeutic doses.[6]

Withdrawal seizures have been described with a number of nonbarbiturate/nonbenzodiazepine sedatives, including meprobamate and chloral hydrate. Tolerance and physical dependence are infrequent among users of zolpidem, America's most popular sleeping pill, but tremor, agitation, and seizures are described during withdrawal.[35] Glutethimide-induced seizures were reported as an acute toxic effect, possibly related to the drug's anticholinergic properties.[44] Seizures are also a feature of acute toxicity in recreational users of antihistamines. During the 1980s, parenteral administration of tripelennamine combined with pentazocine was a popular fad ("Ts and blues"), and seizures were a frequent complication.[7]

γ-Hydroxybutyrate, or its precursors γ-butyrolactone or 1,4-butanediol, is popular at "rave" parties and as a "date rape" drug. Acting at its own receptors as well as at GABA receptors, it produces ethanol-like effects, including a life-threatening abstinence syndrome. Myoclonus and seizures can be features of intoxication, however.[38,54]

Marijuana

Marijuana, made from cut tops and leaves of the hemp plant, *Cannabis sativa,* contains many cannabinoid compounds, of which Δ-9-tetrahydrocannabinol (Δ-9-THC) is the principal psychoactive ingredient. A more potent preparation, hashish, is made from resin covering the leaves. Marijuana can be smoked or eaten. In the brain, Δ-9-THC acts at stereospecific cannabinoid receptors (called CB-1) on synaptic terminals containing either excitatory or inhibitory neurotransmitters.[5]

A case-control study found marijuana use protective against new-onset seizures in men ($OR = 0.42$); for women there was a trend toward risk reduction that did not achieve statistical significance.[45]

In animal studies, cannabinoid compounds are variably proconvulsant or anticonvulsant depending on species and seizure model.[50] The nonpsychoactive compound, cannabidiol, is more consistently anticonvulsant.[9,49]

Anecdotal reports describe either improved or worsened seizure control temporally associated with marijuana use.[10,16,17,23] In a placebo-controlled study of 16 epileptics refractory to other drugs, cannabidiol acutely exacerbated EEG abnormalities but not behavioral seizures; after several months, however, seven of eight patients receiving cannabidiol were seizure-free compared to one of eight controls.[11]

Hallucinogens

Worldwide, dozens of hallucinogenic plants are used ritualistically or recreationally for their hallucinogenic properties. In North America and Europe, the most popular agents are peyote cactus containing mescaline, mushrooms containing psilocybin and psilocin, and the synthetic ergot compound D-lysergic acid diethylamide (LSD). The visual illusions and hallucinations produced by these agents—including those that spontaneously recur days or weeks after last use ("flashbacks")—are not considered epileptiform.[1] True seizures can follow very high doses, however.[19]

Inhalants

The recreational inhalation of volatile substances is a popular form of drug abuse, especially among children and adolescents. Products include solvents, cleaning fluids, glues, aerosols, bottled fuel gas, deodorizers, marker pens, petroleum, anesthetics, and nitrites, and the intoxicating compounds include hydrocarbons, esters, and ketones. Despite the variety of agents, the effects they produce resemble ethanol intoxication. A difference is that hallucinations and seizures can occur with overdose and are not features of inhalant withdrawal.[39,53]

Phencyclidine

Phencyclidine ("PCP", "angel dust") and the related compound, ketamine, are classified as "dissociative anesthetics." Their principal pharmacologic action—inhibition at glutamate receptors—is anticonvulsant, yet myoclonus and seizures including SE occur with overdose. Additional signs of intoxication—fever, tachycardia, hypertension, nystagmus, psychosis, delirium, dystonia, and stupor or coma with a blank stare—are likely to precede or accompany the seizures.[31,37]

Anticholinergics

Plants containing scopolamine and atropine are used recreationally worldwide. In North America and Europe, *Datura stramonium* (jimsonweed) is especially popular among adolescents, who ingest the seeds, leaves, or roots. Drugs with anticholinergic properties (e.g., amitriptyline) are also abused. The syndrome of anticholinergic poisoning—hallucinations, delirium, dilated unreactive pupils, hot dry skin—may include myoclonus or seizures.[40]

Ethanol

As with other drugs, seizures associated with ethanol may be the consequence of acute or remote head injury, CNS infection, stroke, or toxic/metabolic derangement. In many heavy drinkers, seizures are a direct effect of the ethanol ("alcohol-related seizures"), especially as a withdrawal phenomenon.

In a study of alcoholics presenting to an emergency room with either incident (new onset) or prevalent seizures, 78% of seizures occurred between 7 and 30 hours after the last drink. Excepting three subjects whose seizures occurred after 2 or more weeks, 99% of seizures occurred within 72 hours. A few seizures happened during active drinking. Forty-one percent of subjects had a single seizure; 21% had more than three, usually within a few hours after the first. SE occurred in 3%. Seizures were generalized in 95%; 5% had a focal onset. These seizures could occur alone or accompanied by other withdrawal signs. One-third of the patients subsequently developed delirium tremens. (Seizures, however, are not commonly present during delirium tremens.) The authors concluded that alcohol-related seizures were a withdrawal phenomenon, and that subjects whose seizures occurred beyond the withdrawal period or had focal signature probably had underlying structural pathology such as a remote cerebral contusion.[57]

In a study of volunteers, six subjects drank ethanol every few hours (including a 3:00 AM dose) for at least 48 days. Withdrawal produced seizures in two subjects and delirium tremens in two.[28] The pattern of drinking in this study would be unusual for most alcoholics, who do not customarily awaken themselves in the middle of the night to have a drink. Moreover, the high percentage of subjects who experienced seizures was not encountered in other studies. For example, of over a thousand alcoholics who were detoxified without pharmacologic support, only 1% developed seizures.[58]

Consistent with the view that withdrawal might not be the sole mechanism for alcohol-related seizures is a case-control study of incident seizures, in which chronic daily ingestion of 50 g absolute ethanol raised the odds ratio (OR) above one, and 200 g daily increased the OR to 20. The minimal duration of drinking necessary to increase seizure risk could not be determined. In that study, many seizures occurred either during active drinking or more than a week after stopping, and statistical analysis failed to demonstrate a clear-cut temporal relationship between seizures and early abstinence. Moreover, those who had recently increased their ethanol consumption tended to have seizures earlier during abstinence than those who had decreased their consumption.[46]

Another case-control study found similar dose relationships for ethanol and incident seizures, with an increased risk appearing at 50 g daily absolute ethanol for men and 25 g for women, but that study did not address temporal relationships between seizures and active drinking.[33]

Animal studies demonstrate the existence of ethanol withdrawal seizures, and selective breeding can produce genetic susceptibility.[22] Alcohol-related seizures in animals, however, often occur with low doses of ethanol, and their variable time courses and semiology suggest multiple mechanisms. In both animals and humans, repeated bouts of ethanol withdrawal increase the risk of eventual alcohol-related seizures.[32]

A common neuropharmacologic mechanism to explain both withdrawal and nonwithdrawal alcohol-related seizures might be glutamate toxicity. Acutely, ethanol blocks glutamate neurotransmission, with receptor upregulation.[14,56] Abrupt abstinence would then produce a hyperglutaminergic state, resulting in withdrawal symptoms, including seizures. Repeated bouts of withdrawal might result in more lasting excitotoxicity, thus lowering the threshold for seizures independent of acute withdrawal.

Should brain imaging be performed in patients with alcohol-related seizures? In a study of 259 patients with incident alcohol-related seizures and no obvious explanation other than ethanol withdrawal, computerized tomography (CT) identified intracranial lesions in 16 (6.2%).[15] Four had subdural hematomas, four subdural hygromas, two vascular malformations, two cysticercosis, and one each aneurysm, possible neoplasm, skull fracture with subarachnoid hemorrhage, and cerebral infarction. Seven (44%) of the 16 patients were alert and had no focal signs or evidence of trauma. In 10 patients, the identified lesions altered management. The answer to the above question is therefore, yes, as far as new-onset seizures are concerned. More problematic is the patient with repeated alcohol-related seizures. Although imaging may not be necessary in every instance, the clinician must consider the possibility of underlying new treatable pathology in such patients.

Should alcohol-related seizures be treated acutely? Because ethanol withdrawal seizures tend to occur singly or in a brief cluster, the likelihood of recurrence has often passed by the time a decision is made whether to treat. In a controlled trial, either intravenous lorazepam 2 mg or placebo was given to alcoholic patients following a single generalized seizure. Over the next 6 hours, 3% of those receiving lorazepam had a second seizure, compared with 24% of those receiving placebo (OR = 10.4). Of those not admitted, one receiving lorazepam and seven receiving placebo had a second seizure within 48 hours.

Should alcohol-related seizures be treated prophylactically? Anticonvulsants for seizure prevention are usually not indicated in alcoholics. Abstainers do not need them, and drinkers do not take them. Phenytoin, carbamazepine, and valproate, moreover, are probably ineffective in preventing withdrawal seizures.[2,26,36] For those whose seizures are not temporally associated with drinking, who have an additional lesion that by itself could account for seizures, or who have epileptiform electroencephalographic (EEG) abnormalities, prophylactic anticonvulsants may be required even though patient compliance is unlikely.

Can epileptics safely drink ethanol? In one report, one or two drinks daily appeared to precipitate seizures in 5% of epileptic patients; five or six drinks daily precipitated seizures in 85%.[36] In another study, however, epileptics given one to three glasses of vodka over a 2-hour period daily for 16 weeks were no more likely to have a seizure than those given orangeade; there was no change in seizure frequency or in EEG epileptiform activity.[27] Although these observations are reassuring, it is probably advisable to discourage ethanol use by an epileptic.

Management Strategies in Substance Abusers with Seizures

Medical or surgical conditions that might be causing or contributing to seizures—trauma, infection, stroke, metabolic derangement—must be identified and treated. For example, cocaine intoxication might entirely explain fever, delirium, and seizures, but not until an image and a spinal tap have excluded meningoencephalitis or intracranial hemorrhage.

Seizures accompanied by other signs of drug toxicity tend to be refractory to treatment. SE in such patients is nonetheless managed in the usual fashion. Other than naloxone for opioid overdose, flumazenil for benzodiazepine overdose, and physostigmine for anticholinergic poisoning, there are no available pharmacologic agents that specifically reverse the signs of recreational drug overdose, including ethanol.

The treatment of drug withdrawal should include an agent from the same pharmacologic class (e.g., methadone for heroin withdrawal) or with a degree of cross-tolerance (e.g., a benzodiazepine for ethanol withdrawal). Seizures observed during neonatal opioid withdrawal respond more predictably to opioid substitution therapy (e.g., methadone or paregoric) than to anticonvulsants.[47] Phenytoin is an inappropriate agent for either preventing or treating seizures during sedative or ethanol withdrawal, and neuroleptics given for anxiety or agitation in such patients may do nothing more than lower seizure threshold. Ethanol itself is a direct neurotoxin and therefore also an inappropriate agent to use in the prevention or treatment of ethanol withdrawal, including seizures.

As with ethanol, prophylactic anticonvulsants are seldom indicated when drug toxicity or withdrawal is the sole explanation for single or even multiple seizures.

SUMMARY AND CONCLUSIONS

Alcohol and recreational drugs can cause seizures by indirect mechanisms such as trauma, stroke, CNS infection, or metabolic derangement. Depending on the agent, seizures can also be the result of either direct toxicity or withdrawal. Such patients should be thoroughly assessed for underlying cerebral pathology, but if toxicity or withdrawal is then considered the sole cause of a seizure, anticonvulsant prophylaxis is usually not indicated.

References

1. Abraham HD, Duffy H. EEG coherence in post-LSD visual hallucinations. *Psychiatry Res.* 2001;107:151–152.
2. Alldredge BK, Lowenstein DH, Simon RP. Placebo-controlled trial of intravenous diphenylhydantoin for short-term treatment of alcohol withdrawal seizures. *Am J Med.* 1989;87:645–648.
3. Alldredge BK, Lowenstein DH, Simon RP. Seizures associated with recreational drug abuse. *Neurology.* 1989;39:1037–1039.
4. Bohme GA, Stutzmann JM, Rouges BP, et al. Effects of selective mu- and delta-opioid peptides on kindled amygdaloid seizures in rats. *Neurosci Lett.* 1987;74:227–231.
5. Brust JCM. *Neurological Aspects of Substance Abuse,* 2nd ed. Boston. Butterworth-Heinemann, 2004.
6. Busto U, Sellers EM, Naranjo CA, et al. Withdrawal reaction after long-term therapeutic use of benzodiazepines. *N Engl J Med.* 1986;315:854–859.
7. Caplan LR, Thomas C, Banks G. Central nervous system complications of addiction to "T's and Blues." *Neurology.* 1982;32:623–628.
8. Choy-Kwong M, Lipton RB. Seizures in hospitalized cocaine users. *Neurology.* 1989;39:425–427.
9. Consroe P, Benedito MA, Leite R, et al. Effects of cannabidiol on behavioral seizures caused by convulsant drugs or current in mice. *Eur J Pharmacol.* 1982;83:293–298.
10. Consroe PF, Wood GC, Buchsbaum A. Anticonvulsant nature of marijuana smoking. *JAMA.* 1975;234:306–307.
11. Cunha JM, Carlini EA, Periera AE, et al. Chronic administration of cannabidiol to healthy volunteers and epileptic patients. *Pharmacology.* 1980;21:175–185.
12. D'Onofrio G, Rathlev NK, Ulrich AS, et al. Lorazepam for the prevention of recurrent alcohol withdrawal seizures. *Ann Emerg Med.* 1994;23:513–518.
13. Dhuna A, Pascual-Leone A, Langendorf F. Chronic habitual cocaine abuse and kindling-induced epilepsy. A case report. *Epilepsia.* 1991;32:890–894.
14. Dodd PR, Beckmann AM, Davidson MS, Wike PA. Glutamate-mediated transmission, alcohol, and alcoholism. *Neurochem Int.* 2000;37:509–533.

15. Earnest MP, Feldman H, Marx JA, et al. Intracranial lesions shown by CT scans in 259 cases of first alcohol-related seizures. *Neurology.* 1988;38: 1561–1565.
16. Ellison JM, Gelwan E, Ogletree J. Complex partial seizure symptoms affected by marijuana abuse. *J Clin Psychiatry.* 1990;51:439–440.
17. Feeney DM. Marijuana use among epileptics. *JAMA.* 1976;235:1105.
18. Fialip J, Aumaitre O, Eschalier A, et al. Benzodiazepine withdrawal seizures. Analysis of 48 case reports. *Clin Neuropharmacol.* 1987;10:538–544.
19. Fisher D, Underleider J. Grand mal seizures following ingestion of LSD. *Calif Med.* 1976;106:210–212.
20. Fraser HF, Wikler A, Essig EF, et al. Degree of physical dependence induced by secobarbital or pentobarbital. *JAMA.* 1958;166:126–129.
21. Fulroth R, Phillips B, Durand DJ. Perinatal outcome of infants exposed to cocaine and/or heroin in utero. *Am J Dis Child.* 1989;143:905–910.
22. Goldstein DB. The alcohol withdrawal syndrome. A view from the laboratory. *Rec Dev Alcohol.* 1986;4:231–240.
23. Gordon E, Devinsky O. Alcohol and marijuana: Effects on epilepsy and use by patients with epilepsy. *Epilepsia.* 2001;42:1266–1272.
24. Haller CA, Benowitz N. Adverse cardiovascular and central nervous system events associated with dietary supplements containing ephedra alkaloids. *N Engl J Med.* 2000;343:1833–1838.
25. Harden CL, Montjo GE, Tuchman AJ, et al. Seizures provoked by cocaine use. *Ann Neurol.* 1990;28:263–264.
26. Hilbom M, Tokola R, Kuusela V, et al. Prevention of alcohol withdrawal seizures with carbamazepine and valproic acid. *Alcohol.* 1989;6:223–226.
27. Hoppener RJ, Kuyer A, van der Lugt PJM. Epilepsy and alcohol. The influence of social alcohol intake on seizures and treatment in epilepsy. *Epilepsia.* 1983;24:459–471.
28. Isbell H, Fraser HF, Wikler A, et al. An experimental study of rum fits and delirium tremens. *QJ Stud Alcohol.* 1955;16:1–33.
29. Kaiko RF, Foley K, Grabinski PY, et al. Central nervous system excitatory effects of meperidine in cancer patients. *Ann Neurol.* 1983;13:180–185.
30. Kalant H. The pharmacology and toxicology of "ecstasy" (MDMA) and related drugs. *Can Med Assoc J.* 2001;165:917–928.
31. Kessler GF, Demers LM, Brennan RW. Phencyclidine and fatal status epilepticus. *N Engl J Med.* 1974;291:979.
32. Lechtenberg R, Warner TM. Seizure risk with recurrent alcohol detoxification. *Arch Neurol.* 1990;47:535–538.
33. Leone M, Bottacchi E, Beghi E, et al. Alcohol use is a risk factor for a first generalized tonic–clonic seizure. *Neurology.* 1997;48:614–620.
34. Lowenstein DH, Masse SM, Rowbotham MC, et al. Acute neurologic and psychiatric complications associated with cocaine. *Am J Med.* 1987;83:841–846.
35. Madrak LN, Rosenberg M. Zolpidem abuse. *Am J Psychiatry.* 2001;158: 1330–1331.
36. Mattson RH, Sturman JK, Gronowski ML, et al. Effect of alcohol intake in nonalcoholic epileptics. *Neurology.* 1975;25:361–362.
37. McCarron MM, Schulze BW, Thompson GA, et al. Acute phencyclidine intoxication. clinical patterns, complications, and treatment. *Ann Emerg Med.* 1981;10:290–297.
38. McGinn CG. Close calls with club drugs. *N Engl J Med.* 2005;352:2671–2672.
39. Meredith TH, Ruprak M, Little A, et al. Diagnosis and treatment of acute poisoning with volatile substances. *Hum Toxicol.* 1989;8:277–286.
40. Mickolich JR, Paulson GW, Cross CJ, et al. Neurologic and electroencephalographic effects of jimson weed intoxication. *Clin Electro-Encephalogr.* 1976;7:49–57.
41. Miller KA, Witkin JM, Ungard JT, et al. Pharmacological and behavioral characterization of cocaine-kindled seizures in mice. *Psychopharmacology.* 2000;148:74–82.
42. Mueller SM, Solow EB. Seizures associated with a new combination "pick-me-up" pill. *Ann Neurol.* 1982;11:322.
43. Myers JA, Earnest MP. Generalized seizures and cocaine abuse. *Neurology.* 1984;35:675–676.
44. Myers RR, Stockard JJ. Neurologic and electroencephalographic correlates in glutethimide intoxication. *Clin Pharmacol Ther.* 1975;17:212–220.
45. Ng SKC, Brust JCM, Hauser WA, et al. Illicit drug use and the risk of new onset seizures. *Am J Epidemiol.* 1990;132:47–57.
46. Ng SKC, Hauser WA, Brust JCM, et al. Alcohol consumption and withdrawal in new-onset seizures. *N Engl J Med.* 1988;319:666–673.
47. Osborn DA, Jeffrey HE, Cole MJ, et al. Sedatives for opiate withdrawal in newborn infants. *Cochrane Database Syst Rev.* 2002;(3):CD002053.
48. Pascual-Leone A, Dhuna A, Altafallah I, et al. Cocaine-induced seizures. *Neurology.* 1990;40:404–407.
49. Perez-Reyes M, Winfield M. Cannabidiol and electroencephalographic epileptic activity. *JAMA.* 1974;230:1635.
50. Pertwee RG. The central neuropharmacology of psychotropic cannabinoids. *Pharmacol Ther.* 1988;36:189–261.
51. Reynolds K, Lewis LB, Nolen JDL, et al. Alcohol consumption and risk of stroke. A meta-analysis. *JAMA.* 2003;289:579–588.
52. Schwartz RH, Luxenberg MG, Hoffman NG. Crack use by American middle-class adolescent polydrug abusers. *J Pediatr.* 1991;118:150–155.
53. Skuse D, Burrell S. A review of solvent abusers and their management by a child psychiatric outpatient service. *Hum Toxicol.* 1982;1:321–329.
54. Snead OC, Gibson KM. Gamma-hydroxybutyric acid. *N Engl J Med.* 2005; 352:2721–2732.
55. Tortella FC. Endogenous opioid peptides and epilepsy. quieting the seizing brain? *Trends Pharmacol Sci.* 1988;9:366–372.
56. Tsai G, Coyle JT. The role of glutamatergic neurotransmission in the pathophysiology of alcoholism. *Annu Rev Med.* 1998;49:173–184.
57. Victor M, Brausch CC. The role of abstinence in the genesis of alcoholic epilepsy. *Epilepsia.* 1967;8:1–20.
58. Whitfield CL, Thompson G, Lamb A, et al. Detoxification of 1024 alcoholic patients without psychoactive drugs. *JAMA.* 1978;239:1409–1410.
59. Zagnoni PG, Albano C. Psychostimulants and epilepsy. *Epilepsia.* 2002; 43(Suppl 2):28–31.

CHAPTER 269 ■ DISORDERS OF PREGNANCY

MARTHA J. MORRELL AND MAURICE L. DRUZIN

INTRODUCTION

Few conditions occurring during pregnancy give rise to epilepsy, but some pregnancy-associated conditions give rise to seizures. Seizures developing during pregnancy may herald an acute central nervous system (CNS) event, such as cerebrovascular disease, neoplasia, or infection. Fortunately, these occurrences are rare. Most commonly, new-onset seizures in later pregnancy are associated with eclampsia. This chapter reviews the pregnancy-related disorders that may present with seizures; the clinical presentation of each is described, along with a suggested diagnostic evaluation and treatment approach. Because of their frequent occurrence and the controversy regarding the treatment of seizures associated with pre-eclampsia and eclampsia, much of the chapter is devoted to a discussion of the approach to these seizures.

PREGNANCY AND EPILEPSY: APPROACH TO THE FIRST SEIZURE

Seizures may first appear during pregnancy in women who later are given a diagnosis of epilepsy. How often this occurs is not known, although Suter (as described by Lennox and Lennox[33]), in a study of 200 women with epilepsy, found that seizures had begun during pregnancy in 40. It is not clear how many of these women actually experienced eclampsia. Some women with epilepsy have seizures only during pregnancy (gestational epilepsy), but the frequency with which this occurs also is not known. Sleep deprivation and the physiologic stresses associated with pregnancy may lower the seizure threshold and precipitate the first seizure in women with an underlying epileptogenic lesion or genetic predisposition to epilepsy. The hormonal changes of pregnancy may also provoke seizures. The pregnant woman experiences a dramatic increase in the production of estrogens and progestogens. The population of sex steroid hormones also changes during pregnancy; whereas estradiol is the principal sex steroid hormone in women who are not pregnant, estriol is the most prevalent hormone of pregnancy. Some women may be susceptible to changes in cortical excitability triggered by these endocrine changes.[43]

Recommended Evaluation Strategy for the Pregnant Woman With a First Seizure

The appropriate neurologic evaluation for a pregnant woman with a first seizure does not substantially differ from the evaluation indicated for any patient with a first-time seizure. A careful neurologic history is taken and an examination performed to detect any neurologic symptoms or signs that would indicate increased intracranial pressure, a CNS infection or hemorrhage, or a focal CNS lesion. The history is explored for risk factors for seizures and for epilepsy. The basic evaluation should include a complete blood cell count, measurement of electrolytes, liver and renal function tests, and a toxicology screen—particularly to detect cocaine or alcohol, which are the most common substances of abuse associated with seizures.[42] The obstetric history includes determination of dates and an evaluation for hypertension, proteinuria, and edema to exclude pre-eclampsia and eclampsia.

Electroencephalogram (EEG) and neuroimaging are indicated in any woman seen with a seizure in the absence of eclampsia. If it has been determined that the seizure arose from pre-eclampsia/eclampsia and the presentation is otherwise not complicated, then EEG and neuroimaging are not usually required. However, if the patient with pre-eclampsia/eclampsia has focal neurologic symptoms or signs and partial seizures, EEG and neuroimaging should be obtained. Magnetic resonance imaging (MRI) is generally preferred to computed tomography (CT). Magnetic resonance imaging is the most sensitive technology for detecting CNS pathology and is safer for the pregnant woman. There is no known risk to humans from MRI scans using <2.0 tesla.[56] The remainder of the evaluation is guided by the differential diagnosis.

When an antiepileptic drug is used in pregnant women, a dosage adjustment may be required from what is customary in the nonpregnant woman. Because of a reduction in protein binding during pregnancy, highly protein-bound antiepileptic drugs may have higher free, or non–protein-bound, fractions than would usually be anticipated. This translates into a higher CNS concentration. For example, during pregnancy the non–protein-bound fraction of phenytoin may represent 15% of the total fraction, in contrast to 10% in the nongravid state. The standard load of phenytoin (20 mg/kg) may prove excessive for the pregnant woman. A suggested regimen for pregnant women is to give 10 mg/kg and repeat with 5 mg/kg in 2 to 6 hours.[54]

DISORDERS OF PREGNANCY ASSOCIATED WITH SEIZURES

Cerebral Ischemia

Seizures may be a sign of cerebral ischemia. The risk that a pregnant woman will experience a cerebral infarction varies from 1/481 in India to 1/26,099 in Rochester, Minnesota.[68] In one retrospective and prospective study of strokes associated with pregnancy and the puerperium in women delivering in public hospitals in Ile de France, 31 cases of stroke were identified among 348,295 deliveries.[57] Arterial occlusion represents 50% to 80% of all cerebral infarctions occurring during pregnancy, with central venous thrombosis next most common. Arterial infarctions tend to occur in the second and third trimesters, whereas venous infarctions are more likely to occur in the first trimester. In the Ile de France study, nonhemorrhagic strokes (47%) and intracranial hemorrhage (44%) were most likely to occur in association with eclampsia.[57]

Stroke during pregnancy resulting from an arterial thrombosis usually arises in individuals with an identifiable risk factor for stroke. Most arterial infarctions are a consequence of arteropathy associated with premature atherosclerosis, moyamoya disease, Takayasu arteritis, fibromuscular dysplasia, and, rarely, isolated CNS vasculitis. Stroke and seizures may also be the initial manifestation of hematologic disorders, such as hemoglobinopathy (sickle cell disease), antiphospholipid antibody syndrome, thrombotic thrombocytopenic purpura, and deficiencies in antithrombin III and proteins C and S. The factor V Leiden mutation is a hereditary abnormality of the coagulation system that appears to enhance resistance to activated protein C, which inhibits coagulation. Up to 5% of the population exhibits resistance to activated protein C, and about 20% of patients with venous thromboembolism carry the factor V Leiden mutation.[30,71] Evaluation of a patient with stroke and seizures would also consider cardioembolism and paradoxic embolism from a patent foramen ovale, deep venous thrombosis, thrombosis of the pelvic or ovarian vein, or fat embolism. During labor and delivery, amniotic fluid and air embolism are considered in the differential diagnosis.

The clinical syndrome of cerebral venous thrombosis is characterized by headache, nausea and vomiting, visual symptoms, encephalopathy, lateralized neurologic deficits, and focal or generalized seizures.[21] Unlike arterial thrombosis, cerebral venous thrombosis develops in pregnant women who have no other specific risk for stroke. Cerebral venous thrombosis appears to be caused by the combination of the hypercoagulable state of pregnancy and the decrease in cerebral blood flow consequent to blood loss during labor and delivery. Other conditions associated with cerebral venous thrombosis include infection; hyperviscosity syndromes; sickle cell anemia; leukemia; antiphospholipid antibody syndrome; protein C, S, and antithrombin III deficiency; and factor V Leiden mutation. Malignancies and arteriovenous malformations should also be considered.[68] Although cerebral venous thrombosis may require acute treatment for seizures, the long-term prognosis is good. In one series of 77 patients with cerebral venous thrombosis, of 28 patients who experienced seizures acutely, seizures recurred in only four.[45]

Cerebral Hemorrhage

Cerebral hemorrhage occurs in between 1 and 5 pregnancies per 10,000. Associated mortality is 30% to 40%.[69] The risk for intracranial hemorrhage appears to be increased in pregnant women,[57,70] although data from Rochester, Minnesota, found no evidence of a gestational increase.[67] Pregnant women are likely to experience conditions that increase the risk for hemorrhage, however, such as eclampsia, metastatic choriocarcinoma, cerebral emboli, and coagulopathies. In addition, physiologic changes occur in pregnancy that predispose to intracranial hemorrhage, such as hypertension and increases in cardiac output, blood volume, and venous pressure. High concentrations of circulating estrogens may cause arterial dilation and be an additional risk factor for cerebral hemorrhage.[69]

Subarachnoid hemorrhage in the pregnant woman is most likely to be caused by cerebral aneurysms and arteriovenous malformations. Other causes of subarachnoid hemorrhage are eclampsia, cocaine abuse, coagulopathy, subacute bacterial endocarditis, and choriocarcinoma.[69] Aneurysmal bleeding is most likely to occur in older patients (25–35 years of age) and in the second and third trimesters of gestation. Bleeding is unlikely to occur in the postpartum period. In contrast, hemorrhages from arteriovenous malformations are more likely to occur in younger women (18–25 years) and are uniformly distributed throughout gestation, with a higher risk during labor and the puerperium.

Subarachnoid hemorrhage in a pregnant woman, as in a patient who is not pregnant, may be associated with severe headache, nausea, vomiting, focal neurologic signs, and seizures. Transient hypertension and proteinuria are often present and must be differentiated from pre-eclampsia/eclampsia. Diagnosis is established based on the clinical presentation and CT of the brain. If the brain CT findings are negative and intracranial hemorrhage is still suspected, then a lumbar puncture to detect hemorrhage is indicated. If hemorrhage is detected, the patient requires either an MR angiogram or four-vessel angiography, depending on the institution's technical capabilities and experience, and a brain MRI to evaluate for aneurysms and arteriovenous malformations.

Intracerebral hemorrhage in pregnancy is most often attributable to hypertension occurring in the setting of eclampsia. Other causes include bleeding from an arteriovenous malformation, hemorrhagic transformation of an ischemic stroke, cocaine or alcohol abuse, and coagulopathies. The presenting symptoms of intracerebral hemorrhage are usually focal neurologic deficits, headache, nausea, vomiting, and seizures. A noncontrast CT of the head is generally the imaging test of first choice, followed by MRI to detect any structural lesion underlying the hemorrhage.

Treatment of seizures in the setting of subarachnoid or intracranial hemorrhage does not differ in pregnant and nonpregnant patients. The risk for teratogenic effects of antiepileptic drugs is far outweighed by the risk for repeated hemorrhage following a major motor seizure.

Rheumatologic Disease

Patients with immunologic and rheumatologic diseases, such as systemic lupus erythematosus (SLE), may experience an exacerbation of CNS disease during pregnancy.[41] Unlike most rheumatologic disorders, which spare the CNS, SLE involves the CNS in as many as one half of patients.[12] Neurologic disease is the second-leading cause of death in SLE[53] and frequently causes neuropsychiatric disturbances such as seizures, encephalopathies, psychosis, and lateralized motor deficits.[20] The risk for development of pre-eclampsia, hypercoagulability, and antiphospholipid antibodies is also increased in SLE. The CNS lesion in SLE is principally a small-vessel vasculitis with vascular hyalinization, endothelial proliferation, thrombosis, and capillary wall thickening.[1] Low-dose corticosteroids are the preferred treatment for SLE, with or without aspirin or heparin. Lupus of the CNS may require treatment with higher doses of corticosteroids. Antiepileptic drugs for seizures may be required only during acute flares.

Antiphospholipid antibodies may be associated with neurologic disease, either in the context of SLE (30% of patients) or within the primary antiphospholipid antibody syndrome.[35] The syndrome is characterized by deep venous and arterial thrombosis and stroke, repeated miscarriages, and thrombocytopenia. Seizures may occur. Cerebral events during pregnancy associated with anticardiolipin antibodies are generally treated with heparin anticoagulation. Seizures usually require antiepileptic treatment.

Thrombotic thrombocytopenic purpura is a rare disorder that may occur more frequently during pregnancy. Presenting features are thrombocytopenic purpura, microangiopathic hemolytic anemia, renal disease, and neurologic symptoms, which may include headache, encephalopathy, paresis, visual disturbance, and paresthesias. Seizures occur in 20% of patients and are treated acutely with antiepileptic drugs.[48] The outcome of thrombotic thrombocytopenic purpura has substantially improved with plasmapheresis and plasma exchange.[55]

Neoplasia

The types of brain tumors that occur in pregnant women are not different from those in nonpregnant women—most commonly gliomas, then meningiomas and acoustic neuromas.[11] Pregnancy does not appear to be a risk for development of a specific neoplasm, but it can exacerbate tumor growth. Symptoms associated with increased intracranial pressure, such as nausea and vomiting, may be confused with "morning sickness," especially during the first trimester. However, persistent headache and neurologic deficits should raise concern for neoplasia. Seizures are a common presenting symptom of cranial neoplasms and may be partial or generalized. Any patient who has a seizure and in whom neurologic signs and symptoms are present warrants evaluation with an MRI.

Infections

Seizures may be the presenting symptom of infections of the CNS during pregnancy. The frequency of viral meningitis and encephalitis is not increased during pregnancy. However, pregnant women are at higher risk for infections caused by intracellular organisms because specific immune responses are altered to permit maternal adaptation to fetal and placental antigens.[23] The agents most likely to cause CNS infections and seizures during pregnancy include bacteria (*Mycobacterium tuberculosis*, *Listeria monocytogenes*), fungi (*Coccidioides immitus*), protozoa (*Toxoplasma*, *Plasmodium*), and viruses (influenza, varicella-zoster [chicken pox only], and polio).[27] The increased incidence of HIV seropositivity and AIDS in pregnancy should prompt consideration of this entity in any pregnant patient with opportunistic infections of the CNS. Treatment of these infections is the same as for nonpregnant women, with choice of antibiotic guided by information regarding the relative teratogenicity. Seizures are treated with antiepileptic drugs as required during the acute illness.

Pre-eclampsia and Eclampsia

Pre-eclampsia and eclampsia are diseases of pregnancy that occur most often in nulliparous women. Most seizures occurring during pregnancy are a sign of eclampsia. Eclampsia is defined as the development of convulsions and/or unexplained coma during pregnancy or postpartum in patients with signs or symptoms of pre-eclampsia. Pre-eclampsia is a multisystem disorder associated with hypertension, proteinuria, edema, hemoconcentration, hypoalbuminemia, abnormalities of hepatic function or coagulation, and increased urate levels.[32] In a recent study, 3.9% of 467 women with untreated pre-eclampsia progressed to seizures (eclampsia).[7]

Eclampsia is associated with seizures, cerebral bleeding, and death. The diagnosis of eclampsia is made when an antepartum or postpartum woman presents with generalized edema, hypertension, proteinuria, and convulsions. The spectrum of presentation, however, includes severe to minimal or even no hypertension, proteinuria, or edema.

Eclampsia most commonly occurs at or beyond week 28 of pregnancy. However, some cases occur between weeks 21 and 27 (7.5%) or at 20 weeks' or earlier (1.5%). Eclampsia occurring before 20 weeks' gestation is usually associated with molar or hydropic degeneration of the placenta. Eclampsia may also present within 48 hours postpartum and even as late as 4 weeks postpartum.

The incidence of eclampsia in Europe and other developed countries is 1/2,000 deliveries. In developing countries, estimates vary from 1/100 to 1/1,700. Maternal mortality ranges from 1.8% to 5%.[10,16] Eclampsia accounts for approximately 50,000 maternal deaths and is a leading cause of maternal deaths in the United States, Scandinavia, Iceland, Finland, and the United Kingdom.[50]

In the classification scheme of hypertension in pregnancy of the National Institutes of Health, pre-eclampsia and eclampsia are diagnosed according to the following criteria: increase in blood pressure to 140/90 mm Hg or greater in late pregnancy if no early reading is available, plus proteinuria (>300 mg/24 h), edema, or both.[32] Pathologic changes in pre-eclampsia and eclampsia involve multiple organ systems and arise because of vasospasm caused by exaggerated vascular responsiveness to circulating angiotensin II and catecholamines. Cardiac output, intravascular volume, and renal hemodynamics may be decreased. Uteroplacental perfusion may be compromised, leading to fetal growth retardation. A subset of pre-eclampsia is designated the HELLP syndrome: H for hemolysis, EL for elevated liver enzymes, and LP for low platelets.[61]

Neurologic abnormalities associated with eclampsia are usually acute and transient. These may include cortical blindness, focal motor deficits, and coma, although there is usually no permanent neurologic deficit. Seizures are most often generalized, but they may be partial.

During an eclamptic convulsion, the EEG shows spike-and-wave discharges. In one series of 65 patients with eclampsia,[60] a transient neurologic deficit was the presenting symptom in 5% of cases, and another 5% had transient cortical blindness. Electroencephalographic abnormalities were present acutely in 75% of cases, consisting primarily of excessive diffuse slow activity (67%), focal slow activity (33%), and paroxysmal spike activity (10%). These abnormalities were evident during administration of therapeutic doses of magnesium. The EEG abnormalities resolved at follow-up between 1 week and 6 months in all the patients. Other authors have described similar transient EEG abnormalities.[64]

Brain imaging in eclampsia shows vasogenic cerebral edema in 93% to 100% of women.[36,71] Extensive bilateral abnormalities of white matter are described in the posterior regions of the cerebral hemispheres as well as cerebellum and brainstem.[25] In addition, foci of infarction may be present. Angiography has shown spasm in large and medium-caliber arteries.[15] Results of CT are usually normal, but scans may show regions of decreased density corresponding to areas of cerebral edema.[15] The findings are similar to results with imaging in hypertensive encephalopathy. MRI abnormalities can persist for 6 to 8 weeks after resolution of symptoms.[36,71]

Pathologic examination of eclamptic brains usually reveals multiple petechial hemorrhages in cortical patches or subcortical hematomas. Areas predisposed to hemorrhages are the parietooccipital regions and the occipital lobes. Microscopically, these lesions correspond to ring hemorrhages about capillaries that are occluded by fibrinoid material.[15]

The treatment of eclamptic seizures associated with maternal hypertension has been controversial. There is wide consensus that the therapy for pre-eclampsia is delivery if the pregnancy is appropriately advanced. Hypertension is treated as necessary with antihypertensive drugs. The prevention of and treatment of seizures associated with pre-eclampsia and eclampsia has varied across countries and medical centers. The National High Blood Pressure Education Program Working Group on High Blood Pressure in Pregnancy[32] recommends the use of magnesium sulfate for women with pregnancy-induced hypertension to prevent eclamptic seizures during labor and the immediate puerperium. Although most obstetricians in the

United States have traditionally used magnesium sulfate to prevent eclamptic seizures in pregnant women with hypertension, obstetricians in the United Kingdom have favored diazepam and phenytoin.[18,26,47] A number of clinical studies have found magnesium sulfate treatment to be efficacious in preventing recurrent seizures in women with eclampsia.[24,46,58]

A randomized, placebo-controlled trial was performed in women from 33 countries diagnosed with preeclampsia and randomized to receive magnesium (5,071) or placebo (5,070).[2] Primary outcomes were eclampsia and, for women randomized before delivery, death of the infants. A total of 1,201 of 4,999 (24%) women given magnesium sulfate reported side effects versus 228 of 4,993 (5%) given placebo. Women allocated magnesium sulfate had a 58% lower risk of eclampsia (95% confidence interval [CI] 40–71) than those allocated placebo (40, 0.8%, vs. 96, 1.9%; 11 fewer women with eclampsia per 1,000 women). Maternal mortality was also lower among women allocated magnesium sulfate (relative risk 0.55, 0.26–1.14). For women randomized before delivery, there was no clear difference in the risk of the infant dying (576, 12.7%, vs. 558, 12.4%; relative risk 1.02, 99% CI 0.92–1.14). This trial established that magnesium sulfate halves the risk of eclampsia and probably reduces the risk of maternal death. There do not appear to be substantive harmful effects to mother or infant in the short term.

Whether antiepileptic drugs are appropriate to use in the treatment of seizures in this population has been debated. Arguments in favor of using antiepileptic drugs have stressed that magnesium is not antiepileptic, and it affects only the overt manifestations of seizures through neuromuscular blockade without altering the epileptic discharge.[14,28,29] Magnesium may have some unwanted obstetric effects as well. Inhibition of labor and impairment of postpartum hemostasis as a consequence of uterine smooth muscle relaxation have been described,[22] although others have not found that use of magnesium (or phenytoin) is associated with prolonged labor or an increased number of cesarean deliveries.[4]

A number of small trials have evaluated obstetric and seizure outcomes after phenytoin treatment in pre-eclamptic and eclamptic patients. Phenytoin was associated with more rapid cervical dilation and a smaller fall in hemocrit compared with magnesium in 105 pre-eclamptic and eclamptic women.[22] Slater et al.[62] treated 26 women who had eclampsia or pre-eclampsia with intravenous phenytoin and reported no convulsions. Robson et al.[52] treated 5 women who had eclampsia and 67 women who had severe pre-eclampsia with a phenytoin dose of 15 mg/kg or a loading dose of 17.5 mg/kg and found that some women had seizures despite therapeutic levels. Dommisse[13] assigned 22 women with eclampsia to receive either intravenous phenytoin or magnesium. Four of the women on phenytoin (levels of 10–25 mg/mL) had seizures, but none of the women on magnesium had seizures. Appleton et al.[3] randomized 50 patients with pre-eclampsia to phenytoin or magnesium for seizure prophylaxis. No differences were found in patient tolerance, adverse reactions, or neonatal outcomes between groups. No patient in either group had seizures.

Small trials have also evaluated the efficacy of prophylactic benzodiazepine treatment. Fifty-one women with eclampsia were randomized to magnesium or diazepam as an anticonvulsant.[9] Convulsions occurred in about one fourth of the women in each group, and there was no statistically significant difference in maternal morbidity, although significantly fewer infants in the magnesium group had low Apgar scores compared with those in the diazepam group.

Recently, several randomized, large-scale trials have permitted objective comparison of the efficacy of alternative medical treatments for pre-eclampsia/eclampsia. These represent the best information concerning the relative efficacy of magnesium and phenytoin for seizure prophylaxis and improving maternal and fetal outcome.

The Eclampsia Trial Collaborative Group[19] was an international multicenter, randomized trial that compared magnesium sulfate, diazepam, and phenytoin as treatment for eclampsia. This trial included 1,687 women with eclampsia from South Africa, Argentina, Colombia, Zimbabwe, Uganda, Brazil, Ghana, India, and Venezuela. Women were randomized to receive either magnesium or diazepam, or magnesium or phenytoin. Each center chose the comparison pair. Women receiving magnesium had a 54% lower risk of recurrent convulsions than did those receiving diazepam. There was no difference in maternal morbidity or perinatal morbidity and mortality. Women receiving magnesium had a 67% lower risk of recurrent convulsions than did women receiving phenytoin. Maternal mortality was not significantly lower in the women receiving magnesium. However, women on magnesium were less likely to be ventilated, contract pneumonia, and be admitted to an intensive care unit than were those receiving phenytoin. The infants of the mothers on magnesium were less likely to be intubated and to require admission to a special care nursery. Infant mortality remained high in the trial. Overall, 27% of infants died, with a mortality rate of 49% to 58% for those delivered before 34 weeks' gestation. This high infant mortality rate may be a reflection of the multinational nature of the trial. In the United States, mortality rates at 28 weeks or more are 10% or less.[51]

A second trial,[37] based in the United States, evaluated magnesium and phenytoin as prophylaxis for eclampsia in hypertensive pregnant women. Women admitted to labor and delivery with hypertension received either magnesium or phenytoin. Magnesium was administered as 4 g intravenously, followed by 10 g intramuscularly and 5 g intramuscularly every 4 hours thereafter as needed and as tolerated by protocol. Phenytoin was given as 1,000 mg intravenously, then at a maintenance dose 10 hours later of 500 mg orally. In this intention-to-treat analysis, 178 women randomized to the phenytoin group were given no phenytoin or received only partial loading doses. None of these women experienced an eclamptic seizure. Although there were no significant differences in any risk factors for eclampsia between the two groups or in maternal and fetal outcomes, 10 of 1,089 women receiving phenytoin had convulsions, compared with none of the 1,049 women receiving magnesium sulfate. These women had a number of peripartum complications: 5 had cesarean sections, 6 had infants with low birth weight, 1 had abruptio placentae, and 2 required transfusions. Several women who underwent neuroimaging had areas of low density, a finding that has been previously described with eclampsia,[8] but otherwise showed no structural abnormalities. Phenytoin levels in the women who had seizures ranged from 5.8 to 24 mg/mL; 9 of the 10 women with seizures had phenytoin levels of at least 10 mg/mL. The past experience of this center[37] predicted that the incidence of eclampsia after admission for hypertension and during magnesium sulfate prophylaxis would be 1/750 women. In this study, the observed incidence in the magnesium-treated group was 1/1,384, whereas the phenytoin failure rate was 1/100. This can also be compared with an incidence of 1/78 in one study in which women with proteinuric hypertension received no treatment.[8]

Magnesium sulfate may have other beneficial effects in high-risk infants and after neuronal injury in other patient populations. Magnesium is associated with improved survival in infants weighing <1,000 g.[6] Magnesium also appears to protect against hemorrhage into the germinal matrix or ventricles in infants of very low birth weight.[31] In an experimental model of birth asphyxia, magnesium was associated with less evidence of brain injury.[39,65] In one observational study, in utero exposure to magnesium sulfate appeared to be associated with a protective effect against cerebral palsy in infants of very low birth weight.[44] Magnesium administration also decreases secondary neuronal damage after experimental traumatic brain injury.[40,66]

What are the mechanisms by which magnesium effectively treats seizures in these patient populations? Seizures are an expression of dysfunctional cortical excitability and arise in a variety of pathophysiologic conditions. Magnesium may be most effective against seizures and brain injury that arise as a result of increased excitatory neurotransmitters.[34] Magnesium suppresses activity at the *N*-methyl-D-aspartate (NMDA) receptor, blocks calcium influx at the NMDA receptor, and reduces calcium-dependent presynaptic neurotransmitter release. Phenytoin blocks sodium channels but has no significant effect on calcium channels. Although there is no accepted animal model for eclampsia, stimulation at the NMDA receptor may reproduce some of the neurochemical events responsible for the eclamptic seizure. In one experimental model of eclamptic seizures, rats were cannulated in the lateral cerebral ventricle and given NMDA to elicit seizures. Magnesium sulfate was more effective in terminating these seizures than was phenytoin.[38] Seizures in amygdala-kindled rats, however, representing a model more typical of human localization-related epilepsy, responded to phenytoin but not to magnesium in terms of seizure duration, duration of postictal depression, and behavioral seizure stage.[63] Sibai et al.[59] also found that magnesium did not suppress epileptiform potentials as recorded on the EEG.

Seizures in pre-eclampsia and eclampsia may also occur in response to intense vasospasm. Magnesium sulfate is a potent vasodilator and increases cerebral blood flow as measured by Doppler ultrasonography of intracranial vessels.[5] Vasodilation appears to be greatest in the smaller-diameter intracranial vessels distal to the middle cerebral artery. This effect would be anticipated to relieve cerebral ischemia. The vasospasm in pre-eclampsia and eclampsia is thought to be partly related to endothelial dysfunction. Magnesium increases the production of prostacyclin, an endothelial vasodilator, and also protects against endothelial injury mediated by free radicals—perhaps by substituting for calcium and preventing the influx of calcium that is induced by free radicals.[49]

Magnesium has been the standard treatment for pre-eclampsia and eclampsia, reducing maternal and neonatal morbidity and mortality.[49] The largest number of fetal deaths occur as a consequence of maternal hypertension, which is associated with retardation of intrauterine growth, low birth weight, and prematurity as well as a significant rise in fetal death rate.[17] Magnesium addresses the maternal hypertension and improves fetal outcome. It appears that in most cases, magnesium also effectively treats eclamptic seizures. This should not be surprising. The optimal treatment of any seizure corrects the specific neurochemical events triggering the epileptic discharge. The events in seizures arising with pre-eclampsia/eclampsia appear to differ from those in seizures arising with epilepsy. Whether treating eclamptic seizures with magnesium and an antiepileptic drug confers additional benefit has not been directly evaluated. Further understanding of the pathophysiology of seizures associated with pre-eclampsia/eclampsia will better define the best therapy.

SUMMARY AND CONCLUSIONS

The diagnostic and treatment approach to the pregnant woman with seizures follows the same basic principles as the approach to any patient with a first seizure, although the diagnostic differential must be expanded. The need for emergent antiepileptic treatment is assessed. Results of the medical and neurologic history and the physical and neurologic examination are combined with findings of a comprehensive obstetric history and examination. Laboratory examinations include urinalysis for proteinuria, complete blood cell count with platelets to exclude infection and evaluate for a hematologic disorder or HELLP syndrome, determination of electrolytes, liver function tests, and a toxicology screen for cocaine and alcohol. Except in situations in which the diagnosis is clearly pre-eclampsia/eclampsia, EEG and MRI are indicated. In cases of complicated eclampsia or in the setting of focal neurologic deficits, neuroimaging should also be obtained.

Seizures occurring in the later part of gestation in a hypertensive woman are most likely a manifestation of pre-eclampsia/eclampsia. Other potential causes of seizures during pregnancy include acute cerebrovascular disease, infection, exacerbation of a neoplastic lesion or SLE, or hematologic disorders.

In a pregnant woman with seizures in whom the diagnosis of pre-eclampsia/eclampsia has been excluded, treatment of seizures proceeds as would be appropriate for a nonpregnant woman. Although antiepileptic drugs are teratogenic, seizures—particularly convulsive or prolonged seizures—pose a greater risk to the well-being of both mother and fetus. Care should be taken in figuring the doses of highly protein-bound drugs because the non–protein-bound fraction active in the CNS is relatively higher in a pregnant woman.

In the pre-eclamptic patient, magnesium sulfate is indicated for both prophylaxis and treatment of seizures. The question of whether an antiepileptic drug should be administered as well must be answered by future research. In the meantime, it appears prudent to obtain an EEG (or EEG monitoring) in any woman in whom seizures recur after treatment with magnesium sulfate or in any woman whose mental status is not normal. The EEG permits persistent electrographic seizures to be detected; these may be difficult to diagnose clinically in a patient with obtundation and neuromuscular blockade. Patients with clinical or electrographic seizures who are receiving magnesium should be treated with an antiepileptic drug as well. Phenytoin or a benzodiazepine appears to be an acceptable choice because of the relatively good safety profile in both mother and fetus.

References

1. Adelman DC, Saltiel E, Klinenberg JR. The neuropsychiatric manifestations of systemic lupus erythematosis: an overview. *Semin Arthritis Rheum.* 1986;15:185–199.
2. Altman D, Carroli G, Duley L, et al.; Magpie Trial Collaboration Group. Do women with pre-eclampsia, and their babies, benefit from magnesium sulphate? The Magpie Trial: a randomised placebo-controlled trial. *Lancet.* 2002;359(9321):1877–1890.
3. Appleton MP, Kuehle TJ, Raebel MA, et al. Magnesium sulfate versus phenytoin for seizure prophylaxis in pregnancy-induced hypertension. *Am J Obstet Gynecol.* 1991;165:907–913.
4. Atkinson MW, Guinn D, Owen J, et al. Does magnesium sulfate affect the length of labor induction in women with pregnancy-associated hypertension? *Am J Obstet Gynecol.* 1995;173:1219–1222.
5. Belfort MA, Moise KJ. Effect of magnesium sulfate on maternal brain blood flow in preeclampsia: a randomized, placebo-controlled study. *Am J Obstet Gynecol.* 1992;167:661–666.
6. Bottoms S, Paul R, Iams J, et al. Obstetrical determinants of neonatal survival in extremely low birth weight infants. *Am J Obstet Gynecol.* 1994;170(Pt 2):383.
7. Burrows RF, Burrows EA. The feasibility of a control population for a randomized control trial of seizure prophylaxis in the hypertensive disorders of pregnancy. *Am J Obstet Gynecol.* 1995;173:929–935.
8. Chua S, Redman CW. Are prophylactic anticonvulsants required in severe preeclampsia? *Lancet.* 1991;337:250–251.
9. Crowther C. Magnesium sulphate versus diazepam in the management of eclampsia: a randomized controlled trial. *Br J Obstet Gynaecol.* 1990;97:110–117.
10. Cunningham FG, MacDonald PC, Gant NF, et al. Hypertensive disorders in pregnancy. In: *Williams Obstetrics,* 19th ed. Norwalk, CT: Appleton & Lange; 1993: 763–817.
11. DeAngelis LM. Central nervous system neoplasms in pregnancy. In: Devinsky O, Feldmann E, Hainline B. *Neurological Complications of Pregnancy.* New York: Raven Press; 1994: 139–152.

12. Devinsky O, Petito CK, Alonso DR. Clinical and neuropathological findings in systemic lupus erythematosis: the role of vasculitis, heart emboli, and thrombotic thrombocytopenic purpura. *Ann Neurol.* 1988;23:380–384.
13. Dommisse J. Phenytoin sodium and magnesium sulphate in the management of eclampsia. *Br J Obstet Gynaecol.* 1990;97:104–109.
14. Donaldson JO. Does magnesium sulfate treat eclamptic convulsions? *Clin Neuropharmacol.* 1986;9:37–45.
15. Donaldson JO. Eclampsia. In: Devinsky O, Feldmann E, Hainline B. *Neurological Complications of Pregnancy.* New York: Raven Press; 1994: 25–33.
16. Douglas KA, Redman CW. Eclampsia in the United Kingdom. *BMJ* 1994;309(6966):1395–1400.
17. Druzin ML. Pregnancy-induced hypertension and pre-eclampsia: the fetus and the neonate. In: Rubin PC, ed. *Handbook of Hypertension, Vol. 10. Hypertension in Pregnancy.* New York: Elsevier; 1988: 267–289.
18. Duley L, Johanson R. Magnesium sulphate for pre-eclampsia and eclampsia: the evidence so far. *Br J Obstet Gynaecol.* 1994;101:565–567.
19. Eclampsia Trial Collaborative Group. Which anticonvulsant for women with eclampsia? Evidence from the Collaborative Eclampsia Trial. *Lancet.* 1995;345:1455–1463.
20. Estes D, Christian CL. The natural history of systemic lupus erythematosis by prospective analysis. *Medicine.* 1971;50:85–95.
21. Evevoldson T, Ross Russell R. Cerebral venous thrombosis: new causes for an old syndrome? *Q J Med.* 1990;77:1255–1275.
22. Friedman SA, Lim KH, Baker CA, et al. Phenytoin versus magnesium sulfate in preeclampsia: a pilot study. *Am J Perinatol.* 1993;20:233–238.
23. Gall SA. Maternal adjustments in the immune system in normal pregnancy. *Clin Obstet Gynecol.* 1983;26:521–536.
24. Gedekoh RH, Hayashi TT, McDonald HM. Eclampsia at Magee-Womens Hospital, 1970 to 1980. *Am J Obstet Gynecol.* 1981;140:860–866.
25. Hinchey J, Chaves C, Appignani B, et al. A reversible posterior leukoencephalopathy syndrome. *N Engl J Med.* 1996;334:494–500.
26. Hutton JD, James DK, Stirrat GM, et al. Management of severe pre-eclampsia and eclampsia by UK consultants. *Br J Obstet Gynaecol.* 1992;99:554–556.
27. Johnson RT. Infections during pregnancy. In: Devinsky O, Feldmann E, Hainline B. *Neurological Complications of Pregnancy.* New York: Raven Press; 1994: 153–162.
28. Kaplan PW, Lesser RP, Fisher RS, et al. No, magnesium sulfate should not be used in treating eclamptic seizures. *Arch Neurol.* 1988;45:1361–1364.
29. Kaplan PW, Lesser RP, Fisher RS, et al. A continuing controversy: magnesium sulfate in the treatment of eclamptic seizures. *Arch Neurol.* 1990;47:1031–1032.
30. Koster T, Rosendaal FR, deRonde H, et al. Venous thrombosis due to poor anticoagulant response to activated protein C: Leiden Thrombophilia Study. *Lancet.* 1993;342:1503–1506.
31. Kuban KCK, Leviton A, Pagano M, et al. Maternal toxemia is associated with reduced incidence of germinal matrix hemorrhage in premature babies. *J Child Neurol.* 1992;7:70–76.
32. Lenfant C, Gifford RW, Zuspan FP. Report of the National High Blood Pressure Education Program Working Group on High Blood Pressure in Pregnancy. *Am J Obstet Gynecol.* 1990;163:1691–1712.
33. Lennox WG, Lennox MA. *Epilepsy and Related Disorders.* Boston: Little, Brown; 1960: 649–650.
34. Lipton SA, Rosenberg PA. Excitatory amino acids as a final common pathway for neurologic disorders. *N Engl J Med.* 1994;330:613–622.
35. Lockwood CJ, Romero R, Feinberg RF, et al. The prevalence and biologic significance of lupus anticoagulant and anticardiolipin antibodies in a general obstetric population. *Am J Obstet Gynecol.* 1989;161:369–373.
36. Loureiro R, Leite CC, Kahhale S, et al. Diffusion imaging may predict reversible brain lesions in eclampsia and severe eclampsia: initial experience. *Am J Obstet Gynecol.* 2003;189:1350–1355.
37. Lucas MJ, Leveno KJ, Cunningham FG. A comparison of magnesium sulfate with phenytoin for the prevention of eclampsia. *N Engl J Med.* 1995;333:201–205.
38. Mason BA, Standley CA, Irtenkauf SM, et al. Magnesium is more efficacious than phenytoin in reducing *N*-methyl-D-aspartate (NMDA) seizures in rats. *Am J Obstet Gynecol.* 1994;171:999–1002.
39. McDonald JW, Silverstein FS, Johnston MV. Magnesium reduces *N*-methyl-D-aspartate (NMDA)-mediated brain injury in perinatal rats. *Neurosci Lett.* 1990;109:234–238.
40. McIntosh TK. Novel pharmacologic therapies in the treatment of experimental traumatic brain injury: a review. *J Neurotrauma.* 1993;10:215–261.
41. Mintz G, Niz J, Gutierrez G, et al. Prospective study of pregnancy in systemic lupus erythematosis. *J Rheumatol.* 1986;13:732–739.
42. Moroney JT, Allen MH. Cocaine and alcohol use in pregnancy. *Adv Neurol.* 1994;64:231–242.
43. Morrell MJ. Hormones and epilepsy through the lifetime. *Epilepsia.* 1992;33(Suppl 4):49–61.
44. Nelson KB, Grether JK. Can magnesium sulfate reduce the risk of cerebral palsy in very low birthweight infants? *Pediatrics.* 1995;95:263–269.
45. Preter M, Tzourio C, Ameri A, et al. Long-term prognosis in cerebral venous thrombosis. Follow-up of 77 patients. *Stroke.* 1996;27:243–246.
46. Pritchard JA, Cunningham FG, Pritchard SA. The Parkland Memorial Hospital protocol for the treatment of eclampsia: evaluation of 245 cases. *Am J Obstet Gynecol.* 1984;148:951–963.
47. Repke JT, Friedman SA, Kaplan PW. Prophylaxis of eclamptic seizures: current controversies. *Clin Obstet Gynecol.* 1992;35:365–374.
48. Ridolfi RL, Bell WR. Thrombotic thrombocytopenic purpura: report of 25 cases and review of the literature. *Medicine.* 1981;60:413–428.
49. Roberts JM. Magnesium for preeclampsia and eclampsia. *N Engl J Med.* 1995;333:250–251.
50. Roberts JM, Redman CWG. Pre-eclampsia: more than pregnancy-induced hypertension. *Lancet.* 1993;341:1447–1451.
51. Robertson PA, Sniderman SH, Laros RK, et al. Neonatal morbidity according to gestational age and birthweight from five tertiary centers in the United States, 1983–1986. *Am J Obstet Gynecol.* 1992;166:1629–1631.
52. Robson SC, Redfern N, Seviour J, et al. Phenytoin prophylaxis in severe pre-eclampsia and eclampsia. *Br J Obstet Gynaecol.* 1993;100:623–628.
53. Rosner S, Ginzler EM, Diamond HS, et al. A multicenter study of outcome in systemic lupus erythematosis. II: Causes of death. *Arthritis Rheum.* 1982;25:612–619.
54. Ryan G, Lange IR, Naugler MA. Clinical experience with phenytoin prophylaxis in severe preeclampsia. *Am J Obstet Gynecol.* 1989;161:1297–1304.
55. Sammaritano LR. Neurologic aspects of rheumatologic disorders during pregnancy. In: Devinsky O, Feldmann E, Hainline B. *Neurological Complications of Pregnancy.* New York: Raven Press; 1994: 97–130.
56. Schwartz RB. Neurodiagnostic imaging of the pregnant patient. In: Devinsky O, Feldmann E, Hainline B. *Neurological Complications of Pregnancy.* New York: Raven Press; 1994: 243–248.
57. Sharshar T, Lamy C, Mas JL. Incidence and causes of stroke associated with pregnancy and puerperium. A study in public hospitals of Ile de France. Stroke in Pregnancy Study Group. *Stroke.* 1995;25:930–936.
58. Sibai BM. Diagnosis, prevention and management of eclampsia. *Obstet Gynecol.* 2005;105:402–410.
59. Sibai BM, Spinnato JA, Watson DL, et al. Effect of magnesium sulfate on electroencephalographic findings in preeclampsia-eclampsia. *Obstet Gynecol.* 1984;64:261–266.
60. Sibai BM, Spinnato JA, Watson DL, et al. Eclampsia. IV. Neurological findings and future outcome. *Am J Obstet Gynecol.* 1985;152:184–192.
61. Sibai BM, Taslimi MM, el Nazer A, et al. Maternal-perinatal outcome associated with the syndrome of hemolysis, elevated liver enzymes and low platelets in severe preeclampsia-eclampsia. *Am J Obstet Gynecol.* 1986;155:501–509.
62. Slater RM, Wilcox FL, Smith WD, et al. Phenytoin infusion in severe pre-eclampsia. *Lancet.* 1987;1:1417–1421.
63. Standley CA, Irtenkauf SM, Stwart L, et al. MgSO4 versus phenytoin for seizure prevention in amygdala kindled rats. *Am J Obstet Gynecol.* 1994;171:948–951.
64. Thomas SV, Somanathan N, Radhakumari R. Interictal EEG changes in eclampsia. *Electroencephalogr Clin Neurophysiol.* 1995;94:271–275.
65. Thordstein M, Bagenholm R, Thiringer K, et al. Scavengers of free oxygen radicals in combination with magnesium ameliorate perinatal hypoxic-ischemic brain damage in the rat. *Pediatr Res.* 1993;34:23–26.
66. Vink R, McIntosh TK, Faden AI. Mg2+ in neurotrauma: its role and therapeutic implications. In: Strata P, Carbone E, eds. *Mg2+ and Excitable Membranes.* Berlin: Springer-Verlag; 1991: 125–145.
67. Weibers D, Whisnant J. The incidence of stroke among pregnant women in Rochester, Minnesota, 1955 through 1979. *JAMA.* 1985;254:3055–3057.
68. Wilterdink JL, Easton HD. Cerebral ischemia. In: Devinsky O, Feldmann E, Hainline B. *Neurological Complications of Pregnancy.* New York: Raven Press; 1994: 1–11.
69. Wilterdink JL, Feldmann E. Cerebral hemorrhage. In: Devinsky O, Feldmann E, Hainline B. *Neurological Complications of Pregnancy.* New York: Raven Press; 1994: 13–23.
70. Wong C, Giuliani M, Haley E. Cerebrovascular disease and stroke in women. *Cardiology.* 1990;77(Suppl 2):80–90.
71. Zeeman GG, Fleckenstein JL, Twickler DM, et al. Cerebral infarction in eclampsia. *Am J Obstet Gynecol.* 2004;190:714–720.
72. Zoller B, Dahlback B. Linkage between inherited resistance to activated protein C and factor V gene mutation in venous thrombosis. *Lancet.* 1994;343:1536–1538.

CHAPTER 270 ■ OVERVIEW: DISORDERS THAT CAN BE CONFUSED WITH EPILEPSY

FRÉDÉRICK ANDERMANN

INTRODUCTION

The history is crucial in suggesting a diagnosis of epilepsy. The value of the interview hinges largely on the availability of an accurate history from both the patient and a witness to the event. In the absence of either of these essential features, the information is usually incomplete or inadequate, and every effort should be made to obtain a complete and detailed account before attempting to formulate a diagnosis.[2]

The last quarter-century has witnessed a great increase in the number of neurologists sophisticated in the treatment of epilepsy, and such neurologists are now available in many practice groups and academic departments. Many neurologists developed sophisticated monitoring units, to which patients with unexplained paroxysmal events are often referred. It soon became obvious that many of these individuals did not have epileptic seizures, and this led epileptologists and other neurologists to focus on the wide range of disorders presenting for differential diagnosis. More recently this increased awareness and accuracy in diagnosis by referring physicians has led to a reduction in the number of patients with clinically recognizable nonepileptic paroxysmal events who are referred to epilepsy centers.

Nonepileptic seizures present the most common problem in differential diagnosis (see Chapter 282). Increasingly available information and sophistication coupled with ready access to medical literature and the Internet, along with the individual's ability to learn from previous interviewers and examiners, has led to the appearance of complex accounts of what might be called "pseudoepileptic nonepileptic seizures." Thus, such patients often provide a history that contains many features of temporal lobe epilepsy or of other specific epileptic disorders. They may have a background of study in a field related to epilepsy, which obviously makes diagnosis difficult. The patients' social and cultural backgrounds are important determinants not only of the pattern of nonepileptic seizures, but also of their response to treatment. In many settings and localities the majority of patients respond to appropriate psychiatric treatment with remission of the attacks. In other environments with different levels of psychiatric sophistication and social problems, the disorder is much more refractory and the percentage of patients who cannot be relieved of their nonepileptic attacks is higher.[43]

SYSTEMIC DISTURBANCES

Anoxic convulsions, or "ischemic convulsions" as they are sometimes termed, continue to present a diagnostic problem. They occur most often as a sequel to syncope and are related usually to the person being kept in an upright or standing position. Sometimes, however, syncope may occur in individuals who are recumbent. The circumstances of the event and the family history will provide clues to the diagnosis.[18,21,29,43] Not only might patients with asthma during an acute attack have cerebral ischemia, but they also might present with tonic episodes, whose mechanism is analogous to that of anoxic convulsions.[27] When there is some lateralization, the differential diagnosis is, of course, more difficult. However, lateralization of clinical features is not uncommon and has long been recognized in generalized processes such as idiopathic epilepsy.[24] It may be erroneously inferred by the observer, depending on the patient's position during the attack. It is important to distinguish between persistent or habitual lateralization and less significant and inconstant asymmetries in body and limb postures and movements.

Many individuals with migraine present features that make diagnosis difficult (Chapter 274). Acephalgic migraine occurring in older individuals is often not accompanied by headache, and these patients are not infrequently referred for diagnosis because of the suspicion of intermittent cerebral ischemic attacks or an epileptic etiology. Acephalgic migraine, however, does also occur in younger individuals and children.[45]

The march of the migrainous aura has a time course that frequently is different from that of the recruitment of symptoms in epilepsy, and in a majority of individuals distinguishing between the two is not difficult.[12,38,45] After the migrainous aura, however, the patient may have convulsive seizures, so-called intercalated attacks.[3,47] These are most likely related to spreading depression crossing the central sulcus, but proof of the specific mechanism is lacking. Whether these attacks require treatment with antiepileptic medication is not clear. Patients with a habitual tendency to develop such epileptic manifestations in the course of their migraine attacks eventually may develop seizures, usually temporal in pattern, which no longer occur in relation to clear-cut migrainous events. The mechanism of this form of secondary epileptogenesis is not clear.[1] Confusional migraine may also result in an epileptic seizure occurring during the acute event.[1,19] Here, too, the possibility of eventual development of independent epileptic attacks exists.

Patients with basilar migraine not infrequently present difficult diagnostic problems. It is usually the sequence of symptoms pointing to brainstem involvement, such as diplopia and ataxia, that provides clues to the diagnosis.[9,39,46] Neuro-otologic investigation during an attack documenting the very prominent nystagmus is also helpful.

Patients with basilar migraine also may have epileptic events or in rare instances status epilepticus. Here, too, the account of symptoms preceding the seizure will lead to clarification.[14]

The unresponsiveness that is not uncommon during basilar migraine attacks may be interpreted as loss of consciousness; however, the patients generally can be aroused by vigorous stimulation, only to relapse into stupor when stimulation ceases.[9]

In addition to the clinical problems, the recognition that the migraine aura may be manifested by electroencephalographic (EEG) spike discharge (usually over posterior head regions) may lead to diagnostic difficulty.[6,33,44]

Migraine is an extraordinarily common disorder, and despite the efforts of the International Migraine Society, there is still considerable disparity in deciding on its prevalence. It seems fairly clear that migraine and epilepsy have different mechanisms but that relationships between the two conditions, at times of a causal nature, exist. An interesting example is the association between benign rolandic epilepsy or benign occipital epilepsy and migraine.[10] Surprisingly, there is no unanimity among pediatric neurologists and epileptologists about the high and probably consistent association of these two disorders. Clarification must await advances in molecular genetics, which, it is hoped, will provide markers for these conditions.

Recent advances in molecular biology have shed some light on the nature of hemiplegic migraine with coma; it is notable that these patients do not have clear epileptic events. The hallucinations that occur as they recover from the coma are similar to those of peduncular hallucinosis.[26,36,50]

Patients with peduncular hallucinations are often considered to have epilepsy and are so treated. The hallucinations are usually vivid, stereotyped, prolonged, and not associated with overt epileptic manifestations. They are caused by mesencephalic lesions or abnormalities and do not respond to antiepileptic drugs.[15,25,37] The hallucinations of patients with parkinsonism are probably similar to if not identical to those of peduncular hallucinosis and also may raise questions as to their nature.[16,20] The auditory hallucinations of the deaf or the visual hallucinations of the blind are occasionally misinterpreted as epileptic in nature.

NEUROLOGIC DISTURBANCES

Patients with episodic hypothalamic dysfunction or the Kleine-Levin syndrome have varied behavioral abnormalities, including hallucinations and excessive sleep. The patients often have some disturbance of awareness and memory, although they remain fully conscious.[11,42] An epileptic twilight state is at times suspected, but when the examiner is aware of the condition, a detailed history stressing associated features such as excessive eating and inappropriate sexual behavior should lead to the diagnosis.

Paroxysmal events occurring exclusively during sleep have led to diagnostic difficulties for some time (see Chapter 276).[22,35] The identification of nocturnal paroxysmal dystonia as a specific entity arose at a time when there was little awareness of the various patterns found in frontal lobe epilepsy. It now appears that paroxysmal nocturnal dystonia is not an entity that can be distinguished from partial epilepsy of frontal origin. The recent recognition of familial frontal epilepsy has further helped to clarify the diagnosis in a number of individuals.[41] It is not a homogeneous condition, however, and although in some families the attacks are always nocturnal and easily controlled by antiepileptic medication, in others there is variation in the occurrence of attacks in relation to the sleep/waking cycle, and medical control is difficult to achieve. This disorder, or rather this group of disorders, occurs in the absence of visible lesions and most likely is related to regional disorders of channel function or other, unidentified molecular abnormalities.[32,41]

Rapid-eye-movement (REM)–related sleep disorder may be mistaken for epileptic or postepileptic confusion and aggression but has become increasingly recognized as a consequence of the development of sleep medicine.[22] Hypnagogic and hypnapompic myoclonus is often misinterpreted as epileptic by patients with epilepsy and their families. The nature of myoclonus occurring during sleep is often difficult to interpret and to relate to a patient's known epileptic disorder.

Myoclonus has recently been intensively studied by epileptologists and movement disorder specialists, and its neurophysiologic basis is much better understood, but gaps still exist (see Chapter 277). Although the myoclonic component of idiopathic generalized epilepsy is usually easy to recognize, the diagnosis is often missed until generalized tonic–clonic or clonic–tonic–clonic seizures supervene.

The progressive myoclonic epilepsies subsume a number of disorders that share an association with generalized seizures, photosensitivity, and sometimes occipital epileptic discharge, ataxia, and some degree of neurologic deterioration (see Chapter 252). The most common disorders are Lafora disease, Unverricht-Lundborg disease, neuronal ceroid lipofuscinosis, myoclonus epilepsy with ragged red fibers (MERRF), and sialidosis. There are also several other entities that may present in this way.[8,13,30,40,49] Despite recent progress, particularly in the area of molecular biology, the neuronal networks in brainstem and cerebellar structures leading to these manifestations have not been identified. This is surprising considering the great disparity in their biochemical and neuropathologic abnormalities.

Myoclonic ataxia as defined by Marsden et al.[34] implies that these patients do not have overt epileptic seizures. It is likely that at least a percentage of these individuals suffer from MERRF or a related mitochondrial disorder (Chapter 262). Patients presenting in this way should have a detailed investigation of mitochondrial function.[34]

Benign essential myoclonus is an ill-defined disorder. Affected family members may have an occasional seizure, which casts doubt on the nonepileptic nature of the syndrome.[17]

The nature of some of the paroxysmal movement disorders has been intensely debated recently. Benign paroxysmal kinesigenic choreoathetosis (PKC), perhaps the most common of these, is easily recognized if one is aware of the clinical symptomatology. Attacks are classically induced by initiation of movement, are brief, and are not associated with any impairment of awareness. The disorder gradually improves with age. The episodes respond remarkably to low levels of antiepileptic medications such as carbamazepine and phenytoin. However, stopping the small dose of medication usually leads to recurrence.[28] This disorder is clearly not epileptic in the classical sense. Until its mechanism is more clearly understood, the relationship to epilepsy will remain uncertain (see Chapter 278).[7,31]

Symptomatic choreoathetosis may well have a different pathophysiologic basis.[23] The symptoms are more varied than in PKC, triggers are less obvious and not stereotyped, and an epileptic etiology is more frequently assumed. Examination with depth electrode recording in one patient showed spike discharges, which prompted the investigator to assume a relationship of the disorder to epilepsy, at least in the patient so studied.[7] Certainly the presence of such spiking in subcortical structures may be related in some way to the effectiveness of antiepileptic drugs in low doses in some of the individuals with paroxysmal movement disorders.

Alternating hemiplegia of childhood is almost invariably still diagnosed initially as an epileptic disorder. The progressive deterioration and the lack of response to antiepileptic drugs eventually lead to the diagnosis. Perhaps as many as half the children later develop epileptic seizures as well, and in most instances these are easily controlled. This disorder is probably also migraine related, although its cause remains a mystery. The attacks of hemiplegia are associated with only mild or no definite slow-wave electroencephalographic changes during the event. This pattern of alternating hemiplegia is not limited to the classical syndrome, and several disorders may manifest in this way. Benign nocturnal alternating hemiplegia is not associated with mental deterioration and is even more clearly migraine related. Pyruvate dehydrogenase deficiency, undiagnosed basal ganglia disorders, and episodic dystonic attacks in infancy also may present with similar motor symptoms and share what seems to be a common subcortical or brainstem mechanism.[4]

Shuddering attacks are not uncommon in children and are often considered to be myoclonic or epileptic. They may be related to a family history of essential or familial tremor, and this has again been suggested in the recent literature.[5,48] Benign nocturnal myoclonus recently was recognized in infants who continue to develop normally (see Chapter 280).

SUMMARY AND CONCLUSIONS

The clinical features of the epilepsies and of epileptic seizures and epileptic syndromes have been well delineated in recent years. This has led in turn to more accurate diagnosis and increasing recognition of a variety of paroxysmal events of a nonepileptic nature. The progress reported in this overview and in the following chapters is not merely an idle theoretical exercise; rather, it has prevented the needless use of antiepileptic drugs with their known side effects in situations in which these agents cannot be expected to be helpful.

References

1. Andermann F. Clinical features of migraine-epilepsy syndromes. In: Andermann F, Lugaresi E, eds. *Migraine and Epilepsy*. Boston: Butterworths; 1987: 3–30.
2. Andermann F. Identification of candidates for surgical treatment of epilepsy. In: Engel J Jr, ed. *Surgical Treatment of the Epilepsies*. New York: Raven; 1987.
3. Andermann F. Migraine and epilepsy: an overview. In: Andermann F, Lugaresi E, eds. *Migraine and Epilepsy*. Boston: Butterworths; 1987: 405–422.
4. Andermann F, Beaumanoir A, Mira L, et al., eds. *Alternating Hemiplegia of Childhood*. London: John Libbey; 1993.
5. Barron TF, Younkin DP. Propranolol therapy for shuddering attacks. *Neurology*. 1992;42:258–259.
6. Beaumanoir A, Grandjean E. Occipital spikes, migraine and epilepsy. In: Andermann F, Lugaresi E, eds. *Migraine and Epilepsy*. Boston: Butterworths; 1987: 97–110.
7. Beaumanoir A, Mira L, Vanlierde A. Epilepsy or paroxysmal kinesigenic choreoathetosis. *Brain Dev*. 1996;18:139–141.
8. Berkovic SF, Andermann F, Carpenter S, et al. Progressive myoclonus epilepsies: specific causes and diagnosis. *N Engl J Med*. 1986;315:296–305.
9. Bickerstaff ER. Basilar artery migraine. *Lancet*. 1961;1:15–17.
10. Bladin PF. The association of benign rolandic epilepsy with migraine. In: Andermann F, Lugaresi E, eds. *Migraine and Epilepsy*. Boston: Butterworths; 1987: 145–152.
11. Bonnet F, Thibaut F, Levillain D, et al. Kleine-Levin syndrome misdiagnosed as schizophrenia. *Eur Psychiatry*. 1996;11:104–105.
12. Brown AD, Dodson PM, Ainsworth JR. Diagnosis and management of migraine—differential diagnosis may be different in patients presenting to an ophthalmologist. *Br Med J*. 1996;313:691.
13. Buchhalter JR. Inherited epilepsies of childhood. *J Child Neurol*. 1994;9(Suppl 1):12–19.
14. Camfield PR, Metrakos K, Andermann F. Basilar migraine, seizures and severe epileptiform EEG abnormalities. *Neurology*. 1978;28:584–588.
15. Chen JH, Lui CC. Peduncular hallucinosis following microvascular decompression for trigeminal neuralgia: report of a case. *J Formosan Med Assoc*. 1995;94:503–505.
16. de la Fuente Fernandez R, Lopez J, Rey del Corral P, et al. Peduncular hallucinosis and right hemiparkinsonism caused by left mesencephalic infarction. *J Neurol Neurosurg Psychiatry*. 1994;57:870.
17. Delecluse F, Waldamar G, Vestermark S, et al. Cerebral blood flow deficits in hereditary essential myoclonus. *Arch Neurol*. 1992;49:179–182.
18. Farrehi PM, Santinga JT, Eagle KA. Syncope—diagnosis of cardiac and noncardiac causes. *Geriatrics*. 1995;50:24–30.
19. Ferrera PC, Reicho PR. Acute confusional migraine and trauma-triggered migraine. *Am J Emerg Med*. 1996;14:276–278.
20. Goetz CG, Stebbins GT. Mortality and hallucinations in nursing home patients with advanced Parkinson's disease. *Neurology*. 1995;45:669–671.
21. Grubb BP, Kosinski D. Current trends in etiology, diagnosis, and management of neurocardiogenic syncope. *Curr Opin Cardiol*. 1996;11:32–41.
22. Guilleminault C, Moscovitch A, Leger D. Forensic sleep medicine—nocturnal wandering and violence. *Sleep*. 1995;18:740–748.
23. Hamano S, Tanaka Y, Nara T, et al. Paroxysmal kinesigenic choreoathetosis associated with prenatal brain damage. *Acta Paediatr Jpn*. 1995;37:401–404.
24. Howell DA. Unusual centrencephalic seizure patterns. *Brain*. 1955;78:199–208.
25. Howlett DC, Downie AC, Banerjee AK, et al. MRI of an unusual case of peduncular hallucinosis (L'Hermitte's syndrome). *Neuroradiology*. 1994;36:121–122.
26. Joutel A, Bousser MG, Biousse V, et al. Familial hemiplegic migraine. Localisation of a responsible gene on chromosome 19. *Rev Neurol*. 1994;150:340–345.
27. Keene DL, Melmed CA, Andermann F, et al. Anoxic tonic seizures due to asthma: a serious complication in adults. *J Can Sci Neurol*. 1981;8:177–179.
28. Kertesz A. Paroxysmal kinesigenic choreoathetosis. An entity with the paroxysmal choreoathetosis syndrome. Description of 10 cases, including 1 autopsied. *Neurology*. 1967;17:680–690.
29. Lazarus JC, Maura VF. Syncope—pathophysiology, diagnosis, and pharmacotherapy source. *Ann Pharmacother*. 1996;30:994–1005.
30. Lehesjoki AE, Tassinari CA, Avanzini G, et al. PME of Unverricht-Lundborg type in the Mediterranean region: linkage and linkage disequilibrium confirm the assignment to the EPM1 locus. *Hum Genet*. 1994;93:66B–74.
31. Lombroso CT. Paroxysmal choreoathetosis: an epileptic or non-epileptic disorder? *Ital J Neurol Sci*. 1995;16:271–277.
32. Lopes Cendes I, Phillips HA, Scheffer IE, et al. Genetic linkage studies in familial frontal epilepsy—exclusion of the human chromosome regions homologous to the EL-1 mouse locus. *Epilepsy Res*. 1995;22:227–233.
33. Marks DA, Ehrenberg BL. Migraine-related seizures in adults with epilepsy with EEG correlation. *Neurology*. 1993;43:2476–2483.
34. Marsden CD, Harding AE, Obeso JA, et al. Progressive myoclonic ataxia (the Ramsay Hunt syndrome). *Arch Neurol*. 1990;47:1121–1125.
35. Montagna P, Cirignotta F, Giovanardi Rossi P, et al. Dystonic attacks related to sleep and exercise. *Eur Neurol*. 1992;32:185–189.
36. Motta E, Roscisewska D, Miller K. Hemiplegic migraine with CSF abnormalities [Review]. *Headache*. 1995;35:368–370.
37. Nicolai A, Lazzarino LG. Peduncular hallucinosis as the first manifestation of multiple sclerosis [Letter]. *Eur Neurol*. 1995;35:241–242.
38. Panayiotopoulos CP. Elementary visual hallucinations in migraine and epilepsy. *J Neurol Neurosurg Psychiatry*. 1994;57:1371–1374.
39. Passier PE, Vredeveld JW, de Krom MC. Basilar migraine with severe EEG abnormalities. *Headache*. 1994;34:56–58.
40. Pennacchio LA, Lehesjoki AE, Stone NE, et al. Mutations in the gene encoding cystatin B in progressive myoclonus epilepsy. *Science*. 1996;271:1731–1734.
41. Phillips HA, Scheffer IE, Berkovic SF, et al. Localization of a gene for autosomal dominant nocturnal frontal lobe epilepsy to chromosome 20q 13.2 [Letter]. *Nat Genet*. 1995;10:117–118.
42. Pike M, Stores G. Kleine-Levin syndrome: a cause of diagnostic confusion. *Arch Dis Child*. 1994;71:355–357.
43. Rowan AJ, Gates JR. *Non-epileptic Seizures*. Boston: Butterworth-Heinemann; 1993.
44. Sacquegna T, Cortelli P, Baldrati A, et al. Electrographic observations on migraine and transient global amnesia, confusional migraine, and migraine and epilepsy. In: Andermann F, Lugaresi E, eds. *Migraine and Epilepsy*. Boston: Butterworths; 1987: 153–161.
45. Shevell MI. Acephalgic migraines of childhood. *Pediatr Neurol*. 1996;14:211–215.
46. Sudo K, Tashiro K. Psychogenic basilar migraine. *Neurology*. 1996;46:1786.
47. Terzano MG, Manzoni GC, Parrino L. Benign epilepsy with occipital paroxysms and migraine: the question of intercalated attacks. In: Andermann F, Lugaresi E, eds. *Migraine and Epilepsy*. Boston: Butterworths; 1987: 83–96.
48. Vanasse M, Bedard P, Andermann F. Shuddering attacks in children: an early clinical manifestation of essential tremor. *Neurology*. 1976;26:1027–1030.
49. Virtaneva K, Miao JM, Traskelin AL, et al. Progressive myoclonus epilepsy EPMI locus maps to a 175-KB interval in distal 21Q. *Am J Hum Genet*. 1996;58:1247–1253.
50. Zifkin B, Andermann E, Andermann F, et al. Autosomal dominant syndrome of hemiplegic migraine, nystagmus and tremor. *Ann Neurol*. 1980;8:329–332.

CHAPTER 271 ■ SYNCOPE

MARK S. QUIGG AND THOMAS P. BLECK

INTRODUCTION

The term *syncope*, from the Greek for "cutting short," refers to an abrupt and transient loss of consciousness accompanied by loss of muscular tone. It is usually caused by a sudden, global reduction in cerebral perfusion, and clinical recovery occurs with restoration of normal cerebral blood flow. The very transience of this syndrome and the variety of medical disorders that can cause or mimic it are at the core of the diagnostic problems that the neurologist faces.

Definitions

Patients and physicians alike use a variety of terms to describe an occurrence of syncope. The term *fainting* is often used synonymously with syncope and captures the essential criteria—loss of consciousness and muscle tone. If the symptoms differ only in degree, so that there is partial loss of consciousness with a near fall, the term *presyncope* is often used. Less specific terms, such as *passing out*, *blackout*, or *dizziness*, need further clarification to become diagnostically useful. Some clinicians restrict the meaning of *drop attacks* to episodes of transient loss of tone with preservation of consciousness, a definition that carries a different burden of etiologies than does syncope.

INCIDENCE AND PROGNOSIS

When measured in studies of consecutive emergency room visits, syncope prompts about 3% of emergency room evaluations, a proportion that has changed little over the last 25 years.[9,14,56] Multicenter surveys estimate that of 865 million emergency room visits between 1992 and 2000, 6.7 million (0.77%) were related to syncope.[78]

Although no age is spared, the incidence of syncope is highest among the elderly. A study of 711 elderly patients revealed a 10-year prevalence of 23% and a yearly incidence of 7%.[52] Of those who are admitted to hospital, 59.9% are age 70 years or older.[79] In addition to increasing age, other factors leading to higher rates of hospitalization are female gender and white race.[78]

The incidence of syncope among children and adolescents is 1.25%, peaking in the 15- to 19-year-old group.[20] Young athletes at a mean age of 16 years report that 6.2% had syncope within the last 5 years.[10]

Diagnosis is important because the mortality of syncope varies widely with the underlying etiology. Kapoor determined the 5-year outcome of 433 patients evaluated for syncope.[41] Mortality is >50% in patients with a cardiac cause of syncope, compared to 30% in patients with a noncardiac cause and 22% with an unknown cause.

Data from the Framingham Heart Study emphasize that syncope from cardiac causes is often a harbinger of significant coronary disease.[76] In this study, 822/7,814 (10.5%) individuals reported syncope over a 24-year period, for an overall incidence of first report of syncope of 6.2/1,000 person-yr. The relative hazard rate experienced by those with syncope from any cause compared to those without syncope is 1.31. Cardiac syncope has the highest relative risk of death than any other cause of syncope at 2.01 and an especially high risk of death related to coronary artery disease (relative risk 2.66). The Framingham study also emphasizes that those whose etiology of syncope remains unknown do not necessarily experience a benign course, having a relative risk of death from any cause of 1.32.

Older age appears to increase the risk of mortality in cardiac syncope. Another study by Kapoor that compared mortality rates of patients <60 and >60 years of age found that although the 2-year mortality rate was 27% in the older and 8% in the younger group, cardiovascular causes remained the most significant risk factor for mortality in either.[43] In the elderly, syncope carries a greater mortality despite etiology. In elderly patients hospitalized for syncope, the 4-year mortality was 41%, with the relative risk of cardiac syncope not varying significantly from that of noncardiac syncope.[30]

Morbidity associated with trauma from syncopal falls also contributes to the costs related to syncope. Between 16% and 36% of patients presenting with syncope experience a range of injuries from minor lacerations and bruises to fractures of the hip, face, or limbs.[14,41]

The morbidity of syncope goes beyond the physical. Assessments of the functional status of patients with chronic syncope show degrees of psychosocial impairment similar to those experienced by patients suffering from other disabling diseases such as rheumatoid arthritis or low back pain.[51]

The frequency of recurrence of syncope is not especially helpful in characterizing patients by etiology or prognosis,[41] although each syncopal episode increases the probability of serious injury. In Kapoor's study of 433 syncopal patients followed for 5 years, 153 had one or more recurrences, and the mean number of recurrences was greater than six.[41] Whether the diagnosis was cardiac, noncardiac, or unknown, recurrences were common in every category.

The 2000 Healthcare and Utilization Project estimates the annual cost of syncope-related hospital admissions in the United States at $2.4 billion, placing syncope on par with asthma ($2.8 billion) and human immunodeficiency virus ($2.2 billion).[78] The estimated cost per patient is $5,400. The high cost reflects the difficulties in establishing a diagnosis of a syndrome having both a wide range of possible etiologies and a high rate of studies returning nondiagnostic results. These problems have led to the publication of guidelines on evaluation and hospitalization of syncope, the adherence to which, some report, leads to higher yields in diagnostic accuracy but to no clear reductions in cost.[16,26] Other clinicians, however, report success in cost reduction, test reduction, and health benefits in the use of specialized syncope units and protocols of risk stratification and evaluation.[45,74]

CLINICAL DESCRIPTION

Classic Symptoms

The prodromal symptoms of classic syncope are familiar to most physicians and consist of nausea, "clammy" sweating, visual blurring and "graying out," tinnitus, lightheadedness, and dizziness. The patient appears ashen or pale and becomes diaphoretic. Mydriasis may occur with tachypnea and bradycardia. Witnesses frequently note that the victim's "eyes rolled back into the head," reflecting fading extraocular muscle tone. The patient becomes diffusely weak and hypotonic and, as consciousness is lost, falls to the ground with lack of protective reflexes if unsupported. Within seconds to minutes, once the patient is horizontal, color, pulse, and consciousness return. During the anoxic phase, before the patient recovers consciousness, a few myoclonic jerks or even more rhythmic, clonic movements may appear. Such a syncopal convulsion is common and often leads to erroneous reports of epileptic seizures. Sequelae include continued nausea and generalized malaise, but drowsiness, confusion, and amnesia are limited.

Syncopal Myoclonus

These common clinical features have been confirmed by video analysis of syncope induced in healthy volunteers through ocular pressure, hyperventilation, and Valsalva maneuver.[49] Typical prodromal symptoms were blurred vision, dizziness, vertigo, and nausea. Average duration of loss of consciousness was about 12 seconds, and myoclonic activity (syncopal convulsions) occurred in 38/42 syncopal episodes. Automatisms were observed in nearly 80%. Opened eyes and upward eye deviation were also common. Auditory and visual hallucinations, not usually elicited in previous studies, were reported in 60%. Postictally, transient amnesia occurred in 1 of 42 individuals, but cognitive sequelae were otherwise unremarkable. In none of these normal individuals nor in other studies of induced syncopal convulsions in patients did incontinence occur.[2,34,49]

Of the manifestations of syncope, convulsive movements are potentially the most confounding because they raise the question of epileptic seizures. Studies of syncopal convulsions induced in patients during cardiac electrophysiology studies,[2] positive tilt-table studies,[34] and in healthy volunteers[49] describe a prevalence of 45% to 90%.

Myoclonic activity during a syncopal convulsion is usually multifocal and arrhythmic, but generalized, rhythmic myoclonus is also common.[36,49] In our experience, biased by patients admitted for diagnosis in epilepsy monitoring units, dystonic posturing similar to that of a complex partial seizure is not unusual and adds further difficulty in the purely visual distinction between syncopal and epileptic motor activity. This opinion is supported by a large study (694 individuals) of symptoms provoked by tilt-table testing; 8% of participants with positive results ($n = 222$) had "neurologic events" consistent with the clinical behaviors of tonic–clonic seizures, focal seizures, or dysarthria or aphasia.[63]

Electroencephalographic Appearance

Electroencephalographic recordings document the electrophysiologic correlates of syncopal convulsions. In patients with vasovagal syncope who have attacks induced by tilt-table, the electroencephalogram (EEG) demonstrates gradual development of high-amplitude 3- to 5-Hz slowing during prodromal symptoms. Slow-wave frequency decreases to 1- to 3-Hz activity with loss of consciousness.[36] In recordings of cardiac syncope caused by ventricular arrhythmias,[2] electrographic findings are more variable and sometimes feature marked attenuation of cortical activity with loss of consciousness, although in most cases, rhythmic slowing occurs before voltage attenuation. The changes in EEG occur about 10 to 15 seconds after development of arrhythmia. It is of interest that brain-slice preparations deprived of oxygen show a time of onset to isoelectric activity of about 7 minutes,[64] which implies that corticothalamic activity comprising scalp EEG is more susceptible to hypoxia than individual cortical neurons. Normal background activity returns quickly with restoration of circulation and return of consciousness. Myoclonic activity has no consistent relationship with the EEG changes, and could occur either before or after EEG attenuation.[2] In neither study were epileptiform or ictal discharges observed.[2,36] Both the duration of loss of consciousness and postsyncopal confusion are linearly related to the duration of cardiac dysfunction.[2] Figures 1 and 2 demonstrate typical EEG accompaniments in syncope induced by cardiac asystole and in reflex bradycardia induced by breath-holding.

DIFFERENTIAL DIAGNOSIS

Because neurologists and epileptologists can be expected to see a more selected patient group than cardiologists, general practitioners, and emergency room physicians, the bulk of this discussion focuses on the separation of neurologic causes of syncope from other etiologies. However, because neurologic causes are relatively infrequent, a discussion of the differential diagnosis of syncope is undertaken first.

As Table 1 shows, even a brief listing of causes of syncope can be daunting. A more concise method is to group the myriad causes onto five main categories: (a) disorders of orthostatic intolerance; (b) primary cardiac dysfunction; (c) transient neurologic dysfunction; (d) metabolic derangement; and (e) psychiatric syndromes. The relative frequency of these diagnostic groups as they present in emergency rooms and other primary care facilities is shown in Table 2.

Disorders of Orthostatic Intolerance

Disorders of the homeostatic mechanisms of blood pressure maintenance comprise a large portion of syncope seen by physicians. In these disorders, the unifying pathophysiology is the abnormal or insufficient response of the peripheral vascular system and in reflex cardiac mechanisms to internal or external stimuli.

To briefly review, on standing, about 300 to 800 mL (about 25% of total blood volume) is displaced downward from the thorax. Reduced pressure is detected by receptors in the carotid sinus and aortic arch and within cardiac and pulmonary tissues. Tonic central sympathetic inhibition decreases, which allows an increase in peripheral vascular resistance and an increase in heart rate as mediated by medullary cardiovascular control centers.[81] Defects in this regulatory system lead to orthostatic hypotension, which can be due to degeneration of the autonomic nervous system either centrally, as in Shy-Drager syndrome, or peripherally as the result of acquired or hereditary neuropathies. An intact autonomic nervous system, on the other hand, may be unable to compensate for conditions causing hypovolemia, such as anemia or dehydration. Elderly patients have particular problems with compensatory cardiovascular regulation and are vulnerable to orthostasis whatever the cause.[43]

One of the more important causes of syncope in older people is orthostatic hypotension induced by drugs. In a study of elderly, institutionalized patients, hypotensive adverse effects

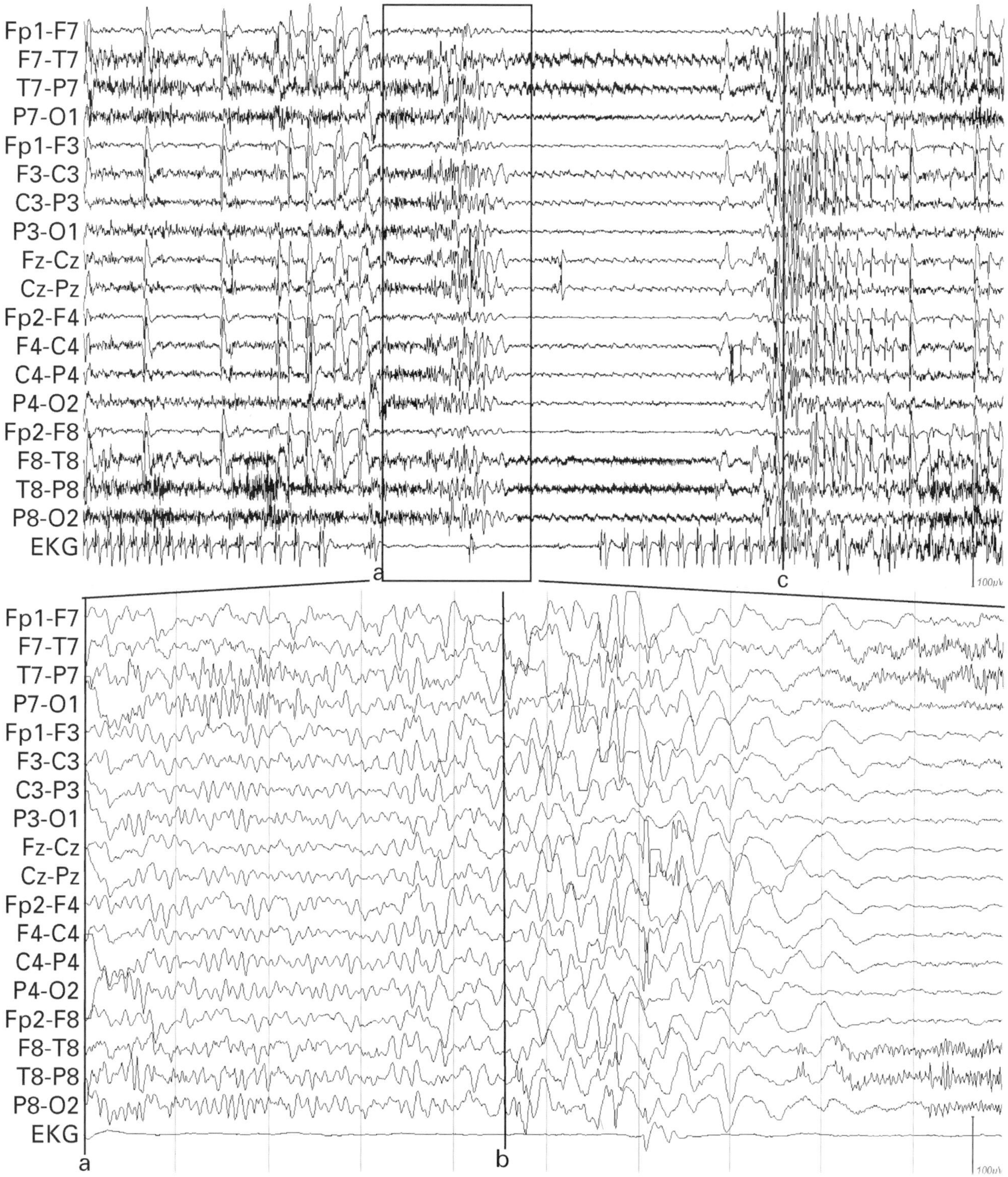

FIGURE 1. Electroencephalographic (EEG) excerpts from intensive video-EEG diagnosis of syncopal convulsion following spontaneous asystole in a patient who had undergone treatment for 1 year for presumptive epileptic seizures. The top panel shows a 60-second page with the box indicating the 10-second page excerpt in the bottom panel. The EEG starts with the patient in her normal, awake state while lying in bed. At time point a, the ECG channel shows the onset of asystole. The patient experiences clinical onset at point b marked by behavioral arrest and bilateral, dystonic posturing. The EEG, typical in response to cerebral hypoperfusion, develops abrupt, generalized slowing approximately 5 seconds after the last heartbeat, followed by generalized attenuation. Note the lack of epileptiform discharges despite the apparent motor activities of a complex partial seizure. Symptoms resolve at point c about 10 seconds following the return of normal sinus rhythm. The lags from ECG to EEG and clinical changes are typical for syncope and represent a combination of cardiac output and cerebral perfusion volume.

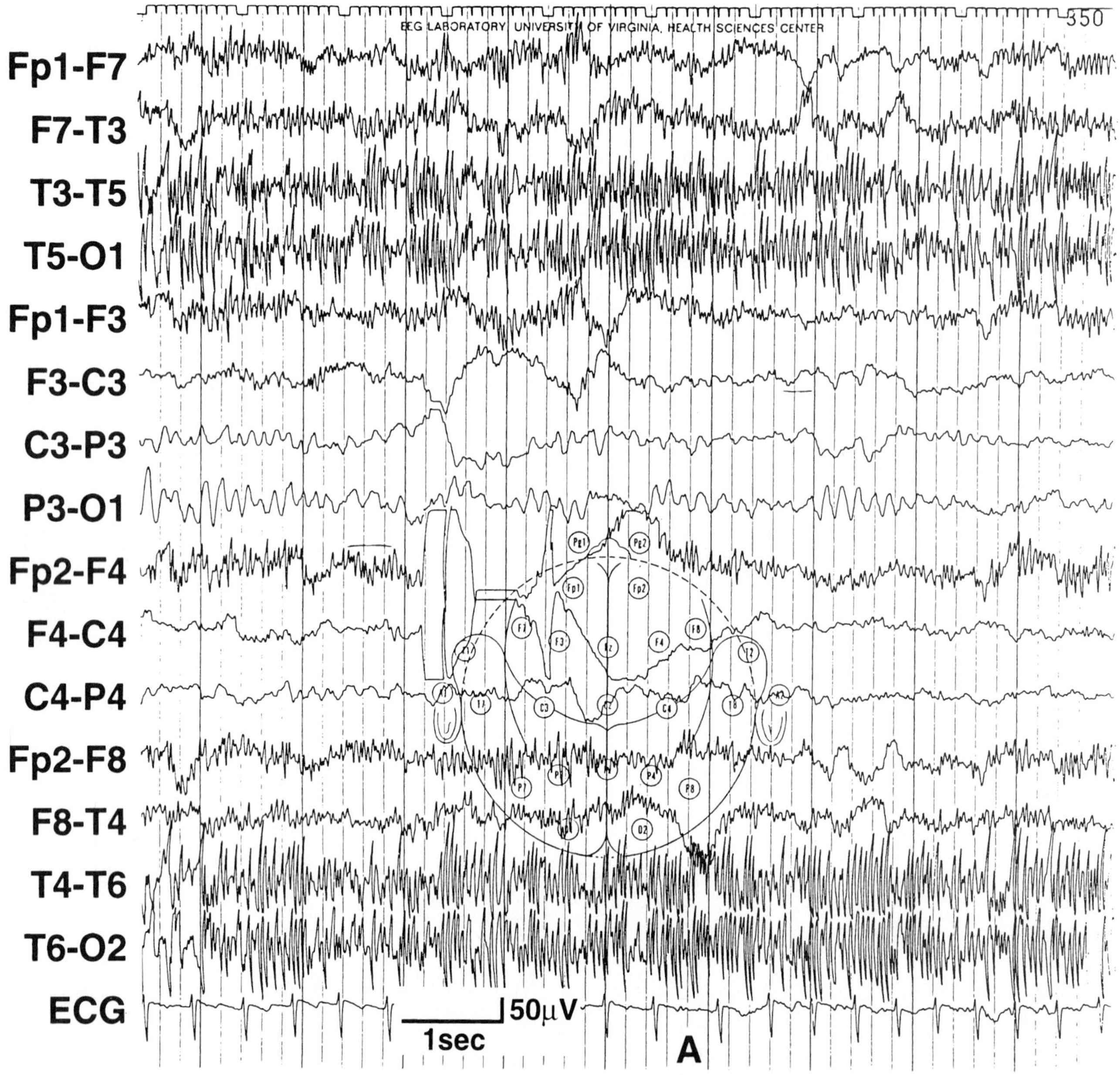

FIGURE 2. Breath-holding spell in a 15-month-old resulting in asystole, syncope, and brief convulsion recorded with continuous-telemetry electroencephalogram and simultaneous video recording. **A:** Patient, held in mother's arms, is crying while the technician re-gels the electrodes. (*Continued*)

of drugs caused 8 of 32 cases of noncardiogenic syncope.[52] Nitrates, levodopa, and thioridazine were cited this study, but any new medication, especially one that antagonizes the alpha-1 receptor such as amitriptyline or chlorpromazine, should be suspect in any elderly patient with syncope.

Current consensus divides disorders of orthostatic intolerance into three groups, as follows.[3]

Reflex Syncope

Reflex syncope is a group of disorders that occur because of a sudden failure of the cardioregulatory system to maintain adequate vascular tone during orthostatic stress, resulting in hypotension that is frequently associated with bradycardia.

Neurocardiogenic syncope (or vasovagal syncope) is a reflex syncope believed to result from an inappropriately hypercontractile response of the heart to abrupt venous pooling. The resulting state mimics hypertension and causes a compensatory but pathologic bradycardia, initiating syncope.[35] In susceptible individuals, neurocardiogenic syncope is triggered by strong emotions such as fear or follows painful stimuli such as venipuncture, dental procedures,[22] or prostate exams.[5] Sometimes the precipitating event is merely a prolonged upright stance, as is frequently required of soldiers standing at attention. In this situation, there is also the confounding variable of venous pooling in the legs because gastrocnemius and soleus muscle contraction ceases. Soldiers who are taught to keep their knees slightly flexed and to intermittently contract their leg muscles are at much lower risk of syncope.

Hypersensitivity of peripheral visceral afferents, whether idiopathic or the result of trauma or tumor, is another mechanism of reflex syncope. Asystole after carotid massage is the hallmark of carotid sinus hypersensitivity. Neuralgic syncope is associated with tumors or other pathology of the

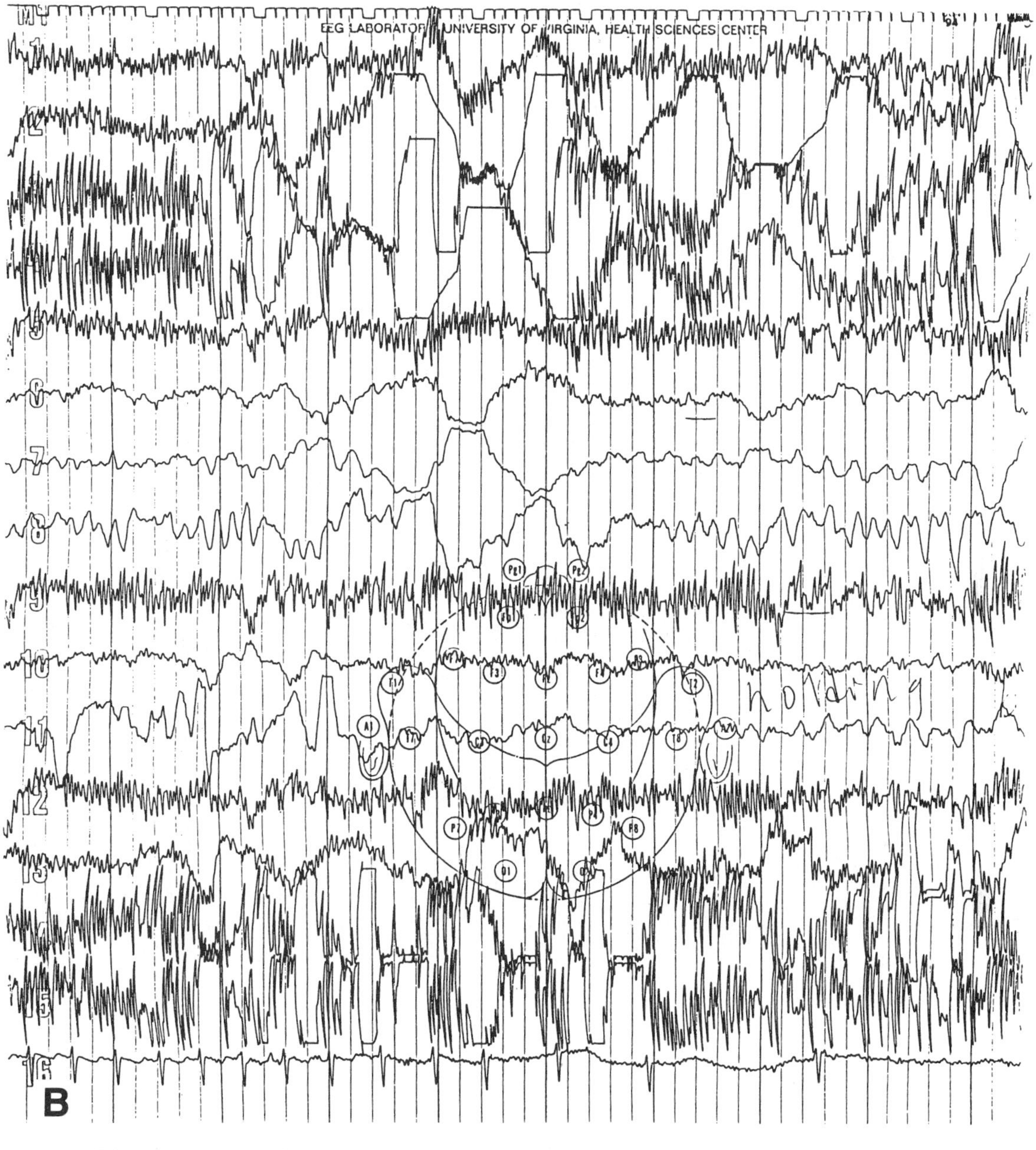

FIGURE 2. (*Continued*) **B:** Crying abruptly stops, and several seconds later, the technician notes that the patient is not breathing. (*Continued*)

glossopharyngeal nerve, and there are rare cases of syncope associated with trigeminal neuralgia well.[40]

A variety of seemingly prosaic activities such as coughing, micturition, defecation, and breath-holding are all subsumed under the term situational syncope. Each stimulus, as in the Valsalva maneuver, leads to syncope through neurally mediated vasodepression analogous to vasovagal syncope. Micturition syncope may in addition reflect the relief of pressure exerted by the bladder on the inferior vena cava producing a transient decrease in venous return.

Autonomic Failure

Autonomic failure, either from primary degeneration of the autonomic nervous system, as in Shy-Drager syndrome (multiple-system atrophy) or that secondary to peripheral neuropathies, is the second major category of disorders of orthostatic intolerance.

Pure autonomic failure syndrome[27] is a chronic, insidious-onset disease with syncope as one major symptom accompanied by other failures of the autonomic nervous system (anhydrosis, impotence, etc.) that, unlike multiple-system atrophy, is not accompanied by a movement disorder or cognitive deficits.[27]

Other autonomic failure syndromes are usually attributable to small-fiber peripheral neuropathies resulting from such diseases as diabetes mellitus or paraneoplastic syndromes. In the case of diabetes mellitus, autonomic neuropathies can present quite early and severely coincident with other evidence of the disease.[72]

Postural Orthostatic Tachycardia Syndrome

Postural orthostatic tachycardia syndrome (POTS) is the third major category of orthostatic intolerance and consists of excessive increases in heart rate in the upright position.[35] The

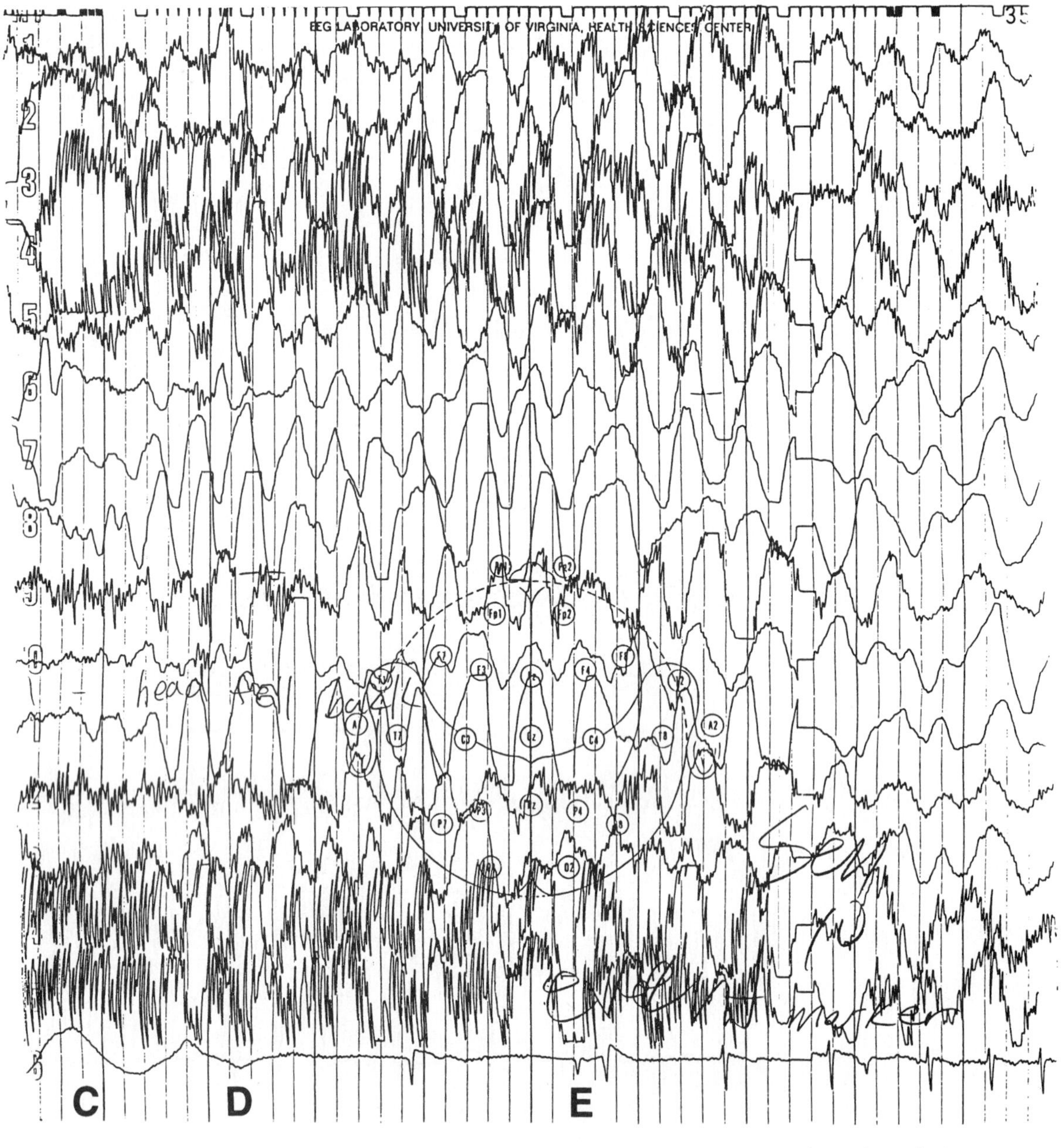

FIGURE 2. (*Continued*) **C:** The patient becomes limp and is unresponsive. **D:** A single axial myoclonic jerk is seen. **E:** The patient abruptly resumes crying. (*Continued*)

partial dysautonomic form is believed to be due to insufficient increases in peripheral vascular resistance on standing and may be a precursor to more severe primary autonomic failure. The second form consists of an initially appropriate tachycardic response to standing that does not "turn off," thus causing symptoms of presyncope and palpitations along with postural hypertension and tachycardia. The latter is often called beta-hypersensitivity syndrome because isoproterenol infusion causes a marked increase in heart rate. Investigation is underway to confirm a genetically mediated basis for these disorders.[73]

Primary Cardiac Dysfunction

Cardiac causes comprise disorders of pump failure caused by obstructed outflow, impaired cardiac filling, shunting, myocardial ischemia, or arrhythmias. The large but not all-inclusive list shown in Table 1 includes typical primary and secondary causes of episodic pump failure. Most of these disorders are distinguished from epilepsy by standard and invasive electrophysiologic tests or by specific aspects of the history or physical examination.[41]

The long-QT syndrome of Romano-Ward is an autosomal-dominant disorder of cardiac repolarization that results in ventricular tachycardias leading to palpitations, syncope, and sudden death. It is a channelopathy of cardiac hERG potassium or voltage-gated sodium channels[71] that is easily confused with epilepsy because patients are often young and usually have had unprovoked syncopal convulsions and the family history reveals similarly affected relatives. Other genetic long-QT syndromes, such as the Jervell-Lange-Nielsen syndrome, have different modes of inheritance and different channel abnormalities.[1] The electrocardiogram (ECG) is diagnostic, demonstrating a long, corrected QT interval. A large number of drugs and other precipitants have more recently been associated with acquired prolonged-QT syndromes.[69] These latter patients may not have prolongation of repolarization at

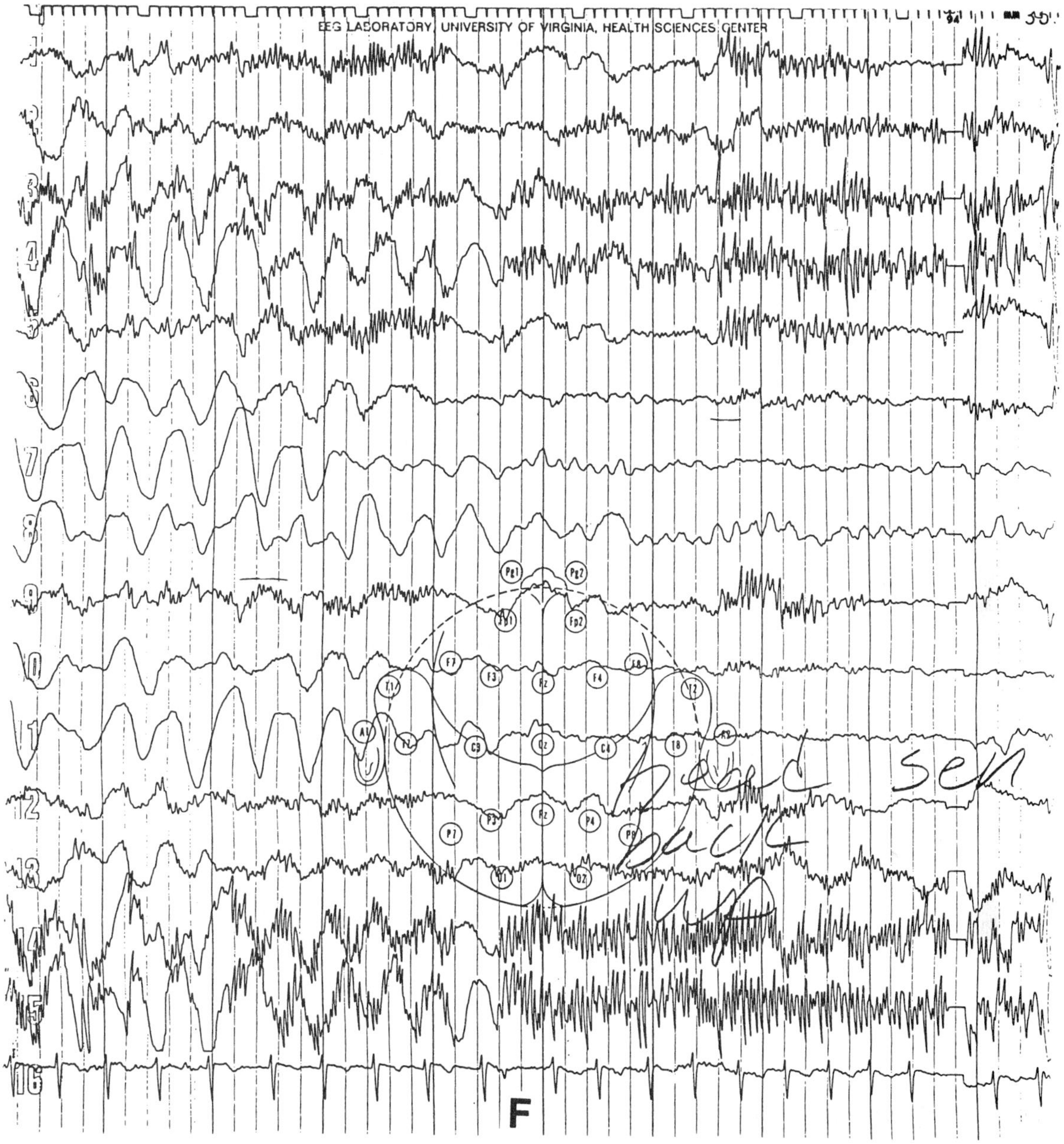

FIGURE 2. (*Continued*) **F:** Normal tone returns. The tracing demonstrates that breath-holding precedes bradycardia/asystole by approximately 6 seconds. Generalized rhythmic delta activity gradually builds up during the event and, after ECG activity and crying resume, gradually resolves. (Adapted from figures provided courtesy of Ted Burns, M.D., Neuromuscular/Autonomic Testing Division, Department of Neurology, University of Virginia.)

baseline. One should also consider the Brugada syndrome, an autosomal-dominant disorder consisting of syncope, sudden death, ECG with ST-segment elevation, and an appearance similar to a right-bundle-branch block in the anterior leads.[80]

Especially in adolescents and young adults, one should also consider arrhythmogenic right ventricular dysplasia as a cause of syncope.[12]

Metabolic Disorders

Metabolic disorders usually cause loss or alteration of consciousness that is more indolent and longer lasting than the relatively abrupt, transient impairment with rapid, spontaneous resolution that characterizes typical syncope. As a correlate of this observation, brain-slice preparations take five times longer to reach isoelectric potentials when deprived of glucose as opposed to oxygen.[64] Thus, most metabolic disorders are more suited to a discussion of delirium or coma. For example, although hypoglycemia is frequently cited as a cause of syncope, reports of proved hypoglycemic syncope are rare.[7] Glucose tolerance tests were not positive in any of 121 patients tested in one study.[42] More common in the modern emergency room is intoxication due to alcohol or other drugs presenting as syncope.[1,21,41]

Psychiatric Disorders

Psychiatric disorders, especially depression and panic disorder, were the cause of syncope in 24% of patients referred to a specialized syncope clinic.[50] Conversion reaction and somatization are other psychiatric causes of syncope.[14,21,41] In contrast to patients with physiologic syncope, psychiatric patients are said to be relatively younger, have a higher recurrence rate, and are more often disabled by attacks.[50] Vertigo, rather than lightheadedness and disequilibrium, is more frequent in younger patients with psychiatric syncope.[75]

TABLE 1

CAUSES OF SYNCOPE BY ETIOLOGY

- Disorders of orthostatic intolerance
  - Reflex syncope
    - Neurocardiogenic/vasovagal
    - Carotid hypersensitivity syndrome
    - Neuralgic
    - Situational
      - Micturation
      - Deglutation
      - Tussive
      - Breath-holding
      - Postexercise/postprandial
  - Autonomic failure
    - Shy-Drager/multiple-system atrophy
    - Parkinson disease
    - Pure autonomic failure
    - Peripheral and autonomic neuropathies
    - Postural orthostatic tachycardia syndrome
    - Partial dysautonomia
    - Primary beta-hypersensitivity
    - Hypovolemia
    - Drug induced
- Disorders of cardiac function
  - Impaired outflow
    - Idiopathic hypertrophic subaortic stenosis
    - Atrial myxoma
    - Aortic stenosis/dissection
    - Pulmonary hypertension
  - Impaired filling
    - Pericardial effusion
    - Pulmonary embolus
  - Shunt
    - R → L Shunt (tetrology of Fallot)
  - Ischemia
  - Bradyarrhythmias
    - Sick sinus
    - Second-degree heart block
    - Atrioventricular heart block
  - Tachyarrhythmias
    - Supraventricular
    - Ventricular
  - Long-QT syndromes
    - Familial (Romano-Ward, Lang-Jervell-Nielsen)
    - Drug induced
- Transient neurologic dysfunction
  - Seizure
  - Seizure-induced bradycardia/asystole
  - Migraine
  - Transient ischemic attack
- Transient metabolic dysfunction and other
  - Drug effects or intoxication
  - Hypocapnia/hyperventilation
  - Hypoglycemia
  - Psychiatric
    - Conversion disorder
    - Panic disorder

Epilepsy and Other Neurologic Disorders

Epileptic Seizures That Mimic Syncope

Transient neurologic causes of syncope, especially epileptic seizures, are relatively infrequent. In a study of cost-effectiveness, tests of neurologic function in 121 occurrences of syncope were not diagnostic in any.[42] Nevertheless, the more unusual neurologic causes of syncope must be differentiated from the more common nonneurologic etiologies.

Complicating the differential diagnosis is the fact that convulsions following syncope are commonplace.[2,36,49] Syncopal convulsions are briefer than generalized tonic–clonic seizures, do not have extended rhythmic clonic jerking, recover rapidly, and lack postictal symptoms.[36] Normal orientation immediately or shortly after the event is a helpful clue to the diagnosis of syncope,[37] although recovery after atonic or frontal lobe seizures may be rapid. Conversely, if hypoxia produced by syncope is more severe or prolonged than usual, recovery may be slower than anticipated.

A variety of epileptic seizures may mimic the loss of tone and consciousness that are salient features of syncope. Some seizure types are more frequently confused with syncope than others. A subset of complex partial seizures, misleadingly termed temporal lobe syncope, can present with sudden drops or falls with or without prodromal symptoms but are followed by confusion, amnesia, and gradual recovery.[15] Scalp recordings suggest that temporal lobe syncope may have an extratemporal localization despite the name.[15] For example, six of seven epilepsy surgery patients who experienced drop attacks and who also suffered from focal motor seizures of the face and arm had seizures localized to the sensorimotor facial area.[48] On the other hand, temporal localization has been described in patients with temporal lobe epilepsy who developed drops and falls late in the course of previously manageable complex partial seizures.[28,67] The development of epileptic drop attacks is a poor prognostic sign, not only of the morbidity from fall-related injuries, but in its implication for future seizure control in the face of loss of inhibitory mechanisms that mediate rapid secondary propagation of seizure activity. Studies of volumetric magnetic resonance imaging (MRI) in patients with mesial atrophy demonstrate that extensive mesial atrophy, especially amygdalar atrophy, correlate with secondary generalization and temporal lobe syncope.[32]

Patients with the Lennox-Gastaut syndrome and other epileptic encephalopathies commonly have atonic seizures. These are frequently the source of greatest morbidity and are usually refractory to antiepileptic drug treatment. They can take the form of brief head nods or of sudden myoclonic jerks followed by atonia (myoclonic–astatic seizures).[19] EEG/video recordings of epileptic drop attacks reveal that the majority take the form of tonic "axial spasms," analogous to an adult version of infantile spasms, with rapid, moderate flexion axially followed by a tonic phase during the fall. The anatomic substrate for these events may be the lower brainstem.[23] Care must be taken in evaluating an exacerbation of epileptic drop attacks because drug intoxication or vasovagal syncope and other form of syncope can coexist.

Seizure-induced Asystole, Bradyarythmias, or Ventricular Tachycardias

A rare cause of syncope is a seizure-induced cardiac asystole or arrhythmia. Simultaneous EEG/ECG recordings have documented cases of asystole following photic-stimulation–induced spike-wave[60] and asystole, supraventricular tachycardia, and bradyarrhythmias following temporal lobe ictal discharges,[11,31,66,68,70] to give a few examples. Asystole

TABLE 2

CAUSES OF SYNCOPE BY FREQUENCY AS SEEN IN EMERGENCY ROOMS

	Kapoor 1990[41]	Eagle et al. 1985[21]	Day et al. 1982[14]	Total	Percent
Cardiovascular volume/tone					
Vasovagal	35	64	57	156	19.3
Other	89	16	9	114	14.1
Cardiac	110	15	17	142	17.6
Neurologic					
Seizure	7	2	58	67	8.3
Other	8	3	5	16	2.0
Metabolic/other	5	7	27	39	4.8
Unknown	179	69	25	273	33.8
Total	433	176	198	807	100.0

during seizures is probably more frequent with left hemispheric foci.[68]

The pathophysiology of ictal arrhythmias is not well understood but may involve cardiac efferents that are stimulated by insular, limbic, and midbrain cardiopedal pathways.[58] Autonomic instability and subsequent cardiac arrest induced by an ictal discharge has been invoked as a mechanism of sudden unexpected death in epilepsy,[46] a finding supported by animal studies that show that epileptic triggering of hypothalamic and mesencephalic cardiovascular control centers by focal application of penicillin G causes cardiovascular instability and bradyarrhythmias.[53]

Ambulatory EEG/ECG monitoring of patients with epilepsy, however, has demonstrated that cardiac dysrhythmias do not occur at an increased rate compared to the general population.[44] The frequency of ictal and interictal discharges has little relation to the generation of cardiac rhythm abnormalities.[44] The usual cardiac response to a seizure is sinus tachycardia that seems to be more dependent on the volume of brain involved in the ictal discharge than on the location of seizure onset.[25] Thus, despite well-documented "epileptic syncope," such cases appear to be more like unlucky exceptions rather than useful models for sudden epileptic death.

One epileptic syndrome in which syncope is a frequent complication is Panayiotopoulos syndrome.[61] In this idiopathic, childhood epilepsy, autonomic seizures start with emesis and may proceed to ictal syncope. Because symptoms may last >30 minutes (thus qualifying as autonomic status epilepticus),[61] the prolonged course and prominent parasympathetic involvement are helpful in differentiating it from the shorter course of typical syncope. It is not clear whether syncope in Panayiotopoulos syndrome results from bradycardia, decreases in peripheral resistance, or both.

Hypoperfusion-induced Seizures

The inverse problem to seizure-induced arrhythmias is the occasional seizure that is provoked by a cardiac arrhythmia,[39,57] presumably from the triggering of a latent seizure focus by decreased cerebral perfusion. Review of both confirmed and suspected cases of hypoperfusion-induced seizures in children shows that rare cases of prolonged bilateral clonus following syncope can be epileptic in origin rather than strictly limited to more typical, brief nonepileptic convulsions.[39] Because nonepileptic syncopal convulsions often mimic epileptic seizures,[63] simultaneous EEG/ECG recordings are the only way reliably to make these diagnoses.

Cerebrovascular Attacks

Neurologic syndromes other than epilepsy can be confused with syncope. Cerebrovascular disease and, specifically, transient ischemic attacks of vertebral-basilar origin can cause abrupt and transient loss of consciousness following interruption of blood flow to the brainstem. Concurrent symptoms helpful in diagnosis are vertigo, ataxia, and parasthesias. Although the posterior circulation is often the site for such symptomatic ischemic disease, bilateral carotid atherosclerosis has also been described.[13] As in cortical stroke syndromes, such patients have a high incidence of hypertension and heart disease.[13]

Basilar migraine is a syndrome that is most common in adolescents and young adults. Some patients have syncope before a severe occipital or vertex headache, but they usually have a variety of associated symptoms, including dizziness, visual phenomena, nausea, disequilibrium, and ataxia. The EEG occasionally shows occipital spikes or intermittent rhythmic delta activity.[17] Patients with basilar migraine can be confused with those with Panayiotopoulos syndrome[61] or other forms of benign occipital epilepsy.[29]

Cataplexy

Finally, cataplexy may occasionally be confused with syncope. As with vasovagal syncope, an emotional trigger sets off a typical attack. Unlike syncope, however, the loss of tone in cataplexy is not clearly accompanied by loss of consciousness. The other hallmarks of narcolepsy—daytime somnolence, hypnogogic hallucinations, and sleep paralysis—help to identify cataplexy as well.

DIAGNOSTIC EVALUATION

History

Because of the significant morbidity and mortality of cardiac syncope, the acute, emergency room evaluation of syncope centers on the distinction between cardiac and noncardiac causes. Risk stratification and protocols have come to bear on syncope evaluation. Table 3 divides syncope into high-, intermediate-, and low-risk groups based on history, physical, and baseline ECG findings used in prospective studies of the efficacy and cost–benefit relation of syncope protocols and specialized syncope units.[74]

Eliciting the critical elements of loss of consciousness and tone of a putative syncopal spell are important during

TABLE 3

EMERGENCY ROOM RISK STRATIFICATION OF SYNCOPE BASED ON HISTORY, PHYSICAL EXAMINATION, AND ELECTROCARDIOGRAM FINDINGS

High-risk group
Chest pain compatible with acute myocardial infarction
Signs of congestive heart failure
Valvular disease
History of ventricular arrhythmias
Electrocardiogram findings of ischemia
Prolonged QTc (>500 ms)
Trifascicular block
Persistent sinus bradycardia between 40 and 60 bpm
Atrial fibrillation and nonsustained ventricular tachycardia without symptoms
Cardiac devices (pacemaker or defibrillator) with dysfunction
Intermediate-risk group
Age ≥50 yr
With previous history of:
Coronary artery disease
Myocardial infarction
Congestive heart failure
Stable cardiomyopathy
Bundle-branch block or Q wave without acute changes on electrocardiogram
Family history of unexplained sudden death
Symptoms not consistent with a vasovagal cause
Cardiac devices without evidence of dysfunction
Physician's judgment that suspicion of cardiac syncope is reasonable
Low-risk group
Age <50 yr
With no previous history of:
Cardiovascular disease
Symptoms consistent with reflex-mediated or vasovagal syncope
Normal cardiovascular examination
Normal electrocardiogram findings

Source: Adapted from Shen WK, Decker WW, Smars PA, et al. Syncope Evaluation in the Emergency Department Study (SEEDS): a multidisciplinary approach to syncope management. *Circulation*. 2004;110:3636–3645, with permission.

tertiary evaluation. Certain clinical characteristics indicate particular syndromes. In a comparison of historical features that distinguished among ventricular tachycardia, atrioventricular block, and vasovagal syncope,[8] cardiac etiologies were suggested by male gender, old age, infrequent recurrence, and short or no prodromal symptoms. On the other hand, vasovagal syncope was more likely when prodromal symptoms were complex, including palpitations. Symptoms from vasovagal syncope tended to persist longer than those from cardiac syncope.

A key to distinguishing reflex syncope from other disorders is a "trigger," that is, an event such as sudden standing, fright, or pain that can initiate an abnormal or insufficient response of the autonomic nervous system. Other triggers may be elusive, and diagnosis may hinge on uncovering subtle signs such as grunting before episodes, as occasionally happens with children who have breath-holding spells.

The timing of certain triggers, specifically exercise, in relationship to syncope is a particularly important historical feature. In a study of 474 young athletes who were surveyed on aspects of syncope, syncope was nonexertional in 87%, postexertional in 12%, and exertional in 1.3%. Two of the 6 athletes with exertional syncope had structural cardiac disease, and the remaining 4 had positive tilt-table tests. In contrast, no adverse events occurred in nonexertional or postexertional syncope despite recurrence rates of ~20 events per 1,000 person-years.[10]

One confounding factor is that patients often cannot provide important historical details and witnesses may be lacking. Retrograde amnesia for the event, especially in the elderly, may be severe enough to have the patient present with falling with no memory of loss of consciousness.[62] In one study of carotid hypersensitivity syndrome, 95% of patients who presented with falling rather than syncope could not recall loss of consciousness following symptomatic carotid massage. In comparison, 12% of patients who presented with syncope recalled loss of consciousness. Similarly, in the evaluation of 65 patients in a specialty syncope clinic, 15% denied loss of consciousness despite subsequent typical syncopal episodes induced by a tilt table. Furthermore, only 58% of patients could recall events immediately before the attack, suggesting that retrograde amnesia may be frequent,[55] although postictal confusion is either brief or absent following syncope in contrast to an epileptic seizure.[36,49]

The presence and quality of prodromal symptoms can be confounding. Falls, lightheadedness, and vertigo often overlap in the presenting symptoms.[55,75] "Dizziness," for example, is a confusing term both linguistically and diagnostically, and patients mean different things by them, as do physicians.[55,75] Up to two thirds of patients with syncope say that their main problem is "dizziness."[75] When prompted by a standard questionnaire, 68% of patients with proved syncope had presyncopal lightheadedness, 55% reported disequilibrium, and 35% had vertigo, with some patients having more than one symptom.[75] Patients who complained solely of vertigo tended to be young and have a psychiatric cause for their symptoms.[75]

Some clinicians emphasize that the predictive value of prodromal symptoms are too low to usefully distinguish cardiac from other causes. Instead, they emphasize event triggers. Of note, no prospective assessment of the predictive value of history has been performed.

Physical Examination

Findings on physical examination help to diagnose some cases of syncope. Orthostatic hypotension is defined as a 20-mm Hg drop in systolic pressure or sinus bradycardia when standing.[55] Carotid massage followed by 3 or more seconds of asystole or a 50-mm Hg drop in blood pressure suggests carotid hypersensitivity.[55] Although one should be cautious in the patient with carotid bruits or at a high risk for carotid atherosclerosis, carotid massage is generally a safe procedure under supervised circumstances with appropriate monitoring. Bárány or Hallpike maneuvers can help to identify patients with vestibular dysfunction and vertigo. Nystagmus may suggest drugs or indicate central or peripheral vesicular dysfunction, depending on the direction, latency, and reproducibility.

The ECG is the significant helpful screening electrophysiologic test for cardiac causes of syncope.[41] Although one half of 433 patients with syncope had ECG abnormalities, these were diagnostic in only a small number of cases. In patients with arrhythmias, the routine ECG was diagnostic in 30% of cases.

Prolonged ECG monitoring using a Holter monitor, event recorder, or loop recorder is another common diagnostic test. Although <5% of patients have symptomatic arrhythmias during extended ECG, Kapoor[41] reported a diagnostic yield of 22% when screening for arrhythmias.

Implantable loop recorders have recently become available and marketed to neurologists. These devices have a battery life of approximately 14 months and record and store a

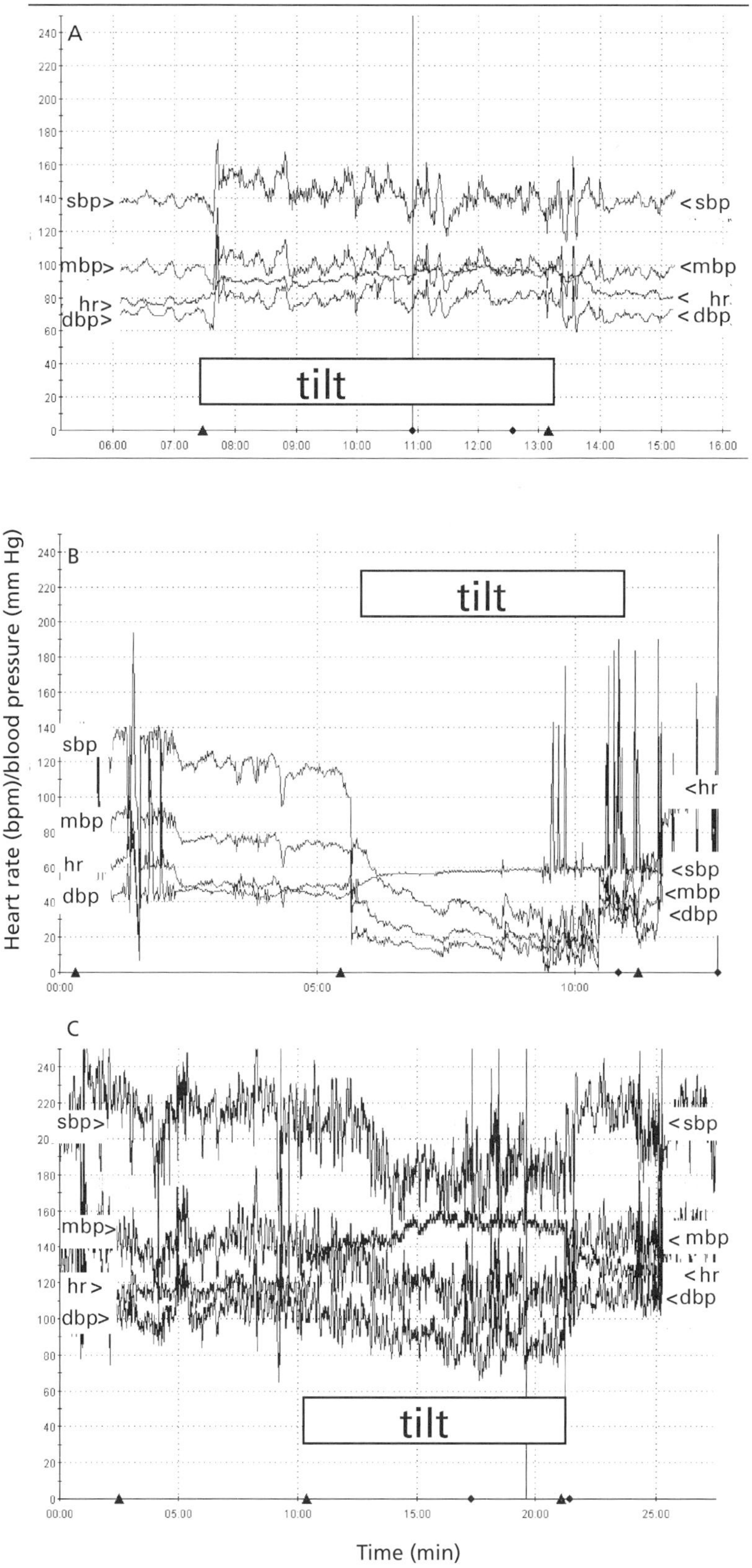

FIGURE 3. Findings in tilt-table testing. **A:** Normal tilt-table response. In response to abrupt vertical positioning of the tilt table, heart rate (hr) increases are limited to 15% to 30% of the horizontal rate because of the appropriate compensatory increase of peripheral vascular resistance, as denoted by the ~10% increase in diastolic blood pressure (dbp). **B:** A patient with Parkinsonism demonstrates central and peripheral postural hypotension marked by a severe drop in peripheral vascular resistance (with corresponding drops in systolic [sbp], mean [mbp], and diastolic blood pressures) accompanied by insufficient compensatory tachycardic response. **C:** A woman with small-cell breast cancer demonstrates positional tachycardia syndrome (POTS) marked by baseline hypertension, a relative hypotension with tilt, and an excessive tachycardic response. (Adapted from figures provided courtesy of Ted Burns, M.D., Neuromuscular/Autonomic Testing Division, Department of Neurology, University of Virginia.)

single-lead ECG when activated by a patient event button at the time of symptoms. Some clinicians recommend early use of implantable loop recorders when cardiac syncope is suspected and when events are rare rather than withholding it until other modes of testing have been exhausted. In early use, implantable recorders yield positive diagnoses in >50% of cases after a 1-year recording duration and in >80% after 2 years.[54]

Invasive electrophysiologic testing has been advocated in the subset of syncopal patients with heart disease[41] because these patients are most likely to have a positive test and the worst prognosis if untreated. With any of the electrophysiologic tests, the diagnostic value of an arrhythmia that does not reproduce symptoms is debatable.

Echocardiography, although frequently used in the diagnostic evaluation of patients with syncope, is best reserved for patients found to have cardiac abnormalities on physical examination or in the course of other studies.[65]

Head-up tilt-table testing, with or without augmentation using isoproterenol, has gained favor because of its usefulness in diagnosing vasovagal syncope.[36] Tilt-table testing (Fig. 3), performed in combination with testing of vagal function, allows localization of orthostatic insufficiency into sympathetic or parasympathetic systems. Although controversies surround its specificity and sensitivity, tilt-table testing is safe in experienced hands. Guidelines for its application have been published.[4]

In most cases, routine EEG has a low diagnostic yield, especially in initial screening.[41] In those patients in whom a seizure is suspected, however, the EEG is of course a useful tool. In one study, the EEG provided useful information in only 12% of patients with suspected nonneurologic causes. On the other hand, the EEG yielded diagnostically helpful findings in 41% of patients suspected of having neurologic disease.[14] A comparison of patients with either epilepsy or syncope demonstrated that findings of focal epileptiform discharges, generalized epileptiform discharges, or focal slowing offered a sensitivity of 40% and a specificity of 95% in distinguishing between these two groups.[38]

The utility of routine brain imaging is also limited. Most studies evaluating the emergent diagnosis of syncope[14,21,41] have found that head computed tomography, when not guided by clinical data, had a poor diagnostic yield. Information is not available, however, regarding MRI, MR angiography, and functional MR.

If the clinical event occurred within 1 hour, elevated serum prolactin levels have been proposed to aid in the distinction between seizure and syncope,[18,82] but the most recent studies give conflicting results, suggesting that this assay may not reliably aid in differential diagnosis.[59]

Finally, as mentioned earlier, intensive telemetry with simultaneous EEG/ECG recording may establish a definitive diagnosis if the events are frequent and confounding enough to merit the costs incurred in such a study. Of note, most cases in which unusual cardioarrhythmic seizures have been documented were captured fortuitously, not through purposeful prolonged monitoring. With the development of implantable electrocortigraphy devices, perhaps long-term monitoring analogous to that of implantable ECG loop recorders will fill this clinical need.

TREATMENT

Treatment of syncope is as varied as the range of possible etiologies. A few statements regarding the treatment of autonomic insufficiency, such as found in the Shy-Drager syndrome, severe polyneuropathy, or idiopathic orthostatic hypotension, deserve mention. Measures to expand volume, such as increased fluid intake and salt ingestion, are often sufficient to ameliorate mild cases. The addition of compression stockings or, with more severe cases, of leg-to-waist customized support garments may be necessary. Fludrocortisone, a mineralocorticoid, will aid in volume expansion provided that due caution is allowed for possible congestive heart failure or recumbent hypertension. Biofeedback training may occasionally be a useful adjunct to more traditional measures.[6]

The development of the tilt-table test has led to a variety of pharmacologic treatments for refractory vasovagal syncope.[77] Beta-blockade is usually tried first, although the use of a beta-blocker for syncope seems at first counterintuitive. Nonetheless, the strategy works in a majority of patients with tilt-table–positive vasovagal syncope,[77] although the mechanism of efficacy is not clearly understood. Beta-blockade may attenuate the hyperactive response of cardiac mechanoreceptors thought to be in part responsible for vasovagal syncope.[36,77] Disopyramide has combined inotropic, anticholinergic, and vasoconstrictive effects and is occasionally used.[77] Anticholinergic drugs such as scopolamine are sometimes efficacious but are poorly tolerated by the elderly as a rule. A double-blind clinical trial failed to show efficacy of transdermal scopolamine.[47] Cardiac pacing is sometimes performed for severe and refractory cases but is often ineffective.[77] Methylphenidate is occasionally worth trying.[33]

When syncope is unpredictable, the patient and other people may be placed at risk by common activities such as driving. A position statement on this issue is available.[24]

SUMMARY AND CONCLUSIONS

In conclusion, syncope consists of loss of consciousness and muscle tone that is abrupt in onset, of short duration, and followed by rapid recovery. Syncope occurs in response to transient impairment of cerebral perfusion. Typical prodromal symptoms often herald onset of syncope, and postictal symptoms are minimal. Syncopal convulsions, resulting from cerebral anoxia, are common but are not a form of epilepsy, nor are there any accompanying EEG ictal discharges. Diagnosis is based on the history, physical, examination, and ECG findings. A major emphasis should be on distinguishing cardiac from noncardiac causes of syncope because of excess mortality of the former. Despite intensive study, one third of all syncope cases remain undiagnosed.

References

1. Ackerman MJ. Cardiac causes of sudden unexpected death in children and their relationship to seizures and syncope: Genetic testing for cardiac electropathies. *Semin Pediatr Neurol.* 2005;12:52–58.
2. Aminoff MJ, Scheinman MM, Griffin JC, et al. Electrocerebral accompaniments of syncope associated with malignant ventricular arrhythmias. *Ann Intern Med.* 1988;108:791–796.
3. Anonymous. Consensus Committee of the American Autonomic Society and the American Academy of Neurology on the Definition of Orthostatic Hypotension, Pure Autonomic Failure and Multiple System Atrophy. *Neurology.* 1996;46:1470–1471.
4. Benditt D, Ferguson D, Grubb B. Tilt table testing for assessing syncope. *J Am Coll Cardiol.* 1996;28:263–275.
5. Bilbro RH. Syncope after prostatic examination. *N Engl J Med.* 1970; 282:167–168.
6. Bouvette CM, McPhee BR, Opfer-Gehrking TL, et al. Role of physical countermeasures in the management of orthostatic hypotension: efficacy and biofeedback augmentation. *Mayo Clin Proc.* 1996;71:847–853.
7. Burman WJ, McDermott MT, Bornemann M. Familial hyperinsulinism presenting in adults. *Arch Intern Med.* 1992;152:2125–2127.
8. Calkins H, Shyr Y, Frumin H, et al. The value of the clinical history in the differentiation of syncope due to ventricular tachycardia, atrioventricular block, and neurocardiogenic syncope. *Am J Med.* 1995;98:365–373.
9. Casini-Raggi V, Bandinelli G, Lagi A. Vasovagal syncope in emergency room patients: analysis of a metropolitan area registry. *Neuroepidemiology.* 2002;21:287–291.
10. Colivicchi F, Ammirati F, Santini M. Epidemiology and prognostic implications of syncope in young competing athletes. *Eur Heart J.* 2004;25:1749–1753.
11. Constantin L, Martins JB, Fincham RW, et al. Bradycardia and syncope as manifestations of partial epilepsy. *J Am Coll Cardiol.* 1990;15:900–905.
12. Dalal D, Nasir K, Bomma C, et al. Arrhythmogenic right ventricular dysplasia: a United States experience. *Circulation.* 2005;112:3823–3832.
13. Davidson E, Rotenbeg Z, Fuchs J, et al. Transient ischemic attack–related syncope. *Clin Cardiol.* 1991;14:141–144.
14. Day S, Cook E, Funkenstein H. Evaluation and outcome of emergency room patients with transient loss of consciousness. *Am J Med.* 1982;73:15.
15. Delgado-Escueta AV, Bascal FE, Treiman DM. Complex partial seizures on closed circuit television and EEG: a study of 691 attacks in 79 patients. *Ann Neurol.* 1982;57:292–300.

16. Del Greco M, Cozzio S, Scillieri M, et al. Diagnostic pathway of syncope and analysis of the impact of guidelines in a district general hospital. The ECSIT study (Epidemiology and Costs of Syncope in Trento). *Ital Heart J.* 2003;4:99–106.
17. De Romanis F, Buzzi MG, Assenza S. Basilar migraine with electroencephalographic findings of occipital spike-wave complexes; a long-term study in seven children. *Cephalalgia.* 1993;13:192–196.
18. Dirik E, Sen A, Anal O, et al. Serum cortisol and prolactin levels in childhood paroxysmal disorders. *Acta Paediatr Jpn.* 1996;38:118–120.
19. Dreifuss FE. Lennox-Gastaut syndrome. In: Dreifuss FE, ed. *Pediatric Epileptology: Classification and Management of Seizures in the Child.* Boston: Wright PSG; 1983.
20. Driscoll DJ, Jacobsen SJ, Porter CJ, et al. Syncope in children and adolescents. *J Am Coll Cardiol.* 1997;29:1039–1045.
21. Eagle K, Black H, Cook E, et al. Evaluation of prognostic classifications for patients with syncope. *Am J Med.* 1985;79:455–460.
22. Edmondson H, Gordon P, Lloyd J, et al. Vasovagal episodes in the dental surgery. *J Dentistry.* 1978;6:189–195.
23. Egli M, Mothersill I, O'Kane M, et al. The axial spasm—the predominant type of drop seizure in patients with secondarily generalized epilepsy. *Epilepsia.* 1985;26:401–415.
24. Epstein AE, Miles WM, Benditt DG. Personal and public safety issues related to arrhythmias that may affect consciousness: implications for regulation and physician recommendations. A medical/scientific statement from the American Heart Association and the North American Society of Pacing and Electrophysiology. *Circulation.* 1996;94:1147–1166.
25. Epstein MA, Sperling MR, O'Connor MJ. Cardiac rhythm during temporal lobe seizure. *Neurology.* 1992;42:50–53.
26. Farwell DJ, Sulke AN. Does the use of a syncope diagnostic protocol improve the investigation and management of syncope? *Heart.* 2004;90:52–58.
27. Freeman R. Pure autonomic failure. In Robertson D, Biaggiona I, eds. *Disorders of the Autonomic Nervous System.* Luxembourg: Harwood Academic; 1995:83–106.
28. Gambardella A, Reutens D, Andermann F. Late-onset drop attacks in temporal lobe epilepsy: a reevaluation of the concept of temporal lobe syncope. *Neurology.* 1994;44:1074–1078.
29. Gastaut H. Benign epilepsy of childhood with occipital paroxysms. In: Roger J, Dravet C, Bureau F, eds. *Epileptic Syndromes in Infancy, Childhood and Adolescence.* London: John Libby; 1985:170–179.
30. Getchell WS, Larsen GC, Morris CD, et al. Epidemiology of syncope in hospitalized patients. *J Gen Intern Med.* 1999;14:677–687.
31. Gilchrist J. Arrythmiogenic seizures: diagnosis by simultaneous EEG/ECG recording. *Neurology.* 1985;35:1503–1506.
32. Gotman J, Cendes F, Andermann F. The relation of spike foci and of clinical seizure characteristics to different patterns of mesial temporal atrophy. *Arch Neurol.* 1995;52:287–293.
33. Grubb B, Kosinski D, Mouhaffel A, et al. The use of methylphenydate in the treatment of refractory neurocardiogenic syncope. *Pacing Clin Electrophysiol.* 1996;19:836–840.
34. Grubb B, Kosinski D, Samoil D. Recurrent unexplained syncope: the role of head-upright tilt table testing. *Heart Lung.* 1993;22:502–508.
35. Grubb BP. Neurocardiogenic syncope and related disorders of orthostatic intolerance. *Circulation.* 2005;111:2997–3006.
36. Grubb BP, Gerard G, Roush K, et al. Differentiation of convulsive syncope and epilepsy with head-up tilt testing. *Ann Intern Med.* 1991;115:871–876.
37. Hoefnagels W, Padberg G, Overweg J, et al. Transient loss of consciousness: the value of the history for distinguishing seizure from syncope. *J Neurol.* 1991;238:39–43.
38. Hoefnagels WA, Padberg GW, Overweg J, et al. Syncope or seizure? The diagnostic value of the EEG and hyperventilation test in transient loss of consciousness. *J Neurol Neurosurg Psychiatry.* 1991;54:953–956.
39. Horrocks A, Nechay A, Stephenson JBP. Anoxic epileptic seizures: observational study of epileptic seizures induced by syncope. *Arch Dis Child.* In press.
40. Kapoor W, Jannetta P. Trigeminal neuralgia associated with seizure and syncope. Case report. *J Neurosurg.* 1984;61:594–595.
41. Kapoor WN. Evaluation and outcome of patients with syncope. *Medicine.* 1990;69:160–175.
42. Kapoor WN, Hanusa BH. Is syncope a risk factor for poor outcomes? Comparison of patients with and without syncope. *Am J Med.* 1996;100:646–655.
43. Kapoor WN, Snustad D, Peterson J, et al. Syncope in the elderly. *Am J Med.* 1986;80:419–428.
44. Keilson MJ, Hauser WA, Magrill JP. ECG abnormalities in patients with epilepsy. *Neurology.* 1987;37:1624–1626.
45. Krahn AD, Klein GJ, Yee R, et al. Cost implications of testing strategy in patients with syncope: randomized assessment of syncope trial. *J Am Coll Cardiol.* 2003;42:495–501.
46. Lathers CM, Schraeder PL. Autonomic dysfunction in epilepsy: characterization of autonomic cardiac neural discharges associated with PTZ-induced epileptogenic activity. *Epilepsia.* 1982;23:633–647.
47. Lee TM, Su SF, Chen MF, et al. Usefulness of transdermal scopolamine for vasovagal syncope. *Am J Cardiol.* 1996;78:480–482.
48. Lehman R, Andermann F, Tandon P, et al. Seizures with onset in the sensorimotor face area: Clinical patterns and results of surgical treatment in 20 patients. *Epilepsia.* 1994;35:1117–1124.
49. Lempert T, Bauer M, Schmidt D. Syncope: a videometric analysis of 56 episodes of transient cerebral hypoxia. *Ann Neurol.* 1994;36:233–237.
50. Linzer M, Perry AJ, Varia I, et al. Psychiatric syncope: A new look at an old disease. *Psychosomatics.* 1990;31:181–188.
51. Linzer M, Pontinen M, Gold DT, et al. Impairment of physical and psychosocial function in recurrent syncope. *J Clin Epidemiol.* 1991;44:1037–1043.
52. Lipsitz L, Wei J, Rowe J. Syncope in an elderly, institutionalised population: prevalence, incidence, and associated risk. *Q J Med.* 1985;55:45–54.
53. Mameli O, Melis F, Giraudi D, et al. The brainstem cardioarrhythmogenic triggers and their possible role in sudden epileptic death. *Epilepsy Res.* 1993;15:171–178.
54. Mason PK, Wood MA, Reese DB, et al. Usefulness of implantable loop recorders in office-based practice for evaluation of syncope in patients with and without structural heart disease. *Am J Cardiol.* 2003;92:1127–1129.
55. McIntosh S, DaCosta D, Kenny RA. Outcome of an integrated approach to the investigation of dizziness, falls and syncope in elderly patients referred to a 'syncope' clinic. *Age Ageing.* 1993;22:53–58.
56. McLaren AJ, Lear J, Daniels RG. Collapse in an accident and emergency department. *J of R Soc Med.* 1994;87:138–139.
57. Mendes LA, Davidoff R. Cardiogenic seizure with bradyarrhythmia: documentation of the mechanism during asystole. *Am Heart J.* 1993;125:1786–1788.
58. Oppenheimer S. The anatomy and physiology of cortical mechanisms of cardiac control. *Stroke.* 1993;24(12 Suppl):I3–15.
59. Oribe E, Amini R, Nissenbaum E, et al. Serum prolactin concentrations are elevated after syncope. *Neurology.* 1996;47:60–62.
60. Ossentjuk E, Sterk CJO, van Leeeuwan S. Flicker-induced cardiac arrest in a patient with epilepsy. *Electroencephalogr Clin Neurophysiol.* 1966;20:257–259.
61. Panayiotopoulos CP. Autonomic seizures and autonomic status epilepticus peculiar to childhood: diagnosis and management. *Epilepsy Behav.* 2004;5:286–295.
62. Parry SW, Steen N, Baptist M, et al. Amnesia for loss of consciousness in carotid sinus syndrome. *J Am Coll Cardiol.* 2005;45:1840–1843.
63. Passman R, Horvath G, Thomas J, et al. Clinical spectrum and prevalence of neurologic events provoked by tilt table testing. *Arch Intern Med.* 2003;163:1945–1948.
64. Rabinovici GD, Lukatch HS, MacIver MB. Hypoglycemic and hypoxic modulation of cortical micro-EEG activity in rat brain slices. *Clin Neurophysiol.* 2000;111:112–121.
65. Recchia D, Barzilai B. Echocardiography in the evaluation of patients with syncope. *J Gen Intern Med.* 1995;10:649–655.
66. Reeves AL, Nollet KE, Klass DW, et al. The ictal bradycardia syndrome. *Epilepsia.* 1996;37:983–987.
67. Reutens DC, Andermann F, Cendes F, et al. Late-onset drop attacks in temporal lobe epilepsy: a reevaluation of the concept of temporal lobe syncope. *Neurology.* 1994;44:1074–1078.
68. Rocamora R, Kurthen M, Lickfett L, et al. Cardiac asystole in epilepsy: Clinical and neurophysiologic features. *Epilepsia.* 2005;44:179–185.
69. Roden DM, Viswanathan PC. Genetics of acquired long qt syndrome. *J Clin Invest.* 2005;115:2025–2032.
70. Rossetti AO, Dworetzky BA, Madsen JR, et al. Ictal asystole with convulsive syncope mimicking secondary generalisation: a depth electrode study. *J Neurol Neurosurg Psychiatry.* 2005;76:885–887.
71. Russell MW, Dick M. The molecular genetics of the congenital long QT syndromes. *Curr Opin Cardiol.* 1996;11:45–51.
72. Said G, Goulon-Goeau C, Slama G, et al. Severe early-onset polyneuropathy in insulin-dependent diabetes mellitus. A clinical and pathological study. *N Engl J Med.* 1992;326:1257–1263.
73. Shannon J, Flatten NL, Jordan T, et al. Orthostatic intolerance and tachycardia associated with norepinephrine-transporter deficiency. *N Engl J Med.* 2000;342:541–549.
74. Shen WK, Decker WW, Smars PA, et al. Syncope Evaluation in the Emergency Department Study (SEEDS): a multidisciplinary approach to syncope management. *Circulation.* 2004;110:3636–3645.
75. Sloane PD, Linzer M, Pontinen M, et al. Clinical significance of a dizziness history in medical patients with syncope. *Arch Intern Med.* 1991;151:1625–1628.
76. Soteriades ES, Evans JC, Larson MG, et al. Incidence and prognosis of syncope. *N Engl J Med.* 2002;347:878–885.
77. Sra JS, Jazayeri MR, Dhala A. Neurocardiogenic syncope: diagnosis, mechanisms and treatment. *Cardiol Clin.* 1993;11:183–191.
78. Sun BC, Emond JA, Camargo CA Jr. Characteristics and admission patterns of patients presenting with syncope to U.S. emergency departments, 1992–2000. *Acad Emerg Med.* 2004;11:1029–1034.
79. Sun BC, Emond JA, Camargo CA Jr. Direct medical costs of syncope-related hospitalizations in the United States. *Am J Cardiol.* 2005;95:668–671.
80. Vincent GM. The long QT and Brugada syndromes: causes of unexpected syncope and sudden cardiac death in children and young adults. *Semin Pediatr Neurol.* 2005;12:12–24.
81. Wieling W, VanLieshout JJ. Maintenance of postural normotension in humans. In: Low P, ed. *Clinical Autonomic Disorder.* Philadelphia: Lippincott-Raven; 1997:73–82.
82. Zelnik N, Kahana L, Rafael A, et al. Prolactin and cortisol levels in various paroxysmal disorders in childhood. *Pediatrics.* 1991;88:486–489.

CHAPTER 272 ■ METABOLIC AND ENDOCRINE DISORDERS RESEMBLING SEIZURES

PETER W. KAPLAN AND SHEHZAD BASARIA

INTRODUCTION

Patients frequently consult a physician because of alarming "spells." These may consist of symptoms such as sudden malaise, a feeling of faintness, flushing, a perceptibly irregular or rapid heart beat, dizziness, sweating, confusion, as well as myriad other alarming complaints. The physician's task is to differentiate psychological from organic complaints and potentially dangerous from benign symptoms and to localize the symptoms to a particular system of the body—cerebrovascular, neurologic, endocrine, or other. When patients are seen with lip smacking, loss of consciousness, prolonged jerking movements, and tongue biting, the diagnosis of a tonic–clonic seizure is straightforward. More difficult diagnostic problems occur when the complaints are subjective, as with symptoms of autonomic or sensory origin, because objective confirmation of disease may be lacking, and the subjective perceptions (e.g., feelings of dissociation, anxiety, or panic) are often difficult to put into words.

Among the many entities considered in the differential diagnosis of "spells" are those associated with metabolic and endocrine disturbances, some of which have proved to be among the "great imitators" of other diseases, including hysteria. Endocrine or metabolic disturbances may in themselves cause seizures, or they may exacerbate epilepsies by lowering seizure thresholds. The primary emphasis of this chapter is on metabolic and endocrine disturbances that result in symptoms that may be mistaken for seizures.

GENERAL COMMENTS REGARDING PATIENT HISTORY

Spells associated with many endocrine disturbances are characteristically accompanied by other features of the endocrine disease. For example, patients with spells caused by thyrotoxicosis usually have tremulousness, weight loss, and sweating in addition to palpitations and anxiety attacks. In other endocrine or metabolic disturbances, however, few clinical signs may be present. In such cases, attention must be paid to the particular precipitating factors, pattern, course, duration, and resolution of the spell in the context of the patient's medical history. For example, in a patient who has undergone gastric surgery, the malaise, sweating, and light-headedness occurring at fixed intervals after meals should alert the physician to the possibility of reactive hypoglycemia with "dumping syndrome." Similarly, patients with diabetes who are taking oral hypoglycemic agents or insulin may have the same symptomatology resulting from episodic hypoglycemia. Typical settings would be a lower-than-usual caloric intake, or unanticipated exercise without appropriate changes in insulin. In these cases, symptomatic hypoglycemia may supervene over the ensuing hours. Conversely, hyperglycemia may appear with intercurrent illness and decreased insulin dosage.

Particular inquiry into dietary habits, medications, and prior medical problems or surgery, therefore, is essential in making the appropriate diagnosis.

With some diseases, the constellation of signs and symptoms may provide the physician with a diagnosis through "pattern recognition." For example, intermittent severe abdominal pain and episodes of limb paralysis, delirium, and "port wine"–colored urine are typical features of an acute intermittent porphyric crisis. A history of previous similar attacks, possibly triggered by drugs, should be sought. In a similar vein, the simultaneous occurrence of paroxysmal headache, facial flushing, and hypertension will evoke the diagnosis of pheochromocytoma.

SPECIFIC METABOLIC AND ENDOCRINE DISORDERS

Hypoglycemia

Because the central nervous system requires a constant supply of glucose, hypoglycemia may produce transient neurologic dysfunction[51] that can be mistaken for or even precipitate seizures. When delivery of glucose to the central nervous system is insufficient, a number of signs and symptoms may appear (Table 1). The particular array of clinical features may vary with the rapidity of development of hypoglycemia and the depth of hypoglycemia, as may the degree of impairment and level of consciousness. The symptoms of hypoglycemia are generally divided into adrenergic symptoms and neuroglycopenic symptoms. The former include anxiety, nervousness, palpitations, diaphoresis, and tremors. Neuroglycopenic symptoms include lethargy, disorientation, confusion, blurry vision, stupor, and in severe cases seizures and coma. In rare cases, focal weakness may also be seen.

The symptoms of falling levels of blood glucose usually occur episodically, and the diagnosis rests on demonstrating subnormal levels of blood sugar in the symptomatic patient. Some patients may lose the warning symptoms[17] and adapt to the sensations that accompany hypoglycemia. This is known as "hypoglycemia unawareness." Patients particularly at risk are the elderly,[70] those taking adrenergic blocking agents,[47] and patients who have a history of frequent hypoglycemic attacks. The variability in the threshold at which particular patients experience symptoms is marked. Normal individuals when fasting may have a blood glucose concentration that falls below 45 mg/dL and remain asymptomatic; in contrast, some patients who have insulin-dependent diabetes mellitus and certain elderly patients become symptomatic when blood glucose

TABLE 1

SYMPTOMS OF HYPOGLYCEMIA IN INSULIN-DEPENDENT DIABETES MELLITUS

Sweating	Tremor
Blurred/double vision	Weakness
Confusion	Vertigo
Odd behavior	Anxiety
Perioral paresthesias	Hunger
Sensation of cold	Ataxia
Slurred speech	Palpitations

Source: From Bouloux P, Kaplan PW. *Imitators of Epilepsy.* New York: Demos; 1994:201, with permission.

levels descend toward 45 mg/dL.[50,51] Diagnosis of symptomatic hypoglycemia, therefore, lies in determining a low plasma glucose level in the symptomatic patient, with relief effected when blood glucose concentrations are normalized (Whipple's triad).[73] It is important to appreciate that some poorly controlled diabetics (who have marked hyperglycemia) experience hypoglycemic symptoms (mostly adrenergic symptoms) even when their glucose levels are lowered toward normal. It is interesting that with better glycemic control, these symptoms resolve.

Causes of Hypoglycemia

The differential diagnosis of hypoglycemia includes the array of causes leading to the condition (Table 2). Because plasma glucose concentrations are affected by a number of agents, imbalance in these dynamic forces may cause hypoglycemia. In humans, there is a dynamic and often delicate balance between factors that increase blood glucose levels, such as epinephrine, cortisol, growth hormone, and glucagon, and factors that decrease glucose levels, including oral hypoglycemic agents, exogenous or endogenous insulin, and concurrent hepatic or renal disease. An excess of glucose-lowering agents or insufficiency of gluconeogenic mechanisms may result in symptomatic hypoglycemia. Common causes are oral hypoglycemic agents, excess exogenous or endogenous insulin, hepatic or renal disease, heavy alcohol use, a decrease in food intake, or unanticipated exercise in an insulin-dependent diabetic patient.[45] A number of drugs when taken concurrently may enhance or prolong the hypoglycemic effect of oral hypoglycemic agents or inhibit compensatory mechanisms of hepatic glucose release.[2] These include anticoagulants, beta-blockers, clofibrate, isoniazid, phenylbutazone, salicylates, and sulfonamides. Other drugs may precipitate hypoglycemia, including colchicine, disopyramide, haloperidol, paracetamol, pentamidine, perhexiline, and quinine. Insulin-treated patients may have hypoglycemic attacks as a result of missed meals, excess insulin dose, and exercise not compensated for by an increase in food intake or adjustment in insulin dose.

TABLE 2

CAUSES OF HYPOGLYCEMIA

Fasting hypoglycemia
- Exogenous hyperinsulinism
  - Sulfonylureas
  - Alcohol
- Endogenous hyperinsulinism
  - Insulinomas
  - Tumor production of insulin-like activity (IGF-2)
- Endocrine causes
- Adrenal insufficiency
- Growth hormone deficiency
- Miscellaneous disorders
  - Hepatic disease
  - Renal disease
- Hypoglycemias of infancy and childhood
  - Neonatal hypoglycemias
  - Congenital deficiencies of glucogenic enzymes
  - Ketotic hypoglycemia of childhood

Reactive hypoglycemia
- Enzyme deficiency of carbohydrate metabolism
  - Galactosemia
  - Hereditary fructose intolerance
  - Functional postprandial hypoglycemia

Source: Adapted from Bouloux P, Kaplan PW. *Imitators of Epilepsy.* New York: Demos; 1994:202, with permission.

Of the oral hypoglycemic agents, the sulfonylureas are the most notorious in causing hypoglycemia. The elderly and the patients with renal disease are particularly sensitive to sulfonylurea-induced hypoglycemia (due to decreased clearance of the drug). They are also the most common cause of factitious hypoglycemia. This surreptitious use is most commonly seen in medical personnel and persons with family members on these agents.[15]

Excessive long-term alcohol intake, resulting in chronic disease of the liver, also predisposes to hypoglycemia because glycogen stores are depleted.[42] Similarly, patients who have not eaten for several days and who have a binge of moderate to heavy drinking may also experience transient or even prolonged hypoglycemia up to 1 day after the end of the binge.

Hypoglycemia may occur in patients after gastric surgery, later than the symptoms of "dumping syndrome." Overactivity of the "enteroinsular axis" is thought to result in excessive release of glucose-dependent insulinotropic peptide (GIP) and other hormones, which in turn increase insulin secretion after ingestion of glucose.[66]

Other rare causes of hypoglycemia include endogenous hyperinsulinism caused by insulin-secreting tumors (insulinomas) of the pancreas.[34] Of such tumors, 10% are malignant, 10% are of questionable malignancy, and the rest are benign.[53] Patients with multiple endocrine neoplasia type I may have multiple tumors that secrete a variety of hormones, including pancreatic polypeptide, glucagon, gastrin, and somatostatin. Symptoms typically include blurred vision, double vision, sweating, palpitations, weakness, confusion, behavioral changes, obtundation, and tonic–clonic seizures. Patients with adrenal insufficiency and growth hormone deficiency may also present with hypoglycemia. Finally, tumor (nonislet)-induced hypoglycemia is seen in rare retroperitoneal mesenchymal tumors that elaborate insulin-like growth factor II (IGF-II). Surgical resection is the treatment of choice in these patients.

Diagnostic Investigation

When the diagnosis of symptomatic hypoglycemia has been made, determination of the particular cause depends largely on the medical and surgical history, evaluation of medications that are known to impair glucose regulation, and a physical examination.

In insulin-treated patients, the query is directed at the dose, timing, method, and location of subcutaneous administration (e.g., thigh, which has greater absorption, especially if the patient exercises). A frequent cause of inappropriate dosing is self-administration of insulin by patients with impaired vision. Syringes with larger writing are now available. Attention should also be directed at patients taking oral hypoglycemic agents or other newly introduced drugs that may interfere with glucose regulation. Surreptitious injection of insulin may be deduced by a high plasma insulin level with a low plasma C-peptide concentration. This contrasts with excessive endogenous insulin production, in which a high plasma insulin level is accompanied by an appropriately high C-peptide level. Both sulfonylureas and insulinomas result in elevated levels of plasma insulin and C-peptide levels. Hence, measurement of serum levels of sulfonylureas is an important part of the workup of hypoglycemia. If insulinoma is suspected, endoscopic ultrasound, magnetic resonance imaging of the abdomen, and arteriography are the main imaging modalities. Octreotide scan is not very sensitive. Percutaneous transhepatic portal venous sampling may be needed in some cases.

Treatment

Treatment of episodic hypoglycemia is based on treatment of the underlying cause. In patients treated with insulin and hypoglycemic agents, careful attention to modification of the regimen may prevent hypoglycemic dips. The aid of a specialist in diabetes should be sought. After gastric surgery, "dumping syndrome" may be avoided by more frequent and smaller meals containing complex carbohydrates. Insulin-secreting tumors are usually resected; if they are inoperable, octreotide, a long-acting somatostatin analog, may be used. If hypoglycemia is a manifestation of adrenal insufficiency, physiologic glucocorticoid replacement results in the resolution of hypoglycemia.

Association with Epileptic Seizures

Hypoglycemia itself may be the cause of seizures. In infants, these usually occur on the second postnatal day in newborns who are small for gestational age. Occasionally, hypoglycemia may be seen in infants of diabetic mothers and in cases of syndromes associated with defects of gluconeogenesis, defects of organic or amino acid metabolism, and mitochondrial dysfunction. Hypoglycemia may trigger tonic–clonic seizures and cause paroxysmal electroencephalographic (EEG) activity that can be confused with seizure activity.

Hyperglycemia

Hyperglycemia is a state that develops gradually, typically during a period of days to weeks. Because changes are gradual and usually progressive, these events are not often mistaken for an epileptic disturbance. Hyperglycemia in the absence of ketosis, however, may be associated with a number of abnormal movements, including asterixis, paroxysmal choreoathetosis, hemiplegia, and partial epileptic seizures.[38,56] Such partial seizures are typically motor, often exhibit a jacksonian march, and may be reflex seizures or effort induced. The seizures are resistant to antiepileptic drugs, but they usually regress on treatment of the hyperglycemia within a few hours to a few days.[7] Occasionally, partial seizures may continue for long periods in the state of epilepsia partialis continua.[22,56] Ketotic hyperglycemia is much less frequently associated with seizures, possibly because of the antiepileptic effect of ketosis.

Hypocalcemia

The predominant clinical features of hypocalcemia are the consequence of a decrease in ionized serum calcium, which in turn leads to an increase in neuromuscular excitability. This may be accompanied by numbness and tingling in the fingers, paresthesias, stiffness, muscle cramps, carpopedal spasm, and perioral numbness. Associated clinical features include papilledema, cataracts, developmental defects, and mental retardation in the congenital forms of the disease and calcification of the basal ganglia with dyskinesias. The electrocardiogram may show prolonged QT_c intervals and T-wave changes.

Several conditions may be accompanied by hypocalcemia, each with its own constellation of clinical features. Well-described causes include thyroid and parathyroid surgery, chronic renal failure, renal tubular acidosis, malabsorption, hypomagnesemia, blood transfusion, acute pancreatitis, osteomalacia or rickets, vitamin D deficiency, intake of chelating agents, and pseudohypoparathyroidism.

Bedside diagnostic features include the Chvostek sign (twitching of the lips or nasal alae, or even of the entire half of the face, produced by tapping the branches of the facial nerve as it passes through the parotid gland above the angle of the jaw). The diagnostic indicator is a low level of ionized serum calcium. The underlying cause of hypocalcemia should be sought.

Tetany is characterized by flexor spasms in the arms and extensor spasms in the legs; it may resemble tonic–clonic seizures and can be induced by hyperventilation. Both tetany and partial or tonic–clonic seizures may supervene.[18] Tonic–clonic seizures can be treated by administering a slow intravenous infusion of 15 mL of 10% calcium gluconate under cardiac monitoring.

Hypercalcemia

The most common cause of hypercalcemia is primary hyperparathyroidism. In this condition, hypercalcemia is generally mild and typically develops over a period of months to years; in most cases, patients are asymptomatic. In contrast, malignancy-induced hypercalcemia usually develops rapidly and can be severe and is accompanied variably by anorexia, nausea, vomiting, weight loss, and constipation. Neurologic symptoms are general fatigue, muscular weakness, and proximal myopathy, with mental status changes that include personality changes, depression, stupor, coma, and tonic–clonic seizures. The major causes of hypercalcemia are primary or tertiary hyperparathyroidism, humoral hypercalcemia of malignancy, multiple myeloma, paraneoplastic disorders, bone metastases, thyrotoxicosis, milk-alkali syndrome, vitamin D intoxication, immobilization, and rarely Paget disease of bone. Adrenal insufficiency and acromegaly are other rare endocrine causes of hypercalcemia.

Occasionally, a more acute hypercalcemia is characterized by paroxysmal headache, nausea, vomiting, abdominal pain, and constipation. Muscle weakness, lethargy, and coma may supervene. There may be visual impairment, tonic–clonic seizures, and spike-and-wave discharges over the occipital regions.[26]

The diagnosis of hypercalcemia is based on the finding of a raised level of ionized calcium. The next step is to measure serum levels of intact parathyroid hormone (iPTH). This test is fundamental to differentiating between parathyroid and non-parathyroid causes of hypercalcemia. An electrocardiogram may show a shortened QT_c duration.

The underlying cause should be sought and treated. Acute management of hypercalcemia includes hydration with saline, subcutaneous calcitonin, and intravenous bisphosphonates.

Excess of Growth Hormone

Paroxysmal attacks of sweating that occur with excess levels of growth hormone may be mistaken for autonomic seizures.[25] Sweating occurs due to increased concentration of sweat glands as a result of growth hormone excess. In contrast to autonomic seizures, paroxysms are not associated with other ictal manifestations.

Hyperthyroidism

The acute malaise, anxiety, sweating, tremulousness, and tachycardia of hyperthyroidism may mimic partial seizures,[52] as may choreiform movements and encephalopathy.[1,24] Features of the illness that suggest thyrotoxicosis include heat intolerance, weight loss despite a healthy appetite, hyperdefecation, goiter, exophthalmos, palpitations, atrial fibrillation, and muscle wasting and weakness. Proximal myopathy is the classical presentation of Graves disease. Patients with severe thyrotoxicosis (thyroid storm) may present with fever, stupor or coma, pyramidal and bulbar dysfunction, and convulsions.[31,41] It is important to appreciate that many elderly patients may not have any of the typical clinical features of hyperthyroidism (apathetic hyperthyroidism). Cardiac arrhythmias, like atrial fibrillation, may be the initial presentation in these subjects.

The most common causes of hyperthyroidism include Graves disease, solitary toxic adenoma, and toxic multinodular goiter (Plummer disease) Other etiologies of thyrotoxicosis include iodine-induced thyrotoxicosis, various thyroiditides, factitious thyrotoxicosis, and central hyperthyroidism (TSHomas). Large metastases of follicular thyroid cancer are a rare cause of thyrotoxicosis. The diagnosis is based on finding an undetectable or suppressed thyroid-stimulating hormone (TSH and increased T_3 or free T_4 levels. Imaging with radioactive iodine is the gold standard in determining the etiology of thyrotoxicosis.

Occasionally, choreiform movements and encephalopathies occur. Clinical seizures may rarely supervene, and partial motor, adversive, and tonic–clonic seizures are reported. A rare manifestation of hyperthyroidism is hypokalemic periodic paralysis, which may be confused with a seizure. This entity is predominantly seen in individuals of Asian decent, and Graves disease is the most common underlying etiology. The attacks may last for minutes to hours. Ingestion of a carbohydrate meal is a well-known trigger (the release of insulin being responsible for shifts in potassium).

Hypothyroidism

Hashimoto thyroiditis is the most common cause of primary hypothyroidism. Other causes include history of thyroid surgery, neck radiation, lithium therapy, and central hypothyroidism. General symptoms include dry skin, constipation, cold intolerance, sallow skin discoloration, ovulatory dysfunction, and minimal weight gain. Hypothyroidism may be accompanied by neurologic complaints, including neuropathy, myopathy, choreoathetosis, dementia, or even coma.[10,37,57] Sudden falls from arrhythmias secondary to hypothyroidism rarely occur.[40] There may be nocturnal jerking movements from obstructive sleep apnea and, more rarely, central sleep apnea. Comatose, hypothyroid patients may have tonic–clonic seizures. In severe hypothyroidism, patients may develop psychosis with hallucinations (myxedema madness). Myxedema coma remains the dreaded complication of severe hypothyroidism. It usually occurs in the elderly and has a high mortality rate. Intravenous thyroxine therapy is indicated in these cases.

Diagnosis rests on finding elevated TSH and low T_3 or free T_4 levels in cases of primary hypothyroidism. In secondary hypothyroidism due to pituitary dysfunction, TSH levels are low or inappropriately normal. Imaging of the pituitary with magnetic resonance imaging (MRI) is mandatory in such cases to rule out mass lesions. Treatment involves replacement of thyroid hormone.

Hashimoto Encephalopathy

Very few entities in neurology and endocrinology have puzzled and at the same time fascinated clinicians (more neurologists than endocrinologists). Hashimoto encephalopathy is one such entity. The story began in 1966 when Lord Brain, a famous English neurologist, described a case of a man with confusion, disorientation, and seizures.[6] The patient also had transient episodes of fluctuating hemiparesis of different extremities and aphasia, which completely resolved. Investigations revealed abnormalities in EEG, and cerebrospinal fluid (CSF) showed elevated levels of protein. Brain antibodies were not detected in the serum. This patient had known Hashimoto thyroiditis with positive antithyroid antibodies and was on optimal thyroxine therapy during these episodes. According to Lord Brain, "the apparent onset of Hashimoto's disease—was followed by an extraordinary and puzzling neurological illness which waxed and waned for over a year." He concluded, "antibody studies in future cases of unexplained encephalopathy should show whether we have described a syndrome or a coincidence."

Hashimoto encephalopathy remains a diagnosis of exclusion, which is usually entertained by a neurologist when a case of acute or subacute encephalopathy is seen in a patient with no evidence of other etiologies (infectious and metabolic causes excluded), positive antithyroid antibodies, and good clinical response to steroids. It is important, however, to appreciate that positive antithyroid antibodies are present in 10% of the U.S. population.[23] Hence, it is debatable whether Hashimoto encephalopathy is a distinct clinical entity or a coincidence of a rare encephalopathy that occurs in an individual with a common endocrinologic condition and a not uncommon circulating antibody. Furthermore, there is no evidence that antithyroid antibodies are directly responsible for the encephalopathy. As a result, some have suggested that this entity should be called "steroid-responsive encephalopathy associated with Hashimoto thyroiditis."

Three fourths of the cases of Hashimoto encephalopathy occur in women. Although many cases have mild hypothyroidism, many patients with encephalopathy are adequately treated with thyroxine. Furthermore, there is no correlation between the degree of hypothyroidism and the severity of encephalopathy. Clinical manifestations include headaches, fatigue, memory loss, confusion, and transient aphasia. Movement disorders like tremors, myoclonus, ataxia, and choreiform movements may be seen. Some patients experience auditory hallucinations. It is important that, as described by Lord Brain, many patients have signs and symptoms suggestive of stroke. The majority of these symptoms are episodic, with most of them resolving either spontaneously or with glucocorticoid therapy. Approximately 80% of the patients have elevated levels of protein in the CSF; however, pleocytosis is only seen rarely.[9] Abnormalities in the EEG are present almost universally and include diffuse slowing of the waves or epileptiform abnormality. The findings on MRI are nonspecific and include white matter changes. In some cases, cerebral angiography shows perfusion abnormalities of the cortex and basal ganglia.[16] The majority of the cases respond to steroids, an important aspect of this condition.

Carcinoid Tumors

The carcinoid syndrome is characterized by paroxysmal flushing, gastrointestinal hypermobility, bronchoconstriction, and right-sided cardiac valvular disease.[63] The paroxysmal flushing typically involves the face, neck, and upper trunk, producing a transient erythema and sensation of warmth, occasionally with palpitations. With more severe paroxysms, dizziness and rarely syncope can occur.[12] Other associated symptoms of gastrointestinal origin include diarrhea and abdominal cramps. This syndrome is produced by the release of serotonin from carcinoid tumors located in structures of the embryonic foregut (bronchus, pancreas, and stomach), midgut (duodenum and transverse colon), or hindgut (descending colon and rectum).[74] Rarely, carcinoid tumors only produce histamine, in which case, pruritis is the most common manifestation.

Carcinoid attacks may be induced by exertion, eating, emotional upset, and alcohol. The diagnosis is made by the finding of elevated levels of 5-hydroxyindoleacetic acid (5-HIAA), a serotonin metabolite, in the urine.[43] Recently, assays have been developed that measure serotonin levels in blood. Differentiation from simple partial seizures or auras in patients who experience flushing or heat sensation is made by the absence of subsequent confusion, automatisms, and convulsions that typify the progression of simple partial seizures to complex partial seizures; further distinguishing characteristics are the absence of bronchoconstriction, cardiac disease, diarrhea, and abdominal cramps. Nonetheless, ill-defined flushing or sensations of heat with upper gastrointestinal discomfort are seen with epileptic auras, and diagnostic confusion may occur.

Spiral computerized tomography (CT) of the chest and abdomen and an octreotide scan are the imaging modalities available. Treatment involves excision of the carcinoid tumors, when possible. Medical treatment, which is disappointing, involves blockade of the effects of secreted 5-hydroxyindoles with serotonin antagonists such as methysergide, α-methyldopa reduction of 5-hydroxytryptophan, or chemotherapy.

Pheochromocytomas

Pheochromocytomas are tumors that produce catecholamines, including norepinephrine, epinephrine, l-dopa, and dopamine. Ninety percent of these tumors arise in the adrenal medulla; the remaining 10% arise from extramedullary chromaffin tissue and are known as paragangliomas. In 10% of the cases the tumors occur bilaterally and may be malignant. Some are inherited as part of a multiglandular neoplastic syndrome (multiple endocrine neoplasia type II [MEN II]), von Hippel-Lindau disease, and von Recklinghausen disease.

Clinical presentation is typified by sudden headache, blurring of vision, hypertension, pallor, sweating, and malaise (Table 3).[59]

Poorly definable symptoms of sudden onset are suggestive of autonomic partial seizures or anxiety or panic attacks. The absence of confusional states, automatisms, and tonic–clonic seizures differentiates the spells from complex partial seizures and secondarily generalized tonic–clonic seizures. The clinical manifestations of pheochromocytoma, caused by tumor secretion of catecholamine,[32,54] which in turn stimulates adrenergic receptors, depend on the catecholamine or vasoactive neuropeptide produced: vasoactive intestinal peptide (VIP), calcitonin gene–related peptide (CGRP) and endothelin, neuropeptide Y, angiotensin II, and rarely corticotropin-releasing factor (CRF) and corticotropin (ACTH). Headaches occur in 80% of patients and are often accompanied by a sense of apprehension, tightness in the chest and abdomen, palpitations, and sweating.[62] Less frequently, nausea, vomiting, and generalized paresthesias occur. During the paroxysms, pallor or flushing and a sensation of warmth may occur with changes in heart rate. In rare cases in which the tumor preferentially secretes epinephrine or dopamine, the patients are normotensive and may even experience episodes of hypotension.

TABLE 3

SYMPTOM COMPLEX IN PHEOCHROMOCYTOMA

Headache	Sweating
Palpitations	Pallor
Tremor/trembling	Feeling of exhaustion
Anxiety	Epigastric and chest discomfort
Dyspnea	Flushing/warm feeling
Paresthesias	Tightness of throat
Convulsions	Nonspecific dizziness
Syncope	Faintness

Source: From Bouloux P, Kaplan PW. *Imitators of Epilepsy.* New York: Demos; 1994:205, with permission.

With their sudden brief onset (typically 15–20 minutes), often associated with a sensation of impending doom, these spells may resemble complex partial seizures, but the absence of true confusional states and the more frequent occurrence of sudden headache, hypertension, visual dysfunction, and vomiting differentiate the symptoms of pheochromocytoma from those of complex partial seizures.

The diagnosis of pheochromocytoma is based on the demonstration of inappropriate catecholamine secretion in blood and urine or abnormal secretion of urinary metabolites. Computed tomography or magnetic resonance imaging may localize tumors, as may the chromaffin-seeking radioactive nuclide ^{131}I-metaiodobenzyl guanidine.[55]

Paroxysms may occur spontaneously or with movement that induces release of vasoactive peptides/catecholamine from the tumors. Movements that displace abdominal contents including straining, lifting, and bending forward, and any strenuous exercise may precipitate spells.

Treatment is by surgical excision of the tumors after complete pharmacologic alpha- and beta-blockade.

Menopausal Vasomotor Flushes

Menopause is frequently accompanied by agitation, anxiety, depression, and hot flushes, associated with increases in levels of gonadotropins.[8] Flushes are not accompanied by impaired consciousness or other features of complex partial seizures. Autonomic seizures, for which they may be mistaken, are usually accompanied by sweating, dilated pupils, salivation, and changes in heart rate, respiration rate, and blood pressure, and they rarely occur without other seizure manifestations. Symptoms may be alleviated by estrogen replacement therapy.

Porphyrias

Porphyrias are disorders of porphyrin metabolism and heme biosynthesis caused by inherited enzyme defects.[5,35] The absence of particular enzymes in heme synthesis leads to the accumulation of psychoactive and neurotoxic metabolites that produce a wide spectrum of acute, subacute, and chronic neurologic changes. The manifestations of subacute changes may resemble seizures.

TABLE 4

CLINICAL FEATURES OF ACUTE INTERMITTENT PORPHYRIA: COMPARISON OF PERCENTAGE INCIDENCE BEFORE PUBERTY, IN ADOLESCENCE, AND IN ADULTHOOD

	Adult cases				Pediatric cases	
	Waldenström[68] (321 cases)	Markovitz[33] (69 cases)	Goldberg[19] (50 cases)	Stein and Tschudy[58] (46 cases)	0–14 yr (37 cases)	15–19 yr (35 cases)
Male patients	40	39	38	26	57	26
Female patients	60	61	62	74	43	74
Abdominal pain	85	95	94	95	97	94
Vomiting	59	52	78	43	70	49
Constipation	48	46	74	48	46	37
Limb pain				50	22	40
Fever	37	36	14	9[a]	51	43
Hypertension	40	49	54	36	38	57
Tachycardia	28	51	64	80[a]	68	66
Mental changes	55	80[b]	58	40[a]	51	74
Limb paresis	42	72	68	60[a]	51	74
Bulbar/respiratory paresis		37		10	14	34
Hyporeflexia	16[c]		54	29[a]	57	69
Seizures	10		16	20[a]	30	34
Death	30	58	24	9.5	16	37

[a]Based on 34 cases.
[b]Includes seizures.
[c]Areflexia.
Source: From Kaplan PW, Lewis DV. Juvenile acute intermittent porphyria with hypercholesterolemia and epilepsy: a case report and review of the literature. *J Child Neurol.* 1986;1:38–45, with permission.

Acute Intermittent Porphyria

Acute intermittent porphyria (AIP), the porphyric syndrome most frequently confused with seizures, is most commonly seen in Sweden.[68,69] Inherited as a mendelian dominant trait, the syndrome can occur with a number of mutations that result in defectiveness of the enzyme porphobilinogen deaminase (PBGD). Although it was originally described in young adults after the onset of puberty, it has been increasingly recognized in children. Among adults, it affects women twice as often as men, whereas in children, it affects both sexes equally.[27] The incidence of clinical features and seizures in pediatric and adult patients undergoing medical treatment is given in Table 4.

Acute attacks may be heralded for years by "nervousness" and tiredness. Attacks may last for days to weeks and are characterized by symptoms that can be referred to psychic, autonomic, and peripheral nerve dysfunction.[68] Dominating the clinical picture are abdominal pain, constipation, and tachycardia. Other clinical features are optic atrophy, ocular palsies, hoarseness, general malaise, lethargy, and coma. During the attack, there may be an agitated delirium with hallucinations and psychosis. Isolated neuropathies, with wrist or foot drop progressing to a flaccid limb paralysis, may supervene and take months to regress.

In the early stages of the crisis, the psychosis and encephalopathy may dominate in the absence of the other typical features of porphyria, although the classic "port wine"–colored urine may appear.[35,65,71]

Porphyria Cutanea Tarda

Porphyria cutanea tarda (PCT), caused by a deficiency of uroporphyrinogen decarboxylase in the liver, is characterized by the presence of urocarboxylic and heptacarboxylic porphyrins in the urine and isocoproporphyrin in the feces. It usually does not occur with acute neuropsychiatric symptoms, but it may be associated with hallucinations and dysphoria and, occasionally, seizures.[29,30] Seizures may be precipitated in patients with epilepsy from other causes who are being treated with porphyrinogenic antiepileptic drugs. It is differentiated clinically from AIP by the presence of skin lesions. Exposed areas of the skin, face, and hands are photosensitive, resulting in ulcerative vesicular eruptions. Coexisting liver disease and diabetes further complicate the diagnosis, which is based on a urinary porphyrin screen. Valproate and gabapentin have been safely used to treat seizures in PCT,[11,29] but valproate has precipitated attacks in AIP.

Variegate Porphyria

Variegate porphyria is the term used by Dean and Barnes[13] to denote the condition of patients from South Africa, who have a mixed clinical picture of photosensitivity, as in PCT, and neurologic episodes, as in AIP. Variegate porphyria is associated with urinary porphobilinogen and D-aminolevulinic acid (D-ALA) and fecal protoporphyrin and coproporphyrin. Episodes can result in sudden hallucinosis, psychosis, and catatonic states, as well as seizures.[13,44] It may be precipitated by oral contraceptives.

Hereditary Coproporphyria

Hereditary coproporphyria (HC), the rarest of the hepatic porphyrias, is characterized by fecal and urinary excretion of coproporphyrin. It may start in childhood, be precipitated by barbiturates and sulfonamides, and be manifested in crises with hypertension, abdominal pain, tachycardia, constipation, confusion, and delirium.[4] Subacute and acute neuropathies may lead to limb paralysis. Epileptic seizures frequently occur, often predating the first diagnosed porphyric crisis.[20]

Treatment

There are three aspects to the treatment of porphyria: (a) avoidance of all drugs known to be porphyrinogenic; (b) interruption of an attack by preventing induction of D-ALA synthetase with a high intake of carbohydrate or administration of intravenous glucose and reducing porphyrin production by the administration of intravenous hematin, and (c) symptomatic management of autonomic symptoms and pain with propranolol, chlorpromazine, meperidine, and morphine.

Porphyric crises can be precipitated by many drugs, including most antiepileptic drugs (AEDs), estrogens, alcohol, and oral contraceptives.[65] Some AEDs without porphygenic effect in a rodent model are levetiracetam, gabapentin, zonisamide, and possibly low doses of oxcarbazepine. The diagnosis is made with the Watson-Schwartz test and enzyme assays that reveal decreased activity of PBGD.

Problems in Diagnosis of Seizures and Management

Although porphyric crises may resemble simple partial sensory seizures, simple partial psychic seizures, and complex partial seizures, the prominence of abdominal pain, tachycardia, constipation, and paralysis distinguish them from ictal syndromes. The porphyric crisis itself, however, may precipitate partial or tonic–clonic seizures. In children, AIP and HC may be associated with mental retardation, itself a risk factor for epilepsy.[27,68] The cause of the psychic and epileptogenic manifestations is unknown, but some investigators have suggested that toxicity is a consequence of the structural similarity of porphobilinogen and D-ALA to γ-aminobutyric acid (GABA) and glutamate.[39] Some authors suggest that porphyrins are endogenous ligands for mitochondrial benzodiazepine receptors.[67]

The management of patients with porphyria who are in or between crises is complicated by the frequently marked porphyrinogenic qualities of most antiepileptic drugs. Barbiturates, carbamazepine, clonazepam, diazepam, ethosuximide, the hydantoins, primidone, paraldehyde, and valproate may all induce crises and are porphyrinogenic in chick embryo hepatocyte cultures.[46,49,60,61] Triggering of the first porphyric crisis around puberty derives from the fact that steroids, including estradiol, containing a 5-β configuration induce D-ALA synthetase, thus precipitating the porphyric crisis.[28,72] Oral contraceptives also increase urinary enzyme excretion in normal patients, and asymptomatic relatives of patients with porphyria should avoid contraceptive pills.[14] The cyclic nature of AIP attacks of varying severity, usually late in the luteal phase or during ovulation, may simulate the catamenial exacerbation of seizure disorders.[65] As with catamenial seizures, attempts to suppress ovarian cycling by oral contraception to reduce porphyric crises have met with variable success.[3]

The chick embryo hepatic cell culture has been used to test the potential of antiepileptic drugs to induce porphyria.[21,46] Reynolds and Miska[46] found that phenytoin, phenobarbital, carbamazepine, clonazepam, and valproate may all increase porphyrin levels. Benzodiazepines (diazepam), bromides, magnesium sulfate, and gabapentin have been suggested as alternatives in the treatment of porphyria based on single case reports and small reviews of the literature.[27,46,49,60,61]

Independent of the acute porphyric attack per se, partial or generalized seizures in children[27] or adults may supervene in about 1% to 30% of hospitalized patients or patients brought to medical attention. In genetically susceptible individuals, the incidental intake of one of the many drugs thought to precipitate porphyria may induce a porphyric crisis, which may, in turn, be associated acutely with partial or generalized seizures. However, seizure onset may appear after the original crisis or even between crises. Some patients may have both conditions, apparently occurring independently, with the onset of epilepsy preceding the first porphyric attack. Common drugs and antiepileptic agents that can usually be safely used in porphyria are listed in Table 5.

TABLE 5

SAFE DRUGS FOR PATIENTS WITH PORPHYRIA

Analgesics
Codeine
Narcotic analgesics
Antibiotics
Penicillins
Streptomycin
Tetracycline
Antiemetics
Chlorpromazine
Prochlorperazine
Promethazine
Diphenhydramine
Trifluoperazine
Anticonvulsants
Bromides
Clonazepam
Diazepam
Gabapentin
Levetiracetam
Zonisamide
Vigabatrin
Others
Chloral hydrate
Corticosteroids
Propranolol

Idiopathic Recurring Stupor

Idiopathic recurring stupor (IRS) is a rare disease that has only recently been elucidated. It is a syndrome of recurring obtundation or coma unassociated with a known toxic, metabolic, or structural abnormality.[48,64] Events in the few cases described occur in early middle age or in older male patients who are light drinkers. Characteristics are drowsiness that is not associated with alcohol intake, slurred speech, drunken gait, and aggressiveness upon challenge. Lethargy deepens to sleep, from which the patient can be briefly aroused only with vigorous stimuli. Spells, which may occur weekly but are usually infrequent, can last up to 3 days, after which the patient may appear stunned and be amnestic.

During stupor, there may be up to a 300-fold increase in levels of endozepine-4, an endogenous ligand for benzodiazepine recognition sites on $GABA_A$ central nervous system receptors, with normalization of levels between attacks.[48] Ictal EEGs reveal a fast (14- to 16-Hz) unreactive background activity without apparent epileptiform activity.[64]

The stuporous state can be reversed by the pure benzodiazepine antagonist flumazenil.

Movement Disorders

A marked tremor may be confused with an epileptic seizure. Several metabolic and endocrine disorders include tremor, such as hypoglycemia and pheochromocytoma. Choreiform movements may be seen with hypocalcemia, hypoglycemia, hyperglycemia, hyperthyroidism, and porphyria. Hypoglycemia and hyperglycemia may induce myoclonus.

TABLE 6

METABOLIC AND ENDOCRINE IMITATORS OF EPILEPSY

Hypoglycemia	Relation to meals or fasting Hunger Characteristic prodrome Hypoglycemia correlated with symptoms Response to glucose
Hyperglycemia	Elevated blood glucose and osmolarity Prolonged confusion Movement disorder syndromes Epilepsia partialis continua
Hypocalcemia	Acral and perioral paresthesias Tetanic spasms and Chvostek sign Low serum calcium Response to calcium
Hyperthyroidism	Anxiety, tremor, sweating, weight loss, tachycardia Choreiform movements Rare periodic paralysis Suppressed thyroid-stimulating hormone, elevated serum T_4, T_3
Hypothyroidism	Choreoathetoid movements Confusion, stupor, or coma Sleep apnea Decreased serum T_4, elevated thyroid-stimulating hormone
Pheochromocytoma	Hypertension, headache, malaise, pallor Episodes resembling panic attacks Secretion of catecholamines Computed tomography, magnetic resonance imaging, or radionuclide tumor identification
Carcinoid	Flushing with transient erythema Bronchoconstriction, diarrhea Increased serotonin metabolites in urine Radiologic localization of gastrointestinal or bronchial tumor
Porphyria	Paroxysmal hyperautonomic symptoms Abdominal pain, delirium, neuropathy Generalized seizures, provoked by drugs Porphyrins in the urine
Hyponatremia	Fluctuating confusion or stupor Generalized seizures Low serum sodium and osmolarity Syndrome of inappropriate antidiuretic hormone

Source: From Bouloux P, Kaplan PW. *Imitators of Epilepsy*. New York: Demos; 1994:210, with permission.

Acute Confusional States

Acute confusional states or delirium may also resemble complex partial seizures. Many metabolic and endocrine disorders, including hyponatremia and hypernatremia, hypocalcemia and hypercalcemia, hypothyroidism and hyperthyroidism, hypocortisolemia and hypercortisolemia, hypoparathyroidism and hyperparathyroidism, hepatic insufficiency, and porphyria, may cause delirium.

SUMMARY AND CONCLUSIONS

Many metabolic, endocrine, and vasoactive/autonomic disturbances share clinical features with simple partial and some complex partial seizures. Differentiating them from myoclonic or tonic–clonic seizures usually poses little difficulty. The key to differentiating partial seizures from metabolic, endocrine, and vasoactive/autonomic dysfunctions is usually the constellation of signs and symptoms associated with the two respective categories. Although rare, simple psychic, autonomic, or sensory seizures not infrequently progress to complex partial seizures or secondarily generalized tonic–clonic seizures. Metabolic or endocrine conditions may lower seizure thresholds, but typically they cause generalized tonic–clonic seizures that are not preceded by partial symptomatology. Similarly, most endocrine and metabolic dysfunctions are associated with other clinical features that distinguish them from partial seizures. Prominent malaise, sweating, anxiety and palpitations, diarrhea or constipation, and abdominal pain or cramping occur relatively infrequently with partial seizures.

Hypoglycemia is one of the most important mimics of epilepsy. The temporal relationship of the cardinal features of hypoglycemia to fasting, food intake, or intake of hypoglycemic drugs should alert the physician to the correct diagnosis, despite the fact that the symptoms of anxiety, clamminess, tachycardia, sweating, and confusion are also associated with anxiety states, hyperventilation, and rare conditions such as pheochromocytoma and carcinoid syndrome. Differentiation rests on demonstration of hypoglycemia and the symptomatic relief provided by reestablishment of normal glucose levels. Rarer causes, including carcinoid syndrome, pheochromocytoma, and porphyria, may be tested for on an individual basis, with a higher diagnostic probability during an attack. Typically, the array of multisystem features, including sudden headache, hypertension, and marked sweating (pheochromocytomas), diarrhea and abdominal cramps (carcinoid syndrome), and abdominal pain, constipation, and paralysis (acute porphyrias), helps to differentiate these conditions.

A more complex issue is the coincidence of epileptic seizures. Carcinoid tumors and pheochromocytomas are rarely associated with seizures. Tonic–clonic seizures, however, are seen with hypoglycemia, as are characteristic partial motor seizures and epilepsia partialis continua in nonketotic hyperglycemia. Similarly, the porphyric syndromes, in addition to resembling certain seizure types, may be associated with epileptic seizures or be precipitated by antiepileptic drugs. The management of these conditions, therefore, involves not only diagnostic differentiation, but also the appropriate management of metabolic and endocrine disorders on the one hand and intercurrent seizures on the other.

Blanket testing for rare endocrine or metabolic disorders is neither justified nor cost-effective. The tests are frequently invasive. It is only with justifiable suspicion of the rare entities that costly and morbid investigation should be undertaken. Table 6 summarizes the characteristic presentations of endocrine and metabolic disorders.

References

1. Ahronheim JC. Hyperthyroid chorea in an elderly woman associated with sole elevation of T_3. *J Am Geriatr Soc*. 1988;36:242–244.
2. Anderson J. Disorders of metabolism I. In: Davis DM, ed. *Textbook of Adverse Drug Reactions*. New York: Oxford University Press; 1977.

3. Anderson K, Spitz I, Sassa S, et al. Prevention of cyclical attacks of acute intermittent porphyria with a long-acting agonist of luteinizing hormone-releasing hormone. *N Engl J Med.* 1984;311:643.
4. Berger H, Goldberg A. Hereditary coproporphyria. *Br Med J.* 1955;2:85–88.
5. Bloomer JR. The hepatic porphyrias; pathogenesis, manifestations and management. *Gastroenterology.* 1976;71:689–701.
6. Brain L, Jellinek EH, Ball K. Hashimoto's disease and encephalopathy. *Lancet.* 1966;2:512–514.
7. Brick JF, Gutrecht JA, Ringel RA. Reflex epilepsy and nonketotic hyperglycemia in the elderly: a specific neuroendocrine syndrome. *Neurology.* 1989;39:394–399.
8. Casper RF, Yen, SSC, Wilkes MM. Menopausal flushes. A neuroendocrine link with pulsatile luteinizing hormone secretion. *Science.* 1979;205:823–825.
9. Chong JY, Rowland LP, Utiger R. Hashimoto's encephalopathy: syndrome or myth? *Arch Neurol.* 2003;60:164–171.
10. Chotmongkol V, Bhuripanyo P. Movement disorder in hypothyroidism: a case report. *J Med Assoc Thai.* 1989;85:775–779.
11. D'Alessandro R, Rocchi E, Cristina E, et al. Safety of valproate in porphyria cutanea tarda. *Epilepsia.* 1988;29:159–162.
12. Davis Z, Moertel CJ, McIlrath DC. The malignant carcinoid syndrome. *Surg Gynecol Obstet.* 1973;137:637–644.
13. Dean G, Barnes HD. Porphyria in Sweden and South Africa. *S Afr Med J.* 1959;33:246–253.
14. Editorial. The pill and porphyria. *Br Med J.* 1972;3:603–604.
15. Editorial. *Lancet.* 1978;2:1293.
16. Forchetti CM, Katsamakis G, Garron DC. Autoimmune thyroiditis and a rapidly progressive dementia: global hypoperfusion on SPECT scanning suggests a possible mechanism. *Neurology.* 1997;49:623–626.
17. Gerich JE, Mokan M, Veneman T, et al. Hypoglycemia unawareness. *Endocrine Rev.* 1991;12:356–371.
18. Glazer GH, Levy LL. Seizures and idiopathic hypoparathyroidism. A clinical-electroencephalographic study. *Epilepsia.* 1960;1:454–465.
19. Goldberg A. Acute intermittent porphyria: a study of 50 cases. *Q J Med.* 1959;28:183–209.
20. Haeger-Aronsen B, Stathers G, Swahn G. Hereditary coproporphyria. *Ann Intern Med.* 1968;69:221–227.
21. Hahn M, Gildemeister OS, Krauss GL, et al. Effects of new anticonvulsant medications on porphyrin synthesis in cultured liver cells: potential implications for patients with acute porphyria. *Neurology.* 1997;49(1):97–106.
22. Hennis A, Corbin D, Fraser H. Focal seizures and non-ketotic hyperglycaemia. *J Neurol Neurosurg Psychiatry.* 1992;55:195–197.
23. Hollowell JG, Staehling NW, Flanders WD, et al. Serum TSH, T4 and thyroid antibodies in the United States population (1988–1994): National Health and Nutrition Examination Survey (NHANES III). *J Clin Endocrinol Metab.* 2002;87:489–499.
24. Ingbar S. The thyroid. In: Williams RH, Foster DW. *Williams Textbook of Endocrinology,* 7th ed. Philadelphia: WB Saunders; 1985:682–815.
25. Jadresic A, Banks LM, Childs DF, et al. The acromegaly syndrome—relation between clinical features, growth hormone values and radiological characteristics of the pituitary tumours. *Q J Med.* 1982;51:189–204.
26. Kaplan PW. Reversible hypercalcemic cerebral vasoconstriction with seizures and blindness: a paradigm for eclampsia? *Clin EEG.* 1998;29:120–123.
27. Kaplan PW, Lewis DV. Juvenile acute intermittent porphyria with hypercholesterolemia and epilepsy: a case report and review of the literature. *J Child Neurol.* 1986;1:38–45.
28. Kappas A, Sassa S, Granick S, et al. Endocrine–gene interactions in the pathogenesis of acute intermittent porphyria. *Res Publ Assoc Res Nerv Ment Dis.* 1974;53:225.
29. Krauss GL, Simmonds-O'Brien E, Campbell M. Successful treatment of seizures and porphyria with gabapentin. *Neurology.* 1995;45:594–595.
30. Kushner JP, Barbuto AJ, Lee GR. An inherited enzymatic defect in porphyria cutanea tarda. Decreased uroporphobilinogen decarboxylase activity. *J Clin Invest.* 1976;58:1089.
31. Laurent LPE. Acute thyrotoxic bulbar palsy. *Lancet.* 1944;1:87–88.
32. Manger WM, Gifford RW. *Pheochromocytoma.* New York: Springer-Verlag; 1977.
33. Markovitz M. Acute intermittent porphyria: A report of five cases and review of the literature. *Ann Intern Med.* 1954;41:1170–1188.
34. Marks V, Rose FC, eds. *Hypoglycemia.* Oxford: Blackwell Scientific; 1981.
35. Kappas A, Sassa S, Galbraith RA, Nordmann V. The porphyrias. In: Scriver CR, Beandet AL, Sly WS, et al. *The Metabolic Basis of Inherited Disease.* 7th ed. New York: McGraw Hill. 1995;2103–2159.
36. Millichap JG. Metabolic and endocrine factors. In: Vinken PJ, Bruyn GW, eds. *Handbook of Clinical Neurology,* Vol. 15. Amsterdam: North-Holland; 1974:311.
37. Mitchell JM. Thyroid disease in the emergency department. Thyroid function tests and hypothyroidism and myxedema coma. *Emerg Med Clin North Am.* 1989;7:885–902.
38. Morres CA, Dire DJ. Movement disorders as a manifestation of nonketotic hyperglycemia. *J Emerg Med.* 1989;7:359–364.
39. Muller WE, Snyder SH. Delta-aminolevulinic acid: influences on synaptic GABA receptor binding may explain CNS symptoms of porphyria. *Ann Neurol.* 1977;2:340–342.
40. Nesher G, Zion MM. Recurrent ventricular tachycardia in hypothyroidism—report of a case and review of the literature. *Cardiology.* 1988;75:301–306.
41. Newcomer J, Haire W, Hartman CR. Coma and thyrotoxicosis. *Ann Neurol.* 1983;14:689–690.
42. O'Keefe SJD, Marks V. Lunchtime gin and tonic a cause of reactive hypoglycemia. *Lancet.* 1977;1:1286–1288.
43. Page IH, Corcoran AC, Udenfriend S, et al. Argentaffinoma as an endocrine tumour. *Lancet.* 1955;1:198–199.
44. Pepplinhuizen L, Bruinvels J, Blom W, et al. Schizophrenia-like psychosis caused by a metabolic disorder. *Lancet.* 1980;1:454–456.
45. Polonsky KS. A practical approach to fasting hypoglycemia. *N Engl J Med.* 1992;326:1020–1021.
46. Reynolds NC Jr, Miska RM. Safety of anticonvulsants in hepatic porphyrias. *Neurology.* 1981;31:480–484.
47. Rizza RA, Cryer PE, Gerich JE, et al. Role of glucagon, epinephrine and growth hormone in human glucose counterregulation. Effects of somatostatin and adrenergic blockade on plasma glucose recovery and glucose flux rates following insulin-induced hypoglycemia. *J Clin Invest.* 1979;64:62–71.
48. Rothstein JD, Guidotti A, Tinuper P, et al. Endogenous benzodiazepine receptor ligands in idiopathic recurring stupor. *Lancet.* 1992;340:1002–1004.
49. Sadeh M, Blatt I, Martonovits G, et al. Treatment of porphyric convulsions with magnesium sulfate. *Epilepsia.* 1991;32:712–715.
50. Santiago JV, Clarke WL, Shah SD, et al. Epinephrine, norepinephrine, glucagon and growth hormone release in association with physiologic decrements in the plasma glucose concentration in normal and diabetic man. *J Clin Endocrinol Metab.* 1980;51:877–883.
51. Santiago JV, White NH, Skor DA, et al. Defective glucose counterregulation due to deficient glucagon and epinephrine secretory responses limits the intensive therapy of insulin-dependent diabetes mellitus. *Am J Physiol.* 1984;247:E215–E220.
52. Schimke RN. Hyperthyroidism. The clinical spectrum. *Postgrad Med.* 1992;91:229–236.
53. Service FJ, McMahon MM, O'Brien PC, et al. Functioning insulinoma—incidence, recurrence and long-term survival of patients. A 60-year study. *Mayo Clin Proc.* 1991;66:711–719.
54. Sheldon G, Sheps MD, Jiang NS, et al. The diagnosis of pheochromocytoma. *Endocrinol Metab Clin North Am.* 1988;2:397–414.
55. Sheps SG, Jiang NS, Klee GG, et al. Recent developments in the diagnosis and treatment of pheochromocytoma. *Mayo Clin Proc.* 1990;65:88–95.
56. Singh BM, Gupta DR, Strobos RJ. Non-ketotic hyperglycemia and epilepsia partialis continua. *Arch Neurol.* 1973;29:187–190.
57. Smith CL, Granger CV. Hypothyroidism producing reversible dementia. A challenge for medical rehabilitation. *Am J Phys Med Rehabil.* 1992;71:28–30.
58. Stein JA, Tschudy DP. Acute intermittent porphyria: a clinical and biochemical study of 46 patients. *Medicine.* 1970;49:1–16.
59. Stein PP, Black HR. A simplified diagnostic approach to pheochromocytoma. A review of the literature and report of one institution's experience. *Medicine.* 1991;70:46–66.
60. Suzuki A, Aso K, Ariyoshi C, et al. Acute intermittent porphyria and epilepsy: safety of clonazepam. *Epilepsia.* 1992;33:108–111.
61. Tatum WO, Zachariah SB. Gabapentin treatment of seizures in acute intermittent porphyria. *Neurology.* 1995;45:1216–1217.
62. Thomas JE, Rooke ED, Kvale WF. The neurologist's experience with pheochromocytoma. A review of 100 cases. *JAMA.* 1966;197:754–758.
63. Thorson G, York G, Bjorkman G, et al. Malignant carcinoid of small intestine with metastasis to liver, valvular disease of the right side of the heart (pulmonary stenosis and tricuspid regurgitation without septal defects). Peripheral vasomotor symptoms, bronchoconstriction and an unusual type of cyanosis. *Am Heart J.* 1954;47:795–817.
64. Tinuper P, Montagna P, Plazzi G, et al. Idiopathic recurring stupor. *Neurology.* 1994;44:621–625.
65. Tschudy DP, Valsamis M, Magnussen CR. Acute intermittent porphyria: clinical and selected research aspects. *Ann Intern Med.* 1974;83:851–864.
66. Vance JE, Stoll RW, Fariss BL, et al. Exaggerated intestinal glucagon and insulin in human subjects. *Metabolism.* 1972;21:405–412.
67. Verma A, Nye JS, Snyder SH. Porphyrins are endogenous ligands for the mitochondrial (peripheral-type) benzodiazepine receptor. *Proc Natl Acad Sci U S A.* 1987;84:2256–2260.
68. Waldenström J. Neurological symptoms caused by so-called acute porphyria. *Acta Psychiatr Neurol.* 1939;14:375–383.
69. Waldenström J. The porphyrias as inborn errors of metabolism. *Am J Med.* 1957;22:758–773.
70. Walter RM Jr. Hypoglycemia: still a risk in the elderly. *Geriatrics.* 1990;45:69–71, 74–75.
71. Watson CJ. Porphyria. *Adv Intern Med.* 1954;6:235–299.
72. Welland F, Hellman E, Collins A, et al. Factors affecting the excretion of porphyrin precursors by patients with acute intermittent porphyria. II. The effect of ethinyl estradiol. *Metabolism.* 1964;13:251.
73. Whipple AO. The surgical therapy of hyperinsulinism. *J Int Surg.* 1938;3:237–276.
74. Williams ED, Sandler M. The classification of carcinoid tumours. *Lancet.* 1963;1:238–239.

CHAPTER 273 ■ SYSTEMIC NONEPILEPTIC PAROXYSMAL DISORDERS FROM NEONATAL TO CHILDHOOD PERIODS

MARK S. SCHER AND FEDERICO VIGEVANO

INTRODUCTION

Paroxysmal phenomena during neonatal and childhood periods cause intermittent or recurrent motor or behavioral signs or symptoms that must be distinguished from epileptic disorders. The clinician's diagnostic acumen can be especially challenged by specific behaviors. Nonepileptic paroxysmal disorders can be on either a neurologic or a systemic basis. The clinical context may help to distinguish paroxysmal nonepileptic disorders from epileptic seizures. Before committing to a specific pharmacologic intervention with medications, which may both be unnecessary and place the child at risk for adverse effects, alternative etiologies first must be considered. Home videography of the suspicious event can be pivotal for the clinician to reach a prompt and correct diagnosis with minimal investment in time and resources. Synchronous video-neurophysiologic monitoring either in the inpatient or outpatient setting[1,65,70] may also be necessary more definitively to categorize the event as epileptic or nonepileptic.

The child's age, state of arousal, and organ system involvement and an accurate description of the event by a witness will lead, in most cases, to the correct diagnosis. One must always be alert to nonepileptic disorders that occur in the context of a child who also has epilepsy. An early classification by Prensky[53] utilized functional categories to subdivide disorders: Disease-related behaviors, altered tone or consciousness, respiratory disturbances, perceptual disturbances, behavioral disorders, and unusual movements (see Table 1). Recent reviews further highlight selected disorders in young children.[18,19,22,48] Discussion of specific epileptic and nonepileptic paroxysmal events of neurologic origin such as nocturnal frontal lobe epilepsy, migraine, tic disorders, sleep disorders, psychogenic seizures, and cerebrovascular events are reviewed elsewhere in this book.

Relative to maturation, these paroxysmal disorders can be referred to as transient, paroxysmal, and/or chronic in presentation.[19] The proportion of transient events is highest during childhood, with the preponderance occurring during the first year of life. Many disorders remain idiopathic and unassociated with other neurologic diseases. When investigations are performed, test results are often normal. The clinician must therefore rely on clinical experience and consider a functional mechanism without known pathophysiologic explanations. Knowledge of these conditions is essential for the pediatric neurologist to avoid unnecessary tests and treatment while alleviating family anxiety (Table 1).

DISEASE-RELATED BEHAVIORS

Various systemic disease states present with recurrent signs and symptoms during infancy and childhood that may be misdiagnosed as epilepsy. Alteration of consciousness or muscle tone, focal neurologic deficits, and diffuse weakness may be clinical signs of systemic nonepileptic paroxysmal disorders.

Tetralogy Spells

This phenomenon is characterized by episodes of cyanosis, dyspnea, and unconsciousness and can present during the first several years. The repertoire of events occurs in 10% to 20% of children with congenital heart disease and may result in seizures. Anoxia-induced seizures occur in such individuals who suffer chronic and significant hypoxemia. Such episodes are labeled "tet spells" because young children with the especially cyanotic congenital heart lesions (such as tetralogy of Fallot) usually present in this manner. The pathogenesis for "tet spells" is the sudden increase in right-to-left shunting of blood through the heart with sudden oxygen desaturation. On careful history taking, attacks of hyperpnea and cyanosis are seldom misinterpreted as epileptic seizures. Loss of consciousness may result from anoxia or hypoxia, however, which then may precipitate seizures in certain children and, therefore, may be confusing to the clinician. For those children old enough to be ambulatory, taking a squatting position and then remaining nearly motionless is a maneuver for recovering cardiac reserve.[49]

Cardiac Arrhythmias

Children with recurrent episodes of loss of consciousness or alterations in arousal may suffer from cardiac arrhythmias. Disturbances of cardiac conduction of either intracardiac or extracardiac origin include sick sinus syndrome,[60] Jervell-Lange-Nelson syndrome, which is genetically determined and includes an associated deafness,[29] and Ward-Romano syndrome.[51] Therefore, careful history taking and examination may reveal characteristic features such as hair hypopigmentation, hearing loss, or dysmorphea. Syncope may frequently include convulsive movements similar to an Adams-Stokes attack. The prolonged-QT syndrome should be suspected in children particularly with underlying cardiac disease on a genetic basis such as the velocardiofacial syndrome (i.e., chromosomal 22q 11.2 deletion).[31] Prolonged-QT syndrome may be benign and transient or prolonged with risk for sudden death.[67] Prognosis is guarded because sudden unexpected death may occur at any time. True epileptic seizures may ensue in affected children as a result of asphyxia-induced brain injury incurred during prolonged episodes of hypoxemia during cardiac arrest. A cardiologic evaluation, including a prolonged electrocardiographic (ECG) recording and/or ECG during exercise may be required.

TABLE 1

SYSTEMIC NONEPILEPTIC PAROXYSMAL DISORDERS

Disease-related behaviors	**Behavioral disorders**
Tetrology spells	Head banging or nodding
Cardiac arrhythmias	Rumination
Poststreptococcal autoimmune disorders	Nightmares
Hypoglycemia	Night terrors
Hypocalcemia	Sleepwalking
Hydrocephalic spells	Confusional states
Hyperthyroidism	Panic attacks
Periodic paralysis	Dyscontrol syndrome or rage attacks
Gastroesophageal reflux	Munchausen syndrome by proxy
Drug poisoning (e.g., neuroleptics)	Psychotic states (i.e., fugue spells, hallucinations)
Cerebrovascular events	Stereotypic behavior
Loss of tone or consciousness	**Unusual movements**
Syncope	Jitteriness or tremulousness
Drop attacks	Shuddering
Narcolepsy/cataplexy	Benign sleep myoclonus (neonate or infant)
Attention-deficit hyperactivity syndrome	Exaggerated startle responses (i.e., hyperekplexia)
Respiratory disturbances	**Other unusual self-stimulator behaviors**
Infant apnea	Paroxysmal torticollis
Apparent life-threatening events	Masturbation
Breath-holding (including vagotomy)	Withholding, constipation
Hyperventilation	Transient dystonia, choreoathetosis
Perceptual Disturbances	Paroxysmal choreoathetosis or dystonic spasms
Headache (i.e., migraine)	Kinesigenic or nonkinesigenic
Abdominal pain	Tic disorder or Tourette syndrome
Vertigo, dizziness	Paroxysmal tonic up gaze

In a recent study of adults, 20% of patients referred to a neurologic department with possible idiopathic epilepsy were subsequently found to have cardiac arrhythmias that caused or significantly contributed to their symptoms.[60] Pediatric populations referred to neurology or epilepsy clinics may reflect comparable percentages, but few studies are available for comparisons with older populations. A report of sudden death in the young presenting with presumed cardiac arrhythmias was the most common cause of mortality in people 5 to 35 years of age. The two most common noncardiac causes of sudden death were epilepsy (23.8%) and intracerebral hemorrhage (23.8%).[55] In another study of adult epileptic patients, one third showed ictal bradycardia, with greater than one half experiencing serious cardiac events meriting pacemaker placement.[58] In general, sinus tachycardia accompanies approximately 90% and bradycardia or asystole 0.5% of all seizures.[72]

Metabolic Abnormalities: Hypoglycemia and Hypocalcemia

Hypoglycemia may occasionally challenge the clinician because of its association with unusual symptomatology. Both seizures and nonepileptic behaviors occur with hypoglycemia at any age, including the neonatal period. Neonates with hypoglycemia may present with tremulous behavior. Rare metabolic disorders can present early in life with hypoglycemia associated with, for example, hyperammonemic states, leucine intolerance, and hereditary fructose intolerance. Particularly after 1 year of age, unusual episodes of unconsciousness, stupor, or even seizures may occur during the early morning hours after an all-night fast. Postevent confusion or stupor can be prolonged after hypoglycemia-induced seizures. Such events may occur after episodes of vomiting, diarrhea, or transient reduced food intake, sometimes in the setting of a transient illness. The combination of symptoms associated with the condition of ketotic hypoglycemia[8] accounts for approximately 50% of cases of hypoglycemia that occur during early childhood. The child appears grossly ketotic during the attack and may exhibit marked hyperventilation. Acetonuria is an essential feature, which is rapidly corrected by administration of glucose. Hospitalization with carefully controlled provocation tests are suggested to induce hypoglycemia, such as with the administration of a ketogenic diet. Treatment consists primarily in preventing ketosis by adhering to regular mealtimes, particularly during times of illness, together with glucose supplementation. Of course, hypoglycemia and seizures may coexist; children may have epileptiform discharges on electroencephalogram (EEG), which may support a seizure diagnosis but not be interpreted in the context of the patient's clinical history. For example, neonatal hypoglycemia can result in injury to parietal-occipital cortical regions, which may later present as one form of focal epilepsy, involving posterior pathways.

Hypocalcemic stress usually results in seizures and can be secondary to primary or secondary hypoparathyroidism (with or without genetic cardiac syndromes). Severe nutritional deficiencies may be associated with poor feeding practices, starvation, or chronic diseases such as malabsorption syndromes or rickets.[2] A rare genetic disease of familial hypomagnesemia may be associated with hypocalcemia.[68] Rarely, profound hypocalcemia can result in nonepileptic tetanic spells, including generalized clonic activity, jaw rigors, and tremulousness.

Gastroesophageal Reflux

Infants may demonstrate episodic extension and lateral flexion of the head, usually in association with feeding. This syndrome was first described by Kinsbourne[34] and is sometimes termed "Sandifer syndrome" because the first patient described by Kinsbourne was under the care of Dr. Paul Sandifer. Although these seizure-like episodes suggest epilepsy, gastroesophageal reflux disorder (GERD) should be suspected after a careful history is obtained. In a retrospective review of 342 infants presenting with symptoms suggestive of GERD, all were <1 year of age; they presented with regurgitation, choking, irritability, failure to thrive, an apparent life-threatening event (ALTE), or wheezing.[64] In a study of 69 infants with ALTE, GERD was diagnosed in 38 cases and gastric volvulus in 21.[45]

Gastrointestinal radiographs, such as barium swallow study, document reflux with or without hiatal hernia or other morphologic abnormalities of the upper airway or gastrointestinal tract. Surgical correction is sometimes required to correct such attacks. The age range for these events is wide, beginning during the neonatal period and extending into adolescence. For infants, choking, apnea, laryngospasm, and opisthotonos also commonly occur,[25] whereas other gastrointestinal complaints, weight loss, or sleep disturbances are noted for older children.

ALTERED MUSCLE TONE OR CONSCIOUSNESS

The following discussion of syncope does not include neurologic conditions, such as cataplexy associated with the sleep disturbance of narcolepsy, or the inattention associated with attention-deficit hyperactivity disorder.

Syncope

Syncope is a common occurrence for adults and older children and is usually distinguished from true epileptic seizures by the historical description of a witness (see Chapter 271).[5] Patients describe warning signs of lightheadedness, dizziness, or visual dimming, such as graying out or browning out. Nausea may also be described after the event. Subjective feelings of temperature change and profuse sweating are also described. Sometimes a specific stimulus such as the sight of blood, minor trauma, or enclosure in a confined space may precipitate an attack. Orthostatic syncope may follow after prolonged standing or sudden change in posture. A careful review of a family history may document similar events in other relatives.[6]

Reflex syncope may also be described with certain physiologic maneuvers such as coughing, swallowing, or micturition.[32] Table 2 lists some causes of syncope, some of which are described elsewhere in this chapter, such as cardiac arrhythmias.

Syncopal events in the neonate, infant, or preverbal children have unique diagnostic challenges. Events may occur precipitously following surprise, pain, or prolonged crying. Breath-holding spells are discussed later, given the prominent respiratory component to this event. Underlying illnesses such as cardiorespiratory or metabolic-genetic causes may suggest a pathophysiologic mechanism. Neurocardiogenic syncope and neurologic disorders (80% and 9%, respectively) are the most common diagnoses for pediatric patients presenting to an emergency department.[41] Cardiogenic studies such as prolonged ECG monitoring, ultrasonography of the heart, or a tilt-table test may help to document associated abnormalities or capture events. Serum studies during an attack may document metabolic disturbances, such as hypoglycemia. Rarely, syncope triggers epileptic seizures, requiring both cardiologic treatment such as antiarrhythmic medication or cardiac pacing, as well as antiepileptic medications.[28] Patients with syncope, however, may have a few clonic jerks or even incontinence during or following the syncopal event[52] without evolving to seizures.

TABLE 2

CAUSES OF SYNCOPE

Menstruation in females Anemia	Decreased blood volume
Vasovagal	Fear Pain Unpleasant sights
Reflex	Cough Micturition Swallowing Carotid sinus pressure
Decreased venous return	Orthostatic with Valsalva maneuver
Disease states Cardiac Cerebrovascular insufficiency	Arrhythmia, obstructive outflow
Familial undetermined causes	

The physical examination of syncopal patients yields normal results. Blood pressure changes from supine to standing positions, however, may demonstrate a substantial drop in the diastolic component, supporting the diagnosis of orthostatic syncope. A tilt-table test may also be helpful. If one documents a blood pressure reduction of more than 15 points or the presence of a sinus bradycardia on standing, orthostatic hypotension should be suspected. A cardiologic evaluation including investigation for a heart murmur or dysrhythmia should be considered. Exceptional cases of congenital heart block have been associated in children with chronic myopathy, ophthalmoplegia, deafness, and ataxia, termed the Kearne-Sayne syndrome.[3]

If an attack is prolonged, a tonic motor seizure may occur. In a review of 77 patients appearing in an emergency room, 40 had syncope, 17 had near-syncope, and 20 did not have a syncopal episode. Vasovagal (50%) and orthostatic hypertension (20%) were the most common causes of syncope. Near-syncopal episodes occurred with lightheadedness (29%), seizures (18%), tension headaches (12%), and migraine (6%).[52] Adolescents, particularly those who lift weights or perform gymnastics, may induce syncope by stretching or straining the musculature, including inducing a neck-hyperextended position.

Children with recurrent symptoms should be evaluated by a cardiologist. Autonomic functioning of patients with beta-adrenergic hypersensitivity should be tested. A tilt-table test is particularly useful, sometimes with administration of isoprotosenol infusion as a provocative agent to induce blood pressure changes.[23]

RESPIRATORY DISTURBANCES

Primary respiratory disorders most commonly occur without associated seizures. These symptoms, however, may be confused with seizures. At times, clonic jerks or isolated seizures may follow primary apnea.[69] An electroencephalogram or polysomnogram during such events will help to distinguish a respiratory disorder from a true seizure.

Infant Apnea or Apparent Life-threatening Events

Apnea usually occurs during sleep and may be associated with centrally mediated hypoventilation, airway obstruction, or aspiration. Paroxysmal events are sometimes commonly referred to as apparent life-threatening events (ALTEs). On polysomnography, central apnea is defined as the absence of both chest and abdominal movements, as well as a cessation of airflow at the nares. Obstructive apnea usually involves movement of the chest and abdomen without airflow at the nares. Clonic or myoclonic jerks may occur during the apnea episode but do not represent true epileptic seizures. Most do not define apnea until it reaches durations of 15 to 20 seconds. Apnea associated with preterm infants is the most common presentation, but it also may occur in older infants.

If apnea occurs while a child is fully awake, this may be associated with gastroesophageal reflux.[26,63] Such an event is common usually when the infant is laid supine after a feeding, and aspiration may result following the reflux event.

Apparent life-threatening events predominantly affect children younger <1 year of age. This syndrome is characterized by a frightening constellation of symptoms in which the child exhibits some combination of apnea, color change, change in muscle tone, coughing, or gagging.[24] Recent studies highlight that a diagnostic testing strategy should depend on the outcome of the initial clinical assessment.[4,42] Together the two studies found that 50% to 70% of patients were correctly diagnosed based on the history and examination. Suggested algorithms follow a stepwise approach, with investigations initially directed by historical and clinical findings. The first step is consideration of child abuse. Based on information from six studies, baseline studies were suggested as follows: (a) basic blood tests, (b) infection screens, (c) metabolic workup, (d) cardiologic evaluations or ancillary organ system monitoring such as EEG, (e) polysomnography, and (f) pH probe studies.[42] It has also been recently emphasized that there are clear differences in epidemiology and risk factors between ALTE and sudden infant death syndrome (SIDS).[33]

Breath-holding Spells

This phenomenon is common between 6 months and 6 years and is often confused with tonic seizures. The child is described as falling, followed by tremulousness or convulsive, clonic-like movements. Two forms—cyanotic and pallid spells—have been reported, both resulting from reflex vagal changes that produce bradycardia and decrease cerebral blood flow. The cyanotic form of breath-holding spell is typically more common, beginning during the second or third year of life in response to anger, fear, excitement, or minor injury. The child will cry and suddenly stop breathing, often during expiration. Cyanosis ensues within seconds, followed by a loss of consciousness, limpness, and loss of postural tone. After 1 to 2 minutes of unresponsiveness, consciousness rapidly returns with the resumption of normal activities without postictal alterations in arousal.

The pallid form of breath-holding spells (BHS) often follows minor trauma or surprise, but crying is minimal or absent. There is rapid loss of consciousness or limpness as with the cyanotic form. Attacks may be longer, however, and frequently involve clonic movements associated with cerebral hypoxia.[39] Children with the pallid form may have more profound bradycardia or even asystole. Both cyanotic and pallid forms of BHS can be associated with autonomic nervous system dysregulation,[14] and children with myelodysplasia and Arnold-Chiari malformations exhibit various brainstem abnormalities manifesting in abnormal control of breathing, upper airway dysfunction, aspiration, pneumonia, and cor pulmonale. Severe and sudden bradyarrhythmia or asystole may also result, necessitating treatment with beta-adrenergic antagonists such as atropine.

Unwitnessed attacks may be difficult to distinguish from seizures, but observers often describe an association between precipitating causes as the historical key to the diagnosis. Electroencephalographic recordings do not demonstrate epileptiform discharges, but may show paroxysmal slowing of background EEG activities during an induced syncopal episode.

The optimal treatment is usually behavioral modification without the need for medication, although atropine may be rarely recommended for frequent pallid spells and a trial of iron supplementation is usually recommended for children with BHS and hematologic evidence of iron-deficiency anemia.[9,47]

The presumed pathogenesis of breath-holding spells involves an acute reduction of cerebral blood flow because of increased intrathoracic pressure. This mechanism is analogous to syncope induced by the Valsalva maneuver, which occurs in addition to acute oxygen desaturation caused by respiratory arrest. Some clinicians describe the pallid form as "vagotonia," which may reveal genetic transmission after obtaining a family history. Children with posterior fossa malformations, such as the Arnold-Chiari anomaly, have also been described as having this physiologic abnormality.[46]

For a typical pediatric population who present with breath-holding spells, 76% of the attacks occur between 6 and 18 months of age.[38] Eighty-five percent of affected children are free from attacks by the age of 5 years. There is generally no relationship with mental retardation and later epilepsy, but it can occur in children with developmental disorders, in whom such attacks are repetitive and stereotypic.

Hyperventilation Syndrome

This phenomenon is most commonly noted in older children, particularly during adolescence. Children with the complete clinical presentation breathe rapidly with shallow, irregular breathing, whereas others complain of an inability to obtain satisfying deep breaths. The initial complaints are commonly dyspnea, chest pain, and lightheadedness. Syncope or pseudoabsence seizures have been described and may be mistaken for true epileptic events. The clinician must have a high index of suspicion in the presence of the typical symptoms, which often include thoracic pain, shortness of breath, and muscle pain. Having the patient rebreathe in a paper bag permits the clinician quickly to control the symptoms of the impending attack. Such a syndrome, however, should alert the clinician to the presence of an anxiety disorder or other significant psychological disturbance. For recurring or chronicity of events, antianxiety medications may help; long-term psychiatric intervention may also be required.

BEHAVIORAL DISORDERS

Rumination

These attacks involve hyperextension of the neck, repetitive swallowing, and protrusion of the tongue and may overlap with the syndrome of gastroesophageal reflux. Although some situations may be due to abnormalities of esophageal peristalsis on an anatomic basis, other patients manifest this behavior as a developmental disturbance because of a dysfunctional relationship between the caretaker and child. The child is usually described as alert but sometimes appears under stress and uncomfortable. Variable feeding techniques are helpful to correct this disorder, depending on the etiologic possibilities. Intensive psychotherapy with both the caretaker and child may be required before long-term benefits result.

Panic Attacks

Panic attacks occur as acute events associated with a chronic anxiety disorder (see Chapter 285). Patients suffering from depression, schizophrenia, or hyperthyroidism may present with these events. The possibility of substance abuse should also be considered. Attacks last from minutes to hours and are accompanied by palpitations, sweating, dizziness or vertigo, and feelings of unreality. Other symptoms have also been described such as dyspnea or a smothering sensation, unsteadiness or faintness, palpitations or tachycardia, trembling or shaking, choking, nausea or abdominal distress, depersonalization or derealization, numbness or tingling, flushes or chills, chest pain or discomfort, and fears of dying, aura, going crazy, or losing control.[50] Specific situational experiences may bring on panic attacks, such as agoraphobia. Children with developmental disturbances, such as those with pervasive developmental disorders with autistic signs, may also manifest stereotypic behaviors that suggest seizures.[12]

Episodic Dyscontrol Syndrome (Rage Attacks)

Episodic dyscontrol syndrome is characterized by recurrent attacks of uncontrollable rage. Such attacks occur despite minimal or absent provocation, often totally out of context with the personality of the patient or the situation.[17] Although this can be seen in younger children, this is more often noted in teenagers and young adults. Younger children with specific language delay or developmental disorders in multiple domains may present with rages. Many patients may have impaired mental status and other neurologic abnormalities on examination, but the history provided by a family or witnesses document that such attacks occur suddenly, are explosive, and are characterized by uncontrollable behavior. Behavior may include primitive physical violence such as kicking, striking, or biting, or even verbal abuse with profanity. Patients display uncharacteristic strength and speed and appear to be psychotic, claiming amnesia, fatigue, or remorse following the episode. At times, such attacks may be difficult to distinguish from complex partial seizures; however, directed violence is very unusual during a true epileptic seizure. Patients rarely describe an aura, and their EEG examination is noncontributory. Some authors indicate that patients with complex partial seizures also have a higher-than-expected incidence of rage attacks.[36,54]

Munchausen Syndrome by Proxy

Clinicians must be cognizant of children with false events or illnesses invented or induced by a relative or caretaker. Meadow[43,44] described children whose mothers fabricated signs and symptoms of illness; a false history of seizures ranging from 1 month to 20 years with an average of 4 years was described. These "seizures" are reported to occur as generalized events at night during sleep, poorly controlled by a wide variety of antiepileptic medications, leading to repeated hospitalizations and multiple diagnostic studies.

The physical examination of these children is usually completely normal. In addition to the commitment and expense of diagnostic studies and prolonged hospitalizations, emotional trauma, prolonged absence from school, and unnecessary restrictions in sports and recreational activities are the consequences to the child of this condition.

The mothers of children with Munchausen syndrome by proxy are medically sophisticated and spend long hours in hospital settings. Knowledge about medical procedures and other factual minutiae allows these individuals to be conversant in sophisticated discussions involving different diagnoses. Fathers, on the other hand, keep a low profile, rarely visit the child in the hospital, and are quite passive by description.[20]

It is essential to diagnose this condition promptly because it is considered a form of child neglect or abuse. The clinician must maintain a high index of suspicion and conduct a methodical review of all medical records with a case conference with as many health care providers as possible.[59] Covert video surveillance of infants in pediatric hospitals is now more widely recommended, although ethical and legal dilemmas have been discussed.[21] Some children are at risk of being asphyxiated or poisoned to induce spells, and mortality is estimated at 10%. Prompt psychiatric intervention for the caretaker is required.

UNUSUAL MOVEMENTS

Tremulousness or Jitteriness

Neonates and young infants commonly present with rapid generalized tremulousness. Infants appear alert, and gentle flexion of the affected body part will extinguish or diminish these movements. The movement is a to-and-fro movement of the limb, which is contrasted with the fast and slow movement phases characterized by clonic activity. Tremors or jitteriness may persist up to 4 to 6 weeks postconceptional age but usually resolve after this time. This movement is a benign pattern during infancy, with a high rate of normal neurodevelopmental outcome.[62] The movements may occur spontaneously or be provoked by stimulation. Older children may also exhibit tremors. In the absence of cerebellar or motor neuron signs, dystonia, family history of cerebellar disease, or a history of hyperthyroidism, childhood essential tremor can be considered. Other entities such as drugs with tremor-inducing properties must be considered. One in 20 essential tremor cases arise during childhood, with an age range at onset of 1 to 14 years.[40] Neonates who are small for gestational age, hypoglycemic infants, infants of diabetic mothers, and infants withdrawing from prenatal substance exposure may present with jitteriness.

Shuddering, Myoclonus, Hyperekplexia, Dyskinesias

Shuddering is an exaggerated movement resembling shivering. Events occur both during waking and sleep states. Video-EEG monitoring may be required to capture the events.[30] There is a rapid tremor involved in the head, arms, and trunk or even the lower extremities. Such episodes have been described as early as 3 to 4 months of age but decrease gradually in frequency and intensity by 10 to 11 months of age. Essential tremor may be more common in families of children with shuddering spells.[27,66] Young children show an abrupt onset of shuddering movements with flexion of the head, elbows, trunk, and knees and abduction of the elbows and knees. Some describe provocation with excitement, fear, anger, or an urge to void.

A more frequent nonepileptic condition described in infants is benign neonatal myoclonus (BNM)[56] or benign myoclonus of early infancy (BMEI),[18] which may include shuddering of the upper limbs in approximately 50% of children. Fejerman[18] suggested that shuddering attacks are a variant of BMEI. Children with BNM resolve by 6 months of age. Myoclonic jerks are only present during sleep and mainly during non–rapid-eye-movement sleep. Arousal always terminates the jerks. By definition, the neurologic examination and electroencephalogram are normal.

Hyperexplexia or hyperekplexia is a relatively benign disorder consisting of exaggerated startle responses and hypertonicity that may occur during the first year of life, and in severe cases presents during the neonatal period. As a relatively uncommon disorder, it is usually sporadic, but familial inheritance has been reported. Thirty-nine patients were recently reported[61] with an average age at onset of 3.3 months. Children usually present with marked irritability and recurrent startles in response to handling or sounds. Severely affected infants had severe jerks and stiffening, sometimes with breath-holding spells. Symptoms gradually resolved by 2 years of age with normal neurodevelopment.

Paroxysmal dyskinesia is a general descriptive term that encompasses a number of clinical phenomena of adults and children.[10] Abnormal movements may be induced by sudden voluntary movements (i.e., paroxysmal kinesigenic choreoathetosis). Some movements may be dystonic, choreic, ballistic, or choreoathetotic. Three other dyskinesias are nonkinesigenic, exertion induced, or hypnogenic. Seven children were recently described, with the earliest onset at 18 months.[35] Most cases are idiopathic with a benign course, diminishing in frequency and severity with age. Video-EEG monitoring may be required to exclude epilepsy, but antiepileptic medications may be required for the specific child.

Paroxysmal Eye Movements: Spasm Nutans, Benign Paroxysmal Tonic Upward Gaze, Eye Fluttering

Spasm nutans is a syndrome occurring in early childhood. It consists of a triad of symptoms: (a) head nodding, (b) ocular oscillations, and (c) anomalous head position. Ophthalmologic and neurologic findings are otherwise normal. This syndrome is benign and has spontaneous resolution.[16] Age of onset ranges from 1 to 15 months, with both head nodding and nystagmus, which most of the time are intermittent. Neuroimaging is required for the rare association of brainstem masses or malformations.

Benign paroxysmal tonic upgaze is an ill-defined neuro-ophthalmologic disorder with onset in infancy.[11] It consists of sudden ocular movements with sustained upward deviation of the eyes. Episodes disappear with time with normal neurodevelopment,[57] although ataxia has been reported in a child.[37]

Although eye fluttering may be part of typical childhood absence epilepsy, nonepileptic eyelid movements have been described in 19 children and adults with well-controlled generalized epilepsy.[7] Eye movements in children began 2 to 4 years before epilepsy was noted and did not resolve with age. Twelve patients had a family history of the eyelid disorder without epilepsy.

Self-stimulatory Behavior

Some behaviors may be mistaken for seizures, especially in neurologically impaired children. Donat and Wright[15] described head shaking and nodding, lateral and vertical nystagmus, staring, tongue thrusting, chewing movements, periodic hyperventilation, tonic postures, ticks, and excessive startle reactions in some children. Self-stimulatory behavior, such as rhythmic hand shaking, body rocking, and head swaying performed during a time of apparent unawareness of the surroundings, are commonly noted in children with mental deficits, as well as those with pervasive developmental disorders such as autism. The clinical syndrome Rett syndrome should be suspected in young girls who are delayed in development and exhibit "hand washing" movements. Deaf and blind children frequently resort to self-stimulatory behavior, such as hitting their ears or eyes. Developmentally normal children with constipation or refusal to urinate may present with unusual behaviors that may appear to be seizure-like or self-stimulatory but instead reflect the child's discomfort and distraction because of his or her resistance to voiding or defecating.

Finally, masturbatory behavior, even in the very young, may give the appearance of seizures. Referrals for neurologic consultation may have requested evaluations for seizures or movement disorders. Infantile masturbation may mimic pain, inattention, or fear. Infants of either gender, for instance, may be found in a sitting position with their legs held tight together or straddling bars of the crib or playpen and rocking back and forth.[71] Direct observation is crucial, and video-monitoring at home or by the neurology team can be diagnostic.

DIAGNOSTIC METHODS AND DIFFERENTIAL DIAGNOSIS

The paroxysmal events discussed here represent, for the most part, transitory functional disorders not associated with any particular disease. As already mentioned, specific investigations should be performed only for organ-specific clues by history and examination, such as cardiopathies causing syncope or gastrointestinal pathologies causing gastroesophageal reflux. In other situations, there are no particular examinations that can lead to an etiologic diagnosis.

The cardinal element for diagnosis is a precise history of the event. It is important to investigate favoring or triggering factors that preceded the event and the patient's subjective sensations, motor manifestations, and postictal state. Differential diagnosis with tonic–clonic generalized epileptic seizures can be particularly difficult in a syncope that can present a tonic contraction of the entire body and sometimes arrhythmic myoclonic limb jerks. Family history must be reviewed for the presence of nonepileptic paroxysmal disorders, such as syncopes or other paroxysmal events. Careful attention must paid to discover any family history of sudden death. The objective examination will be normal, except in cases with cardiopathy, as will the neurologic examination.

The clinician must consider that patients with a suspected convulsive seizure should undergo an EEG or video-EEG study that can provide additional information. Home videography can also prove helpful.

The EEG will characteristically show an absence of interictal epileptogenic abnormalities or the presence of abnormalities not relevant to the symptomatology, for example, rolandic spike discharges in children with episodes of loss of consciousness.

An optimal routine should always include a recording of cardiac activity, by which it is sometimes possible to detect cardiac arrhythmias, especially during a hyperventilation test. There should be an increase in heart rate during the hyperventilation test that can favor the triggering of arrhythmias (Fig. 1).

Even more useful is the polysomnographic study with recording of EEG, ECG, and nasal, oral, and chest breathing, in addition to other parameters. In cases of ALTE, this test is mandatory while the patient is awake and asleep because it helps to identify any central or obstructive apnea.

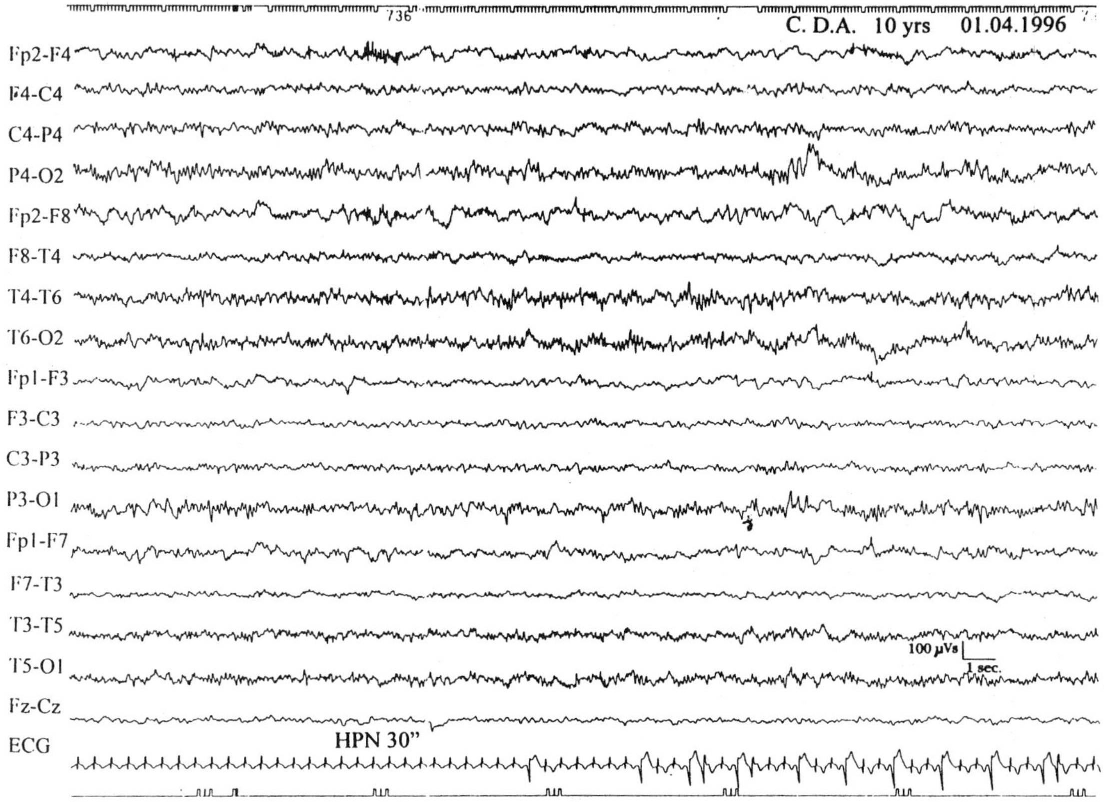

FIGURE 1. A 10-year-old girl who presented with a seizure with loss of consciousness and diffuse tonic contraction. A sister died suddenly at age 13 years. The electroencephalogram is normal; extra systoles appear after 30 seconds of hyperventilation (HPN). Diagnosis: exercise-induced ventricular tachycardia.

The best diagnostic method is undoubtedly the documentation of the paroxysmal manifestation. In cases of frequent and unprovoked paroxysmal manifestations, it could be useful to ask the parent to try to record the phenomenon with a video camera at home.

One can try to provoke the event in the neurophysiology laboratory. Use of the tilt table can provoke syncopes caused by orthostatic hypotension; crying can provoke either a cyanotic or pallid type of breath-holding spell (Fig. 2); contraction of the scapular girdle muscles can provoke a stretching syncope.

When it is possible to record the event, EEG generally does not evidence any change or only nonepileptic changes (Fig. 3).

The first observation during the syncope is a slowing in background activity, then a diffuse synchronization with appearance of diffuse, wide-amplitude 1- to 2-c/s waves. Clinical manifestations include dizziness and visual dimming, pallor with cold sweating, and loss of consciousness. If the syncope is

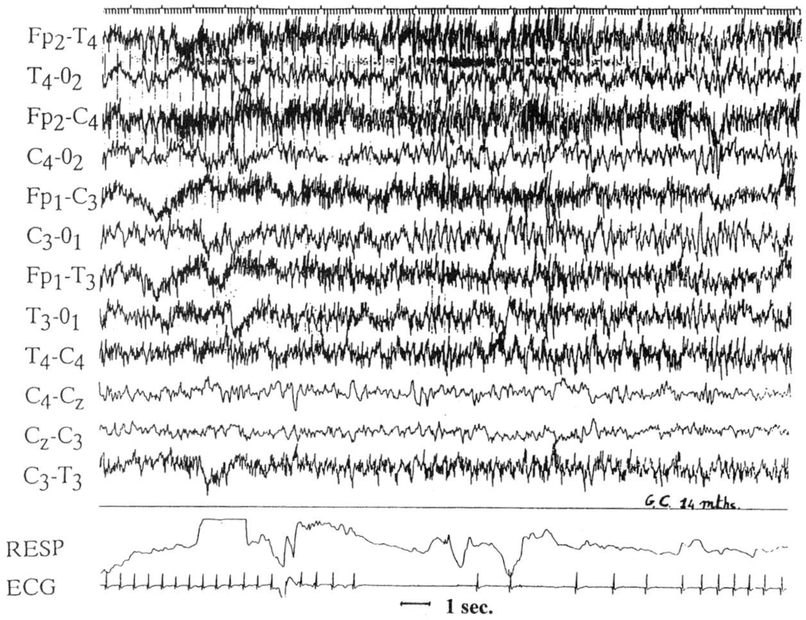

FIGURE 2. A 14-year-old boy with pallid form of breath-holding spells, triggered by emotion or fear. His brother presented with the same phenomenon. A strong emotion (the father leaving the recording room) provoked crying and, after a few seconds, bradycardia to a cardiac pause of 7 seconds. This type of reaction is an expression of "vagotonia."

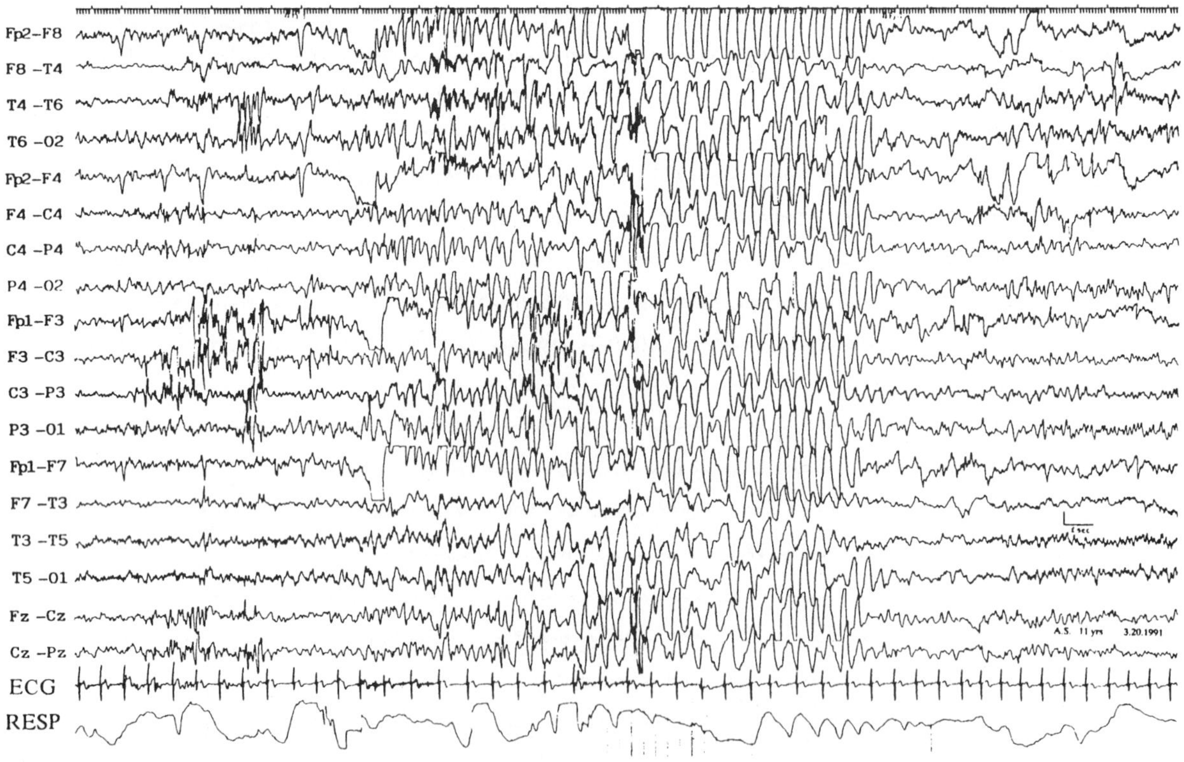

FIGURE 3. An 11-year-old girl with a history of loss of consciousness. The electroencephalogram is performed standing. The patient presented a syncope caused by orthostatic hypotension. Cerebral electrical activity synchronized progressively to 1 to 2 c/s, then progressively desynchronized as symptoms disappeared.

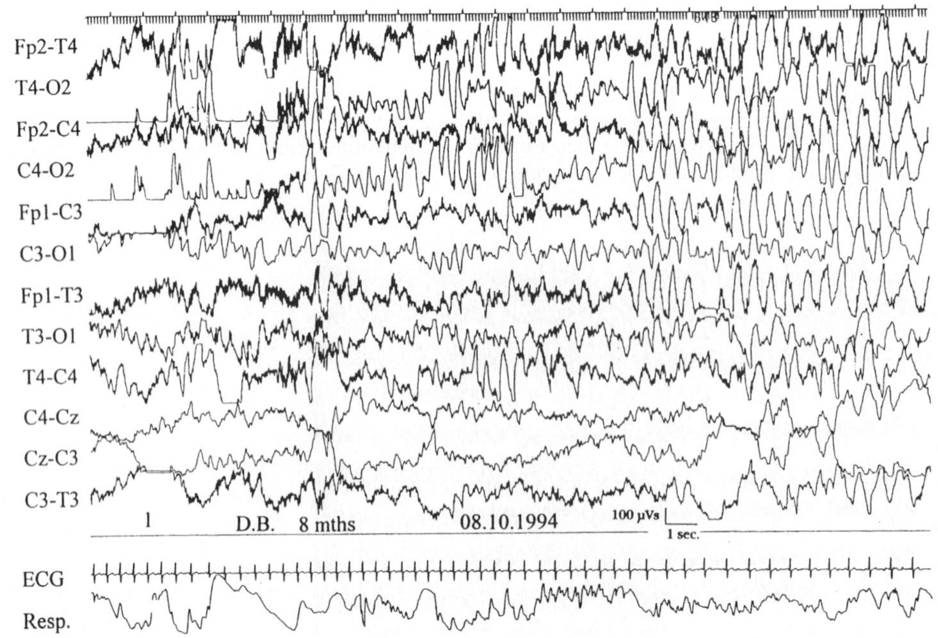

FIGURE 4. An 8-month-old boy with tetralogy of Fallot and frequent cyanotic spells. **A:** After crying briefly, the child stops breathing and rapidly becomes cyanotic. Polygraphic recording shows progressive synchronization of background activity and bradycardia. (*Continued*)

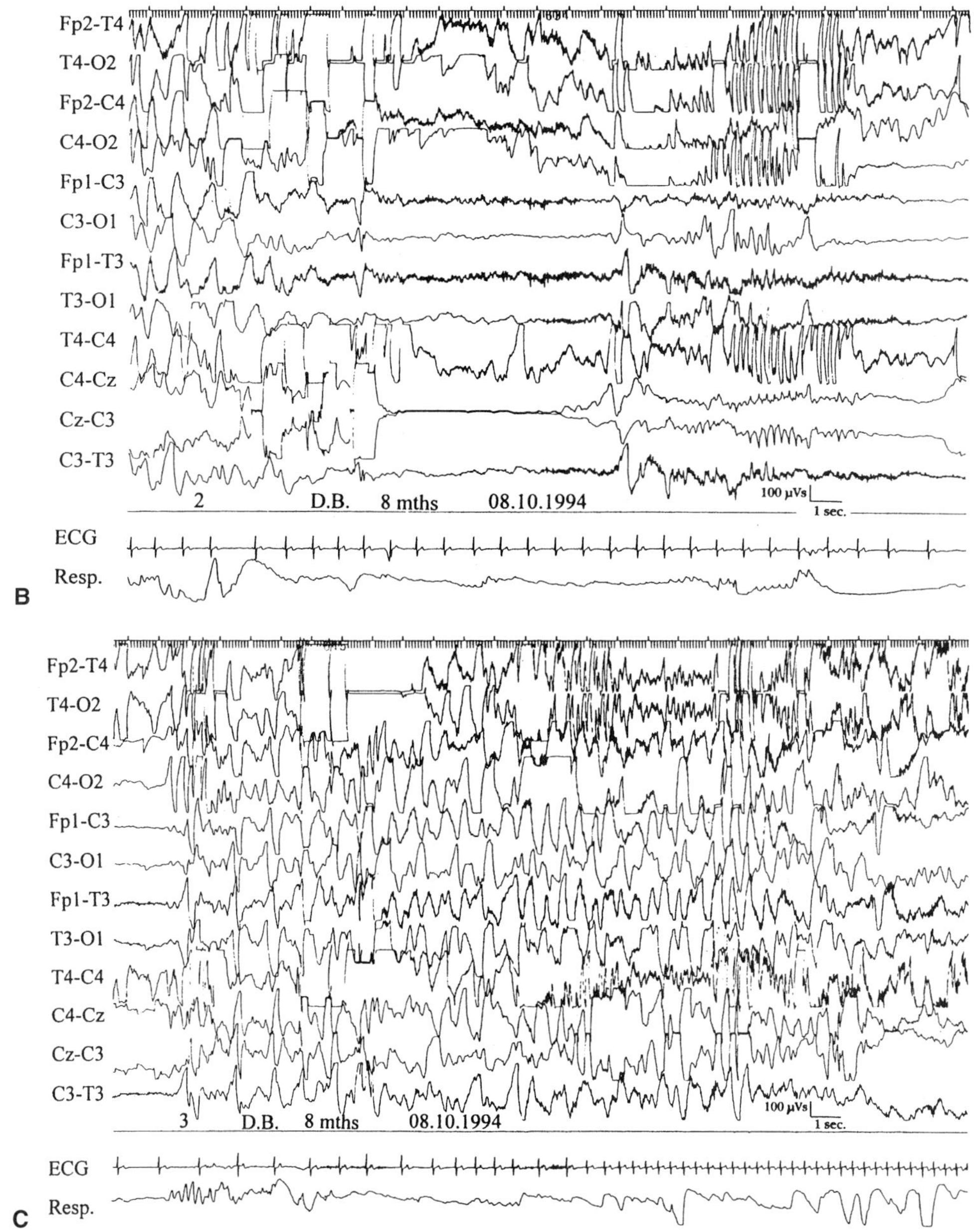

FIGURE 4. (*Continued*) B: The child shows diffuse tonic contraction with apnea and cyanosis. The electroencephalogram (EEG) shows an isoelectric-type pattern; bradycardia is always very significant. There are some artefacts on the EEG due to resuscitation maneuver. C: Respiratory and cardiac activities slowly return to normal and the child regains consciousness. The EEG shows slow, wide-amplitude electrical activity that progressively desynchronizes.

prolonged and there is significant decrease in arterial pressure or severe bradycardia, electrical activity decreases abruptly until an isoelectric pattern is reached. In this phase, the patient is unconscious and can have a diffuse tonic contraction, generally in extension with cyanosis and sometimes even clonic jerks. Subsequently, with the return to baseline cardiac activity and arterial pressure, slow electrical activity with wide amplitude reappears and progressively desynchronizes until normal characteristics are resumed. From a clinical point of view, the patient returns to normal respiration and coloring and regains consciousness (Fig. 4). Epileptic-type abnormalities should not be noted in any phase.

SUMMARY AND CONCLUSIONS

This overview describes nonepileptic systemic paroxysmal disorders during neonatal and childhood periods. Some of these nonepileptic phenomena may be challenging to the clinician. In most situations, however, a careful history by a reliable observer leads the clinician to a successful diagnosis. Home video recordings, synchronous video-neurophysiologic monitoring, or cardiologic testing in the hospital or clinic may document the episodes in question for the clinician, who can then make an accurate diagnosis.

References

1. Asano E, Pawlak C, Shah A, et al. The diagnostic value of initial video-EEG monitoring in children—review of 1,000 cases. *Epil Res*. 2005;66:129–135.
2. Bellazzini MA, Howes DS. Pediatric hypocalcemic seizures: a case of rickets. *J Emerg Med*. 2005;28(2):161–164.
3. Berenberg RA, Pellock JM, DiMauro S, et al. Lumping or splitting? Ophthalmoplegia plus or Kearns-Sayre syndrome. *Ann Neurol*. 1977;1:37–54.
4. Brand DA, Altman RL, Purtill K, et al. Yield of diagnostic testing in infants who have had an apparent life-threatening event. *Pediatrics*. 2005;115(4):885–893.
5. Britton JW. Syncope and seizures differential diagnosis and evaluation. *Clin Auton Res*. 2004;14:148–159.
6. Camfield PR, Camfield CS. Syncope in childhood: A case control clinical study of the familiar tendency to faint. *Clin J Neurol Sci*. 1990;17:306–308.
7. Camfield CS, Camfield PR, Sadler M, et al. Paroxysmal eyelid movements. A confusing feature of generalized photosensitive epilepsy. *Neurology*. 2004;63:40–42.
8. Colle E, Ulstrom RA. Ketotic hypoglycemia. *J Pediatr*. 1964;64:632–681.
9. Daoud AS, Batieha A, Al-Sheyyab M, et al. Effectiveness of iron therapy on breath-holding spells. *J Pediatr*. 1997;130:547–550.
10. Demirkiran M, Jankovic J. Paroxysmal dyskinesias: clinical features and classification. *Ann Neurol*. 1995;38(4):571–579.
11. Deonna T, Roulet E, Meyer HU. Benign paroxysmal tonic upgaze of childhood—a new syndrome. *Neuropediatrics*. 1990;21(4):213–214.
12. *Diagnostic and Statistical Manual of Mental Disorders*, 3rd ed., rev. Washington, DC: American Psychiatric Association; 1987.
13. DiMario FJ. Prospective study of children with cyanotic and pallid breath-holding spells. *Pediatrics*. 2001;107(2):265–269.
14. DiMario FJ, Burleson JA. Autonomic nervous system function in severe breath-holding spells. *Pediatr Neurol*. 1993;9:268–274.
15. Donat JF, Wright FS. Episodic symptoms mistaken for seizures in the neurologically impaired child. *Neurology*. 1990;40:156–157.
16. Doummar D, Roussat B, Beauvais P, et al. Spasmus nutans: apropos of 16 cases. *Arch Pediatr*. 1998;5(3):264–268.
17. Elliott FA. The episodic dyscontrol syndrome and aggression. *Neurol Clin*. 1984;2:113–125.
18. Fejerman N. Nonepileptic disorders imitating generalized idiopathic epilepsies. *Epilepsia*. 2005;46(Suppl 9):80–83.
19. Fernandez-Alvarez E. Transient movement disorders in children. *J Neurol*. 1998;245:1–5.
20. Ferry PC, Banner W, Wolf RA. *Seizure Disorders in Children. Classifying Seizures, the Epilepsies, and Nonseizure States*. Philadelphia: Lippincott; 1986.
21. Foreman DM. Detecting fabricated or induced illness in children may now necessitate controversial surveillance tools. *BMJ*. 2005;331:978–979.
22. Fusco L, Specchio N. Nonepileptic paroxysmal manifestations during sleep in infancy and childhood. *Neurol Sci*. 2005: 26:s205–s209.
23. Grubb BP, Orecchio E, Kurczyski TW. Head upright tilt table testing in an evaluation of recurrent unexplained syncope. *Pediatr Neurol*. 1992;8:423–427.
24. Hall KL, Zalman B. Evaluation and management of apparent life-threatening events in children. *Am Fam Physician*. 2005;71:2301–2308.
25. Herbst JJ. Gastroesophageal reflux. *J Pediatr*. 1981;98:859–870.
26. Herbst JJ, Minton SD, Book LS. Gastroesophageal reflux causing respiratory distress and apnea in newborn infants. *J Pediatr*. 1979;95:763–768.
27. Holmes GL. *Diagnosis and Management of Seizures in Children*. Philadelphia: WB Saunders; 1987.
28. Horrocks A, Nechay A, Stephenson JBP, et al. Anoxic–epileptic seizures: observational study of epileptic seizures induced by syncopes. *Arch Dis Child*. 2005;90:1283–1287.
29. Jervell A, Lange-Nelson F. Congenital deaf mutism, functional heart disease with prolongation of the QT interval and sudden death. *Am Heart J*. 1957;54:59–67.
30. Kanazawa O. Shuddering attacks—report of four children. *Pediatr Neurol*. 2000;23:421–424.
31. Kao A, Mariani J, McDonald-McGinn DM, et al. Increased prevalence of unprovoked seizures in patients with a 22q11.2 deletion. *Am J Med Genet*. 2004;129A:29–34.
32. Katz RM. Cough syncope in children with asthma. *J Pediatr*. 1970;77:48–51.
33. Kiechl-Kohlendorfer U, Hof D, Peglow U, et al. Epidemiology of apparent life threatening events. *Arch Dis Child*. 2004;90:297–300.
34. Kinsbourne M. Hiatus hernia with contortions of the neck. *Lancet*. 1964;1:1058.
35. Li Z, Turner RP, Smith G. Childhood paroxysmal kinesigenic dyskinesia: report of seven cases with onset at an early age. *Brief Commun Epil Behav*. 2005;6:435–439.
36. Lindsay J, Ounsted C, Richards P. Long-term outcome in children with temporal lobe seizures. III. Psychiatric aspects in childhood and adult life. *Dev Med Child Neurol*. 1979;21:630–636.
37. Lispi ML, Vigevano F. Benign paroxysmal tonic upgaze of childhood with ataxia. *Epileptic Disord*. 2001;3(4):2003–2006.
38. Lombroso CT, Fejerman N. Benign myoclonus of early infancy. *Ann Neurol*. 1977;1:138–143.
39. Lombroso CT, Lerman P. Breathholding spells (cyanotic and pallid infantile syncope). *Pediatrics*. 1967;39:563–581.
40. Louis ED, Dure LS, Pullman S. Essential tremor in childhood: a series of nineteen cases. *Mov Disord*. 2001;16(5):921–923.
41. Massin MM, Bourguignont A, Coremans C, et al. Syncope in pediatric patients presenting to an emergency department. *J Pediatr*. 2004;145:223–228.
42. McGovern MC, Smith MBH. Causes of apparent life threatening events in infants: a systematic review. *Arch Dis Child*. 2004;89:1043–1048.
43. Meadow R. Munchausen's syndrome by proxy—the hinterland of child abuse. *Lancet*. 1977;2:343.
44. Meadow R. Munchausen's syndrome by proxy. *Arch Dis Child*. 1982;57:92–97.
45. Okada K, Miyako M, Honma S, et al. Discharge diagnoses in infants with apparent life-threatening event. *Pediatr Int*. 2003;45(5):560–563.
46. Oren J, Kelly DH, Todres D, et al. Respiratory complications in patients with myelodysplasia and Arnold-Chiari malformation. *Am J Dis Child*. 1986;140:221–224.
47. Orii KE, Kato Z, Osamu F, et al. Changes of autonomic nervous system function in patients with breath-holding spells treated with iron. *J Child Neurol*. 2002;17(5):337–340.
48. Paolicchi JM. The spectrum of nonepileptic events in children. *Epilepsia*. 2002;43(Suppl 3):60–64.
49. Paul MH. Tetralogy of Fallot. In: *Rudolph's Pediatrics*, 10th ed. Rudolph AM, ed. Norwalk, CT: Appleton & Lange; 1991:1397–1398.
50. Pellock JM. The differential diagnosis of epilepsy: nonepileptic paroxysmal disorders. In: Wyllie E, ed. *The Treatment of Epilepsy: Principles and Practice*. Philadelphia: Lea & Febiger; 1993.
51. Pignata C, Ferrina V, Andrea G, et al. Prolonged QT interval syndrome presenting as idiopathic epilepsy. *Neuropediatrics*. 1983;14:235–236.
52. Pratt JL, Fleisher GR. Syncope in children and adolescents. *Pediatr Emerg Care*. 1989;5:80–82.
53. Prensky AL. An approach to the child with paroxysmal phenomenon with emphasis on nonepileptic disorders. In: Dotson WE, Pellock JW, eds. *Pediatric Epilepsy: Diagnosis and Therapy*. New York: Demos; 1992.
54. Pritchard PB III, Lombroso CT, McIntyre M. Psychological complications of temporal lobe epilepsy. *Neurology*. 1980;30:277–232.
55. Puranik R, Chow CK, Duflou JA, et al.*Heart Rhythm*. 2005;2(12):1277–1282.
56. Resnick TJ, Moshe SL, Perotta L, et al. Benign neonatal sleep myoclonus: relationship to sleep states. *Arch Neurol*. 1986;43:266–268.
57. Rouveyrol F, Stephan JL. Élévation paroxystique des globes oculaires du nourrisson: à propos de 2 observations. Benign paroxysmal tonic upgaze of infancy: 2 additional cases. *Arch Pediatr*. 2003;10:527–529.
58. Rugg-Gunn F, Simister RJ, Squirrell M, et al. Cardiac arrhythmias in focal epilepsy: a prospective long-term study. *Lancet*. 2004;364:2212–2219.
59. Schreier H. Munchausen by proxy defined. Special article. *Pediatrics*. 2002;110(5):985–988.
60. Scott O, Macartney FJ, Deverall PB. Sick sinus syndrome in children. *Arch Dis Child*. 1976;51:100–105.
61. Shahar E, Raviv R. Sporadic major hyperekplexia in neonates and infants: clinical manifestations and outcome. *Pediatr Neurol*. 2004;31:30–34.
62. Shuper A, Zalzberg J, Weitz R, et al. Jitteriness beyond the neonatal period: a benign pattern of movement in infancy. *J Child Neurol*. 1986;6:243–245.
63. Spitzer AR, Boyle JT, Tuchman DN, et al. Awake apnea associated with gastroesophageal reflux: a specific clinical syndrome. *J Pediatr*. 1984;104:200–205.
64. Tolia V, Wuerth A, Thomas R. Gastroesophageal reflux disease: review of presenting symptoms, evaluation, management, and outcome in infants. *Dig Dis Sci*. 2003;48(9):1723–1729.
65. Valente KD, Freitas A, Fiore LA, et al. The diagnostic role of short duration outpatient V-EEG monitoring in children. *Pediatr Neurol*. 2003;28(4):285–291.
66. Vanasse M, Bedard P, Anderson F. Shuddering attacks in children: an early clinical manifestation of essential tremor. *Neurology*. 1976;26:1027–1030.
67. Villain E, Levy M, Kachaner J, et al. Prolonged QT interval in neonates: benign, transient, or prolonged risk of sudden death. *Am Heart J*. 1992;124:194–197.
68. Visudhiphan P, Visudtibhan A, Chiemchanya S, et al. Neonatal seizures and familial hypomagnesemia with secondary hypocalcemia. *Pediatr Neurol*. 2005;33:202–205.
69. Watanabe K, Hara K, Hakamada S, et al. Seizures with apnea in children. *Pediatrics*. 1982;79:87–90.
70. Watemberg N, Tziperman B, Dabby R, et al. *Epilepsia*. 2005;46(5):716–719.
71. Yang ML, Fullwood E, Goldstein J, et al. Masturbation in infancy and early childhood presenting as a movement disorder: 12 cases and a review of the literature. *Pediatrics*. 2005;116(6):1427–1432.
72. Zijlmans M, Flanagan D, Gotman J. Heart rate changes and ECG abnormalities during epileptic seizures: prevalence and definition of an objective clinical sign. *Epilepsia*. 2002;43(8):847–854.

CHAPTER 274 ■ MIGRAINE

STEPHEN D. SILBERSTEIN, RICHARD B. LIPTON, AND SHERYL HAUT

INTRODUCTION

Migraine and epilepsy are the most common of the chronic neurologic disorders with episodic manifestations. Each group includes a highly variable family of clinical features, natural histories, and patterns of treatment response.[6,99] Therefore, there are many types of migraine, as there are many types of epilepsy. Both disorders are characterized by episodes of neurologic dysfunction that are sometimes accompanied by headache, as well as gastrointestinal, autonomic, and psychologic features.

This chapter focuses on the relationship between migraine and epilepsy for several reasons. First, abundant clinical and epidemiologic data demonstrate that migraine and epilepsy are highly comorbid, in that individuals with one disorder are at least twice as likely to have the other.[5–7,60,61,67] Secondly, the clinical presentation of migraine and epilepsy may overlap, creating a challenge in differential diagnosis. Finally, the disorders share overlapping risk factors, brain mechanisms, and treatments.[61] We will begin by describing the migraine attack, dividing it into four traditional stages—the premonitory phase, the aura, the headache phase, and the resolution phase[31]—and contrast the seizure using this framework. We will then review the diagnosis of migraine using the International Classification of Headache Disorders (ICHD)-2 criteria, emphasizing the variants of migraine most frequently mistaken for epilepsy. Finally, we will summarize the epidemiologic evidence that migraine and epilepsy are associated, and provide treatment considerations.

CLASSIFICATION

Each family of disorders has an internationally recognized classification system. The classification system for headache, developed by international consensus, was updated in 2004, and will be referred to herein as the ICHD-2.[40] The classification system utilized in epilepsy was developed by the International League Against Epilepsy (ILAE).

The ICHD-2 criteria divide headache disorders into two broad groups: Primary headache disorders and secondary headache disorders.[40] In a somewhat similar manner, epilepsies are regarded as idiopathic, symptomatic, or cryptogenic by ILAE criteria. In the secondary headache disorders, the headache is symptomatic of an underlying condition, such as a stroke or a mass lesion. This group is analogous to the symptomatic epilepsies in that an underlying cause has been identified. In the primary headache disorders, the headache does not have an identifiable underlying cause. Primary headaches are divided into four major categories: Migraine; tension-type headache; the trigeminal autonomic cephalgias, including cluster headache; and a group of headache disorders analogous to the idiopathic epilepsies. There is no group of headache disorders akin to cryptogenic epilepsies. Furthermore, there is no classification of headache types analogous to the classification of seizure types.

MIGRAINE

Migraine is an extremely common disorder. Recent population-based studies have yielded remarkably consistent 1-year period prevalence estimates of about 6% in men and 15% to 18% in women.[87,62,97] Most studies find that migraine is about three times more common in women than in men.[62,64,97]

Headache diagnosis is usually based on the retrospective reporting of attack characteristics. The results of general medical and neurologic examinations, as well as laboratory studies, are usually normal and serve to exclude other, more ominous, causes of headache. The ICHD-2 classification of migraine subtypes is presented in Table 1. The most important International Headache Society (IHS) subtypes of migraine are "migraine without aura" (formerly common migraine) (Table 2) and "migraine with aura" (formerly classic migraine) (Table 3). In migraine, the aura is a complex of focal neurologic symptoms that precedes or accompanies an attack.[116] About 20% to 30% of migraineurs have migraine with aura.[63] The same patient may have headache without aura, headache with aura, and aura without headache.

The migraine attack can be divided into four phases: The premonitory phase, which occurs hours or days before the headache; the aura, which comes immediately before the headache; the headache itself; and the postdrome. Although most people experience more than one phase, no one phase is absolutely required for a diagnosis of migraine, and most people do not experience all four phases.[17] The epilepsy attack may also have a premonitory, aura, attack, and postictal phase. The similarity in terminology does not imply similarity in mechanisms.

Premonitory, or prodromal, phenomena occur in approximately 60% of migraineurs, often hours to days before the onset of headache.[3,4,17] The phenomena of the premonitory phase has been elucidated using an electronic diary.[33] Features include constitutional, autonomic, psychological (depression, euphoria, irritability, restlessness, mental slowness, hyperactivity, fatigue, and drowsiness), and neurologic (photophobia, phonophobia, and hyperosmia) features. Some patients report a poorly characterized feeling that a migraine attack is coming. Although features vary widely among individuals, they are often consistent within an individual. The most common premonitory symptoms were feeling tired/weary (72%), difficulty concentrating (51%), and stiff neck (50%). Poor functioning commonly predicted headache.[35] Migraineurs who reported premonitory symptoms accurately predicted their full-blown headaches 72% of the time. Among patients who were almost certain that attacks would occur, 93% had attacks.

Premonitory symptoms have also been reported prior to seizure onset.[30] Although less commonly present than in migraine, patients with epilepsy often report a constellation of symptoms prior to a seizure, including irritability, gastrointestinal upset, heaviness, or depression.

TABLE 1

INTERNATIONAL CLASSIFICATION OF HEADACHE DISORDERS (ICHD)-2 MIGRAINE CLASSIFICATION

1. Migraine
   - 1.1 Migraine without aura
   - 1.2 Migraine with aura
     - 1.2.1 Typical aura with migraine headache
     - 1.2.2 Typical aura with nonmigraine headache
     - 1.2.3 Typical aura without headache
     - 1.2.4 Familial hemiplegic migraine
     - 1.2.5 Sporadic hemiplegic migraine
     - 1.2.6 Basilar-type migraine
   - 1.3 Childhood periodic syndromes that are commonly precursors of migraine
     - 1.3.1 Cyclical vomiting
     - 1.3.2 Abdominal migraine
     - 1.3.3 Benign paroxysmal vertigo of childhood
   - 1.4 Retinal migraine
   - 1.5 Complications of migraine
     - 1.5.1 Chronic migraine
     - 1.5.2 Status migrainosus
     - 1.5.3 Persistent aura without infarction
     - 1.5.4 Migrainous infarction
     - 1.5.5 Migraine-triggered seizures
   - 1.6 Probable migraine
     - 1.6.1 Probable migraine without aura
     - 1.6.2 Probable migraine with aura
     - 1.6.3 Probable chronic migraine

From Headache Classification Committee. The International Classification of Headache Disorders. 2nd ed. *Cephalalgia.* 2004;24:1–160.

Aura

The migraine aura consists of focal neurologic symptoms that precede or accompany an attack. Approximately 20% to 30% of migraineurs experience auras. Most aura symptoms develop slowly over 5 to 20 minutes and usually last for <60 minutes.

TABLE 2

1.1 MIGRAINE WITHOUT AURA

DIAGNOSTIC CRITERIA

A. At least five attacks[87] fulfilling criteria B–D
B. Headache attacks lasting 4–72 hours (untreated or unsuccessfully treated)
C. Headache has at least two of the following characteristics:
   1. Unilateral location
   2. Pulsating quality
   3. Moderate or severe pain intensity
   4. Aggravation by or causing avoidance of routine physical activity (e.g., walking or climbing stairs)
D. During headache at least one of the following:
   1. Nausea and/or vomiting
   2. Photophobia and phonophobia
E. Not attributed to another disorder

From Headache Classification Committee. The International Classification of Headache Disorders. 2nd ed. *Cephalalgia.* 2004;24:1–160.

TABLE 3

MIGRAINE WITH AURA (41)

DIAGNOSTIC CRITERIA

A. At least two attacks fulfilling criterion B
B. Migraine aura fulfilling criteria B and C for one of the subforms 1.2.1–1.2.6
C. Not attributed to another disorder

Typical aura with migraine headache
DIAGNOSTIC CRITERIA

A. At least two attacks fulfilling criteria B–D
B. Aura consisting of at least one of the following, but no motor weakness:
   1. Fully reversible visual symptoms including positive features (e.g., flickering lights, spots, or lines) and/or negative features (i.e., loss of vision)
   2. Fully reversible sensory symptoms including positive features (i.e., pins and needles) and/or negative features (i.e., numbness)
   3. Fully reversible dysphasic speech disturbance
C. At least two of the following:
   1. Homonymous visual symptoms and/or unilateral sensory symptoms
   2. At least one aura symptom develops gradually over ≥5 minutes and/or different aura symptoms occur in succession over ≥5 minutes
   3. Each symptom lasts ≥5 and ≤60 minutes
D. Headache fulfilling criteria B–D for 1.1 *Migraine without aura* begins during the aura or follows aura within 60 minutes
E. Not attributed to another disorder

From Headache Classification Committee. The International Classification of Headache Disorders. 2nd ed. *Cephalalgia.* 2004;24:1–160.

The aura almost always includes visual features but somatosensory, motor, language, and brainstem disturbances are not rare.

The visual aura often has a hemianoptic distribution and includes both positive (scintillations, fortification spectra, photopsia) and negative (scotoma) features. Elementary visual disturbances include colorless scotoma, photopsia, or phosphenes. Simple flashes, specks, or hallucinations of geometric forms (points, stars, lines, curves, circles, sparks, flashes, or flames) occur and may be single or number in the hundreds. More complicated hallucinations include teichopsia, or fortification spectrum, which is the most characteristic visual aura and is almost diagnostic of migraine. An arc of scintillating lights classically begins near the point of fixation and may form a herringbone-like pattern that expands to encompass an increasing portion of a visual hemifield. It migrates across the visual field with a scintillating edge of zigzag or flashing lights that are often black and white; on occasion colored dots appear at the end of the white stripe. A scotoma is a negative phenomenon consisting of a blanking or graying out of vision. Scotomas are usually accompanied by a positive visual display, but may occur independently. Complex disorders of visual perception include metamorphopsia, micropsia, macropsia, zoom vision, and mosaic vision.[99,100]

Numbness or tingling (paresthesia) over one side of the face and in the ipsilateral hand or arm is the most common somatosensory phenomena. Hemiparesis and dysphasia or aphasia may develop. Olfactory hallucinations are rare, unpleasant, and short lived (5 minutes to 24 hours). Anxiety, déjà vu, and jamais vu have been reported as migraine auras and are presumably of temporal lobe origin.[90] One type of aura may follow another: Sensory phenomena may occur as visual phenomena fade, or motor phenomena may develop as sensory phenomena dissipate. Although visual auras are relatively specific for migraine, related phenomena may occur in cerebrovascular disease, including carotid dissection, and in epilepsy, especially of the occipital lobes.

Nonvisual association cortex symptoms also occur; these include complex difficulties in the perception and use of the body (apraxia and agnosia), speech and language disturbances, states of double or multiple consciousness associated with déjà vu or jamais vu, and elaborate, dreamy, nightmarish, trancelike or delirious states.[38,51,59,90,95]

In epilepsy, the aura, representing an actual seizure discharge, is typically rapid in development and brief. In contrast to the common visual auras of migraine, epileptic auras are often associated with more unusual symptoms. Auras are estimated to precede up to 80% of temporal lobe seizures; in this setting, autonomic and psychic phenomena, such as a rising abdominal sensation, nausea, fear, or déjà vu, are common.[103]

Mechanisms of Aura

Cortical spreading depression (CSD) is believed to underlie the migraine aura. CSD consists of a wave of excitation followed by a wave of inhibition that moves across the cortical mantle at a rate of 3 mm/min. Best studied as an animal phenomenon, it can be induced by pricking the cerebral cortex with a pin, by applying potassium chloride, and in other ways.[56] CSD is characterized by transient increases in metabolic and electrical activity and transient increases in cerebral blood flow (CBF), followed by sustained decreases.[75] The aura is associated with an initial hyperemic phase followed by reduced CBF, which moves across the cortex (spreading oligemia).[76]

Several lines of evidence in humans suggest that CSD is a mechanistic substrate of migraine aura. Olesen and Lauritzen[74,76] found 17% to 35% reductions in posterior CBF, which spread anteriorly at 2 to 3 mm/min. It crossed brain areas supplied by separate vessels and is, thus, not due to segmental vasoconstriction.[74] Reduced CBF persisted from 30 minutes to 6 hours, then slowly returned to baseline or even increased. The rates of progression of spreading oligemia could account for the rate of expansion of the scotoma in migraine, suggesting that they are related.[55,56,69,77]

Magnetoencephalographic studies show similar profiles in humans during migraine aura and in experimental animals during CSD,[101] implying that spreading depression may be the mechanism that produces the aura.[18,53,86,87,111] Subjects with spontaneous migraine visual auras have also been studied with functional magnetic resonance imaging (fMRI).[23] Interictally, using perfusion-weighted imaging, CBF, cerebral blood volume, and mean transit time were normal and symmetric. During visual auras, CBF decreased 15% to 53%, cerebral blood volume decreased 6% to 33%, and mean transit time increased 10% to 54% in the occipital cortex gray matter contralateral to the affected visual hemifield. When multiple perfusion images were obtained during the same aura, the margin of the perfusion defect moved anteriorly. The absence of diffusion abnormalities in these patients suggests that ischemia does not occur during the migraine aura.[22]

Blood oxygenation level–dependent (BOLD) fMRI reflects the relative concentration of deoxyhemoglobin in venous blood. Visual stimulation was used to trigger headache in migraineurs.[20] A wave of increased (hyperoxygenated blood) and then decreased (possibly reflecting neuronal metabolic-flow coupling) BOLD signals propagated into the contiguous occipital cortex at 3 to 6 mm/min. When visual stimulation was used to test the visual cortex response, the BOLD signal and the BOLD response to visual activation diminished following progression of the visual aura.[39]

Using transcranial magnetic stimulation–applied magnetic fields of increasing intensity to evaluate occipital cortex excitability, Aurora et al.[9] and Young et al.,[115] but not Afra et al.,[1] found that phosphenes were generated in migraineurs at lower thresholds than controls, and that it was easier to visually trigger headaches in those with lower thresholds. Other evidence of increased central nervous system (CNS) excitability comes from studies of visual and brainstem auditory-evoked potentials.[93] Migraine with aura may be due to neuronal hyperexcitability, perhaps due to cortical disinhibition.

The aura of epilepsy is a simple partial nonmotor seizure that typically precedes an observable seizure, but may occur alone. The patient experiences the aura prior to loss of consciousness, and memory of it may be retained. The aura is associated with the electroencephalographic correlate of the seizure type in which it occurs[27]; however, the EEG pattern is often not evident on surface recording until the seizure has progressed to involve a larger area of cortex.

Headache Phase

The typical migraine headache is unilateral and described as throbbing by 85% of patients. Headache severity ranges from moderate to marked and is aggravated by head movement or physical activity. The onset is usually gradual and the attack usually lasts 4 to 72 hours in adults and 2 to 48 hours in children.[99] Anorexia is common, although food cravings can occur. Nausea occurs in up to 90% of patients, and vomiting occurs in about one third of migraineurs.[63] Many patients experience sensory hyperexcitability manifested by photophobia, phonophobia, and osmophobia, and seek a dark, quiet room.[28,95] To make a diagnosis of migraine, the pain must be accompanied by other features. The ICHD-2 selects particular associated features as cardinal manifestations for diagnosis (Table 2).[98]

Postdrome or Postictal Phase

With migraine, the patient may feel tired, washed out, irritable, and listless and may have impaired concentration. Many patients report scalp tenderness. Some people feel unusually refreshed or euphoric after an attack, whereas others note depression and malaise. In epilepsy, during the postictal phase, there may be a depressed level of awareness or focal neurologic deficits that sometimes provide clues to the site of seizure onset.

FORMAL INTERNATIONAL CLASSIFICATION OF HEADACHE DISORDERS-2 CLASSIFICATION

Migraine without Aura (Common Migraine) (Table 2)

To establish a diagnosis of ICHD-2 migraine without aura (1.1), five attacks lasting from 4 to 72 hours are required. The attacks must have two of the following four pain characteristics: Unilateral location, pulsating quality, moderate to severe intensity, and aggravation by or causing avoidance of routine physical activity. In addition, the attacks must be associated with at least one of the following: Nausea or vomiting or photophobia and phonophobia. No single characteristic is mandatory for a diagnosis of migraine. A patient who has photophobia, phonophobia, and severe pain aggravated by routine activity meets these criteria, as does the more typical patient with unilateral throbbing pain and nausea.[98] Attacks that persist for more than 3 days define status migrainosus. Although the frequency of attacks varies widely, the average migraineur experiences one to three headaches a month. Like epilepsy, migraine is, by definition, a recurrent phenomenon. The requirement for at least five attacks is imposed because headaches simulating migraine may be caused by such organic diseases as brain tumors, sinusitis, or glaucoma.[98]

Migraine with Aura (Classic Migraine) (Table 3)

Descriptively, auras are focal neurologic symptoms that usually develop gradually over 5 to 20 minutes and last for <60 minutes. The diagnosis of migraine with aura (1.2) requires at least two attacks meeting the criteria of one of the subforms. In addition, it cannot be attributed to another disorder. Migraine with aura is subclassified into typical aura with migraine headache (1.2.1) (homonymous visual disturbance, unilateral numbness or aphasia); typical aura with nonmigraine headache (1.2.2); typical aura without headache (1.2.3); familial hemiplegic migraine (FHM) (1.2.4); sporadic hemiplegic migraine (1.2.5) (see Table 6); and basilar-type migraine (1.2.5). Some of these variants will be discussed in detail since they may be confused with epilepsy.

Typical aura with migraine headache (1.2.1) requires at least two attacks with the aura consisting of at least one of the following (but no motor weakness): Fully reversible visual symptoms including positive; fully reversible sensory symptoms including positive; and fully reversible dysphasic speech disturbance. Additionally, it requires at least two of the following: Homonymous visual symptoms and/or unilateral sensory symptoms; at least one aura symptom developing gradually over ≥5 minutes and/or different aura symptoms occurring in succession over ≥5 minutes; and each symptom lasting ≥5 and ≤60 minutes. Fewer attacks are required to make a diagnosis of migraine with aura because a typical aura is highly specific for migraine. Headache with the features of migraine without aura usually follows the aura symptoms. Less commonly, headache lacks migrainous features or is completely absent.[40,98]

If the aura includes motor weakness, it is coded as 1.2.4 *Familial hemiplegic migraine* or 1.2.5 *Sporadic hemiplegic migraine*.

The headache and associated symptoms of migraine with aura are similar to those of migraine without aura but may be less severe and/or of shorter duration. Most people who have migraine with aura also have migraine without aura. The aura usually lasts 20 to 30 minutes and typically precedes the headache, but occasionally it occurs only during the headache.

MIGRAINE VARIANTS

The variants of migraine as classified by the ICHD-2 have been discussed in detail elsewhere.[40] In this section we will describe the migraine variants that are most commonly confused with epilepsy, using ICHD-2 terminology when possible.

Basilar-type Migraine

Originally called basilar or basilar artery migraine,[40] the term *Bickerstaff syndrome* has also been applied to this disorder.[13] It affects all age groups and both sexes, with the usual female predominance. The aura often lasts <1 hour and is usually followed by a headache. In basilar-type migraine, the visual aura is usually followed by at least one of the following: Ataxia, vertigo, tinnitus, diplopia, nystagmus, dysarthria, bilateral paresthesia, or a change in the levels of consciousness and cognition. If marked, these alterations in consciousness define confusional migraine.

The aura symptoms described above are often, but not always, followed by a severe, throbbing occipital headache and vomiting. Although attacks are usually infrequent, they can last for 1 to 3 days. These headaches can be very frightening and difficult to diagnose. On occasion, the attacks can lead to cardiac arrhythmias and brainstem stroke. A diagnosis of basilar migraine should be considered in patients with paroxysmal brainstem disturbances. Basilar migraine may be difficult to differentiate from simple or complex partial seizures and the postictal state following a primary or secondary generalized seizure. The differential diagnosis, besides occipital lobe epilepsy, includes posterior fossa tumor or malformation, urea cycle defects, and mitochondrial disorders.[84]

Confusional Migraine[40,43]

No longer part of the ICHD-2 classification, confusional migraine is probably a form of basilar-type migraine or hemiplegic migraine. It is characterized by a typical migraine aura, a headache (which may be insignificant), and confusion, which may precede or follow the headache. During the confused period the patient is inattentive, is distracted, and has difficulty maintaining speech and other motor activities. The electroencephalogram (EEG) may be abnormal during the attack. Agitation, memory disturbances, obscene utterances, and violent behavior have been reported. Single attacks are most common; multiple attacks rare. Attacks may be triggered by mild head trauma. A more profoundly disturbed level of consciousness may lead to migraine stupor, which can last from hours up to 5 days. The confusional state is usually followed by sleep, resembling postictal depression of mental status. Confusional migraine may be difficult to diagnose. The differential diagnosis includes drug ingestion, metabolic encephalopathies (Reye syndrome, hypoglycemia), viral encephalitis, and acute psychosis. Acute confusional states also occur during complex partial seizures and in the postictal state. The patient may be delirious, hyperactive, restless, and, on occasion, combative. Acute migraine confusional states may recur over a period of days or months and then evolve into typical migraine episodes. A history of typical migraine aura supports a diagnosis of migraine.[52]

Benign Paroxysmal Vertigo of Childhood

Now classified as one of the "childhood periodic syndromes," this condition is a precursor of migraine (1.3.3). This disorder is characterized by recurrent, brief episodic attacks of vertigo. Attacks occur without warning and resolve spontaneously in otherwise healthy children. Children with this disorder cannot stand, and lie silently on the floor or wish to be held during attacks. Attacks last a few minutes and tend to recur at irregular intervals over a period of 6 to 12 months. While headache may not be present at the onset, as the disorder evolves the vertigo may be replaced by attacks of headache and vomiting, facilitating diagnosis. When simple partial seizures give rise to vertigo, the vertigo is usually less prominent than it is in migraine.

Aura without Headache

Migraine aura can occur without headache,[112] although diagnosis is more difficult in this setting. These periodic neurologic phenomena (scintillating scotomata or recurrent sensory, motor, or mental phenomena) should be accepted as migraine only after a full investigation. Headache occurring in association with some attacks will help confirm the diagnosis.[88] Ziegler and Hassanein[116] reported that 44% of their patients who had headache with aura had aura without headache at some time.

Late-life migrainous accompaniments are characterized by attacks of aura without headache beginning in late life.[31,32] Many patients have a history of migraine in early or midlife, often with an attack-free hiatus. Because focal neurologic defects occur without headache, they can be confused with transient ischemic attacks (TIAs) or seizures. Late-life migrainous accompaniment remains a diagnosis of exclusion.

Migraine-triggered Seizure

New to the ICHD-2 is a seizure triggered by a migraine aura (1.5.5). This diagnosis requires migraine that fulfills the criteria for 1.2 Migraine with aura and a seizure fulfilling diagnostic criteria for one type of epileptic attack that occurs during or within 1 hour after a migraine aura. This phenomenon is sometimes referred to as *migralepsy*.

EPIDEMIOLOGIC CONNECTIONS BETWEEN MIGRAINE AND EPILEPSY

Andermann and Andermann[5] summarized a number of studies that examined the association between migraine and epilepsy. The prevalence of epilepsy in persons with migraine ranged from 1% to 17% with a median of 5.9%, substantially higher than epilepsy's population prevalence of 0.5%. Migraine prevalence in patients with epilepsy ranged from 8% to 15%. Many of these studies were limited by the method of patient identification, the lack of appropriate control groups, and poorly specified definitions of migraine and epilepsy. Nonetheless, these studies powerfully argue that migraine and epilepsy are associated.

Ottman and Lipton[79] examined the association between migraine and epilepsy using data from Columbia University's Epilepsy Family Study. Subjects with epilepsy (probands) who were over 18 years of age were identified and recruited from voluntary organizations for persons with epilepsy. Among the probands with epilepsy, migraine prevalence was 24%. Migraine prevalence was 26% in the relatives with epilepsy. In the control group of relatives without epilepsy, only 15% had migraine. The gender-adjusted rate ratio for migraine in probands with epilepsy compared with relatives without epilepsy was 2.4 (95% confidence interval [CI]: 2.0 to 2.9). For relatives with epilepsy compared with relatives without epilepsy the rate ratio was also 2.4 (95% CI: 1.6 to 3.8). These statistics indicate that the incidence of migraine is 2.4 times higher in persons with epilepsy than in persons without epilepsy.

Risk of migraine was not associated with the age of onset of epilepsy. The risk of migraine was elevated in both partial and generalized seizures, although the risk was higher for probands with partial-onset versus those with generalized-onset seizures (relative risk [RR] = 1.3; 95% CI: 1.00 to 1.86). The risk of migraine was elevated in both idiopathic and symptomatic epilepsy. Probands with epilepsy caused by head trauma had a higher risk of migraine than probands with idiopathic/cryptogenic epilepsy (RR = 1.8, 95% CI: 1.32 to 2.43). Nonetheless, migraine risk was elevated in every subgroup of epilepsy defined by seizure type, age of onset, and etiology of epilepsy.[70]

Although migraine and epilepsy are associated, the mechanisms of the association are complex and may be multifactorial. One possibility is a simple unidirectional causal explanation. For example, migraine may cause epilepsy by inducing brain ischemia and injury. Under this hypothesis, we would expect the incidence of migraine to be elevated before, but not after, the onset of epilepsy. Alternatively, epilepsy may cause migraine by activating the trigeminovascular system. This hypothesis leads us to expect an excess risk of migraine after, but not before, the onset of epilepsy. The data show that there is an excess risk of migraine both before and after seizure onset, leading to the rejection of both unidirectional causal models.

Marks and Ehrenberg[67] explored the timing and features of headache in patients with epilepsy. They found that of 79 of 395 patients with epilepsy, 20% also had IHS migraine. In 84% of patients with both migraine and epilepsy (66 of 79), the attacks were completely independent. In 16% of patients (13 of 79), a seizure immediately followed the migraine aura (migralepsy); 11 of 13 were women, seven of whom had a catamenial pattern. Migralepsy was also seen in refractory patients with both migraine and epilepsy in Andermann's series,[6] although this phenomenon does not account for the majority of the comorbidity.

Velioglu and Ozmenoglu[109] studied the relationship between migraine and epilepsy in 412 adults with epilepsy. Fourteen percent of adults with seizures had IHS migraine. Migraine-induced epilepsy (migralepsy) was found in seven patients (1.7%); all had migraine with aura. The authors at times found it difficult clinically to distinguish the aura of migraine from the aura of epilepsy. Patients were at increased risk for both conditions if they had migraine with aura and catamenial epilepsy. Three of the patients with refractory seizures had improved control with the combination of antimigraine and antiepilepsy drugs.

Lenaerts[57] evaluated the degree of comorbidity and tried to establish the pattern of temporal relationship between migraine and epilepsy in 201 patients from tertiary care clinics. He systematically reviewed charts, obtained additional information by telephone interviews where necessary, and applied IHS and ILAE diagnostic criteria. Two-tier grouping according to reason for referral (migraine or epilepsy) was done. Adequate information was obtained from 185 patients (113 females, 72 males). In the epilepsy-referred patient group ($n = 103$), 23% had migraine, a risk ratio of 1.9 ($p = 0.01$). In the migraine-referred group ($n = 82$), 11% had epilepsy, a risk ratio of 21 ($p = 0.05$). Of the 33 comorbid cases, 21 had their attacks in close temporal relation. The migraine attack preceded the seizure in 12 patients (nine migraine with aura) (57%) and followed it in nine (six migraine with aura) (43%). Migraine attacks equally precede or follow seizures, but migraine aura more often precedes the seizure (migralepsy).

Shared environmental risk factors may contribute to comorbidity. The risk of migraine is higher in subjects with epilepsy caused by head injury. Since head injury is also a risk factor for migraine,[8] comorbidity may result, in part, from an effect of head injury on the risk of both disorders. Because risk is also significantly increased in persons with idiopathic/cryptogenic epilepsy, known environmental risk factors cannot account for all of the comorbidity.

Ottman and Lipton[79] tested the alternative hypothesis, that shared genetic risk factors might account for comorbidity. They argued that the risk of migraine should be higher in families with genetic versus nongenetic forms of epilepsy if genetic factors account for comorbidity. They further argued that the risk of epilepsy should be greater in the relatives of probands with migraine and epilepsy versus the relatives of probands with epilepsy alone. In a series of analyses, they adjusted for a number of potentially confounding factors including age, gender, the familial aggregation of migraine, and the comorbidity of migraine and epilepsy. The analyses failed to confirm either of the authors' hypotheses, leading them to reject the idea that genetic susceptibility accounts for comorbidity.[79]

Having rejected the unidirectional model, the environmental model, and the genetic hypothesis, they proposed that an altered brain state (increased excitability) might increase the risk of both migraine and epilepsy and account for comorbidity. Enhanced neuronal hyperexcitability and a reduced threshold to attacks figure prominently in the pathophysiologic models of migraine and epilepsy. Reduction in brain magnesium or perturbations in neurotransmitter systems may provide a basis for these alterations in brain excitability. In theory, genetic or environmental factors could produce these alterations. Regardless of mechanisms, these findings are important for clinical practice.

INTERRELATIONSHIPS BETWEEN HEADACHE AND EPILEPSY

Apart from the causal epidemiologic issues discussed above, there are many possible clinical interrelationships between headache and epilepsy (Table 4). The disorders may exist independently. Migraine may trigger epilepsy (migralepsy) or epilepsy may initiate headache. Seizure and headache seem to be associated in certain syndromes, such as benign occipital epilepsy of childhood with occipital paroxysms (BOEP). In addition, both disorders may have a common underlying cause such as head trauma, an arteriovenous malformation,[66] or neurofibromatosis.[21,85] Finally, migraine may be a predictor of poor outcome in persons with epilepsy. We will now consider some of these interrelationships.

TABLE 4

MIGRAINE AND EPILEPSY RELATIONSHIPS

1. Coexisting epilepsy and migraine
   Both disorders occur together at an increased prevalence, but attacks occur independently
2. Migraine-induced epilepsy (migralepsy)
   Seizures are triggered by migraine aura
3. Epilepsy-induced headache (ictal or postictal)
   Headache occurs as part of seizure or postictal state
4. Primary epilepsy–migraine syndromes
   Syndromes with features of both migraine and epilepsy without a specific underlying cause
   - Occipital epilepsies (e.g., benign occipital epilepsy)
   - Benign rolandic epilepsy
5. Secondary epilepsy–migraine syndromes
   Both migraine and epilepsy occur in the same individual with a common underlying cause
   - Mitochondrial disorders (MELAS)
   - Symptomatic (e.g., arteriovenous malformation of occipital lobe)
     - Neurofibromatosis
     - Stürge-Weber

Modified from Andermann F. Migraine and epilepsy: an overview. In: Andermann F, Lugaresi E, eds. *Migraine and Epilepsy*. Boston: Butterworths, 1987:405–421; and Welch KM, Lewis D. Migraine and epilepsy. *Neurol Clin.* 1997;15:107–114.

Headache as a Consequence of Seizures

Although headache is commonly associated with seizures as a preictal, ictal, or postictal phenomenon, it is often neglected because of the dramatic neurologic manifestations of the seizure. Patients with migraine-triggered epilepsy seek medical attention because of seizures, which may overshadow the migraine and be overlooked by the patient and physician.

Preictal and Ictal Headache

Palmini and Gloor[80] presented a descriptive study of auras in partial seizures. Cephalic auras, defined by the symptoms of nonvertiginous dizziness, lightheadedness, or head pressure, occurred in 22 of 196 patients. In Blume and Young's epilepsy unit, 2.8% of 858 patients had brief ictal pain and 1.3% (11 patients) had headache. Only two patients described the pain as throbbing; the others described it as sharp or steady. Headache preceded the seizure in eight patients and accompanied the other ictal symptoms in three; all three of these patients had partial seizures, although the nature and location of EEG abnormalities varied considerably from patient to patient.

Isler et al.[47] found that hemicranial attacks of pain coincided with seizure activity and lasted for seconds to minutes (hemicrania epileptica). Two exceptions were noted: One a case of complex partial status in which the headache lasted for hours and another in which the headache lasted most of the 20 minutes of a recorded seizure. Overall, 20% of this group of drug-resistant epileptics had cephalic symptoms.

In a more recent study,[114] nearly half of patients undergoing continuous EEG monitoring for intractable epilepsy experienced peri-ictal headache, the majority being postictal. Interestingly, preictal headache lateralized to the side of seizure focus in 9 of 10 patients.

Headache can also be the sole or most predominant clinical manifestation of epileptic seizures, although this is a relatively rare situation.[54] Headache was noted to be a true ictal manifestation during intracranial monitoring, in two cases relieved by resective epilepsy surgery.[54]

Postictal Headache

In a telephone interview of 372 patients attending an epilepsy clinic, 45% had experienced postictal headache (PIH) and 21% always had PIH. Of those who always had PIH, headache was severe 39% of the time; in contrast, it was severe in only 10% of patients with occasional PIH. Twenty-seven percent of patients had independent headaches that were usually similar to their seizure-related headache. Headaches lasted <6 hours in 81% of patients, 12 to 24 hours in 11%, and >24 hours in 8%.[92] The headache was throbbing in over two thirds.

Schön and Blau[94] reported on 100 epileptic patients, 51 of whom had PIH either always ($n = 35$), usually ($n = 5$), or 25% to 50% of the time ($n = 11$). PIH was more commonly associated with generalized tonic–clonic seizures than with focal seizures; 9% of the patients with PIH also had independent migraine attacks. The headaches were either bilateral or unilateral. They were associated with photophobia and phonophobia, throbbing pain, vomiting, nausea, and visual aura, and lasted 6 to 72 hours. Epileptic migraineurs recognized these headaches as being similar to their migraine. Postictal headaches with migraine features respond to triptans.[49]

Ito et al. reported that 40% of 364 patients with partial epilepsies had PIH and that 26% had postictal migraine.

Migraine-like PIH was more likely in temporal and occipital lobe epilepsy and less likely in frontal lobe epilepsy.[48]

The mechanism of ictal and postictal headaches is uncertain. In recent years, the theory of migraine pathogenesis has focused on the trigeminovascular system; activation of this system gives rise to neurogenic inflammation of cranial blood vessels and pain.[70] In animal models, Moskowitz et al. have shown that seizures activate the trigeminovascular system, providing a potential mechanism for the associated headaches. This mechanism would account for the triptan response in postictal headache.[46] Velioglu et al. examined the effect of migraine on the prognosis of epilepsy in a prospective study of 59 patients with both disorders and a control group of 56 patients with epilepsy but not migraine. The group with migraine and epilepsy was less likely to become seizure free and more likely to have intractable seizures and medication problems than patients with epilepsy alone. Thus, comorbid migraine may be a predictor of poor outcome in epilepsy.[108]

In summary, preictal and ictal headaches are relatively rare and short lived. The seizure itself may limit the patient's ability to observe or recall the manifestations of these headaches. In contrast, PIH is common and can impact the quality of life of the person with epilepsy. It is most common with generalized tonic–clonic seizures, but is also common in complex partial seizures; it is less common with simple partial seizures.[92]

Migraine–epilepsy Syndromes

Benign Epilepsy of Childhood with Occipital Paroxysms

BEOP is a clinical syndrome characterized by a partial seizure with visual symptoms, followed by postictal migraine and occipital spikes on EEG. A rare disorder, it accounts for <5% of epilepsy in children (mean age of onset 7.5 years).[24,33,82] BEOP has features of both epilepsy and migraine.[33,35,105] The visual symptoms may include amaurosis, elementary visual hallucinations (phosphenes), complex visual hallucinations, or visual illusions, including micropsia, metamorphopsia, or palinopsia.[11,33,73] The visual symptoms are often followed by hemiclonic, complex partial, or secondarily generalized tonic–clonic seizures. Following the seizure, approximately 25% to 40% of the patients develop migraine-like headaches.[105]

The interictal EEG is characterized by normal background activity and distinct occipital discharges. The occipital spikes typically have a high voltage (200 to 300 μV), diphasic morphology, and a unilateral or bilateral occipital and posterior temporal distribution. The spikes disappear with eye opening and reappear 1 to 20 seconds after eye closure.

Gastaut reviewed the clinical and EEG features of 53 patients with BOEP. Only 55% had the "complete" syndrome of occipital spikes, ictal visual symptoms followed by a partial seizure, and postictal migraine. In patients with nocturnal seizures, motor symptoms predominated; in those with daytime seizures, visual symptoms were more common. Nocturnal seizures are more common in younger children and bear a good prognosis.[33,82] Seizures starting after 8 years of age are more likely to be frequent, diurnal, and persistent,[33,82] although overall, complete seizure control is achievable in about 60% of patients.

Occipital spikes are not specific for BOEP. They have been reported in people with migraine, and in children under 4 they may not be associated with epilepsy or any other defined disorders.[41,58,102] Occipital spikes can also be seen in other disorders, including myoclonic, absence, and photosensitive epilepsies, as well as celiac disease.[19,33]

Benign Rolandic Epilepsy

Benign rolandic epilepsy is characterized by unilateral somatosensory or motor seizures and centrotemporal spikes; both clinical and electrographic features can shift from side to side. Speech arrest, pooling of saliva, and (usually) preservation of consciousness are also typical, although secondary generalization may occur. Most patients respond well to anticonvulsant medication. In one series, 75% of patients were seizure free after 5 years.[10] The seizures almost invariably disappear by age 15. An association with migraine has been reported in some, but not all, studies.[15,16] Rossi et al.[89] found that migraine prevalence in male controls (11.1%) was much higher than one would expect in boys between the age of 6 and 15 years. Giroud et al.,[36] in a control study, found that epilepsy with rolandic paroxysms and migraine were associated. Migraine incidence was studied in four groups of patients: Patients with centrotemporal epilepsy, patients with absence epilepsy, patients with partial epilepsy, and nonepileptic patients with a history of cranial trauma. Migraine was present in 62% of the patients with centrotemporal epilepsy, 34% of the patients with absence epilepsy, 8% of the patients with partial epilepsy, and 6% of the patients with cranial trauma. These results suggest that centrotemporal epilepsy and, to a lesser degree, absence epilepsy are associated with migraine.[36] The association between benign rolandic epilepsy and migraine may be part of the comorbidity of migraine with all forms of epilepsy.[85]

DIFFERENTIAL DIAGNOSIS AND CONCOMITANT DIAGNOSIS OF MIGRAINE AND EPILEPSY: CLINICAL AND ELECTROENCEPHALOGRAPHIC FEATURES

The most important tool in differentiating between migraine without aura and epilepsy is the history.[82] Table 5 illustrates high levels of symptomatic overlap between migraine and epilepsy. Tables 6 and 7 present the features most useful in distinguishing them. In general, in comparison with epilepsy, attacks of migraine are more gradual in onset and of longer duration. Nausea and vomiting are more commonly associated with migraine, while prolonged confusion or lethargy after the attack favors epilepsy.

At times, differentiating migraine with aura from epilepsy can be difficult, particularly when motor manifestations such as tonic or clonic movements are absent. The characteristics of the aura may help[29]: The migraine aura is longer (5+ minutes) and the aura of epilepsy is brief (usually <1 minute).[5] In addition, the aura symptom profiles differ. Autonomic, psychic, or somatosensory features favor epileptic auras, while a mix of positive and negative visual features, such as a scintillating scotoma, favors migraine.[81]

The characteristics of the visual features present in migraine and epilepsy bear further discussion. Colorless glittering scotomata are typical of migraine, as are black-and-white zigzag patterns that appear concentrically around the point of fixation, usually unilaterally. (These are also termed fortification spectra.) The phenomenon of a geometric pattern with expansion from the center to the periphery of the visual field (rarely in the reverse direction) and a simultaneous increase in size over a period of several minutes suggests CSD and migraine. The regular angular patterns in the photopsias that accompany migraine correspond to the cortical structures that generate them.[44–46] Photopsias in migraine may evolve into a scotoma or a temporary homonymous hemianopia. Resolution of the visual field

TABLE 5

SYMPTOMS COMMON TO BOTH MIGRAINE AND EPILEPSY

Symptom	Migraine	Epilepsy
Systemic		
Vomiting	+	+/–
Nausea	+	+/–
Diarrhea	+/–	–
Headache	+	+/–
Visual disturbances		
Colored circles	–	+
Black and white lines	+	–
Blindness	+/–	+/–
Blurred vision	+	+
Visual triggering factors	+	+
Other neurologic		
Olfactory	+/–	+
Vertigo	+	+/–
Confusion	+/–	+
Loss of consciousness	+/–**	+
Impaired consciousness	+/–	+
Loss of memory	+/–	+
Postevent lethargy	+	+
Depersonalization	+/–	+
Paresthesias	+	+
Hemiparesis	+/–**	+
Hemisensory loss	+/–**	+
Aphasia	+/–**	+

*More complex. **Hemiplegic migraine.

defect typically occurs without any positive visual phenomena. Colors may be seen as well, or spots, circles, and beads with or without colors. When these occur, they are usually part of the scintillating scotoma or teichopsia and not a predominant independent feature of the migrainous visual hallucination.

In contrast, visual epileptic auras are predominantly multicolored, with a circular or spherical pattern, as opposed to the predominantly black-and-white zigzag pattern of migraine.[83] During a seizure, hallucinations that begin unilaterally may later encompass the whole visual field, and simple hallucinations may develop into complex forms. In contrast to migraine, epileptic visual auras last for only seconds (with the rare exception of persistent visual auras),[113] thus limiting the patient's opportunity to observe and describe the hallucinations. The auras are often associated with head or eye movement and alteration of consciousness. Formed visual hallucinations are rare in migraine; when present in epilepsy, this manifestation may localize the seizure onset to the temporal or temporo-occipital region.[14]

The sensory auras of migraine and epilepsy also differ. In migraine, the auras are paresthesias (pins and needles) that typically begin in the hand, move up the arm, skip the shoulder, and move into the face and tongue over a period of 10 to 15 minutes. They are often associated with a visual aura.[92] The sensory aura of epilepsy is typically briefer and is often described as burning, cramping, stinging, aching, electric, or throbbing.

Correctly diagnosing and separating epilepsy and migraine can be more difficult in children than in adults. Young children may give incomplete descriptions of their symptoms; features useful in diagnosing epilepsy or migraine in adults may be absent or difficult to elicit in children. Hemicranial pain and visual auras occur less often in children with migraine than in adults. In children, the first symptoms of migraine may not even be associated with headaches.[42] Children are also less likely to experience feelings of déjà vu or to have olfactory hallucinations as part of a simple partial seizure or temporal lobe epilepsy. Furthermore, the epilepsies most commonly mistaken for migraine are childhood syndromes, as discussed above.

While the EEG is extraordinarily useful in diagnosing epilepsy and differentiating subtypes, it is less valuable in diagnosing migraine. EEGs recorded during an attack of migraine with aura, unlike those recorded during a clinical seizure, are usually normal. Focal slowing sometimes occurs during migraine auras, although this is not a consistent finding. Previously recommended EEG markers of migraine, such as robust photic driving at high flash frequencies and slowing with hyperventilation, can be seen in children without a history of migraine and are not very specific.[37]

The incidence of epileptiform activity in patients with migraine appears to be higher than that of the general population. In a large multicenter study, the incidences of spikes and paroxysmal rhythmic events in 10-hour overnight EEGs of normal adult volunteers ($n = 135$) was 0.7%, as compared to 12.5% for subjects with a history of migraine and 13.3% for subjects with a family history of epilepsy.[86] However, this finding does

TABLE 6

PRODROME AND AURA IN MIGRAINE AND EPILEPSY

Symptom	Migraine	Epilepsy
Premonitory	Common	Often
Duration of aura	15–60 min	Brief, often <1 min
Automatisms	Unusual	Absent in aura, present in complex partial seizures
Gastrointestinal aura	Abdominal pain (rare); nausea (common)	"Butterflies"—rising epigastric sensation
Visual disturbances	Positive/negative	Complicated visual phenomenon
Paresthesias	Common (5–60 min)	Common (seconds to minutes)
Altered consciousness	Usually responsive	Responsive during aura, altered responsiveness during complex partial seizure
Olfactory	Very uncommon	More common
Aphasia	Common	Common
Déjà vu	Rare	Common

TABLE 7

FEATURES OF EPILEPSY AND MIGRAINE

Clinical features	Migraine	Epilepsy
Consciousness	Usually clear	Usually clouded
Duration	Hours	Minutes
Family history	Often positive for migraine	Sometimes positive for epilepsy
Onset	Gradual	Sudden
Electroencephalogram	Nonspecific abnormalities	Spikes and sharp waves, ictal patterns

not contribute to the diagnosis of patients with migraine, and may in fact confuse the issue. Currently, the Quality Standards Subcommittee of the American Academy of Neurology has concluded that the EEG is not useful in the routine assessment of headache patients.[2] It does not identify headache subtypes or effectively screen for structural causes of headache. The EEG is useful if headache patients have symptoms that suggest a seizure disorder, such as atypical migrainous aura or episodic loss of consciousness. Assuming head-imaging capabilities are readily available, EEG is not recommended to exclude a structural cause for headache.[2,91]

There is, however, clearly a role for 24-hour closed-circuit television EEG recording; when differentiating migraine aura from epileptic aura is difficult on clinical grounds, these procedures can also facilitate the diagnosis of comorbid epilepsy and migraine as well as the migralepsy syndrome. Marks and Ehrenberg[29] studied patients with migralepsy using multiple 24-hour video EEG telemetry recordings. The entire migraine–epilepsy sequence of two patients was captured, showing changes during the clinical migraine aura that were atypical for electrographic epilepsy. During migraine aura, bursts of spike activity may resemble the ictal EEG during an epileptic seizure. In most reported cases, however, the EEG does not show the usual temporal evolution with progressive increases and declines in the frequency and amplitude of rhythmic, repetitive epileptiform activity typical of ictal EEGs in epilepsy. In addition, the EEG during migraine aura may show "waxing and waning" patterns, separated by completely normal EEG activity despite the persistence of clinical symptoms.

Manzoni et al.[65] and Terzano et al.[106,107] coined the term intercalated seizures to denote epileptic seizures occurring between the migrainous aura and the headache phase of migraine. They found that 16 of 450 patients with migraine (3.6%) also had seizures. The two conditions appeared to be coincidental in 4 of the 16 patients. In another five patients, the two types of attacks were quite distinct, but often an epileptic seizure was followed by a migraine attack and vice versa. The remaining seven patients had intercalated seizures. All had a family history of migraine and two also had relatives with epilepsy. All had visual seizures consisting of highly stylized contours of plain figures, or single or multicolored spots that often rotated. The seizures lasted for 1 to 2 minutes and came out of a scintillating scotoma, slowly developing in the visual field and evolving into unilateral or bilateral hemianopia. DeRomanis et al.[25,26] studied patients who had brief ictal visual hallucinations of "colored dots or discs" and interictal occipital paroxysms on EEG. EEG during a seizure showed that they had occipital epilepsy and not migraine with aura.[85]

Striking EEG patterns have been described in specific subtypes of migraine.[12] The brain regions most often involved in the published EEG samples in basilar-type migraine include the posterior temporal, parietal, and occipital regions. The posterior electrographic localization may not pertain to other forms of migraine.[71] Paroxysmal lateralized epileptiform discharges (PLEDs) or PLED-like activity has been associated with hemiplegic migraine, prolonged migraine aura, or incipient migrainous infarction. Those patients with PLED-like activity did not have any of the usual entities associated with PLEDs, such as stroke, brain abscess, glioblastoma, or viral encephalitis; their PLEDs usually resolved within 24 hours. Certain migralepsy patients had clinical seizures when PLEDs were present on their EEGs.[67]

TREATMENT CONSIDERATIONS

Because migraine and epilepsy are associated, clinicians should be sensitive to the issue of concomitant diagnoses. When diseases are comorbid, the principle of diagnostic parsimony does not apply. Individuals with one disorder are more likely, not less likely, to have the other. In the Epilepsy Family Study, only 44% of probands with epilepsy who were classified as having migraine on the basis of their self-reported symptoms reported physician-diagnosed migraine.[78] In the general population, 29% of men and 40% of women with migraine reported a medical diagnosis.[63] The proportion of probands reporting a physician's diagnosis of migraine was surprisingly low, given that all were already being treated for epilepsy.

Why is the comorbidity of migraine and epilepsy not recognized? Epilepsy may be viewed as a more serious disorder than migraine. As a result, the migrainous symptoms of patients with a diagnosis of epilepsy may have been overlooked or attributed to the seizure disorder. In addition, the diagnosis of atypical migraine symptoms can be quite difficult, and a number of epileptic and nonepileptic syndromes may mimic migraine. Some patients with epilepsy and migraine may not report their headaches because the headaches are being effectively treated with an antiepileptic drug without a diagnosis of migraine. Finally, the interview used in the Epilepsy Family Study may lead to overdiagnosing migraine in some patients.

When planning treatment strategies for epilepsy and migraine, the possibility of comorbid disease should be considered. Although tricyclic antidepressants and neuroleptic drugs are often used to treat migraine in patients with comorbid epilepsy, caution is advisable, as these medications may lower seizure thresholds. When selecting drugs for migraine prophylaxis, it is sometimes advantageous to treat comorbid conditions with a single agent; for example, when migraine and hypertension occur concomitantly, a beta-blocker or calcium channel blocker is commonly used.[97] In the same way, anticonvulsants with efficacy for both migraine and epilepsy (divalproex sodium and topiramate) should be considered in patients with both disorders.

Divalproex sodium is a Food and Drug Administration (FDA)-approved anticonvulsant for migraine prophylaxis. The efficacy of divalproex has been supported by recent open and double-blind, placebo-controlled studies.[50,68,96,104] The doses that are effective in migraine are generally lower than those used for epilepsy; 500 mg/day is often sufficient. Topiramate is a second FDA-approved anticonvulsant for migraine prophylaxis. In both open and small, placebo-controlled, double-blind trials, doses of 50 to 100 mg/day have been shown to be effective for migraine.[99] Other antiepileptic drugs that have been shown to be superior to placebo for migraine include gabapentin, levetiracetam, tiagabine, and zonisamide, but large-scale studies are needed. Lamotrigine may be effective for migraine aura, but not headache.

An advantage to the use of anticonvulsants as migraine prophylactic agents is that they can be administered to patients with depression, Raynaud disease, asthma, and diabetes, circumventing the contraindications to beta-blockers.[98]

In addition, the recognition of potentially similar mechanisms and response to therapy between the disorders has led to crossover of other treatment modalities. For example, the vagal nerve stimulator, an FDA-approved device for the add-on treatment of intractable partial epilepsy, is under investigation for migraine.[72] Similar efforts are likely to continue.

SUMMARY AND CONCLUSIONS

In summary, migraine and epilepsy are comorbid conditions, and the presence of one disorder increases the likelihood of the other. Because of its greater prevalence, migraine is very common in persons with epilepsy, while epilepsy is rare in migraineurs. The comorbidity of migraine and epilepsy presents both pitfalls and opportunities, and the diagnosis and treatment of each disorder must take into account the potential presence of the other.

References

1. Afra J, Mascia A, Gerard P, et al. Interictal cortical excitability in migraine: a study using transcranial magnetic stimulation of motor and visual cortices. *Ann Neurol.* 1998;44:209–215.
2. American Academy of Neurology Quality Standards Subcommittee. Practice parameter: the electroencephalogram in the evaluation of headache (summary statement). Report of the Quality Standards Subcommittee. *Neurology.* 1995;45:1411–1413.
3. Amery WK, Waelkens J, Caers I. Dopaminergic mechanisms in premonitory phenomena. In: Amery WK, Wauquier A, eds. *The Prelude to the Migraine Attack.* London: Bailliere Tindall; 1986:64–77.
4. Amery WK, Waelkens J, Van den Bergh V. Migraine warnings. *Headache.* 1986;26:60–66.
5. Andermann E, Andermann FA. Migraine-epilepsy relationships: epidemiological and genetic aspects. In: Andermann FA, Lugaresi E, eds. *Migraine and Epilepsy.* Boston: Butterworths; 1987:281–291.
6. Andermann F. Clinical features of migraine-epilepsy syndrome. In: Andermann F, Lugaresi E, eds. *Migraine and Epilepsy.* Boston: Butterworths; 1987:3–30.
7. Andermann F. Migraine and epilepsy: an overview. In: Andermann F, Lugaresi E, eds. *Migraine and Epilepsy.* Boston: Butterworths; 1987:405–421.
8. Appenzeller O. Posttraumatic headaches. In: Dalessio DJ, Silberstein SD, eds. *Wolff's Headache and Other Head Pain.* 6th ed. New York: Oxford University Press; 1993:365–383.
9. Aurora SK, Cao Y, Bowyer SM, et al. The occipital cortex is hyperexcitable in migraine: experimental evidence. *Headache.* 1999;39:469–476.
10. Bazil CW. Migraine and epilepsy. *Neurol Clin.* 1994;12:115–128.
11. Beaumanoir A. Infantile epilepsy with occipital focus and good prognosis. *Eur Neurol.* 1983;22:43–52.
12. Beaumanoir A, Jekiel M. Electrographic observations during attacks of classical migraine. In: Andermann F, Lugaresi E, eds. *Migraine and Epilepsy.* Boston: Butterworths; 1987:163–180.
13. Bickerstaff ER. Migraine variants and complications. In: Blau JN, ed. *Migraine: Clinical and Research Aspects.* Baltimore: Johns Hopkins University Press; 1987:55–75.
14. Bien CG, Benninger FO, Urbach H, et al. Localizing value of epileptic visual auras. *Brain.* 2000;123(Pt 2):244–253.
15. Bladin PF. The association of benign rolandic epilepsy with migraine. In: Andermann F, Lugaresi E, eds. *Migraine and Epilepsy.* Boston: Butterworth; 1987:145–152.
16. Bladin PF, Papworth G. "Chuckling and glugging" seizures at night-sylvian spike epilepsy. *Proc Australian Assoc Neurol.* 1974;11:171–175.
17. Blau JN. Migraine prodromes separated from the aura: complete migraine. *BMJ.* 1980;281:658–660.
18. Blau JN. Migraine pathogenesis: the neural hypothesis reexamined. *J Neurol Neurosurg Psychiatry.* 1984;47:437–442.
19. Bye ME, Andermann F, Robitaille Y, et al. Cortical vascular abnormalities in the syndrome of celiac disease, epilepsy, bilateral occipital calcifications, and folate deficiency. *Ann Neurol.* 1993;34:399–404.
20. Cao Y, Welch KM, Aurora S, et al. Functional MRI-BOLD of visually triggered headache in patients with migraine. *Arch Neurol.* 1999;56:548–554.
21. Creange A, Zeller J, Rostaing-Rigattieri S, et al. Neurological complications of neurofibromatosis type 1 in adulthood. *Brain.* 1999;122:373–381.
22. Cutrer FM, O'Donnell A. Recent advances in functional neuroimaging. *Cur Opin Neurol.* 1999;12:255–259.
23. Cutrer FM, Sorenson AG, Weisskoff RM, et al. Perfusion-weighted imaging defects during spontaneous migrainous aura. *Ann Neurol.* 1998;43:25–31.
24. Deonna T, Ziegler AL, Despland PA, et al. Partial epilepsy in neurologically normal children: clinical syndromes and prognosis. *Epilepsia.* 1986;27:241–247.
25. DeRomanis F, Buzzi MG, Cerbo R, et al. Migraine and epilepsy with infantile onset and electroencephalographic findings of occipital spike-wave complexes. *Headache.* 1991;31:378–383.
26. DeRomanis F, Feliciani M, Cerbo R. Migraine and other clinical syndromes in children affected by EEG occipital spike-wave complexes. *Funct Neurol.* 1988;3:187–203.
27. Dreifuss R. Classification of epileptic seizures. In: Engel J, Pedley T, eds. *Epilepsy: Comprehensive Textbook.* Philadelphia: Lippincott-Raven; 1998;517–524.
28. Drummond PD. A quantitative assessment of photophobia in migraine and tension headache. *Headache.* 1986;26:465–469.
29. Ehrenberg BL. Unusual clinical manifestations of migraine, and "the borderland of epilepsy" re-explored. *Semin Neurol.* 1991;11:118–127.
30. Fenwick P. Episodic dyscontrol. In: Engel J, Pedley T, eds. *Epilepsy: Comprehensive Textbook.* Philadelphia: Lippincott-Raven; 1998:2767–2774.
31. Fisher CM. Late life migraine accompaniments as a cause of unexplained transient ischemic attacks. *Can J Neurol Sci.* 1980;7:9–17.
32. Fisher CM. Late-life migraine accompaniments–further experience. *Stroke.* 1986;17:1033–1042.
33. Gastaut H. A new type of epilepsy: benign partial epilepsy childhood with occipital spike-waves. *Clin Electroencephalogr.* 1982;13:13–22.
34. Gastaut H. Benign epilepsy of childhood with occipital paroxysms. In: Roger J, Dravet C, Bureau M, et al., eds. *Epileptic Syndromes in Infancy, Childhood, and Adolescence.* London: John Livvey, Eurotext Ltd.; 1985: 150–158.
35. Giffin NJ, Ruggiero L, Lipton RB, et al. A novel approach to the study of premonitory symptoms in migraine using an electronic diary. *Neurology.* 2003;60:935–940.
36. Giroud M, Couillaut G, Arnould S, et al. Epilepsy with Rolandic paroxysms and migraine; a nonfortuitous association. Results of a controlled study. *Pediatrie.* 1989;44:659–664.
37. Gronseth GS, Greenberg MK. The utility of the electroencephalogram in the evaluation of patients presenting with headache: a review of the literature. *Neurology.* 1995;45:1263–1267.
38. Haas DC. Prolonged migraine aura status. *Ann Neurol.* 1982;11:197–199.
39. Hadjikhani N, Sanchez del Rio M, Wu O, et al. Mechanisms of migraine aura revealed by functional MRI in human visual cortex. *Proc Nat Acad Sci U S A.* 2001;98:4687–4692.
40. Headache Classification Committee. The International Classification of Headache Disorders. 2nd ed. *Cephalalgia.* 2004;24:1–160.
41. Herranz FT, Saenz LP, Cristobal SS. Occipital spike-wave with and without benign epilepsy in the child. *Rev Electroencephalogr Neurophysiol Clin.* 1984;14:1–17.
42. Hockaday JM. Equivalents of childhood migraine. In: Hockaday JM, ed. *Migraine in Childhood.* Boston: Butterworths; 1988:54–62.
43. Hosking G. Special forms: variants of migraine in childhood. In: Hockaday JM, ed. *Migraine in Childhood.* Boston: Butterworths; 1988:35–53.
44. Hubel DH, Wiesel TN. Receptive fields and functional architecture in two nonstriate visual areas (18 and 19) of the cat. *J Neurophysiol.* 1965;195:229–289.
45. Hubel DH, Wiesel TN. Receptive fields and functional architecture of monkey striate cortex. *J Physiol.* 1968;195:214–243.
46. Hubel DH, Wiesel TN. Laminar and columnar distribution of geniculocortical fibers in the macaque monkey. *J Comp Neurol.* 1972;146:421–450.
47. Isler H, Wirsen ML, Elli N. Hemicrania epileptica: synchronous ipsilateral ictal headache with migraine features. In: Andermann F, Lugaresi E, eds. *Migraine and Epilepsy.* Boston: Butterworths; 1987:246–263.
48. Ito M, Adachi N, Nakamura F, et al. Characteristics of postictal headache in patients with partial epilepsy. *Cephalalgia.* 2004;24:23–28.
49. Jacob J, Goadsby PJ, Duncan JS. Use of sumatriptan in postictal migraine headache. *Neurology.* 1996;47:1104.

50. Jensen R, Brinck T, Olesen J. Sodium valproate has a prophylactic effect in migraine without aura. *Neurology*. 1994;44:647–651.
51. Klee A, Willanger R. Disturbances of visual perception in migraine. *Acta Neurol Scand*. 1966;42:400–414.
52. Kors EE, Haan J, Giffin NJ, et al. Expanding the phenotypic spectrum of the CACNA1A gene T666M mutation: a description of 5 families with familial hemiplegic migraine. *Arch Neurol*. 2003;60:684–688.
53. Lance JW. The pathophysiology of migraine. In: Dalessio D, Silberstein SD, eds. *Wolff's Headache and Other Head Pain*. 6th ed. New York: Oxford University Press; 1993:59–95.
54. Laplante P, Saint JH, Bouvier G. Headache as an epileptic manifestation. *Neurology*. 1983;33:1493–1495.
55. Lauritzen M, Olesen J. Regional cerebral blood flow during migraine attacks by xenon-133 inhalation and emission tomography. *Brain*. 1984;107:447–461.
56. Leão AAP. Spreading depression of activity in cerebral cortex. *J Neurophysiol*. 1944;7:359–390.
57. Lenaerts ME. Migraine and epilepsy: comorbidity and temporal relationship [Abstract]. *Cephalalgia*. 1999;19:418(abst).
58. Lerman P, Kivity SE. Focal epileptic EEG discharges in children not suffering from clinical epilepsy: etiology, clinical significance, and management. *Epilepsia*. 1981;22:551–558.
59. Lippman CV. Certain hallucinations peculiar to migraine. *J Nerv Ment Dis*. 1952;116:346.
60. Lipton RB, Ottman R, Ehrenberg BL, et al. Comorbidity of migraine: the connection between migraine and epilepsy. *Neurology*. 1994;44:28–32.
61. Lipton RB, Silberstein SD. Why study the comorbidity of migraine? *Neurology*. 1994;44:4–5.
62. Lipton RB, Silberstein SD, Stewart WF. An update on the epidemiology of migraine. *Headache*. 1994;34:319–328.
63. Lipton RB, Stewart WF, Celentano DD, et al. Undiagnosed migraine headaches: a comparison of symptom-based and reported physician diagnosis. *Arch Intern Med*. 1992;156:1273–1278.
64. Lipton RB, Stewart WF, Diamond S, et al. Prevalence and burden of migraine in the United States: data from the American Migraine Study II. *Headache*. 2001;41:646–657.
65. Manzoni GC, Terzano MG, Mancia D. Possible interference between migrainous and epileptic mechanisms in intercalated attacks. Case report. *Eur Neurol*. 1979;18:124–129.
66. Maria BL, Neufeld JA, Rosainz LC, et al. Central nervous system structure and function in Sturge-Weber syndrome: evidence of neurologic and radiologic progression. *J Child Neurol*. 1998;13:606–618.
67. Marks DA, Ehrenberg BL. Migraine related seizures in adults with epilepsy, with EEG correlation. *Neurology*. 1993;43:2476–2483.
68. Mathew NT. Valproate in the treatment of persistent chronic daily headache. *Headache*. 1990;30:301.
69. Milner PM. Note on a possible correspondence between the scotomas of migraine and spreading depression of Leão. *Electroencephalogr Clin Neurophysiol*. 1958;10:705.
70. Moskowitz MA. The trigeminovascular system. In: Olesen J, Tfelt-Hansen P, Welch KMA, eds. *The Headaches*. New York: Raven Press; 1993:97–104.
71. Muelbacher W, Mamoli B. Prolonged impaired consciousness in basilar artery migraine. *Headache*. 1994;34:282–285.
72. Multon S, Schoenen J. Pain control by vagus nerve stimulation: from animal to man . . . and back. *Acta Neurol Belg*. 2005;105:62–67.
73. Newton R, Aicardi J. Clinical findings in children with occipital spike-wave complexes suppressed by eye-opening. *Neurology*. 1983;33:1526–1529.
74. Olesen J. Cerebral and extracranial circulatory disturbances in migraine: pathophysiological implications. *Cerebrovasc Brain Metab Rev*. 1991;3:1–28.
75. Olesen J, Friberg L, Skyhoj-Olsen T. Timing and topography of cerebral blood flow, aura and headache during migraine attacks. *Ann Neurol*. 1990;28:791–798.
76. Olesen J, Larsen B, Lauritzen M. Focal hyperemia followed by spreading oligemia and impaired activation of RCBF in classic migraine. *Ann Neurol*. 1981;9:344–352.
77. Olesen J, Lauritzen M, Tfelt-Hansen PK, et al. Spreading cerebral oligemia in classical and normal cerebral blood flow in common migraine. *Headache*. 1982;22:242–248.
78. Ottman R, Lipton RB. Comorbidity of migraine and epilepsy. *Neurology*. 1994;44:2105–2110.
79. Ottman R, Lipton RB. Is the comorbidity of epilepsy and migraine due to a shared genetic susceptibility? *Neurology*. 1996;47:918–924.
80. Palmini A, Gloor P. The localizing value of auras in partial seizures: a prospective and retrospective study. *Neurology*. 1992;42:801–808.
81. Panayiotopoulos CP. Difficulties in differentiating migraine and epilepsy based on clinical and EEG findings. In: Andermann F, Lugaresi E, eds. *Migraine and Epilepsy*. Boston: Butterworth; 1987:31–46.
82. Panayiotopoulos CP. Benign childhood epilepsy with occipital paroxysms: a 15-year prospective study. *Ann Neurol*. 1989;26:51–56.
83. Panayiotopoulos CP. Elementary visual hallucinations in migraine and epilepsy. *J Neurol Neurosurg Psychiatry*. 1991;57:1371–1374.
84. Panayiotopoulos CP. Basilar migraine: a review. In: Panayiotopoulos CP, ed. *Benign Childhood Partial Seizures and Related Epileptic Syndromes*. London: John Libbey & Company Ltd.; 1999:303–308.
85. Panayiotopoulos CP. Differentiating occipital epilepsies from migraine with aura, acephalgic migraine and basilar migraine. In: Panayiotopoulos CP, ed. *Benign Childhood Partial Seizures and Related Epileptic Syndromes*. London: John Libbey & Company Ltd.; 1999:281–302.
86. Pearce JMS. Migraine: a cerebral disorder. *Lancet*. 1984;11:86–89.
87. Proposal for revised classification of epilepsies and epileptic syndromes. Commission on Classification and Terminology of the International League Against Epilepsy. *Epilepsia*. 1989;30:389–399.
88. Raskin NH. Conclusions. *Headache*. 1990;30:24.
89. Rossi PG, Santucci M, Giuseppe G, et al. Epidemiologic study of migraine in epileptic patients. In: Andermann F, Lugaresi E, eds. *Migraine and Epilepsy*. Boston: Butterworths; 1987: 313–321.
90. Sacks O. *Migraine: Understanding a Common Disorder*. Berkeley, CA: University of California Press; 1985.
91. Schachter SC, Ito M, Wannamaker BB, et al. Incidence of spikes and paroxysmal rhythmic events in overnight ambulatory computer-assisted EEGs of normal subjects: a multicenter study. *J Clin Neurophysiol*. 1998;15:251–255.
92. Schacter SC, Richman K, Loder E, et al. Self-reported characteristics of postictal headaches. *J Epilepsy*. 1995;8:41–43.
93. Schoenen J, Thomsen LL. Neurophysiology and autonomic dysfunction in migraine. In: Olesen J, Tfelt-Hansen P, Welch KMA, eds. *The Headaches*. 2nd ed. Philadelphia: Lippincott Williams & Wilkins; 2000: 301–312.
94. Schon F, Blau JN. Postepileptic headache and migraine. *J Neurol Neurosurg Psychiatry*. 1987;50:1148–1152.
95. Selby G, Lance JW. Observation on 500 cases of migraine and allied vascular headaches. *J Neurol Neurosurg Psychiatry*. 1960;23:23–32.
96. Sianard-Gainko J, Lenaerts M, Bastings E, et al. Sodium valproate in severe migraine and tension-type headache: clinical efficacy and correlations with blood levels. *Cephalalgia*. 1993;13:252.
97. Silberstein SD, Lipton RB. Epidemiology of migraine. *Neuroepidemiology*. 1993;12:179–194.
98. Silberstein SD, Lipton RB. Overview of diagnosis and treatment of migraine. *Neurology*. 1994;44:6–16.
99. Silberstein SD, Saper JR, Freitag F. Migraine: diagnosis and treatment. In: Silberstein SD, Lipton RB, Dalessio DJ, eds. *Wolff's Headache and Other Head Pain*. 7th ed. New York: Oxford University Press; 2001:121–237.
100. Silberstein SD, Young WB. Migraine aura and prodrome. *Semin Neurol*. 1995;45:175–182.
101. Simkins RT, Tepley N, Barkley GL, et al. Spontaneous neuromagnetic fields in migraine: possible link to spreading cortical depression. *Neurology*. 1989;39:325.
102. Smith JM, Kellaway P. The natural history and clinical correlates of occipital foci in children. In: Kellaway P, Petersen I, eds. *Neurologic and Electroencephalographic Correlative Studies in Infancy*. New York: Grune & Stratton; 1965:230–249.
103. So NK, Andermann F. Differential diagnosis. In: Engel J, Pedley TA, eds. *Epilepsy: A Comprehensive Textbook*. Philadelphia: Lippincott-Raven Publishers; 1997:791.
104. Sorensen KV. Valproate: a new drug in migraine prophylaxis. *Acta Neurol Scand*. 1988;78:346–348.
105. Talwar D, Rask CA, Torres F. Clinical manifestations in children with occipital spike-wave paroxysms. *Epilepsia*. 1992;33:667–674.
106. Terzano MG, Manzoni GC, Parrino L. Benign epilepsy with occipital paroxysms and migraine: the question of intercalated attacks. In: Andermann F, Lugaresi E, eds. *Migraine and Epilepsy*. Boston: Butterworths; 1987:83–96.
107. Terzano MG, Parrino L, Pietrini V, et al. Migraine-epilepsy syndrome: intercalated seizures in benign occipital epilepsy. In: Andermann F, Beaumanoir A, Mira L, et al., eds. *Occipital Seizures and Epilepsies in Children*. London: John Libbey & Company Ltd.; 1993:93–99.
108. Velioglu SK, Boz C, Ozmenoglu M. The impact of migraine on epilepsy: a prospective prognosis study. *Cephalalgia*. 2005;25:528–535.
109. Velioglu SK, Ozmenoglu M. Migraine-related seizures in an epileptic population. *Cephalalgia*. 1999;19:801.
110. Welch KM, Lewis D. Migraine and epilepsy. *Neurol Clin*. 1997;15:107–114.
111. Welch KMA, D'Andrea G, Tepley N, et al. The concept of migraine as a state of central neuronal hyperexcitability. *Neurol Clin*. 1990;8:817–828.
112. Whitty CWM. Migraine without headache. *Lancet*. 1967;ii:283–285.
113. Wolf P. Systematik von satus kleiner anfalle in psychopathologischer hinsicht. In: Wolf P, Kohler GK, eds. *Psychopathologische und Pathogenetische Probleme Psychotischer Syndrome bei Epilepsie*. Vienna: Huber; 1980:32–52.
114. Yankovsky AE, Andermann F, Bernasconi A. Characteristics of headache associated with intractable partial epilepsy. *Epilepsia*. 2005;46:1241–1245.
115. Young WB, Oshinsky ML, Shechter AL, et al. Consecutive transcranial magnetic stimulation induced phosphene thresholds in migraineurs and controls [Abstract]. *Neurology*. 2001;56:A142(abst).
116. Ziegler DK, Hassanein RS. Specific headache phenomena: their frequency and coincidence. *Headache*. 1990;30:152–156.

CHAPTER 275 ■ CEREBROVASCULAR DISORDERS

CLINTON B. WRIGHT, JOAN T. MORONEY, AND RALPH L. SACCO

INTRODUCTION

The relationship between cerebrovascular disease and epilepsy has long been appreciated since Hughlings Jackson first reported partial seizures in the setting of acute stroke.[7] Indeed, cerebrovascular disease has been found to be the most common cause of secondary epilepsy. In a population-based study from Rochester, Minnesota, cerebrovascular disease accounted for 11% of cases.[37] This chapter will review the limited data on the epidemiology and treatment of poststroke seizures and epilepsy. Because the differentiation between cerebrovascular disorders and seizures is sometimes difficult, the chapter will also aim to make the clinical distinction between epileptic syndromes, transient ischemic attacks (TIAs), and other minor ischemic stroke syndromes. The nosology and natural history of TIAs, the more common TIA syndromes, and some less common clinical syndromes of TIAs and minor strokes that might be confused with paroxysmal epileptic syndromes will be discussed.

EPIDEMIOLOGY

Seizures can be a complication of an acute stroke. Traditionally, poststroke seizures have been divided into early and late based on presumed differences in pathophysiology.[41] Early seizures are thought to result from acute biochemical disturbances and may result in part from the damaging effects of the excitatory neurotransmitter glutamate in response to ischemia.[14,17,58] In contrast, late seizures are attributed to gliosis and cortical scarring with resulting selective neuronal loss and hyperexcitability of the surrounding tissue.[39,58] Some authors have argued that early seizures are not reliably related to the strokes themselves because of other concurrent metabolic problems.[38,57] The International League Against Epilepsy (ILAE) defines early poststroke seizures as those that occur before 1 week, but studies have used widely varying definitions, from under 24 hours up to 1 month after stroke.[46,49] Despite varying definitions of what constitutes an early poststroke seizure, several studies have found that the risk of epilepsy is significantly increased among those patients who have seizures within 2 weeks of the onset of a stroke.[71] Late poststroke seizures have also been associated with an increased risk of epilepsy.[10,15,48,71]

Data from five prospective studies have shown that the rate of epilepsy after ischemic stroke ranges from about 2% to 4%.[10,15,48,57,71] However, the reported incidence of epilepsy varies between studies with the definition. Using the ILAE definition of two or more unprovoked seizures more than 1 week after stroke, a study from Rochester, Minnesota, found an overall rate of poststroke epilepsy of 3.3%, and 66% of those that developed an initial late seizure after ischemic stroke went on to develop epilepsy by 4.5 years.[71] In a study from Norway, the overall incidence of poststroke epilepsy was 3.1%, while 11 of 28 subjects with poststroke seizures developed epilepsy (55%).[57]

Limited data are available regarding risk factors for poststroke seizures and more is known about those that occur early than late. Involvement of the cortex is the most well-recognized predictor of early seizure occurrence, having been found to be an independent risk factor in several prospective studies.[8,10,15,47,48,71] Stroke severity and infarct size have also been found to be independent risk factors.[10,48,57,65] Few studies have examined independent predictors of late poststroke seizures or epilepsy.[17] Early seizures appear to be a risk factor for late seizures and possibly epilepsy, and a few studies have found that infarct size, cortical involvement, and recurrent stroke have been independent predictors.[10,48,71] However, in a large prospective study from Norway, stroke severity was an independent risk factor for epilepsy while cortical location was not.[57] Thus, further data are needed to clarify the relative importance of these modifying factors.

TREATMENT

Treatment of poststroke seizures and epilepsy is complicated by a lack of clinical trial data to support the use of a particular antiepileptic drug on the one hand, and evidence that some commonly used drugs may be detrimental to stroke recovery on the other. For example, treatment with antihypertensive drugs that block the adrenergic system, such as prazosin and clonidine, or those that stimulate γ-aminobutyric acid (GABA) receptors, such as benzodiazepines, have been shown to impair recovery after brain injury in the rat, and the antiepileptic drugs phenytoin and phenobarbital have been implicated as well.[33] Less is known about the effect of these drugs on recovery in humans. One study examining the control group of an acute ischemic stroke treatment trial found that subjects administered any of a group of "detrimental drugs" including benzodiazepines, dopamine receptor antagonists, α-1 blockers, α-2 agonists, phenobarbital, or phenytoin had worse motor recovery and less independence in activities of daily living than those that did not receive any of these drugs.[33] Recovery after subarachnoid hemorrhage may also be impeded by such treatment. In a prospective case series, greater phenytoin exposure was associated with worse functional outcome at 14 days and worse cognitive outcome at 3 months.[60] However, treatment after experimental ischemia in rodents has shown that many antiepileptics may be neuroprotective if given very early.[17] For example, phenytoin when given 30 minutes after experimental occlusion of the rat middle cerebral artery was neuroprotective, but not if given after 2 hours.[22] Separately, diazepam given 30 and 90 minutes after induced forebrain ischemia in the gerbil resulted in protection of hippocampal neurons.[69] Neuroprotective properties have also been reported for lamotrigine, topiramate, levetiracetam, and zonisamide.[17] Thus, further data are needed to clarify the importance after stroke of the doses, timing, and length of treatment with antiepileptic drugs that may be helpful or harmful to patients.

NOSOLOGY OF TRANSIENT ISCHEMIC ATTACKS

The term *stroke* generally describes a group of vascular disorders diverse in etiology and includes ischemic brain infarction, intracerebral hemorrhage, and subarachnoid hemorrhage.[4] The term *transient ischemic attack* has been limited to the description of a brief episode of neurologic dysfunction resulting from ischemia and was introduced in 1957 by C. Miller Fisher. TIA is formally defined as "an abrupt onset of focal loss of brain function lasting less than 24 hours that localizes to a portion of the brain supplied by one vascular system and for which no other cause can be found."[2] The arbitrary 24-hour time limit was selected on the basis of prospective studies in the 1970s prior to the widespread use of brain imaging.[3] It was thought that focal deficits lasting beyond 24 hours would be expected to result from a focus of ischemic infarction. This definition now requires revision, based upon recent brain imaging evidence of infarction in a substantial proportion of episodes classified by the 24-hour time limit as TIAs.[11,24] The term *reversible ischemic neurologic deficit* (RIND) was created to define those patients with neurologic dysfunction lasting longer than 24 hours but resolving completely within 1 to 3 weeks.[4] Neurologic deficits in the minor ischemic stroke syndromes conversely persist beyond these arbitrary time periods. Ischemic stroke may be more appropriately viewed as a continuum that encompasses TIA, RIND, and minor ischemic stroke.[18] As similar risk factors and vascular pathologies underlie these diagnostic subgroups, their continued separate distinction from each other is employed primarily for the purposes of differential diagnosis and prognostic risk stratification.[23]

PREVALENCE AND INCIDENCE OF TRANSIENT ISCHEMIC ATTACKS

Differing methods and ambiguities of definition have resulted in a wide disparity in reported prevalence and incidence rates of TIAs.[13] Estimated prevalence has varied from 1.1 to 77 per 1,000 persons, but three recent studies have dealt more effectively with the ascertainment bias inherent in capturing transient episodes, and data have shown incidence rates that are more consistent. Population-based data from Rochester, Minnesota, for the period 1985 to 1989 led to a calculated annual age- and sex-adjusted incidence rate of 68 per 100,000 population.[13] The incidence rate was somewhat higher in the Greater Cincinnati/Northern Kentucky Stroke Study at 83 per 100,000, but 15% of the sample is of black race and may be at higher risk of cerebrovascular disease.[42] Similar rates were seen in the United Kingdom. In the Oxfordshire study the overall age- and sex-adjusted incidence rate for TIA was 51 per 100,000.[66] In addition, annual incidence rates for TIA appear to be reasonably stable over time, taking into account lower ascertainment in earlier studies. The incidence rate did not change appreciably in Rochester between the periods 1960 and 1972 and 1985 and 1989, although the rate increased slightly in Oxfordshire, U.K., between 1981 and 2004 (relative incidence 1.27).[13,66] The incidence of TIA was strongly related to age in all three studies.

NATURAL HISTORY OF TRANSIENT ISCHEMIC ATTACKS

Transient ischemic attacks precede 11% to 50% of strokes, depending on the specific stroke subtype.[3] They have been reported most frequently in association with large artery atherothrombotic disease and less commonly with small vessel disease.[30,59] Approximately 50% to 75% of patients who experience a stroke from extracranial carotid atheromatous disease have a prior TIA.[59] Perhaps the most important finding in recent studies has been the very high rate of stroke following TIA. Data from a large health maintenance organization in California found that roughly 10% of those presenting with TIA went on to have an ischemic stroke within 90 days and half of these occurred within the first 48 hours after the index event.[40] Similarly, data from the Greater Cincinnati/Northern Kentucky Stroke Study found a 17% ischemic stroke rate within 6 months after TIA, 65% of which occurred within the first month.[42] The results from the North American Symptomatic Carotid Endarterectomy Trial (NASCET) helped clarify the outcomes for TIA patients.[1] Patients with TIAs and symptomatic extracranial carotid stenosis exceeding 70% were followed prospectively over a period of 18 months. During this time period, 24% of the medically treated group had a stroke or died, compared with a 7% rate in the endarterectomy-treated group. This striking difference proved that surgery was effective in reducing the risk of stroke after TIA and that TIAs should be regarded as a marker of significantly increased stroke risk. Certain subgroups of TIAs carry a higher stroke risk than do others. Data from NASCET showed that hemispheric TIAs with known high-grade ipsilateral carotid stenosis had a stroke risk exceeding 40% over 2 years.[75] Early stroke risk is probably greater in those patients with "crescendo" TIAs (multiple and frequent) and in the subgroup with ventricular thrombi.[2]

Clinical discrimination between TIAs and nonvascular causes of transient neurologic dysfunction is crucial as the occurrence of a TIA is a reliable warning signal of an impending stroke. An episode consistent with a TIA should be rapidly evaluated to determine the cause. Prompt clinical recognition of TIAs and timely institution of appropriate therapy can help prevent stroke. Furthermore, the possibility of occult coronary artery pathology should be considered in the workup of these patients as the occurrence of TIAs may indicate generalized atherosclerosis; ischemic heart disease is the leading cause of death in elderly TIA patients.[2,25]

DIAGNOSTIC DIFFICULTY

Less than one in ten TIAs are witnessed by a physician; therefore, accurate diagnosis usually depends on a careful interpretation of the patient's history.[26] Health care professionals tend to formulate a preliminary diagnosis within the first few minutes of history taking, which works well when the symptoms follow classic textbook descriptions.[68] However, many patients cannot offer a clear, concise account of abrupt onset of focal neurologic dysfunction, as required for the diagnosis of TIA. Details are often forgotten or unappreciated regarding time, mode of onset, and subsequent course of symptomatology. Historical reliability becomes more questionable when patients consult a physician weeks or months following the event. Nondominant hemispheric TIAs are particularly susceptible to misclassification because the event may be ignored or misinterpreted by the patient.[78] The lack of uniform diagnostic criteria for TIA is reflected in significant interobserver disagreement. The Cooperative Group for the study of TIA found that 30% of patients hospitalized with a diagnosis of TIA had been misclassified.[16]

TABLE 1

FREQUENCY AND TYPE OF SYMPTOMS[a] IN CAROTID TRANSIENT ISCHEMIC ATTACKS

Frequency left carotid[b]		Frequency right carotid[c]	
67%	Sensorimotor (arm)	70%	Sensorimotor (arm)
56%	Weakness (face, arm, or leg)	50%	Weakness (face, arm, or leg)
45%	Aphasia	N/A	
44%	Sensory (arm)	53%	Sensory (arm)
21%	Dysarthria	24%	Dysarthria
20%	TMB	27%	TMB

N/A, not applicable; TMB, transient monocular blindness.
[a]Only symptoms reported by at least 20% of patients are tabulated.
[b]n = 171.
[c]n = 142.
Data derived from Futty DE, Conneally M, Dyken ML, et al. Cooperative study of hospital frequency and character of transient ischemic attacks. V. Symptom analysis. *JAMA*. 1977;238(22):2386–2390.

This finding has been confirmed in other series.[43] Questionnaires on TIA symptomatology have documented a high positive response rate, both in the elderly and in a group of young adults.[56,81] These surveys indicate that episodes of transient central nervous system dysfunction are common. Follow-up of those patients whose transient symptoms were considered too vague to represent TIA has revealed a stroke rate comparable to the TIA group, suggesting that current empiric criteria for TIA are too narrow.[82] Standardized checklists using nonmedical terminology and computer-based diagnostic algorithms offer useful alternatives to enhance diagnostic consistency.[44,63] There is a need for improved diagnostic guidelines for TIAs with enhanced reliability, sensitivity, and specificity.

TYPICAL TRANSIENT ISCHEMIC ATTACK SYMPTOMS

Traditionally, TIAs have been classified according to the vascular territory involved: Carotid or vertebrobasilar. This differentiation is important for management and prognosis.[55] Carotid territory TIAs occur more frequently and may result in the following: Weakness, paralysis, or clumsiness of one side of the body or face; numbness or paresthesias affecting one side of the face or body; loss of vision affecting one eye or, less frequently, one visual field; language disturbance (aphasia); and dysarthria.[4] Analysis of a large series of carotid TIAs has proved helpful in determining the relative frequencies of various symptoms typical of TIAs (Table 1).[31]

Mixed sensorimotor disturbances of the distal arm and hand were the most frequent carotid TIA symptoms, followed by motor weakness variably affecting the face, arm, or leg; aphasia with left carotid territory syndromes; and isolated sensory dysfunction of the arm. Transient monocular blindness (TMB) or amaurosis fugax and dysarthria were less frequent manifestations. Neurologic evaluations during the occurrence of TIAs confirmed the presence of motor or language disturbance. Sensory complaints were found to have less objective associated signs on examination, and reflex asymmetry or Babinski signs were found infrequently. Patients with visual field deficits were often unaware of their deficit, and the examiner found evidence for deficits in addition to the presenting symptom.

Vertebrobasilar TIAs may cause the following symptoms: Weakness, paralysis, or clumsiness with or without sensory deficit affecting the face or limbs; gait imbalance; vertigo; diplopia; dysarthria; or dysphagia.[4] Complaints may alternate from side to side, be bilateral from onset, or affect one side of the face and the opposite body (crossed syndromes). Symptom analysis from a large series of vertebrobasilar TIA patients is presented in Table 2.[31] Vertigo, diplopia, dysarthria, dysphagia, and disequilibrium occurring alone were considered less likely to be a TIA. Whether nonrotatory dizziness may have a vascular etiology remains unclear.

These large clinical series have demonstrated that motor symptoms accompany most TIAs, that typical TIA symptoms are "negative" (loss of function), and that dysarthria can result from either anterior or posterior circulation dysfunction. Symptoms considered unlikely to represent TIAs include loss of consciousness without other vertebrobasilar signs, tonic or clonic activity, light-headedness, syncope, incontinence, and focal symptomatology with migraine headache (e.g., "march" of a sensory deficit, scintillating scotomata). Less typical TIA symptoms that include positive clinical manifestations and can cause diagnostic confusion will be discussed further (Table 3).

TABLE 2

FREQUENCY AND TYPE OF SYMPTOMS[a] IN 97 VERTEBROBASILAR TRANSIENT ISCHEMIC ATTACKS

60%	Ataxia (appendicular or gait)
43%	Vertigo
39%	Diplopia
37%	Blurry vision
27%	Dysarthria

[a]Only symptoms reported by at least 20% of patients are tabulated. Data derived from Futty DE, Conneally M, Dyken ML, et al. Cooperative study of hospital frequency and character of transient ischemic attacks. V. Symptom analysis. *JAMA*. 1977;238(22):2386–2390.

TYPICAL TIME COURSE OF TRANSIENT ISCHEMIC ATTACKS

Eliciting historical information regarding the temporal course of the TIA symptoms is as important as the nature of the actual

TABLE 3

ATYPICAL TRANSIENT ISCHEMIC ATTACK SYNDROMES THAT MAY MIMIC EPILEPTIC ACTIVITY

Syndrome	Vascular territory	Localization
Limb shaking	Carotid	Hemisphere
Asterixis	Vertebrobasilar	Diencephalon
Dyskinesia	Carotid	Hemisphere
	Vertebrobasilar	Diencephalon
Pure sensory	Vertebrobasilar	Diencephalon
	Carotid	Hemisphere
Speech arrest	Carotid	Hemisphere
Visual inversion	Vertebrobasilar	Brainstem
Auditory hallucinosis	Vertebrobasilar	Brainstem
Anosognosia	Carotid	Hemisphere
Akinetic mutism	Carotid	Hemisphere
Drop attacks	Vertebrobasilar	Brainstem

symptoms in making an accurate diagnosis. There is now general acceptance that the arbitrarily defined time period of 24 hours for the definition of TIAs is too long.[55] Most TIAs are rapid in onset and extremely brief, with one series reporting that 24% resolved within 5 minutes, 39% within 15 minutes, and 50% within 30 minutes.[56] Only 40% of TIAs in this series lasted longer than 1 hour. The Cooperative Group for the study of TIAs found that carotid TIAs lasted, on average, 14 minutes, whereas vertebrobasilar events lasted approximately 8 minutes.[5] The prognosis of those patients with longer-lasting TIAs may differ from the subset with brief spells, with reports suggesting that longer-duration TIAs are more likely to exhibit ischemic infarction on more sensitive brain imaging.[11,24] The term *cerebral infarction with transient signs* (CITS) has been developed to describe this subgroup.[79]

ATYPICAL TRANSIENT ISCHEMIC ATTACK PRESENTATIONS

Limb-shaking Carotid Transient Ischemic Attacks

It is generally assumed by physicians that motor TIAs cause limb weakness, whereas focal motor seizures produce convulsive limb movements; however, focal limb shaking resembling a partial motor seizure has been described in association with carotid occlusive disease. Fisher first recognized this unusual manifestation in his observations on carotid TIAs.[27] He noted that the patients described the involved limb as "trembling, shaking, twisting, drawing up, or moving irregularly." His observations have since been corroborated by several investigators.[9,36,84] Russell and Page reported one patient who had involuntary jerking movements affecting the left arm and leg in association with carotid occlusive disease.[66a] Yanagihara and Klass described six patients with involuntary limb jerking, all in association with high-grade stenosis or occlusion of the contralateral carotid artery.[84] They concluded that cerebral ischemia due to diminished cerebral perfusion was the underlying pathogenic mechanism. All of their patients benefited from cerebral revascularization, either carotid endarterectomy (CEA) or extracerebral-intracerebral (EC-IC) bypass grafting. Eight patients were described by Baquis et al. in whom involuntary repetitive movements affected the arm/hand alone or arm and leg opposite to a diseased carotid.[9] The movements had a coarse, wavering, nonrhythmic character with a frequency of 3 to 12 Hz, and seven of the patients had additionally experienced more typical carotid TIAs. In one of their patients, the episodic limb shaking was temporarily related to postural changes in the absence of documented orthostatic hypotension. Cerebral revascularization procedures performed in six of eight patients produced resolution or reduction in the episodic limb-shaking spells. The authors suggested that ischemia affecting the distal field of the atheromatous carotid artery and resulting in perfusion insufficiency was the pathogenic mechanism.

Subsequent investigators have confirmed the mechanism of perfusion insufficiency as the probable cause of focal limb shaking. Levine et al. studied cerebral blood flow (CBF) reactivity to induced hypercapnia using fluoromethane positron emission tomography (PET) scanning in 32 patients with carotid TIAs.[54] Reactivity was found to be significantly diminished in a hemodynamic subset of eight patients whose clinical manifestations included orthostatic limb shaking. Tatemichi et al. reported on a patient whose limb-shaking episodes occurred repeatedly on standing up. Cerebral blood flow was measured using inhaled Xenon-133, and a focal decrease was observed in the right frontal convexity, representing the distal fields between the anterior cerebral artery and the middle cerebral artery.[77] Impaired reactivity was demonstrated in response to hypercapnic challenge using CBF and transcranial Doppler (TCD). A circumscribed loss of cerebral autoregulation was also demonstrated in the same patient, with exacerbation of the perfusion deficit in the right frontal region during hypotension (Fig. 1). The abnormal CBF response to both hypercapnia and hypotension was felt to reflect maximum vasodilation in the distal fields or watershed territory of the involved hemisphere with poor hemodynamic reserve.

These cases illustrate that limb shaking as the first manifestation of a carotid TIA correlates with hemodynamically significant carotid artery disease, with perfusion failure being the most likely mechanism. The patients typically have risk factors for cerebrovascular disease, and the spells are often triggered by postural change or exertion. The movements tend to be coarse and irregular, lasting minutes, and occurring from once a week to several times a day. Other neurologic deficits

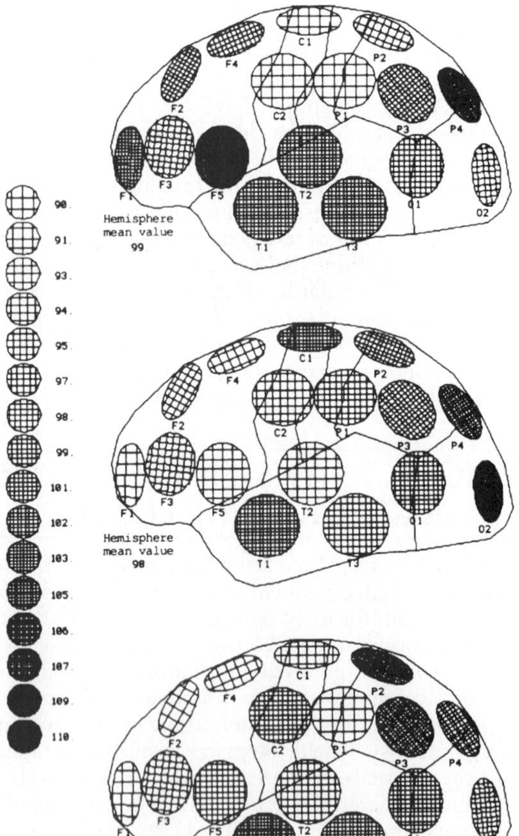

FIGURE 1. Map of cerebral blood flow asymmetry (right initial slope index ([ISI] ÷ left ISI × 100) before carotid endarterectomy under normocapnic (**upper**), hypercapnic (**middle**), and hypotensive (**lower**) conditions. Asymmetry is indicated by intensity of shading, quantified by scale (**left**), given as a percentage. Under normocapnic conditions, there was hypofrontality and reduced perfusion focally in right dorsofrontal and upper rolandic regions (detectors *C1*, *C2*, *P1*, and *P2*). With hypercapnia, more extensive zone in right dorsofrontal region was apparent, extending to superior and inferior frontal regions (detectors *F4*, *F2*, *F1*, *F3*, *F5*, and *T2*). During hypotension, blood flow deficit in right dorsofrontal and prerolandic regions (detectors *C1*, *P1*, *F4*, *F2*, *F1*, and *F3*) was further accentuated. (From Tatemichi TK, Young WL, Prohovnik I, et al. Perfusion insufficiency in limb-shaking transient ischemic attacks. *Stroke.* 1990;21(2):341–347.)

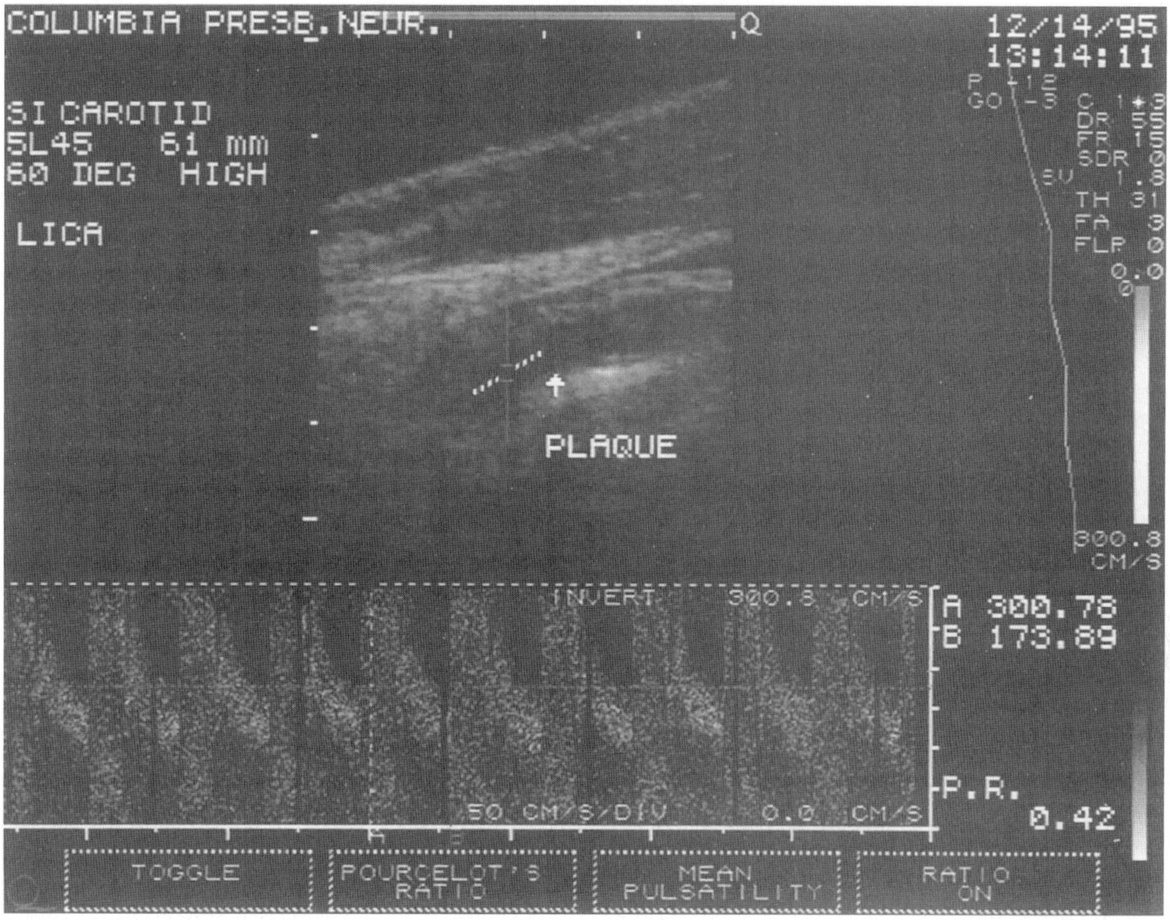

FIGURE 2. Duplex Doppler of the left internal carotid artery showing severe stenosis with plaque obstructing the lumen (*arrow*, **upper**). The Doppler wave form spectra confirm the hemodynamically significant stenosis (**lower**).

rarely occur during the spells, and the interepisode examination is usually normal. A seizure mechanism is not supported in these patients, based on the following observations: No associated clinical seizure phenomena (e.g., impairment of consciousness, rhythmic tonic–clonic jerking, head or eye deviation); no epileptiform activity recorded on electroencephalograms (EEGs) between and during such attacks; a lack of response to trials of antiepileptic medication when such a mechanism was entertained; and, finally, the prompt and favorable response to cerebral revascularization. It remains unclear how ischemia produces the positive motor symptoms, with release of subcortical motor pathways proposed as a possible explanation. Failure to recognize that focal limb shaking can occur secondary to ischemia could lead to delay in diagnosis of the associated severe carotid atheromatous disease (Fig. 2).

The converse situation, where focal seizure activity may cause limb weakness and be misdiagnosed as a TIA, has also been described.[53,64] Fisher referred to this situation as "nonconvulsive seizure paralysis," and noted that it may give rise to diagnostic confusion.[29] Lee and Lerner reported on a 70-year-old diabetic man who presented with recurrent episodes of short-lived right arm weakness and numbness.[53] These spells lasted from 3 to 5 minutes and occurred without warning or other obvious precipitating factors. The patient also noted some speech difficulty during these spells. Neurologic evaluation at the time of admission revealed only a mild right pronator drift, and a computed tomography (CT) scan of the brain was normal. An initial diagnosis of crescendo left carotid TIAs was made, and the patient was anticoagulated with intravenous heparin. Despite therapeutic heparin, the patient continued to have spells at a frequency of three or four hourly. During a typical attack, the patient was noted to first complain of vague right arm discomfort, followed by right arm paralysis; he was described as alert throughout the episode, but with mild word-finding difficulty. An EEG obtained during one such episode demonstrated intermixed spike-and-sharp-wave activity in the left parietal region, which resolved after return of motor function to the affected arm. The presence of these EEG abnormalities was confirmed during subsequent spells. The patient was treated with phenytoin, and the spells decreased in frequency and resolved completely over several days. The authors proposed that a seizure discharge involving the motor region of the left parietal lobe was responsible for the limb paralysis in their patient.

Primavera et al. described a 56-year-old woman with multiple vascular risk factors who presented with recurrent bouts of weakness affecting the right face and arm.[64] Neurologic examination disclosed a right pronator drift, and a CT scan showed multiple old lacunar infarcts. Anticoagulation was begun for a presumptive diagnosis of carotid TIAs, but the intermittent attacks of limb weakness continued. An EEG obtained during a typical attack revealed intermittent high-amplitude slow-wave activity of 2 to 3 Hz intermixed with spikes and sharp waves in the left frontotemporal regions. The attacks decreased in frequency and eventually ceased after treatment with phenobarbital.

These case reports emphasize that the differential diagnosis between TIA and seizure is not always straightforward, even in the presence of vascular risk factors and established ischemic cerebrovascular disease. High-grade carotid stenosis may produce limb shaking, mimicking a focal motor seizure, whereas somatic inhibitory seizures can result in motor weakness, simulating an ischemic TIA.

Unilateral Asterixis

Asterixis is the sudden failure in maintenance of posture, characterized by transient electrical silence in muscles activated to maintain the posture.[80] Clinically it is manifested by asynchronous jerky or flapping movements of the outstretched hands. It was first described by Adams and Foley in a group of patients with hepatic encephalopathy.[6] However, unilateral intermittent asterixis may occur in association with focal cerebral ischemia and be confused with partial motor epilepsy.

Lazzarino and Nicolai described a 56-year-old man who presented 5 months after a left posterior cerebral artery stroke with sudden onset of involuntary movements of the right hand:

> The right hand, when outstretched, showed a movement characterized by sudden flexion of the wrist with loss of position, followed by its sudden restoration. This movement was repeated intermittently at regular intervals, but brief periods of sustained posture between the flaps were present. Active movements abolished these involuntary movements.[52]

Another report described the onset of unilateral asterixis in a 73-year-old man during his recovery from a right ventral thalamic infarct, where the unusual nature of the movements led to a misdiagnosis of epilepsia partialis continua:

> In the left arm, involuntary semi-rhythmic abduction and flexion movements of the fingers and flexion of the wrist were present regardless of the posture of the limb. In contrast, with the left wrist held in extension and the arms pronated, rhythmic loss of posture resulted in wrist flexion movements typical of those seen in asterixis.[74]

The precise mechanism for the asterixis due to ischemia remains uncertain, but it is thought to be related to lapses of sustained muscular contraction secondary to episodic disturbances in the responsible neuronal circuits.[80] The movements may appear at rest, but gravity is the most effective stimulus to elicit asterixis. Failure to consider ischemia as a diagnostic possibility in the evaluation of episodic unilateral involuntary movements may result in the unwarranted administration of anticonvulsant medication.

Episodic Dyskinesia

Acute hemiballism or choreoathetosis is known to occur from infarcts of the subthalamic nucleus of Luys, striatal and thalamic nuclei.[55] The involuntary movements are usually of sudden onset, without accompanying deficits. The following case report serves to illustrate the clinical presentation:

> An 81-year-old, right-handed woman suddenly developed involuntary movements of the left limbs.... On neurologic examination, she showed choreic and ballistic movements of the left limbs. There was almost constant, small-amplitude, proximal and distal choreic movements, with superimposed brisk, large-amplitude proximal movements, primarily related to action. Magnetic resonance imaging (MRI) revealed a small area of hypointense T1 signal in the right thalamus.[45]

Episodic dyskinesias, while less frequently reported, have been described in association with both vertebrobasilar and carotid occlusive disease. Margolin and Marsden reported on four patients with episodic abnormal involuntary movements affecting the limbs opposite to carotid atheromatous disease.[58a] The clinical spectrum included both choreoathetoid and ballistic involuntary movements, lasting from minutes to 1 hour. The patients used the terms *writhing, wild gyrations*, and *snakelike* to describe the involuntary movements. Cerebral revascularization with carotid endarterectomy resulted in resolution of the movements. Stark described recurrent brief attacks of snakelike movements affecting the left arm in a 53-year-old woman with high-grade stenosis of the right internal carotid artery that responded to endarterectomy:

> She had three attacks within 1 month; each was characterized as sudden inability to "control my left arm." When she was asked to demonstrate the attacks, she raised her left arm and made snakelike movements, proximally and distally, characteristic of choreoathetosis.[72]

Unilateral dyskinetic movements may be mistaken for convulsive phenomena unless a vascular etiology is given careful consideration. Witnessed accounts of such episodic involuntary movements may not be available, and if the nondominant hemisphere is involved, the patient may ignore or trivialize the episode. The presence of vascular risk factors and evidence for infarction on brain imaging should be specifically sought. Both the carotid and vertebrobasilar circulation have been implicated in previous reports, and ultrasound examination using duplex Doppler may reveal abnormalities.

Pure Sensory Spells

Sensory disturbances affecting part or all of the contralateral body are frequent manifestations of hemispheric TIAs. Although TIAs are usually considered to result from large-artery atherothrombotic disease, they may also occur from small penetrating vessel disease. Awareness of these so-called lacunar TIAs is critical to any discussion of pure sensory phenomena. The Stroke Data Bank (SDB) found that lacunar syndromes had a preceding TIA in 13% of the cases versus 40% for large-artery syndromes.[30] Thus, both large- and small-vessel pathology need to be considered in the differential of focal sensory complaints. Isolated fleeting sensory dysfunction can also be the result of a partial seizure syndrome, and it is a diagnostic challenge to separate an ischemic from an ictal mechanism.

Pure sensory symptoms involving the arm occurred in approximately 50% of the cases from a large series of carotid TIAs.[31] The distal arm and hand were the sites most frequently affected in the attacks, with the sensory deficit thought to result from ischemia of the sensory cortex in the distal field of the diseased carotid territory. To confidently attribute pure sensory disturbances in the individual patient to a hemispheric TIA, a search using duplex and transcranial Doppler to find an appropriate carotid lesion should be performed. Failure to document hemodynamically significant stenosis of the extracranial carotid artery or its intracranial branches suggests that large-vessel stenosis is less likely to account for the sensory spells.[55]

Pure sensory stroke (PSS) is a well-recognized vascular syndrome resulting from lacunar infarction of the ventral tier thalamic nuclei. Fisher's case 9 in his original collection of PSS cases was characterized by transient attacks of sensory disturbance affecting the fingers of the right hand; the right side of the lips along with the right side of the tongue were affected, in addition to the fingers, during subsequent spells. At autopsy, a lacune in the ventral posterior thalamic nucleus, measuring 7 mm in diameter, was found. Another case in his collection had intermittent sensory spells affecting the left lower lip, fingers of the left hand, and sole of the left foot. Other patterns of sensory involvement described in PSS cases by Fisher were as follows: Face, arm, and leg; head, cheek, lips, and hand; face, fingers, and foot; shoulder tip and lower jaw; distal forearm alone; fingers alone; and leg alone.[28]

The peculiar nature of sensory complaints in thalamic ischemia may lead the unsuspecting to fail to consider a vascular etiology. The patients may describe the affected body part as feeling stretched, hot, swollen, sunburnt, larger, smaller, or heavier. Eyeglasses, jewelry, and clothing may feel heavier on the affected part, and contact may transiently exacerbate the dysesthetic sensations. Thalamic-origin TIAs can give rise to either a sensory disturbance restricted to a few digits or an extensive abnormality splitting the entire body, including the scalp, neck, trunk, and genitalia.[55] It may not be readily appreciated that such midline splitting can be produced by an ischemic mechanism unless the unique somatosensory organization of the thalamus and the thalamocortical connections is considered in the approach to differential diagnosis.

Speech Arrest

Isolated episodes of language disturbance due to left carotid TIAs must be distinguished from those secondary to seizure activity. Cascino et al. described three patients in whom transient episodes of speech arrest were initially attributed to TIAs, but in which subsequent EEG recordings demonstrated bifrontal seizure activity.[20]

Case 1 was a 66-year-old woman with end-stage renal disease admitted for shunt placement. During her hospitalization, she experienced spells in which she would abruptly stop talking and stare aimlessly. She remained alert throughout the episodes and followed verbal commands.

Case 2 was a 72-year-old hypertensive male admitted with a diagnosis of TIAs. Multiple spells lasting minutes were observed, during which he said he could understand speech but "could not get the words out."

The final case they described involved an 87-year-old man on long-term warfarin therapy for an artificial heart valve admitted with abdominal complaints. He was noted to experience several spells of "expressive aphasia," where he could not speak but would follow commands. In all of the cases, the episodes resolved following treatment with anticonvulsants.

Peled et al. provide a further insightful case description of a 65-year-old man with multiple stroke risk factors (smoking, diabetes, hypercholesterolemia) evaluated for transient episodes of sudden inability to talk.[62] These spells lasted from 2 to 5 minutes and occurred up to four times daily. Clinical observation of the spells during the patient's period of hospitalization was remarkable for sudden onset of mutism with preserved comprehension and absence of any forced head, gaze deviation, or focal motor activity. EEG obtained between the episodes proved normal, and a seizure diagnosis was not entertained until the patient was noted to raise his right hand and turn his head to the right during one of his characteristic spells. Closer observation revealed involuntary gaze deviation and clonic motor activity affecting the right face and limbs during some of his spells. Brain imaging demonstrated a probable metastatic lesion in the medial dominant frontal lobe corresponding to supplementary motor area (SMA). Treatment with phenytoin was begun, and the spells resolved.

This case material helps to emphasize that although cerebral ischemia commonly underlies the sudden onset of language disturbances in the elderly, infrequently seizures may be the cause.

Penfield and Roberts have reported that electrical stimulation of the SMA region anterior to the leg representation can produce speech arrest in humans.[63] Proposed pathogenetic mechanisms include interference with the motor pathway subserving vocalization or a true ictal "aphasic" speech arrest from a primary language disorder. Certainly, when dominant SMA lesions produce this latter type of aphasic speech arrest without accompanying eye-head deviation or tonic posturing, the epileptic nature of the spells may be missed, and an incorrect diagnosis of dominant carotid territory TIA may result. Such a misdiagnosis may lead to inappropriate investigations and a decision to commence long-term anticoagulation, with its attendant risks.

Visual Inversion

Momentary vertical inversion of images has been described in Wallenberg syndrome and vertebrobasilar TIAs and can sometimes be confused with the visual phenomena of seizures.[67,73] Patients present with the unusual complaint of acute "upside-down" vision, their world appearing 180 degrees reversed. The entire visual field is affected, with color and shape perception generally preserved, which helps distinguish it from the visual phenomena (e.g., macro- or micropsia, visual hallucinations) that can be associated with temporal or occipital lobe epilepsy. The following case report of an 83-year-old man serves to illustrate the features of this novel visual illusion:

> He was awakened by severe nausea and vertigo. When he switched on the light next to his bed . . . the telephone and bedside table appeared 180 degrees reversed, hanging down from the ceiling. This visual experience lasted only a few minutes. Neurologic exam 5 hours later was normal. The inversion of vision recurred several hours later and the patient again graphically described the experience: people surrounding his bed appeared inverted, with their legs up and heads down, the floor became the ceiling.[73]

This unique visual symptomatology may occur in isolation or be accompanied by nausea, vertigo, gait instability, and examination findings (Horner syndrome, limb ataxia, hemihypalgesia) consistent with lateral medullary infarction (Fig. 3).[67] The 180-degree reversal of vision has been attributed to transient ischemia of central vestibulo-ocular integrative control mechanisms, particularly dysfunction of vestibular inflow, which may disturb visual space orientation and result in aberrant egocentric orientation.[73] Such visual field complaints occur infrequently with vertebrobasilar ischemia but, when present, should alert the physician to the possibility of brainstem ischemia.

Brainstem Auditory Hallucinosis

Intermittent auditory hallucinations, which can raise the suspicion of epileptic activity, have been reported in patients with radiologic evidence of vascular lesions affecting the pontine tegmentum.[19,50] The phenomenon is illustrated by the following case description:

> A 55-year-old hypertensive man . . . complained of hearing low-pitched musical sounds in both ears. The sounds were localized externally but were not associated with any auditory stimuli. He recognized these sounds as abnormal. Examination demonstrated a left Horner's syndrome, nystagmus, and long tract signs. Over the following several days . . . the auditory hallucinations became like people talking and later like the sound of rain falling on a roof.[50]

There was no alteration in consciousness or other positive motor or sensory phenomena, and an EEG had mild slowing but no epileptiform activity. Audiometry found moderate bilateral sensorineural hearing loss with poor speech discrimination affecting the left ear. Magnetic resonance imaging of the brain demonstrated a left caudal pontine tegmental hemorrhage involving the superior olivary nucleus, the trapezoid body, and the dorsal and intermediate acoustic striae. The

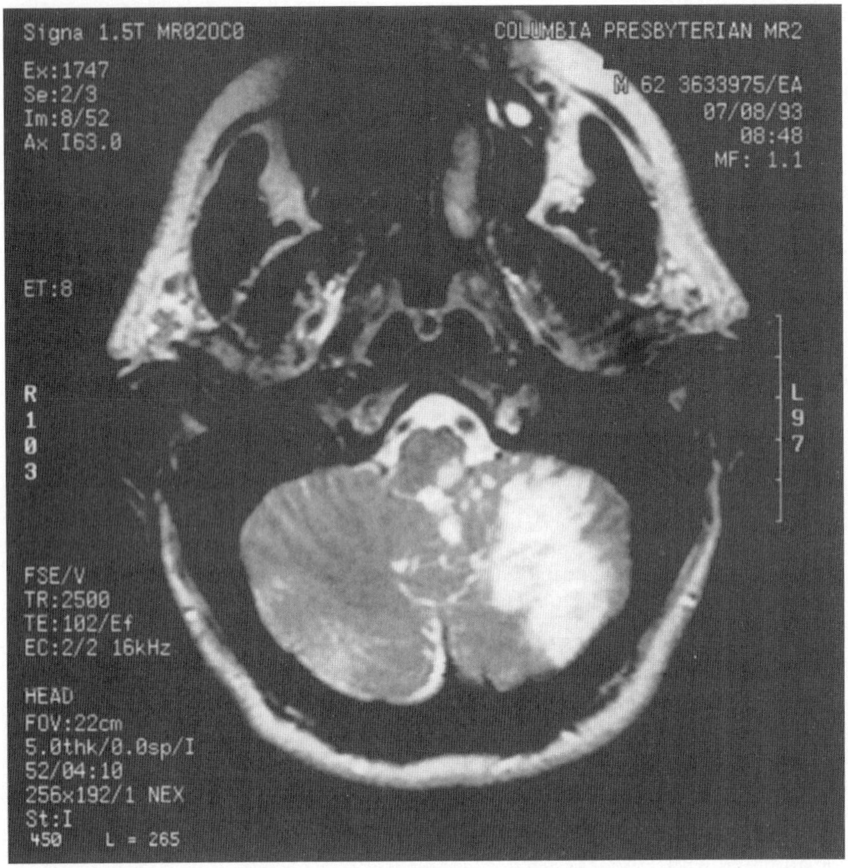

FIGURE 3. Axial (1.5-T) T2-weighted magnetic resonance image in a patient with lateral medullary syndrome showing infarction of the left inferior cerebellar hemisphere and the left lateral medulla.

authors postulated a "release" mechanism for the hallucinations from hearing loss caused by dysfunction of the central auditory pathways.[50] Although rare, the occurrence of auditory hallucinosis, accompanied by other brainstem findings, should prompt an investigation for a vascular etiology.

Auditory Aprosodia

Episodic loss of pitch perception is another auditory aberration that could be attributed to epileptic phenomena and has been described in right hemisphere cerebral ischemia. The following case illustrates the syndrome:

> A 52-year-old man was well until he experienced the first of two episodes of transient loss of pitch perception. The patient was at a party when he noticed that all of the voices that he heard sounded as if they were spoken in a monotone. He recalled no confusion at that time, nor did he recall experiencing any difficulty comprehending the content of what was said. This episode reportedly lasted less than 20 minutes, and was regarded as a curiosity by the patient. Several days later, a second 20-minute episode occurred while the patient was at home in his kitchen.... The patient noted that the music on the radio lost its melodic quality, sounding flat and monotonous. The patient indicated that the loudness and rhythm sounded normal.... Approximately two weeks after...the patient suffered transient spells of left facial droop, slurred speech, and left-sided weakness. Finally, he experienced the sudden onset of left hemiparesis, and a left hemianopsia. CT scan revealed a right middle cerebral artery territory infarct and angiography revealed a total occlusion at the origin of the right internal carotid artery.[70]

These recurrent spells, during which the patient was unable to perceive normal variations in pitch of conversation and music, were thought to represent transient ischemia affecting the auditory cortex of the nondominant hemisphere.

Transient Anosognosia

Transient anosognosia or failure to appreciate neurologic deficits, which may be confused with postictal behavioral disturbances, have been reported in six patients in association with transitory hemiparesis, paresthesias, and visual field cuts.[34] This unusual behavioral syndrome is illustrated by the following case description:

> A 68-year-old man came out of his room unaware of being improperly dressed with his buttons and belt undone, and his shirttail hanging out. He nevertheless declared himself ready to attend a planned choir practice at church. Upon inquiry, he denied being sloppily dressed despite confrontation before a mirror. Intrigued at first, his wife became alarmed after noticing, a few minutes later, an obvious dysarthria and left-sided weakness. Pointing out these deficits to him met with emphatic denial once more. Upon arrival at the hospital he had completely recovered from this initial one-hour episode. An identical 30-minute episode was later witnessed the same evening in our Emergency Room. A head computed tomography (CT) scan was normal. Angiography revealed bilateral internal carotid fibromuscular dysplasia. He remained asymptomatic under anticoagulants, and was discharged 7 days after admission.[34]

The authors concluded that a nondominant hemispheric syndrome from carotid occlusive disease accounted for the change in behavior observed in their patient. Although behavior disturbance can be seen with epileptic phenomena, a vascular etiology should be strongly considered in patients who present with abrupt changes in behavior or personality.

Akinetic Mutism

Akinetic mutism describes patients who appear awake and alert, yet remain mute and motionless, despite intact motor and sensory pathways.[7] This behavioral syndrome may resemble nonconvulsive or absence status, but the differential also includes a vascular etiology.

The disturbance has been described with bilateral frontal lobe lesions and has been attributed to an impaired psychic drive (abulia). Gugliotta et al. described a patient who experienced abrupt onset of akinetic mutism in association with spontaneous bilateral anterior cerebral artery (ACA) occlusion:

> A 65-year-old male had been suffering from sudden mild headache, followed by gait difficulty and limb paresthesia. The day of admission he was found unconscious in bed, with eyes open and rotated upward; he was unable to speak or follow commands. On admission the patient had an alert appearance but was unresponsive to any auditory or visual command. His eyes were open and moved spontaneously as though he was looking around the room, without however following a moving object or person. CT scan of the brain revealed the presence of low density foci, which were localized in the mesial frontal region bilaterally.[35]

Unilateral ACA territory infarction can also present with severe apathy, abulia, and mutism or acute confusional states, and must be considered when the clinical presentation involves transient confusion or stuporous states.[12]

Drop Attacks

Typical drop attacks are characterized by a sudden falling spell that occurs without warning and without loss of consciousness. Drop attacks must be distinguished from akinetic seizures.[7] The patient suddenly falls to the ground while walking or standing and is usually able to get up immediately. The falling spells may recur over a period of years, EEGs obtained are usually normal, and an identifiable mechanism is difficult to find. Such attacks in isolation are not considered typical vertebrobasilar TIAs; however, when associated with other symptomatology, they may suggest brainstem ischemia. The following case illustrates an example:

> A married woman of 52 had a drop attack; she suddenly fell to the ground, hit her face, picking herself up immediately and saying she was all right. There was no loss of consciousness, no warning and no sequels. Since that time there have been repeated attacks of vertigo, some of intense severity, with ataxia. These are associated with occipital headaches, and pains in the neck, which may last up to half an hour. There are intermittent sensory disturbances unrelated to these attacks of vertigo, of a cold sensation and pins and needles over the scalp and upper neck on either side independently. There are also episodes of dysaesthesiae in either arm independently or together.[83]

Carotid occlusive disease may rarely result in spells of transient paraparesis simulating drop attacks. Ho et al. reported a patient with recurrent episodes of transient paraparesis in the setting of a high-grade right internal carotid stenosis and a hypoplastic A1 segment of the left anterior cerebral artery.[51] This vascular anatomy meant that both anterior cerebral artery territories subserving motor control of both legs suffered ischemia from perfusion failure due to the right-sided carotid occlusive disease. In another case reported by the author, a bihemispheric anterior cerebral artery above a left carotid stenosis of 90% led to drop attacks. Shaking of the right arm on reaching for objects provided a clue to the perfusion failure in this case.[32] The spells in both these patients were abolished by revascularization with carotid endarterectomy.

Moyamoya Disease

Moyamoya disease is characterized by chronic progressive multiple stenoses or occlusions of the intracranial arteries of the carotid system.[78] The angiographic hallmark of the condition is the presence of abnormal anastomotic vessels at the base of the brain. It is a form of cerebrovascular disease that predominantly affects children and young adults, where its clinical manifestations may be mistaken for paroxysmal epileptic events. Accurate diagnosis of intermittent spells in this population is hindered by the observation that moyamoya disease may also present with seizures.

The Cooperative Group for the study of moyamoya disease in Japan has described the clinical features of the disease in children and adults. Among 155 children (<15 years), TIAs (39%) and strokes (39%) were the most common presentations, followed by seizures (14%) and hemorrhage (7%).[61] Conversely, the clinical presentation in adults (<15 years) was dominated by hemorrhage (65%), with TIAs (6%) and seizures (6%) occurring less commonly. The recurring ischemic attacks seen in children have certain characteristic features. Hemiplegia and monoplegia are common manifestations at the onset, though sensory, speech, or visual disturbances may also occur. The attacks are typically triggered by crying, coughing, or straining—circumstances that may not immediately suggest an ischemic basis to those unfamiliar with this condition. The hyperventilation associated with these activities results in CBF reductions that are sufficient to induce cerebral ischemia. This observation is consistent with the theory that marginal hemodynamic reserve and perfusion failure affecting the watershed or distal field territory is the underlying mechanism for the ischemic attacks.[76]

SUMMARY AND CONCLUSIONS

TIAs are a powerful marker of increased stroke risk, myocardial infarction, and death. Accurate clinical identification of TIAs depends on recognizing typical, as well as less typical, symptoms and an awareness of mimicking conditions. A reliable history may prove difficult to obtain because the episodes are usually unwitnessed and tend to be brief and frightening, and nondominant hemisphere ischemic attacks may be ignored by the patient. The neurologic examination is generally not helpful, as it is often normal by the time the physician has the opportunity to assess the patient. The proven value of antiplatelet therapy and carotid endarterectomy and the rapid proliferation of hyperacute stroke protocols emphasize the need for the rapid detection of TIAs. The diagnostic evaluation in the individual patient needs to consider that small-vessel disease may also produce ischemic attacks, in addition to the more accepted large-artery atherothrombotic mechanism. The currently accepted definition of TIA regarding time course and the assumption of no persistent cerebral injury have been proven incorrect and will require revision.

The differential diagnosis of patients presenting with focal neurologic disturbances is broad and includes TIAs, seizures, migraine, syncope, and brain tumors. Each requires specific diagnosis and management. Wider use of event detection questionnaires that have been validated in epidemiologic studies is an attractive option that may improve interobserver reliability in the diagnosis of TIAs. Data from large TIA series have helped to identify particular symptoms that are not typical of ischemic attacks, such as isolated dizziness, unconsciousness or drop attacks without accompanying vertebrobasilar symptoms, scintillating scotomata, and "march" of symptoms over body parts. The occurrence of these symptoms should encourage physicians to consider alternative diagnoses. Atypical TIA symptoms such as limb shaking, other adventitious movements, visual phenomena, and behavioral change pose a particular dilemma for the physician faced with discriminating TIA from epileptic phenomena. Physician and public awareness that these less frequent clinical features may have an ischemic etiology should enhance diagnostic accuracy and improve selection of the proper therapy.

References

1. Beneficial effect of carotid endarterectomy in symptomatic patients with high-grade carotid stenosis. North American Symptomatic Carotid Endarterectomy Trial Collaborators. *N Engl J Med.* 1991;325(7):445–453.
2. Guidelines for the management of transient ischemic attacks. From the Ad Hoc Committee on Guidelines for the Management of Transient Ischemic Attacks of the Stroke Council of the American Heart Association. *Stroke.* 1994;25(6):1320–1335.
3. Joint Committee for Stroke Facilities. *Stroke.* 1974;5(2):275–287.
4. Special report from the National Institute of Neurological Disorders and Stroke. Classification of cerebrovascular diseases III. *Stroke.* 1990;21(4):637–676.
5. The Study Group on TIA Criteria and Detection. XI. Transient focal cerebral ischemia: epidemiological and clinical aspects. *Stroke.* 1974;5:277–284.
6. Adams RD, Foley JM. The neurological changes in the more common types of severe liver disease. *Trans Am Neurol Assoc.* 1949;74:217–219.
7. Adams RD, Victor M. *Principles of Neurology.* 5th ed. New York: McGraw-Hill; 1993.
8. Arboix A, Garcia-Eroles L, Massons JB, et al. Predictive factors of early seizures after acute cerebrovascular disease. *Stroke.* 1997;28(8):1590–1594.
9. Baquis GD, Pessin MS, Scott RM. Limb shaking—a carotid TIA. *Stroke.* 1985;16(3):444–448.
10. Bladin CF, Alexandrov AV, Bellavance A, et al. Seizures after stroke: a prospective multicenter study. *Arch Neurol.* 2000;57(11):1617–1622.
11. Bogousslavsky J, Regli F. Cerebral infarct in apparent transient ischemic attack. *Neurology.* 1985;35(10):1501–1503.
12. Bogousslavsky J, Van Melle G, Despland PA, et al. Alcohol consumption and carotid atherosclerosis in the Lausanne Stroke Registry. *Stroke.* 1990;21(5):715–720.
13. Brown RD Jr, Petty GW, O'Fallon WM, et al. Incidence of transient ischemic attack in Rochester, Minnesota, 1985–1989. *Stroke.* 1998;29(10):2109–2113.
14. Buchkremer-Ratzmann I, August M, Hagemann G, et al. Epileptiform discharges to extracellular stimuli in rat neocortical slices after photothrombotic infarction. *J Neurol Sci.* 1998;156(2):133–137.
15. Burn J, Dennis M, Bamford J, et al. Epileptic seizures after a first stroke: the Oxfordshire community stroke project. *BMJ.* 1997;315(7122):1582–1587.
16. Calanchini PR, Swanson PD, Gotshall RA, et al. Cooperative study of hospital frequency and character of transient ischemic attacks. IV. The reliability of diagnosis. *JAMA.* 1977;238(19):2029–2033.
17. Camilo O, Goldstein LB. Seizures and epilepsy after ischemic stroke. *Stroke.* 2004;35(7):1769–1775.
18. Caplan LR. Are terms such as completed stroke or RIND of continued usefulness? *Stroke.* 1983;14(3):431–433.
19. Cascino GD, Adams RD. Brainstem auditory hallucinosis. *Neurology.* 1986;36(8):1042–1047.
20. Cascino GD, Westmoreland BF, Swanson TH, et al. Seizure-associated speech arrest in elderly patients. *Mayo Clin Proc.* 1991;66(3):254–258.
21. Chui HC, Victoroff JI, Margolin D, et al. Criteria for the diagnosis of ischemic vascular dementia proposed by the State of California Alzheimer's Disease Diagnostic and Treatment Centers.[comment]. *Neurology.* 1992;42(3 Pt 1):473–480.
22. Ciesielski-Carlucci C, Lee BK, Boxer LM, et al. A woman who had a stroke, then a myocardial infarction [erratum appears in *Lancet.* 1997;350(9074):372]. *Lancet.* 1997;349(9060):1218.
23. Dennis MS, Bamford JM, Sandercock PA, et al. Incidence of transient ischemic attacks in Oxfordshire, England. *Stroke.* 1989;20(3):333–339.
24. Eliasziw M, Streifler JY, Spence JD, et al. Prognosis for patients following a transient ischemic attack with and without a cerebral infarction on brain CT. North American Symptomatic Carotid Endarterectomy Trial (NASCET) Group. *Neurology.* 1995;45(3 Pt 1):428–431.
25. Eriksson M, Asplund K, Glader EL, et al. Self-reported depression and use of antidepressants after stroke: a national survey [see comment]. *Stroke.* 2004;35(4):936–941.
26. Feldmann E, Wilterdink J. The symptoms of transient cerebral ischemic attacks. *Semin Neurol.* 1991;11(2):135–145.
27. Fisher CM. Concerning recurrent transient cerebral ischemic attacks. *Can Med Assoc J.* 1962;86:1091–1099.
28. Fisher CM. Thalamic pure sensory stroke: a pathologic study. *Neurology.* 1978;28(11):1141–1144.
29. Fisher CM. Transient paralytic attacks of obscure nature: the question of non-convulsive seizure paralysis. *Can J Neurol Sci.* 1978;5(3):267–273.
30. Foulkes MA, Wolf PA, Price TR, et al. The Stroke Data Bank: design, methods, and baseline characteristics. *Stroke.* 1988;19(5):547–554.
31. Futty DE, Conneally M, Dyken ML, et al. Cooperative study of hospital frequency and character of transient ischemic attacks. V. Symptom analysis. *JAMA.* 1977;238(22):2386–2390.
32. Gerstner E, Liberato B, Wright CB. Bi-hemispheric anterior cerebral artery with drop attacks and limb shaking TIAs. *Neurology.* 2005;65(1):174.
33. Goldstein LB. Common drugs may influence motor recovery after stroke. The Sygen In Acute Stroke Study Investigators [see comment]. *Neurology.* 1995;45(5):865–871.
34. Grand'Maison F, Reiher J, Lebel ML, et al. Transient anosognosia for episodic hemiparesis: a singular manifestation of TIAs and epileptic seizures. *Can J Neurol Sci.* 1989;16(2):203–205.
35. Gugliotta MA, Silvestri R, De Domenico P, et al. Spontaneous bilateral anterior cerebral artery occlusion resulting in akinetic mutism. A case report. *Acta Neurol (Napoli).* 1989;11(4):252–258.
36. Hachinski VC, Iliff LD, Zilhka E, et al. Cerebral blood flow in dementia. *Arch Neurol.* 1975;32(9):632–637.
37. Hauser WA, Annegers JF, Kurland LT. Incidence of epilepsy and unprovoked seizures in Rochester, Minnesota: 1935–1984. *Epilepsia.* 1993;34(3):453–468.
38. Heuts-van Raak L, Lodder J, Kessels F. Late seizures following a first symptomatic brain infarct are related to large infarcts involving the posterior area around the lateral sulcus. *Seizure.* 1996;5(3):185–194.
38a. Ho RT, Harrison MJ, Earl CJ. Transient paraparesis—a manifestation of ischaemic episodes in the anterior cerebral artery territory. *J Neurol Neurosurg Psychiatry.* 1986; Jan;49:101–102.
39. Jennett B. Posttraumatic epilepsy. *Adv Neurol.* 1979;22:137–147.
40. Johnston SC, Gress DR, Browner WS, et al. Short-term prognosis after emergency department diagnosis of TIA. *JAMA.* 2000;284(22):2901–2906.
41. Kilpatrick CJ, Davis SM, Tress BM, et al. Epileptic seizures in acute stroke. *Arch Neurol.* 1990;47(2):157–160.
42. Kleindorfer D, Panagos P, Pancioli A, et al. Incidence and short-term prognosis of transient ischemic attack in a population-based study [see comment]. *Stroke.* 2005;36(4):720–723.
43. Koudstaal PJ, Gerritsma JG, van Gijn J. Clinical disagreement on the diagnosis of transient ischemic attack: is the patient or the doctor to blame? *Stroke.* 1989;20(2):300–301.
44. Koudstaal PJ, van Gijn J, Staal A, et al. Diagnosis of transient ischemic attacks: improvement of interobserver agreement by a check-list in ordinary language. *Stroke.* 1986;17(4):723–728.
45. Kulisevsky J, Berthier ML, Pujol J. Hemiballismus and secondary mania following a right thalamic infarction. *Neurology.* 1993;43(7):1422–1424.
46. Labovitz DL, Hauser WA. Preventing stroke-related seizures: when should anticonvulsant drugs be started? *Neurology.* 2003;60(3):365–366.
47. Labovitz DL, Hauser WA, Sacco RL. Prevalence and predictors of early seizure and status epilepticus after first stroke. *Neurology.* 2001;57(2):200–206.
48. Lamy C, Domigo V, Semah F, et al. Early and late seizures after cryptogenic ischemic stroke in young adults. *Neurology.* 2003;60(3):400–404.
49. Lancman ME, Golimstok A, Norscini J, et al. Risk factors for developing seizures after a stroke. *Epilepsia.* 1993;34(1):141–143.
50. Lanska DJ, Kryscio RJ. Endarterectomy for asymptomatic internal carotid artery stenosis. *Neurology.* 1997;48(6):1481–1490.
51. Launes J, Iivanainen M, Erkinjuntti T, et al. Isolated angiitis of the central nervous system. *Acta Neurol Scand.* 1986;74(2):108–114.
52. Lazzarino LG, Nicolai A. Late onset unilateral asterixis secondary to posterior cerebral artery infarction. *Ital J Neurol Sci.* 1992;13(4):361–364.
53. Lee H, Lerner A. Transient inhibitory seizures mimicking crescendo TIAs. *Neurology.* 1990;40(1):165–166.
54. Levine RL, Lagreze HL, Dobkin JA, et al. Cerebral vasocapacitance and TIAs. *Neurology.* 1989;39(1):25–29.
55. Levine SR, Brey RL, Tilley BC, et al. Antiphospholipid antibodies and subsequent thrombo-occlusive events in patients with ischemic stroke [see comment]. *JAMA.* 2004;291(5):576–584.
56. Levy DE. Transient CNS deficits: a common, benign syndrome in young adults. *Neurology.* 1988;38(6):831–836.
57. Lossius MI, Ronning OM, Slapo GD, et al. Poststroke epilepsy: occurrence and predictors—a long-term prospective controlled study (Akershus Stroke Study). *Epilepsia.* 2005;46(8):1246–1251.
58. Luhmann HJ. Ischemia and lesion induced imbalances in cortical function. *Prog Neurobiol.* 1996;48(2):131–166.
58a. Margolin DI, Marsden CD. Episodic dyskinesias and transient cerebral ischemia. *Neurology.* 1982;32:1379–1380.
59. Mohr JP, Caplan LR, Melski JW, et al. The Harvard Cooperative Stroke Registry: a prospective registry. *Neurology.* 1978;28(8):754–762.
60. Naidech AM, Kreiter KT, Janjua N, et al. Phenytoin exposure is associated with functional and cognitive disability after subarachnoid hemorrhage. *Stroke.* 2005;36(3):583–587.
61. Nishimoto A, Ueta A, Onbe H. Cooperative study of moyamoya disease in Japan. *Neurol Med Chir.* 1981;19:221–228.
62. Peled R, Harnes B, Borovich B, et al. Speech arrest and supplementary motor area seizures. *Neurology.* 1984;34(1):110–111.

63. Penfield W, Roberts L. *Speech and Brain-Mechanisms*. Princeton, NJ: Princeton University Press; 1959.
64. Primavera A, Giberti L, Cocito L. Focal inhibitory seizures as the presenting sign of ischemic cerebrovascular disease. *Ital J Neurol Sci*. 1993;14(5):381–384.
65. Reith J, Jorgensen HS, Nakayama H, et al. Seizures in acute stroke: predictors and prognostic significance: the Copenhagen Stroke Study. *Stroke*. 1997;28(8):1585–1589.
66. Rothwell PM, Coull AJ, Giles MF, et al. Change in stroke incidence, mortality, case-fatality, severity, and risk factors in Oxfordshire, UK from 1981 to 2004 (Oxford Vascular Study) [see comment]. *Lancet*. 2004;363(9425):1925–1933.
66a. Russell RW, Page NG. Critical perfusion of brain and retina. *Brain*. 1983;106:419–434.
67. Sacco RL, Freddo L, Bello JA, et al. Wallenberg's lateral medullary syndrome. Clinical-magnetic resonance imaging correlations. *Arch Neurol*. 1993;50(6):609–614.
68. Sandercock P. Recent developments in the diagnosis and management of patients with transient ischaemic attacks and minor ischaemic strokes. *Q J Med*. 1991;78(286):101–112.
69. Schwartz-Bloom RD, McDonough KJ, Chase PJ, et al. Long-term neuroprotection by benzodiazepine full versus partial agonists after transient cerebral ischemia in the gerbil [corrected]. *J Cereb Blood Flow Metab*. 1998;18(5):548–558.
70. Sidtis JJ, Feldmann E. Transient ischemic attacks presenting with a loss of pitch perception. *Cortex*. 1990;26(3):469–471.
71. So EL, Annegers JF, Hauser WA, et al. Population-based study of seizure disorders after cerebral infarction. *Neurology*. 1996;46(2):350–355.
72. Stark SR. Transient dyskinesia and cerebral ischemia. *Neurology*. 1985;35(3):445.
73. Steiner I, Shahin R, Melamed E. Acute "upside down" reversal of vision in transient vertebrobasilar ischemia. *Neurology*. 1987;37(10):1685–1686.
74. Stell R, Davis S, Carroll WM. Unilateral asterixis due to a lesion of the ventrolateral thalamus. *J Neurol Neurosurg Psychiatry*. 1994;57(7):878–880.
75. Streifler JY, Eliasziw M, Benavente OR, et al. The risk of stroke in patients with first-ever retinal vs hemispheric transient ischemic attacks and high-grade carotid stenosis. North American Symptomatic Carotid Endarterectomy Trial [comment]. *Arch Neurol*. 1995;52(3):246–249.
76. Tatemichi TK, Prohovnik I, Mohr JP, et al. Reduced hypercapnic vasoreactivity in moyamoya disease. *Neurology*. 1988;38(10):1575–1581.
77. Tatemichi TK, Young WL, Prohovnik I, et al. Perfusion insufficiency in limb-shaking transient ischemic attacks. *Stroke*. 1990;21(2):341–347.
78. Toole JF. The Willis lecture: transient ischemic attacks, scientific method, and new realities. *Stroke*. 1991;22(1):99–104.
79. Waxman SG, Toole JF. Temporal profile resembling TIA in the setting of cerebral infarction. *Stroke*. 1983;14(3):433–437.
80. Wee AS. Unilateral asterixis: case report and comments. *Eur Neurol*. 1986;25(3):208–211.
81. Wilkinson WE, Heyman A, Burch JG, et al. Use of a self-administered questionnaire for detection of transient cerebral ischemic attacks: I. Survey of elderly persons living in retirement facilities. *Ann Neurol*. 1979;6(1):40–46.
82. Wilkinson WE, Heyman A, Pfeffer RI, et al. A questionnaire for TIA symptoms: a predictor of subsequent stroke. In: Reivich M, Hurtig HI, eds. *Cerebrovascular Diseases*. New York: Raven Press; 1983:71–89.
83. Williams D, Wilson TG. The diagnosis of the major and minor syndromes of basilar insufficiency. *Brain*. 1962;85:741–774.
84. Yanagihara T, et al. Clinical characteristics of senile dementia in Japan. *Rinsho Shinkeigaku* 1999;39(1):45–46.

CHAPTER 276 ■ SLEEP DISORDERS

MARK W. MAHOWALD AND CARLOS H. SCHENCK

INTRODUCTION

Since sleep and epilepsy are common bedfellows, it stands to reason that sleep disorders may mimic, cause, or even be triggered by epileptic phenomena, and vice versa. It is known that, in some individuals, sleep promotes seizures, as does sleep deprivation.[25,86] Conversely, seizure disorders can affect the wake–sleep cycle.[114] As discussed in Chapter 188, in most cases, epilepsy is highly state–dependent: Non-rapid eye movement (NRM) sleep promotes seizures, while rapid eye movement (REM) sleep is a relatively antiepileptic state.[132,134] This fact reflects the dramatic reorganization of the entire central nervous system (CNS) as it moves across the three states of being: Wakefulness, NREM sleep, and REM sleep.

There are certain predisposing factors in NREM sleep that facilitate epileptic discharges. There may be a relationship between sleep spindles and spike-and-wave bursts in human epilepsy.[57] There may also be a relationship between the cyclic alternating pattern (CAP) of "fluctuating cortical excitability" with both sleep-related epilepsy and a number of other sleep disorders.[136,145]

In simpler times, it was felt that sleep was a unitary phenomenon—the passive absence of wakefulness. In the first half of this century, it was discovered that sleep was an active state. Then, in 1953, it was discovered that sleep was actually composed of two completely different states of being: NREM and REM sleep. We, as humans, as most mammals, spend our lives in three completely different states of being: Wakefulness, REM sleep, and NREM sleep. Each of these states has its unique neuroanatomic, neurophysiologic, neurochemical, and neuropharmacologic correlates and substrates.[55,135] It took centuries to determine that sleep is actually a bimodal process because (a) superficially and from a distance, REM and NREM sleep look similar, and (b) these two states cycle back to back, giving the illusion of homogeneity.

There are five primary determinants of the quality of nighttime sleep and of daytime alertness[117]:

1. Homeostatic (duration of prior wakefulness)
2. Circadian (biologic clock influence)
3. Age
4. Drugs
5. CNS pathology

These factors determine the overall wake–sleep pattern, upon which the parasomnias are superimposed. These same factors also play an integral role in epileptic events.

With the advent of neurophysiologic monitoring techniques, it has become obvious that state determination is a very complex and dynamic phenomenon, involving multiple neural networks, neurotransmitters, neuropeptides, neurohormones, and myriad sleep-promoting substances. Given these complexities, it has become clear that the determination of state may be inexact, with components of two or all three states occurring simultaneously or oscillating rapidly. This concept of state dissociation in animals and humans has been extensively reviewed.[73,74,76]

Parasomnia is the term given to undesirable motor, verbal, or experiential phenomena that occur during the sleep period. It is these sleep disorders that are most commonly confused with epileptic phenomena. Parasomnias may be conveniently categorized as primary (disorders of sleep states per se) and secondary (disorders of other organ systems manifesting themselves during sleep). The primary sleep parasomnias can be classified according to the sleep state of origin: REM sleep, NREM sleep, or miscellaneous (those not respecting sleep state). The secondary sleep parasomnias can be further classified by the organ system involved.[72] Many parasomnias are manifestations of state dissociation. These mixed states result in fascinating and perplexing clinical phenomena that may easily be confused with epileptic events, and conversely, these sleep disorders may be perfectly imitated by epileptic events. Furthermore, other primary sleep disorders may trigger seizures, and, conversely, seizures may trigger abnormal sleep phenomena. In addition to the parasomnias, there is impressive overlap among epileptic, sleep, and psychiatric phenomena (Table 1).

CLINICAL DESCRIPTION

The following is a listing of various areas of overlap and confusion between sleep disorders and seizures ranging from normal events to hypersomnia, insomnia, and parasomnias.

Normal Sleep Phenomena

Sleep Starts

Sleep starts (hypnic jerks) are experienced by many normal individuals during the transition from wake to sleep. The most common is the motor sleep start, a sudden jerk of all or part of the body, occasionally awakening the victim or bed partner.[106] Variations on this theme include the visual (flashes of light, fragmentary visual hallucinations), auditory (loud bangs, snapping noises), or somesthetic (pain, floating, something flowing through the body) sleep start, occurring without the body jerk.[20,42,70,101,122] Sleep starts represent a normal (although not understood) physiologic event, and should not be confused with seizures or other neurologic conditions. It is likely that the "exploding head syndrome," characterized by a sensation of a loud sound like an explosion or a sensation of "bursting" of the head, and "explosive tinnitus" are variants of sensory sleep starts.[22,108,121,144,152] Similar phenomena may represent the sole manifestation of a seizure.[37]

Nightmares

Nightmares are frightening dreams that usually awaken the sleeper from REM sleep. Unlike disorders of arousal (see below), they are not usually associated with prominent motor or vocal behavior or autonomic excitation, and the arousal

TABLE 1

OVERLAP AMONG EPILEPTIC, SLEEP, AND PSYCHIATRIC PHENOMENA

Symptom	Sleep disorder	Seizure
Normal sleep phenomena	Sleep starts (hypnic jerks) Nightmares	Seizures manifesting as sleep-onset sensory/motor phenomena or nightmares
Hypersomnia	Sleep deprivation Idiopathic CNS hyperinsomnia	Hypersomnia as a manifestation of having frequent nocturnal seizures resulting in recurrent arousals or hypersomnia as an accompaniment of epilepsy
	Narcolepsy	Akinetic
	Cataplexy	Fugue states
	Sleep paralysis	Partial complex seizures
	Hypnagogic hallucinations	Subclinical status
	Automatic behavior	Poriomania
	Recurrent hypersomnia Kleine-Levin Menstruation-related	Recurrent seizures resulting in prolonged periods of "sleepiness"
	Sleep apnea triggering seizures	Seizures resulting in apnea
Insomnia	Medical Psychiatric Psychological Constitutional	Seizures whose sole manifestation is recurrent arousals
Parasomnias	Disorders of arousal Confusional arousals Sleepwalking Sleep terrors Sleep-eating RBD Dreams/nightmares Enuresis Rhythmic movement disorder Periodic limb movement disorder Posttraumatic stress disorder Cardiopulmonary Cardiac arrhythmias Respiratory dyskinesias Gastrointestinal-paroxysmal choking Panic disorder Psychogenic dissociative disorders	Mesial frontal, temporal lobe seizures presenting with complex, bizarre behaviors, hypnogenic (nocturnal) paroxysmal dystonia, or autonomic (diencephalic) seizures

CNS, central nervous system; RBD, rapid-eye-movement sleep behavior disorder.

results in immediate full wakefulness, with memory for the dream sequence of events that caused the awakening.[72] Seizures manifest as recurrent dreams, nightmares, or disorders of arousal such as sleepwalking, and sleep terrors have been well described in both adults and children. The diagnosis of seizure-related dreams and nightmares may be overlooked, as the symptom is misinterpreted as a primary sleep phenomenon.[12,28,29,39,138] Autosomal dominant frontal epilepsy may also present as recurrent "nightmares."[124,125]

Hypersomnia

Epilepsy

Nocturnal seizures may cause severe sleep fragmentation, if the sole manifestation is arousal (which may not be appreciated by the patient). The end result is excessive daytime sleepiness.[130] Some patients with seizures are hypersomnolent during the day—even after antiepileptic medication discontinuation. Seizure-free preadolescent children with epilepsy are sleepier than healthy controls. In one study, there was no difference in objective sleepiness in children with epilepsy on or off medication, suggesting that use of antiepileptic drugs does not necessarily result in daytime sleepiness.[103] The complaint of daytime sleepiness in patients with epilepsy may be due to a number of different conditions (sleep deprivation, sleep-related seizure-induced arousals, coexisting sleep disorders such as sleep apnea or narcolepsy, or medication effect). Thoughtful evaluation of this complaint is encouraged; hypersomnia in patients with epilepsy should not summarily be attributed to the effect of antiepileptic medications.[7,35]

Narcolepsy

Narcolepsy is a genetically determined disorder characterized by excessive daytime sleepiness, cataplexy (the sudden loss of muscle tone triggered by emotionally laden events), sleep paralysis, hypnagogic hallucinations, and automatic behavior during which prolonged, complex activities may be performed without conscious awareness or recall.[1] The "spell-like" nature of some sleep attacks, cataplexy, and sleep paralysis may be mistaken for seizures. Conversely, atonic or inhibitory seizures may mimic cataplexy,[3,41,45,56,66,139] and the periods of automatic behavior are often misdiagnosed as partial complex seizures, postictal confusion, or poriomania.[32,60,80] The incomplete and waxing and waning nature of cataplexy can imitate tonic–clonic seizure activity.

Periodic Hypersomnia (Kleine-Levin Syndrome)

The Kleine-Levin syndrome is a poorly understood condition characterized by recurrent periods of hypersomnia. The often-cited association with adolescent males and unusual behaviors such as hypersexuality and megaphagia has been overrated.[6,137] Menstruation–related periodic hypersomnia may represent a variant of the Kleine-Levin syndrome.[11] Similar recurrent episodes of hypersomnia may be caused by "ictal sleep" lasting 1 to 3 days at 10- to 60-day intervals.[94,156]

Sleep-disordered Breathing

There is an interesting and important relationship between sleep-disordered breathing and seizures. Nocturnal seizures, probably triggered by periods of hypoxemia, may be the presenting symptom in some individuals with obstructive sleep apnea or sleep-related hypoventilation.[62] Furthermore, sleep apnea may exacerbate seizures in patients with epilepsy due to sleep disruption, sleep deprivation, hypoxemia, or decreased cerebral blood flow. As would be expected, patients who have both epilepsy and sleep-disordered breathing may have better control of their seizures following effective treatment for the sleep-disordered breathing.[79,148] Not all "spells" associated with sleep apnea are epileptic manifestations. They may be due to episodes of cerebral anoxia.[16]

In yet other cases, seizures may cause apnea, often repetitive, and may closely mimic the conditions of obstructive or central sleep apnea.[17,90,146,151,153] Figure 1 shows repetitive apneas as the sole manifestation of seizures.

Insomnia

Paroxysmal, otherwise unexplained awakenings may be the sole manifestation of nocturnal seizures, and will result in the complaint of insomnia.[8,30,31,97,110] Some patients with occasional paroxysmal periodic motor attacks during sleep have very frequent (every 20 to 60 seconds) subclinical arousals resulting in severe sleep fragmentation.[130] These paroxysmal arousals may be due to deep epileptic foci.[92] The arousal preceding nocturnal seizures may be the initial manifestation of the seizure.[78] Animal studies support the concept of frequent arousals as the manifestation of seizures.[133] This may explain the fact that some patients with epilepsy report frequent, otherwise unexplained, nocturnal awakenings and excessive daytime sleepiness.[50]

Parasomnias

Disorders of Arousal

Disorders of arousal are the most common and impressive of the NREM sleep parasomnias, and may readily be confused with epileptic phenomena. These occur on a continuum ranging from confusional arousals to sleepwalking to sleep terrors. The disorders of arousal share common features: A positive family history, suggesting a genetic component; they tend to arise from slow-wave sleep (stages 3 and 4 of NREM sleep), therefore usually occurring in the first third of the sleep cycle (and rarely during naps); and they are common in childhood, usually decreasing in frequency with increasing age.[77] Although they most frequently occur during slow-wave sleep, they may occur during any stage of NREM sleep, and may occur late in the sleep period. Contrary to popular opinion, the

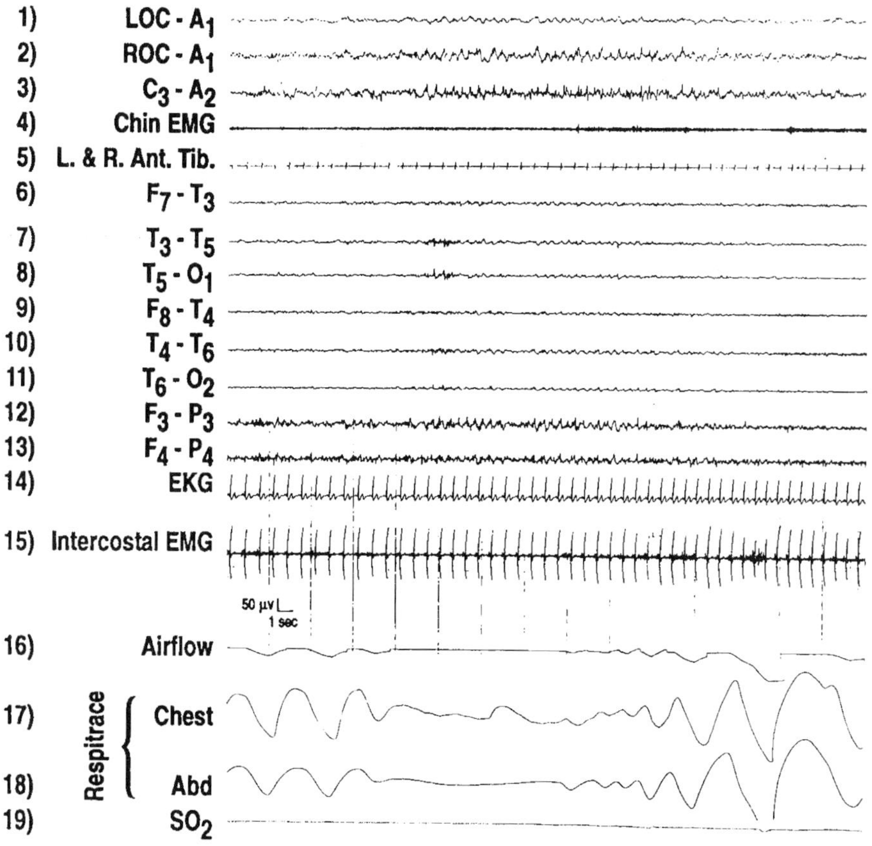

FIGURE 1. Polysomnographic tracing of a 56-year-old male with a long-standing history of well-controlled generalized seizures who developed severe progressive excessive daytime sleepiness. The polysomnogram revealed 22 central apneas per hour as the sole manifestation of seizures. Aggressive medical management was unsuccessful. There was marked improvement in his excessive daytime sleepiness following a right frontal lobectomy.

appearance or persistence of these events into adulthood is usually not associated with significant psychiatric disease. Specialized forms of arousal disorders may manifest as sleep-related eating or sleep-related sexual activity.[126,131]

The disorders of arousal may be difficult to differentiate from nocturnal seizures, and vice versa.[68,109] Preservation of consciousness during seizures may lead to confusion with disorders of arousal or psychogenic conditions.[26] Crying (dacrystic) or laughing (gelastic) seizures may be misinterpreted as confusional arousals or sleep terrors.[5,69] Both disorders of arousal and seizures may be menstrual related.[52,96,127]

The disorders of arousal may be triggered by arousals induced by other sleep disorders such as sleep apnea or seizures, so the clinical event of a sleepwalking or sleep terror episode may, in fact, represent an epiphenomenon of yet a different underlying sleep disorder.[46] It is common clinical experience to see an improvement in disorders of arousal following effective treatment of obstructive sleep apnea (OSA). Conversely, effective treatment of OSA with nasal continuous positive airway pressure (CPAP) may result in disorders of arousal, presumably associated with deep NREM sleep rebound.[34,89] Sleep terrors and seizures can coexist in the same individual.[143]

Rapid Eye Movement Sleep Behavior Disorder

REM sleep behavior disorder (RBD) is a recently described condition in which the anticipated atonia of REM sleep is absent, hypothetically allowing patients to "act out their dreams," often with violent or injurious results. It typically is a disorder of older males, and is frequently misdiagnosed as a nocturnal seizure or psychogenic event. RBD is readily diagnosable by formal sleep studies, which reveal the absence of somatic muscle atonia that normally accompanies REM sleep. RBD responds exquisitely to clonazepam.[128] Nocturnal seizures or obstructive sleep apnea may mimic RBD.[19,53]

Dream/Nightmare Disturbances

As mentioned above, recurrent dreams or nightmares as the primary manifestation of nocturnal seizures have been well documented.

Enuresis

Enuresis was formerly classified as a "disorder of arousal," implying a relationship with NREM or slow-wave sleep.[13] However, enuresis does not respect sleep stage, and may occur during either NREM or REM sleep.[44,88] Enuresis may be the sole manifestation of nocturnal seizures.[4,33,46]

Bruxism

Rarely, bruxism may be the manifestation of a seizure.[84]

Rhythmic Movement Disorder

Rhythmic movement disorder (RMD) refers to a number of behaviors characterized by stereotyped movements (rhythmic oscillation of the head or limbs, head banging or body rocking during sleep) seen most frequently in childhood and, rarely, in adults. RMD may arise from any stage of sleep, may be familial, and is usually not associated with underlying psychiatric or psychological conditions.[118] Rarely, it may be the sole manifestation of a seizure.[46]

Periodic Limb Movements of Sleep

Periodic limb movement of sleep (PLM) is a polysomnographically determined diagnosis. It is characterized by periodic (every 20 to 30 seconds) dorsiflexion of the great toe, foot, or even flexion of the entire leg. These movements are not perceived by the patient, and may be associated with the complaint of excessive daytime sleepiness or insomnia. These movements may also be asymptomatic.[93] When prominent, these movements may be confused with myoclonic seizure activity, or may actually represent epileptic phenomena.[71] These movements may be particularly dramatic in patients with underlying renal failure.[58,111]

Posttraumatic Stress Disorder

Posttraumatic stress disorder (PTSD) is often associated with subjective sleep complaints including "nightmares" and sleep terrorlike experiences.[2] PTSD may be confused with nocturnal panic or seizures manifesting solely as arousals with fearful affect.

Seizures

The behaviors associated with nocturnal seizures are often bizarre, and masquerade as primary sleep parasomnias, secondary sleep parasomnias, or psychiatric conditions.[141] The following are particularly apt to result in diagnostic dilemmas:

1. *Conventional seizures* occur frequently during sleep. In many individuals with epilepsy, seizures occur exclusively during sleep, increasing the likelihood of a misdiagnosis of a primary sleep disorder. Approximately 10% of patients with seizures experience seizures exclusively or predominantly during sleep.[157]
2. *Nocturnal frontal lobe epilepsy* (NFLE), sometimes autosomal dominant, presents a broad spectrum of behaviors, including frequent isolated paroxysmal arousals, episodic nocturnal wanderings, and nocturnal paroxysmal dystonia.[99,112,113,124] NFLE may present as other sleep disorders, particularly disorders of arousal or sleep apnea.[100,125] Nocturnal and diurnal paroxysmal dystonia may exist in the same patient, as can reflex and hypnogenic paroxysmal dystonia. There is considerable overlap among the different clinical categories of paroxysmal dyskinesias.[23,67,91,149] NFLE may be posttraumatic[9] and may coexist with panic disorder.[142] Temporal lobe seizures may also result in hyperkinetic behaviors.[98] Vigilance level-dependent tonic seizures[115] and familial paroxysmal hypnogenic dystonia[65] likely represent variants of this condition. Carbamazepine is often very effective in eliminating these spells.
3. *Pure tonic seizures with arousal* (or paroxysmal polyspike activity with arousal) were mentioned above as seizures presenting as insomnia or hypersomnia due to seizure-induced arousals or sleep fragmentation. An interesting subtype of hypnic tonic postural seizures has been described in ten children, many with a positive family history. This may be a benign epilepsy syndrome similar to benign childhood epilepsy with centrotemporal spikes,[51] and childhood epilepsy with occipital paroxysms.[61,104,105]
4. *Autonomic/diencephalic seizures* are rare, and could present from sleep with such manifestations as intermittent or paroxysmal apnea,[123,151] stridor,[81] coughing,[155] laryngospasm,[116] chest pain and arrhythmias,[24,43,49,59] paroxysmal flushing, localized hyperhidrosis,[63,87] and piloerection,[120] which are easily confused with other primary or secondary sleep parasomnias. Isolated autonomic symptoms are a well-documented manifestation of seizures, and are probably much more common than generally suspected.
5. *Electrical status epilepticus of sleep* (ESES) may be detected during a polysomnogram (PSG) performed for other reasons, and is characterized by continuous spike-and-wave activity during NREM sleep. ESES is seen in

children who usually, but not always, have a history of seizures or neurologic dysfunction. The prognosis is variable inasmuch as it may be an asymptomatic finding. This pattern occurs on a broad spectrum including the Landau-Kleffner syndrome and benign childhood epilepsy with centrotemporal spikes.[40]

Cardiopulmonary

1. *Cardiac arrhythmias* may be a manifestation of seizures, masquerading as nocturnal cardiac abnormalities and possibly playing a role in sudden unexplained death in epilepsy.[54,95] Ictal cardiorespiratory arrest in Panayiotopoulos syndrome has recently been reported.[150] Seizures may also result in stunned myocardium and pulmonary edema.[15,36] Conversely, primary cardiac (prolonged QT interval) or respiratory events (REM sleep-related hypoventilation) may present as seizures.[62,102]
2. *Respiratory dyskinesias* may occur or persist during the sleep period. These include (a) segmental myoclonus such as palatal myoclonus or diaphragmatic flutter and (b) paroxysmal dystonia. Respiratory dyskinesias may also be the manifestation of neuroleptic-induced dyskinesias, and may or may not persist during sleep.[64] These should be differentiated from unusual nocturnal seizures that present with primarily or exclusively respiratory symptoms.[146,151,154]

Gastrointestinal

The sole manifestation of nocturnal seizures may be paroxysmal choking.[14]

Nocturnal Panic Attacks

Nocturnal panic attacks (NPAs) may occur in patients with diurnal panic, or, rarely, may precede the appearance of diurnal panic, or may be exclusively nocturnal in nature.[18,85,119] The striking similarity of the symptoms of dream anxiety attack, sleep terror, nocturnal seizures, and nighttime panic urges caution in diagnosis. Obstructive sleep apnea can also cause symptoms of NPAs.[27] The common association of the affect of "fear" as an accompaniment of nocturnal seizures intensifies their confusion with nocturnal panic.[21,47,48,82] It must be remembered that seizures and panic may coexist.[83,140]

Psychogenic Dissociative States

Complex and potentially injurious behaviors, occasionally confined to the sleep period, may be the manifestation of a psychogenic dissociative state. A history of childhood physical and/or sexual abuse is virtually always present (but may be difficult to elicit). In this condition, unlike other parasomnias or nocturnal seizures, the complex behavior, during electroencephalographic (EEG) monitoring, is seen to arise from clear EEG-determined wakefulness.[129] Pseudoseizures may also arise from apparent sleep.[147]

DIFFERENTIAL DIAGNOSIS

It should be clear from the above that the clinical differentiation between sleep disorders and epileptic events may often be difficult, if not impossible, as primary or secondary sleep phenomena may perfectly mimic epileptic phenomena, and vice versa. Both epileptic and sleep phenomena should be considered in any case of recurrent unusual sleep-related events.

DIAGNOSTIC INVESTIGATION

The decision to investigate further unusual nocturnal events will depend upon the clinical situation. The most common condition is the disorder of arousal, which is very common (and normal) in the general population. Simple sleepwalking or sleep terrors can readily be diagnosed clinically. Indications for formal evaluation include behaviors that (a) are potentially injurious or violent, (b) cause disruption for other household members, (c) result in excessive daytime sleepiness, or (d) display unusual clinical features.

Clinical differentiation between sleep and epileptic phenomena may be most difficult, and misdiagnosis in both directions is common. The diagnosis of nocturnal seizures may be enigmatic if there is no history of diurnal spells. Both waking and sleep-deprived EEGs may not reveal the diagnosis,[10,107] necessitating all-night polysomnographic study using a full seizure montage and continuous video recording. Although exclusively nocturnal seizures may be uncommon, they are routinely misdiagnosed, and should never be overlooked as possibly etiologic in any sleep-related behavior that is recurrent, stereotyped, or inappropriate—regardless of the specific nature of that behavior. "Ambulatory" EEG monitoring has led to the misdiagnosis of functional psychiatric disease in a number of our patients subsequently demonstrated to have bona fide nocturnal seizures. Erroneous psychogenic labeling is enhanced by the bizarre nature of the spells and the fact that environmental clues may play a role in the context of psychomotor seizure.[38] Misdiagnosis is common even following formal and appropriate PSG evaluation. Reasons for misdiagnosis include[75]:

1. Obscuration of the scalp EEG by movement artifact
2. Absence of scalp EEG manifestation of the seizure activity
3. EEG seizure manifestation appearing to be an "arousal" pattern
4. Absence of EEG or clinical postictal period

Extensive polysomnographic monitoring employing a full scalp EEG montage is mandatory. Multiple studies may be necessary to capture an event. Continuous audio/visual monitoring and recording are indicated, and detailed technician observation may be invaluable. The difficulties in evaluating unusual sleep-related events emphasize the necessity of extensive, in-person laboratory monitoring with interpretation of all data (clinical, EEG, sleep, video, and technologist-provided information) by personnel experienced in both sleep medicine and epileptology.

TREATMENT

Effective treatment is available for most sleep disorders and for seizures, and is predicated upon an accurate diagnosis. If seizures are responsible for the sleep–wake complaint, treatment is similar to that for other seizure disorders. If a primary sleep disorder (such as narcolepsy, sleep apnea, or parasomnia) is identified, therapy is dictated by the specific diagnosis.

SUMMARY AND CONCLUSIONS

The interface between sleep disorders and epileptic phenomena is vast and inexorable, as sleep affects seizures, and seizures affect sleep. The myriad sleep and epileptic phenomena may perfectly counterfeit one another. A high index of suspicion and a full awareness of the broad spectrum of both sleep and epileptic phenomena is instrumental to an accurate diagnosis. A thorough clinical and laboratory evaluation of unusual phenomena that could be either sleep- or seizure-related will usually lead to a specific diagnosis, with important and effective therapeutic implications.

From a broader perspective, the intriguing relationship among these conditions is fertile ground commanding further investigation, the results of which will greatly expand our knowledge of brain function, sleep, and epilepsy, and which will undoubtedly result in deeper understanding and better classification, and identification of yet unknown, unusual clinical events. Close cooperation among the fields of sleep medicine, epileptology, and basic neuroscience in this arena of fascinating interface will be most productive—both from a clinical/therapeutic and scientific standpoint.

ACKNOWLEDGMENTS

We are indebted to the unyielding support of our technical, secretarial, and nursing staff.

References

1. Aldrich MS. The neurobiology of narcolepsy. *Prog Neurobiol.* 1992; 41:538–541.
2. American Psychiatric Association. *Diagnostic and Statistical Manual of Mental Disorders Text Revsion (DSM-IV-TR).* Washington, DC: American Psychiatric Pub, Inc.; 2000.
3. Andermann F, Tenembaum S. Negative motor phenomena in generalized epilepsies. A study of atonic seizures. In: Fahn S, Hallett M, Luders HO, et al., eds. *Negative Motor Phenomena.* Philadelphia: Lippincott-Raven; 1995:9–28.
4. Arguner A, Baybas S, Gozukirmizi E, et al. Focal and generalized abnormalities during sleep in cases of enuresis nocturna. In: Popoviciu L, Asgian B, Badiu G, eds. *Sleep 1978 Fourth European Congress on Sleep Research, Tirgu-Mures.* Basel: Karger; 1980:717–720.
5. Armstrong SC, Watters MR, Pearce JW. A case of nocturnal gelastic epilepsy. *Neuropsychiatry Neuropsychol Behav Neurol.* 1990;3:213–216.
6. Arnulf I, Zeitzer JM, File J, et al. Kleine-Levin syndrome: a systematic review of 186 cases in the literature. *Brain.* 2005;128:2763–2776.
7. Becker DA, Fennell EB, Carney PR. Daytime behavior and sleep disturbance in childhood epilepsy. *Epilepsy Behav.* 2004;5:708–715.
8. Benner RP, Atkinson R. Generalized paroxysmal fast activity: electroencephalographic and clinical features. *Ann Neurol.* 1982;11:386–390.
9. Biary N, Singh B, Bahou Y, et al. Posttraumatic paroxysmal nocturnal hemidystonia. *Mov Disord.* 1994;9:98–99.
10. Billiard M, Echenne B, Besset A, et al. All-night polygraphic recordings in the child with suspected epileptic seizures, in spite of normal routine and post-sleep deprivation EEGs. *Electroencephalogr Clin Neurophysiol.* 1981;11:450–460.
11. Billiard M, Guilleminault C, Dement WC. A menstruation-linked periodic hypersomnia. *Neurology.* 1975;255:436–443.
12. Boller F, Wright DG, Cavalieri R, et al. Paroxysmal "nightmares." *Neurology.* 1975;25:1026–1028.
13. Broughton RJ. Sleep disorders: disorders of arousal? *Science.* 1968;159: 1070–1078.
14. Brown LW, Fry JM. Paroxysmal nocturnal choking: a newly described manifestation of sleep-related epilepsy. *Sleep Res.* 1988;17:153.
15. Chin PS, Branch KR, Becker KJ. Postictal neurogenic stunned myocardium. *Neurology.* 2005;64:1977–1978.
16. Cirignotta F, Zucconi M, Mondini S, et al. Cerebral anoxic attacks in sleep apnea syndrome. *Sleep.* 1989;12:400–404.
17. Coulter DL. Partial seizures with apnea and bradycardia. *Arch Neurol.* 1984;41:173–174.
18. Craske MG, Kreuger MT. Prevalence of nocturnal panic in a college population. *J Anxiety Disord.* 1990;4:125–139.
19. D' Cruz OF, Vaughn BV. Nocturnal seizures mimic REM behavior disorder. *Am J End Technol.* 1997;37:258–264.
20. Dagnino N, Loeb C, Massazza G, et al. Hypnic physiological myoclonus in man: an EEG-EMG study in normals and neurological patients. *Eur Neurol.* 1969;2:47–58.
21. Daly D. Ictal affect. *Am J Psychiatry.* 1958;115:97–108.
22. Declerck AC, Arends JB. An exceptional case of parasomnia: the exploding head syndrome. *Sleep-Wake Res (Netherlands).* 1994;5:41–43.
23. Demirkiran M, Jankovic J. Paroxysmal dyskinesias: clinical features and classification. *Ann Neurol.* 1995;38:571–579.
24. Devinsky O, Price BH, Cohen SI. Cardiac manifestations of complex partial seizures. *Am J Med.* 1986;80:195–202.
25. Dinner D. Effect of sleep on epilepsy. *J Clin Neurophysiol.* 2002;19:504–513.
26. Ebner A, Dinner DS, Noachtar S, et al. Automatisms with preserved responsiveness: a lateralizing sign in psychomotor seizures. *Neurology.* 1995;45:61–64.
27. Edlund MJ, McNamara ME, Millman RP. Sleep apnea and panic attacks. *Compr Psychiatry.* 1991;32:130–132.
28. Epstein AW. Recurrent dreams. Their relationship to temporal lobe seizures. *Arch Gen Psychiatry.* 1964;10:49–54.
29. Epstein AW, Hill W. Ictal phenomena during REM sleep of a temporal lobe epileptic. *Arch Neurol.* 1966;15:367–375.
30. Erba G, Cavazzuti V. Pure tonic seizures with arousal. *Sleep Res.* 1981;10:164.
31. Erba G, Ferber R. Sleep disruption by subclinical seizure activity as a cause of increased waking seizures and decreased daytime function. *Sleep Res.* 1983;12:307.
32. Fagan KJ, Lee SI. Prolonged confusion following convulsions due to generalized nonconvulsive status epilepticus. *Neurology.* 1990;40:1689–1694.
33. Fermaglich JL. Electroencephalographic study of enuretics. *Am J Dis Child.* 1969;118:473–477.
34. Fietze I, Warmuth R, Witt C, et al. Sleep-related breathing disorder and pavor nocturnus. *Sleep Res.* 1995;24A:301.
35. Foldvary-Schaefer N. Sleep complaints and epilepsy: the role of seizures, antiepileptic drugs and sleep disorders. *J Clin Neurophysiol.* 2002;19:514–521.
36. Fontes RBV, Aguiar PH, Zanetti MV, et al. Acute neurogenic pulmonary edema: case reports and literature review. *J Neurosurg Anesthesiol.* 2003;15:144–150.
37. Fornazzari L, Farcnik K, Smith I, et al. Violent visual hallucinations and aggression in frontal lobe dysfunction: clinical manifestations of deep orbitofrontal foci. *J Neuropsychiatry Clin Neurosci.* 1992;4:42–44.
38. Forster FM, Liske E. Role of environmental clues in temporal lobe epilepsy. *Neurology.* 1963;13:301–305.
39. Fuster B, Castells C, Etcheverry M. Epileptic sleep terrors. *Neurology.* 1954;4:531–540.
40. Galanopoulou AS, Bojko A, Lado F, et al. The spectrum of neuropsychiatric abnormalities associated with electrical status epilepticus of sleep. *Brain Dev.* 2000;22:279–295.
41. Gambardella A, Reutens DC, Andermann F, et al. Late-onset drop attacks in temporal lobe epilepsy: a reevaluation of the concept of temporal lobe syncope. *Neurology.* 1994;44:1074–1078.
42. Gastaut H, Broughton R. A clinical and polygraphic study of episodic phenomena during sleep. *Recent Adv Biol Psychiatry.* 1967;7:197–221.
43. Gilchrist JM. Arrhythmogenic seizures: diagnosis by simultaneous EEG/ECG recording. *Neurology.* 1985;35:1503–1506.
44. Gillin JC, Rapoport JL, Mikkelsen EJ, et al. EEG sleep patterns in enuresis: a further analysis and comparison with normal controls. *Biol Psychiatry.* 1982;17:947–953.
45. Guerrini R, Dravet C, Genton P, et al. Epileptic negative myoclonus. *Neurology.* 1993;43:1078–1083.
46. Guilleminault C, Silvestri R. Disorders of arousal and epilepsy during sleep. In: Sterman MB, Shouse MN, Passouant PP, eds. *Sleep and Epilepsy.* New York: Academic Press; 1982:513–531.
47. Henriksen GF. Status epilepticus partialis with fear as clinical expression. *Epilepsia.* 1973;14:39–46.
48. Hermann BP, Melyn M. Effects of carbamazepine on interictal psychopathology in TLE with ictal fear. *J Clin Psychiatry.* 1984;45: 169–171.
49. Hockman CH, Mauch HP, Hoff EC. ECG changes resulting from cerebral stimulation. II. A spectrum of ventricular arrhythmias of sympathetic origin. *Am Heart J.* 1966;71:695–700.
50. Hoeppner JB, Garron DC, Cartwright RD. Self-reported sleep disorder symptoms in epilepsy. *Epilepsia.* 1984;25:434–437.
51. Holmes GL. Rolandic epilepsy: clinical and electroencephalographic features. In: Degen R, Dreifuss FE, eds. *Benign Localized and Generalized Epilepsies of Early Childhood.* Amsterdam: Elsevier Science Publishers; 1992:29–43.
52. Ichida M, Gomi A, Hiranouchi N, et al. A case of cerebral endometriosis causing catamenial epilepsy. *Neurology.* 1993;43:2708–2709.
53. Iranzo A, Santamaria J. Severe obstructive sleep apnea/hypopnea mimicking REM sleep behavior disorder. *Sleep.* 2005;28:203–206.
54. Jallon P. Arrythmogenic seizures. *Epilepsia.* 1997;38(Suppl 11):S43–S47.
55. Jones BE. Basic mechanisms of sleep-wake states. In: Kryger MH, Roth T, Dement WC, eds. *Principles and Practice of Sleep Medicine.* 4th ed. Philadelphia: Elsevier Saunders; 2005:136–153.
56. Kanazawa O, Kawai I. Status epilepticus characterized by repetitive asymmetrical atonia: two cases accompanied by partial seizures. *Epilepsia.* 1990;31:536–543.
57. Kellaway P, Frost-Jr JD, Crawley JW. The relationship between sleep spindles and spike-and-wave bursts in human epilepsy. In: Avoli M, Gloor P, Kostopoulos G, et al., eds. *Generalized Epilepsy Neurobiological Approaches.* Boston: Birkhauser; 1990:36–48.
58. Kimmel PL. Sleep disorders in chronic renal disease. *J Nephrol.* 1989;1: 59–65.

59. Kiok MC, Terrence CF, Fromm GH, et al. Sinus arrest in epilepsy. *Neurology.* 1986;36:115–116.
60. Kitagawa T, Takahashi K, Matsushima K, et al. A case of prolonged confusion after temporal lobe psychomotor status. *Folia Psychiatrica Neurol.* 1979;33:279–284.
61. Kivity S, Lerman P. Benign partial epilepsy of childhood with occipital discharges. *Adv Epileptol.* 1989;17:371–373.
62. Kryger MH, Steljes DG, Yee W-C, et al. Central sleep apnoea in congenital muscular dystrophy. *J Neurol Neurosurg Psychiatry.* 1991;54:710–712.
63. Kuritzky A, Hering R, Goldhammer G, et al. Clonidine treatment in paroxysmal localized hyperhidrosis. *Arch Neurol.* 1984;41:1210–1211.
64. Larner AJ. Antony Van Leeuwenhoek and the description of diaphragmatic flutter (respiratory myoclonus). *Mov Disord.* 2005;20:917–918.
65. Lee BI, Lesser RP, Pippenger CE, et al. Familial paroxysmal hypnogenic dystonia. *Neurology.* 1985;35:1357–1360.
66. Lee H, Lerner A. Transient inhibitory seizures mimicking crescendo TIAs. *Neurology.* 1990;40:165–166.
67. Lehkuniec E, Micheli F, De-Abelaiz R, et al. Concurrent hypnogenic and reflex paroxysmal dystonia. *Mov Disord.* 1988;3:290–294.
68. Lombroso CT. Pavor nocturnus of proven epileptic origin. *Epilepsia.* 2000;41:1221–1226.
69. Luciano D, Devinsky O, Perrine K. Crying seizures. *Neurology.* 1993;43: 2113–2117.
70. Lugaresi E, Coccagna G, Cirignotta F. Phenomena occurring during sleep onset in man. In: Popoviciu L, Asgian B, Badiu G, eds. *Sleep 1978 Fourth European Congress on Sleep Research, Tirgu-Mures.* Basel: S. Karger; 1980:24–27.
71. Lugaresi E, Coccagna G, Mantovani M, et al. The evolution of different types of myoclonus during sleep. A polygraphic study. *Eur Neurol.* 1970;4:321–331.
72. Mahowald MW, Ettinger MG. Things that go bump in the night—the parasomnias revisited. *J Clin Neurophysiol.* 1990;7:119–143.
73. Mahowald MW, Schenck CH. Status dissociatus—a perspective on states of being. *Sleep.* 1991;14:69–79.
74. Mahowald MW, Schenck CH. Dissociated states of wakefulness and sleep. *Neurology.* 1992;42:44–52.
75. Mahowald MW, Schenck CH. Parasomnia purgatory—the epileptic/non-epileptic interface. In: Rowan AJ, Gates JR, eds. *Non-Epileptic Seizures.* 2nd ed. Boston: Butterworth-Heinemann; 2000:71–94.
76. Mahowald MW, Schenck CH. Evolving concepts of human state dissociation. *Arch Ital Biol.* 2001;139:269–300.
77. Mahowald MW, Schenck CH. NREM sleep parasomnias. *Neurol Clin.* 2005;23:1077–1106.
78. Malow BA, Varma NK. Seizures and arousals from sleep - which comes first? *Sleep.* 1995;18:783–786.
79. Malow BA, Weatherwax KJ, Chervin RD, et al. Identification and treatment of obstructive sleep apnea in adults and children with epilepsy: a prospective pilot study. *Sleep Med.* 2003;4:509–515.
80. Mayeux R, Alexander MP, Benson DF, et al. Poriomania. *Neurology.* 1979;29:1616–1619.
81. Maytal J, Resnick TH. Stridor presenting as the sole manifestation of seizures. *Ann Neurol.* 1985;18:414–415.
82. McLachlan RS, Blume WT. Isolated fear in complex partial status. *Ann Neurol.* 1980;8:639–641.
83. McNamara ME. Absence seizures associated with panic attacks initially misdiagnosed as temporal lobe epilepsy: the importance of prolonged EEG monitoring in diagnosis. *J Psychiatry Neurosci.* 1993;18:46–48.
84. Meletti S, Cantalupo G, Volpi L, et al. Rhythmic teeth grinding induced by temporal lobe seizures. *Neurology.* 2004;62:2306–2309.
85. Mellman TA, Uhde TW. Patients with frequent sleep panic: clinical findings and response to medication treatment. *J Clin Psychiatry.* 1990;51:513–516.
86. Mendez M, Radtke RA. Interactions between sleep and epilepsy. *J Clin Neurophysiol.* 2001;18:106–127.
87. Metz SA, Halter JB, Porte-Jr D, et al. Autonomic epilepsy: clonidine blockade of paroxysmal catecholamine release and flushing. *Ann Intern Med.* 1978;88:189–193.
88. Mikkelsen EJ, Rapoport JL, Nee L, et al. Childhood enuresis. I. Sleep patterns and psychopathology. *Arch Gen Psychiatry.* 1980;37:1139–1144.
89. Millman RP, Kipp GR, Carskadon MA. Sleepwalking precipitated by treatment of sleep apnea with nasal CPAP. *Chest.* 1991;99:750–751.
90. Monod N, Peirano P, Plouin P, et al. Seizure-induced apnea. *Ann N Y Acad Sci.* 1988;533:411–420.
91. Montagna P, Cirignotta F, Giovanardi-Rossi P, et al. Dystonic attacks related to sleep and exercise. *Eur Neurol.* 1992;32:185–189.
92. Montagna P, Sforza E, Tinuper F, et al. Paroxysmal arousals during sleep. *Neurology.* 1990;40:1063–1066.
93. Montplaisir J, Nicholas A, Godbout R, et al. Restless legs syndrome and periodic limb movement disorder. In: Kryger MH, Roth T, Dement WC, eds. *Principles and Practice of Sleep Medicine.* 3rd ed. Philadelphia: WB Saunders; 2000:742–752.
94. Mothersill IW, Vogt H, Hilfiker P. Epileptic seizures manifesting as sleep, ictal sleep. *Sleep Res.* 1995;24:410.
95. Nei M, Ho RT, Abou-Khalil BW, et al. EEG and ECG in sudden unexplained death in epilepsy. *Epilepsia.* 2004;45:338–345.
96. Newmark ME, Penry JK. Catamenial epilepsy: a review. *Epilepsia.* 1980;21:281–300.
97. Niedermeyer E, Walker AE. Mesio-frontal epilepsy. *EEG Clin Neurophysiol.* 1971;31:104–105.
98. Nobili L, Cossu M, Mai R, et al. Sleep-related hyperkinetic seizures of temporal lobe origin. *Neurology.* 2004;62:482–485.
99. Oldani A, Zucconi M, Asselta R, et al. Autosomal dominant nocturnal frontal lobe epilepsy. A video-polysomnographic and genetic appraisal of 40 patients and delineation of the epileptic syndrome. *Brain.* 1998;121:205–223.
100. Oldani A, Zucconi M, Castronovo C, et al. Nocturnal frontal lobe epilepsy misdiagnosed as sleep apnea syndrome. *Acta Neurol Scand.* 1998;98:67–71.
101. Oswald I. Sudden bodily jerks on falling asleep. *Brain.* 1959;82:92–103.
102. Pacia SV, Devinsky O, Luciano DJ, et al. The prolonged QT syndrome presenting as epilepsy: a report of two cases and literature review. *Neurology.* 1994;44:1408–1410.
103. Palm L, Anderson H, Elmqvist D, et al. Daytime sleep tendency before and after discontinuation of antiepileptic drugs in preadolescent children with epilepsy. *Epilepsia.* 1992;33:687–691.
104. Panayiotopoulos CP. Benign nocturnal childhood occipital epilepsy: a new syndrome with nocturnal seizures, tonic deviation of the eyes, and vomiting. *J Child Neurol.* 1989;4:43–48.
105. Panayiotopoulos CP. Benign childhood epilepsy with occipital paroxysms. In: Andermann F, Beaumanoir A, Mira L, et al., eds. *Occipital Seizures and Epilepsy in Children.* London: John Libbey and Co. Ltd.; 1993: 151–164.
106. Parkes JD. The parasomnias. *Lancet.* 1986;2:1021–1025.
107. Passouant P. Historical views on sleep and epilepsy. In: Sterman MB, Shouse MN, Passouant P, eds. *Sleep and Epilepsy.* New York: Academic Press; 1982:1–6.
108. Pearce JMS. Clinical features of the exploding head syndrome. *J Neurol Neurosurg Psychiatry.* 1989;52:907–910.
109. Pedley TA. Differential diagnosis of episodic symptoms. *Epilepsia.* 1983;24(Suppl 1):S31–S44.
110. Peled R, Lavie P. Paroxysmal awakenings from sleep associated with excessive daytime somnolence: a form of nocturnal epilepsy. *Neurology.* 1986;36:95–98.
111. Pressman MR, Benz RL, Peterson DD. High incidence of sleep disorders in end stage renal disease. *Sleep Res.* 1995;24:417.
112. Provini F, Plazzi G, Montagna P, et al. The wide clinical spectrum of nocturnal frontal lobe epilepsy. *Sleep Med Rev.* 2000;4:375–386.
113. Provini F, Plazzi G, Tinuper P, et al. Nocturnal frontal lobe epilepsy: a clinical and polygraphic overview of 100 consecutive cases. *Brain.* 1999;122(Pt 6):1017–1031.
114. Quigg M. Circadian rhythms: interactions with seizures and epilepsy. *Epilepsy Res.* 2000;42:43–55.
115. Rajna P, Kundra O, Halasz P. Vigilance level-dependent tonic seizures-epilepsy or sleep disorder? A case report. *Epilepsia.* 1983;24:725–733.
116. Ravindran M. Temporal lobe seizure presenting as "laryngospasm." *Clin Electroencephalogr.* 1981;12:139–140.
117. Roehrs TA, Carskadon MA, Dement WC, et al. Daytime sleepiness and alertness. In: Kryger MH, Roth T, Dement WC, eds. *Principles and Practice of Sleep Medicine.* 4th ed. Philadelphia: Elsevier Saunders; 2005: 39–50.
118. Rosen GM, Mahowald MW. Disorders of arousal in children. In: Sheldon SH, Ferber R, Kryger MH, eds. *Principles and Practice of Pediatric Sleep Medicine.* Philadelphia: Elsevier Saunders; 2005:293–304.
119. Rosenfeld DS, Furman Y. Pure sleep panic: two case reports and a review of the literature. *Sleep.* 1994;17:462–465.
120. Roze E, Oubary P, Chedru F. Status-like recurrent pilomotor seizures: a case report and review of the literature. *J Neurol Neurosurg Psychiatry.* 2000;68:647–649.
121. Sachs C, Svanborg E. The exploding head syndrome: polysomnographic recordings and therapeutic suggestions. *Sleep.* 1991;14:263–266.
122. Sander HW, Geisse H, Quinto C, et al. Sensory sleep starts. *J Neurol Neurosurg Psychiatry.* 1998;64:690.
123. Sanmarti FX, Estivial E, Campistol J, et al. Apneic episodes in an infant: exceptional epileptic seizures. *Electroencephalogr Clin Neurophysiol.* 1985;60:16p.
124. Scheffer IE, Bhatia KP, Lopes-Cendes I, et al. Autosomal dominant nocturnal frontal lobe epilepsy. A distinctive clinical disorder. *Brain.* 1995;118(Pt 1):61–73.
125. Scheffer IE, Bhatia KP, Lopes-Cendes I, et al. Autosomal dominant frontal epilepsy misdiagnosed as sleep disorder. *Lancet.* 1994;343:515–517.
126. Schenck CH, Mahowald MW. Review of nocturnal sleep-related eating disorders. *Int J Eat Disord.* 1994;15:343–356.
127. Schenck CH, Mahowald MW. Two cases of premenstrual sleep terrors and injurious sleep-walking. *J Psychosom Obstet Gynecol.* 1995;16: 79–84.
128. Schenck CH, Mahowald MW. REM sleep parasomnias. *Neurol Clin.* 2005;23:1107–1126.
129. Schenck CS, Milner DM, Hurwitz TD, et al. Dissociative disorders presenting as somnambulism: polysomnographic, video, and clinical documentation (8 cases). *Dissociation.* 1989;4:194–204.
130. Sforza E, Montagna P, Rinaldi R, et al. Paroxysmal periodic motor attacks during sleep: clinical and polygraphic features. *EEG Clin Neurophysiol.* 1993;86:161–166.

131. Shapiro CM, Trajanovic NN, Fedoroff JP. Sexsomnia—a new parasomnia? *Can J Psychiatry*. 2003;48:311–317.
132. Shouse MN, da Silva AM, Sammaritano M. Circadian rhythm, sleep, and epilepsy. *J Clin Neurophysiol*. 1996;13:32–50.
133. Shouse MN, Siegel JM. Pontine regulation of REM sleep components in cats: integrity of the pedunculopontine tegmentum (PPT) is important for phasic events but unnecessary for atonia during REM sleep. *Brain Res*. 1992;571:50–63.
134. Shouse MN, Siegel JM, Wu FM, et al. Mechanisms of seizure suppression during rapid-eye-movement (REM) sleep in cats. *Brain Res*. 1989;505:271–282.
135. Siegel J. REM sleep. In: Kryger MH, Roth T, Dement WC, eds. *Principles and Practice of Sleep Medicine*. 4th ed. Philadelphia: Elsevier Saunders; 2005:120–135.
136. Sinforiani E, Zangaglia R, Manni R, et al. REM sleep behavior disorder, hallucinations, and cognitive impairment in Parkinson's disease. *Mov Disord*. 2006;21:462–466.
137. Smolik P, Roth B. Kleine-Levin syndrome: etiopathogenesis and treatment. *Acta Univ Carol Med Monogr*. 1988;CXXVIII:1–94.
138. Snyder CH. Epileptic equivalents in children. *Pediatrics*. 1958;21:308–318.
139. So NK. Atonic phenomena and partial seizures. In: Fahn S, Hallett M, Luders HO, et al., eds. *Negative Motor Phenomena*. Philadelphia: Lippincott-Raven; 1995:29–39.
140. Spitz MC. Panic disorder in seizure patients: a diagnostic pitfall. *Epilepsia*. 1991;32:33–38.
141. Stores G. Confusions concerning sleep disorders and the epilepsies in children and adolescents. *Br J Psychiatry*. 1991;158:1–7.
142. Stoudemire A, Ninan PT, Wooten V. Hypnogenic paroxysmal dystonia with panic attacks responsive to drug therapy. *Psychosomatics*. 1987;28:280–281.
143. Tassinari CA, Mancia D, Dalla-Bernardina B, et al. Pavor nocturnus of non-epileptic nature in epileptic children. *EEG Clin Neurophysiol*. 1972;33:603–607.
144. Teixido MT, Connolly K. Explosive tinnitus: an underrecognized disorder. *Otolaryngol Head Neck Surg*. 1998;118:108–109.
145. Terzano MG, Parrino L. Origin and significance of the cyclic alternating pattern (CAP). *Sleep Med Rev*. 2000;4:101–123.
146. Thach BT. Sleep apnea in infancy and childhood. *Med Clin North Am*. 1985;69:1289–1315.
147. Thacker K, Devinsky O, Perrine K, et al. Nonepileptic seizures during apparent sleep. *Ann Neurol*. 1993;33:414–418.
148. Vaughn BV, D'Cruz OF. Obstructive sleep apnea in epilepsy. *Clin Chest Med*. 2003;24:239–248.
149. Veggiotti P, Zambrino CA, Balottin U, et al. Concurrent nocturnal and diurnal paroxysmal dystonia. *Childs Nerv Syst*. 1993;9:458–461.
150. Verrotti A, Salladini C, Trotta D, et al. Ictal cardiorespiratory arrest in Panayiotopoulos syndrome. *Neurology*. 2005;64:1816–1817.
151. Walls TJ, Newman PK, Cumming WJK. Recurrent apnoeic attacks as a manifestation of epilepsy. *Postgrad Med J*. 1981;57:575–576.
152. Walsleben JA, O'Malley EB, Freeman J, et al. Polysomnographic and topographic mapping of EEG in the exploding head syndrome. *Sleep Res*. 1993;22:284.
153. Wanatabe K, Hara K, Hakamada S, et al. Seizures with apnea in children. *Pediatrics*. 1982;70:87–90.
154. Wantanabe K, Hara K, Hakamada S, et al. Seizures with apnea in children. *Pediatrics*. 1982;70:87–90.
155. Winans HM. Epileptic equivalents, a cause for somatic symptoms. *Am J Med*. 1949;7:150–152.
156. Wszolek ZK, Groover RV, Klass DW. Seizures presenting as episodic hypersomnolence. *Epilepsia*. 1995;36:108–110.
157. Young GB, Blume WT, Wells GA, et al. Differential aspects of sleep epilepsy. *Can J Neurol Sci*. 1985;12:317–320.

CHAPTER 277 ■ MYOCLONUS AND MYOCLONIC SYNDROMES

MARK HALLETT AND HIROSHI SHIBASAKI

INTRODUCTION

The history of myoclonus has been described by Marsden et al.[25] and Hallett.[17] Friedreich first defined myoclonus as a discrete entity in a case report published in 1881 of a patient with essential myoclonus. He wanted to separate the involuntary movement that he saw from epileptic clonus, a single jerk in patients with epilepsy, and chorea. For the next 10 to 20 years, many other types of involuntary movements, such as tic and myokymia, were also called myoclonus, but in 1903 Lundborg[23] proposed a classification of myoclonus that cleared up much of the confusion. Lundborg classified myoclonus into three groups: Symptomatic myoclonus, essential myoclonus, and familial myoclonic epilepsy.

It is important to recognize that certain types of myoclonus are essentially identical to epilepsy. Single jerks in patients with epilepsy have been recognized since ancient times. In the phrase of Muskens,[30] myoclonus can be a "fragment of epilepsy." One of the tasks for the clinician is to determine what is epilepsy and what is not.

CLINICAL DESCRIPTION

Myoclonus is characterized by quick muscle jerks, either irregular or rhythmic.[19] Myoclonic movements are always simple in nature, and this is often a critical feature separating myoclonus from other types of involuntary movements. Myoclonus can be focal, involving only a few adjacent muscles; generalized, involving many or most of the muscles in the body; or multifocal, involving many muscles but in different jerks. Myoclonus can be spontaneous, can be activated or accentuated by voluntary movement (action myoclonus), and can be activated or accentuated by sensory stimulation (reflex myoclonus).

In differentiating myoclonus from other movement disorders, in addition to the simplicity, the principal features that favor myoclonus are the quickness of the movement and the absence of ability for voluntary suppression. Some simple tics look identical to myoclonus and cannot be visually distinguished. A point in favor of tic is the ability to suppress the movements voluntarily, with a frequent concomitant rise in psychic tension dispelled when the movements resume. Some movements of chorea are quick, but slower movements and sustained postures are also present. The major differential diagnosis for rhythmic myoclonus is tremor and the distinction here is often just convention.

Some disorders of the peripheral nervous system can be confused with myoclonus. Electrodiagnosis can help make the diagnosis since these disorders all show characteristic physiologic findings. Fasciculation is the spontaneous firing of a single motor unit. Myokymia typically looks like an irregular oscillation of a muscle, but it can have the appearance of small jerks. Hemifacial spasm is characterized by jerks of the facial muscles and occasional tonic spasms.

A brief, paroxysmal pause of tonic muscular activity may also give rise to a jerk in the affected body part that is often visually indistinguishable from a movement produced by a burst of electromyographic (EMG) activity. This is called negative myoclonus, and the most commonly encountered form is asterixis. Negative myoclonus, like positive myoclonus, can also arise as an epileptic event.[36,40]

There are many types of myoclonus, and there are no common etiologic, physiologic, or therapeutic features. For this reason, recognizing that an involuntary movement is myoclonic in nature is only the beginning of the investigation. In those patients with epileptic seizures, it would be reasonable to suspect that the myoclonus would be related.

CLASSIFICATION

There have been many schemes proposed for classifying the large number of myoclonic disorders, and there are at least two useful approaches, etiologic and physiologic, that have usually been discussed separately.[19] From the point of view of differential diagnosis, the physiologic classification is most relevant, and it can help guide symptomatic treatment. The first consideration of therapy, however, should take the etiologic classification into account since the cause should be dealt with first, if possible. Here, the classifications will be combined using the physiologic classification as the primary index and the etiologic classification as a secondary index.

The starting point for a physiologic classification is to decide whether the myoclonus is a fragment of epilepsy. On this basis, the myoclonus is said to be epileptic or nonepileptic.[16,43] There are a number of subtypes in each category.

EPILEPTIC MYOCLONUS

A significant feature in favor of epileptic myoclonus is if the patient has epileptic seizures. This would be more definitive, of course, if the myoclonus was clearly a fragment of the seizure including a part of the aura. The association of the myoclonus with paroxysmal activity in the electroencephalogram (EEG) is also indicative, and more will be said about the electrophysiologic evaluation in the next section.

Three types of epileptic myoclonus are now recognized: Cortical myoclonus, reticular myoclonus, and primary generalized epileptic myoclonus.[19,37,43] Cortical myoclonus is a fragment of focal or partial epilepsy, and can be subclassified as spontaneous cortical myoclonus, cortical reflex myoclonus, and epilepsia partialis continua. Each myoclonic jerk involves only a few adjacent muscles, but larger jerks with more muscles involved can be seen. The disorder is commonly multifocal and accentuated by action and sensory stimulation.

Reticular reflex myoclonus is a fragment of a type of generalized epilepsy. These jerks are usually generalized with predominance, which is proximal more than distal and flexor more than extensor. Voluntary action and sensory stimulation increase the jerking. Primary generalized epileptic myoclonus is a fragment of primary generalized epilepsy. The most common clinical manifestation is small, focal jerks, often involving only the fingers; thus, the myoclonus is sometimes called minipolymyoclonus. The term minipolymyoclonus was originally coined to refer to small jerks seen in patients with motor neuron disease. Minipolymyoclonus of central origin and minipolymyoclonus of peripheral origin have a similar clinical appearance and are probably most easily separated by the company they keep: Epilepsy and muscle denervation, respectively. A second clinical presentation of primary generalized epileptic myoclonus is generalized, synchronized whole body jerks, not unlike those seen with reticular reflex myoclonus. Electrodiagnosis can help define the type of epileptic myoclonus (see below).

Negative myoclonus can be isolated, but it usually occurs together with positive myoclonus.[15,36,40,43] Clinically, the appearance is called asterixis, and there can be large movements, small multifocal movements, and such frequent movements that the appearance is of an irregular tremor or tremulousness. Negative myoclonus can have a similar physiology to cortical myoclonus with electrophysiologic correlates and production by sensory stimulation. There may be associated seizures.

Myoclonus resulting from a defined pathologic process, the etiologic category of "symptomatic myoclonus," is usually epileptic in type. The principal conditions follow, along with a brief consideration of their treatment.

Progressive Myoclonus Epilepsies

Progressive myoclonus epilepsy with the principal features of slowly progressive myoclonus and epilepsy is most frequently secondary to a degenerative disorder with some involvement of the cerebellum or cerebellar pathways (see also Chapter 252). The disorder can be sporadic, but is often familial. Typically the symptoms begin between 7 and 15 years of age and include action and reflex myoclonus and grand mal seizures. Cerebellar ataxia is said to be common, but differentiation of ataxia and intention myoclonus is often very difficult. Occasional features include dementia, spasticity, myopathy, neuropathy, and deafness. The syndrome is clearly heterogeneous. Cases have been described under the names Unverricht-Lundborg syndrome, Ramsay Hunt syndrome, and "Baltic myoclonus epilepsy." The gene for Unverricht-Lundborg disease (EPM1) has now been linked to the long arm of chromosome 21q22.3 in a number of families, and the gene involved codes for cystatin B, a small protein that is a member of a superfamily of cysteine protease inhibitors.[21] Familial cortical myoclonic tremor with epilepsy or familial adult myoclonic epilepsy has been reported from Japan and Europe. This condition is characterized by autosomal dominant inheritance, late onset, benign course, and only infrequent epileptic seizures. Recently van Rootselaar et al.[45] reported an autopsy case of this condition, in which the pathologic changes similar to those seen in spinocerebellar ataxia (SCA) type 6 were found in the cerebellum.

There are no treatments for degenerative conditions, but there are some important therapeutic implications. It is of critical importance in these cases to recognize that phenytoin treatment may be associated with worsening of the condition.[10] Patients can be treated successfully with other anticonvulsants as described below. Storage diseases may also give rise to the syndrome of progressive myoclonus epilepsy, and for this reason the patients may be thought to have a degenerative condition. The most well-known entity is Lafora body disease. Other entities include lipidoses such as GM_2 gangliosidosis (Tay-Sachs disease), ceroid-lipofuscinosis (Batten disease), and sialidosis (cherry red-spot-myoclonus syndrome).

There are at least two clinical differences between Lafora body disease and Baltic myoclonus epilepsy.[10] Age of onset in Lafora body disease is 11 to 18 years, while the age of onset in Baltic myoclonus epilepsy is earlier, 6 to 16 years. For Lafora body disease dementia is present in two thirds of cases by 2 years after onset, and in all by 5 years; in contrast, in Baltic myoclonic epilepsy, only a rare patient shows dementia in the first 5 years (provided the patients do not receive phenytoin). Occipital seizures are frequent in Lafora body disease. The diagnostic feature of Lafora body disease is the periodic acid-Schiff (PAS)-positive inclusion body found in neurons throughout the gray matter of the brain including the dentate nucleus of the cerebellum. These inclusions can sometimes be found in liver, skeletal muscle, and skin. For clinical purposes, the method of first choice for confirming the diagnosis is skin biopsy, particularly of axillary skin. The gene responsible in about 75% of Lafora body cases (EPM2) has been localized to chromosome 6q and has been identified as encoding a protein tyrosine phosphatase (PTP) now called laforin.[27,35] With these storage diseases, there is no treatment, but screening and prenatal detection can be used for prevention.

Noninfantile neuronopathic Gaucher disease can cause myoclonus. There are rapid advances in Gaucher disease, with enzyme replacement therapy already available for the non-neuronopathic forms and gene replacement treatment on the horizon.

Biotin deficiency is especially important to keep in mind since replacement with biotin can lead to cure.[3]

Mitochondrial disorders are increasingly recognized as common causes of myoclonus and the "Ramsay Hunt syndrome" in particular. Indeed, most patients with progressive myoclonus epilepsy may have a mitochondrial abnormality.[2] One well-defined syndrome is MERRF (myoclonus epilepsy and ragged red fiber syndrome). A muscle biopsy looking for ragged red fibers might be helpful. Presently, there is no good treatment for mitochondrial diseases.

Dementias

Creutzfeldt-Jacob disease (subacute spongiform encephalopathy) frequently exhibits myoclonus as a relatively early feature. The myoclonus can be produced by external stimuli, such as noise, or can be spontaneous and rhythmic associated with a periodic EEG. Patients with Alzheimer disease can also exhibit myoclonus, although this feature typically occurs late in the illness. The myoclonus is multifocal and can be stimulus induced. Electrophysiologic investigations of these two disorders show distinctive results, but both are similar to cortical reflex myoclonus. Myoclonus also is seen in patients with the AIDS–dementia complex.[24]

Viral Encephalopathies

A variety of viruses and postviral syndromes cause myoclonus. Herpes simplex encephalitis is probably the most common example. Subacute sclerosing panencephalitis (SSPE) is frequently characterized by a slow periodic movement often called myoclonus, but its duration is on the order of 1 second and it does not fit the definition. At the first International Congress of Movement Disorders in 1990, the attendees voted to no longer use the term *myoclonus* to describe the involuntary movement in SSPE.

Metabolic Encephalopathies Including Endocrine Disorders

Disorders such as hepatic failure, renal failure, hyponatremia, hypoglycemia, and nonketotic hyperglycemia can give rise to myoclonus. Treatment should be directed to the underlying condition. For example, myoclonus in patients with chronic renal failure on hemodialysis can be due to aluminum toxicity and can be successfully treated with chelation therapy with deferoxamine mesylate.[39]

The opsoclonus-myoclonus syndrome is easy to diagnose because of the dramatic clinical feature of opsoclonus.[34,41] It may arise in a variety of settings including infections, toxins, and a paraneoplastic syndrome. In childhood the syndrome is often associated with neuroblastoma. If there is a tumor, it should be treated, and there may be symptomatic relief, but the disorder might be unaffected or even worsened. Symptomatic therapy that should be considered includes steroids or adrenocorticotropic hormone (ACTH). Trazodone may also be helpful.

Toxic Encephalopathies Including Drug Side Effects

Toxic causes include bismuth, heavy metals, methyl bromide, and drugs. Offending drugs include tricyclic antidepressants, opioids, and lithium.

Physical Encephalopathies Including Hypoxia

These conditions include trauma, heat stroke, electric shock, decompression injury, and hypoxia. Posthypoxic myoclonus, the Lance-Adams syndrome,[20] has received a great deal of attention since the demonstration that the myoclonus could be successfully treated with 5-hydroxytryptophan. The clinical syndrome as reported by Lance and Adams noted the precipitating feature of action and the association with cerebellar ataxia, postural lapses, gait disturbance, and grand mal seizures. The site of the responsible lesion in the brain is not certain, but there does appear to be a disorder of serotonin metabolism supported not only by the therapeutic response to 5-hydroxytryptophan, but also by the reduction in cerebrospinal fluid (CSF) levels of 5-HIAA, which improves with successful therapy.

Focal Brain Damage

The etiology of focal cortical myoclonus can be almost any type of focal cortical lesion; tumors, angiomas, and encephalitis should be suspected. Curiously, particularly in patients with epilepsia partialis continua, the cortex can appear normal to pathologic examination. With recent application of diffusion magnetic resonance imaging (MRI), increasing attention has been drawn to focal cortical dysplasia as a cause of neocortical epilepsy including epilepsia partialis continua.[28] In a number of patients, surgical excision of the excitable tissue has cured the myoclonus,[33] and this approach should be considered.

NONEPILEPTIC MYOCLONUS

The types of nonepileptic myoclonus are particularly heterogeneous. It is important to recognize them, because each has its own treatment, and, in general, use of anticonvulsants is not valuable. Some physiologic phenomena are included in this group including hiccough, sneeze, and the hypnic jerk.

Dystonic Myoclonus and Fragments of Other Involuntary Movement Disorders

Patients with dystonia or chorea, for example, may have quick jerks as well as more prolonged involuntary movements. Other "basal ganglia" disorders such as Wilson disease, neuroaxonal dystrophy, pantothenate kinase-associated neurodegeneration (PKAN; formerly known as Hallervorden-Spatz disease), progressive supranuclear palsy, and Parkinson disease all may manifest myoclonus. The diagnosis is made on the basis of other clinical features. Treatments are available for Parkinson disease, of course. Myoclonus in Huntington disease can be improved with valproic acid, perhaps because of the involvement of the γ-aminobutyric acid (GABA) system in this disorder.[5] Focal myoclonus in the setting of dystonia can often be treated with focal injections with botulinum toxin. Myoclonus dystonia (DYT11) is an autosomal dominant syndrome where symptoms include dystonic myoclonus as well as more prolonged spasms.[13] Tremor, similar to essential tremor, may also be present. There is often a marked response to ethanol. In many families, the genetic abnormality has been identified to be in the protein epsilon-sarcoglycan.[1] In this condition, myoclonus involves mainly proximal or truncal muscles and occurs independently of dystonia in terms of the body sites involved and the time of occurrence.

Essential Myoclonus

This term can be utilized for those patients whose sole neurologic abnormality is myoclonus and specifically do not have seizures, dementia, or ataxia. The EEG and other laboratory investigations should be normal. Familial cases as well as sporadic cases are seen. The most common features of the familial cases are autosomal dominant inheritance with variable severity, equal involvement of males and females, onset in the first or second decade of life, and benign course compatible with normal life span. Essential myoclonus can be generalized or multifocal. The myoclonus is variable in amplitude, and in some cases, the jerks are so small that the disability can be minimal. Jerks can be present at rest and may be improved or worsened by action. Reflex myoclonus has not been described in this group.

In some families with essential myoclonus some involved patients also have essential tremor, and some family members had essential tremor without myoclonus. Some of these patients also may exhibit elements of dystonia, and the diagnosis in these cases may well be myoclonus dystonia (DYT11). The essential tremor, myoclonus, and dystonia may all be sensitive to alcohol in these patients.

Exaggerated Startle

Startle is a normal phenomenon that can be exaggerated if an excessive response occurs to a startling stimulus or if a startle response occurs to a stimulus that ordinarily would not be startling.[26] There are a number of startle syndromes including hereditary hyperekplexia, symptomatic hyperekplexia, startle epilepsy, and Latah syndrome. Startle epilepsy is principally characterized by epileptic seizures triggered by sudden, unexpected stimuli and initiated by a startle.

Periodic Movements in Sleep

There are a variety of types of myoclonus that occur during drowsiness or sleep. There are two physiologic forms, the hypnic jerk and "physiologic fragmentary myoclonus," characterized by small, multifocal jerks maximal in the hands and face but present diffusely. Pathologic types of myoclonus include isolated periodic movements in sleep, restless legs and periodic movements in sleep, and excessive fragmentary myoclonus in non–rapid eye movement (NREM) sleep. Myoclonus associated with epilepsy, intention myoclonus associated with semivolitional movements, and segmental myoclonus also occur in sleep, but are not primarily nocturnal.

Periodic movements in sleep (PMS) occurs in virtually all groups of patients referred to a sleep disorders laboratory, and the clinical correlation is not always clear. Patients with the restless legs syndrome often have PMS. Certainly, PMS can be asymptomatic for the patient, although, as with all types of nocturnal myoclonus, the disorder may cause distress to the patient's spouse. On some occasions, however, PMS can induce sleep fragmentation and excessive daytime sleepiness (see Chapter 276).

Segmental Myoclonus Including Spinal Myoclonus and Palatal Myoclonus

In this disorder, a segment of the spinal cord or brainstem produces persistent rhythmic repetitive discharges usually unaffected by sleep. A number of contiguous muscles produce synchronous contractions at a rate of 0.5 to 3 Hz. Involved regions can be one limb, one limb and adjacent trunk, or both legs. Lesions of the spinal cord giving rise to focal movements include infection, degenerative disease, tumor, cervical myelopathy, and demyelinating disease, and it may follow spinal anesthesia or the introduction of contrast media into the CSF. Unlike palatal myoclonus, spinal myoclonus would only rarely be idiopathic. Spinal myoclonus usually occurs spontaneously and may persist during sleep.

Another form of spinal myoclonus is propriospinal myoclonus.[4,6] This is clinically characterized by axial jerks that are nonrhythmic and that lead to symmetric flexion of the neck, trunk, hips, and knees. Jerks can be spontaneous or stimulus induced. The myoclonus is identified with electrodiagnostic studies that show the myoclonus starting in the midthoracic region and propagating slowly, about 5 meters/sec, both rostrally and caudally.

Palatal myoclonus, now preferably called palatal tremor, is most common in this group, and has now been shown to consist of two separate disorders, essential palatal tremor, which manifests an ear click, and symptomatic palatal tremor, which is associated with cerebellar disturbances.[8] The ear click in essential palatal tremor is the symptom that requires therapy.

Asterixis

Negative myoclonus may well have a subcortical origin as well as a cortical origin (epileptic), although there are no clinical rules for separating them. The distinction is made on the basis of electrophysiologic studies that may show EEG correlates with the cortical form, but this may not be a definite qualitative difference. Certainly, subcortical lesions may cause asterixis, but that does not necessarily imply where the movement is generated. For example, unilateral asterixis is caused by a vascular lesion in the contralateral thalamus, but this does not necessarily mean that this type of asterixis originates from the thalamus.[42] It is difficult to treat asterixis whether cortical or subcortical, and a search for a metabolic or toxic cause should be the first course of action.

Psychogenic Myoclonus

Myoclonus can also be psychogenic. Monday and Jankovic[29] reported the clinical features of 18 such patients. There were 13 women and five men with an age range of 22 to 75 years. The myoclonus was present for 1 to 110 months; it was segmental in ten, generalized in seven, and focal in one. Stress precipitated or exacerbated the myoclonic movements in 15 patients; 14 had a definite increase in myoclonic activity during periods of anxiety. The following findings helped to establish the psychogenic nature of the myoclonus: Clinical features incongruous with "organic" myoclonus, evidence of underlying psychopathology, an improvement with distraction or placebo, and the presence of incongruous sensory loss or false weakness. Over half of all patients with adequate follow-up improved after gaining insight into the psychogenic mechanisms of their movement disorder.

DIAGNOSTIC INVESTIGATION

Clearly the first issue is to seek an underlying cause for the condition. This would imply a full neurologic evaluation including blood studies, neuroimaging, and CSF evaluation.

Electrophysiologic assessment can be a significant help in deciding whether the movement is myoclonus, and, if so, which type.[19,37,43] Techniques to be employed include EMG to evaluate the EMG activity associated with the movement, EEG to determine if there is an EEG event related to the movement (averaging of activity may be needed), analysis of whether the involuntary movement can be produced reflexly, and evaluation of the evoked response in the EEG to stimulation that produces reflex involuntary movements. The physiologic characteristics of epileptic myoclonus are EMG burst length of 10 to 50 msec, synchronous antagonist activity, and an EEG correlate. Nonepileptic myoclonus shows EMG burst lengths of 50 to 300 msec, synchronous or asynchronous antagonist activity, and no EEG correlate.

With cortical reflex myoclonus, the EEG reveals a focal positive–negative event over the sensorimotor cortex contralateral to the jerk preceding both spontaneous and reflex-induced myoclonic jerks. With stimulus sensitivity, C-reflexes are seen and are correlated with giant somatosensory-evoked potentials. Some myoclonus is sensitive to flash stimulus, and in this case photic-evoked potential is markedly enhanced. The EEG event associated with reflex jerks is a giant P1–N2 component of the somatosensory-evoked potential. Often the P1–N2 has exactly the same topography as the positive–negative event preceding the spontaneous myoclonus, but at times there are some differences. A final feature is that if the cranial nerve muscles are active, then the timing of onset of activation is from above downward; that is, the masseter (fifth cranial nerve) is active before the orbicularis oculi (seventh cranial nerve), which is itself active before the sternocleidomastoid (11th cranial nerve). With reticular reflex myoclonus, there are brief generalized EMG bursts lasting 10 to 30 msec triggered by sensory stimulation such as touch or muscle stretch or by action; the EEG correlates, if present, are not time locked to the muscle activation, and the pattern of EMG activation in cranial nerve muscles is with the sternocleidomastoid muscle activated first and the other cranial nerve muscles activated in reverse numeric order. In primary generalized epileptic myoclonus, the EEG correlate is a slow, bilateral frontocentrally predominant negativity similar to the wave of a primary generalized paroxysm.

If an EEG event cannot be found with back-averaging, it might be valuable to look at EEG-EMG coherence during the jerking. This technique was used, for example, to identify the cortical involvement in a series of patients with cortical myoclonic tremor.[44]

TREATMENT

The first approach, as has been emphasized, is to try to find an etiology that can be reversed. Failing that, the myoclonus can be approached symptomatically.

Epileptic Myoclonus

If the myoclonus is part of a defined epileptic syndrome, it should be treated as the syndrome. If the myoclonus needs to be approached by itself, the first approach is anticonvulsants. The most useful agents are clonazepam and valproate, both of which work by promoting GABA action in brain. Primidone may also play a role. Serotonergic agents such as 5-hydroxytryptophan (5-HTP) may also be effective. Piracetam and levetiracetam can be very effective for epileptic myoclonus.[12,14,31] Zonisamide may also be a useful agent.[46] Obeso et al.[32] have pointed out that two or three drugs in combination may well be better than a single drug.

Posthypoxic myoclonus is a special condition to consider because of the specific deficiency of serotonin. 5-HTP, either alone or with carbidopa, is often beneficial in this condition. On the other hand, however, it is not often used as a drug of first choice because of adverse effects. Most patients will respond just as well to clonazepam, valproate, or clonazepam plus valproate. In some cases, posthypoxic myoclonus dramatically responds to levetiracetam.

Essential Myoclonus

Essential myoclonus is a heterogeneous disorder and therapy is largely empiric. Alcohol is most likely to be beneficial, but cannot be recommended for regular use. Sodium oxybate may be successful for alcohol-responsive patients.[11] There are also reports suggesting propranolol, 5-HTP, and clonazepam. Some patients have responded dramatically to benztropine.[9]

Exaggerated Startle

Clonazepam is the therapy of choice.[26] Other benzodiazepines, such as diazepam and chlordiazepoxide, have been used with similar results.

Periodic Movements in Sleep

Treatment of choice is now either dopaminergic therapy or opiate therapy.[22,38] For some patients clonazepam may be helpful.

Segmental Myoclonus

For spinal myoclonus, treatment should be directed to the underlying cause if possible. For example, surgery can ameliorate myoclonus caused by cervical cord compression. Antiviral therapy may improve segmental myoclonus associated with herpes zoster. On the other hand, sometimes drug treatment can be helpful, such as clonazepam, valproate, and L-5-HTP, or trihexyphenidyl. For the ear click of essential palatal myoclonus, a number of drugs may be useful in individual cases, such as clonazepam, tryptophan, carbamazepine, trihexyphenidyl, or ceruletide, but most seem refractory. The ear click can be successfully treated with focal injection of botulinum toxin.[7]

SUMMARY AND CONCLUSIONS

Myoclonus is a simple, quick involuntary movement that can be seen in a large variety of disorders. There are many types of myoclonus, and it is crucial to make a clear diagnosis before beginning therapy. Hopefully, an underlying cause might be uncovered that could be treated. In many cases myoclonus may be a fragment of epilepsy. If it is a feature of a well-defined epileptic syndrome, then treatment of the myoclonus is the same as the syndrome. If the epileptic myoclonus is not a part of a recognized syndrome, the first approach is still anticonvulsants. If the myoclonus is nonepileptic, then symptomatic treatment needs to be individualized to the particular disorder.

ACKNOWLEDGMENTS

This chapter drew heavily on previous reviews including references 18, 19, and 43.

References

1. Asmus F, Zimprich A, Tezenas Du Montcel S, et al. Myoclonus-dystonia syndrome: epsilon-sarcoglycan mutations and phenotype. *Ann Neurol.* 2002;52(4):489–492.
2. Berkovic SF, Andermann F, Carpenter S, et al. Progressive myoclonic epilepsies: specific causes and diagnosis. *N Engl J Med.* 1986;315:296–305.
3. Bressman S, Fahn S, Eisenberg M, et al. Adult onset encephalopathy with myoclonus, ataxia, deafness, hemianopsia and hemiparesis responsive to biotin. *Ann Neurol.* 1983;14:109–110.
4. Brown P, Thompson PD, Rothwell JC, et al. Axial myoclonus of propriospinal origin. *Brain.* 1991;114:197–214.
5. Carella F, Scaioli V, Ciano C, et al. Adult onset myoclonic Huntington's disease. *Mov Disord.* 1993;8:201–205.
6. Chokroverty S, Walters A, Zimmerman T, et al. Propriospinal myoclonus: a neurophysiologic analysis. *Neurology.* 1992;42:1591–1595.
7. Deuschl G, Löhle E, Heinen F, et al. Ear click in palatal tremor: its origin and treatment with botulinum toxin. *Neurology.* 1991;41:1677–1679.
8. Deuschl G, Toro C, Valls-Solé J, et al. Symptomatic and essential palatal tremor. 1. Clinical, physiological, and MRI analysis. *Brain.* 1994;117:775–788.
9. Duvoisin RC. Essential myoclonus: response to anticholinergic therapy. *Clin Neuropharmacol.* 1984;7:141–147.
10. Eldridge R, Iivanainen M, Stern R, et al. Baltic myoclonus epilepsy: hereditary disorder of childhood made worse by phenytoin. *Lancet.* 1983;2:838–842.
11. Frucht SJ, Houghton WC, Bordelon Y, et al. A single-blind, open-label trial of sodium oxybate for myoclonus and essential tremor. *Neurology.* 2005;65:1967–1969.
12. Frucht SJ, Louis ED, Chuang C, et al. A pilot tolerability and efficacy study of levetiracetam in patients with chronic myoclonus. *Neurology.* 2001;57(6):1112–1114.
13. Gasser T, Bereznai B, Muller B, et al. Linkage studies in alcohol-responsive myoclonic dystonia. *Mov Disord.* 1996;11:363–370.
14. Genton P, Gelisse P. Antimyoclonic effect of levetiracetam. *Epileptic Disord.* 2000;2(4):209–212.
15. Guerrini R, Dravet C, Genton P, et al. Epileptic negative myoclonus. *Neurology.* 1993;43:1078–1083.
16. Hallett M. Myoclonus: relation to epilepsy. *Epilepsia.* 1985;26(Suppl 1): S67–S77.
17. Hallett M. Early history of myoclonus. In: Fahn S, Marsden CD,Van Woert MH, eds. *Myoclonus.* New York: Raven Press; 1986:7–10.
18. Hallett M. Diagnosis and treatment of myoclonus. In: Defer G, ed. *Mouvements Anormaux et Douleurs D'Origine Neurologique. Thérapeutique et Neurologie.* Paris: DERN; 1994:55–68.
19. Hallett M, Marsden CD, Fahn S. Myoclonus. In: Vinken PJ, Bruyn GW, Klawans HL, eds. *Handbook of Clinical Neurology.* Amsterdam: Elsevier Science Publishers; 1987:609–625.
20. Lance JW, Adams RD. The syndrome of intention or action myoclonus as a sequel to hypoxic encephalopathy. *Brain.* 1963;86:111–136.
21. Lehesjoki AE. Molecular background of progressive myoclonus epilepsy. *EMBO J.* 2003;22(14):3473–3478.

22. Littner MR, Kushida C, Anderson WM, et al. Practice parameters for the dopaminergic treatment of restless legs syndrome and periodic limb movement disorder. *Sleep*. 2004;27(3):557–559.
23. Lundborg H. *Die progressive Myoklonus-Epilepsie*. Uppsala: Almqvist and Wiksell; 1903.
24. Maher J, Choudhri S, Halliday W, et al. AIDS dementia complex with generalized myoclonus. *Mov Disord*. 1997;12(4):593–597.
25. Marsden CD, Hallett M, Fahn S. The nosology and pathophysiology of myoclonus. In: Marsden CD, Fahn S, eds. *Movement Disorders*. London: Butterworth Scientific; 1982:196–248.
26. Matsumoto J, Hallett M. Startle syndromes. In: Marsden CD, Fahn S, eds. *Movement Disorders 3*. Oxford: Butterworth-Heinemann; 1994:418–433.
27. Minassian BA, Sainz J, Serratosa JM, et al. Genetic locus heterogeneity in Lafora's progressive myoclonus epilepsy. *Ann Neurol*. 1999;45(2):262–265.
28. Misawa S, Kuwabara S, Shibuya K, et al. Low-frequency transcranial magnetic stimulation for epilepsia partialis continua due to cortical dysplasia. *J Neurol Sci*. 2005;234(1–2):37–39.
29. Monday K, Jankovic J. Psychogenic myoclonus. *Neurology*. 1993;43:349–352.
30. Muskens LJJ. *Epilepsy: Comparative Pathogenesis, Symptoms, Treatment*. New York: William Wood; 1928.
31. Obeso JA, Artieda J, Quinn N, et al. Piracetam in the treatment of different types of myoclonus. *Clin Neuropharmacol*. 1988;11:529–536.
32. Obeso JA, Artieda J, Rothwell JC, et al. The treatment of severe action myoclonus. *Brain*. 1989;112:765–777.
33. Obeso JA, Rothwell JC, Marsden CD. The spectrum of cortical myoclonus: from focal reflex jerks to spontaneous motor epilepsy. *Brain*. 1985;108:193–224.
34. Pranzatelli MR. The immunopharmacology of the opsoclonus-myoclonus syndrome. *Clin Neuropharmacol*. 1996;19(1):1–47.
35. Serratosa JM, Gomez-Garre P, Gallardo ME, et al. A novel protein tyrosine phosphatase gene is mutated in progressive myoclonus epilepsy of the Lafora type (EPM2). *Hum Mol Genet*. 1999;8(2):345–352.
36. Shibasaki H. Pathophysiology of negative myoclonus and asterixis. In: Fahn S, Hallett M, Lüders HO, et al., eds. *Negative Motor Phenomena*. Philadelphia: Lippincott-Raven Publishers; 1995:199–209.
37. Shibasaki H, Hallett M. Electrophysiological studies of myoclonus. *Muscle Nerve*. 2005;31(2):157–174.
38. Silber MH, Ehrenberg BL, Allen RP, et al. An algorithm for the management of restless legs syndrome. *Mayo Clin Proc*. 2004;79(7):916–922.
39. Sprague SM, Corwin HL, Wilson RS, et al. Encephalopathy in chronic renal failure responsive to deferoxamine therapy. Another manifestation of aluminum neurotoxicity. *Arch Intern Med*. 1986;146:2063–2064.
40. Tassinari CA, Rubboli G, Parmeggiani L, et al. Epileptic negative myoclonus. In: Fahn S, Hallett M, Lüders HO, et al., eds. *Negative Motor Phenomena*. Philadelphia: Lippincott-Raven Publishers; 1995:181–197.
41. Tate ED, Allison TJ, Pranzatelli MR, et al. Neuroepidemiologic trends in 105 US cases of pediatric opsoclonus-myoclonus syndrome. *J Pediatr Oncol Nurs*. 2005;22(1):8–19.
42. Tatu L, Moulin T, Martin V, et al. Unilateral pure thalamic asterixis: clinical, electromyographic, and topographic patterns. *Neurology*. 2000;54(12):2339–2342.
43. Toro C, Hallett M. Pathophysiology of myoclonic disorders. In: Watts RL, Koller WC, eds. *Movement Disorders*. 2nd ed. New York: McGraw-Hill; 2004:671–681.
44. van Rootselaar AF, Maurits NM, Koelman JH, et al. Coherence analysis differentiates between cortical myoclonic tremor and essential tremor. *Mov Disord*. 2005;21(2):133–135.
45. van Rootselaar AF, van Schaik IN, van den Maagdenberg AM, et al. Familial cortical myoclonic tremor with epilepsy: a single syndromic classification for a group of pedigrees bearing common features. *Mov Disord*. 2005;20(6):665–673.
46. Yoshimura I, Kaneko S, Yoshimura N, et al. Long-term observations of two siblings with Lafora disease treated with zonisamide. *Epilepsy Res*. 2001;46(3):283–287.

CHAPTER 278 ■ MOVEMENT DISORDERS

STANLEY FAHN AND STEVEN J. FRUCHT

INTRODUCTION

As early as the late nineteenth century, neurologists noted overlap between certain movement disorders and epilepsy. This is perhaps most apparent in patients with myoclonus, as discussed in the preceding chapter in this book. Many patients afflicted with chronic myoclonus also have epilepsy, and forms of focal epilepsy can precisely mimic myoclonus. Most of the drugs effective at treating myoclonus (clonazepam, valproic acid, levetiracetam, zonisamide, acetazolamide) are antiepileptics. Besides myoclonus, there are other disorders that occur in brief or sustained paroxysms, without alteration in arousal or consciousness; these disorders are the subject of this chapter. Often these patients are referred for evaluation to epileptologists or movement disorder specialists. Video-electroencephalogram (EEG) monitoring may be necessary to rule out an epileptic cause, although most of these disorders can be recognized once the physician is familiar with the syndrome.

Several paroxysmal movement disorders that may be confused with epilepsy are considered elsewhere in this book. Myoclonus, as mentioned previously, is the closest mimic. Patients with hyperekplexia have an inherited disorder of exaggerated startle and sustained tonic contractions due to mutations in the glycine receptor. These patients usually present in the nursery with exaggerated startle, abnormal tone, and lack of habituation to startle. Recognition is critical because appropriate treatment with clonazepam prevents potentially life-threatening apneic episodes. Paroxysmal torticollis is another disorder beginning in early childhood, with episodes of sustained tonic contraction of neck muscles producing sustained head postures for hours or days. Events typically occur periodically, and alertness and arousal are preserved. This migraine variant is also usually easily distinguished from epilepsy. Infants may sometimes evidence paroxysmal, brief episodes of upward gaze, so-called tonic upgaze of infancy, which may raise the notion of epilepsy. These episodes are brief, typically last seconds, are unassociated with other abnormalities, and, although they are disconcerting to parents, usually disappear by early childhood.

Four other movement disorders mimicking epilepsy are considered further in this chapter: (a) stereotypies (complex tics), (b) episodic ataxia, (c) self-stimulatory behavior, and (d) the paroxysmal dyskinesias.

Stereotypies are highly patterned, complex, sustained movements, often lasting seconds, which are typically repeated multiple times. Examples of stereotypic movements include truncal rocking, skin picking, hand clapping, hand twirling, and complex hand-to-mouth routines (feeding, blowing, touching). Phenomenologically, there is little difference between a complex motor tic, that is, a complex sequence of involuntary movements performed in response to an inner urge, and stereotypies. Stereotypies are most commonly seen in patients with autism, pervasive development delay, and Asperger syndrome, but they may also occur in developmentally disabled individuals, in Rett syndrome, and in otherwise normal children.[19,45,87,116] Because these events are brief, involve complex involuntary movements, and may affect patients' ability to interact with the examiner, they may be mistaken for supplementary motor area seizures. It is not uncommon for video-EEG monitoring to be ordered to differentiate long-duration stereotypies from seizures, particularly when they occur in neurologically abnormal individuals.

Episodic ataxia is a rare, genetic paroxysmal movement disorder that should be easy to distinguish from epilepsy. The disorder occurs in two forms, types 1 and 2. Episodic ataxia type 1 is an autosomal-dominant disorder characterized by paroxysms of ataxia lasting several minutes, often with myokymia between attacks. The disorder has been linked to mutations in the voltage-gated K^+ channel gene, *KCNA1*.[14,27,48] Episodic ataxia type 2 is an autosomal-dominant disorder characterized by paroxysms of ataxia lasting hours, often with interictal symptoms of nystagmus or cerebellar dysfunction. The disorder is linked to mutations in the alpha 1A voltage-dependent calcium channel subunit, CACNA1A. Acetazolamide and 4-aminopyridine have been shown to be beneficial in affected patients.[59,60,125,128]

Self-stimulatory behavior is not infrequently encountered at centers that perform video-EEG monitoring. This condition typically begins in early childhood, affects girls more than boys, and is usually first noticed by parents. In a typical event the child crosses his or her legs, lies flat on the floor, or applies pressure to the groin or perineum against furniture. Children can be distracted during an episode, and there may be accompanying autonomic signs such as facial flushing or sweating. Videorecording is extremely useful in documenting the nature of these events. If the clinical appearance is classic, investigative studies are unnecessary. The term "infantile masturbation" should be avoided when discussing this condition with parents because there is significant stigma associated with it. We have encountered parents who refuse to accept this diagnosis, persisting in extensive evaluations to prove a different etiology for the condition. Most children respond to redirection and support.[32,96,103,149]

In the remainder of this chapter, we discuss the paroxysmal dyskinesias, a complex and unusual group of disorders that bear relation to epilepsy. Because the literature of paroxysmal disorders is extensive and often confusing, we first offer a historical review of the development of these disorders and then present current concepts related to their nosology and etiology.

PAROXSYMAL DYSKINESIAS—HISTORY

Gowers[44] was probably the first to report "movement-induced seizures," in this case, in an 11-year-old girl who developed brief attacks that occurred when she suddenly arose after prolonged sitting. Numerous reports of "movement-induced seizures" followed, published under the designations of *reflex epilepsy* or *tonic seizures induced by movement*. Some cases

TABLE 1

CLINICAL FEATURES OF PAROXYSMAL KINESIGENIC, NONKINESIGENIC, AND EXERTIONAL DYSKINESIA

Feature	PKD	PNKD	PED
Inheritance	AD	AD	AD
Male-to-female ratio	4:1	1.4:1	4:8 ($n = 12$)
Age at onset			
Range	<1–40	<1–30	2–20
Median	12	12	9.5
Mean	12	12	9
Attacks			
Duration	<5 min	2 min–4 h	5–30 min
Frequency	100/d–1/min	3/d–2/y	1/d–2/min
Trigger	Sudden movement, startle, hyperventilation	Nil	Prolonged exercise
Precipitant	Stress	Alcohol, stress, caffeine, excitement, fatigue	Stress, caffeine, fatigue
Treatment	Anticonvulsants (acetazolamide), antimuscarinics	Clonazepam, benzodiazepines	?

AD, autosomal dominant; PED, paroxysmal exertion-induced dyskinesia; PKD, paroxysmal kinesigenic dyskinesia; PNKD, paroxysmal nonkinesigenic dyskinesia.

demonstrated more than tonic contractions—namely, sustained twisting, athetosis, and chorea. Even the presence of choreoathetosis, however, did not lead the earliest interpreters of these brief attacks to conclude that they represented a movement disorder. Rather, they considered them to be a form of epilepsy, with the cerebral site of the "seizures" in the basal ganglia or subcortical region.

After Gowers, the next report of movement-induced paroxysmal movements appears to be that of Spiller in 1927.[126] He described two patients with brief tonic spasms brought on by voluntary movement of the involved limbs, and in one of them by passive manipulation. Contractions were painful and accompanied by sensations of heat or burning. Wilson[145] later described a 5-year-old boy who had brief attacks of unilateral torsion and tonic spasm that lasted up to 3 minutes and were precipitated by pain. Wilson considered this to be reflex tonic epilepsy, and also thought it to be subcortical in origin.

The concept of attacks of tonic, often twisting, contractions without loss of consciousness as uncommon seizure disorders continued. Lishman et al.[80] described seven patients with tonic and athetoid spasms induced by movement while remaining conscious. Abnormal sensations of numbness, vibration, and tightness were noted in the affected limbs before the attacks. Two years later they reported an additional five cases of movement-induced "seizures,"[143] and Burger et al.[15] described two patients with this label. Some also referred to these cases as forms of epilepsy.[38,52]

In 1940, Mount and Reback[99] introduced a new concept—attacks of tonic spasms plus choreic and athetotic movements with unusual triggers. They described a 23-year-old man who had had "spells" since infancy, both "large" and "small." Both types were preceded by a sensory aura of tightness in parts of the body or by a feeling of tiredness. Movements involved the arms and legs, usually a combination of sustained twisted posturing and chorea. The "small" attacks lasted from 5 to 10 minutes; longer attacks were considered "large" and also involved the neck (retrocollis), eyes (upward gaze), face (ipsilateral to the limbs, if the limb involvement was unilateral), and speech. These "large" attacks lasted for as long as 2 hours. Drinking alcohol, coffee, tea, or cola would usually precipitate an attack, as would fatigue, smoking, and intense concentration. The attacks cleared more rapidly if the patient lay down, and they were aborted by sleep. Between attacks, the neurologic examination was normal, and there was never loss of consciousness, clonic convulsive movements, biting of the tongue, or loss of sphincter control. Phenytoin and phenobarbital were without effect, and scopolamine was the only drug found to reduce the frequency, severity, and duration of attacks. The family history revealed 27 other members with similar attacks, with a pedigree showing autosomal-dominant inheritance with complete penetrance. Mount and Reback called this disorder *familial paroxysmal choreoathetosis*.

This paper by Mount and Reback became the seminal report in the field of paroxysmal dyskinesias. After its publication, it was referenced by most reports in the literature over the next five decades, although the next report of a large family with similar attacks of muscle spasms did not reference it. In 1961 Forssman[33] described a family whose members had attacks lasting from 4 minutes to 3 hours; inheritance was autosomal dominant. Attacks were induced by cold, mental tension, irritation, fatigue, lack of sleep, alcohol, and caffeine. Onset of symptoms was in early childhood; an attack might begin with a tonic spasm in one hand and spread up the arm to the other arm, to both legs, and then to the cranial muscles, including the tongue, so that the affected person could not speak during a severe attack. Forssman considered the disorder to be new, possibly related to myotonia and paramyotonia, and did not consider it a form of epilepsy because no alteration of consciousness was involved.

In 1963, Lance[73] reported eight similar patients with attacks of tonic (dystonic) spasms, some with choreoathetosis, usually affecting only one side of the body and often preceded by pain or tingling. Two patients had secondary attacks (static encephalopathy and multiple sclerosis), one case was idiopathic and sporadic, and the remaining five were members of the same family. The attacks lasted <1 minute in two patients, 2 to

5 minutes in the patient with multiple sclerosis, and 5 to 60 minutes in the five familial cases. They were not precipitated by movement, and the familial cases were exacerbated by excitement and fatigue. No EEG abnormality was recorded between attacks.

After the 1963 article by Lance,[73] Weber[142] reported a family of four affected members with nonkinesigenic paroxysmal dystonia and used the term *familial paroxysmal dystonia*. Richards and Barnett[114] reported the next big family with the same type of paroxysmal dyskinesia as Mount and Reback's and thought that Lance's family[73] represented a variant because its members had only tonic spasms and no movements. The family of Richards and Barnett consisted of nine affected members with the trait inherited in an autosomal-dominant pattern. They emphasized the nonkinesigenic nature of the attacks and felt that a wide array of terms could describe the attacks, depending on the severity of each one. Richards and Barnett coined the term *paroxysmal dystonic choreoathetosis* (PDC), which was later adopted by Lance in 1977.[74] The terms *paroxysmal nonkinesigenic choreoathetosis* and *paroxysmal dystonia* were sometimes used instead of PDC.[12] The term *paroxysmal nonkinesigenic dyskinesia* (PNKD), proposed by Demirkiran and Jankovic,[23] is currently the accepted designation for this syndrome (Table 1).

In 1967, Kertesz[65] introduced the label *paroxysmal kinesigenic choreoathetosis* (PKC). This label developed into a most useful and widely accepted designation. Kinesigenicity has an important place in the classification of the paroxysmal dyskinesias, and Demirkiran and Jankovic[23] recommended that the term *paroxysmal kinesigenic dyskinesia* (PKD) be used instead because movements can be dystonic, choreic, or a combination of the two. Rarely, the PKD designation can be applied to certain patients whose dyskinesias are not triggered by sudden movement (or startle).

In his paper, Kertesz reported 10 new cases of paroxysmal dyskinesia and reviewed the literature. It is significant that he differentiated the kinesigenic variety from the cases described by Mount and Reback, Forssman, and Lance, which were not exacerbated by movement but by alcohol, caffeine, or fatigue. Although phenytoin was recognized earlier as a very useful agent for PKD, carbamazepine was later found to be equally useful and was introduced as a treatment by Kato and Araki.[64]

The original cases reported as PNKD were idiopathic and usually familial. It was not long before symptomatic cases began to be reported in patients with perinatal encephalopathy,[119] encephalitis,[100] head injury,[117,144] as a manifestation of multiple sclerosis,[61,90,136] and idiopathic hypoparathyroidism.[2]

The next major advance in classification was by Horner and Jackson,[54] who described two families in which several members had attacks of involuntary movements that occurred during sleep. These appear to be the first reported cases of hypnogenic paroxysmal dyskinesia. In one family, some of the affected members had classic paroxysmal kinesigenic dyskinesia, some hypnogenic, and others a combination of the two. Case 3 in this family began with the hypnogenic variety when the patient was 8 years old. By the time he had reached the age of 11 years, daytime attacks were also occurring, sometimes triggered by sudden movement. The hypnogenic episodes gradually disappeared, leaving him with kinesigenic dyskinesia that responded to antiepileptic drugs.

Lugaresi and colleagues[83,84] independently rediscovered and eventually made known the syndrome of hypnogenic paroxysmal dyskinesia. Lugaresi and Cirignotta[84] described five patients with onset of hypnogenic dystonia at ages 5, 7, 26, 30, and 40 years. Attacks occurred almost every night during sleep, with onset in stages 2 to 4 of sleep. They lasted 15 to 45 seconds and might recur several times in the same night. They could awaken the patient, who might even emit a cry. The movements appeared to be a mixture of dystonia, athetosis, and some more rapid flinging movements. The EEG findings were normal during sleep and wakefulness. Carbamazepine was effective. In their article, Lugaresi and Cirignotta described the movements as choreoathetosis and ballism in addition to dystonia. Maccario and Lustman[85] emphasized that tachycardia is a characteristic occurrence during these episodes.

The disorder was originally described in nonfamilial cases but was later reported in three members of a family.[75] Other sporadic cases have been reported as well,[21,41,113,132] including one with a concurrent reflex dystonic reaction provoked by stimulation of the right foot.[77] Another link with PKD is suggested by the report of Morley,[98] who described a father with hypnogenic dyskinetic attacks and a son with PKD. Both responded to phenytoin.

There has long been considerable speculation as to whether the short-duration hypnogenic attacks might be a manifestation of epilepsy because they respond so well to antiepileptic drugs. The lack of abnormal EEG findings during these attacks has been used to argue against this concept. However, evidence accumulated that many hypnogenic paroxysmal dyskinesias are, indeed, caused by seizures. Tinuper et al.[133] described three patients with this disorder who had EEG evidence of frontal lobe seizures as a cause of their attacks. Sellal et al.[121] and Meierkord et al.[92] studied a series of patients with hypnogenic dystonias and concluded that they represent seizure disorders, particularly of frontal lobe epilepsy, because repeated nocturnal EEG recordings often reveal epileptic patterns of abnormalities. Seizures arising near the mesial posterior frontal supplementary sensorimotor area (SSMA) may be a particular culprit in inducing paroxysmal hypnogenic dyskinesias in children.[5] These types of seizures tend to be brief, frequent, and associated with bilateral tonic posturing, gross proximal limb movements, and preserved consciousness. Dystonic and other dyskinetic features may result from spread of epileptic activity from the mesial frontal region to the basal ganglia because the anatomic connections between these areas are close. The subject of epilepsy masquerading as a movement disorder has been reviewed by Hirsch et al.[51] and Fish and Marsden.[31]

Although most patients with paroxysmal dyskinesias fit into one of these classification schemes, it has become clear that some patients defy easy classification. Several patients have been reported with both nocturnal and daytime paroxysmal events without EEG correlate. Daytime attacks may be triggered by movement or may sometimes occur without trigger.[22,111] Results of imaging and EEG monitoring are usually not helpful, and patients are often difficult to treat.

PAROXYSMAL KINESIGENIC DYSKINESIA

Clinical Features

Attacks of PKD consist of any combination of dystonic postures, chorea, athetosis, and ballism. They can be unilateral—always on one side or on either side—or bilateral. Unilateral episodes may be followed by a bilateral episode. The attacks are brief, usually lasting only seconds, but rarely can last up to 5 minutes. A sudden movement or a startle precipitates them, usually after the patient has been sitting quietly for some time. The attacks can be severe enough to cause a patient to fall down and can occur up to 100 times per day. After an attack, there is usually a short refractory period during which an attack cannot be triggered. Speech can sometimes be affected, with an inability to speak resulting from dystonia, but alteration of consciousness never occurs. Attacks can sometimes be aborted if a patient stops moving or warms up slowly. Very often, patients report variable sensations at the beginning of paroxysms. These can consist of paresthesias, a feeling of stiffness, crawling sensations, or a tense feeling.

Equivalent to PKD are equally brief attacks that are not precipitated by sudden movement or startle. Because the duration and therapeutic response are the same as in PKD, these have been included under the PKD rubric rather than in an entirely new category. These attacks lasting a few seconds can often be triggered by hyperventilation.

Plant[109] emphasized the focal and unilateral nature of PKD in many patients. Of the 73 cases of PKD in the literature reviewed by him, he found the following features: unilateral, one side only, 25; unilateral, either side, 12; unilateral and bilateral, 11; bilateral only, 22; not stated, 3.

Idiopathic Paroxysmal Dyskinesias

Most reported cases of PKD are familial, with autosomal-dominant inheritance. The male-to-female ratio is 3.75:1 (75 male patients and 20 female patients reported by Fahn[28]). Symptoms begin in childhood between the ages of 6 and 16 years, but age at onset varies widely, ranging from as early as 6 months to 40 years.[35,78] The mean and median ages at onset are 12 years. Familial cases may be more common among the Japanese[37,64,67] and Chinese.[62] Findings on computed tomography (CT) are also normal[10,43,66,82,129] with a few exceptions: A case reported by Watson and Scott[141] suggested brainstem atrophy and one reported by Gilroy[40] had an ill-defined unilateral hemispheric lesion. EEG findings are generally normal; Hirata et al.,[50] however, demonstrated an abnormal EEG with rhythmic 5-Hz discharges over the entire scalp in a patient during episodes of PKD, raising the possibility of an epileptogenic basis.

Attacks tend to diminish with age. Fortunately, PKD responds dramatically to antiepileptic drugs. The early literature indicates that phenytoin was most popular, followed by phenobarbital and primidone. More recently, carbamazepine appears to be the drug most commonly used. Valproate,[129] oxcarbazepine,[134] and topiramate[55] have also been shown to be effective. Homan et al.[53] reported that children with PKD need doses of phenytoin similar to those used to treat epilepsy, whereas adults may respond to lower doses.

The pathophysiology of PKD is unclear, and its relationship with epilepsy remains speculative. The existence of movement-induced seizures (e.g., the case of Falconer et al.[29]) and the dramatic response of PKD to antiepileptic drugs are not sufficient reasons to consider PKD a form of epilepsy. The retention of consciousness and lack of postictal phenomena, as well as the presence of dystonia and choreoathetosis, should be sufficient to disqualify PKD as epilepsy. Franssen et al.[34] investigated the contingent negative variation (CNV) in one patient. This is a slow cerebral potential that follows a warning stimulus that prepares the subject to expect an imperative stimulus requiring a decision or motor response. The slow negative-wave component of the CNV was more pronounced compared with that of control subjects. It returned to normal after phenytoin treatment. Mir et al.[97] later demonstrated reduced intracortical inhibition, reduced early-phase transcallosal inhibition, and reduced first phase of spinal reciprocal inhibition in PKD patients; treatment with carbamazepine normalized the abnormality of transcallosal inhibition.

Two recent studies suggest that attacks of PKD are associated with contralateral hypermetabolism in subcortical nuclei. Using single photon emission computed tomography (SPECT), Ko et al. studied a 14-year-old patient and demonstrated increased perfusion in the contralateral basal ganglia at onset of attacks.[69] Shirane et al. studied a 6-year-old with PKD, also using SPECT; subtraction of interictal from ictal cerebral blood flow measures showed unilateral increase of thalamic blood flow during an attack.[123]

The differential diagnosis of PKD includes partial epilepsy, tetany, hyperexplexia, and psychogenic disorders, as noted in the misdiagnosis of the case reported by Waller.[140] The clinical features are so distinctive, particularly if triggered by sudden movement, that there is little likelihood of the condition not being diagnosed correctly once the physician is aware of its existence. However, nonkinesigenic brief attacks of hemidystonia, often precipitated by hyperventilation and controlled with antiepileptic drugs, may be a sign of epilepsy.[70] Therefore, each case of suspected nonkinesigenic paroxysmal dyskinesia should be evaluated for a convulsive disorder.

Two autopsies in PKD have been reported. After case 4 of Kertesz[65] died, apparently by suicide, a postmortem examination revealed no clear abnormality in the brain, just the presence of some melanin pigment in macrophages in the locus ceruleus. Stevens[127] had earlier reported the postmortem findings of one of his patients, which were also essentially normal, showing only a slight asymmetry of the substantia nigra.

Recent studies have linked PKD to two separate loci on chromosome 16.[7,50,130,135] In some families, PKD cosegregates with infantile convulsions, whereas in others, it does not.

Symptomatic Paroxysmal Dyskinesias

The overwhelming majority of reported cases of PKD are idiopathic or familial. Occasional cases of symptomatic PKD have been reported, most frequently in association with multiple sclerosis and head injury. Although sudden movement does not trigger most of the paroxysmal dyskinesias associated with multiple sclerosis, sometimes a patient with multiple sclerosis manifests typical PKD.[90] In fact, PKD can be the presenting symptom of multiple sclerosis, as in the case reported by Roos et al.[118]; the patient's attacks were associated with a lesion in the caudate nucleus and responded to phenytoin. In three of the eight patients reported by Berger et al.[8] with paroxysmal dyskinesia associated with multiple sclerosis, attacks were induced by sudden movement and were relieved with antiepileptic drugs.

As mentioned earlier, attacks lasting for seconds are sometimes induced not by sudden movement but by hyperventilation. These also usually respond to antiepileptic drugs, such as carbamazepine, and may be seen in multiple sclerosis.[122,136] Sethi et al.[122] reported successfully treating three patients who had paroxysmal dystonia (not induced by movement, but triggered by hyperventilation and lasting many seconds) using acetazolamide with or without a combination of carbamazepine. The case of PKD with multiple sclerosis reported by Burguera et al.[16] had a lesion in the left thalamus demonstrated by magnetic resonance imaging (MRI). Paroxysmal kinesigenic dyskinesia was the presenting symptom, as in other cases of demyelinating disease. Case 3 of Whitty et al.[143] was a 13-year-old boy with onset 9 months after mild head trauma. Robin[117] reported a 33-year-old man with severe head injury in whom PKD developed 8 months later. In two of the three cases of posttraumatic paroxysmal dyskinesias reported by Drake et al.,[25] movements were induced by sudden movement of the affected body part. Another posttraumatic case was reported by Richardson et al.[115] Like idiopathic PKD, these posttraumatic cases of PKD responded to antiepileptic drugs. Attacks of dystonia lasting several seconds and induced by tactile stimulation were reported secondary to a head injury; they disappeared within 2 months without treatment.[39] Another case of tactilely induced dyskinesias was reported by Nijssen and Tijssen[105] as a result of a thalamic infarct.

In case 2 of the five cases described by Kinast et al.,[66] attacks of left hemidystonia lasted 1 minute and occurred up to

50 times a day. The major precipitating factor was not sudden movement, but rather stress and the anticipation of movement. Technically, this patient does not fulfill the criterion of attacks induced by sudden movement. However, because of their brief duration, frequency, and response to phenytoin, which are features resembling those of PKD, they are placed under the PKD rubric in the classification scheme of this chapter. Examination revealed left-sided hemiatrophy and hyperreflexia, with normal findings on CT. Gilroy[40] reported a 32-year-old man with an abnormal right hemisphere on CT who had had multiple daily brief attacks of left hemidystonia since the age of 5 years that were typical of PKD.

With the advent of MRI, more cases of PKD have been reported as a result of cerebral infarcts—putaminal,[93] thalamic,[99,101,102] and cortical.[36] Paroxysmal kinesigenic dyskinesia has also been reported in patients with progressive supranuclear palsy,[1] calcifications of the basal ganglia with or without hypoparathyroidism,[41,105,106] and hyperglycemia in the presence of a lenticular vascular malformation.[137]

In one family with X-linked mutations in the thyroid hormone transporter gene *MCT8*, paroxysmal dyskinesias accompanied global mental retardation.[13]

PAROXYSMAL NONKINESIGENIC DYSKINESIA

Clinical Features

Like attacks of PKD, attacks of PNKD consist of any combination of dystonic postures, chorea, athetosis, and ballism. They can be unilateral or bilateral, and unilateral episodes can be followed by a bilateral episode. They can affect a single region of the body or be generalized. The neck can be affected by a combination of torticollis and head tremor.[57] Features that distinguish these attacks from those of PKD are the longer duration, lesser frequency, and different aggravating factors. Attacks last minutes to hours, sometimes longer than a day. Usual duration ranges from 5 minutes to 4 hours. Attacks are triggered by consumption of alcohol, coffee, or tea, and also by psychologic stress or excitement and fatigue. There are usually no more than three attacks per day, and often attacks are spaced months apart. The attacks can be severe enough to cause a patient to fall down. Speech is often affected, with inability to speak caused by dystonia, but alteration of consciousness never occurs. The attacks can sometimes be aborted if a patient goes to sleep. As in PKD, patients very often report variable sensations at the beginning of the paroxysms. These can consist of paresthesias, a feeling of stiffness, crawling sensations, or a tense feeling.

Idiopathic Nonkinesigenic Dyskinesias

The initial reports of PNKD were familial with autosomal-dominant transmission. Kinast et al.[66] in 1980 (case 4) and Dunn[26] in 1981 each described a child with PNKD without a positive family history. Since then, Bressman et al.[12] described seven sporadic cases of PNKD, and Nardocci et al.[101] added another one. The familial cases of idiopathic PNKD still greatly outnumber sporadic cases according to the reports in the literature. The sporadic cases are much more difficult to diagnose, however, and they present the added difficulty of having to be differentiated from psychogenic etiology. Based on the experience of Bressman et al.,[12] the sporadic form may actually be more common than the familial form, but is just rarely reported.

There is a slight preponderance of male patients, with a male-to-female ratio of 1.4:1. Onset is usually in childhood between the ages of 6 and 16 years, but age at onset varies widely, ranging from 2 months to 30 years. The mean and median ages at onset are 12 years. Results of CT are normal.[58,91] The EEGs are also generally normal, but the case of Jacome and Risko[58] may be of interest. The patient had unilateral PNKD and normal interictal EEGs. Photic stimulation at low frequencies induced paroxysmal lateralized epileptiform discharges from the contralateral hemisphere. Two patients with PNKD have been studied with functional imaging. del Carmen Garcia et al.[22] performed an ictal SPECT in a 16-year-old patient with PNKD, showing hyperperfusion in the contralateral caudate and thalamus during an attack. Lombroso et al.[81] used fluorodeoxyglucose positron emission tomography (PET) in a patient with PNKD to show no metabolic asymmetry; flurodopa and raclopride PET, however, showed a reduction in presynaptic dopa decarboxylase activity in the striatum and increased postsynaptic D2 dopamine receptors.[81]

The attacks may diminish spontaneously with age. Unfortunately, the attacks of most patients are persistent and are difficult to treat. As a general rule, PNKD does not respond to the antiepileptic drugs that so effectively treat PKD. An occasional patient responds to such agents as carbamazepine and valproate. Clonazepam, as introduced for PNKD by Lance,[74] appears to be the most successful agent, both for idiopathic PNKD and symptomatic PNKD. A number of other drugs have been tried, sometimes with success. These include antimuscarinics,[99] chlordiazepoxide,[106,139] acetazolamide,[12,91] oxazepam and other benzodiazepines,[71,72] and l-tryptophan.[71] Kurlan and Shoulson[72] treated one patient with familial PNKD with clonazepam and oxazepam with relief for 2 to 3 weeks each, and he was placed on a regimen of 40 mg of oxazepam given on alternate days. Trials of the dopamine-receptor antagonist haloperidol were carried out by Przuntek and Monninger[112] and Coulter and Donofrio[20] with benefit; they also found that levodopa worsened the condition of one patient. At least one patient with PNKD has been treated successfully with deep brain stimulation of the globus pallidus interna.[147]

Lance[74] reported autopsies performed on two patients with PNKD with no pathology. Macroscopic findings in his case II.4 were normal. His case IV.2 died of crib death; macroscopic and microscopic findings were normal.

The gene for familial PNKD was cloned in 2004 by a collaborative consortium lead by Ptacek.[76] In 50 individual from eight families, PNKD was shown to be caused by mutations in the myofibrillogenesis regulator gene. The protein product of this gene may be involved in detoxification of methylglyoxal, a compound present in coffee and alcoholic beverages, perhaps explaining the triggering of attacks by these agents.

Symptomatic Paroxysmal Nonkinesigenic Dyskinesia

The overwhelming majority of reported cases of PNKD are idiopathic or familial. A number of cases of symptomatic PNKD have been reported, most frequently in association with multiple sclerosis and perinatal encephalopathy. In multiple sclerosis, the paroxysmal movements may affect only the eyes, lasting several minutes.[86] Other causes of PNKD are encephalitis,[12,100] cystinuria,[18] hypoparathyroidism,[124,148] basal ganglia calcifications without altered serum calcium,[94] thyrotoxicosis,[30] transient ischemic attacks,[6,89] infantile hemiplegia,[56] head trauma,[25,107] hypoglycemia, AIDS,[102] diabetes,[47] moyamoya,[42] anoxia,[12] and brain tumor.[12]

Paroxysmal nonkinesigenic dyskinesia caused by endocrine disorders responds to appropriate treatment. In general, however, treatment of symptomatic PNKD is often ineffective. Positron emission tomography performed in one patient with posttraumatic paroxysmal hemidystonia revealed decreased oxygen metabolism, decreased oxygen extraction, increased blood volume, and increased blood flow in the contralateral basal ganglia.[107]

PAROXYSMAL EXERTIONAL DYSKINESIA

Lance[74] was the first to describe what he called an intermediate form of PDC (now better known as exercise-induced or exertional dyskinesia). It affected members of a family with attacks briefer than those of classic PNKD, typically lasting from 5 to 30 minutes. Attacks were precipitated by prolonged exercise but not by cold, heat, stress, ethanol, excitement, or anxiety. The spasms affected mainly the legs. A second family was reported by Plant et al.[110] In both families, the inheritance pattern was autosomal dominant. No one in either family derived any benefit from barbiturate, levodopa, or clonazepam. More recently, three other families have been reported with exercise-induced paroxysmal dyskinesia, each with different accompanying neurologic abnormalities. Guerrini et al.[46] reported a family with autosomal-recessive rolandic epilepsy, paroxysmal exercise-induced dystonia, and writer's cramp. Affected patients developed symptoms in childhood, and the disorder was linked to a locus adjacent to that of autosomal-dominant infantile convulsions and paroxysmal choreoathetosis.[46] Margari et al.[88] described a family with exercise-induced dyskinesias and generalized epilepsy, and Perniola et al.[108] reported a similar family autosomal-dominant inheritance.

A sporadic case (case 3) was later reported by Nardocci et al.[101] This patient, with no family history of a similar condition, also had interictal chorea. Treatment with clonazepam proved helpful. Another sporadic case was reported by Wali[138]; an 18-year-old youth had attacks of right hemidystonia lasting about 10 minutes that were precipitated by prolonged running (about 10 minutes) or by cold. The EEG and CT findings were normal; antiepileptic drugs were not helpful. Demirkiran and Jankovic[23] saw five patients, three of them female. Bhatia et al.[9] reported eight sporadic cases, with age of onset 2 to 30 years. A posttraumatic case has also been reported,[79] which was responsive to oral baclofen.

Paroxysmal exercise-induced dyskinesia is probably a heterogeneous disorder, and the underlying etiologies have not been fully discovered. It is worth noting that rare patients with young-onset Parkinson's disease may present in this manner before any other signs of bradykinesia or rigidity are evident.[11] Of note, a patient with exercise-induced dyskinesias without parkinsonism had increased cerebrospinal fluid levels of homovanillic acid and 5-hydroxyindoleacetic acid after an attack, suggesting that dopaminergic transmission is increased during an attack.[4] Ictal SPECT during attacks in two familial cases showed decreased frontal and striatal perfusion, with increased cerebellar perfusion.[68]

SUMMARY AND CONCLUSIONS

Overlap between paroxysmal movement disorders and epilepsy has been noted since the end of the nineteenth century. This reflects not only the shared phenomenology of paroxysmal movement disorders and movements that occur in epilepsy, but also a common etiology of subcortical hyperexcitability. Differentiating paroxysmal movement disorders from epilepsy can be challenging, sometimes requires video-EEG monitoring, and, as demonstrated in this chapter, allows for appropriate evaluation and treatment of these patients.

References

1. Adam AM, Orinda D. Focal paroxysmal kinesigenic choreoathetosis preceding the development of Steele-Richardson-Olszewski syndrome. *J Neurol Neurosurg Psychiatry*. 1986;49:957–968.
2. Arden F. Idiopathic hypoparathyroidism. *Med J Aust*. 1953;2:217–219.
3. Barabas G, Tucker SM. Idiopathic hypoparathyroidism and paroxysmal dystonic choreoathetosis (Letter). *Ann Neurol*. 1988;24:585.
4. Barnett MH, Jarman PR, Heales SJ, et al. Further case of paroxysmal exercise-induced dystonia and some insights into pathogenesis. *Mov Disord*. 2002;17:1386–1387.
5. Bass N, Wyllie E, Comair Y, et al. Supplementary sensorimotor area seizures in children and adolescents. *J Pediatr*. 1995;126:537–544.
6. Bennett DA, Fox JH. Paroxysmal dyskinesias secondary to cerebral vascular disease—reversal with aspirin. *Clin Neuropharmacol*. 1989;12:215–216.
7. Bennett LB, Roach ES, Bowcock AM. A locus for paroxysmal kinesigenic dyskinesia maps to human chromosome 16. *Neuology*. 2000;54:125–130.
8. Berger JR, Sheremata WA, Melamed E. Paroxysmal dystonia as the initial manifestation of multiple sclerosis. *Arch Neurol*. 1984;41:747–750.
9. Bhatia KP, Soland VL, Bhatt MH, et al. Paroxysmal exercise-induced dystonia: eight new sporadic cases and a review of the literature. *Mov Disord*. 1997;12:1007–1012.
10. Bortolotti P, Schoenhuber R. Paroxysmal kinesigenic choreoathetosis. *Arch Neurol*. 1983;40:529.
11. Bozi M, Bhatia KP. Paroxysmal exercise-induced dystonia as a presenting feature of young-onset Parkinson's disease. *Mov Disord*. 2003;18:1545–1547.
12. Bressman SB, Fahn S, Burke RE. Paroxysmal non-kinesigenic dystonia. *Adv Neurol*. 1988;50:403–413.
13. Brockmann K, Dumitrescu AM, Best TT, et al. X-linked paroxysmal dyskinesia and severe global retardation caused by defective MCT8 gene. *J Neurol*. 2005;252:663–666.
14. Browne DL, Gancher ST, Nutt JG, et al. Episodic ataxia/myokymia syndrome is associated with point mutations in the human potassium channel gene, KCNA1. *Nat Genet*. 1994;8:111–112.
15. Burger LJ, Lopez RI, Elliott FA. Tonic seizures induced by movement. *Neurology*. 1972;22:656–659.
16. Burguera JA, Catala J, Casanova B. Thalamic demyelination and paroxysmal dystonia in multiple sclerosis. *Mov Disord*. 1991;6:379–381.
17. Camac A, Greene P, Khandji A. Paroxysmal kinesigenic dystonic choreoathetosis associated with a thalamic infarct. *Mov Disord*. 1990;5:235–238.
18. Cavanagh NP, Bicknell J, Howard F. Cystinuria with mental retardation and paroxysmal dyskinesia in two brothers. *Arch Dis Child*. 1974;49:662–664.
19. Collins MS, Cornish K. A survey of the prevalence of stereotypy, self-injury and aggression in children and young adults with cri du chat syndrome. *J Intellect Disabil Res*. 2002;46:133–140.
20. Coulter DL, Donofrio P. Haloperidol for nonkinesiogenic paroxysmal dyskinesia. *Arch Neurol*. 1980;37:325–326.
21. Crowell JA, Anders TF. Hypnogenic paroxysmal dystonia. *J Am Acad Child Psychiatry*. 1985;24:353–358.
22. del Carmen Garcia M, Intruvini S, Vazquez S, et al. Ictal SPECT in paroxysmal non-kinesigenic dyskinesia. Case report and review of the literature. *Parkinsonism Relat Disord*. 2000;6:119–121.
23. Demirkiran M, Jankovic J. Paroxysmal dyskinesias: clinical features and classification. *Ann Neurol*. 1995;38:571–579.
24. de Saint-Martin A, Badinand N, Picard F, et al. Diurnal and nocturnal paroxysmal dyskinesia in young children: a new entity? *Rev Neurol (Paris)*. 1997;153:262–267.
25. Drake ME Jr, Jackson RD, Miller CA. Paroxysmal choreoathetosis after head injury. *J Neurol Neurosurg Psychiatry*. 1986;49:837–843.
26. Dunn DW. Paroxysmal dystonia. *Am J Dis Child*. 1981;135:381–382.
27. Eunson LH, Rea R, Zuberi SM et al. Clinical, genetic, and expression studies of mutations in the potassium channel gene KCNA1 reveal new phenotypic variability. *Ann Neurol*. 2000;48:647–656.
28. Fahn S. The paroxysmal dyskinesias. In: Marsden CD, Fahn S, eds. *Movement Disorders 3*. Oxford: Butterworth-Heinemann; 1994:310–345.
29. Falconer M, Driver M, Serafetinides E. Seizures induced by movement: report of a case relieved by operation. *J Neurol Neurosurg Psychiatry*. 1963;26:300–307.
30. Fischbeck KH, Layzer RB. Paroxysmal choreoathetosis associated with thyrotoxicosis. *Ann Neurol*. 1979;6:453–454.
31. Fish DR, Marsden CD. Epilepsy masquerading as a movement disorder. In: Marsden CD, Fahn S, eds. *Movement Disorders 3*. Oxford: Butterworth-Heinemann; 1994:346–358.
32. Fleisher DR, Morrison A. Masturbation mimicking abdominal pain or seizures in young girls. *J Pediatr*. 1990;116:810–814.
33. Forssman H. Hereditary disorder characterized by attacks of muscular contractions, induced by alcohol amongst other factors. *Acta Med Scand*. 1961;170:517–533.

34. Franssen H, Fortgens C, Wattendorff AR, et al. Paroxysmal kinesigenic choreoathetosis and abnormal contingent negative variation. A case report. *Arch Neurol*. 1983;40:381–385.
35. Frucht S, Fahn S. Paroxysmal kinesigenic dyskinesia in infancy. *Mov Disord*. 1999;14:694–695.
36. Fuh JL, Chang DB, Wang SJ, et al. Painful tonic spasms: an interesting phenomenon in cerebral ischemia. *Acta Neurol Scand*. 1991;84:534–536.
37. Fukuyama S, Okada R. Hereditary kinesthetic reflex eilepsy; report of five families of peculiar seizures induced by sudden movements. *Adv Neurol Sci (Tokyo)*. 1967;11:168–197.
38. Fukuyama S, Okada R. Hereditary kinesthetic reflex epilepsy. Report of five families of peculiar seizures induced by sudden movements. *Adv Neurol Sci (Tokyo)*. 1967;11:168–197.
39. George MS, Pickett JB, Kohli H, et al. Paroxysmal dystonic reflex choreoathetosis after minor closed head injury. *Lancet*. 1990;336:1134–1135.
40. Gilroy J. Abnormal computed tomograms in paroxysmal kinesigenic choreoathetosis. *Arch Neurol*. 1982;39:779–780.
41. Godbout R, Montplaisir J, Rouleau I. Hypnogenic paroxysmal dystonia: epilepsy or sleep disorder? A case report. *Clin Electroencephalogr*. 1985;16:136–142.
42. Gonzalez-Alegre P, Ammache Z, Davis PH, et al. Moyamoya-induced paroxysmal dyskinesia. *Mov Disord*. 2003;18:1051–1056.
43. Goodenough DJ, Fariello RG, Annis BL, et al. Familial and acquired paroxysmal dyskinesias. A proposed classification with delineation of clinical features. *Arch Neurol*. 1978;35:827–831.
44. Gowers WR. *Epilepsy and Other Chronic Convulsive Diseases. Their Causes, Symptoms and Treatment*. New York: Dover; 1964: 75–76 [reprint of 1885 edition].
45. Gritti A, Bove D, Di Sarno AM, et al. Stereotyped movements in a group of autistic children. *Funct Neurol*. 2003;18:89–94.
46. Guerrini R, Bonanni P, Nardocci N, et al. Autosomal recessive rolandic epilepsy with paroxysmal exercise-induced dystonia and writer's cramp: delineation of the syndrome and gene mapping to chromosome 16p12–11.2. *Ann Neurol*. 1999;45:344–352.
47. Haan J, Kremer HPH, Padberg G. Paroxysmal choreoathetosis as presenting symptom of diabetes mellitus. *J Neurol Neurosurg Psychiatry*. 1988;52:133.
48. Hand PJ, McKinlay RJ, Knight MA, et al. Clinical features of a large Australian pedigree with episodic ataxia type I. *Mov Disord*. 2001;16:938–939.
49. Hattori H, Fujji T, Nigami H, et al. Co-segregation of benign infantile convulsions and paroxysmal kinesigenic choreoathetosis. *Brain Dev*. 2000;22:432–435.
50. Hirata K, Katayama S, Saito T, et al. Paroxysmal kinesigenic choreoathetosis with abnormal electroencephalogram during attacks. *Epilepsia*. 1991;32:492–494.
51. Hirsch E, Sellal F, Maton B, et al. Nocturnal paroxysmal dystonia: a clinical form of focal epilepsy. *Neurophysiol Clin*. 1994;24:207–217.
52. Hishikawa Y, Furuya E, Yamamoto J, Nan'no H. Dystonic seizures induced by movement. *Arch Psychiatr Nervenkr*. 1973;217:113–138.
53. Homan RW, Vasko MR, Blaw M. Phenytoin plasma concentrations in paroxysmal kinesigenic choreoathetosis. *Neurology*. 1980;30:673–676.
54. Horner FH, Jackson LC. Familial paroxysmal choreoathetosis. In: Barbeau A, Brunette JR, eds. *Progress in Neuro-genetics*. Amsterdam: Excerpta Medica; 1969:745–751.
55. Huang YG, Chen YC, Du F, et al. Topiramate therapy for paroxysmal kinesigenic choreoathetosis. *Movement Disord* 2005;20:75–77.
56. Huffstutter WM, Myers GJ. Paroxysmal motor dysfunction. *Ala J Med Sci*. 1983;20:311–313.
57. Hughes AJ, Lees AJ, Marsden CD. Paroxysmal dystonic head tremor. *Mov Disord*. 1991;6:85–86.
58. Jacome DE, Risko M. Photic induced-driven PLEDs in paroxysmal dystonic choreoathetosis. *Clin Electroencephalogr*. 1984;15:151–154.
59. Jen J, Kim GW, Baloh RW. Clinical spectrum of episodic ataxia type 2. *Neurology*. 2004;62:17–22.
60. Jodice C, Mantuano E, Veneziano L, et al. Episodic ataxia type 2 (EA2) and spinocerebellar ataxia type 6 (SCA6) due to CAG repeat expansion in the CACNA1A gene on chromosome 19p. *Hum Mol Genet*. 1997;6:1973–1978.
61. Joynt RJ, Green D. Tonic seizures as a manifestation of multiple sclerosis. *Arch Neurol*. 1962;6:293–299.
62. Jung SS, Chen KM, Brody JA. Paroxysmal choreoathetosis: report of Chinese cases. *Neurology*. 1973;23:749–755.
63. Kato M, Araki S. Paroxysmal kinesigenic choreoathetosis. Report of a case relieved by carbamazepine. *Arch Neurol*. 1969;20:508–513.
64. Kato M, Araki S. Paroxysmal kinesigenic choreoathetosis: report of a case relieved by carbamazepine. *Arch Neurol*. 1969;20:508–513.
65. Kertesz A. Paroxysmal kinesigenic choreoathetosis. An entity within the paroxysmal choreoathetosis syndrome. Description of 10 cases, including one autopsied. *Neurology*. 1967;17:680–690.
66. Kinast M, Erenberg G, Rothner AD. Paroxysmal choreoathetosis: report of five cases and review of the literature. *Pediatrics*. 1980;65:74–77.
67. Kishimoto K. A novel case of conditionally responsive extrapyramidal syndrome. *Ann Rep Res Inst Environ Med Nagoya Univ*. 1957;6:91–101.
68. Kluge A, Kettner B, Zschenderlein R, et al. Changes in perfusion pattern using ECD-SPECT indicate frontal lobe and cerebellar involvement in exercise-induced paroxysmal dystonia. *Mov Disord*. 1998;13:125–134.
69. Ko CH, Kong CK, Ngai WT, et al. Ictal (99m)Tc ECD SPECT in paroxysmal kinesigenic choreoathetosis. *Pediatr Neurol*. 2001;24:225–227.
70. Kotagal P, Lüders H, Morris HH, et al. Dystonic posturing in complex partial seizures of temporal lobe onset: a new lateralizing sign. *Neurology*. 1989;39:196–201.
71. Kurlan R, Behr J, Medved L, et al. Familial paroxysmal dystonic choreoathetosis: a family study. *Mov Disord*. 1987;2:187–192.
72. Kurlan R, Shoulson I. Familial paroxysmal dystonic choreoathetosis and response to alternate-day oxazepam therapy. *Ann Neurol*. 1983;13:456–457.
73. Lance JW. Sporadic and familial varieties of tonic seizures. *J Neurol Neurosurg Psychiatry*. 1963;26:51–59.
74. Lance JW. Familial paroxysmal dystonic choreoathetosis and its differentiation from related syndromes. *Ann Neurol*. 1977;2:285–293.
75. Lee BI, Lesser RP, Pippenger CE, et al. Familial paroxysmal hypnogenic dystonia. *Neurology*. 1985;35:1357–1360.
76. Lee HY, Xu Y, Huang Y, et al. The gene for paroxysmal non-kinesigenic dyskinesia encodes an enzyme in a stress response pathway. *Hum Mol Genet*. 2004;13:3161–3170.
77. Lehkuniec E, Micheli F, De Arbelaiz R, et al. Concurrent hypnogenic and reflex paroxysmal dystonia. *Mov Disord*. 1988;3:290–294.
78. Li Z, Turner RP, Smith G. Childhood paroxysmal kinesigenic dyskinesia: report of seven cases with onset at an early age. *Epilepsy Behav*. 2005;6:435–439.
79. Lim EC, Wong YS. Post-traumatic paroxysmal exercise-induced dystonia: case report and review of the literature. *Parkinsonism Relat Disord*. 2003;9:371–373.
80. Lishman WA, Symonds CD, Whitty CW, et al. Seizures induced by movement. *Brain* 1962;85:93–108.
81. Lombroso CT, Fischman A. Paroxysmal non-kinesigenic dyskinesia: pathophysiological investigations. *Epileptic Disord*. 1999;1:187–193.
82. Lou HC. Flunarizine in paroxysmal choreoathetosis. *Neuropediatrics*. 1989;20:112.
83. Lugaresi E, Cirignotta F. Hypnogenic paroxysmal dystonia: epileptic seizure or a new syndrome? *Sleep*. 1981;4:129–138.
84. Lugaresi E, Cirignotta F, Montagna P. Nocturnal paroxysmal dystonia. *J Neurol Neurosurg Psychiatry*. 1986;49:375–380.
85. Maccario M, Lustman LI. Paroxysmal nocturnal dystonia presenting as excessive daytime somnolence. *Arch Neurol*. 1990;47:291–294.
86. MacLean JB, Sassin JF. Paroxysmal vertical ocular dyskinesia. *Arch Neurol*. 1973;29:117–119.
87. Mahone EM, Bridges D, Prahme C, et al. Repetitive arm and hand movmenst (complex motor stereotypies) in children. *J Pediatr*. 2004;145:391–395.
88. Margari L, Perniola T, Illiceto G, et al. Familial paroxysmal exercise-induced dyskinesia and benign epilepsy: a clinical and neurophysiological study of an uncommon disorder. *Neuro Sci*. 2000;21:165–172.
89. Margolin DL, Marsden CD. Episodic dyskinesias and transient cerebral ischemia. *Neurology*. 1982;32:1379–1380.
90. Matthews WB. Tonic seizures in disseminated sclerosis. *Brain*. 1958;81:193–206.
91. Mayeux R, Fahn S. Paroxysmal dystonic choreoathetosis in a patient with familial ataxia. *Neurology*. 1982;32:1184–1186.
92. Meierkord H, Fish DR, Smith SJM, et al. Is nocturnal paroxysmal dystonia a form of frontal lobe epilepsy? *Mov Disord*. 1992;7:38–42.
93. Merchut MP, Brumlik J. Painful tonic spasms caused by putaminal infarction. *Stroke*. 1986;17:1319–1321.
94. Micheli F, Fernandez Pardal MM, Casas Parera I, et al. Sporadic paroxysmal dystonic choreoathetosis associated with basal ganglia calcifications. *Ann Neurol*. 1986;20:750.
95. Milandre L, Brosset C, Gabriel B, et al. Mouvements involontaires transitoires et infarctus thalamiques. (Transient dyskinesias associated with thalamic infarcts—report of five cases.) *Rev Neurol (Paris)*. 1993;149:402–406.
96. Mink JW, Neil JJ. Masturbation mimicking paroxysmal dystonia or dyskinesia in a young girl. *Mov Disord*. 1995;10:518–520.
97. Mir P, Huang YZ, Gilio F, et al. Abnormal cortical and spinal inhibition in paroxysmal kinesigenic dyskinesia. *Brain*. 2005;128:291–299.
98. Morley JB. Movement-induced epilepsy: three case reports and comparison with a case of hemiballismus. *Proc Aust Assoc Neurol*. 1970;7:19–24.
99. Mount LA, Reback S. Familial paroxysmal choreoathetosis. *Arch Neurol Psychiatry*. 1940;44:841–847.
100. Mushet GR, Dreifuss FE. Paroxysmal dyskinesia. A case responsive to benztropine mesylate. *Arch Dis Child*. 1967;42:654–656.
101. Nardocci N, Lamperti E, Rumi V, et al. Typical and atypical forms of paroxysmal choreoathetosis. *Dev Med Child Neurol*. 1989;31:670–674.
102. Nath A, Jankovic J, Pettigrew LC. Movement disorders and AIDS. *Neurology*. 1987;37:37–41.
103. Nechay A, Ross LM, Stephenson JBP, et al. Gratification disorder ("infantile masturbation"): a review. *Arch Dis Child*. 2004;89:225–226.
104. Newman RP, Kinkel WR. Paroxysmal choreoathetosis due to hypoglycemia. *Arch Neurol*. 1984;41:341–342.
105. Nijssen PCG, Tijssen CC. Stimulus-sensitive paroxysmal dyskinesias associated with a thalamic infarct. *Mov Disord*. 1992;7:364–366.
106. Perez-Borja C, Tassinari AC, Swanson AG. Paroxysmal choreoathetosis and seizure induced by movement (reflex epilepsy). *Epilepsia*. 1967;8:260–270.

107. Perlmutter JS, Raichle ME. Pure hemidystonia with basal ganglion abnormalities on positron emission tomography. *Ann Neurol.* 1984;15:228–233.
108. Perniola T, Margari L, de Iaco MG, et al. Familial paroxysmal exercise-induced dyskinesia, epilepsy, and mental retardation in a family with autosomal dominant inheritance. *Mov Disord.* 2001;16:724–730.
109. Plant G. Focal paroxysmal kinesigenic choreoathetosis. *J Neurol Neurosurg Psychiatry.* 1983;46:345–348.
110. Plant GT, Williams AC, Earl CJ, et al. Familial paroxysmal dystonia induced by exercise. *J Neurol Neurosurg Psychiatry.* 1984;47:275–279.
111. Pourfar M, Guerrini R, Parain D, et al. Classification conundrums in paroxysmal dyskinesias: a new subtype or variations on classic themes? *Mov Disord.* 2005;20:1047–1051.
112. Przuntek H, Monninger P. Therapeutic aspects of kinesigenic paroxysmal choreoathetosis and familial paroxysmal choreoathetosis of the Mount and Reback type. *J Neurol.* 1983;230:163–169.
113. Rajna P, Kundra O, Halasz P. Vigilance level-dependent tonic seizures: epilepsy or sleep disorder? A case report. *Epilepsia.* 1983;24:725–733.
114. Richards RN, Barnett HJ. Paroxysmal dystonic choreoathetosis. A family study and review of the literature. *Neurology.* 1968;18:461–469.
115. Richardson JC, Howes JL, Celinski MJ, et al. Kinesigenic choreoathetosis due to brain injury. *Can J Neurol Sci.* 1987;14:626–628.
116. Ringman JM, Jankovic J. Occurrence of tics in Asperger's syndrome and autistic disorder. *J Child Neurol.* 2000;15:394–400.
117. Robin JJ. Paroxysmal choreoathetosis following head injury. *Ann Neurol.* 1977;2:447–448.
118. Roos R, Wintzen AR, Vielvoye G, et al. Paroxysmal kinesiogenic choreoathetosis as presenting symptom of multiple sclerosis. *J Neurol Neurosurg Psychiatry.* 1991;54:657–658.
119. Rosen JA. Paroxysmal choreoathetosis associated with perinatal hypoxic encephalopathy. *Arch Neurol.* 1964;11:385–387.
120. Schmidt BJ, Pillay N. Paroxysmal dyskinesia associated with hypoglycemia. *Can J Neurol Sci.* 1993;20:151–153.
121. Sellal F, Hirsch E, Maquet P, et al. Postures et mouvements anormaux paroxystiques au cours du sommeil: dystonie paroxystique hypnogenique ou epilepsie partielle ? (Abnormal paroxysmal movements during sleep: hypnogeneic paroxysmal dystonia or focal epilesy?). *Rev Neurol (Paris).* 1991;147:121–128.
122. Sethi KD, Hess DC, Huffnagle VH, et al. Acetazolamide treatment of paroxysmal dystonia in central demyelinating disease. *Neurology.* 1992;42:919–921.
123. Shirane S, Sasaki M, Kogure D, et al. *J Neurol Neurosurg Psychiatry.* 2001;71:408–410.
124. Soffer D, Licht A, Yaar I, et al. Paroxysmal choreoathetosis as a presenting symptom in idiopathic hypoparathyroidism. *J Neurol Neurosurg Psychiatry.* 1977;40:692–694.
125. Spacey S, Materek LA, Szczgielski BI, et al. Two novel CACNA1A gene mutations associated with episodic ataxia type 2 and interictal dystonia. *Arch Neurol.* 2005;62:314–316.
126. Spiller WG. Subcortical epilepsy. *Brain.* 1927;50:171–187.
127. Stevens H. Paroxysmal choreo-athetosis. *Arch Neurol.* 1966;14:415–420.
128. Strupp M, Kalla R, Dichgans M, et al. Treatment of episodic ataxia type 2 with the potassium channel blocker 4-aminopyridine. *Neurology.* 2004;62:1623–1625.
129. Suber DA, Riley TL. Valproic acid and normal computerized tomographic scan in kinesigenic familial paroxysmal choreoathetosis. *Arch Neurol.* 1980;37:327.
130. Swoboda KJ, Soong B, McKenna C, et al. Paroxysmal kinesigenic dyskinesia and infantile convulsions: clinical and linkage sutides. *Neurology* 2000;55:224–230.
131. Tabaee-Zadeh MJ, Frame B, Kapphahn K. Kinesiogenic choreoathetosis and idiopathic hypoparathyroidism. *N Engl J Med.* 1972;286:762–763.
132. Tartara A, Manni R, Piccolo G. A long-lasting CBZ-controlled case of hypnogenic paroxysmal dystonia. *Ital J Neurol Sci.* 1988;9:73–76.
133. Tinuper P, Cerullo A, Cirignotta F, et al. Nocturnal paroxysmal dystonia with short-lasting attacks: three cases with evidence for an epileptic frontal lobe origin of seizures. *Epilepsia.* 1990;31:549–556.
134. Tsao CY. Effective treatment with oxcarbazepine in paroxysmal kinesigenic choreoathetosis. *J Child Neurol.* 2004;19:300–301.
135. Valente EM, Spacey SD, Wali GM, et al. A second paroxysmal kinesigenic choreoathetosis locus (EKD2) mapping on 16q13–q22.1 indicates a family of genes which give rise to paroxysmal disorders on human chromosome 16. *Brain.* 2000;123:2040–2045.
136. Verheul GAM, Tyssen CC. Multiple sclerosis occurring with paroxysmal unilateral dystonia. *Mov Disord.* 1990;5:352–353.
137. Vincent FM. Hyperglycemia-induced hemichoreoathetosis: the presenting manifestation of a vascular malformation of the lenticular nucleus. *Neurosurgery.* 1986;18:787–790.
138. Wali GM. Paroxysmal hemidystonia induced by prolonged exercise and cold. *J Neurol Neurosurg Psychiatry.* 1992;55:236–237.
139. Walker ES. Familial paroxysmal dystonic choreoathetosis: a neurologic disorder simulating psychiatric illness. *Johns Hopkins Med J.* 1981;148:108–113.
140. Waller DA. Paroxysmal kinesigenic choreoathetosis or hysteria? *Am J Psychiatry.* 1977;134:1439–1440.
141. Watson RT, Scott WR. Paroxysmal kinesigenic choreoathetosis and brainstem atrophy. *Arch Neurol.* 1979;36:522.
142. Weber MB. Familial paroxysmal dystonia. *J Nerv Ment Dis.* 1967;145:221–226.
143. Whitty CWM, Lishman WA, FitzGibbon JP. Seizures induced by movement: a form of reflex epilepsy. *Lancet.* 1964;1:1403–1406.
144. Whitty CWM, Lishman WA, FitzGibbon JP. Seizures induced by movement: a form of reflex epilepsy. *Lancet.* 1964;1:1405–1406.
145. Wilson SAK. The Morrison lectures on nervous semeiology, with special reference to epilepsy. Lecture III. Symptoms indicating increase of neural function. *Br Med J.* 1930;2:90–94.
146. Winer JB, Fish DR, Sawyers D, et al. A movement disorder as a presenting feature of recurrent hypoglycemia. *Mov Disord.* 1990;5:176–177.
147. Yamada K, Goto S, Soyama N, et al. Complete suppression of paroxysmal nonkinesigenic dyskinesia by globus pallidus internus pallidal stimulation. *Mov Disord.* 2006;21:576–580.
148. Yamamoto K, Kawazawa S. Basal ganglion calcification in paroxysmal dystonic choreoathetosis. *Ann Neurol.* 1987;22:556.
149. Yang ML, Fullwood E, Goldstein J, Mink JM. Masturbation in infancy and early childhood presenting as a movement disorder: 12 cases and a review of the literature. *Pediatrics.* 2005;116:1427–1432.

CHAPTER 279 ■ SENSORY DISORDERS

CARL W. BAZIL

INTRODUCTION

Because partial seizures can begin anywhere in the cerebral cortex, their manifestations are diverse, and because large portions of the cortex are devoted to primary and secondary interpretation of sensory stimuli, a wide variety of visual, auditory, vestibular, gustatory, and tactile symptoms can be features of epilepsy. Because seizure-related sensory manifestations are so varied, other sensory abnormalities may sometimes be confused with epilepsy. In distinguishing epileptic from nonepileptic sensory symptoms on clinical grounds, a few general principles are important. First, the context of the symptom must be considered. Purely sensory seizures, without other manifestations at least some of the time, are uncommon, so a careful search for other symptoms or signs supportive of epilepsy should be performed. For example, if a single secondarily generalized seizure begins with focal numbness, it is much more likely that the preceding dozens of similar episodes of isolated numbness were actually simple partial seizures. Second, the time course of the patient's sensory event must be considered. Is it truly paroxysmal? Is the symptom recurrent and unprovoked? How long do the symptoms last? In general, epileptic seizures are unprovoked, paroxysmal, and 1 to 3 minutes in duration. Third, the quality of the sensory experience is relevant. Seizures typically consist of "positive" changes rather than "negative" ones, and this may be helpful in identifying nonepileptic sensory phenomena. For example, visions of swirling colors and shapes are more likely to have an epileptic origin than loss of vision, and localized tingling paresthesias are more likely to be epilepsy than diffuse numbness. Finally, the distribution of the sensory disturbance must be considered and whether it makes anatomic sense. Partial seizures arise from the cerebral cortex, and initial symptoms can therefore often be localized to a fairly discrete brain area. Subsequent evolution of symptoms generally involves adjacent cortex. Thus, visual symptoms typically involve one hemifield. Somatosensory seizures are more likely to involve the face and hand (because these have large areas of representation in the cortex) and should be restricted to one side of the body, at least at onset (insular seizures are an exception[7]).

It is clear that an accurate, detailed description of paroxysmal sensory changes is critical in separating epileptic events from a wide variety of nonepileptic conditions. Important sensory conditions that may be confused with epilepsy are listed in Table 1, and additional testing useful in distinguishing these conditions from epilepsy is listed in Table 2. This chapter describes all of these conditions in further detail and explains how they can best be distinguished from epilepsy.

DISORDERS OF OLFACTION

One of the classic (although not the most common) initial symptoms of seizures originating in the medial temporal lobe is a paroxysmal episode involving an unpleasant odor. Typical descriptions include references to burnt rubber, sulfur, and organic solvents,[39] although more commonly the patient is unable to provide a specific analogy. Such "auras" may occur in the absence of other seizure manifestations as an isolated simple partial seizure. However, virtually all such patients experience a complex partial or secondarily generalized seizure at some point, especially if untreated, and this event resolves any diagnostic uncertainty.

Because virtually all abnormalities of the olfactory system result in loss of smell rather than an abnormal sensation of smell, these are not commonly mistaken for epilepsy. The one important exception is psychiatric illness. In such cases, patients will frequently report abnormal smells in association with psychogenic seizures. Although these may superficially resemble the foul odors of temporal lobe epilepsy, more commonly they are described much more precisely and are even reported as pleasant. Thus, a floral scent has been described,[33] as have smells of "perfume," "food," and "pure oxygen." For a more extensive discussion of these seizures, the reader is referred to the section on psychiatric disturbances.

DISORDERS OF VISION

The sudden visual loss that accompanies a *vertebrobasilar transient ischemic attack* (TIA) is not easily confused with an epileptic seizure. Transient ischemic attacks usually last longer than typical seizures. Both, however, may be associated with vertigo, impaired speech, or altered consciousness. The distinction is discussed more fully in Chapter 275. Recurrent, sometimes stereotyped visual hallucinations may also occur in cases of *cerebral amyloid angiopathy*[20] (see also later discussion).

The complex and sometimes confusing relationship between *migraine* and epilepsy is also discussed more fully elsewhere (see Chapter 274). Because of its high prevalence, the visual symptoms of migraine represent a common situation in which the sensory symptoms of another disease may be mistaken for epilepsy. The phenomena of the two disorders can be similar, although the classic hemifield scotoma seen in migraine is rare with epilepsy. On the other hand, patients with migraine may see stars, colored lights, or patterns similar to those seen by patients with epileptic seizures arising from the occipital or posterior temporal lobe.

Other unusual causes of visual hallucinations that can occasionally be confused with epilepsy include withdrawal from alcohol or sedative drugs and psychiatric disease. In both, the images are typically well formed, but their variability and long duration (hours to days rather than minutes) usually distinguish them from epilepsy, even in the absence of other clinical information. Hallucinations occurring exclusively during the transitions between sleep and wakefulness (hypnic hallucinations) are often visual. These can be associated with narcolepsy, but also occur sporadically in otherwise normal individuals and can be precipitated by sleep deprivation.[2]

Peduncular hallucinations, a more unusual cause of paroxysmal visual symptoms, were first described by Lhermitte.[32] These typically occur in the evening and may last for hours. They are quite vivid and well formed; examples include

TABLE 1

SENSORY DISTURBANCES THAT CAN MIMIC SEIZURES

Olfactory disorders
Visual disorders
Migraine
Transient ischemic attack
Peduncular hallucination
Other visual hallucinations
Hearing and vestibular disorders
Auditory hallucination
Dizziness
Benign positional vertigo
Paroxysmal vertigo of childhood
Ménière disease
Somatosensory disorders
Transient ischemic attack
Headache
Transient compression neuropathies
Trigeminal neuralgia
Paroxysmal sensory symptoms of multiple sclerosis
Amyloid angiopathy
Gastrointestinal symptoms
Psychogenic sensory symptoms

a brightly colored parrot[9] or other animals.[1,32,41] Affected patients may have alterations in consciousness, adding to the confusion with seizures. Associated symptoms such as cranial nerve palsies, hemiplegia, hemianesthesia, or ataxia are seen in many patients. Hypomania and increased tone occur often,[41] which may also help to distinguish peduncular hallucinations from seizures. The condition results from infarction of the thalamus or the pars reticulata of the substantia nigra.[9]

DISORDERS OF HEARING AND THE VESTIBULAR SYSTEM

As with olfactory disturbances, most seizures that affect hearing and balance manifest the "positive" features of auditory hallucinations or distortions and vertigo. Therefore, it is these symptoms that are most often mistaken for epilepsy. Auditory hallucinations are common in schizophrenia (see Chapter 287) and also occur occasionally in acute withdrawal states from alcohol and other sedative drugs. In both cases, the variability of the hallucinations in any single patient and the particular clinical setting usually make the distinction from epilepsy fairly easy. Auditory hallucinations are rare in vascular disease. These may be transient, and the absence of psychiatric disease can lead to confusion with epilepsy. Auditory hallucinations, including musical hallucinations, can occur with hearing loss, drug intoxication, or drug withdrawal.[14]

Episodes of dizziness and, in particular, paroxysmal vertigo are more likely to be confused with epilepsy. Dizziness is a very common complaint, especially in the elderly, and although only a small fraction of cases may be confused with epilepsy, this still represents a substantial number. The causes of vertigo are quite diverse and may involve either central or peripheral vestibular mechanisms. Peripheral vertigo can result from cupulolithiasis, head trauma, acceleration injuries, and middle ear infections and typically lasts seconds to minutes. Central vertigo can be caused by drugs, cerebrovascular disease, tumors, and multiple sclerosis and typically lasts several days,[17] and therefore these would not typically be confused with epilepsy. The most common disorder is *benign positional vertigo*, which is usually idiopathic, the result of head trauma, or related to a viral infection.[5] Unlike vertigo associated with seizures, paroxysmal nonepileptic vertigo is rarely unprovoked. The diagnosis is made when positional changes (including Hallpike and Barany maneuvers) elicit the patient's typical symptoms with accompanying nystagmus. Paroxysmal vertigo is also usually of longer duration than vertiginous symptoms seen with epilepsy.

Benign paroxysmal vertigo of childhood is characterized by sudden, brief episodes of vertigo and nystagmus. It was first described by Basser.[6] The syndrome occurs most often in children, usually beginning after 4 years of age, but occasionally before age 1 year; it typically resolves by age 10 years. Episodes last from 20 seconds to 3 minutes and may be accompanied by nausea, vomiting, or headache. The child may stumble or fall because of disequilibrium and, not surprisingly, becomes frightened or confused, features that may further suggest a complex partial seizure. The typical frequency is one to five spells per month.[13] Results of audiologic, otologic, and neurologic examinations are normal. Findings of caloric/rotatory tests may be normal[13] or abnormal.[12] The electroencephalogram (EEG) is uniformly normal. Nystagmus occurs during the actual episodes and, if observed, helps in the distinction from seizures. Benign paroxysmal vertigo is associated with migraine[13,15,26] and may perhaps be a variant of basilar migraine. The disorder most likely results from a transient disturbance in the vertebrobasilar circulation that produces central vestibular dysfunction.[16]

In adults, *Ménière disease*, especially in its early stages, is sometimes confused with epilepsy. In the famous case of Vincent van Gogh, debate continues about whether he had Ménière disease or epilepsy.[4,35] Like seizures, attacks of Ménière disease are often preceded by a warning, typically a nonspecific feeling of fullness in the ears. Unlike seizures, attacks are usually accompanied by nystagmus, hearing loss, and tinnitus. Episodes of vertigo may last for hours but occasionally last only a few minutes. Patients may feel weak and unsteady after the episode, but there is never any alteration in consciousness during or after the attacks.[44] Spells may be so sudden and so severe that the patient actually falls to the ground (although without loss of consciousness). Diagnostic tests such as electronystagmography, audiometry, or auditory-evoked potentials may be helpful in confirming a peripheral vestibular disorder.

TABLE 2

ADDITIONAL DIAGNOSTIC TESTING USEFUL IN SENSORY DISORDERS

Test	Useful condition(s)
MRI	Stroke, TIA, multiple scerosis, brainstem lesion; cerebral amyloid angiopathy
Audiometry	Hearing loss, BPV, Ménière disease
Electronysagmography; rotary chair testing	BPV
BAER	Brainstem lesion
EMG/nerve conduction testing	Peripheral nerve diseases

BAER, brainstem auditory-evoked potentials; BPV, benign positional vertigo; EMG, electromyography; TIA, transient ischemic attack.

DISORDERS OF THE SOMATOSENSORY SYSTEM

Purely sensory transient ischemic attacks (TIAs) are not uncommon and are manifested by a variety of sensory complaints involving the face and limbs. Although patients usually report numbness, they may also describe a variety of "positive" symptoms, such as pain, tingling, heat, or paresthesias. Because many TIAs resolve within 5 minutes, shorter attacks may be confused with epilepsy. The reader is referred to Chapter 275 for a more complete description of TIAs.

Similar symptoms may be seen in *cerebral amyloid angiopathy* (CAA), a common cause of lobar hemorrhage in older, normotensive patients.[24,42] The disease is characterized by deposition of β-amyloid in the media of small and medium-sized cerebral arteries. Confusion with epilepsy may occur in the prodromal stages, when the patient has recurrent spells of numbness or tingling that spread over the body in minutes. Transient sensory symptoms can occur repeatedly in the same area,[20] mimicking the stereotypy found in partial seizures. Some authors have suggested that "CAA spells" are actually seizures, but most have concluded that they are more likely to be the result of spreading depression,[20] perhaps triggered by small hemorrhages. Although definitive diagnosis requires histologic confirmation, patients with CAA frequently have multiple cortical hemorrhages and are more likely to show the apolipoprotein E e-2 allele than is a population-based sample.[19] Distinction from seizures is clearly important, but CAA must also be differentiated from TIAs because anticoagulation leads to an increased risk for lobar hemorrhage. Finally, patients with CAA can also have true epileptic seizures,[8,20,23] which poses further diagnostic problems for the clinician.

Neuropathies rarely produce symptoms that are confused with seizures. The manifestations of neuropathies are typically indolent rather than paroxysmal, progressive or static rather than recurrent, and involve areas that are uncommonly symptomatic during seizures (e.g., stocking-glove distribution, mononeuritis multiplex). In unusual cases, a particular nerve may be recurrently and reversibly affected, and a patient may offer a description of repeated numbness or tingling in a particular area, which may seem paroxysmal. Examples include meralgia paresthetica, ulnar neuropathy, and carpal tunnel syndrome. These cases can usually be distinguished from epilepsy by careful history; if diagnostic uncertainty persists, electromyographic evaluation will resolve the issue.

Patients occasionally complain of paroxysmal head pain that can resemble a seizure. Headache as a sole manifestation of seizure is, however, exceedingly rare.[25,29] More commonly, headache occurs as a nonspecific prodrome, aura, or postictal phenomenon. Because ictal headache is so uncommon, even unusual types of headache are not usually confused with epilepsy.

Trigeminal neuralgia (*tic douloureux*) is a relatively common condition characterized by paroxysmal attacks of severe pain in the distribution of one or more branches of the trigeminal nerve. As in epilepsy, attacks are sudden and unpredictable, and are usually brief in duration. Sometimes, however, attacks of trigeminal neuralgia last for hours, a duration that is very atypical of seizures. Unlike epileptic seizures, attacks of trigeminal neuralgia occur frequently in clusters. The maxillary branch of the trigeminal nerve is involved most often; the ophthalmic division is rarely involved in isolation.[28] Carbamazepine is the most effective medical treatment; phenytoin can also be used. Attacks of trigeminal neuralgia are frequently provoked by sensory stimuli (e.g., touch, cold) to the affected region, which may suggest a form of "stimulus-sensitive" epilepsy. In fact, Pagni[36] proposed that trigeminal neuralgia represents a form of stimulus-evoked epilepsy. Classic trigeminal neuralgia is easily distinguished from epilepsy by the distribution, time course, and quality of the attacks. Atypical presentations, however, are occasionally mistaken for simple partial seizures, and the incorrect diagnosis seems to be further supported by a good response to antiepileptic drugs.

Paroxysmal sensory symptoms, including trigeminal neuralgia, can occur in patients with *multiple sclerosis* (MS). A common paroxysmal disturbance is burning dysesthesia, often restricted to one limb, that lasts <1 minute and often only a few seconds. There are no associated convulsive movements. Attacks may be induced by voluntary movements and respond well to carbamazepine.[46] Episodes of painful chorea, dystonia, and various tonic postures also occur in MS.[27,34,38] These probably arise from an ectopic generation of action potentials in demyelinated axons, with subsequent spread along sensorimotor pathways.[46]

Gastrointestinal symptoms, such as nausea and vomiting, are treated first by general practitioners or internists, although these can be manifestations of simple partial seizures. Gastrointestinal reflux is unlikely to be confused with epilepsy in adults from whom an accurate history may be obtained. It can pose a diagnostic problem in young children, in whom episodes of reflux may be accompanied by vomiting, cyanosis, and posturing simulating epilepsy.[37] In children, recurrent abdominal pain may develop at about 5 years of age. Episodes usually last several hours and are not associated with any gastrointestinal diagnostic abnormalities.[3] Cyclic vomiting is seen at the age of 2 years and disappears after 3 to 4 years.[22] These episodes are frequently accompanied by severe nausea and abdominal pain. Both recurrent abdominal pain and cyclic vomiting are associated with migraine[37] but not epilepsy. They were formerly often misdiagnosed as "abdominal epilepsy."

PSYCHOGENIC SENSORY SYMPTOMS

Psychiatric disorders are discussed in Chapters 281 through 287; however, they deserve special mention in a discussion of sensory phenomena. Because sensory symptoms are usually not accompanied by objective changes, the clinician often must rely entirely on the history for an initial diagnosis. Particularly in the case of a patient with psychiatric illness, this description may be vague and unhelpful, adding to the difficulty in distinguishing epileptic from nonepileptic events.

Psychogenic nonepileptic seizures (PNES) are paroxysmal alterations in movement, sensation, or experience that resemble epileptic seizures but arise from purely psychological causes (see also Chapter 282). Although up to 80% of patients with PNES have motor manifestations,[18,21,30] in other cases, PNES are characterized by sensory changes,[43] including numbness, paresthesias, pain, odors, tastes, and visual/auditory hallucinations.[21,31,33] Psychogenic nonepileptic seizures usually have a more gradual onset and longer duration than epileptic seizures, but these features alone cannot reliably be used to make the distinction from epilepsy.[31]

The presenting symptoms of *panic disorder*, with or without hyperventilation, may include dizziness, vertigo, perioral tingling, numbness or tingling of the hands, generalized weakness, or syncope, and panic disorder may be confused with epilepsy.[40,] Paroxysms of unexplained fear are typical in panic disorder; these may be confused with a limbic seizure. For a more complete discussion, see Chapter 285.

Distinguishing PNES or panic disorder from epileptic seizures may be difficult. Stereotyped attacks favor epileptic seizures, although subjective descriptions of purely sensory symptoms are often difficult to interpret. When diagnosis remains unclear following a careful history, video-EEG monitoring may be required to make the distinction.

SUMMARY AND CONCLUSIONS

Many sensory symptoms and disorders have some resemblance to epilepsy and, in certain circumstances, may be confused with it. In most cases, careful history taking supplemented by appropriate diagnostic testing provides a reliable basis for making the distinction. In some patients, recording one or more of the patient's habitual events with concurrent electroencephalography (video-EEG monitoring) may be required to distinguish epileptic from nonepileptic events reliably. A time-linked ictal discharge during an episode is diagnostic of epilepsy. False-negative results may occur with simple partial seizures, which have no scalp EEG correlate in the majority of cases.[11] In such instances, however, video recording and careful clinical testing should reliably establish the clinical semiology and determine whether this is consistent with an epileptic seizure. Prolonged EEG recordings may also show interictal epileptiform discharges; these strongly suggest a diagnosis of epilepsy,[10,47] but their detection is not equivalent to demonstration of a seizure discharge occurring simultaneously with the symptom in question. When spells occur on a daily basis, 6- to 8-hour EEG with video monitoring on an outpatient basis is a reasonable alternative. Infrequent attacks usually require inpatient video-EEG monitoring, and antiepileptic drugs (if used) may need to be withdrawn. Recent advances in extended outpatient EEG monitoring are making this an alternative to inpatient monitoring in selected cases, although these still suffer from the lack of trained personel to ensure proper recording at all times and to test the patient appropriately during spells.

References

1. Alajouanine TH, Thurel R, Durupt L. Lésion protubérantielle basse d'origine vasculaire et hallucinose. *Rev Neurol (Paris)*. 1944;76:90–91.
2. Aldrich M. The clinical spectrum of narcolepsy and idiopathic hypersomnia. *Neurology*. 1996;46:393–401.
3. Apley J, Naish N. Recurrent abdominal pains: a field survey of 1000 school children. *Arch Dis Child*. 1958;33:165–170.
4. Arenberg IK, Countryman LF, Bernstein LH, et al. Van Gogh had Meniere's disease and not epilepsy. *JAMA*. 1990;264:491–493.
5. Baloh RW, Honrubia V, Jacobson K. Benign positional vertigo: clinical and oculographic features in 240 cases. *Neurology*. 1987;37:371–378.
6. Basser LS. Benign paroxysmal vertigo of childhood (a variety of vestibular neuronitis). *Brain*. 1964;87:141–152.
7. Berthier ML, Starkstein SE, Nogues MA, et al. Bilateral sensory seizures in a patient with pain asymbolia. *Ann Neurol*. 1990;27:109.
8. Briceno CE, Resch L, Bernstein M. Cerebral amyloid angiopathy presenting as a mass lesion. *Stroke*. 1987;18:234–239.
9. Caplan LR. "Top of the basilar" syndrome. *Neurology*. 1980;30:72–79.
10. Delgado-Escueta AV. Epileptogenic paroxysms: modern approaches and clinical correlations. *Neurology*. 1979;29:1014–1022.
11. Devinsky O, Sato S, Kufta CV, et al. Electroencephalographic studies of simple partial seizures with subdural electrode recordings. *Neurology*. 1989;39:527–533.
12. Dunn DW, Snyder CH. Benign paroxysmal vertigo of childhood. *Am J Dis Child*. 1976;130:1099–1100.
13. Eeg-Olofsson O, Lindskog U, Andersson B. Benign paroxysmal vertigo in childhood. *Acta Otolaryngol*. 1982;93:283–289.
14. Evers S, Ellger T. The clinical spectrum of musical hallucinations. *J Neurol Sci*. 2004;227:55–65.
15. Fenichel GM. Migraine as a cause of benign paroxysmal vertigo of childhood. *J Pediatr*. 1967;71:114–115.
16. Finkelhor BK, Harker LA. Benign paroxysmal vertigo of childhood. *Laryngoscope*. 1987;97:1161–1163.
17. Gizzi M, Diamond SP. Dizziness or vestibular problems resembling seizures. In: Kaplan PW, Fisher RS, eds. *Imitators of Epilepsy*, 2nd ed. New York: Demos; 2005:145–161.
18. Gates JR, Ramani V, Whalen S, et al. Ictal characteristics of pseudoseizures. *Arch Neurol*. 1985;42:1183–1187.
19. Greenberg SM, Briggs ME, Hyman BT, et al. Apolipoprotein E E-2 is associated with the presence and earlier onset of hemorrhage in cerebral amyloid angiopathy. *Stroke*. 1996;27:1333–1337.
20. Greenberg SM, Vonsattel JPG, Stakes JW, et al. The clinical spectrum of cerebral amyloid angiopathy: presentations without lobar hemorrhage. *Neurology*. 1993;43:2073–2079.
21. Gulick TA, Spinks IP, King DW. Pseudoseizures: ictal phenomena. *Neurology*. 1982;32:24–30.
22. Hammond J. The late sequelae of recurrent vomiting of childhood. *Dev Med Child Neurol*. 1974;16:15–22.
23. Hendricks HT, Franke CL, Theunissen PHMH. Cerebral amyloid angiopathy: diagnosis by MRI and brain biopsy. *Neurology*. 1990;40:1308–1310.
24. Ishii N, Nishihara Y, Horie A. Amyloid angiopathy and lobar cerebral haemorrhage. *J Neurol Neurosurg Psychiatry*. 1984;47:1203–1210.
25. Jonas AD. Headaches as seizure equivalents. *Headache*. 1966;6:78–87.
26. Koehler B. Benign paroxysmal vertigo of childhood: a migraine equivalent. *Eur J Pediatr*. 1980;134:149–151.
27. Kuroiwa Y, Shibasaki H. Painful tonic seizures in multiple sclerosis. Treatment with diphenylhydantoin and carbamazepine. *Folia Psychiatr Neurol Jpn*. 1968;22:107–119.
28. Lange DJ, Trojaborg W, Rowland LP. Peripheral and cranial nerve lesions. In: Rowland LP, ed. *Merritt's Textbook of Neurology*. Baltimore: Williams & Wilkins; 1995:461–484.
29. Laplante P, Saint-Hilaire JM, Bouvier G. Headache as an epileptic manifestation. *Neurology*. 1983;33:1493–1495.
30. Lempert T, Schmidt D. Natural history and outcome of psychogenic seizures: a clinical study in 50 patients. *J Neurol*. 1990;237:35–38.
31. Lesser RP. Psychogenic seizures. *Neurology*. 1996;46:1499–1507.
32. Lhermitte S. Syndrome de la calotte du pédoncule cérébral: les troubles psycho-sensoriels dans les lésions du mésocéphale. *Rev Neurol (Paris)*. 1922;38:1359–1365.
33. Luther JS, McNamara JO, Carwile S, et al. Pseudoepileptic seizures: methods and video analysis to aid diagnosis. *Ann Neurol*. 1982;12:458–462.
34. Matthews WB. Tonic seizure in disseminated sclerosis. *Brain*. 1958;81:193–206.
35. Monroe RR. The episodic psychoses of Vincent van Gogh. *J Nerv Ment Dis*. 1978;166:480–488.
36. Pagni CA. The origin of tic douloureux: a unified view. *J Neurosurg Sci*. 1993;37:185–194.
37. Rothner AD. Not everything that shakes is epilepsy. *Cleve Clin J Med*. 1989;56(Suppl Pt 2):S206–S213.
38. Shibasaki H, Kiroiwa Y. Painful tonic seizure in multiple sclerosis. *Arch Neurol*. 1974;30:47–51.
39. So NK. Epileptic auras. In: Wyllie E, ed. *The Treatment of Epilepsy: Principles and Practices*. Philadelphia: Lea & Febiger; 1993:369–377.
40. Trimble MR. Pseudoseizures. *Neurol Clin*. 1986;4:449–531.
41. van Bogaert L. L'hallucinose pédonculaire. *Rev Neurol (Paris)*. 1927;48:608–617.
42. Vinters HV. Cerebral amyloid angiopathy: a critical review. *Stroke*. 1987;18:311–324.
43. Volow MR. Pseudoseizures: an overview. *South Med J*. 1986;79:600–607.
44. Wazen JJ. Meniere syndrome. In: Rowland LP, ed. *Merritt's Textbook of Neurology*. Baltimore: Williams & Wilkins; 1995:873–874.
45. Williams D. The borderland of epilepsy revisited. *Brain*. 1975;98:1–12.
46. Yabuki S, Hayabara T. Paroxysmal dysesthesia in multiple sclerosis. *Folia Psychiatr Neurol Jpn*. 1979;33:97–104.
47. Zivin L, Ajmone-Marsan C. Incidence and prognostic significance of "epileptiform" activity in the EEG of nonepileptic subjects. *Brain*. 1968;91:751–778.

CHAPTER 280 ■ NONEPILEPTIC NEUROLOGIC PAROXYSMAL DISORDERS AND EPISODIC SYMPTOMS IN INFANTS

NATALIO FEJERMAN

INTRODUCTION

Misdiagnosis of epileptic seizures in young children is frequent and generally due to considering various paroxysmal or episodic symptoms as epileptic when they are not.[12,59,61,107]

Nonneurologic paroxysmal disorders, such as breath-holding spells, syncope, and psychogenic events, are discussed in Chapter 273. Most of the neurologic conditions listed in Table 1 are uncommon. Nevertheless, they can be an important part of the differential diagnoses of epileptic seizures. Table 1 groups various symptoms and conditions according to their general nature.[116]

ENHANCED NORMAL PHENOMENA

Sporadic Myoclonic Jerks During Sleep (Hypnic Jerks) or Physiologic Sleep Myoclonus

These are universally present in normal people. They appear during the initial stages of sleep and also during rapid eye movement (REM) sleep. Typically, they manifest as slight contractions of face muscles and brief movements of the fingers or toes. There are no electroencephalographic (EEG) correlates.[69] Massive bilateral jerks, mainly involving the legs, can occur during the initial stages of sleep in association with a change in sleep state or arousal.[114]

Localized Myoclonus During Wakefulness

This represents a rare physiologic phenomenon that usually occurs during and after muscular fatigue and when the linear or a particular group of muscles are placed in unsupported postures. The affected muscle groups may vary, but in any individual, each episode of myoclonus involves the same muscles. The myoclonic jerks last a few seconds to several minutes. There are no EEG changes accompanying the myoclonus, and a spinal origin has been suggested.[69] Even hiccoughs, considered a physiologic phenomenon, may occasionally be intense and simulate a paroxysmal disorder in small infants.

Startle Responses

These have been called *sursaut diurne* in the French literature[69] and are sudden, bilateral myoclonic jerks that may be either tight or massive and appear as a surprise reaction to a sudden sensory stimulus. Although segmental myoclonus is rare in young children, startle responses are very common. The Moro reflex has a startle component, and some kind of startle response can be demonstrated in most normal infants. These normal physiologic responses must be distinguished from the exaggerated Moro reflex and pathologic stimulus-induced myoclonus, often with opisthotonus seen in children with static or progressive encephalopathy.[58]

Bruxism

The majority of adults and children have nocturnal bruxism at some point in their lives.[13] In children with autistic behavior and mental retardation, bruxism also occurs in the waking state and may lead to severe dental attrition.[109]

Parasomnias

More common disorders are considered in Chapter 276 (see also Hanson and Peck[79]).

TRANSIENT OR BENIGN MOVEMENT DISORDERS

Benign Neonatal Sleep Myoclonus

In 1982, Coulter and Allen[35] reported three infants who had sleep myoclonus that began in the first month of life. The myoclonic jerks were bilateral, repetitive, and located mainly in the forearm and hands. Neurologic examinations and EEG were normal and continued to be normal during follow-up. Coulter and Allen coined the term *benign neonatal sleep myoclonus* (BNSM) for this phenomenon.

Subsequently, several other small series of cases were published that emphasized the importance of distinguishing BNSM from seizures.[123,143] This condition is probably quite frequent, as suggested in more recent, larger series.[37,42,43]

Benign neonatal sleep myoclonus appears in term newborns during the first few weeks of life. One infant born prematurely developed BNSM at 42 weeks of conceptional age,[120] and the earliest reported onset is in a 5-hour-old newborn.[35] The intensity and frequency of the muscle jerks increase up to the third week of life; more subtle myoclonus appearing earlier may go unnoticed. Myoclonic jerks are mainly present during non–rapid eye movement (NREM) sleep; they are less frequent during REM sleep. In some children, BNSM occurs exclusively during NREM sleep.[42] In most cases, jerks predominately

TABLE 1

NONEPILEPTIC NEUROLOGIC PAROXYSMAL DISORDERS AND EPISODIC SYMPTOMS IN INFANCY

Disorder	Symptoms
Enhanced normal phenomena	Hypnic jerks and waking myoclonic jerks Bruxism
Transient or benign movement disorders	Benign neonatal sleep myoclonus Tonic reflex seizures of early infancy Benign myoclonus of early infancy (benign nonepileptic infantile spasms) Benign paroxysmal tonic upward gaze Transient paroxysmal dystonia Benign paroxysmal torticollis Shuddering attacks Adverse reactions to exogenous agents
Habit-type movements and self-gratification phenomena	Head banging Head or body rocking Other stereotypic movements Masturbation-like episodes
Symptomatic abnormal movements	Neonatal posturing and other nonepileptic episodes Opsoclonus-myoclonus syndrome Bobble-head doll syndrome Encephalopathic nonepileptic myoclonus
Other paroxysmal episodes or neurologic conditions	Nonepileptic apnea Hyperexplexia Cogan oculomotor apraxia Benign paroxysmal vertigo Spasmus nutans Alternating hemiplegia of childhood Paroxysmal dystonia and choreoathetosis

involve the arms, but the feet, face, axial, and abdominal muscles can also be affected.[29,37,42,118,123] Myoclonic jerks may be bilateral; localized or multifocal; rhythmic or arrhythmic. The jerks occur frequently in clusters repeating at 1 to 5/sec for several seconds. Clusters of jerks usually recur irregularly in series lasting 20 to 30 minutes[42] or up to 90 minutes.[20] Longer-lasting episodes of BNSM have been mistaken for convulsive status epilepticus.[5,148]

Sleep state does not change during the episodes, and arousal always terminates the jerks. Occasionally, BNSM is stimulus sensitive and can be elicited, for instance, by noise.[35] Crib rocking can provoke BNSM, which is helpful diagnostically.[5] Curiously, benzodiazepines may increase the intensity of BNSM.[120]

Benign neonatal sleep myoclonus subsides spontaneously beginning with the second month of life and usually disappears before the sixth month. Ictal EEG is, by definition, normal in BNSM. However, one series reported a higher-than-normal incidence of interictal sharp transients in 4 of 10 newborns.[37] Benign neonatal sleep myoclonus may be genetically determined because affected siblings have been reported in two small series of patients, and a history of night jerks in one of the parents has also been found in several cases.[29,143]

Although Coulter and Allen[35] attributed BNSM to an arousal response, EEG recordings have not demonstrated this. Benign neonatal sleep myoclonus shares some features with nocturnal myoclonus seen in adults,[100] and it may reflect transient immaturity or imbalance of the serotonergic system.[123] In our last series of 21 patients, myoclonus disappeared before the age of 7 months, and 2 cases subsequently developed benign myoclonus of early infancy. Prognosis is uniformly good, and no treatment other than reassurance is necessary.[56]

Tonic Reflex Seizures of Early Infancy

This disorder was described in 1996, and a second series of 13 cases was published in 2001.[153,154] Onset occurs between the first and third month of life, with spontaneous remission 2 to 3 months after onset. These are normal infants presenting diffuse tonic contractions with extension of the four limbs, apnea and cyanosis, without loss of consciousness, lasting 3 to 10 seconds. Seizures occur only during wakefulness and with the child being held in an upright position. Because tactile stimulation often triggers the episodes, reflex myoclonic seizures come to mind. Normal interictal and ictal EEGs help to rule out brief tonic or myoclonic seizures and infantile spasms. The main differential diagnosis is with benign myoclonus of early infancy.

Benign Myoclonus of Early Infancy (Benign Nonepileptic Infantile Spasms)

In 1976, Fejerman[54] reported 10 infants with recurrent spells that resembled infantile spasms but in whom neurologic status, EEG, and outcomes were normal, allowing clear differentiation from West syndrome. Additional cases were added in subsequent reports.[16,30,55,56,67,74,75,98,101,102] Fejerman termed their conditions *benign myoclonus of early infancy* (BMEI).

We have now followed a total of 41 patients (26 male, 15 female) for 2 to 27 years.[60] In general, a diagnosis of West syndrome had been made, even with normal EEGs[137]; the correct diagnosis was established only in retrospect. Infants came to attention because of repeated jerks of the neck or upper limb muscles, causing abrupt flexion or rotation of the head with extension and abduction of the arms. Movements are often described as shuddering of the head and shoulders. In a minority of cases, only the arms are involved; sometimes, shuddering movements alternate with unequivocal myoclonic jerks. Occasionally, the only feature is symmetric or asymmetric extension of one or both arms with abduction, head rotation, or head drops. The jerks may be isolated or repeat in a series. They typically occur multiple times a day.

Consciousness is not affected, even when the myoclonic jerks last as long as 30 minutes. Benign myoclonus of early infancy occurs only rarely during sleep.[45] Although feeding may trigger attacks, this does not justify a separate designation, as has been proposed.[53] Benign myoclonus of early infancy is not related to anger or frustration. Myoclonus appears between 1 and 12 months of age, with onset in 90% of cases between 3 and 9 months. This overlap with the peak occurrence of infantile spasms further confounds diagnosis (Table 2) (see Chapter 229). Furthermore, we reported 4 infants who were normal until onset of typical infantile spasms without hypsarrythmia or other abnormalities in their EEGs. Thus, ictal EEG is very important in differential diagnosis.[27]

Neurologic examination is always normal, as are interictal and ictal EEG recordings. There are no other laboratory

TABLE 2

DIFFERENTIAL DIAGNOSIS BETWEEN CRYPTOGENIC WEST SYNDROME AND BENIGN MYOCLONUS OF EARLY INFANCY (BMEI)

Coincidences	Age of onset 3–9 mo Normal neuropsychic development (until onset) Myoclonic or brief tonic contraction in neck, shoulders, and upper limbs Occurring in series Several fits per day	
Differences	**West syndrome**	**BMEI**
Seizures	During waking and during sleep	During waking, exceptionally during sleep
Electroencephalogram	Always abnormal, almost always hypsarrhythmia	Always normal
Psychomotor retardation	In all nontreated cases	Never

abnormalities, and behavioral and neurologic development is normal.

Symptoms, once present, may increase for several weeks, but they gradually subside over a few months. Most children are free of attacks by the end of their second year and always by the end of their third. Other conditions that used to be considered in the differential diagnosis of BMEI are listed in Table 3.[2,49,56,57,133]

Some authors consider shuddering attacks to be different from benign myoclonus of early infancy, and they were initially described as associated with essential tremor.[82,87,150] In fact, I consider that the syndrome named BMEI includes always normal infants who start with fits frequently repeated in bursts, consisting in myoclonic jerks, brief tonic contractions, or shuddering episodes. We do not know the neurochemical basis of this disorder, but we do know that it is a transient phenomenon that may have different neurophysiologic expressions. This interpretation allows the inclusion of some neurophysiologic findings within the spectrum of BMEI.[108]

TABLE 3

DIFFERENTIAL DIAGNOSIS OF BENIGN MYOCLONUS OF EARLY INFANCY

1. Other nonepileptic phenomena
   a. Hyperexplexia
   b. Sandifer syndrome
   c. Tonic reflex seizures of early infancy
   d. Adverse reactions or intolerance to exogenous agents (monosodium glutamate, metoclopramide, etc.)
   e. Shuddering attacks (early symptom of familial essential tremor)
   f. Paroxysmal dystonia or choreoathetosis (paroxysmal torticollis, kinesigenic paroxysmal choreoathetosis, benign infantile dystonia)
2. Epileptic seizures
   a. Early myoclonic and tonic epileptic seizures
   b. Benign familial and nonfamilial infantile convulsions
   c. Infantile spasms (West syndrome)

Transient immaturity or imbalance of the serotonergic system might underlie various myoclonic phenomena, as has been postulated for BNSM,[123] and which could be genetic, thus accounting for occasional familial cases of both BNSM and BMEI.[29,68] We have seen one child with both BNSM and BMEI. Defining pharmacologic subgroups of the various myoclonic disorders is important, not only for understanding the clinical and neurophysiologic heterogeneity of myoclonus,[112] but also for providing rational pharmacotherapy. The areas of brain involved in BMEI are unknown.

Benign Paroxysmal Tonic Upward Gaze

This syndrome is characterized by bouts of tonic upward eye deviation accompanied by ataxia.[106] Age of onset is between 6 and 24 months, and children are otherwise healthy. The episodes of upward eye deviation occur in clusters every 2 to 8 seconds over a period of several minutes.[37,51] During episodes, consciousness is preserved, and attempts visually to track objects downward produce vertical nystagmus. Affected children usually exhibit a compensatory tilt of the head with the chin down. Symptoms occur only during wakefulness. During attacks, EEG recordings are normal. The frequency of the episodes gradually declines, and attacks disappear after 1 to 2 years. Even when the episodes disappear, patients may show slow motor development.[127] Three cases have shown a familial incidence.[23] The brain of one child who died accidentally was normal.[106]

Some children have benefited from treatment with dopa, and this has suggested a possible relationship to Segawa syndrome.[23,40]

Transient Paroxysmal Dystonia

Episodes of paroxysmal dystonia beginning at 3 to 5 months of age were reported in a group of nine infants. The attacks, which occurred only when the children were awake, were characterized by opisthotonus, symmetric or asymmetric increased tone in the arms with extreme pronation of the wrists, and preserved consciousness. Attacks usually lasted several minutes and occurred from once per month to several per day. Sometimes, however, episodes increased in duration to several hours or even days. In all cases, attacks disappeared in the second year of life.[10]

A similar picture had been described earlier as "benign idiopathic dystonia with onset in the first year of life." These infants had dystonic postures, mainly of the hands, lasting seconds to minutes and associated with intention tremor of the arms.[38,41,157]

Benign Paroxysmal Torticollis

Of all of these paroxysmal nonepileptic neurologic disorders, benign paroxysmal torticollis probably least resembles epileptic seizures. Benign paroxysmal torticollis is characterized by recurrent episodes of cervical dystonia lasting a few hours or days. Attacks are frequently associated with vomiting, pallor, irritability, and, sometimes, drowsiness or ataxia.[33,39]

Onset occurs in the first year of life, and attacks repeat several times per year. Over time, they decrease in severity and disappear after a few years. Electroencephalography is always normal. Gastroesophageal reflux, brainstem/cerebellar, or vestibular dysfunction should be excluded. The benignity of the condition has been emphasized in new series of 22 and 11 cases each.[46,6] In another report, two of the four cases came from a kindred with familial hemiplegic migraine linked to CACNA1A mutation.[73] Benign paroxysmal torticollis is now regarded as a migraine equivalent.

Adverse Reactions to Exogenous Agents

Adverse reactions or intolerance to various exogenous agents can include dystonic posturing, shuddering, tonic postures, and myoclonic jerks. Drug ingestion should be sought by careful inquiry, and blood or urine drug screens may be necessary. Metoclopramide,[71] carbamazepine,[110] phenothiazines (especially prochlorperazine), droperidol, and trimeprazine[138] have all been implicated. Intolerance to food additives has also been incriminated as a cause of shuddering attacks.[121]

HABIT-TYPE MOVEMENT AND SELF-GRATIFICATION EPISODES

Head Banging, Head Rolling, Rocking, and Other Stereotypic Movements

These represent a group of repetitive motor behaviors in children that are typically rhythmic and persistent. They are usually not paroxysmal and, therefore, rarely suggest epilepsy.

Head banging and head turning are common in normal infants at the time of going to bed, especially during the first year of life. Occasionally, children seem withdrawn and inattentive, which may suggest a seizure with automatisms. In some children, the rhythmic head movements persist during sleep (jactatio capitis nocturna). Generally, such movements disappear before 3 years of age, and neurologic development is normal.[1] Similar, often exaggerated motor behaviors occur during wakefulness in children with autistic behavior and mental retardation. A unique case of a parasomnia with rhythmic head and body movements and with tongue biting was reported in a 2-year-old girl.[149]

Rocking is less common in normal children and occurs most often in children with mental retardation, developmental disorders, or sensory deficits. The abnormal behavior starts during the first year of life when the child is sitting. Later, lateral or to-and-fro rhythmic movements of the head or body occur while standing as well.[124] A small proportion of normal children has similar behavior.[38,63,129]

Other stereotypic behaviors such as buccal and lingual movements may be mistaken for the oral automatisms of partial seizures, and hand flapping and related mannerisms may be confused with myoclonus.[24] In older children, repetitive hand waving in front of the eyes is used to self-induce photosensitive seizures. In young children, psychogenic seizures can manifest as brief staring episodes that are not easily distinguished from atypical absence seizures. In such cases, video-EEG monitoring will allow definitive diagnosis.[48,103]

Masturbation-like Episodes

Infants, usually girls, are sometimes referred because of brief episodes of staring, adducted thighs, rhythmic contractions of the leg and trunk, flushing, perspiration, and a dazed appearance. Such episodes are frequently mistaken for epileptic seizures, but self-gratification episodes and masturbation should be considered, despite the child's young age.[3,58,135,138] A helpful differential point is that the child is awake and may resist or resent being interrupted.

SYMPTOMATIC ABNORMAL MOVEMENTS

Neonatal Posturing and Other Nonepileptic Episodes

Motor automatisms and tonic postures are the most common paroxysmal events in newborns who do not have a consistent EEG abnormality. They are usually seen in infants with severe encephalopathies and depression of forebrain function. Kellaway and Hrachovy[88] hypothesized that these behaviors are mediated at a brainstem level due to failure of normal cortical inhibition and proposed that they represent "brain stem release phenomena."[88,104] Similar motor activities can be epileptic; however, EEG monitoring is usually necessary to define the underlying pathophysiologic mechanisms.[155,156]

Tonic postures in the newborn may be focal or generalized, and some may have myoclonic components. Many of these motor behaviors were formerly classified as "subtle" or "minimal" seizures, but their inconsistent relation to EEG ictal patterns have called their association into question (see Chapter 56). Other nonepileptic motor behaviors in newborns include oral-buccal-lingual movements such as chewing and sucking, random eye movements, rhythmic blinking, and peculiar limb movements like pedaling or swimming. In older infants, such activities may be part of an epileptic ictal event. The argument persists, however, and the question of whether dissociation between scalp EEG findings and stereotypical paroxysmal motor behavior excludes the possibility of an epileptic mechanism can probably never be answered definitively to everyone's satisfaction.[31,99,104] Nonetheless, therapeutic decisions (e.g., whether to use antiepileptic drugs) require an operational decision to be made in individual cases[155,156] (see Chapter 123).

Thus, several observations that can be made at cribside help to distinguish an epileptic seizure from a nonepileptic event with a strong degree of probability for therapeutic purposes. The following criteria reinforce the presumption that a particular event is nonepileptic: (a) It increases with sensory stimulation (spatial or temporal summation, irradiation); (b) it can be suppressed by gentle passive restraint; and (c) it is not accompanied by autonomic features (tachycardia, apnea, changes in blood pressure).[155] In such newborns, antiepileptic drugs are generally neither necessary nor desirable.

Independent of therapeutic decisions or nosologic questions, motor automatisms and tonic postures in newborns have significance in terms of etiology and prognosis. In one study, 53% of infants with tonic postures and 54% of those with automatisms had hypoxic-ischemic encephalopathy, and, of these, only about 25% were normal at hospital discharge.[104]

Segmental or spinal myoclonus in early infancy can be seen with sepsis, birth trauma, and various degenerative diseases. Isolated cases of spinal myoclonus have been reported in a child with hyperglycorrhachia secondary to parenteral nutrition administered through an improperly placed, indwelling femoral catheter[14] and in a 2-month-old infant with a spinal cord tumor.[122]

Opsoclonus-myoclonus Syndrome

Several years after the initial description of opsoclonus-myoclonus syndrome (OMS),[90] its frequent association with neuroblastoma was recognized.[50,136] Mean age of onset is around 14 months, and symptoms usually appear a few days after an apparent viral infection.[64] The following features are typical: (a) ataxia with marked tremor leading to inability to walk; (b) opsoclonus ("eye dancing") with episodes of rapid eyelid flutter; (c) myoclonus of the face of limbs; and (d) marked irritability and excitability. Brain imaging studies, EEG, and cerebrospinal fluid are normal. Brainstem auditory-evoked potentials can be abnormal early in the course.[86]

Some authors have argued that OMS is always associated with neuroblastoma and that such tumors may regress spontaneously,[22] but this is not true. Nonetheless, emphasis must be placed on a systematic search for neuroblastoma. Routine laboratory tests, including catecholamine levels, may be normal. Abdominal computed tomography (CT) may be necessary to detect small (1.5–2.0 cm) neuroblastomas arising from the abdominal sympathetic chain.

Several cases associated with different acute viral infections have been reported.[68,85,94,132] It is clear that there is still much to learn about the neurobiology of OMS.[113] Low concentrations of 5-hydroxyindoleacetic acid and homovanillic acid were found in the cerebrospinal fluid of 27 children with OMS.[115] There are three main etiologic groups for OMS: (a) OMS associated with neuroblastoma, (b) OMS associated with special viral infections, and (c) OMS without a definable etiology. Acute immune pathogenesis is surely involved, and there are new advances in this sense. Autoimmune antibodies binding to the surface of isolated rat cerebellar neurons were found in 10 of 14 children.[19] Children with OMS manifested a four- to sevenfold higher percentage of total B cells in cerebrospinal fluid compared with controls, and its determination is proposed as a biologic marker of the disease.[117]

Some children show a prompt and persistent response to corticosteroids or adrenocorticotropic hormone (ACTH), but most cases follow a chronic course with remissions and relapses often related to new viral infections.[90] Intravenously administered immune globulin seemed to produce remarkable improvement in an 18-month-old infant with OMS associated with a nonresectable abdominal ganglioneuroblastoma.[111]

Long-term follow-up reveals that some children, especially those with neuroblastoma, become symptom free. The majority, however, have chronic neurologic deficits, including cognitive and motor delays, language deficits, and behavioral abnormalities, regardless of etiology.[78,92]

Bobble-head Doll Syndrome

This is a rare disorder associated with obstructive hydrocephalus due to lesions in the region of the third ventricle and aqueduct.[146] In most of the reported cases, head movements have been characteristically to-and-fro nodding, which creates a peculiar 2- to 3-Hz rhythmic head nodding similar to that seen in dolls with weighted heads attached to coil-spring necks. The movement can be stopped voluntarily and is most obvious when the child is in the upright position. It disappears during sleep and when the head is supported. Pendular movements of the arms may also be seen.

Onset can occur in infancy or up to the fourth year of life.[146] Macrocephaly is a constant finding, and remarkable improvement follows treatment of the hydrocephalus. Ventriculocisternostomy through endoscopic treatment was recommended in cases associated with arachnoid cysts.[65,77] The condition is less often confused with epilepsy than with tremors, habit spasms, or even hysterical disorders.[79,146] Eight cases with head stereotypies resembling bobble-head doll syndrome, in association with axial hypotonia, ataxia, oculomotor abnormalities, and motor delay, were reported. In two of them, a congenital cerebellar abnormality without hydrocephalus was found.[83]

Encephalopathic Nonepileptic Myoclonus

Nonepileptic myoclonic jerks often appear in children with static or progressive encephalopathies, including some storage diseases, various toxic encephalopathies, and encephalopathies secondary to physical agents.[53] Different subcortical lesions that affect the basal ganglia may lead to myoclonus with or without dystonic features.

OTHER NEUROLOGIC CONDITIONS WITH PAROXYSMAL OR EPISODIC SYMPTOMS

Nonepileptic Apnea

Detailed analysis of nonepileptic apnea in newborns is beyond the scope of this chapter. Apnea during sleep is a common, normal phenomenon in premature and term newborns; it is more common in REM sleep than in NREM sleep.[72] The frequency of these normal respiratory pauses decreases after the neonatal period; apnea is rare in normal infants after a few months of age.[76] Video-EEG and polygraphic studies are fundamental tools for differential diagnosis between epileptic and nonepileptic apnea in newborns. Although apnea is common in the course of neonatal and infantile seizures, it is rare for apnea to be the sole manifestation of an epileptic seizure.[32,104]

Most of the information about infantile apnea has been obtained from polygraphic studies of infants diagnosed as having had near-miss for sudden infant death syndrome (near-miss SIDS). This term defines the infant who is found limp, blue, and not breathing, and who presumably would have died without intervention and resuscitation. Most children with SIDS have had a previous near-miss SIDS event.[76] Sudden infant death syndrome and near-miss SIDS have their peak incidence between 2 and 4 months of age, and different etiologies have been implicated.[12] Gastroesophageal reflux is frequently associated with episodes of apnea and can be confused with epilepsy, especially when apnea, choking, and cyanosis are accompanied by unusual head and neck postures and even opisthotonus (Sandifer syndrome).[140] A near-miss SIDS episode can be complicated by a convulsion due to hypoxia.[12,66]

Hyperekplexia

Hyperekplexia ("startle disease") is a rare condition that is often confused with epilepsy in the first year of life. Both major and minor variants have been reported. Most cases are familial, and both autosomal-dominant[9,139] and recessive[128] transmission have been reported. Other cases are sporadic.[70] Hyperekplexia was linked to the short arm of chromosome 5.[119] Several mutations were later found, and data seem to show a direct relationship between the mechanisms of inheritance and the location of the molecular defect. For instance, mutations in the domain of GLRA1 (alpha subunit of the glycine receptor) are frequent in autosomal dominant hyperekplexia.[96] A report of recessive hyperekplexia with a new mutation in the GLRA1 gene was recently presented.[34] In my experience, however, sporadic hyperekplexia was more frequent than the familial forms.[62] This finding is ratified with a recent series of 39 sporadic cases in neonates and infants.[131]

Most cases involve infants with marked muscular hypertonia and severe jerks induced by sound or tactile stimuli. Touching the dorsum of the nose is especially effective in eliciting symmetric myoclonic jerks of the arms and legs. Tonic and clonic generalized attacks with cyanosis occur during sleep. Such children are usually misdiagnosed as having spastic quadriparesis with stimulus-sensitive myoclonic epilepsy, and artifacts in the EEG are commonly misinterpreted as abnormal discharges. The hypertonia decreases with time, and open pyramidal signs are not present. Affected children walk at 2 to 3 years of age and usually have mild mental retardation.

Clonazepam is the drug of choice, effectively reducing the paroxysmal episodes that occur during sleep and drop attacks due to stimulus-induced myoclonus.[62] "Minor" and atypical cases may lack early hypertonia or a clear response to tactile stimuli.[56,105]

The condition usually improves, although rarely an infant may die from cardiopulmonary arrest during an episode occurring in sleep. This type of attack can be stopped by forced flexion of the head and legs.[151] We reported four sporadic cases with the conviction that they were malignant forms of hyperekplexia.[11] Following this line, two children with hyperekplexia associated with refractory status epilepticus who died were recently reported, suggesting that they might represent a new autosomal-recessive syndrome.[97]

Cogan Oculomotor Apraxia

Oculomotor apraxia may be symptomatic of different congenital and acquired conditions, including brain malformations, mesencephalic-diencephalic lesions, and genetic diseases associated with other neurologic signs and mental retardation.[3]

The form of oculomotor apraxia known as Cogan syndrome is usually recognized after 6 months of age by the peculiar head thrusts and impaired saccadic eye movements. These abnormal movements of the eyes and head are usually horizontal and may be mistaken for tics or even epileptic seizures.[138] There is a tendency for the eyes to improve with time, although persistent clumsiness and learning difficulties are frequent.

In two children with this condition, a newly recognized association with nephronophthisis type 1 was reported. Both patients carried the lesions in the NPHP1 gene.[18] Familial occurrence of congenital oculomotor apraxia was also reported in four patients.[84]

Benign Paroxysmal Vertigo

Benign paroxysmal vertigo (BPV) must be considered in the differential diagnosis of seizures in children from 1 to 4 years of age.[15,58,91] The child usually begins crying, clings to the nearest person, or falls to the floor. Pallor and a frightened expression are constant features, but nystagmus occurs in only 35% to 40% of cases. Vomiting is infrequent.[91]

Children old enough to have developed language express fear of falling and a rotational sensation: "The room is turning around," "the floor is moving," "the walls are falling."[61] Episodes last about 1 minute, and recovery is prompt. Attacks usually recur monthly and tend to disappear in a few years. Electroencephalography and neurologic examination between attacks and development are normal.

According to some investigators, vestibular function tests have been consistently abnormal, with labyrinthine dysfunction on one or both sides.[91] In a more recent series, however, such abnormalities were not found.[47] Relation to migraine, instead, seems to be strong: A family history of migraine in 53% of 19 cases and a family history of kinetosis in 83% of the same series were reported.[47] Cyclic vomiting may be associated and was considered together with BPV as part of the so-called periodic syndrome that may be a precursor to migraine.[47,80] More recently, serum creatine kinase-MB (CK-MB) levels were elevated in 22 children with BPV, and the authors suggested that CK-MP may be a diagnostic marker for this condition.[125]

Benign paroxysmal vertigo must be distinguished from other causes of recurrent vertigo in childhood. When attacks last more than a few minutes and are associated with ataxia and other neurologic symptoms, the diagnosis of BPV is unlikely, and other etiologies should be considered.[61,145]

Spasmus Nutans

Spasmus nutans is characterized by the triad of nystagmus, head nodding, and head tilt. Head nodding is most frequently horizontal and may occur in bursts; nystagmus is more constant and usually monocular. Age of onset is usually from 6 to 18 months.[3,63]

Spasmus nutans tends to disappear within a few months or years. The incidence of new cases seems to have declined in the last few decades.[61] The etiology is unknown. However, a recent comparative study of 23 patients with spasms nutans (SN) and 24 patients with idiopathic infantile nystagmus (IIN) demonstrated significant differences between SN and IIN patients and their families with regard to socioeconomic status and exposure to light early in life, concluding that low socioeconomic status is a factor of risk for spasmus nutans.[158] Normal complete neurologic and ophthalomologic examination as well as normal brain magnetic resonance imagining (MRI) are necessary to confirm diagnosis.[44] Differential diagnosis with such pathologies as optic glioma and congenital retinopathies is mandatory.[44,89]

Alternating Hemiplegia

The initial description of alternating hemiplegia (AH) of childhood included eight children described as having complicated migraine beginning in infancy.[151] The condition was later identified as a distinct entity[93] and has been thoroughly reviewed and reconsidered.[7]

A relation of AH with familial hemiplegic migraine (FHM) has been recently suggested, with a novel ATP1A2 mutation reported in a kindred with features in common between AH and FHM.

Differentiation from epilepsy is not easy early because the initial manifestations are usually partial tonic attacks beginning in infancy or even in the neonatal period. Paroxysmal nystagmus, especially monocular nystagmus, is frequently associated with the episodes of unilateral tonic attacks.

Hemiplegia is not usually the first symptom, but it almost always appears during the first year of life. Hemiplegia occurs suddenly and may be preceded by screaming and fussiness. The affected side is hypotonic, with persistent tendon reflexes, and each attack lasts from 30 minutes to several days. A distinct feature of alternating hemiplegia of childhood is the disappearance of all abnormalities when the child falls asleep. Paralysis recurs on awakening in prolonged episodes. Although the hemiplegia, by definition, alternates from side to side in successive attacks, bilateral weakness and variations in tone are not unusual.[4]

Seizures occur in 50% of cases, and partial status epilepticus may occur. The seizures occur independent of, but sometimes in close relationship to, a hemiplegic attack.[4,36]

The episodes of alternating hemiplegia recur at variable intervals but seem to become less severe over time. However, most children develop some degree of ataxia with choreoathetosis and are left with significant mental retardation. Cases of benign familial alternating hemiplegia of childhood are exceptions to this usual evolution.[8]

Flunarizine has benefited some children with alternating hemiplegia by reducing the duration but not the frequency of hemiplegic attacks. Only rarely has flunarizine abolished attacks completely.[7,134]

The etiology and pathogenesis are still debated. Although a possible relationship to migraine has not been completely rejected, there are abnormalities of energy metabolism and mitochondrial function that merit further investigation.[7]

Paroxysmal Dystonia and Choreoathetosis

Two rare familial conditions are *paroxysmal dystonia and choreoathetosis* and *paroxysmal kinesigenic choreoathetosis*.[95,144] In the former, onset is usually between 1 and 2 years of age, and attacks are mainly of dystonia, which lasts from 2 minutes to a few hours. The frequency of attacks ranges from several per day to one every 2 months.[21] Familial cases must be distinguished from the sporadic transient paroxysmal dystonic episodes already discussed.

Paroxysmal kinesigenic choreoathetosis is also an autosomal-dominant disease, but it starts after 5 years of age.[126] A constant feature is that attacks are precipitated by sudden movement, and episodes last only a few seconds to several minutes; they occur several times a day.[138] Antiepileptic drugs usually suppress attacks, but EEGs have been abnormal in only one case.[81]

A genetic bridge between paroxysmal choreoathetosis and benign familial infantile convulsions was established in 1997 in describing a new neurologic syndrome linked to chromosome 16.[142] Caraballo et al. later reported linkage to chromosome 16 in children with benign familial infantile convulsions. Our group was actively involved in this search, and in our cases, paroxysmal choreoathetosis appeared years after onset of benign familial infantile convulsions.[25,26,28] Paroxysmal kinesigenic choreoathetosis also seems to map to chromosome 16.[17,147]

Acquired nonepileptic paroxysmal dystonia is associated with static encephalopathies, but it begins outside infancy.[52] It probably represents different forms of "delayed-onset dystonia."[63] The differential diagnosis includes hereditary progressive dystonia with marked diurnal fluctuation and other dopa-responsive dystonias.[130]

SUMMARY AND CONCLUSIONS

All of the conditions reviewed in this chapter are intermittent, often paroxysmal, and have been confused with epileptic seizures. On one extreme are abnormal movements that are symptomatic of severe brain pathologies requiring specific treatments, such as the opsoclonus-myoclonus syndrome and the bobble-head doll syndrome. Alternating hemiplegia includes both abnormal movements early on and, later, negative phenomenon, namely, hemiplegia.

On the other end of the spectrum are exaggerations of movement and conditions that can be collectively considered "transient or benign movement disorders" because they disappear spontaneously in the course of months or a few years without neurologic sequelae.

All of these conditions should be known to pediatricians and neurologists because misdiagnosing them as epilepsy delays appropriate treatment, exposes small children to the risks of antiepileptic drugs, and creates unnecessary physiologic burdens.[59]

EEG is almost always required to rule out epilepsy, and adding video-EEG recordings increases its value in the study of children with frequent paroxysmal events.[157]

References

1. Abe K, Oda N, Amatomi M. Natural history and predictive significance of head-banging, head-rolling and breath-holding spells. *Dev Med Child Neurol.* 1984;26;5:644–648.
2. Aicardi J. Early myoclonic encephalopathy In: Roger J, Bureau M, Dravet C, et al., eds. *Epileptic Syndromes in Infancy, Childhood and Adolescence,* 2nd ed. London: John Libbey; 1992:13–24.
3. Aicardi J. *Diseases of the Nervous System in Childhood.* Oxford: MacKeith Press; 1992;1053–1054.
4. Aicardi J, Bourgeois M, Fusco L, et al. Alternating hemiplegia of childhood. An overview. In: Andermann F, Aicardi J, Vigevano F, eds. *Alternating Hemiplegia of Childhood.* New York: Raven Press; 1995:207–212.
5. Alfonso Y, Papazian O, Jeffries H, et al. Simple maneuver to provoke benign neonatal sleep myoclonus. *Pediatrics.* 1995;96(6):1161–1163.
6. Al-Twaijri WA, Shevell MI. Pediatric migraine equivalents: occurrence and clinical features in practice. *Pediatr Neurol.* 2002;26(5):365–368.
7. Andermann F, Aicardi J, Vigevano F, eds. *Alternating Hemiplegia of Childhood.* New York: Raven Press; 1995.
8. Andermann E, Andermann F, Silver K, et al. Benign familial nocturnal alternating hemiplegia of childhood. *Neurology.* 1994;44:1812–1814.
9. Andermann F, Keene DL, Andermann E, et al. Startle disease or hyperexplexia. Further delineation of the syndrome. *Brain.* 1980;103:985–997.
10. Angelini L, Rumi V, Lamperti E, et al. Transient paroxysmal dystonia in infancy. *Neuropediatrics.* 1988;19:171–174.
11. Arroyo HA, Caraballo RH, Yepez I, et al. Hyperekplexia: is there a malignant variant? [Abstract]. *Neurology.* 2000;54(7/Suppl 3):294.
12. Arzimanoglou A, Guerrini R, Aicardi J. *Aicardi's Epilepsy in Children,* 3rd ed. Philadelphia: Lippincott Williams & Wilkins; 2004.
13. Attanasis R. Nocturnal bruxism and its clinical management. *Dent Clin North Am.* 1991;35:245–252.
14. Bass WT, Lewis DW. Neonatal segmental myoclonus associated with hyperglycorrhachia. *Pediatr Neurol.* 1995;13(1):77–79.
15. Basser LS. Benign paroxysmal vertigo of childhood. *Brain.* 1964;87:141–152.
16. Beltramino JC. Mioclonias benignas de la infancia temprana o mioclonias de Fejerman. *Arch Arg Pediatr.* 1987;85:119–124.
17. Bennett LB, Roach ES, Bowcock AM. A locus for paroxysmal kinesigenic dyskinesia maps to human chromosome 16. *Neurology.* 2000;54(1):125–130.
18. Betz R, Rensing C, Otto E, et al. Children with ocular motor apraxia type Cogan carry deletions in the gene (*NPHP1*) for juvenile nephronophthisis. *J Pediatr.* 2000;136(6):828–831.
19. Blaes F, Fuhlhuber V, Korfei M, et al. Surface-binding autoantibodies to cerebellar neurons in opsoclonus syndrome. *Ann Neurol.* 2005;58(2):313–317.
20. Blennow G. Benign infantile nocturnal myoclonus. *Acta Paediatr Scand.* 1985;74:505–507.
21. Boel M, Casaer P. Paroxysmal kinesigenic choreoathetosis. *Neuropediatrics.* 1986;15(4):215–217.
22. Brandt S, Carlsen N, Glanting P, et al. Encephalopathia myoclonica infantillis (Kinsbourne) and neuroblastoma in children. *Dev Med Child Neurol.* 1974;16:286–294.
23. Campistol J, Prats JM, Garaizar C. Benign paroxysmal tonic upgaze of childhood with ataxia. A neuro ophthalmological syndrome of familial origin? *Dev Med Child Neurol.* 1993;35;5:436–438.
24. Campos-Castelló J. Estereotipias. *Rev Neurol (Barcelona).* 1995;23(Suppl 3):S363–S367.
25. Caraballo R. Convulsiones familiares y no familiares benignas del lactante. In: Ruggieri V, Caraballo R, Arroyo H, eds. *Temas de Neuropediatría: Homenaje al Dr. Natalio Fejerman.* Buenos Aires: Panamericana; 2005: 53–68.

26. Caraballo R, Cersósimo R, Espeche A, et al. Benign familial and nonfamilial infantile seizure: study of 64 cases. *Epileptic Disord.* 2003;5(1):45–49.
27. Caraballo R, Fejerman N, DallaBernardina B, et al. Epileptic spasms in cluster without hypsarrhythmia in infancy. *Epileptic Disord.* 2003;5(2):109–113.
28. Caraballo R, Pavel S, Lemainque A, et al. Linkage of benign convulsions to chromosome 16p12–q12 suggests allelism to the infantile convulsions and choreoathetosis syndrome. *Am J Hum Genet.* 2001;3:788–794.
29. Caraballo R, Yepez I, Cersosimo R, et al. Benign neonatal sleep myoclonus. *Rev Neurol.* 1998;26(152):540–544.
30. Caviedes Altable BE, Moreno Belzue C, Arteaga R, et al. Mioclonías benignas de la infanica temprana. *An Esp Pediatr.* 1992;36(6):496–497.
31. Clancy R, Legido A, Lewis D. Occult neonatal seizures. *Epilepsia.* 1982;29(3):256–261.
32. Clancy RR, Spitzer AR. Cerebral cortical function in infants at risk for sudden infant death syndrome. *Ann Neurol.* 1985;18:41–47.
33. Cohen HA, Nussinovitch M, Ashkenasi A, et al. Benign paroxysmal torticollis in infancy *Pediatr Neurol.* 1993;9;6:488–490.
34. Coto E, Armenta D, Espinosa R, et al. Recessive hyperekplexia due to a new mutation (R100H) in the *GLRA1* gene. *Mov Disord.* 2005;20(12):1626–1629.
35. Coulter DL, Allen RJ. Benign neonatal myoclonus. *Arch Neurol.* 1982;39:191–192.
36. Dalla Bernardina B, Fontana E, Colamaría V, et al. Alternating hemiplegia of childhood: epilepsy and electroencephalographic investigations. In: Andermann F, Aicardi J, Vigevano F, eds. *Alternating Hemiplegia of Childhood.* New York: Raven Press; 1995:75–88.
37. Daoust-Roy J, Seshia SS. Benign neonatal sleep myoclonus. *Am J Dis Child.* 1992;146:1236–1241.
38. Deonna T. Benign movement disorders. In: Fejerman N, Chamoles NA, eds. *New Trends in Pediatric Neurology.* Amsterdam: Excerpta Medica; 1993:129–136.
39. Deonna T, Martin D. Benign paroxysmal torticollis in infancy. *Arch Dis Child.* 1981;56:956–959.
40. Deonna T, Roulet E, Meyer HU. Benign paroxysmal tonic upgaze of childhood. A new syndrome. *Neuropediatrics.* 1990;21(4):213–214.
41. Deonna T, Ziegler L, Niesen J. Transient idiopathic dystonia in infancy. *Neuropediatrics.* 1991;22(4):220–224.
42. Di Capua M, Fusco L, Ricci S, et al. Benign neonatal sleep myoclonus: clinical features and video-polygraphic recordings. *Mov Disord.* 1993;8(2):191–194.
43. Donat JF, Wright FS. Clinical imitators of infantile spasms. *J Child Neurol.* 1992;7:395–399.
44. Doummar D, Roussat B, Beauvais P, et al. Spasmus nutans: apropos of 16 cases. *Arch Pediatr.* 1998;5(3):264–268.
45. Dravet C, Giraud N, Bureau M, et al. Benign myoclonus of early infancy or benign non-epileptic infantile spasm. *Neuropediatrics.* 1986;17(1):33–38.
46. Drigo P, Carli G, Laverda AM. Benign paroxysmal torticollis of infancy. *Brain Dev.* 2000;22(3):169–172.
47. Drigo P, Carli G, Laverda AM. Benign paroxysmal vertigo of childhood. *Brain Dev.* 2001;23(1):38–41.
48. Duchowny MS, Resnick TJ, Deray MJ, et al. Video EEG diagnosis of repetitive behavior in early childhood and its relationship to seizures. *Pediatr Neurol.* 1988;4(3):162–164.
49. Dulac O, Plouin P, Jambaqué, et al. Spasmes infantiles epileptiques benins. *Rev EEG Neurophysiol Clin.* 1986;16:371–382.
50. Dyken P, Kolar O. Dancing eyes, dancing feet: infantile polyioclinia. *Brain.* 1968;91:305–320.
51. Echenne B, Rivier F. Benign paroxysmal tonic upward gaze. *Pediatr Neurol.* 1992;8(2):154–155.
52. Erickson GR, Chun RWM. Acquired paroxysmal movement disorders. *Pediatr Neurol.* 1987;3(4):226–229.
53. Fahn S, Marsden CD, Van Woert MH. Definition and classification of myoclonus. In: Fahn S, Marsden CD,Van Woert MH, eds. *Myoclonus. Advances in Neurology*, Vol. 43. New York: Raven Press; 1986:1–5.
54. Fejerman N. Mioclonias benignas de la infancia temprana. Comunicacion peliminar. In: *Actas IV Jornadas Rioplatenses de Neurologia Infantile. Neuropediatria Latinoamericana.* Montevideo: Delta; 1976:131–134.
55. Fejerman N. Mioclonias benignas de la infancia temprana. *An Esp Ped.* 1984;21(8):725–731.
56. Fejerman N. Myoclonus and epilepsies. In: Ohtahara S, Roger J, eds. *New Trends in Pediatric Epileptology.* Okayama, Japan: Department of Child Neurology, Okayama University Medical School; 1991:94–110.
57. Fejerman N. Differential diagnosis. In Dulac O, Chugani HT, Dalla Bernardina B, eds. *Infantile Spasms and West Syndrome.* London: WB Saunders; 1994:88–98.
58. Fejerman N. Nonepileptic neurologic paroxysmal disorders and episodic symptoms in infancy and early childhood. *Int Pediatr.* 1996;11(6):364–371.
59. Fejerman N. Nonepileptic disorders imitating generalized idiopathic epilepsies. *Epilepsia.* 2005;46(Suppl 9):1–4.
60. Fejerman N, Caraballo R. Appendix to: Pachatz C, Fusco L, Vigevano F. Shuddering and benign myoclonus of early infancy. In: Guerrini R, Aicardi J, Andermann F, et al., eds. *Epilepsy and Movement Disorders.* Cambridge: Cambridge University Press; 2002:349–351.
61. Fejerman N, Medina CS. *Convulsiones en la infancia,* 2nd ed. Buenos Aires: El Ateneo; 1986.
62. Fejerman N, Medina CS, Caraballo R. Hiperecplexia. In: Fejerman N, Fernandez Alvarez E, eds. *Neurología Pediátrica,* 2nd ed. Buenos Aires: Panamericana; 1997:597.
63. Fernandez Alvarez E. Encefalopatía mioclónica del lactante (Sindrome de Kinsbourne). *Int Pediatr.* 1989;4(2/Suppl):44–46.
64. Fernandez Alvarez E. Transtornos del movimiento In: Fejerman N, Fernandez Alvarez E, eds. *Neurología Pediátrica,* 2nd ed. Buenos Aires: Panamericana; 1997:446–478.
65. Fioravanti A, Godano U, Consales A, et al. Bobble-head doll syndrome due to a suprasellar arachnoid cyst: endoscopic treatment in two cases. *Child's Nerv Syst.* 2004;20(10):770–773.
66. Freed GE, Steinschneider A, Glassman M, et al. Sudden infant death syndrome: prevention and understanding of selected clinical issues. *Pediatr Clin North Am.* 1994;41;5,967–990.
67. Fujikawa Y, Sugai K, Iwasaki Y. Three cases of benign myoclonus of early infancy. *No To Hattatsu.* 2003;35(3):243–248.
68. Galletti F, Brinciotti M, Emanuelli O. Familial occurrence of benign myoclonus of early infancy. *Epilepsia.* 1989;30(5):579–581.
69. Gastaut H. Sémiologie des myoclonies et nosologie analytique des syndromes myocloniques. In: Bonduelle M, Gastaut H, eds. *Les Myoclonies.* Paris: Masson & Co.; 1968:1–30.
70. Gastaut H, Villeneuve A. The startle disease or hyperexplexia: pathological surprise reaction. *J Neurol Sci.* 1967;5:523–542.
71. Gatrad AR. Dystonic reactions to metoclopramide. *Dev Med Child Neurol.* 1976;18:767–769.
72. Gaultier C. Respiratory adaptation during sleep from the neonatal period to adolescence. In: Guilleminault C, ed. *Sleep and Its Disorders in Children.* New York: Raven Press; 1987:67–98.
73. Giffin NJ, Benton S, Goadsby PJ. Benign paroxysmal torticollis of infancy: four new cases and linkage to CACNA1A mutation. *Dev Med Child Neurol.* 2002;44(7):490–493.
74. Giraud N. *Les spasmes infantiles bénins non epileptiques.* Thesis, Marseille, Faculté de Medicine; 1982.
75. Gobbi G, Dravet C, Bureau M, et al. Les spasms bénins du nourrisson (syndrome de Lombroso et Fejerman). *Boll Lega Ital Epil.* 1982;3(Suppl):S17.
76. Guilleminault C. Sleep apnea in the full-term infant In: Guilleminault C, ed. *Sleep and Its Disorders in Children.* New York: Raven Press; 1987:195–212.
77. Hagebeuk EE, Kloet A, Grotenhuis JA, et al. Bobble-head doll syndrome successfully treated with an endoscopic ventriculocystocisternostomy. *J Neurosurg.* 2005;103(Suppl 3):253–259.
78. Hammer MS, Larsen MB, Stack CU. Outcome of children with opsoclonus-myoclonus regardless of etiology. *Pediatr Neurol.* 1995;13(1):21–24.
79. Hanson PA, Peck F. Bizarre posture and movement disorder with third ventricle astrocytoma. *Dev Med Child Neurol.* 1977;19(1):54–57.
80. Headache Classification Committee of the International Headache Society. Classification and diagnostic criteria for headache disorders, cranial neuralgias and facial pain. *Cephalalgia.* 1988;8(Suppl 7):10–73.
81. Hirata K, Katayama S, Saito T, et al. Paroxysmal kinesigenic choreoathetosis with abnormal electroencephalogram during attacks. *Epilepsia.* 1991;32(4)492–494.
82. Holmes GL, Russman BS. Shuddering attacks. *Am J Dis Child.* 1986;140:72–74.
83. Hottinger-Blanc PM, Ziegler AL, Deonna T. A special type of head stereotypies in children with developmental (?cerebellar) disorder: description of 8 cases and literature review. *Pediatr Neurol.* 2002;6(3):143–152.
84. Hsu HN, Yang ML, Lai HC. Familial congenital ocular motor apraxia. *Chang Gung Med J.* 2002;25(6):411–414.
85. Ichiba N, Miyake Y, Sato K, et al. Mumps induced opsoclonus-myoclonus and ataxia. *Pediatr Neurol.* 1988;4(4):224–227.
86. Kalmanchey R, Veres E. Dancing eyes syndrome—brainstem acoustic evoked potential approach. *Neuropediatrics.* 1988;18:193–196.
87. Kanazawa O. Shuddering attacks—report of 4 children. *Pediatr Neurol.* 2000;23(5):421–424.
88. Kellaway P, Hrachovy RA. Status epilepticus in newborns: a perspective on neonatal seizures. In: Delgado-Escueta AV, Wasterlain CG, Treiman DM, et al., eds. *Status Epilepticus. Advances in Neurology*, Vol. 34. New York: Raven Press; 1983:93–99.
89. King RA, Nelson LB, Wagner RS. Spasmus nutans. A benign clinical entity? *Arch Ophthalmol.* 1986;104:1501–1504.
90. Kinsbourne M. Myoclonic encephalopathy in infants. *J Neurol Neurosurg Psychiatry.* 1962;25:271.
91. Koenigsberger MR, Chutorian AM, Gold AP, et al. Benign paroxysmal vertigo of childhood. *Neurology.* 1970;20:1108–1113.
92. Koh PS, Raffeusperger JG, Berry S, et al. Long-term outcome in children with opsoclonus-myoclonus and ataxia and coincident neuroblastoma. *J Pediatr.* 1994;125(5):712–716.
93. Krägeloh I, Aicardi J. Alternating hemiplegia in infants: report of five cases. *Dev Med Child Neurol.* 1980;22:784–791.
94. Kuban KC, Ephros MA, Freeman RL, et al. Syndrome of opsoclonus-myoclonus caused by Coxsackie B3 infection. *Ann Neurol.* 1983;13:69–71.
95. Lance JW. Familiar paroxysmal dystonic choreoathetosis and its differentiation from related syndromes. *Ann Neurol.* 1977;2:285–293.

96. Lapunzina P, Sanchez JM, Cabrera M, et al. Hyperekplexia (startle disease): a novel mutation (S270T) in the M2 domain of the *GLRA1* gene and a molecular review of the disorder. *Mol Diagn.* 20037:125–128.
97. Lerman-Sagie T, Watemberg N, Vinkler C, et al. Familial hyperekplexia and refractory status epilepticus: a new autosomal recessive syndrome. *J Child Neurol.* 2004;19(7):522–525.
98. Lombroso CT, Fejerman N. Benign myoclonus of early infancy. *Ann Neurol.* 1977;1(2):138–148.
99. Lombroso CT, Holmes G. Value of the EEG in neonatal seizures. *J Epilepsy.* 1993;6(1):39–70.
100. Lugaresi E, Cirignota F, Coccagna, et al. Nocturnal myoclonus and restless legs syndrome. In: Fahn S, Marsden CD,Van Woert MH, eds. *Myoclonus. Advances in Neurology*, Vol. 43. New York: Raven Press; 1986:295–308.
101. Martinez Pastor P, Diez Domingo J, Ausina Gomez A, et al. Mioclonías benignas de la infancia. *An Esp Pediatr.* 1993:38:369–370.
102. Maydell BV, Berenson F, Rothner AD, et al. Benign myoclonus of early infancy: an imitator of West's syndrome. *J Child Neurol.* 2001;16(2):109–112.
103. Metrick ME, Ritter FJ, Gates JR, et al. Non-epileptic events in childhood. *Epilepsia.* 1991;32(3):322–328.
104. Mizrahi EM. Neonatal seizures: problems in diagnosis and classification. *Epilepsia.* 1987;28(Suppl 1):S46–S55.
105. Obeso JA, Artieda J, Luquin MR, et al. Antimyoclonic action of piracetam. *Clin Neuropharmacol.* 1986;9(1):58–64.
106. Ouvrier RA, Billson MD. Benign paroxysmal tonic upgaze of childhood. *J Child Neurol.* 1988;3:177–180.
107. Paolicchi JM. The spectrum of nonepileptic events in children. *Epilepsia.* 2002;43(Suppl 3):60–64.
108. Pachatz C, Fusco L, Vigevano F. Benign myoclonus of early infancy. *Epileptic Disord.* 1999;1(1):57–61.
109. Peak J, Eveson JW, Scully C. Oral manifestation of Rett's syndrome. *Br Dent J.* 1992;172:6,248–249.
110. Pellock JM. Carbamazepine side effects in children and in adults. *Epilepsia.* 1987;28(Suppl 3):S64–S70.
111. Petruzzi MJ, De Alarcon PA. Neuroblastoma-associated opsoclonus-myoclonus treated with intravenously administered immune globulin G. *J Pediatr.* 1995;127(2):328–329.
112. Pranzatelli MR. The proposed role of neurotransmitter receptors in the pathophysiology of human myoclonic disorders. *Med Hypotheses.* 1989:30:55–60.
113. Pranzatelli MR. The neurobiology of the opsoclonus-myoclonus syndrome. *Clin Neuropharmacol.* 1992;15(3):186–228.
114. Pranzatelli MR. Myoclonus in childhood. *Semin Pediatr Neurol.* 2003; 10(1):41–51.
115. Pranzatelli MR, Huang Y, Tate E, et al. Cerebrospinal fluid 5-hydroxyindoleacetic acid and homovanillic acid in the pediatric opsoclonus-myoclonus syndrome. *Ann Neurol.* 1995;37(2):189–197.
116. Pranzatelli MR, Pedley TA. Differential diagnoses of epilepsy and seizures in childhood. In: Dam M, Gram L, eds. *Comprehensive Epileptology.* New York: Raven Press; 1991:423–447.
117. Pranzatelli MR, Travelstead AL, Tate ED, et al. CSF B-cell expansion in opsoclonus-myoclonus syndrome: a biomarker of disease activity. *Mov Disord.* 2004;19(7):770–777.
118. Ramelli GP, Sozzo AB, Vella S, et al. Benign neonatal sleep myoclonus: an under-recognized non-epileptic condition. *Acta Paediatr.* 2005;94(7):962–963
119. Rayn SG, Sherman SL, Terry JL, et al. Startle disease or hyperexplexia: response to clonazepam and assignment to the gene (STHE) to chromosome 5q by linkage analysis. *Ann Neurol.* 1992;31:663–668.
120. Reggin JD, Johnson MI. Exacerbation of benign sleep myoclonus by benzodiazepines [Abstract]. *Ann Neurol.* 1989;26:455.
121. Reif-Lehrer L, Stemmermann MG. Monosodium glutamate intolerance in children. *N Engl J Med.* 1975;293:1204.
122. Renault F, Flores-Guevara R, D'Allest AM. Segmental myoclonus in a child with spinal cord tumor. *Dev Med Child Neurol.* 1995;37(4):354–361.
123. Resnick TJ, Moshe SL, Perotta L et al. Benign neonatal sleep myoclonus. Relationship to sleep states. *Arch Neurol.* 1986;43:266–268.
124. Ritvo ER, Ornitz EM, Lafranchi S. Frequency of repetitive behaviors in early infantile autism and its variants. *Arch Gen Psychiatr.* 1968;19:341–347.
125. Rodoo P, Hellberg D. Creatine kinase MK (CK-MB) in benign paroxysmal vertigo of childhood: a new diagnostic marker. *J Pediatr.* 2005;146(4):548–551.
126. Rothner AD. Not everything that shakes is epilepsy: the differential diagnosis of paroxysmal nonepileptiform disorders. *Cleve Clin J Med.* 1989;56(P2):S206–S213.
127. Ruggieri VL, Yepez I, Fejerman N. Benign paroxysmal tonic upward gaze syndrome. *Rev Neurol.* 1998;27(155):88–91.
128. Saenz-Lope, Herranz-Tanarro FJ, Masdeu JC, et al. Hyperexplexia: a syndrome of pathological startle responses. *Ann Neurol.* 1984;15:36–41.
129. Sallustro C, Atwell F. Body rocking, head-banging, and head-rolling in normal children. *J Pediatr.* 1978;93:704–708.
130. Segawa M, Nomura Y, Vetake K. Hereditary progressive dystonia with marked diurnal fluctuation (HPD) and dopa responsive dystonia (DRD): variation of symptoms and pathophysiology. In: Fejerman N, Chamoles NA, eds. *New Trends in Pediatric Neurology.* Amsterdam: Excerpta Medica; 1993:137–142.
131. Shahar E, Raviv R. Sporadic major hyperekplexia in neonates and infants: clinical manifestations and outcome. *Pediatr Neurol.* 2004;31(1):30–34.
132. Sheth RD, Horwitz SJ, Aronoff S, et al. Opsoclonus myoclonus syndrome secondary to Epstein-Barr virus infection. *J Child Neurol.* 1995;10:4,297–299.
133. Shuper A, Mimouni M. Problems of differentiation between epilepsy and non-epileptic paroxysmal events in the first year of life. *Arch Dis Child.* 1995;73(4):342–344.
134. Silver K, Andermann F. Alternating hemiplegia of childhood: treatment with flunarizine. In: Andermann F, Aicardi J, Vigevano F, eds. *Alternating Hemiplegia of Childhood.* New York: Raven Press; 1995:195–198.
135. Snyder CH. Conditions that simulate epilepsy in children. *Clin Pediatr.* 1972;11:487–491.
136. Solomon GE, Chutorian AM. Opsoclonus and occult neuroblastoma. *N Engl J Med.* 1968;279:475–482.
137. Sorel L. Le syndrome de West atypique ou incomplet: á propos de 80 observations. *Boll Lega Ital Epil.* 1978;22/23:181–182.
138. Stephenson JBP. *Fits and Faints. Clinics in Developmental Medicine*, No. 109. London: MacKeith Press; 1990.
139. Suhren O, Bruyn GW, Tuynman JA. Hyperexplexia: a hereditary startle syndrome. *J Neurol Sci.* 1966;3:577–605.
140. Sutcliffe J. Torsion spasms and abnormal postures in children with hiatus hernia. *Sandifer's syndrome. Prog Pediatr Radiol.* 1969;2:190–197.
141. Swoboda KJ, Kanavakis E, Xsaidara A, et al. Alternating hemiplegia of childhood or familial hemiplegic migraine? A novel ATP1A2 mutation. *Ann Neurol.* 2004;55(6):884–887.
142. Szepetowski P, Rochette J, Berquin P, et al. Familial infantile convulsions and paroxysmal choreoathetosis: a new neurological syndrome linked to the pericentromeric region of human chromosome 16. *Am J Hum Genet.* 1997;61(4):889–898.
143. Tardieu M, Khoury W, Navelet Y, et al. Un syndrome spectaculaire et bénin de convulsions néonatales: les myoclonies du sommeil profond. *Arch Fr Pediatr.* 1986;43:259–260.
144. Tibbles JAR, Barnes SE. Paroxysmal dystonic choreoathetosis of Mount and Reback. *Pediatrics.* 1980;65:149–151.
145. Tibbles JAR, Camfield PR, Cron CC, et al. Dominant recurrent ataxia and vertigo of childhood. *Pediatr Neurol.* 1986;2:35–38.
146. Tomasovic JA, Nellhaus G, Moe PG. The bobble-head doll syndrome: an early sign of hydrocephalus. Two new cases and a review of the literature. *Dev Med Child Neurol.* 1975;17:777–792.
147. Tomita H, Nagamitsu S, Wakui K, et al. Paroxysmal kinesigenic choreoathetosis locus maps to chromosome 16p11.2–q12.1. *Am J Hum Genet.* 1999;65(6):1688–1697.
148. Turanli G, Senbil N, Altunbasak S, et al. Benign neonatal sleep myoclonus mimicking status epilepticus. *J Child Neurol.* 2004;19(1):62–63.
149. Tuxhorn Y, Hoppe M. Parasomnia with rhythmic movements manifesting as nocturnal tongue biting. *Neuropediatrics.* 1993;24(3):167–168.
150. Vanasse M, Bedard P, Andermann F. Shuddering attacks in children: an early clinical manifestation of essential tremor. *Neurology.* 1976;26:1027–1030.
151. Verret S, Steele JC. Alternating hemiplegia in childhood: a report of eight patients with complicated migraine beginning in infancy. *Pediatrics.* 1971;47:675–680.
152. Vigevano F, Di Capua M, Dalla Bernardina B. Startle disease: an avoidable cause of sudden infant death. *Lancet.* 1989;1(8631):216.
153. Vigevano F, Fusco L, Cusmai R, et al. Tonic reflex seizures of early infancy: an undescribed nonepileptic paroxysmal disorder [Abstract]. *Epilepsia.* 1996;37(Suppl 4):87.
154. Vigevano F, Lispi ML. Tonic reflex seizures of early infancy: an age-related nonepileptic paroxysmal disorder. *Epileptic Disord.* 2001;3(3):133–136.
155. Volpe JJ. Neonatal seizures: current concepts and revised classification. *Pediatrics.* 1989;84(3):422–428.
156. Volpe JJ. *Neurology of the Newborn,* 3rd ed. Philadelphia: WB Saunders; 1995:172–207.
157. Watemberg N, Tziperman B, Dabby R, et al. Adding video recording increases the diagnostic yield of routine electroencephalograms in children with frequent paroxysmal events. *Epilepsia.* 2005;46(5):716–719.
158. Wizov SS, Reineck RD, Bocarnea M, et al. A comparative demographic and socioeconomic study of spasms nutans and infantile nystagmus. *Am J Ophthalmol.* 2002;133(2):256–262.

CHAPTER 281 ■ OVERVIEW: PSYCHIATRIC DISTURBANCES

MICHAEL R. TRIMBLE

INTRODUCTION

This section is dedicated to the many thousands, probably millions, of people who still receive an erroneous diagnosis of epilepsy, even several years after the publication of the first edition of this book. It is a testament to the broad view of the editors that they have again allotted so much space to this topic, but it also reflects the recognition of the serious clinical issues that surround it.

Historical Perspective

The problem of patients with pseudoneurologic symptoms seen by physicians is as old as the history of medicine,[2] and it became of special interest to neurologists around the end of the nineteenth century, notably with the works of Charcot. Patients with seizures have always been of special interest, so much so that the Salpêtrière school reserved a specific category for such attacks, denoted by the term *hysteria major*. For the first three fourths of the twentieth century, however, interest seems to have dwindled. Even those with a great interest in hysteria, such as Freud and succeeding psychoanalysts, wrote little about seizures, and the borderlands between epilepsy and psychiatry for a long time attracted little in the way of clinical or research interest. Things changed in the last quarter of the twentieth century (see Chapter 199), and with this renewed interest, the question of the misdiagnosis of epilepsy for symptomatically related syndromes, especially psychiatry disorders, was reborn.

CURRENT PROBLEMS OF DIFFERENTIAL DIAGNOSIS

The introduction of new techniques of investigating seizure disorder patients, but especially videotelemetry, led to the realization that many patients who at first sight appeared to have epilepsy and who were given that diagnosis along with prescriptions for anticonvulsant drugs with pronounced sedative effects in fact did not have epilepsy at all.

How frequently this problem occurs is hard to say. It has been estimated, however, that the attacks of up to 20% of patients attending clinics for chronic seizure disorders are nonepileptic in nature, but the epidemiologic studies on this vary, as reviewed by Kanner and colleagues in Chapter 282. The important point is that the figures are not going down with time, in spite of the growing clinical awareness of the problem. These patients often attend for many years, consume large amounts of antiepileptic drugs, and have huge social burdens that in part derive from having been given the label of "epileptic." Why should these errors of diagnosis be so frequent? It is difficult to conceive of a medical diagnosis other than epilepsy that has such important consequences for the patient and that is so frequently incorrectly given.

The problems may be said to begin with terminology. If the words used by physicians are unclear, ambiguous, or misleading, then the concepts that relate to those words will likewise be obscured. The term *pseudoseizures* is popular, but it is problematic. The Oxford English Dictionary defines *pseudo* as "that which is false, counterfeit, pretended or spurious." However, the seizures that are being discussed for the most part have none of these characteristics; they are real. They are experienced by patients, observed by bystanders, and thought about by physicians.

Alternative terms, such as *hysterical seizures* or *hysterical pseudoseizures*, *hysteroepilepsy*, and *psychogenic seizures*, all seem to imply pejoratively that the episodes are false and feigned by a patient for motives apparently unknown, although deception of the doctor essentially is one of them. The designation *psychogenic seizures* entails further difficulties. As Fenwick[1] correctly pointed out, this term should logically be reserved for a form of reflex epilepsy induced by mental activity.

For many, the preferred term for the seizures discussed in the following chapters is *nonepileptic seizures*, thereby acknowledging that these episodes are different from epilepsy, but also that the sudden paroxysmal attacks may resemble epilepsy. The preferred term used in this section is *psychogenic nonepileptic seizures* (PNES), but whatever term is used, it is important that the user have a clear idea of why the label is being given and exactly what is meant. Clarification of concepts, and therefore of patients' problems, cannot be achieved in the middle of a semantic muddle.

The semantic problem leads directly to the problem of differential diagnosis and why the seizures of so many patients are misdiagnosed. Thus, the phenomenon of seizures, not epilepsy, should be at the top of the diagnostic tree (Fig. 1). Many people still confuse seizures and epilepsy and can only equate the two. However, patients come to a seizure rather than an epilepsy clinic (however it is labeled), and during the initial differential diagnosis of a seizure, epilepsy can be considered as only one branch of a diagnostic tree; the other options are numerous. The ready acceptance of the notion that paroxysmal episodes of altered consciousness must be epilepsy is a clinical faux pas on a grand scale, and is in part responsible for the diagnostic errors discussed in the following chapters.

As Figure 1 illustrates, the diagnostic possibilities in patients with seizures are considerable. Thus, anyone professing to assess and manage patients with seizure disorders needs more than a passing knowledge of this spectrum of disorders. Because many conditions represented fall within a category of psychopathology, psychiatric experience should be seen as central.

The chapters in this section cover most of the topics in this diagnostic area, although cross-references are made to some other sections of the book. Although in most cases of epilepsy

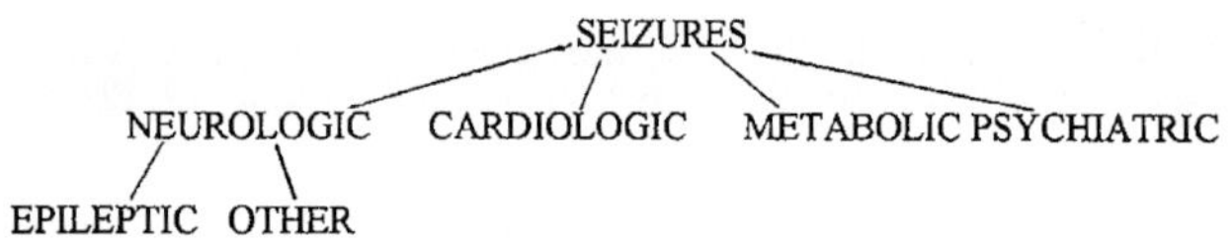

FIGURE 1. Differential diagnosis of seizures.

a clear diagnosis can be given, it is apparent that this is not so for a significant proportion of patients, who are poorly treated as the consequence of an inadequate diagnostic process. Confusions with psychotic disorders are not frequent, and more often the clinical dilemma falls within the personality disorder/anxiety disorder spectrums. Aggression and its link to epilepsy is an old but important chestnut, and it still remains a problem in psychiatric clinics, where people with spontaneous aggressive outbursts are seen, whose electroencephalogram may be abnormal, and in whom the diagnosis of epilepsy is entertained. The diagnosis rarely turns out to be epilepsy (see Chapter 212), but the referring psychiatrist will need reassurance on diagnosis, and the clinical conclusion may well have important forensic relevance. The space devoted to hyperventilation, panic attacks, dissociation, and PNES reflects both the importance of these overlapping areas for neuropsychiatry and the complexities of the underlying concepts and clinical constructs. Different clinical syndromes within this *olla podrida* of presentations may direct different treatments, and familiarity of referral patterns is therefore important for anyone in a seizure disorder clinic with a broad view on their practice. To simply label someone as having a psychiatric problem and to discharge them from the clinic is simply not helpful because they will appear again sooner or later at another clinic with the same problem, and the expense and morbidity simply increase.

SUMMARY AND CONCLUSIONS

It is sometimes said that it is better to err on the side of caution and give an uncertain diagnosis of epilepsy if presence of the disorder is suspected but not confirmed. Uncertainties arise, for example, when an electroencephalographic report makes use of the much abused word *epileptiform* or contains unhelpful comments such as "This record does not rule out temporal lobe epilepsy." An uncertainty becomes a probability, and the patient with suspected epilepsy becomes "the epileptic." Ten years later, this has been transformed to "this well-known epileptic." Actually, if the diagnosis is uncertain, it should remain so until further evidence allows clarification. In reality, from a patient's point of view, if an incorrect diagnosis is to be made, it is better to err in favor of a psychiatric diagnosis. The social stigma is rather less, and the drugs given probably have fewer side effects, than if the patient is mistakenly given the diagnosis of epilepsy and treatment based on that diagnosis.

It is hoped that the information in the following chapters will provide helpful information for those wishing to explore the world of seizures beyond epilepsy and for psychiatrists who deal at the interface of epilepsy and psychiatry as well as neurologists. If the seizures of fewer patients are misdiagnosed, the inclusion of this section in a comprehensive textbook of epilepsy will have been justified.

References

1. Fenwick P. Precipitation and inhibition of seizures. In: Reynolds EH, Trimble MR, eds. *Epilepsy and Psychiatry*. Edinburgh: Churchill Livingstone; 1981: 306–321.
2. Veith I. *Hysteria, the History of a Disease*. Chicago: University of Chicago Press; 1965.

CHAPTER 282 ■ PSYCHOGENIC NON-EPILEPTIC SEIZURES

ANDRES M. KANNER, W. CURT LAFRANCE, JR., AND TIM BETTS

INTRODUCTION

It has been known since the earliest recorded medical writings[51,100,141,148] that not all seizures in humans are of epileptic origin. From ancient times onward, instruction was given in medical texts about how to determine the clinical difference between epileptic and nonepileptic events. Many modern authorities make an assumption that it is only in recent years, with the advent of the electroencephalogram (EEG), that we have been able to detect this difference, but this is not so. Our forbearers had their own conception of what was epilepsy and what was not. Gowers' meticulous description of the hysterical convulsion bears a close relationship to a type of nonepileptic seizure that we recognize today.

The advent of the EEG and, from the late 1960s, continuous EEG monitoring (with or without video recording) led to an increased interest in distinguishing between seizures of epileptic and nonepileptic origin. It is undoubtedly true that the ability to monitor an EEG over a long period of time and register an EEG during a seizure (and to be able, in tranquility, using video, to retrospectively look at the behavior that the patient displayed during a seizure) has enormously helped our ability to distinguish between events that are epileptic and those that are not.

Nonepileptic seizures (NESs) are paroxysmal events that mimic (or are confused with) epileptic seizures, but which do not result from epileptic activity. NESs can be the expression of organic or psychogenic processes. The type of organic disorders often confused with epileptic seizures include convulsive syncope, various forms of sleep and movement disorders, and migrainous processes and are reviewed in Section XI of this book. The decision as to whether a patient's seizures belong in the domain of epilepsy or nonepileptic events may have to be based on various sets of criteria, in addition to the EEG data. The distinction between epilepsy and nonepilepsy cannot always be made with complete confidence, and the physician working in this field must be able to tolerate some degree of uncertainty. Epileptic and nonepileptic seizures also may coexist. This chapter will focus on nonepileptic seizures of psychogenic origin.

NOMENCLATURE

The most commonly used term for nonepileptic seizures is *pseudoseizure*; this term first came into use in the 1960s and was widely used in the 1970s and 1980s. Yet, psychogenic NESs have been labeled with various eponyms over the last two centuries. For example, Charcot referred to these attacks as "hysteroepilepsy"[77] in the 19th century, and he had recommended the use of ovarian compressors for their treatment, based largely on the theory of the ancient Greeks that such attacks were due to the "wandering of the uterus throughout the body, away from its normal location in the pelvis." Other terms used more recently have included *nonepileptic seizures, psychogenic seizures,* and *hysterical seizures.*

There is an increasing tendency to abandon the term *pseudoseizure* as it is considered to have a pejorative connotation and to imply falseness. Deliberate deceit plays only a small part in the genesis of most nonepileptic seizures (i.e., cases of malingering),[22] although, sadly, many clinicians think otherwise. The term *pseudoseizure* also conveys the implication that anything that is not epilepsy is not interesting and that no further attention need be paid to the attacks.

There is an ongoing debate on the use of the term *seizure* as many patients are unable to discriminate between the concepts of *psychogenic* versus *epileptic* processes and get fixated on the word *seizure*. To avert such potential confusion the term *psychogenic nonepileptic event* has been suggested. Such terms help differentiate the nonepileptic nature of these attacks from epileptic seizures and convey their probable psychogenic cause.

Psychogenic seizures is a term much used in the United States and on the continent of Europe to describe psychologically based nonepileptic seizures. It is correct providing that there is agreement about what it means and the range of disorders it covers. Unfortunately, the term also has been used to refer to those epileptic seizures that are triggered by an emotional experience.[44] Potential confusion could be avoided by using the terms *nonepileptic psychogenic seizure* and *epileptic psychogenic seizure*.

The terms *hysterical seizure*, *hysterical epilepsy*, and *hysterical convulsion* should not be used. The word *hysteria* is no longer used in psychiatric parlance because it is meaningless. It has been so much abused and misused that it should be abandoned,[100] and the term *conversion disorder* should be used instead. Not all nonepileptic attacks are related to conversion disorder.

Functional seizure is also sometimes used, but the term is imprecise and has more than one meaning. An epileptic seizure, for instance, that occurs or is precipitated at a propitious time (e.g., before a stressful event) so that the patient avoids a threatening situation could legitimately be called functional. Blumer[36] has suggested the term *paroxysmal somatoform disorder*. In some ways this is an attractive term. However, it does imply that all nonepileptic events of psychological origin relate to the somatoform disorders when they clearly do not. The term could be used as part of a classification of psychologically based nonepileptic seizures, and this would be more acceptable.

Psychogenic nonepileptic seizure (PNES) is the term that has been chosen for this chapter and is coming into common use. It may not be ideal, but it is less pejorative and more meaningful than *pseudoseizure*; however, clinicians must always ensure that the patients and family understand that the inclusion of the term *seizure* does not imply a diagnosis of epilepsy.

EPIDEMIOLOGY OF PSYCHOGENIC NONEPILEPTIC SEIZURES

There are relatively little data on the incidence and prevalence rates of PNESs. Various estimates of prevalence have been given by various investigators in different settings. It is important to try to determine the influence that the setting has both on the way that seizures present and on their frequency. Prevalence will be different if patients with new-onset seizures are being assessed in a primary care setting compared with reassessment of patients who have an intractable seizure disorder in a tertiary referral center.

An indirect estimate of the possible incidence of nonepileptic seizures in a primary care setting can be derived from the work of Sander et al.,[121] which was a careful phenomenologic study of patients presenting to their general practitioner with a seizure disorder and who were carefully assessed and followed. It was shown that some 28% of patients suspected of having epilepsy after presentation to their general practitioner either did not have it (7%) or the diagnosis could not be substantiated even a year after the initial presentation (21%). In the only nationwide population-based study done to date, Sigurdardottir and Olafsson found the population-based incidence of PNESs to be 1.4 per 100,000 in Iceland, compared to an incidence of 35 per 100,000 for true epilepsy among persons older than 15 years.[129] In a retrospective study carried out in Hamilton County, OH, investigators established the incidence of PNESs between 1995 and 1998. They found a mean incidence of 3.03 per 100,000, with the highest incidence in 1998 (4.6 per 100,000). Most patients with the diagnosis of PNES were aged 25 to 45 years (4.38 per 100,000).[138]

The prevalence rates of PNESs have been estimated to range from 10% to 40% among patients referred to epilepsy centers for the evaluation of poorly controlled seizures.[26,30,74,77] The prevalence of comorbid PNES and epilepsy varies according to the type of population studied. For example, in a study of 1,590 patients who underwent a video-EEG (V-EEG) monitoring study at the Epilepsy Center of the University of Alabama in Birmingham, 514 (32.3%) were diagnosed with PNES and 29 (5.3%) of these patients were found to have both PNES and epilepsy.[96] Henry and Drury conducted a V-EEG in 145 patients who had temporal interictal EEG spikes and reported ictal semiology characteristic of temporal lobe seizures for presurgical evaluation of medically refractory seizures. PNESs were unexpectedly identified in 12 (8%) of these patients.[57] On the other hand, a study from Germany found that among 329 consecutive patients in whom the diagnosis of PNES was established, 206 (62%) had only PNES, and 123 (37%) had PNES and epilepsy.[118] In a critical review of the literature, Ramsey et al. came to the conclusion that the comorbid occurrence of epilepsy and PNES was rare with prevalence rates ranging between 4% and 10%.[116] Relatively high prevalence rates can be expected when studies are carried out in populations of cognitively impaired or in pediatric patients, however. Neill and Alvarez, for example, reported prevalence rates of up to 40%.[104] Kotagal et al. found that 25% of pediatric patients with PNES also suffered from epilepsy.[75] Higher prevalence rates of comorbid PNES and epilepsy in these two patient populations is not surprising, as they learn that fewer demands are placed on them when they have a seizure. Hence, they are likely to experience a PNES when facing situations that cause distress or that they consciously or unconsciously are trying to avoid.

PNESs are much more common in women than men; in most series 60% to 75% of patients are women.[12,58,77,78,91,93,110,117] The onset of PNESs most often occurs in the third and fourth decades of life,[12,53,77,89] though they have been described in both children and the elderly.[7,42,68,152,153]

CLINICAL MANIFESTATIONS

PNESs can mimic convulsive and nonconvulsive epileptic seizures; they may present as isolated events or occur in clusters and, often, may mimic status epilepticus. The advent of V-EEG has facilitated the recognition of PNESs among neurologists and epileptologists, and it appears that nonneurologists are increasingly becoming more aware of this type of paroxysmal event. There have been multiple review articles on the diagnosis of PNES[7,21,54,66,68,71,92,126] and various investigators have tried to emphasize the clinical differences between PNESs and epileptic seizures with lists and tables of distinguishing features.[53,78,89] While certain features of convulsive PNESs may be highly suggestive of this diagnosis, there are no clinical phenomena that are 100% specific to one or the other.[151] Because our ability to recognize PNESs is not infallible and in some patients, with different kinds of events, it is impossible to decide if they have epilepsy or not, a diagnosis cannot be established on the bases of clinical phenomena alone, but has to be corroborated with electrographic recordings, and occasionally, functional neuroimaging studies with ictal single photon emission computed tomography (SPECT) may be necessary to reach a correct diagnosis (see below). In short, the diagnosis of a PNES is based on a considered judgment of all relevant history, seizure phenomena, electrophysiologic data, and results of other investigations and remains a clinical one. Using one or two phenomena in a differential diagnosis table to make a rapid diagnosis would be injudicious and could lead to inadvertent misdiagnosis. Furthermore, several studies published in the last 15 years have demonstrated that clinical phenomena associated with PNESs can occur in certain types of epileptic seizures, a fact that still remains underrecognized by many clinicians, including neurologists, and has often lead to the inverse diagnostic problem (i.e., patients with epilepsy being falsely diagnosed with PNES). For example, in a study of 100 consecutive patients that were undergoing a diagnostic V-EEG, Parra et al.[110] found that referring physicians correctly suspected a diagnosis of epileptic seizures in only 9 (43%) of 21 patients, while 12 (57%) patients were incorrectly thought to have PNESs. This misdiagnosis was especially likely in patients with clinical seizures of mesial frontal or parietal lobe origin. To confuse matters further, there are a number of patients who suffer from both epileptic seizures and PNESs, with coexistence of both types of disorders ranging from 7% to 37%. Most studies have found incidence rates ranging between 10% and 20%.[14,38,58,72,90] This point is examined in greater detail in Chapter 208.

Needless to say, reaching a correct diagnosis is of the essence as a misdiagnosis of PNESs as epileptic seizures, and vice versa, exposes patients to ineffective, costly, and potentially dangerous treatments. Indeed, several investigators have found that 69% to 78% of patients with PNESs have been treated with antiepileptic drugs (AEDs)[14,120] and up to 30% of patients have been misdiagnosed at some point with status epilepticus and admitted to an intensive care unit where they were treated with parenteral medications that are associated with potential serious adverse events, and which in some cases caused respiratory arrest.[59,117,120]

In general, a diagnosis of PNES is easier to suspect in convulsivelike events, while in nonconvulsive events a diagnosis of PNES may be impossible without concurrent electrographic recordings. In the next section we review the value and limitations of clinical phenomena in suspecting the diagnosis of PNES.

Convulsive Psychogenic Nonepileptic Seizures

Motor Phenomena

In convulsivelike PNES, motor signs include cloniclike, myocloniclike, and toniclike movements of the extremities and trunk. However, violent thrashing of the extremities and/or of the entire body, opisthotonic arching of the back, pelvic thrusting motions, and side-to-side head movements are the typical motor phenomena associated with PNESs. Frontal lobe seizures have been shown to present with the same type of motor phenomena; for example, Geyer et al. found pelvic thrusting to be equally common in frontal lobe seizures and PNESs[48] (also see below).

Out-of-phase and asynchronous cloniclike movements in the upper extremities (as opposed to in-phase and synchronous during epileptic seizures) is another "typical" motor sign suggestive of PNESs.[46] However, Leis et al. were not able to make this same distinction in their analysis of the motor phenomena of PNESs.[89]

The absence of any facial cloniclike activity in the presence of generalized cloniclike activity can be another "helpful" sign in suspecting a diagnosis of PNES. Family members need to be instructed ahead of time to look for such sign, however.

Incontinence and Self-injury

Contrary to old beliefs, patients with PNES *do get hurt*. Indeed, in a study by Reuber et al., almost 60% of patients had experienced PNES-related injuries, 32.3% had reported urinary incontinence, and 31.5% tongue biting (patients with both PNESs and epileptic seizures were not included in these percentages).[120] Incontinence has been reported to range between 10% and 44% in PNESs, most of which consist of urinary incontinence, but fecal incontinence has been also described.[95,112,120] Bruising and minor lacerations from falls followed by tongue biting (that may be severe enough to cause bleeding) are among the more common injuries reported in patients with PNESs. Tongue biting, which often does occur in a tonic–clonic seizure, also can occur in complex partial seizures, in faints (if the patient falls and bites the tongue as a result of the fall), and in PNESs (either as a result of falling or as a result of deliberate injurious behavior, not necessarily to simulate a seizure but because the patient is responding to inwardly driven motivation to try to hurt himself or herself). The site of the bite may yield clues but can be misleading. In a tonic–clonic seizure the bite is usually on the side of the tongue and is deep, although it may occur at the tip of it. In tongue injury as a result of falling, the bite is usually at the tip. In complex partial seizures the bite may be at the tip or occasionally at the side of the tongue or may involve the cheek. However, patients having PNESs also can bite the side of the tongue, tip of the tongue, and cheek. Finally, serious injuries, including facial bone fractures, are less common but have also been reported and tend to occur in patients with a psychiatric history of suicide attempts.[112]

Vocalizations

Vocalizations can be often seen in convulsivelike PNESs, but occasionally occur in non–convulsivelike events. Vocalizations associated with shedding of tears tend to suggest a strong possibility of PNESs.[17] In convulsivelike events, vocalizations consist of shouting, screaming, and sobbing often associated with understandable speech.[46,53,89,95] In contrast, in epileptic seizures, vocalizations are typically more primitive, such as grunting or a simple shout.[46] Vocalizations are more likely to occur in the middle of PNESs, unlike epileptic seizures, where vocalizations usually occur at the onset of the event.

Nonconvulsive Psychogenic Nonepileptic Seizures

Nonconvulsive PNESs can mimic either absence and/or partial complex seizures; more often than not, a correct diagnosis is unlikely to be reached until patients are referred for V-EEG with a presumed diagnosis of "intractable epilepsy." Patients may be unresponsive while exhibiting a motionless stare and they may exhibit semipurposeful movements simulating motor automatisms of complex partial seizures.[53] Maintenance of eyes closed and responsiveness to "selective" external stimulation, including verbally, in the course of an event during which they "appear" to be unresponsive are two clinical "clues" that should raise the suspicion of a PNES. More commonly, patients remain nonverbal but display active avoidance to both noxious and nonnoxious stimuli and/or resist attempts at eye opening, but this type of avoidant behavior may also be identified in complex partial seizures.

Other Clinical Characteristics of Psychogenic Nonepileptic Seizures

Sudden collapse to the ground with apparent unconsciousness but no movement can be part of epilepsy and can occur without warning. It is usually a primary generalized seizure (either a tonic seizure in which the patient falls stiffly or an atonic one in which the patient collapses with sudden loss of muscle tone). In both seizures recovery of consciousness (unless the patient has injured the head in falling) is swift and there is little postictal confusion (unless, again, the patient's head has been struck in the fall). Occasionally sudden loss of consciousness with falling can be seen in seizures originating in the temporal or frontal lobe.[28] The fall may be flaccid (but can occur with a tonic spasm), and consciousness usually is regained fairly quickly. The patient who falls in a flaccid way and remains apparently unconscious for some time is unlikely to have epilepsy. Epileptic seizures with falls, if monitored via EEG, may not be detected either because the patient is in bed and the characteristic falling is therefore not seen, or because the fall itself produces such artifact in the recording device that the ictal nature of the event is obscured. It also is possible that the preliminary collapse was due to epilepsy but the subsequent withdrawn behavior is a psychological elaboration of the brief epileptic experience. This may not be an uncommon occurrence.

Psychogenic Nonepileptic Seizures as "Drop Attack"

Physical and emotional causes of collapse are considered in other chapters (e.g., syncope in Chapter 271 and hyperventilation in Chapter 285). A not-uncommon cause of collapse and flaccid unconsciousness of a psychological type of nonepileptic seizure is the so-called swoon.[19] Here the patient, when threatened by external events or unpleasant memories or by a situation reminiscent of an unpleasant experience, will close the eyes, sink to the floor, and lie inert and not moving for various lengths of time, sometimes for over an hour. Passive movement and eye opening may be resisted, but usually the patient just lies inert and unresponsive and comes to quite quickly with little in the way of postictal symptoms. Presumably this is a form of learned behavior; it is a common childhood behavior that may have persisted into adult life. There is some evidence[20,61] that it also may be a common mechanism for avoiding flashbacks and reawakened memories in adults with a chronic posttraumatic stress disorder related to previous childhood sexual abuse, particularly if it was the way that the individual dealt with the abuse at the time it was occurring. Some abused people cope with their abuse by lying inert and retreating into themselves or by splitting their consciousness so that they almost seem to be watching events from a corner of the room and become passive observers of themselves; this may become a persistent unconscious learned pattern of behavior to deal with stressful events and later may be mistaken for epilepsy.

Deliberate Simulation of Unconsciousness

Deliberate simulation of unconsciousness, which may involve falling, is part of the repertoire of people with somatoform disorders or with factitious disorder or malingering (deliberately simulated disease). In the case of factitious disorder, individuals simulate illness to maintain the sick role; malingerers do so for social or financial gain. It is easy to sustain for long periods of time and difficult to detect, particularly if the patient does not resist passive movement or eye opening and does not respond to noxious stimuli. Such behavior (often seen as attention-seeking behavior in nurses and other caring professionals who are particularly prone to factitious disorder) is sometimes mistaken for epilepsy. Some professional simulators may inject themselves with insulin beforehand to add further authenticity to their performance.

Nonstereotypic Events?

PNESs have typically been thought of as nonstereotypic events (within patients), while the reverse has been considered to be a clinical sign supportive of a diagnosis of epileptic seizures. While the absence of a stereotypic semiology within patients should raise suspicions of a diagnosis of PNES, the reverse does not rule out this diagnosis. In fact, in four studies, 60% to 90% of patients with PNESs had spells that varied little from event to event.[38,48,53,99] However, even when clinical features and their sequence is relatively stereotypic, the duration of seizures in patients with PENSs tends to be more variable than in those with epileptic seizures.

Events of Long Duration

PNESs are more often than not significantly longer in duration than epileptic seizures and often lead to a misdiagnosis of status epilepticus (see below). A rapid recovery of cognitive functions following a prolonged convulsivelike or non–convulsivelike event should raise suspicions of possible PNESs (see below).

Psychogenic Nonepileptic Seizures Only Occur in Awake State

PNESs can only occur when the patient is awake, and events occurring out of sleep, documented with electrographic recordings, cannot be considered as PNESs. Having said that, clinicians cannot accept the patients' assertion of events occurring out of sleep without electrographic corroboration, as PNESs have been described in patients that "appear to be asleep" but in reality are awake.[16]

Psychogenic Nonepileptic Seizures Mimicking Status Epilepticus

One of the most serious consequences of PNES is their mimicking "status epilepticus" that is not properly diagnosed, which in turn results in unnecessary admissions to intensive care units, aggressive use of parenteral AEDs, and placement of endotracheal tubes. Iatrogenic damage (respiratory arrests, toxic effects from anticonvulsants) are common, and because PNESs do not respond to AEDs, prolonged hospital stays with expensive and dangerous treatments (including paralysis, anesthesia, and assisted ventilation) often occur.[59,117,120] For example, in a study by Reuber et al., 51% of patients with PNESs presented as "pseudostatus" (lasting more than 30 minutes) and 27.8% were admitted to intensive care units.[120] Howell et al.[59] suggested that perhaps 50% of patients admitted to emergency care in the United Kingdom in status epilepticus do not actually have epilepsy.

Some investigators have suggested that PNES mimicking status epilepticus occurs mainly in women whose seizures relate to a posttraumatic stress disorder from previous sexual abuse,[20,29] in individuals with hyperventilation attacks that are easily prolonged by inadvertent reinforcement, or in patients with conversion or factitious disorder (e.g., Münchhausen syndrome or malingering). Accordingly, emergency room staff should be encouraged to observe seizures critically before starting treatment, to use a pulse oximeter to distinguish patients who need immediate intubation from those who can be safely left to breathe without assistance, and to obtain arterial blood gases, which may also detect those who are hyperventilating.

Epileptic Seizures Mimicking Psychogenic Nonepileptic Seizures

As stated above, a study by Parra et al.[110] suggested that as clinicians have become increasingly aware of PNESs, epileptic seizures with atypical features are being misdiagnosed as PNESs. The error rate in diagnosing nonepileptic seizures in patients who clearly have epilepsy probably lies between 5% and 10%.[116,151] Complex partial seizures of mesial frontal origin can present with complex automatisms, very often with "bizarre" features that mimic the typical phenomena of PNESs. These include kicking or pedaling motions of the lower extremities; thrashing and flailing motions of the extremities or entire body, at times with very violent thrusts; and affect-laden vocalizations, such as screams and loud cries. Other phenomena that may contribute to the diagnostic confusion include a preserved consciousness in seizures originating in supplementary sensory motor area, despite a bilateral tonic posturing, and the absence of postictal lethargy or confusion. Kanner et al.[70] compared the clinical phenomena of supplementary sensory motor seizures with those of PNESs and found clinical phenomena suggestive of PNESs in 82% of all seizures recorded in 91% of the frontal lobe epilepsy patients studied.

The atypical clinical phenomena of these seizures are frequently coupled with undetected interictal and ictal epileptiform activity on scalp recordings. The difficulty in identifying any epileptiform discharges results from the great amount of muscle and movement artifact masking the underlying electrical activity. The inability of the angle subtended by scalp electrodes to identify the source of the epileptic activity in mesial or orbitofrontal regions is another contributing cause to this problem. Thus, it is not surprising that these seizures are frequently confused with PNESs.[70,103,123,147,151] Morris et al.[103] have demonstrated the presence of a subtle rhythmic theta pattern in parasagittal leads, buried within muscle and movement artifact. The use of high-frequency filters may be necessary to recognize such pattern. In addition, the presence of a structural lesion on magnetic resonance imaging (MRI) in mesial or orbitofrontal regions should raise suspicions of epileptic seizures in patients diagnosed with PNESs.

There are certain clinical features that may help the clinician distinguish this type of frontal lobe seizure from PNES: (a) frontal lobe seizures are very short in duration (<30 seconds); (b) they are stereotypic, including the complex automatisms; (c) they often occur out of sleep, whereas PNESa *always* occur in the awake state; and (d) they often display a tonic posturing in abduction of the upper extremities, a sign that was found to be specific to epileptic seizures involving the supplementary sensory-motor area and never seen in PNES.[70,103,147] A cautionary note is in order: PNESs may be reported by patients to arise out of sleep, but V-EEG monitoring demonstrates an awake EEG pattern preceding the onset of the PNESs.[16,139] Benbadis et al.[16] coined the term "pre-ictal pseudosleep" to describe the state of wakefulness while appearing asleep in these patients with PNES.

COMORBIDITY OF EPILEPSY AND PSYCHOGENIC NONEPILEPTIC SEIZURES

This topic is reviewed in great detail in Chapter 208. Briefly, quoted rates for the coexistence of epilepsy and PNES vary from <10% to >90% of the population studied.[66,68,71,92,116] The literature is confusing because different populations of patients have been studied by different investigators and because of the uncertainty about the diagnosis of PNESs. It is impossible to be dogmatic about how commonly patients with established epilepsy develop PNESs, particularly because the association at times must be purely coincidental, but coexistence of epilepsy with PNESs is not a common problem. Probably no more than 5% of people with established epilepsy develop nonepileptic seizures.

In the literature, completely different methods have been used for diagnosing nonepileptic seizures, based sometimes on EEG criteria (but not necessarily EEGs recorded during the ictus itself), on clinical criteria, or on a mixture of both. It is also sometimes not clear, when the prevalence of the two conditions is compared, whether the investigator is referring to patients with nonepileptic seizures and present epilepsy or merely a history of it in the past. It is likely, as Ramsey et al. have concluded,[116] that if the history is one of past as opposed to present epilepsy, the proportion of patients with both epilepsy and nonepilepsy is likely to be higher, particularly in patients with learning difficulty.[104]

Sometimes the question can only be answered by withdrawing the antiepileptic medication and seeing if epilepsy reemerges. If it does, one must pose the question, "Was this all epilepsy that I was trying to treat, or am I dealing with somebody who has controllable epilepsy but who has a psychological need for it?"

A review of the literature suggests that 10% to 30% of patients who appear to have established nonepileptic seizures also have a past history of epileptic seizures, which means that even when it is obvious that a patient's seizures are nonepileptic, slow and cautious reduction of anticonvulsant medication is indicated.[66,71] Rapid reduction of anticonvulsant medication, even in patients who do not have epilepsy, may precipitate pharmacologic withdrawal seizures, which will make the picture even more difficult to assess. A final consideration: The literature suggests that if one is assessing a patient with an unknown attack disorder that has two different presentations, 5% to 30% of the time one may be dealing both with epilepsy and a nonepileptic seizure.[116]

DIAGNOSTIC EVALUATION OF PSYCHOGENIC NONEPILEPTIC SEIZURES

Neurologic Workup

The diagnostic workup of PNES consists first and foremost of neurophysiologic studies aimed at capturing the patient's typical events and documenting the absence of a concurrent epileptic ictal pattern. However, the fact that a patient has PNES does not rule out the presence of comorbid neurologic disorders, including a coexisting or past epileptic seizure disorder. In fact, people with a correct diagnosis of NES have been found to have a clearcut history or evidence on examination of cerebral injury,[72,78,118] whereas a significant percentage of people with epilepsy have no such history. Once the diagnosis of NES is established, a psychogenic cause must be investigated with psychiatric and neuropsychological evaluations. Yet, although many people with proven NES have a recognizable psychiatric illness or history or evidence of emotional precipitation of seizures, so do many people with epilepsy. The diagnosis of an NES cannot depend solely on these features but is based on the judicious and considered review of all the evidence available to the clinician. This is particularly important when certain psychological or psychiatric conditions are present in a patient who has an undiagnosed attack disorder. For example, a history of sexual abuse is not uncommon in people with proven epilepsy and may be pathoplastic in the seizure content.[19,52]

The neurologic evaluation of patients with suspected PNES must include V-EEG or ambulatory EEG studies to capture the typical event, and neuroimaging studies including brain MRI to rule out the presence of structural pathology that may be associated with a past or present comorbid neurologic disorder. In addition, the presence of a structural lesion in mesial-frontal regions of the brain may alert the clinician to be cautious on reaching a false-positive diagnosis of PNES and rule out the presence of epileptic seizures mimicking PNESs. In some patients functional neuroimaging studies such as ictal SPECT may be necessary when the distinction between PNES and epileptic seizures with atypical features may be difficult.

Video-electroencephalographic Monitoring

The electrographic diagnosis of PNESs is based on the recording of one of the patient's typical events in the absence of any electrographic change from their baseline "awake" activity. To ensure that a typical event has been captured, the recordings have to be shown to family members who have witnessed the patient's events. Furthermore, it is important to enquire from these family members about the occurrence (in the present or in the past) of events different than those captured during the V-EEG. This will minimize the risk of failing to identify a comorbid epileptic seizure disorder that may be either occurring simultaneously with PNES or a prior seizure disorder that may have remitted with AEDs. Clearly, such information is pivotal on the decision to discontinue AEDs.

When Should Antiepileptic Drug Dosages be Lowered during the Video-electroencephalogram?

PNESs are likely to occur in the early stages of a V-EEG. For example, Parra et al. found that up to 96% of patients with PNESs had a typical event within the first 48 hours of V-EEG.[111] Accordingly, it is reasonable to maintain the patients' usual AED doses during the initial 2 days of the study so as to minimize the risk of facilitating the occurrence of an epileptic seizure early in the monitoring study of patients with both PNES and epilepsy. It has been our experience that once an epileptic seizure has been recorded, clinicians prematurely conclude that all the events are epileptic, leading to a false-negative diagnosis of PNES.

Benzodiazepines should not be discontinued during V-EEG of patients with suspected PNESs, as their abrupt discontinuation may trigger withdrawal seizures or withdrawal psychiatric symptoms, particularly panic attacks and anxiety, resulting in false-negative or false-positive data.

AEDs can be lowered or even discontinued to establish the existence of suspected concurrent epileptic seizures. Such can be the case in patients with documented PNESs whose V-EEG recordings reveal interictal epileptiform activity and who are reported to exhibit other paroxysmal events that by their semiology may be suspected of being epileptic seizures. In the case of suspected epileptic seizures that preceded the onset of PNESs and remitted with pharmacotherapy, discontinuation of AEDs may not necessarily result in their occurrence during the course of a typical V-EEG.

The Significance of Interictal Epileptiform Activity

Interictal EEGs are reported to be abnormal in 23% to 50% of patients with PNESs; although diffuse or focal slowing is the most common abnormality, interictal epileptiform activity is seen in 35% to 50% of patients with PNESs.[14,38,58,72,78,90,104,116,118] The presence of interictal epileptiform activity in recordings of patients with a documented PNES raises the possibility of comorbid occurrence of PNESs and epileptic seizures, or of a prior history of epileptic seizures. As stated above, this comorbidity has been reported in 5% to 40% of patients with PNESs. Devinsky et al. have shown that the semiology of PNESs and epileptic seizures differ from each other in patients with comorbid disorders.[38]

Ictal Recordings

The absence of any electrographic ictal patterns while the patient is unresponsive documents a diagnosis of PNES in most patients. However, 10% of patients with epileptic seizures may not show any ictal pattern on scalp recordings, especially when the ictal activity originates from mesial frontal, mesial parietal, and, occasionally, mesial temporal structures.[70,103,123,147,151] In addition, scalp recordings will fail to reveal any electrographic changes in up to 75% of simple partial seizures,[39] given that scalp electrodes are able to detect epileptiform activity only if a cortical area of 6 cm^2 or more has been synchronously activated. Thus, reliance solely on EEG recordings to make a diagnosis of PNES may yield false-positive data. Accordingly, in the presence of paroxysmal events that are not associated with any loss of consciousness and normal concurrent EEG recordings, clinicians must consider the possibility of a diagnosis of simple partial seizures before concluding that they are PNESs. In the presence of events with unresponsiveness, bizarre clinical phenomena, and concurrent undetectable electrographic ictal patterns, a diagnosis of mesial frontal or parietal lobe seizures should be considered in the presence of the clinical characteristics described above. A diagnosis of PNES is more likely in the absence of clinical signs typical of frontal lobe seizures and if these events can be induced and stopped with the use of suggestive techniques.

Special electrodes have been used during the V-EEG to facilitate the detection of electrographic ictal patterns. These include orbitofrontal electrodes and the use of the 10-10 electrodes over parasagittal areas to identify ictal activity of mesial and orbitofrontal origin.[9,67] In these seizures, the electrographic ictal pattern consists of a very subtle rhythmic theta activity over parasagittal regions.[103] Sphenoidal electrodes inserted under fluoroscopic guidance can identify interictal and ictal activity of mesial temporal origin with a very restricted electric field.[69,73]

Induction of Psychogenic Nonepileptic Seizures

The use of induction protocols to trigger a PNES has been the source of much controversy, first with respect to the potential of a false-positive diagnosis (either by provoking atypical events or by facilitating epileptic seizures) and second with respect to the "ethical" use of many of the protocols used that ultimately can lead the patient to feel that he or she was lied to.

There is a general agreement that induction protocols do facilitate the occurrence of PNESs.[11,32,38,87,89,95,111,131,145] Among the different studies, the sensitivity of various protocols has ranged between 37% and 91%, with most studies reporting a successful induction in 77% to 84%.[11,32,38,87,89,131,145] While most studies report the specificity of induction of PNESs to be 100%,[32,38,87,131] there have been reports of epileptic seizures triggered by induction. Walczak et al.[145] reported that 10% of patients with epilepsy experienced seizures after induction; others have also reported similar findings.[92,111] Therefore, a positive induction does not document a diagnosis of PNES, and to avert this type of error, induction protocols should not be carried out in the absence of concurrent electrographic recordings. The study by Parra et al.[111] previously cited is particularly noteworthy as it addresses the question of whether induction protocols are necessary during V-EEG. Indeed, of 100 patients admitted for V-EEG monitoring studies, 87 experienced their typical event and 82 of these did so spontaneously, without induction. Among the patients with PNESs, 96% experienced their typical event without induction in the initial 48 hours. Slater et al.[131] reported similar findings in which 75% of patients with PNESs had spontaneous events without induction.

Several induction protocols have been suggested. Every protocol is based on the use of a "placebo," which raises serious ethical issues and may jeopardize the patient–physician relationship, the patient's trust of all physicians, and the patient's acceptance of the diagnosis of PNESs. The most frequently used protocol consists of intravenous infusion of a saline solution after the patient is told that he or she will be given a medication likely to induce seizures.[32,38,131,145] Other protocols have relied on the placement of an alcohol-soaked patch on the patient's neck after informing the patient that this was likely to provoke a seizure,[87] while other protocols consist of having the patient undergo photic stimulation and hyperventilation, as performed in any routine EEG study. Clearly, with the former two protocols patients may realize that they have been deceived, while the use of hyperventilation and/or photic stimulation does not carry this risk as these are established maneuvers used in all EEG studies to facilitate the occurrence of seizures.

The potential ethical problems associated with induction protocols may put in jeopardy the entire treatment process, as the nature of the protocol precludes informing patients on the true nature of the procedure, and with the exception of protocols using hyperventilation and photic stimulation, clinicians are in essence lying to patients as to the potential effect of the stimulus on seizure activity. Such misrepresentation of the facts can compromise the patient–physician relationship and trust and give the patient reasons to reject outright the diagnosis of PNES and the suggested treatment. Despite these concerns, several authors have defended the use of induction protocols arguing that by aiding in the accurate diagnosis of PNES, induction may help prevent the patient from receiving inappropriate, potentially harmful AEDs and the incorrect diagnosis of epilepsy, with its potential psychological and social hardships, and that therefore the use of induction techniques is ethically justifiable.[37] While no one questions the value of induction protocols, the use of techniques that may lead patients to feel deceived should be a deterrent to the use of induction protocols relying on a "placebo," as the same results can be reached with protocols relying on the use of regular activation methods in EEG such as photic stimulation, hyperventilation, or both combined.[13,111] Finally, the use of hypnosis as a trigger of PNESs has been gaining increasing interest among psychiatrists.[97] Experts in hypnosis, following full disclosure of the technique, should be the only ones attempting such procedures, however.

Outpatient Electroencephalographic Studies

Attempts to avoid inpatient evaluations and to rely on outpatient diagnostic studies have become necessary with greater frequency in patients suspected of having PNESs, given an increase in medical costs and greater limitations of resources faced by governmental and private third-party payers. Two modalities of outpatient EEG studies have been used: (a) outpatient V-EEG of 2 to 8 hours' duration and (2) ambulatory EEG studies.

Outpatient Video-electroencephalography

There is an increasing body of literature documenting the value of using this type of diagnostic studies. Patients with daily events and those with suspected PNESs are potential candidates. For example, in a prospective study of 37 children with daily paroxysmal episodes, with outpatient V-EEG averaging 3 hours typical events were recorded in 23 patients; in 11 the study allowed clinicians to distinguish epileptic from nonepileptic seizures.[3] In a study of 50 consecutive patients with suspected PNESs, Bahtia et al. used ambulatory V-EEG with the use of an induction protocol consisting of saline infusion.[24] Fifteen patients had a spontaneous event and another 15 had an event induced with induction.

This type of study has an important limitation, as it may fail to record interictal epileptiform activity in patients who may have coexisting rare epileptic seizures or who suffered from epileptic seizures in the past that remitted with AEDs. Clearly, if this type of study is to be used, a detailed history of the patient's present and past events is of the essence, above all when the decision to discontinue AEDs is being considered. Furthermore, some patients may need to undergo a prolonged V-EEG before a definite diagnosis is reached.

Ambulatory Electroencephalography

The advantage of these studies is that the EEG recordings are obtained while the patient is in his or her habitual environment. The disadvantage is that EEG recordings are often masked by movement and muscle artifact during the event, and in the absence of any video, it is impossible for the clinician to establish the nature of the event. Aminoff et al.[6] and Berkovic et al.[18] had concluded that ambulatory EEG studies are useful to identify epileptic seizures. However, events without an electrographic ictal pattern cannot necessarily be considered nonepileptic. Nevertheless, with the availability of ambulatory V-EEG home systems and the ability to use a larger number of channels, and to reformat recordings, ambulatory studies may end up replacing inpatient V-EEG in the future in a significant percentage of cases.

Neuroimaging Studies

Magnetic Resonance Imaging Studies

As stated above, patients with PNES may have abnormal neurologic examinations, EEG studies, and MRI studies. For example, in a study of 45 patients with PNESs, 43% had an abnormal MRI.[72] In these patients, an abnormal MRI finding may identify comorbid neurologic disorders that may explain some of their symptomatology, not related to PNES. More importantly, however, a structural lesion in mesial frontal or parietal regions should lead the physician to seriously reconsider the diagnosis of PNES.

Single Photon Emission Computed Tomography

The use of this type of study can be of great assistance in clarifying whether a paroxysmal event with atypical clinical phenomena is in fact an epileptic seizure mimicking PNES (i.e., partial seizure of mesial frontal origin), provided that the radionuclear marker is injected at the time of the event (ictal SPECT). The epileptogenic zone is represented by an area of hyperperfusion on ictal SPECT. While, the sole use of interictal SPECT yields unreliable data in patients with epilepsy and is of no diagnostic value,[40,105,114,133,135,149] its use in conjunction with an ictal SPECT (SISCOM study) has enhanced the diagnostic yield of data obtained with ictal SPECT. A negative SISCOM or ictal SPECT, however, does not imply a diagnosis of PNES. Conversely, an abnormal SPECT scan does not mean epilepsy is always present. Studies of small series of ictal and interictal SPECT scans in NES revealed a small number of patients with lateralized perfusion abnormalities. The findings did not change, however, when comparing the ictal and the interictal images.[41]

Laboratory Tests

Two blood tests have been used in the differential diagnosis between epileptic and nonepileptic seizures: Prolactin (PRL) and creatine phosphokinase (CPK) serum concentrations.

Serum prolactin levels are commonly elevated following generalized tonic–clonic seizures and complex partial seizures of temporal lobe origin, provided that levels are drawn within 20 to 30 minutes of seizure onset. Prolactin levels are generally not elevated following simple partial seizures, complex partial seizures of frontal lobe origin, or PNESs,[33,35,88,98] though Alving et al. reported a statistically significant increase in prolactin levels in patients following PNESs.[5] Another study reported a significant rise in serum prolactin levels following episodes of hypotensive syncope.[108] The Therapeutics and Technology Assessment Subcommittee of the American Academy of Neurology recently published its report on the use of serum PRL in differentiating epileptic seizures from NESs. The authors reviewed the PRL seizure literature and concluded that a twice normal relative or absolute serum PRL rise, drawn 10 to 20 minutes after the onset of the ictus, compared against a baseline nonictal PRL, is a useful adjunct in the differentiation of generalized tonic–clonic seizures or complex partial seizures from NESs.[31] Unfortunately, this test is not useful for differentiating the epileptic seizures that are more likely to be confused with NESs (i.e., frontal lobe seizures) from NES proper, which limits the utility of this test when it is most needed.

Wyllie et al. have reported an increase in serum CPK levels following 15% of generalized tonic–clonic seizures, but not after partial seizures or PNESs.[154] The levels of CPK peak between 18 and 24 hours postictally. Thus, a high serum CPK following a convulsive event is suggestive of an epileptic seizure, but normal CPK *does not confirm* the diagnosis of PNESs. The gap of 18 to 24 hours between event and peak serum concentrations makes this a useful test to consider in outpatients.

PSYCHIATRIC DISORDERS ASSOCIATED WITH PSYCHOGENIC NONEPILEPTIC SEIZURES

General Considerations

Two considerations in reviewing the psychiatric diagnoses in PNES are (a) etiologic and (b) epidemiologic. The etiologic question is, "What is causing the PNES?" The epidemiologic question that arises is, "What are the psychiatric comorbidities in patients with PNES?" We are gaining in our knowledge of the latter, but presently, we have only theoretical approaches for the former issue of etiology. Both etiology and epidemiology of comorbidities are of great importance, as they influence prognosis and may be treatment targets for patients with PNESs.

No single psychopathogenic process is known to cause PNESs. PNESs are clinically classified under different *Diagnostic and Statistical Manual of Mental Disorders,* fourth edition (DSM-IV) diagnoses, including conversion, somatization, and dissociation disorders, and a much smaller percentage as factitious disorder and malingering. A psychosocial stressor (e.g., sexual or physical abuse, loss of a relationship, work stress, parental divorce)[153] is often identified but may take months to uncover.

The presence of a structural lesion in the brain does not preclude a diagnosis of nonepileptic seizures,[90,94] and the presence of a psychological disorder does not preclude a diagnosis of epilepsy. Many psychiatric conditions are overrepresented in the population of people with epilepsy.[85] Thus, mood and anxiety disorders are pervasive both in epilepsy and in PNESs. Neurologists have underrecognized patients who have a severe anxiety or depressive disorder along with their neurologic disorder.[63]

Etiologic Diagnostic Considerations

Somatoform Disorders

These are a group of disorders in which physical symptoms or signs present without any apparent physical cause and which have an assumed psychological cause. They are distinguished from factitious disorder and malingering. There are several subdivisions of the somatoform disorders, of which two are particularly important in patients with PNESs, conversion and somatization disorders.

Conversion Disorder. The DSM-IV diagnostic criteria for conversion disorder are the presence of one or more symptoms or deficits affecting voluntary motor or sensory function that suggest a neurologic or other general medical condition; psychological factors are judged to be associated with the symptom or deficit because the initiation or exacerbation of the symptom or deficit is preceded by conflicts or other stressors. The symptom or deficit is not intentionally produced or feigned (as in factitious disorder or malingering).

The diagnosis, now, is based not on psychological guesswork as to what is going on in the patient's mind, but on observable phenomena. This laudable attempt to simplify the definition of conversion disorder and therefore make it easier to diagnose has unfortunately resulted in the concept of dissociation (which many European psychiatrists would feel is an essential part of conversion disorder) being relegated to a completely different diagnostic category that will be briefly considered later.

Conversion disorder (unlike the old concept of hysteria and Briquet syndrome) has therefore become almost exclusively neurologic, and seizures feature prominently in its definition. A large proportion of people with PNESs fall into this diagnostic category. It is a diagnosis that is easy to make but one that psychiatrists and neurologists find difficult to substantiate because of each profession's discomfort with the elements of "the other profession." While it is open to misuse (because it is partly based on subjective criteria), a positive diagnosis of conversion disorder can be made in the context of acknowledging the diagnostic criteria; a thorough history, oftentimes uncovering a series of medically unexplained symptoms; and a nonneuroanatomically based examination.

The emotional problems that are causing the conversion disorder are often discoverable, particularly in the early stages of the condition, but not always. Many people with genuine physical symptoms also have psychological problems that may sometimes exacerbate their symptoms. Examples include patients with multiple sclerosis who might embellish their responses on physical examination, in order to "help" the examiner. It is important for patients to see the connection between the symptom and problem for themselves rather than having someone else's explanation being forced on them.

Somatization Disorder (Previously Known as Briquet Syndrome). The full DSM-IV diagnostic criteria are basically related to a history of many sustained, relentless, multisystem physical complaints without neuroanatomic basis, but which are not intentionally produced, occurring over a long period of time with many treatment requests and significant social impairment. Some patients whose primary presenting symptoms are PNESs fall into the category of somatization disorder if a careful assessment is made and a complete medical and surgical history is taken. Care must be taken, however, realizing that some somatic and psychiatric disorders (e.g., connective tissue disorders, depression) can cause widespread somatic complaints, often over long periods of time, which can be mistaken for a somatoform disorder.

Dissociative Disorders

Dissociation is defined as disruption in the usually integrated functions of consciousness, memory, identity, and perception. Splitting of apparent consciousness from present experience can present as amnesia, as a fugue state, as an identity disorder, or as depersonalization and thus may enter into the differential diagnosis of paroxysmal behavior. Depersonalization, amnesia, and, occasionally, fuguelike behavior also may occur as symptoms of epileptic activity.[127,134,155] Dissociative amnesia is currently much associated with theories about repression of later recovered memories of previous childhood abuse. There is some evidence[20] that some particular types of PNESs (swoons and abreactive attacks) are more common in people who have disclosed a previous history of sexual abuse as a child. Swoons can be described as a kind of dissociative state related to avoiding unpleasant memories; abreactive attacks can be seen as an acting out of unpleasant memory flashbacks. Some clinicians argue that dissociation is the underlying mechanism in PNESs based on studies showing that patients with PNESs score higher on dissociative experiences scales than patients with epilepsy.[2,115]

Factitious Disorder

Factitious disorder is a deliberately simulated disease, the simulation of which does not appear to convey any advantage except that of assuming the sick role. External incentives, unlike in malingering, are absent. The condition is therefore inwardly driven by psychological forces, although the patient is aware of the deception. Patients may display considerable ingenuity in maintaining the deception and often deny deception. A smaller proportion of people with NESs belong to this group. Their performance may be polished and practiced. They may, in the interests of verisimilitude, even inflict physical damage on themselves and repeatedly present to different emergency rooms, apparently in status epilepticus. This is sometimes referred to as Münchhausen syndrome.[122]

Diagnosis can be difficult and should not be made until the team managing the patient is absolutely certain that it is correct. Premature diagnosis without concrete evidence, based purely on the puzzling nature of the patient's symptoms, can be a costly mistake.

A variant of factitious disorder is Münchhausen disorder by proxy, in which factitious symptoms of a disorder (often a seizure disorder) are produced in a dependent (usually a child) of the complainant.[4] The actual victim is usually a child, but it is the parent or caregiver who has the factitious disorder and the kind of personality that wants not so much to be in the sick role, but to have someone dependent on them in the sick role. In caregivers (such as nurses) who exhibit this behavior, there is also often a compulsive need not just to have people dependent on them, but to be seen as the dramatic rescuer of the victim. Unfortunately, such personality types are often attracted to nursing, and nurses are particularly likely to show factitious disorder or to initiate Münchhausen syndrome by proxy. This can have an unfortunate rebound effect on nurses with genuine illnesses.

Malingering

Malingering is not a psychiatric disorder, but one where there is a voluntary and conscious production of symptoms (and signs) for gain. The motivation might be to avoid a court case or to obtain disability payments or medication. Nonepileptic seizures are infrequently part of the repertoire of someone who is deliberately malingering.[55] Here the false symptoms and signs are being produced to change external circumstances rather than being internally driven and are usually easier to understand. People who use seizures for malingering purposes are often practiced and accomplished and much harder to detect. Unfortunately, some people who have had a chronic disability such as epilepsy and who have gained financial support as a result (as is only right and proper) may be reluctant to abandon their symptoms because they will lose the benefit if they do. Some people in such a situation may unconsciously or consciously simulate their seizures, long after the seizures themselves have stopped, in order to continue to gain benefit.

A clear distinction cannot always be made between somatization disorder, conversion disorder, factitious disorder, and malingering as the conditions blur into each other (it can be difficult to decide sometimes whether someone's motivation is truly unconscious). Apparent motivation is also based to some extent on a clinician's subjective interpretation. Currently, there are no diagnostic tests that definitely rule in or rule out conscious or unconscious motivation.[80]

Epidemiologic Considerations: Comorbid Diagnoses in Psychogenic Nonepileptic Seizures

Bowman's review revealed that many patients with PNESs also suffer from mood (12% to 100%), anxiety (11% to 80%), personality (33% to 66%), nonseizure conversion/somatoform (20% to 100%), and nonseizure dissociative disorders (up to 90%) co-occurring with their primary PNES diagnosis of conversion, somatoform, or dissociative disorder.[25] The diagnostic frequencies noted in Bowman's PNES population studies using the DSM-III-R were confirmed in a French study using the DSM-IV criteria.[102] Axis II personality disorders also are found in patients with PNES, largely, but not exclusively, of the impulsive, cluster B personality.

Mood Disorder

Mood disorders are common in people with epilepsy. Both depression and hypomania are probably more common than would be expected by chance.[62] The prevalence of mood disorder, particularly depression, is also high in people who have PNESs.[27] It is unlikely that depression itself causes nonepileptic seizures, but the onset of depression is well known for releasing psychopathologic behavior, including conversion disorder.[113] Depression in some patients with PNESs may be related to the environmental stressors and life circumstances that have caused the seizures themselves. Mood disorder is also prominent in somatoform disorder (which may independently be associated with PNESs) and may need to be treated independently.[132]

Anxiety

Nonepileptic seizures are often associated with panic disorder with or without agoraphobia. The DSM-IV defines a panic attack as a discreet period of intense fear or discomfort in which four or more autonomic symptoms develop abruptly and reach a peak within 10 minutes, including palpitations, tachycardia, diaphoresis, tremulousness, dyspnea, feelings of choking, angina, dyspepsia, feeling dizzy, feeling lightheaded, feeling faint, paresthesias, and temperature changes, along with derealization, feelings of unreality, feelings of depersonalization, feelings of being detached from oneself, fear of losing control or going crazy, or fear of dying.

Some panic attacks are, of course, accompanied by hyperventilation (indeed, some of the above panic symptoms are related to hyperventilation) and at times can lead to apparent unconsciousness and be mistaken for epilepsy.[23] Panic attacks also may be mistaken for epilepsy if they occur in the context of agoraphobia or a specific phobia.[124] The agoraphobia or other anxiety symptoms may be mistaken for an emotional reaction to the mistakenly diagnosed epileptic seizure.[47] Patients with generalized anxiety disorder also may be mistakenly diagnosed as having epilepsy if the symptoms of their anxiety are such as to suggest a temporal lobe origin for them.[130] Anxiety also can coexist with a somatoform disorder, which may itself give rise to nonepileptic seizures.

Panic disorder, agoraphobia, specific phobias, anxiety disorder due to epilepsy, or adjustment disorder with anxiety related to epilepsy can all occur in people with genuine epilepsy, making differentiation difficult.[125]

Posttraumatic stress disorder (PTSD), in which sudden intrusive memories (flashbacks) or dissociative experiences occur, can be mistaken for epilepsy, particularly if the flashback leads to an alteration in behavior.[29] Occasionally patients can develop a posttraumatic stress disorder related to their epilepsy if they had a seizure in a particularly frightening or life-threatening situation (e.g., a patient who had a tonic–clonic seizure in the bath and had to be rescued by strangers). Related to their histories of trauma and abuse, patients with PNESs have high frequencies of PTSD.[27] There is a significant literature on the association between childhood or adult trauma and abuse and the development of PNESs with PTSD.[45]

Finally, anxiety commonly co-occurs with a mood disorder, and it can sometimes be difficult to decide which is which. Both can occur in epilepsy, and both may be present in people with PNESs.

Psychotic Illness

A few patients with PNESs also may have a coexistent psychosis, and the seizures may sometimes have a relationship to the patient's disordered psychopathology. Psychoses occur in people with epilepsy, and sometimes the phenomena of schizophrenia (catatonia, made movements) can be mistaken for epilepsy.[142]

THE ROLE OF PSYCHOMETRIC TESTING IN THE DIAGNOSIS OF PSYCHOGENIC NONEPILEPTIC SEIZURES

Psychological Tests

As an adjunct to the gold standard V-EEG diagnosis of PNES, some clinicians use psychological tests. When used with V-EEG, the Minnesota Multiphasic Personality Inventory (MMPI) is a useful predictor of PNESs[136]; however, its reliability and validity in detecting patients with PNESs also has been criticized.[65] Derry and McLachlan[36] have shown that the revised version of the MMPI (the MMPI-2) discriminated with a 92% rate of accuracy between patients with epilepsy and patients with PNESs. They also felt it useful in detecting those patients who have epileptic seizures but who have marked psychopathology, and who, therefore, also may have PNESs. People with PNESs demonstrate a personality profile suggestive of a conversion or somatoform disorder.

Hypnosis also has been used as a diagnostic tool for PNES for over half a century.[137] Kuyk et al. used the technique for recovering memory in psychogenic amnesia and recalling memory of events taking place during the seizure itself with the premise that if ictal memory can be recovered, then the event is a nonepileptic one, and found 100% specificity and 85% sensitivity for a diagnosis of PNES.[79] Barry found that using the hypnotic induction profile reliably distinguished patients with PNES from those with epilepsy.[10]

Cragar et al. reviewed the literature on adjunctive tests for diagnosing PNES and reported sensitivity and specificity of the different measures.[34] A summary of their findings noted that PNES and ES patients did not differ on intelligence tests or on neuropsychological (NP) measures consistently. Both PNES and ES groups did have cognitive deficits when compared to normal controls, and the PNES group tended to perform better than patients with ES on various NP tests. Similarities and differences in these tests are discussed more fully in Chapter 208.

Prognosis/Predictors of Psychogenic Nonepileptic Seizures Outcome

Depending on the psychiatric makeup of the individual with NES, outcomes vary. Kanner et al. found that the presence of a mood disorder, a history of abuse, and a personality disorder were associated with a higher frequency of a patient having persistent PNESs.[72] Betts and Boden suggested that the short-term prognosis of nonepileptic seizures was relatively good, but that relapse, once the patient was discharged into the community, was frequent.[19] Also, a significant number of patients continue to have PNES, even with the institution of therapy.[1] Walczak et al. investigated the outcome of 72 patients with V-EEG–diagnosed PNESs, followed for a mean period of 15 months (range, 12 to 22 months). Patients were asked about the frequency of PNESs in the last 6 months, AED use, occupational status, and extent of psychotherapeutic treatments. PNESs had ceased in 18 patients (35%), decreased >80% in 21 (41%), and decreased <80% in 12 of 51 (24%). Thirty-three patients (65%) were not taking AEDs. Occupational status improved in 20% and did not change in 75%. Overall, 29 of 51 (57%) rated themselves markedly improved and 15 of 51 (29%) rated themselves unchanged or worse. Persisting PNESs were significantly associated with longer duration of PNES before diagnosis and presence of additional psychiatric disease. Persisting PNESs were not associated with gender, presence of epileptic seizures, or extent of psychotherapeutic treatments after diagnosis.[144]

A handful of studies have demonstrated that a certain population of patients with PNESs experience complete remission of their events after their diagnosis is given, even in the absence of any therapeutic interventions. One group reported that 18 of 22 patients with PNESs had a reduction of PNESs in the 24 hours postdelivery of their V-EEG diagnosis.[43] One-year follow-up, however, revealed that 87% of patients with PNES had the return and persistence of their PNESs.[146] In the study by Kanner et al.,[72] 13 of 45 (29%) patients stopped having PNESs after the diagnosis was established and remained free of events until the last follow-up 6 months later. Unfortunately, most of the studies published to date suggest that only about one third of patients had stopped experiencing PNESs at the time of follow-up, 1 to 5 years after diagnosis.[120]

Long-term outcome studies yield disappointing outcomes. Krumholz and Neidermeyer evaluated the prognosis of PNES in 41 patients discharged from the Johns Hopkins Hospital who had follow-up data of 5 years or longer after discharge.[78] Among these 41 patients, there were coexisting organic neurologic disorders in 18 (44%) and mental retardation was identified in 17%. Concurrent epileptic seizures were found in 37% and EEG abnormalities found in 38%. Persistence of PNESs was found in 56% of patients, which was associated with psychosocial problems.

On the other hand, a significantly better outcome has been found in outcome studies of children and adolescents. For example, Wyllie et al. compared the outcome of PNESs documented by V-EEG in 18 nonepileptic children and adolescents (ages 8 to 18; median, 14.5 years old) and 20 adults (ages 25 to 56; median, 34.0 years old).[152] The outcome was significantly better for the younger patients at 1 year, 2 years, and 3 years after diagnosis, as 73%, 75%, and 81% of children and adolescents were free of events at these follow-up times, respectively; at the same follow-up times, the percentages of adults free of psychogenic attacks were only 25%, 25%, and 40%.

In a recent study of 147 patients with PNESs contacted after a mean of 4.2 years after diagnosis (mean age at follow-up, 38.1 years), Reuber et al. found that 71.4% continued to have PNESs, and 28.6% had achieved seizure remission[119]; 60.0% of patients with continuing PNESs and 42.7% of patients in remission were "unproductive." More severe psychopathology was associated with persistence of PNES and unemployment.

Understanding the role of certain psychiatric and neuropsychological variables in the PNES outcome of our patients can be of paramount importance in planning treatment strategies. For example, in a prospective study of neurologic and psychiatric predictors of PNES outcome in 45 patients carried out at the Rush Epilepsy Center, the persistence of PNESs was investigated at 1 month and 6 months after diagnosis.[72] Three outcome patterns were identified: (a) uninterrupted PNESs ($n = 20$), (b) transient cessation of PNESs for a period of at least 3 months with subsequent recurrence ($n = 12$), and (c) cessation of PNESs since diagnosis ($n = 13$). The 20 patients that continued with uninterrupted PNESs were significantly more likely to have a history of abuse (physical, emotional, sexual, mixed), a history of recurrent major depression, a personality disorder, and a history of dissociative disorder (not presenting as PNESs). Given the frequent history of abuse, it is reasonable to expect that PNESs are an expression of a dissociative process. This observation is further supported by the higher frequency of a history of dissociative disorder that preceded and presented in forms other than PNESs. Thus, the uninterrupted persistence of PNESs in these patients is not surprising, since the mere fact of being told that they do not have epilepsy is meaningless to them. Indeed, as long as their events are the expression of a "dissociative state" and patients have not found other means of dealing with stress, PNESs are expected to persist. Furthermore, having made the connection that their events constitute a dissociative process does not necessarily result in their cessation. Of interest is the fact that, despite their severe psychopathology, 17 of these 20 patients readily accepted the psychogenic nature of their events, and were able to recognize their PNESs as a form of dissociation soon after their diagnosis was discussed with them.

Twelve of the 45 patients experienced a transient cessation of PNESs following the diagnostic V-EEG for a period of at least 3 months. They differed from those with the two other outcomes in two areas: They were more likely to deny the presence of any psychiatric or psychological problems. In fact, 8 of the 12 patients with this outcome refused a recommendation to start psychiatric treatment. All patients accepted that their events were not epileptic, however. In addition, patients in this group were more likely to develop new somatic complaints after the diagnosis of PNES was established. In these patients we suspect that somatoform/conversive disorders are mediating their PNESs, in contrast to patients with persistent events who were more likely to have a dissociative disorder.

Thirteen patients stopped experiencing PNES after diagnosis. Paradoxically, this group of patients is the most puzzling from a psychiatric standpoint. Most had psychiatric disorders of mild severity, but in 5 of the 13 patients, *no current psychopathology* was identified during the psychiatric and neuropsychological evaluations. In those cases, no psychiatric treatment was suggested and they were followed in the clinic with visits every 3 months initially and then every 6 months. In the other patients, treatment was tailored to the nature of the identified psychiatric disorder. One of the 13 patients refused referral for psychiatric treatment; yet, there was no PNES recurrence up to the time of the last follow-up visit. The findings of this study provide relevant information to clinicians. Patients who stop having PNESs after disclosure of diagnosis differ significantly in their psychiatric profile from those who experience PNES recurrence. Among the latter patients, a distinct psychiatric profile can be associated with a particular PNES recurrence pattern. These findings suggest that more than one psychopathogenic mechanism is operable in PNES. Second, the psychiatric variables identified commonly in these patients can be predictive of PNES recurrence.

PRESENTATION OF THE DIAGNOSIS OF PSYCHOGENIC NONEPILEPTIC SEIZURES

In any medical disorder, acceptance of the diagnosis is the first step in the therapeutic process. In the case of PNESs, presentation of the diagnosis of PNESs is a pivotal step in helping the patient "come to terms" with a diagnosis that implies a "psychogenic cause." Reluctance to accept the diagnosis of a psychogenic process on the part of the patient may be based on concerns that family members and friends will think that he or she is "crazy" or that he or she is "faking" the spells to get attention or avoid responsibilities. Yet acceptance that the patient's events are not epileptic seizures or events of organic origin is of the essence as the biggest potential source of morbidity and mortality are the physicians in emergency rooms who may not recognize the true nature of the events and treat the patient as one in status epilepticus.

Often the way the diagnosis is presented to the patient and family members accounts for their refusal to accept it and by the same token to refuse recommendation for psychiatric treatment. Interestingly enough, there is no consensus among experts on what is the best way of presenting the diagnosis. At a treatment workshop on PNESs sponsored by the National Institutes of Health and the American Epilepsy Society held in May 2005, it became very clear that there are no systematic data to determine the best protocol to follow in discussing the diagnosis of PNES with patients and family.[140] For example, the following questions were raised: (a) Should a psychogenic cause be implied automatically if no organic cause can be identified, even before a psychogenic cause or evidence of psychopathology has been established? (b) Should the diagnosis be presented by the neurologist or should the psychiatrist (or the psychologist) be present at the meeting?

Shen et al. developed a protocol for the presentation of the diagnosis of PNESs that is now considered classic by many epilepsy centers.[128] This protocol contains six main points:

1. A review of the recorded events with the patient and family to ensure that the captured event is typical for the patient.
2. Explanation in "positive terms" of the nature of the spells (i.e., their nonepileptic cause), and hence the possibility of discontinuing AEDs.
3. An acknowledgement that the nature of the event is yet to be established, and that its cause may not always be found.
4. The observation that in many cases, such events may be of psychogenic origin (with an added explanation that the causes may be related to "upsetting emotions" that remain unconscious (i.e., and therefore the patient is unaware of) and that an evaluation by a psychiatrist, psychologist, or counselor may be indicated. Shen et al. emphasized that having these types of conflicts in no way implies that the patient may be "crazy."
5. Making the observation that a history of sexual abuse is often encountered in patients with these events.
6. A statement to the effect that the spells may spontaneously resolve on their own and that, although one component is subconscious in nature, "one can exert a conscious voluntary effort to abort these attacks."

We have borrowed on most of the points raised in Shen's protocol when discussing the diagnosis of PNES with patients and family members at the Rush Epilepsy Center. We are careful, however, not to impute a psychogenic cause in the absence of evidence obtained in the course of a psychiatric evaluation, informal discussion with the patient and/or family, or neuropsychological data. Furthermore, while we also tell our patients that their spells may stop occurring just by knowing that they are not epileptic in nature, we do not suggest to them that they can exert a conscious voluntary effort to abort these attacks. Our reasons are threefold: First, unless the patient is malingering (which is a minority of the cases), we do not believe that the patients have a conscious control over the occurrence of their events, at least at the beginning. Second, patients (and family members) may often interpret such observation as a suggestion that they are voluntarily faking the events, which in turn raises their resistance to accept the diagnosis further. Third, we are convinced that the exertion of control of the events occur eventually, as a result of the treatment (see later).

It is only after the above-cited explanations that we ask patients if they think that their episodes may be related to a psychogenic process, if they have not volunteered that observation on their own. From this point on, we guide the discussion according to the answer we get from the patient:

1. If patients accept the possibility of a psychogenic process as a cause of their spells, we encourage them to elaborate on their reasons and to cite examples that may illustrate potential conflicts, and we suggest that they undergo a complete neuropsychological and psychiatric evaluation.
2. If patients acknowledge a history of abuse or having been victims of traumatic experiences, we ask them to recall

how they "dealt" with such situations at the time of their occurrence. It has been our experience, and that of others, that most patients have no recollection of the actual traumatic event(s). We use that "personal" experience to illustrate the phenomenon of dissociation, by again reiterating the fact that "when individuals is facing a traumatic experience, their mind will automatically protect itself by blocking any awareness of their surroundings." We then add, "This is similar to what may happen when you are having a spell" and go on to explain that after repeated traumatic experiences, one's mind may learn to automatically "shut out" the outside world, *even in the presence of less traumatic situations*. We repeat the statement, "There is only so much trauma one person can endure before fending the traumatic experience off one's mind." Usually, patients with a history of abuse can easily relate to these observations. This, in fact, becomes the beginning of the therapeutic process. We emphasize to these patients that their process of dissociation will most likely continue until they learn, with the assistance of a counselor, to identify the precipitants, which by now need not be necessarily of a traumatic nature.

3. In the case where patients *adamantly refute* the possibility of any psychogenic cause to their events, we suggest that they undergo a neuropsychological and neuropsychiatric evaluation to rule out that possibility. We reiterate the unconscious nature of these processes, which may preclude patients from recognizing an underlying psychological process. At the same time, we acknowledge the possibility that their spells may not have a psychogenic cause and that we may not be able to find a cause by the completion of the evaluation. We always add, "If we don't look for it, we'll never find it. It's better to rule out completely a possible psychogenic cause." Patients are told that we would like to continue following them in the clinic and we ask them to keep a diary in which they are to write down the circumstances surrounding the occurrence of future events, were they to continue. Note that we do not push patients to accept a psychogenic cause of their spells when it becomes obvious that they are not ready. In our opinion, the best course to take with such patients is to continue following them in the clinic, strengthening our relationship and their trust in us, while at the same time we continue reminding them that their spells are not epileptic (and that no other organic cause has been identified). In our experience, patients eventually end up accepting our recommendation for psychiatric treatment after a few months. During that time we continue achieving our primary therapeutic goal: Averting that their spells be treated as epileptic seizures by other physicians.
4. Occasionally patients may be adamant about their certainty of some organic or epileptic process triggering their spells, and that we may have erred in our evaluation. While in such patients we are likely to suspect a factitious disorder or malingering, we try to keep an "open mind." We review the diagnostic process with patients, show the captured events and recordings of epileptic seizures, and graphically demonstrate on the actual paper to both patients and family the differences between the two. If the diagnosis was based on an ambulatory EEG study, we repeat the evaluation in an inpatient V-EEG monitoring unit, with the use of sphenoidal electrodes. In fact, we have had three patients in whom an erroneous diagnosis of PPS was reached with ambulatory EEG studies. Two of the three patients had neuropsychological testing that failed to reveal any propensity for conversive disorder. A correct diagnosis of epilepsy was established during V-EEG. In short, we must *always* consider the fact that patients may be correct. After all, they know themselves better, notwithstanding the unconscious nature of a potential psychogenic process.

TREATMENT OF PSYCHOGENIC NONEPILEPTIC SEIZURES

General Considerations

In the treatment section, we address the transition from neurologist to psychiatrist, the use/withdrawal of AEDs, pharmacotherapy, and psychotherapy for PNESs. Before examining the various aspects of the treatment modalities, there are certain important general points that must always be borne in mind in conceptualizing the treatment of patients with PNESs.

The first point is that patients (and their families) may well have been living with the assumed diagnosis of epilepsy for a considerable period. When patients who have been treated for epilepsy are diagnosed with PNESs, they are immediately transformed from a "neurologic" patient to a "psychiatric" one.[81] Suddenly changing the diagnosis, however justified it may be, can have a profound psychological effect on the person who receives the new diagnosis, particularly because that person may already have a recognizable psychiatric disorder and may be living with a dysfunctional family. We have frequently encountered the patients who react with, "So, you are saying I'm crazy?!?" From the epilepsy monitoring unit, a number of patients are referred, then lost to follow-up. Therefore, the confrontation process must be handled tactfully and appropriately.[22]

Neurologic Treatment (or, "How Long Should the Neurologist Follow the Patient with Psychogenic Nonepileptic Seizures?")

The neurologist's task, once a firm diagnosis of nonepileptic seizures has been made, does not suddenly cease. The neurologist should continue to offer support to the patient while arrangements are being made for ongoing care. The parting of the ways between the patient and the neurologic specialist should certainly not be an abrupt one. The neurologist should certainly remain available for consultation in case new seizure types develop or there remains some doubt about the certainty of the diagnosis (particularly as new investigatory methods emerge). Although reinvestigation can be justified on occasion, this should only be undertaken if there are clear clinical indications that the diagnosis may have been wrong.

In our opinion, discharge of patients with PNESs from their neurologist's practice should not take place before they have had an opportunity to complete the transition of their care to the psychiatrist or psychologist to whom they were referred. Furthermore, the neurologist may well need to remain in contact with the patient while a slow reduction is made in anticonvulsant medication. Reducing medication on which the patient may have become psychologically and pharmacologically dependent should always be slow. Abrupt termination of some anticonvulsants will lead to pharmacologic withdrawal seizures, which complicates the diagnostic picture. As a matter of ethical necessity, the neurologist should make certain that his or her patient has been appropriately placed with another care team or facility that is competent to manage the nonepileptic seizures. Abrupt termination of the relationship between the neurologist and the patient will make the next doctor's job much harder.

Communication and collaboration between neurology, psychiatry, and psychology in the process of diagnosing and treating the patient with PNESs is an essential part of the multidisciplinary approach needed to assess and manage these patients. Harden et al. noted psychiatrists' lack of confidence in the V-EEG diagnosis as compared to neurologists,[56] and interdisciplinary discussion may improve management of PNESs. A model of PNES treatment has been proposed, composed of accurate diagnosis with V-EEG by the epileptologist; presenting the diagnosis to patients and their family; constructing a problem list of precursors, precipitants, and perpetuating factors of PNES; and prescribing psychotropics, with discontinuing AEDs in lone PNESs, or adjusting appropriately in mixed ESs/PNESs.[83] While no single treatment has been shown to treat all NES patients, the National Institutes of Health and the American Epilepsy Society have supported an international PNES treatment workshop where neurologists, psychiatrists, and psychologists convened to discuss and develop various models to be systematically tested.[140]

Psychiatric Treatment

Ideally, a psychiatrist asked to manage a patient with nonepileptic seizures should have had some experience in this area, should be part of the team that has been assessing the patient, should have confidence in the diagnosis of nonepileptic seizures, and, in particular, should not feel (as sometimes happens) that a difficult patient has been dumped in his or her lap by a neurologic service eager to be rid of the patient. Patients being dismissed sometimes results in the rapid return of the patient to the neurologic facility or, worse, the patient being abandoned by everybody and the whole diagnostic process having to be reundertaken.

Psychiatric assessment of the patient should start long before the diagnosis of PNES is finally given so that the patient's upbringing, social background, personality development, present living circumstances, and relationships with other family members (plus the presence or absence of contributing traumas such as abuse) are already established.

Pharmacotherapy

Barbiturates have been used in diagnosing and treating patients with conversion disorder effectively for over a half a century.[86] Open-label trials of antidepressants in patients with conversion disorders have shown some response.[107,143] Controlled studies of the benefit of psychotropics in PNESs, however, have not been completed, and apart from anecdotal reports, their effect in PNES is unknown.[84] Formal medical psychiatric treatment is necessary for the treatment of any underlying psychotic disorder or depression. Whether antidepressants directly treat PNESs has not been studied in a controlled fashion. Another approach being studied in NES treatment is to treat the comorbid psychiatric disorders (depression and anxiety frequently occur with PNESs) to reduce PNESs. A pilot randomized controlled trial of a selective serotonin reuptake inhibitor (SSRI) for depression and anxiety in patients with PNESs is under way.[82] Benzodiazepines have also been shown to reduce PNES in open-label studies.[8] When pharmacotherapy of the patient's mental state is used, it should be accompanied by psychological support, if not formal psychotherapy.

Clarifying the role of AEDs in patients with PNESs is another major pharmacotherapy issue to be addressed by the treating neurologist and psychiatrist. During the process of withdrawing anticonvulsant medication, psychological symptoms may emerge (e.g., a previously undiagnosed mood disorder with carbamazepine withdrawal or significant anxiety symptoms with benzodiazepine withdrawal). Oto et al. showed that AEDs could be safely discontinued in patients with lone PNESs after V-EEG monitoring.[109] Some have argued for the mood-stabilizing benefits of AEDs as a reason to continue the antiseizure medications. AEDs, however, do not treat PNESs, and toxicity may exacerbate PNESs.[106]

Psychotherapies

If the psychiatrist is not delivering the psychotherapy personally, he or she may work in collaboration with psychologists and nurse practitioners who administer the therapy. The various therapies for PNES are described below.

Cognitive and Behavioral Techniques

The general principle of the behavioral techniques used in managing PNESs is to prevent the reinforcement of seizure activity and to reward and reinforce nonseizure activity (operant conditioning).[60] A randomized controlled trial of cognitive behavioral therapy (CBT) for NESs is being conducted based on an open-label CBT trial in the United Kingdom.[50] It is important to recognize that all the behavioral and cognitive techniques described below are equally applicable to epilepsy itself.[49] This is one reason why (in neuropsychiatric practice) people with PNESs continue to be managed within the seizure clinic, particularly if by doing so they can save face. Operant conditioning infrequently causes a sharp increase in seizure frequency of a temporary nature (often with an equally dramatic decrease). This is actually a good prognostic sign but can disrupt the treatment plan if not anticipated.

Specific behavioral techniques exist for the management of nonepileptic seizures.[22] They are based on anxiety control measures to help the patient to recognize the early stages of an impending anxiety attack and then to apply control techniques based on suddenly lowering arousal or on cognitive techniques to interrupt negative thinking so that seizure progression is interrupted. The patient need no longer be afraid of the seizures because he or she is confident they can be stopped. This can be an effective treatment technique for nonepileptic attacks related to panic or hyperventilation and may have a more general use in some of the seizures related to somatoform disorders.

Psychotherapy

Psychotherapy in the sense of dynamic psychoanalytically based therapy probably has little part to play nowadays in the management of PNESs. Kalogjera-Sackellares published her book describing the use of psychodynamic psychotherapy in PNESs, giving a thorough presentation of the psychotherapeutic technique for patients with PNESs.[64] Psychodynamic psychotherapy, however, is relatively unproven in terms of its efficacy, given the limitation that it is a difficult technique to analyze by controlled trials.

Family Therapy

Patients with PNESs and their family members score in the unhealthy range on measures of family functioning.[76,150] Therapeutic work with the patient's family is extremely important in the management of these disorders because, even if family dynamics are not the prime cause of the seizures, often family tension may be conspiring to keep the patient in the sick role. Family anxiety may reinforce seizure behavior. Under those circumstances, managing the patient and the seizures without also managing the family may well be a fruitless exercise. An open trial of family therapy is being conducted in the United States presently. There has been little written about the use of family therapy in PNESs, and it is an area that needs extensive study.

Other

Hypnosis has been recommended for some patients as a treatment strategy.[101] Particularly for those patients in whom the seizure can be seen as a conversion or dissociative disorder, hypnosis might be helpful, although it would usually be used in conjunction with other therapies. It sometimes can be used as an abreactive agent.

Pilot trials of group psychoeducation (Zaroff 2004) and group psychotherapy (Wittenberg 2004) have been reported, and may provide a general support in anxiety reduction or more specifically a support while the patient is transitioning from neurologic care to psychiatric care.

Additional Considerations

Driving and Nonepileptic Seizures

Benbadis et al. found that 49% of neurologists surveyed applied the same restrictions to patients with PNESs as for patients with epilepsy. Driving records of a sample of PNES patients revealed no statistically significant difference compared with the expected number of motor vehicle crashes for the sample. The authors concluded that their small series did not support the use of driving restrictions for patients with PNESs.[15] Kanner has found that restricting driving privileges to patients with PNESs until they become seizure free is a motivational factor for patients to seek psychiatric treatment (Kanner AM, unpublished data). In our opinion, the decision to lift up the usual "seizure precautions" has to be individualized.

SUMMARY AND CONCLUSIONS

PNESs are commonly mistaken for epilepsy and are often difficult to recognize. Their investigation requires obtaining a thorough history, capturing one of the typical events on V-EEG, and a team prepared to think and act holistically. Like epilepsy, PNESs lie in the disputed territory between the provinces of neurology and psychiatry, and their successful recognition and management require careful and considerate liaison between the two disciplines. This is of particular importance in the small percentage of patients where PNESs and actual epilepsy exist concurrently in the same individual (see Chapter 208). In summarizing the treatment of lone PNESs, along with AED discontinuation, addressing the underlying psychological factors with psychotherapy, with adjunctive antianxiety/antidepressant medication to treat the comorbid axis I disorders, is currently thought to be the preferable treatment regimen for PNESs. Controlled studies are being conducted using pharmacotherapy for the comorbid depression and anxiety found in PNESs, and with cognitive behavioral therapy.

References

1. Aboukasm A, Mahr G, Gahry BR, et al. Retrospective analysis of the effects of psychotherapeutic interventions on outcomes of psychogenic nonepileptic seizures. *Epilepsia.* 1998;39(5):470–473.
2. Akyuz G, Kugu N, Akyuz A, et al. Dissociation and childhood abuse history in epileptic and pseudoseizure patients. *Epileptic Disord.* 2004;6(3):187–192.
3. Al-Qudah AA, Abu-Sheik S, Tamimi AF. Diagnostic value of short duration outpatient video electroencephalographic monitoring. *Pediatr Neurol.* 1999;21(3):622–625.
4. Alving J. Munchhausen's syndrome by proxy: case reports. In: Gram L, Johannessen SI, Osterman PE, et al., eds. *Pseudo-Epileptic Seizures.* Petersfield, UK: Wrighston Biomedical Publishing Ltd.; 1993:67–74.
5. Alving J. Serum prolactin levels are elevated also after pseudo-epileptic seizures. *Seizure.* 1998;7(2):85–89.
6. Aminoff MJ, Goodin DS, Berg BO, et al. Ambulatory EEG recordings in epileptic and nonepileptic children. *Neurology.* 1988;38(4):558–562.
7. Andriola MR, Ettinger AB. Pseudoseizures and other nonepileptic paroxysmal disorders in children and adolescents. *Neurology.* 1999;53(5 Suppl 2):S89–95.
8. Ataoglu A, Ozcetin A, Icmeli C, et al. Paradoxical therapy in conversion reaction. *J Korean Med Sci.* 2003;18(4):581–584.
9. Bare MA, Burnstine TH, Fisher RS, et al. Electroencephalographic changes during simple partial seizures. *Epilepsia.* 1994;35(4):715–720.
10. Barry JJ, Atzman O, Morrell MJ. Discriminating between epileptic and nonepileptic events: the utility of hypnotic seizure induction. *Epilepsia.* 2000;41(1):81–84.
11. Bazil CW, Kothari M, Luciano D, et al. Provocation of nonepileptic seizures by suggestion in a general seizure population. *Epilepsia.* 1994;35(4):768–770.
12. Benbadis SR. How many patients with pseudoseizures receive antiepileptic drugs prior to diagnosis? *Eur Neurol.* 1999;41(2):114–115.
13. Benbadis SR. Provocative techniques should be used for the diagnosis of psychogenic nonepileptic seizures. *Arch Neurol.* 2001;58(12):2063–2065.
14. Benbadis SR, Agrawal V, Tatum IV WO. How many patients with psychogenic nonepileptic seizures also have epilepsy? *Neurology.* 2001; 57(5):915–917.
15. Benbadis SR, Blustein JN, Sunstad L. Should patients with psychogenic nonepileptic seizures be allowed to drive? *Epilepsia.* 2000;41(7):895–897.
16. Benbadis SR, Lancman ME, King LM, et al. Preictal pseudosleep: a new finding in psychogenic seizures. *Neurology.* 1996;47(1):63–67.
17. Bergen D, Ristanovic R. Weeping as a common element of pseudoseizures. *Arch Neurol.* 1993;50(10):1059–1060.
18. Berkovic SF, Bladin PF, Conneely MD, et al. Experience with continuous ambulatory EEG monitoring. *Clin Exp Neurol.* 1984;20:37–46.
19. Betts T, Boden S. Diagnosis, management and prognosis of a group of 128 patients with non-epileptic attack disorder. Part I. *Seizure.* 1992;1(1):19–26.
20. Betts T, Boden S. Diagnosis, management and prognosis of a group of 128 patients with non-epileptic attack disorder. Part II. Previous childhood sexual abuse in the aetiology of these disorders. *Seizure.* 1992;1(1):27–32.
21. Betts T, Boden S. Pseudoseizures (non-epileptic attack disorder). In: Trimble M, ed. *Women and Epilepsy.* Chichester, UK: John Wiley and Sons Ltd.; 1991:237–254.
22. Betts TA. Neuropsychiatry. In: Laidlaw J, Richens A, Chadwick D, eds. *A Textbook of Epilepsy.* 4th ed. Edinburgh; London: Churchill Livingstone; 1993:397–457.
23. Beyenburg S, Mitchell AJ, Schmidt D, et al. Anxiety in patients with epilepsy: systematic review and suggestions for clinical management. *Epilepsy Behav.* 2005;7(2):161–171.
24. Bhatia M, Sinha PK, Jain S, et al. Usefulness of short-term video EEG recording with saline induction in pseudoseizures. *Acta Neurol Scand.* 1997;95(6):363–366.
25. Bowman ES. Nonepileptic seizures: psychiatric framework, treatment, and outcome. *Neurology.* 1999;53(5 Suppl 2):S84–88.
26. Bowman ES. Pseudoseizures. *Psychiatr Clin North Am.* 1998;21(3):649–657, vii.
27. Bowman ES, Markand ON. Psychodynamics and psychiatric diagnoses of pseudoseizure subjects. *Am J Psychiatry.* 1996;153(1):57–63.
28. Broglin D, Delgado-Escueta AV, Walsh GO, et al. Clinical approach to the patient with seizures and epilepsies of frontal origin. *Adv Neurol.* 1992;57:59–88.
29. Cartmill A, Betts T. Seizure behaviour in a patient with post-traumatic stress disorder following rape. Notes on the aetiology of 'pseudoseizures.' *Seizure.* 1992;1(1):33–36.
30. Chabolla DR, Krahn LE, So EL, et al. Psychogenic nonepileptic seizures. *Mayo Clin Proc.* 1996;71(5):493–500.
31. Chen DK, So YT, Fisher RS. Use of serum prolactin in diagnosing epileptic seizures: report of the Therapeutics and Technology Assessment Subcommittee of the American Academy of Neurology. *Neurology.* 2005;65(5):668–675.
32. Cohen RJ, Suter C. Hysterical seizures: suggestion as a provocative EEG test. *Ann Neurol.* 1982;11(4):391–395.
33. Collins WC, Lanigan O, Callaghan N. Plasma prolactin concentrations following epileptic and pseudoseizures. *J Neurol Neurosurg Psychiatry.* 1983;46(6):505–508.
34. Cragar DE, Berry DT, Fakhoury TA, et al. A review of diagnostic techniques in the differential diagnosis of epileptic and nonepileptic seizures. *Neuropsychol Rev.* 2002;12(1):31–64.
35. Dana-Haeri J, Trimble M, Oxley J. Prolactin and gonadotrophin changes following generalised and partial seizures. *J Neurol Neurosurg Psychiatry.* 1983;46(4):331–335.
36. Derry PA, McLachlan RS. The MMPI-2 as an adjunct to the diagnosis of pseudoseizures. *Seizure.* 1996;5(1):35–40.
37. Devinsky O, Fisher R. Ethical use of placebos and provocative testing in diagnosing nonepileptic seizures. *Neurology.* 1996;47(4):866–870.
38. Devinsky O, Sanchez-Villasenor F, Vazquez B, et al. Clinical profile of patients with epileptic and nonepileptic seizures. *Neurology.* 1996; 46(6):1530–1533.

39. Devinsky O, Sato S, Kufta CV, et al. Electroencephalographic studies of simple partial seizures with subdural electrode recordings. *Neurology.* 1989;39(4):527–533.
40. Duncan R. The Clinical use of SPECT in focal epilepsy. *Epilepsia.* 1997;38(s10):39–41.
41. Ettinger AB, Coyle PK, Jandorf L, et al. Postictal SPECT in epileptic versus nonepileptic seizures. *J Epilepsy.* 1998;11:67–73.
42. Fakhoury T, Abou-Khalil B, Newman K. Psychogenic seizures in old age: a case report. *Epilepsia.* 1993;34(6):1049–1051.
43. Farias ST, Thieman C, Alsaadi TM. Psychogenic nonepileptic seizures: acute change in event frequency after presentation of the diagnosis. *Epilepsy Behav.* 2003;4(4):424–429.
44. Fenwick P. Evocation and inhibition of seizures. Behavioral treatment. *Adv Neurol.* 1991;55:163–183.
45. Fleisher W, Staley D, Krawetz P, et al. Comparative study of trauma-related phenomena in subjects with pseudoseizures and subjects with epilepsy. *Am J Psychiatry.* 2002;159(4):660–663.
46. Gates JR, Ramani V, Whalen S, et al. Ictal characteristics of pseudoseizures. *Arch Neurol.* 1985;42(12):1183–1187.
47. Genton P, Bartolomei F, Guerrini R. Panic attacks mistaken for relapse of epilepsy. *Epilepsia.* 1995;36(1):48–51.
48. Geyer JD, Payne TA, Drury I. The value of pelvic thrusting in the diagnosis of seizures and pseudoseizures. *Neurology.* 2000;54(1):227–229.
49. Goldstein LH. Behavioural and cognitive-behavioural treatments for epilepsy: a progress review. *Br J Clin Psychol.* 1990;29(Pt 3):257–269.
50. Goldstein LH, Deale AC, Mitchell-O'Malley SJ, et al. An evaluation of cognitive behavioral therapy as a treatment for dissociative seizures: a pilot study. *Cogn Behav Neurol.* 2004;17(1):41–49.
51. Gowers WR. *Epilepsy and Other Chronic Convulsive Diseases: Their Causes, Symptoms, and Treatment.* 2nd ed. Brinklow, MD: Old Hickory Bookshop; 1963.
52. Greig E, Betts T. Epileptic seizures induced by sexual abuse. Pathogenic and pathoplastic factors. *Seizure.* 1992;1(4):269–274.
53. Gulick TA, Spinks IP, King DW. Pseudoseizures: ictal phenomena. *Neurology.* 1982;32(1):24–30.
54. Gumnit RJ, Gates JR. Psychogenic seizures. *Epilepsia.* 1986;27(Suppl 2):S124–129.
55. Hammond RD. Simulated epilepsy: report of a case. *Arch Neurol Psychiatry.* 1948;60:327–328.
56. Harden CL, Burgut FT, Kanner AM. The diagnostic significance of video-EEG monitoring findings on pseudoseizure patients differs between neurologists and psychiatrists. *Epilepsia.* 2003;44(3):453–456.
57. Henry TR, Drury I. Non-epileptic seizures in temporal lobectomy candidates with medically refractory seizures. *Neurology.* 1997;48(5):1374–1382.
58. Holmes MD, Wilkus RJ, Dodrill CB. Coexistence of epilepsy in patients with nonepileptic seizures. *Epilepsia.* 1993;34(Suppl 2):13.
59. Howell SJ, Owen L, Chadwick DW. Pseudostatus epilepticus. *Q J Med.* 1989;71(266):507–519.
60. Iwata BA, Lorentzson AM. Operant control of seizure-like behavior in an institutionalized retarded adult. *Behav Ther.* 1976;7:247–251.
61. Jehu D. Post-traumatic stress reactions among adults molested as children. *Sexual Marital Ther.* 1991;6(3):227–243.
62. Jones JE, Hermann BP, Barry JJ, et al. Clinical assessment of Axis I psychiatric morbidity in chronic epilepsy: a multicenter investigation. *J Neuropsychiatry Clin Neurosci.* 2005;17(2):172–179.
63. Jones JE, Hermann BP, Woodard JL, et al. Screening for major depression in epilepsy with common self-report depression inventories. *Epilepsia.* 2005;46(5):731–735.
64. Kalogjera-Sackellares D. *Psychodynamics and Psychotherapy of Pseudoseizures. Carmarthen,* Wales, UK: Crown House Publishing, Ltd.; 2004.
65. Kalogjera-Sackellares D, Sackellares JC. Analysis of MMPI patterns in patients with psychogenic pseudoseizures. *Seizure.* 1997;6(6):419–427.
66. Kanner AM. Pseudoseizures. In: Lüders H, ed. *Epilepsy: Comprehensive Review and Case Discussions.* London; Malden, MA: Martin Dunitz; 2001:181–194.
67. Kanner AM. Psychogenic seizures and the supplementary sensorimotor area. *Adv Neurol.* 1996;70:461–466.
68. Kanner AM, Iriarte J. Psychogenic pseudoseizures: semiology and differential diagnosis. In: Kotagal P, Lüders H, eds. *The Epilepsies: Etiologies and Prevention.* San Diego: Academic Press; 1999:509–517.
69. Kanner AM, Jones JC. When do sphenoidal electrodes yield additional data to that obtained with antero-temporal electrodes? *Electroencephalogr Clin Neurophysiol.* 1997;102(1):12–19.
70. Kanner AM, Morris HH, Luders H, et al. Supplementary motor seizures mimicking pseudoseizures: some clinical differences. *Neurology.* 1990;40(9):1404–1407.
71. Kanner AM, Parra J. Psychogenic pseudoseizures: semiology and pathogenic mechanisms. In: Lüders H, Noachtar S, eds. *Epileptic Seizures: Pathophysiology and Clinical Semiology.* 1st ed. New York: Churchill Livingstone; 2000:766–773.
72. Kanner AM, Parra J, Frey M, et al. Psychiatric and neurologic predictors of psychogenic pseudoseizure outcome. *Neurology.* 1999;53(5):933–938.
73. Kanner AM, Ramirez L, Jones JC. The utility of placing sphenoidal electrodes under the foramen ovale with fluoroscopic guidance. *J Clin Neurophysiol.* 1995;12(1):72–81.
74. King DW, Gallagher BB, Murvin AJ, et al. Pseudoseizures: diagnostic evaluation. *Neurology.* 1982;32(1):18–23.
75. Kotagal P, Costa M, Wyllie E, et al. Paroxysmal nonepileptic events in children and adolescents. *Pediatrics.* 2002;110(4):e46, 1–5.
76. Krawetz P, Fleisher W, Pillay N, et al. Family functioning in subjects with pseudoseizures and epilepsy. *J Nerv Ment Dis.* 2001;189(1):38–43.
77. Krumholz A. Nonepileptic seizures: diagnosis and management. *Neurology.* 1999;53(5 Suppl 2):S76–83.
78. Krumholz A, Niedermeyer E. Psychogenic seizures: a clinical study with follow-up data. *Neurology.* 1983;33(4):498–502.
79. Kuyk J, Spinhoven P, van Dyck R. Hypnotic recall: a positive criterion in the differential diagnosis between epileptic and pseudoepileptic seizures. *Epilepsia.* 1999;40(4):485–491.
80. LaFrance WC Jr, Gates JR, Trimble MR. Psychogenic unresponsiveness and nonepileptic seizures. In: Young GB, Wijdicks EF, eds. *Disorders of Consciousness.* 3rd ed. Edinburgh: Elsevier; 2006.
81. LaFrance WC. How many patients with psychogenic nonepileptic seizures also have epilepsy? *Neurology.* 2002;58(6):990–991.
82. LaFrance WC Jr, Barry JJ. Update on treatments of psychological nonepileptic seizures. *Epilepsy Behav.* 2005;7(3):364–374.
83. LaFrance WC Jr, Devinsky O. Treatment of nonepileptic seizures. *Epilepsy Behav.* 2002;3(5 Suppl 1):S19–23.
84. LaFrance WC Jr, Devinsky O. The treatment of nonepileptic seizures: historical perspectives and future directions. *Epilepsia.* 2004;45(Suppl 2):15–21.
85. LaFrance WC Jr, Kanner AM. Epilepsy. In: Jeste DV, Friedman JH, eds. *Psychiatry for Neurologists.* Totowa, NJ: Humana Press; 2006:191–208.
86. Lambert C, Rees WL. Intravenous barbiturates in the treatment of hysteria. *BMJ.* 1944;2:70–73.
87. Lancman ME, Asconape JJ, Craven WJ, et al. Predictive value of induction of psychogenic seizures by suggestion. *Ann Neurol.* 1994;35(3):359–361.
88. Laxer KD, Mullooly JP, Howell B. Prolactin changes after seizures classified by EEG monitoring. *Neurology.* 1985;35(1):31–35.
89. Leis AA, Ross MA, Summers AK. Psychogenic seizures: ictal characteristics and diagnostic pitfalls. *Neurology.* 1992;42(1):95–99.
90. Lelliott PT, Fenwick P. Cerebral pathology in pseudoseizures. *Acta Neurol Scand.* 1991;83(2):129–132.
91. Lempert T, Schmidt D. Natural history and outcome of psychogenic seizures: a clinical study in 50 patients. *J Neurol.* 1990;237(1):35–38.
92. Lesser RP. Psychogenic seizures. *Neurology.* 1996;46(6):1499–1507.
93. Lesser RP, Lueders H, Dinner DS. Evidence for epilepsy is rare in patients with psychogenic seizures. *Neurology.* 1983;33(4):502–504.
94. Lowe MR, De Toledo JC, Rabinstein AA, et al. Correspondence: MRI evidence of mesial temporal sclerosis in patients with psychogenic nonepileptic seizures. *Neurology.* 2001;56(6):821–823.
95. Luther JS, McNamara JO, Carwile S, et al. Pseudoepileptic seizures: methods and video analysis to aid diagnosis. *Ann Neurol.* 1982;12(5):458–462.
96. Martin R, Burneo JG, Prasad A, et al. Frequency of epilepsy in patients with psychogenic seizures monitored by video-EEG. *Neurology.* 2003;61(12):1791–1792.
97. Martinez-Taboas A. The role of hypnosis in the detection of psychogenic seizures. *Am J Clin Hypn.* 2002;45(1):11–20.
98. Meierkord H, Shorvon S, Lightman S, et al. Comparison of the effects of frontal and temporal lobe partial seizures on prolactin levels. *Arch Neurol.* 1992;49(3):225–230.
99. Meierkord H, Will B, Fish D, et al. The clinical features and prognosis of pseudoseizures diagnosed using video-EEG telemetry. *Neurology.* 1991;41(10):1643–1646.
100. Micale MS. *Approaching Hysteria: Disease and its Interpretations.* Princeton, NJ: Princeton University Press; 1995.
101. Miller HR. Psychogenic seizures treated by hypnosis. *Am J Clin Hypn.* 1983;25(4):248–252.
102. Mondon K, de Toffol B, Praline J, et al. Comorbidité psychiatrique au cours des événements non épileptiques: étude rétrospective dans un centre de vidéo-EEG [Psychiatric comorbidity in patients with pseudoseizures: retrospective study conducted in a video-EEG center. *Rev Neurol (Paris).* 2005;161(11):1061–1069.
103. Morris HH 3rd, Dinner DS, Luders H, et al. Supplementary motor seizures: clinical and electroencephalographic findings. *Neurology.* 1988;38(7):1075–1082.
104. Neill JC, Alvarez N. Differential diagnosis of epileptic versus pseudoepileptic seizures in developmentally disabled persons. *Appl Res Ment Retard.* 1986;7(3):285–298.
105. Newton MR, Berkovic SF, Austin MC, et al. SPECT in the localisation of extratemporal and temporal seizure foci. *J Neurol Neurosurg Psychiatry.* 1995;59(1):26–30.
106. Niedermeyer E, Blumer D, Holscher E, et al. Classical hysterical seizures facilitated by anticonvulsant toxicity. *Psychiatr Clin (Basel).* 1970;3(2):71–84.
107. O'Malley PG, Jackson JL, Santoro J, et al. Antidepressant therapy for unexplained symptoms and symptom syndromes. *J Fam Pract.* 1999;48(12):980–990.
108. Oribe E, Amini R, Nissenbaum E, et al. Serum prolactin concentrations are elevated after syncope. *Neurology.* 1996;47(1):60–62.

109. Oto M, Espie C, Pelosi A, et al. The safety of antiepileptic drug withdrawal in patients with non-epileptic seizures. *J Neurol Neurosurg Psychiatry*. 2005;76(12):1682–1685.
110. Parra J, Iriarte J, Kanner AM. Are we overusing the diagnosis of psychogenic non-epileptic events? *Seizure*. 1999;8(4):223–227.
111. Parra J, Kanner AM, Iriarte J, et al. When should induction protocols be used in the diagnostic evaluation of patients with paroxysmal events? *Epilepsia*. 1998;39(8):863–867.
112. Peguero E, Abou-Khalil B, Fakhoury T, et al. Self-injury and incontinence in psychogenic seizures. *Epilepsia*. 1995;36(6):586–591.
113. Pehlivanturk B, Unal F. Conversion disorder in children and adolescents: clinical features and comorbidity with depressive and anxiety disorders. *Turk J Pediatr*. 2000;42(2):132–137.
114. Price HE, Rosenbaum DH, Rowan AJ, et al. Measurement of regional cerebral blood flow by SPECT in nonepileptic seizure disorder patients [Abstract]. *Epilepsia*. 1992;33(Suppl 3):54(abst).
115. Prueter C, Schultz-Venrath U, Rimpau W. Dissociative and associated psychopathological symptoms in patients with epilepsy, pseudoseizures, and both seizure forms. *Epilepsia*. 2002;43(2):188–192.
116. Ramsay RE, Cohen A, Brown MC. Coexisting epilepsy and non-epileptic seizures. In: Rowan AJ, Gates JR, eds. *Non-Epileptic Seizures*. 1st ed. Stoneham, MA: Butterworth-Heinemann; 1993:47–54.
117. Rechlin T, Loew TH, Joraschky P. Pseudoseizure "status." *J Psychosom Res*. 1997;42(5):495–498.
118. Reuber M, Fernandez G, Bauer J, et al. Interictal EEG abnormalities in patients with psychogenic nonepileptic seizures. *Epilepsia*. 2002;43(9):1013–1020.
119. Reuber M, Mitchell AJ, Howlett S, et al. Measuring outcome in psychogenic nonepileptic seizures: how relevant is seizure remission? *Epilepsia*. 2005;46(11):1788–1795.
120. Reuber M, Pukrop R, Bauer J, et al. Outcome in psychogenic nonepileptic seizures: 1 to 10-year follow-up in 164 patients. *Ann Neurol*. 2003;53(3):305–311.
121. Sander JW, Hart YM, Johnson AL, et al. National general practice study of epilepsy: newly diagnosed epileptic seizures in a general population. *Lancet*. 1990;336(8726):1267–1271.
122. Savard G, Andermann F, Teitelbaum J, et al. Epileptic Munchausen's syndrome: a form of pseudoseizures distinct from hysteria and malingering. *Neurology*. 1988;38(10):1628–1629.
123. Saygi S, Katz A, Marks DA, et al. Frontal lobe partial seizures and psychogenic seizures: comparison of clinical and ictal characteristics. *Neurology*. 1992;42(7):1274–1277.
124. Scicutella A. Anxiety disorders in epilepsy. In: Ettinger AB, Kanner AM, eds. *Psychiatry Issues in Epilepsy: A Practical Guide to Diagnosis and Treatment*. 1st ed. Philadelphia: Lippincott Williams & Wilkins; 2001:95–109.
125. Scicutella A, Ettinger AB. Treatment of anxiety in epilepsy. *Epilepsy Behav*. 2002;3(5 Suppl 1):S10–12.
126. Scott DF. Recognition and diagnostic aspects of nonepileptic seizures. In: Riley TL, Roy A, eds. *Pseudoseizures*. Baltimore: Williams & Wilkins; 1982:21–33.
127. Sethi PK, Rao TS. Gelastic, quiritarian, and cursive epilepsy. A clinicopathological appraisal. *J Neurol Neurosurg Psychiatry*. 1976;39(9):823–828.
128. Shen W, Bowman ES, Markand ON. Presenting the diagnosis of pseudoseizure. *Neurology*. 1990;40(5):756–759.
129. Sigurdardottir KR, Olafsson E. Incidence of psychogenic seizures in adults: a population-based study in Iceland. *Epilepsia*. 1998;39(7):749–752.
130. Silberman EK, Post RM, Nurnberger J, et al. Transient sensory, cognitive and affective phenomena in affective illness. A comparison with complex partial epilepsy. *Br J Psychiatry*. 1985;146:81–89.
131. Slater JD, Brown MC, Jacobs W, et al. Induction of pseudoseizures with intravenous saline placebo. *Epilepsia*. 1995;36(6):580–585.
132. Smith GR. The epidemiology and treatment of depression when it coexists with somatoform disorders, somatization, or pain. *Gen Hosp Psychiatry*. 1992;14(4):265–272.
133. Spanaki MV, Spencer SS, Corsi M, et al. The role of quantitative ictal SPECT analysis in the evaluation of nonepileptic seizures. *J Neuroimaging*. 1999;9(4):210–216.
134. Spatt J. Deja vu: possible parahippocampal mechanisms. *J Neuropsychiatry Clin Neurosci*. 2002;14(1):6–10.
135. Spencer SS. The relative contributions of MRI, SPECT, and PET imaging in epilepsy. *Epilepsia*. 1994;35(Suppl 6):S72–89.
136. Storzbach D, Binder LM, Salinsky MC, et al. Improved prediction of nonepileptic seizures with combined MMPI and EEG measures. *Epilepsia*. 2000;41(3):332–337.
137. Sumner JW Jr, Cameron RR, Peterson DB. Hypnosis in differentiation of epileptic from convulsive-like seizures. *Neurology*. 1952;2:395–402.
138. Szaflarski JP, Ficker DM, Cahill WT, et al. Four-year incidence of psychogenic nonepileptic seizures in adults in Hamilton County, OH. *Neurology*. 2000;55(10):1561–1563.
139. Thacker K, Devinsky O, Perrine K, et al. Nonepileptic seizures during apparent sleep. *Ann Neurol*. 1993;33(4):414–418.
140. The NES Treatment Workshop Committee, LaFrance WC Jr, Alper K, Babcock D, et al. Nonepileptic Seizure Treatment Workshop summary. *Epilepsy Behav*. 2006;8:451–461.
141. Trimble MR. Pseudoseizures. *Neurol Clin*. 1986;4(3):531–548.
142. Trimble MR. *The Psychoses of Epilepsy*. New York: Raven Press; 1991.
143. Voon V. Treatment of psychogenic movement disorder: psychotropic medications. In: Hallett M, Fahn S, Jankovic J, et al., eds. *Psychogenic Movement Disorders: Neurology and Neuropsychiatry*. Philadelphia: Lippincott Williams & Wilkins, and American Academy of Neurology Press; 2005: 302–310.
144. Walczak TS, Papacostas S, Williams DT, et al. Outcome after diagnosis of psychogenic nonepileptic seizures. *Epilepsia*. 1995;36(11):1131–1137.
145. Walczak TS, Williams DT, Berten W. Utility and reliability of placebo infusion in the evaluation of patients with seizures. *Neurology*. 1994;44(3 Pt 1):394–399.
146. Wilder C, Marquez AV, Farias ST, et al. Abstract 2.469. Long-term follow-up study of patients with PNES. *Epilepsia*. 2004;45(Suppl 7):349.
147. Williamson PD, Spencer DD, Spencer SS, et al. Complex partial seizures of frontal lobe origin. *Ann Neurol*. 1985;18(4):497–504.
148. Wilson JVK, Reynolds EH. Texts and documents. Translation and analysis of a cuneiform text forming part of a Babylonian treatise on epilepsy. *Med Hist*. 1990;34(2):185–198.
149. Won HJ, Chang KH, Cheon JE, et al. Comparison of MR imaging with PET and ictal SPECT in 118 patients with intractable epilepsy. *AJNR Am J Neuroradiol*. 1999;20(4):593–599.
150. Wood BL, McDaniel S, Burchfiel K, et al. Factors distinguishing families of patients with psychogenic seizures from families of patients with epilepsy. *Epilepsia*. 1998;39(4):432–437.
151. Wyler AR, Hermann BP, Blumer D, et al. Pseudo-pseudoepileptic seizures. In: Rowan AJ, Gates JR, eds. *Non-Epileptic Seizures*. 1st ed. Stoneham, MA: Butterworth-Heinemann; 1993:73–84.
152. Wyllie E, Friedman D, Luders H, et al. Outcome of psychogenic seizures in children and adolescents compared with adults. *Neurology*. 1991;41(5):742–744.
153. Wyllie E, Glazer JP, Benbadis S, et al. Psychiatric features of children and adolescents with pseudoseizures. *Arch Pediatr Adolesc Med*. 1999; 153(3):244–248.
154. Wyllie E, Lueders H, Pippenger C, et al. Postictal serum creatine kinase in the diagnosis of seizure disorders. *Arch Neurol*. 1985;42(2):123–126.
155. Zeman AZ, Boniface SJ, Hodges JR. Transient epileptic amnesia: a description of the clinical and neuropsychological features in 10 cases and a review of the literature. *J Neurol Neurosurg Psychiatry*. 1998;64(4):435–443.

CHAPTER 283 ■ EPISODIC DYSCONTROL

LUDGER TEBARTZ VAN ELST AND MICHAEL R. TRIMBLE

INTRODUCTION

Episodic dyscontrol (ED) is a rare but severe form of human aggressive behavior. The following case report illustrates the phenomenology of such troubling paroxysmal behaviors.

- A.E. was a 33-year-old white carpenter who was one participant of our study into episodic dyscontrol or intermittent explosive disorder in epilepsy at the Institute of Neurology.[77] A.E. was completely healthy and did not suffer from any major medical, neurologic, or psychiatric condition up to the age of 28 years, when he developed herpes encephalitis and subsequently suffered from temporal lobe epilepsy (TLE). He presented to the Chalfont Centre with complex partial seizures with a frequency of two to three clusters of up to six seizures a day. On these occasions, he would feel agitated somewhat 2 to 3 hours prior to the seizure. He then typically would feel odd; both sides of his face would start twitching, followed by salivation. During these seizures, which lasted 2 to 3 minutes, he would be awake but unresponsive to other people, with eyes wide open. Once to twice a month, a classic secondary–generalized tonic–clonic seizure evolved out of such a complex partial seizure. Neuropsychiatric assessment revealed a normal interictal electroencephalogram (EEG) with no ictal EEG available at time of presentation. Structural magnetic resonance imaging (MRI) displayed bilateral hippocampal and amygdala volume loss and increased hippocampal signal in T2 images. On psychiatric assessment, there was no formal diagnosis, and in particular no evidence for any affective, psychotic, or personality disorder or attention-deficit hyperactivity disorder (ADHD) apart from episodic dyscontrol.
- With a frequency of two to three episodes a year and a duration of 30 to 60 minutes, A.E. could behave in a very aggressive and violent way. Typically, there were no adequate triggers and a sudden onset of severe arousal, anger, and rage. The patient then became physically aggressive, attacking people and objects. The attack did not follow any obvious premeditated plan, and the behavior was poorly organized, with A.E. attacking every person or object at hand.
- On one such occasion at the tertiary referral center, A.E. was queuing for his medication when suddenly he gripped a nearby billiard stick, hitting the nurses and fellow patients at hand. He then left the ward and destroyed three cars before he could be restricted by the police. During this episode, there was no obvious evidence for an epileptic seizure and no evidence for hallucinations or persecutory delusions. The day before the attack, the he had had a pint of lager beer; apart from that, however, there was no evidence for any other drug abuse. The day after the attack, the patient felt extremely ashamed for this behavior. He could not recall and describe his feelings and thoughts during the episode in detail and remained vague in his recollection of the scene. At the same time, he was not absolutely amnesic and felt very guilty and depressed because of this behavior.

This case illustrates the complexity and danger of episodic dyscontrol and illustrates why many authors believe that ED might be related to epilepsy in particular because of its paroxysmal nature. Before we discuss the precise phenomenology and neurobiology of ED, however, we first have to clarify the relationship of this special form of aggressive behavior to aggression and violence as a general phenomenon of human life.

Human aggression is an important social and clinical problem.[32,67,75,82] The phenomenologic and probably neurobiologic heterogeneity of aggressive and violent behaviors is a major scientific problem leading to difficulties in assessment and classification. An important distinction has emerged between the terms *violence* and *aggression*. Treiman defined violence as forceful infliction of abuse or damage on another individual or object.[81] However, according to this concept, violence is not necessarily the result of intentional aggression. Aggression, in contrast, is defined as an offensive action directed toward another individual or object with the premeditated intention to harm, threaten, or control other subjects, groups, or situations.[81]

An advantage of this distinction is that it can be used to describe different destructive behaviors more precisely by referring to a special mental state, that is, the intentionality that does or does not motivate the destructive behavior. It leaves researchers with the problem of assessing intentionality, however, which in clinical practice is often impossible.

Therefore, it seems to be desirable to define phenomenologic criteria of specific behavioral syndromes of interest to obtain a nontheoretical approach to classifying aggressive and violent behaviors.

CLASSIFYING AGGRESSION

One approach to doing this is to refer to basic research on animals. Here, aggressive behavior is classified according to the context in which it is observed. Authors like Moyer distinguished different subtypes of aggressive behavior in animals based on a precise characterization of the behavioral context in which such behavior is observed.[55] For example, predatory aggression is defined as violent behavior in which a predator kills its prey. It is characterized by a calm and very concentrated mental state of the aggressive animal and behavior that is well structured and goal directed. Maternal aggression, in contrast, is characterized by high arousal of the aggressive animal and a specific situational trigger when its offspring is menaced by predator. Table 1 summarizes the context-specific classification of aggressive behavior in animals.

Contrary to animal behavior, human behavior depends less on external cues and stimuli, and behavioral programs are less preformed. Therefore a simple transfer of the context-based classification of animal aggression to human behavior is not

TABLE 1

SUBTYPES OF ANIMAL AGGRESSION

Aggression type	Example of animal behavior	Behavioral characteristic
Predatory aggression	Cat kills mouse	Calm, concentrated, goal directed, well structured
Intermale (territorial) aggression	Two lions fight for supremacy	Arousal, concentrated, goal directed, well structured
Maternal aggression	Bird attacks cat when it approaches the nest	Arousal, concentrated, goal directed, well structured
Sex-related aggression	Mantis kills male after copulation	Calm, behavioral stereotypes
Fear-induced aggression	Flight–fight Reaction Buffalo fight predator	Arousal, vocalization, less well structured, diverse behavioral pattern, reactive behavior

Source: Modifed from Moyer KE. *Violence and Aggression—A Physiological Perspective*. New York: Paragon House; 1987.

possible.[42] Nevertheless, there is general agreement that at least two different phenomenologic and neurobiologic subtypes of aggressive behavior can be differentiated in humans: (a) predatory and (b) defensive aggression.[35,42,55,56,85]

Predatory aggression as described earlier is characterized semiologically as a well-structured and goal-directed behavior performed in an emotionally calm and concentrated state of mind. Defensive aggression, in contrast, is generally seen in the context of high emotional arousal and is associated with vocalizations and signs of anger or fear. The behavioral pattern itself is less structured and is defensive.[83]

Most forms of human aggression that are generally seen in a clinical context are considered to be defensive, that is, the behavior is generally poorly structured and a reaction toward a perceived threat, be it adequate or not.[2] Obviously, the perception of whether a stimulus is threatening is decisive in the information processing leading to this kind of aggressive behavior. However, there are also forms of offensive aggression that are often seen in criminals or patients with a diagnosis of dissocial personality disorder (ICD-10 Classification of Mental and Behavioural Disorders [ICD 10] F60.2), conduct disorder in adolescents, or hyperkinetic disorder of social behavior (ICD-10 F90.1).

AGGRESSIVE BEHAVIOR IN CLINICAL PRACTICE

In clinical practice, aggressive behavior can be observed in the context of different medical, neurologic, and psychiatric disorders and diseases. In patients with mental retardation, it is a common problem, possibly as a consequence of impaired social perception or deficits in expressing personal needs.[9,37,44,67] Furthermore, aggression is often seen in the context of organic brain disease such as frontal or hypothalamic brain tumors, neurodegenerative disease, delirium, or drug abuse. These common forms of aggression in the clinical setting tend to be malstructured, defensive, and generally occur in the context of states of confusion and diffuse emotional arousal.

Well-structured, premeditated, and goal-directed aggressive behaviors can occur on the background of psychiatric disorders such as psychosis with delusional states, ADHD, or bipolar disorder. It is frequently observed in patients with antisocial personality disorder (APD), in which it is part of the characteristic traitlike behavior.[9,53,71]

The only clinical syndrome of aggression that has been identified as a distinct category in the international classificatory system is intermittent explosive disorder (IED) according to the guidelines of the *Diagnostic and Statistical Manual of Mental Disorders*, 4th ed. (DSM–IV).[5] The concept of IED has been modeled on the clinical descriptions of episodic dyscontrol.[8]

PHENOMENOLOGY OF EPISODIC DYSCONTROL

As mentioned, IED is basically a synonym for episodic dyscontrol. Because IED is an internationally accepted diagnostic construct, we will use this term in this chapter rather than ED. Both entities are characterized by several discrete episodes of failure to resist aggressive impulses that result in serious assaults or destruction of property. The behavior is out of proportion to any apparent precipitating psychosocial stressors and is not due to substance abuse, another mental disorder such as personality disorder, any other first-axis psychiatric disorder, or a general medical condition such as head trauma or neurodegenerative diseases. Consequently and in spite of the sometimes suggestive paroxysmal semiology, IED cannot be regarded as a special semiology of epilepsy. Whether this distinctive conception will stand the test of time, however, remains to be seen.

EPIDEMIOLOGY OF INTERMITTENT EXPLOSIVE DISORDER

There are only a few studies analyzing the prevalence of IED in primary medical settings. One study aimed at determining the lifetime and current prevalence of IED along with other demographic characteristics and patterns of comorbidity in an outpatient psychiatric sample of 1,300 individuals presenting for outpatient psychiatric treatment.[21] Following structured diagnostic assessment for axis I and II disorders, the authors reported a lifetime prevalence of IED of 6.3% (SE, ±0.7%) and a cross-sectional prevalence of 3.1% ± 0.5% of psychiatric patients. IED was the current principal diagnosis in only 0.6% ± 0.2% of patients. Most of these patients (80%) were interested in treatment for their intermittent aggressive behavior. The authors concluded that DSM-IV IED in psychiatric samples is far more common than previously thought and pointed out that IED develops early in life, especially in male patients.

NEUROBIOLOGY OF INTERMITTENT EXPLOSIVE DISORDER

There are few studies looking at neurobiologic mechanisms specifically in IED. The fact that there is some controversy as to the reliability of the clinical diagnosis aggravates the problem of neurobiologic research into this entity.[54] Nevertheless, there is some evidence that disturbances of the functional integrity of frontotemporal brain circuits might play an important role in the genesis of IED and ED.

Clinical Studies

There are numerous studies addressing the relationship between focal lesional brain pathology and aggressive and impulsive behavior. Prefrontal brain damage and in particular orbitofrontal brain pathology have been closely associated with aggressive dyscontrol.[17] The specific entity of ED or IED has scarcely been addressed in any of these studies, however, although there are a few cases in which ED has been related to hypothalamic or basal ganglia lesions.[27,80]

With respect to neurochemical brain pathology, there is some vague evidence that functional disturbances of the serotonergic system might play a critical role in impulsive aggression in general.[43] In fact, one consistent finding in biologic psychiatry is an association between low cerebrospinal fluid 5-hydroxyindole acetic acid levels and impulsive aggressive acts, suggesting a decreased serotonin turnover. Again, however, there no specific studies in IED or ED.

Electroencephalographic and Imaging Studies

EEG studies point to an increased prevalence of unspecific EEG abnormalities in disorders with disturbed impulse control in general and ED in particular.[12,30] Drake et al., for example, reported a significant increase of diffuse or focal slowing in the EEGs of ED patients as compared to healthy volunteers or depressed patients.[30] N100 and P160 auditory-evoked potential amplitudes were lower in episodic-dyscontrol patients than in controls, but the difference was not significant. The authors concluded that such findings suggest that nonspecific cerebral dysfunction and EEG changes may be associated with disordered impulse or behavior control.[30]

A systematic literature review based on PubMed searches did not reveal any positron emission tomography, single photon emission computed tomography, or functional MRI study that specifically looked at neurobiologic mechanisms of ED or IED. There are two studies by our group, however, in which we addressed IED in the context of epilepsy, using structural MRI techniques.[78,88]

In these studies we hypothesized that, in patients with TLE and intermittent affective aggression, amygdala sclerosis in the context of hippocampal sclerosis would be more common as compared to control patients. In addition, we aimed to analyze a possible association between aggression on one hand and hippocampal sclerosis, low IQ, and poor social adjustment on the other in patients with TLE. In a further approach, we analyzed cortical gray matter abnormalities in these patients to gather evidence for frontal lobe pathology in patients with TLE and IED.

Amygdala Pathology in Patients With Temporal Lobe Epilepsy and Episodic Dyscontrol

For that purpose, we compared 25 patients with TLE and IED with 25 control patients with TLE without any psychopathology and 20 healthy volunteers.[78] Both patient groups were matched for age, gender, demographic background, duration of epilepsy, and seizure severity. There was no significant group difference regarding the history of birth complications, febrile convulsions, or status epilepticus. In the IED group, however, the incidence of encephalitic brain disease (Fisher's exact test: $p = .05$) and left-handedness (chi-square test: $p < .05$) was significantly increased. There was less right-sided focal EEG abnormality and more bilateral EEG abnormality in the aggressive group, and hippocampal sclerosis was significantly less common in patients with TLE and IED. Other left temporal pathology, including 3 patients with amygdala pathology (amygdala sclerosis, amygdala glioma, amygdala dysembryoplastic neuroepithelial tumor), 2 patients with multiple small temporal infarctions, and 2 patients with diffuse left temporal atrophy of unknown origin, was significantly more common in patients with TLE plus IED. In the aggressive patients, a subgroup of 5 patients (20%) showed amygdala atrophy as compared to only 1 in the nonaggressive group (chi-square test: $p = .04$). An increased incidence of encephalitis (chi-square test: $p < .005$; Fisher's exact test: $p = 0.1$) was the only clinical feature that distinguished patients with amygdala atrophy from those with normal amygdala volumes. In 12 of 25 patients, we could prove some evidence of amygdala-related brain pathology as compared to only 1 in the nonaggressive group. Furthermore, there was a highly significant group difference in IQ figures, with the verbal IQ (VIQ), the performance IQ (PIQ), and hence the full IQ (FIQ) all being lower in the aggressive group. In addition, there was a significant group difference in Beck Depression Inventory and Spielberger State Trait Anxiety Index scores, with the aggressive group rating much higher in depression ($p < 0.05$), state ($p < 0.05$), and trait anxiety ($p < 0.01$).[78]

Cortical Abnormalities in Patients With Temporal Lobe Epilepsy and Episodic Dyscontrol

In a second analysis, we employed the method of voxel-based morphometry to detect possible subtle cortical brain pathology that was not present on visual assessment of the MRI scans analyzing the same study sample.[88] Both TLE patient groups were compared with each other and with the control subjects on a voxel-by-voxel basis for increases and decreases of gray matter. Details of the methodology are published elsewhere.[88,89] In this study, we were able to demonstrate reductions of gray matter density over large areas of the left extratemporal neocortex with maxima in the left frontal neocortex; one maximum difference projection had a Z score of 5.67 at Talairach coordinates $x = 58$, $y = 36$, $z = 9$ mm (left anterior frontolateral cortex), the other a Z score of 4.78 in a more-posterior left frontal lobe location (Talairach coordinates $x = 66$, $y = 0$, $z = 28$ mm). Patients with TLE who did not have IED showed no significant decrease of cortical gray matter compared with control individuals. Patients with TLE with IED also had reduction of left frontal gray matter compared with patients with TLE without IED, although this was less marked than when compared with control individuals (Z score of 3.49 at Talairach coordinates $x = 66$, $y = 2$, $z = 26$ mm). The statistical parametric mapping–based voxelwise correlation of social dysfunction and aggression scale scores and automatically segmented gray matter in all patients with TLE showed a left frontal gray matter area

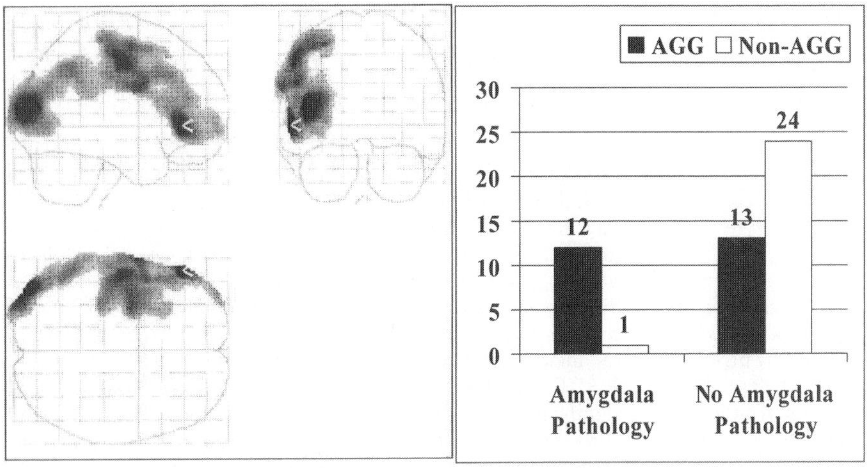

FIGURE 1. Prevalence of amygdala-related brain pathology and cortical gray matter density loss in 25 patients with temporal lobe epilepsy and episodic dyscontrol. AGG, aggression. (Redrawn after Tebartz van Elst L. Aggression and epilepsy. In: Trimble M, Schmitz B, eds. *The Neuropsychiatry of Epilepsy*. Cambridge: Cambridge University Press; 2002:81–106.)

being negatively correlated with these scores, which expressed social consequences of interictal affective aggression (Z score of 3.65 at Talairach coordinates $x = 66$, $y = 2$, $z = 26$ mm). Age, scores of depression and anxiety, IQ measures, or scores of verbal fluency did not significantly correlate with specific decreases in gray matter in all patients with TLE.[88] Figure 1 illustrates the main findings from these two studies.

NEUROBIOLOGY OF AGGRESSION IN GENERAL AND INTERMITTENT EXPLOSIVE DISORDER IN PARTICULAR

Various brain structures are known to play an important role in the generation of aggressive behavior in animals and humans. The most important of these structures are the periaqueductal gray,[10,16] the hypothalamus,[7] the amygdala and associated limbic structures,[1,29,39,45,66] and the frontal lobes.[23,53,61]

Even though the precise function of the aforementioned structures and their role in the complex interplay of the different brain circuits in regulating different aggressive behaviors is unclear, the first elements of a functional anatomy of aggression can be identified (Table 2). Brainstem structures like the periaquaductal gray are crucial for the activation of evolutionarily preformed behavioral programs like attacking or defensive behavior in animals.[10,16] These structures are controlled by higher neuronal centers in the hypothalamus,[13,84] which in addition to controlling these behavioral brainstem programs, adjust the internal endocrinologic and immunologic environment to aggressive behavior in flight-or-fight situations.[50,63,69,90]

The frontal lobes are known to play a critical role in the ability to suppress behavioral impulses. Thus, patients with frontal lobe lesion often lose the ability to suppress aggressive impulses and therefore might present with severe aggressive and violent psychopathology.[23,46,59,71]

The amygdala is thought to play a crucial role in the mediation of fear-induced aggression, a subtype of defensive aggression.[1,20,33,48] They receive input from various levels of sensory information processing and project to most of the other critical brain structures, including the brainstem, hypothalamus, thalamus, and frontal lobe.[3,4] From a neurophysiologic perspective, they are in a key position for the affective evaluation of multimodal sensory input. Thus, pathology within the circuits affecting the amygdala might lead to mental states in which the misinterpretation of sensory input as threatening leads to aggressive outbursts. In agreement with this assumption, electrical stimulation of the amygdala can lead to experiences like fear, anxiety, or anger,[19,34] and lesioning of the amygdala severely impairs fear conditioning in animals[25] and humans.[47] Furthermore, in an open retrospective study of 481 cases of bilateral amygdalotomies performed for the control of conservatively untreatable aggressiveness, moderate to excellent improvement of aggressive behavior was reported in 70% to 76% of cases.[62]

DUAL BRAIN PATHOLOGY IN PATIENTS WITH EPISODIC DYSCONTROL

Based on our findings in patients with TLE and IED in which significant brain pathology could be observed in amygdala-related circuits on one hand and the prefrontal lobe on the other, we suggested that a dual brain pathology affecting limbic brain structures and prefrontal areas at the same time might be a critical pathogenetic element in the genesis of episodic

TABLE 2

FUNCTIONAL RELEVANCE OF DIFFERENT BRAIN STRUCTURES FOR AGGRESSIVE BEHAVIOR

Brain structure	Assumed function
Frontal lobe	Inhibitory function Suppression of aggressive behavioral drive
Amygdala and limbic circuits	Emotional evaluation of multimodal sensory and cognitive input Emotional drive and arousal
Hypothalamus	Control of brainstem behavioral programs Regulation of internal environment Coordination of behavioual programs and internal environment in flight–fightsituations
Brainstem structures, i.e., periaqueductal gray	Evolutionarily preformed behavioral flight–fight programs

Source: Modified from Tebartz van Elst L. Aggression and epilepsy. In: Trimble M, Schmitz B, eds. *The Neuropsychiatry of Epilepsy*. Cambridge: Cambridge University Press; 2002:81–106.

dyscontrol and intermittent explosive disorder.[77] Within this concept, both clinical entities are understood as hyperarousal-dyscontrol syndromes. The clinical phenomenology of hyperarousal, that is, the sudden onset of extreme arousal, fear, and rage, is probably related to some sort of amygdala-network instability. Following this line of thought, we associate the failure to control the aggressive impulses resulting from emotional arousal in the context of functional amygdala instability with prefrontal lobe dysfunction.

The observations of our study support this notion. Brain pathology in patients with epilepsy and aggression was more diverse in nature and more diffuse in distribution. We found an increased prevalence of a history of encephalitis in patients with epilepsy plus aggression. Encephalitis in the past might have been a pathogenetic element for the more diffuse and widespread pathology in the temporal lobe seen in our aggressive patients. Furthermore, the increased prevalence of left-handedness in our aggressive patients may indicate early brain pathology such as encephalitis affecting the left hemisphere (i.e., lateralization of dominance to the right hemisphere).

Eleven of 12 patients with amygdala-related brain pathology displayed this pathology on the left-hand side, and the only patient with right-sided amygdala atrophy alone was left-handed. Thus, the dominant hemisphere seems to play a more important role in the mediation of affective aggression than the nondominant hemisphere.

The finding of frontal cortical gray matter loss was clearly lateralized too. Patients with TLE plus IED displayed highly significant left frontal gray matter loss that correlated with the aggression psychometry scores. This, together with the left-lateralized finding of amygdala-related brain pathology, could support a theory of left-lateralized dual brain pathology in IED.[77]

This theory is further supported by earlier functional imaging and MR spectroscopy studies showing a reduced prefrontal glucose metabolism in those convicted of murder and significantly lower neuronal markers in the frontal lobes of repetitively violent patients with learning disabilities, although without clear lateralizing effects.[60,61]

Figure 2 illustrates this pathogenetic model of hyperarousal-dyscontrol syndromes. Pathology within the amygdala or amygdaloid circuits might result in hyperarousal states in which patients become angry and aroused without a sufficient external stimulus (hyperarousal syndrome). This dysfunctional arousal resulting in aggressive behavioral impulses normally can be suppressed by learned behavioral rules. In the case of additional frontal lobe pathology, however, the capacity of the affected patients to suppress behavioral impulses arising from the "emotional brain" is limited, and thus an additional dyscontrol syndrome leaves the patients vulnerable to the development of hyperarousal-dyscontrol syndromes, that is, episodic dyscontrol or intermittent explosive disorder.[77]

INTERMITTENT EXPLOSIVE DISORDER—IS IT EPILEPSY?

When analyzing the phenomenology of episodic aggressive behavior as illustrated in the case report at the beginning of this chapter, the question arises as to whether this episodic aggressive behavior might be understood as some form of frontal or limbic lobe epilepsy. The ictal nature of the aggressive outbursts, the lack of adequate psychosocial triggers, and the discrepancy with the interictal undisturbed personality all support this suspicion. Because frontal or limbic lobe epilepsy can be observed without pathologic findings in the surface EEG and it is difficult anyway to obtain an EEG during the aggressive episodes from the affected patients, this hypothesis is very difficult to investigate.

The observation that antiepileptics often are very effective in controlling impulsive aggression (see later comments) further supports the notion of a link between ED and epilepsy. The fact that they do not help in another substantial subgroup of patients with IED or ED does not contradict the hypothesis because many patients with classical epilepsy do not respond to antiepileptic treatment either.

From deep brain recording in patients with postictal psychosis we know, however, that there are other nonictal but still epilepsy-related pathomechanisms that can result in severe psychiatric symptoms including aggression that are not truly ictal in nature.[68] Therefore, although the hypothesis that IED might be some form of undiagnosed limbic or frontal epileptic attack disorder is far from being falsified, it is not proven either, and other epilepsy-related pathomechamisms could also explain the paroxysmal behavioral dysfunction. Further studies comparing patients with and without various neurologic diseases using even more sophisticated methods of functional brain assessment will be necessary to solve this question.

SOCIAL AND PSYCHOLOGICAL ASPECTS OF AGGRESSION IN EPILEPSY

Another important observation that arose from our studies was that there was a strong link between aggression and high levels

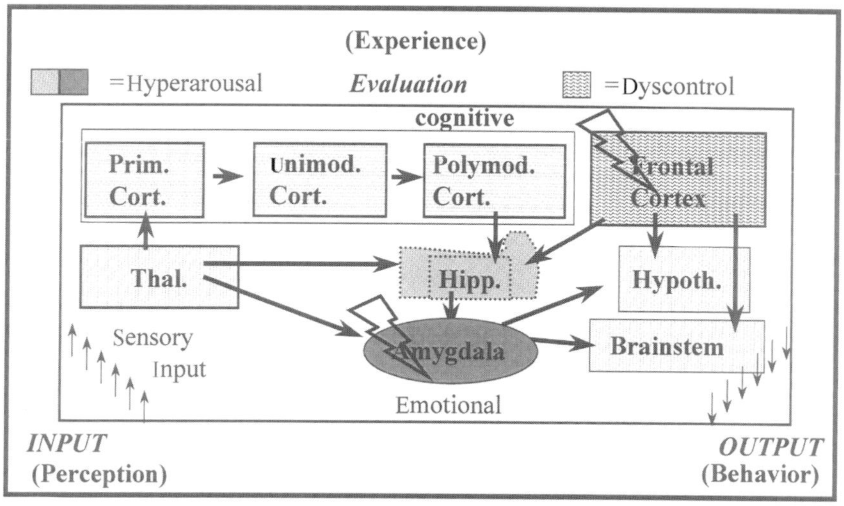

FIGURE 2. Dual brain pathology in hyperarousal-dyscontrol syndromes. Thal, thalamus; Prim Cort, primary cortex; Unimod Cort, unimodal cortex; Polymod Cort, polymodal cortex; Hipp, hippocampus; Hypoth, hypothalamus. (Redrawn after Tebartz van Elst L. Aggression and epilepsy. In: Trimble M, Schmitz B, eds. *The Neuropsychiatry of Epilepsy*. Cambridge: Cambridge University Press; 2002:81–106; and Tebartz van Elst L, Trimble MR, Ebert D, et al. Dual brain pathology in patients with affective aggressive episodes. *Arch Gen Psychiatry.* 2001;58;1187–1188.)

of depression and anxiety, confirming other reports of such an association in the non–psychiatrically ill population.[14] It seems plausible that high levels of anxiety result in states of hyperarousal that might be facilitated by amygdala pathology, as suggested by other authors.[18] Regarding the relationship between depression and aggression, there are only few and inconclusive reports in the general literature.[15] Our findings point to a clear association among depression, anxiety, and hyperarousal-dyscontrol states at least in TLE.

Social disadvantage, prejudice, poor housing, poverty, and poor communication skills are further factors that make hyperarousal states and states of discontentment and anger more likely and thus might increase the probability of aggressive behavior. Disentangling the complex interaction among these different psychobiologic elements, however, is often not possible.

THERAPY OF AGGRESSION AND EPISODIC DYSCONTROL

Intermittent explosive disorder and episodic dyscontrol are not unitary nosologic entities; they are essentially clusters of symptoms or syndromes that may occur in quite different medical, psychological, or social contexts. The most important point for an adequate therapy of ED and IED is a thorough medical and psychosocial diagnosis. Care should be taken to investigate any possible medical, neurologic, or psychiatric problem or comorbidity that might contribute to these most devastating and distressing behavioral syndromes. In case such diagnoses or comorbidities do exist, they have to be treated properly because this might in some cases solve the problem. For those patients in whom IED occurs in the context of established or suspected epilepsy, we refer to Chapter 212, where we outline the treatment principles for aggression in the context of epilepsy. The treatment of IED in the context of other psychiatric disorders such as schizophrenia, bipolar disorder, ADHD, borderline personality disorder, or conduct disorder should basically follow the treatment guideline of these respective disorders (see the standard psychiatric textbooks).

In case there are no medical, neurologic, or psychiatric comorbid or contributing diseases or disorders (which is probably a rare constellation), a symptomatic treatment should be started. To our knowledge, there are no systematic double-blind, placebo-controlled therapy studies in IED or ED. However, there are many case reports of successful therapy of this condition.

The two pharmacologic agents that are most often reported to be successful in IED are selective serotonin reuptake inhibitors (SSRIs)[26,31,38,64] and antiepileptic agents.[6,49,51,58,73,74] Carbamazepine in particular has been reported to be successful in as many as 65% of patients with IED.[28] The latter observation further supports the assumption that IED might be pathogenetically related to epilepsy. An alternative explanation of this observation, however, is the notion that IED might be pathogenetically related to bipolar disorder because most antiepileptics—carbamazepine in particular—are potent mood stabilizers. Following this line of thought, we could see episodic dyscontrol as a brief quasi-manic episode.[52] In line with this assumption, there is some evidence that lithium might be helpful in treating ED or IED.[41,72] Apart from that, there are reports of successful treatment of IED with beta-blockers such as propanolol[36,65] and antipsychotic agents.[40,57,86]

Finally, it must be stressed that anger management, contingency management, and psychotherapy all can be very helpful and successful in treating impulsive aggressive behavior. In particular, in the context of mental handicap and personality disorders, aggression and impulsivity might be part of attention-seeking behavior and role testing. In these cases, the feedback strategies and the reactions of relatives and caregivers are very important, and methods of contingency management may be a critical element of any successful treatment.[11,22] Apart from that, different methods of anger management, cognitive–behavioral therapy, or skills training that have been developed irrespective of whether impulsive behavior is seen in the context of ED or epilepsy or not may be very helpful in the therapy of aggression in whatever context.[24,70,79,87]

It should be stressed again, however, that there are no well-designed treatment studies and that all recommendations basically follow expert opinions.

SUMMARY AND CONCLUSIONS

Episodic dyscontrol and its DSM-IV correspondent intermittent explosive disorder represent severe forms of a paroxysmal aggressive attack disorder. In contrast to premeditated antisocial aggression, IED is characterized by high levels of arousal, anxiety, anger, and fear. The behavior is generally poorly structured, but it can be very dangerous.

The question of whether IED is pathogenetically related to epilepsy is unresolved. There is evidence that frontolimbic brain pathology does play an important role in the pathogenesis of IED. IED often is accompanied by other neurologic or psychiatric disorders such as epilepsy, other organic brain disorders, or bipolar or schizophreniform disorder even though these are exclusion criteria following DSM-IV. In these cases, basic treatment should follow the principles for the respective disorders. The epilepsy and bipolar or schizophreniform disorders should be treated first. Often, depressive symptoms in the context of IED are undiagnosed, and in these cases, depression again should be treated.

If IED persists in spite of up-to-date treatment of all comorbid conditions or if none of these are recognizable, the clinician should try to implement a symptomatic treatment of the aggressive behavior itself. Although there are no well-designed treatment studies, there is evidence to support attempts for symptomatic relief using antidepressants and SSRIs in particular, antiepileptics, lithium, antipsychotic agents, and even beta-blockers. In these cases, the decision of which of these different drugs should be used first depends on the specific history, family history, response to earlier medication attempts, comorbid and possibly subsyndromal psychopathologic findings, and experience of the specialist. In any case, the target syndrome is of sufficient importance to support systematic trials of all therapeutic options even if they are off-label as is generally the case. If therapists feel unfamiliar with this approach, they should consider referral to specialists or ask for advice from tertiary referral centers. Our experience that some of these interventions in fact help even though all other substances failed to bring any relief motivates this approach.

References

1. Aggleton JP. The contribution of the amygdala to normal and abnormal emotional states. *Trends Neurosci.* 1993;16:328–333.
2. Albert DJ, Walsh ML, Jonik RH. Aggression in humans: what is its biological foundation? *Neurosci Biobehav Rev.* 1993;17:405–425.
3. Alheid GF, de Olmos JS, Beltramino CA. Amygdala and extended amygdala. In: Paxinos G, ed. *The Rat Nervous System.* San Diego, CA: Academic Press; 1995:495–578.
4. Amaral DG, Price JL, Pitkänen A, et al. Anatomical organisation of the primate amygdaloid complex. In: Aggleton, JP, ed. *The Amygdala: Neurobiological Aspects of Emotion, Memory, and Mental Dysfunction.* New York: Wiley-Liss; 1992:1–66.
5. American Psychiatric Association. *Diagnostic and Statistical Manual of Mental Disorders,* 4th ed. Washington DC: American Psychiatric Association; 1994.

6. Andrulonis PA, Donnelly J, Glueck BC, et al. Preliminary data on ethosuximide and the episodic dyscontrol syndrome. *Am J Psychiatry.* 1980;137:1455–1456.
7. Andy OJ, Jurko MF. Hyperresponsive syndrome. In: Hitchcock E, Laitinen L, Vaernet K, eds. *Psychosurgery.* Springfield, IL: Charles C Thomas; 1972: 117–126.
8. Bach-Y-Rita G, Lion JR, Climent CE, et al. Episodic dyscontrol: a study of 130 violent patients. *Am J Psychiatry.* 1971;127:1473–1478.
9. Barratt ES, Stanford MS, Kent TA, et al. Neuropsychological and cognitive psychophysiological substrates of impulsive aggression. *Biol Psychiatry.* 1997;4:1045–1061.
10. Behbehani MM. Functional characteristics of the midbrain periaquaductal gray. *Prog Neurobiol.* 1995;46:573–605.
11. Berryman J, Evans IM, Kalbag A. The effects of training in nonaversive behavior management on the attitudes and understanding of direct care staff. *J Behav Ther Exp Psychiatry.* 1994;25:241–250.
12. Beshai JA. Behavioral correlates of the EEG in delinquents. *J Psychol.* 1971;79:141–146.
13. Bhatnagar S, Dallman M. Neuroanatomical basis for facilitation of hypothalamic-pituitary-adrenal responses to a novel stressor after chronic stress. *Neuroscience.* 1998;84:1025–1039.
14. Bjork JM, Dougherty DM, Moeller FG. A positive correlation between self-ratings of depression and laboratory-measured aggression. *Psychiatry Res.* 1997;69:33–38.
15. Braconnier A, Jeanneau A. Anxiety, aggression, agitation and depression: psychopathologic aspects. *Encephale.* 1997;23(Spec Iss No 3):43–47.
16. Brandao ML, Cardoso SH, Melo LL, et al. Neural substrate of defensive behavior in the midbrain tectum. *Neurosci Biobehav Rev.* 1994;18:339–346.
17. Brower MC, Price BH. Neuropsychiatry of frontal lobe dysfunction in violent and criminal behaviour: a critical review. *J Neurol Neurosurg Psychiatry.* 2001;71:720–726.
18. Cendes F, Andermann F, Gloor P, et al. Relationship between atrophy of the amygdala and ictal fear in temporal lobe epilepsy. *Brain.* 1994;117:739–746.
19. Chapman WP, Schroeder HR, Geyer G, et al. Physiological evidence concerning importance of amygdala nuclear region in the integration of circulatory functions and emotion in man. *Science.* 1954;120:949–954.
20. Charney DS, Deutch A. A functional neuroanatomy of anxiety and fear: implications for the pathophysiology and treatment of anxiety disorders. *Crit Rev Neurobiol.* 1996;10:419–446.
21. Coccaro EF, Posternak MA, Zimmerman M. Prevalence and features of intermittent explosive disorder in a clinical setting. *J Clin Psychiatry.* 2005;66:1221–1227.
22. Connor DF, Steingard RJ. A clinical approach to the pharmacotherapy of aggression in children and adolescents. *Ann N Y Acad Sci.* 1996;794:290–307.
23. Damasio AR, Tranel D, Damasio H. Individuals with sociopathic behavior caused by frontal damage fail to respond autonomically to social stimuli. *Behav Brain Res.* 1990;41:81–94.
24. Davis GR, Armstrong HE Jr, Donovan DM, et al. Cognitive–behavioral treatment of depressed affect among epileptics: preliminary findings. *J Clin Psychol.* 1984;40:930–935.
25. Davis M, Rainnie D, Cassell M. Neurotransmission in the rat amygdala related to fear and anxiety. *Trends Neurosci.* 1994;17:208–214.
26. de Dios PC, Santo-Domingo CJ, Lozano SM. Pharmacological treatment of the intermittent explosive disorder. Report of three cases and literature review [in Spanish]. *Actas Luso Esp Neurol Psiquiatr Cienc Afines.* 1995;23:74–77.
27. DeLong GR. Mid-gestation right basal ganglia lesion: clinical observations in two children. *Neurology.* 2002;59:54–58.
28. Denicoff KD, Meglathery SB, Post RM, et al. Efficacy of carbamazepine compared with other agents: a clinical practice survey. *J Clin Psychiatry.* 1994;55:70–76.
29. Dicks P, Myers RE, Kling A. Uncus and amygdala lesions: effects on social behavior in the free ranging rhesus monkey. *Science.* 1969;165:69–71.
30. Drake ME Jr, Hietter SA, Pakalnis A. EEG and evoked potentials in episodic-dyscontrol syndrome. *Neuropsychobiology.* 1992;26:125–128.
31. Feder R. Treatment of intermittent explosive disorder with sertraline in 3 patients. *J Clin Psychiatry.* 1999;60:195–196.
32. Fenwick PBC. Aggression and epilepsy. In: Trimble MR, Bolwig T, eds. *Epilepsy and Psychiatry.* Chichester, UK: John Wiley; 1986:31–60.
33. Gallagher M, Chiba AA. The amygdala and emotion. *Curr Opin Neurobiol.* 1996;6:221–227.
34. Gloor P, Olivier A, Quesney LF, et al. The role of the limbic system in experiential phenomena of temporal lobe epilepsy. *Ann Neurol.* 1982;12:129–144.
35. Goldstein M. Brain research and violent behavior: a summary and evaluation of the status of biomedical research on brain and aggressive violent behavior. *Arch Neurol.* 1974;30:1–35.
36. Grizenko N, Vida S. Propranolol treatment of episodic dyscontrol and aggressive behavior in children. *Can J Psychiatry.* 1988;33:776–778.
37. Gunn J. Criminal behaviour and mental disorder. *Br J Psychiatry.* 1977;130:317–329.
38. Hadi F, Franco K, Hermida T, et al. Citalopram for impulsive aggression. *J Am Acad Child Adolesc Psychiatry.* 2003;42:749–750.
39. Halgren E. Emotional neurophysiology of the amygdala within the context of human cognition. In: Aggleton JP, ed. *The Amygdala: Neurobiological Aspects of Emotion, Memory, and Mental Dysfunction.* New York: Wiley-Liss; 1992:191–228.
40. Hirose S. Effective treatment of aggression and impulsivity in antisocial personality disorder with risperidone. *Psychiatry Clin Neurosci.* 2001;55:161–162.
41. Hollander E, Pallanti S, Allen A, et al. Does sustained-release lithium reduce impulsive gambling and affective instability versus placebo in pathological gamblers with bipolar spectrum disorders? *Am J Psychiatry.* 2005;162:137–145.
42. Kalin NH. Primate models to understand human aggression [Review]. *J Clin Psychiatry.* 1999;60(Suppl 15):29–32.
43. Kavoussi R, Armstead P, Coccaro E. The neurobiology of impulsive aggression. *Psychiatr Clin North Am.* 1997;20:395–403.
44. Kligman D, Goldberg DA. Temporal lobe epilepsy and aggression. *J Nerv Ment Dis.* 1975;160:324–341.
45. Kling AS, Brothers LA. The amygdala and social behavior. In: Aggleton JP, ed. *The Amygdala: Neurobiological Aspects of Emotion, Memory, and Mental Dysfunction.* New York: Wiley-Liss; 1992:353–377.
46. Krakowski M, Czobor P. Violence in psychiatric patients: the role of psychosis, frontal lobe impairment, and ward turmoil. *Comprehens Psychiatry.* 1997;38:230–236.
47. LaBar KS, LeDoux JE, Spencer DD, et al. Impaired fear conditioning following unilateral temporal lobectomy in humans. *J Neurosci.* 1995;15:6846–6855.
48. LeDoux JE. Emotions: clues from the brain. *Annu Rev Psychol.* 1995; 46:209–235.
49. Lewin J, Sumners D. Successful treatment of episodic dyscontrol with carbamazepine. *Br J Psychiatry.* 1992;161:261–262.
50. Luo B. Cholecystokinin B receptors in the periaqueductal gray potentiate defensive rage behavior elicited from the medial hypothalamus of the cat. *Brain Res.* 1998;796:27–37.
51. Maletzky BM. The episodic dyscontrol syndrome. *Dis Nerv Syst.* 1973; 34:178–185.
52. McElroy SL. Recognition and treatment of DSM-IV intermittent explosive disorder. *J Clin Psychiatry.* 1999;60(Suppl 15):12–16.
53. Miller BL, Darby A, Benson DF, et al. Aggressive, and socially disruptive and antisocial behaviour associated with fronto-temporal dementia. *Br J Psychiatry.* 1997;170:150–155.
54. Monopolis S, Lion JR. Problems in the diagnosis of intermittent explosive disorder. *Am J Psychiatry.* 1983;140:1200–1202.
55. Moyer KE. *Violence and Aggression—A Physiological Perspective.* New York: Paragon House; 1987.
56. Mungas D. An empirical analysis of specific syndromes of violent behavior. *J Nerv Ment Dis.* 1983;171:354–361.
57. Olvera RL. Intermittent explosive disorder: epidemiology, diagnosis and management. *CNS Drugs.* 2002;16:517–526.
58. Payne SD. Carbamazepine and episodic dyscontrol. *Br J Psychiatry.* 1993;162:425–426.
59. Petty RG, Bonner D, Mouratoglou V, et al. Acute frontal lobe syndrome and dyscontrol associated with bilateral caudate nucleus infarctions. *Br J Psychiatry.* 1996;168:237–240.
60. Raine A, Buchsbaum M, LaCasse L. Brain abnormalities in murderers indicated by positron emission tomography. *Biol Psychiatry.* 1997;42:495–508.
61. Raine A, Stoddard J, Bihrle S, et al. Prefrontal glucose deficits in murderers lacking psychosocial deprivation. *Neuropsychiatry Neuropsychol Behav Neurol.* 1998;11:1–7.
62. Ramamurthi B. Stereotactic operation in behaviour disorders. Amygdalotomy and hypothalamotomy. *Acta Neurochirurg Suppl.* 1988;44:152–157.
63. Reis DJ. Brain norepinephrine: evidence that neuronal release is essential for sham rage behavior following brainstem transection in cat. *Proc Natl Acad Sci USA.* 1969;64:108–112.
64. Reist C, Nakamura K, Sagart E, et al. Impulsive aggressive behavior: open-label treatment with citalopram. *J Clin Psychiatry.* 2003;64:81–85.
65. Roach NE, George MD, Skoch MG. Propranolol for episodic dyscontrol syndrome. *J Kans Med Soc.* 1984;85:240–241, 247.
66. Rolls ET. Neurophysiology and functions of the primate amygdala. In: Aggleton JP, ed. *The Amygdala: Neurobiological Aspects of Emotion, Memory, and Mental Dysfunction.* New York: Wiley-Liss; 1992:143–165.
67. Saver JL, Salloway SP, Devinsky O, et al. Neuropsychiatry of aggression. In: Fogel BS, Schiffer RB, Rao SM, eds. *Neuropsychiatry.* Baltimore: Williams & Wilkins; 1996:523–548.
68. Schulze-Bonage A, Ostertag C, Fröscher W, et al. *Bitemporal depth electrode recordings in an epilepsy patient with postictal psychosis: additional evidence for a genuine postictal psychotic pathophysiology.* Unpublished; 2005.
69. Shaikh MB. Serotonin 5-HT1A and 5-HT2/1C receptors in the midbrain periaqueductal gray differentially modulate defensive rage behavior elicited from the medial hypothalamus of the cat. *Brain Res.* 1997;765:198–207.
70. Stanley B, Bundy E, Beberman R. Skills training as an adjunctive treatment for personality disorders. *J Psychiatr Pract.* 2001;7:324–335.
71. Stein DJ, Hollander E, Cohen L, et al. Neuropsychiatric impairment in impulsive personality disorders. *Psychiatry Res.* 1993;48:257–266.
72. Stein G. Drug treatment of the personality disorders. *Br J Psychiatry.* 1992;161:167–184.
73. Stone JL, McDaniel KD, Hughes JR, et al. Episodic dyscontrol disorder and paroxysmal EEG abnormalities: successful treatment with carbamazepine. *Biol Psychiatry.* 1986;21:208–212.

74. Sugarman P. Carbamazepine and episodic dyscontrol. *Br J Psychiatry.* 1992;161:721.
75. Swartz MS, Swanson JW, Hiday VA, et al. Violence and severe mental illness: the effects of substance abuse and nonadherence to medication. *Am J Psychiatry.* 1998;155:226–231.
76. Tebartz van Elst L. Aggression and epilepsy. In: Trimble M, Schmitz B, eds. *The Neuropsychiatry of Epilepsy.* Cambridge: Cambridge University Press; 2002:81–106.
77. Tebartz van Elst L, Trimble MR, Ebert D, et al. Dual brain pathology in patients with affective aggressive episodes. *Arch Gen Psychiatry.* 2001;58:1187–1188.
78. Tebartz van Elst L, Woermann F, Lemieux L, et al. Affective aggression in patients with temporal lobe epilepsy—a quantitative magnetic resonance study of the amygdala. *Brain.* 2000;123:234–243.
79. Thomas SP. Teaching healthy anger management. *Perspect Psychiatr Care.* 2001;37:41–48.
80. Tonkonogy JM, Geller JL. Hypothalamic lesions and intermittent explosive disorder. *J. Neuropsychiatry Clin Neurosci.* 1992;4:45–50.
81. Treiman DM. *Psychobiology of Ictal Aggression.* New York: Raven Press; 1991:341–356.
82. Trimble MR. *Biological Psychiatry.* Chichester, UK: John Wiley; 1996.
83. Valzelli L. *Psychobiology of Aggression and Violence.* New York: Raven Press; 1981.
84. Van de Poll NE, Van Goozen SHM. Hypothalamic involvement in sexuality and hostility: comparative psychological aspects. *Prog Brain Res.* 1992;93:343–361.
85. Vitiello B, Stoff DM. Subtypes of aggression and their relevance to child psychiatry. *J Am Acad Child Adolesc Psychiatry.* 1997;36:307–315.
86. Walker C, Thomas J, Allen TS. Treating impulsivity, irritability, and aggression of antisocial personality disorder with quetiapine. *Int J Offender Ther Comp Criminol.* 2003;47:556–567.
87. Willner P, Brace N, Phillips J. Assessment of anger coping skills in individuals with intellectual disabilities. *J Intellect Disabil Res.* 2005;49:329–339.
88. Woermann F, Tebartz van Elst L, Koepp MJ, et al. Reduction of frontal neocortical grey matter associated with affective aggression in patients with temporal lobe epilepsy. An objective voxel-by-voxel analysis of automatically segmented MRI. *J Neurol Neurosurg Psychiatry.* 2000;68:162–169.
89. Woermann FG. Voxel-by-voxel comparison of automatically segmented cerebral gray matter—a rater-independent comparison of structural MRI in patients with epilepsy. *NeuroImage.* 1999;10:373–384.
90. Zanchetti A. Reflex and brain stem inhibition of sham rage behaviour. *Prog Brain Res.* 1968;22:195–205.

CHAPTER 284 ■ DISSOCIATIVE DISORDERS

RICHARD J. BROWN AND MICHAEL R. TRIMBLE

INTRODUCTION

Within the context of psychiatry and neurology, the term *dissociation* is extremely difficult to define satisfactorily. Since its introduction in the late nineteenth century, the term has been applied to a wide range of neurologic, psychiatric, and psychological phenomena. As a result, there is considerable confusion over what actually constitutes dissociation, and the concept is frequently misapplied. This is particularly true within the field of epilepsy. Many epileptic phenomena have been labeled as dissociative, including the sensory, affective, and cognitive features of partial seizures, behavioral automatisms, postictal amnesia, and fugue.[27] Similarly, certain psychiatric phenomena that mimic epileptic events, so-called "nonepileptic seizures," have been identified as primarily dissociative in nature. Indeed, many authorities have argued that the dissociative nature of nonepileptic seizures could provide the basis for their conceptual and practical differentiation from "genuine" epileptic events.[44] If, however, dissociation is experienced both by individuals with epilepsy and by those with pseudo-epileptic seizures, how can its occurrence aid in the differential diagnosis of these conditions?

HISTORICAL ASPECTS

The term *dissociation* originates in the work of Pierre Janet, who proposed one of the earliest systematic accounts of the psychological mechanisms underlying hysteria. According to Janet,[36,38] a fundamental weakness in the hysterical individual's mental character makes the person susceptible to a breakdown in the normally integrated functions of consciousness when faced by environmental stress or trauma. As a result, organized sets of knowledge pertaining to the trauma may become "dissociated" from the main body of consciousness and may serve to take control of behavior and experience if activated by environmental events. The automatic activation of these dissociated memories results in a hysterical reaction (or "somnambulism") that, in some instances, takes the form of a nonepileptic attack. Following Charcot's demonstrations at the Salpêtrière in which hysterical symptoms were shown to be both induced and removed by hypnosis, Janet's dissociation theory assumed that this process of dissociation was driven by an autohypnotic state. According to this view, two aspects of the hysterical individual's psychophysiologic makeup are responsible for the processes of dissociation and somnambulism. First, the hysterical individual possesses an abnormally high degree of suggestibility that allows ideas from the external environment to develop within him or her in the absence of his or her effort or awareness. Second, the hysterical individual suffers from an attentional dysfunction or "retraction of the field of consciousness" (Janet,[38] p. 314), which prevents them from entertaining alternative states of mind, thereby accentuating their responsivity to external suggestion. The resulting process of dissociation leads to "dedoublément," or double consciousness, whereby two or more discrete but conscious modes of being existed alongside one other, separated by amnesia. In extreme cases, the autonomy of this dissociative consciousness gave rise to one or more alter personalities.[54]

Although it was originally assumed that these processes were triggered by external traumas, subsequent psychoanalytic theory gravitated from external happenings to an inner efficient causation based on traumatic conflict arising from the patient's psychically unacceptable desires and fantasies. Thus, the etiology was expanded to include subjective traumatization or "vehement emotions" whereby "every memory, every thought, competent to arouse strong and lasting emotions, can play the part of a fixed idea, and may originate hysterical symptoms."[39] In these terms, symptomatology became a composite of fact and fantasy, metaphor and symbolism. This was the case even when there was an association with objective traumatic events because, in classical Freudian theory, before the onset of symptoms, there is a reconstruction in memory overlaid with fantasy (Freud,[23] p. 625). Freud also proposed that falsifications are introduced into memory in order "to interrupt disagreeable and causal connections" (Freud,[24] p. 446, footnotes).

These discoveries led Freud to view hysterical etiology as fantastic, so that, as with dreams, the symptoms became the "the royal road" to the unconscious:

> Hysterical symptoms are nothing other than fantasies brought into view through *"conversion."*... So far as the symptoms are somatic ones, they are often enough taken from the circle of the same sexual sensations and motor innervation as those [that] originally accompanied the fantasy when it was still conscious. (Freud,[21] p. 90; italics added)

This move from fact to fantasy is evident in Freud's revision of his early seduction theory,[35] which suggested that some hysterical patients suffered from unconscious memories of childhood seduction. Later he asserted that such memories were infantile wish fulfillments, although not always: "So often they are not fantasies but real memories.... A fantasy of being seduced when no seduction has occurred is usually employed by a child to screen the autoerotic period of his sexual activity" (Freud,[22] p. 417).

Although popular for nearly a century, recent interest in the prevalence of childhood abuse has led to a backlash against Freudian theory, coincidental with a renewed interest in Janet's work on dissociation,[19] adaptations of his theory in cognitive psychology,[30,31] and a mushrooming of publications linking objective traumatic experiences to dissociative psychopathology. This is particularly relevant for the evaluation of nonepileptic seizures. Indeed, both the *Diagnostic and Statistical Manual for Mental Disorders*, 4th edition (DSM-IV),[2] and the *International Classification of Diseases* (ICD-10)[65] make an explicit link between traumatic events and the onset of dissociative symptoms. Moreover, a number of studies have found disproportionately high rates of physical, sexual, and emotional abuse in patients with dissociative disorders.[16,34,53] Bowman,[7] for example, found that 70% and 77% of her sample of 27 nonepileptic seizure patients had experienced physical or sexual abuse, respectively. Similarly, Betts and Boden[6] obtained positive sexual abuse histories from 54% of 96 patients with nonepileptic seizures.

Thus, 100 years of thought about hysteria has brought the traumagenic theory full circle, and yet the difficulties encountered by nineteenth century investigators remain. Trauma is ill conceived and now tends to be exclusively considered only as an objectively measurable event, ranging from natural disasters to childhood abuse. As a result, there is a lack of consideration given to inner efficient causes, such as an individual's perceptions of events, which would seem important in the process of traumatization. Not only could this explain the obvious lack of psychopathology in some victims of abuse,[66] but it might also account for the presence of psychopathology following relatively harmless events. For example, in LaBarbera and Dozier's study of pseudoseizures,[45] three of the four girls reported no history of sexual abuse but had experienced minor sexual events perceived as traumatic. Equally, in cases in which there have been false allegations of serious trauma,[14] there is often an incidence of minor sexual traumatization. Finally, the determinism of trauma in the development of nonepileptic attacks and psychopathologically related disorders is problematic in terms of the unquestioned and overgeneralized evocation of dissociation as a defense mechanism as well as the lack of explanations for its prolonged use, even years after the event.[63]

CLASSIFICATION OF DISSOCIATIVE DISORDERS

The Dissociative disorders category in the latest edition of the *Diagnostic and Statistical Manual*[2] encompasses dissociative amnesia, dissociative fugue, dissociative identity disorder (formally multiple personality disorder), depersonalization disorder and dissociative disorder not otherwise specified (see Table 1). According to DSM-IV,[2] "the essential feature of the dissociative disorders is a disruption in the usually integrated functions of consciousness, memory, identity, or perception of the environment" (p. 477). A slightly broader definition is offered in the latest edition of the *International Classification of Diseases*,[65] which identifies the loss of control over bodily movements as an additional dissociative phenomenon. As such, the ICD-10 Dissociative (conversion) disorders category encompasses dissociative amnesia, dissociative fugue, dissociative motor disorders, dissociative convulsions, dissociative anesthesia and sensory loss, dissociative stupor, mixed dissociative (conversion) disorders, other dissociative (conversion) disorders, and dissociative (conversion) disorders, unspecified (Table 1). The Somatoform and Dissociative disorders are related in that these phenomena are characterized by symptoms that, on the face of it, resemble those that occur in certain physical conditions but are presumed to be psychological in origin. Dissociative and somatoform phenomena differ in that the symptoms of the former resemble those of neurologic illness, whereas the symptoms of the latter are more akin to those encountered in internal medicine. As Kihlstrom[40] cogently argued, all of the phenomena identified as dissociative disorders within DSM-IV and ICD-10 are linked by the fact that each has a temporary disruption in consciousness or volition as its primary defining feature.

The differences between DSM-IV and ICD-10 in their classification of the Dissociative and Somatoform disorders are readily apparent. First, unlike ICD-10, DSM-IV places nonepileptic attacks in the Somatoform rather than the Dissociative disorders category along with other so-called "conversion" phenomena, such as unexplained motor and sensory symptoms, that are identified as dissociative in ICD-10. This difference is more practical than conceptual, with DSM-IV placing greater emphasis on the importance of excluding physical illness in the differential diagnosis of these phenomena.[2] Second, unlike DSM-IV, ICD-10 does not identify depersonalization as a dissociative phenomenon, due to the lack of any significant loss of control over sensation, memory, or movement in this condition and its limited affect on personal identity. Third, DSM-IV identifies a distinct category for multiple personality disorder, relabeled dissociative identity disorder in the latest edition of this scheme. In contrast, ICD-10 places multiple personality disorder in the other dissociative (conversion) disorders category, reflecting controversy over whether this syndrome is iatrogenic or culturally bound to North America. Inconsistencies aside, both DSM-IV and ICD-10 explicitly state that physical conditions such as epilepsy should be excluded in the differential diagnosis of the Dissociative and Somatoform disorders.

TABLE 1

CLASSIFICATION OF DISSOCIATIVE DISORDERS IN ICD-10 AND DSM-IV

ICD-10 dissociative (conversion) disorders	DSM-IV dissociative disorders
Dissociative amnesia	Dissociative amnesia
Dissociative fugue	Dissociative fugue
Dissociative motor disorders	Dissociative identity disorder
Dissociative convulsions	Depersonalization disorder
Dissociative anaesthesia and sensory loss	Dissociative disorder not otherwise specified
Dissociative stupor	
Trance and possession disorders	
Mixed dissociative (conversion) disorders	
Other dissociative (conversion) disorders	
Dissociative (conversion) disorder, unspecified	

ICD-10, *International Classification of Diseases* (ICD-10)[65]; DSM-IV, *Diagnostic and Statistical Manual for Mental Disorders*, 4th edition.[2]

CONTEMPORARY VIEWS OF DISSOCIATION

To some extent, the differences between DSM-IV and ICD-10 demonstrate ongoing controversy about the definition of the term "dissociation." When the term was originally introduced in the nineteenth century, it was used to refer to a specific mental mechanism thought to be associated with a relatively limited set of psychological symptoms. Over the years, however, the number of phenomena thought to be attributable to dissociation has expanded considerably, and the dissociation label is now applied to an extraordinary range of psychological symptoms, states, and processes. Cardeña[15] described a useful taxonomy that captures the different ways in which the concept of dissociation has been used. According to this scheme, there are three major facets of the dissociation construct: (a) dissociation as nonconscious or nonintegrated mental modules or systems;

(b) dissociation as an alteration in consciousness; and (c) dissociation as a defense mechanism.

Dissociation as Nonintegrated Mental Modules or Systems ("Compartmentalization")

Dissociation in this sense reflects the original meaning of the concept introduced by Janet[36,38] as the basic psychopathologic mechanism underlying hysterical symptoms. This concept encompasses the medically unexplained symptoms characteristic of the DSM-IV conversion disorders, as well as dissociative amnesia, dissociative fugue, and dissociative identity disorder.[33] Holmes et al.[33] used the term *compartmentalization* to refer to the putative process involved in the generation of these conditions.

These phenomena should be distinguished from other pathologic phenomena characterized by a lack of integration between mental modules or systems that are caused by neurologic rather than psychiatric events. Blindsight, a rare condition in which the sufferer displays above-chance visual discrimination despite reporting a lack of visual experience, provides one example of how normally integrated functions can become dissociated through neurologic damage. Many of the unusual behaviors often displayed by patients following commissurotomy also fall within this category, as do those exhibited by individuals suffering from hemi-neglect. In each of these cases, the dissociation is between the individual's ongoing behavior and his or her introspective verbal report.

Neurologic dissociations such as blindsight are superficially analogous to those observed in psychiatric instances of dissociation, such as the preservation of implicit perception[a] in the context of dissociative blindness (see, e.g., Kihlstrom[40]). Neurologic and psychiatric dissociation differ, however, in that the former is often permanent, reflecting irreversible damage to the underlying neurologic subsystems in question.[40] Psychiatric instances of dissociation, in contrast, are thought to be the product of an alteration in the parameters governing otherwise intact psychological functions; they are, therefore, reversible by definition. Similarly, neurologic and psychiatric dissociations differ in that, unlike the former, the latter involves symptoms (e.g., "glove" anesthesia) that need not, and typically do not, relate to the actual organization of the nervous system and its many distributed components. On these grounds, it is apparent the "dissociation" in these cases is an entirely different phenomenon, and the two must not be confused.

The idea that normally integrated psychological processes can become temporarily dissociated and exist in isolation of one another has also been cited as the basis for other, less pathologic, phenomena.[15,32,64] Many apparently "hypnotic" phenomena fall within this category, including profound amnesia, the loss of perceptual experience, and complex behaviors characterized by a sense of involuntariness, all of which can be temporarily produced by appropriate suggestions in certain individuals. The extent to which similar processes are involved in these phenomena and those displayed by individuals with dissociative psychopathology has been a matter of debate since the time of Janet. Conceptually, there are good grounds to assume a common mechanism in hypnotic and dissociative phenomena[11,12] and recent functional imaging evidence provides some support for a link between the two.[29]

According to Cardeña,[15] this particular definition of dissociation has also been inappropriately applied to a number of other normal psychological phenomena. Following Hilgard,[32] the execution of complex behaviors with only minimal conscious awareness, such as the action of driving a car while holding a conversation, has often been identified as a dissociative phenomenon. As Cardeña pointed out, however, the dissociation label should not simply be applied to any behavior or psychological process that, for whatever reason, occurs without full awareness. Such a practice ignores the fact that, in many such cases, the individual can bring the apparently "dissociated" process into awareness by an act of selective attention. Other such cases involve "dissociation" between systems or processes that one would not normally expect to operate in an integrated fashion. According to Cardeña, mental modules or systems should only be regarded as truly dissociated from one another if their dissociation is (a) in contrast to a normal state of integration and (b) cannot be overcome by an act of will.

[a]Implicit perception is evidenced when an external stimulus produces psychological effects despite not being perceived consciously.[40] The phenomenon of blindsight provides one such example. Implicit perception is akin to the concept of implicit memory, in which behavior is influenced by learned information that the individual cannot consciously recall.

Dissociation as an Alteration in Consciousness ("Detachment")

A second use of the dissociation concept refers to an altered state of consciousness characterized specifically by a disengagement from the self or the environment.[15,33] Holmes et al.[33] used the term *detachment* to refer to this category of conditions. As Cardeña pointed out, this sense of the dissociation concept should not be applied to everyday phenomena, such as daydreaming and other states of distraction, in which engagement with the environment is less than complete. Instead, it should be reserved specifically for states that are regarded by the experiencing individual as qualitatively different from their normal state of awareness. Although a number of different phenomena fall within the bounds of this definition (e.g., "trance" and "possession" states), probably the most commonly reported are depersonalization and derealization. In depersonalization, the individual experiences a profound feeling of detachment from his or her thoughts, perceptions, actions, and emotions, often characterized by a sense of numbness or disembodiment. In derealization, the individual experiences an intact sense of self coupled with a feeling of detachment from the external environment, which often feels unreal or at a distance. Such feelings are extremely common, and frequently occur in the context of psychiatric illnesses such as depression and anxiety; they also occur as a circumscribed problem in their own right, such as in depersonalization disorder.

Although DSM-IV identifies depersonalization disorder as a dissociative phenomenon, this condition clearly relates to a different sense of dissociation than that which applies to the other members of this category; this difference further justifies the separation of depersonalization disorder from the Dissociative disorders category in ICD-10. Depersonalization and derealization are also found in certain drug states (e.g., those produced by marijuana, LSD, and ketamine) and neurologic conditions such as temporal lobe epilepsy and can occur spontaneously in the context of stress or fatigue.

Dissociation as a Defense Mechanism

Finally, dissociation has been described as a defense mechanism that protects the individual from potentially overwhelming pain or anxiety. In many respects, this account of dissociation is indistinguishable from the Freudian concept of repression.[20]

This sense of the dissociation concept is typically used to describe the psychological *function* served by the creation of a detached state or the compartmentalization of mental modules or systems.[15] In this view, exposure to a traumatic situation may trigger the compartmentalization of memories, which preserves psychological integrity by preventing the distressing material from entering consciousness after the event. Alternatively, such traumatic exposure may spontaneously elicit a depersonalized state that prevents extreme emotion from inhibiting an appropriate behavioral response. As such, this definition of dissociative may relate to either of the definitions described previously. In both cases, dissociation of this sort could be either an acute response to an isolated traumatic event or a trait-like characteristic acquired as a result of repeated exposure to trauma.

EPILEPSY AND DISSOCIATION

Although the differential diagnosis of ICD-10 and DSM-IV Dissociative disorders explicitly requires the exclusion of symptoms with an identifiable neurologic basis, many of the phenomena associated with epilepsy, particularly temporal lobe epilepsy, have been regarded as dissociative in nature (Table 2).[18,27] Indeed, ICD-10 includes a specific category for Dissociative disorders due to a general medical condition, which encompasses many of the symptoms exhibited by those with epilepsy. The absence of such a category from DSM-IV, however, reflects doubt concerning the value of attaching the dissociative label to these phenomena. In our view, such doubt is well justified in many cases.

The notion that many epileptic phenomena can be regarded as dissociative is based, to a considerable extent, on the frequent occurrence of amnesia in epilepsy (see, e.g., Good[27]). Complex partial and generalized seizures typically provoke profound amnesia for events occurring during the ictus. Moreover, certain individuals experience a postictal fugue state characterized by apparently purposeful behavior for which they are subsequently amnesic, much like dissociative fugue. Despite their prima facie resemblance to dissociative phenomena, however, these events should *not* be regarded as episodes of dissociation.[27] Dissociative amnesia is characterized by an inability to retrieve information that has been learned and is present in memory despite its inaccessibility.[2] Amnesia for ictal events, in contrast, reflects a disruption in normal information processing, resulting from uncontrolled neural activity, that prevents the encoding of new material during the ictus. The ictal amnesia is not a product of a retrieval failure, therefore, but simply the absence of memories to retrieve. It is for this reason that this form of amnesia is irreversible, unlike most cases of dissociative amnesia.[2]

TABLE 2

DISSOCIATIVE DISORDERS AND DISSOCIATIVE EVENTS[a]

Neurologic	Psychologic
Temporal lobe epilepsy	Dissociative identity disorder
Transient global amnesia	Dissociative amnesia
Epileptic fugues	Dissociative fugues
Body image disorders	Dissociative (conversion) disorders
Somnambulisms	Depersonalization
Drug-dependent learning	Derealization
Sleep amnesia	Déjà-vu
	Hypnosis
	Out-of-body experiences

[a]Showing the main neurologic and psychological states associated with dissociation, with decreasing levels of pathology in descending order. *Source*: Adapted from Cardeña. The domain of dissociation. In: Lynn SJ, Rhue JW, eds. *Dissociation. Clinical and Theoretical Perspectives.* New York: Guilford Press; 1994:15–31, with permission.

Postictal fugue should not be regarded as a dissociative episode for similar reasons. Unlike dissociative fugue, postictal fugue is characterized by a disruption in consciousness associated with significant confusion and an abnormal electroencephalogram (EEG).[62] The apparently purposeful behavior displayed in postictal fugue is not dissociated from ongoing cognitive activity as it is in dissociative fugue; rather, it occurs in the relative *absence* of such activity. The inability to reverse the amnesia associated with postictal fugue serves as an illustration of this fact. The behavioral automatisms often observed in the context of complex partial seizures and regarded as a dissociative phenomenon by some (e.g., Good[27]) are amenable to a similar interpretation. As with the behaviors exhibited during postictal fugue, ictal automatisms only occur in the context of a disruption in consciousness and disturbed behavioral control; genuinely dissociated behaviors are noteworthy because they occur despite an otherwise intact ability to control action.[b] In both cases, it is likely that these behaviors result from the uncontrolled activation of circumscribed motor programs by epileptic discharges in neural sites associated with behavioral control. The fact that such automatisms are particularly characteristic of seizures originating in the frontal lobes lends support to this view.

Many of the phenomena associated with partial seizures originating in the temporal lobes, such as hallucinations, sensory and cognitive auras, déjà-vu, and déjà-veçu, should also be distinguished from true episodes of dissociation. Although hallucinations and auras have a phenomenology that departs from external reality, these phenomena involve the paradoxical *integration* of information within conscious awareness. As such, they may be more appropriately regarded as phenomena of *association* rather than dissociation.[40] The phenomenology of epileptic hallucinations and auras probably originates in the activation of representational structures in the temporal lobes, either directly, by seizure activity in representational networks, or indirectly, through seizure-related stimulation of limbic structures such as the amygdala and anterior cingulate.[3] Experiences of epileptic déjà-vu and déjà-veçu are also more associative than dissociative and may involve a similar neurophysiologic process. For example, stimulation of the amygdala by seizure-related discharges could imbue current perceptions and cognitions with an unwarranted emotional coloring that may be experienced as a sense of having encountered the situation before (see, e.g., Bancaud et al.[3] and Sierra and Berrios[58]).

Certain phenomena associated with temporal lobe epilepsy, however, can be regarded as examples of dissociation according to the scheme described by Cardeña.[15] Depersonalization and derealization commonly occur in the context of temporal lobe epilepsy and involve an alteration in consciousness characterized by dissociation from the self and/or the environment. According to Sierra and Berrios,[58] depersonalization and derealization are the products of a vestigial defense mechanism evolved to provide the optimum processing conditions for adaptive behavior in the face of threat. By this view, extreme anxiety triggers an inhibitory response from the left prefrontal cortex that dampens output from the sympathetic nervous system via the inhibition of the amygdala and anterior cingulate.

[b]"Dissociated" behaviors should be distinguished from normal automatic behaviors because the latter are generally in accord with system goals and can therefore be considered voluntary (Brown and Oakley[12]; see also Cardeña[15]).

In turn, the right prefrontal cortex is activated by ascending arousal systems controlled by uninhibited amygdala circuits, generating further inhibition of the cingulate. As a result, the individual experiences a sense of vigilant alertness devoid of any emotional or cognitive content, a state that is ideally adapted for the control of action in the face of extreme and potentially debilitating danger. If this response is triggered in the absence of threat, however, the resulting sense of depersonalization and derealization can be highly unpleasant and incapacitating. Given the validity of this account, depersonalization and derealization in the context of temporal lobe epilepsy may be the result of seizure activity in the amygdala that prevents the emotional tagging of perceptual and cognitive information prior to its entry into conscious awareness.[c] Alternatively, it may reflect an indirect defensive response in the face of anxiety elicited by seizure-based stimulation of the amygdala. Intuitively, one suspects that the former is the more plausible possibility, although the latter cannot be ruled out a priori. Following this account of depersonalization and derealization, these phenomena can be regarded as dissociative in sense (b) of the term; whether they should, in the context of epilepsy, be regarded as the result of a dissociative defense mechanism remains an empirical issue.[3]

The fact that few epileptic phenomena can be regarded as dissociative in any strict sense reflects widespread confusion over what actually constitutes dissociation. Although widely endorsed, the idea that any breakdown in memory, consciousness, identity, perception, or behavioral control is dissociative overextends the term and diminishes its descriptive validity.[15] Amnesia cannot be considered dissociative unless it involves an inability to retrieve intact information that should, under normal circumstances, be available for recall.[40] Amnesia resulting from a failure to encode information, including that which occurs in the context of epilepsy, does not fall within this category. Loss of behavioral control can only be considered dissociative if it is within the context of an otherwise intact ability to control action. Seizure-related motor phenomena, including complex automatisms, are not dissociative because they occur only in the context of reduced behavioral control in general. Current psychiatric taxonomies do not make these distinctions clearly enough, and rely instead on a purely descriptive approach that precludes precise classification based on the mechanisms underlying different phenomena.

NONEPILEPTIC SEIZURES AND DISSOCIATION

The concept of dissociation is particularly important in relation to nonepileptic attacks because it sheds light on both the mechanisms and, potentially, the differential diagnosis of these phenomena.

In all cases, nonepileptic attacks involve a temporary loss of behavioral, sensory, or cognitive control that occurs in the context of intact neuropsychological functioning, as evidenced by a normal EEG during the nonepileptic ictus. The absence of paroxysmal brain discharges serves as the principal feature that distinguishes nonepileptic from "genuine" epileptic events. By itself, however, the EEG cannot provide a completely reliable basis for the identification of epileptic and nonepileptic seizures,[13] which underlines the potential value of dissociation as a criterion for an inclusive diagnosis of nonepileptic attack disorder.

Several converging lines of evidence indicate that these events involve a dissociative psychological mechanism, namely compartmentalization.[44] In the first instance, nonepileptic seizures are commonly found in the context of other forms of dissociative psychopathology. Bowman[7] and Bowman and Markand[8] found that the vast majority of those with nonepileptic attacks meet criteria for DSM-IV dissociative disorders such as dissociative amnesia and identity disturbance. Posttraumatic stress disorder, commonly assumed to involve a dissociative mechanism, was also particularly common in this group of patients.[7,8] Other studies have found that nonepileptic seizures frequently occur alongside other unexplained physical symptoms (e.g., Krishnamoorthy et al.[41] and Maldonada and Spiegel[47]), suggesting that they may be one aspect of a broader tendency to express psychological distress somatically, so-called "somatization."[46] A number of authorities have suggested that compartmentalization is an important aspect of this phenomenon also (e.g., Brown[11]). Eating disorder symptoms, which have been linked to a dissociative process (e.g., Pettinati et al.[51]), also appear to be particularly common in patients with nonepileptic seizures.[41]

The frequent cooccurrence of dissociative psychopathology in patients with nonepileptic attacks appears to indicate a general propensity for dissociative experiences in this population. Consistent with this notion is a study by Kuyk et al.[43] showing that individuals with nonepileptic attacks display elevated levels of hypnotic susceptibility. In a related vein, in many cases, nonepileptic attacks can be provoked using suggestion, placebo. or hypnosis (e.g., Dericioglu et al.[17]). High hypnotic susceptibility is commonly found in patients with dissociative psychopathology,[25,57,60] and a dissociative interpretation of hypnosis has been offered by a number of authorities (e.g., Hilgard[32] and Woody and Bowers[64]). Bowman[7] also found that individuals with nonepileptic seizures had elevated scores on the Dissociative Experiences Scale (DES),[5] a self-report measure assessing everyday occurrences of dissociation compared to nonclinical controls. However, in a more recent study, Alper et al.[1] found that DES scores are also elevated in patients with complex partial seizures (see also Devinsky et al.[18]); indeed, there was no significant difference in overall DES scores between these patients and a group with nonepileptic seizures. Nevertheless, both epileptic and nonepileptic groups scored higher on the DES than typically observed in nonclinical populations. This finding demonstrates the danger of conflating the various definitions of dissociation within a single measure such as the DES. Because the DES treats dissociation as a unitary concept, it cannot differentiate between conditions that are characterized by different forms of dissociative phenomena, such as epilepsy and nonepileptic attack disorder.

Evidence implicating high dissociative comorbidity, hypnotic susceptibility, and exposure to trauma in individuals with nonepileptic seizures provides only indirect evidence for a dissociative interpretation of this phenomenon. Although such evidence suggests that a tendency to dissociate may be a common feature of these individuals, it does not constitute conclusive proof that nonepileptic attacks are themselves dissociative. A recent study by Kuyk et al.[43] places such an interpretation on a firmer footing. Like epileptic seizures, nonepileptic attacks are often associated with a dense amnesia for events occurring during the ictus. We have already stated that epileptic amnesia should not be considered a dissociative phenomenon, because it arises from a seizure-related disruption in memory encoding rather than an inability to retrieve intact memory traces. However, Kuyk et al.[43] showed that the amnesia associated with nonepileptic attacks may actually be the product of such a retrieval deficit. They compared a group of individuals with amnesia for events occurring during well-documented nonepileptic attacks with a group displaying amnesia following complex partial and generalized epileptic seizures. All individuals were hypnotized and given suggestions designed to facilitate the recovery of ictal events; the experimenter remained blind to

[c]Such a process could also be responsible for the paradoxical sense of unfamiliarity that characterizes *jamais-vu*, a phenomenon commonly observed in epilepsy.

group status at all times. Using a free-recall paradigm, 17 of 20 patients with nonepileptic seizures recovered significant information concerning the designated attack; this information was verified by video recordings or third-party reports. In contrast, not one of the 17 patients with epilepsy retrieved information concerning their attack during hypnosis. Such a finding appears to demonstrate that, unlike that found in epilepsy, nonepileptic amnesia results from a process that prevents the individual from accessing memories successfully encoded during the attack. This apparent separation of intact memorial information from conscious awareness following a nonepileptic attack, coupled with the phenomenologic character of these events, clearly identifies these phenomena as examples of dissociative compartmentalization.

DIFFERENTIAL DIAGNOSIS OF EPILEPSY AND DISSOCIATIVE PHENOMENA

The differential diagnosis of epilepsy and nonepileptic attack disorder is considered elsewhere in this book. In this section, we describe the nature and differential diagnosis of other conditions that are often confused with epilepsy.

Dissociative Amnesia

Dissociative amnesia is one variant of psychogenic amnesia; a list of the differential diagnoses for these conditions is given in Table 3. Dissociative amnesia is often overlooked and mistaken for a diagnosis of complex partial seizures. Thus, it is important to reemphasize that loss of awareness and amnesia should not automatically lead to a diagnosis of epilepsy.

Fugues

Fugues are characterized by the patient "coming to" in a strange place and professing no knowledge of how he or she arrived there. Again, there is a profound amnesia, sometimes extending backward in the patient's life for many years. Patients may adopt a different identity, which may be of brief duration, but in some cases may be retained in a remarkable way for a number of years.[52]

Such fugues are often a clinical manifestation of depression, but they often seem to come on after a trauma, and head injury is frequently reported. Some points of differential diagnosis between psychogenic fugue and postictal fugue are given in Table 4. Psychogenic fugues also need to be distinguished from transient global amnesia, poiromania, somnambulism, and postconcussional amnesia.

TABLE 3

PSYCHOGENIC AMNESIAS IN APPROXIMATE ORDER OF CHRONICITY

Situational amnesia
Posttraumatic stress syndrome[a,b]
Ganser syndrome[c]
Psychogenic fugue[b]
Hysterical dementia
Depressive dementia
Multiple personality disorder[b,c]
Histrionic personality disorder[a]

[a] Amnesia is not always a feature.
[b] Those disorders are most likely to be confused with epilepsy.
[c] Nosologic validity of these syndromes is in doubt.

TABLE 4

CLINICAL ASSESSMENT OF FUGUE STATES

Psychogenic fugues	Postictal fugues
Identifiable emotional precipitant	Unlikely to be first presentation of epilepsy
Wandering is socially appropriate	Associated with obvious confusion
Gradual recovery of orientation	Rapid recovery
Electroencephalogram is usually normal	Abnormal electroencephalogram

Somnambulism

Somnambulism implies sleepwalking, and this is much more common in childhood. In adults, it has distinct psychopathologic significance. It is one of the parasomnias, usually arising in non–rapid eye movement (REM) sleep. There may be only brief wandering or lengthier episodes, with the completion of quite complex but purposeless tasks, for which there is profound amnesia. During the attack, the eyes are open; the patient seems confused and expresses surprise if awakened. Its onset in adulthood is usually associated with emotional trauma.

A family history of sleepwalking or night terrors is reported in 80% of somnambulists, and many children have isolated and clinically nonsignificant sleepwalking episodes. It is often considered one of the neurotic traits of childhood, alongside nailbiting, phobias, enuresis, food faddisms, tics, and mannerisms. In themselves they have little import, but they may cluster and suggest a tendency to later neurotic breakdown. Certainly the onset of somnambulism in adult life suggests some underlying psychopathology, often depressive, and, in association with seizures, suggests that the latter will be nonepileptic.

Sometimes the somnambulism can be distinguished from epilepsy only with polysomnography and telemetry, and third-party accounts of the attacks may be misleading.

Dissociative Identity Disorder (Formerly Multiple Personality Disorder)

Dissociative identity disorder is characterized by the presence of two or more identities or personality states. Each state is often, although not always, amnesic for the other. Patients typically complain of an inability to remember the full sequence of their personal history. The sudden switch from one state to another may give rise to a suspicion of epilepsy, and nonspecific EEG changes may add further confusion. Many reported cases give histories of earlier physical and mental deprivation, abuse, and head injuries. The fact that multiple personalities are described in association with epilepsy,[4] especially temporal lobe epilepsy,[56] adds confusion because the nosologic status of this condition is held in doubt by some authors.[49]

TABLE 5

CRITERIA FOR POSTTRAUMATIC STRESS DISORDER[a]

Exposure to a traumatic event
Experienced, witnessed, or confronted with event(s) involving actual or threatened death, serious injury, or threat to integrity of self or others
Response of intense fear, helplessness, or horror
Persistent reexperiencing of the trauma
Recurrent and intrusive distressing recollections
Recurrent and distressing dreams of the event
Acting or feeling as if the traumatic event were recurring
Intense psychological distress at exposure to internal or external cues
Physiologic reactivity on exposure to internal or external cues
Persistent avoidance of stimuli associated with the trauma and numbing of general responsiveness
Efforts to avoid associated thoughts, feelings, or conversations
Efforts to avoid associated activities, places, or people
Inability to recall an important aspect of the trauma
Markedly diminished interest in significant activities
Feeling of detachment from others
Restricted range of affect
Sense of a foreshortened future
Persistent symptoms of increased arousal
Difficulty falling or staying asleep
Irritability or outbursts of anger
Difficulty concentrating
Hypervigilance
Exaggerated startle response
Duration of the disturbance >1 mo
The disturbance causes clinically significant distress or impairment in social, occupational, or other important areas of functioning

[a] 309.81 in *Diagnostic and Statistical Manual for Mental Disorders*, 4th edition.[2]

Posttraumatic Stress Disorder

Posttraumatic stress disorder (PTSD) has assumed considerable importance in recent years, yet it is an easily missed diagnosis. The current criteria, as laid down by DSM-IV,[2] are given in Table 5. Obviously, the precipitating trauma is the significant criterion for entry, but in many cases the trauma may have occurred in the past and perhaps been reactivated by recent events. The similarity between PTSD and nonepileptic seizure disorder patients has been commented on by some authors (see Chapters 207 and 282), and the hyperexplexia of PTSD may be mistaken for myoclonic seizures. In such cases, the patient's seizures are seen as the central and often only complaint, and the accident that may have preceded them provided a head injury as an etiology for the attacks. However, typically, the posttraumatic amnesia will be brief, and the accident terrifying. Careful history taking will unravel the pervasive underlying symptoms of a PTSD, although in some patients there may be extreme reluctance to discuss the accident. Psychogenic amnesia is a cardinal clinical symptom of this condition.

Déjà-vu

Déjà-vu and its associated states such as jamais-vu and déjà-veçu are experienced by many people and do not necessarily signify psychopathology. The most common medical association with déjà-vu is an anxiety disorder, in which setting the experience fails to have the vivid and clearly repetitive nature that the aura of a temporal lobe focus brings.

Posttraumatic Amnesia

Posttraumatic amnesia is distinguished by the clear relationship to a head injury, although in some cases this is clinically obscure. For example, a patient may deny any such injury, or, more commonly, a seemingly trivial injury may provoke a profound loss of memory that seems enduring. Such cases are unlikely to be taken for a seizure disorder, but if they are associated with some apparent confusion, a partial status needs to be excluded. A prolonged retrograde amnesia, especially with loss of personal identity, in the presence of normal learning abilities or minimal posttraumatic amnesia is usually indicative of a psychogenic amnesia.

MEASUREMENT OF DISSOCIATION

Several scales to measure symptoms of dissociation have been developed, but few have been evaluated in neurologic populations, such as those with epilepsy. Moreover, the descriptive nature of the scales means that they are unable to separate out the mechanisms responsible for the dissociative symptoms in question. As such, they cannot be used to aid in the differential diagnosis of epilepsy, although they can be useful for determining the extent and nature of dissociative symptoms in research settings.

The Dissociative Experiences Scale (DES) is a brief self-report questionnaire designed to elicit information regarding lifetime experiences of "dissociation" in normal and clinical populations.[5] Although the DES is the most widely used measure of dissociation, the use of total scores on the scale is problematic because they conflate different types of dissociation (e.g., detachment and compartmentalization) within the same measure. It is more appropriate to identify and use separate subscales pertaining to the types of dissociation under scrutiny. Most factor-analytic research suggests that the scale comprises three subscales measuring amnesia, depersonalization–derealization, and absorption.[3] Alternatively, scales specifically developed to assess different types of dissociation, such as the Cambridge Depersonalization Scale,[59] the Multidimensional Dissociation Inventory,[10] or the Somatoform Dissociation Questionnaire,[50] can be used.

The Structured Clinical Interview for DSM-IV Dissociative Disorders (SCID-D) is more specific for diagnosis of DSM-IV dissociative conditions than the DES, having separate subscales for symptoms of dissociative amnesia, depersonalization, derealization, identity confusion, and identity alteration.[61]

TREATMENT

Pharmacotherapy

When there is an indication for pharmacotherapy, for example, antidepressants with an affective disorder, these should be prescribed. In addition, antidepressants are helpful in countering the symptoms of other disorders such as the intrusive events of posttraumatic stress.[47]

In nonepileptic seizures, anticonvulsants are unnecessary and should be withdrawn. Although some physicians maintain patients on anticonvulsants such as carbamazepine for their mood-enhancing properties, there is evidence that the prescription of anticonvulsants for pseudoseizures without epilepsy may aggravate such attacks.[28] In many cases, slow withdrawal of anticonvulsants, with reassurance that patients do not have epilepsy, in a supportive clinical environment will lead to a resolution of attacks without further intervention.

For many patients with dissociative disorders, the nonmedical therapeutic interventions described in what follows are the most appropriate.

Hypnotherapy

Both Janet and Freud used hypnosis to access the isolated memories in patients and make "associative corrections." In other words, they attempted to reproduce the supposed hysterical action of autohypnosis under controlled conditions and "disinfect" the dissociated traumatic memories, either by direct countersuggestion or, more indirectly, catharsis. Freud soon abandoned this practice, however, because of its lack of success. He found that patients were either unable to be hypnotized, in spite of the apparent autohypnotizability of such patients, or, more important, they were cured but later produced another set of symptoms (symptom substitution).

Today hypnosis is still used in two ways. It is sometimes used to induce an attack, in other words, to help with the diagnosis. This has variable success and in part relates to the effectiveness of the person doing the hypnosis as a hypnotist. It is not widely used and not recommended to the inexperienced. Furthermore, as with other induction methods, outcome should be viewed with caution because epileptic seizures can also be triggered in this way.[42]

Hypnosis is also used to elicit the traumagenic events of dissociative disorders isolated in memory as part of treatment. It is a controversial option, however, not least because "lost truths" and discovered fantasies are difficult to differentiate, especially in an altered state of consciousness. Evidence gathered by both the British False Memory Syndrome Association and its American equivalent suggests that hypnotherapy and "recovered memory therapy" are major instigators of false allegations.[14]

Psychotherapy

Colloquially known as "the talking cure," psychotherapy encompasses a vast array of theoretical orientations and practices, ranging from individuals to groups. Psychodynamic psychotherapy views dissociative symptoms as signals of individual and/or family distress. As such, they are not the focus of psychotherapeutic treatment but are indirectly alleviated by allowing patients to explore the factors that have contributed to their disorders, including past history and interpersonal difficulties. Cognitive behavior therapy (CBT) aims to identify and alter maladaptive thoughts and behaviors that are contributing to the maintenance of symptoms.[26]

The choice of treatment for the patient depends on a number of factors, including an identifiable cause such as past trauma, age, family dynamics, intellectual impairment, compliance, patient preference, and psychological mindedness. In addition, this is not such an easy option as it at first sounds. Patients with nonepileptic attacks are often difficult to manage, and the combination of apparent neurology with psychopathology is confusing for the inexperienced. It is recommended that patients be referred to therapists with special knowledge, experience, and interest in conversion and dissociative disorders.

There is only very limited evidence demonstrating the efficacy of psychotherapeutic intervention in patients with dissociative disorders, and substantial randomized, controlled trials are urgently needed.

SUMMARY AND CONCLUSIONS

Dissociation is a complex and multifaceted concept that is frequently misapplied within the field of epilepsy. In this chapter, we have explored the various components of the dissociation concept and how they relate to the phenomena of epilepsy and nonepileptic seizures. We have demonstrated why many epileptic phenomena often thought to be instances of dissociation, such as amnesia, postictal fugue, behavioral automatisms, aura and hallucinations, should not be regarded as dissociative at all. We have also argued, however, that depersonalization and derealization occurring in the context of epilepsy can be regarded as dissociative, in the sense that they involve an altered state of consciousness characterized by disengagement from the self or environment. We have also presented evidence indicating that nonepileptic attacks should be considered dissociative phenomena, in this case involving a temporary disruption in behavioral control and subjective awareness despite intact neuropsychological functioning. Although certain aspects of epilepsy are dissociative, therefore, they do not involve the same type of dissociation as that underlying nonepileptic attacks.

If the dissociation concept is to prove useful in this area, much greater precision, both conceptual and methodologic, is required. Researchers and clinicians should be explicit about which definition of dissociation they are referring to, and efforts should be made to use measures of dissociation that, unlike total scores on the DES, are "phenomenon pure." Assessing the reversibility of nonepileptic amnesia, which may prove to be invaluable as an aid to differential diagnosis in this area, provides one illustration of the potential utility of such an endeavor.

References

1. Alper K, Devinsky O, Perrine K, et al. Dissociation in epilepsy and conversion nonepileptic seizures. *Epilepsia*. 1997;38:991–997.
2. American Psychiatric Association. *Diagnostic and Statistical Manual for Mental Disorders,* 4th ed. Washington, DC: American Psychiatric Association; 1994.
3. Bancaud J, Brunet-Bourgin F, Chavel P, et al. Anatomical origin of déjà-vu and vivid memories in human temporal lobe epilepsy. *Brain*. 1994;127:71–90.
4. Benson DF, Miller BL, Signer SF. Dual personality associated with epilepsy. *Arch Neurol*. 1986;43:471–474.
5. Bernstein EM, Putnam FW. Development reliability and validity of a dissociation scale. *J Nerv Ment Dis*. 1986;174(12):727–735.
6. Betts T, Boden S. Diagnosis, management and prognosis of 128 patients with nonepileptic attack disorder. Part I. *Seizure*. 1992;1:19–26.
7. Bowman ES. Etiology and clinical course of pseudoseizures: relationship to trauma, depression and dissociation. *Psychosomatics*. 1993;4:333–342.
8. Bowman ES, Markand ON. Psychodynamics and psychiatric diagnoses of pseudoseizure patients. *Am J Psychiatry*. 1996;153:57–63.
9. Bowman ES, Markand ON. Psychodynamics and psychiatric diagnoses of pseudoseizure patients. *Am J Psychiatry*. 1996;153:57–63.
10. Brier J. *Multiscale Dissociation Inventory*. Odessa, FL: Psychological Assessment Resources; 2002.
11. Brown RJ. Psychological mechanisms of medically unexplained symptoms: an integrative conceptual model. *Psychol Bull*. 2004;130:793–812.
12. Brown RJ, Oakley DA. An integrative cognitive theory of hypnosis and high hypnotizability. In: Heap M, Brown RJ, Oakley DA, eds. *The Highly Hypnotizable Person: Theoretical, Experimental and Clinical Issues*. London: Brunner-Routledge; 2004:152–186.
13. Brown RJ, Trimble MR. Dissociative psychopathology, non-epileptic seizures and neurology. *J Neurol Neurosurg Psychiatry*. 2000;69:285–291.
14. Byrne P, Sheppard N. Allegations of child sexual abuse: delayed reporting and false memory. *Ir J Psychol Med*. 1995;12(3):103–106.
15. Cardeña E. The domain of dissociation. In: Lynn SJ, Rhue JW, eds. *Dissociation. Clinical and Theoretical Perspectives*. New York: Guilford Press; 1994:15–31.

16. Chu JA, Dill DL. Dissociative symptoms in relation to childhood physical and sexual abuse. *Am J Psychiatry*. 1990;147:887–892.
17. Dericioglu N, Saygi S, Ciger A. The value of provocation methods in patients suspected of having non-epileptic seizures. *Seizure*. 1999;8:152–156.
18. Devinsky O, Putnam F, Grafman J, et al. Dissociative states and epilepsy. *Neurology*. 1989;39:835–840.
19. Ellenberger HF. *The Discovery of the Unconscious*. New York: Basic Books; 1970.
20. Erdelyi MH. *Psychoanalysis: Freud's Cognitive Psychology*. New York: WH Freeman; 1985.
21. Freud S. Hysterical phantasies and their relation to bisexuality. In: *The Pelican Freud Library,* Vol. 10: *On Psychopathology*. London: Pelican Books; 1908; reprinted 1979:83–94.
22. Freud S. The paths to the formation of symptoms. In: *The Pelican Freud Library,* Vol. 1: *Introductory Lectures on Psychoanalysis*. London: Pelican Books; 1916–1917; reprinted 1982.
23. Freud S. Inhibitions, symptoms and anxiety. In: *The Pelican Freud Library,* Vol. 10: *On Psychopathology*. London: Pelican Books; 1926; reprinted 1979:229–329.
24. Freud S. Dostoevsky and parricide. In: *The Penguin Freud Library,* Vol. 14: *Art and Literature*. London: Penguin Books; 1928; reprinted 1991:435–469.
25. Frischholz EJ, Lipman LS, Braun BG, et al. Psychopathology, hypnotizability, and dissociation. *Am J Psychiatry*. 1992;149:1521–1525.
26. Goldstein LH, Deale AC, Mitchell-O'Malley SJ, et al. An evaluation of cognitive behavioral therapy as a treatment for dissociative seizures. *Cogn Behav Neurol*. 2004;1:41–49.
27. Good MI. The concept of an organic dissociative syndrome. *Harvard Rev Psychiatry*. 1993;1(3):145–157, 435–469.
28. Gumnit RJ, Gates JR. Psychogenic seizures. *Epilepsia*. 1986;27(Suppl 2):S124–S129.
29. Halligan PW, Athwal BS, Oakley DA, et al. Imaging hypnotic paralysis: Implications for conversion hysteria. *Lancet*. 2000;355:986–987.
30. Hilgard ER. Towards a neo-dissociation theory. *Perspect Biol Med*. 1974;17:301–316.
31. Hilgard ER. Neodissociation theory. In: Lynn SJ, Rhue JW, eds. *Dissociation*. London: Guilford Press; 1995:32–52.
32. Hilgard ER. *Divided Consciousness: Multiple Controls in Human Thought and Action*. New York: Wiley; 1997.
33. Holmes E, Brown RJ, Mansell W, et al. Are there two qualitatively distinct forms of dissociation? A review and some clinical implications. *Clin Psychol Rev*. 2005;25:1–23.
34. Irwin HJ. Proneness to dissociation and traumatic childhood events. *J Nerv Ment Dis*. 1994;8:456–460.
35. Israels H, Schatzman M. The seduction theory. *Hist Psychiatry*. 1993; IV:23–59.
36. Janet P. *L'automatisme psychologique*. Paris: Felix Alcan; 1889.
37. Janet P. *The Major Symptoms of Hysteria*. London: Macmillan; 1907.
38. Janet P. *The Major Symptoms of Hysteria,* 2nd ed. New York: Macmillan; 1924.
39. Janet P. *Psychological Healing,* Vol. 1. London: George Allen and Unwin; 1925.
40. Kihlstrom JF. One hundred years of hysteria. In: Lynn SJ, Rhue JW, eds. *Dissociation: Clinical and Theoretical Perspectives*. New York: Guilford Press; 1994:365–394.
41. Krishnamoorthy ES, Brown RJ, Trimble MR. Personality and psychopathology in non-epileptic attack disorder (NEAD): A prospective study. *Epilepsy Behav*. 2004;2:418–422.
42. Kuyk J, Jacobs LD, Aldenkamp AP, et al. Pseudoepileptic seizures: Hypnosis as a diagnostic tool. *Seizure*. 1995;4:123–128.
43. Kuyk J, Spinhoven P, van Dyck R. Hypnotic recall: A positive criterion in the differential diagnosis between epileptic and pseudoepileptic seizures. *Epilepsia*. 1999;40:485–491.
44. Kuyk J, van Dyck R, Spinhoven P. The case for a dissociative interpretation of pseudoepileptic seizures. *J Nerv Ment Dis*. 1997;18:468–474.
45. LaBarbera JD, Dozier JE. Hysterical seizures: The role of sexual exploitation. *Psychosomatics*. 1980;21:897–903.
46. Lipowski ZJ. Review of consultation psychiatry and psychosomatic medicine. III. Theoretical issues. *Psychosom Med*. 1968;30:395–422.
47. Maldonada JR, Spiegel D. The treatment of post-traumatic stress disorder. In: Lynn SJ, Rhue JW, eds. *Dissociation*. London: Guilford Press; 1995:215–242.
48. Meierkord H, Will B, Fish D, et al. The clinical features and prognosis of pseudoseizures diagnosed using video-EEG telemetry. *Neurology*. 1991;41:1643–1646.
49. Merskey H. The manufacture of personalities. *Br J Psychiatry*. 1992; 160:327–340.
50. Nijenhuis ERS, Spinhoven P, Van Dyck R, et al. The development and the psychometric characteristics of the Somatoform Dissociation Questionnaire (SDQ–20). *J Nerv Ment Dis*. 1996;184:688–694.
51. Pettinati HM, Horne RL, Staats, JM. Hypnotizability in patients with anorexia nervosa and bulimia. *Arch Gen Psychiatry*. 1085;42: 1014–1016.
52. Pratt RTC. Psychogenic loss of memory. In Whitty CWM, Zanwill OL, eds. *Amnesia*. London: Butterworths; 1977:224–232.
53. Pribor EE, Yutzi SH, Dean TJ, et al. Briquet's syndrome, dissociation, and abuse. *Am J Psychiatry*. 1993;150:1507–1511.
54. Prince M. *The Dissociation of a Personality*. Oxford: Oxford University Press; 1905; reprinted 1978.
55. Putnam F. Dissociation and disturbances of self. In: Cicchetti D, Toth SL, eds. *Disorders and Dysfunctions of the Self*. Rochester, NY: University of Rochester Press; 1994:251–265.
56. Schenk L, Bear D. Multiple personality and related dissociative phenomena in patients with temporal lobe epilepsy. *Am J Psychiatry*. 1981;138:1311–1316.
57. Schilder P. *The Image and Appearance of the Human Body*. London: Kegan Paul Trench and Trubner; 1950.
58. Sierra M, Berrios GE. Depersonalization: Neurobiological perspectives. *Biol Psychiatry*. 1998;44:898–908.
59. Sierra M, Berrios GE. The Cambridge Depersonalisation Scale: A new instrument for the measurement of depersonalisation. *Psychiatry Res*. 2000;93:153–164.
60. Spiegel D, Hunt T, Dondershine HE. Dissociation and hypnotizability in post-traumatic stress disorder. *Am J Psychiatry*. 1988;145:301–305.
61. Steinberg M. *Interviewers Guide to the Structured Clinical Interview for DSM–IV Dissociative Disorders (SCID–D)*. Washington, DC: American Psychiatric Association; 1993.
62. Thomas L, Trimble MR. Dissociative disorders. In Engel J, Pedley TA, eds. *Epilepsy: A Comprehensive Textbook*. Philadelphia: Lippincott-Raven; 1997:2775–2784.
63. van der Kolk BA, ed. *Psychological Trauma*. Washington, DC: American Psychiatric Association; 1987.
64. Woody EZ, Bowers KS. A frontal assault on dissociated control. In Lynn SJ, Rhue JW, eds. *Dissociation: Clinical and Theoretical Perspectives*. New York: Guilford Press; 1994:52–79.
65. World Health Organisation. *The ICD-10 Classification of Mental and Behavioural Disorders: Clinical Descriptions and Diagnostic Guidelines*. Geneva: World Health Organisation; 1992.
66. Yorokoglu A, Kemph J. Children not severely damaged by incest with a parent. *J Am Acad Child Psychiatry*. 1966;5:14–124.

CHAPTER 285 ■ PANIC DISORDER AND HYPERVENTILATION SYNDROME

ALAN B. ETTINGER, JONATHAN M. BIRD, AND ANDRES M. KANNER

INTRODUCTION

Panic disorder and hyperventilation syndrome (HVS) are frequently underrecognized conditions that are easily mistaken for epileptic seizures. This chapter highlights practical diagnostic strategies for distinguishing these disorders. We explore etiologies of HVS and conclude with a discussion of the effects of hyperventilation on seizures and the EEG because these issues may arise in the context of the evaluation of hyperventilation symptoms. Potential areas of commonality in the pathogenesis of panic disorder and epilepsy are discussed in Chapter 206.

PANIC ATTACKS AND PANIC DISORDER

A 28-year-old woman had undergone a subtotal resection of a right temporal ganglioglioma at 11 years of age. This had presented with complex partial seizures associated with déjà-vu sensation followed by altered responsiveness. She was seizure free until 8 years later, when typical seizures recurred, but now with secondary generalization. A further resection of a large part of the right temporal lobe was undertaken. This resulted in significant improvement in the epilepsy, but the patient continued to have occasional complex partial seizures with a rising epigastric aura, déjà-vu sensations, and complex motor automatisms.

She subsequently developed new episodes, different from her typical complex partial seizures. These began with a sense of shortness of breath and a choking feeling. She experienced nausea that was distinct from the earlier rising epigastric aura. The episodes also included dizziness and a perception that things were unreal around her. She also had an overwhelming feeling that she was going to die. With great concern about these episodes, the husband gave up his job to be constantly by her side.

Video-electroencephalographic (EEG) monitoring demonstrated that, although the patient has had ongoing epileptiform discharges and slow waves over the right temporal region, the new episodes were unassociated with electrographic correlate. A diagnosis of panic attacks was rendered. The patient has undergone a process of psychoeducation, reassurance, and discussion with the appropriate neurosurgeons. She began to articulate her fear of dying from her tumor. Panic attacks improved significantly with this treatment but occasionally recurred without clear provocation. Her husband was trained to be observant but not overindulgent in response to the episodes, and he ultimately returned to work.

One of the most common episodic symptoms that can be confused with a seizure is a *panic attack*. Numerous series attest to the common misdiagnosis of seizures in patients with panic attacks[26,38] and the erroneous diagnosis of panic attacks among patients with seizures.[1,14,51,78] Recurrent unexpected panic attacks define the condition termed *panic disorder*.[66] Diagnostic criteria for panic attacks and panic disorder are listed in Table 1. Significant morbidity associated with epilepsy or panic disorder and with the failure to allocate appropriate treatment makes the need to distinguish these two disorders especially crucial.

Epilepsy has a lifetime prevalence of 3% to 4%,[36] and panic disorder has a lifetime prevalence of 1% to 2%.[64] Although there is a fairly equal overall rate of epilepsy in men and women, panic disorder is twice as likely in women.

According to the *Diagnostic and Statistical Manual of Mental Disorders*, 4th edition (DSM-IV),[3] a panic attack is a "discrete period of intense fear or discomfort" in which four or more of the symptoms listed in Table 1 "develop abruptly and reach a peak within 10 minutes." Many of the symptoms of panic attacks are reminiscent of symptoms that may appear during some types of epileptic seizures. Differences between panic attacks and seizures are highlighted in Table 2 and elaborated on in the following discussion.

Fear is a commonly encountered component of partial seizures and is the most common ictal psychiatric symptom.[13,81] The importance of the temporal lobe as a site of localization for fear auras is validated by electrical stimulation of mesial temporal structures such as the amygdala, which produces many of the symptoms reminiscent of panic attacks (intense fear, dizziness, nausea, tachycardia, chest pain, and depersonalization).[29] Gloor argued that "the aura of fear in a temporal lobe seizure may take exactly the form of a typical panic attack."[29] He further contended that this "situation is further compounded in those patients with epilepsy who also have panic attacks that may provoke their epileptic seizures, either by hyperventilation or by some direct effect of the CNS arousal."[29]

The fear aura tends to be associated more with a typical rising epigastric aura, whereas panic attacks are associated more with a spreading abdominal discomfort. The aura tends to be described as if it has a "harder," more organic feel. Williams[81] described ictal fear as unnatural rather than seeming more reality based. The intensity of ictal fear sensation is mild to moderate and rarely reaches the intensity of a panic attack.

Anxiety symptoms in panic attacks vary in nature among different individuals. Some experience a nonspecific sensation of "impending doom," whereas others may experience a fear of having incurred a devastating medical problem such as a heart attack or stroke. Sometimes, the anxiety is less prominent than the other features, such as palpitations or chest discomfort, noted in Table 1. It is thus of little wonder that most patients with a panic attack present initially to an emergency room or a nonpsychiatric medical clinician rather than to a psychiatrist.[34]

In panic attacks, autonomic symptoms and other bodily symptoms appear such as palpitations, sweating paresthesias, dizziness, nausea, feeling faint, and a sense of abdominal or central chest discomfort, and it is not uncommon for patients experiencing a panic attack to be thought of as having an acute

TABLE 1

SYMPTOMS OF PANIC ATTACK AND PANIC DISORDER

Panic attack (summary of DSM-IV criteria)
A discrete period of intense fear or discomfort, in which four (or more) of the following symptoms develop abruptly and reach a peak within 10 min

Cardiopulmonary symptoms
- Chest pain or discomfort
- Sensations of shortness of breath or smothering
- Palpitations, pounding heart, or accelerated heart rate

Neurologic symptoms
- Trembling or shaking
- Paresthesias (numbness or tingling sensation)
- Feeling dizzy, unsteady, light-headed, or faint

Psychiatric symptoms
- Derealization (feelings of unreality) or depersonalization (being detached from onself)
- Fear of losing control or going crazy
- Fear of dying

Automic symptoms
- Sweating
- Chills or hot flushes

Gastrointestinal symptoms
- Feeling of choking
- Nausea or abdominal distress

Panic disorder (summary of DSM-IV criteria)

With agoraphobia
- A. Recurrent, unexpected panic attacks
- B. At least one of the attacks has been followed by 1 mo or more of persistent concern about having additional attacks; worry about the implications of the attack or its consequences; a significant change in behavior related to the attack
- C. The presence of agoraphobia, i.e., anxiety about being in places or situations in which escape might be difficult (or embarrassing) or in which help might not be available in the event of having a panic attack

Without agoraphobia
- A. Both A and B above
- B. Absence of agoraphobia

DSM-IV, *Diagnostic and Statistical Manual for Mental Disorders*, 4th edition.

coronary attack or a stroke. Autonomic symptomatology is also common in seizures, but these are of lesser "subjective" intensity than in panic attacks. Of note, paroxysmal salivation is a typical autonomic symptom in seizures of mesial temporal or insular origin and not of panic attacks. Salivation may often be copious and associated with nausea and vomiting.

Subjective dyspnea often experienced during a panic attack led to the earlier confusion and often mislabeling of panic attacks as hyperventilation syndrome, although some might argue that they are intimately related (see later discussion).[28] Alteration in breathing pattern is very common to both seizures and panic attacks, so that the documentation of hyperventilation has limited distinguishing value. If hyperventilation is severe, tetany may occur, which could be confused with seizures associated with tonic activity.

In contrast to complex partial seizures, distinct confusion or loss of consciousness is unusual in a panic attack, although patients may become completely absorbed by the panic experience to the point at which they are unable to report what is going on around them. A panic attack associated with profound hyperventilation could also conceivably lead to a "subjective perception" of loss of consciousness. Symptoms of derealization, depersonalization, and déjà-vu may occur in both conditions.[73] The patient with panic attacks associated with these symptoms could end up undergoing an extraordinarily extensive testing if panic is not considered in the differential diagnosis by the medical clinician. Because of dissociation during panic attacks and subsequent claims of amnesia for the episodes, the patient may never make it to a psychiatrist for treatment (M. Trimble, personal communication). Distortion of perception should raise additional suspicion for partial seizures.

"Reported" preservation of awareness of surroundings and responsiveness during the ictus are usually interpreted as supportive evidence of a panic attack. It is important to remember, however, that in seizures of nondominant mesial temporal origin, patients may continue to follow commands and interact with the examiner or other interlocutors during the ictus, giving the appearance of "intact" consciousness.[23] Careful testing of these patients, however, after the event reveals that they do not recall what happened during it. In such cases, recording of these events with video-EEG may be the only way of establishing a correct diagnosis.

Ictal fear usually lasts <30 seconds and is usually more stereotyped than panic attacks. A partial complex seizure during which ictal fear may occur usually lasts only 2 minutes. However, partial complex status epilepticus associated with isolated fear has been reported.[62] In contrast, panic attacks usually last from 5 to 20 minutes and have a longer buildup of anxieties.

Postictal symptoms of panic and symptoms of primary panic disorder can often lead to confusion. For example, in a study of 100 patients with refractory epilepsy, Kanner et al.[44] found that 10% of patients experienced postictal symptoms of panic after >50% of their seizures. The median duration of these symptoms was 24 hours. A careful history of the context in which symptoms occur as well as a review of other clues (Table 2) should help to avoid militate against this potential confusion.

Seizures can begin at any age, although certain forms of seizures, such as absence seizures, are much likelier to begin in childhood. Panic disorder usually begins in late adolescence or early adulthood, although onset in the 30s and even 40s can occur.[64] Symptoms suggestive of panic attacks that begin in older age groups should be vigorously investigated for the possibility of a seizure disorder.

The value of performing a detailed history (including contacting witnesses of an episode) when distinguishing seizures from panic attacks cannot be overemphasized. Anecdotal experience and review of case series of seizures[79] mistaken to be panic attacks often reveals some evidence of associated classic ictal phenomenology during some of the attacks such as automatisms or motor activity suggestive of spread of seizure activity. Patients often fail to recognize or report such associated symptoms such as transient confusion or subtle automatisms, and therefore it behooves the clinician to search for these clues. Sometimes, a frank convulsion following fear symptomatology clinches the epileptic diagnosis. Identifying a past medical history of febrile seizures or other risk factors for spontaneous seizures provides additional diagnostic clues.

Panic attacks tend to be somewhat less stereotyped than seizures, although this is best documented on video-EEG because historical accounts of observers may not necessarily emphasize the obvious replicability of ictal episodes.

Although some panic attacks may be linked to specific situations, panic disorder comprises at least two spontaneous panic attacks, at least one of which is associated with worry about subsequent attacks or avoidance behavior. Controversy

TABLE 2

DIFFERENTIAL DIAGNOSIS OF SEIZURE VERSUS PANIC ATTACK

Characteristics	Seizure	Panic attack
Signs and symptoms		
DSM-IV–based panic symptoms	Less common	Common
Repetitive, highly stereotyped presentations	More common	Rare
Atypical symptoms (aphasia, perceptual distortions)	More common	Less common
Association with rising epigastric sensation	More common	Not present
Disturbed behavior in sleep	More common	Less common
Altered consciousness	May occur	Usually preserved, patient may report it though
Fear duration	Usually 30 s; entire seizure usually <2 min; postictal fear may occur	Usually 5–10 min, up to 20 min
Agoraphobia	Less common, but may occur	More common
Rapid onset of episodes	More common	Less common
Postepisode confusion	Can occur	Not present
Postepisode fatigue	More common	Less common
History		
History of seizure risk factors (e.g., febrile seizures, head trauma)	Common	Less common
Family history of panic	Uncommon	Common
Anticipatory anxiety	Uncommon	Common
Findings		
Interictal neurologic deficits	Common	Uncommon
Abnormal sleep-deprived interictal electroencephalogram	Often present	Usually absent
Electrographic seizure activity during episode	Common, but "surface–negative events" may occur	Not present
Automatisms during episode	Common	Not present
Treatment		
Response to anxiolytics (nonbenzodiazepine)	Not helpful	Helpful
Response to antidepressants	Rarely worsens	Helpful
Response to antiepileptic drugs	Usually	Occasionally and depending on agent

DSM-IV, *Diagnostic and Statistical Manual for Mental Disorders*, 4th edition.
Source: Modified from Lee DO, Helmers SL, Steingard RJ, et al. Case study: seizure disorder presenting as panic disorder with agoraphobia. *J Am Acad Child Adolesc Psychiatry.* 1997;36(9):1295–1298.

exists whether agoraphobia (a common comorbid condition consisting of fear related to places from which escape may be difficult)[48,64,76] is a component of panic disorder or represents an independent condition that may be provoked by a panic attack. Similar to epilepsy, anticipatory anxiety may become so severe that the individual begins to restrict travel and activity for fear of finding himself or herself in the midst of an attack. Social phobias are common in panic disorder, but agoraphobia may also occur in epilepsy.

Although sleep can be provocative for many types of seizures, it is worth remembering that two thirds of patients with panic attacks have had one or more events at night. Polysomnography has demonstrated panic attacks occurring at sleep onset during stage 2 sleep or slow-wave sleep, but most commonly after awakening.[10,53,61,63]

The EEG may be helpful in suggesting an epileptic disorder both interictally, if epileptiform abnormalities or other focal cerebral abnormalities are found, or ictally, if an episode is caught during an episode while the EEG is running. Not uncommonly, the epileptologist is consulted to help to distinguish a seizure disorder from panic disorder and extended EEG monitoring such as video-EEG is ordered. Video-EEG has the advantage of permitting a detailed review of recorded clinical behavior in addition to detailed EEG analysis. Experienced electroencephalographers are aware, however, of the limitations of the EEG, in that simple partial and sometimes even complex partial seizures may not reveal an obvious correlate on scalp EEG[14] and that, therefore, the absence of an obvious electrographic seizure during an episode does not necessarily exclude seizures.[18] Supplementation of routine EEG recording with meticulously placed sphenoidal electrodes may enhance the yield on EEG.[43] Elevated serum prolactin levels 15 to 20 minutes after an episode may help to point to a seizure as the etiology, even when there is no obvious change on the surface EEG recording.[9]

It has been suggested that lactate infusion could be used as a diagnostic tool to provoke panic if it is present, but this is rarely necessary or even feasible.[57,70] Hyperventilation may provoke a panic attack in those prone to panic disorder, but evidence suggests that such provoked attacks are subjectively different from natural panic attacks.[31] It is generally considered that both these procedures have their effects by causing alterations in pCO_2 and pH.[66]

As in epilepsy,[19] comorbid depression and possibly bipolar disorder[20,64] are commonly found in panic disorder, as is the development of secondary psychosocial problems.[50] Whereas the risk of suicide among epilepsy patients is five times that in the general population,[5] the combination of panic attacks with major depression raises the risk of suicide beyond that encountered in major depression alone.[64]

Patients with ictal panic may also suffer from interictal panic attacks. However, studies of the comorbidity of panic disorder and epilepsy are limited. One of the few available surveys[68] suggests that up to 21% of epilepsy patients experience panic attacks compared to only 3.8% of the population.[45] Although the timing of the panic attacks in relation to the onset of epilepsy was not revealed by this study, the assumption that panic attacks were reactive to developing epilepsy cannot be made, especially in light of studies of other psychiatric comorbidity (i.e., depression) in epilepsy, which showed that depression may often precede the first seizure.[15,37] Agoraphobia, however, may develop in epilepsy due to the fear of having a seizure while crossing the street or in a public place. Mechanisms of potential commonality between panic disorder and epilepsy are described in Chapter 206.

Long-term outcome studies are lacking in panic disorder, although studies and anecdotal experience suggest that many patients will have a waxing and waning of episode frequency, whereas others may have more prolonged episode-free periods, which is again similar to the variability of outcomes seen among some epilepsy patients.

Similar to the risks among epilepsy patients of seizure exacerbation following abrupt withdrawal of benzodiazepines,[35] misuse of benzodiazepines by patients with panic disorder attempting to relieve their symptoms may be associated with worsened panic attacks during benzodiazepine withdrawal.

Panic disorder should also be distinguished from numerous medical conditions that may give rise to similar symptomatology, such as cardiac dysrhythmias in younger people (e.g., Romano-Ward syndrome; prolonged-QT syndrome) and paroxysmal metabolic disorders (e.g., carcinoid syndrome, hypoglycemia, pheochromocytoma, and Cushing syndrome). All of these disorders, however, are relatively rare. Other conditions to consider include alcohol drug withdrawal, illicit drug effects (amphetamines, cocaine, marijuana-induced tachycardia), vertigo-related disorders, and asthma.[21,46] Such alternative conditions should be strongly considered when panic attacks are unresponsive to the usual treatments or do represent seizures.

As discussed in Chapter 206, treatments for panic disorder (benzodiazepines, selective serotonin reuptake inhibitors, tricyclic antidepressants, and, more rarely, monoamine oxidase inhibitors) may affect the same neurotransmitters (e.g., γ-aminobutyric acid, norepinephrine, and serotonin) that are also crucial in aborting or promoting epileptogenesis. Other treatments for panic disorder include cognitive–behavioral therapy[4] and psychotherapeutic approaches.

Panic symptoms may often be identified in psychogenic nonepileptic events (PNES) that often are misdiagnosed as epileptic seizures. This topic is reviewed in great detail in Chapters 207 and 282.

HYPERVENTILATION SYNDROME

A 20-year-old student of environmental studies presented with episodes occurring several times per day in which she would complain of feeling very light-headed and then fall backward. She would appear confused and express uncertainty as to where she was. She would feel cold and numb and experience tingling sensations in her hands. Her hands would subsequently begin to shake with a coarse tremor, which would then evolve into profound hand stiffness. In the most severe episodes, she would experience tetanic contraction of the hands accompanied by considerable distress and crying. After the event, the patient remained distressed and complained of headache.

Video-EEG monitoring demonstrated no epileptiform discharges, but there was notable hyperventilation observed before and during each episode, resulting in diffuse slow wave changes. During an EEG study, hyperventilating volitionally on command reproduced her typical symptoms completely. This case illustrates the clinical expressions of the hyperventilation syndrome (HVS).

Successful treatment involved demonstrating the video-EEG carefully to her and taking her through a course of relaxation training, including exercises in controlled breathing. The episodes of hyperventilation reduced significantly, although it was possible that they could recur during stressful moments. Overall, the patient felt more in control of her symptoms and found them much less disabling. She was able to return to her routine course of studies.

The hyperventilation syndrome is another challenging diagnosis that overlaps with but is distinct from panic disorder. Although some believe that HVS is simply one variety of panic or anxiety disorder, others argue for recognizing it as an independent entity.

The evolution of the recognition of this syndrome is nicely described by Evans.[22] As early as the Civil War, a mysterious condition characterized by palpitations, shortness of breath, dizziness, and headaches afflicting Union soldiers was described by DaCosta.[11,22] Similar symptoms were noted among soldiers in World War I.[56] Gowers described a similar syndrome of difficulty breathing, yawning, reduced concentration, and a sense of unreality influenced by emotion and more commonly seen among women.[32] Goldman identified the relationship of "forced ventilation" with tetany as well as dizziness, paresthesias, and attacks of nervousness and crying associated with hysteria.[30] The term "hyperventilation syndrome" was introduced in the late 1930s to describe diverse symptoms associated with anxiety and often reproduced by having patients willfully hyperventilate. Lewis argued that acute and chronic hyperventilation syndrome presented frequently and ubiquitously.[69a]

Since at least 1929,[80] it has been recognized that some individuals may hyperventilate chronically. White and Hahn[80] called this "sighing dyspnoea"; this is not quite an accurate description, however, because, although "sighing" can describe the form of breathing, patients rarely complain of discomfort of breathing (dyspnea). Some may, however, complain of an inability to breath deeply enough.

Pincus[55] drew neurologic attention to the condition of chronic hyperventilation syndrome in his influential book *Behavioural Neurology*. He commented, "of all psychophysiological reactions, probably the most common one dealt with by physicians is the hyperventilation syndrome." Lum[58] observed that the typical and known cases of HVS were just the

TABLE 3

SYMPTOMS AND SIGNS OF THE HYPERVENTILATION SYNDROME

General	
Fatiguability, exhaustion, weakness, sleep disturbance, nausea, sweating	
Cardiovascular	
Chest pain, palpitations, tachycardia, Raynaud phenomenon	
Gastrointestinal	
Aerophagia, dry mouth, pressure in throat, dysphagia, globus hystericus, epigastric fullness or pain, belching, flatulence	
Neurologic	
Headache, pressure in the head, fullness in the head, head warmth	
Blurred vision, tunnel vision, momentary flashing lights, diplopia	
Dizziness, faintness, vertigo, giddiness, unsteadiness	
Tinnitus	
Numbness, tingling, coldness of face, extremities, trunk	
Muscle spasms, muscle stiffness, carpopedal spasm, generalized tetany, tremor	
Ataxia, weakness	
Syncope and seizures	
Psychological	
Impairment of concentration and memory	
Feelings of unreality, disorientation, confused or dreamlike feeling, déjà-vu	
Hallucinations	
Anxiety, apprehension, nervousness, tension, fits of crying, agoraphobia, neuroses, phobia, panic	
Respiratory	
Shortness of breath, suffocating feeling, smothering spell, unable to get a good breath or breathe deeply enough, frequent sighing, yawning	

Source: From Evans RW. Hyperventilation syndrome. In: Kaplan PW, Fisher RS, eds. *Imitators of Epilepsy*. New York: Demos; 2005: 241–252, Table 18.1.

"tip of the iceberg" and that as many as 6% of general medical outpatients may have the syndrome.

HVS occurs in most age groups, with a peak between ages 15 to 55 years[65]; it occurs predominantly in women. It presents as one of two varieties—a less common but much more obvious acute form and a less obvious but more common type termed chronic HVS. Acute HVS presents with obvious overbreathing and tachypnea and may have associated chest pain, dyspnea, dizziness, palpitations, and muscle spasms related to tetany, paresthesias, and syncope.[65] Chronic HVS is more challenging to recognize because it is associated with a diverse array of somatic complaints that are often misdiagnosed based on the organ system suggested by the symptomatology. Furthermore, overbreathing is usually not apparent; instead, intermittent deep sighs and frequent yawning may be seen. Symptoms of chronic HVS are best categorized according to bodily symptoms (Table 3).

The neurologist is likely to encounter HVS in the context of one or more diverse symptoms including general dizziness, diffuse weakness, confusion or agitation, paresthesias in the extremities or periorally, and depersonalization sensations. Pincus[69] studied 550 neurologic outpatients and found 30 to suffer from this syndrome. These patients were asked to hyperventilate voluntarily to see if they could evoke the symptoms of which they were complaining. The typical clinical features were light-headedness, headache, paresthesias, giddiness, weakness, and difficulty concentrating. They tended to be aged between 15 and 30 years, to be female, and to have a history of psychosomatic illnesses. The majority (80%) showed some episodes of alteration of consciousness, and 6% had episodes of loss of consciousness, whereas 3% had episodes of tetany. Twenty percent had been given a diagnosis of epilepsy at some stage. Some patients also had gastrointestinal complaints, such as difficulty swallowing and abdominal pain or of chest symptoms such as chest pain, palpitations, and dyspnea.

HVS-related symptoms affecting thinking function and mood are the most likely symptoms to lead to a referral to the epileptologist. Complaints of déjà-vu or hallucinations are rare but have been reported.[2]

Hyperventilation is characterized by ventilation exceeding metabolic demand, leading to hemodynamic and chemical alterations that foster diverse symptomatology. Although a reduction in pCO_2 from willful hyperventilation can often reproduce these symptoms, many individuals with HVS do not in fact have reduced pCO_2 during HVS episodes. The terms "behavioral breathlessness" or "psychogenic dyspnea" have been proposed as alternatives.[65]

Breathing may be atypical in HVS, in which a more thoracic (as opposed to abdominal) breathing occurs. Typically, there is heaving of the upper sternum and a lack of lateral costal expansion—like a normal sigh. This may, therefore, be a learned behavior (a habit). In depression, there may be evident sighing hyperventilation, and chronic hyperventilation may be associated with depression. If chronic, hyperventilation will result in diminished reserve due to chronic mild hypocapnia, and, thus, a slight exacerbation under mild stress may lead to decompensation and marked symptoms. Patients with chronic hyperventilation syndrome are found to have a tendency to a childhood history of emotional problems, a family history of anxiety disorders, and a relative failure of psychosexual adjustment.[71]

Conflict thus may lead to worsening of hyperventilation, which is part of a preparation for "fight or flight." Hyperventilation may also be a learned way of avoiding conflict in an individual with a strong sense of personal vulnerability. If, however, hyperventilation occurs when the individual is actually at rest (as is often the case, possibly the result of inner conflict), the preparation, as if for fight or flight is physiologically unnecessary.

Although the etiology of HVS is not definitively clear, one theory suggests that some individuals are prone to specific abnormal respiratory responses to stimuli like stress (or chemical or other triggers) that result in excessive and disordered breathing, emphasizing thoracic rather than normal diaphragmatic respiration, thereby producing an expanded chest and increased residual lung volume. This then precludes inspiring the normal volume and produces a sensation of dyspnea. A "suffocation alarm" then leads to an autonomic response with symptoms including palpitations, anxiety, and diaphoresis.[65]

HVS may be medically more benign than some of the alternative diagnoses suggested by its symptoms (e.g., myocardial infarction); therefore some HVS sufferers incur significant morbidity from the numerous testing procedures often performed in search of an explanation for symptoms. Furthermore, HVS patients experience genuine discomfort and psychological distress related to their symptoms.

The most critical aspect of making a diagnosis of HVS is to consider it when considering a differential diagnosis; this helps to temper an otherwise excessive laboratory testing plan. In the face of acute HVS, the clinician may want to exclude internal or external organic causes, including lesions in the pons or midbrain tegmentum, liver disease, and salicylate poisoning. Occasionally, complex partial seizures (arising particularly from the insular cortex) may involve hyperventilation as part of the aura, although this is usually accompanied by automatisms and other obvious signs of a seizure. In the face of presentation with chest pain, diagnoses like pulmonary embolus and myocardial infarction may need to be ruled out.

Diagnosis of chronic hyperventilation syndrome may be made from a careful history taking, possibly combined with an attempt to precipitate or exacerbate the symptoms by voluntary hyperventilation typically by increasing respiration to 60 per minute or encouraging sustained deep breaths for 3 minutes.[59] The validity of this "hyperventilation test" has been challenged more recently.[41] Antecedent anxiety may be more compelling than the hyperventilation itself in bringing about the symptoms A negative test does not necessarily exclude this diagnosis.

Knowledge about the treatment of HVS is based predominantly on small case series and anecdotal experience. The management of acute hyperventilation by the time-honored method of rebreathing from a paper bag should be prescribed with caution because severe complications may arise if the diagnosis is wrong and a more serious condition exists. Some argue that this technique sometimes exacerbates anxiety through retention of CO_2. Simple reassurance alone is often sufficient to attenuate an acute episode. For the longer term, teaching patients how to use abdominal (diaphragmatic) breathing or other breathing retraining techniques (including reducing depth of ventilation) are often effective. Stress reduction methods, sometimes in conjunction with psychotherapy, biofeedback, or hypnosis, have been used. Psychotropic agents for potentially associated anxiety or depression include benzodiazepines, tricyclic antidepressants, and selective serotonin reuptake inhibitors.

Hyperventilation and the Electroencephalogram

Normal and common central manifestations of hyperventilation include light-headedness, a sense of unreality, and, eventually, loss of consciousness. The psychological effects of acute hyperventilation are marked. At first, heightened perception may be reported and may be a partial explanation for certain beatific visions and spiritual experiences in states of religious excitement.[42] However, this is then followed by dulling of consciousness and diminished awareness of the environment. As the dominant rhythm of the EEG drops below 5 Hz, there is increasing impairment of reaction time, memory, and calculation abilities. On recovery, there may be amnesia for the episode. If hyperventilation is prolonged, mental confusion, myoclonic jerking, convulsions, and loss of consciousness may ensue.[27,75]

The quality and nature of respiration have a profound effect on the brain. Two deep breaths significantly reduce arterial carbon dioxide; further hyperventilation results in respiratory alkalosis. There is a direct relationship between pCO_2 and the caliber of the cerebral blood vessels. During hyperventilation, Doppler ultrasound measurements of the mean flow velocity in the middle and posterior cerebral arteries drop by up to 50% after 4 minutes.[7] After cessation of hyperventilation, the mean flow velocity increases briefly to 130% to 140% of normal.

Hyperventilation is a well-established procedure during the performance of the EEG[39] and it is considered helpful for producing focal slow-wave abnormalities suggestive of regions of focal disturbance, as well as generalized epileptiform abnormalities (especially idiopathic generalized epilepsies in the young such as typical absence).[12,40] It is much less useful for bringing out focal interictal epileptiform abnormalities.[49] Hyperventilation results in slowing of EEG rhythms in normal individuals, independent of the inspired oxygen concentration.[47] It is the hypocapnia that causes the decreased cerebral blood flow, as well as increased hemoglobin affinity for oxygen, and results in cerebral tissue hypoxia. Hyperventilation also leads to a marked surface negative direct current shift, possibly due to depolarization of the apical dendritic trees of the cortical pyramidal cells.[72,77] This surface negative shift is likely to represent increased excitability of the cortical neuronal networks and may explain the resultant potential epileptogenicity. It is of interest that certain antiepileptic drugs have the opposing effect of reducing surface negativity in normal controls.[72]

Hyperventilation and hypocapnia significantly increase the length of seizures evoked by electroconvulsive therapy in a progressive fashion[6] directly related to decreasing pCO_2. Thus, hyperventilation has effects in the human cerebral cortex that might be expected to produce epileptic activity.

Hyperventilation-induced Seizures

Voluntary hyperventilation was proposed as a means of eliciting epileptic seizures as early as 1924.[24] There are many case reports in the literature in which a variety of forms of epileptic attack are provoked by this means.[8,25,60,67] Many of these reports involve individuals (adults or children) with mental retardation and often with absence or atypical absence attacks.[8,60] The report by Bruno-Golden and Holmes[8] describes two children with severe mental impairment and a history of infantile spasms followed by tonic seizures. Observation demonstrated that the seizures were often preceded by hyperarousal and hyperventilation. Management involved a behavioral approach, training in uninostril breathing (more successfully completed than training in diaphragmatic breathing in this population), and a program of physical exercise. Very considerable reduction in seizure frequency was recorded. A similar story is described by Magarian and Olney,[60] this time in a 66-year-old man with a 20-year history of absence spells. Educational and behavioral therapy was again successful; however, there remains doubt as to whether these "absence spells" were epileptic. Fried et al.[25] described a group of 18 patients with undoubted intractable epilepsy who were given diaphragmatic breathing training. Ten of them completed the training and had significantly reduced seizure frequency and severity.

As early as 1947 Engel et al.[16] raised doubts that hyperventilation resulted in tonic–clonic or partial seizures. This issue remains controversial. Although Holmes et al.[40] found that hyperventilation elicited a clinical seizure in only 2 of 433 consecutive patients with proven epilepsy, Guaranha et al.[33] found that up to 24 of 97 patients had hyperventilation-induced seizure activation (although in the context of reduction of antiepileptic medications in patients with the most severe seizure disorders undergoing presurgical evaluations.)

There has been debate about whether physical exercise induces seizures or reduces their frequency. In general, exercise is seen as a good thing, and, although it results in fast breathing, this is not regarded as a problem because alkalosis does not ensue. Esquivel et al.[17]compared exercise with voluntary hyperventilation in a group of 12 children with absence epilepsy undergoing EEG monitoring. They found a decrease in the number of absence attacks during the physical exercise and an increase during hyperventilation. Plasma pH was also measured and showed a positive correlation with seizure frequency. In general, therefore, it is felt that moderate exercise is good for epilepsy control. In some individuals, however, seizures are clearly induced by exercise[67,74] but not necessarily by voluntary hyperventilation. The mechanisms of seizure induction in these cases are unclear, nor is it known why some people have seizures during the "let-down" period after physical exercise. Careful history taking, possibly with EEG monitoring during exercise, will be required to give the patient appropriate advice about exercise.

Peripheral physiologic effects of hyperventilation may be as important to the epileptologist as are central effects. Respiratory alkalosis reduces the proportion of ionized calcium in the blood and causes tetany. Peripheral neuromuscular manifestations, short of tetany, include paresthesia, weakness, and muscular cramps. These symptoms and signs may be misdiagnosed as a seizure by the unwary. Nonspecific ST- and T-wave changes will be provoked on the ECG, causing confusion to the cardiologist reviewing an ECG in the absence of careful history taking and observation, especially because an increased pulse rate and palpitations are common autonomic concomitants of hyperventilation, along with epigastric distress and swallowing difficulties.

Finally, hyperventilation is a frequent procedure used to elicit suspected PNES during the course of a diagnostic video-EEG. In fact, the use of hyperventilation and photic stimulation is favored over other induction techniques (e.g., intravenous saline infusions). Given that hyperventilation can induce epileptic seizures and PNES, the diagnosis should not be based solely on clinical observations, but must also be documented with concurrent EEG recordings (see also Chapters 74 and 282).

SUMMARY AND CONCLUSIONS

Panic disorders and HVS are common conditions that are misdiagnosed as epileptic seizures. A careful history is very often sufficient to reach a correct diagnosis, although in some instances a recording of the paroxysmal episodes with video-EEG may be necessary. Some patients may experience epileptic seizures and panic disorder and/or HVS, and, hence, the presence of one condition should not automatically exclude the other(s). As with any other neurologic or psychiatric disorder, treatment of paroxysmal episodes presenting as panic attacks or recurrent episodes of hyperventilation should be based on robust diagnostic evidence.

References

1. Alemayehu S, Bergey GK, Barry E, et al. Panic attacks as ictal manifestations of parietal lobe seizures. *Epilepsia.* 1995;36:824–830.
2. Allen TE, Agus B. Hyperventilation leading to hallucinations. *Am J Psychiatry.* 1968;125:632–637.
3. American Psychiatric Association. *Diagnostic and Statistical Manual of Mental Disorders,* 4th ed. Washington DC: American Psychiatric Association; 1994.
4. Barlow D, Gorman JM, Shear MK, et al. Cognitive–behavioral therapy, imipramine, or their combination for panic disorder: A randomized controlled trial. *JAMA.* 2000;283:2529.
5. Barraclough B, ed. *Suicide and Epilepsy.* London: Churchill Livingstone; 1981.
6. Bergsholm P, Gran L, Bleie H. Seizure duration in unilateral electroconvulsive therapy. The effect of hypocapnia induced by hyperventilation and the effect of ventilation with oxygen. *Acta Psychiatr Scand.* 1984;69(2):121–128.
7. Bode H, Puglia E. Intra-individual variation of cerebral blood flow velocity in sleeping and awake children [in German]. *Ultraschall Med.* 1992;13(5):204–207.
8. Bruno-Golden B, Holmes GL. Hyperventilation-induced seizures in mentally impaired children. *Seizure.* 1993;2(3):229–233.
9. Chen DK, So YT, Fisher RS. Use of serum prolactin in diagnosing epileptic seizures: Report of the Therapeutics and Technology Assessment Subcommittee of the American Academy of Neurology. *Neurology.* 200513;65(5):668–675.
10. Craske M, Barlow D. Nocturnal panic. *J Nerv Ment Dis.* 1989;177:160–167.
11. Da Costa JM. On irritable heart; a clinical study of a form of functional cardiac disorder and its consequences. *Am J Med Sci.* 1871;71:2–52.
12. Dalby MA. Epilepsy and 3 per second spike and wave rhythms. A clinical, electrographic and prognostic analysis of 346 patients. *Acta Neurol Scand.* 1969;45(Suppl 40):1–183.
13. Daly D. Ictal affect. *Am J Psychiatry.* 1958;115:97–108.
14. Devinsky O, Sato S, Theodore WH, et al. Fear episodes due to limbic seizures with normal scalp EEG. A subdural electrographic study. *J Clin Psychiatry.* 1989;50:28–30.
15. Dunn DW, Austin JK. Symptoms of depression in adolescents with epilepsy. *J Am Acad Child Adolesc Psychiatry.* 1999;38(9):1132–1138.
16. Engel GL, Ferriss EB, Logan M. Hyperventilation: Analysis of clinical symptomatology. *Ann Int Med.* 1947;27:683–704.
17. Esquivel E, Chaussain M, Plouin P, et al. Physical exercise and voluntary hyperventilation in childhood absence epilepsy. *Electroencephalogr Clin Neurophysiol.* 1991;79(2):127–132.
18. Ettinger AB, Jandorf L, Cabahug CJ, et al. Post-ictal SPECT in epileptic vs. non-epileptic seizures. *J Epilepsy.* 1998;11:67–73.
19. Ettinger AB, Reed M, Cramer J, for the Epilepsy Impact Project Group. Depression and Co-morbidity in community-based patients with epilepsy or asthma. *Neurology.* 2004;63(6):1008–1014.
20. Ettinger AB, Reed ML, Goldberg JF, et al. Prevalence of bipolar symptoms in epilepsy vs other chronic health disorders. *Neurology.* 2005;65:535–540.
21. Ettinger AB, Weisbrot DM. Potential causes of commonly encountered symptoms. In: Ettinger AB, Weisbrot DM, eds. *The Essential Patient Handbook; Getting the Health Care You Need—From Doctors Who Know.* New York: Demos; 2004:256–258
22. Evans RW. Hyperventilation syndrome. In: Kaplan PW, Fisher RS, eds. *Imitators of Epilepsy.* New York: Demos; 2005:241–252.
23. Fakhoury T, Abou-Khalil B, Peguero E. Differentiating clinical features of right and left temporal lobe seizures. *Epilepsia.* 1994;35(5):1038–1044.
24. Foerster O. Hypervventilationjspilepsie. *Dtsch Z Nervenheilkd.* 1924;83: 347–356.
25. Fried R, Rubin SR, Carlton RM, et al. Behavioral control of intractable idiopathic seizures: I. Self-regulation of end-tidal carbon dioxide. *Psychosom Med.* 1984;46(4):315–331.
26. Genton P, Bartolomei F, Guerrini R. Panic attacks mistaken for relapse of epilepsy. *Epilepsia.* 1995;36(1):48–51.
27. Gibbs EL, Lennox WG, Gibbs FA. Variations of carbon dioxide content of blood in epilepsy. *Arch Neurol Psychol.* 1940;43:223–241.
28. Glass RM. Panic disorder—it's real and it's treatable. *JAMA.* 2000;283(19): 2573–2574.
29. Gloor P. Experiential phenomena of temporal lobe epilepsy: Facts and hypotheses. *Brain.* 1990;113:1673–1694.
30. Goldman A. Clinical tetany by forced respiration. *JAMA.* 1922;78:1193–1195.
31. Gorman JM, Liebowitz MR, Fryer AJ, et al. A neuroanatomical hypothesis for panic disorder. *Am J Psychiatry.* 1989;146:148–161.
32. Gowers WR. *The Border-land of Epilepsy. Faints, Vagal Attacks, Vertigo, Migraine, Sleep Symptoms and Their Treatment.* London: J and A Churchill; 1907.
33. Guaranha MSB, Garzon E, Buckpiguel CA, et al. Hyperventilation revisited: Physiologic effects and efficacy on focal seizure activation in the era of video-EEG monitoring. *Epilepsia.* 2005;46(1):69–75.
34. Ham P, Waters DB, Oliver MN. Treatment of panic disorder. *Am Fam Physician.* 2005;71(4):733–740.
35. Hauser P, Devinsky O, DeBellis M, et. al. Benzodiazepine withdrawal delirium with catatonic features. *Arch Neurol.* 1989;46:696–699.
36. Hauser W, Annegers J, Kurland L. Prevalence of epilepsy in Rochester, Minnesota: 1940–1980. *Epilepsia.* 1991;32(4):429–445.
37. Hesdorffer DC, Hauser WA, Annegers JF, et al. Major depression is a risk factor for seizures in older adults. *Ann Neurol.* 2000;47(2):246–249.
38. Hirsch E, Peretti S, Boulay C, et al. Panic attacks misdiagnosed as partial epileptic seizures. *Epilepsia.* 1990;31:636.
39. Hoefnagels WA, Padberg GW, Overweg J, et al. Syncope or seizure? The diagnostic value of the EEG and hyperventilation test in transient loss of consciousness. *J Neurol Neurosurg Psychiatry.* 1991;54(11):953–956.
40. Holmes MD, Dwaraja AS, Vanhatalo S. Does hyperventilation elicit epileptic seizures? *Epilepsia.* 2004;45(6):618–620.
41. Hornsveld H, Garssen B, van Spiegel P. Voluntary hyperventilation: The influence of duration and depth on the development of symptoms. *Biol Psychol.* 1995;40:299–312.
42. Huxley A. *Doors of Perception.* London: HarperCollins; 1954.
43. Kanner AM, Jones JC. When do sphenoidal electrodes yield additional data to that obtained with antero-temporal electrodes? *Electroencephalogr Clin Neurophysiol.* 1997;102(1):12–19.
44. Kanner AM, Soto A, Gross-Kanner H. Prevalence and clinical characteristics of postictal psychiatric symptoms in partial epilepsy. *Neurology.* 2004;62:708–713.
45. Katerndahl DA, Realini JP. Lifetime prevalence of panic states. *Am J Psychiatry.* 1993;150:246–249.
46. Katon W. *Panic Disorder in the Medical Setting.* Washington, DC: U.S. Government Printing Office; 1989.
47. Kennealy JA, Penovich PE, Moore-Nease SE. EEG and spectral analysis in acute hyperventilation. *Electroencephalogr Clin Neurophysiol.* 1986;63:98–106.
48. Klein DF. *Anxiety Reconceptualized.* New York: Raven Press; 1981.
49. Klein KM, Knake S, Hamer HM, et al. Sleep but not hyperventilation increases the sensitivity of the EEG in patients with temporal lobe epilepsy. *Epilepsy Res.* 2003;56(1):43–49.
50. Kokkonen J, Kokkonen ER, Saukkonen AL, et al. Psychosocial outcome of young adults with epilepsy in childhood. *J Neurol Neurosurg Psychiatry.* 1997;62(3):265–268.

51. Laidlaw JDD, Khin-Maung-Zaw. Epilepsy mistaken for panic attacks in an adolescent girl. *BMJ*. 1993;306:709–710.
52. Lee DO, Helmers SL, Steingard RJ, et al. Case study: Seizure disorder presenting as panic disorder with agoraphobia. *J Am Acad Child Adolesc Psychiatry*. 1997;36(9):1295–1298.
53. Lesser I, Poland R, Holcomb C, et al. Electroencephalographic study of nighttime panic attacks. *J Nerv Ment Dis*. 1990;173:744–46.
54. Lewis BI. The hyperventilation syndrome. *Ann Int Med*. 1953;38:918–927.
55. Lewis DO, Pincus J, Shanok S, et al. Psychomotor epilepsy and violence in a group of incarcerated adolescent boys. *Am J Psychiatry*. 1982;139:882–887.
56. Lewis T. *The Soldier's Heart and the Effort Syndrome*. New York: Paul B. Hoeber; 1919.
57. Liebowitz MR, Gorman JM, Fyer A, et al. Possible mechanisms for lactate's induction of panic. *Am J Psychiatry*. 1986;143(4):495–502.
58. Lum LC. Hyperventilation: The tip and the iceberg. *J Psychosom Res*. 1975;19(5–6):375–383.
59. Lum LC. Hyperventilation syndromes in medicine and psychiatry: A review. *J R Soc Med*. 1987;80:229–231.
60. Magarian GJ, Olney RK. Absence spells. Hyperventilation syndrome as a previously unrecognized cause. *Am J Med*. 1984;76(5):905–909.
61. Malow BA, Vaughn BV. Sleep disorders and epilepsy. In: Ettinger AB, Devinsky O, eds. *Managing Epilepsy and Co-Existing Disorders*. Boston: Butterworth Heinemann; 2002:255–267.
62. McLachlan RS, Blume WT. Isolated fear in complex partial status epilepticus. *Ann Neurol*. 1980;8:639–641.
63. Mellman TA, Uhde TW. Sleep panic attacks: New clinical findings and theoretical implications. *Am J Psychiatry*. 1989;146:1204–1207.
64. Moore D, Jefferson J. *Panic Disorder*, 2nd ed. St. Louis, MO: Mosby; 2004.
65. Newton E. Hyperventilation syndrome. *e-medicine*. 2005(9-26-05).
66. Nutt D, Lawson C. Panic attacks. A neurochemical overview of models and mechanisms. *Br J Psychiatry*. 1992;160:165–178.
67. Ogunyemi AO, Gomez MR, Klass DW. Seizures induced by exercise. *Neurology*. 1988;38(4):633–634.
68. Pariente PD, Lepine JP, Lellouch J. Lifetime history of panic attacks and epilepsy: An association from a general population survey. *J Clin Psychiatry*. 1991;52(2):88–89.
69. Pincus JH. Disorders of conscious awareness. Hyperventilation syndrome. *Br J Hosp Med*. 1978;19:312–313.
69a. Pincus JH, Tucker GJ. *Behavioural Neurology*. Oxford: Oxford University Press, 1985.
70. Pitts RN, McClure JN. Lactate metabolism in anxiety neurosis. *N Engl J Med*. 1967;227:1329–1339.
71. Riley TL, ed. *Syncope and Hyperventilation*. Baltimore: Williams & Wilkins; 1982.
72. Rockstroh B. Hyperventilation-induced EEG changes in humans and their modulation by an anticonvulsant drug. *Epilepsy Res*. 1990;7(2):146–154.
73. Roth M, Harper M. Temporal lobe epilepsy and the phobic anxiety-depersonalisation syndrome, Part II: Practical and theoretical considerations. *Comprehens Psychiatry*. 1962;3:215–226.
74. Schmitt B, ThunHohenstein L, Vontobel H, et al. Seizures induced by physical exercise: Report of two cases. *Neuropaediatrics*. 1994;25:51–53.
75. Schuler P, Claus D, Stefan H. Hyperventilation and transcranial magnetic stimulation: Two methods of activation of epileptiform EEG activity in comparison. *J Clin Neurophysiol*. 1993;10:111–115.
76. Uhde TW, Boulenger JP, Roy-Byrne PP, et al. Longitudinal course of panic disorder: Clinical and biological considerations. *Prog Neuropsychopharmacol Biol Psychiatry*. 1985;9(1):39–51.
77. Von Bulow I, Elbert T, Rockstroh B, et al. Effects of hyperventilation on EEG-frequency and slow cortical potentials in relation to an anticonvulsant and epilepsy. *J Psychophysiol*. 1989;3:147–154.
78. Weilburg J, Bear D, Sachs G. Three patients with concomitant panic attacks and seizure disorder: Possible clues to the neurology of anxiety. *Am J Psychiatry*. 1987;144:1053.
79. Weilburg JB, Schachter S, Worth J, et al. EEG abnormalities in patients with atypical panic attacks. *J Clin Psychiatry*. 1995;56(8):358–362.
80. White PD, Hahn RG. Symptoms of sighing in cardiovascular diagnosis. *Am J Sci*. 1929;177:179–188.
81. Williams D. The structure of emotions reflected in epileptic experiences. *Brain*. 1956;79:29–67.

CHAPTER 286 ■ OBSESSIVE-COMPULSIVE BEHAVIOR

MARK S. GEORGE AND MARCO MULA

INTRODUCTION

The neuropsychiatric syndrome of obsessive-compulsive disorder (OCD) was discovered and described >150 years ago. Unfortunately, for many years, OCD was thought to be rare, untreatable, and result from hidden conflicts. All of these notions now appear to be mistaken. Occurring in about 2% of all adults, OCD consists of recurrent intrusive thoughts (obsessions), senseless repetitive actions (compulsions), or both. Although the etiology of OCD is unclear, recent neuroimaging studies and cases of secondary OCD implicate the basal ganglia, cingulate gyrus, and orbital and prefrontal cortex as crucial structures in the pathogenesis of OCD. A true cure for this disorder is elusive. However, OCD symptoms partially respond to treatment with antidepressants, especially selective serotonin reuptake inhibitors (SSRIs),[10,17,25,28,44] and, among tricyclics, clomipramine,[40] and behavioral therapy is effective for some patients in stopping rituals and compulsions.[11] Once thought to be the quintessential psychoanalytic disorder, OCD is now viewed as a largely biologic illness arising from abnormal brain function.

In this chapter, we discuss interesting new findings in OCD, paying particular attention to how OCD patients might be distinguished from patients with epilepsy. The symptoms of senseless repetitive actions (compulsions) or recurrent intrusive thoughts (obsessions) on some occasions might resemble the automatisms that occur with complex partial seizures arising from the temporal or frontal lobes. To make a proper differential diagnosis, the practicing epileptologist must be familiar with both primary OCD and other disorders that might have obsessive-compulsive behaviors (OCB) as part of their presenting symptomatology.

CLINICAL PRESENTATION

Obsessive-compulsive Disorder

Primary OCD, as defined by the *Diagnostic and Statistical Manual of Mental Disorders*, 4th edition (DSM-IV),[2] consists of recurrent urges to perform an action (compulsions) or recurrent intrusive thoughts (obsessions), or both. Furthermore, for the symptoms to qualify as true OCD, the compulsions or obsessions must cause significant dysfunction, be recognized by the sufferer as coming from his or her mind (not externally planted), and be egodystonic (i.e., unpleasant and not pleasurable).

An important clinical point is that the obsessions in OCD must be recognized by the individual as senseless, at least at some point in the disorder. A patient with OCD realizes that his or her compulsions do not result from mind control or from some other form of thought insertion, such as might be seen in schizophrenia. Because the obsessions are unpleasant and often of a violent or sexual nature, OCD sufferers attempt to ignore, control, or suppress the obsessions, often with a compulsion. For example, a husband with an obsessional worry about harming his new bride might be forced or compelled to repeatedly check on her welfare to assure himself that he has not harmed her. To summarize, obsessions are recurrent, persistent, resisted by the individual, and unpleasant. Often, obsessions center on certain themes such as contamination, aggressive thoughts concerning harming others or oneself, the need for symmetry or exactness, excessive somatic worries such as about AIDS or terminal cancer, and sexual or religious worries. A common feature of OCD is pathologic doubt and the person's inability to convince himself or herself that he or she has made a correct decision or that the environment is safe.

In contrast, compulsions are repetitive, purposeful, intentional actions sometimes performed in response to an obsession. It is important that the person recognizes or has recognized the senselessness of the actions. Performing the behavior often reduces anxiety. If an OCD sufferer resists performing a compulsion, invariably inner tension mounts until the compulsion is yielded to and the tension disappears. Common compulsions include checking, cleaning, ordering, counting, repeating, and hoarding. The DSM-IV has placed qualifying criteria on compulsions, which must be distressing to the individual, time consuming (>1 hour/d), and cause impairment in function. The phenomenology of obsessions and compulsions varies, depending on whether a person has pure OCD, OCD accompanied by motor tics, or OCD with motor and vocal tics [a disorder known as *Gilles de la Tourette syndrome* (GTS)].[15,21] For example, OCD/GTS subjects have increased touching compulsions and only rarely have washing compulsions—the most common compulsion in pure OCD.

Most cases of OCD begin in middle to late adolescence. The course can vary from chronic and unremitting to a more episodic illness featuring episodes of remission and relapse. Obsessive-compulsive behavior was, until the last few decades, thought to be rare; however, the National Institute of Mental Health (NIMH) Epidemiologic Catchment Area Survey revealed a U.S. prevalence of 2% to 3%.[26,46] Obsessive-compulsive behavior is also often accompanied by other psychiatric disorders. For example, one study found that 30% of OCD patients suffered from a major depressive episode, 27% had simple phobias, 14% had panic disorder, 9% had agoraphobia, and 5% had GTS. The exact gene or genes for OCD and its pattern of transmission are unknown. However, Pauls et al.[41–43] established that OCD is linked to GTS and chronic motor tics. OCD in GTS seems to respond in a similar fashion as primary OCD to drug treatment with SSRIs and behavioral therapy.[16,48]

Obsessive-compulsive Disorder Spectrum

In addition to pure OCD as defined earlier, there are many OCD-related disorders that some have labeled an *OCD spectrum*. This spectrum includes a collection of disorders or behaviors that resemble OCD in some way and often respond to treatment with antiobsessional agents. Dysmorphophobia is the fixed idea that a part of one's anatomy is disfigured or wrongly proportioned.[20] Trichotillomania is the compulsive pulling of one's hair, often seen in young to middle-aged women.[1,53] There is interesting research into the relationships between the eating disorders, particularly anorexia nervosa, and OCD. In addition, some obsessions involve sexual themes, and some forms of fetishism respond to treatment with serotonin-reuptake inhibitors.[56] Similarly, some obsessions involve violent, aggressive themes, and new research has shown that periodic impulse dyscontrol disorders respond to treatment (or, paradoxically, can be made worse by) serotonin-reuptake inhibitors.[8,35,37]

The Neuroanatomy of Obsessive-compulsive Behavior—Results of Neuroimaging Studies in Obsessive-compulsive Disorder

Structural studies of OCD subjects have yielded inconsistent but intriguing results. Luxenberg et al. in 1988,[33] using computed tomography (CT) scans, found decreased volume of the caudate heads in OCD subjects compared with controls. Follow-up studies by Garber et al.[12] and Kellner et al.,[27] however, using more sophisticated magnetic resonance imaging (MRI), failed to confirm these initial findings.

With regard to functional neuroimaging studies [positron emission tomography (PET), single photon emission computed tomography (SPECT)], a fairly consistent picture emerges. Numerous studies conducted in different centers with both PET[3–6,34,39,50,54] and SPECT[19] have consistently found *abnormalities in the orbitofrontal white matter and basal ganglia that change with pharmacologic or behavioral treatment.* This is one of the more consistent and remarkable findings in the recent history of biologic psychiatry and serves as the foundation for the ongoing revolution in understanding OCD.

It is important to realize that the differences noted in OCD are always found only on comparing group means. Unfortunately, we lack the ability to diagnose OCD on an individual basis using PET or SPECT. In addition, for almost all patients studied, as their OCD symptoms improve with either pharmacologic or behavioral treatment, the brain metabolism also changes to a more "normal" pattern.[19] The changes in brain metabolism thus appear to mirror the clinical improvement.

Recently, using oxygen PET and then in a later study with fast MRI, Rauch et al.[47] imaged regional brain activity in OCD patients before and during symptom provocation. Compared with before they are exposed to a provoking stimulus (such as a dirty rag for someone with a cleaning compulsion), OCD patients, when actively obsessing, show greatly increased activity in the right orbitofrontal lobe. At the NIMH, Greenberg et al.[18] attempted to expand on these studies and used noninvasive, repeated transcranial magnetic stimulation (rTMS) over the dorsolateral prefrontal cortex in an attempt to influence OC symptomatology. Results in OCD patients have been mixed with this promising technique of probing brain function.

Putative Neuroanatomic Model

These imaging studies begin to outline a tentative neuroanatomic model of primary OCD. This model may, in turn, help us to understand and organize the secondary causes of OCB. The circuit involved links the orbitofrontal region with the caudate nucleus, which projects to the globus pallidus, which then sends inhibitory fibers to the thalamus. The thalamus then sends excitatory fibers back to the prefrontal cortex, forming a closed loop. The final common pathway for OCD symptoms results from increased thalamofrontal activity. This fronto-caudate-pallidal-thalamo-frontal loop explains most of the cases of secondary OCD. According to this model, irritative lesions (e.g., epilepsy) of the frontal cortex or cingulate gyrus might produce OCD symptoms. Similarly, destructive lesions of the basal ganglia would also be predicted to worsen OCD symptoms by releasing the brake on the thalamus.

DIFFERENTIAL DIAGNOSIS

Primary or idiopathic OCD is, by definition, not associated with any known gross structural brain pathology. Obsessions or compulsions can, nevertheless, sometimes arise in other conditions or diseases that affect the critical brain regions just outlined (see Table 1) (for review, see George et al.[14]). When evaluating a patient with repetitive senseless actions, it is important to exclude obsessions or compulsions that may arise due to Sydenham chorea,[52] vascular or toxic basal ganglia lesions,[31,32,36,38,45,51,55,57] postencephalitic Parkinson disease (Von Economo encephalitis—encephalitis lethargica),[23,24,49] and central nervous system stimulant use.[9,29] Most of these disorders involve the *prefrontal lobes*, the *cingulate gyrus*, or the *basal ganglia*. These are the same regions that behave abnormally in recent neuroimaging studies of primary OCD subjects.

Properly evaluating the symptom of repetitive behavior can be a diagnostic challenge. Table 2 is an aid in determining whether the behavior is due to OCD or to localization-related epilepsy.

Patients with seizure discharges in the prefrontal or cingulate gyrus can present with OC symptoms. Ward described three patients with no past psychiatric or neurologic history who reported the new onset of the "feeling of compulsion" with no associated movement.[56] A 59-year-old woman suddenly developed an urge to walk to the left that she could not resist. Several weeks later, she developed a mild left hemiparesis. The electroencephalogram (EEG) showed a focal abnormality in the right frontal region, and CT scan revealed a *right frontoparietal glioblastoma.* A 43-year-old man experienced eight episodes over 2 months of a strong urge to shake his right arm, sometimes accompanied by an urge to shout, blurry

TABLE 1

DIFFERENTIAL DIAGNOSIS OF OBSESSIVE-COMPULSIVE BEHAVIOR

Primary or idiopathic obsessive–compulsive disorder
Gilles de la Tourette syndrome[15]
Sydenham chorea[52]
Postencephalitic Parkinsons disease[24]
Stimulant abuse (particularly amphetamines)[9]
Tumors and infarctions of the orbitofrontal lobe [55,57]
Multiple sclerosis[13]
Following closed-head injury with damage to prefrontal, cingulate, or basal ganglia[36]
Manganese toxicity[38]
Epilepsy[32,56]

TABLE 2

DIFFERENTIAL DIAGNOSIS OF OBSESSIVE-COMPULSIVE BEHAVIOR (OCB): PRIMARY OBSESSIVE-COMPULSIVE DISORDER (OCD) VERSUS OCB RELATED TO FOCAL EPILEPSY

	Primary OCD	OCB related to focal epilepsy
History	Chronic, remitting	Acute onset
Family history of OCD	+	–
Other OCD symptoms	+	–
Accompanying mental state	Clear, totally aware	Cloudy, +/– amnestic
Aware of senselessness of action	+	–
Clinical tests		
Neuropsychological tests	++	
Electroancephalogram	–	Slowing, localized discharge[a]
Single photon emission camputed tomography	–	Abnormal[a]
Serum prolactin	–	Increased[a]
Magnetic resonance imaging	–	Possible mesial temporal sclerosis
Clinical neurologic exam	Normal	Possible localization-related signs

[a]These may often be normal as well in patients with epilepsy.[2]

vision, or spatial disorientation. He later developed speech arrest and right arm weakness. EEG abnormalities were found in the left frontal and temporal areas, and a CT scan revealed a *left frontal glioblastoma*. Finally, a 62-year-old woman suddenly developed episodes in which she had the urge to shake her right arm, sometimes accompanied by an expressive dysphasia. An EEG showed left temporal slowing but no definite discharges or spikes. A CT scan showed *small lacunar infarcts in the right superior cerebellar peduncle and the left basal ganglia*. Kroll and Drummond[30] reported an interesting case of a 26-year-old man with a 6-year history of bizarre behavior who had been diagnosed as paranoid schizophrenic and was refractory to standard neuroleptic treatment. He had staring episodes, along with left shoulder and arm twitching. During these episodes, he described his thoughts as muddled or blocked, with increases in anxiety and obsessive thoughts, sometimes with an associated smell of sulfur. He had obsessive, intrusive thoughts about harming his mother, women, and babies. His neurologic exam and MRI scan were normal. An unmedicated EEG showed irregular activity at 5 to 7 Hz and focal slowing in the left temporal area. A presumptive diagnosis of *left-sided complex partial seizures* was made, and he was successfully treated with carbamazepine with resolution of the spells and obsessive thoughts.

These cases illustrate that obsessive-compulsive behaviors may arise in the setting of localization-related epilepsy, although this is rare. In all of the reported cases of OCB arising in the setting of epilepsy, key points in the history or physical or clinical investigations point toward the proper diagnosis and away from primary OCD. Thus, in contrast to primary OCD, localization-related seizures with OCB usually have an abrupt onset with no other associated OC behaviors and a negative family history for OCD. Often, focal seizures with OCB are found in someone with a clouded mental state who exhibits other behaviors that are not found in OCD (motor or sensory changes, smells, etc.). In almost all cases, the EEG or brain imaging studies were abnormal. EEG changes are not commonly seen in primary OCD,[22] and, as reviewed earlier, brain imaging studies in individual patients are normal. If the diagnosis remains unclear even after a thorough history, physical examination, and clinical workup, a treatment trial with an anticonvulsant may be in order. In general, anticonvulsants have not been found to be effective in primary OCD.

INVESTIGATIONS

There is no definitive clinical test for primary OCD. Thus, it is quite important to perform a thorough history and physical examination and to use the appropriate diagnostic tests to exclude the other diseases in the clinical differential (Table 1). To distinguish primary OCD from localization-related seizures with OCB, one would likely perform an MRI scan of the head, as well as an EEG (Table 2). Neuropsychological testing does not distinguish between idiopathic OCD and OCB in epilepsy because it is similar in both cases, showing a specific frontal-subcortical dysfunction.[7] If the diagnosis is still unclear, one could possibly obtain a serum prolactin after an OC event (probably elevated in epilepsy, normal in OCD) or even a SPECT scan (focally abnormal in seizures).

SUMMARY AND CONCLUSIONS

Recurrent obsessions and compulsions arise in a variety of clinical disorders that affect key brain regions (the cingulate, frontal and temporal lobes, and basal ganglia). Localization-related epilepsy is an infrequent cause of obsessions or compulsions. Much more commonly, OCB is due to primary OCD, although other neurologic illnesses must be excluded. In most cases of a patient presenting with obsessions or compulsions, a thorough history, physical exam, and associated diagnostic tests will lead to the proper diagnosis and treatment.

References

1. Alexander RC. Fluoxetine treatment of trichotillomania. *J Clin Psychiatry.* 1991;52:88.
2. American Psychiatric Association. *Diagnostic and Statistical Manual of Mental Disorders,* 4th ed. Washington DC: American Psychiatric Association; 1994.
3. Baxter LR, Phelps ME, Mazziotta JC, et al. Local cerebral glucose metabolic rates in obsessive-compulsive disorder. *Arch Gen Psychiatry.* 1987;44:211–218.

4. Baxter LR, Schwartz JM, Guze BH, et al. PET imaging in obsessive compulsive disorder with and without depression. *J Clin Psychiatry*. 1990;51:61–69.
5. Baxter LR, Schwartz JM, Mazziotta JC, et al. Cerebral glucose metabolic rates in non-depressed patients with obsessive-compulsive disorder. *Am J Psychiatry*. 1988;145:1560–1563.
6. Benkelfat C, Nordahl TE, Semple WE, et al. Local cerebral glucose metabolic rates in obsessive-compulsive disorder. *Arch Gen Psychiatry*. 1990;47:840–848.
7. Berthier ML, Kulisevsky J, Gironell A, et al. Obsessive compulsive disorder associated with brain lesions: Clinical phenomenology, cognitive function, and anatomic correlates. *Neurology*. 1996;47(2):353–361.
8. Bitler DA, Linnoila M, George DT. Psychosocial and diagnostic characteristics of individuals initiating domestic violence. *J Nerv Ment Dis*. 1994;182:583–585.
9. Ellinwood EH Jr. Amphetamine psychosis I. Description of the individuals and process. *J Nerv Ment Dis*. 1967;144:273–283.
10. Fineberg NA, Bullock T, Montgomery DB, et al. Serotonin reuptake inhibitors are the treatment of choice in obsessive compulsive disorder. *Int Clin Psychopharmacol*. 1992;7:43–47.
11. Foa EB, Goldstein A. Continuous exposure and complete response prevention in the treatment of obsessive compulsive neurosis. *Behav Ther*. 1978;9:821–829.
12. Garber HJ, Ananth JV, Chiu LC, et al. Nuclear magnetic resonance study of obsessive-compulsive disorder. *Am J Psychiatry*. 1989;146:1001–1005.
13. George MS, Kellner CH, Fossey MD. Obsessive-compulsive symptoms in a patient with multiple sclerosis. *J Nerv Ment Dis*. 1989;177:304–305.
14. George MS, Melvin JA, Kellner CH. Obsessive-compulsive symptoms in neurologic disease: A review. *Behav Neurol*. 1992;5:19–30.
15. George MS, Trimble MR, Ring HA, et al. Obsessions in obsessive-compulsive disorder (OCD) with and without Gilles de la Tourette syndrome (GTS). *Am J Psychiatry*. 1993;150:93–97.
16. George MS, Trimble MR, Robertson MM. Fluvoxamine and sulpiride in comorbid obsessive-compulsive disorder and Gilles de la Tourette syndrome. *Hum Psychopharmacol*. 1993;8:327–334.
17. Goodman WK, Price LH, Rasmussen SA, et al. Fluvoxamine as an antiobsessional agent. *Psychopharmacol Bull*. 1989;25:31–35.
18. Greenberg B, George MS, Dearing J, et al. Transcranial magnetic stimulation in OCD [Abstract]. In: *APA New Research Abstracts*. Washington, DC: APA Press; 1995.
19. Hoehn-Saric R, Pearlson GD, Harris GJ, et al. Effects of fluoxetine on regional cerebral blood flow in obsessive-compulsive patients. *Am J Psychiatry*. 1991;148:1243–1245.
20. Hollander E, Liebowitz MR, Winchel R, et al. Treatment of body-dysmorphic disorder with serotonin reuptake blockers. *Am J Psychiatry*. 1989;146:768–770.
21. Holzer JC, Goodman WK, McDougle CJ, et al. Obsessive-compulsive disorder with and without a chronic tic disorder. A comparison of symptoms in 70 patients. *Br J Psychiatry*. 1994;164:469–473.
22. Insel TR, Donnelly EF, Lalakea ML, et al. Neurological and neuropsychological studies of patients with obsessive-compulsive disorder. *Biol Psychiatry*. 1983;18:741–751.
23. Jelliffe SE. *Postencephalitic Respiratory Disorders*. Washington, DC: Nervous and Mental Disease Publishing; 1927.
24. Jelliffe SE. *Psychopathology of Forced Movements and the Oculogyric Crises of Lethargic Encephalitis*. Washington, DC: Nervous and Mental Disease Publishing; 1932.
25. Jenike MA, Hyman S, Baer L, et al. A controlled trial of fluvoxamine in obsessive-compulsive disorder: Implications for a serotonergic theory. *Am J Psychiatry*. 1990;147:1209–1215.
26. Karno M, Golding JM, Sorenson SB, et al. The epidemiology of obsessive compulsive disorder in five U.S. communities. *Arch Gen Psychiatry*. 1988;45:1094–1099.
27. Kellner CH, Jolley RR, Holgate RC, et al. Brain MRI in obsessive-compulsive disorder. *Psychol Res*. 1991;36:45–49.
28. Kelly A, Moriarty J, George MS. Fluvoxamine vs. clomipramine in OCD: A multi-center, randomized, double-blind study [Abstract]. *Neuropsychopharmacology*. 1994;10:27, 47, 13s.
29. Koizumi HM. Obsessive compulsive symptoms following stimulants. *Biol Psychiatry*. 1985;20:1332–1337.
30. Kroll L, Drummond LM. Temporal lobe epilepsy and obsessive-compulsive symptoms. *J Nerv Ment Dis*. 1993;181:457–458.
31. Laplane D, Levasseur M, Pillon B, et al. Obsessive-compulsive and other behavioural changes with bilateral basal ganglia lesions. *Brain*. 1989;112:699–725.
32. Laplane D, Widlocher D, Pillon B, et al. Comportement compulsif d'allure obsessionnelle par necrose circonscrite bilaterale pallido-striatale. *Rev Neurol*. 1981;137:269–276.
33. Luxenberg JS, Swedo SE, Flament MF, et al. Neuroanatomic abnormalities in obsessive compulsive disorder with quantitative x-ray computed tomography. *Am J Psychiatry*. 1988;145:1089–1093.
34. Martinot JL, Allilaire JF, Mazoyer BM, et al. Obsessive-compulsive disorder: A clinical, neuropsychological and positron emission tomography study. *Acta Psychiatr Scand*. 1990;82:233–242.
35. McElroy SL, Phillips KA, Keck PE. Obsessive compulsive spectrum disorder. *J Clin Psychiatry*. 1994;55s:33–51.
36. McKeon J, McGuffin P, Robinson P. Obsessive-compulsive neurosis following head injury: A report of four cases. *Br J Psychiatry*. 1984;144:190–192.
37. Mehlman PT, Higley JD, Faucher I, et al. Low CSF 5-HIAA concentrations and severe aggression and impaired impulse control in nonhuman primates. *Am J Psychiatry*. 1994;151:1485–1491.
38. Mena I, Marik O, Fuenzalida S, et al. Chronic manganese poisoning. *Neurology*. 1967;17:128–136.
39. Nordahl TE, Benkelfat C, Semple WE, et al. Cerebral glucose metabolic rates in obsessive-compulsive disorder. *Neuropsychopharmacology*. 1989;2:23–28.
40. Pato MT, Zohar-Kadouch R, Zohar J, et al. Return of symptoms after discontinuation of clomipramine in patients with obsessive-compulsive disorder. *Am J Psychiatry*. 1988;145:1521–1525.
41. Pauls DL, Leckman JF. The inheritance of Gilles de la Tourette syndrome and associated behaviors. *N Engl J Med*. 1986;315:993–997.
42. Pauls DL, Leckman JF, Towbin KE, et al. A possible genetic relationship exists between Tourette's syndrome and obsessive-compulsive disorder. *Psychopharmacol Bull*. 1986;22:730–733.
43. Pauls DL, Towbin KE, Leckman JF, et al. Gilles de la Tourette's syndrome and obsessive-compulsive disorder: Evidence supporting a genetic relationship. *Arch Gen Psychiatry*. 1986;43:1180–1182.
44. Perse TL, Greist JH, Jefferson JW, et al. Fluvoxamine treatment of obsessive-compulsive disorder. *Am J Psychiatry*. 1987;144:1543–1548.
45. Pulst S, Walshe TM, Romero JA. Carbon monoxide poisoning with features of Gilles de la Tourette syndrome. *Arch Neurol*. 1983;40:443–444.
46. Rasmussen SA, Eisen JA. Epidemiology of obsessive-compulsive disorder. *J Clin Psychiatry*. 1990;51:10–15.
47. Rauch SL, Jenike MA, Alpert NM, et al. Regional cerebral blood flow measured during symptom provocation in obsessive-compulsive disorder using 15O-labelled CO_2 and positron emission tomography. *Arch Gen Psychiatry*. 1994;51:62.
48. Riddle MA, Leckman JF, Hardin MT, et al. Fluoxetine treatment of obsessions and compulsions in patients with Tourette's syndrome. *Am J Psychiatr*. 1988;145:1173–1174.
49. Sacks O. *Awakenings*. New York: Doubleday; 1974.
50. Sawle GV, Hymas NF, Lees AJ, et al. Obsessional slowness: Functional studies with positron emission tomography. *Brain*. 1991;114:2191–2202.
51. Seibyl JP, Krystal JH, Goodman WK, et al. Obsessive-compulsive symptoms in a patient with a right frontal lobe lesion. *Neuropsychiatr Neuropsychol Behav Neurol*. 1989;1:295–299.
52. Swedo SE. Sydenham's chorea: A model for childhood autoimmune neuropsychiatric disorders. *JAMA*. 1994;272:1788–1791.
53. Swedo SE, Leonard HL, Rapoport JL, et al. A double-blind comparison of clomipramine and desipramine in the treatment of trichotillomania (hair pulling). *N Engl J Med*. 1989;32:497–501.
54. Swedo SE, Schapiro MB, Grady CL, et al. Cerebral glucose metabolism in childhood onset obsessive-compulsive disorder. *Arch Gen Psychiatry*. 1989;46:518–523.
55. Tonkonogy J, Barriera P. Obsessive-compulsive disorder and caudate-frontal lesion. *Neuropsychiatr Neuropsychol Behav Neurol*. 1989;2:203–209.
56. Ward CD. Transient feelings of compulsion caused by hemispheric lesions: Three cases. *J Neurol Neurosurg Psychiatry*. 1988;51:266–268.
57. Weilburg JB, Mesulam M, Weintraub S, et al. Focal striatal abnormalities in a patient with obsessive-compulsive disorder. *Arch Neurol*. 1989;46:233–235.
58. Zohar J, Kaplan Z, Benjamin J. Compulsive exhibitionism successfully treated with fluvoxamine: A controlled case study. *J Clin Psychiatry*. 1994;55:86–88.

CHAPTER 287 ■ NONAFFECTIVE PSYCHOSES, SCHIZOPHRENIA, AND SCHIZOPHRENIA-LIKE PSYCHOSES

MICHAEL R. TRIMBLE AND BETTINA SCHMITZ

INTRODUCTION

In this chapter, in contrast to Chapter 204, we consider the clinical occasions in which some of the symptoms of schizophrenia may be mistaken for those of epilepsy. In reality, there are very few situations in which this arises, and when they do, there are usually obvious causes for the confusion. We do not discuss the clinical phenomenology, investigations, and treatment of schizophrenia per se, and refer the interested reader to Chapter 270 by Jadresic in the first edition of this work.[9a]

In contrast to disorders of affect, psychotic states, although they imply a severe disturbance of neurologic function, are less frequently encountered than disturbances of mood in neurologic practice. There are many reasons for this, not the least being that many people with neurologic disorders and reduced quality of life experience depression as a consequence, and, in general, a number of neurologic disorders influence areas of the brain that are linked to the regulation of mood, emphasizing the frontal-striatal axis.

The brain must allow the individual to interpret the world in which he or she lives in an orderly manner so that he or she can behave in a logical and adaptive way. The symptoms of psychosis, however, such as hallucinations and delusions, suggest deviant neurologic processing, and underlying this will be disturbances of neurologic function, often secondary to structural disease. The close association between some neurologic disorders and psychoses suggests neurochemical and or neuroanatomic bases for the abnormal mental states, for example, the psychoses associated with Parkinson disease and l-dopa therapies. There are biologic underpinnings to the psychotic disorders of epilepsy, and these are discussed in Chapter 204. It is interesting that, as noted, the discussions revolve around similar anatomic deviations as in schizophrenia in the absence of epilepsy and involve medial temporal structures, the amygdala and hippocampus in particular, and their efferent projections.[17]

TERMINOLOGY

The term *psychosis* generally refers to a condition in which there are hallucinations and delusions associated with abnormalities in behavior such as excitement and overactivity or psychomotor retardation, or catatonia, in which insight is diminished or lost.

A *hallucination* is a perception in the absence of an adequate sensory stimulus, and it must be distinguished from an *illusion*, which is due to a misinterpretation of perceptions. *Pseudo-hallucinations* are hallucinatory experiences that occur in subjective rather than objective space, are less clearly delineated, and thus lack the objectivity of hallucinations proper. The latter have concrete reality and are linked to a lack of insight into their nature.

Delusions are unshakable convictions that are manifestly incorrect. They have to be interpreted within the patients' cultural setting, but it is the tenacity with which patients hold onto their beliefs against all logic that inevitably reveals the delusion. They need to be distinguished from overvalued ideas, which are strongly held beliefs that are not incorrigible.

Delusions are the hallmark of a paranoid illness and occur in a spectrum of psychiatric disorders, including schizophrenia. In the affective disorders, they are characteristically mood congruent, whereas mood-incongruent delusions are typical for schizophrenia. In the *Capgras syndrome*, a significant person in the patient's life is replaced by a supposed identical double, and in the *Fregoli syndrome*, a supposed persecutor can change his or her appearance and appear as other people. These are referred to as *misidentification syndromes*.

Hallucinations that occur in clear consciousness for which there is no insight and that are mood incongruent are very suggestive of schizophrenia. In this condition, they are usually auditory, although patients may experience them in any modality. Specific auditory hallucinations noted in association with schizophrenia are referred to as being among the Schneiderian first-rank symptoms. These are listed in Table 1. When present in clear consciousness, they usually signify schizophrenia, although this is not diagnostic because they are sometimes noted in other psychotic disorders—for example, in mania. Furthermore, the diagnosis of schizophrenia can be made in their absence based on history and other observed abnormal behavior.

Olfactory hallucinations are reported in schizophrenia and in simple partial seizures of the uncinate variety. In epilepsy, these experiences are typically brief, unpleasant, hard to characterize, and consistent in their phenomenology. In schizophrenia, they are much more variable and may last for considerable periods of time, and they are usually accompanied by a delusional interpretation. In coenesthetic hallucinations, the body or part of the body feels altered or distorted, often in quite fantastic ways. Although often reported in schizophrenia, they may occur in migraine or following cerebrovascular accidents.

A characteristic feature of schizophrenia is alteration of thought and language. This may vary from a subtle flattening of the expression and concrete thinking to a florid schizaphasia. In the latter, neologisms (paraphasias) emerge, there are loose connections between thoughts and tangential thinking, and intrusive delusional content can lead to a veritable "word salad."

TABLE 1

THE FIRST-RANK SYMPTOMS OF SCHNEIDER[a]

Thought withdrawal
Thought broadcasting
Hearing one's thoughts spoken aloud
Hearing voices arguing about or discussing one
Hearing voices comment on one's actions
Delusional perception[b]
Experiencing bodily sensations as if imposed from outside
Experiencing affects as if imposed and controlled from outside
Experiencing impulses as if imposed and controlled from outside
Experiencing motor actions as if imposed and controlled from outside

[a]These are not diagnostic of anything, but when present in the setting of clear consciousness, support a diagnosis of schizophrenia.
[b]Abnormal significance is attached to a real perception without any logical explanation.

PAROXYSMAL SYMPTOMS IN SCHIZOPHRENIA

The diagnosis of schizophrenia is usually not difficult to make in the advanced case, especially with knowledge of the patient's history. However, by the time the patient has revealed his or her aberrant behavior and psychotic thinking, the underlying disorder will be well advanced. There is often evidence of difficult and unusual behavior going back to childhood, with comments about the person being different, a loner, and the like, and perhaps using unusual language or manifesting unusual thought processes for several years. A family history may be revealed (but is often concealed), and typically academic decline becomes apparent in the teenage years, often blamed on either stress or illicit drug taking.

Such cases usually first go to a psychiatrist for diagnostic evaluation, and if the diagnosis is clear, these patients may remain under psychiatric care for many years. In the early, uncertain stages of the disorder, however, patients with a developing schizophrenia may be referred to a neurologist, but usually on the grounds of academic failure and personality change, suggestive of a developing organic brain syndrome—the dementia praecox of Kraepelin. Such referrals, however, are not usually in reference to epilepsy.

The signs and symptoms of schizophrenia that are most likely to be confused with epilepsy are quite limited. They relate especially to the paroxysmal nature of the presentations and to the neurologic-soundingness of them. The signs are those of the motor disturbances of catatonia, and the symptoms are usually hallucinations, especially affecting the body image. Certain first-rank symptoms are also relevant, especially thought withdrawal and thought insertion.

MOVEMENT DISORDERS

The classic motor disorder of schizophrenia is catatonia, and for Kraepelin this deserved a separate nosologic category.[10] It seems that catatonic forms are much less apparent now than 100 years ago; one reason may be the effective intervention of psychotic disorders with neuroleptic drugs. The original descriptions of these movement abnormalities revealed a wide range of motoric instability, from tics and dyskinesias to frank dystonia. Stereotypies, echophenomena, mannerisms, and special signs such as automatic obedience and negativism were reported, and such abnormal movements were thought to be integral to the condition. This was before the introduction of neuroleptic drugs and the later widespread reporting of tardive motor syndromes. It is estimated that around 50% of untreated schizophrenics display such motor abnormalities.[11,12]

Cutting referred to catatonia as follows[6]:

> Catatonia is the generic name for about eight separate disorders of movement and posture, which have in common a tendency to be intermittent, to defy classification as disorders of power, tone, co-ordination, praxis or involuntary movement, and in a general sense to involve the surrender of the affected person's will. (p. 277)

The paradigmatic picture is of immobility, and the classic picture of catatonia with unresponsiveness and postures held sometimes for hours, which may reveal a waxy flexibility, was often illustrated in early pictures and film clips of schizophrenia. However, this represents only a part of the catatonic spectrum. More relevant for the diagnostic issues of epilepsy are the sudden episodes of catatonic excitement. These can vary from brief to longer disruptions of behavior (seconds to hours), in which the patient suddenly becomes overactive with hyperkinesis, even violent, as if being strung from their motoric slumber by the sudden onset of a seizure. These episodes seem free from environmental or emotional precipitants, and after the period of overexcitement, there is a resumption of the status quo.

Other abnormal movements that may occasionally lead to diagnostic confusion are tics. These will only very rarely be myoclonic in form, however, and are much more often brief but repetitive, associated with other behavior changes of the type noted earlier such as in habits and mannerisms.

After noting that patients may have seizures (and in his time epileptic seizures were reported quite often in schizophrenia, presumably because of the number of secondary forms he was witnessing from, e.g., encephalitis and syphilis), Kraepelin continued[10]:

> There are spasms in single muscle groups (face, arm), tetany or even apoplectic seizures with paralysis which last for a considerable time.... In a whole series of patients (6% of the men and 3% of the women) spasms and fainting fits occurred previously in youth.... The spasmodic phenomena in the musculature of the face and of speech ... resemble movements of expression, wrinkling of the forehead, distortion of the corners of the mouth, irregular movements of the tongues and lips, twisting of the eyes, opening them wide and shutting them tight. (p. 83) The patient who has been senselessly excited may suddenly become mute and motionless; the patient who has been stuporous, perhaps for weeks, abruptly begins to utter unintelligible screams ... or he leaps with long bounds through the room ... and then remains again inaccessible, or possibly even passes through a longer period of excitement. (p. 148)

These paroxysmal bursts of abnormal behavior, which were so well described in the past, are much rarer today, and are not recognized by a generation of psychiatrists and neurologists poorly versed in the intricacies of phenomenologic psychiatry. When they do occur, they often lead to a question of an underlying seizure disorder and a request for neurologic evaluation. It is then not uncommon to ask for an electroencephalogram (EEG), which may then be reported as abnormal, raising further the suspicion of epilepsy (see later discussion).

A good history will confirm the diagnosis of schizophrenia, but a clear description of the abnormal behavior from a nurse, physician, or caregiver can be revealing by fairly quickly establishing that the paroxysms are simply not like epileptic seizures in their semiology. There is no clear seizure as such, no alteration or loss of consciousness, and no repetition of the progression of the attack with each recurrence as there is with epileptic seizures. The earlier history is that of schizophrenia, as outlined previously, and not that of epilepsy. In fact, careful questions about attacks resembling complex partial or secondary generalized seizures note an absence of such a background: There are no febrile convulsions, no clear episodes of loss of consciousness, and no suggestions of a localizing neurologic sign.

Further questioning will reveal the diagnosis; it is the company that such symptoms keep that is relevant. There will be ongoing delusions, a failure of the patient to explain or even describe his or her attacks, and a lack of insight.

HALLUCINATIONS

Hallucinations may be in any modality, but the coenesthetic and olfactory ones are the most likely to cause diagnostic confusion. Olfactory hallucinations are reported in patients with simple partial seizures and very rarely as the sole manifestation of the seizure. No more than about 7% to 10% of patients with temporal lobe epilepsy, however, report olfactory hallucinations,[4] and the classification of the seizure is often referred to as an uncinate seizure. In reality, the site of origin of the episode may be in the hippocampal uncinate, but it may arise from elsewhere, such as the insula. The experience, however, is vivid, repeated, unpleasant, and evanescent. It is not usually accompanied by an abnormal taste, but the latter is not perhaps unexpected. In clinical practice, the question is often put to a patient, "Do you have any unusual tastes or smells that accompany your attacks?" The answer is often given in the affirmative, and such replies as "a metallic taste" or a variant of that are given. This is recorded in the patient's notes as an uncinate event, in spite of the fact that it is nothing like the descriptions of patients with epilepsy with established smell auras. Such fleeting metallic tastes and other variant smells are commonly reported in patients who are then misdiagnosed as having epilepsy and are later rediagnosed as nonepileptic.

In a similar way, the smell hallucinations in schizophrenia may be misinterpreted. These are the third-most-common form of hallucination reported in schizophrenia (after auditory and visual ones), but gustatory hallucinations are less frequent. Cutting[5] gave a figure of 6% reporting of olfactory hallucinations in schizophrenia. The latter are rather diffuse; sometimes good and sometimes bad; may be flitting or lasting in an individual patient; and are often characterized, unlike those of the uncinate seizures, which are hard to specify and describe. The schizophrenic smells himself or herself, others, food, or evidence of good or evil, whereas the patient with epilepsy refers to unpleasant smells as unpleasant, perhaps like burning rubber. As with the aberrant motoric behaviors described earlier, further questioning will reveal the psychotic attachments to the smell experience, and the underling schizophrenic disorder.

Coenesthetic hallucinations relate to disturbances of the body and the body image. For probable historical reasons, they are poorly discussed in English-language texts on psychopathology, but they have attracted much more attention on the European continent. Fleeting sensory disturbances, shots of pain, pulling, squeezing, twisting, and the like of the body or parts of the body are described, and their paroxysmal nature gives rise to the suspicion of a simple partial seizure. Many physicians are unaware of the relative frequency of such hallucinations, tending to identify only visual and auditory events with hallucinations proper. Corporeal sensations are common in schizophrenia, however, and like olfactory hallucinations, have a different quality from the equivalent epileptic event. They are usually unpleasant or painful, and may be sexual. They last for varying lengths of time and vary with each description. They come and go over time, without the stereotyped nature of the experiences of a simple partial seizure. Again, a few questions will reveal the attached delusional thinking.

Formal thought disorder refers to patterns of thinking seen in schizophrenia and other psychoses, central to which is disorganization and concretization of thought. Such terms as fusion, derailment, lack of association, and interpenetration of thoughts are self-explanatory, however these are revealed by the patients during history taking, and would not relate to any diagnostic confusion with epilepsy.

The three symptoms that are sometimes confused are thought insertion, in which ideas or words are interpenetrated into the patient's mind; thought blocking; and thought withdrawal. In the latter two, patients claim that their thoughts are being interfered with by some outside agency, with sudden stoppages to the flow of the thoughts. The patient suddenly ceases to speak, his or her line of thought is interrupted, and he or she may momentarily appear blank or confused. The paroxysmal and brief nature of this may make it seem like an epileptic seizure, and the episodes can be frequently repeated, but clinical perception soon reveals the psychotic form underlying these events.

ELECTROENCEPHALOGRAPHIC FINDINGS IN SCHIZOPHRENIA

Hill[7] reviewed the results of early EEG findings of abnormalities in schizophrenia. Schizophrenic patients typically exhibit low-amplitude irregular EEGs, described as "choppy,"[7] and numerous qualitative studies indicate abnormal conventional EEG findings in 20% to 60% of schizophrenic patients. The abnormalities described in schizophrenia included left-sided slow-wave asymmetries, especially at the left anterior temporal area and occasionally involving the left frontal and parietal areas, slow bursts, and spikes or sharp waves.[13,14] Stevens et al.[15] showed by 24-hour telemetry recordings that temporal EEG abnormalities occur in 30% of schizophrenic patients. Schizophrenic patients with EEG abnormalities that appeared either before or during neuroleptic treatment had more evidence of brain dysfunction than did patients without such EEG abnormalities.

Considerable attention has been devoted to the hypothesis that schizophrenia is primarily associated with dominant hemispheric dysfunction. Abrahams and Taylor[1] showed that schizophrenic patients had twice as many, mostly left-sided, temporal abnormalities compared to patients with affective disorders, who have more right-sided EEG findings.

A recent study by Inui et al.[9] looked into electroencephalographic abnormalities in 143 patients whose discharge diagnoses met the *Diagnostic and Statistical Manual of Mental Disorders*, 4th edition,[2] criteria for mood disorder, schizophrenia, and other psychotic disorders. The study revealed that the frequency of epileptiform variants, including the phantom spike and wave, positive spikes, and small sharp spikes, was significantly higher among patients with mood-incongruent psychotic mood disorder (33%), schizoaffective disorder (33%), and schizophreniform disorder (30%) as compared with patients with nonpsychotic mood disorder (3.2%) and schizophrenia (0%). The results implied that patients with "atypical" psychoses, which are located between typical mood disorder and schizophrenia, might have a biologic vulnerability to seizures, as represented by these epileptiform EEG variants. These associations also pose diagnostic challenges, however, because patients with atypical presentations are the ones most likely to lead to diagnostic confusion.

STRUCTURAL ABNORMALITIES

Another potential source of confusion arises in cases in which a patient with schizophrenia has some paroxysmal behavior disorder and, in addition to the EEG, a brain scan is performed. It has been known for a long time that schizophrenia is associated with changes on scans, both computed tomography and magnetic resonance imaging, the main findings being ventricular dilation and tissue loss, including loss of hippocampal neurons. Thus, some dilation of the temporal horns of the lateral ventricles may be noted, with decreased temporal lobe volume, increasing the suspicion that the case may be one of epilepsy.[16] This rarely relates to a hippocampal sclerosis, however, and in fact one of the consistent differences in the neuropathology of temporal lobe epilepsy in comparison to schizophrenia is the absence of gliosis in the schizophrenic hippocampus. Nonetheless, cases of hippocampal sclerosis are rarely described in patients with schizophrenia who do not have overt epileptic seizures, and the links between the sclerosis and the subsequent psychosis are unclear.

COMORBIDITY OF EPILEPSY AND PSYCHOSIS DUE TO A COMMON UNDERLYING CONDITION

There are a number of disorders in which epilepsy and psychosis both develop secondary to an underlying usually progressive neurologic disorder. The causes are legion although each individual disorder itself is quite rare. The reader is referred to Cummings and Mega[3] for an extended list of neurologic disorders that can be linked to the development of schizophrenia-like states, but most are not also linked to epilepsy. However, encephalitides, some storage disorders, endocrine disorders such as hypoparathyroidism, and inflammatory conditions such as systemic lupus erythematosis may all occasionally cause diagnostic confusion as to whether the developing psychosis is somehow linked to an underlying epilepsy, although the progressive nature of the disease will likely soon be revealed.

SUMMARY AND CONCLUSIONS

In clinical practice, schizophrenia is not often confused with epilepsy, but the reasons that this sometimes does occur are clear. Many physicians who manage epilepsy are unfamiliar with the polymorphous presentations of schizophrenia and are unaware of the paroxysmal nature of many of the symptoms, especially the motor disorders. Further confusion may arise with misinterpretations of the EEG and, occasionally, any brain imaging. Careful clinical evaluation should resolve diagnostic confusion, however, although neuropsychiatric evaluation will most likely be essential to this endeavor.

References

1. Abrahams R, Taylor MA. Differential EEG patterns in affective disorder and schizophrenia. *Arch Gen Psychiatry*. 1979;36:1355–1358.
2. American Psychiatric Association. *Diagnostic and Statistical Manual of Mental Disorders,* 4th ed. Washington DC: American Psychiatric Association; 1994.
3. Cummings JL, Mega MS. *Neuropsychiatry and Behavioural Neuroscience*. Oxford: Oxford University Press; 2003.
4. Currie S, Heathfield KWG, Henson RA, et al. Clinical course and prognosis of temporal lobe epilepsy: A survey of 666 patients. *Brain*. 1971;94:173–190.
5. Cutting J. *Principles of Psychopathology*. Oxford: Oxford University Press; 1997.
6. Cutting J. *The Psychology of Schizophrenia*. Edinburgh: Churchill Livingstone; 1985.
7. Davies PA. Evaluation of the electroencephalogram of schizophrenic patients. *Am J Psychiatry*. 1940;96:851.
8. Hill D. Psychiatry. In Hill D, Parr G, eds. *Electroencephalography*. London: MacDonald; 1950:319–363.
9. Inui K, Motomura E, Okushima R, et al. Electroencephalographic findings in patients with DSM IV mood disorder, schizophrenia, and other psychotic disorders. *Biol Psychiatry*. 1998;43:69–75.

9a. Jadresic D. Nonaffective Psychoses: Schizophrenia and schizophreniative psychoses. In: Engle J. Jr., Pedley TA (eds.) *Epilepsy: A Comprehensive Textbook*. Philadelphia, Lippincott-Raven; 1998:2797–2804.

10. Kraepelin E. *Dementia Praecox*. Edinburgh: E and S Livingston; 1919.
11. Owens DGC, Johnstone EC, Frith CO. Spontaneous involuntary disorders of movement. *Arch Gen Psychiatry*. 1982;39:452–561.
12. Rogers D. The movement disorders of severe psychiatric illness: A conflict of paradigms. *Br J Psychiatry*. 1985;147:221–232.
13. Small JG, Milstein V, Sharpley PH. Electroencephalographic findings in relation to diagnostic constructs in psychiatry. *Biol Psychiatry*. 1984;19:471–487.
14. Small JG. Psychiatric disorders and EEG. In: Niedermeyer E, Lopes da Silva F, eds. *Electroencephalography: Basic Principles, Clinical Applications, and Related Fields*. Baltimore, Williams & Wilkins; 1993:581–596.
15. Stevens JR, Bigelow L, Denney D, et al. Telemetered EEG-EEG during psychotic behaviours of schizophrenia. *Arch Gen Psychiatry*. 1979;36:251–262.
16. Sudath RL, Casanova MF, Goldberg TE, et al. Temporal lobe pathology in schizophrenia: A quantitative MRI study. *Am J Psychiatry*. 1989;146:464–472.
17. Trimble MR. *Biological Psychiatry,* 2nd ed. Chichester, UK: John Wiley; 1996.

CHAPTER 288 ■ OVERVIEW: DELIVERY OF HEALTH CARE AND SOCIOECONOMIC ISSUES

ROBERT J. GUMNIT, JOSEMIR W. SANDER, AND SIMON D. SHORVON

INTRODUCTION

As medical care becomes more sophisticated and thus more expensive, people and governments find that they must make difficult choices about where money earmarked for health will be spent. The expectations for care of people may vary from country to country and from culture to culture, although the desire for good treatment and cure will not. The duties of a conventional health care delivery system in relation to epilepsy, regardless of location, are similar (Table 1). The means to deliver care and the way it is organized, however, differ from country to country.

This section explores the ways in which different countries seek to meet the health needs of people with epilepsy. Before beginning a country-by-country survey, it is worthwhile defining, as far as possible, the general issues that each country must face. This section also reviews the socioeconomic issues that confront epilepsy care. Full socioeconomic appraisals of different epilepsy treatments and health delivery have not been undertaken, and therefore there are many remaining questions in this area.

LEVELS OF CARE

Primary Care

Primary care is defined as the care given by the first physician whom the patient ordinarily consults. The primary care physician is expected to possess some knowledge of a broad range of medical problems. Primary care physicians provide excellent care for many medical conditions, especially common problems. It is more difficult, however, for a primary care physician to keep abreast of modern methods of diagnosis and treatment of diseases with a low incidence. For example, in the United States, the average primary care physician sees one new case of epilepsy every 2 years. In the United Kingdom, a general medical practitioner (GP) might expect to diagnose one or two new cases each year, as well as having a caseload of 8 to 12 people with active epilepsy. The responsibility for long-term prescribing for patients varies from country to country. In the United Kingdom, this is an important responsibility of primary care physicians, but in other settings it is usually devolved to secondary care providers.

The ratio of primary care physicians to specialty physicians varies widely from country to country and within countries, especially between urban and rural areas. This ratio affects national policy regarding the management of chronic disease of relatively low incidence. In some countries, primary care is provided by nurses, health visitors, and also by other health care workers. In some resource-poor countries, practitioners of traditional medicine may also play a role.

Secondary Care

Secondary care denotes the most common type of specialty care. A general surgeon, general internist (physician), pediatrician, and, in some parts of the world, a neurologist would be considered to provide secondary care. In some countries, the dividing line is not sharp; in the United States, a general internist may practice some primary care medicine. Nonetheless, the underlying concept is that the practice is limited to certain problems so as to allow for greater in-depth knowledge on the part of the physician. Even so, in secondary care, the range of problems dealt with is relatively broad.

Tertiary Care

Tertiary care is the most specialized level. In epilepsy care, physicians with a prior qualification in neurology usually provide this, although physicians from other specialties are often involved (notably neurosurgery, psychiatry, clinical neurophysiology, and internal medicine). In most countries, tertiary care is available in teaching or university settings.

Specialized Centers or Fourth-level Care

With the increasing complexity of medicine, a fourth level of specialized care is developing in many countries. Patients with complex forms of blood dyscrasias or who require bone marrow transplantation or heart, lung, or liver transplantation are examples of people who receive fourth-level care in highly specialized centers. Epilepsy is one of few chronic diseases for which highly specialized centers have developed, although these are usually restricted to developed countries, with only a few in resource-poor countries.

ORGANIZATION OF HEALTH CARE SYSTEMS

The organization of systems by which care is delivered varies widely from country to country and often even within countries. In most countries, a mix of systems is found. In some countries, however, practitioners no longer practice alone, and in other, particularly resource-poor countries, multispecialty clinics have not developed, again largely because of socioeconomic factors.

TABLE 1

THE DUTIES OF A HEALTH CARE SYSTEM IN RELATION TO EPILEPSY

1. Identification of people with the condition
2. Diagnostic evaluation
3. Choice of drug treatment at all stages of the condition
4. Initial management, reevaluation of patients who have not responded to the initial choice of therapy, and long-term management of the disease
5. Management of emergencies
6. Management of complications and secondary consequences of the condition
7. Delivery of preventive care

Individual Practitioners

Classically, in the United States, physicians were in private practice, often alone in a solo practice. For reasons of convenience (sharing night calls) or expense (sharing overhead costs), groups of physicians began to practice together in a single office. In the United Kingdom, at the start of the National Health Service in 1948 many GPs were "single handed," but currently GPs are more likely to work in partnerships of three to six doctors.

Single-specialty Groups

All members of these groups of physicians are ordinarily engaged in a single specialty, for example, family practice or pediatrics. Groups of this sort are found in many parts of the world where there is a private system of medicine, but in the United Kingdom they are generally only found in the case of GP partnerships.

Polyclinics

The term *polyclinic* has different meanings in different countries. It is used here to mean a highly organized group of physicians, usually on a salaried basis, who provide a full range of services, from primary through specialized care. The degree of specialization, of course, varies widely.

Multispecialty Clinics

Much more commonly found in European countries and the United States, multispecialty clinics often do not include primary care physicians. Rather, aggregations or departments based on specialty are housed under an umbrella organization. In most parts of the world, these multispecialty clinics are organized about major hospital centers or universities.

Forms of Hospital-based Practice

There is great variability in the way that hospital-based care is provided throughout the world. In some countries, primary care physicians can admit patients directly to a hospital and decide whether to consult a specialist. In other places, only a specialist can admit a patient to a hospital where specialized care is available, and the primary care physician relinquishes control over the patient. In some countries, these hospital-based practices are essentially run by the government, either through a health authority or under the aegis of a university.

SOCIOECONOMIC CONSIDERATIONS

In most countries, health care delivery is often limited by financial considerations and the availability of resources. In each country, therefore, decisions are made about priorities. For instance, in resource-poor countries, the treatment of infection may be more of a priority than the treatment of chronic diseases.

A logical decision on health care provision may involve the most cost-effective treatment for any condition. The cost-effectiveness of delivery of epilepsy care in different systems, however, has not been carried out. For example, surgery is often viewed as a most cost-effective treatment for some forms of epilepsy, but little is known about its use and cost-effectiveness in resource-poor countries.

Government Versus Private Bureaucracy

As soon as medical care involves more than a single doctor, a bureaucratic structure begins to develop. When medical care involves many physicians and large support staffs, bureaucratic considerations become a primary issue. Decisions may be based on health care priorities or other political reasons. In democratic settings, there is at least some degree of accountability, but in many parts of the world, political decisions are made for personal or self-interested reasons. In some parts of the world, government is trusted and the decisions of government authorities respected, but in others, government is mistrusted and the decisions of government authorities are seen at best as a barrier and at worst as malevolent. These same themes exist whether the bureaucracy is part of government or is apparently of a private nature.

In most systems of health services, the allocation of resources becomes a political matter. In some cases, the politics involves the government and health ministers, whereas in other cases, it depend on relationships that exist within a private bureaucracy.

The major difference between public and private bureaucracies is that, in public bureaucracies, decisions are often influenced by broad governmental priorities, for example, the need to win the next election. In private bureaucracies, decisions are influenced usually by primarily financial considerations. Whether high-quality care and serving patients are primary goals varies from provider to provider.

These differences in care are seen in purest form in the private bureaucracies that run large health care systems in a capitalistic market economy, such as that of the United States. The large health service organizations in the United States struggle continuously to instill a customer-oriented attitude in their employees. Although to some extent this orientation toward customer service is altruistically motivated, for the most part it is motivated by the desire to increase market share and expand the business. To do so, the health service organization must offer a low price and, it is hoped, high value to the purchaser of the contract; it must also please the patient. The extent to which the patient can exercise free choice and take business from one group to another is the extent to which the patient can influence the quality of care provided.

SUMMARY AND CONCLUSIONS

In most areas of the world, care is provided in a tiered system. The ways in which the systems are funded and the funding available vary widely from country to country and particularly between industrialized and resource-poor countries. This section provides a snapshot of service provision for people with epilepsy in a number of countries as well as a brief review of the socioeconomic issues that affect epilepsy.

CHAPTER 289 ■ BRAZIL

CARLOS A. M. GUERREIRO

INTRODUCTION

Brazil is a country of continental dimensions (8,511,965 km^2), divided into 26 states and a federal district. In 2004, its population was estimated to be 178.4 million inhabitants; life expectancy at birth (male/female), 66.0/73.0 years; gross domestic product (GDP) per capita (international $, 2002), U.S. $7,762; health life expectancy at birth (male/female), 57.2/62.4; child mortality (male/female) per 1,000, 39/32; adult mortality (male/female) per 1,000, 240/129; and total health expenditure per capita (international $, 2002), 611; and total health expenditure as percentage of GDP (2002), 7.9.[53] In October 2005 the estimated population was 184.7 million inhabitants.

Brazil has achieved dramatic results in improving living conditions: Infant mortality declined from around 50 per 1,000 live births in 1990 to 33 per 1,000 in 2000, and net enrollment in basic education rose from 84% in 1991 to 97% in 2002. Brazilians with access to an improved water source rose from 73% of the population in 1986 to 87% in 2001.

Despite Brazil's impressive advances, the poorest one fifth of Brazil's 184.7 million people account for only a 2.2% share of the national income. Brazil is second only to South Africa in a world ranking of income inequality. More than one quarter of the population live on <$2 a day and 13% live on <$1 a day. Brazil's northeast contains the single largest concentration of rural poverty in Latin America. Past development programs have failed to make a major dent in a region in which 49% of the population is classified as poor.

Crime is plaguing urban Brazil. Political corruption is also a serious problem in the country.

In global terms, Brazil rates 13th in economic strength and among the first group of countries in agricultural production.[54]

Information related to demographic, socioeconomic, and health indicators of the country is listed in Tables 1 and 2.[16,54]

GENERAL DATA ON THE HEALTH SYSTEM

Some states in the country suffer more than others, particularly from some long-standing endemic diseases such as dengue, cholera, Chagas disease, schistosomiasis, and malaria. New diseases, such as AIDS, are also a growing problem.

The rate of reported AIDS cases increased from 10.6 per 100,000 in 1992 to a high of 18.7 per 100,000 in 1998. Brazil has experienced a stabilizing trend with rates of 16.5, 16.4, and 14.8 per 100,000 in 1999, 2000, and 2001, respectively. In the last decade, heterosexual transmission of reported AIDS cases grew from 25.8% in 1991 to 56.1% in 2002. Since 1998, the death rate from AIDS has stabilized at 6.3 per 100,000. This tendency is attributed to Brazil's guarantee of access to free antiretroviral drugs since 1996.

The country also rose to the challenge posed by the single biggest health threat in the modern world, pioneering an anti-HIV/AIDS strategy that became an international model by guaranteeing universal access to retroviral medication.[15]

Brazil has a constitution that states that health is the right of every citizen and the duty of the state to provide. A law was passed on September 19, 1990, creating the Unified Health System (Sistema Único de Saúde [SUS]). The SUS is composed of the health activities and services provided by municipal, state, and federal organizations and institutions. This same law assumed the coexistence of private medicine in its various forms.

Despite this legislation, a great number of problems remain. These range from the social policies practiced by the federal government to the management of responsibility at the different levels and the effective management of rendering services.

Although SUS theoretically offers total coverage to everyone, in reality, only 77% of the population is covered, according to an estimate that we have applied using data from the federal government from 1994 (from the Bulletin of Ministry of Economy, 1994). Of those not covered, 22% were unassisted, and another 55% received some assistance. The remaining 23% sought assistance from the private sector: Medical insurance, health maintenance organizations (HMOs), traditional fee-for-service providers, and others.

Large portions of citizens receiving private medical care eventually seek, or are directed to, public health services. This happens especially in cases of chronic or terminal diseases and those involving complex and costly procedures. In these cases, there is no reimbursement from the public sector.

Epilepsy Data

An epidemiologic study with a selected sample size of 17,293 individuals revealed that the cumulative prevalence of epilepsy in São José do Rio Preto, a 350,000-inhabitant city in São Paulo state, was 18.6 per 1,000 inhabitants with 8.2 being active, defined as at least one seizure within the last 2 years. The prevalence per 1,000 inhabitants for the age groups (years) was 4.9 (0 to 4), 11.7 (5 to 14), 20.3 (15 to 64), and 32.8 (65 or over).[12]

Very recent data from the Demonstration Project of Global Campaign Against Epilepsy, in Brazil, supported by the International League Against Epilepsy, the International Bureau for Epilepsy, and the World Health Organization, revealed that the prevalence of cumulative and active epilepsy, respectively, was 9.1 per 1,000 and 5.3 per 1,000 people in Campinas and São José do Rio Preto, both in São Paulo state.[40] The prevalence of active epilepsy was higher in the more deprived social classes (range from A = richest to E = poorest) in Campinas and in São José do Rio Preto (Class D + E = 7.4 vs. Class A = 1.6 per 1,000). Over one third of patients with active epilepsy had inadequate treatment, including 19% who were on no medication. These data illustrate the treatment gap in the area.[40] In another study based on data from the central municipal pharmacy of Campinas and São José do Rio Preto in 2003, it was estimated that in the best-case scenario, 50% of patients with epilepsy were not on medication on a regular basis.[41]

TABLE 1

SOCIOECONOMIC, DEMOGRAPHIC, AND HEALTH INDICATORS DATA ABOUT BRAZIL

	Most recent year	Data
Socioeconomic context		
Total population (000s)	2003	176,596
GNI per capita, Atlas method (U.S.$)	2003	2,760
Expected years of schooling	2002	15
Adult literacy rate (% of population ages 15+)	2003	88
Demographic indicators		
Average annual population growth rate (%)	1990–2003	1.4
Age dependency ratio (dependents as a proportion of working-age population)	2003	0.5
Total fertility rate (births per woman)	2003	2.1
Adolescent fertility rate (births per 1,000 women ages 15–19)	2003	68
Contraceptive prevalence rate (% of women ages 15–49), any method	1996	76.7
Health status indicators		
Life expectancy at birth (yr)	2003	69
Infant mortality rate (per 1,000 live births)	2003	33
Under 5 yr of age mortality rate (per 1,000)	2003	35
Maternal mortality ratio (per 100,000 live births), modeled estimates	2000	260
Prevalence of child malnutrition—underweight (% of children under age 5)	1996	6
Health care indicators		
Child immunization rate, measles (% of ages 12–23 months)	2003	99
Child immunization rate, DPT3 (% of ages 12–23 months)	2003	96
Births attended by skilled health staff (% of total)	1996	87.6
Physicians (per 1,000 people)	2001	2.1
Hospital beds (per 1,000 people)	1996	3.1
Tuberculosis treatment success rate (% of registered cases)	2002	75
DOTS detection rate (% of estimated cases)	2003	18
Health finance indicators		
Health expenditure, total (% of GDP)	2002	7.9
Health expenditure, public (% of GDP)	2002	3.6
Health expenditure, public (% of total health expenditure)	2002	45.9
Health expenditure per capita (U.S.$)	2002	206.0
Risk factors and future challenges		
Prevalence of HIV, total (% of population ages 15–49)	2003	0.70
Prevalence of HIV, female (% of population ages 15–24)	2001	0.50
Tuberculosis incidence (per 100,000 people)	2003	62
Tuberculosis death rate (per 100,000 people)	2002	8

DOTS, directly observed treatment strategy; DPT3, three doses of the combined vaccination against diphtheria, pertussis, and tetanus; GDP, gross domestic product. GNI, gross national income.
From World Bank. Health Nutrition Population. Available at: http://web.worldbank.org/WBSITE/EXTERNAL/COUNTRIES/LACEXT/BRAZILEXTN/0, contentMDK:20189430~pagePK:141137~piPK:141127~theSitePK:322341,00.html. Accessed: August, 2005.

Campinas and São José do Rio Preto are two cities located in one of the wealthier regions of Brazil, where there is a good public and private health care system and where the population has easy access to treatment.

Neurologists

Based on data furnished by a Novartis profile, 4,863 neurologists were identified in Brazil in 2005. This probably included clinical neurologists, pediatric neurologists, and some neurosurgeons who practice clinical neurology. According to the Brazilian Academy of Neurology, there are 1,197 members, and the Brazilian Epilepsy Society had 477 members in 2005. The distribution of the number of neurologists per 100,000 inhabitants in the different states is shown in Figure 1. An analysis of Figure 1 reveals a distinct relationship between the per capita income of the state and the number of accessible neurologists. The higher-income areas have more neurologists,

TABLE 2

GENERAL INFORMATION ABOUT BRAZIL IN 2000, 2003, AND 2004

	2000	2003	2004
People			
Population, total	170.1 million	176.6 million	178.7 million
Population growth (annual %)	1.2	1.2	1.2
National poverty rate (% of population)	..	..	..
Life expectancy (yr)	..	68.7	..
Fertility rate (births per woman)	..	2.1	..
Infant mortality rate (per 1,000 live births)	35.0	33.0	..
Under 5 yr of age mortality rate (per 1,000 children)	39.0	35.0	..
Births attended by skilled health staff (% of total)	..	..	..
Child malnutrition, weight for age (% of children under age 5)	..	..	..
Child immunization, measles (% of under 12 mo)	99.0	99.0	..
Prevalence of HIV, total (% of population aged 15–49)	..	0.7	..
Literacy rate, adult male (% of males ages 15 and above)	..	88.3	..
Literacy rate, adult female (% of females aged 15 and above)	..	88.6	..
Primary completion rate, total (% age group)	111.0	112.0	..
Primary completion rate, female (% age group)	111.0	..	..
Net primary enrollment (% relevant age group)	94.6	..	..
Net secondary enrollment (% relevant age group)	69.2	..	..
Environment			
Surface area (km^2)	8.5 million	8.5 million	..
Forests (1,000 km^2)	5.4 million	..	..
Deforestation (average annual % 1990–2000)	0.4	..	..
Internal freshwater resources per capita (cubic meters)	..	30,680.2	..
CO_2 emissions (metric tons per capita)	1.8	..	..
Access to improved water source (% of total population)	..	..	..
Access to improved sanitation (% of urban population)	..	..	..
Energy use per capita (kg of oil equivalent)	1,091.3	..	..
Electricity use per capita (kWh)	1,877.5	..	..
Economy			
GNI, Atlas method (current U.S.$)	620.8 billion	486.9 billion	552.1 billion
GNI per capita, Atlas method (current U.S.$)	3,650.0	2,760.0	3,090.0
GDP (current U.S.$)	601.7 billion	505.7 billion	604.9 billion
GDP growth (annual %)	4.4	0.5	5.2
GDP implicit price deflator (annual % growth)	9.8	15.0	8.1
Value added in agriculture (% of GDP)	7.3	5.8	5.2
Value added in industry (% of GDP)	28.0	19.1	17.2
Value added in services (% of GDP)	64.7	75.1	77.7
Exports of goods and services (% of GDP)	10.7	16.9	22.5
Imports of goods and services (% of GDP)	12.2	13.1	17.0
Gross capital formation (% of GDP)	21.5	17.3	19.2
Revenue, excluding grants (% of GDP)	..	..	..
Cash surplus/deficit (% of GDP)	..	..	..
Technology and infrastructure			
Fixed lines and mobile telephones (per 1,000 people)	318.7	486.5	..
Telephone average cost of local call (U.S.$ per 3 minutes)	0.0	..	..
Personal computers (per 1,000 people)	50.1	..	..
Internet users (per 1,000 people)	29.4	..	..
Paved roads (% of total)	5.5	..	..
Aircraft departures	617.8 thousand	486.8 thousand	..
Trade and finance			
Trade in goods as a share of GDP (%)	18.9	25.1	..
High-technology exports (% of manufactured exports)	18.6	12.0	..
Net barter terms of trade (1995 = 100)	100.0	..	..
Foreign direct investment, net inflows in reporting country (current U.S.$)	32.8 billion	10.1 billion	..
Present value of debt (current U.S.$)	223.8 billion	254.1 billion	..
Total debt service (% of exports of goods and services)	93.5	63.8	..
Short-term debt outstanding (current U.S.$)	31.0 billion	19.6 billion	..
Aid per capita (current U.S.$)	1.9	1.7	..

GDP, gross domestic product; GNI, gross national income.
From Development Indicators Database. Available at: http://devdata.worldbank.org/external/CPProfile.asp?SelectedCountry=BRA&CCODE+BRA&CNAME=Brazil&PTYPE=CP. Accessed August 2005.

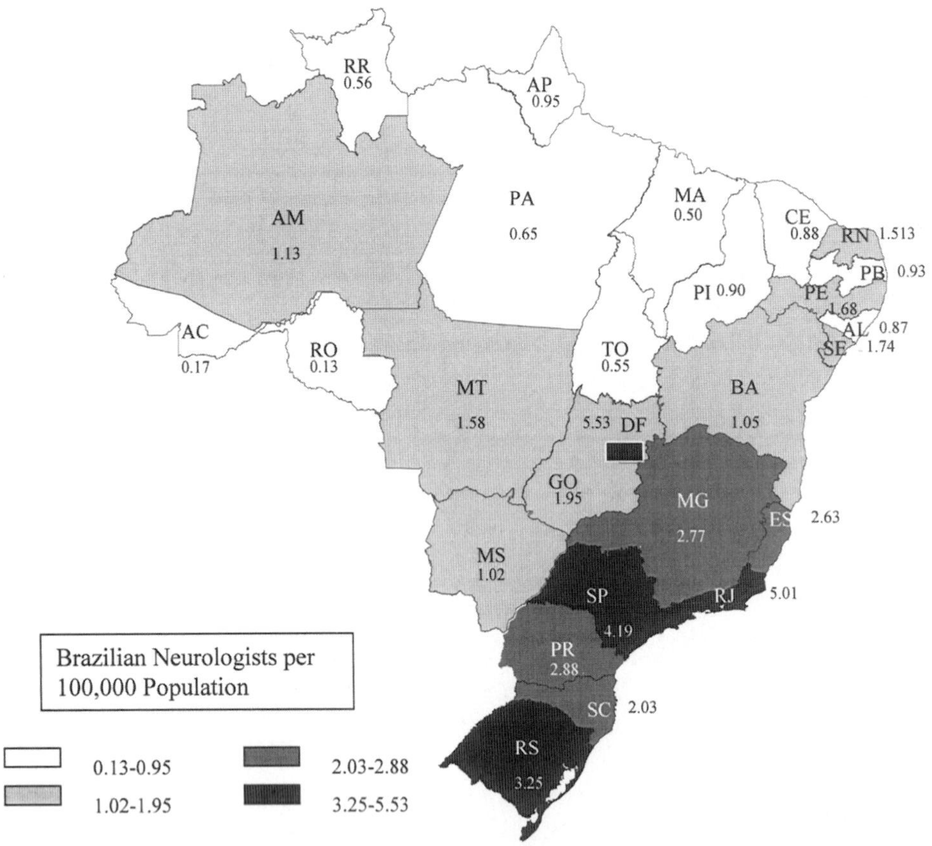

FIGURE 1. The distribution of neurologists per 100,000 inhabitants in the different states of the federation.

as in the case of the Federal District and the states of Rio de Janeiro, São Paulo, and Rio Grande do Sul. The latter state's rates are close to those of the northeastern states in the United States.[38]

Neurologists practice principally in the private sector (52%), in specialized outpatient clinics or HMOs (22%), in hospitals (23%), and in the federal health system (3%).

Drugs

Clinicians and Neurologists

In clinical practice, the drugs most prescribed (almost a third of prescriptions) by neurologists are antiepileptic drugs (AEDs). General practitioners and pediatricians are also responsible for a good number of AED prescriptions in Brazil.

Recent research conducted at the end of 2004 and beginning of 2005 in the private sector in Brazil and the relative sales of some basic antiepileptic drugs in private practice are shown in Figure 2.[14]

Drug Consumption and Treatment

Recently, there has been a tendency to decrease the use of sedative drugs and to substitute them for carbamazepine or valproate. This indicates a change in the AED prescribing patterns described in 1979 and 1980.[32]

There are few quantitative data about compliance in patients with epilepsy in Brazil.[1] To evaluate adherence, tolerance, and efficacy of the first AED prescribed, the author and colleagues followed 78 diagnosed epilepsy patients, ranging in age from 6 to 61 years (average, 17.96 years) for up to 29 months (average, 12.68 months). It was found that 11 patients (14.10%) did not adhere to the prescribed treatment, and 14 (17.94%) did not tolerate the first drug. Sixty-six percent of the patients were seizure free after 8 weeks of treatment, and 63.8% were seizure free after 56 weeks.[28] These data are consistent with the international literature.[9,13,18]

Brazil is a good example of many intermediate-economy countries where there is unequal wealth distribution and low-income areas where only phenobarbital is available. In other areas, the four basic AEDs (carbamazepine, phenytoin, phenobarbital, and valproate) are available in public health care, and in some more organized parts of the country, the new drugs (gabapentin, lamotrigine, topiramate, and vigabatrin) are available, sponsored by the federal government. The latter scenario is probably found in the black areas of the Brazilian map shown in the Figure 1.

THE SISTEMA ÚNICO DE SAÚDE REFERENCE SYSTEM

The data mentioned above demonstrate the political, social, and economic heterogeneity of the country's diverse regions. The public health system in one of the country's most populous and prosperous regions, the state of São Paulo, illustrates this.

The state of São Paulo is divided into five large regions (macroregions). The following will focus on the region of Campinas, which comprises 19 urban communities and a population of approximately 3 million. This region is responsible for approximately 9% of the gross national product (GNP), being three times higher than the Brazilian GNP and twice the state average. Despite this, social inequities such as growing slum areas and urban violence have been revealed.

Health care is divided into three areas: Primary, secondary, and tertiary care. Primary care consists of home care, health

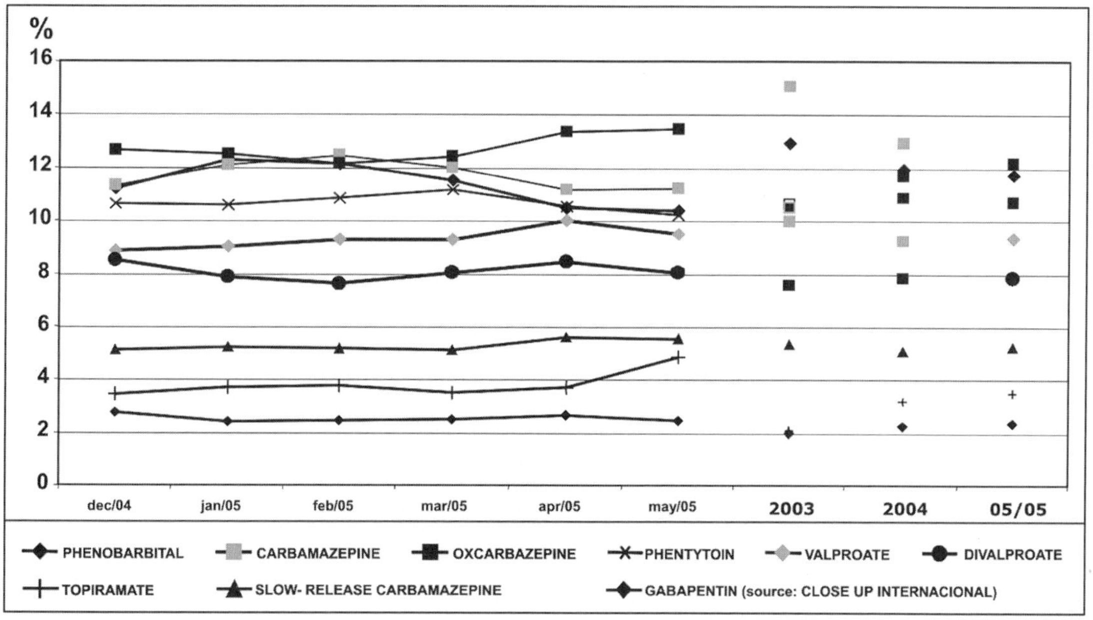

FIGURE 2. Sales of the main antiepileptic drugs available in Brazil by private practices (averages through May 2005).

centers that support general clinics, and diagnostic and therapeutic support services (SADTs). On a secondary level, besides SADT, there are specialized outpatient clinics and local and macroregional hospitals. Tertiary care includes specialized outpatient clinics (university hospitals), regional hospitals, and SADTs.

Federal government financial resources cover approximately 70% of medical expenditures. The remaining 30% is supplied by the municipalities and the state.

From a neurology practice point of view, electroencephalogram testing and computed tomography scanning are currently available in medium-sized cities, but magnetic resonance imaging is performed by federal services in large cities only.

ASPECTS RELATED TO EPILEPSY IN BRAZIL

Types of Seizures and Epilepsy

In Brazil, there appears to be no significant difference to developed countries in the incidence of the diverse types of epileptic seizures and syndromes.[27,44]

Etiologies

The high incidence of parasitic diseases is one of the factors that contribute to the greater prevalence of epilepsy in Brazil. Neurocysticercosis is the most common of these parasites, and it is the most frequently diagnosed cause of epilepsy in adults.[3,4,10,43,50,51] Seizures often start in childhood,[35,42] and specific clinical and computed tomography findings have been described in children.[24,30]

Malaria, when it presents with cerebral complications, may result in epilepsy. It is also a cause of febrile convulsions in children in tropical regions, in the northern part of the country.[45]

Perinatal brain damage is another factor suggested as a cause for the high incidence of epilepsy. This is possibly true in regions with inadequate prenatal care. However, Sakamoto[46] found that 14% of epilepsy cases were caused by perinatal lesions, which is no different from data collected by the Collaborative Perinatal Project of the National Institute of Neurological Diseases and Stroke in the United States.[37]

Because the incidence of motor vehicle accidents is high in Brazil, craniocerebral trauma is likely to be an important cause of epilepsy.[11] Sakamoto[46] found trauma to be the etiology of epilepsy in 3% of children and adolescents; Gorz et al.[26] found trauma to be the etiology in 13% of adolescents and adults with epilepsy.

In a country like Brazil, basic strategies for the prevention of epilepsy should include prenatal care, safe childbirth, control of infections—especially parasitic diseases—and reduction of brain injury due to trauma and stroke.

Psychosocial Aspects

Lay knowledge of epilepsy in Brazil is clearly unsatisfactory. When evaluating the knowledge of public and private school teachers and those in medical areas, Simonatto et al.[48] found it inadequate. The high rate of illiteracy and low cultural standards help perpetuate old prejudices about epilepsy. A comprehensive educational effort to inform the patients and their families about epilepsy is a basic step in successfully managing this condition.[2]

Epilepsy is clearly associated with psychosocial difficulties.[7,21,47] Prejudice and discrimination are often worse than the seizure itself[7,36] with impact on the daily lives of people with epilepsy. According to studies carried out in Europe[7,25,52] and North America,[5,6,17] epilepsy stigma has been considered one of the most important negative factors on the quality of life of people with epilepsy. The definition of stigma in these studies[8,33] is portrayed slightly differently and, in most cases, is based on qualitative assessment expressed in proportions. Fernandes[23] has developed a scale to measure perception of stigma in epilepsy that consists of ten questions that provide a total score ranging from 0 (no stigma) to 100 (highest level of stigma). In a study carried out in Campinas, 1,850 people were interviewed and the results showed that the magnitude of stigma is different within demographics, such as gender, religion, and level of education, in an urban area. This finding is

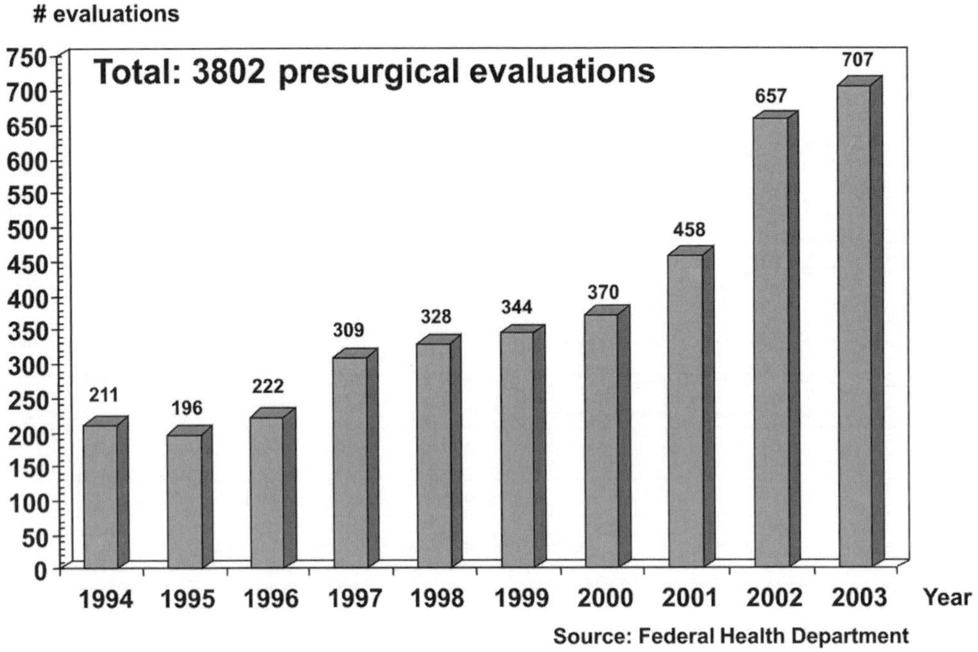

FIGURE 3. The number of presurgical evaluations registered by the Brazilian Epilepsy Program between 1994 and 2003.

relevant as a reference for mass media campaigns to fight prejudice and improve social acceptance of people with epilepsy.

In southeast Brazil, Guerreiro et al.[31] evaluated the impact of epilepsy on the quality of life in 17 recently diagnosed children. The relationship between parents and children was found to be significantly altered. However, culturally and socially, the interaction of these children in school and with their families did not show significant changes after the manifestation of epilepsy.[49]

A famous Brazilian with epilepsy is the writer Machado de Assis. He is considered by some to be the most important 19th-century writer in Latin America; in Brazil, he is considered the greatest of all time. Despite having cryptogenic localization-related epilepsy with complex partial seizures of right temporal lobe origin and despite the strong prejudices existing in the second half of the last century, he made good use of his genius through writing.[29] His life serves as an example to other people with epilepsy and to those who may be prejudiced against the condition.

SPECIALIZED CENTERS

Considering the size of Brazil, there are few centers for the social rehabilitation of people with epilepsy. The ones that do exist have a multidisciplinary structure, are generally affiliated with a university, and are located mainly in the southern and southeastern regions of the country.

Brazilian National Epilepsy Surgery Program

Epilepsy surgery started with Niemeyer in Rio de Janeiro in the late 1950s. Indeed, he was the first to propose amygdalohippocampectomy to treat temporal lobe epilepsy and he described the technique in detail.[39] In the 1970s, São Paulo University Medical School (USP) started a surgical program, followed by the Neurological Institute at Goiânia in the 1980s. In the 1990s, three epilepsy centers joined the group: Catholic University (PUC, Porto Alegre), University of São Paulo (USP-Ribeirão Preto), and State University of Campinas (UNICAMP).

In 1994, the Federal Health Department started the National Epilepsy Program within the Program of High Complexity Medical Procedures. Some of the program's data over 10 years (1994 to 2003) in the eight approved centers are shown in Figures 3, 4, and 5.

Positive aspects of this public health policy were technical criteria for accreditation of epilepsy surgery centers, strong partnership between the Health Department and national medical societies, and a reimbursement policy granting epilepsy surgery the same status as renal transplantation. Of note are that seven of the eight epilepsy surgery centers are university institutions; presurgical investigation and surgeries are at internationally accepted standards; morbidity, mortality, and outcome figures are similar to major epilepsy surgery centers; and there is progressive development of new epilepsy surgery centers and a network of epilepsy centers with potential for collaborative research and training. The limitations observed were that the distribution of centers does not parallel demographic data; a national center for regulation of patient access is still preliminary; and there is a lack of specific policies for more complex cases (invasive procedures) and a lack of long-term planning for the expansion of new epilepsy centers. New challenges of this program include improvement of the current system for referrals of patients from less privileged regions and stimulation of greater cooperation between epilepsy surgery centers, patient care, and scientific cooperation.

THE ROLE OF SOCIETIES

The Brazilian Epilepsy League plays an important role in advising the Ministry of Health on issues regarding epilepsy and in providing education to physicians. The Brazilian Epilepsy

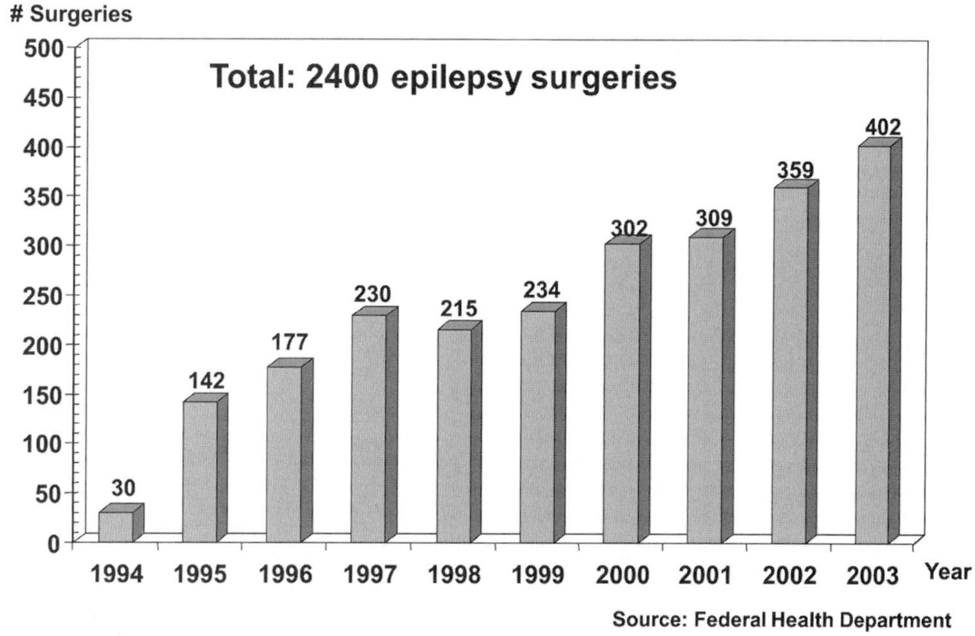

FIGURE 4. The number of epilepsy surgeries registered by the Brazilian Epilepsy Program between 1994 and 2003.

League sends out videos, booklets, and books to its nearly 300 members and to medical schools. It organizes scientific meetings and courses in its various regional chapters and has an annual national scientific meeting.

The National Demonstration Project on Epilepsy in Brazil has galvanized lay epilepsy associations across the country since 2002 in a joint effort to help drive epilepsy out of the shadows in Brazil.[34] The main activities are (a) the National Week of Epilepsy, which takes place in all regions of the country,[22] and (b) the National Meeting of Associations and Support Group of People with Epilepsy, where the achievements and resolutions to drive epilepsy out of the shadows are discussed.[19,20,23] These activities have been coordinated by the ASPE (Assistência à Saúde de Pacientes com Epilepsia) and EPI-Brasil (Federation of Associations of People with Epilepsy of Brazil) and represent an important step toward promoting an awareness of epilepsy, diminishing the associated stigma and improving the quality of life of people with epilepsy and their families.

SUMMARY AND CONCLUSIONS

The organization of the country's medical system for epilepsy care reflects the low socioeconomic development of the nation.

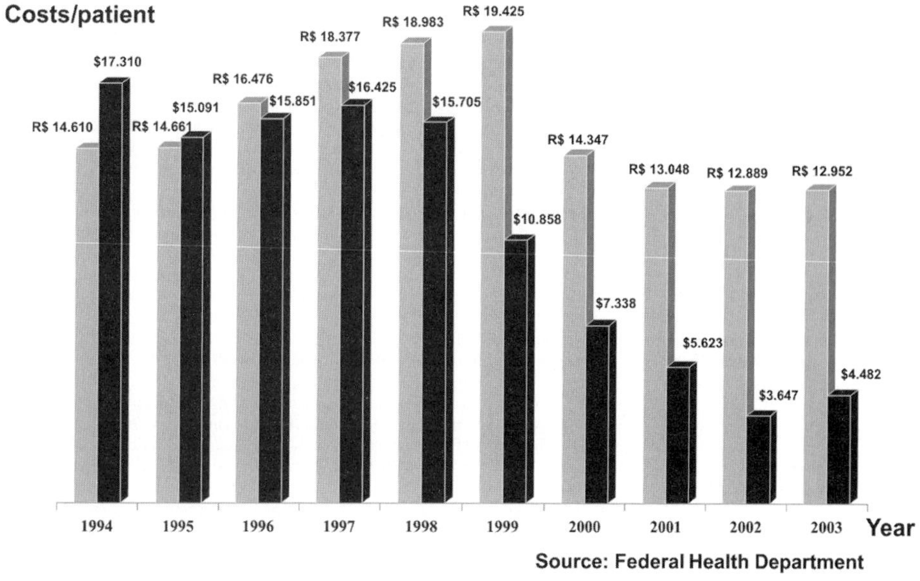

FIGURE 5. Costs per patient of the presurgical evaluation plus surgery in reais (R$) and in U.S.$ ($) between 1994 and 2003.

Some factors that are causing or contributing to the high rate of epilepsy in the country are the high incidence of infectious diseases, mainly parasitic (especially neurocysticercosis); the poor quality of maternal–infant care in the low socioeconomic regions (particularly in the interior of the northeast and in the misery belts around the large cities); and the high rate of traffic accidents with resulting head trauma. Improved health care, basic education, and sanitation can greatly improve these conditions. The role of nongovernmental agencies in educating the public has produced encouraging results, although their efforts are currently limited to a few segments of society.

Basic measures should be taken to bring about a more efficient health care system. With regard to patients with epilepsy, the governmental policies related to epilepsy with referential and counterreferential centers should be reformed. Low-income patients all over the country, and not just in certain areas, should receive AEDs at no cost.

The official recognition of epilepsy surgery by the Ministry of Health is helping organize an algorithm in this increasingly complex medical care field. It is crucial that the Ministry of Health includes epilepsy in the public health priorities as proposed by International League Against Epilepsy.[34] In this setting, the World Health Organization, the International League Against Epilepsy, and the International Bureau for Epilepsy launched the Global Campaign Against Epilepsy in 1997.

ACKNOWLEDGMENTS

The author thanks Dr. Américo C. Sakamoto, who provided data on the National Epilepsy Surgery Program, and Drs. Li Li Min, Ana L. Noronha, and Paula T. Fernandes for data related to the Demonstration Project in Brazil.

References

1. Alonso NB, Silva DF, Campos CJR. Aderência em epilepsias. I. Aspectos conceituais e factores de influência. *Arq Neuropsiquiatr.* 1991;49(2):147–149.
2. Alonso, NB, Albuquerque M, Pinto THB, et al. Evaluation of patients' perceptions regarding epilepsy and treatment. *Epilepsia.* 1993;34 (Suppl 2):1.
3. Arruda WO, Camargo NJ, Coelho RC. Neurocysticercosis. An epidemiological survey in two small rural communities. *Arq Neuropsiquiatr.* 1990;48(4):419–424.
4. Arruda WO. Etiology of epilepsy. A prospective study of 210 cases. *Arq Neuropsiquiatr.* 1990;49(3):251–254.
5. Austin JK, Dunn DW, Huster GA, et al. Development of scales to measure psychosocial care needs of children with seizures and their parents. *J Neurosci Nurs.* 1998;30:155–160.
6. Austin JK, Shafer PO, Deering JB. Epilepsy familiarity, knowledge, and perceptions of stigma: report from a survey of adolescents in the general population. *Epilepsy Behav.* 2002;3(4):368–375.
7. Baker G. The psychosocial burden of epilepsy. *Epilepsia.* 2002;43(Suppl 6): 26–30.
8. Baker GA, Jacoby A, Buck D, et al. Quality of life of people with epilepsy: a European study. *Epilepsia.* 1997;38(3):353–362.
9. Beghi E, Tognoni G. Prognosis of epilepsy in the newly referred patient: a multicenter prospective study. Collaborative Group for the Study of Epilepsy. *Epilepsia.* 1988;29(3):440–445.
10. Bittencourt PRM, Gracia CM, Lorenzana P. Epilepsy and parasitosis of the central nervous system. In: Pedley T, Meldrum B, eds. *Recent Advances in Epilepsy,* Vol 4. Edinburgh: Churchill-Livingstone; 1988:123–160.
11. Bittencourt PRM, Turner M. Epilepsy in the third world: Latin American aspects. In: Dam M, Gram L, eds. *Comprehensive Epileptology.* New York: Raven Press; 1991:807–820.
12. Borges MA, Min LL, Guerreiro CA, et al. Urban prevalence of epilepsy: populational study in São Jose do Rio Preto, a medium-sized city in Brazil. *Arq Neuropsiquiatr.* 2004;62:199–204.
13. Camfield PR, Camfield CS, Smith EC, et al. Newly treated childhood epilepsy: a prospective study of recurrences and side effects. *Neurology.* 1985;35:722–725.
14. Close Up International. Technical Statistical Books and Reports edition on the Prescription Markets. Available at: http://www.close-upinternational.com/, Brazilian Branch. Accessed August, 2005.
15. Department of Health and Human Services, Centers for Disease Control and Prevention. Available at: http://www.cdc.gov/nchstp/od/gap/countries/brazil.htm. Accessed August, 2005.
16. Development Indicators Database. Available at: http://devdata.worldbank.org/external/CPProfile.asp?SelectedCountry=BRA&CCODE+BRA&CNAME=Brazil&PTYPE=CP. Accessed August 2005.
17. DiIorio C, Osborne SP, Letz R, et al. The association of stigma with self-management and perceptions of health care among adults with epilepsy. *Epilepsy Behav.* 2003;4(3):259–267.
18. Elwes RDC, Johnson AL, Shorvon SD, et al. The prognosis for seizure control in newly diagnosed epilepsy. *N Engl J Med.* 1984;311:944–947.
19. Fernandes PT, Leitão L, Souza RJ, et al. Relatório do II Encontro Nacional de Associações e Grupos de Pacientes com Epilepsia. *J Epilepsy Clin Neurophysiol.* 2004;10(2):117–120.
20. Fernandes PT, Noronha ALA, Cendes F, et al. Relatório do I Encontro Nacional de Associações e Grupos de Pacientes com Epilepsia. *J Epilepsy Clin Neurophysiol.* 2003;9(2):93–96.
21. Fernandes PT, Salgado PC, Noronha ALA, et al. Stigma scale of epilepsy: conceptual issues. *J Epilepsy Clin Neurophysiol.* 2004;10:213–218.
22. Fernandes PT, Souza RJ, Li LM. Relatório do II Semana Nacional de Epilepsia. *J Epilepsy Clin Neurophysiol.* 2004;10(4):245–247.
23. Fernandes PT, Souza RJ, Li LM. Relatório do III Encontro Nacional de Associações e Grupos de Pacientes com Epilepsia. *J Epilepsy Clin Neurophysiol.* 2005;11(2):97–99.
24. Ferreira LS, Zanardi VA, Scotoni AE, et al. Childhood epilepsy due to neurocysticercosis: a comparative study. *Epilepsia.* 2001;42:1438–1444.
25. Fisher RS, Vickrey BG, Gibson P, et al. The impact of epilepsy from the patient's perspective I. Descriptions and subjective perceptions. *Epilepsy Res.* 2000;41(1):39–51.
26. Gorz AM, Silvado CES, Bittencourt PRM. Barbiturate-refractory epilepsy: safe schedule for therapeutic substitution. *Arq Neuropsiquiatr.* 1986;44:225–231.
27. Guerreiro CAM, Silveira, DC, Costa ALC, et al. Classification and etiology of newly diagnosed epilepsies in Southeast Brazil. *Epilepsia.* 1993;34(Suppl 2):14.
28. Guerreiro CAM, Voestsch B, Montenegro MA, et al. Epilepsias recém-diagnosticadas: aderência, tolerância e prognóstico com a primeira droga. *J Liga Brasileira Epilepsia.* 1995;1:15–17.
29. Guerreiro CAM. Machado de Assis's epilepsy. *Arq Neuropsiquiatr.* 1992;50(3):378–382.
30. Guerreiro MM, Facure NO, Guerreiro CAM. Aspectos da tomografia computadorizada craniana na neurocisticercose na infância. *Arq Neuropsiquiatr.* 1989;47(2):153–158.
31. Guerreiro MM, Silva EA, Scotoni AE, et al. Qualidade de vida em epilepsia. *J Liga Brasileira Epilepsia.* 1994;7(1):21–26.
32. III and IV Commissions on Antiepileptic Drugs of the International League Against Epilepsy. Availability and distribution of antiepileptic drugs in developing countries. *Epilepsia.* 1985;117–121.
33. Jacoby A, Gorry J, Gamble C, et al. Public knowledge, private grief: a study of public attitudes to epilepsy in the United Kingdom and implications for stigma. *Epilepsia.* 2004;45(11):1405–1415.
34. Li LM, Sander JW. National demonstration project on epilepsy in Brazil. *Arq Neuropsiquiatr.* 2003;61:153–156.
35. Manreza MLG, Barros NG, Andrade JQ, et al. Epilepsy secondary to childhood neurocysticercosis. *Epilepsia.* 1993;34(Suppl 2):102–103.
36. Morrell MJ. Stigma and epilepsy. *Epilepsy Behav.* 2002;3:21–25.
37. Nelson KB, Ellenberg JH. Predisposing and causative factors in childhood epilepsy. *Epilepsia.* 1987;28(Suppl):16–24.
38. Neurologists 2004, AAN Member Demographic and Practice Characteristics. Henry K, Lawyer BL, and members of the AAN Member Demographics Subcommittee. 2005 American Academy of Neurology 1080 Montreal Avenue, St. Paul, MN 55116.
39. Niemeyer P. The transventricular amygdalo-hippocampectomy in temporal lobe epilepsy. In: Baldwin M, Bailey P, eds. *Temporal Lobe Epilepsy.* Springfield, IL: CC Thomas; 1958:461–482.
40. Noronha AL, Borges MA, Marques LH, et al. Prevalence and pattern of epilepsy treatment in different socio-economic classes in Brazil. *Epilepsia.* 2007;48:880–885.
41. Noronha AL, Marques LH, Borges MA, et al. Assessment of the epilepsy treatment gap in two cities of south-east Brazil. *Arq Neuropsiquiatr.* 2004;62:761–763.
42. Quagliato EMAB. Epilepsia e neurocisticercose. In: Guerreiro CAM, Guerreiro MM, eds. *Epilepsia.* São Paulo: Lemos Editorial; 1993:97–102.
43. Quagliato EMAB. Forma epiléptica da cisticercose encefálica—análise de 96 casos. *Tese de Doutoramento.* Campinas: Faculdade de Ciências Médicas da UNICAMP; 1987.
44. Román GC, Senanayake N. Epilepsy in Latin America. *J Liga Brasileira Epilepsia.* 1993;6(2):47–52.
45. Román GC, Senanayake N. Neurological manifestations of malaria. *Arq Neuropsiquiatr.* 1992;50(1):3–9.

46. Sakamoto AC. Estudo clínico e prognóstico das crises epilépticas que iniciam no infância numa populacão brasileira. *Tese de Doutorado*. Ribeirão Preto: Universidade de São Paulo; 1985:74.
47. Salgado PC, Fernandes PT, Noronha ALA, et al. The second step in the construction of a stigma scale of epilepsy. *Arq Neuropsiquiatr*. 2005;63 (2-B):395–398.
48. Simonatto D, Dias MD, Pinto THB, Albuquerque M. Epilepsia e educacão pblica. *Arq Neuropsiquiatr*. 1992;50(3):309–312.
49. Souza EAP, Silva EA, Scotoni AE, et al. Impact of recently diagnosed epilepsy in children's lives. *Epilepsia*. 1993;34(Suppl 2):3.
50. Takayanagui OM, Jardim E. Aspectos clínicos da neurocisticercose. Análise de 500 casos. *Arq Neuropsiquiatr*. 1993;41(1):50–63.
51. Takayanagui OM. Neurocisticercose. I. Evolucão clínico-laboratorial de 151 casos. *Arq Neuropsiquiatr*. 1990;48(1):1–10.
52. Vickrey BG, Hays RD, Graber J, et al. A health-related quality of life instrument for patients evaluated for epilepsy surgery. *Med Care*. 1992;30(4):299–319.
53. World Health Organization. World Health Report, 2005. Available at: http://www.who.int/countries/bra/en/. Accessed August, 2005.
54. World Bank. Available at: http://web.worldbank.org/WBSITE/EXTERNAL/COUNTRIES/LACEXT/BRAZILEXTN/0,,contentMDK:20189430~pagePK:141137~piPK:141127~theSitePK:322341,00.html. Accessed August, 2005.

CHAPTER 290 ■ CANADA

SAMUEL WIEBE

INTRODUCTION

This monograph describes broadly the health services for epilepsy in Canada. A brief overview of the Canadian health care system provides the basis for a portrayal of services covered, challenges to epilepsy care in Canada, and specific epilepsy health care services by province.

A depiction of the Canadian geography is pertinent as this is directly relevant to health care delivery. Canada spans an area of approximately 10 million km^2, of which a substantial proportion is north of 60th parallel and in the arctic regions. Approximately 31 million people inhabit ten provinces and three territories, with a population density of 3.1 residents per km^2, one of the lowest in the American Continent. The boundaries of the vast Canadian expanse comprise the Atlantic, Pacific, and Arctic oceans. Two thirds of the population (20 million) live in metropolitan areas, most of which are located in proximity to the southern national border. The large northern areas encompassing the Yukon, Northwest Territories, and Nunavik have only 100,000 inhabitants.[7] It is readily apparent that geography poses a gargantuan challenge to equal access to health care services.

THE CANADIAN HEALTH CARE SYSTEM

The Canadian Health Care system rests on the principles enshrined in the Canada Health Act, whose tenets are equity and solidarity. Its objective is to ensure that all eligible Canadian residents have reasonable access to insured health services on a prepaid basis, without direct charges at the point of service. Canada's National Health Insurance Program consists of 13 interlocking provincial and territorial health insurance plans, all of which share certain common features and basic standards of coverage. The roles and responsibilities for Canada's health care system are shared between the federal and provincial-territorial governments. The latter are responsible for the management, organization, and delivery of health services for their residents. Essentially, each province or territory has a list of insured services covered by the national insurance program. These comprise the great majority of medically necessary physician and hospital services. There is interprovincial reciprocity of services with the exception of the province of Quebec. Physicians can refer anywhere in Canada if services are not available locally or if they are justified by complexity. There is variable coverage of medication, eye care, dental care, and allied health care services. In general, medications are not covered except in special populations, such as the elderly, disabled or unemployed, and registered natives and Inuits. Each province has a medication list whose contents vary by province. Restricted use is specified if other drugs fail. A special application is required for unlisted drugs. In jurisdictions that have drug coverage, a copayment by the patient is required. This is widely variable, ranging from the prescription cost up to a maximum yearly of $850 CDN, and then a portion of the excess in some provinces. This coverage may take income into account. A few groups have complete coverage without copayment, including children. All consults to specialists require referral by general practitioners or family doctors, and some allied health care services also require referrals.

ACCESS TO HEALTH CARE

Statistics Canada carries out national surveys that evaluate access to health care.[6] In 2003, 20% of the general population reported some difficulty accessing specialized care and 15% had some difficulty accessing diagnostic tests. The main barriers to access were long wait times for service, reported by approximately 60% of those patients who identified any type of difficulty. The health access survey also assessed the effect of waiting for specialized care. The main effect of waiting was worry or stress (60% of individuals), whereas only 20% reported worsening of health status as a result of waiting. Interestingly, people with epilepsy in rural areas report fewer barriers to health care than those in urban areas.[9] This somewhat counterintuitive finding may have two possible explanations. Epilepsy care in rural areas occurs mostly through family physicians and emergency rooms, which are more readily accessible than urban specialists with long waiting lists. Alternatively, more complex patients requiring multiple levels of health care, which are often less accessible, may migrate to urban settings. Population surveys in Canada have also shown that patients with epilepsy have a higher use of specialists, nursing, and allied health services than patients with other common chronic conditions.[9]

According to Statistics Canada and the Canadian Institute of Health Information, the ratio of population per hospital in Canada is approximately 31,000, and there is approximately one hospital per 9,260 km^2.[2] The latter varies substantially among regions and provinces, from a low of 3,000 km^2 per hospital in Ontario to a high of 450,000 km^2 per hospital in the northern territories. In general, populated provinces have more and busier hospitals that are often nearly fully occupied, whereas provinces and territories with few inhabitants have fewer hospitals per area, distributed over vast and remote geographic regions, and with more challenging access.

According to a 1996 survey of specialist manpower, the mean distance from a general practitioner to a neurologist was 102 km, and it was 135 km for a neurosurgeon. This is highly variable among regions. In 2002, there were 694 neurologists in Canada, resulting in a ratio of 44,700 people per neurologist. This also is highly variable among regions, ranging from zero neurologists in the three vast northern territories to 218 in Ontario, and resulting in the following population-to-neurologist ratios: British Columbia, 43,000; Alberta, 43,200; Saskatchewan/Manitoba, 74,700; Ontario, 50,100; Quebec, 33,400; and Maritime Provinces, 61,000.[1] In most provinces the ratio has decreased over time (e.g., more neurologists per population), with the exception of Saskatchewan and Manitoba, where the number of neurologists has actually decreased over the last few years.

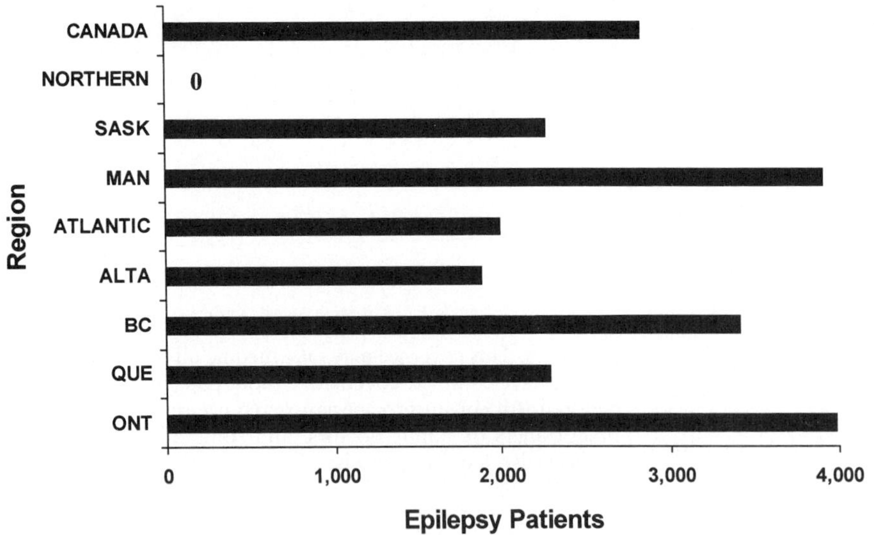

FIGURE 1. Epilepsy patients per epileptologist. In 2004, the ratio of patients with epilepsy to epilepsy neurologists varied across provinces, but with the exception of the Northern territories, it was always <4,000. Northern, Nunavut, Northwest Territories, Yukon; Sask, Saskatchewan; Man, Manitoba; Atlantic, Nova Scotia, Newfoundland & Labrador, New Brunswick, Prince Edward Island; Alta, Alberta; BC, British Columbia; Que, Quebec; Ont, Ontario. (Source: Wiebe, unpublished survey; and Tellez-Zenteno JF, Pondal-Sordo M, Matijevic S, et al. National and regional prevalence of self-reported epilepsy in Canada. *Epilepsia.* 2004;45(12):1623–1629.)

EPILEPSY-SPECIFIC HEALTH CARE RESOURCES

The only existing Canadian study of the epidemiology of epilepsy in the general population reports a prevalence of active epilepsy of 5.6 per 1,000.[8] The prevalence of epilepsy is higher in groups with lower educational level and income, and in the unemployed. Although the prevalence of active epilepsy is fairly constant across provinces, and translates into approximately 210,000 patients with epilepsy nationally, there are minor interprovincial differences (e.g., the prevalence is somewhat lower in the Pacific than in the Atlantic provinces).[8]

The approximate ratio of epilepsy patients per neurologist in Canada is 300, based on a prevalence of epilepsy of 7 per 1,000 and a total of 694 neurologists.[1] Again, this ranges from zero in the northern territories to 245 patients per neurologist in Quebec. Bailey's national survey found that 104 (15%) neurologists in Canada reported an interest in epilepsy.[1] However, a 2004 survey by the author identified only 74 neurologists focusing in adult or pediatric epilepsy, with a provincial median of eight and a range of zero in the vast northern territories to 22 in Quebec. The ratio of adult to pediatric epileptologists in Canada is approximately 3:1, which is remarkable given that a large number of the epilepsies are of childhood onset. This survey also identified 23 neurosurgeons focusing on epilepsy surgery in Canada, with a provincial median of 3.5, ranging from zero in the north to six in Alberta. According to these data, the national ratio of patients with epilepsy per epileptologist is 2,843, the provincial median ratio is 2,300, and the range is zero in the north to 1,800 in Alberta (Fig. 1). The national ratio of patients with epilepsy per epilepsy neurosurgeon is 9,000, with a provincial median ratio of 7,000, and a range of zero neurosurgeons in the northern territories to 3,000 patients per neurosurgeon in the more abundantly served Atlantic provinces and Alberta.

Our 2004 survey identified approximately 45 video-electroencephalographic (V-EEG) monitoring beds in the country. This results in a national ratio of 4,600 patients with epilepsy per monitored bed, and a provincial median ratio of 5,300, ranging from zero monitored beds in the north to 3,000 patients per monitored bed in Alberta (Fig. 2). The Canadian Institute of Health Information reported a total of 326 computed tomography (CT) scanners nationally, which translates into a ratio of 645 patients with epilepsy per CT scanner, and a provincial median ratio of 600 patients with epilepsy per CT scanner (range: 325 in the northern territories to 840 in Ontario) (Fig. 3).[3] Similar sources revealed a total of 147 magnetic resonance imaging (MRI) scanners nationally, which is equivalent to a national ratio of 1,400 patients with epilepsy

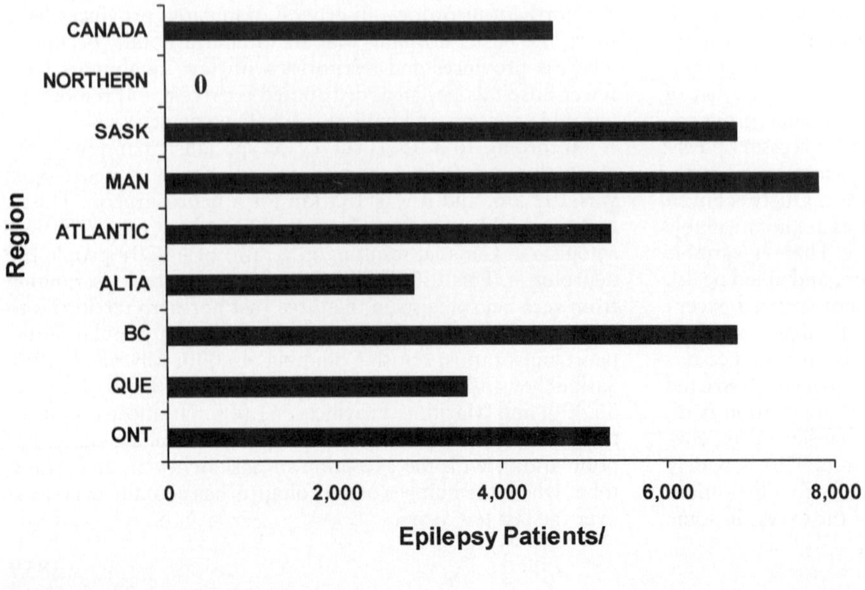

FIGURE 2. Epilepsy patients per electroencephalographic (EEG) monitoring bed. The number of patients with epilepsy per video-EEG monitored bed ranged from 2,500 to 8,000 in different provinces, and there were none in the Northern territories. Northern, Nunavut, Northwest Territories, Yukon; Sask, Saskatchewan; Man, Manitoba; Atlantic, Nova Scotia, Newfoundland & Labrador, New Brunswick, Prince Edward Island; Alta, Alberta; BC, British Columbia; Que, Quebec; Ont, Ontario. (Source: Wiebe, unpublished survey; and Tellez-Zenteno JF, Pondal-Sordo M, Matijevic S, et al. National and regional prevalence of self-reported epilepsy in Canada. *Epilepsia.* 2004;45(12):1623–1629.)

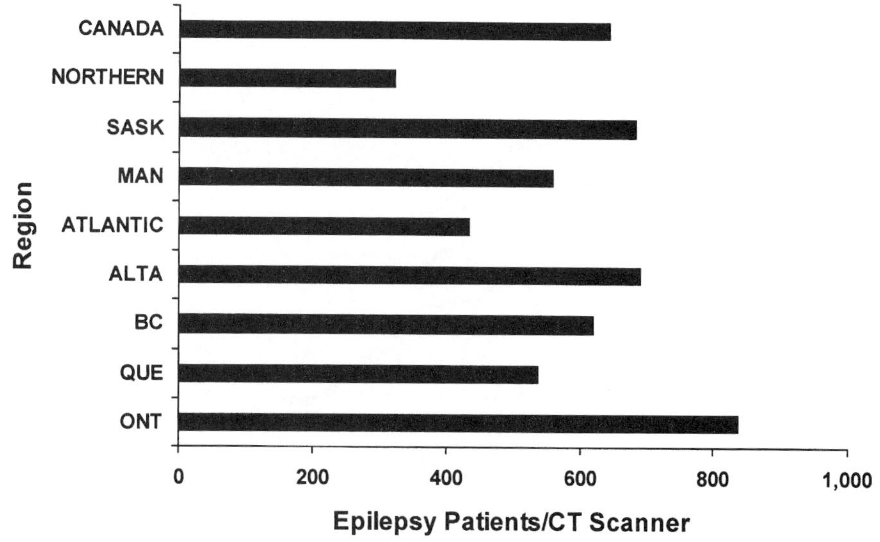

FIGURE 3. Epilepsy patients per computed tomography (CT) scanner. All Canadian provinces have CT scanners. The ratio of patients to scanner is lowest in the North because of its sparse population. Northern, Nunavut, Northwest Territories, Yukon; Sask, Saskatchewan; Man, Manitoba; Atlantic, Nova Scotia, Newfoundland & Labrador, New Brunswick, Prince Edward Island; Alta, Alberta; BC, British Columbia; Que, Quebec; Ont, Ontario. (Source: Canadian Institute for Health Information. *Medical Imaging in Canada: 2004*. Ottawa, Canada: Canadian Institutes for Health Information; 2004; and Tellez-Zenteno JF, Pondal-Sordo M, Matijevic S, et al. National and regional prevalence of self-reported epilepsy in Canada. *Epilepsia*. 2004;45(12):1623–1629.)

per MRI scanner, and a provincial median ratio of 1,500 patients per scanner (range: zero in the North to 900 in Alberta) (Figs. 4 and 5).[3] According to the Canadian Institute of Health Information, in 2004 there were eight positron emission tomography (PET) scanners in the country.[3]

In 2003 there were approximately 17 adult epilepsy clinics and 18 pediatric epilepsy clinics in Canada. These clinics had access to a total of approximately 30 clinical psychologists or social workers and less than two dozen nurses.

EPILEPSY NURSES

Best available data revealed that in 2003 in Canada there were less than two dozen nurses working part or full time in epilepsy. Furthermore, three large Canadian provinces have no access to dedicated epilepsy nurses. A recent survey conducted across Canada showed that 68% of epilepsy centers/clinics have dedicated epilepsy nurses, with a median of 1.7 nurses per epilepsy center.[5] Only 58% of centers have dedicated funding for epilepsy nurses. The role of epilepsy nurses is described in Table 1.

ANTIEPILEPTIC DRUGS

Most of the frequently used antiepileptic drugs (AEDs) are included in provincial drug formularies. The latter determine which drugs are available at no cost to special populations, such as the elderly, disabled, unemployed, registered Aboriginals, and Inuits. New AEDs take time to reach provincial formularies and special application can be made for these drugs. In Canada, drugs are licensed by a federal agency following a rigorous process that is similar to that of the Food and Drug Administration in the United States. At the time of this writing, the following commonly used AEDs are licensed and available for use in Canada: Phenytoin, phenobarbital, carbamazepine and carbamazepine controlled release, valproate, ethosuximide, primidone, clobazam, lorazepam, lamotrigine, topiramate, vigabatrin, levetiracetam, and oxcarbazepine. AEDs not available in Canada include zonisamide, tiagabine, and felbamate.

NATIONAL EPILEPSY ORGANIZATIONS

The Canadian League Against Epilepsy is the country's professional organization and is the national chapter of the International League Against Epilepsy. Epilepsy Canada is a national organization whose focus is on research and education, and it is the national chapter of the International Bureau for Epilepsy. The Canadian Epilepsy Alliance is a lay organization, which focuses on patient and public education and support. Regional epilepsy associations often serve the functions

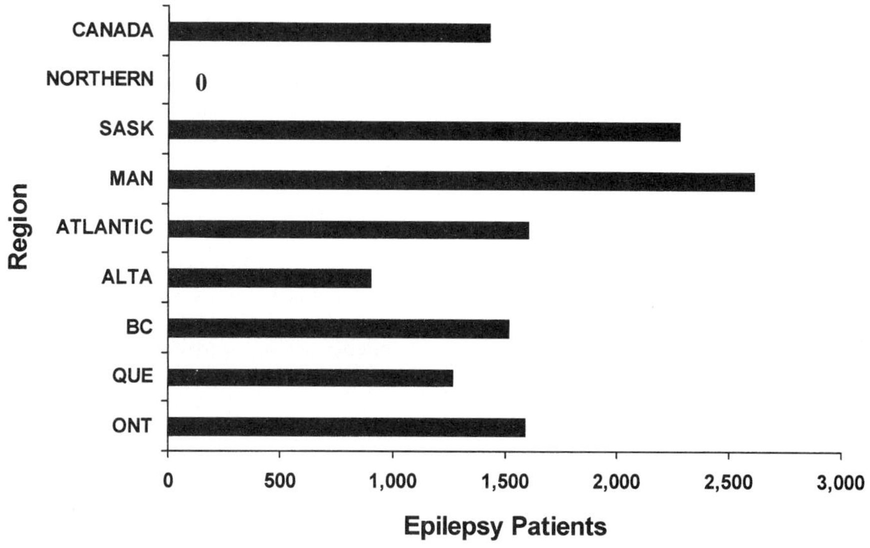

FIGURE 4. Epilepsy patients per magnetic resonance imaging (MRI) scanner. In 2004 there were 167 MRI scanners in Canada. The ratio of patients with epilepsy to MRI scanner was approximately twice that of CT scanners. There was no MRI scanner in the vast North. Northern, Nunavut, Northwest Territories, Yukon; Sask, Saskatchewan; Man, Manitoba; Atlantic, Nova Scotia, Newfoundland & Labrador, New Brunswick, Prince Edward Island; Alta, Alberta; BC, British Columbia; Que, Quebec; Ont, Ontario. (Source: Canadian Institute for Health Information. *Medical Imaging in Canada: 2004*. Ottawa, Canada: Canadian Institutes for Health Information; 2004; and Tellez-Zenteno JF, Pondal-Sordo M, Matijevic S, et al. National and regional prevalence of self-reported epilepsy in Canada. *Epilepsia*. 2004;45(12):1623–1629.)

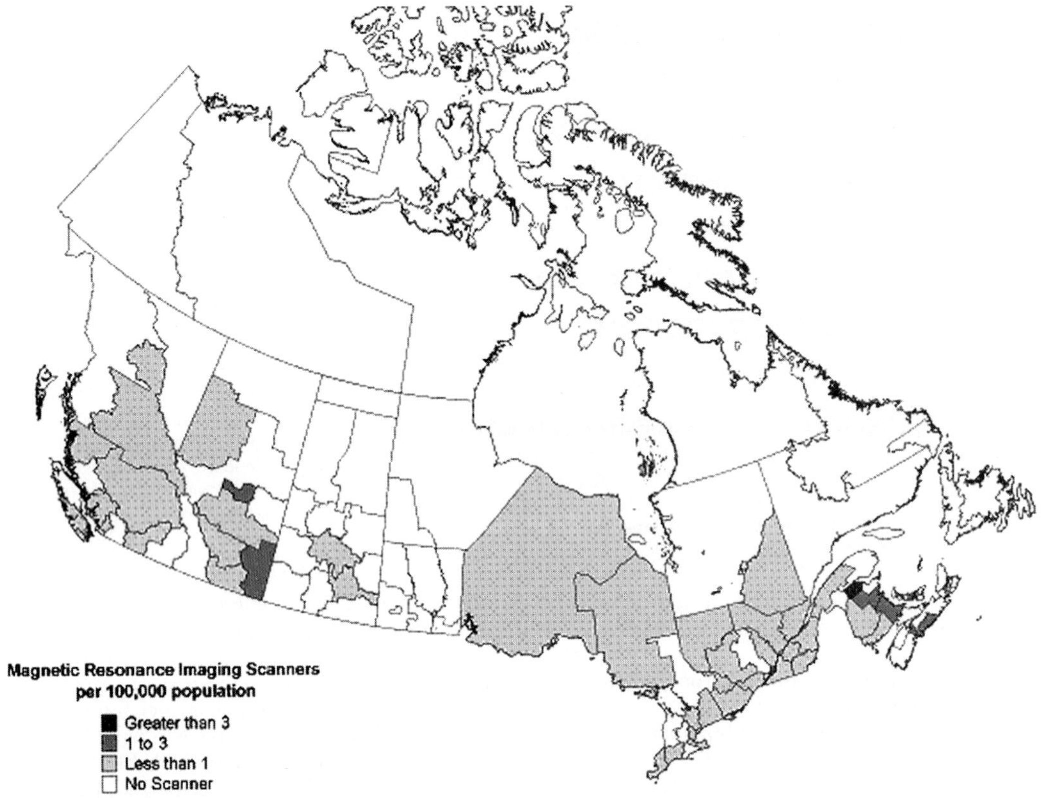

FIGURE 5. Magnetic resonance imaging (MRI) scanners per 100,000 population, 2004. Canadian map illustrating the distribution of MRI scanners in the country in 2004. Notice the distribution of scanners toward the Southern border, and also the clustering around specific large centers located in more heavily populated areas. (Source: Medical Imaging in Canada, 2004. Reprinted with permission from the Canadian Institute for Health Information.)

of epilepsy support groups and have variable degrees of interaction with epilepsy clinicians. The distribution of regional epilepsy support groups follows closely that of the population density across the country. All of the epilepsy support organizations function as not-for-profit charities.

ABORIGINAL POPULATIONS

Canada has the second largest aboriginal population (3.3% of the total population) after New Zealand. For comparison, the percentage of aboriginal population in Australia is 2.2% and in the United States is 1.5%. Little is known about access to health care in general and to epilepsy care in particular in aboriginal populations. However, Canadian national surveys reveal that contact with physicians or with traditional healers varies even within the aboriginal population. Aboriginals residing in urban settings have more frequent contact with physicians than those residing in rural settings. In turn, Aboriginals in the arctic regions have the least contact with physicians or traditional healers (about half as often as those in urban dwellings).[7] This is important because the aboriginal population has higher mortality rate, infant mortality, hospitalization rates, and potential years of life lost from injury than the nonaboriginal Canadian population.[4] Although the incidence and prevalence of epilepsy in aboriginal populations in Canada has not been studied, it is conceivable that lower health indices and a high rate of injuries may have an impact on epilepsy and on access to health care resources for epilepsy.

TABLE 1

EPILEPSY NURSES' CLINICAL ACTIVITIES

Activity	Number (%)
Clinical education	14 (76%)
Seizure monitoring unit	12 (65%)
Presurgical evaluation (outpatient)	10 (58%)
Other patient care	15 (82%)
Patient telephone education	15 (82%)

SUMMARY AND CONCLUSIONS

The Canadian health care system is based on the principles of equity and solidarity, as embodied in the Canadian Health Act, whose objectives are to ensure that all eligible Canadian residents have reasonable access to insured health services, on a prepaid basis, without direct charges at the point of service delivery. The current main barriers to care, according to Statistics Canada (2), are long waiting lists to access elective specialized care and elective diagnostic tests. Another important challenge is the enormous geographic expanse of the country, which also impacts on access to care.

The availability of epilepsy services across the country differs substantially between more and less densely populated areas, which is often a South-North gradient. Among more populated areas, there is some variability in services, especially in regards to the level of specialization, however access is generally adequate. The ratio of adult to paediatric epileptologists is approximately 3:1, which is remarkable given the large number of epilepsies of childhood onset. Facilities for the investigation and treatment of complex epilepsies are available throughout the country and several provinces have more than one centre. Patients can be referred across centres and across provinces throughout the country, as needed.

Most of the frequently used AEDs are included in provincial drug formularies, which determine availability at no cost to special populations such as the elderly, disabled and unemployed. There is no national insurance plan for AEDs, and each province has a different level of insurance. At the time of this writing, AEDs not marketed in Canada include zonisamide, tiagabine, piracetam, and feldamate.

Funding for research in epilepsy derives mostly from the Canadian Institutes of Health Research, which is a federal health research organization. In addition, provincial agencies have smaller opportunities to fund research in epilepsy in some areas. Canada has representative chapters from the International League Against Epilepsy and from the International Bureau for Epilepsy, with corresponding professional and lay memberships, and it is also a member of the North American Region of the International League Against Epilepsy.

References

1. Bailey P, Buske L, Warren S. Highlights of the 2002 Canadian Neurological Society (CNS) Manpower Survey. *Can J Neurol Sci.* 2005;32(4):425–432.
2. Canadian Institute for Health Information. *Canada's Health Care Providers: 2005 Chartbook.* Ottawa, Canada: Canadian Institute for Health Information; 2005.
3. Canadian Institute for Health Information. *Medical Imaging in Canada: 2004.* Ottawa, Canada: Canadian Institutes for Health Information; 2004.
4. Health Canada. *A Statistical Profile on the Health of First Nations in Canada for the Year 2000.* Ottawa, Canada: Health Canada; 2001.
5. Penney S, Robertson M, Martini J, et al. The role and value of specialized epilepsy nurses in Canada. *Epilepsia.* 2005;46(Suppl 8):20.
6. Sanmartin C, Gendron F, Berthelot J, et al. *Access to Health Care Services in Canada: 2003.* Ottawa, Canada: Statistics Canada; 2004.
7. Statistics Canada. *2001 Census of Canada.* Ottawa, Canada: Statistics Canada; 2001. Available at: http://www12.statcan.ca/english/census01/home/index.cfm. Accessed.
8. Tellez-Zenteno JF, Pondal-Sordo M, Matijevic S, et al. National and regional prevalence of self-reported epilepsy in Canada. *Epilepsia.* 2004;45(12):1623–1629.
9. Wiebe S, Bellhouse DR, Fallahay C, et al. Burden of epilepsy: the Ontario Health Survey. *Can J Neurol Sci.* 1999;26(4):263–270.

CHAPTER 291 ■ CHINA

SHICHUO LI, LIWEN WU, GUOMING LUAN, WEIPING LIAO, WENZHI WANG, JIANZHONG WU, AND LIYUN HE

INTRODUCTION

The People's Republic of China (hereinafter referred to as China) is located in East Asia and on the West Coast of the Pacific Ocean. China has 9.6 million km^2 of area and 1.3 billion of population with 56 ethnic groups. Urban population accounts for 42% of the total. The administrative division of the mainland China is 22 provinces, five autonomous regions, and four municipalities directly under the central government.

The following are some public health indicators in China: National health expenditure (2003) of $63.3 (U.S.) per capita and total of $818.7 hundred million (U.S.), which accounted for 5.6% of the gross domestic product (GDP) and 11% of the central government's expenditure allocated to health; life expectancy at birth (2000), 71, 69, and 73 years for total, male, and female, respectively; birth rate (2003), 12.29 per 1,000; death rate (2003), 6.42 per 1,000; infant mortality rate (2004), 25.5 per 1,000; maternal mortality rate (2004), 50.2 per 100,000; and mortality rate under 5 years of age (2004), 30 per 1,000 live births.

Statistics for public health resources are as follows: doctors per 1,000 inhabitants, 1.7; hospital beds per 1,000 inhabitants, 2.4; total number of health institutes in 2004, 296,492, and among them, 18,396 hospitals; and total number of health personnel in 2004, 5,353,628, and among them, 1,904,771 doctors and assistant doctors.

Since the establishment of the People's Republic of China in 1949, remarkable advances have been made in the public health system and in employment. These include the following: (a) There has been an extraordinary improvement in measures of people's health. The life expectancy at birth in 1949 was 35 years, but in 2004 it was 71.8 years. The infant mortality rate in 1949 was 200 per 1,000 live births, but in 2004 it was 25.5. The maternal mortality rate in 1949 was 1,500 per 100,000, but in 2004 it was 50.2. (b) A medical service system has been established that covers the whole nation. The three-tier healthcare system, in rural (county–township–village) and urban areas (city–district–neighborhood) has made great contributions to the improvement of people's health. (c) A medical insurance system is in development. In urban areas, there are four types of medical insurance systems: (i) "free-of-charge system," which covers about 50 million public servants, university students, etc.; (ii) basic medical insurance and (iii) supplementary medical insurance, both of which cover about 130 million workers; and (iv) commercialized insurance, which covers part of private enterprises employees. In rural areas, a new "cooperative medical service system" has just been implemented in a pilot stage, and this presently covers about 156 million farmers. (d) There has been great improvement in the prevention and control of communicable diseases. For example, deaths caused by communicable/parasitic diseases fell from first (in the 1950s) to the ninth (in 2004) place as a cause of death; smallpox, poliomyelitis, etc., have been eradicated; there has been effective control of severe acute respiratory syndrome (SARS) and avian influenza; and effective measures and networks have been put in place to control HIV/AIDS, tuberculosis, hepatitis B and schistosomiasis. (e) Remarkable improvements have been made in maternal and child healthcare. The prenatal examination rate has now reached 90%; the hospitalized delivery rate has reached 83%; and the mortality rate of children under 5 years of age has reached 29.9 per 1,000, whereas in 1949, it was 250 to 300 per 1,000.

Beginning in the late 1970s, China implemented an "open-door and reform" policy. Since then, public health work has further improved and in a number of diseases controlled. The medical service system is now under reform and the medical/health services are expanding coverage. The Chinese government has made great efforts toward the strategic goal of "health for all."

Epilepsy was recognized and described 2,200 years ago in the oldest Chinese medical monograph *Medical Classic of the Yellow Emperor* (Huang Di Nei Jing). In China, epilepsy has long been treated by traditional Chinese medicine (TCM, meaning herbal medicine, acupuncture/moxibustion, and other folk therapies), and a long experience with epilepsy treatment has accumulated. However, the most effective control of epilepsy has resulted from modern medical practices, including surgical treatment. From the 1950s, clinical diagnosis and treatment of epilepsy in China has improved steadily, but very little research on its public health aspects occured until the 1970s.

What is described in this chapter—that is, the epidemiology, clinical neurologic diagnosis and treatment, epilepsy surgery, basic research, sociopsychological problems, rural community control programs, and TCM recognition of epilepsy in China—covers about the last three decades.

EPIDEMIOLOGY

Epidemiology is the study of the distribution and determinants of disease in human populations. Recently, psychosocial and economic indicators, such as quality of life and standards of care, have been incorporated into epidemiologic research, as their relationship to morbidity became evident.

There are several key difficulties in conducting epidemiologic research on epilepsy and in interpreting the epidemiologic literature.[32,47] These include:

- Variations in the definitions and classification of seizures and of epilepsies
- Poor case ascertainment due to ignorance or concealment by patients or their families, or due to the fact that some patients are not aware of having seizures
- Diagnostic imprecision, even when potential patients are identified
- Differences between studies in the age distribution of study populations, or in the place or mode of recruitment of subjects

These and other factors all limit the precision and validity of data and comparability among studies. Despite these difficulties, sufficient data are available from a number of studies

TABLE 1

PREVALENCE RATIO AND INCIDENCE RATE OF EPILEPSY IN CHINA

Year	Study	Reporter	Sample population	Prevalence (per 1,000)	Incidence (per 100,000)
1981	Sichuan		426,789	4.8	35
1983	6 cities	Li	63,195	4.4	35
1985	22 provinces	Li	246,812	3.6	26
1992	Jiangsu	Shan	(0–14 yr)	5.9	200
2003	6 rural areas	Wang	55,616	7.0	(active 4.6)

to give a useful profile of the epidemiologic characteristics of epilepsy in China.

Prevalence Ratio

Researchers use lifetime prevalence to express the magnitude and scope of the burden of a defined disorder in the population. Point prevalence is the proportion of a defined population with a disease at a given point in time (usually the first or last day of a year). The point lifetime prevalence ratio results for epilepsy in China from some studies are shown in Table 1. We may see that the prevalence for epilepsy in China is about 4 to 6 per 1,000, which is similar to the average figure in industrialized countries. In Wang's study, patients with epilepsy who had seizures in the past year were categorized as "active epilepsy"; for those cases, the prevalence ratio was found to be 4.6 per 1,000.[41]

Incidence Rate

Incidence rate is the rate of occurrence of new cases of epilepsy in a defined population in a specified time period (usually 1 year). Table 1 also shows the incidence rates for epilepsy in China as 26 to 35 per 100,000 individuals per year.

Mortality Rate

Unfortunately in most countries epilepsy is not listed in "cause of death" statistics as an independent disease. Deaths of persons with epilepsy (PWE) are always registered as caused by the underlying disease or some other reason, such as "accident." Reports from China showed 7.9 per 100,000 per year in urban areas and 6.9 per 100,000 per year in rural areas. The figure from China is higher than that from other countries, and this difference is not explained.[47]

In recent years, the *standardized mortality rate* (SMR) has been used in the epidemiologic literature to analyze deaths in epilepsy. These analyses show that the SMR for epilepsy patients is more than twice that for the general population. Causes of mortality include (a) underlying brain diseases, such as tumor or infection; (b) seizure-related deaths (status epilepticus; drowning, burns, or other trauma; severe aspiration or airway obstruction by food, etc.; deaths caused by habitual seizures when coexisting with cardiorespiratory disease); (c) suicide; (d) death as a consequence of medical or surgical treatment of epilepsy; and (e) sudden unexplained death in epilepsy (SUDEP), whose causes remain ill-understood.[29,47]

Research and data on SUDEP are very rare in China. From 1994 to 2004, only three papers on this topic were published, and two of them were literature reviews. Wang et al.[44] analyzed the clinical and pathologic information of seven cases of SUDEP. They found that all seven cases had edema of the brain and lungs. Some of the patients had reduction of neurons and increase of glial cells. There were no tumors or injuries. All seven died when they had a general tonic–clonic seizure. Two occurred in sleep and four had agitation or fright before death.

One hundred and twenty PWE from four provinces in China who had been part of a project, "community control of epilepsy," in the late 1980s were followed up 5 years later. Thirteen had died. The mortality rate of this group was 2.2% per year and around 3.4 times higher than the rate in the general population. Among the 13 deceased, two (15.4%) might be categorized as SUDEP. This may be the only epidemiologic information for SUDEP in China.[40]

Distribution by Sex and Age

As reported from most of other countries, in China, the prevalence and incidence of epilepsy is more frequent in men than in women. The prevalence in men and women in urban areas is 1.3:1 and the incidence is 1.7:1; in rural areas, it is 1.1:1 and 1.4:1, respectively. These differences are probably related to the more social and physical activities of men than of women and thus more frequently risk factors and causes for epilepsy are encountered by men. For age-specific prevalence, data from China showed that it is rising with age in childhood and adolescence, then plateauing in middle age, and decreasing in old age. As for age-specific incidence, there are two peaks: in childhood and the elderly. A study from Sichuan province indicated that 80% of epilepsy occurred before 15 years of age. Cerebrovascular disease, brain tumors, and other identifiable causes are responsible for the second peak of incidence in the older age group.[23]

Subtypes of Seizures

Table 2 shows the relative frequency of subtypes of seizures reported from China and some other countries.[23] Much of the variation among countries is probably related to differences in methods of data collection, sample size, classification scheme, and certainty of clinical diagnosis. Therefore, it is difficult to compare them or draw inferences. For example, the apparent high proportions of generalized seizures in the two studies from China reflect the fact that those studies focused on convulsive seizures rather than nonconvulsive seizures.

Risk Factors

In epidemiologic studies, scientists usually use retrospective methods (typically case-control studies) to identify risk factors

TABLE 2

RELATIVE FREQUENCY OF SUBTYPES OF SEIZURE

Subtype	China 1	China 2	Singapore	Turkey	Tanzania	United States
GS	89.6	77.3	65.2	78.9	58	40
GTCS	81	71.8	56.3	65.4	54.1	23
Absence	4.8	3.9	2.2	4.9	1	6
Other	3.8	1.6	6.7	8.6	2.9	11
PS[a]	7.6	18.6	34.8	19.7	31.9	57
SPS	4.8	4.4	2.2	7.4	0.5	21
CPS	2.8	5.9	4.5	12.3	9.2	36
PS > GS	—	8.3	28.1	—	22.2	—
Other	2.8	4.1	—	1.2	10.1	3

CPS, complex partial seizure; GS, generalized seizure; GTCS, generalized tonic–clonic seizure; PS, partial seizure; PS > GS, partial seizure with secondary generalization; SPS, simple partial seizure.

for epilepsy. For a number of practical reasons, prospective (cohort) methods, although theoretically preferable, are rarely used.

Table 3 shows the results of two case-control studies that were conducted in six cities of China in 1983 and in rural areas of 22 provinces in 1985.[23] The findings generally match those of a number of studies in other countries.[47] Many epidemiologic studies implicate genetic factors, perinatal factors, and a history of febrile seizures as risk factors for various major kinds of epilepsy, although some controversy persists.

The discovery of epilepsy genes has benefitted from the success of the Human Genome Project, a multinational endeavor that has produced detailed maps of the human chromosomes. The genes responsible for particular genetic epilepsies can now be identified and localized to specific chromosomal regions, ultimately allowing researchers to determine the structure of the encoded molecules. This requires the study of families in which several members are affected with well-characterized epilepsies. The *genetic "lesions"* responsible for idiopathic epilepsies give rise to various familial epilepsy syndromes.[3] A genetic etiology is indicated by, for example, familial incidence and frequent clinical concordance in twin studies.

In most studies, populations with *poor perinatal health care*, high incidence of premature births and head trauma during delivery, and high infant mortality are at high risk for epilepsy. The major perinatal factors include short gestation, low birth weight, prolonged labor, neonatal asphyxia, and assisted delivery.

Febrile illness of any kind can trigger seizures in young children. About 3% of children who have *febrile convulsions* go on to develop epilepsy in later life.

Some investigations suggest that rural populations with poor health services and disadvantaged urban populations should be included in the epilepsy high-risk group: The relevant factors here are almost certainly poverty and low socioeconomic status, which are themselves associated with high rates of epilepsy, as they are with so many other diseases.

Causes of Symptomatic Epilepsy

When epilepsy appears to be caused by an identifiable brain disease, it is categorized as *symptomatic epilepsy*. These causes include head injury; intracranial infection (e.g., neurocysticercosis, malaria); cerebrovascular disease; brain tumor; drugs and alcohol; carbon monoxide poisoning; and effects of ionizing radiation.

Table 4 shows the results of a retrospective study in six cities of China in 1983.[3]

Prognosis and Remission

There are very few research reports on the natural history of epilepsy in China. In a survey conducted in the rural areas of 22 provinces in the 1980s, there were 904 cases of epilepsy, 417 of

TABLE 3

RISK FACTORS FOR IDIOPATHIC EPILEPSY (CASE-CONTROL STUDIES IN SIX CITIES AND RURAL AREAS OF 22 PROVINCES OF PEOPLE'S REPUBLIC OF CHINA)

	6 cities		22 rural areas	
Expected risk factor	RR[a]	$p <$	RR	$p <$
Parents' intermarriage	—	(>0.05)	9	0.001
Epileptics in family	2.5	0.01	15.4	0.001
Previous febrile seizures	7.5	0.01	32.2	0.001
Premature or difficult labor	3.2	0.025	13	0.001
Born when mother >30 yr of age	1.5	0.05	1.4	0.025

[a] RR (relative risk) = B/C; B, case (+), control (–); C, case (–), control (+).

TABLE 4

PUTATIVE CAUSES OF SYMPTOMATIC EPILEPSY CASES IN SIX CHINESE CITIES

Putative cause	No. of cases	%
Head injury	29	47.5
Intracranial infection	15	24.6
Cerebrovascular disease	10	16.4
Intracranial tumor	2	3.3
Other	5	8.2
Total	**61**	**100.0**

them were treated, 448 were not, and 39 were unclear. Among the untreated 448 cases, spontaneous remission rate (SRR) at 2 years was 40.4% and at 5 years was 27.4%. Studies showed that SRRs ranged from 20% to 39%. These figures are similar to what Zielinski reported (5-year remission rates of 28.6% to 30.6%).

Factors relative to the prognosis or remission rate (RR) include: (a) *Age of onset.* The highest RR was reported if onset was between 7 and 9 years old. The RR for those whose onset was before 14 years was 71%, and before 20 years, 42%. For those whose onset was before 1 year and after 40 years, the RR is low because of one increase in number of organic disorders that cause epilepsy in those age groups. (b) Seizure types: Generalized tonic–clonic seizures (GTCSs) had a higher RR (38% to 62%). (c) Frequency of seizures: Low frequency of seizures had a higher RR. More than one seizure per day had an RR of 20% to 27%, fewer than ten seizures per year had an RR of 50% to 57%, and fewer than one seizure per year had an RR of 67%. This indicates that seizure frequency before treatment is an important factor that affects prognosis, but it is an exception for absence seizures. (d) Idiopathic or symptomatic epilepsy: The former (RR of 47% to 63%) has a higher RR than the latter (RR of 24% to 27%). (e) Course of the disorder: Shorter course had a higher RR: <1 year, RR 53%; >5 years, RR 17%. (f) Neuropsychological defects: There were higher RRs if the patients were without these defects.[10,23]

The impacts of antiepileptic drug (AED) treatment on prognosis are evident. Regular treatment with AEDs may control 70% to 80% of epileptic seizures, whereas with AEDs taken irregularly the RR is similar to untreated. Good compliance with AED treatment leads to good prognosis. One study showed a 92% control rate in a compliant treatment group of children patients, but 56% in the noncompliant group. Recurrence after stopping AED treatment is a major concern of epileptologists. A report from China showed a 24% recurrence rate for 8 years after stopping AEDs, and 55% of the recurrence occurred in the first 1 years.[10]

CLINICAL DIAGNOSIS AND TREATMENT

The diagnosis and treatment of epilepsy in China has improved greatly in the past 50 years, which may be attributed to the practical efforts of neurologists/epileptologists, the development of the electroencephalography (EEG) and other diagnostic equipment and technology, and the broad international academic exchanges.[49]

Diagnosis of Epilepsy

Adequately Using the International Seizure and Epilepsy Classification to Diagnose Epilepsy

The accurate categorization and recognition of seizures and epilepsies are the foundation of correct diagnosis and further in-depth research and communication, and are also reflected in the progressive knowledge about epilepsy. The international classifications in the 1980s have been wildly used, including the Seizure Classification in 1981, the Epilepsy and Epilepsy Syndrome Classification in 1985, and its revision in 1989 proposed by the International League Against Epilepsy (ILAE). These have received common acceptance by most epileptologists. The introduction of the 1981 ILAE seizure classification into China occurred at the first National Epilepsy Conference in 1985, and it was revised somewhat to make it suitable to the practical situation in China.[37] The Chinese Classification of Epilepsy and Epilepsy Syndromes, referring to ILAE's proposal, was recommended in the seventh National Pediatric Neurology Conference in 1995.[8] The aforementioned classifications of the 1980s are now wildly used in the clinical and research work in China, as well as in research about mesial temporal lobe epilepsy and absence epilepsy, the study of the relationship between mesial temporal epilepsy and hippocampal sclerosis, and clinical observation on uncommon epilepsy syndromes, such as the acquired epileptic aphasia and West syndrome. Since the 1990s, more attention has been given to the clinical research and EEG analysis of frontal lobe epilepsy, which has complex clinical manifestations, and the recognition and diagnosis level to it has been thus much improved.

For the past few decades, much progress has been made in understanding epilepsy symptomatology, etiology, pathology, diagnosis, and treatment. The same progress can be observed in China. In 2001, the ILAE Task Force, led by Prof. Engel, proposed a new classification of epilepsy that reflected the new knowledge in epileptology and influenced the clinical practice greatly. It introduced some new concepts as "axis" in diagnosis, which was helpful to standardize the clinical diagnosis. The proposal was introduced in China soon after its publication and is now used widely.[1] There have been great changes in the classification of epileptic seizures, which rely mostly on the symptoms reflecting the relationship between the symptom and anatomic location that gives clues about the epilepsy syndrome. In addition, classification now emphasizes the psychosocial impacts on the quality of life of epileptic patients in diagnostic procedures. We found that the new proposal was not easy to use with in clinical practice because of lack of detailed explanation in some parts. Epileptic seizures and their semiology, are the core of epilepsy classification. In some degree the new classification ignores changes in high-level cortical function, for example, by excluding classification criteria based on changes in consciousness and neglecting mental manifestations, which are important features of some epileptic seizures. Furthermore, it is difficult to classify occasional seizures observed in clinical work.

The Development of the Electrophysiological Techniques

There are two key features in epilepsy: Clinical seizure and EEG manifestations. EEG is one of the most important auxiliary examinations in epilepsy diagnosis. With no doubt, the emergence of EEG is a milestone that divided the history of epilepsy diagnosis into two stages.

The first EEG machine in China was imported into the Nanjing Brain Disease Hospital in 1949 in China and used in clinical examinations in 1951. Then a series of training courses about epilepsy and EEG were held by Feng Yingkun from the Peking Union Medical College (PUMC) Hospital. Now EEG testing is used in most hospitals in China. The international system of 10- to 20-electrode placement is used and includes both referential and bipolar recordings. Activating procedures, such as open/close eyes, hyperventilation, intermittent photic stimulation, and sedated sleep are routinely applied in most hospitals. The recording and interpretation of EEG requires expertise, but there are not yet standardized training and qualification systems for EEG technicians in China.

Mesial temporal lobe epilepsy is the most common epilepsy type. Feng Yingkun found that acupuncture pins could be used as substitutes for sphenoidal electrodes with good effect and easy acceptance.[11] There have now been more than 30,000 patients who had acupuncture pins used as sphenoidal electrodes in the PUMC Hospital.

Since the 1990s, video-EEG has been performed in many EEG labs in China. The electrocorticogram and deep electrode EEG have been used in some hospitals, which can give more information in locating the epileptogenic foci.

Other Examination Methods

In addition to electrophysiology, some new diagnostic techniques have been introduced in recent years. Imaging the hippocampus is now performed in China. Hippocampus volumetric quantitative measurement techniques are also very helpful in diagnosing and treating mesial temporal epilepsy.

The Establishment of Epilepsy Centers and Epilepsy Clinics

Since the 1990s, specialized epilepsy clinics and centers have been established in the bigger hospitals. These kinds of centers usually include neurologists, pediatric neurologists, neurosurgeons, psychiatrists and social workers. Sophisticated equipment for diagnosis is available and an operating theater equipped. Multidiscipline cooperation is the most important characteristic of such centers/clinics. They serve not only as clinical work sites, but also as sites for research, training, and public education. These centers are important developments in the prevention and control of epilepsy in China.

Drugs for Epilepsy

Medication is still the most important treatment option for patients with epilepsy. Selection of AEDs depends on the type of seizure and syndrome classification. The common AEDs used in China are valproate, carbamazepine, phenytoin, and phenobarbital. Approximately 60% to 70% of epilepsy patients can achieve remission using monotherapy. Polytherapy is chosen when patients' seizures cannot be controlled by monotherapy. We have found that side effects of rash and neutropenia occur in about 5% to 10% of patients on carbamazepine. Valproate needs careful consideration when it is used in women of child bearing age because of weight-gain and polycystic ovary syndrome effects. Phenytoin and phenobarbital have similar efficacy to carbamazepine but are no longer the first choice because of their adverse effects. However, they are still used as first-line AEDs in rural and poor regions in China. Valproate is drug of first choice in treating generalized seizure, and carbamazepine for focal seizures. Since the 1990s blood levels of AEDs have been available in big hospitals and epilepsy centers.

Since the 1990s, there have become available more than ten new AEDs on the international market, and most of them are useful in cases of intractable epilepsy. With relatively wide spectra, fewer adverse effects, fewer interactions, and better tolerance, the new AEDs offer, more choices for refractory patients. Presently, lamotrigine, topiramate, vigabatrin, gabapentin, and oxcarbazepine are available in China, and zonisamide and levetiracetam are going to be on the market soon. Most new AEDs serve as add-on drugs. The combination of lamotrigine and valproate is better for some refractory epilepsies, but skin rash has occurred.

EPILEPSY SURGERY: A REVIEW

Although the trephenation opening found on a skull unearthed in Shandong province indicates that the history of surgical treatment of brain disease in China is more than 5,000 years old, modern epilepsy surgery has been available only in recent years. There is no record of epilepsy surgery in the literature or in hospitals' records before the People's Republic of China was established in 1949. The earliest record of epilepsy surgery in China may date to the 1950s to 1960s, for example, "traumatic epilepsy" written by Guosheng Duan, "hemispherectomy for West Syndrome" by Yuquan Shi, and "epilepsy surgery" by Yadu Zhao. In the following two decades, some political and social factors resulted in temporary delay in further development of epilepsy surgery.

In the late 1980s, following implementation of reform and open-door policy, scientific and technologic exchanges between China and Western developed countries resumed quickly. Advanced medical equipment and new techniques were introduced to China. A number of senior neurosurgeons restarted surgical treatment for epilepsy including anterior temporal lobe resection, callosotomy, multiple subpial transection (MST), stereotactic neurosurgery, and cerebellar stimulation. The method of lower-power electrocoagulation of eloquent areas in or adjacent to epileptogenic foci, advocated by Guoming Luan, added a new way to treat eloquent areas in epilepsy.

Localization of Epileptogenic Foci

The effectiveness of epilepsy surgery is mainly based on a precise localization of epileptogenic foci. Currently, many provincial and municipal level hospitals have electrophysiologic examination and sophisticated equipment such as CT, MRI, and even SPECT, PET, and MEG for the diagnosis of epilepsy and synthetic localization of epileptogenic foci. The introduction of MEG has improved the synthetic preoperative evaluation for epilepsy to a new stage. Furthermore, the development of electrophysiologic examination manifested not only in the noninvasion, but also in the invasion technique of using strip or grid or depth electrode. They can give further explanations about which areas have eloquent and noneloquent functions and which areas can be identified as irritating and epileptogenic areas.

The Basic Study Related to Epilepsy Surgery

In recent years, basic scientific research has made great progress, such as the epileptic nets and stereotactic atlas of epileptogenic foci and tissues around them. The various epileptic animal models made by chemical and electrical methods can help neurosurgeons prepare all kinds of operations; the electrophysiologic studies of cerebral cells and tissues can make a ground for treating the intractable epilepsy using electrostimulation methods; the chemical studies of neurosynapse and neuroreceptors in the excitable and suppressive neurotransmitters filed can theoretically support the method of cerebral tissue and neurostem cell transplantation to treat refractory epilepsy;

the microstructure studies of epileptogenic foci such as amygdalohippocampus tissues can further expound dual epileptic pathology and its relation to postoperative effects; the neuroimaging studies such as MRI and MRS can clearly define the side and site of epileptogenic foci; and the anatomy studies of epileptic surgical approaches can increase the surgical safety coefficient and reduce the probability of postoperative complications.

The Clinical Studies of Epilepsy Surgery

Most types of epilepsy operations performed elsewhere have been successfully done in China. The number of operations has increased year by year. For example, only 1,840 epilepsy cases were reported in the first epilepsy surgery congress held in 1991, among which there were 933 cases of stereotactic ablation and only half of patients had resections with craniotomy. In the sixth congress of stereotactic and functional neurosurgery in 2004, a total of 2,077 operated cases were reported, among which there were 2,029 epilepsy cases with craniotomy treatment (more than two times the number of 13 years ago) and 48 cases with the stereotactic ablation. There were 680 cases with epileptogenic lesion and neocortical resection reported in the *Chinese Journal of Stereotactic and Functional Neurosurgery* in 2001 and 2002. By 2004, the number of reported cases of epileptogenic lesion and neocortical resection increased to 1,057. The total proportion of Engel I and II levels reached 65% to 85% among them. With regard to temporal lobe epilepsy, about 400 operations were performed each year, and the Engel levels I and II effectiveness reached 75% to 90%. Approximately 400 cases of hemispherectomy, stereotactic radiosurgery, electrostimulation, and other operations have been done each year. What is worth mentioning is that several hospitals recently used lower-power electrocoagulation to treat eloquent epilepsy, amounting to about 200 cases every year, and the proportion of Engel I and II results is around 65%. This fact indicates that the new method has obtained recognition by our domestic colleagues. The number of hospitals with epilepsy surgery capability increased every year. For example, in Beijing, three hospitals had epilepsy departments in the 1990s, whereas nine hospitals had such departments in 2005. Research on "the basic and clinical studies of intractable epilepsy surgery" has been awarded the second prize of the National Science Technology Progress Award.

Application of Neuroimaging and Gamma Knife

A number of hospitals have bought Gamma Knife equipment and begun epilepsy stereotactic radiosurgery programs. In 2004, 15 Leksell Gamma Knifes and 20 OUT-XGD rotation Gamma Knifes were available in China. However, there are still disputes about choice of treatment-site, dose, and effectiveness.

Academic exchanges on epilepsy surgery have been quite active in China in recent years. The Epilepsy Surgery Association was founded in 1990 with around 150 to 200 epilepsy surgeons as members. Several conferences and workshops on epilepsy surgery have been held in the past two decades. The National Epilepsy Surgery Workshop has been held four times since 1991, and the National Stereotactic and Functional Neurosurgery Congress has been held six times since 1987. International academic exchanges about epilepsy surgery have increased remarkably as well.

Three journals of epilepsy surgery are issued in China: *Chinese Journal of Stereotactic and Functional Neurosurgery*, *Asian Journal of Epilepsy*, and *News Letter of Epilepsy Surgery*. In the past 10 years, five monographs were published: Epilepsy Surgery, Temporal Lobe Epilepsy, Temporal Lobe Epilepsy Surgery, Neurosurgery and Epilepsy, and the second edition of Lüders' *Epilepsy Surgery*, in translation.

BASIC RESEARCH ON GENETICS AND NEUROSCIENCES

In recent years studies on the molecular basis of inherited epilepsy have been performed in China. Tang et al. reported a novel frameshift mutation of the *KCNQ2* gene, 1931delG, in a large Chinese family with benign familial neonatal convulsions (BFNC). This mutation is located in the C-terminus of *KCNQ2*, in codon 644, predicting the replacement of the last 201 amino acids with a stretch of 257 amino acids showing a completely different sequence.[36] In a Chinese family with benign familial infantile convulsions (BFICs), Xiao et al. found that it was not linked to the 19q12.1-13.1, 16p12-q12, or 2q24 loci.[50] The results indicated that BFIC showed genetic heterogeneity and the Chinese BFIC families might be mapped on another new locus.

Childhood absence epilepsy (CAE) is one of the most frequently recognized syndromes among the idiopathic generalized epilepsies (IGEs). CAE is considered a genetic disease with a possible polygenic inheritance pattern, but the genes responsible for CAE have not yet been identified. Lu et al. reported that γ-aminobutyric acid $(GABA)_A$ receptor subunit genes, *GABRA5* and *GABRB3*, may be directly involved either in the etiology of CAE in the Chinese population or in linkage disequilibrium with disease-predisposing sites.[28] Their studies suggest that the *GABBR1*, *GABRG2*, T-type calcium channel gene α (1G), and *T-STAR* might not be susceptibility genes for CAE, at least in the Chinese population studied,[7,27] whereas the T-type calcium channel gene *CACNA1H* might be a susceptibility gene to childhood absence epilepsy.[5] The mutation of G773D has been found in one other Chinese family with CAE. Ge et al. concluded that the CAE gene is transmitted with disequilibrium on locus D8S1783, and the CAE gene may be in the ECA1 area on chromosome 8q24. Heterogeneity of the CAE gene in different populations was suspected.[12]

Familial febrile convulsion (FC) is a common pediatric disorder with an obvious inherent predisposition. Qi et al. concluded that FC is linked with chromosome region 19p13.3, but not with chromosomes 6p and 8q.[31] The *CSNK1G2* gene of the region 19p13.3 appears to be a susceptibility gene for FS in the Han population of northern China.[52]

Liu et al. studied the clinical and inherent characteristics of generalized epilepsy with febrile seizures plus (GEFS+) in a large group of Chinese families. This group is screening mutations of *SCN1A*, *SCN1B*, *SCN2A*, and *GABRG2* in the Han population, and a new mutation of *SCN1A* has recently been discovered. Huang et al. reported a GEFS+ gene mapped to 5q34 in two Chinese families and a single nucleotide polymorphism (SNP) from candidate gene *GANRA6* exon 8.[15,26]

Many laboratory facilities are dedicated to exploring the fundamental mechanisms of epilepsy, including drug resistance and the consequences of repeated seizures on brain function, by using different epilepsy models. A model with pharmacoresistent temporal lobe epilepsy features has been developed by repeated intramuscular injection of Coriaria lactone (CL),[45] an abstract from traditional herbs. This model was demonstrated with high kindling efficiency and typical behavioral and electrophysiologic manifestations. CL is reported to increase the release of glutamate and inhibit the synthesis of GABA in cultured neurons; there is also evidence from cerebrospinal fluid (CSF) of an acute CL-induced epilepsy model. In pathologic studies on the CL model, degeneration of neurons and necrosis of astrocytes appeared widely in different cerebral areas; this was also supported by an increased BCl-2 level in neurons. During the early stage of a CL-induced seizure, an influx of extracellular Ca^{2+} has been found, indicating that Ca^{2+} signals were involved in the CL-induced seizures. One distinct feature of this model was the pharmacoresistance to AEDs, such as carbamazepine, valproate, and phenytoin. An up-regulation of P-GP-multidrug resistance 1 (MDR1) encoded protein P-170 was found in the CL model, especially in the AED-treated CL model, indicating that the mechanism underlying pharmacoresistance to AEDs was associated with overexpression of *MDR1* gene.[8] This model had been widely used in studies of epileptogenesis.

Audiogenic seizure-prone rats were also widely used as epilepsy models. The P77PMC rat has congenital audiogenic seizure (AGS). Zhang et al.[53] found that antisense oligodeoxynucleotides for *N*-methyl-D-aspartate (NMDA) receptor 1 and gap junction protein Cx32 could alleviate AGS and inhibit the frequency and amplitude of neuronal discharges in temporal cortical slices of the P77PMC rat. These results indicate that gap junction protein might play a role in the pathogenesis of epilepsy by controlling functions of electrical synapses. The DBA/2J mouse was another breed of mouse with high-intensity noise-induced audiogenic seizures. Li et al.[24] examined the gene expression profiling of AGS DBA/2J mice by using oligo-microarrays. They specifically tested the effects of Qingyangshenylycosides (QYS), abstracts from TCM, on seizure behavior and gene expression of AGS. Results showed that QYS could effectively prevent AGS and AGS-induced gene expression changes. The antiepileptic effects of some TCM were studied in other research groups. Acorus tatarinowii Schott (ATS), one of the traditional antiepileptic medicines, had been demonstrated to be able to induce sedation, decrease spontaneous activity, and possess anticonvulsive and spasmolytic action in modern pharmacologic studies. Liao et al.[25] reported that both the decoction and volatile oil extracted from ATS exhibited neuroprotection and anticonvulsive effects. Further studies on these Chinese herbs might provide clues for the development of new antiepileptic drugs.

Epileptic seizures might induce neuronal death and secondary epileptic foci. Antiepileptogenesis and neuroprotection may have clinical significance. To evaluate the long-term effects of prolonged neonatal seizures on seizure threshold and neuronal activity in the brain, Ni et al.[30] compared the immunoreactivity changes of c-Fos, NMDA receptor 2C, and $GABA_A$ in single seizure and recurrent seizure models. They found that prolonged seizures had long-term effects on seizure threshold and receptor protein expression, and recurrent seizures could cause obvious neuronal injury. Yin et al.[51] demonstrated that down-regulation of N-ethylmaleimide-sensitive fusion (NSF) protein and the loss of DA neurons were involved in mechanisms underlying the spatial learning memory deficits induced by spontaneous recurrent seizures (SRS). Nitric oxide (NO) is a readily diffusible "intercellular messenger molecule" acting to generate a cascade effect by the second messenger cyclic guanosine monophosphate (cGMP) that mediates excitotoxicity in various brain structures. Sun CK et al.[34] demonstrated that a single injection of kainate (10 mg/kg intraperitoneally) induces progressive seizures with an increased accumulation of nitrite, the stable metabolite of NO, in hippocampal homogenates of rodents, measured by the Griess reaction. L-NG-nitroarginine (NNA), an inhibitor of constitutive NO synthases (cNOS), especially neuronal NOS (nNOS), significantly enhanced the severity of kainate-induced seizures and damage in hippocampal subregions. However, administration of L-arginine (Arg), a substrate for NO synthase, unexpectedly suppressed both seizures and brain damage. The effects of NNA and Arg on kainate-induced seizures and brain damage were accompanied by appositive changes in immunoreactivity of glial fibrillary acidic protein (GFAP) and interleukin-6 in the hippocampus.

The research grants for epilepsy have been increased greatly in China in recent years. As more and more scientists have been interested in epileptology, more detailed discoveries are expected in the future.

PSYCHOSOCIAL ASPECTS OF EPILEPSY IN CHINA

Fear, misunderstanding, and the resulting social stigma and discrimination surrounding epilepsy often force people with this disorder "into the shadows." The social effect may vary from country to country and culture to culture, but it is clear that throughout the world the social consequences of epilepsy are often more difficult to overcome than the seizures themselves.[48]

Cross-cultural studies on epileptic patients revealed high rates of psychological and social problems.[2,18] Epileptic patients are frequently denied schooling, shunned by their peers, find it difficult to marry, and meet active employment discrimination.

In recent years, psychosocial studies on epilepsy have been performed in China. In 1988 a public awareness of epilepsy study was conducted among 1,278 respondents in Henan province. The study found that 93% of interviewees had heard of epilepsy; more than 75% knew someone with epilepsy; and almost 75% had seen someone have a seizure.[21] Furthermore, expressed negative attitudes were extensive. More than 50% of the sample said that they would object to having their children associate or play with persons with epilepsy; more than 50% also believed epileptics should not be employed in the same jobs as others. Notably, 87%, irrespective of their education level, would object to having their children marry a person with epilepsy.

In 1992, in cooperation with Dr. A. Kleinman from Harvard University, the Beijing Neurosurgical Institute conducted a psychosocial study in adult epileptic patients.[19] Forty patients with epilepsy in urban areas and 40 patients with epilepsy in rural areas were selected from the Ningxia and Shanxi provinces. The patients and their family members were interviewed together and separately during home visits by local research teams composed of neurologists who had been trained to use a semi-structured interview schedule in training workshops. The interview canvassed demographics, experiences of illness and treatment, and both family and patient perspectives on local social responses to and consequences of the illness. The interview format used open-ended questions to encourage extended responses.

Great variation exists in the public's ideas of the cause of epilepsy, ranging from heredity, head injury, possession, geomancy, poverty, and overwork to anger and fright. Patients and their family members showed a tendency to increasingly use overwork, strong effects, and a wide range of new explanations to explain why seizures continued (Table 5). Possession and head injury were less frequently named as likely causes.

Table 6 shows respondents' perception of the chief effects of epilepsy on the patients. Emotional, financial, and family/marital burdens were reported to be extensive. Relations with others and overall quality of life also were strongly affected. These effects appear to be greater in rural areas. Stigma affects both the family members and the patients themselves. Most of them felt "loss of face" (conveying the embodied sense of shameful loss of moral status) and feelings of diminished self-esteem were widespread.

TABLE 5

PERCEIVED CAUSES OF SEIZURES BY EPILEPTIC PATIENTS

"Cause"	%	"Cause"	%
Anger	23%	Wrong food	5%
Possession	19%	Retribution	5%
Fright or anxiety	16%	God's will	3%
Head injury	16%	Heredity	4%
Negative geomancy	8%	Infection	3%
Poverty	8%	Congenital	1%
Overworked	8%	Others[a]	25%

[a]Includes weather change, menstruation, smoking, febrile convulsion, carbon monoxide poisoning, etc.
From Wang WZ, et al. *Chin Ment Health J.* 1995;9:129.

The Western tradition's emphasis on the subjective feeling of the afflicted individual, often viewed as isolated and forlorn, is the dominant analytic paradigm for understanding the suffering that results from serious chronic illness and disability.[20] Furthermore, suffering becomes the pain, hurt, loss, and search for meaning of a unique person who alone must bear the deep burden of his or her troubles. According to this view, suffering is a mode of social experience. The point is not to minimize the seriousness of the problems faced by individual patients with epilepsy in our study, but rather to appreciate the importance that they and their families attribute to the interpersonal, relational locus of hardship among the members of the family. Indeed, this intersubjective sensibility frequently leads family members to emphasize their own adversity as equivalent to or even greater than the patient's experience. The study focused on the concerns by the family and its members. What is most at stake in suffering is the abridgement of the family's aspirations, the threat to the life chances of its members, and the loss and hurt of the others. The result showed that suffering is as much the intersubjective experience of parents, spouses, siblings, and children as that of the patient.

For Chinese parents, the presence of a disabled child means that they are both legally and morally responsible for his or her care until that son or daughter gets married or the child dies. With marriage, the responsibility for care is shifted to the spouse and the couple's future children. Thus, there is great pressure to arrange marriage. To do so, parents try to disguise that their child has epilepsy, but if they are unable to, they will barter for a spouse with promises of an urban residence permit or employment. Illness and disability restrict the pool of potential marital partners to those who also have illness or disability and to those who are poorer, more rural, less educated, and physically less attractive. The consequences of disguise and barter are fraught with interpersonal tensions that the parents, patient, and spouse must negotiate over the long term. But to not marry is far worse: It threatens the centrality of family in Chinese society.

Many respondents believe that the financial consequences of epilepsy are serious and even ruinous. Perhaps no other aspect of social life so clearly shows the power of chronic illness to affect local worlds and reciprocally of local worlds to influence the course of illness and treatment. The current economic transformation of Chinese society marks finances as a major issue, especially in the poor regions where our study was conducted. Some farmers in our sample lived at the brink of financial catastrophe. The social welfare net of communal life is no longer

TABLE 6

IMPACTS OF EPILEPSY ON PATIENTS AND FAMILY

	Ningxia		Shanxi		Total (%)	
	Patients	Family	Patients	Family	Patients	Family
Stigma	36	38	35	23	71 (89)	61 (76)
"Loss of face"	28	24	25	10	53 (66)	34 (43)
Self-esteem	33	—	35	—	68 (85)	
Emotional burden	39	40	39	39	78 (98)	79 (99)
School failure	17	—	4	—	21 (26)	
Marital and family conflict	33	30	15	16	48 (60)	46 (58)
Arranging marriage	15	—	6	—	21 (26)	
Work problems	32	15	28	10	60 (75)	25 (31)
Financial problems	33	39	28	26	61 (76)	65 (81)
Relations with others	34	30	24	15	58 (73)	45 (56)
Quality of life	34	38	29	16	63 (79)	54 (68)

From Wang WZ, Li SC, Cheng X, et al. A study on phychological and social aspects in adults with epilepsy. *Chin Ment Health J.* 1995;9:129

available to prevent the poorest in China from falling into extreme poverty. The economic constraints on the social course of epilepsy and other chronic illnesses often means that patients cannot afford proper treatment. The illness, in turn, transforms the economic conditions of everyday life, using up very limited reserves, creating or deepening debt, and forcing families into humiliating and often unavailing negotiations with creditors, who are also under financial pressure. The outcome is illness as the precipitant of end-stage misery. This is a powerful social consequence of illness that deserves far more attention in medical anthropology. Those who are most disadvantaged also appear to suffer the most from discrimination on account of epilepsy.

Recent research in the West challenges the idea that the stigma of epilepsy is unrelenting, and its effects always devastating. In those whose seizures are in remission, psychosocial functioning has been reported as high, with low levels of distress.[17] Public information campaigns in Western societies have improved public attitudes toward epilepsy sufferers. But the situation for epilepsy in China and other low-income regions, is extremely different and has not changed. Those with seizures routinely experience discrimination in schools, in the workplace, and in the community.

Most patients in our sample have chronic epilepsy with frequent seizures. For them and their families, the serious consequences of epilepsy are intensified by Chinese society's prioritizing of social control as the chief concern in the societal response to this and to other chronic conditions in which behavior is affected. The emphasis on social control, rather than patient rights, means that students with epilepsy may be refused to enter colleges, universities, and even middle school; people with epilepsy may not be employed, and some work units may discriminate against patients and their families who are requesting more resources for treatment.

On the other hand, overcontrol can also be viewed in a more positive light as an extreme aspect of families' routine supervision of seriously afflicted members at work, play, and home, which supports many members to participate in daily life activities while protecting them from injury. In Chinese society, institutional assistance for the disabled is largely limited to the family. Thus, the family is at once both the source of nurture and assistance but also a potential source of overcontrol.

Stigma is a moral category, yet in the Chinese context, moral blame is applied to the patient and extends to the entire family. Ideas that attribute the cause of epilepsy to bad fate, heredity, negative geomantic forces, and the malign influences of gods, ghosts, or ancestors are all accusations about the moral status of the family. Inasmuch as Chinese society turns on the individual's kinship circle and social network, families and networks that are morally compromised are perceived as ineffective and indeed actually can become so as members drop out and their social-relational power is lost. The moral status of the person is his or her face; social relations "give face" or "save face." To "lose face" is to carry the social experience of shame into the inner experience of the body/self. The indigenous Chinese model of stigma, however, is sociosomatic and frames intersubjective delegitimation, not spoiled personal identity, as the central process. Because the person is constructed in Chinese culture as a relational self, delegitimation of the family and network is the most fundamental assault the person can experience.

Our findings revealed that epilepsy is best regarded as possessing a social course, and it results in many psychosocial problems in China, which including medical workers and governments, society should pay more attention to.

Another study on developing approaches to reducing stigma of epilepsy[16] organized by Ann Jacoby from Liverpool University, United Kingdom, supported by the National Institutes of Health, has been carried out since 2004 in China and Vietnam. Its first phase finished in June 2005, and the results were published in 2006.

COMMUNITY CONTROL PROGRAMS IN RURAL AREAS

In 1985, the Mental Health Division of the World Health Organization (WHO) began designing a project to manage epilepsy care at a community level, because there were so many PWE in developing countries, especially in rural areas, but a lack of neurologists to treat them. With the similar situation and concern, China joined the efforts of the WHO.

In 1989 and 1993, a feasibility study on "community control of epilepsy" was conducted in China. The basic design of this project was to train village public health workers (PHWs) to use flow charts to administer phenobarbital (PB) to patients with GTCSs. Effects of treatment by village PHWs were compared with effects of treatment by neurologists. Compliance and side effects were also compared between the two groups. There were no statistical differences in the outcomes between the two treatment groups. Therefore it was suggested that the "community control of epilepsy" project was feasible in rural areas of China.[22,39]

In 1997, the WHO, in cooperation with the ILAE and the International Bureau for Epilepsy (IBE), launched the Global Campaign Against Epilepsy (GCAE).[9] As part of the GCAE's activities, a demonstration project to test the pragmatic model was set up in five locations worldwide.[33] The project, entitled Epilepsy Management at a Primary Health Level: Protocol for a Demonstration Project in the People's Republic of China, was successfully conducted in China.[42]

The Chinese project included an epidemiologic survey, an intervention trial, and an educational program in target areas. The study found that 63% of the detected people with active epilepsy (PWAE) had not received antiepileptic medication in the week before the survey (i.e., the treatment gap was 63%).[43] More than 85% of PWAE had GTCSs. Commenced from December 2001, the intervention trial was conducted including identifying patents with GTCSs, PB treatment, follow-up, and management. At the same time, education promotion activities were provided to the patients, their family numbers, and the public to broaden their scientific knowledge about epilepsy and reduce their misunderstanding and discrimination against people with epilepsy. This research involved eight counties in six provinces, with a total investigated target of 3,185,067 inhabitants. A total of 2,455 patients (1,381 males) were recruited into the study (demographic details on baseline are shown in Table 7). Duration of follow-up ranged from 1 day to 32 months (mean 20.5 months; median 25 months).

Methods

Patients with GTCSs were identified at a primary care level and provided with PB monotherapy. The starting dose was 60 mg for adults and 15 mg for children, taken once daily at nighttime, and maintenance dosage was 120 to 180 mg/day for adults and 4 to 5 mg/kg/day for children. Patients attended their local clinic every 2 weeks for the first 2 months and monthly thereafter, for dose adjustments, side effect assessment, and adherence checking, and to receive a further supply of medication. Physicians completed a follow-up form at each visit, recording seizure numbers, compliance, and side effects (using a checklist of common side effects of PB) experienced by the patients. Efficacy was evaluated from the percentage reduction in seizure frequency from baseline and as the retention of patients on treatment.

TABLE 7

PATIENT DEMOGRAPHICS IN THE CHINA DEMONSTRATION PROJECT

Age	Mean 32.6 yr	(SD 20.7 yr)
2–14 years	268	11%
15–44 years	1544	63%
45–59 years	459	19%
≥60 years	184	7%
Age at onset	Mean 17.1 yr	(SD 14.4 yr)
Duration of epilepsy	Mean 15.5 yr	(SD 17.9 yr)
Baseline seizure frequency	Mean 35 seizures per year	

SD, standard deviation.

Findings

Efficacy

The efficacy of PB treatment was evaluated over three periods. The first evaluation included 2,217 patients who were treated for 6 months, the second included 1,897 patients who completed 12 months treatment, and the third included 1,324 patients who completed 24 months treatment. The changes of the seizure frequency in the three periods are listed in Table 8. No evident differences in efficacy of PB treatment were observed among the study sites.

Side Effects of Phenobarbital

Over the treatment period the frequency of all side effects was reduced (Table 9). Most patients, including 189 taking at least 180 mg PB per day, experienced few side effects; only 4% and 0.3%, respectively, experienced moderate and severe side effects; and 32 patients (1%) discontinued medication because of side effects.

Adherence and Withdrawal

Tablet counting proved that over 95% of patients had good compliance to the treatment regimen at each follow-up. By the end of 24 months of treatment, adherence in those continuing in the study was estimated at almost 100%.

A total of 562 patients (23%) withdrew from the study before its completion, and 35 patients died during the study period. The causes of withdrawal are shown in Table 10. In the group who did not complete the study, the most common cause for withdrawal (28% of all withdrawals) was the subjective assumption of cure by the patients. Eighty-one individuals had increased seizure frequency of more than 50% from baseline. The reason for this "increase" needs to be further studied. Eighteen percent of those were withdrawn due to noncompliance.

The above-mentioned project was successfully implemented within the existing services in rural areas of China. It confirmed that in this setting the PB treatment protocol is feasible and that PB has high efficacy and tolerability and can help to reduce the large treatment gap. Because of this study's success the same approach has been extended to ten more locations in China and will become a national program. By September 2005, more than 10,500 individuals with GTCS epilepsy had been treated according to this protocol. This project has given hope and confidence to many PWE in China, but the work should be replicated in other countries before it can be fully recommended. Even the best intervention can only succeed when individuals and communities understand enough of the process and are able to fully participate. Furthermore, the integration of such a program into existing services is essential to ensure its sustainability. These issues should be taken into consideration in any future interventions.

TABLE 8

SEIZURE FREQUENCY AFTER 6, 12, AND 24 MONTHS OF TREATMENT

Change in seizure frequency from baseline	6 Months		12 Months		24 Months	
	N	%	N	%	N	%
Seizure free	919	41	644	34	347	26
Reduced by >75%	305	14	415	22	415	31
Reduced by 51%–75%	245	11	230	12	185	14
Reduced by 26%–50%	162	7	146	8	99	7
Reduced by <25%	217	10	156	8	91	7
Increased by ≥25%	369	17	306	16	187	14
Total	2,217		1,897		1,324	

TABLE 9

SIDE EFFECTS EXPERIENCED AT DIFFERENT TIME POINTS

Side effects	1–3 mo (N = 2,455) N (%)	7–12 mo (N = 2,135) N (%)	19–24 mo (N = 1,495) N (%)
Drowsiness	667 (27)	287 (13)	120 (8)
Dizziness	320 (13)	182 (9)	81 (5)
Headache	185 (8)	108 (5)	41 (3)
Ataxia	182 (7)	87 (4)	30 (2)
Anxiety	154 (6)	94 (4)	31 (2)
Hyperactivity	51 (2)	37 (2)	13 (1)
Gastrointestinal complaints	347 (14)	192 (9)	55 (4)
Skin rash	81 (3)	34 (2)	13 (1)
Others	69 (3)	27 (1)	14 (1)

TRADITIONAL CHINESE MEDICINE AND EPILEPSY

Knowledge of Epilepsy in Traditional Chinese Medicine[46–14]

In traditional Chinese medicine (TCM), epilepsy belongs to the diagnosis "Xian Bing" and is also called "Yang Dian Feng" (goat stroke). It refers to a seizure caused by organic and mental injury, which results in the loss of spirit control. The etiology of epilepsy is due to congenital and acquired factors, especially mental factors. Congenital factors refer to heredity dysfunction, pregnancy disturbance, and bad gift of embryo. It was said in the TCM classical book *Plain Questions* that "epilepsy of baby after birth come[s] from the outside shock, which frightens the mother and cause[s] Qi stasis." Huo You Xin Shu, another pediatrics book of China noted the following: "An overmuch taking in of sour-salty food or mental disturbance of the mother may interfere [with] the embryo and cause epilepsy." Acquired factors include external pathologic factors such as abnormal diet and mental status, injury, and brain parasites. Stroke may also cause epilepsy.

Pathologic Pivots

Generally, deficiency of the liver, kidney, and spleen, which will cause internal wind, phlegm, and blood stagnation, is the basis of epilepsy.

TABLE 10

CAUSES OF WITHDRAWAL

Withdrawal causes	Patient numbers (%)
Patient perception of "cure"	169 (28)
Noncompliance with regimen	104 (18)
Perception of inefficacy	97 (16)
Lost to follow-up	53 (9)
Migrated from study area	38 (6)
Death	35 (6)
Side effects	32 (5)
Others	69 (12)
Total	597 (100)

Seizure Stage

Abnormal circulation of Qi is the pathologic pivot of epilepsy in seizure stage. Every kind of Qi in TCM has its own principle of circulation. If any type of Qi is circulating the wrong way, a reverse flow of Qi will attack and clog the openings of the brain, resulting in dizziness, twitching, or coma.

Truce Stage

Mild epilepsy may have a truce of months or years, while a severe epilepsy may have a truce of only minutes. The truce only means a temporary dissipation of evils, but a recurrence is expectable at any time because of the existence of pathologic factors.

Convalescence Stage

In this stage, epilepsy may stop for more than 3 years. Three outcomes are accessible in this stage: Healing, because of the elimination of pathologic factors and rectification of organic functions; recurrence, only in special conditions such as infections, brain injuries, overeating, fatigue, and menstruation, but with organic function coming back normal; and no recovery of the organs can be expected, especially brain, liver, and kidney.

Treatment in Traditional Chinese Medicine

Treatment Principles

Alerting the consciousness in seizure stage, reinforcing the deficiency, expelling evils in truce and convalescence stages should be the treatment principle. To expel the evils, we should clear the phlegm and repress the internal wind. To reinforce deficiency, we should nourish the spleen, liver, and kidney and calm the heart.

Various TCM therapies are available as medicine, acupuncture and moxibustion, massage, diet, and psychological therapy. For medicinal treatment, we have patent medicine and syndrome-differentiating medicine. For acupuncture, we have body, auricle, and scalp acupuncture. Thread imbedding and fascia cutting are also introduced on the basis of acupuncture.

Recent Development of Treatment on Epilepsy in Traditional Chinese Medicine[4–35]

Pharmacologic Treatment

The controlled clinical trials of the fixed TCM prescriptions for epilepsy treatment developed recently were carried out in China.

Extracts of Chinese Medicine

Extracts of Chinese medicine for epilepsy, which proved to be effective, has been paid more and more attention these days. Distilling of effective ingredients from herbs may help us to better understand their chemical structure and structure activity relationship so that further synthesizing and developing work of new medications can be done. The effective ingredients in some herbs now can already be affirmed, and the mechanism research are now being undertaken.

Nonpharmacological Treatment

Acupuncture and Medicine. Acupuncture is effective economically and harmless for the treatment of epilepsy. Acupuncture combined with medicine proved to be clinically effective in research comparing traditional acupuncture and scalp acupuncture, electroacupuncture, thread imbedding, and acuinjection.

SUMMARY AND CONCLUSIONS

There are approximately 9 million people with epilepsy in the People's Republic of China, including 6 million people with active epilepsy. Moreover, there are an additional 0.4 million new cases each year. A survey suggests that nearly 65% of these patients do not receive appropriate medical treatment. In China, epilepsy has been treated by TCM in a long history. Beginning in the 1950s, the clinical diagnosis and treatment of epilepsy made substantial progress. Epidemiology, clinical neurologic diagnosis and treatment, epilepsy surgery, basic research, sociopsychological problems, rural community control programs, and TCM recognition of epilepsy in China have progressed greatly in recent years.

References

1. A proposed diagnostic scheme for people with epileptic seizure and with epilepsy given by ILAE. *Clin J Neurol.* 2001;36(4):302–307.
2. Alvarado L, et al. Psychosocial evaluation of adults with epilepsy in Chile. *Epilepsia.* 1992;33:651–657.
3. Berkovic SF, et al. Familial temporal lobe epilepsy: a common disorder identified in twins. *Ann Neurol.* 1996;40:227–235.
4. Chen S, Han Z, Chen Y. Dian Xian Pian for spontaneous and secondary epilepsy. *Chin Patent Med.* 2004;26(9):24.
5. Chen Y, Liu J, Pan H, et al. Association between genetic variation of CACNA1H and childhood absence epilepsy. *Ann Neurol.* 2003;54:239–243.
6. Chen Y. Treatment of 174 cases of epilepsy with Taohong Siwu decoction. *Jiang Su TCM J.* 2003;24(12:25.
7. Chen YC, Zhang YH, Lü J, et al. Association of child absence epilepsy with T-STARgene. *Natl Med J China.* 2003;83(13):1134–1137.
8. Chinese Medical Association Paediatrics Neurology Society. A proposed classification about the children with epilepsy and with epilepsy syndrome. *Chin J Pediatr.* 1996;34(2):129.
9. De Boer HM. "Out of the shadows": a global campaign against epilepsy. *Epilepsia.* 2002;43(Suppl 6):7–8.
10. Ding CY, Zhao YQ, Li SC. Summary of literature on natural history and prognosis of epilepsy in China. To be published.
11. Feng Y, ed. *Clinical EEG.* Beijing, China: People's Medical Publishing House; 1984:61–64.
12. Ge X, Wang ZP, Zhang YF, et al. Analysis of haplotype-based haplotype relative risk and transmission disequilibrium test in childhood absence epilepsy. *Chin J Pediatr.* 2003;41(9):675–679.
13. Huang P, Liu M. *TCM Treatment for Neurological Diseases.* Beijing, China: Beijing Peoples' Health Publishing Company; 466–511.
14. Huang W. *Applicated TCM Internal Medicine.* Shang Hai Science and Technology Publishing Company; 370–378.
15. Huang XS, Yin J, Wei J, et al. Linkage mapping of the generalized epilepsy with febrile seizures plus gene. *Chin J Neurol.* 2005;38(4):239–242.
16. Jacoby A, Snape D, Baker GA. Epilepsy and social identity: the stigma of a chronic neurological disorder. *Lancet Neurol.* 2005;4:171–178.
17. Jacoby A. Epilepsy and quality of everyday life: findings from a study of people with well-controlled epilepsy. *Soc Sci Med.* 1992;43(6):657–666.
18. Jensen R, Davis M. Public attitudes toward epilepsy in Denmark. *Epilepsia.* 1992;33:459–464.
19. Kleinman A, WZ Wang, et al. The social course of epilepsy: chronic illness as social experience in interior china. *Soc Sci Med.* 1995;40(10):1319–1330.
20. Kleinman A. *The Illness Narratives: Suffering, Healing and the Hunan Condition.* New York: Basic Books; 1988:3–30.
21. Lai CW, et al. Survey of public awareness, understanding, and attitudes toward epilepsy in Henan Province, China. *Epilepsy.* 1990;31:182–186.
22. Li SC, Wang WZ, Cheng XM, et al. A report of the feasibility test for "community control of epilepsy" proposed by WHO. *Chin J Neurol Psychiatry.* 1989;22:144–147.
23. Li SC, Wu J. Epidemiology of epilepsy. In: Li SC, ed. *Epidemiology of Neurological Diseases.* Beijing, China: People's Health Publishing House; 2001.
24. Li X, Hu Y. Gene expression profiling reveals the mechanism of action of anticonvulsant drug QYS. *Brain Res Bull.* 2005;66(2):99–105.
25. Liao WP, Chen L, Yi YH, et al. Study of antiepileptic effect of extracts from Acorus tatarinowii Schott. *Epilepsia.* 2005;46(Suppl 1):21–24.
26. Liu XR, Deng YH, Liao WP, et al. The clinical and genetic features of generalized epilepsy with febrile seizure plus(GEFS+) in Chinese families. *Neurol Asia.* 2004;9(1):91.
27. Lu J, Chen Y, Pan H, et al. The gene encoding GABBR1 is not associated with childhood absence epilepsy in the Chinese Han population. *Neurosci Lett.* 2003;343(3):151–154.
28. Lu JJ, Zhang YH, Pan H, et al. Case-control study and transmission/disequilibrium tests of the genes encoding GABRA5 and GABRB3 in a Chinese population affected by childhood absence epilepsy. *Chin Med J (Engl).* 2004;117(10):1497–1501.
29. Nashef L. Death from intractable focal epilepsy. In: Oxbury J, Polkey CE, Duchowny M, eds. *Intractable Focal Epilepsy.* London: WB Saunders; 2000: 41–52.
30. Ni H, Jiang YW, Bo T, et al. c-Fos, N-methyl-d-aspartate receptor 2C, GABA-A-alpha1 immunoreactivity, seizure latency and neuronal injury following single or recurrent neonatal seizures in hippocampus of Wistar rat. *Neurosci Lett.* 2005;380(1–2):149–154.
31. Qi Y, Lu J, Wu X. Familial febrile convulsions is supposed to link to human chromosome 19p13.3. *Natl Med J China.* 2001;81(1):27–29.
32. Sander JW, Shorvon SD. Epidemiology of the epilepsies. *J Neurol Neurosurg Psychiatry.* 1996;61(5):433–443.
33. Sander JW. Global Campaign Against Epilepsy. Overview of the demonstration projects. *Epilepsia.* 2002;43(Suppl 6):34–36.
34. Sun CK, Huang YG, Jia YS, et al. A GluRs-NOSs-RNI/ROIs cascade mechanism may be involved in experimental complex partial seizures. In: Moncada S, Stamler J, Gross S, et al., eds. *The Biology of Nitric Oxide (Part 5).* London: Portland Press Ltd.; 1996:329.
35. Sun Q, Wu S. Medicine and acupuncture for 370 cases of epilepsy. *Chin TCM Sci Technol J.* 2003;10(4):251.
36. Tang B, Li H, Xia K, et al. A novel mutation in KCNQ2 gene causes benign familial neonatal convulsions in a Chinese family. *J Neurol Sci.* 2004;221(1–2):31–34.
37. The 1st National Epilepsy Science Conference. The classification of epilepsy seizure (protocol). *Chin J Neurol Psychiatry.* 1986;19:256.
38. The China Topiramate Study Group, China. An open-label multicenter trial of topiramate as add-on therapy for refractory partial-onset seizures in adults. *Clin J Neurol.* 2001;34(3):132–134.
39. Wang WZ, Li SC, Cheng XM, et al. An extended test of the WHO "community control of epilepsy" project. *Chin J Nerv Ment Dis.* 1993;19: 16–19.
40. Wang WZ, Li SC, et al. An extended test for "community control of epilepsy" proposed by WHO. *Chin J Nerv Ment Dis.* 1993;19(1):16–19.
41. Wang WZ, Wu JZ, et al. The prevalence and treatment gap in epilepsy in China, an ILAE/IBE/WHO study. *Neurology.* 2003;60:1544–1545.
42. Wang WZ, Wu JZ, Wang DS, et al. The prevalence and treatment gap in epilepsy in China: an ILAE/IBE/WHO study. *Neurology.* 2003;60:1544–1545.
43. Wang WZ;Wu JZ, et al. The use of phenobarbital in the treatment of convulsive forms of epilepsy in a primary care setting: a large-scale pragmatic open label study in rural China. In press.
44. Wang XF, et al. Clinical and pathological features of SUDEP. *Chin J Neurol.* 2004;37(6):495–498.

45. Wang Y, Zhou D, Wang B, et al. A kindling model of pharmacoresistent temporal lobe epilepsy in Sprague-Dawley rats induced by Coriaria lactone and its possible mechanism. *Epilepsia*. 2003;44(4):475–488.
46. Wang YY. *Chinese Internal Medicine*. Shang Hai Science and Technology Publishing Company 144–149.
47. Western Pacific Region and the GCAE. *Call for Attention and Action*. WHO; 2004.
48. World Health Organization. *Epilepsy: Social Consequences and Economic Aspects*. Fact Sheet No. 165. WHO Information; 2001.
49. Wu L, Ren L. The retrospect and prospect of epilepsy in the 50 years. *Chin J Neurol*. 2005;38(3):144–148.
50. Xiao B, Deng FY, Xiong G, et al. Clinical and genetic study on a new Chinese family with benign familial infantile seizures. *Eur J Neurol*. 2005;12(5):344–349.
51. Yin S, Guan Z, Tang Y, et al. Abnormal expression of epilepsy-related gene ERG1/NSF in the spontaneous recurrent seizure rats with spatial learning memory deficits induced by kainic acid. *Brain Res*. 2005;1053(1–2):195–202.
52. Yinan M, Yu Q, Zhiyue C, et al. Polymorphisms of casein kinase I gamma 2 gene associated with simple febrile seizures in Chinese Han population. *Neurosci Lett*. 2004;368(1):2–6.
53. Zhang YH, Shan WS, Zhang GR, et al. The relation between electrical synapse and the mechanism of epilepsy in genetical epilepsy-prone rat. *J Chin Med*. 1998;78(4):311–313.
54. Zhang Z, Pan Y, Fei Y, et al. An open add-on study with lamotrigine in patients with refractory epilepsy. *Clin J Neurol*. 1996;29(1):33–37.
55. Zhou L, Liu C. Jian Zhong Tang and Shen Tie Lao Yin for epilepsy of children. *Appl TCM Intern Med J*. 2004;18(3:224.

CHAPTER 292 ■ GERMANY

MARGARETE PFÄFFLIN AND RUPPRECHT THORBECKE

INTRODUCTION

The German social welfare system was introduced between 1883 and 1889 by Chancellor Bismarck in an attempt to maintain his authoritative rule by outmaneuvering the rising social democratic movement. This system, which has survived several political eras—the Kaiserreich, the Weimar Republic, and National Socialism—was created to insure general life risks. State legislation on health insurance was passed in 1883, on state accident insurance in 1884, and on old-age and pension insurance in 1889. In 1927, this system was supplemented by legislation on unemployment insurance (including job-creating measures). Subsequent to the increasing number of senior citizens, a fifth pillar of welfare, the nursing insuring act, was enacted in 1994. Currently, more than 90% of the 82 million inhabitants of Germany are covered by the state-provided social welfare system in regard to sickness, accidents at the workplace, occupational disease, disability, unemployment, nursing needs, and motherhood.[9]

OBJECTIVES OF GERMAN SOCIAL WELFARE

The principles of state-provided social welfare are listed as follows:

1. Compulsory membership. All adults with incomes below a certain level (3.375 € per month in 2002) must join. Family members (children, spouses) without income are covered as well. Professionals and people with incomes above this level may opt for the social insurance system or obtain private insurance.
2. Solidarity. Payment depends on one's income; services of social welfare depend on one's needs. Everyone receives the same services, independent of premium, health risks, gender, or age. Public pension plans and unemployment insurance are related to former income level and the length of time insured.
3. Principally, health insurance is financed through the members. Nevertheless, insurance fees are divided (e.g., between employers and employees, between pensioners and the state pension insurance). Low-income groups like students pay a fixed fee. With the exception of state accident insurance, which is paid solely by the employers, each person pays around half of the premium. Because the level of the premium is related to income, the basis of the social welfare system is determined by the sum of all wages. The state subsidizes some of the insurance plans.
4. Social welfare insurance plans are self-governing public corporations under federal supervision. Their boards are composed of elected delegates equally representing employers and employees. Numerous organizations back up the insurance plans. However, all are controlled by state health legislation. Unemployment insurance has only one supporting organization, the federal labor office.

The tasks of different insurance plans partially overlap, which can lead to conflicts with respect to responsibility for measures. Who pays is determined by who has the financial risk in case the measure fails. State pension or unemployment insurance is responsible for vocational rehabilitation; state pension or health insurance is responsible for "medical" (functional) rehabilitation. Apart from this, health insurance covers medical treatment. This "division of responsibility" has strings attached. Vocational training, for example, cannot be started during medical treatment or medical rehabilitation, even though this would be advantageous from the patient's point of view. Therefore, comprehensive care relies on the voluntary cooperation of health professionals beyond the limits of administration.

Community welfare completes the system of social welfare. It is founded on the principle of communal welfare, which existed long before Bismarck. Under this plan, persons who are not able to make their own living, who are unemployed (for more than 1 year, currently), and who are not covered by health insurance can ask for income support or welfare. Social welfare is financed primarily by community taxes. The number of people on welfare is determined mainly by employment opportunities. In the past 20 years this number has grown threefold.

PRIVATE INSURANCE PLANS

Individuals with incomes above a certain limit can obtain private insurance. Private insurance plans charge according to the covered services. Age, gender, health risks, and chronic illnesses influence the level of premium an individual is charged. Private insurers can reject applicants if the insurance risk is assessed as being too high. About 10% of the population had private health insurance in 2003.[9] Persons with epilepsy who cannot insure themselves in the state health insurance system (e.g., self-employed persons, lawyers, and physicians) may have difficulty finding private health insurance. If they are accepted by a private company, they often have to pay high risk premiums or the insurance plan does not include epilepsy as a covered condition. For persons with epilepsy, private accident insurance plans and disability insurance are especially difficult to obtain. Among 236 privately insured patients with epilepsy, none was able to obtain disability insurance.[10]

STATE HEALTH CARE

State Health Insurance: Budget Organization and Development

Originally, state health insurance was established to guarantee medical care and help avoid loss of income due to sickness. Since 1970, members of the state health insurance system generally receive sickness benefits for 6 weeks. In 2003, more than 72 million inhabitants were insured by state health insurance.[9] Of these, about 30% were covered as noncontributing family members, and 22% were pensioners paying minimal contribution. During the past 20 years, the income from premiums has increased at a far slower rate than the expenditure. Although the average membership rate changed from 8.4% to 14% of salary, expenditure increases continuously, especially expenditure on hospital treatment, which increases every year between 1% and 3%.[2,9] Hospital expenditure accounts for one third of all health care expenditures.

In 1993, a law was passed to keep the increase in expenditures equal to that of the income premium. Expenditure has decreased as a result, but not enough. Therefore, numerous laws have been passed to control expenditures. This process is ongoing. Financial barriers between hospital treatment and primary care are partially torn down through "integrative care" such as disease management plans and managed care programs. Administration has blown up to a great extent, not to the advantage of patent care. Insurance plans independent from employment and wages are in discussion. As a result, the idea of the welfare state is being questioned, with some suggesting that state health insurance should be limited to standard treatment, and optional treatment should be paid for privately. Already, since about 8 years, an increasing amount of health care services has to be paid by the patients themselves in addition to the reimbursements of the insurance.

Health Services

Germany has a high density of medical care services, albeit one that is unevenly distributed between urban and rural areas. In 2003, there was one physician for every 370 inhabitants and one hospital bed for every 150 inhabitants, which is a decrease of about 20% within the last 15 years. Of about 300,000 physicians, 41% worked in hospitals, 3% in rehabilitation units, 42% in solo practice, and 13% in scientific institutions, administration, and federal health services (institutions that control epidemics with measures such as vaccinations and hygiene). When a patient decides to be treated, he or she has free choice among doctors in private practice (general practitioners and specialists, e.g., neurologists) who are contractors of health insurance plans. Often the proximity of a practice or the waiting period rather than the quality of treatment is decisive in determining a patient's choice. Doctors in own practice may refer patients to hospitals or to outpatient treatment units at hospitals. The ratio between doctors in hospitals and nonmedical staff members (e.g., nurses, technical staff members, midwives, social workers, psychologists, pharmacists) was 1:7.5 in 2003.[9]

The basic idea of the German health system is that the doctor provides treatment and advice. Newly, therapeutic psychologists in solo practice are included in the treatment service and refunded by the insurance plans comparable to physicians. Despite this rather physician-centered approach, nonmedical health-related services outside the hospitals have expanded greatly during the past 100 years. Such services include advice centers established by churches and welfare associations and health-related services developed outside the state health systems. These services as a rule are either free of charge for the clients (e.g., advice centers of churches or of the state) or clients can use the service at their own expense (e.g., physiotherapy or psychotherapy in solo practice). Reimbursement by the state health insurance for nonmedical health-related services is possible, as an exception, and often requires bureaucratic procedures.[1] Thus, comprehensive care is affected sometimes by a lack of funding but more often by a lack of communication and competition for patients.

Primary Care

Primary care in Germany does not have as clear a structure as it does in other countries, such as the United Kingdom. There are general practitioners and pediatricians in solo practice, specialists or consultants (such as neurologists and internists) in solo practice, and specialists in hospital outpatient clinics. The latter depend on permits given by health insurance and physicians organizations. Apart from university clinics, these are only given in exceptional cases. Outpatient clinics may offer comprehensive care because professionals other than doctors, who are employed in the affiliated hospital, may be called on for their services (e.g., neuropsychologists or social workers). However, these additional services are not always refunded by the patient's insurance. There are no clear rules with respect to treatment of specific diseases. Thus, a general practitioner, an internist, or a neurologist might treat a person with epilepsy.

The structure of primary care is negotiated by doctors' organizations and health insurance providers. Arrangements include the guarantee of medical care in a certain region, guarantee of 24-hour availability, and a basic set of covered services. Physicians prescribe medications, confirm a patient's inability to work, and refer patients to specialists or hospitals. Medical treatment in regard to necessity, implementation, and correct calculation is scrutinized. Economic efficiency is evaluated by the doctors' organizations and health insurance providers, as is compensation. Services of physicians are calculated by evaluating every service. Because of the current law that establishes the formula that costs may not increase more than basic wages, physicians working harder get less for their services than before.[1]

Hospital Treatment

Hospitals are one of the oldest services provided. Although their purpose has not changed over the years, their equipment, size, and specialization have. In 2003 hospitals numbered 2,197, of which 373 had a special department for neurology.[9] Hospitals are financed by a dual system. Capital costs for investment are paid through the public budget, and current costs for treatment are paid by the patients, usually through the state health insurance plans. Until 1992, hospitals had cost-based charges. Since then, hospitals have received a budget that is linked to basic wages. Now a complicated account and contract system is instated, which will mean that hospitals are managed more like businesses. Competition between hospitals leads to fusions of hospitals, closing down of smaller houses, and reduction of the number of hospital beds. The financial frames are set through the German version of the DRG system (diagnose related groups). Patients with high nursing needs (e.g., the elderly or chronically ill persons, including persons with epilepsy) may then become unattractive to hospitals. The average hospital stay has shortened from 14.0 days in 1991 to 8.9 days in 2003, and capacity utilization from 84.1% in 1991 to 77.6% in 2003.[9]

CARE FOR PERSONS WITH EPILEPSY

Care for Children

Primary Care

As a rule, children with epilepsy in Germany are treated by pediatricians. Newly, a number of pediatric neurologists in solo practice have organized themselves. The list of pediatric neurologists sums up to 107 pediatric neurologists in solo practice. In larger cities only with several pediatricians in solo practice, one usually concentrates on epilepsy, and children with seizures can be referred to him or her by his or her colleagues. Children in Germany have the right to nine medical checkups in the first 6 years of life; more than 90% of families take part in these checkups. After the checkups, a doctor may order nonmedical treatment such as psychological therapy and diagnostics, speech therapy, or psychomotor exercises.

The pediatrician can refer children to a pediatric neurologist who works in an outpatient clinic or a medical center. In Germany there are around 170 pediatric outpatient clinics, of which 103 additionally specialized in epilepsy (in 2004). These specialized outpatient clinics usually have access to psychologists, social workers, physiotherapists, and other specialists, of whom quite a few have expertise in epilepsy. Education of staff members in epilepsy is one of the most important issues now. Nonmedical professionals can attend courses to acquire an additional expertise in epileptology certified through the German chapter of the International League Against Epilepsy (ILAE). Therefore, expertise in pediatric (as well as in adult) epilepsy is growing. The pediatrician in solo practice may also refer a child requiring sophisticated treatment to a hospital specializing in pediatric neurology. There are about 200 such departments in Germany; every outpatient clinic for children with epilepsy is affiliated with one of these.

A pediatrician is more likely to refer a child with epilepsy (especially one with complicated epilepsy) to a colleague with expertise in epilepsy at one of the above-mentioned centers if he or she has already established a good working relationship. Referral to such a center ensures that the pediatrician is expanding the patients' treatment options.

Primary care for children in Germany is, with a few exceptions, sufficient and of good quality. A child's development can be closely tracked through the medical checkup system. Somatic illnesses are usually recognized early. Some problems remain, however. It is often not easy to find the level of specialized care adequate to a patient's needs, and persistence is required. Parents may have to test several options before finding the right one. Pediatricians often misjudge the level of development in children with complicated types of epilepsy, falsely assuring concerned parents that nothing is wrong. When children are finally referred to specialized care, they have often experienced delays in diagnosis and treatment of secondary problems.

Hospital Treatment

Children with febrile or afebrile seizures are usually transferred to the pediatric department of the nearest general hospital or to the nearest pediatric neurology department of a university hospital.[3] Diagnosis and proposal for treatment are offered to the pediatrician in solo practice. Children with more complicated forms of epilepsy, including refractory seizures, are transferred to the hospital again and again. Only if treatment is unsuccessful over a long period of time is a child referred to one of five specialized centers for epilepsy. Regular children's hospitals usually do not have the resources to treat complicated types of epilepsy. They lack the experience in helping parents cope with changes in medication, during which children may have more frequent seizures, and also lack expertise in psychosocial problems accompanying difficult-to-treat epilepsies. Staff members in epilepsy centers, in which medical treatment, psychosocial counseling, and special education are offered, usually believe that early referral prevents delays in achieving optimal treatment.

Children can be treated in all of the five epilepsy centers for children in Germany. The centers provide specialized treatment including epilepsy surgery, neuropsychological assessments, counseling for parents, and educational advice. For adolescents, guidance in vocational training is offered. The Bethel Epilepsy Center is one of the most important referral centers for epilepsy surgery in children in Europe. It is *the* referral center for the very young age group in the German-speaking countries. Epilepsy centers also function as advisory centers, transferring their expertise in treatment and rehabilitation into the home communities of the patients. They also serve as educational centers for medical and nonmedical personnel.

Centers for Medical Rehabilitation

There are five rehabilitative centers for children and adolescents with neurologic diseases. They follow a comprehensive approach with the aims to integrate children into school and into professional education. They teach skills to prepare them for independent living. Apart from medical treatment they offer physiotherapy, speech therapy, (neuro-)psychological treatment, counseling, and special work-preparatory courses. All centers have broad experience with children with epilepsy.

Care for Adults

Primary Care for Adults

In Germany little is known about primary care for adults with epilepsy. To remedy this, a widespread survey has been performed.[6] Results show that an average of four to five patients with epilepsy consulted 1 of about 62,000 family doctors per year (Table 1). After the first seizure, in most cases it is the family doctor who is asked for advice and who establishes a diagnosis. Frequently this doctor refers the patient to a neurologist for confirmation of diagnosis, electroencephalography (EEG), and initial treatment. The neurologist usually refers

TABLE 1

PATIENTS WITH EPILEPSY PER GROUP OF PHYSICIANS IN SOLO PRACTICE AND PER YEAR

			No. of epilepsy patients		Percentile	
Physicians	No. of physicians	M ±	SD	25%	50%	75%
Neurologists	4,000	48.19	57.45	10	30	65
General practitioners	61,916	4.83	4.68	2	4	6
Pediatricians	6,000	14.45	29.05	3	7	15

M, mean; SD, standard deviation.
From Pfäfflin M, May TW. Wieviele Patienten mit Epilepsien gibt es in Deutschland und wer behandelt sie? *Neurol Rehabil.* 2000;6(2):77–81.

the patient back to the primary care physician or tries to establish a consulting arrangement. In Germany there are about 4,000 neurologists in solo practice who care for 50% to 60% of patients with epilepsy, the remaining being treated by general practitioners or pediatricians. Within the group of neurologists in solo practice, about 12% concentrate on epilepsy, treating a higher number of patients with epilepsy. They do have a special qualification in the treatment and counseling of persons with epilepsy. Their qualification is certified by the German chapter of the ILAE. The German chapter of the ILAE has established guidelines for the treatment of persons with epilepsy in solo practice specializing in epilepsy treatment. Because of this development, the standard of care for persons with epilepsy has improved in Germany.

The German chapter of the ILAE established guidelines for diagnosis and treatment of epilepsy, which take the position that a division of labor should be established within a multilevel service system. Up to now, the expertise in a multilevel system of care has not been used systematically by physicians or patients. Patients move frequently between family doctors and neurologists. Only a few are treated in outpatient clinics or specialized centers.

In 2005 there were 38 outpatient clinics for adolescents and adults with epilepsy. These clinics have access to EEG and video-EEG, and most of them to computed tomography (CT) and magnetic resonance imaging (MRI). The average waiting period for a first appointment is 1 to 3 months. All outpatient clinics have access to a social worker, who in the some cases has a specialized training in epilepsy. In the last 10 years the social workers have been offered advanced training, and they form a network to support each other in specialized questions. Brochures, leaflets, and Internet information have been developed for patients' service. Problems of prime importance are occupational in nature. About 50% of adult patients with seizures are faced with considerable job problems. They are unemployed, prematurely retired, or employed below their qualifications. Epilepsy was cited as the reason for an inability to work in about half of the cases seen in the outpatient clinic of the Epilepsy Center Bethel in 2003.

Hospital Treatment

The number of hospital treatments and the average length of stay are generally viewed as excessive in Germany (Table 2). Many persons who have seizures with loss of consciousness or body control are admitted to the hospital even when they carry a note stating that no help is necessary. This is because people who witness a seizure may feel that they are providing assistance by taking the person to a hospital. A person who is admitted to a hospital usually has to stay at least 1 night for observation. In theory, patients can leave the hospital on their own volition, but most do not.

In Germany there are eight specialized epilepsy centers, which provide the highest level of care for adults with epilepsy. All these centers provide diagnosis and treatment for in- and outpatients, as well as research and education. Among them four centers have specialized in epilepsy surgery, and three have specialized in social and vocational rehabilitation. The Epilepsy Center Bethel is the only center that combines all functions.[7]

Centers for Medical Rehabilitation

Three centers for medical rehabilitation exist in Germany currently, the first being launched in 1997.[8] Their main aim is to ameliorate the psychological, social, and vocational consequences of epilepsy. All three are run on an inpatient basis. They are funded mainly by the state pension insurances with the aim to reduce early disability in patients with epilepsy. Early retirement in epilepsy patients is prominent and very costly. An evaluation study has shown that such centers are effective in improving quality of life and reducing the frequency of hospital stays and unemployment in those treated.

SUMMARY AND CONCLUSIONS

The future of epilepsy treatment in Germany is hopeful, although there are several problems to be overcome. The German chapter of the ILAE together with voluntary epilepsy organizations has developed standards of care for persons with epilepsy. The underlying philosophy emphasizes the need for comprehensive care for people with epilepsy apart from high-standard medical treatment counseling and support for the various psychiatric and social difficulties often associated with epilepsy. There are standards for physicians as well as for allied health professionals specializing in epileptology ("Zertifikat Epilepsie plus," "Zusatzausbildung Epilepsie"), and there is an ongoing demonstration project for the development of the qualification of an "epilepsy nurse." A standard for outpatient clinics concentrating on epilepsy ("Anfallsambulanzen") has been established for a while, and in 2000 standards for private practices specializing in the care of persons with epilepsy ("Schwerpunktpraxen") were decided. The German chapter of the ILAE enforces these standards by certifying persons and/or institutions for fulfilling them and publishing their addresses. As of the writing of this paper a standard of "epilepsy centers" proposed by the German chapter of the ILAE is under discussion.

Standards for treatment and care including rehabilitation will become even more important as citizens from the European Union can ask for treatment in various European countries. It is important to include self-help groups in the process of developing these standards because they have the most comprehensive perspective and can act without financial dependency.

Information on epilepsy for the general public, for nonmedical professionals (e.g., teachers, facilitators, personnel from rehabilitation or counseling centers), and for persons with epilepsy and their families is produced by the German chapter of the ILAE, by the German Epilepsy Foundation ("Stiftung Michael"), by national self-help organizations

TABLE 2

HOSPITAL TREATMENT IN 2000

	No. of cases	No. of days hospitalized	Days per case
Total	17,313,222 (100%)	65,821,972 (100%)	9.0
Epilepsy	128,698 (0.74%)	1,312,720 (0.84%)	10.2

Included are all cases with the main diagnosis epilepsy (G40 and G41, International classification of Diseases and Related Health Problems (ICD) version 10, WHO); http://www.who.int/classifications/en/ From Statistisches Bundesamt Deutschland 2005 und Fachserie 12 Gesundheitswesen, Reihe 6.1., Jg. 1994–2003.

("Deutsche Epilepsievereinigung," "Epilepsie-Bundes-Elternverband"), and regional self-support groups. One shortcoming in epilepsy information is that it is not developed on a systematic base. In consequence, there are gaps and the quality of information differs highly. There are numerous efforts to use the various possibilities of the Internet for epilepsy information.

Since the end of the 1990s there have been strong efforts to develop patient education programs for adults and children with epilepsy and their families. About 1,500 adult persons with epilepsy are educated with the MOSES program.[4] A version of the program for children and their parents has been ready for administration in the routine medical practice since 2005.[5]

Because counseling and support for psychosocial problems are most often provided by institutions outside the medical systems, various efforts are now under way to bind services closer together to create comprehensive epilepsy networks. Such efforts have been done in Bavaria, North Rhine-Westphalia, and Berlin. Networks serve three functions: First, they facilitate the transfer of new knowledge and experience and reduce competition. Second, they increase the number of referrals (e.g., for early evaluation for surgical treatment or for rehabilitation interventions). A promising development in this field is the installation of specific counseling centers for epilepsy with the function of public education, counseling of schools or other institutions, and individual counseling of persons with epilepsy. Such centers, in which a social worker specialized in epileptology is always present and sometimes also a psychologist, exist in various federal states (e.g., Bavaria, Hessian, Lower Saxony, North Rhine-Westfalia, and Saxony), and hopefully will also be installed in more states.

The most urgent problems in care for people with epilepsy are the following:

- Referring patients much earlier to the most competent institutions and specialized centers
- Developing epilepsy networks for comprehensive care for persons with epilepsy
- Educating and hence empowering more adults and children with epilepsy and their relatives because in the coming structures of our health system, it is even more the patients' responsibility to obtain adequate
- Maintaining specialized epilepsy centers or comparable institutions (even under economic strain) that are experienced in treatment and counseling of patients with difficult-to-treat epilepsy and psychosocial problems.

References

1. Blendon RJ, Donelan K, Leitman R, et al. Physicians' perspectives on caring for patients in the United States, Canada, and West Germany. *N Engl J Med.* 1993;328:1011–1016.
2. Iglehart JK. Germany's health care system. *N Engl J Med.* 1991;324:503–508, 1750–1756.
3. Freitag CM, May TW, Pfäfflin M, et al. Incidence of epilepsies and epileptic syndromes in children and adolescents: a population-based prospective study in Germany. *Epilepsia.* 2001;42(8):979–985.
4. May TW, Pfäfflin M. The efficacy of an educational treatment program for patients with epilepsy (MOSES): results of a controlled, randomized study. *Epilepsia.* 2002;43(5):539–549.
5. May TW, Pfäfflin M. Psychoeducational programs for patients with epilepsy. *Dis Manage Health Outcomes.* 2005;13(3):185–199.
6. Pfäfflin M, May TW. Wieviele Patienten mit Epilepsien gibt es in Deutschland und wer behandelt sie? *Neurol Rehabil.* 2000;6(2):77–81.
7. Pfäfflin M, Fraser RT, Thorbecke R, et al., eds. *Comprehensive Care for People with Epilepsy.* London: John Libbey; 2001.
8. Specht U, Thorbecke R, May TW, et al. Comprehensive short term rehabilitation program for people with epilepsy: positive effects on quality of life and performance. *Epilepsia.* 2004;45(S7):57.
9. Statistisches Bundesamt Deutschland 2005 und Fachserie 12 Gesundheitswesen, Reihe 6.1, Jg. 1994–2003.
10. Thorbecke R. Experience of people with epilepsy hoping to buy an insurance policy. In: Cornaggia C, Beghi E, Hauser AW, et al., eds. *Epilepsy and Risks a First-step Evaluation.* Heemstede: IBE; 1994: 103–108.

CHAPTER 293 ■ INDIA

SATISH JAIN AND P. SATISH CHANDRA

INTRODUCTION

India is the second most populated country in the world with majority of population being rural. Although the economy has been growing at a rapid pace, the per capita expenditure on health, family welfare, water supply and sanitation in recent years has been dismally low. The health services provided by the government are totally free or highly subsidized for the poor and needy. The rapidly emerging private health sector with health insurance facilities is affordable to only a small section of the population.

It is estimated that with a population of more than 1 billion, there are about 6–10 million people living with epilepsy in India, accounting for nearly one fifth of the global burden. The challenge of meeting the needs of the people with epilepsy in a developing country like India is a daunting task for every one involved in the planning and delivery of health care. In a country like India with diverse cultures, castes and low literacy; various myths and misconceptions about epilepsy that exist among the people further add to the societal disease burden and treatment gap. Developing countries such as India need to develop alternative strategies to reach out to the needy people living with epilepsy in different parts of such a vast country. The best approach in a country like India with limited resources for health-care would be to encourage "private-public participation." There is an urgent need to have a separate National Epilepsy Control Programme (NECP) in countries like India. In order to be successful, the proposed NECP must be an initiative of the government and should work in collaboration with the health care providers in the private sector and non-governmental organizations.

DEMOGRAPHIC AND SOCIOECONOMIC INDICATORS

India is the largest country in the Southeast Asian Region of the World Health Organization (WHO) with an estimated population of more than 1 billion living in an area of 3287.3 thousand km^2 with the population density being 325 per km^2. The majority of the population is rural, with only 27.8% living in urban areas. India has 35 states and union territories accounting for 593 districts, 5,161 towns, and 593,643 inhabited villages as of March 31, 2001.[8] The majority of the population as per the 1991 Census was young, with 37.8% being in the 0- to 14-year and 55.5% in 15- to 59-year age group. The national literacy rate for 2001 was 65.5%, with males (75.96%) having a better literacy rate as compared to females (54.28%).

The combined national crude birth rate for 2002 as per the sample registration system of the Registrar General of India was 25.0, the crude death rate being 8.1 and the natural growth rate of 16.9 per 1,000 population. The average annual exponential growth rate of the population is calculated to be 1.96%. The gross per capita net national product at current price for 2003–2004 was estimated to be about U.S. $463 (INR 20860, 1 U.S.$ = INR 45.00). Only 3.97% of the total expenditure in the budget was allocated to the Health, Family Welfare, and Indian System of Medicine and Homeopathy (ISM & H) for the 10th 5-year plan (2002 to 2007). The per capita expenditure on health, family welfare, water supply, and sanitation during 2002–2007 will be about US $2.53 per year.[8]

BASIC STRUCTURE OF HEALTH CARE DELIVERY SYSTEM IN INDIA

The primary and secondary health care in the government sector is delivered through a vast network of subcenters (SCs; one SC for about 5,000 population and manned by health workers); primary health centers (PHCs; one PHC for 30,000 to 50,000 population); and taluk hospitals/community health centers (CHCs; one CHC for 100,000 population) that are under the administrative control of district hospitals (DHs; one DH for 1.5 to 2 million population). The tertiary health care is provided by hospitals attached to medical colleges, apex institutions, and super-specialized centers. Government health services are totally free/highly subsidized for the poor and needy. A rapidly emerging private health sector, in the absence of government health insurance to the majority, is affordable to only a small section of the population. Though allopathy (modern medicine) takes care of the majority, traditional systems of medicine also are widely used in the country.[6]

There were 189 medical colleges (during 2000–2001) and 185 dental colleges (2003–2004) imparting education and health care facilities in the modern system of medicine. In addition, there were 431 colleges providing training and health care facilities in the ISM&H, with the maximum being in Ayurveda (209) followed by homeopathy (180), Unanai (36), and Siddha (six). There were 15,393 hospitals as of January 1, 2002, with 914,543 hospital beds (of all types) accounting for 89 hospital beds per 100,000 population. In addition to the hospitals, there were 137,311 SCs, 22,842 PHCs, and 3,043 CHCs on March 31, 2001. There were 605,800 medical doctors registered with the Medical Council of India as of December 31, 2002, at the rate of 59 doctors per 100,000 population. In addition, 839,862 nurses and midwives were registered with the Nursing Council of India as of March 31, 2003.[8]

While the primary and secondary health care facilities may at the most provide only the basic health care, some of the private and government hospitals and institutions now are providing "state of the art" facilities often at a fraction of the cost that needs to be paid in the hospitals in the developed nations. Although still not adequate, there has been a phenomenal growth in the health care sector in the last few years, especially in the private sector. The private health insurance agencies also have begun to play a role in the country, though not in a big way. Distribution of these health care facilities leaves much to be desired, and despite the fact that many parts of the country may still be without adequate health care facilities, medical tourism is projected to be a major revenue-earning industry in the next few years.

MENTAL HEALTH CARE IN INDIA

India being a land of contrasts, mental health care is provided by a multitude of trained and untrained personnel that include neurologists, neurosurgeons, psychiatrists, physicians, pediatricians, those trained in the ISM&H, and a large number of health and non–health care personnel (registered and unregistered medical practitioners, religious heads, and even faith healers). In urban areas for most people with epilepsy who receive treatment, the expert care is provided mainly by the neurologists and neurosurgeons, though primary care is delivered by family physicians, pediatricians, and internal medicine experts.

SPECIALIST RESOURCES

The challenge of meeting the needs of people with epilepsy in a developing country like India is a daunting task for everyone involved in the planning and delivery of health care. The limited resources and lack of adequate trained manpower complicates the problem further. At present there are about 800 trained neurologists and 1,300 to 1,500 trained neurosurgeons in the country. The paradox of a country like India is that as per the president-elect of the Association for Indo-American Neurologists, there are 600 to 700 neurologists of Indian origin in the United States (personal communication).

A high-powered committee set up by government of India, the Technology, Information, Forecasting, and Assessment Council (TIFAC), examined the technology and manpower requirement for the year 2020. The needs in the discipline of neurology were also assessed by the TIFAC. Assuming even a modest ratio of one neurologist for 200,000 population as against 8,000 in Italy and 18,000 to 50,000 in the United Sates, India would require ≥5,000 neurologists as against the present strength of <1,000 neurologists. Even if a hundred trained neurologists were to be added to the pool annually, giving allowance for outward movement from the country, it would take at least half a century to achieve the goal. A further confounding problem is the distribution of neurologists, because major proportions gravitate to metropolitan cities and big towns, leaving almost 70% of the population in the rural areas deprived of specialists' care. Thus, there is an urgent need to reconsider and conceptualize alternative strategies to organize services at the peripheral, regional, and apex levels, as recommended by the TIFAC.[6]

MAGNITUDE OF THE EPILEPSY PROBLEM IN INDIA

Many studies based on well-accepted methods, valid screening and diagnostic tools, and case confirmation methods have been conducted to identify epilepsy in the community in an inexpensive way in different parts of India. Population-based neuroepidemiologic studies conducted in different regions have shown that epilepsy constitutes nearly a third of all neurologic disorders. The prevalence of epilepsy varies from 2.5 to 11.9 per 1,000 population.[2,3,5–7,9–14] In the Bangalore Urban Rural Neuroepidemiological (BURN) survey, a task force project supported by the Indian Council of Medical Research (ICMR) covering a population of 102,557, a prevalence rate of 8.8 per 1,000 population was observed, with the rate in rural communities (11.9) being twice that of urban areas (5.5). Epilepsy was found to be the second leading neurologic problem in both urban and rural populations, next only to vascular headache.[7] Based on these data and information emanating from various studies, it is estimated that in India (with a population of more than 1 billion), there are about 6 to 10 million people living with epilepsy, accounting for nearly one fifth of the global burden.[2,3,5–7,9–14] Though most of the epidemiologic studies in India estimated prevalence of epilepsy, one study from Yelandur has provided incidence data.[10] Accordingly, 50 new cases per 100,000 population are added annually, giving an additional burden of 500,000 new-onset epilepsy cases every year in India.

Burden of epilepsy as estimated using disability adjusted life years (DALYs) accounts for 1% of the total burden of disease in the world, excluding that due to social stigma and isolation, which is highly prevalent in India and might account for a much higher disease burden. In a country like India with a diverse culture, caste, and low literacy, various myths and misconceptions exist about epilepsy among the people, which further adds to the treatment gap. The treatment gap in epilepsy ranges between 38% and 80%. The lowest figure is from Kerala, which has a high literacy rate and health-conscious people. The BURN data have demonstrated that even in urban areas, the treatment gap is as high as 50%. This large treatment gap is due to multiple factors, including lack of awareness about epilepsy among the people; social stigma; reluctance to accept the diagnosis; improper distribution of the available medical facilities, especially among rural, tribal, and hilly areas of the country; and availability and/or affordability of the long term antiepilepsy drug treatment.[6]

DELIVERY OF EPILEPSY CARE IN INDIA

In India, with its population of more than 1 billion, a dismally low trained neurologist ratio of 1 in 1,250,000, and a very high epilepsy burden, primary care physicians, general practitioners, pediatricians, and psychiatrists provide 60% to 70% of epilepsy care. Hence, it is imperative that developing countries such as India develop alternative strategies to reach out to the needy people living with epilepsy in different parts of such a vast country. Various models of delivery of epilepsy care have been tried and are in practice. Brief accounts of the same are given below.

Satellite Clinic Model

The National Institute of Mental Health & Neuro Sciences (NIMHANS), Bangalore, has developed a satellite clinic model (SCM), which has been implemented for more than two decades, since 1982. This model is successful in delivering neurologic and psychiatric care to the rural community—an example of joint collaborative work between governmental and nongovernmental agency. The NIMHANS provides expert panels; local governmental agencies along with nongovernmental organizations (NGOs) such as the Lions or Rotary conduct the service camps on a "fixed day at fixed place" every month. This approach results in the delivery of expert care at the patient's doorstep.

Epilepsy accounts for 40% to 50% of all the neuropsychiatric patients seen in these camps. The NIMHANS caters to five places located within a 50- to 100-km radius, on 5 fixed days every month. More than 150 to 300 people attend each camp. First-line standard antiepileptic drugs such as phenobarbital, phenytoin, carbamazepine, and valproate are provided free to needy patients and simple medical records are maintained to follow these individuals. The camps are coupled with awareness campaigns about common neurologic disorders such as stroke, epilepsy, and mental retardation through the NGOs using both electronic and print media. Over the last two decades thousands of people made use of this satellite clinic model and have benefited from these camps.

Community Health Center Model

The NIMHANS has also developed another model called the "community health center model" to take care of the patients at the community level in the urban areas in Bangalore. CHCs covering a population of 50,000 to 100,000 work in close liaison with medical colleges. There are nearly 200 medical colleges in India that look after the CHCs via their preventive and social medicine departments. The services of medical colleges and CHCs can be used to look after the epilepsy patients in their jurisdiction and also for the distribution of first-line antiepileptic drugs to the needy. The paramedical staff attached to these CHCs maintains health records. The epilepsy patients can be treated and followed up by this trained workforce at the patient's doorstep. The CHCs also have their mobile health care units reaching out to remote villages and far-flung, unreached areas. It has been demonstrated that the community health center model is successful in reaching out to the people at their doorsteps.

District Epilepsy Care Model

The "epilepsy control program" through a district model was developed by the NIMHANS, Bangalore, with the support of the WHO (SEARO) through the Ministry of Health, Government of India. This was implemented between 1999 and 2001. The program has three main objectives:

1. It would sensitize state health administrators regarding epilepsy as a public health problem.
2. It would train district medical officers in the delivery of epilepsy care. The trained doctors could further train other PHC medical officers.
3. "Nodal neurologists" at the state level would coordinate with these district medical officers to sustain this program.

Districts are used for health care delivery in this model since they have the advantage of being an independent administrative unit. The district medical officer (DMO) is the administrative head that implements and monitors various national health programs at district levels. In addition, all health programs at PHCs and Taluks come under jurisdiction of the district. Districts as models for mental health care have already been successfully implemented in India. There are 593 districts with an average population of 1.5 to 2 million people in each district.

The essential step in the district model is training of DMOs. The internal medicine experts/pediatricians/psychiatrists can also be included in the training of the trainer's program. Training is focused on (a) identification of epilepsy, (b) diagnosis, (c) treatment, (d) counseling, (e) psychosocial aspects of epilepsy, and (f) legal aspects of epilepsy. Training is done using training modules, audiovisual aids, and lectures that also include demonstration of practical aspects of managing acute emergencies in epilepsy. Evaluation of the training course is done using pre- and posttraining questionnaires. The training courses need to be followed by periodic workshops. These medical officers would subsequently train other primary health center doctors and also coordinate with the nodal neurologists. Programs of this nature require support from the government and NGOs in getting an uninterrupted free supply of antiepileptic drugs, maintenance of simple medical records, maintenance of epilepsy diaries, and regular follow-up from the patients. This model has also been successfully tested during the 3-year period by the NIMHANS.

Fortis Epilepsy Control Program Model

The Fortis group of hospitals is a part of the Fortis health care that is fast emerging as a leader in the delivery of health care in the private sector in India. As a part of its commitment to provide affordable health care at the community level, the Fortis Epilepsy Control Program (FECP) was launched on November 18, 2005, with an aim to provide some treatment to those with epilepsy who receive no treatment at all at the community level.

As part of the FECP, 18 practicing doctors from different parts of the state of Uttar Pradesh (UP) and the National Capital Region (NCR) with at least an MBBS degree were invited and trained on November 17, 2005 (the World Epilepsy Day) at Fortis Hospital, NOIDA, to detect grand mal seizures using the protocol prepared under the guidance of the WHO-SEARO.[1] The trained doctors started treating only those patients diagnosed to have grand mal seizures in the area of their practice from January 1, 2006. The doctors trained have been told to exclude and not to treat patients below the age of 10 years and above the age of 60 years; those having any other seizure type or multiple seizure types (probably an epilepsy syndrome); women with a potential to have children or pregnant women; those having serious medical illnesses like hepatic or renal disease; those with known allergies to antiepileptic drugs; and those having any abnormality on neurologic examination like focal deficits and evidence of raised intracranial tension. All patients to be included for treatment under the FECP will be made aware and offered the choice of investigations like electroencephalography, computed tomography scan, or magnetic resonance imaging scan of the brain.

Those epilepsy patients with grand mal seizures selected for treatment will be treated with tablets of Phenytal (100 mg phenytoin and 30 mg phenobarbitone), two tablets once a day at bedtime for an average adult. The participating doctors will provide these tablets to all patients at the nominal cost of about Re 1 per day for two tablets (about U.S. $2 per 3 months of medicinal supply). A complete database of patients with all contact details will be maintained by the treating doctors. The patients included in the treatment plan will be followed up at regular intervals, preferably every month specifically for seizure control and any adverse effects of antiepileptic drugs. Any patient having problems due to poor seizure control or side effects of drugs or any other problem will be referred for an "expert opinion" to Fortis Hospital at NOIDA or any other tertiary care hospital. Neurologists from the Fortis Advanced Centre for Epilepsy, NOIDA, will periodically visit the participating doctor's clinic to review the work being done.

In the first phase, 18 doctors trained are participating in the FECP. During the second phase the plan is to enroll more doctors practicing in 10 to 15 neighboring districts. In the third phase, the program will be extended to all other districts of UP and NCR and also to neighboring states, depending on the resources.

The models outlined above are not exclusive but complementary to one another and will be able to "reach the unreached" with regard to epilepsy.

NATIONAL EPILEPSY CONTROL PROGRAM (NECP)

Launch of the WHO/International League Against Epilepsy (ILAE)/International Bureau of Epilepsy (IBE) joint initiative of the "Global Campaign Against Epilepsy" in 1997[4] has given impetus to start a similar National Epilepsy Control Program

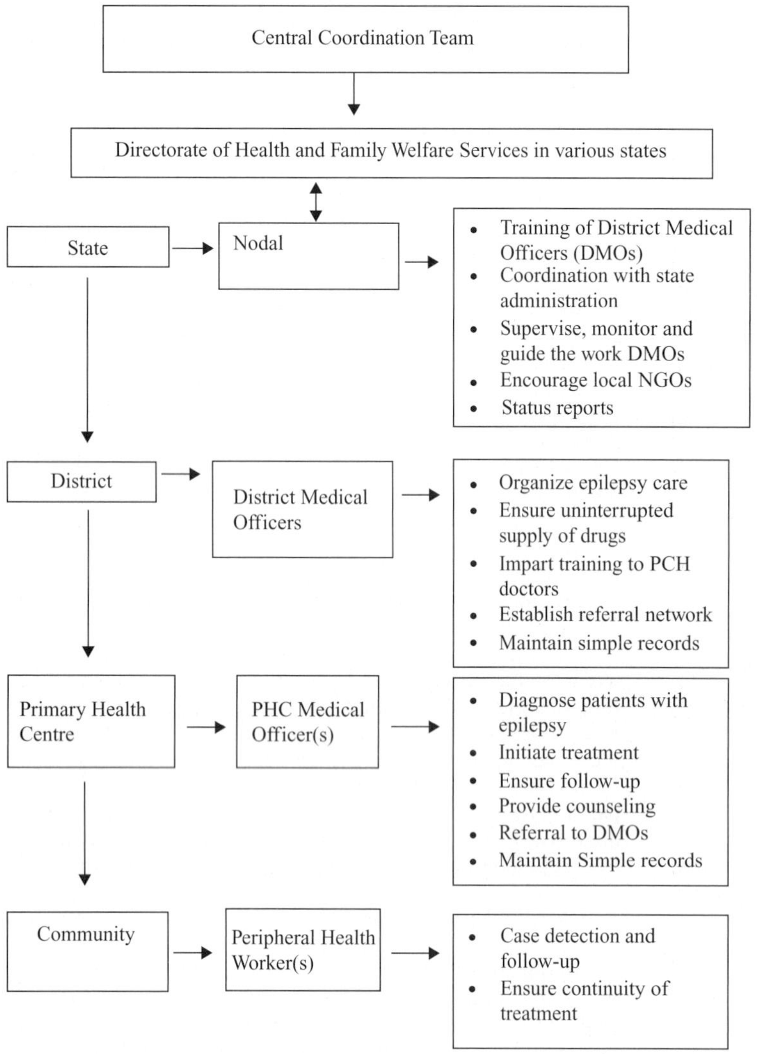

FIGURE 1. National Epilepsy Control Programme: action plan. (Adapted from Gourie-Devi M, Satishchandra P, Gururaj G. Epilepsy control program in India: a district model. *Epilepsia.* 2003;44[Suppl 1]:58–62.)

in India. This needs to be implemented all around the country with the following objectives:

1. To provide accessible and affordable health care to all people living with epilepsy, particularly to the people living in rural and far-flung areas and vulnerable sections of the society
2. To have joint participation of community and nongovernmental agencies in the delivery of comprehensive epilepsy care to people living with epilepsy
3. To ensure integration of people with epilepsy in various spheres of activity through psychosocial and vocational rehabilitation
4. To reduce the prevalence rate of epilepsy in the community by reducing the birth injuries and controlling parasitic diseases (neurocysticercosis) and other neuroinfections and road traffic accidents
5. To create and improve awareness among the people about epilepsy

The proposed action plan of the National Epilepsy Control Program is given in Figure 1. It is proposed to have one national epilepsy center, which will be linked to four or five regional epilepsy centers in different parts of the country to coordinate with state level centers. To achieve the goal of the National Epilepsy Control Program, the Indian Epilepsy Association (IEA), Indian Epilepsy Society (IES), and other nongovernmental agencies need to actively participate together with the main focus being on improving awareness about epilepsy and providing comprehensive epilepsy care to the people with epilepsy. This can be achieved with the "center to periphery" or "periphery to center" approach. The proposed National Epilepsy Control Program should preferably be a separate program. It could also be integrated into an appropriate ongoing vertical national health program in India for easy implementation.

SUMMARY AND CONCLUSIONS

India is a land of contrasts. Until recently the ever-increasing population was proving to be a major handicap for the national growth. The availability of a large trained workforce (as a result of the large population) has changed the apparent "disadvantage" into a big national "advantage." Today, India's economy is rapidly growing and is matched by that of China only. The India growth story has just gotten bigger and better. For the first time, India has emerged stronger on the global investment radar in 2005, overtaking even the most developed economies of the world. India today is one of the most attractive foreign direct investment destinations in the world.

Despite being home to about one fifth of the entire world's population with epilepsy and a rapidly improving economy, there is no national epilepsy control program in India. This is perhaps the right time for the governmental heath planning authorities to take note of the situation and take some remedial steps. There is an urgent need to have a separate NECP in India. Clubbing the epilepsy control program with the National Mental Health Program in India is likely to have serious implications with regard to increased societal stigma. Such a step could be a retrograde action in view of the Global Campaign Against Epilepsy that aims to bring "epilepsy out of the shadows." The best approach in a country like India with limited resources for health care would be to encourage "private–public participation." The models adopted by the NIMHANS and the Fortis group have the potential to be applied at the national level with support from the government in collaboration with the health care providers in the private sector and nongovernmental organizations. There are costs for doing all of this, but the costs of not doing this are perhaps much higher.

References

1. Anand K, Jain S, Paul E, et al. Development of a validated clinical case definition of generalized tonic–clonic seizures for use by community-based health care providers. *Epilepsia*. 2005;46:743–750.
2. Bharucha NE. Epidemiology of epilepsy in India. *Epilepsia*. 2003;44 (Suppl 1):9–11.
3. Das SK, Sanyal K, Neuroepidemiology of major neurological disorders in rural Bengal. *Neurol India*. 1996;44:47–58.
4. Engel J Jr, Birbeck GL, Diop AG, et al. Out of the shadows - ILAE-IBE-WHO global campaign against epilepsy. In: Engel J Jr,Birbeck GL, Diop AG, et al., eds. *Epilepsy Global Issues for the Practicing Neurologist - World Federation of Neurology Seminars in Clinical Neurology*. New York: Demos Medical Publishing, LLC; 2005:125–133.
5. Gourie-Devi M, Rao VN, Prakshi R. Neuroepidemiological study in semiurban and rural areas in south India: pattern of neurological disorders including motor neuron disease. In: Gourie-Devi M, ed. *Motor Neuron Disease: Global Clinical Patterns and International Research*. New Delhi: Oxford and IBH Publishing Company; 1987:11–21.
6. Gourie-Devi M, Satishchandra P, Gururaj G. Epilepsy control program in India: a district model. *Epilepsia*. 2003;44(Suppl 1):58–62.
7. Gourie-Devi M, Gururaj G, Satishchandra P, et al. Prevalence of neurological disorders in Bangalore, India: a community-based study with a comparison between urban and rural areas. *Neuroepidemiology*. 2004;23:261–268.
8. Government of India - Central Bureau of Health Intelligence. Health Information of India. Directorate General of Health Services, Ministry of Health & Family Welfare, New Delhi, India; 2003.
9. Kapoor SK, Chandra V, Banerjee AK, et al. Pilot study of the prevalence of major neurologic disorders in a rural population of India. *Neuroepidemiology*. 1990;9:287–295.
10. Mani KS, Geeta R, Srinivas HV, et al. The Yelandur study: a community based approach to epilepsy in rural South India: epidemiological aspects. *Seizure*. 1998;7:281–288.
11. Mani KS, Geeta R, Srinivas HV, et al. Epilepsy control with phenobarbital or phenytoin in rural South India: the Yelandur study. *Lancet*. 2001;357:1316–1320.
12. Radhakrishnan K, Pandian JF, Santoshkumar T, et al. Prevalence, knowledge, attitude and practice of epilepsy in Kerala, South India. *Epilepsia*. 2000;41:1027–1035.
13. Razdan S, Kaul RL, Motta A, et al. Prevalence and pattern of major neurological disorders in rural Kashmir. *Neuroepidemiology*. 1994;13:113–119.
14. Sridharan R, Murthy BN. Prevalence and pattern of epilepsy in India. *Epilepsia*. 1999;40(5):631–636.

CHAPTER 294 ■ JAPAN

E. ANN YEH AND MASAKAZU SEINO

INTRODUCTION

In 1994, Japanese government officials introduced a new vision of social welfare for the 21st century.[8] Central to this vision was the issue of how to handle problems that stem from the growing population of elderly individuals, many of whom will soon become disabled and utilize health care services to a greater degree than their younger counterparts. These concerns are not limited to the elderly, but extend to all disabled individuals. How these people will be cared for and who will be responsible for their care are questions that need to be addressed.

With these concerns in mind, this chapter examines the current health care policies of the Japanese government, beginning with a review of health insurance in Japan. A discussion of national health care spending follows, along with a description of the organization and distribution of health care personnel. Health care services available to individuals with epilepsy are examined, with special reference to medical specialists treating epilepsy in Japan. The chapter concludes with a brief discussion of the contradictions inherent in current government policy.

HEALTH INSURANCE

The health insurance system of Japan currently operates on the basic premise that all individuals should have access to affordable health care. However, the original impetus of the government for establishing a health insurance system was not the provision of affordable medical care, but rather the maintenance of a strong workforce. It was but one element of government efforts at nation building in the early 20th century.[4] In 1960, the year that universal health care was instituted, 94.2% of the population of Japan was covered by health insurance. Since then, the proportion of insured individuals has increased annually. In 2002, virtually 100% of the Japanese population was covered by health insurance.[10] Health insurance in Japan is of two main types: Employee insurance (60.3%) and National Health Insurance (NHI) (39.7%). Benefits include compensation for clinical visits and drugs.[5]

Employee Insurance

The number of individuals covered by employee insurance (either as a principal policy holder or as a dependent of a policy holder) grew from 48.5% of the population in 1960 to 60.3% of the population in 2002. There are four distinct categories of employee insurance: Government-managed insurance (46.9% of the total number of employee insurance policy holders), large enterprise insurance (40.0%), mutual aid associations (12.8%), and seamen's insurance (0.3%). Insurance premiums of approximately 8.6% of an employee's salary are deducted monthly. At present, 70% of the medical costs of both policy holders and their dependents are covered, while 80% of medical costs for children younger than 3 years of age and 90% of costs for individuals older than 70 years of age are covered.[5]

National Health Insurance

NHI was established in 1938. In 1960, health insurance coverage through NHI was extended to all residents of Japan not eligible for employee insurance—self-employed individuals, students, farmers, unemployed individuals, and part-time workers, among others. Benefits under NHI are far less comprehensive than those available under employee insurance; 70% of medical costs are covered. Premiums are scaled to income and assets, with an average household yearly payment of 163,842 yen. This amounted to 2.8% of the average national income in 2002. In 1984, a pensioner's plan was introduced that increased benefits for retired persons to 80% of all hospital costs and 70% of outpatient costs of policy holders and to 80% of the hospital costs of dependents. In 2002, approximately 50,297,000 people, or 39.7% of the population of Japan, were insured through NHI.[5]

Payment for Hospital Services: Epilepsy and the General Population

According to a 2002 patient survey, on any given day in Japan, an estimated 7,929,000 people were either hospitalized or used outpatient services. Of these patients, 60.3% were covered by employee insurance (split almost evenly between policy holders [30.1%] and dependents [30.2%], and 39.7% by NHI).[9]

The proportions of types of health insurance used in medical consultations related to epilepsy differ somewhat. According to estimates by the Ministry of Health, Labor and Welfare (MHLW), 38% of visits by patients with epilepsy were paid for with NHI. In addition, although employee insurance was used by almost the same proportion of individuals (11.2%) as in the general population (10.7%), insurance for dependents with epilepsy was used with greater frequency (22.5%). As with the general population (1.8%), there were no clinical visits related to epilepsy that were paid for in full by patients. Health services for 9.2% of patients with epilepsy were paid for through publicly funded Medicaid (Seikatsu Hogo Hou) and through other public funds. These numbers are significantly higher than the proportion estimated for all hospital patients (0.5% under the Mental Health Act, 7.5% under the Social Welfare Act, and 6.1% through other public funds).[10]

These figures indicate that a significantly higher proportion of individuals visiting clinics and hospitals for problems related to epilepsy are self-employed or unemployed and receive some sort of public assistance. The relatively higher numbers of patients using insurance for dependents can be explained partially by the large proportion of people <25 years of age using hospital services for problems related to epilepsy (see Specialists Treating Epilepsy).

BUDGET ORGANIZATION AND DEVELOPMENT

National spending on health care in Japan has increased rapidly since 1954, the year the Ministry of Health and Welfare (MHW) began keeping such records.[5] That year, health care spending equaled 215.2 billion yen (1.871 billion U.S. dollars at the 2005 exchange rate of 115 yen per dollar). Medical costs in Japan have increased in tandem with the standard of living and national income. They have remained at approximately 5% to 6% of national income since 1975, ranging from 5.22% in 1975 to 6.42% in 1987.[3] In 2002, 31.1 trillion yen, or 8.58% of the national income, was spent on health care.[5] Normal births, medical checkups and public health measures, costs of prosthetic devices, and costs related to nursing homes are not included in these figures,[5] nor are costs related to research.[4]

Health care spending as a proportion of national income appears to be low compared with the United States (13.9% in 2001), France (9.4%), Canada (9.4%), and Germany (10.8%).[3] However, according to the Organization for Economic Cooperation and Development (OECD), spending in Japan is underestimated by about 25% because figures do not account for spending in categories included in other national estimates.[12] Even with the added 25%, the figures for Japan are low compared with these countries. With respect to the gross national product (GNP), health care spending in Japan, which was 7.4% of the GNP in 1998, was lower than that of countries such as the United States and France.[5]

Sources of payment for health care range from insurance (employee insurance and NHI) (44.9% of total), the Geriatric Act (34.37%), patient payments (15.3%), and government-sponsored plans (including welfare and the Mental Health Act, and others) (5.5%) (2002 figures).[3]

Regarding the sources of money spent on health care, in 2002, 51.7% came from insurance premiums, a figure that has risen steadily from 45.8% in 1954. Spending from public sources has risen from 16% in 1954; the current rate is 33% (25.1% from federal and 7.9% from regional sources). Patient payments account for 15.3%, and 0.2% comes from other sources.[3]

Whereas in 1955 10.2% of all medical payments came from Medicaid (Iryou Hogo/Seikatsu Hogo), the amount has dropped steadily and was 0.8% in 2002. In addition, medical costs borne by patients not using insurance dropped from 20.7% in 1955 to 1.3% in 2002. Employee insurance covered 60.3% of health care, and NHI covered 39.7% in 2002, proportions roughly equivalent to the relative number of individuals insured under these categories.[5]

ORGANIZATION OF HOSPITALS, PHYSICIANS, AND HEALTH CARE WORKERS

Hospitals and Clinics

Medical facilities in Japan (excluding dental facilities) totaled 966,044 in 2002. They are organized into hospitals having more than 20 beds (9,280) and clinics with fewer than 20 beds (86,764).[a]

Most of the facilities fall into one of five major categories, representing ownership: Individual ownership (10.4%); medical juridical persons (nonprofit organizations) (Iryou Houjin) (60.2%); public medical facilities (15.0%); National (3.7%); and employee insurance groups (1%) in 2002. Privately owned clinics and hospitals make up the overwhelming majority of medical facilities, and as the government does not regulate their distribution, the concentration of facilities in different prefectures varies widely. In 2002, the average number of general hospitals was 6.7 per 100,000 people in Japan.[5,b]

In 2002, Japan had one of the highest proportions of medical beds per capita in the world: 1,573 per 100,000 people, which is comparable to Iceland (1,670 per 100,000), Sweden (1,480 per 100,000), and Norway (1,500 per 100,000). The proportion is about twice that of Canada (778 per 100,000) and almost three times that of the United States (586 per 100,000). The percentage of filled hospital beds in Japan was estimated to be 85.3% of general hospital beds and 93.2% of psychiatric beds in 2001.[5]

There were about 1,646,000 hospital beds in 2002 in Japan, with 1,372 general hospital beds per 100,000 people. Of all beds in hospitals with >200 beds, 54% were located in hospitals run by medical juridical persons, 21% in hospitals run by local, and 6% in hospitals run by federal government. As with hospitals, great discrepancies in numbers of beds exist from prefecture to prefecture. The prefecture with the highest concentration of hospital beds, Kagoshima Prefecture, had 2,081 beds per 100,000 people, while the lowest, Saitama Prefecture, had 878 beds per 100,000 people in 2002.[5]

Medical and paramedical services (including physician services and occupational/physical/speech therapies, laboratory testing, and some nursing services) are billed on a fee-for-service basis, with prices for services and drugs regulated by governmental bodies.

Decisions concerning changes in billing rates are highly political. From the mid-20th century to the present, members of the Japanese Medical Association (JMA), the majority of whom operate private clinics, have been extremely powerful in shaping billing decisions, such that current billing decidedly favors clinicians in private practice.[4] In the early 1960s, the JMA was able to bring about an increase in compensation for services by refusing to cooperate with certain public health measures. A second effect of the JMA's lobbying has been that responsibility for chronic, costly health problems has been shifted to the state.

Because physicians working in clinics do not usually have admitting privileges in hospitals, much duplication and fragmentation of medical services takes place in Japan.[4] Referral is only sometimes practiced: According to the MHLW 2002 survey of patients, the majority of patients visiting outpatient services (93.2%) and who were hospitalized (55.2%) did not receive referrals from staff at other hospitals or clinics.[10] The government is attempting to change this practice. Starting in 1988, patients were required to receive referrals to utilize the services of specially designated tertiary care centers. Patients who do not receive referrals to the centers cannot use their health insurance for the first consultation they receive there.

Outpatient services are used with greater frequency in Japan than in the United States. The number of outpatient visits per capita in Japan was more than twice that of the United States in 1996 (16.0 vs. 5.8).[12] On an average day in 2002, 6,478,000

[a]Throughout this chapter, *hospital* refers to a medical facility with 20 beds, and *clinic* indicates a medical facility with 0 to 19 beds.

[b]This number does not include clinics, psychiatric hospitals, dental clinics, or contagious disease beds. If these facilities are included, the total number of medical facilities in Japan in 2001 was 167,555 or approximately 13.9 per 100,000 people. (These figures are noted in the text.)

people, or 5.1% of the general population, visited a hospital or clinic for an outpatient consultation, and 1,451,000 people, or 1.1% of the population, were hospitalized (41.8% in general beds, 17.4% in psychiatric beds, 31.9% in long-term care beds, and the remainder in nursing beds and beds devoted to the care of specific diseases).[10]

Although a relatively small proportion of the population in Japan is admitted to hospitals, Japan has an average length of hospital stay of 37.9 days (24.0 days in general hospital beds, 195 days in rehabilitation hospital beds, and 385.7 days in psychiatric hospital beds).[5] This is just twice the 1998 U.S. average of 20.4 days (7.8 days in acute care hospitals).[11] The staff-to-patient ratio in general hospitals in Japan is low, with an average of 103.3 staff members per 100 beds (including 11.2 physicians, 31.4 nurses, 14.7 assistant nurses, 0.4 occupational therapists, 1.0 physical therapists, and 3.1 technicians). The ratio is even lower at psychiatric hospitals, with an average of 53.2 staff members per 100 beds (including 2.7 physicians, 13.0 nurses, and 14.5 assistant nurses).[5]

Although the staff-to-patient ratio is low in hospitals, technologic apparatus is more readily available in Japan than in other countries.[4] In 1999, 10,693 Japanese medical facilities had either whole-body or head-only computed tomography (CT) scanners. All of the country's 2,938 magnetic resonance imaging (MRI) scanners were located in hospitals.[5]

Physicians

The number of physicians in Japan has nearly doubled since the early 1970s, when the government began its campaign to increase the number of physicians to 150 per 100,000 people. In 2002, there were 255,792 licensed physicians in Japan, or approximately 200 physicians for every 100,000 people.[5] Most physicians in Japan are specialists, the greatest concentration of whom are internists (30.6%), followed by surgeons (10.1%) and pediatricians (5.8%).[5] Because there are almost no general practice physicians in Japan, internists often act as primary care generalists; over one third of all hospital consultations on a given day in 2003 were estimated to be with internists, and 91.3% of all hospitals in Japan had internists on staff.[c] By comparison, 9.7% of all hospital consultations were conducted by surgeons and 66.8% of all general hospitals had surgeons on staff. In general hospitals 4.3% of all consultations were performed by pediatricians and 40.8% of all general hospitals had pediatricians on staff.[5]

Physicians are plentiful in more densely populated areas in Japan. There are, however, regional differences in the distribution of physicians. Saitama prefecture, for example, has the lowest physician-to-population ratio (121.8 per 100,000 people), while Tokushima prefecture has the highest physician-to-population ratio (258 per 10,000 people) in the country.[5]

SERVICES FOR EPILEPSY IN JAPAN

The MHLW estimates that on an average day 26,900 people with epilepsy received treatment at clinics and hospitals around the country in 2002. These visits constituted 0.34% of all clinical encounters.[d] Of the consultations related to epilepsy, approximately 72.5% were outpatient visits. The number of hospitalized patients with epilepsy has decreased over the years, with hospitalized patients with epilepsy totaling 8,997 in 1994, 8,332 in 1996, and 7,400 in 2002.[7,10]

The number of consultations related to epilepsy has risen together with the total estimated number of medical consultations. Estimated figures for all medical consultations between 1984 and 2002 show a decrease in inpatient consultations and a slow rise in outpatient consultations. The number of outpatient consultations for epilepsy increased more significantly than outpatient visits in general, with a rise from 172,000 in the 1980s to 195,000 in the mid-1990s. Ninety-eight to 99% of hospitalizations for patients with epilepsy in any given year began in the previous year.[7,10]

According to MHLW estimates, all hospitalizations and most outpatient consultations related to epilepsy take place in hospitals.[10] The number of patients who received referrals from other hospitals or clinics in 2002 was 55.2% for inpatients and 93.9% for outpatients. The rapid increase in the number of referrals in the 1990s can be attributed to a newly introduced health insurance system that provides physicians with incentives for issuing referrals. Those patients who first visit hospitals or clinics without referrals issued by previous physicians must pay their fees out of pocket. Insurance companies will not cover these visits.

Hospitalizations for individuals with epilepsy represent approximately 0.5% of hospitalizations for all problems. Hospital stays are long, averaging 122.0 days—far longer than the national average of 44.9 days.[10] As with the national average, the average number of days that patients with epilepsy are hospitalized varies greatly from institution to institution. The shortest average length of stay is at company hospitals (14 days). Hospitalizations for epilepsy in other types of hospitals (e.g., nonprofit or public) are similar in length (approximately 16.1 days). The longest average hospitalization for epilepsy is in psychiatric hospitals (688.1 days).[9]

The number of beds in a hospital also determines the length of a hospital stay. In hospitals with between 200 and 699 beds, average stays for problems related to epilepsy range from 131.3 to 254.4 days. In facilities with 20 to 49 beds, epilepsy patients stay an average of 12 days. In 1990, more than half (53%) of the hospitalizations for epilepsy in Japan were estimated to have lasted longer than 5 years. Seventy-three percent of these had lasted longer than 10 years.[9]

SPECIALISTS TREATING EPILEPSY

Although in North America people with epilepsy receive treatment primarily from neurologists or pediatricians, and in some cases general practitioners or family doctors, in Japan neuropsychiatrists and pediatricians are primarily responsible for the treatment of epilepsy. Other specialists who treat epilepsy in significant numbers in Japan are neurologic internists and neurosurgeons. Because internists often act as generalists, they see a significant number of epilepsy patients—10.5% of all cases. Most of these are outpatient visits that are split almost evenly between hospitals and private clinics. Epilepsy cases make up only a small percentage (0.2%) of the total number of cases seen by internists. A small number of consultations for epilepsy are carried out by surgeons (0.9%) and pediatric surgeons (0.3%).[9]

Neuropsychiatrists receive training in areas that in North America would fall under the specialties of psychiatry or neurology. Consequently, they treat conditions that are categorized in North America as psychiatric (i.e., schizophrenia, depression) or neurologic (i.e., stroke, epilepsy, cerebral palsy).[10] Most neuropsychiatrists (92.4%) practice in hospitals. The remaining 7.6% either have their own private clinics or are employees of small clinics.[2]

[c] Internists in private practice act as generalists. However, those affiliated with university hospitals act as specialists.

[d] All figures referring to epilepsy here are taken from MHW sources, which, following the International Classification of Diseases, classify epilepsy as a neurologic disorder. "Epileptic convulsions, fits, or seizures NOS" fall into this category.

According to estimates of the MHLW, approximately 50.1% of patients receiving treatment for epilepsy are seen by neuropsychiatrists. Most of these consultations take place in hospitals (93.9%), and the majorities are inpatient consultations (64%). In 1990, 3.6% of all psychiatric consultations were estimated to be related to epilepsy.[9]

In the 1970s, a new specialty was introduced in Japan—neurologic internal medicine. Specialists in this area make up only a small fraction of all practicing physicians (1.3%). Most neurologic internists are hospital based. They conduct an estimated 3.7% of all medical consultations for epilepsy, which make up approximately 3.3% of their total consultations. In 1990, all consultations were hospital based, and most (75%) were outpatient consultations.

In 1990, children under 15 years of age comprised 23.3% of all patients seen for problems related to epilepsy in Japan. An estimated 24.8% of all medical consultations related to epilepsy were treated by pediatricians.[9] Although most pediatricians are hospital based (68.9%), 20% have their own clinics. However, almost all pediatricians treating epilepsy are employed by hospitals (89%). Of all pediatric consultations related to epilepsy, 91% take place through outpatient services.[9]

Finally, although surgery for epilepsy is not performed frequently in Japan (fewer than 500 cases in 2002), neurosurgeons treat a significant number of people with epilepsy—approximately 10% of the total. These consultations make up about 2.8% of the total number of clinical consultations with neurosurgeons and, for the most part, are outpatient, hospital-based appointments (80.0%). Most neurosurgeons (99%) are hospital employees. They made up 2.5% of all physicians in 2002.[10]

Although most people being treated for epilepsy appear to be covered by health insurance, several additional costs may burden individuals with epilepsy. Travel costs to specialized clinics, particularly for individuals with chronic health problems who must visit them frequently, are often prohibitive.

Because epilepsy in and of itself has only recently been recognized by the government as a disability, subsidized transportation was not provided in the past for people with epilepsy unless the individual also had severe mental disabilities, psychiatric problems, or physical disabilities.[e] This changed in 1995, when epilepsy was included in the Comprehensive Welfare Act for Individuals with Disabilities (Sougou Shougaisha Fukuski Hou), which awarded disability certificates (techou) based on an individual's degree of impairment with respect to daily living and degree of seizure frequency and severity. Financial burdens on individuals with severe disabilities have presumably been reduced by this act. However, individuals who must be accompanied by a parent or friend to doctors' appointments incur even greater costs that are not subsidized by the government.

Finally, people who have been given a diagnosis of active epilepsy are prohibited from driving in Japan, unless the length of time they have been seizure free exceeds 2 years. Thus, many people with epilepsy must rely on friends, family, or public transportation to get to their appointments. These barriers constitute perhaps the greatest obstacles to the utilization of hospital services for people with epilepsy.

[e]Transportation costs *are* provided for individuals on social welfare. In addition, some local communities (*Shi Chou Son*) provide costs for local transport to individuals with epilepsy. All individuals who receive this support also receive support under Mental Hygiene Article 32 for Outpatient Care.

SUMMARY AND CONCLUSIONS

Health care in contemporary Japan operates on the fundamental assumption that all residents should have access to medical services of some sort. However, policies are not blind to an individual's "social contribution," a concept that originated in the early 20th century. This concept linked work with the right to health care. A two-tiered health insurance system continues to exist. It provides full-time company employees with health care benefits that are equivalent to those provided via NHI to the unemployed and people with part-time employment. Premiums for inclusion in NHI are scaled to income and assets. However, payment for medical services is not scaled to income. This therefore constitutes an additional barrier to access to health care for the unemployed and underemployed.

Individuals who are chronically ill, such as those with epilepsy, are most likely to be unemployed or working part time. One result of current policy is that these individuals are therefore more likely to incur larger personal health care bills per hospital visit than the average patient. Individuals with epilepsy who utilize health care services in Japan are far more likely than the average patient to be holders of NHI or to be dependents of policyholders of employee health insurance. When hospitalized, their stays are longer than the national average for all health problems—both chronic and acute. Individuals with epilepsy also incur larger-than-average bills for repeated outpatient visits and long-term drug therapy.

Contemporary political talk in Japan idealizes the concept of welfare, promoting the creation of a society that accommodates individuals who do not necessarily fit into narrow standards of "normalcy." However, these idealistic visions are not realized in current health policy. Indeed, current policy simply reinforces the notion that productive ability is equivalent to social worth and that the valid contributions to society arise entirely through full-time employment. Unless this message is replaced with a more flexible idea of what constitutes valid social contributions, current policy may actually prevent the realization of the government's much touted social "vision."

References

1. *Heisei 4 nen, Iryou shisetsu chousa* (*Survey of Institutions, 2002*). Tokyo: Kousei Toukei Kyoukai; 2004.
2. *Heisei 14 nen, Ishi, shikaishi, yakuzaishi chousa* (*Survey of Physicians, Dentists, and Pharmacists, 2002*). Tokyo: Kousei Toukei Kyoukai; 2004.
3. *Hoken to nenkin no doukou, 2002* (*Trends in Insurance and Pensions, 2002*). Tokyo: Kousei Toukei Kyoukai; 2002.
4. Ikegami N. Japan: maintaining equity through regulated fees. *J Health Polit Policy Law*. 1992;174:689–713.
5. *Kokumin eisei no doukou, 2002* (*Trends in Public Health, 2002*). Tokyo: Kousei Toukei Kyoukai; 2002.
6. Kousei Toukei Kyoukai. *Nihon no kanja to iryoushisetsu* (*Patients and Medical Institutions in Japan*). Tokyo: Kouse Toukei Kyoukai; 2001.
7. Kouseishou. *Wa ga kuni no seishin hoken, Heisei 15 nendo ban* (*Mental Health in Our Country*). Tokyo: Kouseishou; 2003.
8. Kouseishou Daijin Kanbou Seisakuka. *21 seiki fukushi bijhon* (*Welfare Vision for the 21st Century*). Tokyo: Kousei Toukei Kyoukai; 1996.
9. Kouseishou Daijinbou Toukei Jouhou-bu. *Heisei 2nen, Kanja chousa* (*Patient's Survey, 1990*). Tokyo: Kousei Toukei Kyoukai; 1992.
10. Kouseiroudoushou Daijinbou Toukei Jouhou-bu. *Heisei 14 nen, Kanja chousa* (*Patient's Survey, 2002*). Tokyo: Kousei Toukei Kyoukai; 2004.
11. Kouseishou Kenkou Seisakukyoku Soumuka. *Byouin youran 2004 nenpan* (*Hospital Handbook*). Tokyo: Igakushoin; 2004.
12. OECD (Organization for Economic Cooperation and Development). *Health Care Systems in Transition*. Paris: OECD; 1990.

CHAPTER 295 ■ NIGERIA

BOLANLE ADAMOLEKUN

INTRODUCTION

Nigeria is a federation of 36 states and a federal capital territory, with a land mass of almost 1 million km^2. With a population estimated at 128 million in 2005, it is Africa's most populous country. The prevalence of epilepsy in Nigeria varies from 0.53% in areas with well-developed primary health care services to 3.7% in the rural areas with poor health care infrastructures.[2] About 70% of the total population live in the rural areas.

Children under 15 years constitute 48% of the total population.[12] Peak age-specific prevalence rates for epilepsy occur in the first and second decades.[13]

THE DEVELOPMENT OF HEALTH CARE SERVICES IN NIGERIA

Traditional Medicine

Traditional medicine may be defined as the sum total of all knowledge and practices used in the prevention, diagnosis, and therapy of physical or mental illnesses and relying exclusively on practical experience and observations handed down from generation to generation, whether orally or written.[2]

Traditional medicine has evolved over centuries as the indigenous health care system in Nigeria. Genuine indigenous health care practices are usually based on the cultural and religious beliefs of the people. In a multiethnic country like Nigeria with over 250 ethnic groups, there are expectedly some variations in the system of traditional medicine, with each variant being strongly bound to the local ethnic culture and beliefs. However, common to all the variants of traditional medicine are dualist explanations of the etiology of illness in natural and supernatural terms and the therapeutic use of herbs and magico-religious rituals.

Nigeria has more traditional healers than Western-trained doctors. Although traditional medicine is well known to be a popular option for Nigerians, official government involvement has been minimal, being generally limited to sponsorship of conferences on traditional medicine and programs for the training of traditional birth attendants.[16]

The only legal reference to traditional medicine was in the Medical and Dental practitioners' decree of 1988, where the government referred to a traditional healer as "any person acknowledged by the members generally of the community to which he belongs as having been trained in a system of therapeutic medicine traditionally in use in that community." This definition appeared to leave the accreditation of traditional healers to the community. Government boards of traditional medicine were set up first in Lagos in 1981, and subsequently in other states with the purpose of accreditation and attestation of bona fide traditional healers, in response to the endemic problem of infiltration by charlatans. Recently, the Federal Ministry of Health has announced plans to produce a draft traditional medicine policy for Nigeria.

Members or leaders of some of the numerous churches and mosques in Nigeria practice faith healing. They are not officially recognized or funded at any of the three tiers of government because of the constitutional secularity of the Nigerian State, but nevertheless enjoy wide patronage.

Conventional Medicine

Conventional health care services in Nigeria evolved out of the medical services of the British colonial army. The army medical service, initially meant only for its members and dependents, began to provide medical services to government employees and their dependents following the integration of the army with the colonial administration after the Second World War, and later to the public living near such facilities. The colonial government started off the present system of conventional health services with a network of rural dispensaries and maternity homes to which rural health centers and hospitals were subsequently added.

The first national policy on health care services was introduced as part of the 1946–1956 development plan in the colonial era. The second and third development plans included revisions of this national health policy, with the third (1975–1980) containing a provision for primary health care.

The current national health policy[8] was launched in 1989, and provided for a three-tier schedule of responsibilities of the federal, state, and local governments. Under this system, the delivery of primary health care is the responsibility of local governments, while the state governments are responsible for the delivery of secondary health care and the federal government for tertiary health care. This schedule of responsibilities is coordinated by the Federal Ministry of Health. The National Primary Health Care Development Agency (NPHCDA), formed in 1992, is responsible for the delivery of primary health care services and the construction of the new health centers. It establishes and trains local development committees to manage local health care.

Although both traditional and conventional health services form a plural system of health care, they remain functionally unrelated in any way. There are no official avenues for referral between the two systems.

HEALTH CARE FINANCING AND EXPENDITURE

Revenue

Government health services are financed from the consolidated revenue fund. There are no special taxes or levies for generating funds for health care. The Western regional government had introduced government lotteries in 1955 and legislated[10] that all monies received from the sale of tickets be paid into a medical development fund. However, this effort was eventually discouraged by poor receipts.

The nonexistence of a special health fund, tax, or levy and the relatively low fees paid by patients for health services have resulted in a widening gap between expenditure and resources. For example, most states devote up to 10% of their total annual budget to health services, whereas their annual health revenue usually constitutes <1% of the health budget. In federal teaching hospitals, internally generated revenue accounts for only 5% to 8% of the total annual expenditure.

In order to reduce the burden of the provision of health finances on the three tiers of government, a National Health Insurance scheme was launched in 2005. Federal government workers constitute the first core group to be covered by the pilot phase of the program. The program will later be extended to the organized private sector, but is unlikely to cover the majority of Nigerians, who are either self-employed or work for small enterprises.

Cost recovery through revolving funds is consistent with the national policy, which states that users shall pay for curative services but preventive services shall be subsidized.[8] A seed fund is provided to purchase a good stock of drugs and other consumables employed in medical care. Subsequently, further replenishment of stocks is provided for by sales. Provision is made for losses, exemptions, inflation, and overheads by adding 5% to 20% of the actual cost to the amount charged to the patient. The revolving fund scheme has been quite successful in many teaching hospitals.

Expenditure

In 2002, the Nigerian public health expenditure as a percentage of the gross domestic product (GDP) was 1.2%, while the private health expenditure as a percentage of the GDP was 3.5%. State governments devote between 5% and 10% of their total annual budget to health care, while local governments spend 10% to 15%.

Government medical care is labor intensive. For example, 70% to 90% of each federal teaching hospital's annual budget is spent on salaries and emoluments, leaving little for health care services and drugs.

The concept of "managed care" is practiced by all public and private companies and corporations who are obliged by law to provide free health care for their workers and their dependents. The companies enter into contracts with selected private hospital groups as health care providers, or provide limited cash reimbursements for medical expenses purchased by employees in the private health sector. The financial expenditure on health by companies is not usually made explicit in company financial statements, but the contribution to health care by this private sector financing of health is quite substantial, given the number of companies that offer this service and the large number of workers and relatives covered.

Public and institutional spending on health probably constitutes <30% of the total health expenditure in Nigeria. The majority of expenditure is by private individuals who purchase care as needed in private for-profit clinics and hospitals. These clinics and hospitals are commonly regarded as providing prompter, more courteous, and more efficient services.

Acutely ill patients receive substantial financial support from the immediate and extended families, which mitigates considerably the overall costs of health care to the patient and makes it possible for such patients to have access to health care that may otherwise be out of reach from pecuniary constraints. However, this family support tends to wane over time in patients with illnesses requiring chronic therapy, such as epilepsy.

ORGANIZATION OF HEALTH CARE SERVICES

Numeric Strength and Distribution of Health Care Personnel

Doctors

Nigeria attained the recommended doctor-to-population ratio of 1:8,000 in 1982. In 1993, the ratio was 1:4,379, with wide variations between different states.[12] The 1991 doctor-to-population ratio varied from 1:1,614 in urban and affluent Lagos state to 1:114,069 in Katsina state and to 1:235,827 in Jigawa state with a low level of urbanization and weak economic infrastructures. In general, doctors tend to cluster in urban areas, avoiding rural and economically depressed areas, as is the case elsewhere in the world.

There were about 110 specialists in the clinical neurosciences practicing in Nigeria in 2004. These include 75 psychiatrists, 10 neurosurgeons, and about 25 neurologists.

Nurses

Registered nurses and midwives constitute the largest trained workforce in the health care system, with a nurse-to-population ratio of 1:655. They are also much more evenly spread between and within the states than doctors.

Community Health Workers

Community health officers are drawn from the cadres of public health nurses, community health supervisors, nursing sisters, or rural health superintendents and undergo a special 1-year training program in community health. They are the most senior community health workers.

Community health supervisors are drawn from the cadres of community health assistants, staff nurses, or rural health inspectors and undergo a special 1-year training program in community health.

Community health extension workers are responsible for the direct supervision of volunteer village health workers and spend 80% of their working time in the community. In 1993, the community health worker-to-population ratio was 1:2,166.

PRIMARY HEALTH CARE

Traditional Medicine

There are some 200,000 traditional healers in Nigeria.[7] These include specialists such as herbalists, bone setters, traditional birth attendants, and those occupied with simple surgery, mental diseases, and therapeutic occultism.[16] Herbal medicine is the most widely practiced specialty of traditional medicine among Africans. There are also general practitioners who are competent in more than one form of therapy but are not specialized in any.

Herbal Therapy

The traditional mode of treatment of seizures commonly involves consultations with traditional deities in the supernatural world by the rendition of incantations or metaphors, combined with the administration of herbal remedies. The herbal remedies are commonly mixtures of plants with anticonvulsant, antipyretic, or antibacterial activity.

One traditional herbal remedy for generalized convulsions in Western Nigeria is the fruits of *Tetrapleura Tetraptera* Taub and the leaves of *Nicotiana Tabacum* Linn. These plants contain *Scopoletin* and its methyl derivative, *Scoparone*, which have been shown to protect against leptazol-induced convulsions.[1] However, the plants are sometimes extracted into a concoction containing cow's urine or local gin before administration. This concoction has a prolonged hypoglycemic effect, and is known to cause permanent cerebral damage in children.[15]

The health-seeking behavior of patients with epilepsy suggests a strong preference for traditional herbal medicine over conventional medicine, especially in the rural areas. For instance, all of 101 freshly screened patients with epilepsy in a community-based survey in Igbo-Ora, Western Nigeria, had been treated with herbal remedies, while only four (3.9%) were receiving conventional antiepileptic drug therapy.[13] This is particularly remarkable because the village being surveyed had good primary health care facilities, which had been functioning several years prior to the survey.

Spiritual Therapy

Epilepsy is often regarded as a manifestation of visitation of the devil, the effect of witchcraft, or the revenge of an aggrieved ancestral spirit.[14] The management of epilepsy is therefore commonly assumed to be in the domain of spiritual healers who hold out the attractive promise of a complete cure of epilepsy by magico-spiritual therapies. These elaborate therapies include ritual dances, incantations, propitiatory rites, and exorcism. They may take up considerable time, effort, and money, but are of considerable psychotherapeutic value to the patients in view of the deep-rooted beliefs about the supernatural etiology of epilepsy.

An emerging group of spiritual healers are the Islamic and Christian faith healers, who combine the basic concepts of their religions with superstitious customs and practices. They promise an instant and complete cure for epilepsy by exorcism and provide for the psychological needs of their adherents.

Traditional herbal medicine appears to be more popular for epilepsy care than spiritual therapy. Of 265 epileptic patients who have used alternative forms of therapy prior to seeking hospital treatment in one study,[3] 47% had used traditional medicine, 20.4% had used spiritual healing, while the rest had combined both treatments. However, after initiation of drug therapy in hospitals, more than two thirds of patients who had earlier used spiritual therapy tended to continue such therapy, compared with 14.6% of patients who had used traditional herbal medicine. This implies a stronger perception of continuing psychological benefit from spiritual therapy.

Eighty-six percent of patients who chose alternative medicine as their first level of care were influenced to do so by relatives, friends, and neighbors.[3] Most patients with epilepsy reporting for the first time in a conventional hospital facility would have spent between 1 and 5 years in traditional or spiritual therapy before reporting to the hospital. Thus, the intervention of these alternative practitioners often delays the arrival of patients at centers where more adequate therapy may be available.

Government Primary Care Services

The primary health care services of the national health system are provided by the local governments, their combined primary health care clinics, and health center facilities constituting 50% of all health establishments in Nigeria.[12] These facilities are well spread out in rural areas and indeed are often the only access to conventional health care for people domiciled in those areas. Government primary health care is provided at two levels:

1. The Village Health Service is provided by volunteer village health workers under the control and supervision of village health committees.
2. The District Health Center serves as a referral point for the Village Health Service. Services are provided at this level by community health officers, supervisors, and community health extension workers.

The national mental health policy calls for the integration of mental health into the national primary health care program. "Mental health" was used in this context to include the care of major psychosis, epilepsy, mental retardation, and dementia.

Therefore, mental health has been incorporated as the ninth component of primary health care. Standing orders on mental health for community workers have been developed. The orders for the junior community health extension workers at the village level[6] requires that cases of epilepsy be referred to the health center, but kept on the risk register and followed up. Accordingly, there are no antiepileptic drugs on the official drugs list for the village dispensary. The official standing orders for community health officers, supervisors, and assistants working at the district health center,[5] however, only requires the workers to treat acute seizures with paraldehyde or diazepam and to refer suspected cases of epilepsy to the general hospital.

The government primary health care workers are thus not officially required or trained to make a diagnosis of epilepsy or administer drug therapy to patients with epilepsy. Accordingly, most health centers do not have patients with epilepsy on their registers.

General Medical Practitioners

Individuals and private groups own 30.5% of all health establishments in Nigeria. These profit-orientated private health facilities are most often manned by single medical doctors in a solo practice. Some of these doctors are specialists by training, but in practice are general practitioners seeing all cases.

Private hospitals and clinics are most concentrated in the urban areas where they are largely responsible for the availability of health facilities to 75% of the urban Nigerian population within 4 km of their residences.[12] Only 35% of rural dwellers have similar access.

As there are no fee-for-service schemes or other incentives to encourage the participation of private practitioners in government primary care services, they are largely autonomous of the government. Many private hospitals have retainerships with companies and corporations for the primary care of their staff and dependents.

However, most workers will not disclose their history of epilepsy to their employers because of fears about job discrimination[4] and will therefore tend to avoid utilizing health services provided by their employers.

Most cases of epilepsy in urban areas are probably diagnosed and treated by general practitioners in private hospitals and in the general outpatient departments (GOPD) of tertiary hospitals, particularly partial seizures and absences, which are often poorly recognized by nonmedical health care workers.

SECONDARY HEALTH CARE

State governments are responsible for secondary health care. The state general hospitals where secondary care is provided make up 11.6% of all the health establishments in Nigeria. The hospitals serve as a referral center for the district health centers. There is a plan for each local government area to have a general hospital. There are currently 451 general hospitals for the 589 local governments in Nigeria.

The general hospitals have outpatient departments run by general practitioners. The hospitals are also expected to have a full complement of curative care, with specialists in medicine, pediatrics, surgery, and obstetrics. While this complement is often attained in urban general hospitals, it is an exception in general hospitals located in the rural areas. Most rural general hospitals have a single general practitioner to provide services. These may sometimes be young medical doctors on national youth service.

In those where specialist physicians and pediatricians are available, the general hospitals serve as the first level of access to specialist care for patients with epilepsy. The patients are usually referred from private clinics in the catchment area and from the hospitals' own general outpatients department. There are no neurologists at the general hospital level.

There is a full range of routine antiepileptic drugs in the essential drugs list at the secondary care level. Of these, phenobarbitone and phenytoin are readily affordable, but carbamazepine and sodium valproate are more expensive. There are no facilities for therapeutic drug monitoring of serum levels of antiepileptic drugs. There are also no facilities for electroencephalography (EEG) in these hospitals; patients requiring EEG are referred to the teaching hospitals with neurologic services.

There is an increasing number of well-equipped private hospitals in the urban centers that provide a full complement of secondary health care services.

TERTIARY HEALTH CARE

There are 12 neuropsychiatric hospitals and 25 teaching hospitals in Nigeria. The neuropsychiatric hospitals are run by psychiatrists, while epilepsy care in the teaching hospitals is provided by neurologists, psychiatrists, pediatricians, and internists. Access to epilepsy care in the tertiary centers is by referral from general practitioners in private hospitals and the outpatients departments of the tertiary hospitals.

All the teaching hospitals have neurologic units with facilities for EEG and computed tomography scan. One of these, the University College Hospital, Ibadan, was designated as a center for excellence in neurosciences by the federal government in 1986. Six teaching hospitals have facilities for magnetic resonance imaging. Most routine antiepileptic drugs are available but the newer antiepileptic medications are prohibitively expensive. There are no special centers for epilepsy care in Nigeria.

SUMMARY AND CONCLUSIONS

Young adults living in rural areas constitute the majority of Nigerians with epilepsy. There is evidence that the majority of them are receiving traditional therapy rather than conventional antiepileptic drug therapy, even in areas where there are well-established and otherwise efficient primary health care facilities. This preference for traditional medicine has been documented to cause delays of up to 5 years before many patients with epilepsy reach centers where they can be better treated.

A review of the standing orders for epilepsy care at the primary health care level in Nigeria showed that the community health workers are not motivated or trained to treat patients with epilepsy. Nigerians have been shown to demonstrate a pragmatic, efficacy-testing health-seeking behavior for any particular complaint[9,11]; decisions on choice of care depend on, among other things, whether the health care facility in question has a reputation for alleviating such complaints. In order to demonstrate the efficacy of conventional antiepileptic drug therapy in the rural areas, there is a need to fully integrate the management of epilepsy into the national primary health care programs along the lines suggested by the World Health Organization in 1990.[17]

The development of efficient tertiary epilepsy care in Nigeria is hampered by the small numbers of specialists in the clinical neurosciences and by poor funding.

References

1. Adesina SK, Ojewole JAO, Marquis VO. Isolation and identification of an anticonvulsant agent from the fruit of *Tetrapleura Tetraptera Taub Nig J Pharm*. 1980;11:260–262.
2. Akerele O. WHO's traditional medicine programme: progress and perspectives. *WHO Chron*. 1984;38(2):76–81.
3. Danesi MA, Adetunji JB. Use of alternative medicine by patients with epilepsy: a survey of 265 epileptic patients in a developing country. *Epilepsia*. 1994;35(2):344–351.
4. Danesi MA. Patient perspectives on epilepsy in Nigeria. *Epilepsia*. 1984;25(2):184–190.
5. Federal Ministry of Health, Lagos. National Basic health services scheme. Community Health Officers, Supervisors and Assistants' Standing Orders. Lagos: Federal Ministry of Health; 1981.
6. Federal Ministry of Health, Lagos. Primary Health Care Curriculum for Junior Community Health Extension Workers. Lagos: Federal Ministry of Health; 1992.
7. Federal Ministry of Health, Lagos. Report of the National Investigative Committee on Traditional and Alternative Medicine (NICTAM). Lagos: Federal Ministry of Health; 1978.
8. Federal Ministry of Health, Lagos. The National Health Policy and Strategy to Achieve Health for All Nigerians. Lagos: Federal Ministry of Health; 1988.
9. Igun UA. Stages in health-seeking: a descriptive model. *Soc Sci Med*. 1979;1:13.
10. Lotteries (Government) Law of 1955, Chapter 72 of the Laws of Western Nigeria; 1959.
11. Maclean U. *Magical Medicine: A Nigerian Case Study*. London: Allen Lane the Penguin Press; 1971.
12. Nigerian Medical Association. *The National Medical Directory*. 1993.
13. Osuntokun BO, Adeuja AOG, Nottidge VA, et al. Prevalence of the epilepsies in Nigerian Africans: a community-based study. *Epilepsia*. 1987;28(3):272–279.
14. Osuntokun BO. Epilepsy in Africa. *Trop Geog Med*. 1978;30:23–32.
15. Osuntokun BO, Odeku EL. Epilepsy in Ibadan, Nigeria. A study of 522 cases. *Afr J Med Sci*. 1970;1:185–200.
16. Tella A. Traditional Medicine in Quest of Health for All by the Year 2000 AD. University of Maiduguri, Inaugural Lecture Series 51; 1992.
17. WHO/MNH/MND/90,3. *Initiative of Support to Peoples with Epilepsy*. Geneva: World Health Organization; 1990.

CHAPTER 296 ■ SAUDI ARABIA

SONIA KHAN AND ABDUL AZIZ AL SEMARI

INTRODUCTION

Although the Kingdom of Saudi Arabia comprises the largest area of the Arabic peninsula southwest of Asia, it continues to provide high standards in health care. Medical technology is continually upgraded. One of the first initiatives of King Abdul Aziz Al Saud, the founder of modern Saudi Arabia, was to improve health care facilities and to provide free medical treatment to all citizens and to pilgrims who travel to Mecca.[10,11]

The report of the World Health Organization (WHO) in 2006[17] shows that the total population of Saudi Arabia is 24,573,000. Life expectancy at birth is 59.8 years for males and 62.9 years for females. Child mortality per 1,000 is 29 for males and 24 for females. Adult mortality per 1,000 is 196 for males and 120 for females.[17] Saudi Arabia's health care achievements now match those of many developed countries. Saudi Arabians are no longer required to travel abroad to get specialized medical treatment. The country has the facilities to train physicians, nurses, and other medical personnel to staff the infrastructures of the Saudi health care system, which extends today to most remote communities in the country (Table 1). The government of Saudi Arabia continues to provide massive support to existing health projects in order to ensure that health services are accessible to all people at all levels.[9,12]

The Saudi health system has developed strategies to achieve the following objectives[9,12]:

1. Identification and treatments of patients
2. Delivery of preventive medicine
3. Improvement of diagnostic facilities
4. Improvement of treatment modalities
5. Optimum clinical and social follow-up of patients with chronic diseases
6. Availability of high-standard tertiary care centers for expert evaluation of complicated patients
7. Improvement of health education

The Saudi health system faces several challenges[9,12]:

1. Limited epidemiologic studies
2. Large mass of inhabited land
3. Diversity of living environments in urban and rural areas
4. Rapidly proliferating numbers of national and expatriate inhabitants

To overcome these challenges, the Saudi health system developed four phases of planning with shifts, changes in priorities, and overtime organizational arrangements. The proliferation of the health system within a short period of time had brought into focus several health-planning issues such as coordination, health information systems, and the need for establishing national bodies for health planning and accreditation. To achieve the objectives of the Saudi health system, the Kingdom organized the delivery of health care into several levels.[9,12]

PRIMARY CARE

This service is defined as the health care provided by primary care physicians evaluating patients. In Saudi Arabia, the primary care centers are distributed evenly in the country to include variable urban and rural regions. All major health sectors provide primary care centers in the country, but the Ministry of Health (MOH) remains the largest health sector providing primary health care in Saudi Arabia through a number of hospitals and polyclinics established at a standard design to match the numbers and needs of the population served (Table 2).[6,8,12,13]

Primary care physicians can refer patients to a higher level of health service according to their needs.[6,8,12,13]

SECONDARY CARE

This level comprises most of the general hospitals in Saudi Arabia, and the Ministry of Health represents almost 63% of hospital beds in Saudi Arabia, followed by other hospitals (Table 2). Physicians practicing at this level can refer patients to tertiary care hospitals as needed. The Ministry of Defense and Aviation operates a medical evacuation program consisting of assigned equipped executive jets and helicopter aircrafts with flight physicians and nurses to transport patients to tertiary care centers.

TERTIARY CARE AND SPECIALIZED CENTERS

In Saudi Arabia, a number of tertiary care hospitals are available and receive patients with complex medical conditions from different regions of the country. These centers provide advanced facilities for diagnosis and management of various medical and surgical disorders under the supervision of highly trained medical experts. Some of these centers are world famous for referrals, teaching, and research such as the King Faisal Specialist Hospital and Research Center and the Riyadh Military Hospital.

Major health care–providing sectors include government and private hospitals. Governmental sectors include the Ministry of Health, the Ministry of Defense and Aviation, the Ministry of Interior, the National Guard, University Hospitals, the King Faisal Specialist Hospital and Research Center, and the general organization for social insurance hospitals. The private sector hospitals provide a vital contribution to health service and have expanded dramatically over the past decade; there are a number of these hospitals and clinics in Saudi Arabia.[8]

EPILEPSY HEALTH SERVICES IN SAUDI ARABIA

Epilepsy is a major neurologic disorder in Saudi Arabia. The incidence and prevalence of epilepsy in Saudi Arabia are

TABLE 1

LABOR FORCE IN HEALTH SERVICES

Doctors	1989	1993
Ministry of Health	12,617	14,563
Other government agencies	4,298	5,076
Private sector	5,718	8,135
Total	*22,633*	*27,774*
Nursing staff		
Ministry of Health	28,266	33,373
Other government agencies	9,255	12,485
Private sector	8,319	11,232
Total	*45,840*	*57,090*
Health technicians		
Ministry of Health	15,125	17,868
Other government agencies	6,518	6,899
Private sector	3,549	3,895
Total	*25,192*	*28,662*

From the Ministry of Planning, Kingdom of Saudi Arabia.

underestimated. Head trauma due to road traffic accidents remain a major etiology of epilepsy in Saudi Arabia due to the high rate of road traffic accidents. Other etiologies of epilepsy in Saudi Arabia include cerebrovascular diseases, trauma, central nervous system infections, and developmental and genetic disorders. There is a significant reduction in prenatal injury as an etiology of epilepsy due to advanced obstetric and pediatric care.[2–5,7,14–16] Epileptic patients in Saudi Arabia can be treated by primary care physicians, pediatricians, and internists, but more often they are referred to adult and pediatric neurologists in major cities of the country. Facilities for digital electroencephalography (EEG) and neuroimaging with computed tomography (CT) scans or magnetic resonance imaging (MRI) are available in general hospitals distributed throughout the country.

Antiepileptic drugs are widely available in Saudi Arabia in different formulations. Traditional antiepileptic drugs include phenytoin, phenobarbitone, primidone, carbamazepine, sodium valproate, ethosuximide, and clonazepam.[1,3] New antiepileptic drugs such as vigabatrin, lamotrigine, topiramate, oxcarbamazepine, gabapentin, and levetiracetam are available in major hospitals and pharmacies. Carbamazepine remains the most common antiepileptic drug prescribed. Patients with unclassified epilepsy or those with intractable epilepsies are referred to tertiary care epilepsy centers for further evaluation and management. Epilepsy centers have advanced structural and functional neuroimaging techniques and facilities for video-EEG monitoring. Trained epileptologists and neurosurgeons supervising investigations of epileptic patients in those centers are available in Riyadh and Jeddah. The largest and oldest epilepsy center in Saudi Arabia is in the King Faisal Specialist Hospital in Riyadh. The second largest epilepsy center is in the Riyadh Military Hospital. More recently, additional units have been introduced at the King Faisal Specialist Hospital in Jeddah, the National Guard Hospital in Riyadh, and the King Faisal University Hospital in Dammam. Facilities for

TABLE 2

HOSPITALS, HOSPITAL BEDS, AND PRIMARY HEALTH CENTERS

	(1989) (number)	(1993) (number)	Increase (number)	Percent (%)
Hospitals				
Ministry of Health	162	174	12	7.4
Other government agencies	30	32	2	6.7
Private sector	61	75	14	22.9
Total	*253*	*281*	*28*	*11.1*
Hospital beds				
Ministry of Health	25,918	26,974	1,076	4.1
Other government agencies	6,592	7,338	746	11.3
Private sector	6,445	7,477	1,032	16.0
Total	*38,955*	*41,789*	*2,834*	*7.3*
Primary health centers	1,640	1,707	67	4.1

From the Ministry of Health, Kingdom of Saudi Arabia.

video-EEG monitoring are also available in the private sector hospitals such as the Saudi German and Erfan Bagedo hospitals in Jeddah. The numbers of advanced epilepsy units are expected to rise in Saudi Arabia, with increasing numbers of trained national epileptologists and epilepsy surgeons returning to Saudi Arabia after finishing their scholarships. The following section provides an overview of the two largest epilepsy comprehensive programs established in Saudi Arabia.

THE COMPREHENSIVE EPILEPSY PROGRAM OF THE KING FAISAL SPECIALIST HOSPITAL AND RESEARCH CENTER

The comprehensive epilepsy program was established in the year 1998 at the King Faisal Specialist Hospital and Research Center. The major aims of this program are to treat the referred patients medically and surgically in specialized adult and pediatric epilepsy clinics, by adult and pediatric epileptologists, neurophysiologists, and neuropsychologists. The majority of approved antiepileptic medications are available. The existing epilepsy monitoring unit has the capacity to monitor five patients at one time for surgical evaluation and classification. The patients who are admitted for surgical management are discussed during a weekly epilepsy conference. Wada tests, subdural EEG recordings, and electrocorticography are performed routinely. Figures 1 through 5 and Table 3 show data on admissions, surgical procedures, and outcome. Programs for deep brain stimulation and ketogenic diet are being developed to treat refractory cases of epilepsy.

An epilepsy registry has been established, and it is the first of its kind in the Kingdom of Saudi Arabia, thus serving as a resource to improve the understanding of epilepsy and to assess the magnitude and impact of this disorder on the society. The major goals of the epilepsy program are to treat the referred patients and collect, analyze, and disseminate accurate and timely data pertaining to their demographics, medical history of risk factors, type of disease, treatment, and outcome to health care providers and researchers. It is hoped that this will also serve as a model for the establishment of a Kingdom-wide registry for this disease.

The neurophysiology technologists training program was developed in 2002. Its objectives are to train and graduate skilled technicians to perform a quality service in the neurophysiology laboratory, and to provide the society with a role model of a well-trained neurophysiology technologist (Fig. 6).

THE EPILEPSY COMPREHENSIVE PROGRAM AT RIYADH MILITARY HOSPITAL

This epilepsy program was introduced in January 1998 and is the second largest referral program for advanced epilepsy management in the Kingdom of Saudi Arabia. Adult and pediatric epileptic patients are referred to the epilepsy comprehensive program at the Riyadh Military Hospital from all military hospitals as well as from other governmental and private hospitals in all regions of the Kingdom of Saudi Arabia. Through special arrangements, referrals from the Arabic Gulf region and the Middle East can be seen in the Riyadh Military Hospital. The epilepsy comprehensive program receives 15 to 20 new epileptic patients per month in the outpatient clinics,

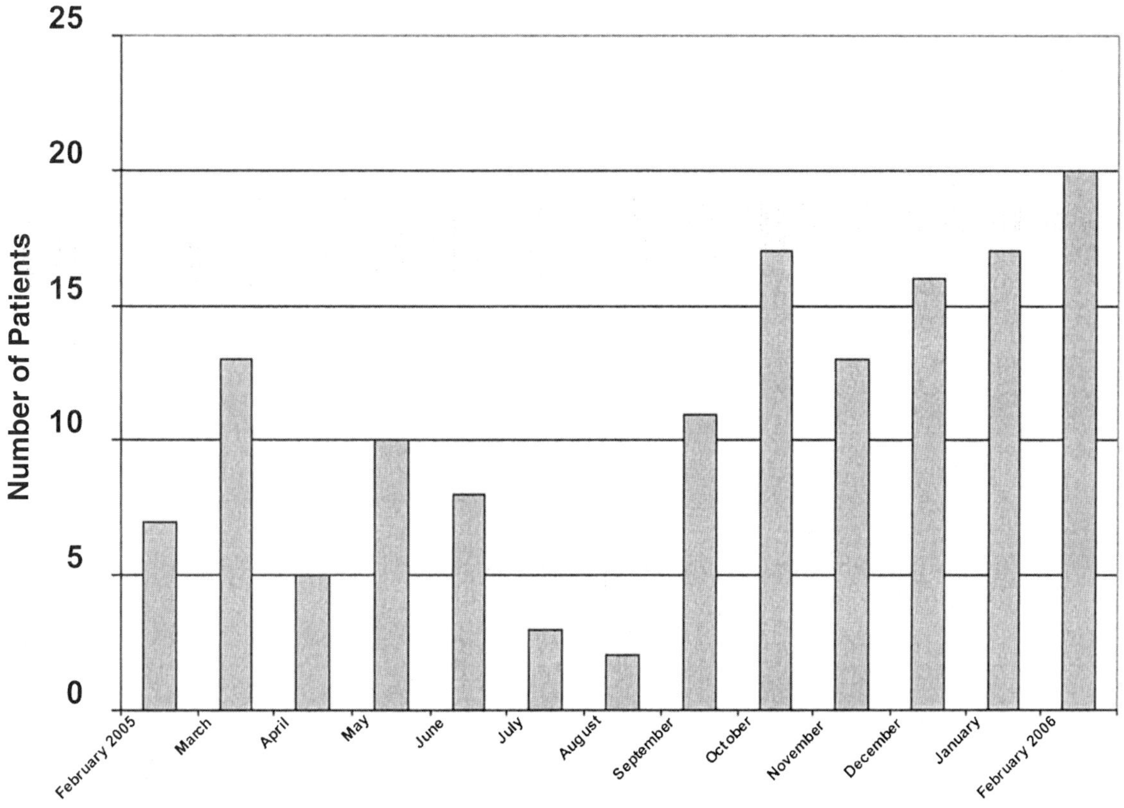

FIGURE 1. Epilepsy monitoring unit admissions (February 2005–present).

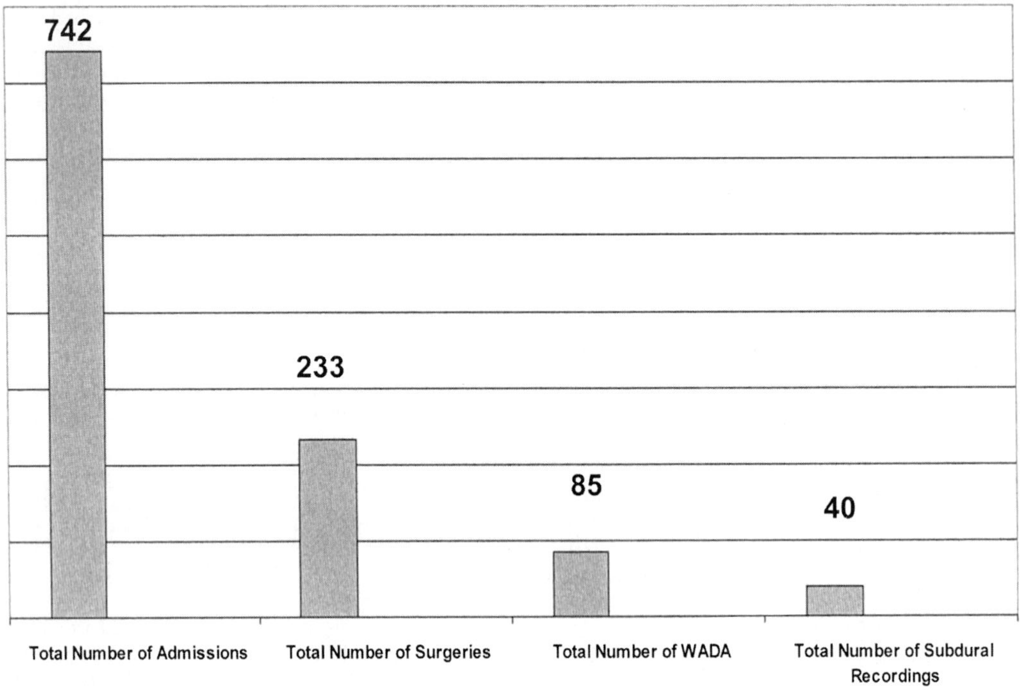

FIGURE 2. Epilepsy monitoring unit statistics.

evaluates ten epileptic patients per month in the epilepsy monitoring unit, and provides long-term video-EEG monitoring for ten patients per month. A total of 1,500 active epilepsy patients are followed by the comprehensive epilepsy program (Fig. 7).

The epilepsy program has two adult epileptologists, two pediatric neurologists, two neurophysiologists, two neuropsychologists, one epilepsy surgeon, and two neuroradiologists, in addition to a number of trained neurophysiology technologists and full-time nurses.

Services of the Epilepsy Comprehensive Program at Riyadh Military Hospital

Diagnosis of Epilepsy

Military and nonmilitary personnel are referred for evaluation of episodes of loss of consciousness. A comprehensive workup of high-resolution MRI scans of the brain,

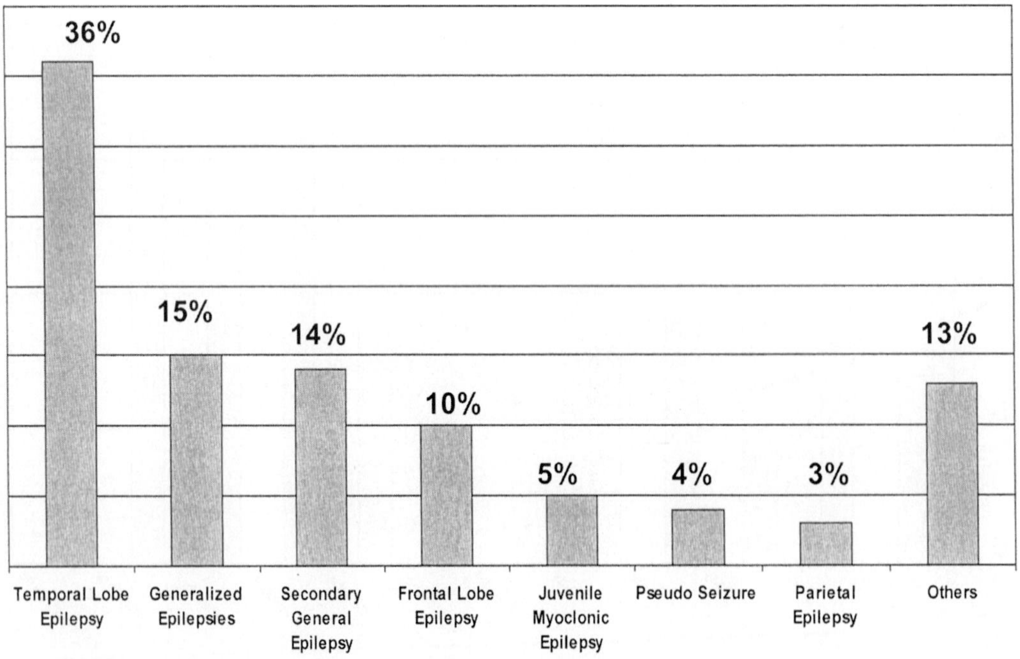

FIGURE 3. Diagnosis based on distribution of epilepsy cases.

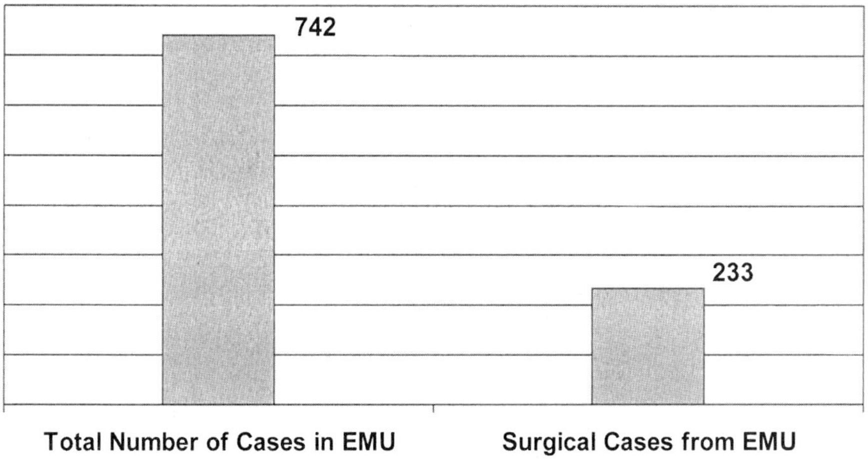

FIGURE 4. Epilepsy monitoring unit (EMU) admissions and surgical cases.

21-electrode digital EEGs, and long-term video-EEG monitoring is performed. Cardiac workup including echocardiography, 24- and 72-hour electrocardiography (ECG) Holter monitoring, advanced electrophysiologic tests of the heart, and other relevant tests are also included in the workup.

A wide variety of epileptic syndromes and nonepileptic conditions such as pseudoseizures, neurocardiac syncope, and other diagnoses are entertained in the epilepsy unit (Table 4).

Medical Management of Epilepsy

Newly diagnosed epileptic patients and epileptic patients not responding to standard antiepileptic drugs are referred to the epilepsy comprehensive program for medical management or adjustment of antiepileptic drugs. In addition to the standard antiepileptic drugs such as phenytoin, carbamazepine, valproate, ethosuximide, phenobarbitone, and primidone, new antiepileptic drugs are available. These include lamotrigine, topiramate, gabapentin, and levetiracetam.

Surgical Management of Epilepsy

A presurgical workup is performed on patients with intractable epilepsies. This include a detailed history and physical examination of the patients; blood investigations including antiepileptic drug levels; 21-channel digital interictal awake, asleep, and sleep-deprived EEG; full neuropsychological and psychological evaluation; and long-term video-EEG monitoring for 5 to 7 days using scalp EEG electrodes with zygomatic (Zg1, Zg2) or sphenoidal electrodes (Sph1, Sph2). The patient is monitored to capture three to five events and to perform ictal single photon emission tomography (SPECT) scans. Additional presurgical tests are performed as needed such as interictal SPECT scans, interictal positron emission tomography-^{18}F-fluorodeoxyglucose (PET-FDG) scans, and functional MRI for language and memory lateralization and motor function mapping. Nonselective intracarotid amobarbital test function (Wada test) in epilepsy surgery patients remains the standard tool to lateralize memory and language at the epilepsy comprehensive program. Recently, propofol replaced amobarbital in the Wada test due to the unavailability of the amobarbital.

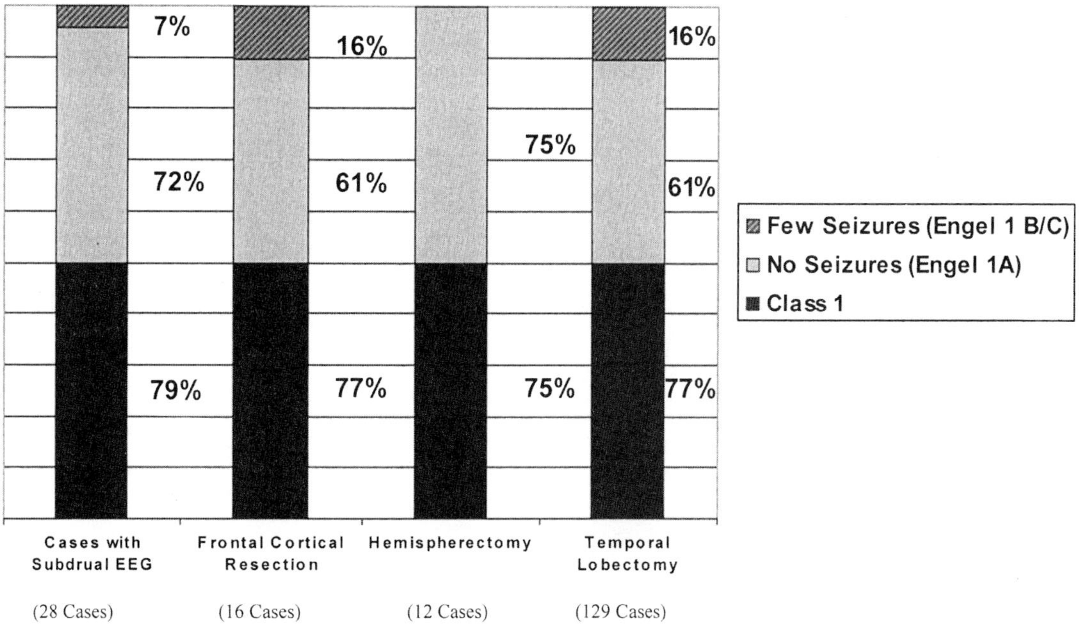

FIGURE 5. First-year outcome by surgical procedure. EEG, electroencephalogram.

TABLE 3

SURGICAL OUTCOME BY SURGICAL PROCEDURE

Surgical procedure	Total Surgical cases	Followed case	Seizure free	
			Cases	Percent
Parietal cortical resection	4	2	1	50%
Parieto-occipital lesionectomy	2	2	2	100%
Multiple subpial transection	1	1	1	100%

A reasonable number of epilepsy surgeries are performed yearly (Table 5). Decisions and plans for epilepsy surgery for each patient take place after finishing the full presurgical workup and discussing the presurgical data at the weekly epilepsy surgery meeting attended by the epilepsy team. Further plans for epilepsy surgery are made in the meeting. The most common intractable epilepsy encountered is temporal lobe epilepsy with hippocampal sclerosis as the most common surgical substrate. The most common epilepsy surgical procedure is anterior temporal lobectomy. Other epilepsy surgical procedures, such as lesionectomies for foreign tissue lesions such as vascular malformations, tumors, and focal cortical dysplasias, are performed. Functional hemispherectomy for diffuse unilateral hemispheric lesions is performed. Facilities for intraoperative monitoring methods such as electrocorticography, cortical stimulations, and somatosensory-evoked potentials for mapping of the motor cortex and other eloquent regions are available. Surgical outcome of lesional epilepsy surgery is comparable to the international literature (Table 6). No epilepsy surgery for nonlesional epilepsy has been performed yet due to technical limitations. Other palliative surgical procedures for intractable epilepsy can be performed at the epilepsy comprehensive program. The first implantation of vagal nerve stimulation in the Kingdom of Saudi Arabia was performed at the epilepsy comprehensive program in 1998 for three patients with intractable epilepsy. Vagal nerve stimulation as a treatment modality for intractable epilepsy at the epilepsy comprehensive program remains restricted for very selective patients.

Epilepsy Registry Data

Locally registered data of 1,000 active epileptic patients are available, which include demographic, clinical, EEG, and MRI data as well as seizure and epilepsy classification according to the International League Against Epilepsy (ILAE) classification.

Women and the Epilepsy Program

Women with epilepsy at different ages are referred to the specialized epilepsy clinics for counseling and follow-up.

Newly diagnosed epileptic young and elderly women are referred to the epilepsy program for the choice of appropriate antiepileptic drugs according to their diagnoses, ages, and comorbid conditions such as menstrual irregularities, osteoporosis, etc. Epileptic women of childbearing age are referred to the specialized epilepsy clinic for pre-pregnancy counseling, choice of contraceptive pills, and comprehensive follow-up during the pregnancy delivery and postpartum periods.

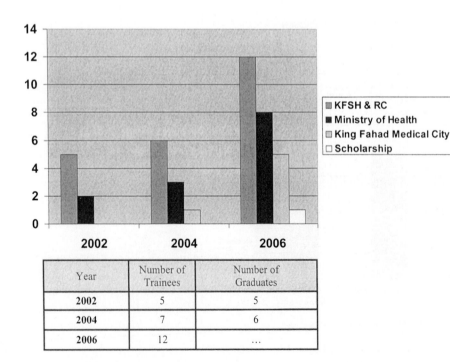

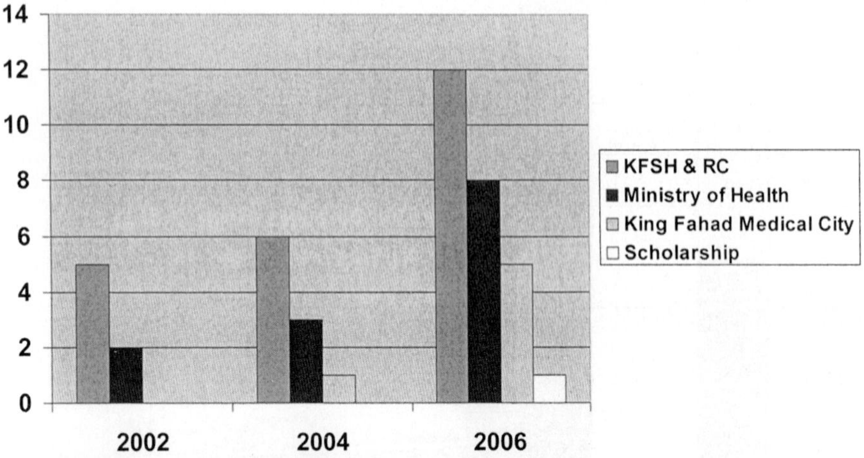

Year	Number of Trainees	Number of Graduates
2002	5	5
2004	7	6
2006	12	...

FIGURE 6. Neurophysiology technology training program. KFSH & RC, King Faisal Specialist Hospital and Research Center.

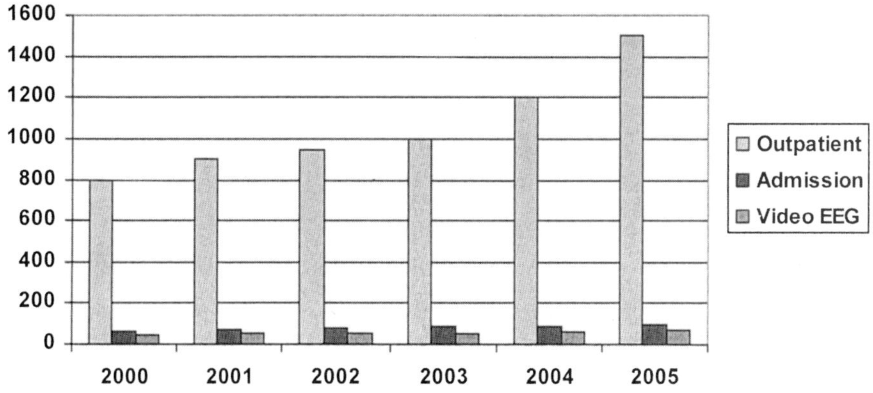

FIGURE 7. Annual statistics of the epilepsy program (2000–2005). EEG, electroencephalogram.

Epilepsy Training

The epilepsy comprehensive program provides regular biannual courses on basic and practical epileptology for nurses, technologists, and other health providers interested in epilepsy. These courses are limited to the hospital staff. In addition, neurology and neurosurgery board residents rotate for a 2-month period during their training in the epilepsy unit to learn basic epileptology related to their specialties.

Epilepsy Education and Training

Due to the small number of trained epileptologists and epilepsy surgeons in Saudi Arabia, the government of Saudi Arabia in general and the Saudi neuroscience society in particular encourage young neurologists and neurosurgeons to pursue higher training in epileptology and epilepsy surgery, respectively.

Through fully sponsored governmental scholarships, national neurologists and neurosurgeons are sent to the most prestigious European and North American epilepsy centers to pursue their subspecialty training and to gain the highest level of expertise in epilepsy. Internationally recognized epilepsy centers and programs in Europe and North America receive neurology and neurosurgery graduates on a regular basis. In addition, the government of Saudi Arabia provides local and international scientific scholarships for paramedical personnel to obtain higher training in their fields.

Major epilepsy centers in Saudi Arabia provide limited medical training in epileptology for the neurology and neurosurgery residents. In addition, high-standard training programs are available locally for nurses and neurophysiology technicians. Regular scientific activities include the full-day annual Saudi epilepsy meeting under the annual Saudi neuroscience symposium and regular half-day workshops, lectures, and seminars for neurologists, neurosurgeons, physicians, board residents, and paramedical staff. Every two years a 2-day Saudi epilepsy course takes place in collaboration with the regional commission of the ILAE and the International Bureau of Epilepsy.

Collaborative clinical and research projects take place regularly between the Saudi epilepsy centers and international recognized epilepsy centers with regular visits from international epileptologists and epilepsy surgeons to the epilepsy centers in Saudi Arabia. The Saudi chapter of the ILAE and the Saudi chapter of the International Bureau of Epilepsy represent the scientific body that supervises all academic epilepsy activities in Saudi Arabia. Regular scientific epilepsy papers and abstracts are presented in local, regional, and international neuroscience and epileptology conferences.

Patient Education in Epilepsy

Lay knowledge of epilepsy is unsatisfactory in Saudi Arabia. Despite the improved standards of general education in the Kingdom, significant misunderstanding and social stigma of epilepsy remain in Saudi Arabia.

Many patients believe in traditional medicine in the form of herbal or spiritual therapies. Other patients avoid medical management to avoid psychosocial stigma. Despite advanced medical and surgical standards in the management of epilepsy in Saudi Arabia, patient education has remained significantly retarded for a long time. The King Faisal Specialist Hospital and Research Center in Riyadh took the first step toward a comprehensive educational program for patients and the

TABLE 4

DIAGNOSES AT THE COMPREHENSIVE EPILEPSY PROGRAM (2002–2005)

Diagnoses	Mean age (yr)	Gender		Total
		Male	Female	
Generalized epilepsy	25	17	30	47 pt (20%)
Partial epilepsy	38	70	60	130 pt (60%)
Pseudo seizure	35	5	30	35 pt (15%)
Others	30	20	3	23 pt (5%)

TABLE 5

EPILEPSY SURGERY AT THE RIYADH MILITARY HOSPITAL (NOVEMBER 1998–JUNE 2006)

Year	Temporal surgery	Extratemporal surgery	Total
1998	1	—	1
1999	10	4	14
2000	12	2	14
2001	8	2	10
2002	8	4	12
2003	13	4	17
2004	10	4	14
2005	8	4	12
2006	3	3	6
Total	73	27	100

public by forming the Epilepsy Support and Information Center (ESIC).

EPILEPSY SUPPORT AND INFORMATION CENTER

The ESIC is a community volunteer group affiliated with the comprehensive epilepsy program at the King Faisal Specialist Hospital and Research Center in Riyadh composed of both community volunteers and medical professionals. The center is dedicated to dispersing information about and understanding of epilepsy in Saudi Arabia and the International Arab Community. ESIC's mission is to promote increased awareness, understanding, and acceptance of epilepsy. Other epilepsy centers and ministries of health are organizing a collaborative patient support group with ESIC to improve epilepsy patient education in Saudi Arabia. ESIC endeavors to promote epilepsy health education and support for individuals with epilepsy and their families through the publication and nationwide distribution of printed materials on epilepsy.

List of Publications

The following is a list of ESIC's publications:

- Questions and Answers about Epilepsy
- Febrile Seizures
- Epilepsy and Children
- Advice on Raising a Child with Epilepsy
- Epilepsy Medications and Epilepsy
- Myth and Misunderstanding about Epilepsy
- Epilepsy and Education: The Role of the Teacher (Booklet)
- Epilepsy and Pregnancy (Booklet)
- Questions and Answers about Epilepsy (Booklet)
- Adil and Epilepsy (Children's Story Booklet)
- Epilepsy Information Fact Sheet
- 12 Antiepileptic Drug Wallet Cards

Patient Information Lectures and Conferences

ESIC offers six public information lectures and three public epilepsy conferences.

Website

The ESIC has established the first comprehensive epilepsy Internet Website (www.epilepsyinarabic.com) in the Arabic language. Visitors to the site contact us on a regular basis through e-mail and ESIC receives regular online requests for Arabic language brochures from many countries, including Saudi Arabia and the other Gulf States, Libya, Jordan, Syria, Egypt, Morocco, Spain, Britain, and the United States, to name a few.

Family Festival for Epilepsy Awareness

To date, the ESIC has organized five annual Family Festivals for Epilepsy Awareness. The sixth annual Family Festival is planned for November 2007.

Teacher Awareness Program

To date, the ESIC has organized ten half-day Teacher Awareness Conferences at schools, universities, and government rehabilitation centers in Saudi Arabia.

Epilepsy News/Media Campaign

In May 2006, the ESIC distributed a four-page Epilepsy Public Information Fact Sheet with basic facts and information about epilepsy. The fact sheet was distributed Kingdom-wide as an insert in the Al-Riyadh Daily National Newspaper. Total distribution was 140,000 newspapers nationwide.

TABLE 6

SURGICAL OUTCOME AT THE RIYADH MILITARY HOSPITAL

	Temporal		Extratemporal	
Surgical outcome	n	%	n	%
Engel I	55	75%	19	70%
Engel II	15	21%	5	19%
Engel III	2	3%	2	7%
Engel IV	1	1%	1	4%

Epilepsy Workshops for Health Care Professionals

To promote enhanced medical care and strengthen the medical emergency response to epilepsy, the ESIC organizes regular accredited full-day epilepsy workshops for primary health care professionals. To date, the ESIC has organized three epilepsy workshops. The last workshop was held March 12, 2005 and was organized in cooperation with the Saudi Arabian Ministry of Health.

Research

To highlight the societal impact of epilepsy and the needs of individuals with epilepsy to national health care planners, the ESIC is cooperating with the King Faisal Specialist Hospital and Research Center comprehensive epilepsy program to provide support and assistance in the establishment of a National Epilepsy Registry. The ESIC is also involved in an ongoing research survey aimed at determining the predominant societal attitudes and general level of knowledge about epilepsy in Saudi Arabia.

Awards

In 2001, the ESIC received the internationally recognized Initiative Prize from the Arab Gulf Funding for United Nations Program. The prize, received in the UN offices in Geneva Switzerland, consisted of a trophy and a $40,000 grant.

International Involvement

The ESIC has been a full chapter member of the International Bureau for Epilepsy since 2001, and has participated in the Eastern Mediterranean Epilepsy Task Force and in the drafting of the Eastern Mediterranean Declaration on Epilepsy in Cairo, Egypt.

SUMMARY AND CONCLUSIONS

Epilepsy is a common neurologic disorder in Saudi Arabia. Delivery of health services in general and of epilepsy in particular in Saudi Arabia is done at the primary care, then secondary care, then tertiary care levels. Despite the rapid proliferation of the population of Saudi Arabia, the advanced epilepsy centers with epilepsy surgery services remain confined to few centers and hospitals with limited capacities. Therefore, the official recognition of the increasing demands on more national epilepsy monitoring units and epilepsy surgical programs should be included in the main health-planning strategies toincrease epilepsy monitoring beds and to advance neurophysiologic and neuroimaging techniques in Saudi Arabia to the highest international standards. Epidemiologic studies are limited on epilepsy in Saudi Arabia. Therefore, national multicenter epidemiologic surveys should be launched to verify the magnitude and demands of epilepsy as a health problem in Saudi Arabia. National multicenter registries for epilepsy patients, pregnancy, and antiepileptic drugs and epilepsy surgery data should be initiated to achieve a better understanding of epilepsy in Saudi Arabia. Patient education of epilepsy is limited; therefore, all efforts should unify to overcome local misconceptions about epilepsy and improve general understanding of epilepsy. General national and local guidelines are needed for various epilepsy-related issues such as driving and pregnancy. Education about epilepsy in the elderly should be generated and approved by higher authorities to reduce morbidity and mortality of epilepsy. Education on epilepsy for health professionals should be optimized to organize a structured algorithm in the management of epilepsy in Saudi Arabia.

References

1. Abduljabbar M, Al Khamis K, Ogunniyi A, et al. Phenytoin dosage adjustment in Saudi epileptics, utilization of study state pharmacokinetics parameters. *Eur J Neurol.* 1999;6(3):331–334.
2. Al Bunayan M, Abo Talib Z. Outcome of pregnancies in epileptic women, a study in Saudi Arabia. *Seizure.* 1999;8(1):26–29.
3. Al Bunyan MA. Random total antiepileptic drug levels and seizure control during pregnancy. *Saudi Med J.* 2001;22(4):355–339.
4. Al Eissa YA. Febrile seizures: rate and risk factors of recurrence. *J Child Neurol.* 1995;10(4):315–319.
5. Al Rajeh S, Awada A, Badimosi O, et al. The prevalence of epilepsy and other seizure disorders in an Arab population, a community-based study. *Seizure.* 2001;10(6):410–414.
6. Al Shammari SA, Khoja TA, Rajeh SA. Role of primary care physician in the care of epileptic patients. *Public Health.* 1996;110(1):47–48.
7. Al Sulaiman AA. Epilepsy in Saudi children with cerebral palsy. *Saudi Med J.* 2001;22(1):19–21.
8. Alnaif MS. Physicians perception of health insurance in Saudi Arabia. *Saudi Med J.* 2006;27(5):693–699.
9. Berti G. Emerging issues in health planning in Saudi Arabia, the effects of organization and development on the healthcare system. *Soc Sci Med.* 1991;33(7):815–824.
10. Brwon G. An up close and personal look at Saudi Arabia (Jeddah and Riyadh) history, culture and healthcare. *ABNF J.* 2005;16(4):83–86.
11. Gumnit RJ. Overview of delivery of healthcare and socioeconomic issues. In: Engel J Jr, Pedley TA, eds. *Epilepsy: A Comprehensive Textbook.* Philadelphia: Lippincott-Raven Publishers; 1997:2807–2809.
12. Littlewood J, Yousuf S. Primary healthcare in Saudi Arabia, applying global aspects of health for all locally. *J Adv Nurs.* 2000;32(3):675–681.
13. Mahfouz AA, Al Sharif AI, El Gama MN, et al. Primary healthcare services utilization and satisfaction among the elderly in Asian region Saudi Arabia. *East Mediterranean Health J.* 2004;10(3):365–371.
14. Obeid T, Awada A, Amene P, et al. The controversy of birth order as a risk factor for epilepsy, a study from Saudi Arabia. *Acta Neurol Scand.* 2002;105(3):174–178.
15. Obeid T, Daif AK, Waheed G, et al. Photosensitive epilepsies and photoconvulsive responses in Arabs. *Epilepsia.* 1991;32(1):77–81.
16. Salih MA, Abdul Gader AG, Al Jarallah AA, et al. Outcome of stroke in Saudi children. *Saudi Med J.* 2006;Suppl:591–596.
17. World Health Organization. Working Together for Health. World Health Organization; Geneva, Switzerland. 2006.

CHAPTER 297 ■ SENEGAL

AMADOU GALLO DIOP AND IBRAHIMA PIERRE NDIAYE

INTRODUCTION

Epilepsy is one the most common neurologic diseases in outpatient and inpatient health management in Senegal, West Africa. It is the same situation in the majority of African and many developing countries, where it constitutes a major public health care problem.[11] From newborns to teenagers, childhood are the most stressed group due to several causes of epilepsy including perinatal problems, febrile convulsions, cerebral malaria, and consanguinity, which is a genetic factor.[1,19,22]

Such as in the majority of African countries, the cultural environment is a limiting factor for early diagnosis and treatment of seizures. Interpreted as a subnatural affliction, epilepsy is mainly managed by traditional healers, reducing the chance for Senegalese people living with seizures to benefit from modern drugs and better opportunities to become seizure free. A heavy burden is generated, leading to school withdrawal, nonemployment, and other social discriminations.

OVERVIEW OF THE COUNTRY

Senegal is a Western African country of 196,722 km^2. It is surrounded by Mauritania (at north), Guinea and Guinea-Bissau (at south), Mali (at east), and the Atlantic Ocean (at west). Gambia Republic is situated inside Senegal. Forty-five percent of the population is younger than 15 years old; 53.5% of the population is female, and 52% of the population is rural. The increasing rate for the general population is 2.6% per year. The population of Senegal is estimated to be near 12 million (Table 1). The general life expectancy is estimated at 54 years for males and 58 years for females. The infantile mortality rate is estimated to be 58 of 1,000 births.

The mean population density is estimated at 54 inhabitants per km^2, but it is very disparate: 3,659 inhabitants per km^2 are living in the capital city Dakar region, versus eight inhabitants per km^2 for the region of Tambacounda in the southeastern region, which represents 30% of the surface of the country. This situation can be explained by the large surface of this region, the low-wealth environment, and its aridity. Sixteen ethnic and language clusters are defined, but the main ethnic group and most spoken language is *Wolof*. It is important to be aware of this diversity because it may be considered in any information and education program, because of specific social and cultural values that are correlated to each. The rate of illiteracy is 43% of 15- to 24-year-old males and 62% of 15- to 24-year-old females. Ninety-two percent of the people in Senegal are Muslim.

Senegal is composed of 11 regions. Regions are divided in departments, themselves divided into districts, then into rural communities. These structures are led, respectively, by governors, prefects, and rural community presidents. Cities are led by a mayor. In their intervention domains are included health in coordination with the ministry of health, education, environment, urbanism, agriculture, youth, sport, and art craft.

Senegal is a low-economy country. The gross national product per inhabitant is estimated to be U.S. $480. The economy is mainly based on exploitation of phosphate, fishing, tourism, and agriculture.

GENERAL DATA ON THE HEALTH SYSTEM

Health Organization and General Data

Senegal guarantees in its constitution that health is a right of every citizen and the duty of the state to provide. The medical and health systems are inherited from French colonization. A recent law is trying to organize traditional medicine, but one can guess how difficult it is to do so because of the secrecy surrounding this mystic and intrafamilial legacy. Despite this legislation, total or partial health insurance or coverage is a reality for about one third of the population represented by public and private workers and their families. The remaining two thirds remain in an informal sector, financing their health fees through their own or indirect supports. The health system is structured like a pyramid constituted from the base to the top by health post (for villages and rural communities), health center (inside cities), regional hospital, and two university hospitals. This represents the following (Table 2):

- 11 medical regions (led by the regional head doctor)
- 56 health districts (with one or more doctors and paramedical staff)
- 59 health centers (with nurses and midwives)
- 813 health posts (with nurses)
- 37 private Catholic health posts located in the suburban area of Dakar

The geographic accessibility to a health structure is theoretically 1.2 km for Dakar's patients, versus 16.2, 12.9, 11.0, and 10.3 km for the regions of Tambacounda, Louga, Saint-Louis, and Kolda, respectively.

In the context of the African continent, Senegal has a very low prevalence rate of HIV/AIDS infection: 0.8%. Heterosexual transmission is the major route. Since the early beginning of the AIDS pandemic, a strong policy of information, prevention, and caring has been developed. Reported AIDS cases increased progressively and remain stable now, estimated to be about 45,000 people. This tendency is attributed to Senegal's initiative of access to free antiretroviral drugs since 1996.

Health Financing

The health annual budget roses to 9% of the global government budget since 2002. But 65% of the budget of the Ministry of Health is dedicated to pay salaries. There is a decreasing participation of the government financing of health and an increase in the population participation. Thirty percent of

TABLE 1

SOCIOECONOMIC, DEMOGRAPHIC, AND HEALTH INDICATOR DATA ABOUT SENEGAL

Population, total	11.9 million
Population growth (annual %)	2.4
Life expectancy at birth, total (yr)	56.1
Fertility rate, total (births per woman)	4.8
Mortality rate, infant (per 1,000 live births)	77.6
Mortality rate, under 5 yr (per 1,000)	136.6
Births attended by skilled health staff (% of total)	57.8
Malnutrition prevalence, weight for age (% of children under 5)	22.7
Immunization, measles (% of children aged 12–23 months)	57.0
Prevalence of HIV, total (% of population aged 15–49)	0.9
Primary completion rate, total (% of relevant age group)	45.2
School enrollment, primary (% gross)	76.0
School enrollment, secondary (% gross)	19.4
School enrollment, tertiary (% gross)	4.9
Ratio of girls to boys in primary and secondary education (%)	89.8
Literacy rate, adult total (% of people aged 15 and above)	39.3

From www.worldbank.org and www.who.int.

credit and expenses are done in the capital region of Dakar. Other sources of finances include development partners and local communities. They contribute in building, training, salary, and daily expenses. But it is difficult to determine their exact contributions. City administrations are also contributing in the health expenses, drugs, and maintenance. Armed forces and police also participate in health expenses of their personnel and families.

Health Personnel

Representing the health personnel are 649 (public and private) doctors and 3,287 paramedical staff (midwives, private nurses, and health agents) (Table 3). The mean general doctor-to-population ratio in Senegal is one doctor for 18,300 inhabitants, one midwife per 6,124 reproductive women and 0- to 4-year-old children, and one nurse for 4,570 inhabitants. The World Health Organization (WHO) recommends one doctor for 5,000 to 10,000 people, one midwife for 300 people, and one nurse for 300 people. There is a wide disparity: 90% of specialized doctors are concentrated in Dakar, the capital. The Dakar region has more than 50% of doctors, pharmacies, surgeons, nurses, and midwives. The national ratio is 11,163 inhabitants per health post. This is not so far from what WHO recommends (10,000 inhabitants).

Excluding two psychiatrists (one at North, one at South), the rest of the neuroscience personnel resides in Dakar: 15 public and two private neurologists, three private and 11 public psychiatrists, and six public neurosurgeons. Postgraduating diplomas in Psychiatry, Neurosurgery, and Neurology have existed in Senegal since 1993, 1998, and 2000, respectively.

Neurologists

Seventeen neurologists were identified in Senegal in 2007, among them eight professors (three with PhDs) and two private. All public-sector neurologists practice in the capital city of Dakar, where the unique service of Neurology of the University Hospital is located. The ratio of one neurologist for 700,000 people, far from the recommended WHO rate of one for 50,000 people, is one the best in the intertropical area of Africa, where the ratio ranges from one neurologist for 1 to 4 million people. This reality demonstrates the strong need to cooperate with psychiatrists, neurosurgeons, general practitioners, pediatricians, and public health staff.

EPILEPSY IN SENEGAL

Epidemiology

The mean national prevalence rate of epilepsy in Senegal was estimated to be 3.1% in 1970,[4,5] then 8.3% in 1986.[19] Different epidemiologic research has stressed the very different disparities from one region to another. In the suburban area near Dakar, Pikine, characterized by promiscuity and problems of hygiene and water supply, the prevalence was estimated at 12% in 1989.[23] A survey conducted in the same area during the demonstration project of the Global Campaign Against Epilepsy revealed a prevalence rate of 14%.[21] It has been remarked that when there is a good concentration of health

TABLE 2

HEALTH INFRASTRUCTURES

Medical regions	Hospitals	Health districts	Health centers	Health posts
Dakar	8	8	11	115
Diourbel	2	4	5	70
Fatick	1	6	6	73
Kaolack	1	4	4	72
Kolda	1	4	3	68
Louga	1	5	5	56
Matam	1	3	3	50
Saint-Louis	2	4	4	81
Tambacounda	1	6	5	58
Thies	2	8	9	91
Ziguinchor	2	4	4	79
Total	22	56	59	813

TABLE 3

HEALTH PERSONNEL DATA IN SENEGAL

Physicians (number)	649
Physicians (density per 1,000 population)	0.06
- Including neurologists	17
- Including psychiatrists	14
- Including neurosurgeons	6
Nurses (number)	3,287
Nurses (density per 1,000 population)	0.32
Dentists (number)	97
Dentists (density per 1,000 population)	0.01
Pharmacists (number)	85
Pharmacists (density per 1,000 population)	0.01
Public and environmental health workers (number)	705
Public and environmental health workers (density per 1,000 population)	0.07
Lab technicians (number)	66
Lab technicians (density per 1,000 population)	0.01
Other health workers (number)	704
Other health workers (density per 1,000 population)	0.07
Health management and support workers (number)	564
Health management and support workers (density per 1,000 population)	0.05

personnel, the rate decreases. This is the case in Saint-Louis (1.9%), the former capital of Senegal, or in Niakhar (3.1%), a village where a hepatitis project is conducted with constant medical visits for the surveillance.[18]

No incidence studies have been conducted, but there is, as described elsewhere, a dramatic presence of epilepsy among children and the elderly.[13] When the results are analyzed regarding age, it is clear that childhood is the most affected group.[2] Epilepsy is the first cause of hospitalization among young patients (16.1% to 32%) in the different hospitals of Dakar.[1,18,22] Among them, 7.46% have been hospitalized for status epilepticus, which is a real problem of public health with a high risk for vital prognosis.[15] Surveys conducted in schools revealed that the mean prevalence rate is 21% in different schools in Dakar and Thies (the second city 75 km from Dakar). The rate is 2.6% in Saint-Louis among 6- to 15-year-old alumni.[2] The question is, Does this reflect a true reality due to the good ratio of health personnel to population? Or is it related to a possible withdrawal of epileptic children from school by their parents and/or teachers because of a frequent cultural allegation of "risk of contamination" to the rest of the classroom?[20]

Concerning the elderly, it has been also demonstrated that the incidence within this group is progressively becoming higher after 50 in Senegal as soon as the life expectancy progressively raises.[14] A prospective follow-up of a group of pregnant epileptic women with a prevalence rate of 1.05% revealed no difference in the occurrence of fetal development versus the nonepileptic group.[16]

The Etiologic Factors

The difficulty to investigate every epilepsy case contributes to enormous bias for the precision of etiologies. Many existing factors can lead to epileptic conditions. It is assumable that leading causes described worldwide and especially in developing countries may be considered in Senegal as well as in other African countries, including pregnancy problems (53% of pregnancies are nonmedically assisted, leading to a possible cause in 10% to 60% of epilepsy due to bad perinatal environment or ischemia from prolonged delivery), febrile convulsions, infections, and febrile diarrhea in children under 5 years old.[11] Bacterial meningitis, cerebral malaria, and other encephalitis were found in 7% to 19% in a hospital study conducted in Senegal. Furthermore, in Senegal, 43% of marriages are celebrated within the (large) family, entertaining the consanguinity and favoring expression of potential genetic epilepsy. A close intrafamilial relation between genitors is reported in 7% to 50% of surveyed people with epilepsy.[3] In the population ever so, vascular factors are reported in 68%, before infections, cerebral tumors, and metabolic factors including diabetes.[6,10]

Diagnosis and investigation of epilepsy in Senegal benefit from a limited number of specialists (the ratio is 1 for 700,000 people, versus 1 for 50,000 people as recommended by the WHO), as described above. In 2007, the available material is composed of six public and five private computed tomography (CT) scans and six public and four private electroencephalograms (EEGs) and two public and two private magnetic resonance imaging (MRI).

Sociocultural Representation

In many developing countries it is estimated that 80% of people with epilepsy are not treated with modern medications. The large majority of Senegalese patients living in rural areas are not consulting modern medical centers. Part of the reason could be geographic and/or economic related to the difficulty of access to health care structures. In a survey conducted in the suburban area of the capital city, Dakar, it has been demonstrated that 35% were taking antiepileptic drugs (AEDs) only, 41% associated them with traditional means, 11% took only traditional means, and 13% were not taking anything. The treatment gap (related to modern AED treatment) was consequently estimated to be 23.3%. But this is just the visible part of the iceberg.[21] The hidden and major part is related to the fact that epilepsy is considered a subnatural affliction and must be managed by traditional healers.[17] In the Senegalese culture, seizures are the manifestation of strong spirits involving the body and shaking it. The various definitions in local language reflect a basic knowledge of epileptic presentations. Some seizures could be considered as a positive but too powerful spirit.[12] In most instances traditional healing is the first treatment sought. In some countries, the traditional belief systems endorse discrimination against people with the condition, leading to their exclusion from mainstream society and restrictions on their accessing basic human and civil rights. However, the role of traditional healing should not be completely discredited as in many instances the person with epilepsy obtains a degree of secondary benefit from this form of intervention in the way of reassurance and emotional support. Efforts should be made to integrate traditional and Western interventions in a way that provides a range of services offering holistic support and care for the person with epilepsy and his or her family.[9] These would include advice, counseling, social support, school-to-work transitioning, job creation and training, rehabilitation, and community integration. The challenge is how to conciliate conflicting convictions that guide the traditional and scientific treatment concepts.[24]

Available Antiepileptic Drugs and Diagnostic Facilities in Senegal

The antiepileptic drugs available in Senegal and the cost of a month's worth of tablets in private pharmacies and in generic public forms are indicated in U.S. dollars (at the rate of December 2006) in Table 4.

TABLE 4

ANTIEPILEPTIC DRUGS AVAILABLE IN SENEGAL

Drug	Strength	Public price[a]	Generic price[a]
Phenobarbitone	10 mg	1	0.4
Phenobarbitone	50 mg	1.02	0.4
Phenobarbitone	100 mg	1.24	0.6
Carbamazepine	200 mg	8.7	NA
Carbamazepine	SR 200 mg	14	NA
Carbamazepine	SR 400 mg	16.5	NA
Ethosuximide	NA	NA	NA
Phenytoin	100 mg	3.18	NA
Valproate	200 mg	9.3	NA
Valproate	500 mg	14.5	NA
Valproate	SR 500 mg	17	NA
Clonazepam	2 mg	9.5	NA
Diazepam	10 mg	7.9	NA
Diazepam	5 mg	6.7	1.24

NA, not available.

Primary health care centers can have all forms of phenobarbitone, phenytoin, and intravenous diazepam. In Dakar's pharmacies and in the capital of the nine other regions, one can find all the drugs cited above. A new generation of AEDs and brand new drugs and intravenous valproate and phenytoin are not available in Senegal.

The Role of the Senegalese League Against Epilepsy

The situation described above led to the creation in 1995 of the Senegalese League Against Epilepsy. Its originality is that this International League Against Epilepsy (ILAE)/International Bureau for Epilepsy (IBE) chapter gathers patients, families, and health and social workers and volunteers, with the purpose to improve the knowledge, awareness, and management of epilepsy.

The Senegalese League Against Epilepsy (SLAE) plays an important role in advising the Ministry of Health on issues regarding epilepsy and in providing education to physicians. The SLAE has created videos, leaflets, surveillance books for patients, training and guideline booklets for health personnel, and posters and T-shirts for public advertising. It organizes scientific meetings and courses in its various regional chapters.

Selected as a site of the Global Campaign Against Epilepsy (GCAE) Demonstration Project on Epilepsy, Senegal had conducted an epidemiologic survey about epilepsy quality care and KAP (Knowledge, Attitude, and Practice) evaluation among the general population and health personnel. These public health operational research projects led to concrete interventions deducted from the results. A weekly epilepsy consultation has been set up since then in the suburban area of the capital city of Dakar. Five regional branches have been installed with training and local care activities. The location of the unique neurology service in Dakar and the research results led to the concept of "Caravan for Epilepsy." It consists of a 3-day intervention: Day 1: Arrival of the neurosciences team, meeting with administrative and health leaders, and media talk show on epilepsy. Day 2: Full-day training course with general practitioners and paramedical staff, while some members of the team meet with schools, women associations, and social workers. Day 3: Full-day consultation of patients coming from villages and small cities surrounding the main regional city and informed about this mission by the day 1 radio talk show. If indicated, some patients can be investigated with a portable EEG. Intensive information and education programs are continually conducted via TV, radio, newspapers, and public conferences on epilepsy. A group of traditional healers of the region of Dakar has benefited also from a training program on epilepsy to develop a better collaboration between modern and traditional medicine, which is utilized by the very large majority of people with epilepsy in Senegal and Africa, whatever their instruction level, residence, and concomitant modern health management.

SUMMARY AND CONCLUSIONS

Describing Senegal realities reflects and summarizes the very common situation of epilepsy in developing countries of the sub-Saharan part of Africa. The management of public health has been dominated since the introduction of modern medicine in Africa via French colonization, many centuries ago. The leading infectious diseases masked the real incidence of nontransmissible disorders, including neurologic ones. Many factors cause a high rate of epilepsy in the country: The high incidence of infectious diseases, the poor quality of maternal–infant care in this low socioeconomic country, consanguineous marriages, and delayed diagnosis and management of tumoral and traumatic causes. Nowadays, more consideration is progressively given to nontransmissible diseases. Many cultural factors maintain epilepsy in the shadows and lead to a dramatic treatment gap. Improved and delocalized epilepsy health care, communication with the different segments of the population, basic education, and intensive training of doctors and paramedical staff, coordinated by a league against epilepsy, raise awareness and begin to give optimism to the improvement of epilepsy management quality and reduction of personal burden and condition of people living with epilepsy. The war will take a long time to win, but step by step, an encouraging and sustainable effort can lead to more success stories for epilepsy in African developing countries such as Senegal.

References

1. Agbere ARD. Analyse de la morbidité et de la mortalité à l'HEAR, 1983–1984. *Thèse Med*. 1986;16.
2. Agbohoui OL. Épilepsie en milieu scolaire Sénégalais. *Thèse Med Dakar*. 1994;18.

3. Bassane B. Aspects étiologiques des affections neurologiques à la Clinique Neurologique de Fann, Bilan de 16 années. *Thèse Med Dakar*. 1986; 73.
4. Collomb H, Dumas M, Ayats H, et al. Epidemiology of epilepsy in Senegal. *Afr J Med Sci*. 1970;1(2):125–148.
5. Collomb H, Dumas M, Girard PL, et al. Neurology in Senegal (10-year report). *Bull Soc Med Afr Noire Lang Fr*. 1971;16(4):575–580.
6. Diagana MB. Épilepsie et Diabète - Aspects cliniques, étiologiques, électrocliniques et thérapeutiques (à propos de 30 observations colligées à la Clinique Neurologique du CHU de Fann). *Thèse Méd Dakar*. 1989; 23.
7. Diallo I. Etude comparative de la mortalité et de la morbidité en 1965 et 1975 dans le Service de Pédiatrie du CHU de Dakar. *Thèse Med Dakar*. 1980;88.
8. Diop AG, de Boer H, Mandlhate C, et al. The Global Campaign against Epilepsy in Africa. *Acta Tropica*. 2003;87(1):149–159.
9. Feksi AT, Kaamugisha J, Gatiti S, et al. A comprehensive community epilepsy programme: the Nakuru project. *Epilepsy Res*. 1991;8(3):252–259.
10. Girard PL, Dumas M, Collomb H. Gliomas (neuroectodermal tumors) in Senegal. *Afr J Med Sci*. 1973;4(2):265–274.
11. Jallon P. Epilepsy in developing countries. *Epilepsia*. 1997;38(10):1143–1151.
12. Karfo K. Vécu de l'Épilepsie Grand Mal au Sénégal. *Thèse Méd Dakar*. 1991;46.
13. Khalil M. Epilepsie au Sénégal. Aspects électro-clinique et thérapeutique. *Thèse Méd Dakar*. 1988;37.
14. Martini L, Stephany F, Jacquin-Cotton L, et al. Epilepsy after 50 in a hospital setting in Dakar. *Dakar Med*. 1981;26(1):89–100.
15. Mbodj I, Ndiaye M, Sene F, et al. Prise en charge de l'état de mal épileptique dans les conditions de pays en développement. *Neurophysiol Clin*. 2000;30:165–169.
16. Mone C. Epilepsie et grossesse. *Thèse Med Dakar*. 1988;19.
17. Ndiaye IP, Ndiaye M, Tap D. Sociocultural aspects of epilepsy in Africa. *Prog Clin Biol Res*. 1983;124:345–351.
18. Ndiaye M. Enquête épidémiologique sur l'épilepsie à Saint-Louis (milieu scolaire). *Thèse Med Dakar*. 1997;52.
19. Ndiaye M, Sene-Diouf F, Diop AG, et al. Epilepsy: first-ranked disorder in Pediatric services of Senegal. *Bull Soc Pathol Exot (France)*. 2000;93(4):268–269.
20. Ndour D, Diop AG, Ndiaye M, et al. Knowledge, Attitudes and Practice survey among teachers in Senegal. *Rev Neurol (France)*. 2004;160(3):338–341.
21. Ndoye NF, Sessouma B, Boissy L, et al. Prevalence rate and Treatment Gap in the Pikine (Senegal) Demonstration Project Site of the Global Campaign *Against Epilepsy*. London: International Epilepsy Congress; 2003.
22. Seck D. L'Hôpital d'Enfants Albert Royer de Dakar: Principales Pathologies et Mortalité hospitalière en 1995. *Thèse Pharm Dakar*. 1997;91.
23. Thiam I. Facteur de risque dans l'Épilepsie (à propos d'enquête en zone sub-urbaine). *Thèse Méd Dakar*. 1989;31.
24. Thiam MH, Gueye M. Clinical aspects of hysteria at the psychiatric clinic of the Fann University Hospital Center. A prospective study of 121 cases. *Dakar Med*. 1998;43(1):41–44.

CHAPTER 298 ■ UNITED KINGDOM

STEPHEN W. BROWN AND FRANK M. C. BESAG

INTRODUCTION

In 1911 a National Health Insurance Scheme was introduced in the United Kingdom that allowed low-paid workers (but not their families) access to primary health care. This was the first intervention by a British government in the area of general health care delivery. There was interest in taking matters further, and at the end of World War I an election pledge to establish a general health service was made by Lloyd George's coalition. A Consultative Council on Medical and Allied Services was set up, headed by the King's physician, Sir Bertrand Dawson (1864–1945, later Viscount Dawson of Penn), which produced an interim report in 1920. This discussion document suggested a framework for a comprehensive service emphasizing primary care and preventive medicine while defining the roles of secondary and tertiary services, in the event no action was taken and there was no further report. However, the philosophy and ideas of the Dawson Report were to influence the development of the National Health Service as World War II drew to a close more than 20 years later.

DEVELOPMENT OF THE PRESENT SYSTEM

Shortly after the outbreak of World War II, the national government in Britain, which included representatives of all main political parties, asked Sir William Beveridge (1879–1963), an economist and master of University College Oxford, to chair an interdepartmental committee on the coordination of the Social Services. This was not expected to be completed until after the war, but the report entitled *Social Insurance and Allied Services* was published in 1942, some 18 months after the work started. It proposed a comprehensive social insurance scheme covering the whole population without income limit. The government response, with other pressing priorities, was initially low key, but the report sold 70,000 copies in 4 days and was popular with the public. An understanding then emerged that with the coming of peace a health care service for the nation would be established, free at the point of entry and financed by national taxation, based on a White Paper of 1944. This policy would be carried out by whichever party won the first postwar general election. In 1945, the Labour Party assumed power between the German and Japanese surrenders. Acts of Parliament in 1946 (covering England and Wales) and in 1947 (Scotland) were passed, and the National Health Service (NHS) was inaugurated on July 5, 1948.

The National Health Service Act (1946) defined ministerial responsibility for establishment in England and Wales of "a comprehensive health service designed to secure improvement in the physical and mental health of the people and the prevention, diagnosis and treatment of illness for that purpose.... Service so provided shall be free of charge.... " Responsibility for ushering in the new age fell on the Labour politician Aneurin Bevan (1897–1960), who was the Minister for Health and Housing. There was initial resistance from the medical profession, but Bevan proved an able negotiator, and in his own words overcame doctors' objections by "filling their mouths with gold." Bevan believed that access to free medical care would improve ordinary people's health to the extent that there would be economic benefits, and in particular that the cost of the new NHS would fall with time as the rate of disease was reduced. This thinking was fortunately not enshrined in statute as history proved him completely wrong. Meanwhile private practice was allowed alongside and within the NHS.

Between 1948 and 1974 the NHS consisted of three main branches: Public health services, which were the responsibility of local government; the hospital-based services; and the primary care service in which family practitioners (general practitioners [GPs]) worked. Difficulties in planning and coordinating services led to considerable consultation and debate between 1968 and 1972, and in 1974 a major reorganization created three administrative tiers—at Regional, Area, and District levels—that sought to overcome these problems. This unfortunately proved bureaucratically inefficient, and in 1982, following a Royal Commission report, the middle tier of Area Health Authorities was abolished.

Up to this point stages in the development of the service were a consequence of consultation and forward planning that took place under governments of both main political parties, and the broad policy was bipartisan. From the mid-1980s onward the Conservative government began to introduce changes that deviated from this consensus. In 1985 the NHS was placed under a management board chaired by its own chief executive, accountable to but with some autonomy from the government Department of Health and Social Security. In the late 1980s the NHS was subjected to a private review by the government, after which a major change in its mode of operating was devised. Against concerted opposition from all those relevant professional bodies who expressed an opinion, as well as from other political parties, an amending act was passed in 1991, and a new, reformed NHS appeared on April 1, 1992.

The main changes reflected the adoption of an internal market strategy. This meant that the old District Health Authorities were allocated a grant based on their individual population needs, to purchase health services from provider units such as hospitals. Provider units were given the opportunity to become self-governing trusts, in competition with each other, obtaining their income from purchasing authorities by selling services to them. Doctors working in primary care were allowed (and encouraged) to take responsibility for managing their own budgets for purchasing secondary services (known as GP Fundholders). This controversial purchaser/provider split appeared to lay the foundation for an increase in the establishment of managerial, accounting, and general administrative staff, with a power shift away from health professionals. Some rationalization was attempted by a drastic reduction in the number of Regional Health Authorities in 1994, together with partial devolving of planning to the periphery. At the time of writing, virtually all provider units have self-governing Trust status, while the commissioning of most services is a function of locality-based Primary Care Trusts. These came about after the Labour Party won the 1997 election with a policy pledge to abolish the internal market of the NHS and to remove the perceived unfair advantage of the fund-holding primary care sector over the non–fund-holding sector. The years since then have seen a series of rapid changes in structure, characterized by the increasing devolution of service commissioning to the primary care level, and a downscaling of the influence of the old Regional Offices, which were eventually abolished. This also happened against a background of devolution of government to Welsh, Scottish, and Northern Irish Assemblies, producing different NHS structures with subtle differences in four jurisdictions. Total spending on health by the government has substantially increased, but not surprisingly some of this has been required to finance the structural reforms and monitoring apparatus that have had to be introduced. In England and Wales recommended treatment guidelines for NHS use are drawn up by a quasi-autonomous government-funded organization, originally called the National Institute for Clinical Excellence, later expanded to the National Institute for Health and Clinical Excellence, but always known by its acronym, NICE. This describes itself as "the independent organization responsible for providing national guidance on the promotion of good health and the prevention and treatment of ill health." NICE also appraises health technologies, including drugs, to make recommendations for use within the NHS based on cost effectiveness, with the economic modeling emphasizing cost to the NHS rather than cost to society as a whole—an approach that has led to considerable criticism; it remains to be seen whether this narrow approach will survive. Nevertheless, NHS organizations in England and Wales are required to audit their practice against NICE guidance, and a degree of performance management is dependent on this. NICE produced comprehensive epilepsy management guidelines in October 2004.[13] In Scotland, some of the equivalent functions of NICE are performed by the Scottish Intercollegiate Guideline Network (SIGN), which produced updated epilepsy guidelines in June 2004.[16] There are some subtle differences in emphasis, which if followed closely could lead to different care pathways being followed by people with epilepsy in the United Kingdom depending on where they live, though whether this is important only time will tell. Both NICE and SIGN guidelines may be accessed through the Internet at www.nice.org.uk and www.sign.ac.uk, respectively. One consequence of current policy is the setting of various clinical and managerial targets (e.g., waiting times) that contribute to performance management of NHS organizations. An early attempt at this in England by a previous government was the publication in 1992 of *The Health of the Nation*.[7] Inclusions and exclusions in this document are somewhat arbitrary. Targets for reduction in HIV and suicide are included, despite the relatively small numbers in England of those affected by HIV and the fact that suicide statistics depend on quality control of coroner's courts. Epilepsy was not mentioned. Later, epilepsy came to move further up the governmental agenda. One of the key influences in this was the National Sentinel Clinical Audit of Epilepsy-related Death, published in 2002.[10] This came about after intensive lobbying of the government by the voluntary sector, and its influence on service development has been significant. The government was moved to produce an Action Plan for epilepsy service improvement, which, although criticized heavily by the voluntary sector and by epilepsy specialists, nevertheless raised the profile of epilepsy considerably.[3] Indeed, much direct representation to government about epilepsy services has been through charitable and voluntary groups, such as the British Epilepsy Association (now called Epilepsy Action), the National Society for Epilepsy, and the Joint Epilepsy Council of Great Britain and Ireland. In the United Kingdom these nonprofit organizations are called charities. In 1994 the government tacitly opposed a Disabled Rights Bill and met with much lobbying and criticism from groups advocating rights for the disabled and from consumer groups. Shortly afterward, the Charity Commission, the government-appointed body that regulates the activities of charities (some of which had been highly critical of the government's failure to support the bill), issued firm guidelines that seemed at first effectively to stop charities from future involvement in political lobbying, unless they were willing to risk losing their charitable status.[6] This advice was subsequently revised.[5] The government then brought forward separate legislation on disability rights, the Disability Discrimination Act, which came into law in 1997.

BUDGET ORGANIZATION AND DEVELOPMENT

National Government

The NHS is financed by taxation. Responsibility for setting and allocating the NHS budget for the United Kingdom lies with the central government. In England this is the responsibility of a politician, the Secretary of State for Health, who heads a ministry, the Department of Health. In Scotland, Wales, and Northern Ireland health issues are the responsibility of different government departments, belonging to the devolved parliamentary assemblies in Scotland, Wales, and, when it is sitting, Northern Ireland.

For the purposes of health administration England was previously divided into a number of Regions, each with a population of approximately 5 million, with strategic overview provided by an NHS Executive Regional outpost, which has replaced the old Regional Health Authority. Each Region contained a number of Health Authorities (HAs), with populations of approximately 250,000 each. NHS Regional outposts were broadly responsible for strategic planning within their areas, but details of service provision were decided and carried out at District level. The process of peripheral devolvement has seen the abolition of Regional outposts and of the old Health Authorities, to be replaced in England by smaller Strategic Health Authorities (SHAs) and Primary Care Trusts (PCTs). At the time of writing there is speculation that many PCTs may be forced to merge for economic and strategic reasons, and SHAs may also combine to larger organizations, which might effectively bring back the old District/Regional boundaries, the process therefore turning full circle within a few years. Not surprisingly many who work in the service find it difficult to embrace these sorts of changes with the same enthusiasm as the politicians.

Board members of NHS organizations are currently appointed by the Secretary of State. There are proposals that may allow some local election to boards in the future, but this has yet to be implemented. Currently PCTs (and to a lesser extent SHAs) in England and their equivalent bodies in other jurisdictions are the authorities with responsibility for purchasing health services on behalf of the community, with funding from central government, the level being fixed by population size and type.

The purchasing authorities, as defined earlier, may contract with health providers such as hospitals, ambulance services, and so on, which are organized as self-governing trusts. There is also the option to purchase from the private sector, so that the public and private sectors become less demarcated.

State Provincial Government

Provincial (local) government below the level of the four jurisdictions (England, Scotland, Wales, Northern Ireland) has no direct role in the United Kingdom as far as health care is concerned. However, local government is responsible for the organization of social services and for the provision of children's education. Therefore long-term care, which can be construed as a social services responsibility, has to be considered in this way, and the special educational needs of children with epilepsy have to be assessed and provided for at this level. Because of this split, opportunities arise for budget holders to attempt to shift financial responsibility away from their own areas, although officially cooperation between different agencies is encouraged.

Insurance Company/Health Schemes by Budget

Since the NHS was founded there has always been a small but flourishing private sector. Only 11% of people have private health insurance.[15] The NHS has traditionally been regarded as superior in emergency care and, until recently, in provision for chronic illness. The private sector offers shorter waiting times for nonurgent surgical procedures, better access to some investigations (especially magnetic resonance imaging), and a more discrete, personalized service.

Finances

In 1987 the United Kingdom spent 6.1% of its gross domestic product (GDP) on health. At first this appears to compare unfavorably with some other industrialized countries (Table 1).

Until 1980 the NHS budget had been increasing by about 4% per year, after inflation. From 1980 to 1986 this rate of increase slowed to 1%, although it increased again after 1986. The slowing of growth in income between 1980 and 1986 was consistent with government policy to increase efficiency in the public sector and to limit public spending. This meant that in 1986 the gap between actual and expected budget was £3.53 billion, a shortfall of nearly 20%. However, increased spending after 1986 had largely closed this gap by 1992. The usual explanation for the discrepancy between GDP spent on health in the United Kingdom and other countries is that the nationalized health system spends less on administration, and so overall costs are kept low. This was especially apparent in the spending squeeze between 1980 and 1986, although evidence from other countries suggests that policy attempts to improve efficiency may have the opposite effect.[18]

TABLE 1

PROPORTION OF GROSS DOMESTIC PRODUCT (%) SPENT ON HEALTH

	1980	1987
United States	9.2	11.2
Sweden	9.5	9.0
Canada	7.4	8.6
France	7.6	8.6
Netherlands	8.2	8.5
Austria	7.9	8.4
Germany	7.9	8.2
Iceland	6.4	7.8
Switzerland	7.3	7.7
Luxembourg	6.8	7.5
Norway	6.6	7.5
Finland	6.5	7.4
Belgium	6.6	7.2
Australia	6.5	7.1
Italy	6.8	6.9
New Zealand	7.2	6.9
Japan	6.4	6.8
Portugal	5.9	6.4
United Kingdom	5.8	6.1
Spain	5.9	6.0
Denmark	6.8	6.0
Greece	4.3	5.3
Mean	7.0	7.5

From Heginbotham C. Leading for health: responses: rationing. *BMJ*. 1982;304:496–499.

CONTROL OF EXPENDITURE BY DIFFERENT SEGMENTS

At the National Level

The total NHS budget is set after Treasury negotiation each year, and decided by the Cabinet. The Secretary of State for Health has the responsibility of making the case in Cabinet for appropriate funding in the context of total government budget, competing with other departments such as education or defense.

In the past, budgets for the main parts of hospital services were then devolved to Regional Health Authorities. Since the complex and changing reforms of the last 10 years, the trend has been toward establishing local health commissioning organizations such as PCTs, which are allocated funds according to a formula based on local population demographics.

People who have private health insurance are still most likely to use the NHS for primary care by choice. Where contact with hospital-based services is concerned, insurers may be reluctant to provide coverage for expensive or long-term treatment, so these are likely to be met from NHS resources too.

ORGANIZATION OF PHYSICIANS

Primary Care

Nurse Practitioners

Epilepsy specialist nurses started appearing as a distinct group in the United Kingdom in the early 1990s. The first appointments came mainly from the charitable sector (the David Lewis Centre, in Manchester, and the National Society for Epilepsy, in London), although NHS funding was involved in an innovative community-based scheme established in Doncaster in Yorkshire.[17] These nurse practitioners bring an added dimension of counseling skills to the clinical team and are able to provide more time to answer patients' questions than physicians. They also assist in liaison between primary and secondary care services, and can supervise previously prescribed changes of medication, thus freeing up the time of doctors. There is now a professional body that sets standards, the Epilepsy Specialist Nurses Association.[8] A major impetus to the development of the specialty has been provided by the British Epilepsy Association (BEA) in collaboration with industrial sponsorship to provide pump-priming finance for the establishment of a number of new posts around the United Kingdom starting in 1995. This project, launched in BEA's 45th anniversary year, is known as the Sapphire Nurses Programme, and represents a potentially major change in the mode of service delivery.

It did not come about by project planning in the NHS, despite published evidence of efficacy of such a service[8] and despite the much-vaunted sensitivity of the NHS reforms to local needs. As in other areas of epilepsy provision in the United Kingdom, the main thrust has come from the voluntary, charitable sector. However, in 1995 the result of raised consumer expectations, pressure from the charitable sector, and interest from within the Department of Health (DOH) combined so that the DOH sponsored a number of pilot projects, mainly in the primary care arena, referred to as the Epilepsy Initiative. Matters altered considerably after the change of government in 1997, and current NICE guidance endorses the value of epilepsy specialist nursing. There are also opportunities for specialist nurses to become prescribers of medication within agreed treatment protocols, although this has yet to have a significant impact in epilepsy.

General Practitioners and Family Practice

In the United Kingdom it is unlikely that antiepileptic drug treatment would be initiated solely by a general practitioner. Where patients present with suspected epilepsy, the primary care physician will virtually always obtain an opinion from a specialist. The United Kingdom has relatively fewer neurologists per capita than other European or North American countries, and so the specialist opinion may be obtained from a general physician (internist) or general pediatrician. Recent data suggest that initiation of treatment for children is carried out by general pediatricians in about 55% of cases, whereas for adults, neurologists initiate treatment in about 66%.[14] The vast majority will be seen in the public (NHS) sector by physicians working in hospital practice. After initial investigation and treatment, most patients are referred back to their GPs for longer-term follow-up.

GPs are mainly organized into partnerships that may be based in health centers providing total primary care services for populations of 12,000 to 20,000 (with six to 10 GPs). A significant number work in smaller partnerships, and there are a few single-handed practitioners. GP partnerships typically employ primary care nurses and other allied professionals. At present in the United Kingdom there is no established model that is equivalent to the polyclinic or multispecialty clinic seen in some other countries, although some areas have commenced a pilot scheme for Primary Care Resource Centres that may fulfill some of these functions, and there is encouragement for the development of specialist GPs (GPSIs—GPs with a Special Interest) in various therapeutic areas and opportunities for this to develop in epilepsy.

GPs have the responsibility to provide all primary care medical services to the whole population registered with them, and so all GPs have a responsibility for epilepsy. Similarly, virtually all people with epilepsy are registered with GPs, although for many the involvement with treatment consists of little more than obtaining repeat prescriptions for antiepileptic drugs. About 20% of patients continue to see hospital physicians.

General Pediatricians and General Physicians (Internists)

General pediatricians and general physicians are hospital-based practitioners. Within the hospital setting there is an increasing trend to specialization, so that a district general hospital will have a group of general physicians that will include some with special interests in cardiology, endocrinology, gastroenterology, and so on. Where there is no staff neurologist, one of the general physicians may take this on as a special interest and will therefore have a broad responsibility for epilepsy. However, it is likely that all general physicians will see some patients with epilepsy, and all will take turns at receiving urgent admissions of patients with epilepsy from accident and emergency departments.

TABLE 2

MEDICAL PRACTITIONERS WHO SEE EPILEPSY PATIENTS REGULARLY

	Percentage of specialists seeing specialty patients with epilepsy
General medicine (internists)	56
Psychiatrists	20
Pediatricians	80
Gerontologists	73

The percentage of the different specialists (other than neurologists) who see epilepsy patients regularly is shown in Table 2.[9]

Neurologists

In the early 1990s the United Kingdom had about 300 trained career neurologists, approximately the same number as Denmark, a country with one-tenth the population. There has been a tendency until recently for neurologic practice to be most concentrated in teaching hospitals. However, the specialty is set for expansion. It is likely that neurologists in the NHS will be concentrated in neuroscience centers, each serving a population of 1.5 to 2.5 million, along with neurosurgeons and neurophysiology services. District hospitals serving much smaller catchments within the neuroscience center areas will obtain neurologic services from the center, on a hub-and-spoke principle. Private practice neurology exists and frequently shares facilities with the NHS service.

Referrals to neurology services will typically be made by GPs or hospital-based physicians. Self-referral is not the usual pattern in the NHS, and is unusual even in the private sector. The main barrier to access is the shortage of neurologists, with the waiting list for nonurgent outpatient appointments varying across the country from 2 to 92 weeks in 1993.[9] Reducing waiting list times such as this has been a high priority of the Labour Government, and it is alleged that the maximum time has been considerably reduced. Data for 2004 suggested that of 84,290 referrals for outpatient neurology consultations in England, only 384 (0.46%) had to wait more than 21 weeks to be seen.[12]

Epilepsy Centers

The term *epilepsy center* has two different meanings in the United Kingdom. It may refer to a residential facility owned and administered by a nonprofit organization specializing in epilepsy, or it may refer to a specialist unit within an NHS neuroscience center. The former typically have close links with the latter, so that there is some integration of service. For example, Chalfont Centre, a residential facility in rural Buckinghamshire run by the nonprofit National Society for Epilepsy, forms part of a service provided also by the National Hospital for Neurology and Neurosurgery in London.

The availability of epilepsy services in different parts of the United Kingdom is a reflection of both the enthusiasm of different local physicians and the local public profile of consumer groups and nonprofit organizations. Epilepsy surgery programs are currently well established at nine major NHS neuroscience centers in the United Kingdom, with several others in development. There are at least four multidisciplinary residential assessment units for adults and two for children, all mainly within the independent nonprofit sector, and there are a larger number of NHS neuroscience centers with specialist hospital-based assessment facilities. The total number of specialist outpatient clinics known to the British Epilepsy Association had increased to 59.[2] The reasons for this increase and the reason why there continues to be a slow but sustained improvement in epilepsy services include:

- New antiepileptic drug licenses and increased activity by the pharmaceutical industry to sponsor continuing medical education, thereby raising awareness among professionals
- Increased consumer expectations and demands
- The BEA Sapphire Nursing scheme (see earlier)
- Continued lobbying from nonprofit organizations, in particular resulting in the National Sentinel Audit of Epilepsy-related Death, the government Action Plan, and the issuing of epilepsy guidance by NICE

As a recognition of and in response to the preceding, the NHS published an Executive Letter (EL 95/120) early in 1996[1] drawing the attention of purchasers and providers to the potential for developing epilepsy services, to the role of voluntary organizations, and to how epilepsy relates to the priorities for service development in the NHS. Needless to say, the voluntary organizations carefully monitored the response and carried out some research into its effectiveness.[4]

SUMMARY AND CONCLUSIONS

The British National Health Service was established in 1948 as a publicly funded service, free to the consumer at the point of access. Private medical practice continues to exist alongside the state sector, but a large majority of citizens use the NHS exclusively for the services that it provides.

Rising costs and the need to establish more effective management caused the government to introduce a number of structural changes, characterized in the 1980s by the establishment of the NHS Executive and in the 1990s by the introduction of an internal market with a purchaser/provider split. A new government was elected in May 1997, which has reversed some but not all these changes and introduced some new ones.

The priorities for the NHS include (among others) an increasing focus on primary care, the effective use of resources, and working with service users and caregivers.

Neurology as a medical specialty was traditionally more diagnostic than therapeutic, and much of the treatment of common neurologic conditions was carried out by general physicians. Epilepsy services therefore tended not to develop exclusively in neurology departments, and indeed have often been supported by the charitable (nonprofit or voluntary) sector. Consequently, epilepsy services remained fragmentary, variable in quality, and difficult for the consumer to find. A number of factors have contributed to an improved outlook, including a greater commitment to develop neuroscience services, greater consumer empowerment, and development of innovative service models, including enhanced primary care liaison and the use of specialist nursing. Nonprofit organizations representing views of service users and professionals, such as the Epilepsy Action (British Epilepsy Association) and the National Society for Epilepsy, have played an important part in establishing epilepsy on the health planning agenda, and these organizations will continue to fulfill this role.

References

1. A positive approach to epilepsy. *NHS Executive Letter EL(95)120*. Leeds: NHS Executive Headquarters; 1996.
2. *British Epilepsy Association Annual Review for 1996*. Leeds: British Epilepsy Association; 1997.
3. Besag FMC. The Department of Health Action Plan "improving services for people with epilepsy": a significant advance or only a first step? *Seizure*. 2004;13:553–564.
4. Brown SW, Lee P. Developments in UK provision for people with epilepsy: the impact of NHS Executive Letter 95/120. *Seizure*. 1998;7:185–187.
5. *CC9a—Political Activities and Campaigning by Local Community Charities*. London: Charity Commission; 1996.
6. *CC9—Political Activities and Campaigning by Charities*. London: Charity Commission; 1996.
7. Department of Health. *The Health of the Nation: A Strategy for Health in England*. London: HMSO; 1992.
8. Epilepsy Specialist Nurses Association c/o Children's Centre, 70 Walker Street, Hull HU3 2HE United Kingdom.
9. Epilepsy Task Force, c/o The Joint Epilepsy Council of the UK and Ireland, P.O. Box 186, Leeds LS20 8WY United Kingdom.
10. Hanna NJ, Black M, Sander JWS, et al. *The National Sentinel Clinical Audit of Epilepsy-Related Death: Epilepsy – Death in the Shadows*. The Stationery Office; 2002.
11. Heginbotham C. Leading for health: responses: rationing. *BMJ*. 1982;304:496–499.
12. Available at: http://www.performance.doh.gov.uk/waitingtimes/2004/q4/qm08y00.html. Accessed September 29, 2005.
13. National Institute for Clinical Excellence. *Clinical Guideline 20. The Epilepsies: The Diagnosis and Management of the Epilepsies in Adults and Children in Primary and Secondary Care*. London: National Institute for Clinical Excellence; 2004.
14. Neurotrak. Wellcome Foundation Market Research (personal communication).
15. Richmond C. Private medicine takes on the NHS in Britain. *Can Med Assoc J*. 1994;150:1459–1460.
16. Scottish Intercollegiate Guideline Network (SIGN). *Diagnosis and Management of Epilepsy in Adult: A National Clinical Guideline* (No. 20). Edinburgh: Scottish Intercollegiate Guideline Network; 2004.
17. Taylor MP, Readman S, Hague B, et al. A district epilepsy service, with community-based specialist liaison nurses and guidelines for shared care. *Seizure*. 1994;3(2):121–127.
18. Wollhandler S, Himmelstein DU. The deteriorating administrative efficiency of the U.S. health care system. *N Engl J Med*. 1991;324(18):1253–1258.

CHAPTER 299 ■ UNITED STATES

ROBERT J. GUMNIT

INTRODUCTION

The organization of health care in the United States has undergone major changes in recent years. In this chapter, the historical background is presented, after which the organization of health care as it exists in 2006 is outlined.

HISTORICAL BACKGROUND

Health care in the United States was initially provided by generalist physicians. During the colonial era, they graduated largely from the medical schools of Great Britain. By the time of the Revolutionary War (1776), however, some physicians in the United States developed expertise in certain areas and were considered specialists. Medical schools were established in the United States along with the earliest universities and tended to follow the Scottish model. Under the Constitution, regulation of medical practice in the United States is relegated to the individual states. As a result, each state has its own licensing authority. During the 19th century, the quality of training and care varied widely, and fraudulent claims to medical training were frequently made. This was particularly a problem in rural areas of the western states.

By the time of the Civil War (1861), specialization in neurology had developed, and some of the earliest research in neurologic disease was done at that time. The specialties of neurology and psychiatry were closely intertwined from the earliest days of the medical system.

At the beginning of the 20th century, under the aegis of a charitable foundation, a study of medical education in the United States was carried out (the Flexner report), and a revolution occurred. A national accreditation authority for medical schools was established, and medical schools were reorganized more along the lines of the German system. Training in basic science was required of all students, and organized clinical training began. Still, up to the beginning of World War II (1939), the overwhelming majority of physicians were in primary care, and specialty care was available only in major cities and in association with university schools of medicine.

The end of World War II, the creation of the GI Bill of Rights, and the establishment of federal subsidies for medical insurance, research, and education produced a second revolution. Large numbers of physicians were trained, many more medical schools were established, and specialty training in the form of residencies became the norm. State licensing authorities no longer permitted physicians to practice after only a single year of postgraduate training (internship), and formal residencies and accreditation boards were created in all specialties, including family practice.

Large numbers of dollars flowed into the health care system as health insurance became a fringe benefit provided by nearly all large employers. Health insurance was readily available for purchase by individuals, and the federal government began subsidizing health care for the poor and elderly.

LEVELS OF CARE

Nonetheless, today, the United States, despite its enormous wealth, fails to provide for the basic health needs of a large part of its population. It has more levels of care than any other major industrialized country.

Level 1: Provisions for the Very Poor, Whether or Not They Are Homeless

The very poor have no money and no health insurance. Historically, they depended on charitable acts of individual physicians. As practices became more highly organized, and the poor became more concentrated in inner cities, finding access to charity care became increasingly more difficult. The federal government provided large amounts of money to hospitals for capital expansion and modernization under the Hill-Burton Act of 1946. A subsequent law required any hospital that received Hill-Burton funds to provide emergency care to all coming to its emergency department, whether or not they could pay. This was the final safety net, but provided only for the most obvious emergencies. However, the educational needs of physicians in training and the sense of local responsibility on the part of cities and counties has led to a system of county hospitals with outpatient facilities of varying completeness. Some of these are now being closed because of fiscal constraints.

Level 2: Medicaid

From 1966 to 1996, the federal government provided money to the states under Title XIX of the Social Security Act. This provided matching funds to the states to care for sick children, mothers of minor children, and the disabled. Strict federal guidelines were enforced. This broad mandate became eroded during the 1990s. The programs of the individual states now have more variability, and the ability of the poor to choose their own physicians is once again becoming compromised.

Level 3: Medicare

In 1965, the federal government initiated the Medicare program (Title XVIII) to provide health insurance for the elderly. Anyone over the age of 65 is eligible. This is a complicated act that provides for inpatient hospital care (Part A). Hospital care is primarily paid for by the federal government, with deductibles and copayments by patients. Voluntary premium payments by eligible patients, with some support from the federal government, provide funding for outpatient hospital care and physician care (Part B).

The payments from both Title XVIII and Title XIX are far below community standards and stress the physician segment more than the hospital segment of the health care system. In January 2006, Medical Part D was implemented, providing for a benefit to assist in the purchase of pharmaceuticals. This law (and its regulations) is extraordinarily complicated, depends upon a multitude of competing private plans, and is partially needs based. Early implementation was poorly planned, and many patients were denied needed medicines. It is too soon to know how this program will eventually develop.

Level 4: Private Insurance

Individuals were able to buy hospitalization insurance beginning in the early 1930s. A few people were able to purchase physician insurance also. The wage freezes imposed at the time of World War II were circumvented by employers and unions that agreed to purchase health insurance for employees. The cost of insurance was not subject to the wage freeze. These payments started a major industry in the United States—private health insurance. For many years, private health insurance was of the indemnity type. Any service prescribed by a physician and provided by a licensed practitioner or facility was covered. To this extent, it was analogous to the collision insurance that one buys for an automobile. The great majority of the people in the United States are still covered by insurance that is purchased by an employer. However, insurance has become increasingly expensive because of increased demand, increased costs, the complexity of medical treatment, and the failure to obey market forces. A major effort to control costs by setting up large bureaucratic organizations to provide medical service took place in the 1990s. These schemes are called *health maintenance organizations (HMOs)*, *preferred provider organizations (PPOs)*, *independent practice organizations (IPOs)*, or *physician-hospital organizations (PHOs)*. Over time, the restrictive nature of the HMOs lost favor, and most employers provide some form of PPOs. This type of plan offers more choice of physician to the patient.

Level 5: Indemnity Insurance and Private Payments

Where it still exists, traditional indemnity insurance permits unlimited access to medical and hospital care. Increasingly, certain services are no longer available, because managed care organizations will not purchase them and there are too few indemnity patients to sustain them.

The policy of the Bush administration (2000–2008) is to shift cost and responsibility to the individual patient. Tax-exempt Medical Savings Accounts are now being promoted heavily. Higher deductibles and copayment requirements are becoming burdensome.

Thus, it is extremely difficult in the United States to understand how decisions are made with respect to health care expenditures. They are made by many different groups at many different levels, in many different locations. The United States has failed to initiate a nationwide health care system and relies instead on competition within the marketplace and multiple individual decisions. As the major sources of money become restricted (national, state, and employer), an increasing portion of the money spent on health care comes from individual persons.

ORGANIZATION OF PHYSICIANS FOR PRIMARY CARE

In the United States, primary care is largely provided by family practitioners, although increasing numbers of nurse practitioners and physician assistants are being used. The general practitioner who also performs surgery and obstetrics is a dying breed, and the average family practice physician refers most surgical cases to specialists.

Family practitioners are found throughout the United States. Only a few are left in solo practice; most practice together in single-specialty groups that in some areas comprise as many as 30 or 40 people. Others work in large family practice departments of multispecialty clinics. From the standpoint of epilepsy care, most patients with epilepsy receive care from primary care physicians (although in urban areas, many patients are also followed routinely by a neurologist).

In the United States, primary care is also often provided by pediatricians and internists. Internists who subspecialize are known as *cardiologists* or *rheumatologists*, for example. They tend to practice in small, single-specialty groups or in departments of multispecialty clinics. The average internist or pediatrician sees no more patients with epilepsy than the average family practitioner. The average primary care physician cares for between five and ten patients with epilepsy. Pediatricians and internists tend to be located in urban areas, including smaller cities with as few as 10,000 to 20,000 people.

There are roughly 750,000 licensed physicians in the United States and only 12,000 neurologists. Most neurologists practice in large urban areas or in association with medical schools. Very few are in solo practice; most are in single-specialty groups or in departments of multispecialty clinics.

In the United States, many people seek out neurologic care directly, although the majority is still referred by primary care physicians. With the development of managed care organizations of various sorts, new barriers have been created to specialty access for people with epilepsy. In addition to the problems of distribution and distance, barriers exist to accessing a neurologist (or any other specialist) without a referral from a primary care physician.

In the United States, primary care physicians frequently admit a patient to a hospital and call a neurologist in consultation. This is in contrast to what occurs in many other countries, where the patient is referred to a hospital group or a neurologist, who then takes on the primary responsibility for hospital care.

Excellent comprehensive epilepsy centers are available throughout the United States (see Chapter 302).

It is important to note that, in the United States, a license to practice medicine is generic. There is no legal restriction to physicians' describing themselves as specialists in any area. Control over quality is a function of hospital staff privileges. In this way, physicians in major hospitals cannot practice in an area for which they have not had appropriate residency training; specific privileges are granted, and these may often relate to something as narrow as whether or not a lumbar puncture can be performed.

However, what takes place in an individual physician's office is completely unregulated. This allows innovative, less expensive treatments to be provided by highly ethical physicians. It also allows opportunities for misrepresentation and less than ideal treatment by others.

SUMMARY AND CONCLUSIONS

The United States has at least five different levels of care, largely driven by economics and barriers erected against those with pre-existing physical conditions. The relatively unregulated practice of medicine and the fact that the license to practice medicine is generic leads to wide disparities in quality of care.

CHAPTER 300 ■ ZAMBIA

GRETCHEN L. BIRBECK AND ELLIE KALICHI

INTRODUCTION

In 2000, epilepsy accounted for 0.5% of the global burden of disease,[22] and appreciation for epilepsy as a public health problem is growing as the full range of medical, psychological, social, and economic morbidities associated with the condition are being recognized and quantified.[20] Use of such measures as the disability-adjusted life year (DALY) to more fully capture the burden of nonfatal, chronic diseases has played an important role in placing epilepsy on the public health agenda in many regions. Of the approximately 50 million people with epilepsy, over 80% reside in developing countries, and less than 10% of these individuals are receiving treatment.[30] A very productive collaboration, The Global Campaign Against Epilepsy, has evolved between the World Health Organization (WHO), International Bureau for Epilepsy (IBE), and the International League Against Epilepsy (ILAE).[14] This consortium's work is aimed at reducing the treatment gap, decreasing the social and physical burden of epilepsy, educating health care personnel, dispelling stigma, and providing support for prevention of epilepsy. These efforts are laudable, but these international efforts rely on individual health care providers working in developing countries to seek and/or accept the role of advocate and push forward the agenda of improving the lives of people epilepsy within their own community, city, country, or region.

No "how to" manual is available to describe the process whereby one would begin to improve epilepsy care for a population. Epilepsy texts typically provide advice on individual case management and sometimes provide guidance on the resources and organization necessary to develop an Epilepsy Surgery Center. Undoubtedly, there are many ways in which a motivated neurologist could approach such a mission, and the most appropriate tactics will vary greatly depending on the physicians' expertise, available time, the burden of disease he faces, the resources and organization of the existing health care system, the local beliefs surrounding epilepsy, and more. Nevertheless, it may prove useful for physicians who have the opportunity and inclination to provide epilepsy care in less developed regions to learn about experiences elsewhere.

The Chikankata Epilepsy Care Team (ECT), located in a rural region of Zambia's Southern Province, has been providing care to a large population of people with epilepsy since 2000. The ECT came into existence after efforts to understand the burden of epilepsy in the region in 1994 eventually resulted in local support (both community- and hospital-based) for the development of such a team. The ECT has since played a significant role in country-wide programs aimed at decreasing epilepsy-associated stigma and narrowing the treatment gap. This chapter provides an overview of our perspective on how care providers "in the trenches" might undertake efforts locally to improve epilepsy care, and goes on to describe the potential to expand such work to a national level under the right circumstances. We will also discuss other "success stories" we've encountered or learned about in the literature.

BARRIERS TO EPILEPSY CARE IN LESS DEVELOPED REGIONS

Epilepsy care provision in less developed regions is negatively influenced by several factors (Table 1).

Barriers to care for people in less developed settings are complex, multifactorial, and depend on economic, social, and cultural factors usually considered outside the realm of medicine. Yet, failure to recognize and address these barriers in the organization of health services delivery as well as in the approach to individual patient care will doom any attempts one makes to provide care to such vulnerable populations.

Consider the role that local health beliefs may play in determining whether a person with epilepsy is *ever* brought to your attention for care. Given the often violent and entirely unpredictable nature of seizures, these events are frequently interpreted as the result of supernatural or spiritual forces. As such, even people who would seek care at a health center for a fever or cough may take their seizure-related problems to a traditional or evangelical healer. Health care providers, who may have little formal education and no training in epilepsy, may hold similar beliefs regarding seizures that occur outside of acute infections. Only educational programs aimed at first-line health care providers and case-finding endeavors in the community will overcome these problems.

Even if someone wishes to seek medical care for their seizure disorder, medical services may not be accessible. Health care centers offering even first-line anticonvulsants may be either prohibitively expensive or too geographically distant from the person's home to be a feasible source of care. Primary health care centers, usually staffed with nonphysician care providers, are often supplied with only the most basic medications, so that even if the health care provider is able to diagnose the condition and knows what treatment is needed, the treatment may not be available. These barriers are only exacerbated by the continuing brain drain. Physicians from regions such as Africa are leaving developing regions in droves as a consequence of the poor working and social conditions in the home country and the wealthy, aging West's need for a larger pool of health care providers. Finally, epilepsy-associated stigma further may decimate the social capital of the person suffering from epilepsy, making it even more difficult for them to garner the community support needed to seek care. For example, women with epilepsy in Zambia often lack the usual male protector, having been largely abandoned by their families. Therefore, these women are particularly vulnerable to sexual assault if they travel alone. So, although most Zambian women can safely seek medical care alone or accompanied only by their children, this is not true for women with epilepsy, who need an adult to travel with them. The barriers to care listed in Table 1 are certainly not exhaustive, and each setting undoubtedly offers unique barriers. These can only be appreciated if one develops a dialogue with experienced, empathetic health care providers,

TABLE 1

BARRIERS TO EPILEPSY CARE DELIVERY IN LESS DEVELOPED REGIONS[25]

Barrier	Example
Health beliefs[4]	People with epilepsy and their families perceive seizures as a supernatural or spiritual problem and therefore care is sought from traditional or evangelical healers. Health care workers may hold supernatural or spiritual beliefs regarding the etiology of seizures.
Lack of available services[10,31]	Health care providers and facilities may be either geographically or financially unavailable to many people with epilepsy.
Health care worker limitations[6,10]	May have no training in the diagnosis and treatment of epilepsy. May not be allowed to prescribe anticonvulsants. May not have recourse to refer patients for physician-level care. May have only a few minutes to spend with each patient.
Lack of physicians	Too few physicians, with most in the private sector
Lack of diagnostic resources	No recourse to neuroimaging, EEG, or basic laboratory services.
Lack of treatment resources	Few treatment options if first-line medications fail or aren't tolerated. Even first-line agents may not be available in some regions.
Stigma[2]	Fear of drawing further attention to the seizures may result in an unwillingness to seek care. Health care workers may avoid providing care to people with epilepsy, given fears of stigma by association, particularly in regions where contagion beliefs regarding epilepsy care common.
Lack of social support[2,3,7]	Devalued persons with epilepsy may not have sufficient social supports to seek care consistently.

community leaders, and most of all people with epilepsy who are actively struggling with the barriers.

DATA GATHERING

Developing or expanding epilepsy care services requires careful planning and input from stakeholders in the health care system. As neurologists, we may simply assume this is a reasonable health care priority. However, this is not always a safe assumption. Recognize that any program must eventually be self-sustaining. And therefore, the program must have enough value to warrant eventual support within a system that is probably chronically underfunded and that encompasses many other competing health care needs. Eventually, any investment in epilepsy care entails a lost opportunity to invest in some other aspect of care. One must ask the key question: Is epilepsy a significant enough problem in this community, given the other health burdens present, to warrant long-term investment?

This is not a trivial question. But before taking the issue to key stakeholders, some objective data is required to assess the true burden of the disease in the population. The most obvious measure of the epilepsy burden in a population is the prevalence of epilepsy. Standard methods have been described that are ideal for epidemiologic purposes.[19] But the burden of epilepsy cannot be captured in a simple prevalence number. One must consider a far broader range of epilepsy-related morbidity and mortality to appreciate and express the full burden of disease (Table 2).

Formal studies to quantify the burden of disease may offer some academic currency and open doors to extramural funding opportunities. But even simple, hospital-based studies may offer data and insights into the burden of disease in a region sufficient to guide decision-making regarding resource allocation. For example, if your hospital has a busy burn center, consider a study to determine the proportion of burn victims who were burned during a seizure. If the number is substantial, then resources presently allocated to the burn center might be partially directed to epilepsy care, with the goal of burn preventions. Improving epilepsy care has been associated with a decrease in severe burns in some regions.

Small, hospital-based studies can yield important information. In the Chikankata catchment area, anecdotal experiences suggested that a substantial burden of neurologic disease was going unrecognized even in the inpatient setting. By conducting a hospital-based, systematic period prevalence study (which had virtually no cost in addition to the time invested by a senior neurology resident), we were able to determine that 10% of hospital admissions were primarily related to a neurologic disorder, and that neurology patients consumed almost one-third of the intensive care unit bed-days.[5] These data allowed those of us interested in expanding neurologic services to capture the attention of hospital administration, which had previously considered neurologic diseases to be esoteric problems irrelevant

TABLE 2

MEASURES OF EPILEPSY MORBIDITY AND MORTALITY

Aspect	Measure
Epidemiologic	Prevalence*
	Incidence
	Treatment gap
Health-related quality of life	KENQOL[27]
	SF-36[9]
	WHOQOL[23]
Functional status	DALY[11]
	Karnofsky score
Epilepsy-related physical morbidity	Burns
	Drowning
	Fractures
Social morbidity (largely mediated by stigma)	Loss of educational opportunities
	Loss of marital opportunities
Economic morbidity	Related to lack of education
	Incapacity to work due to social or physical disability

*Consider age-specific prevalence, given the impact of loss of work-related productivity in young adults.

TABLE 3

STAKEHOLDERS TO CONSULT WHEN DEVELOPING EPILEPSY CARE SERVICES

Entity	Example
Health care providers[16]	Physicians
	Clinical officers
	Nurses
	Community health workers
	Traditional birth attendants
Other healers[1,13]	Traditional healers
	Evangelical healers
Administrators	Hospital administrators
	Nursing directors
	Local representatives of the ministry of health
	Pharmacy directors
	Medical records personnel
Community leaders	Headmen
	Elected community representatives
	Elders
	Church leaders
	Respected businessmen or -women
People effected by epilepsy[21]	People with epilepsy
	Parents of children with epilepsy
	Family members of people with epilepsy
Other important social entities	Clerics
	Teachers
	Employers
	Police

in a large rural bush hospital. Among all the conditions identified, epilepsy appeared to be one that was particularly under-recognized and undertreated. We were then able to leverage matching funds from the administration to conduct a door-to-door survey to determine the prevalence of epilepsy in the region. We found that, although our catchment area of 65,000 people had only 32 individuals with epilepsy registered at the hospital's chronic disease registry, more than 1,000 people with epilepsy eventually came forward for treatment.[8] This deluge of previously under-recognized disease treatable with medications generally available and by existing health care workers allowed us to establish local support for the development of an epilepsy care team.

INVOLVING KEY STAKEHOLDERS

If, after consideration of the full range of epilepsy-related morbidity and mortality in the region of interest, epilepsy appears to be a significant public health problem, further plans to develop or expand neurologic services should only be undertaken in consultation with relevant stakeholders. Only if individuals who are part of the health care system *and* potential recipients of services are part of the process of service development will those services be appropriate for the circumstances and environment. See Table 3 for considerations of who potential stakeholders might be; this is not a comprehensive list.

The importance of persuading these stakeholders to guide the priorities of any evolving epilepsy care program cannot be overestimated. For any program to thrive in a sustainable fashion, many different groups must have a vested interest in the well-being of the program, and the program must be developed in a way that recognizes the most urgent problems at hand. A shared partnership with the community may entail delaying or even abandoning one's own academic interests (e.g., an EEG monitoring unit) for something recognized as more important from the community's perspective (e.g., a community-based care program). If an evolving program can offer what is most needed from the stakeholders' perspective, opportunities usually become available to pursue more academic interests, but these interests must be put in perspective. Even if outside funding is available to support the more academic and/or research-oriented questions, research programs that fail to take into consideration the needs of the community will eventually flounder and/or engender suspicion and animosity in the community under study.

Traditional healers are perhaps one of the most critical groups of stakeholders frequently ignored when health system planning is undertaken in developing countries.[1] Historically, the relationship between traditional healers and physicians has been one of animosity and criticism. However, traditional healers play an important social role, even if their treatments offer little therapeutic benefit (and that has not been formally studied in most instances). In developing regions, physicians and traditional healers witness each others' iatrogenic complications and failures on an almost daily basis. Given that most people with epilepsy in developing countries seek care from healers at least initially and often exclusively, we must work to develop more interactive and collaborative relationships with these care providers if we wish to reduce the treatment gap in areas with the greatest need.

As physicians, most of us have received little training and have even less experience in developing working relationships with such a diverse group of individuals. This is doubly compounded if the physician in question is an expatriate or non-native health care provider. Serious consideration should be given to soliciting assistance from more experienced individuals. Consider the value of involving a sociologist, anthropologist, or health services researcher as you engage key stakeholders. Good intentions for meaningful exchange can be entirely lost if the venue or circumstance for a meeting inadvertently offend or imply a lack of respect for those involved. There may be reasons to meet with some stakeholders separately. And the need to avoid proselytizing is critical. The goal is not to convince stakeholders of your perspective, but to gather theirs.

CARE PLANS

Once health care delivery priorities have been established in a region, one must consider how to deliver those services. This entails consideration of the actual plan for health care providers' interactions with patients as well as developing algorithms for individual care plans. In resource-limited settings, it is neither feasible nor desirable to anticipate that epilepsy care will be primarily provided by a neurologist. It may not even be possible to expect physician-level input into epilepsy care for the vast majority of patients. The skill and training level of the care provider who will diagnose and then provide chronic treatment to people with epilepsy must be determined by the existing capacity of the health care system. It is essential element to assure that health care providers who are likely to initially encounter people with epilepsy and/or people with epilepsy-related injuries are capable of recognizing the condition when they encounter it. Whether these individuals then go on to treat the condition or refer to someone with more expertise will depend on the geographic and fiscal feasibility of such a referral system. Initial programs for expanding epilepsy care may need to focus on expanding the diagnostic skills of health care providers on the front line and streamlining the referral process when they encounter someone with epilepsy.[12,18,24,26,28,30]

Once stable treatment regimens are established for patients, their care should be transferred back to the health care provider most financially and geographically accessible to them, if they are to be expected to maintain adherence to drug therapy over the long term. Clear, written communications to the health care provider who will assume care of the patient is critical. Epilepsy educational materials for physicians and clinical officers in developing regions are available at low-cost through several routes.[15,17]

Although algorithms for health care provision are not popular in much of the developed world, such clearly delineated and simplified care plans are often critical for health care provision in developing regions, where resources and health care expertise are limited. As much as possible, such epilepsy care algorithms should be evidence-based. When an evidence-base is lacking, expert opinion should be acquired. Ideally, an expert panel should be consulted if an epilepsy care algorithms is being developed that will be applied to a large population. E-mail and Internet access have improved substantially in the past few years, and establishing such an expert panel may now be possible with a minimum of fiscal resources. One must not neglect the importance of including local experts who function within the health care system of interest. Critical aspects of routine nursing and pharmacy practices may be inadvertently ignored if only outside opinions are sought. Key stakeholders (purchasers of medications for the public health care system, hospital administration) must also be included in this process.

Many developing regions may only be able to offer phenobarbitone to the majority of people with epilepsy. If second-line agents are not routinely available, some rational process should be put into place to determine criteria whereby people are placed on second-line agents. Inevitably, a two-tiered system will be in place in most health care systems in which people with resources can purchase drugs within the private sector. But within the public health system, medical criteria should determine the allocation of drugs with limited availability. Predetermined criteria for placing patients on a second- or third-line agent will assist health care providers in decision-making and assure some social equity. Unfortunately, within the private sector, inappropriate utilization of complex drug regimens may be unavoidable.[29]

ACQUIRING RESOURCES

Developing, enhancing, or expanding neurologic service in a less developed environment goes beyond simply working as a clinician in a one-on-one patient interaction. Services must include clinical care, infrastructural development of the health system, efforts at outreach, education for health care providers and the lay public, and research. Because the limited budgets of developing countries cannot even sustain the essentials for basic care, optimal expansion of neurologic services will require accessing resources beyond those available through public health funds, although partnership with the appropriate health authorities and appropriate allocations for neurologic disorders should be sought. Many options for accessing additional resources exist for those keen clinicians and/or administrator willing to explore these routes (Table 4).

Developing relationships with clinicians and organizations outside your own region or country can serve as a great source of intellectual stimulation and often results in productive collaborations that benefit both parties. Clinicians from developed regions with an interest in working in less developed regions often struggle to make appropriate contacts and identify opportunities to offer their services. The same is true of researchers. Fostering these relationships at every level will help to build bridges that can lead to future opportunities for expanding neurologic care.

TABLE 4

POTENTIAL SOURCES FOR ADDITIONAL REVENUES AND RESOURCES

Source	Approach
Clinical revenues	An allocated day or half-day for private-pay patients, with revenues directed to the upgrade of clinical service.
Churches or philanthropies in wealthier countries	Fundraising when you are abroad or encouraging visitors who become familiar with your operation to do the same on returning home
Local businesses	Approach local businesses for support.
Educational grants	Seek funding through educational grants: www.cos.com www.grantsnet.com www.WFNeurology.org
Research grants	Seek funding through research grants: www.cos.com www.grantsnet.com www.wellcome.ac.uk www.nih.gov
International collaborations	Contact researchers conducting studies of interest to you: www.ilae.epilepsy.org www.ibe-epilepsy.org

In terms of accessing resources for a growing epilepsy care program, consider clinical revenue streams. Where neurologic expertise is limited and concentrated in academic medical centers, private patients are often willing to pay substantial sums to avoid long waits and queues. Although such services shouldn't be offered to the extent that it is detrimental to publicly available services, setting aside some time for such private patients and applying the resulting revenues to care expansion is one option. Where civil servant salaries are quite low, academic specialists may already provide private services to augment their own salaries to a reasonable level. Consider then that visiting volunteer specialists who do not have work permits might be able to provide services in exchange for donations or other services. Or, possibly, such visitors may assist in the established private clinics, with the additional revenues being directed to expansion of epilepsy care services.

Visiting clinicians and interested individuals who become familiar with your program's goals may also serve as fundraisers and advocates. Developing a simple printed brochure that outlines your activities, goals, and fund-raiser campaign and that can be given out freely may help encapsulate your work in a marketable way. Such materials may even be provided to private patients and representatives of local businesses with philanthropic tendencies.

Funding opportunities for educational and research programs can serve as an important source of revenue for building infrastructure, hiring staff, and purchasing equipment. If one has Internet access, several search engines are quite helpful at identifying potential funding sources. Also, make certain to make inquiries to your local, regional and national medical programs. If you do not have experience writing proposals, this may be another opportunity for collaborations with international colleagues. For example, if you read an article describing research that interests you, consider contacting the investigators. Contact information, usually including an e-mail address, is provided in most journal articles. Never doubt that your expertise, experience, interests, and environment offer a great deal to potential collaborators.

ACKNOWLEDGMENT

This work was supported by grants NIH K23NS046086 and NIH R21NS48060.

SUMMARY AND CONCLUSIONS

The global burden of epilepsy is concentrated in resources poor regions with limited healthcare services. Substantial socioeconomic issues impact the quality of care and quality of life for people with epilepsy, particularly in developing regions. To improve epilepsy care delivery, it is imperative to understand the barriers to care delivery and care-seeking in the local environments and develop pragmatic approaches to overcoming these barriers. Accessing resources for optimizing care can be facilitated by acquiring data regarding the magnitude and consequences of epilepsy as well as the potential cost-effectiveness of treatment. Data dissemination and education of policy makers is paramount. Collaborative partnerships to develop local priorities for care and research require meaningful exchange between clinicians, researchers and key stakeholders. For successful and sustainable programs, community representatives must be included in such endeavors. Unique partnerships between clinicians and scientists in developed and less developed regions will be required to tackle the global problem of epilepsy in resource-poor regions where ~80% of people with epilepsy reside.

References

1. Baskind R, Birbeck G. Epilepsy care in Zambia: a study of traditional healers. *Epilepsia.* 2005;46(7):1121–1126.
2. Baskind R, Birbeck GL. Epilepsy-associated stigma in sub-Saharan Africa: the social landscape of a disease. *Epilepsy Behav.* 2005;7(1):68–73.
3. Birbeck GL. Barriers to care for patients with neurologic disease in rural Zambia. *Arch Neurol.* 2000;57(3):414–417.
4. Birbeck GL. Seizures in rural Zambia. *Epilepsia.* 2000;41(3):277–281.
5. Birbeck GL. Neurologic disease in a rural Zambian hospital. *Trop Doct.* 2001;31(2):82–85.
6. Birbeck GL, Kalichi E. Health services in Zambia: the primary healthcare workers' perspective. *Trop Doct.* 2003; Accepted 1/17/03.
7. Birbeck GL, Kalichi EM. Famine-associated AED toxicity in rural Zambia. *Epilepsia.* 2003;44(8):1127.
8. Birbeck GL, Kalichi EM. Epilepsy prevalence in rural Zambia: A door-to-door survey. *Trop Med Int Health.* 2004;9(1):92–95.
9. Birbeck GL, Kim S, Hays RD, et al. Quality of life measures in epilepsy: how well can they detect change over time? *Neurology.* 2000;54(9):1822–1827.
10. Birbeck GL, Munsat T. Neurologic services in sub-Saharan Africa: a case study among Zambian primary healthcare workers. *J Neurol Sci.* 2002;200(1–2):75–78.
11. Chisholm D. Cost-effectiveness of first-line antiepileptic drug treatments in the developing world: a population-level analysis. *Epilepsia.* 2005;46(5):751–759.
12. Coleman R, Gill G, Wilkinson D. Noncommunicable disease management in resource-poor settings: a primary care model from rural South Africa. *Bull World Health Organ.* 1998;76(6):633–640.
13. Danesi MA, Adetunji JB. Use of alternative medicine by patients with epilepsy: A survey of 265 epileptic patients in a developing country. *Epilepsia.* 1994;35(2):344–351.
14. Diop AG, de Boer HM, Mandlhate C, et al. The global campaign against epilepsy in Africa. *Acta Trop.* 2003;87(1):149–159.
15. Engel J, Birbeck G, Diop A, et al. *Epilepsy: Global Issues for the Practicing Neurologist.* New York: Demos; 2005.
16. Ferri C, Chisholm D, Van Ommeren M, et al. Resource utilisation for neuropsychiatric disorders in developing countries: A multinational Delphi consensus study. *Soc Psychiatry Psychiatr Epidemiol.* 2004;39(3):218–227.
17. GCAE. *Epilepsy: A Manual for Medical and Clinical Officers in Africa,* 2nd ed. Geneva: WHO; 2002.
18. Gourie-Devi M, Satishchandra P, Gururaj G. Epilepsy control program in India: A district model. *Epilepsia.* 2003;44(Suppl 1):58–62.
19. International League Against Epilepsy. Guidelines for epidemiologic studies on epilepsy. Commission on epidemiology and prognosis, International League Against Epilepsy. *Epilepsia.* 1993;34(4):592–596.
20. IOM. *Neurological and Psychiatric Disorders: Meeting the Challenge in the Developing World.* Washington DC: Institute of Medicine; 2001.
21. Kendall S, Thompson D, Couldridge L. The information needs of carers of adults diagnosed with epilepsy. *Seizure.* 2004;13(7):499–508.
22. Leonardi M, Ustun TB. The global burden of epilepsy. *Epilepsia.* 2002;43(Suppl 6):21–25.
23. Liou HH, Chen RC, Chen CC, et al. Health related quality of life in adult patients with epilepsy compared with a general reference population in Taiwan. *Epilepsy Res.* 2005;64(3):151–159.
24. Mani KS, Rangan G, Srinivas HV, et al. Epilepsy control with phenobarbital or phenytoin in rural south India: The Yelandur study. *Lancet.* 2001: 28;357(9265):1316–1320.
25. Murthy JM. Some problems and pitfalls in developing countries. *Epilepsia.* 2003;44 (Suppl 1):38–42.
26. Nimaga K, Desplats D, Doumbo O, et al. Treatment with phenobarbital and monitoring of epileptic patients in rural Mali. *Bull World Health Organ.* 2002;80(7):532–537.
27. Nyandieka LN, Bowden A, Wanjau J, et al. Managing a household survey: A practical example from the KENQOL survey. *Kenya Quality of Life. Health Policy Plan.* 2002;17(2):207–212.
28. Placencia M, Sander JW, Shorvon SD, et al. Antiepileptic drug treatment in a community health care setting in northern Ecuador: A prospective 12-month assessment. *Epilepsy Res.* 1993;14(3):237–244.
29. Radhakrishnan K, Nayak SD, Kumar SP, et al. Profile of antiepileptic pharmacotherapy in a tertiary referral center in South India: A pharmacoepidemiologic and pharmacoeconomic study. *Epilepsia.* 1999;40(2):179–185.
30. Scott RA, Lhatoo SD, Sander JW. The treatment of epilepsy in developing countries: where do we go from here? *Bull World Health Organ.* 2001;79(4):344–351.
31. WHO. *Atlas: Epilepsy Care in the World 2005.* Geneva: WHO; 2005.

CHAPTER 301 ■ COMPARISON OF DIFFERENT SYSTEMS AND THE BURDEN OF EPILEPSY

MATILDE LEONARDI AND CHONG TIN TAN

INTRODUCTION

The aim of this chapter is to compare information and data collected on epilepsy around the world and to find a means of comparing them so as to produce indications for further work.

Several authors in the preceding chapters have highlighted the national situation on epilepsy and epilepsy care. However, despite differences, it is important to define ways to overcome these discrepancies and to note the advancement of care and research that could enhance the care of people with epilepsy worldwide.

The past 10 years have been important for progress in epilepsy care, and many initiatives and much research have contributed to raise a lot of attention on the burden of epilepsy.

THE MAIN PILLARS FOR CHANGE IN THE FIELD OF EPILEPSY

Although some traditional epidemiologic data reported in the chapters in this section do not show major changes in epilepsy course, several factors are contributing to change in the care and course of epilepsy worldwide. The main pillars for change could be identified in the following factors: (a) the Global Burden of Disease study and all the research done in the field of summary measures of the population's health; (b) the World Health Organization (WHO), International Bureau for Epilepsy (IBE), and International League Against Epilepsy (ILAE) Campaign on Epilepsy, with the publication of detailed information in the WHO Atlas on Epilepsy in 2005; (c) the publication of the International Classification of Functioning, Disability, and Health (ICF) classification in 2001 and the shift from diagnosis alone to functioning and disability approach to health; and (d) the increasing attention on innovative methodologies to collect information for policy decision making. All these factors will be analyzed here so as to provide a means for future work at the country as well at international level.

THE BURDEN OF EPILEPSY AND THE GLOBAL BURDEN OF DISEASE

The Global Burden of Disease (GBD) 2000 study was carried out by the World Bank in collaboration with the WHO and the Harvard School of Public Health. Three main goals were addressed: To provide information about nonfatal health outcomes, to develop unbiased epidemiologic assessment for major disorders, and to quantify the burden of diseases with a measure that could also be used for cost-effectiveness analysis. The GBS study provided the true magnitude of the long underestimated impact of neurologic disorders. With mortality indicators alone, mental and neurologic disorders have never been ranked in the top ten priority list of public health significance. Demographic changes and epidemiologic transition, as well as changes in family structure, are projecting the burden due to neurologic and psychiatric disorders to increase up to 15% of the global disease burden.[15]

There is a growing need to combine information on mortality and nonfatal health outcomes to represent the health of a population that reflects health expectancies and health gaps. Summary health measures can be used for comparing the health status of different populations and health of populations at different points of time, and for balancing priorities between fatal and nonfatal outcomes. These are measures that combine information on mortality and nonfatal health outcomes to represent the health of a particular population as a single number. The GBD study provided the DALY (Disability Adjusted Life Year), a measure that added disability to mortality in the evaluation of the burden of diseases. The allocation of limited resources for health care should be based on the relative importance (or burden) of different conditions to the health of the nation. Mortality as major public health indicator has had the effect of limiting the attention given to highly prevalent, seriously disabling but nonfatal disorders. Use of traditional measurement methods has led, in fact, to a serious underestimation of the relative importance of neurologic disorders worldwide, because they rarely cause death and because several of them produce severe and long-term disability but not death. The number of deaths does not take into consideration the nonfatal outcome of illness, and prevalence rates do not take into consideration the severity and duration of disability produced by a disease. There is also increasing attention being given to the shift from communicable diseases to chronic, noncommunicable diseases: The so-called "epidemiologic transition," which is also related to the increase of life expectancy.

Diagnosis alone does not predict service needs, length of hospitalization, level of care, or functional outcomes. The occurrence of a disorder is not an accurate predictor of receipt of disability benefits, work performance, return to work, or likelihood of social integration. This means that if we use a medical classification of diagnosis alone (e.g., the International Classification of Diseases [ICD]) or the ILAE classification, we will not have the information we need for health planning and management purposes. Neurologic disorders contribute substantially to the overall disease burden of developed and developing societies, but this is generally underestimated by the public health community.[27]

Epilepsy is one of the most common serious disorders of the brain, affecting about 50 million people worldwide. Epilepsy accounts for 1% of the global burden of disease; 80% of the burden of epilepsy is in the developing world, where in some areas 80% to 90% of people with epilepsy receive no treatment at all.[30] It is clear that epilepsy is a major public health problem and that it is important to assess its burden as well its cost to persons and to societies so that health care priorities can be set in a rational way. To highlight differences, we analyzed common epidemiologic data as also reported in previous chapters and through literature assessment.

As stated in *Epilepsy: Out of the Shadows* background booklet, "The suffering and the disability caused by the disease are physical and psychosocial, is bringing a huge burden to people with epilepsy, their families and society at large."[9]

The burden of epilepsy is also strongly associated with significant psychological and social consequences for everyday living. This has been clearly highlighted in the previous chapters of this section. People with hidden disabilities such as epilepsy are among the most vulnerable in any society. While their vulnerability may be partly attributed to the disorder itself, the particular stigma associated with epilepsy brings a susceptibility of its own. Stigmatization leads to discrimination, and people with epilepsy experience prejudicial and discriminatory behavior in many spheres of life and across many cultures.[31]

People with epilepsy experience violations and restrictions of both their civil and human rights. Civil rights violations, such as unequal access to health and life insurance or prejudicial weighting of health insurance provisions; withholding of the right to obtain a driving licence; and limitations to the right to enter particular occupations, certain legal agreements, and in some parts of the world even marriage, are severely aggravated by epilepsy. Discrimination against people with epilepsy in the workplace and in respect of access is not uncommon for many. Violations of human rights are often more subtle and include social ostracism, being overlooked for promotion at work, and denial of the right to participate in many of the social activities taken for granted by others in the community. For example, ineligibility for a driving licence frequently imposes restrictions on social participation and choice of employment.[31]

THE WORLD HEALTH ORGANIZATION–INTERNATIONAL BUREAU FOR EPILEPSY–INTERNATIONAL LEAGUE AGAINST EPILEPSY GLOBAL CAMPAIGN AGAINST EPILEPSY

The problems related to provision of care and treatment of people with epilepsy are too complex to be solved by individual organizations; therefore, the three leading international organizations working in the field of epilepsy (the WHO, IBE, and ILAE) joined forces to create the Global Campaign Against Epilepsy. The campaign aims to provide better information about epilepsy and its consequences and to assist governments and those concerned with epilepsy to reduce the burden of the disorders. More than 90 countries worldwide have been involved in the campaign.[31]

Regional conferences have been organized in all WHO regions to raise awareness on the public health impact of epilepsy, and a questionnaire was developed in order to make an inventory of country resources for epilepsy worldwide. Regional reports were developed and the main result of this effort was the publication in 2005 of the *Atlas of Epilepsy Care in the World.* The Global Campaign also had some demonstration projects that consisted of assisting countries in the development of their national epilepsy programs. Much of the information about data comparability on epilepsy has been collected in the *Atlas,* and this chapter summarizes some of the main results.[30] This initiative and its results could be considered another pillar to analyze information on epilepsy from different countries in a different way. The results of the WHO/IBE/ILAE Campaign allow a detailed evaluation of differences between developed and developing countries in several epilepsy indicators.

COMPARISON OF DIFFERENT SYSTEMS: UNDERLYING FACTORS FOR REGIONAL DIFFERENCES AND SALIENT FINDINGS

Epidemiologic indicators needed to construct the diagram of each disease are several and can be listed as prevalence, incidence, mean age of onset, course, natural history, duration, severity breakdown, mortality, and impact of treatment. These indicators are the starting point for data comparison as well as for highlighting information gaps. Salient findings on incidence, prevalence, treatment gap, and socioeconomic data are reported in this chapter as they are crucial to highlighting country differences in the field of epilepsy. While data on incidence, prevalence, and treatment gap are available in several publications and are also reported in this section in detail, it is important to also report here some of the data that have been recently published in the WHO *Atlas*[30] that cover a broader spectrum of items and that are a useful indicator of epilepsy burden and care worldwide.

THE PREVALENCE OF EPILEPSY

The number of people with epilepsy is high in most regions of the world, and 43,704,000 people with epilepsy are reported from 108 countries covering 85.4% of the world population. The mean number of people with epilepsy varies across regions: The prevalence per 1,000 population is 8.93 from 105 responding countries. It is 12.59 and 11.29 in the Americas and Africa, respectively, 9.97 in WHO South East Asia, 9.4 in the Eastern Mediterranean, 8.23 in Europe, and 3.66 in the Western Pacific.[30] The mean number of people with epilepsy per 1,000 population ranges from 7.99 in the high-income countries to 9.5 in the low-income countries.[6,7] The overall prevalence of epilepsy ranges from 2.7 to 41 per 1,000 population, though in the majority of reports the rate of active epilepsy is in the range 4 to 8 per 1,000.[8] The prevalence of active epilepsy is generally lower in industrialized countries than in developing countries, which may reflect a lower prevalence of selected risk factors. In industrialized countries, the prevalence of epilepsy is lower in infancy and tends to increase thereafter, with the highest rate occurring in elderly people.[8] Where available, age-specific prevalence rates of lifetime and active epilepsy from developing countries tend to be higher in the second (254 vs. 148 per 1,000) and third decades of life (94 vs. 145 per 1,000).[1] The differences between industrialized and developing countries may be mostly explained by the differing distribution of the risk factors and by the shorter life expectancy in the latter. Prevalence of epilepsy, as incidence, tends to be higher in men. Socioeconomic background has been found to affect the frequency of epilepsy reports in both industrialized and developing countries, in which prevalence rates have been shown to be greater in the rural compared with the urban context or in the lower compared with the higher socioeconomic classes.[17]

THE INCIDENCE OF EPILEPSY

The annual incidence of unprovoked seizure is 33 to 198 per 100,000, and the incidence of epilepsy is 23 to 190 per

100,000.[10] The overall incidence of epilepsy in Europe and North America ranges from 24 and 53 per 100,000 per year, respectively. In studies from Africa and South America, the peak incidence of epilepsy occurs in young adults, and the dramatic increase in incidence in the elderly has not been identified. It's similar to the patterns of incidence, and therefore risks for epilepsy are different in these populations.

The incidence in children is eventually higher and even more variable, ranging from 25 to 840 per 100,000 per year, most of the differences being explained by the differing populations at risk and by the study design. In developing countries, the incidence of the disease is higher than that in industrialized countries and is up to 190 per 100,000 (the higher incidence of epilepsy may also be explained by the different structure of the populations at risk, which is characterized by a predominant distribution of young individuals and a short life expectancy).

In industrialized countries, epilepsy tends to affect mostly the individuals at the two extremes of the age spectrum. The peak in the elderly is not detected in developing countries, where the disease peaks in the 10- to 20-year-old age group.[1] The incidence of epilepsy and unprovoked seizure has been reported to be higher in men than in women in both industrialized and developing countries.[30]

The incidence of epilepsy is higher in the lower socioeconomic classes. This assumption is supported by the comparison between industrialized and developing countries and by the comparison, within the same population, of people of different ethnic origin.[21]

Several recent studies provide incidence from developing countries. An incidence of epilepsy that is considerably higher than that reported in industrialized countries (114 per 100,000 person-years) has been reported from rural area of Chile.[11] A study in Tanzania reported the incidence of epilepsy to be 77 per 100,000. These data are three times the incidence reported in industrialized countries in which similar definitions have been used.[18] In studies in France and Rochester, Minnesota, at least half of newly occurring afebrile seizures do not fulfil criteria for epilepsy. Nonetheless, the incidence of epilepsy may likely be higher in developing countries then in industrialized countries.[8]

TREATMENT OF EPILEPSY: GAPS AND SERVICES

Worldwide, the proportion of patients with epilepsy who at any given time remain untreated is large, and is greater than 80% in most low-income countries.[19]

The size of this treatment gap reflects either a failure to identify cases or a failure to deliver treatment. In most situations, however, both factors will apply. Inadequate case finding and treatment have various causes, some of which are specific to low-income countries. They include people's attitudes and beliefs, government health policies and priorities (or the lack of them), treatment costs and drug availability, and the attitude, knowledge, and practice of health workers.[31]

Although most epileptic syndromes cannot be prevented, epilepsy can be treated effectively in the majority of cases. The most common treatment is medication, but brain surgery and, very rarely, vagal nerve stimulation may be used as alternatives in some patients failing to achieve seizure control by medication.[4] Therapeutic drug monitoring is available in 45.1% in Africa, 54.6% in the Western Pacific, 55.6% in WHO South East Asia, 85.7% in the Eastern Mediterranean, 93.3% in Europe, and 95.8% in the Americas. Neuropsychological services are available in 37% of low-income countries. Such facilities are present in 88.6% of high-income countries.[30] In developing countries there is often also limited access to antiepileptic drugs (AEDs), particularly new AEDs; irregular supply of drugs; and poor access to investigations such as electroencephalographic (EEG), computed tomography (CT) brain scan, magnetic resonance imaging (MRI), therapeutic drug monitoring, long-term video-EEG monitoring, and single photon emission computed tomography (SPECT). The patients often have to pay for the medications and investigations out of pocket, which can be astronomical when compare with the family income.

There is also a relative lack of use of epilepsy surgery. In 25% to 30% of people with epilepsy the seizure cannot be controlled with drugs. Epilepsy surgery is a safe and effective alternative treatment in selected cases. Investment in epilepsy surgery centers, even in the poorest regions, could greatly reduce the economic and human burden of epilepsy. There is a marked treatment gap with respect to epilepsy surgery, however, even in industrialized countries. In a survey of epilepsy surgery in Asia, 80% of surgery was done in Japan and South Korea, although the two countries account for less than 10% of the Asian populations surveyed.[12]

Epilepsy surgery is not available in 88.6% in Africa, 68.2% in the Western Pacific, 66.7% in WHO South East Asia, 50% in the Americas and the Eastern Mediterranean, and 33.3% in Europe. Epilepsy surgery is not available in 87% of low-income countries. The facility for epilepsy surgery is also absent in 34.3% of high-income countries.[30]

EPILEPSY CARE AND HEALTH PROFESSIONALS

It is difficult to quantify the number of medical professionals involved predominantly in epilepsy care. The figures reported in WHO's *Atlas* are based on best estimates by the respondents. Information about the distribution of the medical professionals in countries is not available, but the majority is likely to be concentrated in urban areas. The median number of neurologic nurses per 1,000,000 population in Europe involved in epilepsy care is 0.7 for low-income countries; it is 1.7 for higher middle-income and 1.1% for high-income countries. The median number of neurologic nurses per 1,000,000 population is 1.9 in Europe and 0.3 in WHO South East Asia.

No facility for training in epileptology exists in countries in WHO South East Asia, while such facilities exists in only 2.6% of the countries in Africa, 6.7% in the Eastern Mediterranean, 17.4% in the Western Pacific, 20.8% in the Americas, and 31.8% in Europe. Few studies report the number of health professionals devoted to epilepsy in many of the developing countries. As is the case in Nigeria, the primary care is manned by medical assistants who do not have the medications or skills in managing epilepsy. At the tertiary care level, there is scarcity of neurologists, even more so pediatric neurologists, and epileptologists. This is worse for regions outside the big cities and for public patients. For example, there are only 25 neurologists and 10 neurosurgeons in Nigeria, with 128 million people (see Chapter 295). All 15 neurologists practicing in the public health sector in Senegal, with 12 million people, are in the capital city of Dakar (see Chapter 297). In India, only 10% of the medical workers are employed by the government.[16] The lack of trained specialists and medical facilities needs to be seen in the context of severe deficiencies in health delivery that apply not only to epilepsy, but also to the whole range of medical conditions. Training medical and paramedical personnel and providing the necessary investigatory and treatment facilities will require tremendous effort and financial expenditures and will take time to achieve. A lack of involvement of paramedical professionals such as neuropsychologists, specialist nurses, occupational therapists, and educators in the care of epilepsy has also been noted in the epilepsy care of the East.[20] Nonscientific concepts of causes and treatment of epilepsy are common. For example, in Nigeria, dualist natural and supernatural terms to explain illness are prevalent, with traditional herbal remedy strongly preferred over conventional antiepileptic drugs in the rural areas (see Chapter 296). A significant proportion of countries does not have professional or patient-based epilepsy societies. Even when these are present, they are often limited to large urban centers. For example, a nationwide epilepsy society for both professionals and patients was formed in China only in 2005. With limited resources, research is of low priority, with limited data related to epilepsy.

SOCIOECONOMIC BURDEN AND COSTS OF EPILEPSY

The lack of uniformity in the available studies on the cost of illness of epilepsy makes it difficult to compare cost figures from different studies. Some findings, however, can be summarized.

Many socioeconomic factors underlie the differences in care of epilepsy between the developed and developing countries. A low level of general education and high illiteracy is seen in some developing countries. For example, in India, the national literacy rate in 2001 was 65.5%, and 54.3% for females (see Chapter 294). The limited government resources generally are made worse by medical care being considered low priority by some governments. For example, Indian state budgets allocate only 2.3% of their money to health care.[16] The per capita expenditure on health, family welfare, water supply, and sanitation during 2002 to 2007 is about U.S. $2.53 per year (see Chapter 294). As such, in many developing countries, the government-subsidized health care is limited to hospital bed stay and medical consultation. Medications, surgery, and investigations are borne by the patients directly. Various disability benefits enjoyed by the developed countries are also not available. Difficulties of transport and communication in the remote area posing problems to access to modern health care facilities are also common. Nongovernmental organizations that play a crucial role in public health and awareness raising are rare in many parts of the world.

These differences are reflected in many aspects of health care structure and management of epilepsy in developing countries. It is thus not surprising that a large treatment gap for epilepsy has been reported in many developing countries, particularly the rural areas, with a large number of undiagnosed and untreated patients. For example, the treatment gap for China was 63%.[24]

Economic assessments of the national burden of epilepsy have been conducted in a number of high-income countries[2] and in India, all of which have clearly shown the significant economic implications the disorder has in terms of health care service needs, premature mortality, and lost work productivity. The Indian study calculated that the total cost per case of these disease consequences for epilepsy amounted to U.S. $344 per year (equivalent to 88% of average income per capita) and the total cost for the estimated 5 million cases in India was equivalent to 0.5% of the gross national product.[23]

As part of a wider WHO cost-effectiveness work program,[22] information has been generated concerning the amount of burden averted by the current or scaled-up use of treatment with AEDs, together with estimates of cost and cost effectiveness. Effectiveness was expressed in terms of DALYs averted and costs were expressed in international dollars. Compared with a "do-nothing" scenario (i.e., the untreated natural history of epilepsy), results from nine developing epidemiologic subregions suggest that extending AED treatment coverage to 50% of primary epilepsy cases would avert 150 to 650 DALYs per million population (equivalent to 13% to 40% of the current burden), at an annual cost per case of international $55 to $192. Older first-line AEDs (phenobarbitone, phenytoin) were most cost effective on account of their similar efficacy but lower acquisition cost (International $800 to $2,000 for each DALY averted). In all nine developing regions, the cost of securing one extra healthy year of life was less than average per capita income. Extending coverage further to 80% or even 95% of the target population would evidently avert more of burden still, and would remain an efficient strategy despite the large-scale investment in manpower, training, and drug supply/distribution that would be required to implement such a program.[31]

In Europe, a separate budget for epilepsy care and services is present in only 6.4% of the responding countries. Private insurance and private foundations constitute only 1.9% and 1%, respectively, of the primary method of financing. While social insurance is the primary method of financing in 55.6% and 56% of higher middle-income and high-income countries, respectively, none of the low-income countries employs it as the primary method of financing. A study by Ekman and Forsgren on the cost of epilepsy in Europe allowed one to see regional differences and provided an estimate of the economic burden of epilepsy.[4]

FUNCTIONING AND DISABILITY IN EPILEPSY AND THE INTERNATIONAL CLASSIFICATION OF FUNCTIONING, DISABILITY, AND HEALTH CLASSIFICATION

As shown, the knowledge about prevalence, incidence, socioeconomic burden, and prognosis of epilepsy is still limited because of the methodologic weakness of many studies. Data on epilepsy, as well as on several other neuropsychiatric disorders, are still scarce in many parts of the world and inconsistent because of the sampling frames and how samples are defined.

Uncertainty about the prevalence distribution as well as about the variation of severity of epilepsy reflects the limitation of instruments for classifying it in a comparable manner across populations and the limitations in the information available to classify, beyond the diagnostic classification, the severity and, mostly, the disability of the disorder.[15]

Up-to-date international comparable data about functioning and disability are simply not available. The primary reason for this is that different countries, for different purposes, define disability differently. As a recent European Commission study on definition of disability in Europe has shown, data on disability are not consistently gathered because some countries define disability in terms of performance levels in employment or other social activities. In the employment sector specifically, for example, coordinated policy across Europe has been undermined by the inability to collect comparable data about rates of disability and employment.[5] As a rule, disability population surveys focus on a limited number of functional domains (e.g., activities of daily living [ADLs]) and ask questions about a limited number of impairments, making it difficult to identify new and emerging populations of persons with disabilities, such as, for example, those associated with HIV, depression, and substance use disorders. Furthermore, often a priori and arbitrary thresholds for identifying impairments are provided, without any evidence of prevalence levels. Finally, disability surveys ask questions that are not easily or directly linked to data from population health surveys, so there is no obvious way of linking health conditions, such as diseases or injuries, to impairments, nor to identify the role of environmental factors in limiting, or expanding, levels of participation across the range of normal activities. It is clear that at the moment, it is almost impossible to evaluate the impact of either demographic changes (such as aging) or social change (such as new legislation, policy change, or changes in lifestyles) on disability.[13]

Though there are international disability data gathering efforts by OECD and UNSTAT, these efforts merely reproduce the same wide disparity in the prevalence rates of disability across countries and regions, created by a lack of a common framework and methodology for defining disability.

The WHO has for several years been aware of this widespread problem of data comparability both in health and disability statistics. Following its mandate for producing standards for international data comparability in the health area, the WHO began as early as 1974 to supplement its ICD International Statistical Classification of Diseases and Related Health Problems[26] with a companion classification of functioning and disability, the International Classification of Impairments, Disability, and Handicap (ICIDH).[25] This classification underwent a revision process that lasted several years. After extensive international field testing, the final version of the International Classification of Functioning, Disability, and Health was endorsed by the World Health Assembly in May 2001. The World Health Organization's ICF has been accepted by 191 countries as the international standard to describe and measure health and disability.[29] The ICF is the product of decades of research, refinement, and testing in an international collaborative setting. Both as a model for structuring health and disability information and as a classification and coding tool for collecting this information, ICF fills the gap in our understanding of disability and its dimensions, causes, and prevalence.

The International Statistical Classification of Diseases and Related Health Problems (ICD-10) and the ICF are the two classifications that currently make up the WHO Family of International Classifications (WHO-FIC).

In the evaluation of differences between countries in the field of epilepsy, the presence of the ICF could be considered as a crucial pillar for a change in perspective. The methodology that ICF proposes to overcome data gaps in epilepsy is a shift from diagnosis alone to functioning and disability.

Disability is a multidimensional phenomenon arising out of an interaction between the individual's health status and the physical and social environment. Disability data, and the instruments to measure them, must reflect this biopsychosocial model of disability. Valid and reliable information are essential to design, implement, or evaluate policies and legislation to combat discrimination and promote social integration and participation and to enhance opportunities.

Data currently being collected, nationally and internationally, embody conceptual confusions, inconsistencies, and ambiguities about disability and the relationship between health conditions, impairments, and environmental factors. What we lack is the knowledge about the level of functioning and disability. The ICF provides the framework for documenting the interaction between health status and environmental features, and the differential distribution of disability among different groups in different contexts.

There is no better conceptual model for the measurement of the types and prevalence of impairments that offers a holistic conception of disability suitable for data collection, clinical measurement, and social policy. Using the ICF framework, the WHO estimates that as much as 500 million healthy life years are lost each year due to disability associated with health conditions. This is more than half the years that are lost annually due to premature death. The ICF provides a common measure about this immense problem and makes possible to collect those vital data in a consistent and internationally comparable manner.

ICF defines disability as "difficulty in functioning at the body, person or societal levels, in one or more life domains, as experienced by an individual with a health condition in interaction with contextual factors." The ICF definition is inclusive of all aspects of disability, captures the interactive dynamic of disability, and acknowledges the equally important contribution of health conditions and environmental factors to disability. In fact, the ICF provides the framework for documenting the interaction between health status and environmental features, and therefore the differential distribution of disability among different groups in different contexts.[13]

This definition includes all aspects of disability, highlights the interactive dynamic nature of disability, and acknowledges the equally important roles of the person's state of health and environmental factors in the production and mediation of the disability experience.

The model described in the ICF will assist in the prediction and understanding of changes in the prevalence and differential distribution of impairments; assess the impact of social, political, demographic, cultural, and environmental factors in the production of disability; and support policy developments for achieving an improved quality of life and equal opportunities for people with disabilities.

Since its endorsement by the World Health Assembly in 2001, the ICF has been applied in a variety of settings at the national and international level and has been translated into 40 languages. ICF-based health and disability surveys have been conducted in many countries worldwide. From these data, population norms can be generated for estimating disability prevalence. At a national level, ICF0-based data sets and questionnaires for census and surveys are being used by numerous countries including Spain, Australia, Canada, Chile, China, Indonesia, Namibia, Nicaragua, and South Africa. Several countries have started the process of streamlining their health and social information standards and legislation within the ICF framework. Development and piloting of ICF-based indicators and reporting systems for use in rehabilitation, home care, age care, and disability evaluation are ongoing in Germany, Italy, Sweden, the Netherlands, the United Kingdom, Australia, Canada, Colombia, India, Mexico, and the United States.

The ICF sets out an internationally comparable language of all dimensions of human functioning at the *body, person, and societal levels*. Difficulties of functioning at the body level, or impairments, can therefore be conceptually and operationally distinguished from difficulties of functioning at the person or societal levels (activity limitations and participation restrictions). The ICF's model of disability is interactive—combining the best of the so-called medical and social models into a fully integrated model. The ICF also contains a classification of environmental factors, that is, the physical, social, and attitudinal factors that, as barriers, contribute to the creation of impairments, activity limitations, and participation restrictions, or as facilitators increase or extend levels of functioning at the body, person, or societal levels. The classification of environmental factors makes it possible, for the first time, to identify, assess, and measure the impact of a person's environment on his or her levels of disability. The underlying theory of the ICF is based on two important principles that directly affect measurement strategies:

1. The principle that disability is a common, indeed universal feature of the human condition, not the mark of a social minority group (universalism)
2. Functioning and disability, both at the population and individual levels, are *continuous* phenomena, matters of "more or less" rather than strict dichotomous categories

Taken together, these principles entail that the measurement of disability must arise from a determination of the range of functioning across all domains, rather than a priori from either self-identification or by allocation into categories merely by the presence of certain bodily impairments such as blindness, deafness, mental retardation, or paralysis.

In the ICF Environmental Factors classification, all discriminatory behaviors and attitudes are included, making it possible for the first time to include questions in surveys and other information-gathering instruments on environmental barriers and facilitators using a common framework that will then make data comparisons more feasible and practical. This might be very relevant for epilepsy because, as previously reported, stigma is still a major issue both in developed and developing countries.

These data can then be compared across countries, populations, and age groups. In addition, the effects of these behaviors and attitudes on individuals' levels of participation can be measured and interventions designed.

POLICY MAKERS AND EPILEPSY

As stated in the previous edition of this book, although the political, economic, and social changes that are occurring globally take many different forms, and although rapid changes in health care delivery are under way in many countries, there is clearly a convergence of ideas toward the fact that health care is part of the glue that holds each society and the international community together, a social good that should be available to all people on the basis of needs.[14] There is a strong interest among policy makers in monitoring the impact of health care measures, reforms, and other interventions by using common cost-effective measures.

The information that health and disability policy makers require—for developing summary measures and other analytic tools for measuring health, which in turn assist in the tasks of proposing and implementing policies and monitoring the performance of policies for subsequent revision—cover at least the following range of data points: Basic prevalence data about diseases and injuries; data about impairments and capacity levels associated with health conditions; data about actual performance levels; data about the presence of environmental barriers and facilitators (as defined and classified in the ICF), and the extent to which these affect observed performance levels.

All these diverse data could not possibly be collected in a single survey or questionnaire, or at least one that could feasibly be put into the field. More plausibly, one can imagine a range of surveys—both on health issues but also on broader social issues such as health determinants, employment, and other social factors—that are coordinated by a common conception of health and disability, and that altogether could collect a substantial portion of these data. Of course, for most countries of the world, even this approach is far beyond available resources. This is leading, then, to the question that is the object of this chapter: What is the state of the art of collecting basic information about epilepsy, the prevalence of its impairments, and their relationship to health outcomes (however construed) on the one hand, and the burden and quality-of-life assessments on the other hand? The interest here has been not merely in listing only what has been done to date, but, more generally, in highlighting the underlying concepts used and the unresolved issues that researchers have faced, either successfully or not, and are facing.

Differences between developed and developing countries are still large; however, there is an increasing recognition that reducing the incidence and severity of disability due to a disease in the population involves modifying the social and physical environment as well as enhancing the level of functioning of the person.

Designed to meet these growing needs, the ICF has potential uses in many sectors, and it is expected that in the future functioning data might allow a better comparison between countries on the burden of the disease and might serve the needs of policy making to improve the quality of life of people with epilepsy worldwide.[15]

SUMMARY AND CONCLUSIONS

This chapter summarized some of the salient findings developed in recent years that allow one to move toward new features in data comparison on epilepsy. Disability data, recently published in the Global Burden of Disease study, allow broader comparability in epilepsy, due to the characteristics of the disease. Traditional epidemiologic information has been supported by a full range of data that are useful for policy development.

The WHO/IBE/ILAE Global Campaign focused on the importance of awareness for filling the gap between developed and developing countries and provided the international community with the *Atlas on Epilepsy* that is showing the path for further work and research.

Finally, after the publication in 2001 of the ICF, it became clear that information about the levels of functioning across all areas of life is essential data for policy purposes. Medical diagnostic data alone do not predict health service needs, length of hospitalization, or level of care required, and the presence of a disease is not an accurate predictor of receipt of disability benefits, work performance, return to work potential, or likelihood of social integration or any other important goal for disability policy that is based on human rights. What is missing are data about the full, lived experience of health, which includes functioning and disability.

Intervention costing, in terms of outlines defined by levels of functioning, will in turn open the door to protocols for comparing the cost-effectiveness of interventions aimed at the individuals (medication, rehabilitation, training) as opposed to those aimed at the environment (e.g., normative, architectural, accessibility, fighting stigma).

One of the most difficult, yet most important, decisions in all areas of disability policy is whether resources are better spent in increasing the functioning levels of the person or in making the environment more accessible and accommodating. In a sense, all of disability policy depends on this incredibly difficult decision. Without reliable and relevant data, however, these decisions are not based on evidence. The overall human rights goals of equality and full participation are not served, and never will be served, without this information. In this sense, the ICF is the most important of all human rights instruments for persons with disabilities.

The ICF in the field of epilepsy can therefore be used to capture and structure holistic and multidimensional data about human functioning for a wide variety of uses, including population surveys, administrative data collection, and clinical assessment. Properly used, it can help us to understand the relationship between impairments and environmental factors that together determine levels of participation in education, employment, and all areas of social involvement.

Only when disability data are collected at the population level in terms of the ICF model of disability will this evidence be available. It is only then that data collected will be relevant to the relationship between environmental, political, social, and cultural factors and the occurrence of impairments. This is a clear indication for future new research in the field of epilepsy.

References

1. Bharucha NE, et al. The epidemiology of epilepsy and its treatment. In: Shorvon S, et al., eds. *The Treatment of Epilepsy*. Blackwell Science; 2004: 21–42.
2. Cockerell OC, et al. The cost of epilepsy in the United Kingdom: an estimation based on the results of two population-based studies. *Epilepsy Res.* 1994;18:249–260.

3. Commission on Epidemiology and Prognosis, International League Against Epilepsy. Guidelines for epidemiological studies on epilepsy. *Epilepsia.* 1993;34:592–596.
4. Ekman M, Forsgren L. Economic evidence in epilepsy: a review. *Eur J Health Econom Suppl.* 2004;1:S36–42.
5. European Commission Directorate-General for Employment and Social Affairs. *Definition of Disability in Europe: A Comparative Analysis.* Study prepared by Brunel University, Unit E.4, Bruxelles; 2002.
6. Forsgren I, et al. The epidemiology of epilepsy in Europe – a systematic review. *Eur J Neurol.* 2005;12:245–253.
7. Forsgren I, et al. Cost of epilepsy in Europe. *Eur J Neurol.* 2005;12(Suppl 1):54–58.
8. Hauser WA. Incidence and prevalence. In: Engel J, Pedley TA, eds. *Epilepsy: A Comprehensive Textbook.* Philadelphia: Lippincott-Raven Publishers; 1997: 47–57.
9. ILAE/IBE/WHO. Out of the Shadow. Global Campaign Against Epilepsy. ILAE/IBE/WHO Annual Report 1999.
10. Kotsopoulus IA, et al. Systematic review and meta-analysis of incidence studies of epilepsy and unprovoked seizures. *Epilepsia.* 2002;43:1402–1409.
11. Lavados PM, et al. A descriptive study of epilepsy in the district of El Salvador, Chile, 1984–1988. *Acta Neurol Scand.* 1992;91:718–729.
12. Lee BI. Current status and future direction of epilepsy surgery in Asia. *Neurol Asia.* 2004;9(Suppl 1):47–48.
13. Leonardi M, et al. The definition of disability: what is in a name? *Lancet.* 2006;368(9543):1219–1221.
14. Leonardi M, Menken M. Comparison of different systems. In: Engel J, Pedley TA, eds. *Epilepsy: A Comprehensive Textbook.* Philadelphia: Lippincott-Raven Publishers; 1997:2859–2863.
15. Leonardi M, Ustun TB. The global burden of epilepsy. *Epilepsia.* 2002;43(Suppl 6):21–25.
16. Mani KS, Rangan G. India. In: Engel J, Pedley TA, eds. *Epilepsy: A Comprehensive Textbook.* Philadelphia: Lippincott-Raven Publishers; 1997:276: 2835–2840.
17. Placencia M, et al. Epileptic seizures in an Andean region of Ecuador. Incidence and prevalence and regional variation. *Brain.* 1992;115:771–782.
18. Rwiza HT, et al. Prevalence and incidence of epilepsy in Ulanga, a rural Tanzanian district: a community-based study. *Epilepsia.* 1992;33:1051–1056.
19. Sander JW. Prevention of epilepsy. In: Shorvon SD, et al., eds. *The Management of Epilepsy in Developing Countries: An ICEBERG Manual. International Congress and Symposium Series, No. 175.* London: Royal Society of Medicine; 1991:19–21.
20. Seino M. Comprehensive epilepsy care: Contributions from para-medical professionals. *Neurol J Southeast Asia.* 2001;6:1–5.
21. Shamansky SL, et al. Socioeconomic characteristics of childhood seizure disorders in the New Haven area: an epidemiologic study. *Epilepsia.* 1979;20:457–474.
22. Tan Torrs T, et al. *Making Choices in Health: A WHO Guide to Cost-Effectiveness Analysis.* Geneva, Switzerland: World Health Organization; 2003.
23. Thomas SV, et al. Economic burden of epilepsy in India. *Epilepsia.* 2001;42:1052–1060.
24. Wang WZ, Wu JZ, Wang DS, et al. The prevalence and treatment gap in epilepsy in China. *Neurology.* 2003;60:1544–1545.
25. World Health Organization. *International Classification of Impairment, Disability and Handicap. A Manual of Classification Relating to Consequences of Diseases.* Geneva, Switzerland: World Health Organization; 1980.
26. World Health Organization. *International Statistical Classification of Disease and Related Health Problems.* 10th Revision. ICD 10 Vols. 1–3. Geneva, Switzerland: World Health Organization; 1992–1994.
27. World Health Organization. Consultative Meeting on Epilepsy Project. Report. MNH/NND/99.3. 1999, Geneva, Switzerland.
28. World Health Organization. Epilepsy out of the Shadow: The Burden of Epilepsy. February 12, 2001, Geneva, Switzerland.
29. World Health Organization. *International Classification of Functioning Disability and Health.* Geneva, Switzerland: World Health Organization; 2001.
30. WHO (2005) Atlas: Epilepsy care in the world, Epilepsy Atlas. *World Health Organization.* Geneva, Switzerland.
31. WHO (2007) Neurological Disorders: public health challenges. *Chapter 3.2: 56–69 World Health Organization.* Geneva, Switzerland.
32. WHO (2004) Epilepsy in the Western Pacific Region, A call to action. Global Campaign Against Epilepsy. WHO Regional Office for the Western Pacific; 2004.

CHAPTER 302 ■ COMPREHENSIVE EPILEPSY PROGRAMS—UNITED STATES

ROBERT J. GUMNIT

INTRODUCTION

The difference between a specialty epilepsy clinic and a comprehensive epilepsy program (CEP) is highlighted in this section. CEPs are different from epilepsy centers. Epilepsy centers can be places for the long-term residential treatment of people with seizures, or they can be places where a patient goes for specialized treatment. Specialized centers for the long-term care of people with epilepsy have essentially disappeared from the United States. When patients with epilepsy require long-term care, it is usually because of associated conditions: Severe brain damage, severe psychiatric problems, or mental retardation. Patients with epilepsy who have these conditions are usually cared for in residential centers or small residential programs whose treatment is directed at the primary problem causing the disability.

In the best sense of the term, a CEP is one in which a multispecialty team (physicians, psychologists, nurses, social workers, and specialized technical help) is brought together to provide an organized approach to the management of people with complex problems related to epilepsy.[1]

There is no organization in the United States that accredits a specialized epilepsy center or a CEP (although efforts are underway to establish one). Any physician with any training can print up stationery that says "Comprehensive Epilepsy Program," mount a sign on the door, and go into business. There are documented cases of physicians without specialized training doing just that. CEPs in the United States vary greatly in quality and organization.

HISTORICAL DEVELOPMENT

CEPs were originally developed under the aegis of the United States Public Health Service as part of the so-called 314(e) program in the early 1960s. One of the first was established in 1964, at the St. Paul Ramsey Hospital in St. Paul, Minnesota, and evolved into what is now called *MINCEP Epilepsy Care*. In that sense, the MINCEP program is the oldest in the United States. Nonetheless, major university centers devoted to specialized treatment (but without the full, comprehensive approach of medical, surgical, educational, psychologic, social, and community organization) have been in existence for many years.

The National Association of Epilepsy Centers (NAEC) was established in 1986 to help with the development of CEPs. A recent survey indicates that more than 130 places in the United States refer to themselves as *epilepsy centers*. Some of these consist of no more than a single neurologist with a particular interest in epilepsy. Others are CEPs in the fullest sense. The NAEC has published guidelines for classifying epilepsy centers and for the services to be rendered. Member centers (there were 116 in 2007) self-designate and affirm that they meet these guidelines. For more information, consult www.naec-epilepsy.org.

MECHANISMS OF REFERRAL

In accordance with the free-market economy underlying health care in the United States, patients historically have been able to reach a CEP by a variety of routes. Some are referred by a neurologist, others by primary care physicians. Some learn about a center from social agencies, and others from friends and neighbors.

With the development of managed care organizations, many patients may no longer have free access to a CEP. They may be restricted to one with which the organization has a contract, or the organization may resist any referral at all. Furthermore, the amount paid for care is set by the individual health plan or insurance company. In some cases (certain state medical assistance programs, for example), the amount is so small that the specialized center cannot afford to provide the necessary treatment.

LOCATION OF CENTERS

Some major urban centers in the United States do not have a comprehensive program. Others have two or more. (Los Angeles has nine groups claiming to be CEPs!) In general, it takes a population base of at least 2 to 3 million to support a CEP. In the case of uncommon conditions (e.g., extratemporal lesions requiring subdural arrays, Landau-Kleffner syndrome), a much larger population is necessary if a center is to develop a reasonable experience.

Nearly all comprehensive programs are associated directly or indirectly with major medical centers, and usually medical schools as well. Because of the unique structure of the U.S. health care system, it is possible for a major medical center to exist in a small, rural community and draw patients from many miles around.

LEADERSHIP AND STAFFING

The leadership and staffing of CEPs vary enormously. The major centers are headed by epileptologists with national reputations, have several physicians who specialize in epilepsy on staff, and provide a full range of support services (psychiatry, psychology, neuropsychology, social work, video-electroencephalographic monitoring). Centers in a developmental phase or those that merely aspire to the name may have far fewer resources.

A lack of uniformity exists among centers in regard to programs, size, and funding. Some centers serve only a few patients, whereas others perform several hundred evaluations a year.

FUNDING

Centers in general are funded on a fee-for-service basis. Some centers offer medical services as a loss leader so as to generate a high volume of surgical cases. Others try not to get involved in the long-term medical management of patients and seek only to evaluate and operate on patients who need simple types of surgery. This latter approach can be criticized as "skimming the cream." For a CEP to survive on a long-term basis, it must earn a sufficient profit by caring for a high volume of routine cases in order to subsidize the care of patients with the most complicated problems.

When the center is part of a large organization, bureaucratic imperatives drive the funding (the regular operating budget as well as capital investment). When the center is free-standing in private practice, ensuring the growth of the center and meeting the needs of patients take priority.

BARRIERS TO ACCESS

In the United States, various barriers to access to care exist. Many people who are poor or totally disabled do not have adequate access to health care. Financial barriers are a major issue. Indeed, this is compounded by the tendency of many physicians to treat some patients unsuccessfully until they are so disabled that they lose their jobs and health insurance, then they turn such patients over to public charity.

A second barrier is ignorance. Many patients are unaware of the existence of comprehensive programs despite the best effort of lay organizations and the centers themselves to educate the public. Many primary care physicians are ignorant of their existence as well, and do not know how or when to refer a patient.

Reluctance to refer can also be a major problem. Pride and refusal to admit that someone else may be able to do something that they cannot do exists among physicians everywhere in the world. In a fee-for-service environment that is under stress because of a reduced number of patients with indemnity insurance, the financial implications of making a referral come into play as well. If the patient is covered by a managed care organization, even if the physician wants to refer, the organization may be unwilling to spend the money.

Many patients are reluctant to travel for care. Some people will journey to the ends of the earth to see a physician with marginally better credentials. Other patients are unwilling to travel across town to consult a physician at a highly specialized center. For patients with epilepsy, travel may be difficult and presents a particular problem.

Perhaps the biggest barrier is the sense of hopelessness that develops in many patients who have had uncontrolled seizures for years. After a while, they simply lose their ability to cope and cease to seek better care.

Competing voices in the marketplace also may serve as a barrier to reaching a CEP. Religious healers and practitioners of alternative medical philosophies (homeopathy, naturopathy, food fads) all create a clamor.

Nonetheless, many fine CEPs exist throughout the United States, and most can find some way to help a patient obtain the care needed if only the patient will apply for help.

SUMMARY AND CONCLUSIONS

The quality of epilepsy care in the United States varies broadly, and CEPs vary widely in quality and distribution. Frequently, socioeconomic factors are a major impediment to patients seeking appropriate help.

References

1. The National Association of Epilepsy Centers. Recommended guidelines for diagnosis and treatment in specialized epilepsy centers. *Epilepsia*. 2001;42(6):804–814.

CHAPTER 303 ■ COMPREHENSIVE EPILEPSY PROGRAMS—NORWAY*

SVEIN I. JOHANNESSEN AND KARL O. NAKKEN

INTRODUCTION

In Norway, with a population of about 4.5 million people, only one specialized center for epilepsy exists. It is designated as a national center of competence in epileptology and comprehensive epilepsy service. Being an institution with nationwide responsibilities, its role in the National Health Service system and its program for activities are defined by the Department of Health and endorsed by the Norwegian Parliament.

NATIONAL CENTER FOR EPILEPSY—HISTORICAL BACKGROUND

At the end of the 19th century, in Kristiania (now Oslo), the deacons established a home for people with epilepsy. In 1910, they bought a farm in Sandvika, 15 kilometers outside Oslo, where they established a nursing home for the residential care of 64 patients with chronic epilepsy. Dr. Monrad Krohn, professor of neurology at the National Hospital (Rikshospitalet) in Oslo was the first medical supervisor. The deacons were inspired by the epilepsy colonies, which at that time had been established in some European countries, including Denmark and Germany.

In 1924, the institution was donated to the State, which for many years ran it as a nursing home/farm for people with severe epilepsy. To the extent possible, the residents took part in the farm work. In 1954, thanks to a donation from the Norwegian Red Cross, a new unit was built for temporary service to 36 children with epilepsy. The new medical director, Dr. Georg F. Henriksen, specializing in neurology, psychiatry, and clinical neurophysiology, had been trained in epileptology in the United States and Canada.

During Dr. Henriksen's tenure (1954–1974), the National Nursing Home for Epileptics developed into the National Hospital for Epileptics with 184 beds: 36 for children, 34 for residential care, and the rest for adolescents and adults with difficult-to-treat epilepsy. The patients were admitted from all over Norway to be diagnosed and treated by a multiprofessional staff of about 150. Most patients had not only epilepsy, but also considerable additional problems, such as mental retardation, psychiatric and behavioral disturbances, and neurologic deficits.

In 1974, Dr. Yngve Løyning, a specialist in neurology and clinical neurophysiology, succeeded Dr. Henriksen. In 1975, the institution was renamed the National Center for Epilepsy (Statens Senter for Epilepsi [SSE]), reflecting its development into a multiprofessional comprehensive service center in epileptology. Residential care was abandoned in 1980.

Epilepsy surgery was introduced in Norway by professor Kristian Kristiansen at the Department of Neurosurgery at Oslo City Hospital (Ullevål) in 1949. He had his training at professor Wilder Penfield's department in Montreal, and Kristiansen was for many years the only Norwegian surgeon who performed epilepsy surgery. In 1976, epilepsy surgery was transferred to the National Hospital (Rikshospitalet) in Oslo. In 1992, the Norwegian Health Authorities decided to centralize this resource-intensive service. Selection of candidates for epilepsy surgery, preoperative investigations, and postoperative follow-up and rehabilitation would take place at the National Center for Epilepsy, whereas neuroradiologic investigations, intracarotid amobarbital (Wada) tests, and diagnostic and therapeutic surgery would be performed at the National Hospital.

In 1971, Norwegian Health Authorities planned to establish additional epilepsy centers in association with the university hospitals in the western, mid, and northern parts of Norway. The center in Sandvika was supposed to serve the southeastern part of the country, increasing its number of beds to 308 (including 92 for residential care) and the number of employees to 340. However, over the next years, it became evident that the additional centers would not be built because (a) the neurologic and pediatric epilepsy service had improved considerably throughout the country, making the need for more centers questionable; (b) the authorities decided that patients in need of permanent care should be treated in their local counties; (c) the economy in all regions had become weaker; and (d) the capacity at the center in Sandvika had improved, owing to the fact that the duration of stays at the center had decreased dramatically. The center would continue its nationwide service with fewer, rather than more beds, provided the staff was increased.

In 2005, the center had 25 buildings, occupying 21,000 m^2 of the 400,000 m^2 land area. There are 87 beds and about 300 employees.

Despite the continuous improvement of medical and psychosocial epilepsy service in Norway, the need for internal and external comprehensive service from the center in Sandvika is still increasing. The average yearly admission of inpatients over the past 30 years (1975–2005) has increased more than fivefold. During the same time, the number of beds was reduced from 183 to 87. This intensification has led to a marked reduction in average length of stay at the center, from 150 days to 17 days.

In the last few years, the center in Sandvika has been designated as a competence center for severely disabled patients with epilepsy, including those with mental retardation, tuberous sclerosis, and autism.

*Dedicated to our former Director Yngve Løyning, MDhc, PhD.

DEVELOPMENT OF THE NORWEGIAN HEALTH-CARE SYSTEM

Regionalized Service

Since 1976, the system for health service in Norway, as in the other Scandinavian countries, has been regionalized. The intention is that each of the five health regions should have the resources to provide its population with most of the medical and psychosocial service needed. Some of the regional hospitals have supraregional or nationwide service functions, which are often resource-intensive and mostly intended for small groups of patients.

In addition, special institutions with supraregional or nationwide service functions exist for special groups of patients: Those with rare diseases or syndromes, those requiring particularly resource-demanding or multiprofessional services (e.g., drug-resistant epilepsies, cerebral palsy, multiple sclerosis), or those with different ailments in need of the same service (e.g., various physical deficits requiring rehabilitation).

Service Levels

Medical and psychosocial service is provided at four levels of increasing competence: In the local district, in the counties, in the regions at university hospitals, and in the special institutions or centers. The goal is to treat patients at the lowest possible service level as close to their own district as possible. A primary care physician, who calls in other professionals as consultants when needed, coordinates all service. Although rehabilitation teams are available in the counties, a complete multiprofessional staff providing the integrated, comprehensive service necessary for patients with difficult-to-treat epilepsy is established at a national epilepsy center at the fourth service level only.

Mechanisms of Referral

According to the outlined service principles, patients with epilepsy should have access to service on all four levels, depending on the severity and complexity of their condition. In Norway, it is recommended that all patients with epilepsy be referred to a specialist in pediatrics or neurology (depending on the age of the patient) to clarify the diagnosis, etiology, and type of seizures and epilepsy, as well as to initiate, change, or terminate antiepileptic drug (AED) treatment. The general practitioner should monitor the patient's AED treatment according to seizure control, side effects, and serum concentrations. The specialist should be available for consultation and renewed investigation when needed. Only those with drug-resistant seizures are referred to the National Center for Epilepsy. The number of referrals is restricted for economic reasons. The expenses are covered by the health regions, which require an approval by a specialist at the local hospital.

Barriers to Care

The service system does not impose any barriers to necessary care except the economic barriers for use of service outside the county (i.e., in the regional hospitals and epilepsy center). However, the numbers of pediatricians and neurologists are not sufficient in all parts of the country to give patients with epilepsy access to a specialist as soon as needed. Rehabilitation teams often do not have the capacity or competence to deal with psychosocial problems associated with seizures.

NATIONAL CENTER FOR EPILEPSY

Geographic Location

The National Center for Epilepsy is located just outside Oslo, which is located in the southeast end of the elongated country. The location causes some difficulties for the follow-up of patients and communication with health personnel in distant parts of the country. This is one of the reasons why we at the center in Sandvika (belonging to Health Region South) have advocated establishment of local epilepsy centers in the other four health regions (Health Region East-, West-, Mid-, and North Norway).

For many years, the center has collaborated closely with the National Hospital in Oslo, where neuroradiologic investigations and surgical interventions are performed.

Leadership and Staffing

In 2002, the epilepsy center became a part of the National Hospital. In 2005, great organizational changes took place within the health service in the Oslo area. The Norwegian Radium Hospital (specialized in cancer treatment) was merged with the National Hospital (Rikshospitalet University Hospital) and organized into eight clinics. The National Center for Epilepsy became a part of the Division of Clinical Neuroscience, which also comprises Departments of Neurology, Neurosurgery, as well as Psychosomatic Medicine. The center no longer has a director of its own, but is now under the medical leadership of the Division of Clinical Neuroscience.

Employees at the center for the time being, nearly 300, represent the necessary disciplines for addressing the various problems of the patients. The staff includes 23 physicians who cover neurology, pediatrics, clinical neurophysiology, and psychiatry, and one clinical pharmacologist. Of these, eight are interns training for any of these specialities. There are nine clinical neuropsychologists, three social workers, six vocational therapists, five physiotherapists, and 13 laboratory technicians. In addition, there are about 100 nurses, of whom many have subspecialized in epileptology and/or psychiatry. The nurses are key persons in the epilepsy education offered to all our patients, and the importance of having structured epilepsy nursing for improved quality of life has recently been documented.[4] The center has its own elementary and secondary school, with 18 specially trained educators, including speech therapists.

Services Available

The service offered by the center is established in accordance with the objectives decided upon by the Health Authorities and the Norwegian Parliament. These include service to inpatients and outpatients, consultative assistance to health professionals and others dealing with patients with epilepsy, education of students and health professionals, information to relevant groups in the society, and distribution of results from clinical research.

Internal Service

Patients are admitted to the center for seizures of an unclear nature or difficult-to-treat seizures, for evaluation of surgical treatment, for postoperative controls, and for psychosocial problems related to the epilepsy or epilepsy treatment. Many patients have multiple medical problems, often with complex causes. Several are in need of family therapy and/or of habilitation and rehabilitation. Most patients profit from a multiprofessional comprehensive service, and some participate in group therapy.

For inpatients, the center has separate wards for children ($n = 32$), 1 to 14 years of age, as well as for adolescents and adults without mental retardation ($n = 34$), with slight retardation ($n = 14$), and with severe retardation ($n = 7$). Other units are designated for intensive monitoring ($n = 5$; $n = 10$ from 2006), vocational observation and training, physiotherapy, and leisure activities. There are as well laboratories for clinical chemistry/clinical pharmacology, clinical neurophysiology, and clinical neuropsychology. The school has a capacity for about 40 children. The center has housing facilities for relatives and guests.

The center also accommodates national centers of competence-related diagnostic groups, such as tuberous sclerosis, autism, and learning disability with epilepsy.

Between 30 and 40 patients undergo epilepsy surgery every year, mostly resective surgery. Analyses of the outcome and its prediction factors have been presented.[1,3] Every year, about 15 drug-resistant patients who were found unsuitable for surgery are offered vagal nerve stimulation.[8]

External Services

External service offered at the center includes preadmission assessment; postdischarge follow-up by long-distance communication and outpatient clinical and laboratory service, visiting service to some residents with learning disabilities, nationwide consultative service to health professionals and authorities, graduate and postgraduate educational service to health personnel and school teachers, and supervision of students in different health professions.

In Norway, two nursing homes are available for patients with severe epilepsy (Kure and Røysumtunet). Physicians from the center serve these two institutions through visits on a regular basis.

Number of Patients Served

In 2004, 1,413 patients were admitted to the National Center for Epilepsy. Their average stay was 16.9 days (1 day–4 months). The number of admissions is increasing slightly year by year. The average waiting time before admission was 110 days. In 2004, about 200 patients were evaluated for epilepsy surgery, but only about 35 of them were actually operated. The need for epilepsy surgery is estimated to be about 50 patients per year.[6]

About 1,400 patients, both children and adults, are admitted to the outpatient clinic for approximately 2,000 consultations per year. Among these, about 50 patients participate in drug trials.

At the Department of Clinical Chemistry/Clinical Pharmacology, about 45,000 blood samples from in- and outpatients were analyzed in 2004, mainly to determine serum concentrations of AEDs.

At the Department of Clinical Neurophysiology, 4,176 recordings were performed in 2004, both standard electroencephalogram and combined video and telemetry, 100 evoked potential studies, 100 electromyograms, and about 20 ictal single-photon emission computed tomograms (SPECT) were recorded.

The Department of Neuropsychology performs about 110 general neuropsychological assessments (including personality inventories) per year, 40 preoperative assessments (including Wada tests), 35 postoperative assessments, 20 online evaluations of cognitive effects of interictal EEG disturbances, and about 15 functional magnetic resonance image (fMRI) scans.

FUNDING

Funding of Health Service

A part of the salaries of all employees in Norway are taxed to fund the National Health Security System. This tax covers all the expenses for all health service and social service, except for a small amount paid by the patient for service from outpatient clinics and private practitioners. Thus, the health regions offer service to patients in hospitals and institutions from funds allocated by the government.

BARRIERS TO CARE

Finances

Because the health regions are underfinanced, the use of service outside the regions is decreasing. This is a concern for special institutions like the epilepsy center. Fortunately, so far, the admissions to the center have not been reduced.

Ignorance

The existence of the epilepsy center is well known to most patients with epilepsy, their relatives, and health care and social service personnel. However, the benefits of comprehensive service, and particularly of surgical treatment, are not sufficiently known. Thus, many patients are referred too late, often when psychosocial problems have become fixed and irreversible.

RESEARCH

In recent years, research activities have been pursued in the following fields: Clinical pharmacokinetics of AEDs, evaluation and monitoring of AED treatment, clinical trials of new AEDs in phase III and IV, epilepsy surgery, intensive observation and differential diagnoses of episodic brain dysfunctions, automatic detection and quantification of epileptiform EEG discharges, neuropsychological testing of performance in relation to epileptiform activity, physical fitness and physical exercise in relation to epilepsy,[7] the influence of drug treatment on psychosocial functioning, genetic aspects of epilepsy, analyses of comprehensive service needs,[5] and benefit evaluation of the center service.

FUTURE EPILEPSY SERVICE

In 1995, Health Region West established high-level medical services to patients with epilepsy at the Departments of Pediatrics and Neurology at Haukeland University Hospital in Bergen. In Health Region North, a comprehensive epilepsy service has for some years been planned at the Department of Neurology at Tromsø University Hospital, but is not yet realized.

However, in Health Region Mid-Norway no plans exist to establish a unit for patients who need to stay for a longer time than is possible in ordinary hospital wards. Therefore, patients requiring comprehensive service will continue to be referred to the National Center for Epilepsy in Sandvika.

In 1981, the National Center for Epilepsy presented a plan for its future service based on analyses of service needs. We renewed our recommendation to establish similar centers in the other health regions. Whether such centers will be realized is open to the gravest doubt and, until further notice, the present center will need 100 beds for a nationwide inpatient service, with a corresponding level of sufficient staffing.

SUMMARY AND CONCLUSIONS

The views from the Norwegian Center for Epilepsy can be summarized as follows:

A person with newly diagnosed epilepsy may face long-lasting problems including seizure susceptibility, drug-related side effects, and the psychosocial burden. Fortunately, most patients have minor problems, but all patients will be in need of some comprehensive service.

Ideally, comprehensive service should be provided at all service levels. Those specialists in pediatrics or neurology who establish the diagnosis of epilepsy and initiate drug therapy should cooperate closely with the local general practitioner, nurse, social worker, and, if necessary, school teachers and a psychologist. According to the patients' requirements, information should be given to all those involved. The patient should be informed about the Norwegian Epilepsy Association (and its local branch) and about other sources of epilepsy information. At the regional hospital, a multidisciplinary team at the Departments of Pediatrics and Neurology provides comprehensive service.

About 30% of patients with epilepsy will be in need of comprehensive service from a specialized center or unit, where they can stay for a longer time than in ordinary hospital wards. At such epilepsy centers/units, they will be offered integrated multidisciplinary services, including physical, social, and vocational habilitation and rehabilitation and, if required, patients can attend school. To meet these demands in an optimal way, an epilepsy center should cover a population of about 1 million, thus serving about 2,500 patients with severe epilepsy.[2]

Ideally, in each Health Region, an epilepsy center/unit for long-term comprehensive service should be established, preferably in close collaboration with the regional hospital.

In a small country like Norway, epilepsy surgery should be coordinated from, and centralized to, one epilepsy center and one collaborating regional hospital. Patients with severe epilepsy and considerable comorbidities may not be able to take care of themselves. Earlier, many of these patients lived in big central institutions. In 1991, such institutions were closed in Norway, and today many of these patients are living in small, local, sheltered homes. In addition to the local comprehensive service, these patients should be followed-up on a regular basis by an epileptologist from the nearest epilepsy center/unit, and be admitted for a temporary stay when necessary.

References

1. Bjørnæs H. *Refractory focal epilepsy and cognition: Effects of age, tratment, laterality, gender, and IQ. Thesis.* Oslo: Oslo University; 2005.
2. Dam M. The future of epilepsy centers. Abstract 67, Golden Jubilee Conference and North European Epilepsy Meeting, York; 1986.
3. Guldvog B, Løyning Y, Hauglie-Hanssen E, et al. Surgical versus medical treatment for epilepsy. I. Outcome related to survival, seizures, and neurologic deficit. *Epilepsia.* 1991;32:375–388.
4. Helde G, Bovim G, Braathen G, et al. A stuctured, nurse-led intervention program improves quality of life in patients with epilepsy: A randomized, controlled trial. *Epilepsy Behav.* 2005;7(3):451–457.
5. Løyning Y. Comprehensive Care. In: Wada JA, Penry JK, eds. *Advances in Epileptology. Xth Epilepsy International Symposium.* New York: Raven; 1980:363–367.
6. Løyning Y, Henriksen O, Hauglie-Hanssen E. Surgery for Epilepsy. The Protocol of the Norwegian Center. In: Engel J Jr, ed. *Surgical Treatment of the Epilepsies.* New York: Raven; 1987.
7. Nakken KO. *Physical exercise in epilepsy. Need, ability, benefit, and risk. Thesis.* Oslo: Oslo University; 1999.
8. Nakken KO, Henriksen O, Røste GK, et al. Vagal nerve stimulation: The Norwegian experience. *Seizure.* 2003;12(1):37–41.

CHAPTER 304 ■ COMPREHENSIVE EPILEPSY PROGRAMS—JAPAN

MASAKAZU SEINO AND E. ANN YEH

INTRODUCTION

Epidemiologic studies of epilepsy, which are indispensable to estimate the magnitude of a problem, are limited in Japan. A 1-day population-based survey of children under the age of 13 years, conducted in Okayama Prefecture in 1999, showed the prevalence rate of seizure disorders to be 8.9 per 1,000 population (2,222 per 250,997). When febrile seizures and other single provoked seizures and acute symptomatic seizures were excluded (848 cases), the rate was 5.5 per 1,000.[14] The figures are comparable with those in the United States and Europe.[5] According to a 1-day survey done by the Ministry of Health in 2002, on the estimated number of patients with epilepsy whose medical fees were subsidized by any one of the governmental health insurance systems, 74,000 patients were hospitalized and 195,000 patients visited outpatient clinics.[7]

The issue of medically refractory epilepsy is a topic of special significance in epilepsy treatment. A series of nationwide surveys was carried out to establish the number of people with refractory epilepsy in Japan. People with refractory epilepsy were defined as those with an increase or no change in seizure frequency despite at least 3 years of intensive medical treatment at either a university hospital or a specialized center. The number of patients identified in these surveys as having refractory epilepsy was over 100,000. Most of these patients also had multiple neurologic and psychosocial problems. Of patients 15 years of age or younger, 13.5% were found to have medically refractory epilepsy,[15] and the epilepsy of 25.3% of patients over 16 years of age was medically refractory.[13]

In Japan, epilepsy patients were treated by psychiatrists until 1950s. For this reason, mental hospitals are the final stop for individuals with most refractory and disabling epilepsy. *The Handbook for Mental Health and Hygiene* reported, in 2002, that 4,243 (1.3%) of 330,050 patients institutionalized in mental hospitals in Japan on a long-term basis had intractable seizures in addition to personality and psychiatric disorders or mental disabilities.[8] The number of patients with epilepsy who were admitted to mental hospitals has decreased markedly over the past decade. The numbers have dropped yearly since 1995. Between 1995 and 1997, respectively, 8,997, 8,574, and 8,332 patients with epilepsy were hospitalized in mental hospitals in Japan. This decrease in numbers of hospitalized patients presumably represents improvements in epilepsy care in general in Japan.[1]

HISTORICAL DEVELOPMENT

In a 1966 article, Wada[20] noted that Japan's progress in the scientific aspects of epileptology was on par with that of North America and Europe, although Japan lagged behind in its support of comprehensive medical services for epilepsy. Unlike the nations of North America and Europe, where custodial facilities for people with epilepsy and other disabilities were established in the middle of the 19th century,[2,3] state-sponsored institutional care for people with disabilities was not introduced in Japan until the mid 20th century. Legislation for the creation of institutions for individuals with severe mental disabilities was introduced in 1959. This legislation was established only after the state was pressured by lay people and professionals to take responsibility for the support for individuals with severe disabilities. Thus, although the influential 1969 Reid Report[2] was shelved for lack of funding and political will in Great Britain,[18] its recommendations concerning the general care and management of patients with epilepsy, as well as for the creation of special epilepsy centers, were welcomed with great enthusiasm by Japanese professionals.

Although the need for establishing comprehensive multidisciplinary treatment programs for people with epilepsy in Japan was advocated by Nakata as early as 1966,[12] it was only in the 1970s that a special center for the treatment of epilepsy was established.[19] Inspired by the Reid Report,[2] the Japanese Ministry of Health and Welfare decided in 1975 to convert a tuberculosis hospital located in Shizuoka into a special center for epilepsy.[23] The center was defined as an integrated organization from which delivery of the following services would be possible: (a) long-term, longitudinal care of individuals with epilepsy from infancy through adolescence to adulthood; (b) multidisciplinary team treatment by neurologists, pediatricians, neurosurgeons, psychiatrists, nurses, and comedical personnel; (c) occupational therapy and rehabilitation activities; and (d) training and research in epileptology. In addition, during the 1980s and 1990s, several governmental sanatoriums Tokyo, Kyoto, Niigata, and Yamagata converted their neurology/psychiatry clinics into epilepsy assessment centers. The total number of these converted beds was approximately 250 in 2005.

THE NATIONAL EPILEPSY CENTER IN SHIZUOKA, JAPAN

The remainder of this chapter is devoted to a description of the current therapeutic activities and demographic features of the National Epilepsy Center in Shizuoka, based on statistics from 1975 to 2002. From 1975 to 2001, a total of 22,950 new patients with epilepsy visited our Center. The number of patients younger than 15 years of age has deceased since the mid 1980s, whereas the number of patients older than 15 years of age has gradually increased. The electroencephalogram (EEG) was the most frequently performed clinical investigation. A total of 187,600 EEGs was performed between 1975 and 2001.

Geographic Distribution of Outpatients

A total of 1,451 new patients visited the center's ambulatory services in 2003, including 27% from Shizuoka Prefecture (where the center is located) and 31% from adjacent prefectures situated between Tokyo and Nagoya (about 200 km away, or a 1-hour trip by bullet train from Shizuoka). The remaining lived in areas beyond the Tokyo and Nagoya metropolitan areas.

Geographic Distribution of Inpatients

The center has four wards for patients with epilepsy. There are 100 beds in the two adult wards and another 100 beds in the two wards for children. On average, 178.1 inpatients/day were hospitalized at the center in 2002. Patients come from every prefecture in Japan. Approximately a quarter of the inpatients are residents of Shizuoka Prefecture. The other patients come from other parts of Japan.

Age Distribution

The age of new outpatients ranged from 1 month to 76 years. The mean age was 18.5 years. Forty-five percent were under the age of 15, and 55% were over the age of 15 years. The age of inpatients ranged from 1 month to 62 years, also with a mean age of 18.5 years.

Patient Referrals to the Outpatient Clinic

The center is an officially recognized tertiary center for epilepsy in Japan. Based on statistics from 1991, 79% of outpatients were referred to the center by other physicians. Pediatricians made 37% of the referrals, neurosurgeons 8%, neurologic internists 8%, and general practitioners 7%. Twenty-one percent of the outpatients visited the center without referrals, of whom 8% were without diagnosis or treatment.

The government is attempting to decrease the number of patient self-referrals. Since 1988, under the Standard for Special Medical Treatment Act, patients have been required to receive referrals to utilize the services of specially designated tertiary care centers. Patients who do not receive referrals to the centers cannot use their health insurance for the first consultation they receive there.

The Diagnosis of Epileptic Syndromes and Epilepsies in 100 Consecutive Inpatients in 2002

The diagnosis of epileptic syndromes and epilepsies in 100 consecutive inpatients in 2002 was as follows: Syndrome identified in 39%, syndrome probable in 19%, other epilepsies in 32%, and nonepilepsy in 10%. Of the 39 patients whose syndromic diagnosis was definite, temporal lobe epilepsy was found in 21, frontal lobe epilepsy in eight, occipital lobe epilepsy in four, West syndrome in two, juvenile myoclonic epilepsy in one, and epilepsy with grand mal on awakening in one. Of the 19 patients whose syndromal diagnosis was probable but not definite, frontal lobe epilepsy was diagnosed in eight, occipital lobe epilepsy in four, temporal lobe epilepsy in three, progressive myoclonus epilepsy in two, familial adult myoclonic epilepsy in one, and Doose syndrome in one.

Of another cohort of 659 of the center's outpatients, 349 (53%) were followed for 3 years at the center's ambulatory services; 310 (47%) were sent back to the referring physicians. Treatment outcomes, expressed by rate of reduction in seizure frequency at 3-year follow-up compared with baseline, were as follows: Complete seizure freedom in 121 patients (35%), greater than 75% reduction in seizure frequency in 76 (22%), and greater than 50% reduction in 58 (17%). In other words, seizure frequency was reduced by at least 50% in almost 75% of outpatients treated at the National Epilepsy Center.[15]

Length of Admission of Inpatients

In 1998, the mean duration of admission was 123 days. One obvious reason for the long hospitalizations is that most of the center's inpatients have seizures that are extremely difficult to control, and because hospitalizations are fairly inexpensive, neither staff physicians nor patients and their families have much incentive to keep stays short. However, more complex social reasons exist. Most of the adult patients who are hospitalized at the center say they would like the treatment they receive to help them lead "normal" lives—lives during the course of which they could work, marry, have children, and so on. Because there are major restrictions on the employment (and thus economic independence and marriage) of individuals with epilepsy in Japan, the only way that many patients imagine this ideal can be realized is through full seizure control. These hopes are often nearly impossible to meet. One result has been long hospitalizations.

Epilepsy Surgery

Seven hundred and thirty nine patients have undergone epilepsy surgery at the center since 1982. Decisions regarding surgeries are made by a multidisciplinary team. Twenty-nine percent of the surgery candidates underwent presurgical evaluations with long-term intracranial EEG-video monitoring. Radiographic surveys, computed tomography (CT), magnetic resonance imaging (MRI), single-photon emission computed tomography (SPECT), and magnetoencephalography (MEG) were also used in the presurgical evaluations. Outcomes of 100 patients who underwent temporal lobe surgery and were followed for more than 2 years were as good as or better than results reported for Europe and North America.[10] After a mean follow-up of 8.0 years, 80.5% of 425 patients receiving temporal lobe surgery had seizure outcomes falling into Engel's Class I. Sixty-two percent of 140 extratemporal cases were classified as Engel's Class I after a mean 6.2-year follow-up.[11]

Mihara concluded that resective surgery provides sustained, positive benefits with a high likelihood for seizure freedom (80%) for most medically refractory patients with discrete lesions. In patients without a clear MRI lesion who underwent extra-temporal lobe resection, however, Engel's class I to II was achieved in less than 50% of patients. High-resolution MRI should be performed early in all patients with partial seizures.[11]

Finances in 2002

The National Epilepsy Center operates under the auspices of the Ministry of Health and Welfare of Japan. All income from medical services is considered governmental income, and the hospital's annual budget is issued by the Ministry independently. The approximate income in 2002 was 4.11 billion Yen, while total expenditures amounted to 4.05 billion Yen. (For the sake of conversion, about 115 Japanese Yen were equivalent to 1 U.S. dollar in 2006.) Thus, the hospital operated at a surplus of 1.6% in 2002, whereas the hospital has operated at a yearly deficit of 10% for the past 10 years.

TABLE 1

COMPREHENSIVE CLASSIFICATION OF PEOPLE WITH EPILEPSY

Group 1: People with epilepsy who (a) have had no seizures for 5 years or longer, (b) do not have associated (physical, intellectual, psychiatric) disabilities, and (c) can do all types of work except for that involving heavy lifting.

Group 2: People with epilepsy who have had no seizures for 3 years, and are able to do certain types of work, even if their associated disabilities are taken into account.

Group 3: People with epilepsy who have been seizure-free for less than 3 years, and who are employable even if hazards caused by seizures and interictal disabilities are taken into account.

Group 4: People with epilepsy who are having several seizures a month or even fewer. The seizures may cause hazards. These individuals are employable only in sheltered situations.

Group 5: People with epilepsy who are having several seizures a week or even fewer. Their seizures cause hazards. These individuals are unable to support themselves because of interictal disabilities, and are therefore in need of occasional help from others.

Group 6: People with epilepsy who are having several seizures a day or more (in some cases, fewer), and are entirely unable to care for themselves and always in need of help from others.

From Yagi and Onuma, ref. 21.

SEVERITY OF EPILEPSY AND COMPREHENSIVE CLASSIFICATION

In 1986, Yagi and Onuma[17] introduced a system to classify individuals with epilepsy according to their ictal and interictal levels of disability. The system was designed to evaluate levels of need for health and special services. The six levels of this classification system are summarized in Table 1.

In this classification system, ratings are based not only on patients' inherent seizure types and frequencies, but also on the severity of seizure-related disabilities. For example, higher ratings are given to seizures that (a) cause abrupt falls and injury, (b) are accompanied by prolonged impairment of consciousness including automatisms, and (c) result in immobility, even if consciousness is not impaired. In a survey of 542 outpatients at the center, the breakdown was as follows: Group 1, 8%; group 2, 16%; group 3, 38%; group 4, 22%; group 5, 11%; and group 6, 4%.

Patients classified in groups 1 through 3 (63%) can be managed as outpatients and, in principle, are employable, whereas those in groups 4 and 5 (33%) have been subjected to short- or long-term hospital admissions, depending on the severity of their seizures. Patient classifications are subject to change. For example, a patient in group 4 whose hospital stay is shorter than expected might be shifted up to group 3, and a patient in group 5 whose condition worsens may be moved down to group 6.

REHABILITATION AND "HABILITATION"

The Reid Report envisaged special centers as being concerned with medical care and rehabilitation, with the ultimate goal of returning people with epilepsy to a normal life in the community. It specified the need for facilities for people with severe epilepsy—individuals whose seizures cannot be adequately controlled and who require long-term accommodation. According to the report, the needs of these patients must be recognized as being different from those of the long-stay resident who is institutionalized for other reasons (mainly custodial care).[2]

With respect to the needs of these patients, Grant argues that specialized services are necessary for individuals "... whose seizures cannot be effectively controlled, and those who require medical supervision under everyday living conditions or in a working setting."[4] These patients would fall into groups 5 and 6 in the comprehensive classification system described above.

Patients who fall into groups 3 and 4 in the system would most nearly approximate the group that Laidlaw and Laidlaw[9] describe as "... people with epilepsy who very nearly but not quite can manage on their own, who are employable, but break down under external environment stresses, who, given just a little bit of support, can be most successful."

In Europe, proposals for the creation of special centers were specifically aimed at the deinstitutionalization of individuals with epilepsy.[2] However, during the years following the North American and European movements for deinstitutionalization, critics have made it clear that deinstitutionalization in itself does not offer a more "humane" solution than institutionalization,[19] and that it must be accompanied by alternatives other than the street and soup kitchens. It is also clear that supportive, residential environments can be of benefit to some individuals. Finally, it is the opinion of the first author (M.S.) of this chapter, based on more than 30 years of experience at the Center, that residential care is necessary for a limited number of individuals who have severe, frequent seizures and intellectual or behavioral problems. The authors suggest that this type of residential care for people with epilepsy be based on a goal of "habilitation"—the provision of schooling (for children) and care (for adults) in livable and supportive environments, rather than on the primary goal of "rehabilitation"—the accommodation of individuals to society. These goals do not conflict with, and indeed may be integrated easily with, the goals of current community care plans.[13]

SUMMARY AND CONCLUSIONS

Over one million people in Japan have epilepsy. One-tenth of them have medically intractable seizures. Most of these individuals have concomitant physical and/or intellectual disabilities.

Although the need for comprehensive services for epilepsy was established before 1975, it was only in 1975 that the Japanese Ministry of Health decided to convert a tuberculosis hospital into a special center for epilepsy. Our experience over the past 30 years at the National Epilepsy Center in Shizuoka suggests that treatment can improve seizure control in approximately two-thirds of patients. Outcomes for patients who underwent epilepsy surgery were as good as or better than results reported for North America and Europe. The management of epilepsy should be oriented toward seizure control, psychological well-being, and social rehabilitation. To satisfy these goals, it is imperative that different types of health care professionals come together to form multidisciplinary treatment teams. However, in Japan, only a small number of these multidisciplinary teams have been established. Furthermore, the need for residential care for individuals who have severe disabilities related to epilepsy must be addressed. This type of residential care should be oriented toward "habilitation"—the provision of schooling and care in livable and supportive environments—rather than the goal of "rehabilitation"—the accommodation of individuals to normal life in the community.

References

1. Akimoto H. A Nationwide Survey on Patients with Epilepsy Admitted to Mental Hospitals. In: *A Nationwide Plan for the Control of Epilepsy*. Tokyo: Japanese Epilepsy Association; 1986:349–379 (in Japanese).
2. Central Health Service Council. *People with epilepsy: Report of the joint subcommittee of the Standing Medical Advisory Committee and the Advisory Committee of the Health and Welfare of Handicapped Persons (IA Reid, Chairman)*. London: HMSO; 1969.
3. *Commission for the Control of Epilepsy and Its Consequences. Plan for nationwide action on epilepsy*. Bethesda, MD: U.S. Department of Health Education and Welfare; DHEW publication No (NIH)78–279 (Vols. 1–4).
4. Grant R. Special Centers. In: Reynolds EH, Trimble MR, eds. *Epilepsy and Psychiatry*. Edinburgh: Churchill Livingstone; 1981:347–358.
5. Hauser WA, Hesdorffer DC. *Epilepsy: Frequency, Causes and Consequences*. New York: Demos, 1990.
6. Japanese Epilepsy Association. *A Nationwide Plan for the Control of Epilepsy*. Tokyo; 1986 (in Japanese).
7. Kouseishou Daijinbou Toukei Jouhou-bu. *Heisei 14 nen, Kanja chousa (Patient's Survey, 2002)*. Tokyo: Kousei Toukei Kyoukai; 2002 (in Japanese).
8. Kouseishou. *Wa ga kuni no seishin hoken, Heisei 15 nendo ban (Mental Health in Our Country)*. Tokyo: Kouseishou; 2003:70–71 (in Japanese).
9. Laidlaw J, Laidlaw MV. People with Epilepsy—Living with Epilepsy. In: Laidlaw J, Richens A, eds. *A Textbook of Epilepsy*. Edinburgh: Churchill Livingstone; 1976:355–384.
10. Mihara T. Comprehensive assessment of outcome in 100 patients followed for over 2 years after resective surgery for temporal lobe epilepsy. *Adv Neurol Res*. 1994;38:771–780.
11. Mihara T. *Surgery, Seizures*. Workshop on Epilepsy Surgery in Asia; 2006. (Abstract).
12. Nakata M. *Two Hundred Years of Epilepsy: Historical Notes on Epilepsy*. Tokyo: Japanese Epilepsy Association; 1984 (in Japanese).
13. Ohtahara S. Pediatric Patients with Refractory Epilepsies. In: Seino M, ed. *Report of a Collaborative Study on the Causes and Treatment of Refractory Epilepsies*. Tokyo: NCNP of the Ministry of Health and Welfare; 1985:13–21 (in Japanese).
14. Oka E, Otsuka Y, Yoshinaga H, et al. Neuroepidemiological Study of Childhood Epilepsy by Application of International Classification of Epilepsy (ILAE 1989) – A Population-based Study in Okayama Prefecture, Japan. In: *Annual Report of the Japan Epilepsy Research Foundation*, 2001:117–124 (in Japanese).
15. Seino M. Adult Patients with Refractory Epilepsies. In: Seino M, ed. *Report of a Collaborative Study on the Causes and Treatment of Refractory Epilepsies*. Tokyo: NCNP of the Ministry of Health and Welfare; 1985:23–28 (in Japanese).
16. Seino M. Classification of Epileptic Syndromes and Seizures: New and Old. The Fourth Asian and Oceanian Epilepsy Congress, 2002:223 (Abstracts).
17. Seino M, Yagi K. Epilepsy rehabilitation. In: *Proceedings of the 18th International Epilepsy Congress*. New Delhi; 1989:36–42 (Abstract).
18. Shorvon SD. Medical Services. In: Laidlaw J, Richens A, Oxley J, eds. *A Textbook of Epilepsy*, 3rd ed. Edinburgh: Churchill Livingstone; 1988:611–630.
19. Skull A. *Decarceration: Community Treatment and the Deviant—A Radical View*. New York: Basil Blackwell; 1984.
20. Wada T. Socio-medical aspects of epilepsy in Japan. *Epilepsia*. 1966;7:73–79.
21. Yagi K, Onuma T. Classification of Impairments of Epilepsy. In: *Plan of Action for the Fight Against Epilepsy*. Tokyo: Japanese Epilepsy Association; 1986:237–249 (in Japanese).
22. Yeh EA. The struggle for and establishment of a comprehensive care treatment center for the treatment of epilepsy in Japan. *International Epilepsy News (International Bureau for Epilepsy)*. 1992;109:7–9.
23. Yeh EA. The measurement of quality: Epilepsy, quality of life and contemporary Japan. *The Japan Foundation Newsletter*. 1994;21:9–16.

CHAPTER 305 ■ RESIDENTIAL EPILEPSY CENTERS—UNITED KINGDOM

FRANK M. C. BESAG AND STEPHEN W. BROWN

INTRODUCTION

The term *epilepsy center* is used to denote two different situations in the United Kingdom: (a) a collection of professionals specializing in epilepsy and offering different aspects of service at a specified geographical site or area and (b) residential centers for children or adults with epilepsy that offer short- to medium-term assessments, longer-term placements, or both. There are two main types of residential centers, sometimes existing together at one site: The adult centers and the epilepsy special schools.

It might be argued that a comprehensive "epilepsy center" should comprise a group of hospital-based professionals, including physicians who specialize in epilepsy neurosurgery and neuroimaging, in close proximity to a residential center that can offer longer-term assessments or indefinite care in selected cases.

HISTORICAL DEVELOPMENT

A major change in attitude has occurred, from the earlier concept of an "epileptic colony" to that of a residential center that has strong community links and emphasizes preparation for living within society. This contrasts sharply with the image of an "asylum" that either protects the individual with epilepsy from the community or protects the community from the person with epilepsy; neither of these aims would be considered acceptable in current practice.

It is interesting to note that the early residential centers were actually referred to as "colonies," for example, the Lingfield Colony and the Chalfont Colony. Both these centers have changed their names to reflect the change in attitude.

The history of epilepsy centers in Europe seems to be relatively short. The monks at the priory of St. Valentine at Rufach in Alsace provided a "hospice for epileptics" at the end of the 15th century. The Bishop of Wurzburg started a home for people with epilepsy in 1773. In the United Kingdom, the National Hospital for the Paralyzed and Epileptic opened in Queen Square, London, in 1860. The Lingfield Colony (now The National Centre for Young People with Epilepsy) was founded in 1898 by a group of Christian people who had been inspired by Pastor Friedrich von Bodelschwingh. This man had taken over the center at Bethel near Bielefeld, Germany, in 1872, 5 years after it had been established. Subsequently, The Chalfont Centre was founded in Buckinghamshire in 1894, and the David Lewis Centre in Cheshire was opened in 1904. The Park Hospital in Oxford later provided medium-term residential assessments for children with epilepsy, and Bootham Park Hospital in York has provided specialist services, primarily for adults. St. Elizabeth's School and Home at Much Hadham in Hertfordshire and the Meath Home in Surrey initially provided only for female patients but now accept patients of both sexes. The Quarriers Homes in Scotland also have a long tradition of providing residential care for adults with epilepsy.

What is the role for these epilepsy centers in a country with an advanced system of medical care, in which the emphasis is on moving services out into the community? People with epilepsy certainly should lead lives that are as normal as possible and, for most, this implies that they should be living in the community. However, there are two situations in which the epilepsy center may play a role. The first of these is for short- or medium-term assessment and treatment. If there is real diagnostic doubt that cannot reasonably be resolved by the hospital services, it may be appropriate to use the specialist residential center to clarify the diagnosis. The center may also be used for complex, protracted changes in antiepileptic drugs, particularly if a significant risk for status epilepticus is involved. The second situation arises when longer-term placement is needed for a very small proportion of people with epilepsy whose needs cannot reasonably be fulfilled using resources available in the community. The number of people with epilepsy in this category has, appropriately, diminished steadily over recent years, both because of better treatment and because of changing attitudes.

REASONS FOR REFERRAL

Some of the possible reasons for referral to a residential center are listed in Tables 1 and 2. It is not simply the presence of these factors but the degree to which they hamper satisfactory management that is likely to determine whether the epilepsy center must play a role or not. The possible reasons for referral have been discussed in detail elsewhere.[2,3]

LOCATION OF CENTERS

It is mandatory that a specialist epilepsy center have a team of doctors, other caregivers, educational specialists, psychologists, physiotherapists, occupational therapists, and speech therapists if it is to provide a full range of services. This necessarily implies that, to be viable, the center has to be of a reasonable size and have a moderately large number of residents at any one time. An alternative would be for the center to share facilities with other establishments. In practice, the centers tend to be moderately large, and consequently they are relatively few in number across the country. The geographical location may not be very convenient. The Winterton Report[7] on services for people with epilepsy recommended that two new special assessment centers be set up, partly to reduce the distances patients have to travel. This document referred to earlier reports by Morgan and Kurtz[5] and Reid,[6] which stated that "special

TABLE 1

REASONS FOR REFERRAL

Difficult epilepsy
Other medical problems
Cognitive problems
Behavioral problems
Peer group problems
Family and social problems
Psychiatric problems
Multiple problems

centres should be provided for those people with epilepsy whose management presents particular problems,"[5] and "the evidence is of a continuing number of young adults, both males and females, requiring a period of inpatient treatment during which they can be observed by trained staff, investigated and started on remedial programmes of treatment—special centres should, therefore, be seen to have a continuing role."[5] In the current financial climate, however, it seems unlikely that additional centers will be initiated. It might be argued that the centers should be placed closer to large populations. For historical reasons, they have tended to be placed in rather rural situations, because they were founded at a time when close links with the local community were not considered to be essential. There was no particular reason why a "colony" needed to be near a heavily populated region. The current philosophy of facilitating close links with the community, however, implies that the centers should ideally be closer to the communities they serve.

Relation to Medical Centers

Notwithstanding the historical reasons for the epilepsy centers being located away from major cities, a clear need exists for them to have very close links with major hospitals. In practice, because the United Kingdom is not very large, it is possible for the centers to be in semirural areas and yet to be relatively close to major hospitals capable of providing specialist services, such as magnetic resonance imaging and neurosurgery.

LEADERSHIP AND STAFFING

Currently, a very healthy trend exists for the residential special centers to be led by professionals who have an international standing in the field of epilepsy. The implication is that they adopt the approach of providing high-quality service, making full use of the multidisciplinary team.

TABLE 2

FEATURES OF DIFFICULT EPILEPSY

Frequent seizures
Injury during seizures
Risk for status epilepticus
Variable seizure frequency
Postictal problems
Problems with antiepileptic drugs
Inadequate control
Difficult-to-recognize epilepsy

SERVICES AVAILABLE

Uniformity Among Epilepsy Residential Centers

If it is accepted that the centers should provide a high-quality, specialist, tertiary referral service, it is essential that they have a full range of therapists, as already indicated. It is also essential that they have links with the appropriate hospital-based investigational and neurosurgical treatment facilities. It could certainly be argued that sophisticated encephalographic (EEG) and video-EEG monitoring should be mandatory at such centers. In the United Kingdom, these services are available at most of the centers, but there is the occasional notable exception. In the United States[4] and Australia,[1] attempts have been made to set minimal standards, but no such consensus has yet emerged in Europe.

Number of Patients Served

Only a very small proportion of people with epilepsy require the services of a residential center. However, the individuals who need these services tend to be the more difficult and demanding patients who would, in any case, require much in the way of resources for their needs to be met. Placement in a specialist residential center may be a very efficient way of fulfilling their needs, particularly if the outcome is a beneficial review of drug therapy or a successful referral for neurosurgery.

FUNDING

In the past, most residents at the special centers have been sponsored by the local authority of their home area. At least for placements in which the department of education plays a role, there appears to be a current trend away from funding by local authorities to a more centralized form of control through the so-called quasi-autonomous nongovernment organizations (QANGOS). In some cases, this may imply that funding is more easily available. However, it is difficult for a central funding agency to have a good appreciation of the needs of individual patients.

There is also an increasing trend to multiagency funding, with, for example, the district health authority and educational and social services all having to contribute toward the payment. This seems to be based on the naïve concept that greater cooperation will be fostered between the actual agencies providing longer-term care. In practice, it often adds to administrative costs and, worse still, delays or jeopardizes placements because of interagency disputes.

BARRIERS TO ACCESS

The families of patients with epilepsy may be faced with a dilemma if they consider that referral to a center represents some failure, on their part, to provide a caring environment. In these circumstances, there is a role for wise professional counsel based on decisions concerning what really is best for the individual with epilepsy.

Professionals may be reluctant to refer because they may view referral as an admission of defeat or because the admission may draw on limited budgets.

The person with epilepsy may also resist referral for a number of reasons, including feelings of hopelessness. What is the point of a further disruption to life if it will not achieve anything? There may also be an understandable fear of changing from the "disabled" role, with its apparent certainties of care, to the less certain role of increasing independence if control of the epilepsy improves. Support of the peer group, both within the center and subsequently through local epilepsy action groups, can be invaluable in this regard.

COMPREHENSIVE EPILEPSY PROGRAMS

Recognition is growing of the need to coordinate all services: Hospital-based services, residential centers, outpatient clinics, and community outreach services. Relatively few groups of professionals anywhere in the world offer this type of comprehensive service. The need has been recognized in the United Kingdom, but much further development is required.

SUMMARY AND CONCLUSIONS

An unfortunate tendency has emerged to leave referral to specialist services until very late, with the result that the patient's life is disrupted in a major way by epilepsy. Late referral may also be associated with increasing difficulties in treatment. Rather than viewing the epilepsy center as a repository for the long-term care of "hopeless" cases, future emphasis should ideally be on early referral and a much higher volume throughput of cases, with intensive medium-term assessment, investigation, presurgical preparation, and postsurgical rehabilitation as appropriate. Above all, the current trend for preparing patients with epilepsy for life outside the residential establishment should be developed further, either through discharge into the community or through part-time involvement in the community for those who continue to require longer-term residential placement.

References

1. Australian Health Ministers' Advisory Council. Superspecialty Services Subcommittee. *Guidelines for Comprehensive Epilepsy Centres*. Canberra: Australian Institute of Health; 1991.
2. Besag FMC. The role of the special centres for children with epilepsy. In: Oxley J, Stores G, eds. *Epilepsy and Education*. London: Education in Practice Medical Tribune Group; 1986:65–71.
3. Besag FMC. Epilepsy, education and the role of mental handicap. In: Ross EM, Woody RC, eds. *Epilepsy*. London: Ballière's Clinical Paediatrics International Practice and Research. 1994;2(3):561–583.
4. The National Association of Epilepsy Centres. Recommended guidelines for diagnosis and treatment in specialized epilepsy centers. *Epilepsia*. 1990;31(Suppl 1):1–16.
5. Morgan JD, Kurtz Z. *Special Services for People with Epilepsy in the 1970s*. London: Her Majesty's Stationery Office; 1987.
6. Reid JJA. *People with Epilepsy. Report of a Joint Subcommittee of the Standing Medical Advisory Committee and the Advisory Committee on the Health and Welfare of Handicapped Persons*. London: Her Majesty's Stationery Office; 1969.
7. Winterton PMC. *Report of the Working Group on Services for People with Epilepsy. A Report to the Department of Health and Social Security, the Department of Education and Science, and the Welsh Office*. London: Her Majesty's Stationery Office; 1986.

CHAPTER 306 ■ COMPREHENSIVE EPILEPSY CENTERS—THE NETHERLANDS

HARRY MEINARDI AND ALBERT P. ALDENKAMP

INTRODUCTION

In the first edition of this handbook, a description of specialized care for epilepsy reflected a rather stable period of health care in The Netherlands. Recent rapid developments in the fields of science, communication, and accessibility with simultaneous changes in demography, and economy however, clash and obstruct the implementation of theoretically feasible improvements in health care. Although most of the objectives of specialized care for people with epilepsy presented in the previous edition are still valid, some must be adapted to present-day requirements. Because this chapter is rewritten during a period in which many of the changes are still in the making, some uncertainties about the future situation are unavoidable.

The objective of special centers for epilepsy are still in essence to (a) offer intramural and extramural care to individuals with epilepsy within the framework of available facilities or facilities to be created in accordance with new developments and knowledge, and (b) promote the control of epilepsy.

Care comprises several elements, including diagnosis, rehabilitation, and temporary or long-term residential care. *Diagnosis*—the examination, observation, and evaluation of the symptoms and signs of disease and the psychic and social functioning of the patient in order to plan assistance—includes one or all of the following:

- Recommendations for the patient and the patient's family, including presentation of all treatment possibilities (drug treatment, diet, surgery, neuro-stimulation, psychological treatment)
- Recommendations for other health care providers to manage or supplement assistance
- A program for continued support by intramural or extramural facilities of the specialized center

Rehabilitation, the second aspect of care, is the integrated treatment of disordered physical, psychic, and social functioning. Finally, as the third element of care, an important precondition for temporary or prolonged residential care is the *verification that the specialized center is the most appropriate provision within the Dutch health care system for the referred patient.*

The second major objective of the specialized epilepsy care center is to promote the control of epilepsy in general by developing conditions that guarantee optimal physical, psychic, and social well-being for people with epilepsy, or that prevent the development of epilepsy. This can be achieved through:

- Research
- Public education
- Assistance of authorities responsible for health care and welfare on a regional, national, and international level

At present, society considers persons with epilepsy and their relatives to be responsible for the management of their own health. In other words, the patient is no longer comparable to a passenger who boards a ship to be transported to his destination. Rather, he has become a private ship's captain, who rents a ship and crew and takes over command, only consulting a trained pilot when the waters get treacherous.

In addition, the cost of illness is usually paid by insurance companies, which feel entitled to make patient care decisions on their behalf. This is exemplified by the way health services presently are paid for based on *diagnosis-treatment combinations.*

HISTORICAL DEVELOPMENT

In a general article on specialized centers for epilepsy, Meinardi and Pachlatko[4] reviewed the history of some of these centers. The oldest specialized center is reputedly the hospice of St. Valentine in Rufach, France. Although the institution is still there, it no longer functions as a hospice for people with epilepsy. This chapter concentrates on specialized centers in The Netherlands.

Specialized centers for epilepsy in The Netherlands play an important role, both scientifically and with regard to patient care. In 1985, Meinardi[3] described the various theses on epilepsy published in The Netherlands since Prince William the Silent offered a university to Leyden in 1575, in recognition of the city's important contribution to the liberation of The Netherlands from despotic Spanish rule. During the years 1955 to 1985, more than a quarter of these theses were produced by the staff of specialized centers for epilepsy.

The first specialized center for epilepsy in The Netherlands was founded on January 26, 1882, in Haarlem, in the Western part of The Netherlands. The society created to enable the development of a hospital for people with epilepsy originated as part of the so-called *Reveille movement*. This movement was started by well-to-do citizens who wanted to put their Christian principles into practice. Years passed before a specialized center was established. The owner and director of a Deaconesses' Hospice in Haarlem, Lady Teding van Berkhout, was approached several times with a request to admit people with epilepsy. This request was usually rejected, and patients were referred to a psychiatric hospital. Finally, two girls were admitted in 1879, but the experiment was a failure. One of the girls was taken by coach to Bielefeld. In that German city, in 1867, the reverend Von Bodelschwingh had started a specialized center for patients with epilepsy. This experience was decisive; with the help of some friends and allies, the Christian Society for the Care of People with Falling Sickness (the Christian Society) was established, and a small building on the grounds of Lady Teding van Berkhout's home was opened for girls with epilepsy, partly supported by staff from her Deaconesses' Hospice. At first, six girls were admitted, but the pressure for appropriate care for people with epilepsy was such that soon other buildings had to be bought to accommodate an increasing number of patients. In 1885, the mansion "Meer en Bosch" was acquired. For many years, the name "Meer en Bosch" was used as *pars pro toto* for all activities of the specialized center.

In 1966, the national regulations regarding the financing of health care made it desirable to put the facilities of the Christian Society into separate foundations. The new name, Instituut voor Epilepsiebestrijding (Institute for the Fight Against Epilepsy), was for public relations considerations expanded to include the names of the major campuses of the institute, "Meer en Bosch" and "De Cruquiushoeve." These campuses, in Heemstede and nearby Vijfhuizen, comprise a total area of 155 acres. Early in the 20th century, outpatient centers were created in parts of The Netherlands too remote for patients to make a one-day consultation with doctors at the major epilepsy centers. These outpatient facilities served for the intake of new patients and after-care for those who could go home after successful reduction or complete suppression of their seizures. During the 1980s, experiments started to expand the services of the outpatient units. Two so-called *Polimides* were created that used the technical developments of portable electroencephalogram (EEG)-machines and automatic video-registration linked with a piezo-electric seizure detection device to observe patients in their home situation and thus reduce the need for hospitalization in the epilepsy center. Finally, during the years 1988 to 1992, the political trend of paying more attention to consumer needs resulted in a decision to require the Instituut voor Epilepsiebestrijding to build an annex for 80 patients in the northeastern region of The Netherlands. In particular, parents of children with epilepsy had protested to the Ministry of Health that, when intramural tertiary care was needed, they had no other option but to go to a specialized center either in the south or the west of The Netherlands. Permission to build a new epilepsy center was constrained by an order of the government not to increase the total number of beds in the specialized centers for epilepsy. In consultation with the three centers in Breda, Heeze, and Heemstede, it was decided that the Instituut voor Epilepsiebestrijding would transfer some of its capacity to Zwolle. This new center opened in October 1999. The name of the organization now responsible for the centers in Heemstede and Zwolle and nine outpatient clinics in a circle of strategic towns north of the Rhine was changed into Stichting Epilepsie Instellingen Nederland (SEIN). Presently, the intramural capacity of the centers in Heemstede and Zwolle is 600 beds, of which 440 are designated for residential (long-term) care, while facilities in the nine consultation centers North of the Rhine care for 9,278 outpatients.

Only relatively recently has Dutch society ceased to be subdivided along ecclesiastical lines. It is therefore not surprising that, following the successful establishment of a Protestant Christian institution, a secular society against falling sickness was established in 1902, and in 1920, a home for Catholic men with epilepsy. The former had as one of its leaders Dr. L. J. J. Muskens, cofounder of the International League Against Epilepsy (ILAE). In 1902, this group it opened a hospital for people with epilepsy in Amsterdam. The catholic center was established in the South in Geldrop. It was not until the 1960s (although the initiative dates from 1953), that a residential center for women was established adjacent to the home for Catholic men. This new center also provided advanced intramural medical care to both men and women. These two organizations gradually merged into the Epilepsy Center Kempenhaeghe in Heeze, near Geldrop; it has an intramural capacity of 525 beds and also outpatient departments in five different cities that care for 3,869 outpatients.

Several interesting phenomena relating to the social forces that affect health provision can be observed in the development of epilepsy services in The Netherlands. The Hospital Muskens built in Amsterdam near the Municipal University Hospital was closed in 1986. Factors contributing to its closure were the impossibility of expanding the building, because costs of building in the center of Amsterdam were prohibitive. So, when specialized centers for epilepsy began to engage in rehabilitation and provide sheltered workshops for their patients, Amsterdam had to default. Furthermore, the neighboring University Hospital was very much in need of referrals of other patients with chronic illnesses in addition to epilepsy. Willy-nilly, these referrals were accepted, and thus the advantages of a specialized center for epilepsy were lost.

Another interesting development was that, as late as the 1960s, a new, small Catholic epilepsy center comprising 132 beds, named Hans Berger Kliniek, was started in Breda. This facility presently also cares for 2,000 patients via outpatient departments in four cities. This center in Breda was started mainly because of the rapid emptying of a large sanatorium for tuberculosis patients in that city. The decreased need for care of patients with respiratory disorders was compensated for by establishing departments of epileptology, cardiac surgery, and child psychiatry. However, at the end of the 20th century, it became government policy to merge smaller hospitals with only a few specialties with larger, more general hospitals. Although the special center for epilepsy remained an independent foundation, it had to move its facilities to a general hospital, the AMPHIA in Breda. Its intramural capacity was reduced to 56 beds, with an additional four beds for day care. To achieve a situation similar to the SEIN-managed centers in Heemstede and Zwolle, a merger between Kempenhaeghe and the Hans Berger Kliniek has recently been established.

Although hospitals had to merge in order to increase in size, residential facilities for the long-term care of persons with epilepsy, psychiatric patients, or the mentally handicapped were stimulated to reduce their size. In the Heemstede epilepsy center, but especially in the Southern epilepsy center Kempenhaeghe, developments started to change chronic intramural care. Whereas in the past all facilities were on the campus of the epilepsy centers, this changed to smaller community houses in the surrounding communities, with services provided by the epilepsy center.

In yet another development, the university hospital of Maastricht in the south of The Netherlands has chosen epilepsy as one of its priorities for patient care and research and is cooperating with the epilepsy center Kempenhaeghe. Negotiations aiming at a similar type of cooperation are ongoing between SEIN and the Christian University Hospital in Amsterdam. In both university hospitals, units for epilepsy surgery are in development. Epilepsy surgery is also continuing in the university hospital of Utrecht, where modern epilepsy surgery was initiated during the 1970s.

Although beyond the scope of this chapter to detail, all Special Centers for Epilepsy provide, on request, incidental and regular consultations in homes and institutions for mentally handicapped patients. Among the persons cared for in these establishments, 20% to 30% may have epilepsy, with a rather high prevalence of refractory epilepsies: Among 172 patients with epilepsy on optimal treatment in a home for the mentally retarded, 61 (35%) were seizure-free, whereas at the other extreme, 23 (13%) had a seizure frequency between several per week and daily.[5]

In summary, the three specialized epilepsy centers located in Heemstede/Zwolle, Heeze/Breda, and their outpatient clinics in Heemstede, Amsterdam, Leeuwarden, Groningen, Zwolle, Enschede, Nijmegen, Heeze, Sittard, Arnhem, Utrecht, Breda, Terneuzen, Goes, Rotterdam, and The Hague, make specialized care for people with refractory epilepsy available in

16 areas, each serving approximately 1 million of the 16 million inhabitants of The Netherlands.

MECHANISMS OF REFERRAL

The specialized centers for epilepsy in The Netherlands must be viewed against the background of health services in that country. In The Netherlands, 16.3 million people inhabit an area of 34,000 square kilometers. One general practitioner is available for every 2,350 inhabitants, and one neurologist for every 22,500 inhabitants. There are 3,015,704 children younger than 14 years old and, for many of them, specialist care is provided by pediatricians. One pediatrician is available for every 2,500 children below the age of 14.

In 2006, a new Health Insurance Act was implemented. Its impact on care for persons with epilepsy can not yet be fully estimated. Under this Act, all Dutch citizens, irrespective of income, must buy a basic package of health insurance. The government has established a list of conditions that must be covered by the basic package. The costs may vary according to the contracts that insurance companies establish with health care providers on the one hand and their clients on the other. The cost will not depend on the age or health of the client. This is made possible through a compensation fund that will reimburse those insurance companies with a higher-than-average proportion of high-risk clients who present extra costs. Once a year, the client can reconsider whether to stay with the same insurance company or switch to one that he expects will better suit his needs. The new Health Insurance Act stipulates that a Netherlands Care Authority be established that will supervise proper execution of the law; it also is mandated with stimulating competition and, where no competition is possible, setting budgets and tariffs for hospitals. (The Netherlands Care Authority absorbs and replaces the present Board for Statutory Control of Health Care Insurances as well as the Board for Health Care Tariffs.)

Many health care items previously covered under the compulsory insurance scheme for low-income people (<31,000 Euro annual income, or those on welfare) are now excluded from basic coverage. Additional insurance to cover these items can be purchased, but is not obligatory.

Consultation with a general practitioner by a person registered as his patient is free of charge. Concomitantly, how insurance companies pay for other services rendered to their clients has drastically changed. A system of diagnosis-treatment combinations has been developed, with input from all parties concerned. Cost elements known to be associated with a particular diagnosis—for example complex partial seizures or appendicitis—are averaged and shown on the bill whether or not all these elements have been utilized for the particular patient named on the bill, such as anesthesia or surgery. How these changes will affect services for people with epilepsy is difficult to predict. An important problem still under debate concerns financing for research needed to optimize diagnosis and treatment. Although special centers for epilepsy in The Netherlands do not have academic hospital status, in the past, the Heemstede center did have permission to include the cost of research personnel in its fees, a practice that has not yet been approved under the new regulations.

An increasing number of neurologists are employed by the hospitals where they practice. Their income is independent of the number of patients seen, or the number of interventions offered. Others are in private practice and have contracts with hospitals for the facilities provided. There are 725 registered neurologists in The Netherlands. There are 90 general hospitals, 85 psychiatric hospitals, ten hospitals for special categories (e.g., three for epilepsy), and ten University hospitals (in all, 22 teaching hospitals). The problem with epilepsy care and the development of a nationwide network of outpatient clinics manned by the staff of specialized centers for epilepsy is rooted in the incompatibility of the needs of teaching hospitals and the quality of care requested by patients with long-term illnesses such as epilepsy. In particular, long-term patients become discouraged by the frequent rotation of the junior physicians directly responsible for their care. In The Netherlands, specialized centers for epilepsy started as hospices at the end of the 19th and beginning of the 20th century. Although located in a semi-rural area, SEIN (Meer en Bosch-de Cruquiushoeve) is surrounded by four universities at distances of 20, 25, 35, and 60 kilometers. It was therefore easy for its staff to keep up with the latest scientific developments and often to take the lead in research. Because epilepsy patients could obtain high-quality care without having to cope with the continuous turnover of physicians inherent in a teaching hospital, they preferred to avoid the university hospitals. As a consequence, interest in epilepsy at the universities slackened, with subsequent deleterious effects on the ability of their graduates to treat patients with chronic epilepsy. In recent years, closer ties have developed between the special centers and university hospitals, Consultative collaboration aimed at the education of neurologic residents has been established between SEIN and the university hospitals of Utrecht, Rotterdam, Amsterdam, and Groningen, and between Kempenhaeghe and the Universities of Nymegen and Maastricht. Both centers offer a short internship to neurologists in training. Furthermore, SEIN has links with the Free University of Amsterdam and is considering moving its short-term care facilities and part of its laboratories to a site adjacent to the Hospital of this University. Kempenhaeghe has established a link with Maastricht University.

The insurance companies cooperated in the development of a nationwide network for tertiary epilepsy care by permitting referrals from neurologists to epileptologists, even though epileptology is not a registered specialty. This was facilitated by the inclusion of epilepsy centers as a special category of hospitals in the law covering hospital provisions. As mentioned, the intramural capacity is presently 1,337 beds, spread over four locations. Furthermore, a network of 17 outpatient clinics is maintained by the specialized centers and cares for 12,300 of the estimated 96,000 people with active epilepsy in The Netherlands.

The epilepsy centers once employed neuropsychiatrists. From the early 1970s on, specialization as a neuropsychiatrist was no longer possible; only the constituent specializations of neurology and psychiatry were thenceforth registered. The medical staff of the epilepsy centers was subsequently selected from neurologists and supplemented with clinical psychologists.

In The Netherlands, epilepsy centers are in fact autonomous organizations, with sometimes divergent interests. However, through the national epilepsy organizations such as the Dutch branch of the ILAE and an umbrella organization (the National Epilepsy Fund), they keep in close contact and work to keep their policies—and, in particular, their relations with the government—consistent.

FUNDING

The possibility of achieving one's objectives is determined by the means available. A specialized center, like all other health care facilities in The Netherlands, is financed by the fees the insurance companies pay for the services rendered. Because the health insurance premium has a pronounced influence on the national economy, tariffs and the services considered acceptable were negotiated on a national level by the Central

Bureau Tariffs Health Care. The state, insurance companies, and health care providers participated in these negotiations. Only after intensive negotiations were most, but not all, financial consequences of the objectives of Special Centers for Epilepsy accepted. In particular, the provision of psychotherapy on an outpatient basis was rejected on the assumption that other existing institutions could serve that purpose. Unfortunately, a lack of familiarity with specific, epilepsy-related factors has repeatedly caused attempts to assist patients along these lines to go wrong. The full impact of The Netherlands Care Authority cannot yet be estimated.

Not all costs for rehabilitation are paid for by health insurance. To reintegrate people with epilepsy who, because of seizures (and often overprotection) have lost or never acquired job experience, the Instituut voor Epilepsiebestrijding was permitted to open a sheltered workshop with the financial assistance of the Ministry of Social Affairs. This was also motivated by the reluctance of the regular regional sheltered workshops to accept people with epilepsy. Because the cost of maintenance of sheltered workshops was increasingly a problem for the government, negotiations were started during the 1990s to terminate the special arrangement with epilepsy centers and refer patients for rehabilitation to the regional sheltered workshops. Interestingly, a few years after this had been achieved, the regional workshops moved from Haarlem to a location immediately adjacent to the campus of the SEIN in Heemstede, which reflects a further removal of the discrimination between persons with epilepsy and persons with other handicaps.

Similarly, the Ministry of Education finances schools on the campuses of the epilepsy centers. Although, according to their charter, the schools were originally established for "children with epilepsy," in the 1980s this was changed to "special schools for the multiply handicapped." This implies that, in addition to epilepsy, another handicap should be present—most often mental retardation. Hospitalized children with normal intelligence and no physical handicap may attend the schools, but the costs are not reimbursed, and therefore the number of children in this category remains small. The Ministry of Education does finance outreach by staff of the schools at the epilepsy centers to other schools, which receive advice on how to manage pupils with epilepsy.

NEUROSURGERY FOR EPILEPSY

In the budget of the Instituut voor Epilepsiebestrijding, a small amount had been made available for research by the Central Bureau Tariffs Health Care. Fortunately, the Christian Society, which formally is no longer connected with the epilepsy centers, does provide financial support for research and development and for recreational facilities for long-term patients. In the period from 1989 to 1993, a 3-year project was cofunded with the government to establish the optimal protocol for functional neurosurgery for patients with epilepsy. Functional neurosurgery for epilepsy in The Netherlands started in 1971 as a collaborative undertaking of the University Hospital at Utrecht and the Instituut voor Epilepsiebestrijding, the latter being responsible for the presurgical analysis, and in particular the monitoring of patients in whom intracranial electrodes have been placed for detailed analysis. Before any final decision to operate, a counsel, The Dutch Epilepsy Surgery Program, in which all major groups concerned with patients with intractable epilepsy participate, reviews the findings. As of 2005, patients go for presurgical analysis to Heeze or Heemstede. After receiving a verdict from the Dutch Epilepsy Surgery Program, epilepsy surgery still mainly takes place in Utrecht, but now is also being performed at the Free University in Amsterdam and at Maastricht University.

The Christian Society has also funded a project to investigate whether the provision of long-term monitoring facilities on an outpatient basis, including monitoring at home, could effectively make intramural observation redundant. Based on its findings, diagnostic and counseling services at home have been greatly expanded. However, during the late 1990s, the Christian Society has also spent some of its funds assisting SEIN to reorganize, thus reducing its ability to support research.

On a national level, research grants for epilepsy are provided annually by the National Epilepsy Fund, which derives its income from charity and legacies. These grants are, however, not restricted for use by the specialized centers. The Christian Society initiated providing monies for an endowed chair in epileptology, which, after prolonged deliberations by the departments of neurology of the Dutch universities, was finally established in 1984, at the University of Nymegen.

After the retirement of the first chair-holder in 2000, this chair was moved to the Free University of Amsterdam. Nijmegen appointed at its own expense a new professor of epileptology; however, this chair will not be continued after his retirement, which is due in 2006. In recent years, the National Epilepsy Fund has established two additional chairs for epileptology at the Universities of Utrecht and Maastricht.

TERTIARY VERSUS SECONDARY CARE

Two articles[2,7] have been published by the Nymegen department of epileptology comparing treatment and outcome in a secondary and tertiary epilepsy care outpatient facility. To compare the two facilities, several characteristics were considered that might influence the course of epilepsy. These were age, gender, type of seizure, duration of epilepsy type, and strength of medication. The strength of medication was determined by the ratio of the prescribed daily dose to the defined daily dose (PDD/DDD ratio). The DDD is the assumed average recommended adult dose for the major indication for prescribing the drug, and it is the unit of comparison recommended by the World Health Organization (WHO) Drug Utilization Research Group.[5] The PDD is the dose actually prescribed for the individual patient. Also, the following indexes have been determined on a clinimetric basis:

- Index of Seizures (IS), indicating seizure type and frequency
- Seizure Activity Index (SA), which modifies the IS to include seizure severity
- Neurotoxicity Index (NTX)
- Systemic Toxicity Index (STX)
- Composite Index of Impairments (CII), reflecting all treatment-related impairments, that is, paroxysmal impairments (seizures) caused by the disorder being treated and drug-induced impairments or adverse effects of treatment (CII = SA + NTX + STX)

These indexes have been extensively described in previous publications.[1,6] Parameters of other effects, such as psychosocial and occupational impacts caused by disabilities and handicaps, were not included.

In the first part of these studies, patients were examined who regularly visited the outpatient departments of the University Hospital in Nymegen (UH), or the outpatient departments of the Instituut voor Epilepsiebestrijding in Utrecht and

Heemstede (EC), literally cross-secting The Netherlands. Selection criteria were as follows:

- Patient files should be well documented, including an accurate history and adequate neurophysiologic data for a firm diagnosis. The patient should have well-defined types of seizures according to the International Classification of the ILAE.
- No factors should be present that might be considered to complicate the evaluation process. These factors included progressive brain disorders, obvious noncompliance in drug use or seizure registration, pseudoseizures, and severe mental retardation.

When the data of 120 patients from the UH and 225 from the EC were analyzed, it became clear that there was no significant difference in sex or age between the two groups. However, a significant difference was noted in duration of epilepsy. The median duration of epilepsy was 20 years for the EC group and 10 years for the UH group ($p = 0.0001$). The groups were also different with respect to seizure types. At the UH, a higher percentage of patients had primarily generalized tonic–clonic seizures (45.8% vs. 11.6% for the EC; $p < 0.001$), whereas at the EC, a higher percentage of patients had secondarily generalized tonic–clonic seizures, although the difference was not significantly different (16.4% vs. 9.2% for the UH; $p = .08$). No difference in partial seizures was noted between the EC and the UH. The patients of the EC had a greater diversity of seizure types. Apart from the above-mentioned types, myoclonic, tonic, and atonic seizures were seen in this group, although mostly in combination with other seizure types. Patients with more than one seizure type were more numerous at the EC than at the UH (45.4% vs. 15.1%; $p < 0.001$).

Treatment

The groups were clearly treated differently. More patients were treated with monotherapy at the UH (62.5% vs. 28.0% at the EC; $p < 0.001$). At both centers, if monotherapy was used, carbamazepine was the preferred drug. The average number of antiepileptic drugs (AEDs) used per patient was 2.0 for the EC and 1.4 for the UH. There was a significant

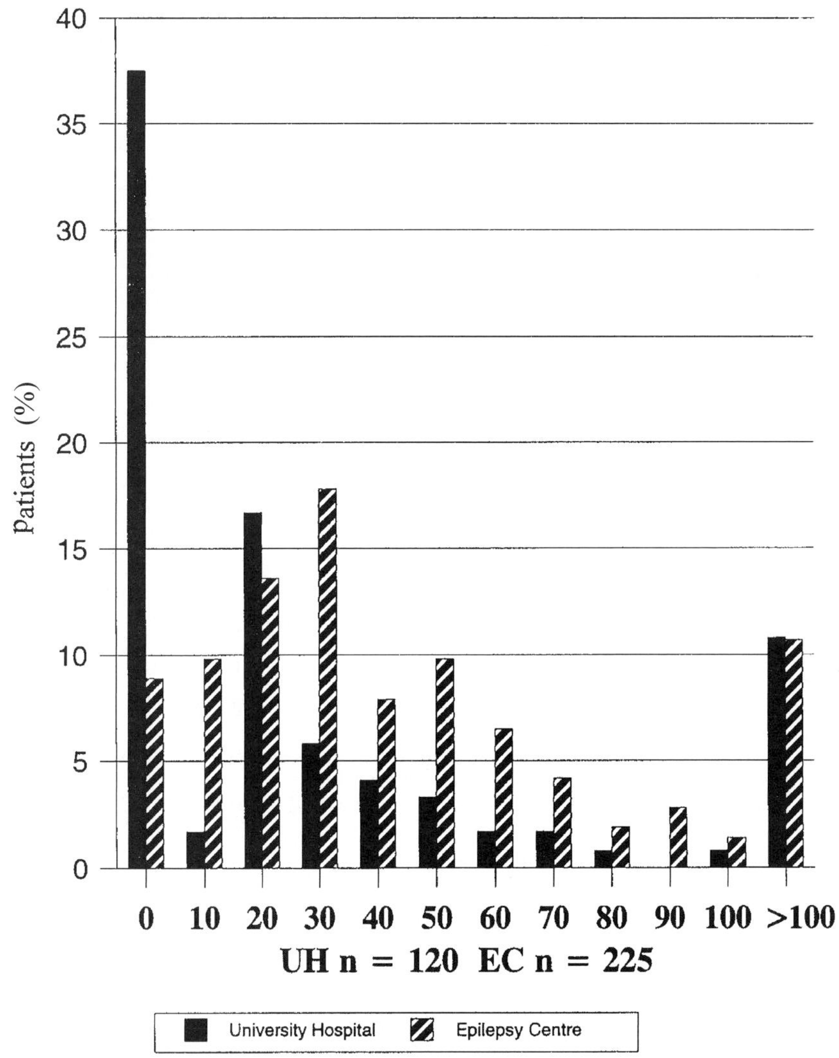

Univ	37.5	1.7	16.7	5.8	4.1	3.3	1.7	1.7	0.8	0	0.8	10.8
Epil	8.9	9.8	13.6	17.8	7.9	9.8	6.5	4.2	1.9	2.8	1.4	10.7

FIGURE 1. Distribution of the CII (abscissa) for the UH ($n = 120$) and the EC ($n = 225$). *White bars*, university clinic; *shaded bars*, epilepsy center.

TABLE 1

DISTRIBUTION OF SEIZURE TYPES (32 MATCHED PAIRS)

Seizure type	Percentage of patients (n)
CPS	28.1 (9)
SGTCS	15.6 (5)
PGTCS	34.4 (11)
SPS + SGTCS	3.1 (1)
CPS + SGTCS	18.8 (6)

CPS, complex partial seizure; SGTCS, secondarily generalized tonic–clonic seizure; PGTCS, primarily generalized tonic–clonic seizure; SPS, simple partial seizure.

difference in the PDD/DDD ratio between the two centers. The median PDD/DDD ratio was 1.7 for the EC and 0.8 for the UH ($p = 0.0001$).

Composite Index of Impairment

The CII was significantly higher at the EC ($p = 0.0001$). At the UH, 37.5% of the patients had complete seizure control and no drug side effects, which resulted in a CII score of 0. This was the case for only 8.9% of patients at the EC ($p < 0.001$). For the group of patients with a CII score of >100, no significant difference was found between the two centers. At the EC, 10.7% had a CII score of >100; at the UH, this was 10.8% ($p = 1.00$) (Fig. 1).

At both centers, no clear correlation was observed between the duration of epilepsy and the outcome of any of the indexes (Spearman correlation coefficient was 0.06 or lower). Also, no significant correlation was seen between the PDD/DDD ratio and the toxicity ratings (Spearman correlation coefficient was 0.49 or lower).

Matched Groups of Patients from Secondary and Tertiary Care Facilities

The first study answered in the affirmative that secondary and tertiary referral centers care for different categories of patients. However, there was also clearly an overlap (Fig. 1). It was therefore decided to re-examine the data of two groups from the UH and the EC matched for seizure type and duration of epilepsy. Only 32 pairs could be collected. The seizure types and duration of epilepsy are shown in Tables 1 and 2.

Although the groups were matched for duration of epilepsy, this does not necessarily bring about a match in age groups. However, concerning age distribution, a significant difference was found only in the age group of 15 to 19 years, with six patients (18.8%) at the EC and one patient (3.1%) at the UH. No great differences were observed in the other age groups.

TABLE 2

DURATION OF EPILEPSY (32 MATCHED PAIRS)

Duration of epilepsy	Percentage of patients (n)
1–5 y	25.0 (8)
6–10 y	43.8 (14)
11–15 y	18.8 (6)
16–20 y	12.5 (4)

Composite Index of Impairments in Matched Groups

Notwithstanding matching, the two groups were significantly different with respect to the CII ($p = 0.014$). Far more patients at the UH than at the EC had a CII score of 0 (45.9% vs. 9.4%; $p = 0.001$), indicating that more patients were seizure-free and had no drug side effects. On the other hand, 18.8% of the patients at the UH had a CII score of >100; this was the case for only 9.4% of the patients at the EC. This difference, however, was not statistically significant (Fig. 2).

Seizure Activity Index and Toxicity Ratings in Matched Groups

For the SA, no significant difference was observed between the two centers ($p = 0.060$). More patients at the UH than at the EC had an SA score of 0, but twice as many patients at the UH as at the EC had an SA score of >100 (18.8% vs. 9.4%), although this by itself was not statistically significant.

The NTX rating was significantly lower for the patients at the UH than at the EC ($p = 0.003$). At the UH, 71.9% of the patients had an NTX of 0, as opposed to 21.9% at the EC.

The STX rating was likewise significantly lower for the patients at the UH than at the EC ($p = 0.016$). At the EC, 18.1% of the patients had an STX >0, as opposed to only 6.2% at the UH.

Treatment Differences of Matched Groups

Although there were some differences in mode of pharmacotherapy, none reached statistical significance. As for the individual drugs prescribed, it was noticed that the drugs ethosuximide and diazepam were prescribed only at the UH. Clobazam and vigabatrin were prescribed only at the EC (Table 3).

At the UH, more patients were treated with monotherapy (56.2%) than at the EC (40.6%), although this difference was not statistically significant. When the patients were treated with monotherapy, carbamazepine was most frequently prescribed at the EC (53.8% of the patients on monotherapy). At the UH, carbamazepine and valproate were prescribed as monotherapy for an equal number of patients (44.4%). At the EC, 56.2% of the patients were treated with polytherapy and, at the UH, this value was 37.5%. This difference was not statistically significant.

The average number of AEDs used per patient was 1.8 for the EC and 1.4 for the UH.

The difference in the PDD/DDD ratio (EC, 0.80; UH, 0.90) between the two centers was statistically insignificant, but only marginally so.

PSYCHOGENIC PSEUDO-EPILEPTIC (NON-EPILEPTIC) SEIZURES

Paradoxically, the diagnosis and treatment of persons with psychogenic nonepileptic seizures is a service that appears best provided by special centers for epilepsy and not in a psychiatric setting. About 30% of the patients referred to a specialized epilepsy center have nonepileptic seizures in addition to epileptic seizures, and about 10% have nonepileptic seizures

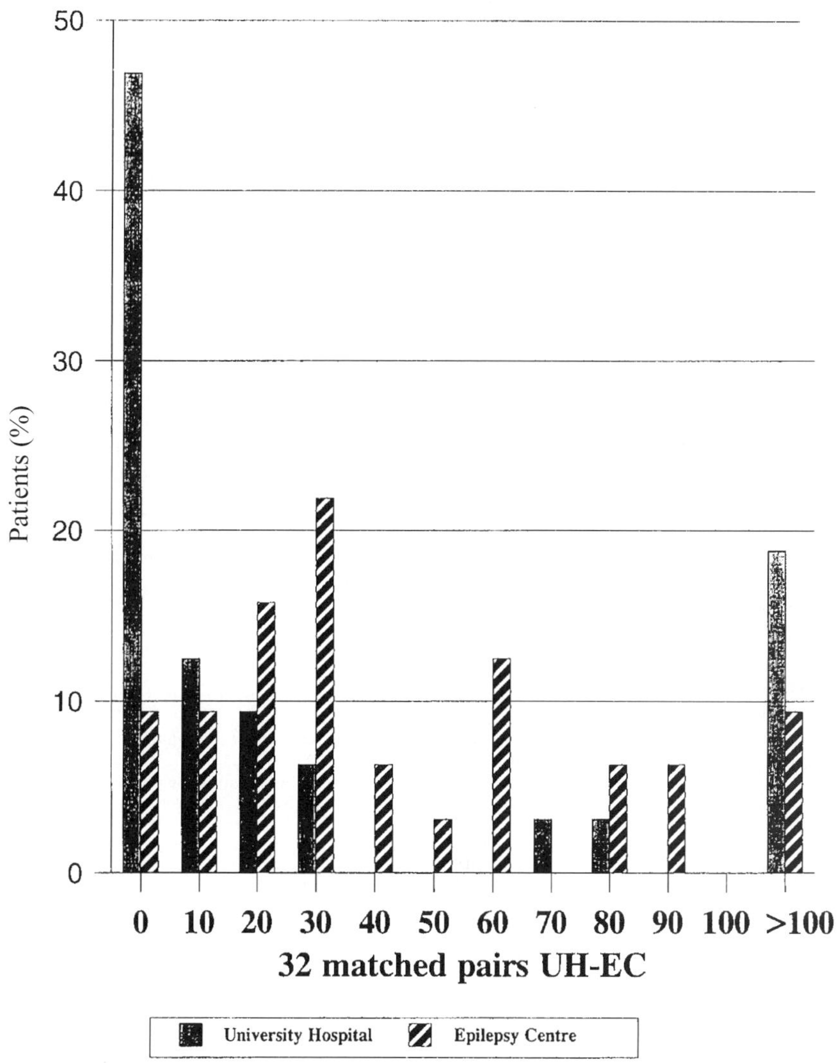

Univ	46.9	12.5	9.4	6.3	0	0	0	3.1	3.1	0	0	18.8
Epil	9.4	9.4	15.8	21.9	6.3	3.1	12.5	0	6.3	6.3	0	9.4

FIGURE 2. Distribution of the CII (abscissa) for 32 matched pairs of the UH and the EC. *Black bars*, university hospital; *cross-hatched bars*, epilepsy center.

TABLE 3

AVERAGE DOSE AND RATIO OF PRESCRIBED DAILY DOSE TO DEFINED DAILY DOSE FOR ANTIEPILEPTIC DRUG PRESCRIBED

	Epilepsy center			University hospital		
Antiepileptic drug	mg	(*n*)	PDD/DDD	mg	(*n*)	PDD/DDD
Carbamazepine	813.64	(22)	0.81	678.33	(16)	0.68
Clobazam	13.33	(3)	0.67	—	—	—
Diazepam	—	—	—	10.00	(1)	1.00
Ethosuximide	—	—	—	1,000.00	(1)	0.80
Phenobarbital	73.33	(3)	0.73	133.00	(7)	1.33
Phenytoin	285.71	(8)	0.95	354.00	(9)	1.18
Primidone	500.00	(2)	0.40	1,250.00	(1)	1.00
Valproate	1250.00	(16)	0.83	1,037.50	(10)	0.69
Vigabatrin	1500.00	(3)	0.75	—	—	—

PDD/DDD, prescribed daily dose/defined daily dose.

only. Within the centers, specialized expert teams are available for the diagnosis, treatment, and referral of these patients.

SUMMARY AND CONCLUSIONS

Through a sometimes obscure process of growth, what began as a local appeal to take pity on people in the unenviable position of being afflicted with epilepsy has expanded into a legally constituted tertiary care system covering The Netherlands. This system cares for 14% of the patients with epilepsy in The Netherlands, presumably those with seizures resistant to therapy or those unable to cope unaided with the psychic or social aftermath of their illness. However, as the attitude of society toward people with disorders changes, and as the need to analyze the epilepsies through careful observation by trained personnel is gradually replaced by technical advances, secondary (specialist) care may eventually make tertiary care redundant. As a first step in analyzing the situation during the 1980s, the care provided by a university hospital and an epilepsy center has been studied. Overall, clear differences were observed in the patient groups. The duration of epilepsy of patients from the epilepsy center was longer, and they were more likely to have several seizure types and a higher composite index of impairment.

No distinct differences were found in the treatment policies between the secondary epilepsy care center and the tertiary epilepsy care center after patients were matched according to seizure type and duration of epilepsy. Nonetheless, distinct differences in treatment outcome were noted, as assessed by the CII. The combination of "same treatment but different outcome" agreed with the expected prevalence of more difficult-to-treat patients in a tertiary referral care center. The matching variables of "seizure type" and "duration of epilepsy" were thought to reflect the severity of epilepsy, but selecting patients by matching for seizure type and duration of epilepsy as evidence of similar severity is clearly insufficient to obtain completely comparable groups. Other factors aside from seizure type and duration of epilepsy are apparently important to the outcome of treatment of epilepsy. It will be a challenge to future researchers to find out which factors make the difference. The answer to that question will help determine whether tertiary epilepsy care will continue to be needed in the future, and suggest the appropriate equipment of such service.

During the 1980s, development started toward implementing information technology in patient care. Kempenhaeghe developed a Medical Information System (MIS) that supports patient care and administration, and this MIS system is now implemented in all epilepsy centers. This will eventually lead to a electronic patient file.

Unfortunately, although it was hoped that the electronic recording of patient's data would facilitate future comparisons between type of services and outcome using clinimetric indices, developments along those lines are still unsatisfactory.

References

1. Cramer JA, Smith DB, Mattson RH, et al. A method of quantification for the evaluation of antiepileptic drug therapy. *Neurology*. 1983;33(Suppl 1):26–37.
2. Lammers MW, Wijsman DJP, Hekster YA, et al. Epilepsy treatment in The Netherlands. Comparison of matched groups of two medical centers. *Acta Neurol Scand*. 1994;89:415–420.
3. Meinardi H. *Epileptology: military art, art of healing or science?* (Inaugural address.) Catholic University of Nymegen; 1985.
4. Meinardi H, Pachlatko C. Special Centers for Epilepsy. In: Dam M, Gram L, eds. *Comprehensive Epileptology*. New York: Raven Press; 1990.
5. WHO Collaborating Center for Drugs Statistics Methodology and Nordic Council on Medicines. *Guidelines for DDD*. Oslo; 1991.
6. Wijsman DJP, Hekster YA, Keyser A, et al. Clinimetrics and epilepsy care. *Pharmaceutisch Weekblad (Sci)*. 1991;13:182–188.
7. Wijsman DJP, Lammers MW, Hekster YA, et al. Epilepsy treatment in The Netherlands. Comparison of two medical centers. *Acta Neurol Scand*. 1993;87:438–442.

CHAPTER 307 ■ ECONOMIC ASPECTS OF EPILEPSY AND ANTIEPILEPTIC TREATMENT

DEMETRIS K. PILLAS, CAROLINE E. SELAI, JOHN T. LANGFITT, AND MARC R. NUWER

INTRODUCTION

Significance of Economic Evaluation of Epilepsy and Its Treatment Modalities

Over the last 15 years there has been a dramatic increase in the therapeutic options available for the treatment of epilepsy. Epilepsy can now be treated with 13 different U.S. Food and Drug Administration (FDA)-approved antiepileptic drugs (AEDs);[37] surgery has now been established as an effective treatment for reducing or eliminating seizures in patients with medically intractable epilepsy.[61] Furthermore, vagal nerve stimulation (VNS), which includes the first implantable device with antiseizure properties, is now considered a safe therapeutic procedure, with clinically useful and sustained benefits.[53]

Many of these developments for treating epilepsy have a higher initial cost than the older treatments they replace. On the other hand, they may offer long-term savings if an increasing number of patients undergoing the new treatments become seizure-free. Therefore, it has become necessary to evaluate the economic burden of health care alternatives as well as their therapeutic efficacy. It is no longer sufficient merely to demonstrate a satisfactory degree of efficacy for a particular treatment if the cost of such therapy would cause the health care system to deny an equivalently efficacious yet cheaper remedy to a wider group of the target population.[10]

In addition, with the growing emphasis on cost containment and managed care in health care delivery, evaluations of the cost of epilepsy and its treatment are increasingly required by government agencies, advocacy groups, and health care payers concerned with the allocation of research and treatment resources among disease conditions.

In such a context, it is of interest to review critically the recently published literature on the economic aspects of epilepsy and its treatment in order to:

- Compare the variance and distribution of costs between and within various countries
- Identify and discuss methodologic issues and limitations in calculating the cost of epilepsy
- Evaluate the cost-effectiveness of the different treatments available

In this chapter, we explore these issues by systematically reviewing all the recent epilepsy-related cost-evaluation studies, analyzing their results, comparing their findings and, discussing their implications.

TYPES OF ECONOMICS STUDIES

We identified studies via Medline and hand-searching English-language, epilepsy-related, and health economics journals. To have been included, studies had to have (a) been published between January 1998 and January 2006, (b) followed one of the standard methods of health economics evaluation (cost of illness [COI], cost-minimization analysis [CMA], cost-effectiveness analysis [CEA], cost-benefit analysis [CBA], cost-utility analysis [CUA]) (Table 1), and (c) aimed to provide estimations on the cost of epilepsy alone, not including comorbidities.

We identified 31 studies: 17 COI studies,[1,3,8,9,11,17,19,21,23,24,31,34,35,41,45,63,64] four studies using a CMA,[29,30,48,58] 10 studies performing a CEA,[16,32,40,42,47,49,55,56,59,65] two studies using a CBA,[12,13] and five studies performing a CUA.[18,25,44,50,51] All studies were classified based on how the primary outcome was reported.

The general, transnational comparative, approach presented here takes into account not only the differences in the studies' methods, but the epidemiologic features (incidence and prevalence of epilepsy), stage of economic development, and organization of health care sector in the countries studied.

Transnational Comparison of Cost-of-illness Studies

COI studies enumerate all costs attributable to a disease to arrive at a total cost of that disease. A COI study can follow a variety of perspectives.[2,5,7,14,28,33,36,38] From an epidemiologic point of view, COI studies can be conducted using either a prevalence- or incidence-based approach, depending on whether an annual or longitudinal horizon is adopted. Also, COI evaluations vary in their study design (i.e., prospective or retrospective study design) and method of data collection (e.g., questionnaire, medical database, case report). The sampling strategy is also a significant parameter when evaluating the cost of a disease. This ranges from collecting data from a general practitioner or a hospital, to estimating costs based on administrative databases or national samples. COI studies also vary as to whether the direct or indirect costs of a disease are calculated. *Direct costs* are the monetary value of resources consumed in the prevention, treatment, or rehabilitation of people with the disorder. *Indirect costs* represent the loss of productivity to society due to a disease and its treatment.[7,14]

To achieve a comprehensive transnational comparison of all recent COI studies, these study perspectives were taken into consideration when analyzing, categorizing, and tabulating the studies and their results. The results appear in Tables, 2, 3, and 4.

Comparison of COI Prevalence-based Studies

Table 2 includes only prevalence-based studies, stating the country of the study, data source, method of data collection, direct or indirect costs estimated by the study, and any additional general information in the study that is of significance.

TABLE 1

TYPES OF ECONOMIC EVALUATION

Type of study	Description
Cost-of-illness studies (COI)	To itemize, value, and sum the costs of a particular problem with the aim of giving an idea of its economic burden
Cost-minimization analysis (CMA)	If the interventions have the same consequences, the economic analysis can concentrate on inputs only. This analysis is concerned with the identification of the intervention with the lowest possible costs
Cost-effectiveness analysis (CEA)	If the outcome of interest is the same in two programs, but they have different success in achieving the outcome
Cost-benefit analysis (CBA)	If neither the consequences nor the outcomes of two programs are the same; cost-benefit analysis aims to compare all social costs and consequences across different interventions or against a do-nothing option
Cost-utility analysis (CUA)	This analysis is preferred by analysts who have reservations about valuing benefits in dollar terms; *utility* refers to the preferences individuals or society may have for any particular set of health outcomes—this approach incorporates quality of life adjustments to treatment outcomes

Comparison of COI Incidence-based Studies

Incidence-based studies are shown in Table 3, with an emphasis on the evolution of costs over time. Only the first 4 years after onset were included, because most studies estimated costs up to the fourth year.

Direct Cost Distribution

Table 4 depicts the breakdown of the direct costs of epilepsy treatment. Three categories are included:

- Hospital costs: In- and outpatient visits, admissions, emergency room visits, and emergency transportation (ambulance) costs
- Drug costs: Prescribed antiepileptic drugs (AEDs), as well as costs attributable to adverse drug reactions from the AEDs
- Other costs: Diagnostic procedures, such as laboratory tests, electroencephalography, computed tomography, and magnetic resonance imaging scans as well as medical consultations that are part of the diagnostic procedures.

Six studies that did not categorize direct costs in this way were excluded from the table.[19,23,34,35,41,63]

Cost-minimization Analysis

CMA provides the simplest economic evaluation when the alternate treatments, in this case AEDs, have equivalent clinical efficacy. To be equivalent, the comparators should be of the same efficacy in all patients, under all conditions, with similar risks of adverse events.[10]

Table 5 displays study duration, the configuration of the treatment pathways followed, and the nature of the direct costs included during the cost estimation procedure for four CMA studies, along with the mean cost per patient for each of the four AEDs that were examined.

Cost-effectiveness Analysis

CEA assesses how efficiently a specific health intervention influences health, compared with the next best alternative. Thus, CEAs specifically account for the costs to health of a disease and treatment that are typically excluded from COI studies (i.e., premature mortality, morbidity, disability, as well as pain and suffering).[36]

Tables 6 and 7 include ten CEA studies. Table 6 focuses on CEA studies on AEDs; Table 7 presents CEA studies of alternative treatments which, in this case, only incorporate surgical treatment of epilepsy. The information included relates to the AEDs/treatments compared, patient population, cost and outcome measures, as well as the general findings/results of each specific study.

Cost-benefit Analysis

CBA primarily attempts to reduce outcome measures to monetary terms. Hence, when costs and benefits are expressed in the same unit of measurement, it is possible to judge whether a specific therapeutic modality is desirable from a societal viewpoint.[26] The two published CBA studies were conducted by the same author. Therefore, a tabulation of the CBA studies is not presented.

Cost-utility Analysis

In CUA, an attempt is made to directly assess the impact of the treatments on patient well being by using a utility indicator. This approach shifts the focus from clinical indicators to the patients themselves and assesses the treatment effects, via various parameters, to determine the quality of life (QoL).[39] Although an increasing number of published studies focus on the QoL of epileptic patients, only five studies, referring to AED treatment of epilepsy, can be considered to be cost-utility studies.[18,25,44,50,51]

Conversion of the Results of Cost-of-epilepsy Studies

In transnational comparisons of health economics evaluations, several monetary issues must be considered, such as fluctuating exchange rates and the rate of inflation.

For purposes of comparison, the estimates from different countries were converted into 2003 US$. The rate of inflation was calculated using the Consumer Price Index. The exchange rate used was the mean exchange rate for the US$ for the year 2003.

FINDINGS AMONG ECONOMICS STUDIES

Cost-of-illness Studies

The literature identified 17 studies performing a COI analysis. Tables 2, 3, and 4 show the results in US$ at the 2003 exchange

TABLE 2

MAIN CHARACTERISTICS OF COST-OF-ILLNESS STUDIES: PREVALENCE-BASED STUDIES

Country	Data sources	Data collection		Annual cost per patient (US$)		Comments (costs in US$)	Ref.
				Direct	Indirect		
U.S.	National sample	Retrospective	Database	1,758	—	2,053 for children	24
U.S.	Multiple MCOs	Retrospective	Database	3,007	—	Adults taking CBZ formulation (n = 1,767)	22
U.S.	MCO and medical center	Retrospective	Database	935	5,994	Total cost from 1,031–12,612 in different severity groups	8
U.S.	MCO	Retrospective	Database	1,575/3,449	—	1,575 (epilepsy-attributable cost) and 3,449 (case-control estimate)	19
U.K.	GP	Retrospective	Provider and population surveys	3,065	—	866–6,855 depending on seizure frequency	31
Italy	EC	Prospective	Questionnaire	1,098	—	547–3,530 in different prognostic categories (aged 18+)	3
Italy	EC	Prospective	Provider and population surveys	1,055	—	371–3,551 in different severity groups	63
Italy	UH, hospital and outpatient service	Prospective	Case report	1,590	—	760–2,941 in different severity groups (childhood epilepsy)	23
Italy	Referral centers	Retrospective	Case report	1,588	224	Total cost from 1,569 for adults to 2,412 for children	11
Italy	Referral centers	Retrospective	Questionnaire	1,290		411–2,941 in different severity groups	21
The Netherlands	GP, UH and EC	Prospective	Questionnaire and cost diary	2,444	—	808 cost at GP, 2,790 cost at UH, and 4,298 cost at EC	34
India	EC	Retrospective	Case report	55	128	117 cost of annual productivity loss	35
India	Medical centers	Retrospective	Questionnaire	105	283	Cost of travel included in direct cost	64
Hong Kong	EC	Retrospective	Database	433	582	Costs derived from dividing the 4-year total cost by 4	41
Burundi	National sample	Retrospective	Questionnaire	1.8	10.5	12 (epileptics), 7.7 (control group)	45
Oman	UH	Prospective	Case report	1,524	—	Only patients aged 13 and over	1

EC, epilepsy center; GP, general practitioner (physician); MCO, managed care organization; UH: University hospital.

TABLE 3

MAIN CHARACTERISTICS OF COST-OF-ILLNESS STUDIES: INCIDENCE-BASED STUDIES

Country	Data sources	Data collection		Annual cost (US$) per patient (direct cost) Year 1	Year 2	Year 3	Year 4	Comments (costs US$)	Ref.
U.S.	Medical center plus HMO	Retrospective	Database	3,813	848	569	496	3,749 to 7,671 depending on seizure frequency (in 4 years)	9
U.S.	National sample	Retrospective	Database	1,317	892	892	892	Top-down analysis	24
U.S.	Expert panel	Retrospective	Questionnaire	6,506	2,282	2,282	2,282	Bottom-up analysis	24
France	Specialists	Prospective	Cohort	2,379	626	—	—	Second year costs were more sensitive to seizure frequency	17

rate. A total of 15 of these studies were included in Table 2, as prevalence-based studies. The vast majority of the studies were conducted in the United States or Europe (three in the United States, one in the United Kingdom, five in Italy, and one in The Netherlands). Only four other countries conducted COI studies (India, Hong Kong, Burundi, and Oman). Table 3 shows that only three studies followed an incidence-based approach (one of which calculated the costs in two different ways). Two of these were based in the United States, and the other in France.

Prevalence Based-studies

Direct Costs of Epilepsy. The estimated annual direct costs of epilepsy vary significantly from study to study and range from US$1.8 to US$3,449 (Table 2). However, a closer look reveals that a smaller disparity of costs tends to exist if they are grouped based on the degree of development of the country in which the studies were conducted. Estimated direct costs vary from US$935 to US$3,449 in the United States, US$3,065 in the United Kingdom, and US$1,055 to US$1,590 in Italy. In the less developed countries, the costs of epilepsy range from US$55 to US$105 in India, to US$1.8 in Burundi (Table 2). Nevertheless, the variation between the costs is large. Heaney et al. found that prices for medical services and AEDs vary widely even between developed countries.[27] In a comparison among eight economically developed European countries, similar medical services were found to vary by as much as 24 times, whereas the prices of similar AEDs varied up to 4.4 times. Previous reviews have speculated on the difficulty of comparing results from COI studies.[2,5,7,14,28,33,36,38] Methodologic issues give rise to such disparities in cost-of-epilepsy estimations. Perhaps future studies could normalize or reduce international disparities; for example, they might be normalized using per capita income, gross domestic product, or some other standard economic indicator.

Indirect Costs of Epilepsy. Most cost studies in epilepsy have focused on direct medical costs because researchers have easier access to records of medical care. Records of nonmedical care are less centralized, and formal records of time costs, which are necessary for calculating indirect costs, rarely exist.[27] As a consequence, out of the 17 COI studies reviewed in this chapter, only six have estimated the indirect costs incurred by a specific society. Out of these six studies, only one found the indirect costs to be less than the direct costs.[11] This study calculated only productivity losses because of hospital visits and hospitalization to derive direct costs. The other studies reached a consensus in finding indirect costs considerably greater than direct costs. In general, four of the six studies found indirect costs to be from two to six times that of the direct costs (Table 2). Once again, the discrepancy between the findings is largely due to differences in the methodology applied.

Distribution of Direct Costs. Considerable variability exists in the findings among COI studies regarding the distribution of direct costs (Table 4). Four studies found hospital costs to be the highest, four others found drug costs to be the most important, and one study positions other general expenses at the top. This can be explained, once again, by the different methods used, and also by the fact that each country has a unique health care system that functions in a different way. For example, Burundi, which has a health care system that is less well developed than most Western countries, has drug costs as the main cost. The U.K.-based study by Jacoby et al. found other general costs to be most significant.[31] This was also the only study to include the cost of inpatient episodes as a separate cost component. Kotsopoulos et al. discovered that using a more comprehensive list of cost components is associated with a decrease in the contribution of drug and hospital costs to the total direct costs.[33]

TABLE 4

DISTRIBUTION OF DIRECT COSTS

Country	Hospital costs (%)	Drug costs costs (%)	Others (%)	Ref.
U.S.	51	24	25	24
U.S.	39	31	30	8
U.K.	32	10	58	31
Italy	23	60	17	3
Italy	82	12	6	11
Italy	34	48	18	21
India	17	58	25	64
Burundi	22	71	7	45
Oman	68	23	9	1

Incidence-based Studies

All three studies that estimated the direct costs of epilepsy from an incidence-based approach indicate high initial health care cost at onset for most patients, followed by lower cost in subsequent years (Table 3). This reflects the high cost of initial diagnostic evaluation and the fact that some patients achieve

TABLE 5

COST-MINIMIZATION STUDIES

Country	Study duration (year)	Treatment pathways	Nature of direct costs	Mean cost (US$) per patient (whole follow-up)				Ref.
				PHT	CBZ	VPA	LTG	
12 European countries	1	First-line switched to second-line mono- or polytherapy	Hospital, drugs, laboratory tests, ADR	30–86	108–328	134–880	683–1,896	29
U.K.	2	First-line switched to second-line mono- or polytherapy	Hospital, ambulatory care, drugs, laboratory tests, ADR	1,337–1,395	1,444–1,506	1,576–1,605	2,770–3,770	30
U.K.	1	If withdrawal, CBZ switched to VPA, and LTG switched to CBZ	Drugs, switching of treatment, ADR	—	337	—	980	58
India	2	First-line switched to second-line mono- or polytherapy	General drug therapy, ADR	—	60	105	—	48

ADR, adverse drug reactions; CBZ, carbamazepine; LTG, lamotrigine; PHT, phenytoin; VPA, valproate.

early remission.[7] Costs in subsequent years tend to stabilize around a fixed amount. De Zélicourt et al. found that costs during the first year were highly sensitive to the severity of seizures, whereas second-year costs had a much lower variance and were sensitive to frequency of seizures.[17]

Comparison of COI Studies: Methodological Issues

Any attempt to compare the findings of the reviewed COI studies is hampered by the methodologic variations among the studies. The methodologic differences arise from a variety of sources.

Differences in the Study Population. Cost estimates will vary according to which population is targeted and how the sample is ascertained. Some studies included the whole spectrum of the epilepsy population, whereas others included only certain specific age groups or severity groups. Certain studies only estimated the cost of childhood epilepsy,[23] whereas others focused entirely on the cost of adult epilepsy.[3] The study by Al-Zakwani et al. only included patients aged 13 years and above.[1] It is not surprising that no study had the same proportion of young/old people in its population, and this in itself can result in cost variation, because clear evidence suggests that childhood epilepsy is associated with greater costs than is adult epilepsy.[11,23,24] In addition to this, the various COI studies include different population groups regarding seizure frequency or seizure type/severity. Begley et al.,[9] de Zélicourt et al.,[17] and Jacoby et al.[31] found that costs differ significantly relative to seizure frequency, thereby demonstrating how populations with dissimilar seizure frequencies can affect the estimated cost. Similarly, Beghi et al.,[3] Begley et al.,[8] Garattini et al.,[21] Guerrini et al.,[23] and Tetto et al.[63] found a notable difference in costs, depending on which severity group the populations belonged.

Estimating the epilepsy costs of patients treated in the community requires careful case ascertainment to ensure representativeness. Retrospective ascertainment of cases contained in administrative databases has the potential to yield larger and more representative samples than does clinic-based sampling, but the validity of this approach can be highly variable. For example, AED use as a proxy for an epilepsy diagnosis has a high-false positive rate, since AEDs are prescribed for other conditions (e.g., pain, bipolar disorder).[57] Rochat et al. estimated the prevalence of epilepsy, using prescription data from the Danish National Health service.[52] Lacking diagnostic information, the authors excluded from their analysis subjects who also were prescribed high-strength analgesics, under the untested assumption that these subjects were using certain AEDs for pain instead of epilepsy. On the other hand, Frost et al. used a three-step approach that identified cases by procedure codes, followed by physician verification and record review of uncertain cases.[20]

Differences in the Methods of Data Collection. COI studies used a variety of methods when collecting their data. Some researchers acquired their cost-estimation data from administrative databases, whereas others used a questionnaire or prepared a case report for each patient (Table 2). Langfitt notes that studies relying on questionnaires sent to patients recruited by physicians are likely to obtain unreliable data.[36] A number of studies gathered their data retrospectively, whereas others followed the patient population prospectively (Table 2). Studies that prospectively attribute episodes of care to epilepsy based on a priori criteria are more likely to provide more accurate estimates than are retrospective assessments that rely on coding algorithms or medical record data that were not designed for this purpose. It is encouraging that the number of prospective studies conducted has increased significantly in recent years. The study by Levy et al. revealed that, out of 13 prevalence-based studies reviewed (conducted between 1993 and 2000), not one was prospective.[38] Among studies from 1998 to 2004, and out of 15 prevalence-based studies, five are prospective (Table 2).

TABLE 6

COST-EFFECTIVENESS OF ANTIEPILEPTIC DRUGS AS ADD-ON THERAPY

Drugs compared	Patients	Cost measures	Outcome measures	Results (costs in US$)	Refs.
LTG and TPM	Intractable epilepsy	AED, routine treatment	50% seizure reduction	200 mg/day TPM dominates 500 mg/day LTG (0.875 probability) 400 mg/day TPM dominates 500 mg/day LTG (0.986 probability)	65
CLB, GBP, LTG, and VGB	Intractable epilepsy	AED, ADR, routine treatment	50% seizure reduction, no ADR	GBP: 14,158 per satisfied patient* LTG: 11,474 per satisfied patient* CLB: 2,363 per satisfied patient* VGB: 2,770 per satisfied patient*	56
LTG and TPM	Intractable epilepsy	AED, ADR, routine treatment	50% seizure reduction, no ADR	LTG: 11,472 per satisfied patient* 3,442 per 50% seizure reduction TPM: 6,050 per satisfied patient 2,823 per 50% seizure reduction	55
CBZ, PB, PHT, and VPA	Idiopathic epilepsy	AED, hospital costs	75% treatment response, 70% adherence	PB: $868–1639 per DALY averted $798–2386 ICER PHT: $903–1690 per DALY averted $836–2496 ICER CBZ: $1194–2106 per DALY averted $1138–3399 ICER VPA: $1708–2845 per DALY averted $1675–5003 ICER	16
LTG and standard therapy (first-line AEDs)	Intractable epilepsy	AED, ADR, routine treatment	50% seizure reduction	ICER of LTG: 715 per year	32
LTG and standard therapy (first-line AEDs)	Intractable epilepsy	AED, ADR, routine treatment	Seizure-free days	ICER of LTG: 7.6 per seizure-free day	42
LEV and standard therapy (first-line AEDs)	Intractable epilepsy	AED, ADR, routine treatment, hospitalization	Seizure-free days	ICER of LEV: 60.7 per seizure-free day	59

ADR, adverse drug reactions; CBZ, carbamazepine; CLB, clobazam; DALYs, disability adjusted life years; GBP, gabapentin; ICER, incremental cost-effectiveness ratio; LEV, levetiracetam; LTG, lamotrigine; PB, phenobarbitone; PHT, phenytoin; TPM, topiramate; VGB, vigabatrin; VPA, valproic acid.
*A patient who achieves 50% reduction in the number of seizures and is not affected by any serious adverse drug reaction.

Differences in Sampling. Some COI studies ascertained epilepsy cases from centers/clinics or general hospitals/medical centers, whereas others gathered their data from general practitioners, administrative databases, or national samples; in some studies, the data were collected from a combination of sources (see Tables 2 and 3).[34] Different sampling strategies result in different case mixes. The cost of the same type of epilepsy differed among three health care settings (clinical research hospital, general hospital, and outpatient services).[23] Clinical samples will have a higher proportion of severe cases. Samples drawn from administrative databases may be more representative of the entire spectrum of epilepsy, but also may contain nonepilepsy cases, depending on how rigorously cases are defined, as noted earlier.

Differences in What is Included in the Costs. Although those studies that estimated the direct costs reached a general level of consensus as to which cost components they should include, this was not the case for studies that estimated indirect costs. Some studies that estimated indirect costs considered lost earnings resulting from excess unemployment and premature mortality,[8] whereas other studies included only work days lost for treatment.[11] One study used a very crude estimation model based on how many patients claimed that epilepsy was the reason they left their jobs or how it generally affected their professional lives.[35] Thomas et al.[64] and Nsengiyumva et al.[45] doubled the estimated indirect costs calculated, arguing that each patient is accompanied by one other person during his transport and admission to the hospital. These different approaches to the measurement of indirect costs illustrate the difficulties in identifying the extent to which epilepsy is to be held responsible for lost productivity. Levy states that the problem is generated by the inherent difficulty of observing the effect of a chronic disease on professional occupation.[38]

Differences in Methods of Calculation. Two studies demonstrated the variability in costs when different methods of calculation are employed, even if the same population is used.[19,24]

TABLE 7

COST-EFFECTIVENESS OF ALTERNATIVE TREATMENTS

Treatments compared	Patients	Cost measures	Outcome measures	Results (costs in US$)	Ref.
Surgery, medical therapy	Refractory temporal lobe epilepsy	Direct costs, indirect costs	Seizure-free patients	Surgical therapy more effective—return of high initial surgery costs—in 7.3–35 years (depending on which costs are included in the analysis) Employment income: 29,961 seizure-free (after surgery) 27,968 improved (after surgery) 18,231 unimproved (after surgery) 21,084 (before surgery)	47
Surgery, medical therapy	Refractory temporal lobe epilepsy	AED, hospital costs, transportation	Seizure-free patients	Total direct costs over life-time: 5,646 (no surgery) Cost of surgery: 1,355 70% of patients become seizure-free after surgery 30% of patients off AED within 3 years of surgery	49
Vagal nerve stimulation, medical therapy	Children with Lennox-Gastaut syndrome	Direct costs, indirect costs	Seizure-free patients	VNS therapy more effective—return of high initial therapy costs in 2.3 years. Costs during 6 postoperative months are 3,370 less than costs during 6 months before VNS	40

VNS, vagal nerve stimulation.

Costs can be estimated using a top-down analysis or a bottom-up analysis. According to the top-down approach, COI is calculated as a percentage of the total health expenditure, whereas the bottom-up approach uses the summation of cost data from individual patients to arrive at total disease costs. The first method is a service-based analysis, whereas the latter is an individual-based analysis.[33] Halpern et al. estimated the costs of epilepsy using both methods and found very different results (US$1,317 using top-down analysis and US$6,506 using bottom-up analysis).[24] Two other approaches to determining the costs of epilepsy are the *epilepsy-attributable cost method* and the *case-control cost method*. Using the epilepsy-attributable cost method, the mean cost per patient is derived by summing all the costs classified a priori as epilepsy related. In the case-control cost method, the overall health care costs of epilepsy patients (cases) are compared with the costs for similar persons without epilepsy (controls), with the difference between cases and controls representing the marginal cost of epilepsy.[38] Frost et al. performed a study comparing the two methods and found very diverse results (US$1,575 for epilepsy-attributable cost and US$3,449 for case-control estimate).[19] Smaller differences between methods (US$1,650 vs. US$1,836) were found in a study of institutionalized mentally retarded persons.[15] This demonstrates that the choice of estimation method can significantly influence the proportion of costs attributed to epilepsy.

Most of these methodologic limitations are not confined to COI studies; they arise in all types of economic analyses.

Cost-minimization Analysis: Methodological Issues

Four studies reported a CMA (see Table 5). Three of those were conducted in Europe (two in the United Kingdom and one a collaborative effort of 12 European countries) and one in India. All four studies restricted their evaluation to include only direct medical costs. Also, all studies used a model relating to the treated patients and treatments prescribed, based on clinical trials specific to each product. Furthermore, all studies took side effects and adverse drug reactions (ADRs) associated with medical treatment into consideration, because it is now established that such ADRs are usually associated with considerable medical costs.[54]

Despite the similarities, the studies differ significantly on many other parameters:

- The studies generally followed differing combinations of treatment pathways, particularly regarding the drugs evaluated. Only the Heaney et al. studies had exactly the same configuration of treatment pathways.[29,30]
- The studies incorporated dissimilar cost components when estimating the total direct costs of the AEDs (Table 5).
- The studies differed in duration. Two of the studies had a drug follow-up period of 1 year,[29,58] whereas the other two lasted for 2 years.[30,48]

Despite the methodologic variations of these studies, there does appear to be a consensus regarding the ranking of the AEDs relevant to their cost. Lamotrigine was by far the most expensive drug, incurring more than twice as many costs as any other drug. Valproate and carbamazepine were the second and third most costly drugs respectively, incurring much more costs than phenytoin, which appears to be the cheapest drug of the four examined.

Equivalent Efficacy in CMA Studies

By definition, CMA studies are only conducted when it can be assumed that the alternate treatments considered are equally effective. All CMA studies of AEDs consider AEDs equally effective when they result an equal proportion of patients achieving at least a 50% reduction in seizures. However, such an outcome measure leads to inconclusive results, because most clinical trials tend to assess efficacy of AEDs based on seizure reduction alone.[38] However, AEDs differ when judged on other criteria. For example, although carbamazepine and lamotrigine do not reportedly differ in their efficacy in controlling seizures, one study has found lamotrigine to be better tolerated and to have positive effects on subjective well-being.[10] Therefore, lamotrigine may be preferred to carbamazepine treatment. In CMA studies, only the cost-effect of AEDs is included in the evaluation, whereas the effect on patient QoL is ignored because an indicator, based on clinical efficacy rather than effectiveness, was used. Recent literature has been in agreement that it is preferable to use CEA rather than CMA when comparing the various treatments of epilepsy, because CEA avoids conclusions being based on clinical efficacy parameters alone.[10,36,38,39]

Cost-effectiveness Analysis: Methodological Issues

Ten CEA studies described in Tables 6 and 7 are indicative of the two areas in which cost-effectiveness analyses have focused recently:

- AED effectiveness: Whether novel AEDs lead to improved tolerability and seizure control, which accumulate cost savings and better health effects that offset the higher cost of the drugs (Table 6).
- Epilepsy surgery: Whether the high initial resource investment for epilepsy surgery reduces long-term costs due to improved seizure control (Table 7).

As in previous studies, a variety of methodologic limitations exist in CEA. In this type of analysis, comparisons can be made since, by definition, CEA studies include comparisons in their analysis. Therefore, a CEA study can facilitate informed decisions about which treatment pathway to follow.

Cost-effectiveness of Antiepileptic Drugs

Table 6 shows that all seven studies used patients with intractable epilepsy, five included adverse drug reactions in their calculations,[32,42,55,56,59] and five studies defined their outcome measures by calculating the proportion of patients who achieved a 50% seizure reduction[32,55,56,65] or a 75% treatment response,[16] whereas two studies focused on seizure-free days gained due to successful AED therapy.[42,59]

In their study, van Hout et al. adopted a Bayesian statistical analysis to calculate the probability that therapy A dominates or weakly dominates therapy B.[65] They found that 200 mg/day of topiramate is more effective than 500 mg/day of lamotrigine by a probability score of 0.875. If the dose of topiramate was to be increased to 400 mg/day, the probability of it being more effective than lamotrigine would rise to 0.986. It is notable that this study does not incorporate costs related to side effects of the AED. This omission may affect the results, because higher dosages of topiramate than those provided in this study have been associated with higher numbers of patients discontinuing therapy.[60]

Selai et al. attempted to estimate the cost attributable to AED use to achieve patient satisfaction.[55,56] Satisfaction was defined as the achievement of a 50% reduction in the number of seizures, as well as absence of any serious adverse drug reactions in the patient. Results, which are illustrated in Table 6, include topiramate being found to be more cost effective than lamotrigine, a finding that is consistent with those of van Hout et al.[65]

Markowitz et al. adopted a different perspective in calculating the cost-effectiveness of a certain AED therapeutic pathway.[42] The incremental cost per extra day without a seizure was calculated. Results showed that the use of lamotrigine is associated with an overall reduction of use in direct medical care resources (hospitalizations, outpatient visits, diagnostic and laboratory tests, and surgery), and that this would result in a US$ 7.6 saving per seizure-free day gained. Sheehy et al. followed a similar approach and found the incremental cost effectiveness ratio (ICER) of levetiracetam to be US$ 60.7 per seizure-free day.[59] A problem that arises from such an analysis is that there is no published evidence of seizure-free days being correlated with economic cost. Only seizure frequency has been found to be related to medical costs, as explained in the COI analysis.

The studies by Chisholm and Knoester et al. also attempted to calculate the cost-effectiveness of AED therapy based on incremental cost effectiveness ratios (ICERs).[16,32] Where as Chisholm estimated the costs required to achieve a 75% treatment response and 70% adherence, Knoester only estimated the costs required to achieve a 50% reduction in seizures. Knoester et al. measured the cost-effectiveness of lamotrigine and estimated an ICER of US$715 per year.[32] The Chisholm study found that, out of four AEDs (carbamazepine, phenobarbitone, phenytoin, and valproic acid), phenobarbitone was found to be the most cost-effective, with a US$868 to US$1,639 cost per disability-adjusted life years (DALYs) averted and an ICER of US$798 to US$2,386.[16] Costs were found to have great variation depending on which region of the developing world the countries belonged to, with African countries having the lowest costs and Eastern Mediterranean countries the highest.[16]

Cost-effectiveness of Temporal Lobectomy

Table 7 presents the three studies that have focused on the cost-effectiveness of epilepsy surgery. It shows that two of the studies examined similar patient populations using similar outcome measures, the latter being the proportion of patients becoming seizure-free after the surgery.[47,49] The third study referred only to children diagnosed with Lennox-Gastaut syndrome.[40]

Platt and Sperling found surgical therapy to be considerably effective.[47] A return of the high initial surgery costs was attained in a period ranging from 7.3 to 35 years, depending on which costs were included in the analysis. This, by itself, is illustrative of how methodologic variation can affect a study's results. It is interesting to note that the mean employment income was found to increase considerably after the surgery (from US$21,084 to US$29,961) in patients who became seizure-free, but decreased (from US$21,084 to US$18,231) in patients who did not improve after surgery.

Similarly, in their study in India, Rao and Radhakrishnan found temporal lobectomy to be very cost effective, as its initial costs were US$1,355, in comparison with total direct lifetime costs of US$5,646.[49] Because 70% of patients became seizure-free after the surgery and 30% discontinued AED use within 3 years of the surgery, the overall lifetime costs after the surgery were reduced compared to the overall lifetime costs had the surgery not taken place.

Majoie et al. focused on vagal nerve stimulation (VNS) therapy, which they found to be considerably cost-effective, as it returns the high initial therapy costs in just 2.3 years. To illustrate this, epilepsy costs during the 6 post-operative months were found to be US$3,370 less than the costs during the 6 months before the therapy was carried out.[40]

Use of Hypothetical Modeling in CEA Studies

CEA studies showed that hypothetical modeling of certain outcomes is the most common method for such an analysis in epilepsy studies. Such outcomes could result from different treatments, services involved in treatment, treatment of ADRs, and other treatment pathways. This involves combining data from various secondary sources, thus comparing the new AEDs through situations that are not relevant to the specific CEA. Heaney offers a characteristic example of a CEA study of lamotrigine, which used data that included patients who may have failed trials of both vigabatrin and clobazam.[26] Because most of the CEA studies reviewed are retrospective and must rely on existing data, such methodologic flaws are commonly incorporated into the estimations and, consequently, the results.

Selai et al. demonstrated the importance of using an accurate model to estimate the cost effectiveness of an antiepileptic therapy.[55] Significant differences were found when presenting data as cost per patient treated, compared with the cost for reducing seizures by more than 50%, compared with cost per patient satisfied. When only the cost of a patient becoming 50% seizure-free was considered (without indices of satisfaction), the costs dropped considerably. Given that most of the CEA studies reviewed estimated cost effectiveness solely on the grounds of patients achieving a 50% seizure reduction, it is conceivable that many of the costs have been underestimated.

Cost-benefit Analysis

Only two studies performed a cost-benefit analysis.[12,13] The earlier study by Boon et al. aimed at estimating the cost-benefits of VNS.[13] A later study by this group went a step further, estimating and comparing costs of daily treatment of patients who were either treated with AED polytherapy only, underwent epilepsy surgery, or had VNS.[12]

VNS was found to be very cost-beneficial on both occasions. The study by Boon et al. estimated that, on average, the annual epilepsy-related direct medical costs dropped from US$10,665 (before the implantation) to US$5,091 (at 12 months after the implantation).[13] This group also found costs reduced from US$5,331 to US$2,757. Both studies reach a consensus, because costs seem to be reduced by half.[12] Direct costs were estimated in dissimilar ways, which might explain the variation in cost figures.

Additionally, the Boon et al. study found that the mean decrease in costs to patients who followed traditional AED polytherapy was minimal.[12] Specifically, costs were reduced from US$2789 to US$2,675 in this patient group. Interestingly, epilepsy surgery was found to be only moderately cost-beneficial, because it reduced average annual costs from US$1,618 to US$1,310. On the other hand, one could argue that a saving of US$308 per patient per year accumulates to a substantial amount over the long term.

In both studies, Boon et al. appear to define CBA idiosyncratically as costs avoided.[12,13] This is a significant shortcoming, since the term benefits should include all types of benefits (e.g., QoL improvements) and not only costs avoided.

It is not surprising that CBA studies are not very favorable to researchers conducting economic evaluations, because they require both costs and consequences to be expressed in monetary terms or ratios. Therefore, CBA studies necessitate the placing of a monetary value even on outcomes that defy economic evaluation in monetary terms. Subsequently, they exclude very important outcome measures that are impossible to equate or express as monetary values.

Cost-utility Analysis

Only five of the studies incorporated a CUA[18,25,44,50,51] (Table 8). All studies utilized the quality adjusted life years (QALY) calculation, which determines the impact of a treatment on both a patient's longevity and on the value of those additional life-years. Messori et al. focused on the use of lamotrigine in refractory epilepsy and estimated the QoL values by prospectively interviewing a group of patients with refractory epilepsy.[44] Clinical data were obtained from a placebo-controlled clinical trial of lamotrigine,[43] and the various costs were derived from Begley's cost-of-illness study.[4] Only direct costs were taken into account.

This study concluded that the use of adjunctive lamotrigine in refractory epilepsy costs, on average, US$49,935 per QALY (year of life in which a patient enjoys perfect health). Because this type of evaluation facilitates a comparison of treatments relating to various diseases, the cost of QALYs produced by AEDs may be compared with QALYs produced by different treatments in different areas. This study found lamotrigine to have a worse pharmacoeconomic profile in comparison to other (nonepilepsy) pharmacologic treatments.

Although this study can be considered pioneering, because it was the first CUA on antiepileptic treatment, its validity is questionable, since the data are obtained from three separate studies. As a result, the QoL data were obtained from an ad hoc study on patients not necessarily taking the drugs under evaluation.

Forbes et al. performed a CUA of VNS for adults with medically refractory epilepsy.[18] The study used a meta-analysis of randomized controlled trials of VNS and estimated that six people require the implantation of VNS devices in order for one person to experience a 50% reduction in seizure frequency. Costs saved from improved epilepsy control were taken from previously published literature. The total cost per QALY was found to be US$52,329 when using the time trade-off method and US$114,275 when EuroQol EQ-5D utility values were used.

In this study, most patients were unable to complete the time-trade off valuations, even in the presence of a research nurse; this raises questions regarding the appropriateness of using this method with epilepsy patients.

Remak et al. focused on five different AEDs (clobazam, gabapentin, lamotrigine, topiramate, and vigabatrin) and found that only topiramate and vigabatrin patients showed an increase in their EQ-5D scores. Topiramate was found to have an ICER of US$11,767 per QALY compared with vigabatrin.[51]

Another study by Remak et al. and the study by Hawkins et al. focused on evaluating the costs incurred from a variety of treatment scenarios.[25,50] Remak et al. evaluated a variety of treatment scenarios in which carbamazepine, lamotrigine, topiramate, and valproic acid were used either as first-line or second-line treatment. They concluded that the best treatment scenario would be to administer topiramate as first-line treatment and lamotrigine as second-line treatment. Such a scenario would cost an additional US$11,372 per additional QALY, compared to the second-best treatment scenario, which would involve administering valproic acid as first-line treatment and topiramate as second-line treatment.[50]

Hawkins et al. focused on the full range of pharmaceutical therapies used in the U.K. health system. They found that,

TABLE 8

COST-UTILITY STUDIES

Treatment evaluated	Patients	Cost measures	Results (costs in US$)	Ref.
LTG	Refractory epilepsy	Direct costs	49,935 per QALY	44
VNS	Refractory epilepsy	Direct costs, indirect costs	52,349 per QALY (using the time trade-off method) 114,275 per QALY (using the EuroQol EQ-5D)	18
CLB, GBP, LTG, TPM, and VGB	Refractory epilepsy	Direct costs	Only TPM and VGB patients show an increase in EQ-5D scores. TPM has an ICER of 11,767 per QALY compared with VGB.	51
CBZ, LTG, TPM, and VPA	Newly diagnosed and refractory epilepsy	Direct costs	Best treatment scenarios: TPM (first-line treatment) and LTG (second-line treatment) cost 11,372 per additional QALY compared to VPA (first-line treatment) and TPM (second-line treatment).	50
The full range of pharmaceutical therapies feasibly used in the U.K. health system	Newly diagnosed and refractory epilepsy	Direct costs	Best treatment scenarios: Partial seizures: CBZ (monotherapy), VPA (monotherapy), CBZ (second-line treatment) and OXC (adjunctive therapy) if willingness to pay >27,685 per QALY. Generalized seizures: VPA (newly diagnosed epilepsy), and TPM (adjunctive therapy) if willingness to pay >53,831 per QALY.	25

CBZ, carbamazepine; CLB, clobazam; GBP, gabapentin; ICER, incremental cost effectiveness ratio; LTG, lamotrigine; OXC, oxcarbazepine; TPM, topiramate; VGB, vigabatrin; VPA, valproic acid; VNS, vagal nerve stimulation; QALY, quality-adjusted life-year.

for partial seizures, the best treatment scenarios would use carbamazepine and valproic acid (administered as monotherapy), lamotrigine (administered as second-line treatment), and oxcarbazepine (administered as adjunctive therapy) if the willingness to pay for additional health benefits exceeded US$27,685 per QALY. Similarly, for generalized seizures, valproic acid was found to be the best treatment scenario for newly diagnosed epilepsy and topiramate for adjunctive therapy, if the willingness to pay for additional health benefits exceeded US$53,831 per QALY.[25]

Caution should be used when interpreting cost-utility studies, because it has already been demonstrated that the choice of utility instrument determines the results to a considerable extent.[62] The Stavem study compared four methods of measuring utility weights (time trade-off, standard gamble, 15D, and the EuroQol EQ-5D visual analog scale) and found that these preference instruments measure different aspects of health-related QoL and, therefore yield different results.[62]

OVERVIEW OF FINDINGS

Over the last 6 years, a plethora of studies have focused on the costs of epilepsy using a number of health cost evaluation methods. In this chapter, the various studies were compared to assess the economic, conceptual, and methodologic issues in this growing literature.

Many of the authors of these studies do not fully explain their methods, which introduces uncertainties into the results and limits their value. This might be partly explained by the researchers' lack of economic expertise, since most studies were performed by medical specialists. Kotsopoulos et al.[33] and Levy[38] observed similar problems in their reviews.

Inevitably, there are many limitations and methodological complexities in epilepsy cost studies, and these limitations should be taken into consideration when interpreting the results. The main issues identified were differences in the study population, differences in the sources used to obtain the data, differences in what is included in the costs, and differences in the methods of cost estimation.

In spite of this methodologic heterogeneity, some interesting interpretations can be made regarding the results of the studies. In particular, COI studies demonstrated a marked difference among costs in various countries and health care systems. Costs tend to be higher in more developed countries in comparison to the lesser developed ones; however, this was an expected outcome (Table 2). Studies found costs in uncontrolled patients to be from 1.5[24] to 3.5[9] times higher in the first year of treatment compared to the second year, when better control is achieved through treatment. Studies examining the longitudinal aspect of epilepsy-related costs found costs to be very high in the year of onset but then decreasing until a steady figure was reached in 2 to 4 years (Table 3). COI studies focusing on the breakdown of costs came to very inconsistent results, but do show that each health care system works in a unique way and has dissimilar cost components (Table 4).

To further our understanding of the total costs of epilepsy, the authors of future COI studies must provide clear methods and analysis of their data. Such studies will continue to be of limited use unless they are conducted with a common set of methods that will allow comparisons across studies. Unfortunately, previous reviews identified the same issues of concern, and only a limited degree of improvement has occurred.[2,5,7,14,28,33,36,38,46]

CMA evaluations, which mainly focused on four drugs, found lamotrigine to be the most costly and carbamazepine the most economical. Nevertheless, such studies inappropriately assumed equivalent clinical efficacy of these drugs to represent equal seizure reduction rates. This resulted in these drugs being equal in all aspects and therefore being compared as such. Should a broader perspective be placed on equivalent drug efficacy, then CMA will no longer be able to be applied to the majority of AEDs, because they will be found to generate different patient outcomes.

CBA studies, which are the least popular within the literature, generally focused on VNS and epilepsy surgery, and found both these treatments to be significantly cost beneficial.[12,13] The limitations of these studies have been outlined earlier.

CEA studies found topiramate to be more cost-effective than lamotrigine, and phenobarbitone to be more cost-effective than carbamazepine, phenytoin, and valproic acid. Surgical lobectomy and VNS were found to be very cost-effective treatments in the long term. In such studies, the common use of hypothetical modeling based on secondary data is very likely to give rise to inaccurate results. Nevertheless, CEA studies, compared to CMA evaluations, avoid the efficacy of drugs being reduced to clinical efficacy parameters alone and therefore include more dimensions of the consequences of treatment.

CUA studies go a step further by assessing the treatment's effect on the patient, incorporating QoL adjustments to the treatment outcomes. This facilitates the comparison of a variety of therapeutic options across the medical spectrum in terms of patient-perceived preferences, and can ensure that resources are allocated fairly among the various diseases.

Within the span of this review (January 1998 to January 2006), only five CUA studies had been performed so far in the epilepsy field. This small number is disappointing, considering that CUA is becoming the favored tool in the economic evaluation of health care. The scarcity of CUA studies can be partially explained by the fact that there is still difficulty and controversy concerning the way the patients' point of view can be incorporated in an economic analysis and eventually expressed in monetary terms.

SUMMARY AND CONCLUSIONS

Despite the methodologic heterogeneity and the difficulties of comparing the studies, there are significant findings. If cost-of-epilepsy studies follow more uniform methodology and data collection, they can offer invaluable information about which therapeutic modalities are most effective. Only then can economic evaluations of epilepsy treatment inform decisions about the allocation of scarce health care resources.

Also, future economic studies in epilepsy must aim to evaluate the variability in costs incurred according to the various case definitions of epilepsy, severity of the disease, cost components, and various demographic influences on the disease. This will provide insights regarding the great variations in costs found by the majority of cost-evaluation studies, and will lead to a greater consensus on which specific methodology should be utilized.

The International League Against Epilepsy (ILAE) has recognized the importance of economic considerations in the development of epilepsy care and has focused on improving the methods used to conduct epilepsy cost studies so that comparisons across studies within epilepsy can be made.[51]

The expertise of economists, health service researchers, and epileptologists must be combined if we hope to overcome the methodologic problems that arise during cost evaluation of this disease. Only then will we be able to adequately document the economic burden of epilepsy and evaluate alternative strategies for its prevention and management.

References

1. Al-Zakwani I, Hanssens Y, Deleu D, et al. Annual direct medical cost and contributing factors to total cost of epilepsy in Oman. *Seizure*. 2003;12:555–560.
2. Annegers JF, Beghi E, Begley CE. Cost of epilepsy: Contrast of methodologies in United States and European studies. *Epilepsia*. 1999;40(8):S14–S18.
3. Beghi E, Garattini L, Ricci E, et al. Direct cost of medical management of epilepsy among adults in Italy: A prospective cost-of-illness study (EPICOS). *Epilepsia*. 2004;45:171–178.
4. Begley CE, Annegers JF, Lairson DR, et al. Cost of epilepsy in the United States: A model based on incidence and prognosis. *Epilepsia*. 1994;35:1230–1243.
5. Begley CE, Annegers JF, Lairson DR, et al. Estimating the cost of epilepsy. *Epilepsia*. 1999;40(8):S8–S13.
6. Begley CE, Beghi E, Beran R, et al. ILAE Commission on the burden of epilepsy, Subcommission on the economic burden of epilepsy: Final report 1998–2001. *Epilepsia*. 2002;43:668–673.
7. Begley CE, Beghi E. The economic cost of epilepsy: A review of the literature. *Epilepsia*. 2002;43(4):S3–S9.
8. Begley CE, Famulari M, Annegers JF, et al. The cost of epilepsy in the United States: An estimate from population-based clinical and survey data. *Epilepsia*. 2000;41:342–351.
9. Begley CE, Lairson DR, Reynolds TF, et al. S. Early treatment cost in epilepsy and how it varies with seizure type and frequency. *Epilepsy Res*. 2001;41:205–215.
10. Beran RG. Economic analysis of epilepsy care. *Epilepsia*. 1999;40(8):19–24.
11. Berto P, Tinuper P, Viaggi S, et al. Cost-of-illness of epilepsy in Italy. Data from a multicentre observational study (Episcreen). *Pharmacoeconomics*. 2000;17:197–208.
12. Boon P, D'Have M, Van Walleghem P, et al. Direct costs of refractory epilepsy incurred by three different treatment modalities: A prospective assessment. *Epilepsia*. 2002;43:96–102.
13. Boon P, Vonck K, Vandekerckhove T, et al. Vagus nerve stimulation for refractory epilepsy; efficacy and cost-benefit analysis. *Acta Neurochir*. 1999;141:447–453.
14. Brunetti M, Pagano E, Garattini L. The economic cost of epilepsy: A review. *Ital J Neurol Sci*. 1998;19:116–119.
15. Burke TA, McKee JR, Pathak D S, et al. Costs of epilepsy in an intermediate care facility for persons with mental retardation. *Am J Ment Retard*. 1999;104(2):148–157.
16. Chisholm D, on behalf of WHO-CHOICE. Cost-effectiveness of first-line antiepileptic drug treatments in the developing world: A population-level analysis. *Epilepsia*. 2005;46(5):751–759.
17. de Zélicourt M, Buteau L, Fagnani F, et al. The contributing factors to medical cost of epilepsy: An estimation based on a French prospective cohort study of patients with newly diagnosed epileptic seizures (the CAROLE study). *Seizure*. 2000;9:88–95.
18. Forbes RB, Macdonald S, Eljamel S, et al. Cost-utility analysis of vagus nerve stimulators for adults with medically refractory epilepsy. *Seizure*. 2003;12:249–256.
19. Frost FJ, Hurley JS, Petersen HV, et al. A comparison of two methods for estimating the health care costs of epilepsy. *Epilepsia*. 2000;41:1020–1026.
20. Frost FJ, Hurley JS, Petersen HV, et al. A comparison of two methods for estimating the health care costs of epilepsy. *Epilepsia*. 2000;41(8):1020–1026.
21. Garattini L, Ricci E, Roggeri D, et al. Costs of epilepsy care in referral centers in Italy. *Eur Jour Health Econ*. 2000;19:87–99.
22. Garnett WR, Gilbert TD, O'Connor P. Patterns of care, outcomes, and direct health plan costs of antiepileptic therapy: A pharmacoeconomic analysis of the available carbamazepine formulations. *Clin Therap*. 2005;27(7):1092–1103.
23. Guerrini R, Battini R, Ferrari AR, et al. The costs of childhood epilepsy in Italy: Comparative findings from three health care settings. *Epilepsia*. 2001;42:641–646.
24. Halpern M, Rentz A, Murray M. Cost of illness of epilepsy in the U.S.: Comparison of patient-based and population-based estimates. *Neuroepidemiology*. 2000;19:87–99.
25. Hawkins N, Epstein D, Drummond M, et al. Assessing the cost-effectiveness of new pharmaceuticals in epilepsy in adults: The results of a probabilistic decision model. *Med Decis Making*. 2005;25(5):493–510.
26. Heaney D. The pharmacoeconomics of the new antiepileptic drugs. *Epilepsia*. 1999;40(8):S25–S31.
27. Heaney DC, Sander JA, Shorvon SD. Comparing the cost of epilepsy across eight European countries. *Epilepsy Res*. 2001;43:89–95.
28. Heaney DC, Sander JW. Ensuring appropriate care in epilepsy: An overview of epidemiological and cost of illness considerations. *Dis Manage Health Outcomes*. 1998;4:303–313.

29. Heaney DC, Shorvon SD, Sander JW, et al. Cost minimization analysis of antiepileptic drugs in newly diagnosed epilepsy in 12 European countries. *Epilepsia.* 2000;41(5):S37–S44.
30. Heaney DC, Shorvon SD, Sander JW. An economic appraisal of carbamazepine, lamotrigine, phenytoin and valproate as initial treatment in adults with newly diagnosed epilepsy. *Epilepsia.* 1998;39(3):S19–S25.
31. Jacoby A, Buck D, Baker G, et al. Uptake and costs of care for epilepsy: Findings from a U.K. regional study. *Epilepsia.* 1998;39:776–786.
32. Knoester PD, Boendermaker, AJ, Egberts ACG, et al. Cost-effectiveness of add-on lamotrigine therapy in clinical practice. *Epilepsy Res.* 2005;67:143–151.
33. Kotsopoulos IA, Evers SM, Ament AJ, et al. Estimating the costs of epilepsy: An international comparison of epilepsy cost studies. *Epilepsia.* 2001;42:634–640.
34. Kotsopoulos IA, Evers SM, Ament AJ, et al. The costs of epilepsy in three different populations of patients with epilepsy. *Epilepsy Res.* 2003;54:131–140.
35. Krishnan A, Sahariah SA, Kapoor SK. Cost of epilepsy in patients attending a secondary-level hospital in India. *Epilepsia.* 2004;45:289–291.
36. Langfitt JT. Cost evaluations in epilepsy: An update. *Epilepsia.* 2000; 41(2):S62–S68.
37. Leary LD, Morrell MJ. Update on new antiepileptic drugs in children. *Primary Psychiatry.* 2004;11(4):40–45.
38. Levy P. Economic evaluation of antiepileptic drug therapy: A methodologic review. *Epilepsia.* 2002;43:550–558.
39. Levy P. Pharmacoeconomic evaluation of medical treatment of epilepsy: Where do we stand? *Acta Neurol Belg.* 1999;99:239–246.
40. Majoie HJ, Berfelo MW, Aldenkamp AP, et al. Vagus nerve stimulation in children with therapy-resistant epilepsy diagnosed as Lennox-Gastaut syndrome: Clinical results, neuropsychological effects, and cost-effectiveness. *J Clin Neurophysiol.* 2001;18:419–428.
41. Mak W, Fong JK, Cheung RT, et al. Cost of epilepsy in Hong Kong: Experience from a regional hospital. *Seizure.* 1999;8:456–464.
42. Markowitz MA, Mauskopf JA, Halpern MT. Cost-effectiveness model of adjunctive lamotrigine for the treatment of epilepsy. *Neurology.* 1998;51:1026–1033.
43. Matsuo F, Bergen D, Faught E, et al. Placebo-controlled study of the efficacy and safety of lamotrigine in patients with partial seizures. *Neurology.* 1993;43:2284–2291.
44. Messori A, Trippoli S, Becagli P, et al. Adjunctive lamotrigine therapy in patients with refractory seizures: A lifetime cost-utility analysis. *Eur J Clin Pharmacol.* 1998;53:421–427.
45. Nsengiyumva G, Druet-Cabanac M, Nzisabira L, et al. Economic evaluation of epilepsy in Kiremba (Burundi): A case-control study. *Epilepsia.* 2004;45:673–677.
46. Pillas D, Selai C. The economic aspects of epilepsy and antiepileptic treatment: A review of the literature. *Expert Rev Pharmacoeconomics Outcomes Res.* 2005;5:327–338.
47. Platt M, Sperling M. A comparison of surgical and medical costs for refractory epilepsy. *Epilepsia.* 2002;43(4):S25–S31.
48. Radhakrishnan K, Nayak S, Kumar S, et al. Profile of antiepileptic pharmacotherapy in a tertiary referral center in South India: A pharmacoepidemiological and pharmacoeconomic study. *Epilepsia.* 1999;40:179–185.
49. Rao MB, Radhakrishnan K. Is epilepsy surgery possible in countries with limited resources? *Epilepsia.* 2000;41(4):S31–S34.
50. Remak E, Hutton J, Price M, et al. A Markov model of treatment of newly diagnosed epilepsy in the UK: An initial assessment of cost-effectiveness of topiramate. *Eur J Health Econom.* 2003;4:271–278.
51. Remak E, Hutton J, Selai CE, et al. A cost-utility analysis of adjunctive treatment with newer anti-epileptic drugs in the U.K. *J Med Econ.* 2004;7: 29–40.
52. Rochat P, Hallas J, Gaist D, et al. Antiepileptic drug utilization: A Danish prescription database analysis. *Acta Neurol Scand.* 2001;104(1):6–11.
53. Schachter SC, Wheless JW. Vagus nerve stimulation 5 years after approval: A comprehensive update. *Neurology.* 2002;59(4):S15–S20.
54. Schlienger RG, Oh PI, Knowles SR, et al. Quantifying the costs of serious adverse drug reactions to antiepileptic drugs. *Epilepsia.* 1998;39(7):S27–S32.
55. Selai CE, Smith K, Trimble MR. Adjunctive therapy in epilepsy: A cost-effectiveness comparison of two AEDs. *Seizure.* 1999;8:8–13.
56. Selai CE, Trimble MR, Lavett J. Pharmacoeconomics: A Cost-Effectiveness Study of Four Antiepileptic Drugs. In: Trimble MR, Hindmarch I eds. *Benzodiazepines.* Petersfield: Wrightson Biomedical Publishing; 2000: 131–146.
57. Shackleton DP, Westendorph R, Kestelijn-Nolst Trenite DGA, et al. Dispensing epilepsy medication: A method of determining the frequency of symptomatic individuals with seizures. *J Clin Epidemiol.* 1997;50:1061–1068.
58. Shakespeare A, Simeon G. Economic analysis of epilepsy treatment: A cost-minimization analysis comparing carbamazepine and lamotrigine in the U.K. *Seizure.* 1998;7:119–125.
59. Sheehy O, St-Hilaire JM, Bernier G, et al. Economic evaluation of levetiracetam as an add-on therapy in patients with refractory epilepsy. *Pharmacoeconomics.* 2005;23(5):493–503.
60. Shorvon SD. Safety of topiramate: Adverse events and relationships to dosing. *Epilepsia.* 1996;37(2):S18–22.
61. Spencer S. Long-term outcome after epilepsy surgery. *Epilepsia.* 1996; 37:807–813.
62. Stavem K. Quality of life in epilepsy: Comparison of four preference measures. *Epilepsy Res.* 1998;29:201–209.
63. Tetto A, Manzoni P, Millul A, et al. The costs of epilepsy in Italy. A prospective cost-of-illness study in referral patients with disease of different severity. *Epilepsy Res.* 2002;48:207–216.
64. Thomas SV, Sarma PS, Alexander M, et al. Economic burden of epilepsy in India. *Epilepsia.* 2001;42:1052–1060.
65. van Hout BA, Gagnon DD, McNulty P, et al. The cost effectiveness of two new antiepileptic therapies in the absence of direct comparative data. *Pharmacoeconomics.* 2003;21:315–326.

CHAPTER 308 ■ THE ECONOMIC IMPACT OF EPILEPSY

CHRISTOPH PACHLATKO, DAN CHISHOLM, HARRY MEINARDI, AND JOSEMIR W. SANDER

INTRODUCTION

Epilepsy imposes a significant clinical, epidemiologic, and economic burden on societies throughout the world. This chapter focuses on the economic dimension of this burden or impact, in particular how it can be measured and, ultimately, how it can be reduced. Three specific questions are addressed: First, what is the relevance of an economic perspective to the management of epilepsy as a public health issue? Second, what is the economic perspective on the burden of epilepsy, and how well do economic studies demonstrate this burden? Third, what is the economic perspective on evaluation, and how does economic evaluation contribute to the evidence on clinical and cost effectiveness? This chapter complements others in this volume that deal with related topics, including the issues surrounding epidemiologic burden and need, treatment effectiveness, and the costs of treatment.

Interest in the economic aspects of epilepsy has been growing in both richer and poorer countries. In the wealthier nations, an ongoing debate continues about how to curb rapidly rising health care costs. State-financed health care systems are facing the problem of an inflation of needs and, therefore, are forced to find ways to limit the expenditures for health care. On the other hand, poorer countries are facing the fact of a tremendous need for health care but inadequate economic resources. The uneven distribution of epilepsy care among countries, and sometimes within countries, does not correspond so much with real needs, but rather with underlying economic conditions. It is a well-known fact that approximately 80% of all health expenditures occur in established market economies, whereas the remaining 20% of financial resources is spent in the rest of the world, where approximately 90% of the people with epilepsy are living.[21] Therefore, it is important to consider the economic aspects of ongoing efforts to improve the situation of people with epilepsy in all regions of the world.

The growing interest in this field has led to an increasing number of publications on economic aspects of epilepsy. Since the early 1990s, attempts have been made to apply general instruments of health care economics to the field of epilepsy care. The first studies mainly concentrated on the calculation of the cost of epilepsy. In a second phase, the economic studies investigated, in particular, selected aspects of the treatment of epilepsy, such as antiepileptic drugs or epilepsy surgery, including its cost-effectiveness.[4,24] In correspondence with the World Health Organization (WHO), the perspective has been broadened once again to the global burden of disease[21] and to the assessment of the performance of different health care systems.[20,32] Furthermore, economic aspects have been included within the Global Campaign on Epilepsy, a joint initiative launched in 1997 by the International League Against Epilepsy, the International Bureau for Epilepsy, and the WHO to improve the situation of people with epilepsy worldwide.

The Rationale and Relevance of an Economic Perspective

Before considering different methods and results from economic analyses of epilepsy and its treatment, it is important to raise the question of why such studies are needed in the first place. In short, the requirement for an economic dimension in planning and evaluating treatments and services for epilepsy stems from a tension between, on the one hand, the epidemiologic or clinical need for intervention, and on the other, the resources available to meet this identified need. In the extreme case of there being no limits on resource availability, there would be little need for an economic dimension, other than to track the steady, unremitting flow of monies being channeled into epilepsy care and prevention. Equally, in the extreme case that care or prevention strategies are entirely ineffective or unavailable, economic considerations might be restricted to considering the economic consequences of the untreated natural history of disease. Of course, the reality for most diseases and most countries is that effective care and/or prevention strategies exist, but the budget is limited, which implies that choices must be made about which interventions to make available within this budget constraint. Assuming that the primary goal of a health system is to optimize potential health improvements in the population, then the choice is made mainly in terms of delivering maximum health gain for least cost. This is in fact a definition of efficiency, and is the concept underlying cost-effectiveness and other forms of economic evaluation (see later sections).

In addition, economic considerations may and certainly should enter into the debate around a number of other components of epilepsy care, including the organization or quality of primary care and neurologic services in a country, plus the financial protection of epilepsy patients and their families from potentially catastrophic payments for drugs and health care services. There is currently very little available epilepsy-specific evidence that can be drawn upon to shed light on these issues, but the experience from comparative international studies undertaken is that reliance on private, out-of-pocket payments by households for health care is a far less equitable financing mechanism than prepayment via taxation or insurance.[34] In countries where there is a high level of out-of-pocket expenditures on health, therefore, an increased likelihood exists of pushing households containing a family member with epilepsy into impoverishment.

The Epidemiologic and Economic Burden of Epilepsy

The "burden" of epilepsy can be considered at a number of levels and from a number of different viewpoints, so it is as well to distinguish between these different perspectives when thinking about what measured burden is likely to show. Most directly, this "burden" will be felt at the individual or household level in terms of the physical pain and psychological stress associated with epileptic seizures, the (potentially catastrophic) financial implications of treatment or lost work opportunities, and, in all too many societies, the social stigma attached to this condition. By contrast, burden at the community or population level is typically expressed in terms of the epidemiologic profile of the disease (numbers of new or existing cases in the population), the financial resources devoted to prevention and treatment, and societal productivity losses resulting from premature mortality or morbidity. The focus here is on population-level estimates of both the epidemiologic and economic burden attributable to epilepsy at the national and international level, but this should not detract from the importance of establishing and sharing better information concerning the household burden of epilepsy, particularly in low-income countries where the risk of catastrophic out-of-pocket expenditures is highest.

Before illustrating the assessment of both the epidemiologic and economic burden of epilepsy, it is important to note that epilepsy is not an uniform disease, but rather a term that summarizes many conditions that have the symptom of an epileptic seizure in common. Policy-makers, such as governments or insurance agents, often do not distinguish between the different forms of epilepsy when evaluating the need for care and the services available, respectively. In economic terms, the consequences of having epilepsy may vary considerably depending on the frequency, severity, and kind of seizures. Furthermore, not all economic consequences may be attributable to epilepsy, because epilepsy is often related to an underlying disease that may continue to exist even after remission of the seizures. Various economic studies in epilepsy have therefore divided up the population with epilepsy into different prognostic groups with similar health care needs.[2]

Epidemiologic Assessment of the Global Burden of Epilepsy

From the epidemiologic perspective, epilepsy is a significant cause of disability and disease burden in the world. Using a metric called the disability-adjusted life years or DALY,[21] which can be thought of as 1 lost year of healthy life, the WHO has calculated the global burden of disease and injury attributable to different causes or risk factors. This measure of burden assesses the gap between current health status and an ideal situation in which everyone lives into old age free of disease and disability. Overall, epilepsy contributed more than 7 million disability-adjusted life years (0.5%) to the global burden of disease in 2000.[15,33] Figure 1 shows the distribution of DALYs or lost years of healthy life attributable to epilepsy, both by age group and by level of economic development. It is apparent that close to 90% of the worldwide burden of epilepsy is to be found in developing regions, with more than half occurring in the 39% of global population living in countries with the highest levels of premature mortality (and lowest levels of income). An age gradient is also apparent, with the vast majority of epilepsy-related deaths and disability in childhood and adolescence occurring in developing regions, whereas later on in the lifecycle, the proportion drops because of relatively greater

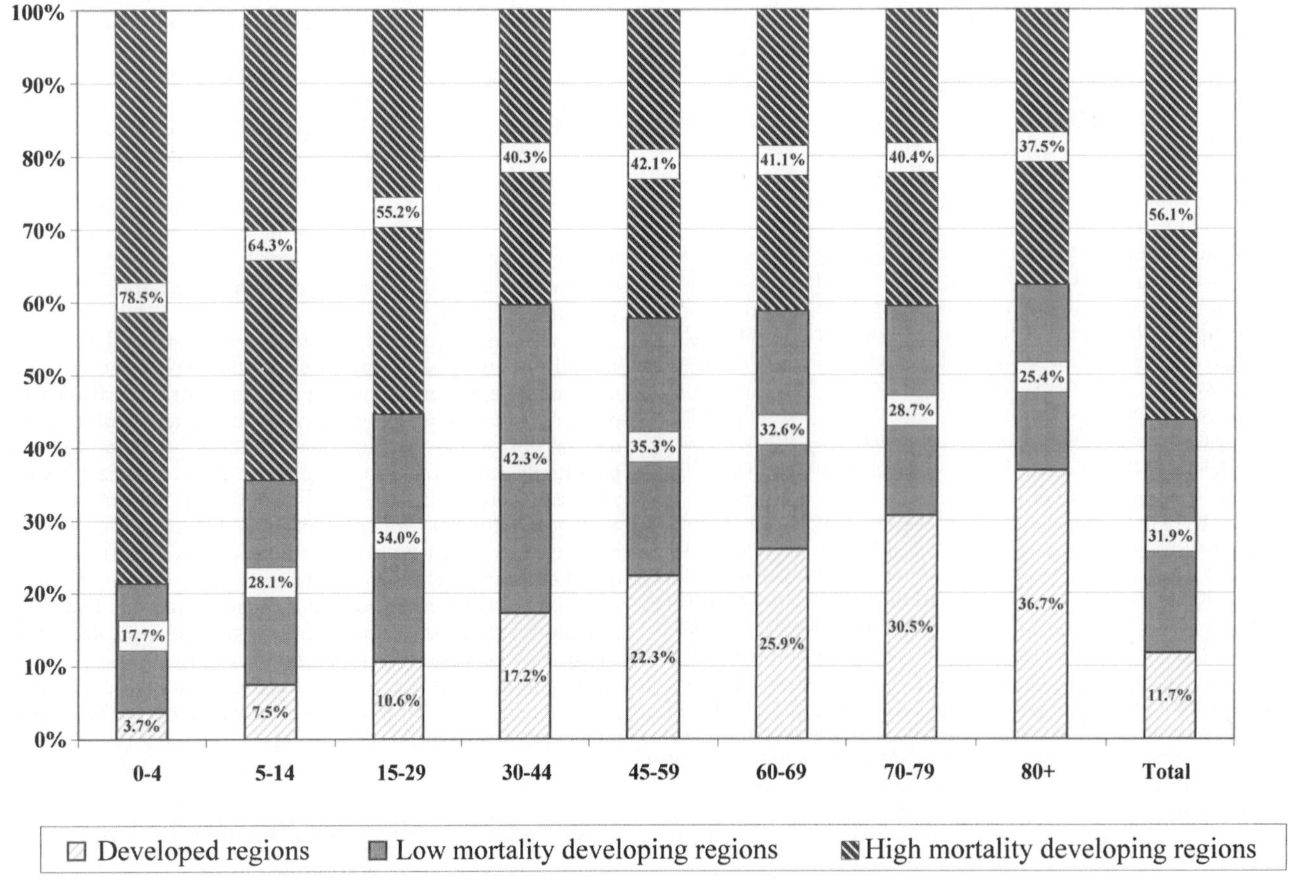

FIGURE 1. Distribution of the global burden of epilepsy by age group and level of economic development. (From World Health Organization. Statistical Annex 3, 2004. In: World Health Report 2004: Changing history (available at http://www.who.int/whr/2004/annex/topic/en/annex_3_en.pdf), with permission.)

survival rates into older age by people living in more economically developed regions. In terms of the absolute number of healthy life years lost per 1 million population, estimates range from less than 500 in early childhood and older age in developed regions to as much as 2,000 in the younger age groups of high-mortality developing regions. Owing to the consistent and comparative nature of this work, summary estimates of population health such as these provide the most appropriate measure of the relative burden of epilepsy at the international level.

That is not to say, however, that such summary measures of population health are not without limitations. For example, good-quality data on basic epidemiologic parameters (such as rates of incidence or recovery) do not exist for many developing countries, such that estimates for whole subregions of the world may be extrapolated from neighboring regions where such data do exist. Just as importantly, and in common with other disease categories, good-quality descriptive data on disability due to epilepsy were lacking at the time of this study. Recent work on the measurement of health state preferences in epilepsy[14] suggests that the disability weights applied to treated and untreated epilepsy in the Global Burden of Disease study may be underestimated. Finally, DALY estimates of the burden of epilepsy take into account neither the potential health consequences on people other than the diagnosed case (such as the burden on family members or caregivers), nor the nonhealth consequences of disease (such as lost ability to work).

Economic Assessment of the National Burden of Epilepsy

Disease burden has also been gauged from an economic perspective for many years in the form of so-called "cost of illness" studies, which have attempted to attach monetary values—as opposed to DALY estimates—to a variety of societal costs associated with a particular disorder, often expressed as an annual estimate aggregated across all involved agencies. Such studies have direct parallels with epidemiologic estimates of disease burden, in the sense that the principal aim is to influence policymaking and resource allocation by demonstrating the relative magnitude or burden associated with a particular disorder (by multiplying case prevalence by cost per case, put very crudely). The potential advantage of cost of illness studies over DALY-based estimates of burden is that they are able to measure in a single metric (money) not only the direct health-related impact of disease (in terms of health care costs, etc.) but also other economic consequences such as lost work or leisure time, and family or caregiver burden.

Economic assessments of the national burden of epilepsy have been conducted in a number of high-income countries such as Italy and the United States[1,3] and also in two developing countries, India and Burundi.[22,29] A number of comparative reviews have also been produced.[2,12,16,25] Each of these studies or reviews have set out to demonstrate the various economic implications the disorder has in terms of health care service needs and lost work productivity. For example, the Indian study calculated that the total cost per case of these disease consequences for epilepsy amounted to US$344 per year (equivalent to 88% of average income per capita), and that the total cost for the estimated 5 million cases resident in India was equivalent to 0.5% of the gross national product.[29]

An extensive array of costs is associated with epilepsy, including so-called "direct" intervention costs such as inpatient and outpatient care, medication, and diagnostic tests, and also "indirect" costs that cover lost time and productivity. The indirect cost of epilepsy, due to unemployment, underemployment, or premature death, is higher than one may assume. Studies have shown, for example, that in Europe, the unemployment rate among people with epilepsy is two or three times higher than among the general population.[9] To face unemployment or underemployment is a severe problem for these patients. At the same time, it is an (often underestimated) economic burden to society.

The wide range of potentially included cost components has resulted in significant heterogeneity in studies that attempt to capture the cost of illness (COI) of epilepsy. Key methodologic discrepancies include the range of services included in direct cost estimates (e.g., surgery, residential care, special education), the valuation of lost time (loss of productivity, loss of caregiver productivity), the inclusion of mortality costs, sampling frames (patients who are seeing specialists, adults, children), data sources (expert panel estimates, medical records, patient surveys), and the handling of comorbidity.

Table 1 provides a summary of the differing methods used in selected COI studies across a number of developed and developing countries. Most studies include inpatient and outpatient fees, drug costs, diagnostic costs, and laboratory costs. Others include the cost of surgery,[8] ambulatory transportation[5,8] and residential care, day care, and social workers costs.[13] Many of these studies use national tariff costs, which may include profits,[1,5,22] while other studies use insurance fee schedules,[8] payments, or charges. Only one study took into account mortality costs,[5] but many studies did take into account productivity losses due to loss of time from medical treatment. However, the methods with which these costs were calculated varied widely, from including only the patients' lost productivity days due to hospital visits and hospitalization, to productivity losses due to travel, to the loss of productivity time of caregivers.

Because such studies differ with respect to the exact methods used, as well as underlying cost structures within the health system, they are currently of most use at the level of individual countries, where they can serve to draw attention to the wide-ranging resource implications and needs of people suffering from epilepsy. However, like epidemiologic estimates using DALYs or some other measure of population health, COI studies are not in themselves appropriate mechanisms for allocating resources to specific treatment strategies.

The Economic Evaluation of Epilepsy Treatment

Having established the *attributable burden* of epilepsy, two subsequent questions for decision-making and priority-setting relate to *avertable burden* (the proportion of attributable burden that is averted currently or could be avoided via scaled-up use of proven efficacious treatments) and *resource efficiency* (determination of the most cost-effective ways of reducing burden). Analysis of these two issues can reveal the technically most efficient response to the attributable burden of a particular disease. Figure 2 provides a schematic overview of these concepts, showing how the total burden of epilepsy can be broken down into the following separate components: (a) disease burden that is already being averted via existing strategies, (b) disease burden that could be avertable via scaled-up implementation of cost-effective interventions such as antiepileptic drug treatment, and (c) disease burden that cannot currently be averted by the set of interventions under consideration.[30]

Economic analysis provides a set of principles and analytical techniques that can be usefully employed to assess the relative costs and consequences of different interventions or treatment strategies.[23] It seeks to address a number of key policy questions about the magnitude of epilepsy, the relative effect and cost of different treatment strategies, and the most appropriate use of scarce resources (Table 2). Economic evidence can be

TABLE 1

SUMMARY OF METHODS USED IN SELECTED COST-OF-ILLNESS STUDIES OF EPILEPSY

First author year country (reference)	Inclusion/exclusion criteria	Direct medical costs	Direct nonmedical and indirect costs	Data sources	Comments
Nsengiyumva 2004, Burundi (22)	Reoccurrence of at least two spontaneous seizures within 24 hours	IP, OP, DT, DG,	PC*2	Survey, retrospective	Inclusion standards are very different from other studies; assumed patients came with attendee and so doubled time costs
Thomas 1998, India (29)	Consecutive cases of epilepsy found in outpatient epilepsy service	IP, OP, DT, DG	PC (OP*2+ SE) NT*2	Retrospective questionnaire	Assumed every patient came with attendee and so doubled time and travel costs; all patients were seeing specialists
Krishnan, 2004, India (16a)	All patients at one epilepsy clinic	IP, OP, DG, EC	AT, PC (estimated)	Clinical records	Small sample, weak study
Beghi 2004, Italy (1)	18 years or older with confirmed case of epilepsy, attending epilepsy centers for over 2 years	IP, OP, DT, DG, SP		12-month prospective, questionnaire and patient-held records	Patients kept details of diagnostic tests and visits; no official records used; only adults at referral clinic included
Berto 2000, Italy (5)	Registered since 1996, diagnosed with epilepsy at last visit and had at least one follow-up, and a follow-up period of at least 12 months	IP, OP, DT, DG	PC, PCT	Clinical Records, retro	Excellent study, takes into account employment rate, working days, differentiates between children and adult costs
Jacoby 1998, UK (13)	Patients of GP and must have had active epilepsy in last 2 years or be on AEDs	IP, OP, DT, DG, EC, HV, PS, NU, RS			
Halpern 2000, USA (8)	Bottom-up approach: Expert panel of neurologists, general physicians and pediatricians	IP, OP, DT, DG, SU, AD	AT	Expert Panel	Panel estimates are subjective. Excluded opinion of generalists but did include cost of surgery
	Top-down approach: Subset of respondents to 1987 National Medical Expenditure Survey	IP, OP, EC		National Survey	No indirect costs
Begley 2000, USA (3)	Patients seeing specialists and generalists	IP, OP, DT, DG, SU, EC, PC, AT, LT	PC, MC, HP	Billing data/medical charts; survey of adult patients in treatment center	Indirect costs may be overestimated because data taken from epilepsy centers, but may be underestimates as based on adults only

Direct Costs: OP, outpatient visits; IP, inpatient visits; SE, seizure events; DT, diagnostic tests; DG, drugs; AD, drug side-effects; SU, surgery; SP, specialists; EC, emergency consultations; AT, ambulatory transportation; LT, lab tests; HV, health visitors; PS, psychiatrists/psychologists; NU, nurses; RS, remedial schooling. **Indirect costs:** PC, productivity costs; PCT, productivity costs due to travel; NT, normal transportation; MC, mortality costs.

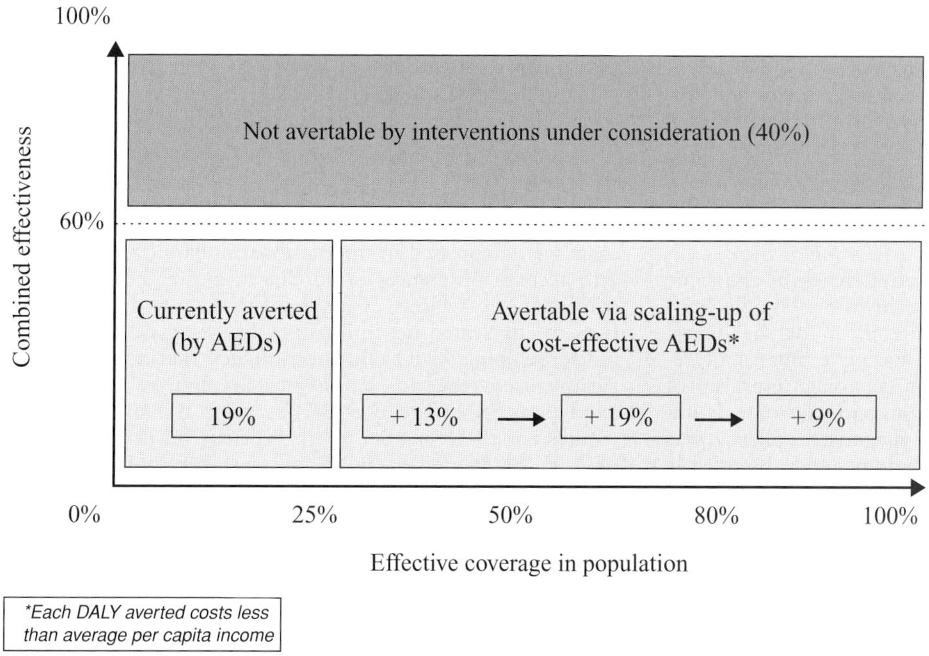

FIGURE 2. Attributable and avertable burden of epilepsy in a WHO African subregion. (Schema is from World Health Organization. *Investing in Health Research and Development: Report of the ad hoc Committee on Health Research Relating to Future Intervention Options.* Geneva: World Health Organization, 1996; data is from Chisholm D. Cost-effectiveness of first-line antiepileptic drug treatments in the developing world: a population-level analysis. *Epilepsia.* 2005;46:751–759, with permission.)

generated in two distinct ways. Preferably, it would be generated on the back of additional empirical studies in a range of socioeconomic settings (particularly in developing countries, where current evidence is most scarce). Well-designed and sufficiently powered economic evaluations of epilepsy treatments are certainly needed and valuable, but they are also difficult, time-consuming, and expensive to carry out (as well as having limited application beyond the immediate confines of the study location). Alternatively, cost-effectiveness information can be generated via appropriate disease modeling of the best available existing data concerning the expected costs and effects of interventions in these different settings. The danger of this latter approach lies in the inevitable assumptions that are required to be made when basing cost-effectiveness estimates on a variety of data sources from different research settings, whereas the obvious attraction is that policy-relevant results can be generated relatively more quickly and cheaply. Over the longer-term, these two approaches can in fact be considered complimentary—empirical studies feed into initial or revised modeling exercises, while modeling studies synthesize and may even stimulate empirical research studies—but this should not detract from the shorter-term need to bring cost-effectiveness arguments into play when arguing for an increased level of resource investment to and prioritization for epilepsy care.

Despite the identified need for cost-effectiveness evidence by, among others, the International League Against Epilepsy[23] and the WHO,[31] there remains a relative paucity of empirically based economic evaluations from developed countries, and a total absence in developing countries. This, despite the likelihood that, due to their low price and established

TABLE 2

POLICY QUESTIONS ADDRESSED BY ECONOMIC ANALYSIS OF EPILEPSY

Policy question	Research task	Evidence generated
1. How significant is the burden of epilepsy?	Estimate burden of disease (DALYs) Identify other social and economic consequences of disorders	% of total disease burden caused by epilepsy Estimates of monetary impact on economy
2. How effective is epilepsy treatment?	Estimate current effective coverage Assess impact of new interventions	Comparative efficacy of interventions % of burden averted with current treatment or avertable with better treatment strategies
3. What will it cost to provide effective care?	Calculate full cost of interventions Estimate cost of scaling-up coverage	Comparative cost of interventions at different levels of treatment coverage
4. What are the most efficient strategies?	Integration of costs and effectiveness Inclusion in essential packages	Evidence-based priorities for the efficient allocation of health care resources

efficacy, use of older AEDs in primary health care settings can be expected to represent a very cost-effective use of health care resources. Most completed economic evaluations have been concerned with specific treatment modalities, in particular the cost-effectiveness of different AEDs—either comparing first-line treatment or considering newer AEDs as add-on pharmacotherapy—and epilepsy surgery.[12,25]

Economic analysis of different first-line AEDs in the context of higher-income countries has been carried out using a form of economic evaluation called *cost-minimization analysis*, which assumes that treatment effectiveness is the same for each comparator, thereby coming down to a simple comparison of which drug produces this effect for the lowest cost. Assuming equal efficacy, and basing estimates of resource use on a consensus panel, an economic appraisal of carbamazepine, lamotrigine, phenytoin, and valproate as initial treatment in adults with newly diagnosed epilepsy was carried out, first in the United Kingdom and subsequently across 12 European countries.[10,11] This study found that lamotrigine was two or three times more expensive in terms of direct health service costs incurred. Assuming equal efficacy remains a contested area, however, with manufacturers of newer AEDs dedicated—and in some cases mandated by regulatory authorities—to showing reduced sedative effects.

A number of economic evaluations have also been carried out in high-income countries for adjuvant pharmacotherapy using newer AEDs, arguably because that is where new market opportunities (and also regulatory standards) are greatest. For example, one study showed that the use of lamotrigine resulted in an overall reduction in the use of health resources,[17] a phenomenon referred to as a *cost-offset* (i.e., additional drug costs are offset by lower service use). The cost-effectiveness measure in this study was the additional cost associated with the newer drug per extra seizure-free day gained over the study period. An alternative measure that has also been used in this context is the Quality Adjusted Life Year (QALY), which combines both the quantity and quality of life into a composite index of health outcome. Economic evaluations of this kind are called *cost-utility analysis*. One such study using this method calculated that the cost of gaining one QALY as a result of using adjunctive lamotrigine amounted to US$50,000.[19]

For the subset of patients with refractory temporal lobe epilepsy, incremental costs per QALY gained have also been computed for surgery (in comparison to medical therapy), with results in the range US$16,000 to US$27,000.[12] Using a lifetime approach, these studies indicate the potential economic advantages of investing in the shorter-term in order to produce long-term improvements in both seizure control and quality of life.[25]

Economic evaluations of different epilepsy treatments from lower-income countries are few and far between. Two of these come from a tertiary referral center in the Indian state of Kerala, where both a study of the cost and effects of surgery plus a pharmacoeconomic study comparing phenobarbitone, phenytoin, carbamazepine, and valproate (plus combinations) were carried out.[26,27] The annual drug cost of phenobarbitone and phenytoin was estimated at US$15 to US$20, significantly lower than the cost of carbamazepine or valproate (US$50 and US$90, respectively). No estimation was made for the cost of health care visits or program management, however. For patients with refractory temporal lobe epilepsy, the cost of anterior temporal lobectomy was estimated at US$1,200 (compared to US$150 for similar patients not undergoing surgery), and the outcome was that 70% were seizure-free 2 years postoperatively (compared to about 10% for medically treated cases).

Another study stems from Colombia, which, based on an epilepsy surgery program established over the last decades in Cartagena.[7] has shown the feasibility of epilepsy surgery in a developing country. Although the cost of the surgical treatment in Colombia is relatively low (<US$2,000 for an operated patient), the program meets international standards. Compared with the high cost of lifelong medication, it is evident that epilepsy surgery may be effective also in economic terms.

More recently, information has been generated as part of a wider WHO cost-effectiveness work program[28] on the amount of burden averted by the current or scaled-up use of AED treatments in low- and middle-income regions of the world, together with estimates of cost and cost-effectiveness.[6] Effectiveness was expressed in terms of DALYs averted, and costs were expressed in international dollars (I$, which take into account differences in purchasing power between countries or world regions). Compared to a do-nothing scenario (i.e., the untreated natural history of epilepsy), results from nine developing WHO subregions suggest that extending AED treatment coverage to 50% of primary epilepsy cases would avert between 150 to 650 DALYs per 1 million population (equivalent to 13%–40% of the current burden). This burden can be averted at an annual cost per capita of I$0.20 to I$0.80 for phenobarbitone and phenytoin (I$70–I$120 per treated case), and I$0.25 to I$1.33 for carbamazepine and valproate (I$105–I$207 per treated case). These cost estimates includes the AED drug itself, health care use, and also program implementation costs such as training and administration.

Older first-line AEDs (phenobarbitone, phenytoin) were most cost-effective because of their similar efficacy but lower acquisition cost (I$800–I$2,000 for each DALY averted). In all nine developing regions, the cost of securing 1 extra healthy year of life was less than average per capita income. Extending coverage further to 80% or even 95% of the target population would evidently avert more of the burden still, and would remain an efficient strategy despite the large-scale investment in manpower, training, and drug supply and distribution that would be required to implement such a program.

The results for one WHO developing subregion in Africa—consisting of 20 countries with a high rate of child mortality and a very high level of adult mortality—are depicted in Figure 2, which divides the total attributable burden of epilepsy as follows: (a) burden that is averted by AEDs at current levels of effective treatment coverage (19% of total burden), (b) burden that could be averted via the scaling-up of AEDs (up to a further 41% of total burden is averted if complete coverage could be reached), and (c) burden that is not avertable via AEDs (estimated to be 40%, although this assumes that the current level of drug compliance would prevail).

It may be argued that the purchase of the low-cost AEDs (like phenobarbitone) does not resolve the whole problem, because it is known that, in various regions of the developing world, epilepsy is not considered to be a medical problem but rather a trouble with social or spiritual implications. In such regions, medical treatment is not asked for unless there is a basic knowledge among the people offering primary health care. In addition there is a need for securing permanent access to AEDs, since an interruption of the treatment may cause a dangerous deterioration of the disease (indeed, if phenobarbitone is not gradually withdrawn but suddenly stopped, life-threatening status epilepticus may ensue). However, these arguments enhance the high impact of economic factors on the development of epilepsy care, especially in remote rural areas. An improvement of the condition will depend on the sustained access to low-cost treatment and improved knowledge of how to use it. From an economic viewpoint, it still is the most cost-effective approach to use low-cost AEDs for a large number of untreated people.

SUMMARY AND CONCLUSIONS

The burden of epilepsy manifests itself at a number of different levels. Taking a population-level approach, both epidemiologic and economic studies have revealed the extent of the negative impact of epilepsy on existing levels of health and health care. It is an unfortunate truth that the current burden, often couched in terms of the "treatment gap in epilepsy,"[18] is most concentrated in regions with the greatest health challenges and the least resources with which to respond to these challenges. More positively, however, one can conclude that, in these very regions, there exists the greatest opportunity to reduce current levels of epilepsy-related deaths and disability, employing efficacious treatments that have been shown to be a highly cost-effective use of scarce resources.

Although the volume of completed studies remains modest, particularly in middle- and low-income countries, increasing economic evidence supports the argument that interventions for epilepsy are not only available and effective but also affordable and cost-effective. This constitutes an important argument both for increased parity with other (noncommunicable) diseases and for increased investment into service development for this condition. This message has been supported and disseminated in all continents by the works and projects of the aforementioned Global Campaign on Epilepsy.

Critical factors in the successful implementation of such a scaled-up level of service delivery, apart from renewed political support and investment, can be expected to relate to appropriate training, continuity of drug supply, and enhanced consumer or community involvement.

ACKNOWLEDGMENT

The authors would like to acknowledge the contribution of Gaurav Banka, who undertook a COI literature review for epilepsy as part of an internship with the WHO in 2005.

References

1. Beghi E, Garattini L, Ricci E, et al. Direct cost of medical management of epilepsy among adults in Italy: A prospective cost-of-illness study (EPICOS). *Epilepsia.* 2004;45:171–178.
2. Begley CE, Annegers JF, Lairson DR, et al. Methodological issues in estimating the cost of epilepsy. *Epilepsy Res.* 1999;33:39–55.
3. Begley CE, Famulari A, Annegers JF, et al. The cost of epilepsy in the United States: An estimate from population-based and survey data. *Epilepsia.* 2000;41:342–352.
4. Begley CE, Beghi E. The economic cost of epilepsy: A review of the literature. *Epilepsia.* 2002;43(Suppl 4):3–9.
5. Berto P, Tinuper P, Viaggi S. Cost-of-illness of epilepsy in Italy. Data from a multicentre observational study (Episcreen). *Pharmacoeconomics.* 2000;17:197–208.
6. Chisholm D. Cost-effectiveness of first-line anti-epileptic drug treatments in the developing world: A population-level analysis. *Epilepsia.* 2005;46:751–759.
7. Fandiño J, Torres M, Vergara J, et al. Low-cost epilepsy surgery in Colombia. In: Pachlatko C, Beran RG. Economic Evaluation of Epilepsy Management. 1996:91–104.
8. Halpern M, Rentz A, Murray M. Cost of illness of epilepsy in the U.S.: Comparison of patient-based and population-based estimates. *Neuroepidemiology.* 2000;19:87–99.
9. Heaney D. Epilepsy at work: Evaluating the cost of epilepsy in the workplace. *Epilepsia.* 1999;40(Suppl 8):44–47.
10. Heaney D, Shorvon S, Sander JW, et al. An economic appraisal of carbamazepine, lamotrigine, phenytoin and valproate as initial treatment in adults with newly diagnosed epilepsy. *Epilepsia.* 1998;39(Suppl 3):S19–S25.
11. Heaney D, Shorvon S, Sander JW, et al. Cost minimization analysis of antiepileptic drugs in newly diagnosed epilepsy in 12 European countries. *Epilepsia.* 2000;41(Suppl 5):S37–S44.
12. Heaney DC, Begley CE. Economic evaluation of epilepsy treatment: A review of the literature. *Epilepsia.* 2002;43(Suppl 4):10–17.
13. Jacoby A, Buck D, Baker G, et al. Uptake and costs of care for epilepsy: Findings from a U.K. regional study. *Epilepsia.* 1998;39:776–786.
14. Langfitt J, Wiebe S. Cost-effectiveness of epilepsy therapy: How should treatment effects be measured? *Epilepsia.* 2002;43(Suppl 4):17–24.
15. Leonardi M, Ustun B. The global burden of epilepsy. *Epilepsia.* 2002;43(Suppl 6):21–25.
16. Levy P. Economic evaluation of antiepileptic drug therapy: A methodologic review. *Epilepsia.* 2002;43:550–558.
16a. Krishnan A, Sahariah SG, Kapoor SK. Cost of epilepsy in patients attending a secondary-level hospital in India. *Epilepsia.* 2004;45(3):289–291.
17. Markowitz M, Mauskopf J, Halpern M. Cost-effectiveness model of adjunctive lamotrigine for the treatment of epilepsy. *Neurology.* 1998;51:1026–1033.
18. Meinardi H, Scott RA, Reis R, et al. The treatment gap in epilepsy: The current situation and ways forward. *Epilepsia.* 2001;42:136–149.
19. Messori A, Trippoli S, Becagli P, et al. Adjunctive lamotrigine therapy in patients with refractory seizures: A lifetime cost-utility analysis. *Eur J Clin Pharmacol.* 1998;53:421–427.
20. Murray CJ, Evans DB, eds. *Health Systems Performance Assessment.* Geneva: World Health Organization; 2003.
21. Murray CJ, Lopez AD, eds. *The Global Burden of Disease.* Geneva: World Health Organization; 1996.
22. Nsengiyumva G, Druet-Cabanac M, Nzisabira L, et al. Economic evaluation of epilepsy in Kiremba (Burundi): A case-control study. *Epilepsia.* 2004;45:673–677.
23. Pachlatko C, Beran RG, eds. *Economic evaluation of epilepsy management: Proceedings of the Symposium on economic aspects of epilepsy at the 21st International Epilepsy Congress, Sydney 1995.* London: John Libbey; 1995.
24. Pachlatko C, Beran RG, eds. The relevance of health economics to epilepsy care. *Epilepsia.* 1999;40(Suppl 8):3–7.
25. Pillas D, Selai C. Economic aspects of epilepsy and antiepileptic treatment: a review of the literature. *Expert Review of Pharmacoeconomics and Outcomes Research.* 2005;5:327–338.
26. Radhakrishnan K, Dinesh Nayak S, Pradeep Kumar S, et al. Profile of antiepileptic pharmacotherapy in a tertiary referral center in South India: a pharmacoepidemiologic and pharmacoeconomic study. *Epilepsia.* 1999;40: 179–185.
27. Rao MB, Radhakrishnan K. Is epilepsy surgery possible in countries with limited resources? *Epilepsia.* 2000;41(Suppl 4):S31–S34.
28. Tan Torres T, Baltussen RM, Adam T, et al. *Making Choices in Health: WHO Guide to Cost-Effectiveness Analysis.* Geneva: World Health Organization; 2003.
29. Thomas SV, Sarma PS, Alexander M, et al. Economic burden of epilepsy in India. *Epilepsia.* 2001;42:1052–1060.
30. World Health Organization. *Investing in Health Research and Development: Report of the ad hoc Committee on Health Research Relating to Future Intervention Options.* Geneva: World Health Organization; 1996.
31. World Health Organization. *Consultation on priority-setting in the field of epilepsy research.* Geneva: World Health Organization; 2000.
32. World Health Organization. *World Health Report 2000: Health Systems, Improving Performance.* Geneva: World Health Organization; 2000.
33. World Health Organization. Statistical Annex 3, 2004. In: World Health Report 2004: Changing history (available at http://www.who.int/whr/2004/annex/topic/en/annex_3_en.pdf).
34. Xu K, Evans DB, Kawabata K, et al. Household catastrophic health expenditure: A multicountry analysis. *Lancet.* 2003;362:111–117.

CHAPTER 309 ■ INFORMATION TRANSFER AND EDUCATION

PATRICIA K. CRUMRINE AND SIMON D. SHORVON

INTRODUCTION

The purpose of an international textbook on epilepsy is to educate as many people as possible about the field of epilepsy, thus enhancing the care of those with this condition. The ability of those working in the field to provide information to each other, their patients, and their patients' families and to the community at large is an important role. This means not only giving information, but also interpreting, comparing, and objectively evaluating the information and its sources. How this is accomplished is constantly changing. The ability to obtain and evaluate new information is critical to the clinician working with epilepsy. Today's clinicians have limited time to read journals and attend out-of-town meetings, yet they have increasing demands to document ongoing educational credits (CMEs). The sources for new information have changed from the time when the physician depended on scientific journals for the main source to the present, when there are many resources available. Industry is now playing a larger role in the information transfer process, and the ability to evaluate the objectivity of this for the health care provider becomes necessary.

The role of information transfer or dissemination affects all persons in the health field. This service is necessary for the ongoing education of physicians, scientists, physicians- and scientists-in-training, medical students, nurses, other health care providers, patients, their families and the community at large. The means for providing this service vary depending on the group that is involved and the specific goal of the information transfer. Technology advances have improved the way that information may be disseminated. Today, larger portions of the population are computer literate and have access to computers. Information provided via this means may be able to reach larger numbers of people.

The physician as an educator has a role in the information transfer process. In the past, most information was provided through written materials (books, journals) and lectures and seminars. Thus, information was often limited to only those within the medical field and was not readily available to lay people and the community at large. Currently, the means of information transfer include not only books, journals, and seminars, but also peer-developed guidelines for evaluation and treatment of specific diseases, Web-based audio/video seminars, online information with detailed discussions of disease processes, video presentations of surgical procedures, and active support groups for many chronic diseases.[3]

It is important for the treating physician and other health care providers to be knowledgeable about the current social and cultural issues pertinent to the populations that they treat. This means being able to apply these issues to the process of information transfer. Information and means of delivery that are acceptable and appropriate for one population may be totally unacceptable for another.

The dissemination of new research in the epilepsy field is critical to the quality of care for patients with epilepsy. This transfer requires the ability to provide health care providers access to information on new diagnostic tools, technology, and treatment options for patients once they have been evaluated as safe and available. This transfer also requires providing the interpretation of this research to the health care provider and the public.

The role of this chapter is to provide the reader with information about information transfer concerning epilepsy, ways of dissemination, self-education, the role that Health Insurance Portability and Accountability Act (HIPAA) regulations play in this information transfer, and ways of evaluating the effectiveness of this transfer.

DISSEMINATION OF INFORMATION PERTINENT TO EPILEPSY

Epilepsy is a chronic condition affecting 2.7 million people in the United States and 50 million people worldwide.[55] It affects individuals of all ages, from the newborn to the elderly; 4% of individuals who reach the age of 85 years will have developed epilepsy. Many of these people will be cared for by health care providers who are not epileptologists and whose primary training in epilepsy consists of what they learned during their educational years in medical school and residency. A report by the National Institute for Clinical Excellence (NICE) in the United Kingdom noted epilepsy misdiagnosis rates of 20% to 31%.[37] This report cited the financial impact of these misdiagnoses as £160,125,000 ≠ British pounds, total cost. Krauss et al.[36] reviewed stories published in the media concerning epilepsy. They found that 31% of the stories contained errors; many of these were inaccurate reports on the science of epilepsy. Even physicians and pharmaceutical spokespeople provided incorrect information concerning drug treatments. These facts emphasize the need for education and dissemination of information to treating physicians and the public.

The National Center for Chronic Disease, Prevention and Health Promotion in the United States gathered experts in the field of epilepsy to develop a public agenda. This meeting led in 1997 to the first major public health conference on epilepsy, Living Well with Epilepsy, and the collaboration of multiple organizations in the United States with defined goals that included the following:

- Assessment of evidence linking elements of care to clinical outcomes in special populations of patients with epilepsy.
- Development of health service purchasing specifications for services related to epilepsy.
- Enhancement of awareness and understanding of epilepsy through targeted education and awareness campaigns and increased support of research.

- Development of a bibliography/database of work related to epilepsy self-management.
- Implementation and evaluation of the self-management interventions in epilepsy.
- Support of population-based epidemiologic studies of epilepsy prevalence, incidence, and health care needs in selected communities.
- Assessment of the utility of existing health care data sets for studying trends in access to care, levels of care, and other demographic variables related to epilepsy.
- Continuing development of a tool to assess public perceptions of epilepsy.
- Support of epidemiologic studies of preventable causes of epilepsy, including traumatic brain injury and infections such as cysticercosis.
- Evaluation of the incidence, prevalence, and patterns of care for epilepsy in a managed care setting.[9]

A second conference, Living Well with Epilepsy II, was held in 2003 to revisit the goals set by the first conference and develop new strategies for improved awareness. The organizers noted that there was still a lack of awareness concerning the seriousness of epilepsy and available treatment options. This lack of information involved all segments of society, including health care providers, patients with epilepsy, and the general public.[10] One of the charges from this conference was to address self-management and assure that those with epilepsy have the information and support needed to manage the condition and its treatment.

LEARNING METHODS

Adult learners have different styles and needs for learning. As students, many of us quickly realized which manner of learning works best for us. Most of us experienced the lecture format as we passed through our educational programs. This method involves listening and comprehending and then processing the information for future retrieval. For some this is easy, whereas for others it is not. For some, the process of note taking enhances learning skills with this method. Others find that what they read and visualize leads to better learning and information retrieval. In the field of health care, learning has often been by demonstration and discussion. Technology has added another dimension to learning tools with the development of audio/video formats. Many lectures today are enhanced with digital slides, audio, and/or video. Another new tool that lends itself to the learning process is the ability to access information over the Internet. All of these methods are applicable to all those who need to learn about epilepsy: medical students, physicians-in -training, physician/specialists, nurses, other health care providers, researchers, patients, family members/caregivers, teachers, employers, and the public. For each of these groups, one or more of the methods may be applicable to the learning process.

INFORMATION TRANSFER TO HEALTH CARE PROVIDERS

Traditional and Current Means of Information Transfer

Historically, physicians and other health care providers obtained information from textbooks, formal lectures offered as part of the educational process, peer-reviewed journal articles, annual meetings of their medical specialty, weekly or monthly "grand rounds" in hospital settings, and, more important, discussion with their peers. Other than the lectures in medical school, for which testing procedures existed, there generally were no means for evaluating the effectiveness of the learning process. Textbooks provide good general scientific and treatment information but may not always have the most up-to-date information on current therapeutic options because the publishing of textbook material may be several years behind current accepted therapy practices. Even journals may be somewhat out of date by the time their new information is published.

Technology advances have increased information resources available to health care providers. Information is available electronically. Journals and textbooks also are available via this format. Thus, physicians spend less time in libraries than in the past. There has also been a tremendous increase in the number of scientific journals being published. Educators have had to learn new ways of presenting information for lectures. The use of 35-mm slides has become a technology of the past. Most presentations now use a Power Point format with digitized video images. The problem sometimes is that of information overload. Lowe and Barnett noted that as of 1994 there were 17,000 new biomedical books and 30,000 biomedical journals published annually.[40] They estimated that a physician would have to read 19 original articles per day to maintain knowledge in a field. They also noted that most physicians in this time period obtained their information, not from books or journals, but from other health professionals. However, there is not always a filtering system in place to provide information that is relevant and up to date for a particular physician and clinical setting.

Traditionally, the exposure of medical students to information has been via lecture and bedside teaching methods. The amount of time devoted to teaching about epilepsy has always been small. Many students may complete their training in medicine without having seen a seizure or treated someone with epilepsy. Many training programs in the Western Hemisphere and Europe have implemented problem-based learning that provides exposure to a wide variety of disease states at all levels of medical school training. However, the amount of time spent on epilepsy remains small.

Information on epilepsy in nursing education and other health care education was a small part of the nursing educational process in the past. With the development of specialties in nursing, nurses with interests and talents in working with patients with epilepsy have become valued members of epilepsy teams. These nurses have become active members of the epilepsy community, working in hospital settings and as educators, researchers, and public health advisors. One example of their activities is the guideline for competencies for epilepsy nurse specialists published by the Royal College of Nursing.[12] Nurses have worked to increase knowledge of epilepsy in the school setting and have developed educational tools for of nurses in this field.[46]

Documentation of continuing medical/nursing education (CME/CNE) and maintenance of certification (MOC) are mandated by many states in the United States and many other countries. The numbers and types of CME credits vary from state to state and country to country. This documentation is often imposed by state licensing renewal processes and hospital accreditation. As with other types of learning, CME can be obtained in various formats, including attending accredited seminars, reviewing journal articles answering questions, and engaging in online activity through a hospital-, university-, CME-accredited organization. Continuing education is now required by many health care professions (e.g., physicians, nurses, pharmacists, dentists.)

The Accreditation Council for Continuing Medical Education (ACCME) in the United States reported in 2004 that they sponsored (directly and jointly) 71,564 activities, with 6.5 million participating physicians and 3.2 million participating nonphysicians. The range of activities included courses, regularly scheduled conferences, Internet enduring materials, other enduring materials, and journal-based CME.[2] Enduring materials are printed, recorded, or computer-assisted instructional materials which may be used over time at various locations. Is continuing education effective in changing the practice of health care providers? Davis et al. reviewed the literature for articles relating to the effectiveness of various educational strategies from 1975 to 1994.[14] They specifically looked for studies that were randomized trials of education strategies that assessed physician performance and/or health care outcomes. Of 99 trials with 160 interventions, they found that 70% demonstrated a change in physician performance and 48% produced a positive change in health care outcomes.

INFORMATION TRANSFER TO STUDENTS AND PHYSICIANS-IN-TRAINING

Traditionally, information transfer and education have been via didactic lectures and bedside demonstration. The younger generation of students and physicians is very technology savvy and uses computers and other technologies easily. They have grown up using computers for most of their educational years and find that information accessible via this mode is to their liking. They incorporate this into other modes of information storage such as handheld devices (personal digital assistants, PDAs). Their learning modes are often different from those of their senior physicians. They are more comfortable in obtaining information electronically than from textbooks, and read this information off computers. They may be less likely to subscribe to printed journals in the future than this generation of physicians.

Time constraints of resident hours in the United States have changed the ways of educating residents and even medical students. There is often less bedside teaching than in the past. Within medical schools there is a renewed interest in providing quality education. Some schools have established academies of medical educators to advance the mission of education.[33]Although initial evaluations of these academies show that schools recognize teaching efforts by their faculty members and promote them for these efforts, it is unclear what the outcome is relative to student learning.

Epilepsy Information/Education

Epilepsy education constitutes a small portion of the curriculum for the typical medical student and resident. A study performed by Mason et al. evaluated three seminars on epilepsy given to third-year medical students.[41] They found that the seminars improved general knowledge of the subject but did not change attitudes about it.

Education about epilepsy for physicians in training is quite variable. Those in surgical specialties probably never receive any education during their training years. Those in primary care specialties such as medicine, pediatrics, and family practice may receive some, but this varies. Unique programs have been developed to teach neurology and child neurology residents about epilepsy. The J. Kiffin Penry Epilepsy Education Program runs two of these. They consist of a several-day minifellowship, with the curriculum consisting of daily lectures, workshops, and case presentations about epilepsy. Participants take pre- and post-tests to assess the knowledge gained.

INFORMATION TRANSFER TO PATIENTS AND CAREGIVERS

Patients, families, and other caregivers traditionally depended on their primary physician for information concerning medical status and treatment. A family might have had a general health care book on the bookshelf at home. Much of their information often came from friends or other family members. The patient accepted what was said to him or her and did not question the treating physician. Medicine has changed and now encourages the patient and family to participate in the care as an active member of the team. The availability of information through various media contributes to this participation. The use of the Internet to access information has increased patient knowledge but has also contributed to patient confusion about which treatment option may be the best. Kind et al. studied the availability of computer and Internet access in a low-income urban population in the United States.[35] In a survey of 260 people they found that 58% had access to a computer and 41% had home Internet access. Ninety-two percent of those surveyed indicated that they would like to discuss information on the Internet with a health professional. A Harris Poll from 2003 surveying Internet use reported that 67% of all adults have been online and that 57% use the Internet at home.[30] The estimate for European usage is 35.5%, and for worldwide usage it is about 15.2%.[42] Harrisinteractive surveyed patients in four countries (United States, France, Germany, and Japan) in January 2002.[28] This report noted that those surveyed in United States and Japan were most concerned about using Web sites not based in their own countries. Americans and Japanese were the most likely to purchase drugs online if they were available from pharmaceutical companies.

Patients and their families desire information about their health problems and treatment. This information contributes to improved compliance with medication, better relationships with health care providers, and a more positive outlook about the patients' medical problem.[27,38,48–49,51–52] The Healthy People 2010 Information Access Project is a collaboration of U.S. government agencies, public health organizations, and health science libraries to assist the public health workforce find and use information effectively.[54–55] A study by Deber asked whether patients wanted their physicians to do the problem solving and whether they wanted to be involved in the decision making.[15] Most of the patients wanted the physician to do the problem solving, but a significant percentage wanted to be involved in the decision making part of the process. Deber discussed the problems that occur with patient education, which included the following issues: (a) the importance of the manner in which information is presented; (b) the potential for overwhelming the patient with large amounts of information; (c) the possible confusion for the patient of conflicting treatment options; and (d) the variability in quality of information, its completeness, and its accuracy.

Besides the Internet, other sources of information and education that have been used in the clinical setting are pamphlets, video tapes, drug information sheets, physician/nurse phone calls, and, more recently, e-mail communications. Many patients express interest in the ability to communicate with their health care provider via email because they can do this on their own time, do not have to wait for a phone call from their provider, and feel freer in asking questions. People's learning styles differ, and what may work for one patient may not be as effective for another. Eaden et al. carried out a randomized trial comparing the efficacy of a video plus an informational leaflet to an informational leaflet alone for patients about surveillance and cancer risk in ulcerative colitis.[18] They noted that there was no clear advantage of the video plus the leaflet over the pamphlet. They suggested that staff time and costs should be weighed in the consideration of which medium to use.

Email has become increasingly popular for patients and their health care providers. A Harrisinteractive telephone survey conducted in March 2002 noted that 110 million adults use the Internet for health information.[52] Many of those surveyed indicated a willingness to pay for these services. What they hoped to obtain from this service was the ability to ask questions of the health care provider without having to make a visit, fix appointments, receive results of medical tests, and obtain prescriptions.[29] The results of a University Pediatric Faculty Practice survey of 1,018 adults accompanying a child reported that 47% used the Internet for medical information.[5] Of these, only 47% considered that the information was good.

Epilepsy Information and Education

How does this information translate into the care of patients with epilepsy? Patients and their families have consistently indicated that they wanted information from their physicians about the disorder and its causes and treatments.[8,43] A U.K. study by Buck et al. in 1996 solicited information via questionnaire from patients with epilepsy concerning their satisfaction with their care.[8] Patients were asked whether they thought that their physician had adequate knowledge about epilepsy and whether he or she provided enough information concerning this. Sixty-seven percent of those responding to the survey stated that their physician, usually a general practitioner, gave them enough information about their epilepsy. On the question of whether they felt that the physician had considered their personal views, 71% felt that the general practitioner was more likely to do so compared to the hospital specialist.

INFORMATION TRANSFER TO THE COMMUNITY AND PUBLIC

The public has become more knowledgeable about diseases, treatments, and outcomes. There are many resources for this knowledge; these include television documentaries, news reports, magazine articles, and the Internet. National organizations and parent support groups play significant roles in the dissemination of this information. With some diseases, there is a stigma attached to the disorder, and education of the public is more difficult. Bagley in 1972 studied the attitudes of the public toward epilepsy, cerebral palsy, and mental illness and found that those with epilepsy were rejected more often than those with the other two illnesses.[4] Even 23 years later Baumann found similar results concerning attitudes toward children with epilepsy compared to those with asthma.[6] The Epilepsy Foundation of America and many other chapters of the International League Against Epilepsy (ILAE) have launched public awareness programs aimed at educating employers, teachers, public servants such as police, and the public at large. The ILAE together with the World Health Organization (WHO) and the International Bureau for Epilepsy (IBE) undertook a joint campaign in 1997 called "Out of the Shadows."[32] The primary goal of this campaign is to increase public and professional awareness of epilepsy and raise epilepsy to a plane of acceptability in the public domain. The Epilepsy Foundation of America has a "Speak Up, Speak Out" campaign encouraging those with epilepsy and their families to advocate for important issues related to epilepsy and health care.[22] They also sponsor a Public Policy Institute each year; children from around the United States travel to Washington, D.C., meet with their representatives, and tell their stories about the impact that epilepsy has had on their lives. The Living Well with Epilepsy II conference in 2003 addressed ways of improving public awareness and acceptance of those with epilepsy.[21] Similar activities are carried out by other affiliates of the ILAE around the world. In third world countries, efforts have been undertaken to improve health access for those with epilepsy and diminish the stigma associated with the disorder.

SELF-EDUCATION AND SELF-MANAGEMENT FOR THOSE WITH EPILEPSY

Self-management implies that a person has a certain amount of knowledge about his or her medical condition. Data from reports of management of chronic diseases in both the United States and the United Kingdom indicate significant benefits of providing patients with information.[25] This resulted in reductions in outpatient visits by 37% and in accidents by 34%.[25] This type of patient–physician role has been studied in various age groups, including adolescents with chronic illness.[47] Self-management begins with the diagnosis of epilepsy and involves establishing a relationship with the treating physician. Self-management was one of the goals of the Living Well with Epilepsy II Conference that took place in 2003.[10] This is a goal that both the treating physician and the patient/caregiver should work toward from the onset of the diagnosis of epilepsy. Although there has not been much research related to the self-management of epilepsy, the few studies that exist demonstrate positive effects of self-management, control, and social support.[26] Part of self-management is understanding and coping with the diagnosis. This may require an understanding of one's feelings of anger, frustration, depression, or guilt.[49] The physician and epilepsy nurse can play an important role in assisting the patient and family through this initial process. Early referral to community support services is also important in assisting the patient and the family in the role of self-management.

The Centers for Disease Control and Prevention in collaboration with the American Epilepsy Society, the Epilepsy Foundation, and the Agency for Healthcare Research and Quality are developing a bibliographic database for the self-management of epilepsy. The sponsored research project includes the development of a computerized epilepsy self-management project.[17] The goals of these researchers are to use such a program to assist patients with treatment issues, improve knowledge, provide information to help with dealing with stress and sleep issues, and improve compliance with taking of their medication.

Many epilepsy associations in the United States and throughout the world have Web sites with self-help information.[19,20,23] The guidelines from *Epilepsy Action* cite four keys to self-management: (a) working knowledge, (b) personal awareness, (c) confidence, and (d) taking responsibility. The last is especially important and involves knowledge of the roles of the environment, stress, sleep, food and alcohol, illness, and hormones in seizure control.[19] This guideline also gives patients some specific instructions on questions that they can pose to their physician during visits.

As with information transfer to others, learning skills and preferences vary relative to the person. These issues should also be discussed with the health care worker. This opens up the opportunity to provide information in formats that enhance the greatest learning, including pamphlets, lectures, support groups, audiotapes, videos, CDs, books, and Internet resources. The ultimate goal for the patient is to accept the diagnosis, work toward the best control possible without side effects of medication, and be able to continue with his or her activities and employment and enjoy a good quality of life.

The ability to self-manage depends on the ability to establish a good working relationship with the health care worker (physician, nurse practitioner, nurse). Physicians have not always been recognized to be the best listeners. Patients and families of patients with chronic illness frequently complain that physicians in acute care settings do not listen to their explanation of the illness or treatment. This lack of understanding occurs in spite of the fact that these people deal with the chronic illness on a daily basis. A study by Braddock et al using audiotapes of primary care office visits to evaluate six criteria for informed decision making reported that discussions leading to informed decision making included fewer than two of six described elements.[7] These elements were as follows: (a) discussion of the clinical issue and nature of the decision, (b) discussion of the alternatives, (c) discussion of the pros (or benefits) and cons (or risks) of the alternatives, (d) discussion of uncertainties associated with the decision, (e) assessment of the patient's understanding, and (e) asking the patient to express a preference.[7] There are still patients who prefer to defer to their physicians for final decisions. A study by Levinson et al. noted that this preference was more likely to occur in populations of older and poorer patients.[39] The physician must be able to read patients, understand their desires, and assist them in the process of understanding and working with their illness.

RESEARCH INFORMATION AND DISSEMINATION

Information concerning new treatments and devices needs to be available to the treating physician and to the public in a timely fashion. In the past, the transfer of this information has been through peer-reviewed journals to physicians and then from physicians to patients and their families. The timeline for this transfer can be months after the availability of a new therapy. The explosion of information now available to physicians limits the time that they can spend reviewing new ideas critically. Information comes from peer-reviewed journals, the Internet, and often from pharmaceutical industry representatives. Physicians still feel that the information that they receive from peer-reviewed journals about new therapies represents the best information. Although many physicians use electronic sources of information, they do not consider these as reliable as the peer-reviewed journals.[3] Other forms of information transfer related to research and new technologies occur at national or international society meetings. In these settings, health care providers have the opportunity to experience new ideas and then share them with their peers at home and their patients. Pollock advocated a system in academic institutions that requires health care providers attending a society meeting to return to their home institution and give a presentation of what they heard and learned.[44] Patients today often search for the newest treatments for complex disorders. They come to their physician visits armed with information that they obtained from the Internet or a magazine or newspaper. It is not uncommon that the information that they bring is something that the physician has not read.

Patients and families see the physician as the primary resource for new information about therapies or diagnostic studies. It is important to find ways in which health care providers can find the time to seek out this information from reliable sources.

ROLE OF EPILEPSY ORGANIZATIONS AND SUPPORT GROUPS

The health care provider, researcher, patient, and patient caregiver have an increasing array of information resources and support groups about epilepsy available to them. Many patients are very resourceful and access these resources without any prompting or difficulties. For others, the health care provider can be very helpful in directing the patient to these services. Among these resources are the following:

1. Epilepsy Foundation of America (EFA)
2. International League Against Epilepsy (ILAE) and it various national chapters
3. World Health Organization
4. International Bureau for Epilepsy (IBE)
5. Centers for Disease Control and Prevention (CDC)

The national chapters of the International League Against Epilepsy provide services to local populations in the form of printed materials, workshops, lectures, support groups, advocacy for employment, information on educational and legal issues, and camps for children with epilepsy. As noted earlier, the ILAE, IBE, and WHO began a joint initiative in 1997 called "Out of the Shadows." This is a global campaign designed to improve the diagnosis, treatment, prevention, and social acceptance of people with epilepsy. The second phase began in 2001 with the goals of promoting public and professional education, identifying the needs of people with epilepsy, and encouraging governments and departments of health to address the needs of people with epilepsy.[16]

In addition to these global activities, the local chapters of these organizations strive to provide services to people with epilepsy on a daily basis. One difficulty for the person with epilepsy and the family is that often they are unaware of these organizations and the opportunities for services. If the medical care of the person with epilepsy is in the hands of a general physician who does not have much contact with epilepsy services, the patient may not be provided with the information about them. The availability of information on the Internet is changing this somewhat, but there are still many people who do not receive services.

These organizations educate the public about epilepsy and advocate for services for persons with epilepsy. In spite of the increased publicity concerning epilepsy, people with epilepsy still perceive a stigma.[34,50]

ROLE OF THE PHARMACEUTICAL INDUSTRY IN INFORMATION TRANSFER AND EDUCATION

The role of the pharmaceutical industry in medical education and information dissemination is very significant in the current market. Figueras and Laporte noted that the marketing budgets for pharmaceutical companies exceeds those for research and development.[24] They also noted that these companies play very important roles in medical societies and continuing medical education, and that because health care systems provide limited access to independent information, the pharmaceutical industry therefore becomes the bigger player in the dissemination of health information both to professionals and the public.[24] Many companies now have an "applied therapeutics" team whose primary goal is the development and dissemination of scientific information both internally and externally.

A report by the Accreditation Council for Continuing Medical Education in 2001 noted that more than half of the funding for CME came from commercial resources.[1] This report also noted that about one third of medical schools in the United States receive about half of their CME funding from the industry. Because of the increasing need for physicians to have mandated CME credits, there will be a need for educational resources. Most responders to a survey taken at a CME conference stated that they were there because of the need for CME and to learn about latest treatments.[13]

The other dilemma related to information from pharmaceutical industries is that many health care providers have been investigators in the clinical trials for the drugs or devices in question. One study recommended that patients be informed of financial and publication agreements between the industry and persons conducting the trials.[11]

There is a need to develop specific relationships with industry that benefit the patient and the health care provider without compromising standards of medical practice.

THE FUTURE OF INFORMATION TRANSFER

Health Insurance Portability and Accountability Act

The passage of the Health Insurance Portability and Accountability Act (HIPAA) in 1996 and its implementation in 2003 has had a profound impact on information transfer in the medical community. It has affected direct patient care and clinical research. Those with chronic illnesses who seek services from multiple health care providers frequently feel the effect of this regulation. Sharing of medical information from one provider to another is more cumbersome than before. Enrolling patients in clinical studies requires several extra steps to ensure that patient confidentiality is maintained. Sharing of information with school officials, employers, and others involved in the day-to care of the patient may be limited unless permission is obtained from the patient or family member. This limitation of information may affect the care that patients receive if an acute medical problem arises. The epilepsy population is particularly impacted by HIPAA. For children with epilepsy, providing school nurses and teachers with information may be difficult. The same applies to employers of patients with epilepsy.

As we move forward with the development of medical record systems, these regulations will play a role in their design and management.

Electronic Records

Medical information is increasingly collected and stored electronically. Inpatient information is placed in electronic systems. Medical records are available on a number of archival systems throughout the United States and Europe. As technology has permitted the conversion of data to digital forms, the ability to store this information electronically has increased. Many hospitals store all patient orders, laboratory studies and results, and inpatient and outpatient records electronically. The thrust is to eliminate the paper medical record. The hypothesis is that use of electronic medical records will save the health industry billions of dollars, with improved health care efficiency and safety.[31] Another potential advantage of electronic records could be to provide patients with their personal electronic record, giving them more opportunity to participate with the health care provider in their care.[53] There are large-scale projects currently looking at ways to transfer computer-based information over the World Wide Web and maintain patient confidentiality.[45] The hope is that this can prevent repetition of tests, aid in identification of patient allergies and medications, and provide good patient care at a savings.

Many physicians use PDAs when they see patients in the hospital or office. Many of the PDAs now have Internet and phone capabilities, permitting access to many sources of information such as drug databases, Current Procedural Terminology codes, and other resources. Information obtained and stored in this manner is commonplace in the Western medical world.

As we move into the next decades, more and more of the information that we obtain and share will probably occur via electronic sources. Less of this will occur via paper sources such as journals, books, and newspapers. Even today, many medical journals offer an online version of the journal as a subscription option. At this stage, it is difficult to evaluate the efficacy of these various forms as they relate to physician learning, patient learning, and patient care. These are projects for the future.

SUMMARY AND CONCLUSIONS

The availability of information relative to epilepsy and other medical conditions is available in many formats. The physician as both a learner and an educator needs to be aware of these resources both for his or her education and for the education of his or her patients. With increasing demands on the heath care provider's time, it becomes important for the provider to be able to find information in places that he or she can access off-hours, such as the Internet, online seminars, and journal articles. The public also is increasingly interested in having more medical information available to them. The patient and caregivers are more facile with using the Internet and seeking out information. It is the responsibility of the health care provider to make appropriate resources available to their patients and guide them through the understanding of the information. In addition to standard methods of information resources, nonprofit organizations and support groups are playing greater roles in providing information to patients and their families. As physicians move forward in their training and practices, it is important to remember that learning is a lifelong process. Methods and tools for learning and the information itself will change, and physicians must be aware of these changes.

References

1. Accreditation Council for Continuing Medical Education. *Annual Report Data 2001*. Chicago: Accreditation Council for Continuing Medical Education; 2002.
2. Accreditation Council for Graduate Medical Education. *2004 Report of the ACGME*. Chicago: Accreditation Council for Graduate Medical Education; 2005.
3. Agency for Health Care Policy and Research. *Information to Guide Physician Practice Overview*. Rockville MD: Agency for Health Care Policy and Research; 1996.
4. Bagley C. Social prejudice and the adjustment of people with epilepsy. *Epilepsia*. 1972;13:33–45.
5. Baraff LJ, Wall SP, Lee TJ, et al. Use of the Internet and e-mail for medical advice and information by parents of a university pediatric faculty practice. *Clin Pediatr*. 2003;42:557–560.
6. Baumann RC. Kentuckians' attitudes toward children with epilepsy. *Epilepsia*. 1995;36(10):1003–1008.
7. Braddock CH III, Fihn SD, Levinson W, et al. How doctors and patients discuss routine clinical decisions: informed decision making in the outpatient setting. *J Gen Intern Med*. 1997;12(6):339–345.
8. Buck D, Jacoby A, Baker GA, et al. Patients' experiences and satisfaction with the care of their epilepsy. *Epilepsia*. 1996;37(9):841–849.
9. Centers for Disease Control and Prevention. *Living Well with Epilepsy: Report of the 1997 National Conference on Public Health and Epilepsy*. Atlanta: Centers for Disease Control and Prevention; 1997.
10. Centers for Disease Control and Prevention. *Living Well with Epilepsy II: Report of the 2003 National Conference on Public Health and Epilepsy*. Atlanta: Centers for Disease Control and Prevention; 2003.
11. Commens CA. Truth in clinical research trials involving pharmaceutical sponsorship. *Med J Aust* 2001;174(12):648–649.
12. Concannon B, Beeston L, Lawrence K, et al. *RCN Competencies: Competencies: A Competency Framework and Guidance for Developing Paediatric Epilepsy Nurse Specialist Services*. London: Royal College of Nursing; 2005: 1–38.
13. Daugherty JM, Sweeney HA. Industry pays the doctor bill for escalating CME costs. *Med Marketing Media*. 2000;35:88–90.
14. Davis DA, Thompson MA, Oxman AD, et al. Changing physician performance. A systematic review of the effect of continuing medical education strategies. *JAMA*. 1995: 274(9):700–705.
15. Deber RB. Shared decision making in the real world. *J Gen Intern Med*. 1996: 11(6)377–378.
16. de Boer HM, Engel J Jr, Prilpko LL. *"Out of the Shadows." A Global Campaign Against Epilepsy*. Geneva: World Health Organization; 2005.

17. Dilorio CW. *Using computers to develop an epilepsy self-management program.* Prevention Research Center, Centers for Disease Control and Prevention; 2006. Available at: http://www.cdc.gov/prc/research_projects/sips/computers_develop_self_management. Accessed January 28, 2006.
18. Eaden J, Abrams K, Shears J, et al. Randomized controlled trial comparing the efficacy of a video and information leaflet versus information leaflet alone on patient knowledge about surveillance and cancer risk in ulcerative colitis. *Inflamm Bowel Dis.* 2002;8(6):407–412.
19. Epilepsy Action. *Epilepsy and self management.* Available: http://www.epilepsy.org.uk/infor/self.html. Accessed January 22, 2006.
20. Epilepsy Foundation. *Answer place–social aspects.* Available: http://www.epilepsyfoundation.org/answerplace/Social/. Accessed January 28, 2006.
21. Epilepsy Foundation. *Living Well with Epilepsy II: Report of the 2003 National Conference on Public Health and Epilepsy.* Landover MD: Epilepsy Foundation; 2003:1–52.
22. Epilepsy Foundation. *Speak Up, Speak Out network.* Available at: http://www.epilepsyfoundation.org/advocacy/. Accessed January 28, 2006.
23. Epilepsy Foundation Australia. *Seizure smart–self management*; 2004. Available: http://www.epilepsy.org.au. Accessed January 28, 2006.
24. Figueras A, Laporte JR, Failures of the therapeutic chain as a cause of drug ineffectiveness. *BMJ.* 2003;326:895–896.
25. Fisher B, Dixon A, Honeyman A. Informed patients; reformed clinicians. *J R Soc Med.* 2005;98:530–531.
26. Gallant MP. The influence of social support on chronic illness self-Management: a review and directions for research. *Health Educ Behav.* 2003;30(2):170–195.
27. Gravois R, Garvin T. Moving from information *transfer* to information *exchange* in health and health care. *Soc Sci Med.* 2003;56(3):449–464.
28. Harrisinteractive. *Harris interactive reports on future use of the Internet in 4 countries in relation to prescriptions, physician communication and health information*; June 1, 2002. Available at: www.harrisinteractive.com/news/allnewsbydate.asp? News ID=467. Accessed January 20, 2006.
29. Harrisinteractive. *Harris interactive reports many patients willing to pay for online communication with their physicians.* Available at: www.harrisinteractive.com/news/allnewsbydate.asp? News ID=446. Accessed April 11, 2002.
30. Harris Poll #8. *Those with Internet access to continue to grow but at a slower rate*; February 4,2003. Available at: http://www.harrisinteractive.com.
31. Hillestad R, Beigelow J, Bower A, et al. Can electronic medical record systems transform health care? Potential health benefits, savings, and cots. The adoption of interoperable EMR systems could produce efficiency and safety savings of $142–$371 billion. *Health Affairs.* 2005;24(5):1103–1117.
32. International League Against Epilepsy, International Bureau of Epilepsy, World Health Organization. *"Out of the Shadows."* Brussels: International League Against Epilepsy; 2004.
33. Irby DM, Cooke M, Lowenstein D, et al. The academy movement: a structural approach to reinvigorating the educational mission. *Acad Med.* 2004;79(8):729–736.
34. Jacoby A. Stigma, epilepsy, and quality of life. *Epilepsy Behav.* 2002;3:S10–S20.
35. Kind T, Huang ZJ, Farr D, et al. Internet and computer access and use for health information in an underserved community. *Ambul Pediatr.* 2005;5(2):117–121.
36. Krauss GL, Gondek S, Krumholz S, et al. The "scarlet E": the presentation of epilepsy in the English-language print media. *Neurology.* 2000;54:1894–1898.
37. Lee P. What is the full cost of epilepsy misdiagnosis in the UK? In: *Epilepsy Action.* Yeadon, Leeds, UK: British Epilepsy Association, 2005.
38. Leino-Kilpi H, Johansson K, Heikkinen K, et al. Patient education and health-related quality of life: surgical hospital patients as a case in point. *J Nurs Care Qual.* 2005;20(4)307–316.
39. Levinson W, Kao A, Kuby A, et al. Not all patients want to participate in decision making. A national study of public preferences. *J Gen Intern Med.* 2005;20(6):531–535.
40. Lowe HJ, Barnett GO. Understanding and using the Medical Subject Headings (MeSH) vocabulary to perform literature searches. *JAMA.* 1994;271(14):1103–1108.
41. Mason C, Fenton GW, Jamieson M. Teaching medical students about epilepsy. *Epilepsia.* 1990;31(1):95–100.
42. Miniwatts International. *Internet usage statistics*; 2005. Available at: http://www.internetworldstats.com.
43. National Center for Health Statistics. *Healthy People 2000: Final Review, National Health Promotion and Disease Prevention Objectives.* Hyattsville, MD: Public Health Service; 2001.
44. Pollock S. Information transfer—the missing step. *J Dent Educ.* 2003;67(3):293.
45. Rind DM, Kohane IS, Szolovits P, et al. Maintaining the confidentiality of medical records shared over the Internet and the World Wide Web. *Ann Intern Med.* 1997;127(2):138–141.
46. Santilli N, Dodson WE, Walton AV. *Students with Seizures: A Manual for School Nurses.* Landover, MD: Epilepsy Foundation of America; 1991.
47. Sawyer SM, Aroni RA. Self-management in adolescents with chronic illness. What does it mean and how can it be achieved? *Med J Aust.* 2005;183:405–409.
48. Schauffler HH, Rodriquez T, Milstein A. Health education and patient satisfaction. *J Fam Pract.* 1996;42(1):62–68.
49. Shafer, PO. Epilepsy and seizures: advances in seizure assessment, treatment, and self-management. *Nurs Clin North Am.* 1999;34(3):743–759.
50. Shafer, PO. Improving the quality of life in epilepsy: nonmedical issues too often overlooked. *Postgrad Med. Online.* 2002;111(1). Available at http://www.postgradmed.com/issues/2002/01_02shafer.htm.
51. Stewart MA. Effective physician–patient communication and health outcomes: a review. *CMAJ.* 1995;153(8):1064–1065.
52. *Survey shows 'cyberchondriacs' at 110 million nationwide*; May 1, 2002. Available at: www.harrisinteractive.com/news/allnewsbydate.asp? News ID=456. Accessed January 2006.
53. Tang PC, Lansky D. The missing link: bridging the patient–provider health information gap. Electronic personal health records could transform the patient–provider relationship in the twenty-first century. *Health Affairs.* 2005;24(5):1290–1295.
54. U.S. Department of Health and Human Services, Office of Disease Prevention and Health Promotion. *Healthy People 2010 Information Access Project.* Washington, DC: U.S. Department of Health and Human Services; 2007.
55. World Health Organization and Epilepsy Foundation of America. *Epilepsy Facts and Figures.* Landover, MD: Epilepsy Foundation of America; 2005.

INDEX

Note: Page numbers followed by *f* indicate figures, page numbers followed by *t* indicate tables.